SPECIAL FEATURES

RESEARCH UTILIZATION BOXES

MEDICATION TABLES

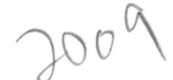

SPECIAL FEATURES

MULTIDISCIPLINARY PLAN OF CARE BOXES

AACN ADVANCED
CRITICAL CARE NURSING

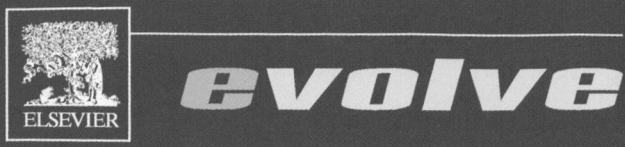

AACN ADVANCED CRITICAL CARE NURSING

KAREN K. CARLSON, RN, MN, CCNS
Critical Care Clinical Nurse Specialist
The Carlson Consulting Group
Bellevue, Washington

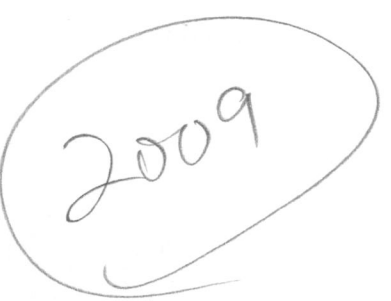

AMERICAN
ASSOCIATION
of CRITICAL-CARE
NURSES

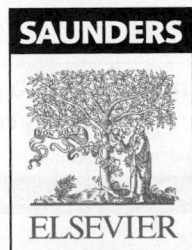

SAUNDERS

ELSEVIER

SAUNDERS
ELSEVIER

11830 Westline Industrial Drive
St. Louis, Missouri 63146

AACN Advanced Critical Care Nursing ISBN: 978-1-4160-3219-9

Notice

Knowledge and best practice in this field are constantly changing. As new research and experience broaden our knowledge, changes in practice, treatment and drug therapy may become necessary or appropriate. Readers are advised to check the most current information provided (i) on procedures featured or (ii) by the manufacturer of each product to be administered, to verify the recommended dose or formula, the method and duration of administration, and contraindications. It is the responsibility of the practitioner, relying on their own experience and knowledge of the patient, to make diagnoses, to determine dosages and the best treatment for each individual patient, and to take all appropriate safety precautions. To the fullest extent of the law, neither the Publisher nor the Editors assume any liability for any injury and/or damage to persons or property arising out of or related to any use of the material contained in this book.

International Standard Book Number: 978-1-4160-3219-9

Managing Editor: Maureen Iannuzzi
Senior Developmental Editor: Jennifer Ehlers
Publishing Services Manager: Deborah L. Vogel
Senior Project Manager: Ann E. Rogers
Design Direction: James Almond
Cover Designer: Steven Stave

Printed in Canada

Last digit is the print number: 9 8 7 6 5 4 3 2 1

To the critical care nursing staff at Virginia Mason Medical Center, Seattle, Washington. Your expertise, knowledge, care, compassion, and collaboration as a team are a model for how it must be done to keep patients and families first. Thank you for showing us the way.

Karen K. Carlson

In Memory
Karen K. Carlson
1956-2007

Our beloved Karen Carlson completed the final chapter of her life as this book's final chapter edits were being completed, illustrations finalized, and permissions obtained. Karen was diagnosed with breast cancer approximately 8 years ago; throughout her disease process Karen remained dedicated to her family, her profession, and most importantly for her, to her God.

One of Karen's singular talents was her gift of mentorship. She touched so many nurses' lives over the past 27 years with an impact that is immeasurable. Karen directly and indirectly educated thousands of critical care nurses, not only in the United States but across the world. She challenged nurses to think differently; her conviction that advancing nursing knowledge is key to providing excellent patient care for vulnerable critical care patients and their families was a cornerstone of her practice. Early in Karen's career, she recognized the value of collaboration and led the development of one of the most successful collaborative educational models in the United States—the Seattle Area Critical Care Education Cooperative, a consortium that continues to provide high-quality education to critical care nurses throughout the Puget Sound area.

From this collaborative model, Karen quickly learned that many areas in the United States (particularly in small and rural hospitals) have neither advanced practice clinicians nor the benefit of a consortium to educate and develop nurses. Intent on reaching out to as many nurses and patients as possible, Karen led a team of writers in developing two editions of AACN's *Acute and Critical Care Orientation Manual*, the original work that prompted development of AACN's highly successful Web-based *Essentials of Critical Care Orientation*.

Karen's contributions to the American Association of Critical-Care Nurses began in the Northeast Louisiana Chapter. They continued in the Puget Sound Chapter from where, after holding numerous leadership positions, she was appointed to national committees and then elected to AACN and AACN Certification Corporation national boards of directors. Karen was also active in the American Heart Association as an ACLS course director and faculty member.

Karen was a force in the development of other major AACN publications. Her editorial leadership, in partnership with coeditor Debra Lynn-McHale Wiegand, brought major enhancements to the fourth and fifth editions of the *AACN Procedure Manual for Critical Care*, which has been adopted as the approved manual by most American hospitals. Karen served as series editor for *AACN Protocols for Practice: Symptom Management*, a seminal work in which content experts present research findings to clinicians in a usable and practical format designed for clinical application.

Karen continued her legacy of providing critical care nurses with exceptional resources to guide their practice with this book, which evolved from the well-respected *AACN Clinical Reference*. Her vision was to offer experienced critical care nurses a new and comprehensive resource that would continue to advance their bedside knowledge. From day one, it was Karen's vision and leadership that made this book what you see before you today.

With each milestone of her life, Karen touched countless lives as a caring friend and mentor who guided our professional careers in ways we find difficult to express in writing. Karen intuitively knew when and how to push practitioners out of their comfort zones so they would pass on their knowledge by way of teaching, writing, editing, publishing, and becoming entrepreneurs. We speak for our many colleagues who would never be where they are today had it not been for Karen's guidance, encouraging us and telling us "Yes, you can do it." For that we all say thank you. We are forever grateful, and nursing is so much richer for it.

Vicki S. Good
Peggy L. Kirkwood
Christine Smith Schulman

Section Editors

Vicki S. Good, RN, MSN, CCRN, CCNS
BHCS Corporate Director of Patient Safety
Baylor Health Care System
Dallas, Texas

Peggy L. Kirkwood, RN, MSN, APRN, BC
Cardiovascular Nurse Practitioner
Mission Hospital
Mission Viejo, California

Christine Smith Schulman, RN, MS, CNS, CCRN
Clinical Nurse Specialist
Trauma & Critical Care Nursing
Portland, Oregon

Contributors

Nancy Albert, RN, PhD, CCNS, CCRN, CAN, FCCM, FAHA
Director, Nursing Research and Innovation
The Cleveland Clinic Foundation
Cleveland, Ohio

Kathleen M. Baldwin, PhD, RN, ANP, GNP, CNS
Director, Graduate Studies in Nursing
Texas Christian University
Fort Worth, Texas

Laurie Baumgartner, RN, MSN, CNS, ACNP, CCRN
Clinical Nurse Specialist, Cardiac Telemetry
Hoag Hospital
Newport Beach, California

Patricia Ann Blissitt, RN, PhD, CCRN, CNRN, CCM, APRN, BC
Staff Nurse
Neuroscience ICU
Duke University Hospital
Durham, North Carolina

Jo Ann Brooks, RN, DNS, FAAN, FCCP
Vice President, Quality
Clarian Health
Indianapolis, Indiana

Denise Buonocore, RN, MSN, APRN-BC, CCRN
Acute Care Nurse Practitioner, The Heart Institute
  at Bridgeport Hospital
Bridgeport, Connecticut
Clinical Faculty Acute Care NP Program
Yale University School of Nursing
New Haven, Connecticut

Suzanne M. Burns, RN, MSN, RRT, ACNP, CCRN, FAAN, FCCM
Professor of Nursing, Acute and Specialty Care
University of Virginia Health System
Charlottesville, Virginia

Diane Byrum, RN, MSN, CCNS, CCRN, FCCM
Critical Care Clinical Nurse Specialist
Presbyterian Hospital
Charlotte, North Carolina

Debra J. Carter, RN, MS, CRNP, CCTC
Cardiac Transplant Nurse Practitioner
Comprehensive Transplant Center
The Johns Hopkins Hospital
Baltimore, Maryland

Dennis J. Cheek, RN, BSN, MSN, PhD, FAHA
Abell-Hanger Professor of Gerontological Nursing
Harris School of Nursing and School of Nursing Anesthesia
Texas Christian University
Fort Worth, Texas

Molly Clark, MS, RD, CD
Clinical Dietician
Department of Nutrition and Foodservices
Harborview Medical Center
Seattle, Washington

Laura M. Criddle, RN, MS, CCRN, CCNS
Clinical Nurse Specialist
Premier Jets/Lifeguard Air Ambulance
Doctoral Student, Oregon Health & Science University
Portland, Oregon

Lori A. Dambaugh, RN-BC, BSN, PCCN
Clinician IV
Rochester General Hospital
Rochester, New York

Michael W. Day, RN, MSN, CCRN
Trauma Nurse Coordinator
Trauma Services
Sacred Heart Medical Center
Spokane, Washington

Sharon Dickinson, RN, MSN, CNS, ANP, CCRN
Clinical Nurse Specialist, Surgical Intensive Care
University of Michigan Health System
Ann Arbor, Michigan

Joni L. Dirks, RN, MS, CCRN
Critical Care Educator
Sacred Heart Medical Center
Spokane, Washington

Diane K. Dressler, RN, MSN, CCRN
Clinical Assistant Professor
Marquette University College of Nursing
Milwaukee, Wisconsin

Margaret M. Ecklund, RN, MS, CCRN, APRN-BC
Clinician VI/Nurse Practitioner
Rochester General Hospital
Rochester, New York

Eleanor Fitzpatrick, RN, MSN, CCRN
Clinical Nurse Specialist
Thomas Jefferson University Hospital
Philadelphia, Pennsylvania

Mary Beth Flynn Makic, RN, PhD, CNS, CCRN
Clinical Nurse Specialist
University of Colorado Hospital
Denver, Colorado

John J. Gallagher, RN, MSN, CCNS, CCRN
Clinical Nurse Specialist, Surgical Critical Care
Hospital of the University of Pennsylvania
Philadelphia, Pennsylvania

Tarek Hassanein, MD
Medical Director of Liver Transplantation and
    Chief of Clinical Hepatology
University of California–San Diego Medical Center
San Diego, California

Richard Henker, RN, PhD, CRNA
Associate Professor and Vice Chairman
Department of Acute/Tertiary Care
University of Pittsburgh School of Nursing
Pittsburgh, Pennsylvania

June Howland-Gradman, RN, MS, MBA
President, JuneRN, Inc.
Nursing Consultant and Educator
Orland Park, Illinois

Carol E. Jacoby, RN, MSN, ANCP
Nurse Practitioner
Center for Hematological Malignancies
Oregon Health & Science University
Portland, Oregon

Roberta Kaplow, PhD, RN, CCNS, CCRN, AOCNS
Clinical Nurse Specialist
DeKalb Medical Center
Decatur, Georgia

Julene B. Kruithof, RN, MSN, CCRN
Critical Care Educator
Spectrum Health
Grand Rapids, Michigan

Dana M. Kyles, RN, BSN
Manager
Transfusion Support and Blood Services
Infection Control Operations
Harborview Medical Center
Seattle, Washington

Denise M. Lawrence, RN, BSN, MS, ACNP
Acute Care Nurse Practitioner, Surgical Intensive Care Unit
Hartford Hospital
Hartford, Connecticut

Barbara Leeper, MN, RN, CCRN, FAHA
Clinical Nurse Specialist, Cardiovascular Services
Baylor University Medical Center
Dallas, Texas

Terry A. Lennie, RN, PhD, FAHA
Associate Professor
College of Nursing
University of Kentucky
Lexington, Kentucky

Carol S. Manchester, RN, MSN, APRN, BC-ADM, CDE
Diabetes Clinical Nurse Specialist
University of Minnesota Medical Center, Fairview
Minneapolis, Minnesota

Andrea P. Marshall, MN (Research), BN, RN, IC Cert
Sesqui Senior Lecturer Critical Care Nursing
Faculty of Nursing and Midwifery
The University of Sydney
Sydney, Australia
Honorary Associate
Faculty of Nursing, Midwifery and Health
University of Technology, Sydney
Sydney, Australia

Rhonda K. Martin, MS, RN, MLT(ASCP), CCRN, CNS/ACNP-C
Nurse Practitioner, Hepatology and Liver Transplantation
University of California San Diego Medical Center
San Diego, California

Rhonda S. Milam, MS, RD, CD, CNSD
Clinical Dietitian
Sacred Heart Medical Center
Spokane, Washington

Nancy C. Molter, RN, MN, PhD, CCRC
Research Nurse, Joint Theater Trauma System
Contractor, AIMUSA, LLC
U.S. Army Institute of Surgical Research
Fort Sam Houston, Texas

Debra K. Moser, DNSc, RN, FAAN
Professor and Gill Endowed Chair of Nursing
University of Kentucky College of Nursing
Lexington, Kentucky

Nancy Munro, RN, MN, CCRN, ACNP
Acute Care Nurse Practitioner, Critical Care
National Institutes of Health
Bethesda, Maryland
Faculty Associate
University of Maryland Graduate School of Nursing
Baltimore, Maryland

Denise O'Brien, RN, MSN, APRN, BC, CPAN, CAPA, FAAN
Clinical Nurse Specialist, Postanesthesia Care Unit
University of Michigan Health System
Ann Arbor, Michigan

Mary Frances D. Pate, RN, DSN
Clinical Nurse Specialist
Assistant Professor
Oregon Health & Science University School of Nursing
Portland, Oregon

Sara Paul, RN, MSN, FNP
Director, Heart Function Clinic
Western Piedmont Heart Centers
Hickory, North Carolina

Kristine J. Peterson, RN, MS, CCNS, CCRN
Clinical Nurse Specialist, CV and Critical Care
Park Nicollet Health Services
Methodist Hospital
St. Louis Park, Minnesota

Jan Powers, RN, MSN, FCCM, CCRN, CCNS, CNRN, CWCN
Director of Clinical Nurse Specialists and Critical Care Clinical
    Nurse Specialist
St. Vincent Hospital
Indianapolis, Indiana

Patricia Radovich, RN, MSN, CNS, FCCM
Clinical Nurse Specialist, Hepatology and Liver Transplantation
Loma Linda University Medical Center
Loma Linda, California

Jeannette Richardson, RN, MS
Clinical Nurse Specialist, Critical Care
Portland Veterans Administration Medical Center
Portland, Oregon

Barbara Riegel, RN, DNSc, FAAN, FAHA
Associate Professor
School of Nursing
University of Pennsylvania
Philadelphia, Pennsylvania

Sophia Chu Rodgers, RN, MSN, ACNP, NP-C
Sophia Rodgers Consulting
Consultant, Educator, Clinician
Albuquerque, New Mexico

Robert Rothwell, RN, MN, CCRN
Clinical Nurse Specialist, Surgical
Veterans Administration Puget Sound Healthcare System
Seattle, Washington

Polly Sather, RN, MSN
Clinical Instructor and Acute Care Nurse Practitioner
ACNP Medical Intensive Care Service
Yale-New Haven Hospital
New Haven, Connecticut

Michael L. Schlicher, RN, MSN, PHN
Trauma Clinical Nurse Specialist
United States Army
Ryder Trauma Center
Miami, Florida

Sandra L. Schutz, RN, MSN
Clinical Nurse Specialist
CHF Program Coordinator
Swedish Heart & Vascular Institute
Seattle, Washington

Brenda K. Shelton, RN, MS, CCRN, AOCN
Critical Care Clinical Nurse Specialist
The Sidney Kimmel Comprehensive Cancer Center
Johns Hopkins University
Baltimore, Maryland

Sandra L. Siedlecki, PhD, RN, CNS
Senior Nurse Researcher
Department of Nursing Research and Innovation
The Cleveland Clinic Foundation
Cleveland, Ohio

Diane Vail Skojec, RN, MS, CRNP
Cardiac Transplant Nurse Practitioner
Comprehensive Transplant Center
The Johns Hopkins Hospital
Baltimore, Maryland

Julie A. Stanik-Hutt, PhD, ACNP, CCNS
Associate Professor and Coordinator, Acute Care Nurse
    Practitioner Track
Johns Hopkins University School of Nursing
Baltimore, Maryland

Louis R. Stout, RN, MS, CEN
Lieutenant Colonel, United States Army Nurse Corps
U.S. Army Institute of Surgical Research
Fort Sam Houston, Texas

Kathleen H. Toto, RN, MSN, ACNP
Acute Care Nurse Practitioner
Parkland Health and Hospital Systems
CHF Clinic
Dallas, Texas

Mary Fran Tracy, RN, PhD, CCRN, CCNS, FAAN
Critical Care Clinical Nurse Specialist
University of Minnesota Medical Center, Fairview
Minneapolis, Minnesota.

Deborah Tuggle, MN, RN, CCNS
Critical Care Clinical Nurse Specialist
Jewish Hospital—St. Mary's Healthcare
President, Critical Care Curriculum
Louisville, Kentucky

Charles A. Walker, PhD, RN
Associate Professor
Harris College of Nursing and Health Sciences
Texas Christian University
Fort Worth, Texas

Debra J. Lynn-McHale Wiegand, RN, MBE, PhD, CCRN, FAAN
Assistant Professor
School of Nursing
University of Maryland
Baltimore, Maryland

Laura D. Williams, RN, MBA, CHPN
Palliative Care Manager
Saint Joseph's Hospital
Atlanta, Georgia

Reviewers

Nancy J. Ames, RN, MSN, CCRN
Critical Care Clinical Nurse Specialist
National Institutes of Health, Clinical Center
Bethesda, Maryland

Richard Blair Arbour, RN, MSN, CCRN, CNRN
Staff Nurse/Clinical Researcher
Albert Einstein Healthcare Network
Philadelphia, Pennsylvania

Marie K. Arnone, RN, MA, CCRN
Clinical Development Specialist
Swedish Medical Center
Seattle, Washington

Karen Ballard, RN, BSN, OCN
Nurse Manager
Oncology and Outpatient Infusion
Providence St. Vincent Medical Center
Portland, Oregon

Connie Barden, RN, MSN, CCRN, CCNS
Cardiovascular Clinical Specialist
Mercy Hospital
Miami, Florida

Laurie Baumgartner, RN, MSN, CNS, ACNP, CCRN
Clinical Nurse Specialist, Cardiac Telemetry
Hoag Hospital
Newport Beach, California

Susan Annette Beaty, RN, BSN, OCN
Staff Nurse
University of Washington Medical Center
Seattle, Washington

Linda Bell, RN, MSN
Clinical Practice Specialist
American Association of Critical-Care Nurses
Aliso Viejo, California

Mary-Liz Bilodeau, RN, MS, CCRN, CCNS, CS, BC
Burn Service Clinical Nurse Specialist
Massachusetts General Hospital
Boston, Massachusetts

Karen Birmingham, PharmD, BCPS
Clinical Pharmacy Coordinator
Allergy, Cardiology, Pulmonology, and Consultative Internal
    Medicine
Group Health Cooperative
Clinical Assistant Professor
University of Washington College of Pharmacy
Seattle, Washington

Pamela J. Bolton, RN, MS, ACNP, CCNS, CCRN, PCCN
Acute Care Nurse Practitioner
Good Samaritan Hospital
Cincinnati, Ohio

Judith A. Borish, RN, MSN
Clinical Nurse Specialist
Kindred Hospital
Seattle, Washington

Zara R. Brenner, RN, MSN, APRN, BC
Assistant Professor, State University of New York at Brockport
Clinical Nurse Specialist, Care Manager
Rochester General Hospital
Rochester, New York

Linda A. Briggs, RN, BC-ANCP, ANP
Clinical Assistant Professor
Georgetown University School of Nursing & Health Studies
Washington, District of Columbia

Kathryn Ann Brush, RN, BSN, MS, CCRN, FCCM
Surgical Critical Care Clinical Specialist
Massachusetts General Hospital
Boston, Massachusetts

Margaret L. Campbell, RN, PhD, FAAN
Nurse Practitioner, Detroit Receiving Hospital
Assistant Professor
College of Nursing
Wayne State University
Detroit, Michigan

Colleen M. Casey, RN, BS, BA
John A. Hartford Foundation Building Academic Geriatric Nursing
Predoctoral Scholar
Oregon Health & Science University School of Nursing
Portland, Oregon

Dennis J. Cheek, RN, PhD, FAHA
Abell-Hanger Professor of Gerontological Nursing
Harris School of Nursing & School of Nursing Anesthesia
Texas Christian University
Fort Worth, Texas

Damon Cottrell, RN, MS, CCNS, CCRN, APRN-BC, CEN
Clinical Nurse Specialist
The Washington Hospital Center
Washington, District of Columbia

Erin Cox, RN, MS, APRN-BC, CCRN
Clinical Nurse Specialist, Vascular Surgery
Massachusetts General Hospital
Boston, Massachusetts

Patricia B. Crane, RN, PhD, FAHA
Associate Professor
School of Nursing
The University of North Carolina at Greensboro
Greensboro, North Carolina

Laura M. Criddle, RN, MS, CCRN, CCNS
Clinical Nurse Specialist
Premier Jets/Lifeguard Air Ambulance
Doctoral Student
Oregon Health & Science University School of Nursing
Portland, Oregon

Michael W. Day, RN, MSN, CCRN
Trauma Nurse Coordinator
Trauma Services
Sacred Heart Medical Center
Spokane, Washington

Linda DeStefano, RN, MSN, CCRN, CCNS, ACNP, FCCM
Clinical Nurse Specialist, Critical Care Services
Saddleback Memorial Medical Center
Clinical Faculty UCLA Acute Care NP/CNS Program
Laguna Hills, California

Sandra B. Dunbar, RN, DSN, FAAN, FAHA
Emory University
Nell Hodgson Woodruff School of Nursing
Atlanta, Georgia

Margaret M. Ecklund, MS, RN, CCRN, APRN-BC
Clinician VI/Nurse Practitioner
Pulmonary Medicine
Rochester General Hospital
Rochester, New York

Maurice H. Espinoza, RN, MSN, CNS
Clinical Nurse Specialist
University of California Irvine Medical Center
Irvine, California

Eleanor Fitzpatrick, RN, MSN, CCRN
Clinical Nurse Specialist
Thomas Jefferson University Hospital
Philadelphia, Pennsylvania

Sonya A. Flanders, RN, BSN, CCRN
Cardiovascular Nurse Clinician
Baylor University Medical Center
Dallas, Texas

Patria Fopiano, RN, BSN
Cardiothoracic Surgery Coordinator
University of California, Irvine
Irvine, California

Marlin Ana Galiano, RN, MSN
Critical Care Educator
Providence St. Vincent Medical Center
Portland, Oregon

Karen K. Giuliano, RN, PhD, FAAN
Clinical Scientist
Philips Medical Systems
Andover, Massachusetts

Cynthia Hambach, RN, MSN, CCRN
Adjunct Clinical Faculty
Drexel University College of Nursing and Health Professions
Philadelphia, Pennsylvania

Linda Harrington, RN, PhD, CNS
Associate Professor
Texas Christian University
Clinical Nurse Specialist
Presbyterian Hospital of Plano, Texas
Dallas, Texas

Joseph Haymore, RN, MS, CNRN, ACNP
Clinical Instructor
Georgetown University School of Nursing and Health Studies
Neurosurgery and Neuro Critical Care Nurse Practitioner
NeuroCare Associates
Washington, District of Columbia

Rosemarie Hirsch, RN, MN, CCRN
Assistant Director/Department Chairperson
Santa Ana College
Santa Ana, California

Traci Ann Hoiting, RN, MS, ACNP-BC
Vice President for Nursing Practice and Clinical Operations
Swedish Medical Center
Seattle, Washington

June Howland-Gradman, RN, MS, MBA, BC, CCNS
President, JuneRN, Inc.
Nursing Consultant and Educator
Orland Park, Illinois

Carol Jacobson, RN, MN
Director, Quality Education Services
Seattle, Washington

Jennifer Mary Joiner, RN, MSN, CSC
Nurse Educator, Cardiac Surgery
Robert Wood Johnson University Hospital
New Brunswick, New Jersey

Ellen D. Jones, ND, FNP, BC, BSN, MN-FNP
Associate Professor
University of North Carolina at Greensboro
Greensboro, North Carolina

Peggy Kalowes, RN, PhD, CNS
Assistant Professor, Department of Nursing
College of Health and Human Services
California State University, Long Beach
Long Beach, California

Deborah G. Klein, RN, MSN, CCRN, CS
Clinical Nurse Specialist
Cardiac ICU and Heart Failure Special Care Unit
The Cleveland Clinic
Cleveland, Ohio

Joseph Krenitsky, MS, RD
Nutrition Support Specialist
University of Virginia
Charlottesville, Virginia

Kristine A. Larison, RN, BS, MBA-HCA, RNC-NCC
Manager
Perinatal Services
Providence St. Vincent Medical Center
Portland, Oregon

Rosemary Koehl Lee, RN, MSN, CCRN, CCNS
Advanced Patient Care Facilitator/Clinical Nurse Specialist
Critical Care Department
Baptist Hospital
Miami, Florida

Suzy Lockwood, RN, PhD
Associate Professor
Texas Christian University
Oncology Clinician
Baylor All Saints Medical Center
Fort Worth, Texas

Jeanne Lowe, BA, RN, CCRN, CWCN
Clinical Nurse Educator
Harborview Medical Center
Achievement Rewards for College Scientists Fellow
NIH/NINR Biobehavioral Nursing Research Predoctoral Fellow
University of Washington School of Nursing
Seattle, Washington

Dea Mahanes, RN, MSN, CCRN, CNRN, CCNS
Neurocritical Care Clinical Nurse Specialist
University of Virginia Health System
Charlottesville, Virginia

Peggy McAtee, RN, MN, CCRN
Cardiovascular Education
Baylor All Saints Medical Center
Fort Worth, Texas

Donald Robert McCaffree, MD, MSHA
University of Oklahoma College of Medicine
Pulmonary Disease and Critical Care Section
Oklahoma City, Oklahoma

Debra R. Metter, RN, BSN, CCRN
Staff Nurse, Critical Care Educator
Burn Intensive Care Unit
Harborview Medical Center
Seattle, Washington

Pat Moloney-Harmon, RN, MS, CCNS, CCRN, FAAN
Clinical Nurse Specialist, Children's Services
Sinai Hospital of Baltimore
Baltimore, Maryland

Keri E. Nasenbeny, RN, MHA
Nurse Manager, Medical-Surgical Transplant Intensive Care
University of Washington
Seattle, Washington

Molly Nunez, RN, MSN, ACNP
Cardiovascular Nurse Practioiner
University of California, Irvine Medical Center
Orange, California

Carol Rees Parrish, RD, MS
Nutrition Support Specialist
University of Virginia Health System
Digestive Health Center of Excellence
Charlottesville, Virginia

Teresa Preuss, RN, MSN, CCRN
Clinical Charge Nurse, Medical Cardiac Care Unit
Thomas Jefferson University Hospital
Philadelphia, Pennsylvania

Jeannette Richardson, RN, MS
Critical Care Clinical Nurse Specialist
Portland Veterans Administration Medical Center
Portland, Oregon

Hildy Schell, RN, MS, CCRN, CCNS
Clinical Nurse Specialist, Adult Critical Care
University of California, San Francisco Medical Center
University of California, San Francisco School of Nursing
San Francisco, California

Linda Schickedanz, RN, MSN
Clinical Nurse Specialist
Baylor All Saints Medical Center
Fort Worth, Texas

Sandra L. Schutz, RN, MSN
Clinical Nurse Specialist
CHF Program Coordinator
Swedish Heart & Vascular Institute
Seattle, Washington

Bonnie Sealey, RN, MSN, ACNP, BC, FHRS
Nurse Practitioner
Florida Heart Associates
Fort Myers, Florida

Rose B. Shaffer, RN, MSN, ACNP-CS, CCRN
Cardiology Nurse Practitioner
Thomas Jefferson University Hospital
Philadelphia, Pennsylvania

Helen Simons, RN, CCRN
Clinical Nurse Educator
Harborview Medical Center
Seattle, Washington

Randi Slatten, MN, ARNP
Cardiology/Gerontology
Department of Veterans Affairs
Puget Sound Healthcare System

Kimberly K. Smith, RN, MS, CCRN
Lieutenant Colonel, United States Army Nurse Corps
Critical Care Clinical Specialist
Brooke Army Medical Center
Fort Sam Houston
San Antonio, Texas

Robert E. St. John, RN, MSN, RRT
Adjunct Clinical Instructor of Nursing
St. Louis University School of Nursing
St. Louis, Missouri

Linda M. Tamburi, RN, MS, APN, C, CCRN
Clinical Nurse Specialist, Critical Care Medicine
Robert Wood Johnson University Hospital
New Brunswick, New Jersey

Denise Thornby, RN, MS, CNAA
Director, Education & Professional Development
Virginia Commonwealth University Health System
Richmond, Virginia

Evangeline N. Veloria, RN, MS, ACNP, CCRN, APRN-BC
Instructor of Clinical Nursing
Nurse Practitioner, Cardiothoracic & Surgical ICU
Columbia University Medical Center
New York, New York

Kathleen M. Vollman, RN, MSN, CCNS, FCCM
Clinical Nurse Specialist/Educator/Consultant
Advancing Nursing
Northville, Michigan

Deborah Webb, RN, MSN, CNRN
Neuroscience Clinical Specialist
Harborview Medical Center
Seattle, Washington

Janice M. Whitman, RN, MSN, CCRN
Advanced Practice Nurse
Overlake Hospital Medical Center
Bellevue, Washington

Margie Whittaker, RN, MSN, CCRN, CNRN
Nurse Manager, Surgical Intensive Care Unit
Mission Hospital Regional Medical Center
Mission Viejo, California

Debra J. Lynn-McHale Wiegand, RN, MBE, PhD, CCRN, FAAN
Assistant Professor, University of Maryland School of Nursing
Baltimore, Maryland;
Staff Nurse, Surgical Cardiac Care Unit
Thomas Jefferson University Hospital
Philadelphia, Pennsylvania

Gerion Williams, RN, BSN, CCRN
Clinical Nurse, CVSICU
Tampa General Hospital
Tampa, Florida

Kathleen Woodruff, RN, BSN
University of Washington Medical Center
Seattle, Washington

Mary Zellinger, RN, MN, ANP-C, CCRN-CSC
Clinical Nurse Specialist
Cardiovascular/Critical Care Services
Emory University Hospital
Atlanta, Georgia

Preface

INTRODUCTION

Written by AACN experts, *AACN Advanced Critical Care Nursing* is a comprehensive, nursing-focused resource that helps experienced staff and nurses in advanced practice roles care effectively for critical care patients in any clinical setting. The book's foundation is the critical thinking process: the comprehension, analysis, synthesis, and application of knowledge. In addressing patient conditions, each body system is considered separately, emphasizing complex scientific, anatomic, pharmacologic, and pathophysiologic concepts. A multidisciplinary, evidence-based approach is taken in determining an appropriate course of action for each condition and potential complication.

Anatomy, physiology, and pathophysiology are presented in an application format, rather than as a dry recitation of facts. Assessment focuses on recognizing unusual or life-threatening signs and symptoms and on interpreting out-of-range laboratory values and other abnormal test results. Then the emphasis shifts to linking those findings to diagnoses and interventions. While the chapter text provides a wealth of background information on each condition and its treatment, the book's approach is hands on and relentlessly practical—it highlights both expected and unexpected clinical events and invites nurses to draw on their own experience and knowledge of the topic in addressing evolving multisystem complications.

ORGANIZATION

AACN Advanced Critical Care Nursing begins with a look at the current critical care environment and the varied settings in which critical care is practiced. Because critical illness generally affects multiple body systems, a chapter on comorbid conditions is included. The often-overlooked topics of pain and sedation are also considered in this introductory section.

The next section of the book underscores its multidisciplinary approach by addressing topics that affect all critical care patients, whether they are being treated for trauma, having an organ transplant, or recovering from surgical complications. A chapter on symptom management covers diarrhea, nausea and vomiting, and dyspnea. Nutrition and thermoregulation in critical care are examined in separate chapters. Finally, a model of family-centered care is introduced and the important concept of prophylaxis is presented as a means of improving patient outcomes.

The next several sections are organized by body system: cardiac, pulmonary, neurologic, gastrointestinal, renal, endocrine, hematologic, immunologic, and multisystem disorders. Within each section, the book's practical, multidisciplinary perspective is reflected in chapters such as those on blood component replacement, electrolyte emergencies, and special neurologic patient populations.

The final section of *AACN Advanced Critical Care Nursing* presents other special patient populations, including critically ill pregnant patients, elderly patients, pediatric patients who are being cared for in adult critical care units, patients with severe neuropsychiatric disorders, bariatric surgery patients, oncology patients, and patients with chemical dependencies. Separate chapters are devoted to caring for postoperative patients and to providing sensitive, appropriate palliative care at the end of life.

Wherever possible, the chapters follow a consistent format. Threaded *Case Studies* in many chapters challenge nurses to think critically in applying the information presented on each topic. *Research Utilization* boxes also give the reader an opportunity to synthesize the chapter content and to apply the principles of evidence-based practice and critical thinking. *Nutrition* boxes, *Medication Tables*, and hundreds of new, full-color illustrations complement the core chapter content. (These features are described in greater detail in the following sections of this preface.) Exhaustive references drawn from the most current research available, as well as from classic studies, have been included for each chapter.

SPECIAL FEATURES

Nutrition Boxes

Rather than focusing solely on how fluid and energy intake affects the critically ill patient, *AACN Advanced*

Critical Care Nursing goes a step further to consider how critical illness itself, as well as medications frequently prescribed in the critical care unit, can compromise the patient's nutritional and metabolic status. For example, should protein be restricted in patients with both liver dysfunction and protein-energy malnutrition, which often go hand in hand? How might organ transplant recipients' serum glucose levels be affected by their medications? *Nutrition* boxes throughout the book allow the reader to explore these topics in detail.

Research Utilization Boxes

Perhaps more than in any other area of nursing, advances in critical care need to be disseminated as soon as research supports their application to practice. Just as important, practices proved ineffective or counterproductive must be abandoned. To further this aim, *Research Utilization* boxes in *AACN Advanced Critical Care Nursing* examine published research studies that may influence clinical practice. Each box follows a consistent format outlining the clinical issue addressed by the study, summarizing the research, discussing its application to practice, and suggesting specific questions to be investigated as research in the area proceeds. This feature not only familiarizes nurses with the research in question but also demonstrates the principles of critical thinking that undergird evidence-based practice in the field.

Threaded *Case Studies* with *Decision Point* Questions

Critical care nurses know that few patients have open-and-shut cases. To reflect this reality, threaded, multi-part *Case Studies* show how the course of a patient's illness unfolds, rather than presenting it in a static snapshot. For example, readers learn about L. M.'s chronic history of alcohol abuse and hepatitis C and his 2-day history of hematemesis and melena, before reviewing his initial assessment parameters and following him through acute respiratory failure, sepsis, and other multisystem complications. At the end of each part of the *Case Study*, *Decision Point* questions ask the reader what factors should be considered or what action should be taken. An appendix in the back of the book offers a thorough analysis of specific points and a discussion of the factors that led to the patient's recovery or precipitated his decline.

Medication Tables

In the critical care setting, it is often useful to summarize data in tabular format. *Medication Tables* throughout the book—for instance, "Medications Used in the Treatment of Renal Failure"—make detailed pharmacologic information accessible to readers at a glance. Consistent column headings show each drug's generic and trade names, summarize its actions in the body, list indications and usual dosages, and point out special considerations regarding dosage, administration, storage, cost, drug interactions, onset of action, half-life, risks, alternatives, and other pertinent facts.

Multidisciplinary Plans of Care

What sets apart a good critical care nurse from a great one may be his or her ability to pull together a capable, collaborative team and use its resources efficiently. To aid the critical care nurse in this effort, *AACN Advanced Critical Care Nursing* includes Multidisciplinary Plans of Care in many chapters. Using a consistent format, common problems are listed in tabular format with corresponding interventions, rationales, and expected outcomes.

FULL-COLOR ILLUSTRATIONS

The artwork in *AACN Advanced Critical Care Nursing* leads the way among critical care textbooks, demonstrating complex concepts with hundreds of beautiful new full-color illustrations. Theoretic principles such as the anion gap and the Frank-Starling mechanism are easier to grasp when illustrated with precision and clarity. The emphasis, however, is on practicality—where to place facial electrodes, for instance, or how to calculate pH. Figures depicting pupil response, Chvostek's sign, and other physiologic responses allow nurses to assess patients more accurately and confidently. Equipment illustrations, such as a tracheostomy speaking valve, an abdominal pressure dressing, and a pediatric crash cart, familiarize readers with the tools of the trade in every area of critical care. Dozens of algorithms help readers troubleshoot unpredictable problems, such as hypotension, and aid clinical decision making in complicated areas like transfusion, trauma, and sepsis.

EVOLVE

The accompanying Evolve site (available at http://evolve.elsevier.com/AACN/advanced/) offers additional resources for users of *AACN Advanced Critical Care Nursing*. Featuring regular updates of timely, evidence-based content, this website helps nurses provide state-of-the-art care. Best of all, online access continues as long as this edition remains in print.

The Evolve website also includes the following resources:

- An image collection that supplies all of the book's illustrations electronically
- Physiologic and procedural animations
- Heart and lung sounds
- PDFs of specially selected AACN procedures
- Patient teaching handouts from Nursing Consult

AACN Procedure Manual for Critical Care

Need a refresher before you debride a pressure ulcer? Want to review ventilator weaning criteria or troubleshoot an intraventricular catheter problem? If *AACN Advanced Critical Care Nursing* explains why and what to do, the *AACN Procedure Manual for Critical Care*, fifth edition, shows how to do it. The manual offers comprehensive, practical coverage of these procedures and hundreds of others unique to the critical care environment. This edition has been thoroughly revised, updated, and expanded to reflect the current state of critical care nursing practice. Information is presented in a meticulously illustrated step-by-step format, complete with supporting rationales for each step of every procedure. This resource also emphasizes evidence-based practice by providing thorough coverage of the latest clinical studies.

Key features are outlined below:

- Each procedure is organized in a consistent, step-by-step format using the following categories: prerequisite nursing knowledge, equipment, patient and family education, patient assessment and preparation, procedure, expected outcomes, unexpected outcomes, patient monitoring and care, and documentation.
- Each procedure is supported by research-based data.
- Advanced-practice procedures are noted with a special AP icon, indicating that these procedures should be performed only by physicians, advanced practice nurses, and other health care professionals (including critical care nurses) with additional knowledge, skills, and demonstrated competence per professional licensure or institutional standard.
- The book concludes with a special section on calculating medication dosages, including flow rates and continuous infusion rates.

Acknowledgments

As I sit on my deck with the sun setting over the Olympic Mountains here in the Pacific Northwest, I contemplate the magnitude of work that has gone into this resource you now hold in your hands. The vision of a few and the insights and contributions of many are evident. I will be long indebted to Ellen French, AACN's publishing director, who approached me with the idea for an advanced textbook and asked me to consider developing a proposal. Her vision for this text and her incredible ongoing support throughout the project set a foundation for its excellence. I would like also to thank the practice and education team at the AACN national office, especially Linda Bell, for their diligent reviews that helped to shape the final product.

As well, this text would not have been possible without the fortitude, diligence, and patience of my section editors: Vicki Good, Peggy Kirkwood, and Christine Schulman. Had they known then what they know now, I would guess that this editorial team might look different. To all three of you, my heartfelt thanks for hanging in there with me as we worked through untold challenges. We have a book to be proud of in spite of references and abbreviations.

It has been my privilege to work with a number of talented editorial staff at Elsevier. The support and encouragement that Barbara Cullen, my initial editor and friend, provided as the project moved forward was outstanding. As she handed the reins to Maureen Iannuzzi, my current editor, that support and encouragement continued. I feel fortunate to have had the expertise of both talented women at my disposal for this project. As well, this work would not have been possible without the incredible knowledge and professionalism of Melissa Kinsey, my developmental editor. On a day-to-day basis, Melissa helped me navigate the uncharted waters of a first edition book with all the inherent challenges it brought. Process queen, this content queen is grateful beyond words for your help. As well, I appreciate Jennifer Ehlers, who is bringing to life the Evolve site for the book and helping in untold ways with the wrap-up details that would be making me crazy. My thanks to Joanna Pellegrini who facilitated the permission process, another editorial detail that has been known to drive editors over the edge.

When one of our beautiful new illustrations catches your eye or helps explain a concept, you will join me in thanking Elsevier's illustration buyer, Kari Wszolek, who was the liaison between Melissa and the art house, along with Victor Ayers and his team at Imagineering who did a fabulous job creating the artwork. As we moved into production, I am grateful to have the support of Ann Rogers, our wonderful production manager; Beth Welch, our copyeditor; and Durrae Johanek, our proofreader, who have all helped massage this massive work into final shape. Without this hard-working team at Elsevier, this text would not be in your hands.

A simple thank you seems inadequate to our critical care colleagues—the experts in this field—who are the real stars in making this book a reality. Your hard work and dedicated effort toward making this book a resource that will be valuable to our colleagues is deeply appreciated. To those of you who wrote, thank you for accepting the challenge to aim for a higher level. To those of you who reviewed, thanks for helping us ensure we were meeting our goal of creating a book that will help the novice move toward expertise.

Last, yet extremely important, I would like to thank those close to me who provided personal support and encouragement throughout this endeavor. To Marianne Chulay and Debra Wiegand, my writing and editing mentors, thank you for helping me mature as an editor. To Jim, the true love of my life, who believes that I can do whatever I set my mind to, thank you for your constant love and support. I thank God for you and our kids every day. To Daniel and Katie, my smaller cheerleaders, I appreciate your positive attitudes when mom needed to work on the book. Katie, I still have the sticker that together we will place on my calendar on the day this book is finished. You are both bright spots in my day. Lastly, I would like to thank nurses from across specialties, especially Jane Tobler-Wolf and Karen Moore, for your compassionate, tender care of my family and me over the past few years. As your colleague, I am so proud to share the profession of nursing with you.

Karen K. Carlson
August 2007

Contents

UNIT 3   CARDIAC

UNIT 11 MULTISYSTEM DISORDERS

Chapter 40 Shock and End Points of Resuscitation, 1067

John J. Gallagher

Chapter 41 Optimizing Hemodynamics: Strategies for Fluid and Medication Titration in Shock, 1099

Deborah Tuggle

Chapter 42 Trauma, 1134

Christine Smith Schulman

CHAPTER 1

The Critical Care Environment

Vicki S. Good

The critical care environment has undergone countless changes since its inception. Historically, nurses have experienced times during which patients were placed in critical care merely to be watched more closely. Today, patients are placed into the critical care environment because of life-threatening conditions and/or the need for complex interventions and treatments.[9,21,49] The critical care patient from years past is now treated on general medical-surgical units, and most of today's critical care patients would not have survived in the past.[30]

Numerous words have been used to describe the critical care environment. These include dynamic, complex, stressful, vulnerable, unstable, high-tech, and fast-paced.[4,9,21,30,31,86] These same words can be used to describe today's critical care patient. In the face of increasing complexity of both the environment and the patient is the fact that the United States is experiencing one of the worst nursing shortages in recorded history. In addition, patients are more educated than ever before. The patient and family are demanding a safe healthcare environment, positive patient outcomes, and quality care. The experienced nurse plays a primary role in meeting these demands. To retain talented experienced nurses at the bedside, a positive healthcare environment must be achieved.[1,21,67,83,86] This and related issues are explored in the Research Utilization box at right.

Throughout its existence, the American Association of Critical-Care Nurses (AACN) has taken an active role in establishing standards for the critical care environment.[88] This chapter will discuss two such initiatives that have resulted in positive changes in the practice environment: the Synergy Model and the Healthy Work Environment Standards.

The Synergy Model was introduced by AACN to provide a conceptual framework for linking critical care nursing practice to the competencies of the critical care nurse in order to optimize patient outcomes.[5,45,88] According to AACN, synergy results when the needs and characteristics of a patient, clinical unit, or system are matched with a nurse's competencies.[5]

AACN continued its work to remodel critical care practice by establishing the Healthy Work Environment

◆ RESEARCH UTILIZATION

The Influence of Work Environment on Retention of Experienced Critical Care Nurses

CLINICAL ISSUE

As the nursing shortage continues, nursing leaders have identified the importance of recruiting additional registered nurses to the critical care bedside. However, of greater importance is the need to retain the experienced critical care registered nurse at the bedside of the critically ill patient. Improving the working environment of registered nurses is one of the keys to retaining experienced clinicians.

SUMMARY

Using the AACN national standards for establishing and sustaining a healthy work environment as the basis of the study, the researchers surveyed more than 4000 registered nurses working in the critical care environment. Specific issues addressed included nurse satisfaction as a career, intent to stay in their current position, reasons for intention to leave, and issues that would encourage the nurse to stay in their current position. The study questions reviewed the organization as a whole (macrosystem) and the specific unit where the registered nurse was employed (microsystem). Overall, the nurses responded that their unit (microsystem) had a greater impact than the organization (macrosystem) on the health of their environment. This study contains several detailed tables displaying the findings of the researchers. The key findings of the research include the following:
- The majority of registered nurses are planning to remain in nursing as a career.
- Issues in the work environment have the greatest impact on job satisfaction.
- Work environment issues on the unit level (microsystem) have a greater impact on the bedside registered nurse than organizational issues (macrosystem).
- Improvements in nursing leadership could greatly impact retention.

Box continues on page 4

Standards in 2005.[7] Although the Synergy Model and the Healthy Work Environment Standards are independent of one another, they are closely linked. In the critical care setting, when both the Synergy Model and Healthy Work Environment Standards are used, the result is exceptional nursing practice in a healthy environment, ultimately leading to positive patient outcomes.[5,7,12,54,65,88]

SYNERGY MODEL OVERVIEW

Attempting to match the skills of caregivers with the needs of patients in any environment is challenging without a model of care on which to base decisions. The Synergy framework is such a model for patient care that matches the competency and skills of the nurse to the needs and the characteristics of the patient (Table 1-1). Eight patient characteristics are identified in the model. These include the following: resiliency, vulnerability, stability, complexity, resource availability, participation in care, participation in decision making, and predictability. Levels of need range from 1 to 5, with 5 representing the highest level. The acutely ill patient demonstrates this higher level of need. These patient and family characteristics, when matched with nurse competencies, will facilitate the best patient outcomes (Figure 1-1).

Nursing characteristics include clinical judgment, clinical inquiry, facilitation of learning, collaboration, systems thinking, advocacy and moral agency, caring practices, and response to diversity (Table 1-2). Levels

again range from 1 to 5; 1 is defined as a competent nurse and 5 is defined as an expert nurse. The underlying principle of the Synergy Model is that positive outcomes will occur when nurses' characteristics and competencies are matched with the needs of the patients for whom they are caring.[25,45,55]

The Synergy Model provides a framework for outcome analysis.[25] The outcomes of patient-nurse synergy are threefold: patient-derived, nurse-derived, and system-derived,[25] as illustrated in Figure 1-2. As a nurse develops within these areas, the natural outcome is an increased ability to create a compassionate, therapeutic environment in which patients are cared for by skilled, knowledgeable professionals. As patients and nurses develop these caring relationships, trust develops and information is then more easily exchanged, allowing for more mutual participation in care. As nurses work to coordinate care for these complex patients, using a high degree of collaboration, mortality is lower, patient satisfaction is higher, and nosocomial complication rates are lower.[26] Continuity of care and strong clinical judgment help to stabilize care within our chaotic critical care environment, which should lead to higher clinical effectiveness and better patient outcomes.

HEALTHY WORK ENVIRONMENT STANDARDS

In early 2005, in a response to the overwhelming concern expressed about providing quality care to critical care patients, the AACN published standards for establishment of a healthy work environment. AACN has defined six fundamental standards for establishing and sustaining healthy work environments (Table 1-3). The standards are a foundation and not considered all-inclusive (i.e., clinical practice, patient outcomes, and regulatory requirements for the environment are not discussed in these standards); however, they must be met to provide safe, quality patient care.[7]

The six standards are interdependent to establish and sustain a healthy work environment. For example, to make effective patient care decisions, the nurse must possess skilled communication and true collaboration. If a critical care unit embraces all six healthy work environment standards, the likelihood of enhancing clinical excellence and achieving optimal patient outcomes increases[7] (Figure 1-3).

To be most effective in implementing and sustaining a healthy work environment, there must be strong organizational commitment. Commitment must occur from all levels of leadership and staff in an organization, from the chief nursing officer to the staff nurse. Without support and commitment, efforts will be in

TABLE 1-1 Patient Characteristics of the AACN Synergy Model for Patient Care

CHARACTERISTIC	↑ neg level LEVEL 1	LEVEL 3	LEVEL 5 ↑ pos. level
Resiliency: Capacity to return to a restorative level of functioning using compensatory coping mechanisms; ability to bounce back quickly after an insult[60]	Minimally resilient	Moderately resilient	Highly resilient
Vulnerability: Susceptibility to actual or potential stressors that may adversely affect patient outcomes[63]	Highly vulnerable	Moderately vulnerable	Minimally vulnerable
Stability: Ability to maintain steady-state equilibrium[62]	Minimally stable	Moderately stable	Highly stable
Complexity: Intricate entanglement of two or more systems (e.g., body, family, therapies)[56]	Highly complex	Moderately complex	Minimally complex
Resource availability: Extent of resources (e.g., psychologic, social) that patient, family, and community bring to situation[61]	Few resources	Moderate resources	Many resources
Participation in care: Extent to which patient and family engage in aspects of care[57]	No participation	Moderate participation	Full participation
Participation in decision making: Extent to which patient and family engage in decision making[58]	No participation	Moderate participation	Full Participation
Predictability: Summative characteristic that allows one to expect a certain trajectory of illness[59]	Not predictable	Moderately predictable	Highly predictable

From references 56-63. American Association of Critical-Care Nurses, Aliso Viejo, Calif. Used with permission.

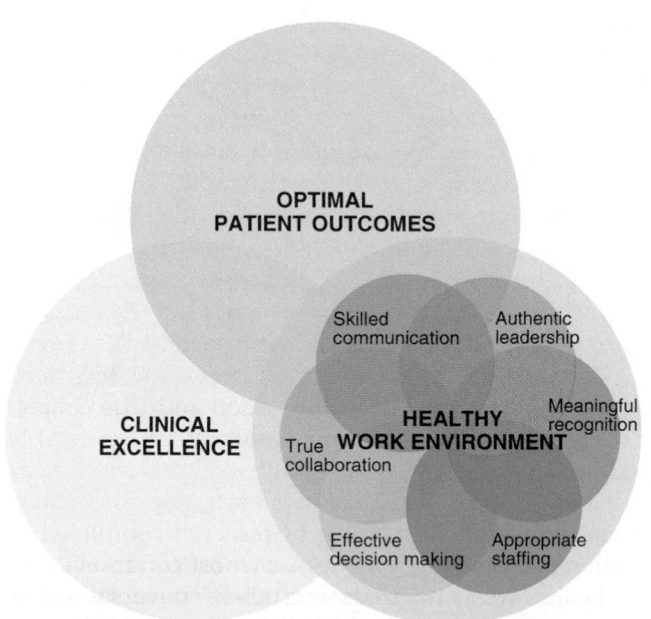

⇕FIGURE 1-1 Interdependence of healthy work environments, clinical excellence, and optimal patient outcomes.

vain.[7,86] The implementation of the healthy work environment standards may require changes in cultural norms, clinical practices, and philosophies of leadership.

Skilled Communication

Nurses must be as proficient in communication skills as they are in clinical skills (Box 1-1). One of the major challenges facing the healthcare team is the lack of effective communication. The Joint Commission (TJC) has determined that the number one root cause of sentinel events is a breakdown in the healthcare team's communication.[14,52] Communication is as critical to the provision of safe patient care as clinically competent staff. Therefore communication (written, spoken, and nonverbal) is the foundation of a healthy work environment.[7,33,37,68]

Crucial Conversations. According to Merriam Webster,[74] communication is defined as "a process by which information is exchanged between individuals

TABLE 1-2 Nurse Characteristics of the AACN Synergy Model for Patient Care

CHARACTERISTIC	Nurses' Competencies Fall Along Continuum Represented by These Three Categories		
	LEVEL 1 (COMPETENT)	LEVEL 3	LEVEL 5 (EXPERT)
Clinical judgment: Clinical reasoning, which includes clinical decision making, critical thinking, and global grasp of situation, coupled with nursing skills acquired through a process of integrating formal and experiential knowledge.[46]			
Advocacy/moral agency: Working on another's behalf and representing concerns of patient, family, and community; serving as a moral agent in identifying and helping to resolve ethical and clinical concerns within clinical setting.[84]			
Caring practices: Constellation of nursing activities that are responsive to uniqueness of patient and family and that create a compassionate and therapeutic environment, with aim of promoting comfort and preventing suffering. These caring behaviors include, but are not limited to, vigilance, engagement, and responsiveness.[39]			
Collaboration: Working with others (e.g., patients, families, and healthcare providers) in a way that promotes and encourages each person's contributions toward achieving optimal and realistic patient goals. Collaboration involves intra- and interdisciplinary work with colleagues.[41]			
Systems thinking: Body of knowledge and tools that allows nurse to appreciate care environment from a perspective that recognizes holistic interrelationship that exists within and across healthcare systems.[44]			
Response to diversity: Sensitivity to recognize, appreciate, and incorporate differences into provision of care. Differences may include, but are not limited to, individuality, cultural differences, spiritual beliefs, gender, race, ethnicity, disability, family configuration, lifestyle, socioeconomic status, age, values, and beliefs surrounding alternative/complementary medicine involving patients, families, and members of healthcare team.[43]			
Clinical inquiry to innovator/evaluator: Ongoing process of questioning and evaluating practice, providing informed practice, and innovating through research and experiential learning. Nurse engages in clinical knowledge development to promote best patient outcomes.[40]			
Facilitator of learning or patient/family educator: Ability to facilitate patient and family learning.[42]			

From references 39-44, 46, 84. American Association of Critical-Care Nurses, Aliso Viejo, Calif. Used with permission.

through a common system of symbols, signs, or behavior." The healthcare environment is full of special symbols and language unique only to the healthcare profession. Within the healthcare environment, numerous pieces of information are exchanged continuously.

The definition seems clear and simple; therefore why do healthcare professionals struggle with communication? According to research completed by VitalSmarts and Kerry Patterson, most communication in healthcare surrounds "crucial conversations"— conversations that can be difficult to handle. According to Patterson, a crucial conversation is a discussion between two or more people where stakes are high, opinions vary, and emotions run strong.[69,76] Each of

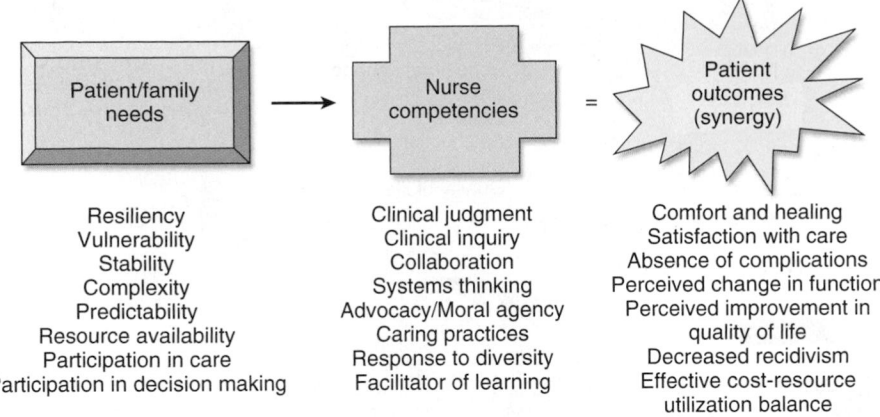

Patient/family needs	Nurse competencies	Patient outcomes (synergy)
Resiliency	Clinical judgment	Comfort and healing
Vulnerability	Clinical inquiry	Satisfaction with care
Stability	Collaboration	Absence of complications
Complexity	Systems thinking	Perceived change in function
Predictability	Advocacy/Moral agency	Perceived improvement in
Resource availability	Caring practices	quality of life
Participation in care	Response to diversity	Decreased recidivism
Participation in decision making	Facilitator of learning	Effective cost-resource
		utilization balance

◆FIGURE 1-2 Patient and family characteristics drive nurse competencies to achieve optimal (synergistic) outcomes.

TABLE 1-3 AACN Standards for Establishing and Sustaining Healthy Work Environments

Skilled communication	Nurses must be as proficient in communication skills as they are in clinical skills.
True collaboration	Nurses must be relentless in pursuing and fostering true collaboration.
Effective decision making	Nurses must be valued and committed partners in making policy, directing and evaluating clinical care, and leading organizational operations.
Appropriate staffing	Staffing must ensure an effective match between patient needs and nurse competencies.
Meaningful recognition	Nurses must be recognized and must recognize others for the value each brings to the work of the organization.
Authentic leadership	Nurse leaders must fully embrace the imperative of a healthy work environment, authentically live it, and engage others in its achievement.

Data from references 7, 76.

these three elements is present every day in the critical care setting and complicates the communication between healthcare professionals. Table 1-4 provides coaching strategies for having crucial conversations.

To make the greatest impact on the critical care environment, institutions should focus on seven areas that impact conversations the most. These include broken rules, mistakes, lack of support, incompetence, poor teamwork, disrespect, and micromanagement.[69,76] Many of these issues involve the need to hold crucial conversations with colleagues who may be at a different hierarchical level than a staff nurse. Crucial conversations are very difficult to hold because of trust and power issues. The important thing to remember is that if these issues are not handled, harm to the patient may occur. Therefore it is important for the healthcare environment to be conducive to open communication *before* problems occur.[69,76,77]

Nurse-physician communication and behavior. Throughout the years, nurses and physicians have pursued ways to become more proficient in their communication surrounding patient care. Nurses and physicians have different roles and therefore approach patients in different manners. Nurses are trained to *care* for the patient while physicians are trained to *cure* the patient.[82] A lack of understanding of these fundamental differences between the nurse and physician roles may contribute to suboptimal workplace collaboration and an increase in tension that may result in disruptive behaviors.[36,67,80]

At a minimum of one time in their professional career, 62% to 96% of nursing staff have witnessed disruptive physician behavior.[21,36,80,82] This behavior can range from a physician with a raised voice to a physician yelling, demonstrating disrespect, berating colleagues, berating patients, or using abusive language.[21,36,80]

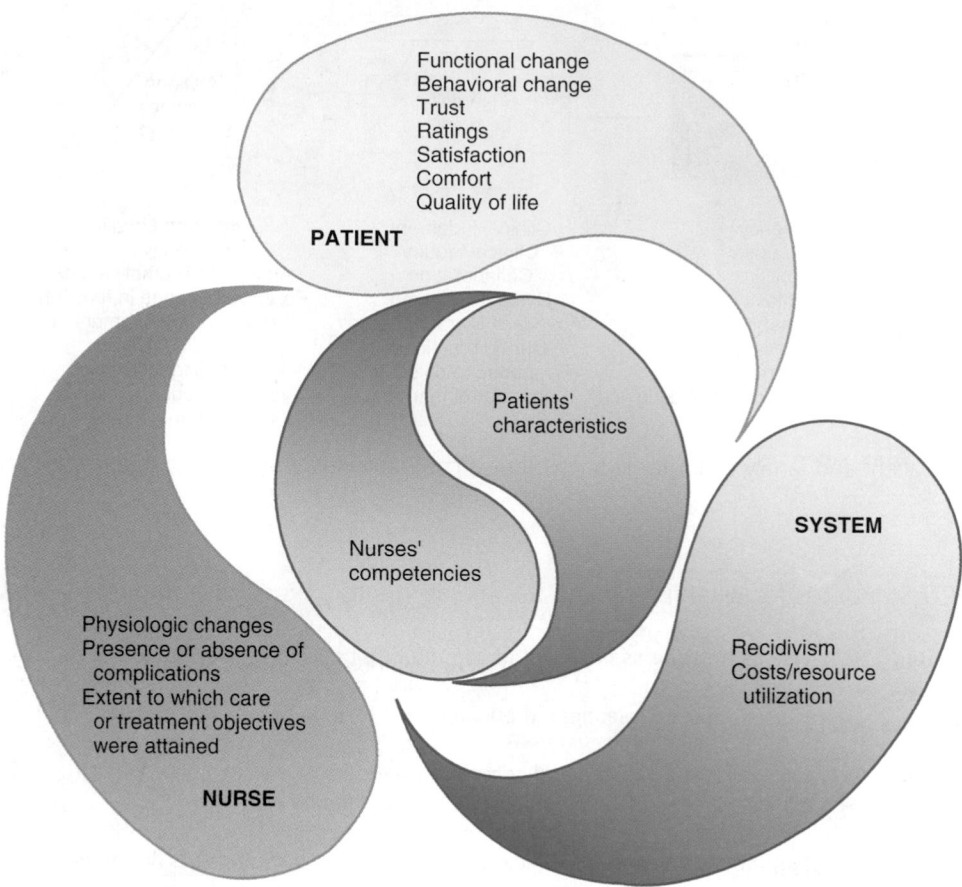

◆FIGURE 1-3 Three levels of outcomes delineated by the *AACN Synergy Model for Patient Care:* those derived from the patient, those derived from the nurse, and those derived from the healthcare system.

Box 1-1

Critical Elements of Skilled Communication

- The healthcare organization provides team members with support for and access to education programs that develop critical communication skills, including self-awareness, inquiry/dialogue, conflict management, negotiation, advocacy, and listening.
- Skilled communicators focus on finding solutions and achieving desirable outcomes.
- Skilled communicators invite and hear all relevant perspectives.
- Skilled communicators call upon goodwill and mutual respect to build consensus and arrive at common understanding.
- Skilled communicators demonstrate congruence between words and actions, holding others accountable for doing the same.

- The healthcare organization establishes formal structures and processes that ensure effective information sharing among patients, families, and the healthcare team.
- Skilled communicators have access to appropriate communication technologies and are proficient in their use.
- The healthcare organization establishes systems that require individuals and teams to formally evaluate the impact of communication on clinical, financial, and work environment outcomes.
- The healthcare organization includes communication as a criterion in its formal performance appraisal system, and team members demonstrate skilled communication to qualify for professional advancement.

From reference 7. American Association of Critical-Care Nurses, Aliso Viejo, Calif. Used with permission.

TABLE 1-4   Coaching for Crucial Conversations

PRINCIPLE	SKILL	CRUCIAL QUESTION

Start with heart.	Focus on what you really want.	What am I acting like I really want?
		What do I really want?
		  For me?
		  For others?
		  For the relationship?
		How would I behave if I really did want this?

	Refuse the sucker's choice.	What do I not want? How should I go about getting what I really want and avoiding what I don't want?
Learn to look.	Look for when the conversation becomes crucial. Look for safety problems. Look for your own style under stress.	Am I going to silence or violence? Are others?

Make it safe.	Apologize when appropriate.
	Contrast to fix misunderstandings.
	CRIB to get to mutual purpose:
	  Commit to seek mutual purpose.
	  Recognize the purpose behind the strategy.
	  Invent a mutual purpose.
	  Brainstorm new strategies.
		Why is safety at risk?
		  Have I established a mutual purpose?
		  Am I maintaining mutual respect?
		What will I do to rebuild safety?

Master my stories.	Retrace my path to action. Separate fact from stories. Watch for three clever stories. Tell the rest of the story.	What is my story? What am I pretending not to know about my role in the problem? Why would a reasonable, rational, and decent person do this? What should I do right now to move toward what I really want?
State my path.	Share your facts. Tell your story. Ask about others' paths. Talk tentatively. Encourage testing.	Am I talking about the real issue? Am I really open to others' views? Am I confidently expressing my own views?
Explore others' paths.	Ask. Mirror. Paraphrase. Prime. Agree. Build. Compare.	Am I actively exploring others' views? Am I avoiding unnecessary disagreement?
Move to action.	Decide how you'll decide. Document decisions and follow up.	How will we make decisions? Who will do what by when? How will we follow up?

Many healthcare systems have successfully implemented programs to address disruptive behavior. For the nursing profession, partnering with our physician colleagues to ensure that the critical care environment supports nondisruptive behavior is essential.

To handle disruptive behavior most effectively, the institution must ensure that all policies, procedures, and actions are in support of a nondisruptive culture. The most important aspect must include defined consequences noted in the policies; they must be consistently followed. These policies must also hold both the physician and the nurse accountable and must dedicate resources to the provision of a nondisruptive environment.[15,80]

Many healthcare professionals do not possess expert skills in handling disruptive behavior. Therefore education and training must occur on how to best handle crucial conversations and confrontations when they occur.[76,77] Leaders must demonstrate the key behaviors they want to have practiced. The leader may need to serve as a mentor to others in these interpersonal skills.

True collaboration and healthy nurse-physician relationships will only occur if the organization maintains open communication regarding these issues and executive leadership fully supports the policies.[15,36,67,80]

Interdisciplinary communication. Many institutions have increased the efficiency of interdisciplinary communication by using the "SBAR" (situation, background, assessment, and recommendation) model. The SBAR model has demonstrated improvement in communication and reduction in patient care errors.[13,38] There are four key elements to the SBAR model[13]:

- **Situation:** This includes patient identification data, code status, vital signs, and the chief complaint or the nurse's concern(s).
- **Background:** Data in this section include the patient's mental status, skin condition, and respiratory status.
- **Assessment:** In this section, the clinician defines what she believes to be the problem.
- **Recommendation:** This includes physician orders and recommended actions.

The key to the success of the SBAR model is the consistent assessment and diagnostic data the clinical staff gather before initiating communication with any other discipline. The SBAR model uses a standardized approach for all communication, thus decreasing the likelihood of omitting key information.[13,38]

Written communication. Patient care is guided by numerous pieces of data coming together and being communicated to all the key players. On the basis of the data, patient care decisions are made. The exchange of the data becomes the key function of the communication processes between team members. A critical objective in the critical care environment is to determine the most effective and efficient way to communicate these patient care data.[29]

Healthcare organizations must continue to partner with industry experts in information systems to ensure a seamless process to exchange patient care information. The degree of use of information systems varies drastically from organization to organization. Some healthcare systems are using voice recognition for charting and order entry, teleradiology, and telemedicine, while others are only using email and possibly an electronic medical record.

The popularity of a variety of clinical information systems continues to increase because of the advantages that these information systems and electronic medical records provide. The electronic medical record has been shown to positively influence the flow of information.[29] When key data are effectively and efficiently communicated, improvements in quality, safety, and efficiency of patient care will result. The electronic medical record improves the multidisciplinary flow of information across the healthcare team by allowing access to the information in a variety of locations in real time as care is delivered. Many organizations have patients' medical records and key monitoring information available to the physician at her home and/or office.

The key requirement of any clinical information system is that all data must be retrievable from one location. The primary components of a clinical information system must include physician order entry, diagnostic testing retrieval, clinical documentation, pharmacy monitoring, and medication documentation. Many of these components are operated from multiple different platforms; therefore there must be one overall information system managing all clinical information in order to provide consistency. Clinical information systems continue to grow in their rate of success in the clinical setting, primarily because all information is in one place, they are easy to use, and they contain web-user interfaces.[20]

Computerized physician order entry (CPOE) is increasing in favor within the healthcare setting. CPOE offers key standardization to the medication delivery process, specifically the communication of medication orders. CPOE is a valuable tool to decrease adverse drug events (ADEs) within the critical care environment compared to a manual team approach with the physician, registered nurse, and pharmacist.[20] The impact of CPOE on ADEs is primarily on the medication delivery component of writing and transmitting orders. After implementation of CPOE, Potts et al.[78] demonstrated a decrease in ADEs by 40.9%.

These two aspects of medication delivery (writing orders and transmitting orders) are the most troublesome for nurses, physicians, and pharmacists. Both writing orders and transmitting orders involve a large potential for human error surrounding illegible handwriting.[20,78] CPOE computerizes these aspects of medication delivery, thereby demonstrating a decrease in ADEs when used.

As with any communication system, caution should be exercised with CPOE. Practitioners can become too dependent on the CPOE and fall into the habit of not verifying information delivered by the system. Examples of potential errors within a CPOE include fragmented displays that prevent visualization of the entire order, pharmacy inventory mistaken for dosage, ignored renewal and stop notices, and incompatible orders. A standardized CPOE system does not allow flexibility. Flexibility must be provided to allow for patient-specific needs.[66]

Despite all the advances in technology, verbal communication remains the most common way to communicate information in the critical care environment.[29] Verbal communication is the most problematic form of communication because of the potential for interpretations, bias, and misperceptions. Therefore hospital leadership must continue to place high priority on the development and maintenance of effective communication. Through effective communication, organizations will experience greater patient safety and increased employee satisfaction.

True Collaboration

Nurses must be relentless in pursuing and fostering true collaboration (Box 1-2). Collaboration among the healthcare team is an essential element in a healthy work environment. The presence of true collaboration in the critical care environment has been directly linked to increased job satisfaction of nursing staff, decreased patient care errors, and increased quality of care delivered to patients.[27,36,67,80] During a recent market research study performed by AACN, 90% of members and constituents reported that collaboration is among the most important elements in creating a healthy work environment.[3] There are three primary opportunities for collaboration within the critical care environment: nurse to physician, nurse to nurse/other clinicians, and nurse to patient/family.

Collaboration is an ongoing process and is developed over time versus a one-time interaction. For a nurse to effectively engage in collaboration, effective communication, trust, knowledge, respect, and integration must be demonstrated.[7,27,79] This challenge sounds simple, but when examining the educational preparation of nursing and physician staff, just like in communication, most practitioners have not received formal training in these skills. Therefore it is essential for nursing and physician leaders to mentor others so that true collaboration can occur.

Nurse-Physician Relationship. It is essential that the critical care environment have a healthy nurse-physician

---

Box 1-2

Critical Elements of True Collaboration

- The healthcare organization provides team members with support for and access to education programs that develop collaboration skills.
- The healthcare organization creates, uses, and evaluates processes that define each team member's accountability for collaboration and how unwillingness to collaborate will be addressed.
- The healthcare organization creates, uses, and evaluates operational structures that ensure the decision-making authority of nurses is acknowledged and incorporated as the norm.
- The healthcare organization ensures unrestricted access to structured forums, such as ethics committees, and makes available the time needed to resolve disputes among all critical participants, including patients, families, and the healthcare team.

- Every team member embraces true collaboration as an ongoing process and invests in its development to ensure a sustained culture of collaboration.
- Every team member contributes to the achievement of common goals by giving power and respect to each person's voice, integrating individual differences, resolving competing interests, and safeguarding the essential contribution each must make.
- Every team member acts with a high level of personal integrity.
- Team members master skilled communication, an essential element of true collaboration.
- Each team member demonstrates competence appropriate to his or her role and responsibilities.
- Nurse managers and medical directors are equal partners in modeling and fostering true collaboration.

From reference 7. American Association of Critical-Care Nurses, Aliso Viejo, Calif. Used with permission.

relationship for true collaboration to grow. If the relationship between the key professionals caring for the critical care patient is unhealthy, this leads to increased errors, decreased quality, and decreased staff retention/satisfaction.[36,67,80] To establish true collaboration, the nurse-physician relationship must be addressed, yet this is a difficult relationship to understand.

Mutual respect between all disciplines is one of the fundamental elements that must be present in order to foster a collaborative work environment. The nurse and physician must demonstrate mutual respect surrounding each other's unique knowledge and competence. Lack of respect for one's colleagues leads to disharmony in the workplace, ultimately leading to decreased quality of care provided to patients.[21,24,36,67,80]

Possessing the mutual respect of our physician colleagues has been cited as one of the top reasons for nurse retention within an organization.[72,89] However, it is essential to recognize that true collaboration will not occur overnight, nor will it be sustained if it is not given constant attention and resources.

Nurse-to-Nurse Collaboration. The ability to collaborate with other nurses before making both clinical and nonclinical decisions has been shown to prevent errors, increase nurse confidence, and increase nurse retention.[21] As the complexity of the critical care patient increases, the need for the critical care nurses to collaborate on decisions increases as well.[21]

Bucknall[21] determined that critical care nurses had an increased confidence level and looked more confident when making decisions when they had the opportunity to collaborate with other nurses. Synergy is built as nurses collaborate together on complex patient issues. That same synergy can be experienced when nurses work together on other issues.

Nurses need to work collaboratively among themselves and with the nursing leadership to resolve issues on the unit. Nurses' ability to collaborate with the nurse administrator on more than just clinical decisions positively impacts employee satisfaction. To increase nurse satisfaction and retention, the bedside critical care nurse must be actively involved in operational issues. Such operational issues include scheduling, quality improvement processes, policy development, and participation in organizational decisions that impact professional nursing practice.[21,67]

The nursing shortage is predicted to reach an RN vacancy rate of 23% by 2008.[6] There continues to be concern throughout the nursing profession about the ability of experienced nurses to mentor graduate nurses entering the nursing profession. Therefore mentoring programs must focus on both the new graduate and the preceptor. Another concern surrounds the fact that the number of experienced bedside clinicians is diminishing. As the new graduate nurse begins a career focused on the bedside care of clinically complex critical care patients, there are fewer experienced nurses to provide key mentoring and collaboration.[21,24,67]

Nurse-to-Family Collaboration. When collaboration is discussed, the immediate thought is the collaboration between the healthcare team. There is a critical element of collaboration that must not be forgotten—the collaborative relationship between the nurse and the patient/family. Research indicates that when there is a harmonious relationship among staff, patient, and family, the patient will experience a decreased length of stay, increased patient satisfaction, and increased overall collaboration.[21,79] Chapter 8 of this textbook addresses Families in Critical Care; it is essential to not overlook their important role in collaboration in patient care.

Effective Decision Making

Nurses must be valued and committed partners in making policy, directing and evaluating clinical care, and leading organizational operations (Box 1-3). The line between collaboration and effective decision making is exceedingly blurred. To make effective decisions, nurses cannot stand alone. The complexity of the critical care environment continues to grow, which necessitates that all practitioners collaboratively engage in clinical decision making. All decisions made surrounding patient care must be sound in reasoning and grounded in the institution's mission, vision, and values as well as available evidence and industry standards of care. Therefore the bedside clinician, ancillary personnel, the physician, and administration personnel all must work together in effective decision making.

Collaborative Interdisciplinary Decision Making. In addition to seeking the opinions of nursing colleagues, the complexity of the critical care patient demands that all disciplines collaborate to make the most effective and efficient decisions. The interdisciplinary critical care team includes, but is not limited to, the staff nurse, the clinical nurse specialist (CNS), and the physician as well as personnel specializing in the following areas: social work, physical therapy, occupational therapy, speech therapy, diet, pharmacy, pastoral care, and anesthesia. Interdisciplinary decision making takes many forms, including clinical pathways, protocols, team meetings, and face-to-face communications.[21,24,79] As reviewed earlier, face-to-face communication causes most practitioners the greatest problems, yet it is essential that focus is given to the further development of this skill.

Box 1-3

Critical Elements of Effective Decision Making

- The healthcare organization provides team members with support for and access to ongoing education and development programs focusing on strategies that ensure collaborative decision making. Program content includes mutual goal setting, negotiation, facilitation, conflict management, systems thinking, and performance improvement.
- The healthcare organization clearly articulates organizational values, and team members incorporate these values when making decisions.
- The healthcare organization has operational structures in place that ensure the perspectives of patients and their families are incorporated into every decision affecting patient care.
- Individual team members share accountability for effective decision making by acquiring necessary skills, mastering relevant content, assessing situations accurately, sharing fact-based information, communicating professional opinions clearly, and inquiring actively.
- The healthcare organization establishes systems, such as structured forums involving all departments and healthcare disciplines, to facilitate data-driven decisions.
- The healthcare organization establishes deliberate decision-making processes that ensure respect for the rights of every individual, incorporate all key perspectives, and designate clear accountability.
- The healthcare organization has fair and effective processes in place at all levels to objectively evaluate the results of decisions, including delayed decisions and indecision.

From reference 7. American Association of Critical-Care Nurses, Aliso Viejo, Calif. Used with permission.

Nurses who have the ability to participate in decision making on their unit are more likely to demonstrate higher job satisfaction.[23,67] When nurses are involved in the decision-making process both of unit operations and of patient care, their job satisfaction and retention will increase. Research has demonstrated a clear relationship between nurse retention and the level in which the registered nurse has a voice in organizational and clinical decision making.[23,67] There are many opportunities for the staff nurse to participate in decision making. Some of the most successful models include staff nurse councils, quality improvement projects, and interdisciplinary team rounds.

Information Systems. The healthcare industry is in a constant state of evolution. Patients in the critical care unit today would never have survived in years past, mostly because of the wealth of knowledge and new treatments that are now available. The current amount of knowledge present in healthcare is humanly impossible to manage. Therefore the healthcare industry is partnering with the information technology industry to provide the most efficient and safe care delivery possible. By partnering with the information systems industry, decision making is becoming more efficient and safer. Clinical pathways and protocols allow the healthcare team to intervene and monitor a patient's progress based on current evidence-based research. To holistically care for the patient, there must be continuous collaboration on decisions for optimal patient outcomes and patient safety. There are numerous examples of how clinical pathways increase the safety of care provided. Clinical pathways guide practitioners throughout the decision-making process, ensuring care is provided consistently on the basis of the latest research.[16,24]

The strength of clinical pathways is their provision of "checks and balances" within patient care delivery.[16,24] The effectiveness of clinical pathways is linked directly to their *consistency* of use and the *efficiency* of use. Many organizations have found that the most effective way to ensure consistency and efficiency with clinical protocols is to link the protocol to a computerized information system.[16,87] Computerized information systems increase efficiency by providing prompts for care providers regarding needed interventions and can also increase the number of automatic referrals to ancillary departments. The reliability of computerized systems can approach 100%, whereas human inspection will have far more variance in their processes.[16] Computerized clinical decision models guide the practitioner through the decision-making process, providing alerts when a practitioner chooses an intervention that might be contraindicated in the patient's particular situation. Through automated clinical pathways, patients are more effectively and efficiently cared for by providing evidence-based protocols to guide all disciplines.[64]

One key advantage of using computerized protocols to guide care for patients is the ease with which the protocol can be updated when new evidence is discovered. Many robust computerized systems are directly linking clinical pathways to practice alerts from national healthcare associations. When new evidence is presented, it is efficiently updated to reflect this change in practice.

A second and equally important advantage is most computerized clinical protocols are directly linked to the patient care documentation record. Therefore as the protocol is implemented, the documentation is completed. This increases compliance with key documentation requirements from regulatory agencies and legal requirements.

As a result of the ever-changing healthcare environment, clinical decision making will continue to be a challenge. The vast amount of new information released in healthcare makes it impossible for healthcare professionals to maintain a current knowledge base. Therefore as critical care clinicians, we must look for ways to make the best decisions to care for our patients in the safest and most efficient ways possible. As discussed, collaboration is a hallmark in effective decision making. Without collaboration from all healthcare disciplines, patient safety will be jeopardized. As information continues to stream into the healthcare field, the use of clinical pathways and computerized automation will be very important. The computer systems can assist clinicians in effective decision making.

Appropriate Staffing

Staffing must ensure an effective match between patient needs and nurse competencies (Box 1-4). When looking to build and maintain a healthy work environment, there is little debate on the impact of appropriate staffing levels. The bedside registered nurse has been referred to as the "front line" in providing patient surveillance, assessing the patient, and intervening when problems develop, as well as the one key person ready to rescue patients when they are in trouble. The registered nurse plays a vital role in patient care and also is the highest expense in the acute care hospital budget. Therefore it is essential for organizations to ensure safe staffing levels with competent practitioners while monitoring expenses.[2,19,51] Because of the complexity of this issue, there are several ways nurses and organizations can work together to ensure appropriate staffing.

Nursing Shortage. Historically, the nursing shortage has had peaks and valleys. What makes this nursing shortage any different from those in the past? Predictions currently estimate a nursing shortage of 400,000 nurses by the year 2020; therefore it is the largest shortage ever recorded.[90]

Staffing levels and patient outcomes. Many regulatory agencies are concerned with patient safety as it relates to nurse staffing levels. As of March 2002, The Joint Commission on Accreditation of Healthcare Organizations (JCAHO) found that staffing levels were a factor in 24% of reported sentinel events.[51] In addition to patient safety, there have been numerous studies directly linking patient outcomes and nurse satisfaction to nurse staffing levels.

In a hallmark study, Needleman and colleagues[75] found a direct link between the number of registered nurse hours per patient day and six patient outcomes. These outcomes were length of stay and rates of urinary tract infections, upper gastrointestinal bleeding, hospital-acquired pneumonia, shock or cardiac arrest, and failure to rescue.[75] Shortly after the release of this study, Aiken and colleagues[2] demonstrated similar findings. Aiken et al.[2] found that in hospitals with

---

Box 1-4

Critical Elements of Appropriate Staffing

- The healthcare organization has staffing policies in place that are solidly grounded in ethical principles and support the professional obligation of nurses to provide high-quality care.
- Nurses participate in all organizational phases of the staffing process from education and planning—including matching nurses' competencies with patients' assessed needs—through evaluation.
- The healthcare organization has formal processes in place to evaluate the effect of staffing decisions on patient outcomes. The evaluation includes analysis of both patient and system outcomes. This evaluation includes analysis of when patient needs and nurse competencies are mismatched and how often contingency plans are implemented.
- The healthcare organization has a system in place that facilitates team members' use of staffing and outcome data to develop more effective staffing models.
- The healthcare organization provides support services at every level of activity to ensure nurses can optimally focus on the priorities and requirements of patient and family care.
- The healthcare organization adopts technologies that increase the effectiveness of nursing care delivery. Nurses are engaged in the selection, adaptation, and evolution of these technologies.

From reference 7. American Association of Critical-Care Nurses, Aliso Viejo, Calif. Used with permission.

high patient to nurse ratios, the surgical patients experienced higher risk-adjusted 30-day mortality and failure to rescue rates, and nurses were more likely to experience burnout and job dissatisfaction. These studies were very powerful and helped to demonstrate the value of the bedside registered nurse to the entire healthcare team.

Staffing requirements. These studies along with California's ground-breaking mandated staffing ratios have encouraged regulatory agencies to begin to evaluate staffing levels and their relationship to patient safety.[2,51,53,75] TJC has recently released staffing effectiveness standards for all acute care hospital settings. Each patient has his/her own unique characteristics. These characteristics, along with the nurse's unique competencies and experience, must guide the staffing requirements for the critical care unit (Box 1-5). Therefore the critical care nurse must work with the nursing leadership team to provide appropriate nurse staffing to meet patient needs and regulatory requirements.[2,53,75]

The critical care unit is a dynamic environment, with patient acuity and patient volume changing drastically within a given shift. Therefore flexibility has to be present in determining the number of nurses required per shift. Staffing requirements are built on the basis of average census and average acuity of a unit. The role of the charge nurse becomes crucial in monitoring adequate staffing. With more and more critical care units having to depend on new graduate nurses and agency/temporary staff, the charge nurse must take a leadership role within the unit to ensure appropriate staffing. The charge nurse must be given the flexibility to staff appropriately to meet patient demands.[35]

Not only is the bedside nurse concerned about the provision of appropriate staffing levels, but many

---

Box 1-5

Considerations for Staffing Requirements

- Acuity of patient
- Availability of assistive personnel (e.g., health unit secretary, monitor technician, patient care technician)
- Availability of other nursing personnel (e.g., CNS, educator)
- Physical facilities
- Presence of a shift supervisor
- Skill competency required
- Skill levels of the interdisciplinary team (e.g., physicians, NP)
- Years of experience of practitioners

From reference 7. American Association of Critical-Care Nurses, Aliso Viejo, Calif. Used with permission.

---

nursing labor unions have advocated for mandated nurse-to-patient ratios. In 1999 California became the first state to mandate nurse-to-patient ratios.[34] Effective July 2003, California mandated a critical care nurse-to-patient ratio as one nurse for every two critical care patients.[34,81]

Many people commended this effort, but there have been a large number of opponents as well. The number of RNs needed to meet the mandates increases the number of RNs at the bedside. With the current nursing shortage, these nurses are difficult to locate, leading to increases in overtime, use of agency nurses, and frustration when there are no nurses to be provided. The California Healthcare Association estimated that it would cost a minimum of $400 million a year in wages and benefits to provide the mandated staffing level.[51] Mandated staffing ratios also negatively impact the ability of the nursing staff to practice flexibility in staffing. Mandated ratios treat every patient and nurse the same and do not allow for variation in either. Some states have followed California's lead, but many states continue to search for a better answer.[34,51,81]

TJC requires every acute care hospital to monitor the effectiveness of its staffing ratios. Each hospital must monitor patient outcomes and compare those outcomes to the staffing levels of the unit. There are a variety of nurse-driven patient outcomes that an institution can choose to monitor. These include, but are not limited to, patient falls, skin breakdown, and adverse drug events. These outcomes are compared to human resource outcomes such as, but not limited to, vacancy rate, nursing hours per patient day, and RN nursing hours per patient day. Each hospital determines which outcomes and which human resource data will be monitored based on typical problems and high-risk issues for the healthcare institution.[53]

Nurse competency. Several years ago, AACN defined a vision of a healthcare system driven by the patient's needs where the critical care nurse makes an optimal contribution. As AACN put this vision into operation, it revealed that the blueprint for the credentialing examinations followed a systems approach to thinking versus being patient centered. To that end, AACN introduced the Synergy Model as discussed earlier in this chapter. According to the Synergy Model, when one links patient characteristics to nurse competencies, optimal patient outcomes will result. The patient is the priority within the Synergy Model and the competencies of the nurse must link directly to the patient.[5,11,28]

New graduate nurses. To meet the demand for the number of needed bedside nurses, critical care units face the challenge of hiring new graduate registered nurses. Research has demonstrated that most new graduate nurses do not exit their educational program at a competent level. New graduate nurses can take up to 1 year following graduation before they feel comfortable at the bedside.[22] Therefore the healthcare organization must have programs to assist the new graduate nurse in his/her transition from new graduate to competent bedside registered nurse. The most successful programs provide a lengthy orientation that includes mentoring, precepting, and critical care classes. Many organizations refer to these programs as internships or residencies. During such programs, the graduate nurses are constantly monitored and given daily formal feedback on their progress. Critical care units that are most successful in transitioning new graduate nurses to competent critical care registered nurses decrease the workload of their experienced nurse preceptor so that he/she can focus on the new graduate. This is becoming more of a challenge in the face of the nursing shortage.[17,21,90]

Physical layout of the critical care unit. Patient flow and efficiency will be determined greatly by the geography of the critical care unit. Therefore the geographic layout of the critical care unit will affect the nurse staffing ratios and skill mix. Units that are designed as individual rooms with doors will require higher nurse-to-patient ratios than those units with an open-bay model. If the unit has large amounts of geographically distant sections, potentially more nursing hours will be needed to provide observation and assessment of the critical care patient.[35,48]

Many institutions are addressing nurse staffing issues and the shortage of hospital beds, specifically critical care and telemetry beds, with a concept called the "acuity adaptable room." During an average hospitalization for a critical care illness, a patient can experience three to six moves from one unit to other units. With each transfer of location, there is an increased risk of patient care errors, miscommunication, and missed or delayed treatments. The acuity adaptable room allows for the provision of all levels of care in one room. The patient moves through each stage of treatment—critical care, progressive care, and medical-surgical care—without leaving the room. Therefore the patient is cared for by the same staff throughout hospitalization, which can lead to increased communication, coordination of care, and ultimately increased patient satisfaction.[47]

Chapter 2 has additional information on how the patient care setting can have an influence on the provision of critical care.

Meaningful Recognition

Nurses must be recognized and must recognize others for the value each person brings to the work of the organization (Box 1-6). One of the fundamental keys to developing a healthy work environment is to ensure satisfied employees.[85] A key human desire is the need to be recognized for our contributions, both in our personal and in our professional lives. The purpose of recognition is to acknowledge, honor, and celebrate the contribution of individuals or groups.[71]

The type of recognition desired by individuals varies from person to person. Recognition can be either tangible or intangible. Examples of tangible recognition

---

Box 1-6

Critical Elements of Meaningful Recognition

- The healthcare organization has a comprehensive system in place that includes formal processes and structured forums that ensure a sustainable focus on recognizing all team members for their contributions and the value they bring to the work of the organization.
- The healthcare organization establishes a systematic process for all team members to learn about the institution's recognition system and how to participate by recognizing the contributions of colleagues and the value they bring to the organization.
- The healthcare organization's recognition system reaches from the bedside to the board table, ensuring individuals receive recognition consistent with their personal definition of meaning, fulfillment, development, and advancement at every stage of their professional career.
- The healthcare organization's recognition system includes processes validating that recognition is meaningful to those being acknowledged.
- Team members understand that everyone is responsible for playing an active role in the organization's recognition program and meaningfully recognizing contributions.
- The healthcare organization regularly and comprehensively evaluates its recognition system, ensuring effective programs that help to move the organization toward a sustainable culture of excellence that values meaningful recognition.

Data from references 2, 7, 51, 53, 75. American Association of Critical-Care Nurses, Aliso Viejo, Calif. Used with permission.

include gift cards, bonus payments, and gifts, whereas intangible examples are verbal expressions of thanks, recognition in unit/hospital newsletters, and recognition at department meetings.[85]

A second key form of recognition is group recognition for achievements. Group recognition such as the Magnet Recognition Program from the American Nurses Association and the Beacon Award from AACN are gaining in popularity in recognizing environments superior in the delivery of patient care.[7,8,10,50,73,86]

Key Aspects of Individual Recognition. Why is recognition so important to nurses? The simplest reason is the fact that all individuals appreciate a simple "thank you" for their hard work and dedication to the organization. When an employee feels valued by the organization, that individual is more likely to think favorably of the organization, stay at the organization longer, and have increased productivity.[71,73]

The type of recognition provided is not as important as the fact that recognition is being provided. Simple forms of recognition are the best, such as thank you notes, announcements of achievements in staff meetings, bulletin boards, or emails of key achievements. Many institutions have adopted simple ways to provide staff immediate recognition by patients, families, and co-workers. These include documents for individuals to complete noting the special activities that the staff member has performed as well as small tokens of appreciation such as movie tickets or gift certificates to the cafeteria. All of these items provide instant recognition to the staff member and make a lasting impression on employees of their contribution.[85]

Keys to meaningful recognition include that it must be sincere, timely, and visible. If recognition is performed automatically and routinely, it potentially loses its value with the individual. For example, if an organization requires its leadership to write a thank you note every Friday and the staff is aware of this "requirement," the note may have little value to the employee. Recognition and feedback to the staff must be timely. Staff will not respond well to recognition that occurs several weeks after the event. In addition to timely recognition, the recognition must be visible to others. Nurses want their contributions to be recognized by both their leader and their peers. Therefore it is important for nurses to be recognized in front of their peers.[18,71,73]

As the critical care environment continues to struggle with the nursing shortage, it is crucial to recognize individual nurses for years of service. The value of an experienced bedside nurse is difficult to measure. Many units have developed innovative ways to recognize nurses for years of service. The military recognizes its workforce by rank and assignment.[32] Civilian critical care units recognize nurses in a variety of ways. These include "walls of honor" noting years of service, scheduling preferences, preceptor responsibilities, and continuing educational opportunities plus numerous other incentives.[18,71-73]

Group Recognition. It is equally important to recognize the critical care unit as a whole as it is to recognize the individuals within the critical care unit. There are two key recognition programs that recognize units/hospitals for providing and sustaining a healthy work environment. These are the American Nurses Association's Magnet Recognition Program[10] and the American Association of Critical-Care Nurses' Beacon Award.[8]

The Magnet Recognition Program was developed by the American Nurses Credentialing Center (a division of the American Nurses Association) to recognize healthcare organizations that provide the best in nursing care. This program was started after the ANA studied hospitals that appeared to be a "magnet" in recruiting and retaining registered nurses. Hospitals are evaluated based on nursing quality indicators and their ability to provide nursing care based on the standards of nursing practice defined by the American Nurses Association. Key indicators evaluated include nurse vacancy rates, patient outcome data such as skin breakdown and patient falls, clinical ladder programs, and the percentage of staff with certification and advanced degrees.[10] The recognition is prestigious and exemplifies the provision of a healthy work environment.

AACN launched the Beacon Award for Critical Care Excellence to recognize critical care units and hospitals that have led and sustained the journey toward excellence in the work environment. The Beacon Award is granted to critical care units exhibiting high-quality standards, exceptional care of patients and families, and healthy work environments. The award requires that the unit submit an application demonstrating how they have met and sustained the defined criteria for a Beacon Unit. The application is evaluated by an expert review panel. One of the primary purposes of the Beacon Award is to provide recognition for those units that provided excellence in critical care. Beacon Units are recognized at the National Teaching Institute, in *AACN News,* and in the AACN website. The organization can market itself as a recognized leader in critical care to the public, payers, and regulatory agencies.[8]

Authentic Leadership

Nurse leaders must fully embrace the imperative of a healthy work environment, authentically live it, and engage others in its achievement (Box 1-7). The role of the front line nurse leader is the foundation for a successful healthcare organization. The front line nurse leader is continually balancing the demands of the organizational executive leaders with the needs of the critical care patients and the critical care nursing personnel. The goal before the nurse leader is to provide high-quality care while decreasing the length of patient stay and improving the financial performance of the unit. Additionally, the nurse leader faces the challenging role as the primary influence on staff satisfaction and ultimately staff retention. Therefore the value of an authentic nurse leader is priceless.

Key Characteristics of a Nurse Leader. The first topic that must be addressed is the educational preparation of a nurse entering a leadership position. Many nurse managers were at one time great bedside nurses that were promoted to the position of nurse leader. Some of these individuals have had formal training regarding management and leadership skills, but many of these individuals have had little to no training. Therefore it is essential that organizations make a commitment to ensure adequate development of individuals in this role. This development must include both formal training and mentoring by senior nurse leaders. Skills that must be addressed include financial issues, quality improvement, regulatory requirements, customer service initiatives, and employee satisfaction.[7,19,72,73]

It can take several years for a nurse leader to develop these new skills. To prevent interruption in unit leadership, succession management is important. Succession management encourages hospitals to recognize future leaders and begin their development so they will be ready to take over when a vacancy occurs.

Participative Leadership. Hospitals who have achieved Magnet Recognition have been the subject of much research surrounding the value of nurse leadership on employee satisfaction and retention. A participative leadership style is the most common style in successful organizations such as magnet hospitals. Participative leadership recognizes the value of people and their ability to assist and influence decision making. According to Max DePree,[26] there are five key steps to participative management: respect people; understand that what we believe precedes policy and practice; agree on the rights of work; understand the respective role and relationship of contractual agreements and covenants; and understand that relationships count more than structure. By using these five

---

Box 1-7

Critical Elements of Authentic Leadership

- The healthcare organization provides support for and access to educational programs to ensure that nurse leaders develop and enhance knowledge and abilities in skilled communication, effective decision making, true collaboration, meaningful recognition, and ensuring resources to achieve appropriate staffing.
- Nurse leaders demonstrate an understanding of the requirements and dynamics at the point of care, and within this context successfully translate the vision of a healthy work environment.
- Nurse leaders excel at generating visible enthusiasm for achieving the standards that create and sustain healthy work environments.
- Nurse leaders direct the design of systems necessary to effectively implement and sustain standards for healthy work environments.
- The healthcare organization ensures that nurse leaders are appropriately positioned in their pivotal role in creating and sustaining healthy work environments. This includes participation in key decision-making forums, access to essential information, and the authority to make necessary decisions.

- The healthcare organization facilitates the efforts of nurse leaders to create and sustain a healthy work environment by providing the necessary time and financial and human resources.
- The healthcare organization provides a formal co-mentoring program for all nurse leaders. Nurse leaders actively engage in the co-mentoring program.
- Nurse leaders role model skilled communication, true collaboration, effective decision making, meaningful recognition, and authentic leadership.
- The healthcare organization includes the leadership contribution of creating and sustaining a healthy work environment as a criterion in each nurse leader's performance appraisal. Nurse leaders must demonstrate sustained leadership in creating and sustaining a healthy work environment to achieve professional advancement.
- Nurse leaders and team members mutually and objectively evaluate the impact of leadership processes and decisions on the organization's progress toward creating and sustaining a healthy work environment.

steps, the leader and the follower can raise one another up to higher levels, thereby increasing staff satisfaction and ultimately staff retention.[67]

A participative leader must be committed to empower staff in order to increase effectiveness. Empowered staff have access to resources, information, and support to help them perform their jobs. The nurse leader plays a pivotal role in assisting critical care staff nurses in accessing each of these key items. Not having the resources to care for your critically ill patient is a major source of frustration for a critical care nurse. The resources most wanted can be as small as having a copier on the unit to as large as having enough bedside nurses on a given shift, yet both have equally important roles in staff satisfaction and the provision of safe patient care.[19,67,85,86] A participative leader would encourage staff to work together to define their needs and to develop solutions to those needs. By having increased involvement, the staff nurse will have increased nurse satisfaction and retention.

Role of Accountability. Critical care nurses desire to work with staff that are competent to perform their jobs, are active patient advocates, and have a desire to serve their patients. When nurses encounter other staff members not performing their duties adequately, resulting in compromised patient quality and safety, nurses want to see their colleagues held accountable for their actions.

In a study performed by the Alliance for Health Care Research,[73] it was determined that one of the key factors of success for some of the top "high-performing organizations" was the ability for the leadership team to evaluate and hold staff members accountable, specifically ensuring that behavior standards were met, a "no-excuses" environment was provided, and evaluations were performed promptly and staff held accountable for their actions.[73]

The nurse leader must ensure that the practice expectations of the critical care unit are consistently followed. The practice expectations have been developed by evidence-based research and nursing standards of care from key nursing organizations such as the AACN and ANA. Consequences for not following unit expectations must be defined and implemented. When a nurse leader does not consistently hold staff accountable for practice, the unit's success falters. The foundation for success is consistent accountability within a unit by the designated leader.[19,72] Leaders are often afraid to hold nurses accountable for fear that the staff might leave. Research has demonstrated that a unit will have increased retention if there are consistent performance expectations and staff are held accountable for their actions.[85]

Power of a Nurse Leader. The nurse leader must have a support system and the necessary resources to influence the critical care unit, and ultimately the healthcare organization. The authentic nurse leader must possess skills such as communication, decision making, collaboration, finance, and leadership. The nurse leader becomes the glue holding the critical care unit together and the branch reaching out to other departments in the organization to effectively care for the critically ill patient.

CONCLUSIONS

Healthy work environments are vital for the provision of optimal patient outcomes. Providing and sustaining a healthy work environment is a process that is never ending. The healthcare environment is a dynamic one in which technology, research, and patient disease states are in constant change and growth. As we learn more regarding the nursing care of our critical care patients, we also learn more about how to create a healthy work environment.

The six standards discussed in this chapter merely provide a framework for creating and sustaining a healthy work environment. Each standard is interdependent on the other. A unit cannot demonstrate true collaboration when the unit is lacking skilled communication. Effective decisions cannot be made without having a collaborative team caring for the patient. Therefore as you set out to develop your healthy work environment, do not look at each standard exclusively, but look at them inclusively.

Each individual critical care nurse must accept responsibility for the environment we work in and care for our patients. We must change one person, one unit, one system at a time in order to be most effective. By participating in this process, we can better authentically contribute to critical care nursing and the provision of a healthy work environment.[70]

REFERENCES

1. Adomat, R., & Hicks, C. (2003). Measuring nursing workload in intensive care: an observation study using closed circuit video cameras. *J Adv Nurs, 42*(4), 402–412.
2. Aiken, L. H., et al. (2002). Hospital nurse staffing and patient mortality, nurse burnout, and job dissatisfaction. *JAMA, 288*(16), 1987–1993.
3. American Association of Critical-Care Nurses. (2003). *American Association of Critical-Care Nurses: strategic market research study.* Aliso Viejo, Calif: AACN.
4. American Association of Critical-Care Nurses. (2003). Toxic work environments impede care: AACN submits testimony to IOM committee. *AACN News, 20*(3), 1, 8.

5. American Association of Critical-Care Nurses. (2005). *The AACN synergy model for patient care.* http://www.aacn.org/certcorp/certcorp.nsf/vwdoc/SynModel?opendocument.

6. American Association of Critical-Care Nurses. (2005). *AACN's healthy work environment initiative backgrounder.* www.aacn.org/aacn/pubpolcy.nsf/Files/HWEBackgrounder/$file/HWEBackgrounder.pdf.

7. American Association of Critical-Care Nurses. (2005). AACN standards for establishing and sustaining healthy work environments: a journey to excellence. *Am J Crit Care, 14*(3), 187–197.

8. American Association of Critical-Care Nurses. (2005). *Beacon Award for clinical excellence.* http://www.aacn.org/AACN/ICURecog.nsf/vwdoc/MainPage.

9. American Association of Critical-Care Nurses. (2005). *Critical care nursing: fact sheet.* http://www.aacn.org/_8825651000134c1b.nsf/8/0/818297476d23f9628825692900802d92?.

10. American Nurses Credentialing Center. (2005). *ANCC magnet recognition program: recognizing excellence in nursing services.* http://www.ana.org/ancc/magnet/index.html.

11. Annis, T. D. (2002). The synergy model in practice: the interdisciplinary team across the continuum of care. *Crit Care Nurse, 22*(5), 76–79.

12. Anonymous. (2003). Multihospital system adapts AACN synergy model. *Crit Care Nurse, 23*(5), 86–88.

13. Anonymous. (2005). SBAR initiative to improve staff communication. *Healthcare Benchmarks Qual Improvement, 12*(4), 40–41.

14. Author not available. (2005). SBAR initiative to improve staff communication. *Healthcare Benchmarks Qual Improvement, 12*(4), 40–41.

15. Barnsteiner, J., Madigan, C., & Spray, T. (2001). Instituting a disruptive conduct policy for medical staff. *AACN Clin Issues, 12*(3), 378–382.

16. Bates, D. W., et al. (1995). Incidence of adverse drug events and potential adverse drug events: implications for prevention. *JAMA, 274*(1), 29–34.

17. Beecroft, P. C., et al. (2004). Bridging the gap between school and workplace: developing a new graduate nurse curriculum. *J Nurs Admin, 34*(7-8), 338–345.

18. Bethune, G., Sherrod, D., & Youngblood, L. (2005). 101 tips to retain a happy healthy staff. *Nurs Manag, 36*(4), 24–30.

19. Boyle, S. M. (2004). Nursing unit characteristics and patient outcomes. *Nurs Econ, 22*(3), 111–123.

20. Bria, W. F., & Shabot, M. M. (2005). The electronic medical record, safety, and critical care. *Crit Care Clin, 21*(1), 55–79.

21. Bucknall, T. (2003). The clinical landscape of critical care: nurses' decision-making. *J Adv Nurs, 43*(3), 310–319.

22. Casey, K., et al. (2004). The graduate nurse experience. *J Nurs Admin, 34*(6), 303–311.

23. Chol, J., et al. (2004). Perceived nursing work environment of critical care nurses. *Nurs Res, 53*(6), 370–378.

24. Cook, A. F., et al. (2004). An error by any other name. *Am J Nurs, 104*(6), 32–43.

25. Curley, M. A. Q. (1998). Patient nurse synergy: optimizing patients' outcomes. *Am J Crit Care, 7*, 64–72.

26. DePree, M. (1989). *Leadership is an art* (1st ed.). New York: Dell Trade.

27. Disch, J., & Ingbar, D. (2001). Medical directors as partners in creating healthy work environments. *AACN Clin Issues, 12*(3), 366–377.

28. Edwards, D. F. (1999). The synergy model: linking patient needs to nurse competencies. *Crit Care Nurse, 19*(1), 88–90, 97–99.

29. Erdley, W. S. (2005). Concept development of nursing information: a study of nurses working in critical care. *Computers, Informatics, Nursing, 23*(2), 93–99.

30. Ericksen, A. B. (2004). Delving deeper: subspecialties in critical care. *Healthcare Traveler, 11*(11), 18–19, 22, 24.

31. Ewart, G. W., et al. (2004). The critical care medicine crisis: a call for federal action. *Chest, 125*(4), 1518–1521.

32. Foley, B. J., et al. (2002). Characteristics of nurses and hospitals work environments that foster satisfaction and clinical expertise. *JONA, 32*(5), 273–282.

33. Fontaine, D. (2004). Creating a healthy healthcare environment. *RN, 67*(1), 30ac1–30ac2.

34. Fox, S., Jones, D., & Walker, P., et al. (1999). Strategically planning for the future of nursing in California. *J Nurs Admin, 29*(2), 4–6, 13.

35. Galley, J., & O'Riordan, B. (2003). Royal College of Nursing: guidance for nurse staffing in critical care. *Intensive Crit Care Nurs, 19*(5), 257–266.

36. Greene, J. (2002). The medical workplace: no abuse zone. *H&HN, 76*(3), 26–28.

37. Grover, S. (2005). Shaping effective communication skills and therapeutic relationships at work: the foundation of collaboration. *AAOHN J, 53*(4), 177–187.

38. Haig, K. M., Sutton, S., & Whittington, J. (2006). SBAR: a shared mental model for improving communication between clinicians. *Jt Comm J Qual Patient Saf, 32*(3), 167–175.

39. Hardin, S. R. (2005). Caring practices. In S. R. Hardin & R. Kaplow (Eds.), *Synergy for Clinical Excellence: The AACN Synergy Model for Patient Care* (pp. 69–73). Sudbury, Mass: Jones and Bartlett.

40. Hardin, S. R. (2005). Clinical inquiry. In S. R. Hardin & R. Kaplow (Eds.), *Synergy for Clinical Excellence: The AACN Synergy Model for Patient Care* (pp. 97–101). Sudbury, Mass: Jones and Bartlett.

41. Hardin, S. R. (2005). Collaboration. In S. R. Hardin & R. Kaplow (Eds.), *Synergy for Clinical Excellence: The AACN Synergy Model for Patient Care* (pp. 75–81). Sudbury, Mass: Jones and Bartlett.

42. Hardin, S. R. (2005). Facilitator of learning. In S. R. Hardin & R. Kaplow (Eds.), *Synergy for Clinical Excellence: The AACN Synergy Model for Patient Care* (pp. 103–107). Sudbury, Mass: Jones and Bartlett.

43. Hardin, S. R. (2005). Response to diversity. In S. R. Hardin & R. Kaplow (Eds.), *Synergy for Clinical Excellence: The AACN Synergy Model for Patient Care* (pp. 91–95). Sudbury, Mass: Jones and Bartlett.

44. Hardin, S. R. (2005). Systems thinking. In S. R. Hardin & R. Kaplow (Eds.), *Synergy for Clinical Excellence: The AACN Synergy Model for Patient Care* (pp. 83–89). Sudbury, Mass: Jones and Bartlett.

45. Hardin, S. R., & Kaplow, R. (2005). *Synergy for clinical excellence: the AACN synergy model for patient care.* Sudbury, Mass: Jones and Bartlett.

46. Hardin, S. R., & Stannard, D. (2005). Clinical judgment. In S.R. Hardin & R. Kaplow (Eds.), *Synergy for clinical excellence* (pp. 57–62). Sudbury, Mass: Jones and Bartlett.

47. Hendrich, A., Fay, J., & Sorrells, A. (2004). Effects of acuity-adaptable rooms on flow of patients and delivery of care. *Am J Crit Care, 13*(1), 35–45.

48. Hendrich, A. L., Fay, J., & Sorrells, A. K. (2004). Effects of acuity-adaptable rooms on flow of patients and delivery of care. *Am J Crit Care, 13*(1), 35–45.

49. Hoban, V. (2004). Critical care. Why it is now vital for all nurses. *Nursing Times, 100*(45), 20–22.

50. Hu, J., Herrick, C., & Hodgin, K. A. (2004). Managing the multigenerational nursing team. *Health Care Manager, 23*(4), 334–340.

51. Joint Commission on Accreditation of Healthcare Organizations. (2005). *Health care at the crossroads: strategies for addressing the evolving nursing crisis.* (pp. 1–42). www.jointcommission.org/NR/rdonlyres/5C138711-ED76–4D6F-909F-B06E0309F36D/0/health_care_at_the_crossroads.pdf.

52. Joint Commission on Accreditation of Healthcare Organizations. (2005). *Root causes of sentinel events 1995–2004.* www.jcaho.com/acredited+organizations/ambulatory+care/sentinel+events/root+ca.

53. Joint Commission on Accreditation of Healthcare Organizations. (2005). *Staffing effectiveness*. www.jointcommission.org/Accreditation Programs/AssistedLiving/Standards/FAQs/HRManagement/Planning/staff_effectiveness.htm?HTTP___JCSEARCH. JCAHO.ORG_CGI_BIN_MSMFIND.EXE?RESMASK=MssResEN. mskhttp%3A//jcsearch.jcaho.org/cgi-bin/MsmFind.exe%3Fhttp%3A//jcsearch.jcaho.org/cgi-bin/MsmFind.exe%3FRESMASK%3DMssResEN.msk.

54. Kaplow, R. (2002). Applying the synergy model to nursing education. *Crit Care Nurse, 22*(3), 77–81.

55. Kaplow, R. (2003). AACN synergy model for patient care: a framework to optimize outcomes. *Crit Care Nurse* (suppl), 27–30.

56. Kaplow, R. (2005). Complexity. In S. R. Hardin & R. Kaplow (Eds.), *Synergy for Clinical Excellence: The AACN Synergy Model for Patient Care* (pp. 27–31). Sudbury, Mass: Jones and Bartlett.

57. Kaplow, R. (2005). Participation in care. In S. R. Hardin & R. Kaplow (Eds.), *Synergy for Clinical Excellence: The AACN Synergy Model for Patient Care* (pp. 37–41). Sudbury, Mass: Jones and Bartlett.

58. Kaplow, R. (2005). Participation in decision making. In S. R. Hardin & R. Kaplow (Eds.), *Synergy for Clinical Excellence: The AACN Synergy Model for Patient Care* (pp. 43–48). Sudbury, Mass: Jones and Bartlett.

59. Kaplow, R. (2005). Predictability. In S. R. Hardin & R. Kaplow (Eds.), *Synergy for Clinical Excellence: The AACN Synergy Model for Patient Care* (pp. 49–54). Sudbury, Mass: Jones and Bartlett.

60. Kaplow, R. (2005). Resiliency. In S. R. Hardin & R. Kaplow (Eds.), *Synergy for Clinical Excellence: The AACN Synergy Model for Patient Care* (pp. 13–17). Sudbury, Mass: Jones and Bartlett.

61. Kaplow, R. (2005). Resource availability. In S. R. Hardin & R. Kaplow (Eds.), *Synergy for Clinical Excellence: The AACN Synergy Model for Patient Care* (pp. 33–36). Sudbury, Mass: Jones and Bartlett.

62. Kaplow, R. (2005). Stability. In S. R. Hardin & R. Kaplow (Eds.), *Synergy for Clinical Excellence: The AACN Synergy Model for Patient Care* (pp. 23–25). Sudbury, Mass: Jones and Bartlett.

63. Kaplow, R. (2005). Vulnerability. In S. R. Hardin & R. Kaplow (Eds.), *Synergy for Clinical Excellence: The AACN Synergy Model for Patient Care* (pp. 19–22). Sudbury, Mass: Jones and Bartlett.

64. Kelley, M. A., et al. (2004). The critical care crisis in the United States: a report from the profession. *Chest, 125*(4), 1514–1517.

65. Kerfoot, K. M., & Lavandero, R. (2005). Healthy work environments: Enroute to excellence. *Crit Care Nurse, 25*(3), 71–72.

66. Koppel, R., et al. (2005). Role of computerized physician order entry systems in facilitating medication errors. *JAMA, 293*(10), 1197–1203.

67. Larrabee, J. H., et al. (2003). Predicting registered nurse job satisfaction and intent to leave. *JONA, 33*(5), 271–283.

68. Lindeke, L., & Kieckert, A. (2005). Nurse-physician workplace collaboration. *Online J Issues Nurs, 10*(1), http://www.nursingworld.org/ojin/topic26/tpc26_4.htm.

69. Maxfield, D., et al. (2005). *Silence kills: the seven crucial conversations for healthcare.* (pp. 1–16). Provo, Utah: VitalSmarts.

70. McCauley, K. (2005). President's Address: Live your contribution: our quest for excellence. In *National Teaching Institute and Critical Care Exposition.* New Orleans, La: American Association of Critical Care Nurses.

71. McConnell, C. R. (1997). Employee recognition: a little oil on the troubled waters of change. *Health Care Superv, 15*(4), 83–90.

72. McManis & Monsalve Associates. (2003). *Healthy work environments: striving for excellence* (pp. 1–117). American Organization of Nurse Executives.

73. Meade, C. M. (2005). *Organizational change processes in high performing organizations: in-depth case studies with health care facilities* (pp. 1–26). Gulf Breeze, Fla: Alliance for Health Care Research.

74. Merriam Webster. (2006). *Merriam Webster on-line dictionary.*

75. Needleman, J., et al. (2002). Nurse-staffing levels and the quality of care in hospitals. *New Engl J Med, 346*(22), 1715–1722.

76. Patterson, K., et al. (2002). *Crucial conversations: tools for talking when stakes are high* (p. 240). New York: McGraw-Hill.

77. Patterson, K., et al. (2005). *Crucial confrontations: tools for resolving broken promises, violated expectations, and bad behavior.* (p. 284). New York: McGraw-Hill.

78. Potts, A. L., et al. (2004). Computerized physician order entry and medication errors in a pediatric critical care unit. *Pediatrics, 113*, 59–63.

79. Revta, B. (2004). NICU—The "I" stands for integrated. *J Neurosci Nurs, 36*(3), 174–176.

80. Rosenstein, A. H. (2002). Nurse-physician relationships: impact on nurse satisfaction and retention. *Am J Nurs, 102*(6), 26–34.

81. Seago, J. (2002). The California experiment: alternatives for minimum nurse-to-patient ratios. *J Nurs Admin, 32*(1), 48–58.

82. Simms, C. (2000). Stopping the word war. *Nurs Manag, 31*(9), 65–71.

83. Smith, A. P. (2004). Partners at the bedside: the importance of nurse-physician relationships. *Nurs Econ, 22*(3), 161–164.

84. Stannard, D., & Hardin, S. R. (2005). Advocacy/moral agency. In S. R. Hardin & R. Kaplow (Eds.), *Synergy for clinical excellence* (pp. 63–68). Sudbury, Mass: Jones and Bartlett.

85. Studer, Q. (2003). *Hardwiring excellence: purpose, worthwhile work, making a difference* (1st ed.). Gulf Breeze, Fla: Fire Starter Publishing.

86. Tigert, J. A., & Spence, H. K. (2004). Critical care nurses' perceptions of workplace empowerment, magnet hospital traits and mental health. *CACCN, 15*(4), 19–23.

87. Tracy, M. F., & Ceronsky, C. (2001). Creating a collaborative environment to care for complex patients and families. *AACN Clin Issues, 12*(3), 383–400.

88. Triola, N. (2006). Dialogue and discourse: are we having the right conversations? *Crit Care Nurse, 26*(1), 60–66.

88a. Ulrich, B. T., Lavandero, R., Hart, K. A., et al. (2006). Critical care nurses' work environments: a baseline status report. *Crit Care Nurse, 26*(5):46–50, 52–57.

89. Vital Smarts. (2005). *Silence kills: the 7 crucial conversations in healthcare.* Provo, Utah: McGraw-Hill.

90. Yurko, L., Coffee, T., & Yowler, C. J. (2004). The burn nursing shortage: a burn center survey. *J Burn Care Rehabil, 25*(2), 216–218.

Alternative Settings for Critical Care

Margaret M. Ecklund and Lori A. Dambaugh

The use of emerging technology and the increased availability of pharmaceutical options have provided opportunities for increased survival in critically ill patients over the past 15 years. To that end, many individuals who may not have survived the early phases of illness are able to recover to a stable level and leave the boundaries of traditional critical care units. The emergence of progressive care has provided additional venues for care.[5] Characteristics of patients whose clinical stability is appropriate for these venues will be reviewed and the challenges facing caregivers in each setting described. This chapter will focus on the progressive care unit (PCU), the skilled nursing/long term care facility, the ambulatory setting, and home healthcare.

MOVING CRITICAL CARE BEYOND TRADITIONAL CRITICAL CARE

Critical care has roots dating back to the early twentieth century. One of the earliest critical care units was developed in 1923 at the Johns Hopkins Hospital in Baltimore, Maryland.[3] In the 1940s, there was an explosive growth in technology used for the care of the critically ill. These early advancements included increased knowledge of anesthesia, the development of the first successful dialysis machine, new resuscitative measures with intravenous (IV) fluids and blood products, and the introduction of the first external defibrillator. External cardiopulmonary resuscitation (CPR) was first introduced in the 1960s, leading to decreased mortality.[3]

In addition, critical care was developed in response to inadequate staffing and resources on general medical-surgical floors.[14] Evidence demonstrated that closer nursing observation led to better patient outcomes.[3] As a result of the ever-growing number of critical care areas and thus the new specialty of critical care nursing, the American Association of Critical-Care Nurses (AACN) was established in 1971. AACN and its members help develop guidelines and define best practice for critical care nursing. Additionally, in recent years, AACN has expanded its critical care certification program to include progressive care, recognizing progressive care as a critical care specialty. Certification across the critical care continuum has helped to validate knowledge, establish standards, and promote excellence among nurses within the progressive care specialty.

In the late 1980s special care units began to emerge to address the needs of chronically critically ill patients.[7] In addition, a number of factors led healthcare leaders and their institutions to seek other alternatives to delivering critical care, often in environments outside of the traditional critical care areas. While only 5% of all hospital beds are considered critical care, these patients consume almost 25% of all hospital expenses.[3] According to the National Center for Health Statistics, the average life expectancy in the United States in 2002 was 77.3 years.[12] Current technology has enabled treatment of diseases that were considered futile 10 to 20 years ago. Backlogs in critical care have resulted in overcrowded emergency departments (EDs) and the admission of inappropriate patients to general medical-surgical units.[11] Patients may require frequent monitoring and nursing interventions but not need the intensity of critical care or require the invasive monitoring more typically seen in critical care patients.

Progressive care, as defined by AACN, is the care delivered to patients whose needs fall along the acute end of the continuum of care and is used to describe areas that may be referred to as intermediate care units, direct observation units, step-down units, telemetry units, or transitional care units.[1] Box 2-1 lists AACN's core competencies for the progressive care unit nurse.

Progressive care units are an option both to help alleviate the demand for the traditional critical care beds and to transition patients between critical care and general medical-surgical units.[11] These units, also referred to as intermediate care units or step-down units, provide care to the chronically critically ill patient with varying levels of acuity, resiliency, and stability.[2] Progressive care units may specialize in

---

Box 2-1

AACN's Core Competencies for the Progressive Care Nurse

- Dysrhythmia monitoring techniques
  — Basic and advanced life support
  — Basic dysrhythmia interpretation and treatment
- Drug dosage calculation, continuous medication infusion administration, and patient monitoring for medication effects (e.g., nontitrated vasoactive agents, platelet inhibitors, antiarrhythmic agents, and insulin)
- Patient monitoring using standardized procedures for before, during, and after procedures (e.g., cardioversion, transesophageal echocardiography [TEE], cardiac catheterization with percutaneous coronary intervention [PCI], bronchoscopy, esophagogastroduodenoscopy [EGD], percutaneous endoscopic gastrostomy [PEG] tube placement, chest tube insertion)
- Hemodynamic monitoring, including equipment setup, troubleshooting, and monitoring as well as recognition of signs and symptoms of patient instability
- Recognition of the signs and symptoms of cardiopulmonary emergencies and initiation of standandardized interventions to stabilize the patient awaiting transfer to critical care
- Interpretation of arterial blood gases (ABGs) and communication of findings
- Recognition of indications for and management of patients requiring noninvasive O_2 delivery systems including oral airways, BiPAP, and nasal continuous positive airway pressure (CPAP)
- Assessment of the ventilated patient to ensure delivery of the prescribed treatment and patient response
- Assessment and understanding of long-term mechanical ventilation and weaning
- Recognition of the indications for and complications of enteral and parental nutrition
- Assessment, monitoring, and management of patients requiring renal therapeutic interventions (e.g., hemodialysis, peritoneal dialysis, stents, continuous bladder irrigation, and urostomies)
- Recognition of and evaluation of the family's need for enhanced involvement in care to facilitate the transition from hospital to home

---

certain patient populations (e.g., cardiac, surgical, neurologic, or pulmonary) or may encompass a broader continuum of general diagnoses. These units are traditionally multidisciplinary in nature. The patient care team often includes the staff nurse, advanced practice nurse, nurse manager, clinical educator, respiratory therapist, social worker, occupational therapist, physical therapist, speech therapist, dietitian, and chaplain or pastor. The complex nature of these patients is benefited by this multidisciplinary approach. The case presented in Box 2-2 illustrates the complexity of these patients and the effectiveness of the multidisciplinary approach.

Matching the skill of the caregiver with the needs of the patient, in an alternative environment, can be variable without a model of care on which to base decisions. As outlined in Chapter 1, using the Synergy Model[7,8] the progressive care patient is moderately stable with less complexity and requires moderate resources and intermittent nursing vigilance. Characteristics defining the differences in progressive care patients versus traditional critical care patients include decreased risk of a life-threatening event, decreased need for invasive monitoring, increased stability, and increased ability to participate in care. Progressive care patient venues are not limited by geography, but by the needs and required interventions for the patient.

THE PATIENT'S JOURNEY TO PROGRESSIVE CARE

The need for progressive care may occur during a number of points on the acute care illness continuum. One point may occur within the recovery period of illness post critical care, when technology and interventions have brought an individual to a plateau level. The patient is stable with the current high level of interventions, but has failed to progress to wellness. If therapies (e.g., ventilation, airway maintenance, enteral nutrition, and dialysis) are reduced or withdrawn, clinical deterioration will follow. This patient has become "chronically critically ill."

End-of-life discussions are pivotal at this time. It is important to review the intensity of illness and the potential for recovery. These discussions assess the elements of quality and quantity of life with the individual and relevant family/significant others. The primary care team members are all essential contributors to this discussion. Assessing and providing for spiritual support may be helpful.

For the individual who chooses not to continue the chronically critically ill lifestyle, the choices available for end-of-life care are many. Limiting current and future interventions is within the scope of choices. Choices range from allowing natural death to total

---

Box 2-2

Case Example of a Patient Appropriate for the PCU

J.W. is a 67-year-old male diagnosed with Guillain-Barré syndrome. He experienced respiratory failure, and a tracheostomy tube was placed because of his inability to wean off the ventilator. He experiences profound weakness in all of his extremities, is unable to bear weight, and is completely dependent in all areas of activities of daily living. He receives nutrition via a small-bore feeding tube because of his high risk for aspiration. He has a stage II pressure ulcer on his sacrum as a result of his immobility and inadequate nutritional intake. Before his hospitalization, J.W. was a self-employed farmer and now risks losing his livelihood. J.W.'s illness has placed a great strain on his wife and two adult sons.

This is a patient typical of the progressive care population. An example of the multidisciplinary approach follows. The patient's highest priority need is his fragile respiratory status. The nurse practitioner, respiratory therapist, and primary nurse collaborate to implement an appropriate weaning plan for the patient. The weaning process is prolonged, but eventually the patient is able to tolerate tracheostomy plugging with supplemental oxygen and minimal suctioning. Monitoring of the patient during this process may include continuous oximetry and frequent assessment by the primary RN and respiratory therapist. In collaboration with the physical therapist, the patient is able to slowly regain strength and the ability to walk using an assistive device. Ambulation also becomes a joint effort of the physical therapist, primary nurse, and respiratory therapist. The speech therapist works with the patient to assess the safety of oral feeding. Speech therapy and nursing work together to create a safe eating plan for the patient to prevent aspiration. Occupational therapy fits the patient with assistive devices to help him perform his activities of daily living more independently. The bedside nurse is instrumental in helping the patient to use the techniques he has learned. Social work consults with the patient and family to make the appropriate referrals and necessary financial arrangements. Pastoral care helps the family to find coping mechanisms to deal with this life-changing illness. After a 6-month hospital stay, the patient is discharged home after being decannulated and having a short stay in the acute rehabilitation unit.

---

withdrawal of care. Specific issues relative to this can be referenced in Chapter 54, End-of-Life Care.

If patients and their support systems accept the current situation and necessary support, the team begins a plan of care that includes strategies for adaptation to a limited lifestyle with technology for life support. The venue of care in the hospital environment at this point of the illness continuum is either a critical care unit or a PCU. A second point on the acute care illness continuum may occur when patients are directly admitted to a PCU from the ED or other general medical-surgical units. These patients generally require close monitoring or a specific therapy that the general unit is unable to provide. Table 2-1 provides examples of PCU admission criteria. Admission criteria are set to ensure care needs are matched with the nurse competencies and resources available in the progressive care venue.

PROGRESSIVE CARE IN THE HOSPITAL SETTING

Assessment and triage are pivotal for appropriate patient placement in the PCU. In a PCU, the RN-to-patient ratio varies from 1:3 to 1:4.[10] Ratios vary depending on the specific patient population and acuity levels. Usually, different levels of licensed nurses are available to provide care; unlicensed assistive personnel may also be part of the care team.

The delivery models selected for PCUs optimize resources and each caregiver's ability to practice within his or her scope.[7] Successful models implement the team approach. The RN, as charge nurse or team leader, delegates tasks to licensed practical nurses and unlicensed caregivers as appropriate to their ability and within their legal scope of practice. The RN collaborates with members of the multidisciplinary team, including the physical, occupational, speech, and respiratory therapists; dietitian; chaplain or pastor; and social worker. Optimal plans of care revolve around meeting the holistic needs of each patient.

In addition to the multidisciplinary focus, each unit's leadership determines the tools necessary to deliver care. Devices for oximetry, ventilation, and cardiac monitoring are options to assess vital parameters, individualized for each patient. Equipment to assist with lifting, moving, or transferring patients supports the caregiver team and ensures optimal mobility with safety awareness. Many devices that once required a patient to be prescribed bed rest have progressed to allow mobility for the patient, thus enhancing recovery. For example, smaller, more portable mechanical ventilators may enhance mobility.

Competency: **Mechanical Ventilation Savina Intensive Care Ventilator**	Name:
	Date:
Patient Care Unit: **Critical Care Unit and PPCU**	Preceptor/Validator:

Performance Criteria	*Preceptor/Validator Initials*
General Considerations	
1. Verbalizes knowledge of equipment reference	
2. Inspects equipment for safety and cleanliness	
➢ Verbalizes method of cleaning visible soil	
➢ Verbalizes process for reporting equipment in need of repair	
Volume Ventilator Considerations	
1. Demonstrates ability to locate ventilator controls	
➢ Alarm silence	
➢ 100% suction (O_2 suction)	
2. Demonstrates ability to locate ventilator settings (located on front panel)	
➢ Tidal volume	
➢ O_2	
➢ Set rate	
➢ PEEP if applicable to mode	
➢ Ventilator mode (AC/SIMV/CPAP)	
➢ Verbalizes the function and meaning of each mode	
3. Identifies patient data monitors on the display panel (presses the values key and measured values are displayed)	
➢ Airway pressure (P_{aw})	
➢ Tidal volume (Vt)	
➢ Peak airway pressure(P_{peak})	
➢ Rate patient's inspiratory source (assisted, spontaneous)	
Alarm Considerations	
4. Identifies ventilator alarms and conditions causing alarms	
Identifies three levels of alarm (troubleshooting) conditions	
➢ Warning!!! (red LED flashes and five-tone sequence sounds)	
➢ Caution!! (yellow LED flashes and three-tone sequence sounds)	
➢ Advisory! (yellow LED lights and two-tone sequence sounds)	
Informational message will appear in upper-right corner of main screen	
➢ Airway Pressure High! Patient is fighting the ventilator or coughing	
✓ Check patient's condition and ventilation pattern	
➢ Airway Pressure Low! Leaking cuff or disconnection	
✓ Cuff may need inflating. Check patient circuit for tight connections.	
➢ Apnea! Patient's spontaneous breathing has stopped or disconnection has occured.	
✓ Reconnect if necessary. Check patient's condition and notify Respiratory Therapy.	
➢ Apnea Ventilation! Apnea detected—system switched to mandatory ventilation	
✓ Check ventilation mode and notify Respiratory Therapy.	
➢ Device Failure! Ventilator fault	
✓ Disconnect ventilator and ventilate patient with an Ambu bag. Notify Respiratory Therapy.	
➢ Fan Failure!	
✓ Disconnect ventilator and ventilate patient with an Ambu bag. Notify Respiratory Therapy.	
➢ High Frequency! Patient is breathing at a high spontaneous breathing frequency.	
✓ Check patient's condition and ventilation pattern.	
➢ Leakage! Leaking cuff	
✓ Cuff may need inflating. Check tightness of circuit connections.	
Utilize this tool in addition to mechanical ventilation (generic) competency assessments.	

◆FIGURE 2-1 Sample competency checklist for a pulmonary unit. Courtesy Rochester General Hospital, Department of Patient Care Services. AC = Assist control, CPAP = continuous positive airway pressure, P_{aw} = airway pressure, PEEP = positive end-expiratory pressure, P_{peak} = peak airway pressure, SIMV = synchronized intermittent mandatory ventilation, V_t = tidal volume.

TABLE 2-1 Description and Admission Criteria of Selected Types of Progressive Care Units

	PULMONARY PROGRESSIVE CARE UNITS	CARDIOLOGY STEP-DOWN UNITS	GENERAL INTERMEDIATE CARE
Patient population	Patients in respiratory failure, with failure to wean Patients actively weaning from ventilator and requiring frequent monitoring and respiratory interventions by nurses and respiratory therapists Patients with significant suctioning needs and requiring close monitoring Patients requiring noninvasive ventilation (e.g., BiPAP) Patients requiring dialysis, telemetry, or frequent wound care Oxygen needs may be significant, preventing discharge	Patients after cardiac catheterization, stent placement, angioplasty, and peripheral stenting Patients requiring cardioversion, transcutaneous pacing	Patients with low probability or who have been ruled out as having a myocardial infarction (MI) Patients experiencing MI, demonstrating hemodynamic stability Patients who are mildly hypertensive without evidence of impending organ failure Patients requiring noninvasive ventilation with demonstrated home stability on appropriate device (e.g., BiPAP) Patients with resolving sepsis Patients with gastrointestinal bleeding who are responding to therapy Patients requiring frequent nursing interventions (e.g., hyperglycemia, drug withdrawal)
Staffing mix	Skill mix of nurse practitioner, clinical nurse specialist, clinical educator, registered nurses, licensed practical nurses, and unit technicians. Nurse-to-patient ratio: 1:3 to 1:4.	Skill mix of nurse practitioner, clinical nurse specialist, clinical educator, registered nurses, licensed practical nurses, and unit technicians. Nurse-to-patient ratio is 1:4 to 1:5.	Skill mix of nurse practitioner, clinical nurse specialist, clinical educator, registered nurses, licensed practical nurses, and unit technicians. Nurse-to-patient ratio may range from 1:3 to 1:5.
Equipment	Ventilators Telemetry monitoring Wireless ventilator monitors and pulse oximetry Lifting equipment	Hardwire and portable telemetry Arterial line	Telemetry monitoring Pulse oximetry Lifting devices
Accepted medications; some with dosage limitations within unit standard	Nitroglycerin Heparin Dobutamine (Dobutrex) Diltiazem (Cardizem) Insulin Furosemide (Lasix) Morphine Octreotide (Sandostatin)	Nitroglycerin Heparin Dobutamine (Dobutrex) Diltiazem (Cardizem) Amiodarone (Cordarone) Nesiritide (Natrecor)	Nitroglycerin Heparin Diltiazem (Cardizem) Insulin Furosemide (Lasix) Morphine
Intravenous access	Percutaneous inserted central catheters (PICCs) Central lines Dialysis catheters	PICC lines Central lines Dialysis catheters	PICC lines Central lines Dialysis catheters

Table 2-1 Description and Admission Criteria of Selected Types of Progressive Care Units—cont'd

	PULMONARY PROGRESSIVE CARE UNITS	CARDIOLOGY STEP-DOWN UNITS	GENERAL INTERMEDIATE CARE
Not acceptable; must be considered for higher level of care	Femoral lines Patients who require continuous IV sedation Patients on vasoactive continuous IV drips that require hardwire monitoring Patients requiring external pacing Patients requiring vital signs taken more than every 2 hours	Patients requiring continuous external pacing Patients hemodynamically unstable after angiogram Patients in cardiogenic shock	Patients with acute MI who are not hemodynamically stable Patients with acute respiratory failure Patients requiring large amounts of IV sedation Patients requiring vasoactive drips Patients requiring continuous external pacing

Data from references 10, 11.

SELECTED MEDICATIONS USED IN THE PROGRESSIVE CARE UNIT

DRUG CLASS	DRUG NAME	INDICATION FOR USE IN PCU
Antiarrhythmic	Amiodarone (Cordarone)	Loading and maintenance infusions for treatment of supraventricular dysrhythmias Maintenance infusions for treatment of hemodynamically stable ventricular tachycardia
	Lidocaine Vaughn Williams class IB	Initial and maintenance infusions for treatment of hemodynamically stable ventricular tachycardia
	Procainamide Vaughn Williams class IA	Loading and maintenance infusions for treatment of hemodynamically stable supraventricular dysrhythmias or ventricular tachycardia
	Diltiazem (Cardizem) Vaughn Williams class IV	Loading and maintenance infusions to control rate of ventricular response in patients with supraventricular dysrhythmias
	Esmolol (Brevibloc) Vaughn Williams class II	Loading and maintenance infusions to control rate of ventricular response in patients with supraventricular dysrhythmias
Vasoactive	Dopamine	Used in doses to increase renal perfusion Maintenance infusions of 5 mcg/kg per minute for cardiac transplant patients
Vasoactive	Nitroglycerin	Hemodynamically stable patients with anginal signs and symptoms, acute coronary syndrome, uncomplicated non–ST-segment myocardial infarction, or after percutaneous coronary intervention; patients awaiting cardiac surgery; postoperative patients requiring stable dose
Inotropic	Dobutamine	Maintenance infusion to improve cardiac output in patients with chronic heart failure; used primarily for patients awaiting cardiac transplantation
	Milrinone (Primacor)	Maintenance infusion to improve cardiac output in patients with chronic heart failure; used primarily for patients awaiting cardiac transplantation
Natriuretic peptide	Nesiritide (Natrecor)	Loading and maintenance infusions to treat decompensated congestive heart failure

From reference 9.

Pleural drainage, once reserved for acute care settings, can now be used with water seal drainage systems or intermittent sampling of fluid by aspiration. Small, self--sealing chest tubes allow egress from the acute care environment. Standardized plans of care or pathways are useful in this population to guide and then evaluate care and can offer an opportunity for the team to measure success compared to national benchmarks.

Patients transitioning from a traditional critical care to a PCU typically move from a less physically demanding to a more physically demanding environment. The PCU's philosophy is to maximize the patient's own capabilities while promoting increased physical independence. This requires a multidisciplinary approach related to all aspects of care.

Collaboration between unit leadership within the institution can achieve adherence to admission standards among the PCU. The critical care area, ED, and general medical-surgical units must be familiar with admission criteria for this patient population. Admission and discharge criteria should be congruent among all step-down units for consistency. Documentation of these standards can also improve continuity across care units.[9] The result of the coordinated efforts will be effective patient flow.

Nursing competency should be assessed upon hire and on an annual basis for each staff member. Skill competency assessment should be based on the needs of the specific units and patient population (high-risk/low-volume). As outlined previously (see Box 2-1), core competencies for PCUs should include, but not be limited to, the following: mechanical ventilation, telemetry, chest tubes, noninvasive ventilation, and sheath removal (Figure 2-1). In addition, a variety of medications not usually seen outside of critical care is often used in progressive care units. An example of one unit's use of medications is seen in the Medication table on p. 27. Decisions on the level of care and interventions provided on any given PCU will need to be made at the institutional level. Also, AACN has a variety of resources available to support nurses working in progressive care units (Box 2-3).

Box 2-3

AACN Resources for Progressive Care

- *AACN Essentials of Critical Care Nursing* (2005). New York: McGraw-Hill.
- *AACN Essentials of Progressive Care Nursing* (2007). New York: McGraw-Hill.
- *AACN Pocket Essentials of Critical Care Nursing* (2005). New York: McGraw-Hill.
- *AACN Pocket Essentials of Progressive Care Nursing* (2007). New York: McGraw-Hill.
- *AACN Procedure Manual for Critical Care* (5th ed.) (2005). Philadelphia: Saunders.
- *AACN Protocols for Practice: Noninvasive Monitoring* (2nd ed.) (2005). Boston: Jones and Bartlett.
- *AACN Protocols for Practice: Palliative Care and End-of-Life Issues in Critical Care* (2006). Boston: Jones and Bartlett.
- *AACN Protocols for Practice: Caring for Mechanically Ventilated Patients* (2nd ed.) (2006). Boston: Jones and Bartlett.

PUBLISHED BY AACN

- *AACN Protocols for Practice: Care of the Cardiac Patient Series Protocol, 2002*

Care of the Cardiac Patient in Rehabilitation and Recovery
Care of the Patient Undergoing Cardiovascular Surgery
Care of the Patient with an IABP
Care of the Patient with Acute Coronary Syndrome
Care of the Patient with Heart Failure
Care of the Patient with a Ventricular Assist Device
Care of the Patient with an Arrhythmia

- *AACN Protocols for Practice: Symptom Management in Acute and Critical Care Series* (2003)
Management: Diarrhea Protocol
Management: Dyspnea Protocol
Management: Fever Protocol
Management: Nausea and Vomiting Protocol

- *AACN Protocols for Practice: Hemodynamic Monitoring Series* (1998)
Arterial Pressure Monitoring
Cardiac Output Monitoring
Pulmonary Artery Pressure Monitoring
SVo_2 Monitoring

OUT-OF-HOSPITAL VENUES

Skilled Nursing Facilities/Long Term Care Facilities

Reimbursement available to skilled nursing facilities promotes wise resource utilization. Given the nature of long-term, ongoing care, participation in social activities and normalization of activity patterns are important aspects of the plan of care. Registered nurses competent in assessment of needs and delegation of duties are best suited for this venue. Direct care roles can be delegated to an unlicensed individual. The RN or the licensed practical nurse (LPN) is responsible for medication administration. Other care needs, such as airway care and ventilator monitoring, are often a joint responsibility with respiratory therapists. Activities and rehabilitative therapies are jointly accomplished with physical medicine therapists along with activity support personnel or volunteers.

Community resources vary as to skilled nursing/long term care facilities and healthcare venues. When a patient has reached his or her potential of recovery and demonstrates hemodynamic stability even with high technology (e.g., ventilator support), referrals can be initiated to appropriate nursing facilities outside of the hospital setting. Long term care venues that accept the ongoing ventilator-dependent patient have criteria for admission. These criteria are set by using staffing patterns that consider patient characteristics and needs as well as nursing competencies.

When a hospital initiates a patient referral, an admission team from the new venue reviews the patient data submitted. A representative from the admission team visits the hospital to review the record and complete an assessment of patient appropriateness. Careful selection of future residents helps to assure the appropriate match of patient need with caregiver availability and competence. If a patient is too vulnerable or requires excessive resources, the long term care team may suggest plan of care amendments. They may defer acceptance at this point, and offer to reassess the patient at a future time. If the patient is accepted, visits to the facility by the patient's family and a video or internet tour for the patient may be helpful to ease transition. Developing a partnership between patients and families who have made the transition with prospective patients and families may help with questions and acceptance. Skilled nursing facility admission criteria are outlined in Table 2-2.

TABLE 2-2 Skilled Nursing Facility Admission Criteria

CRITERIA	APPROPRIATE FOR ACCEPTANCE
Hemodynamic	Stable
Ventilator support	Stable with minimal changes No recent airway emergencies Adequate oxygenation with Fio_2 less than 40%
Immune system	Up to date on immunizations No active infection Isolation needs known (drug-resistant issues) If IV access, long-term IV line present without infection (PICC)
Hematopoietic	No active blood loss; hematocrit stable with minimal or no need for transfusion
Nutritional	Adequate oral intake or stable feeding access (G-tube or percutaneous endoscopic gastrostomy tube [PEG] placed)
Renal	Adequate function Renal failure requiring hemodialysis is challenging option for skilled nursing facility (SNF) ventilator patients
Advance directives	Written document Patient with needs known to caregivers for future hospitalizations
Psychosocial	Patient and family accepting of long term care option and financial accountability

---

Box 2-4

Patient Transition From Hospital to Skilled Nursing Facility

I.L. is a 75-year-old female with a history of lung cancer and chronic obstructive pulmonary disease (COPD). She was treated with radiation and chemotherapy 5 years before admission. She continued to smoke and was on home oxygen at 2 L/min. She developed respiratory failure secondary to pneumonia and was intubated. After multiple failed attempts at extubation, a tracheostomy tube was placed. While she slowly gained strength, she developed recurrent nonmalignant pleural effusions and required repeated pleural drainage. Hypoxia and dyspnea limited her ventilator weaning. She was a candidate for placement of a self-sealing pleural tube, allowing intermittent drainage of the pleural space. After more than 3 L were removed over the course of 3 weeks, she was weaned from the ventilator and required less oxygen; she was also able to tolerate increased activity. She was moved to a rehabilitation unit at a nursing home. The skill of assessment and drainage of the pleural tube was taught to the nurses caring for her at the hospital and nursing facility. Eventually her husband assumed the skill and she was discharged home.

In this example, some of the details of the patient's transition have been omitted for simplification. Nevertheless, I.L.'s experience offers a broad and instructive illustration of the progressive care continuum.

On the day of discharge, the discharging team may choose to send a nurse and/or respiratory therapist with the individual. This accomplishes three goals: patient safety on the journey, continuity of care, and comfort to the patient during the trip. Patient anxiety is increased during the transfer; therefore having a familiar practitioner is very valuable. The discharge, despite planning, may be a stressful event, so meeting the breathing needs with the most comfortable approach is most helpful for the patient. Collaboration among the respiratory therapists, providers, nurses, and accepting team for meeting ventilation needs helps ensure a comfortable transition. An example of a patient appropriate for transfer to a skilled nursing facility is described in Box 2-4.

Ambulatory Settings

Ambulatory venues can also be considered progressive care. Therapies supporting ongoing or chronic illnesses, and those requiring intermittent administration, can be delivered episodically. For example, positive inotropic drugs (e.g., nesiritide [Natrecor]) can be delivered on an episodic basis to help manage heart failure. These types of drugs have been limited to critical care or hospital settings in the past. With prescribed criteria for the levels of resilience and stability, patients can be seen as an outpatient for assessment and treatment by a team with competence in this skill. This affords disease management with the potential of increased quality of life and potential decreased hospital admissions.[7]

Home Care

The choice of home care is the desire of many (Box 2-5). However, this option creates the most challenges for those delivering care. For example, individuals requiring mechanical ventilation need 24-hour supervision, 7 days a week (unless they are independent enough to manage airway and ventilation needs). Additional therapies that may be managed at home include peritoneal dialysis, TPN (total parenteral nutrition), and complex wound management. Peritoneal dialysis may be initiated in the hospital, and taught to families and caregivers by the dialysis team. Total parenteral nutrition may also be managed at home. Families are instructed how to access and maintain central lines. Training related to dressing changes and site assessment may be managed with the assistance of the home care intravenous nurse. Patients may also return home with complex surgical wounds or existing pressure ulcers. Coordination with the outpatient wound ostomy nurse and home care agency is essential to determine appropriate supplies and insurance coverage for equipment.

Public funds and private insurance do not routinely cover the cost of direct caregivers in the home; the responsibility of care falls to the family or significant others.[15] For covered services, the availability of licensed caregivers (RNs or LPNs) is often at a premium.

An examination of personal resources is necessary to project a healthcare budget. State rules govern Medicaid eligibility. A social worker referral can provide support to the individual/family as they examine financial resources and funding applications. With approved Medicaid, some states will allow funding of durable medical equipment and some caregiver coverage, based on physician appeal to the state governing office.

The hospital, skilled nursing care facility, or long term care institution team assesses the feasibility of discharging the patient to home, using input from patients and their support systems. When home is chosen as the appropriate venue for these complex

Box 2-5

Patient Transition From Hospital to Home

S.F. was a 68-year-old woman initially admitted to critical care. She had a complex medical history including amyotrophic lateral sclerosis (ALS), respiratory failure, and hypertension. Her 73-day hospital stay included respiratory failure, pneumonia, life-threatening infections, and several return admissions to the critical care unit. Following stabilization and extubation failures, she received a tracheostomy tube for ongoing airway management. After being weaned off intravenous sedation and vasoactive medications, she was transferred to a progressive pulmonary unit.

Initially her management out of critical care was complicated by agitation and restlessness, followed by a period of increased strength and poor decision making. Lorazepam (Ativan) was used around the clock and eventually titrated to a lower dose before discharge to help with anxiety management. Her course was complex, but with diligent management and multidisciplinary planning she was able to improve her strength and tolerate a tracheostomy collar (spontaneous breathing) during the daytime hours with ventilator support at night. Her airway was patent with intermittent suction needs (approximately every 3 hours). Oral secretions and dysphagia prevented successful oral intake. She had a jejunostomy tube (J-tube) placed within the months before admission, based on the progressive nature of the ALS. S.F. used the oral suction independently to manage the high volume of clear saliva she produced and could not swallow. Fall prevention strategies were also implemented with supervised out of bed activity. Physical and occupational therapists collaborated with the nursing team to promote independence and strength.

S.F. had a supportive daughter and grandchildren who made the decision to care for S.F. at home. They believed they needed to make the effort for the care at home, as a nursing home was not an option. The feasibility of the plan was discussed with the family, and several difficult financial and personal decisions were made because of the 24-hour daily coverage needed for S.F.'s care. S.F.'s daughter would resign from her job and assume the role of her mother's primary caregiver, with her husband and children assuming backup roles. A family meeting, including the multidisciplinary team and all potential caregivers, was held to discuss a plan of care that would meet the patient's needs.

The nurse practitioner and clinical educator devised a teaching plan individualized for the patient's needs. Teaching included ventilator management, suctioning techniques, nutrition via J-tube, medication management, and wound care. Advanced decision making was also discussed using a decision tree. Teaching sessions were conducted with small groups of family members. Skills were demonstrated and family members performed return demonstrations several times. Teaching was initially performed by the nurse practitioner and clinical educator, and reinforced by staff nurses and respiratory therapists. The respiratory therapist from the home oxygen vendor also met with the caregivers on several occasions to teach the logistics and management of the ventilator. S.F. was discharged to home after all caregivers had demonstrated competence. Follow-up visits at home by the nurse practitioner and clinical educator provided both a social connection and a continuity of care connection. Community home care follow-up continued the plan of care. Figure 2-2 depicts S.F. in the home environment with her smaller, home ventilator.

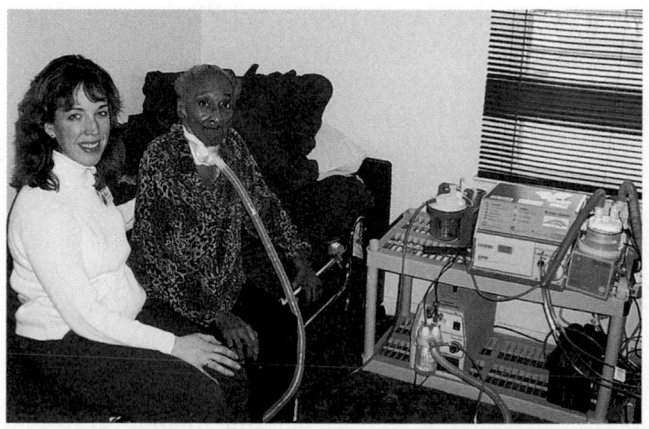

◆FIGURE 2-2 Patient using a home ventilator with the assistance of a home health professional.

patients, extensive education and training must be completed with the patient and family. A teaching plan is established and educational sessions coordinated with patients and their chosen caregivers. A complex discharge plan follows to meet the specialized needs of the patient.

CONCLUSIONS

Complex care is currently delivered in multiple venues outside of the traditional critical care unit as population demographics and healthcare systems change. The constant is patient need matched with caregiver competency to effectively meet needs. An effective plan of care matching patient need with caregiver competency benefits all involved.

REFERENCES

1. American Association of Critical-Care Nurses. (2005). *Progressive care fact sheet*. Retrieved from www.aacn.org.
2. Berke, W. J., & Ecklund, M. M. (2003). Keep pace with step-down care. *Crit Care Nurse, 23*, 56–58.
3. Calvin, J., Habet, K., & Parrillo, J. (1997). Critical care in the United States: who are we and how did we get here? *Crit Care Clin North Am, 13*, 363–376.
4. Curley, M. A. Q. (1998). Patient nurse synergy: optimizing patients' outcomes. *Am J Crit Care, 7*, 64–72.
5. Daly, B. J., et al. (1991). Development of a special care unit for chronically critically ill patients. *Heart Lung, 20*(1), 45–51.
6. Ecklund, M. M. (2006). Homecare management of ventilator-assisted patients. In S. M. Burns (Ed.). *AACN's practice protocols: care of the mechanically ventilated patient*. Sudbury, Mass: Jones and Bartlett.
7. Hardin, S. R. (2005). Introduction to the AACN synergy model for patient care. In S. R. Hardin & R. Kaplow (Eds.), *Synergy for clinical excellence: the AACN synergy model for patient care*. Sudbury, Mass: Jones and Bartlett.
8. Kaplow, R. (2003). AACN synergy model for patient care: a framework to optimize outcomes. *Crit Care Nurse, 23*(suppl), 27–30.
9. McCabe, P. J., & Kalpin, P. (2005). Using shared decision making to implement evidence-based practice in progressive care. *Crit Care Nurse, 25*, 76–87.
10. Meyer, M. (2002). Avoid PCU bottlenecks with proper admission and discharge criteria. *Nurs Manag, 33*, 31–35.
11. Nasraway, S., et al. (1998). Guidelines on admission and discharge for adult intermediate care units. *Crit Care Med, 26*, 607–610.
12. National Center for Health Statistics. (2002). *Life expectancy data*. Available at http:www.cdc.gov/nchs/fastats/lifexpec.htm.
13. Ridley, S. A. (1998). Intermediate care: possibilities, requirements and solutions. *Anaesthesia, 53*, 654–664.
14. Wilson, V. (1990). From sentinels to specialists. *Am J Nurs, 10*, 32–43.
15. www.health.state.ny.us.

CHAPTER 3

Comorbid Conditions

Denise Buonocore and Polly Sather

Admission to critical care and the outcome of that admission are determined by the patient's primary diagnosis and any baseline comorbidities of the patient. In addition, the presence of multiorgan involvement during critical illness plays a role in the morbidity and mortality of the patient. For the purposes of this chapter, comorbid conditions refer to chronic preexisting conditions before the critical care admission. Conditions that arise during the hospitalization are considered to be acute conditions or complications and are not discussed in this chapter.

CRITICAL CARE PREDICTIVE SCORING SYSTEMS

Patients with existing comorbid conditions when they are admitted to critical care have a 2% to 8.4% increase in mortality above patients with no comorbid conditions.[50,53,54] Predictive scoring systems in use in many critical care units attempt to calculate the mortality risk of the critical care patient on the basis of these comorbidities when the patient is admitted to critical care. Predictive scoring systems use a severity of illness score to adjust for mortality risk upon admission to critical care. The overall score given to a patient is calculated based on several factors including, but not limited to, case-mix differences, patient age, physiologic scoring, and preexisting conditions. However, many of these scoring systems have different views about which comorbid conditions have the greatest impact on outcome. The scoring systems described in this chapter are used solely as a starting point for understanding and comprehending the impact and importance of comorbidity in critical care. They are not meant to be all-inclusive in predicting outcomes in critical care. The three most frequently used predictive scoring systems are the APACHE (Acute Physiology and Chronic Health Evaluation, now in its fourth modification), the SAPS II (Simplified Acute Physiology Score II), and the MPM II (Mortality Prediction Model II).

Scoring Systems Defined

The APACHE II to APACHE IV models use the following comorbidities in their scoring system: AIDS, hepatic failure, cirrhosis, lymphoma, metastatic cancer, leukemia or multiple myeloma, and immunosuppression.[15,50] The APACHE IV model equations were built exclusively from a contemporary database of more than 100,000 patients admitted to critical care units in the United States. This was the first time the APACHE equations were updated and recalibrated at the same time. The APACHE II version is perhaps the most widely studied version, probably because of its free access.

The SAPS II model was originally designed to streamline data collection. Data are collected, and a severity score is determined after 24 hours in critical care. Data points include existing risk factors (such as age, type of admission, 12 physiologic variables, and the presence or absence of 3 chronic diseases), physiologic derangement (such as AIDS/HIV with clinical complications such as pneumocystic pneumonia or lymphoma), hematologic malignancy (such as lymphoma, acute leukemia, or multiple myeloma), and metastatic cancer (confirmed by surgery, computerized tomography [CT] scan, or other method).[53]

The MPM II model is less physiologically based than either APACHE or SAPS. It uses 15 variables to derive the severity score. The score is measured on admission but can be updated at 24 hours after admission. The variables include several physiologic variables, type of admission, age, use of cardiopulmonary resuscitation, use of mechanical ventilation, and presence or absence of three chronic disease states. The three chronic diagnoses that impact the score include chronic renal insufficiency, cirrhosis, and metastatic cancer.[55]

Comorbidities Within the Scoring Systems

The specific comorbidities in these scoring systems are listed in Table 3-1. Each of these scoring systems has limitations, one of which is the limited number of comorbidities identified in the scoring system. The APACHE considers the greatest number of

TABLE 3-1 Predictive Scoring Systems and the Comorbidities Identified

APACHE II–IV	SAPS II	MPM II
AIDS	AIDS	
Hepatic failure		
Cirrhosis		Cirrhosis
Lymphoma		
Metastatic cancer	Metastatic cancer	Metastatic malignant neoplasm
Leukemia	Hematologic malignancies	
Multiple myeloma		
Immunosuppression		
		Chronic renal insufficiency

Data from references 15, 50, 53, 55.

comorbidities. The only comorbidity found in all three scoring systems is the presence of metastatic disease. AIDS, cirrhosis, hematologic malignancies, and chronic renal insufficiency are used in two of the three mentioned scoring systems.

Additional Scoring Systems and Their Identified Comorbidities

Additional scoring systems by Elixhauser et al.[27] and Johnston et al.[47] have looked at the impact of comorbidity in acute and critical illness. Elixhauser et al.[27] studied 30 comorbidities using administrative data from California hospitals. They found that the greater the number of comorbidities affecting a patient, the greater the mortality risk as well as resource utilization. The death rate was higher by a factor of 7 if the patient had three or more comorbidities. The comorbidities reaching statistical significance ($P < 0.05$) are listed in Table 3-2. Johnston et al.[47] identified independently weighted comorbid conditions impacting inpatient mortality in a veterans population. This group of researchers used the same 30 comorbidities described by Elixhauser et al.,[27] but only 14 were found to be significant predictors of mortality. Of the 14 predictors, 6 were significant in the medical and surgical

populations and included hypertension ($P < 0.01$), uncomplicated diabetes ($P < 0.01$), complicated diabetes ($P < 0.001$), metastatic cancer ($P < 0.001$), solid tumor without metastasis ($P < 0.01$), and coagulopathy ($P < 0.01$). In the surgical group, three additional risks included pulmonary circulation disorders ($P < 0.05$), peripheral vascular disorders ($P < 0.001$), and fluid or electrolyte disorders ($P < 0.05$). Additionally, five items were significant predictors of mortality in the medical group, including heart failure ($P < 0.001$), liver disease ($P < 0.001$), lymphoma ($P < 0.05$), weight loss ($P < 0.01$), and anemias attributable to nutritional deficiency of iron, vitamin B_{12}, folate, protein, or other nutrients ($P < 0.05$). Several comorbid conditions not significant at baseline analysis demonstrated statistical significance in subanalysis. In the surgical subgroup, these included paralysis ($P < 0.01$), chronic pulmonary disease ($P < 0.01$), and renal failure ($P < 0.01$) and in the medical subgroup blood loss anemia ($P < 0.05$) and drug abuse ($P < 0.01$). The authors' method of analysis using independently weighted Elixhauser comorbidities was found to be a more sensitive predictor of mortality than the APACHE III scoring system in the veterans population.[47]

Impact of Comorbidities on Length of Stay and Treatment

While most of the scoring systems use comorbidities to evaluate mortality risk, there are several studies in which comorbidities are used to predict such factors as length of stay (LOS) or time on a ventilator. Parker et al.[67] found that by using a combination of the Deyo-adapted Charlson Comorbidity Index[26] and the Chronic Disease Score (CDS)[86] both readmission outcomes and LOS in a multivariable model adjusted for patient baseline characteristics could be predicted. The Charlson Comorbidity Index is a measure of the risk of 1-year mortality attributable to comorbidity in a longitudinal study of generalized hospitalized patients and was subsequently adapted for use with ICD-9 codes.[16] The comorbidities are given varying levels of weight in this index and include the following: cardiovascular disease (myocardial infarction [MI], chronic heart failure [HF], peripheral vascular disease, cerebrovascular disease), dementia, chronic pulmonary disease, connective tissue disease, ulcer disease, mild liver disease, diabetes, hemiplegia, moderate or severe renal disease, diabetes with end organ damage, any tumor, leukemia, lymphoma, moderate or severe liver disease, metastatic solid tumor, and AIDS.[16]

The CDS is a comorbidity measure based on medication use.[86] Medications used to treat the following diseases are weighted: heart disease, respiratory

TABLE 3-2 Elixhauser Comorbidities Affecting In-Hospital Mortality

COMORBIDITY	IN-HOSPITAL MORTALITY (ODDS RATIO)*
Congestive heart failure	2.3
Cardiac dysrhythmias	1.4
Valvular disease	0.7
Pulmonary circulation disorders	1.9
Peripheral vascular disorders	1.2
Hypertension	0.6
Paralysis	1.7
Other neurologic disorders	2.8
Chronic pulmonary disease	1.2
Diabetes, complicated	1.1
Hypothyroidism	0.7
Renal failure	2.1
Liver disease	1.9
Peptic ulcer disease excluding bleeding	0.8
AIDS	3.2
Lymphoma	1.8
Metastatic cancer	3.1
Coagulopathy	4.1
Obesity	0.5
Weight loss	3.2
Fluid and electrolyte disorders	2.7
Blood loss anemia	0.9
Alcohol abuse	1.1
Psychosis	1.2
Depression	0.6

Data from reference 27.
*$P < 0.05$.

illness, asthma, rheumatism, rheumatoid arthritis, cancer, Parkinson's disease, hypertension, diabetes, epilepsy, ulcers, glaucoma, gout, hyperuricemia, high cholesterol, migraines, and tuberculosis. In the study by Parker et al.,[67] the CDS was a significant predictor of 30-day hospital readmission and LOS. Additionally, combining pharmacy-based information with information derived from the patient discharge abstract improved prediction of hospital outcomes, although improvements in predictive performance were modest.[67]

While multiple risk factors were studied in the development of all the previously mentioned scoring systems, other comorbidity risk factors have recently been identified as being important in outcome and morbidity in critical illness. For example, diabetes mellitus (DM) concomitant with its relationship to stress-induced hyperglycemia has emerged as a relevant risk factor. Numerous studies have found that elevated blood glucose levels during critical illness are a significant contributor to both morbidity and mortality.[33,45,51,84]

Scoring systems are better at predicting general mortality in critical care as opposed to whether a single particular patient will die.[54] By use of these scoring systems, one can predict that a patient may have a 75% chance of death; however, we do not know if the patient will be in the 25% that will survive the critical illness. Traditional scoring systems may not be adequate predictors in certain patient groups such as trauma, obstetrics, and AIDS.[14,56,81] Tan and colleagues[81] studied the impact of comorbidities in trauma patients and found that comorbidities were common in trauma patients, especially those older than 40 years of age. They concluded that the outcome of trauma patients with comorbidities is difficult to predict using the traditional trauma scoring systems and specifically the APACHE II system.[81]

COMORBIDITIES USED IN SCORING SYSTEMS

Metastatic Cancer/Hematologic Malignancy

If an admission to critical care is required by cancer patients, this admission worsens the prognosis for the inpatient population. Mortality rates of greater than 50% have been demonstrated in cancer patients in the critical care setting.[40,80] In their study of the newly diagnosed cancer patient admitted to critical care for organ failure, Darmon et al.[24] determined that the need for vasopressor therapy ($P < 0.001$) or mechanical ventilation ($P < 0.001$), the development of hepatic failure

($P < 0.01$), or the need for hemodialysis ($P < 0.009$) was predictive of 30-day mortality. Overall, 30-day and 180-day survivals were 60% and 49%, respectively.[24] In cancer patients admitted to critical care with respiratory failure and the need for mechanical ventilation, critical care mortality exceeded 50% overall and invariably exceeded 75% for patients with respiratory failure associated with severe acute lung injury.[80] In one French study of patients with cancer admitted with acute respiratory failure, critical care mortality was 44.8% and in-hospital mortality was 47.8%.[9] In this study, factors associated with increased mortality were documented as follows: invasive aspergillosis (odds ratio [OR], 2.13; 95% confidence interval [CI], 1.05–14.74), no definite diagnosis (OR, 3.85; 95% CI, 1.26–11.70), vasopressors (OR, 3.19; 95% CI, 1.28–7.95), first-line conventional mechanical ventilation (OR, 8.75; 95% CI, 2.35–35.24), conventional mechanical ventilation after noninvasive mechanical ventilation failure (OR, 17.46; 95% CI, 5.04–60.52), and late noninvasive mechanical ventilation failure (OR, 10.64; 95% CI, 1.05–107.83).[9]

Cancer patients who receive bone marrow transplant (BMT) and require mechanical ventilation are especially prone to poor prognosis when admitted to critical care, with a mortality rate as high as 95%.[22,30] BMT recipients who enter critical care but do not undergo mechanical ventilation have a mortality rate of 20% to 50%.[2,22,30,69] The mortality rate is high for patients with hematologic malignancy, with up to 47% of patients not surviving their hospitalization and 75% mortality in the patients requiring critical care.[36] In addition, central nervous system and hepatic failure were both independently associated with poor prognosis in this cohort.[36]

HIV, AIDS, and Immunosuppression

Similar to the critical care mortality rates of patients with cancer, the mortality rates of patients with HIV/AIDS are alarmingly high. Studies report 30% to 77% mortality while in critical care.[14,52,62,73] Patients with HIV/AIDS are frequently admitted to critical care with the primary diagnosis of *Pneumocystis jiroveci* pneumonia (PCP), sepsis, or acute renal failure (ARF).[14,52,73] Rosenberg and colleagues demonstrated that those patients with HIV/AIDS and severe sepsis had a greater mortality than those patients with severe sepsis and no HIV/AIDS (29% versus 20%; $P < 0.0001$).[73] One recent study by Narasimhan et al.[66] demonstrated patients admitted to critical care with HIV/AIDS were more likely to be injection drug users who had been admitted to critical care because of non–HIV-associated conditions. In this study, overall survival was 49%. Another study by Lazard and colleagues[52] demonstrated that

the presence of hypoalbuminemia (albumin level lower than 3 g/dl) and also the length of time between AIDS diagnosis and critical care admission (longer than 1 year) were significant predictors of mortality while these patients were in critical care with HIV/AIDS. Their study used the first SAPS, which was based on the worst values of 14 clinical and biologic variables during the first 24 hours in the medical intensive care unit (MICU). This study identified that a SAPS I score greater than 10 (relative risk [RR], 6.1; 95% CI, 1.5–26.6) was a good predictor of critical care mortality in the HIV/AIDS population.

Hepatic Failure and Cirrhosis

The prognosis of patients who are critically ill with hepatic failure or cirrhosis is poor.[31,35,41,87] Cirrhosis develops late in liver disease. It is not typically recognized early in the course of the disease because there may not be overt signs and symptoms until the disease has extensively progressed. Cirrhosis is generally considered to be irreversible in its advanced stages, at which point the only option may be liver transplantation. Once patients develop complications of cirrhosis, they are considered to have decompensated disease. The complications of cirrhosis include variceal hemorrhage, ascites, spontaneous bacterial peritonitis, hepatorenal syndrome, hepatic encephalopathy, hepatopulmonary syndrome, and hepatocellular carcinoma. The high morbidity and mortality of cirrhosis is secondary to these complications. Mortality in the patient with cirrhosis admitted to a critical care unit has been demonstrated between 63% and 66.6%.[41,87] A large-scale analysis of hospital discharge data from a national survey confirmed that patients with a precondition of cirrhosis do poorly when critically ill. This study by Foreman et al.[31] found that the diagnosis of cirrhosis not only increases in-hospital mortality but also is significantly associated with sepsis and increases the risk of death from sepsis. Similarly, cirrhosis is associated with a higher risk for developing respiratory failure and death from respiratory failure.[31]

The two most common causes of cirrhosis in the United States are alcoholic liver disease and hepatitis C, which together account for almost half of those patients undergoing liver transplantation.[35] The rates of morbidity and mortality in critical care are two to four times greater in patients with a history of chronic abuse of alcohol than in patients without alcohol abuse.[63,79,87] One study by Hudson et al.[42] demonstrated that the incidence of acute respiratory distress syndrome (ARDS) was 71% in patients with a low arterial pH and a history of alcohol-related illness compared with only 39% for those without this history.

In a retrospective chart review, Moss and Burnham[64] found that 50% of the patients who developed ARDS chronically abused alcohol. The in-hospital mortality rate in those patients with ARDS who abused alcohol was 65%, compared with 36% for those patients with ARDS who did not abuse alcohol ($P = 0.001$).[64] Another study by Moss and colleagues[65] demonstrated that in a cohort of patients with septic shock and alcohol abuse the incidence of ARDS was 70% compared with 31% in those without alcohol abuse.

Renal Insufficiency and End-Stage Renal Disease

Both acute and chronic renal disease have been associated with increased mortality in critical care.[21,25,75] Similarly, both end-stage renal disease (ESRD) and chronic renal insufficiency (CRI) have been shown to be associated with increased mortality in critical illness.[19,58,74,75] The primary cause of death in patients with chronic kidney disease is cardiovascular disease—the most frequent admitting diagnosis.[19,74] The second leading cause of death is sepsis.[58,74] Other frequent complications of this population include gastrointestinal bleeding, malnutrition, and anemia.[23]

Renal insufficiency has been shown to be a mortality predictor in several studies of patients admitted to the hospital with acute coronary syndrome (ACS) or for percutaneous coronary angiography (PTCA) with or without stents.[3,49,77] Al Suwaidi et al.[3] found in a meta-analysis of four trials of patients with ACS that abnormal renal function (creatinine clearance rate less than 70 ml/min) is a marker of adverse baseline clinical characteristics and is independently associated with increased risk of death and the combined endpoint of death/myocardial infarction (MI). In their emergency department study of patients presenting with chest discomfort, McCullough et al.[61] found that the presence of chronic kidney disease was a positive marker for in-hospital and 30-day outcomes. Those patients with a corrected creatinine clearance rate of less than 47.0 ml/min at 30 days had the highest rates of cumulative MI, development of heart failure, and death (40.2%). In a Canadian study by Keough-Ryan and colleagues,[49] moderate to severe chronic renal insufficiency (moderate CRI, glomerular filtration rate [GFR] of 30 to 59 ml/min/1.73 m^2 [0.50 to 0.98 ml/sec]; severe CRI, GFR <30 ml/min/1.73 m^2 [<0.50 ml/sec]) independently predicted death (hazard ratio [HR], 1.06; 95% CI, 1.01–1.12; HR, 1.23; 95% CI, 1.18–1.29) in a cohort of consecutive patients admitted with ACS. Shlipak et al.[77] found that in an elderly population admitted with non-ST elevation MI, those with mild or moderate renal insufficiency (mild renal insufficiency creatinine level, 1.5 to 2.4 mg/dl [132 to 212 μmol/L]; moderate renal insufficiency creatinine level, 2.5 to 3.9 mg/dl [221 to 345 μmol/L]) had substantially elevated risk for death during the first month of follow-up. This increased mortality risk continued until 6 months after myocardial infarction.

For those patients with established ESRD admitted to critical care, a recent study found that hospital mortality was actually lower than the previously estimated 9%.[23] This was similar to a study by Clermont et al.[21] in which the mortality risk in patients with ESRD admitted to critical care was 11%, but somewhat dissimilar to the study by Uchino et al.[83] in which the mortality risk was 18%. In the Mayo Clinic study, it was also noted that gastrointestinal bleeding (GIB) was the major cause of mortality.[23] This suggests that preventive measures to reduce the incidence of GIB in this patient population may lead to better outcomes.

OTHER COMORBIDITIES AS PREDICTORS OF OUTCOME

Respiratory Conditions

The need for mechanical ventilation is a known predictor of morbidity and mortality during hospitalization.[13,38] Respiratory conditions such as chronic obstructive pulmonary disease (COPD), interstitial lung disease, pulmonary fibrosis, and smoking history lead to earlier intervention with mechanical ventilation and result in worse outcomes.[4,10,13,38,46,78] In their study of 15 patients with idiopathic pulmonary fibrosis admitted to critical care for respiratory failure, Blivet and colleagues[10] found poor clinical outcomes in this patient population. Eleven patients died before leaving critical care and two died shortly after. The patients died of hypoxemia or from septic shock.

Patients with an admission diagnosis of COPD to critical care have a higher incidence of complications and mortality. In a study of men admitted with acute exacerbation of COPD, Soler-Cataluña and colleagues[78] found that severe exacerbations requiring hospital management are independently associated with all-cause mortality, and the mortality risk increases with exacerbation frequency. The patients with the greatest mortality risk were those with three or more acute COPD exacerbations (HR, 4.13; 95% CI, 1.80-9.41).[78] Another study by Scarduelli et al.[76] demonstrated that heart failure, dysrhythmias, shock, and hypotension occur more frequently in critically ill patients with a prior history of COPD. In a multivariate analysis, the APACHE II score, electrocardiograph (ECG) abnormalities (including supraventricular ectopy, right and/or left ventricular hypertrophy), and digoxin therapy were independent predictors of cardiovascular complications.[76]

Despite advances in infection control and anti-microbial therapy, patients with pneumonias, either community-acquired or nosocomial, have greater morbidity and mortality during critical care hospitalization.[4,68] The mortality rate of community-acquired pneumonia in hospitalized patients can range from 8% to 54%. In a Canadian study of the factors that predict in-hospital mortality among patients who require hospitalization for the treatment of community-acquired pneumonia (CAP), Marrie and Wu[59] found functional status at the time of hospital admission is a powerful predictor of mortality. Hyperkalemia and lymphopenia were associated with early mortality, and the type of antibiotic therapy influenced late mortality. Additionally, in their study of patients with CAP, Pascual and colleagues[68] determined that hospital mortality was 46%. Multivariate logistic regression analysis revealed the independent predictors of hospital mortality were the following: extent of lung injury (as assessed by hypoxemia index), number of nonpulmonary organs that failed, presence of immunosuppression, age greater than 80 years, and medical comorbidity with a prognosis for survival of less than 5 years.

The postoperative pneumonia risk index developed by Arozullah et al.[8] identifies patients at risk for postoperative pneumonia and may be helpful in guiding perioperative care (Table 3-3). The index ascribes points to variables including type of surgery, risk factors related to general health and immune status, and risk factors related to respiratory status, neurologic status, and fluid status. Comorbidities that were significant in this study included age greater than 50 years, functional status (partially or totally dependent), weight loss greater than 10% in past 6 months, COPD, impaired sensorium, history of cerebrovascular accident, blood urea nitrogen level, long-term steroid use, smoking within past year, and alcohol use more than two drinks per day for the previous 2 weeks. These comorbidities are ascribed a point value along with type of surgery to compute a total point score for risk of pneumonia after surgery. Table 3-3 describes the point values and risk classes. Use of a risk tool such as this may be helpful in identifying patients at risk and targeting them for early intervention.

Cardiovascular Disease

Cardiovascular disease may be an important risk factor during critical illness. In the American College of Cardiology (ACC) and the American Heart Association (AHA) guidelines for evaluation of cardiac risk of non–cardiac surgery patients, cardiovascular risk

TABLE 3-3 Postoperative Pneumonia Risk Index	
VARIABLE	RISK INDEX POINTS*
Type of Surgery	
Abdominal aortic aneurysm repair	15
Thoracic	14
Upper abdominal	10
Neck	8
Neurosurgery	8
Vascular	3
Age (years)	
≥80	17
70–79	13
60–69	9
50–59	4
Functional Status	
Totally dependent	10
Partially dependent	6
Weight loss >10%	7
History of COPD	5
General anesthesia	4
Impaired sensorium	4
History of CVA	4
Blood Urea Nitrogen Level (mg/dl)	
<8	4
22–30	2
≥30	3
Other Factors	
Transfusion >4 units	3
Emergency surgery	3
Steroid use for chronic conditions	3
Current smoker within 1 year	3
Alcohol intake >2 drinks/day in past 2 weeks	2

From reference 8.
*To calculate risk of postoperative pneumonia, add total points from right column and use the following probabilities: (1) 0.24%, 0–15 points; (2) 1.19%, 16–25 points; (3) 4.0%, 26–40 points; (4) 9.4%, 41–55 points; (5) 15.8%, >55 points.

factors are considered to be major or intermediate risk clinical predictors for perioperative risk of MI, HF, or death.[6] The major clinical predictors are unstable coronary syndromes, decompensated HF, significant dysrhythmias, and severe valvular disease. Intermediate cardiovascular disease predictors include mild angina pectoris, prior MI, and compensated or prior HF. These intermediate predictors add two additional risk factors that are linked closely with known cardiac disease: DM and renal insufficiency.[6] The stress of critical illness can increase the risk of cardiac sequelae. As noted previously, the study by Scarduelli et al.[76] demonstrated that 39% of patients admitted to respiratory intensive care units with COPD developed cardiovascular complications including hypotension, shock, HF, and/or dysrhythmias. Mortality rates were increased 15.5% in patients that developed cardiovascular complications compared to 4.7% in those without cardiovascular complications ($P = 0.0044$).[76] There have been numerous studies demonstrating that cardiac ischemia may develop during weaning from mechanical ventilation,[1,17,43] and one study by Booker et al.[12] provided data that the extreme metabolic and physiologic demand of critical illness may lead to cardiac events. As discussed in the Research Utilization box at right, detection of myocardial ischemia during critical illness and its impact on morbidity and mortality, especially in critically ill patients without a prior cardiac diagnosis, need further study.

Diabetes Mellitus

Patients with DM can be a challenge in critical care. Patients with DM are at greater risk for poor wound healing, infection, and vascular events that ultimately may lead to worse outcomes. Surprisingly, diabetes is not a chronic condition that is taken into account in the APACHE, SAPS, or MPM scoring systems. The importance of glycemic control in all critically ill patients has been studied extensively in the literature over the past decade.[33,45,84] The goal of controlling blood glucose levels between 80 and 110 mg/dl is now a standard in critical care.[7] Chapter 34 of this textbook addresses the standards of care surrounding glycemic control in the critically ill adult patient.

Age

While age is not a true comorbidity, studies have examined the impact of age on outcome in acute and critical care with varying results.* In most of these studies, age is a predictor of mortality when compared to underlying disease and physiologic status. The assumption is made that in the presence of comorbidities increased age is associated with clinically worse outcomes.[44] The most vulnerable subgroups are the frail elderly, those with loss of functional status or with cognitive impairment, and those older than 85 years of age.[72,85] Elderly patients, more than 85 years of age, admitted to critical care with APACHE scores of greater than 25 have higher mortality rates than those with lower APACHE scores.[85] The most important predictors of mortality in this group are the use of inotropes and the severity of the acute illness.[85]

---

*References 11, 18, 48, 57, 60, 72, 85.

▲ RESEARCH UTILIZATION

Extreme Metabolic and Physiologic Demand of Critical Illness

CLINICAL ISSUE

Extreme metabolic and physiologic demand of critical illness could potentially lead to adverse cardiac events. There has been some evidence that that there is a potential for ischemia during weaning from mechanical ventilation.

SUMMARY

This study does provide some validity to the concept that the extreme metabolic and physiologic demand of critical illness may lead to cardiac events. Critically ill patients who did not have a primary cardiac diagnosis in this study had ischemic events during their critical illness. The researchers found that transient myocardial ischemia occurred in the first 24 to 48 hours in more than 1 in 10 patients. More than 15% had evidence of myocardial injury. Most of these events were silent ischemia or infarction. Transient myocardial ischemia, measured by continuous electrocardiography, and advanced age were predictors of cardiac events. In patients with substantial elevations in troponin levels, 86% had actual cardiac events (unstable angina requiring interventional treatment, acute MI diagnosed by ECG and elevation of serum biomarkers, congestive heart failure, unstable cardiac dysrhythmias, hypotension with compromised organ perfusion, or death because of cardiac disorders such as dysrhythmia, HF, or other primary cardiac cause) during their hospitalization. In multiple regression analysis, myocardial ischemic burden (calculated by multiplying the magnitude of ST segment changes in each lead times the duration in minutes and summing the products for the 12 leads), age, and elevations in troponin I levels together accounted for 39% of the variability of cardiac events ($P < 0.001$).

APPLICATION

Given the potential for adverse cardiac events during critical illness, especially in the older patient (older than 65), it may be prudent to use continuous 12-lead ECG monitoring for this age-group and for patients with increased coronary risk factors or histories of coronary artery disease. Additionally, ST segment monitoring may be of value in these patients.

NEED FOR FURTHER STUDY

Studies are needed to improve the detection of myocardial ischemic events especially in regard to ST segment monitoring.

Booker, K. J., Holm, K., Drew, B. J., et al. (2003). Frequency and outcomes of transient myocardial ischemia in critically ill adults admitted for noncardiac conditions. *Am J Crit Care*, 12(6), 508–516.

Obesity

Obesity is a chronic inflammatory state with effects on several body systems. These include the pulmonary, cardiovascular, gastrointestinal, hematologic, renal, immune, and metabolic systems.[70] Obesity is associated with increased risk for cardiovascular disease, DM, and pulmonary disease, especially sleep apnea and obstructive airway disease.[71] Obesity is often considered to be a risk factor for increased overall mortality, perioperative mortality, and mortality after trauma, and in some studies it is a risk factor of both morbidity and mortality during critical illness.[20,28,34,37] A retrospective study of morbid obesity in the MICU found that obese patients—defined as having a body mass index (BMI) $\geq 40 \, kg/m^2$—were at higher risk of morbidity and mortality.[28] Specifically, the length of mechanical ventilation was significantly longer, which exposes this group to other risks such as ventilator-associated pneumonia, skin breakdown, and deep vein thrombosis from longer time in bed. Multiorgan failure, an arterial partial pressure of oxygen (Pao_2) to fraction of inspired oxygen (Fio_2) ratio less than 200 for greater than 48 hours, and depressed left ventricular ejection fraction were also more prevalent in this group. Goulenok and colleagues[37] found in their prospective study significant differences between obese (BMI >27) and nonobese patients, with obese patients having increased length of intensive care unit (ICU) stay ($P = 0.024$), higher SAPS II scores ($P < 0.001$), and greater ICU mortality ($P < 0.001$). By multivariate analysis, predictive factors for mortality were SAPS II score ($P < 0.0001$) and BMI >27 ($P < 0.01$). There have been other studies that show that morbid obesity is not a predictor of poor outcome in critical care.[32,82] The controversy in the literature may be in part be based on the fact that the definition of "obesity" varies greatly from study to study, from a BMI of 27 to a BMI of 51.[28,32,37,82] Further study in both medical and surgical obese populations is warranted.

Social and Psychological Comorbidities

Social comorbidities that may impact critical care illness include chronic alcohol and tobacco use.* Iribarren and colleagues[46] identified that there is a relationship between cigarette smoking and admission to critical care with ARDS, with approximately 50% of ARDS cases attributable to smoking. As stated previously, morbidity and mortality in critical care are two to four times greater in patients with a history of chronic abuse of alcohol.[63,79,87] There have also been suggestions in the literature that the patient's

psychological state may be a risk for increased mortality. In a study by Ely et al.,[29] delirium was a predictor of mortality in the mechanically ventilated patient. For greater detail on the standards of care related to the critically ill patient with a psychiatric disorder, see Chapter 50; for information about care of the patient with a chemical dependency, see Chapter 53.

CARE OF PATIENTS WITH MULTIPLE COMORBIDITIES

As critical care practitioners, it is readily evident that the addition of multiple comorbidities to an already critical condition increases the complexity of patient care as well as the need for critical thinking in caring for these patients. The impact of comorbidities can be seen in several of the patient characteristics as outlined in the *American Association of Critical-Care Nurses (AACN) Synergy Model for Patient Care.*[5] The model describes the patient characteristic of complexity as the intricate entanglement of two or more systems. Systems can be physiologic or emotional states of the body, family dynamics, or the environment. Resiliency is the patient's capacity to return to a restorative level of functioning and can be affected by age, comorbidities, and compensatory mechanisms. Vulnerability is the level of susceptibility to adverse outcomes and can be impacted by comorbidities. Predictability of the outcome or course of illness can be low if there are multiple comorbidities.[5] Because of the unpredictability and high complexity of illness, patients with multiple comorbidities will require high levels of nursing clinical judgment and expertise. For example, care of a patient that is 40 years old with no comorbidities with severe pneumonia requiring ventilator treatment is far different from that for an 80 year old with diabetes, COPD, angina with minimal activity, and severe pneumonia requiring ventilatory support. As the complexity of the critical care patient increases, so does the need for an advanced level of critical thinking and clinical expertise of the critical care nurse and advanced practitioner.

CONCLUSIONS

Patients with comorbidities, especially those of the magnitude listed previously in this chapter, are at a higher opportunity for increased morbidity and mortality during critical care hospitalization. Risk scoring systems are helpful in providing a starting point as to which comorbidities are important in treating patients with a critical illness, but these scoring systems are

---

*References 39, 49, 63, 64, 65, 79.

not all-inclusive of several important comorbidities. In an attempt to incorporate evidence-based medicine into clinical practice, it is necessary to have an understanding of the specific comorbidities that are the greatest predictors of poor outcome as researched in the literature. However, as demonstrated here, there is paucity of data as well as conflict of data on some comorbidities such as age and obesity. These comorbidities are deserving of further attention and research.

REFERENCES

1. Abalos, A., Leibowitz, A. B., Distefano, D., et al. (1992). Myocardial ischemia during the weaning period. *Am J Crit Care, 1*(1), 32–36.
2. Afessa, B., Tefferi, A., Hoagland, H. C., et al. (1992). Outcome of recipients of bone marrow transplants who require intensive-care unit support. *Mayo Clinic Proc, 67*(2), 117–122.
3. Al Suwaidi, J., Reddan, D. N., Williams, K., et al. (2002). Prognostic implications of abnormalities in renal function in patients with acute coronary syndromes. *Circulation, 106*(8), 974–980.
4. Almirall, J., Mesalles, E., Klamburg, J., et al. (1995). Prognostic factors of pneumonia requiring admission to the intensive care unit. *Chest, 107*, 511–516.
5. American Association of Critical-Care Nurses. (2006). *American Association of Critical-Care Nurses Synergy Model for Patient Care.*
6. American College of Cardiology and American Heart Association. (2005). *ACC/AHA guideline update for perioperative cardiovascular evaluation for noncardiac surgery.*
7. American Diabetes Association, American Association of Clinical Endocrinologists, and American College of Endocrinology. (2006). *Inpatient diabetes mellitus and glycemic control: a call to action consensus development conference position statement.* www.aace.com/meetings/consensus/IIDC/IDGC0207.pdf.
8. Arozullah, A. M., Khuri, S. F., Henderson, W. G., et al. (2001). Development and validation of a multifactorial risk index for predicting postoperative pneumonia after major noncardiac surgery. *Ann Intern Med, 135*(10), 847–857.
9. Azoulay, E., Thiery, G., Chevret, S., et al. (2004). The prognosis of acute respiratory failure in critically ill cancer patients. *Medicine, 83*(6), 360–370.
10. Blivet, S., Pilit, F., Sab, J. M., et al. (2001). Outcome of patients with idiopathic pulmonary fibrosis admitted to the ICU for respiratory failure. *Chest, 120*(1), 209–212.
11. Bo, M., Massaia, M., Raspo, S., et al. (2003). Predictive factors of in-hospital mortality in older patients admitted to a medical intensive care unit. *J Am Geriatr Soc, 51*(4), 529–533.
12. Booker, K. J., Holm, K., Drew, B. J., et al. (2003). Frequency and outcomes of transient myocardial ischemia in critically ill adults admitted for noncardiac conditions. *Am J Crit Care, 12*(6), 508–516.
13. Breen, D., Churches, T., Hawker, F., et al. (2002). Acute respiratory failure secondary to chronic obstructive pulmonary disease treated in the intensive care units: a long term follow up study. *Thorax, 57*(1), 29–33.
14. Brown, M. C., & Crede, W. B. (1995). Predictive ability of acute physiology and chronic health evaluation II scoring applied to human immunodeficiency virus-positive patients. *Crit Care Med, 23*(5), 848–853.
15. Cerner. (2006). *APACHE IV scoring system.* From www.cerner.com.
16. Charlson, M. E., Pompei, P., & MacKenzie, C. R. A. (1987). New method of classifying prognostic co-morbidity in longitudinal studies: development and validation. *J Chronic Dis, 40*, 373–383.
17. Chatila, W., Ani, S., Guaglianone, D., et al. (1996). Cardiac ischemia during weaning from mechanical ventilation. *Chest, 109*, 1557–1583.
18. Chelluri, L., Pinsky, M. R., Donahoe, M. P., et al. (1993). Long-term outcome of critically ill elderly patients requiring intensive care. *J Am Med Assoc, 269*(24), 3119–3123.
19. Cheung, A. K., Sarnak, M. J., Yan, G., et al. (2000). Atherosclerotic cardiovascular disease risks in chronic hemodialysis patients. *Kidney Int, 58*(1), 353–362.
20. Choban, P. S., Weireter, L. J., & Maynes, C. (1991). Obesity and increased mortality in blunt trauma. *J Trauma, 31*, 1253–1257.
21. Clermont, G., Acker, C. G., Angus, D. C., et al. (2002). Renal failure in the ICU: comparison of the impact of acute renal failure and end-stage renal disease on ICU outcomes. *Kidney Int, 62*(3), 986–996.
22. Crawford, S. W., & Petersen, F. B. (1992). Long-term survival from respiratory failure after marrow transplantation for malignancy. *Am Rev Respir Dis, 145*(3), 510–514.
23. Dara, S. I., Afessa, B., Bajwa, A. A., et al. (2004). Outcome of patients with end-stage renal disease admitted to the intensive care unit. *Mayo Clinic Proc, 79*(11), 1385–1390.
24. Darmon, M., Thiery, G., Ciroldi, M., et al. (2005). Intensive care in patients with newly diagnosed malignancies and a need for cancer chemotherapy. *Crit Care Med, 33*(11), 2488–2493.
25. Dember, L. M. (2002). Critical care issues in the patient with chronic renal failure. *Crit Care Clin, 18*(2), 421–440.
26. Deyo, R. A., Cherkin, D. C., & Ciol, M. A. (1992). Adapting a clinical co-morbidity index for use with ICD-9-CM administrative databases. *J Clin Epidemiol, 45*(6), 613–619.
27. Elixhauser, A., Steiner, C., Harris, D. R., et al. (1998). Comorbidity measures for use with administrative data. *Med Care, 36*(1), 8–27.
28. El-Solh, A., Sikka, P., Bozkanat, E., et al. (2001). Morbid obesity in the medical ICU. *Chest, 120*(6), 1989–1997.
29. Ely, E., Shintani, A., Truman, B., et al. (2004). Delirium as a predictor of mortality in mechanically ventilated patients in the intensive care unit. *J Am Med Assoc, 291*(14), 1753–1762.
30. Faber-Langendoen, K., Caplan, A. L., & McGlave, P. B. (1993). Survival of adult bone marrow transplant patients receiving mechanical ventilation: a case for restricted use. *Bone Marrow Transplant, 12*(5), 501–507.
31. Foreman, M. G., Mannino, D. M., & Moss, M. (2003). Cirrhosis as a risk factor for sepsis and death. *Chest, 124*, 1016–1020.
32. Frat, J. (2005). Obesity in ICU patients: increase or decrease in mortality. *Chest, 127*(1), 414.
33. Furnary, A. P., Gao, G., Grunkemeier, G. L., et al. (2003). Continuous insulin infusion reduces mortality in patients with diabetes undergoing coronary artery bypass grafting. *J Thoracic Cardiovasc Surg, 125*(1), 1007–1021.
34. Garrouste-Oregeas, M., Troche, G., Azoulay, E., et al. (2004). Body mass index: an additional prognostic factor in ICU patients. *Intensive Care Med, 30*, 437–443.
35. Goldberg, E., & Chopra, S. (2006). *Diagnostic approach to the patient with cirrhosis,* http://uptodateonline.com/utd/content/topic.do?topicKey=cirrhosi/6052.
36. Gordon, A. C., Oakervee, H. E., Kaya, B., et al. (2005). Incidence and outcome of critical illness amongst hospitalized patients with haematological malignancy: a prospective observational study of ward and intensive care unit based care. *Anesthesia, 60*(1), 340–347.
37. Goulenok, C., Monchi, M., Chiche, J. D., et al. (2004). Influence of overweight on ICU mortality. *Chest, 125*(1), 1441–1445.
38. Groenewegen, K. H., Schols, A. M., & Wouter, E. F. (2003). Mortality and mortality-related factors after hospitalization for acute exacerbation of COPD. *Chest, 124*(2), 459–467.

39. Gross, P. A., DeMauro, P. J., Van Antwerp, C., et al. (1988). Number of comorbidities as a predictor of nosocomial infection acquisition. *Infect Control Hospital Epidemiol, 9*(11), 497–500.

40. Hauser, M. J., Tabak, J., & Baier, H. (1982). Survival of patients with cancer in a medical critical care unit. *Arch Intern Med, 142* (3), 527–529.

41. Ho, Y. P., Chen, C., Yang, C., et al. (2004). Outcome prediction for critically ill cirrhotic patients: a comparison of APACHE II and Child-Pugh scoring systems. *J Intensive Care Med, 19*(2), 105–110.

42. Hudson, L. D., Milberg, J. A., Anardi, D., et al. (1995). Clinical risks for development of the acute respiratory distress syndrome. *Am J Respir Crit Care Med, 151*(1), 293–301.

43. Hurford, W. E., & Favorito, F. (1995). Association of myocardial ischemia with failure to wean from mechanical ventilation. *Crit Care Med, 23*(1), 1475–1480.

44. Incalzi, R. A., Capparella, O., Gemma, A., et al. (1997). The interaction between age and comorbidity contributes to predicting the mortality of geriatric patients in the acute-care hospital. *J Intern Med, 242*, 291–298.

45. Inzucchi, S. (2002). Glycemic management of diabetes in the perioperative setting. *Int Anesthesiol Clin, 40*(2), 77–93.

46. Iribarren, C., Jacobs, D. R., Sidney, S., et al. (2000). Cigarette smoking, alcohol consumption and risk of ARDS: a 15-year cohort study in a managed care setting. *Chest, 117*(1), 163–168.

47. Johnston, J. A., Wagner, D. P., Timmons, S., et al. (2002). Impact of different measures of co-morbid disease on predicted mortality of intensive care unit patients. *Med Care, 40*(10), 929–940.

48. Kass, J. E., Castriotta, R. J., & Malakoff, F. (1992). Intensive care unit outcome in the very elderly. *Crit Care Med, 20*(1), 1666–1671.

49. Keough-Ryan, T. M., Kiberd, B. A., Dipchand, C. S., et al. (2005). Outcomes of acute coronary syndrome in a large Canadian cohort: impact of chronic renal insufficiency, cardiac interventions, and anemia. *Am J Kidney Dis, 46*(5), 845–855.

50. Knaus, W. A., Wagner, D. P., Draper, E. A., et al. (1991). The APACHE III prognostic system: risk prediction of hospital mortality for critically ill hospitalized adults. *Chest, 100*(1), 1619–1636.

51. Krinsley, J. S. (2004). Effect of an intensive glucose management protocol on the mortality of critically ill adult patients. *Mayo Clin Proc, 79*(8), 992–1000.

52. Lazard, T., Retel, O., Guidet, B., et al. (1996). AIDS in a medical intensive care unit: immediate prognosis and long-term survival. *J Am Med Assoc, 276*(20), 1240–1245.

53. LeGall, J. R., Lemeshow, S., & Saulnier, F. (1993). A new simplified acute physiology score (SAPS II) based on a European/North American multicenter study. *J Am Med Assoc, 270*, 2957–2963.

54. Lemeshow, S., & Le Gall, J. R. (1994). Modeling the severity of illness of ICU patients. A systems update. *J Am Med Assoc, 272*(13), 1049–1055.

55. Lemeshow, S., Teres, D., Klar, J., et al. (1993). Mortality probability models (MPM II) based on an international cohort of intensive care unit patients. *J Am Med Assoc, 270*(20), 2478–2486.

56. Lewinsohn, G., Herman, A., Lenonov, Y., et al. (1994). Critically ill obstetrical patients: outcome and predictability. *Crit Care Med, 22*(9), 1412–1414.

57. Mahul, P., Perrot, D., Tempelhoff, G., et al. (1991). Short and long-term prognosis, functional outcome following ICU for elderly. *Intensive Care Med, 17*(1), 7–10.

58. Manhes, G., Heng, A. E., Aublet-Cuvelier, B., et al. (2005). Clinical features and outcome of chronic dialysis patients admitted to an intensive care unit. *Nephrol Dialysis Transplant, 20*(6), 1127–1133.

59. Marrie, T. J., & Wu, L. (2005). Factors influencing in-hospital mortality in community-acquired pneumonia: a prospective study of patients not initially admitted to the ICU. *Chest, 127*, 1260–1270.

60. Mayer-Oakes, S. A., Oye, R. K., & Leake, B. (1991). Predictors of mortality in older patients following medical intensive care: the importance of functional status. *J Am Geriatr Soc, 39*(9), 862–868.

61. McCullough, P. A., Nowak, R. M., Foreback, C., et al. (2002). Emergency evaluation of chest pain in patients with advanced kidney disease. *Arch Intern Med, 162*(21), 2464–2468.

62. Morris, A., Creasman, J., Turner, J., et al. (2002). Intensive care of human immunodeficiency virus-infected patients during the era of highly active antiretroviral therapy. *Am J Respir Crit Care Med, 166*(3), 258–259.

63. Moss, M., Bucher, B., Moore, F. A., et al. (1996). The role of chronic alcohol abuse in the development of acute respiratory distress syndrome in adults. *J Am Med Assoc, 275*(1), 50–54.

64. Moss, M., & Burnham, E. L. (2003). Chronic alcohol abuse, acute respiratory distress syndrome and multiple organ dysfunction. *Crit Care Med, 31*(4), S207–S212.

65. Moss, M., Parsons, P. E., Steinberg, K. P., et al. (2003). Chronic alcohol abuse is associated with an increased incidence of ARDS and severity of multiple organ dysfunction in patients with septic shock. *Crit Care Med, 31*(3), 869–877.

66. Narasimhan, M., Posner, A. J., DePalo, V. A., et al. (2004). Intensive care in patients with HIV infection in the era of highly active antiretroviral therapy. *Chest, 125*(5), 1800–1804.

67. Parker, J. P., McCombs, J. S., & Graddy, E. A. (2003). Can pharmacy data improve prediction of hospital outcomes? Comparisons with a diagnosis-based co-morbidity measure. *Med Care, 41*(3), 407–419.

68. Pascual, F. E., Matthay, M. A., Bacchetti, P., et al. (2000). Assessment of prognosis in patients with community-acquired pneumonia who require mechanical ventilation. *Chest, 117*, 503–512.

69. Paz, H. L., Crilley, P., Weinar, M., et al. (1993). Outcome of patients requiring medical ICU admission following bone marrow transplantation. *Chest, 104*(2), 527–531.

70. Pieracci, F. M., Barie, P. S., & Pomp, A. (2006). Critical care of the bariatric patient. *Crit Care Med, 34*(6), 1796–1804.

71. Pi-Sunyer, F. X. (1991). Health implications of obesity. *Am J Clin Nutr, 53*, 1595S–1603S.

72. Rockwood, K., Noseworthy, T. W., Gibney, R. T., et al. (1993). One-year outcome of elderly and young patients admitted to intensive care units. *Crit Care Med, 21*(5), 687–691.

73. Rosenberg, A. L., Seneff, M. G., Atiyeh, L., et al. (2001). The importance of bacterial sepsis in intensive care unit patients with acquired immunodeficiency syndrome: implications for future care in the age of increasing antiretroviral resistance. *Crit Care Med, 29*(3), 548–556.

74. Sarnak, M. J., & Jaber, B. L. (2000). Mortality caused by sepsis in patients with end-stage renal disease compared with the general population. *Kidney Int, 58*(4), 1758–1764.

75. Sarnak, M. J., & Levey, A. S. (2000). Cardiovascular disease and chronic renal disease: a new paradigm. *Am J Kidney Dis, 35*(4), s117–s131.

76. Scarduelli, C., Ambrosino, N., Confalonieri, M., et al. (2004). Prevalence and prognostic role of cardiovascular complications in patients with exacerbation of chronic obstructive pulmonary disease admitted to Italian respiratory intensive care units. *Italian Heart J, 5*(12), 932–938.

77. Shlipak, M. G., Heidenreich, P. A., Noguchi, H., et al. (2002). Association of renal insufficiency with treatment and outcomes after myocardial infarction in elderly patients. *Ann Intern Med, 137*(7), 555–562.

78. Soler-Cataluña, J. J., Martínez-García, M.Á., Román Sánchez, P., et al. (2005). Severe acute exacerbations and mortality in patients with chronic obstructive pulmonary disease. *Thorax, 60*, 925–931.

79. Spies, C. D., Neuner, B., Neumann, T., et al. (1996). Intercurrent complications in chronic alcoholic men admitted to the intensive care unit following trauma. *Intensive Care Med, 22*(4), 286–293.

80. Staudinger, T., Stoiser, B., Mullner, M., et al. (2000). Outcome and prognostic factors in critically ill cancer patients admitted to the intensive care unit. *Crit Care Med, 28*(5), 1322–1328.

81. Tan, C. P., Ng, A., & Civil, I. (2004). Comorbidities in trauma patients: common and significant. *New Zealand Med J, 117*(1201), U1044.

82. Tremblay, A., & Bandi, V. (2003). Impact of body mass index on outcomes following critical care. *Chest, 123*(4), 1202–1207.

83. Uchino, S., Morimatsu, H., Bellomo, R., et al. (2003). End-stage renal failure patients requiring renal replacement therapy in the intensive care unit: incidence, clinical features, and outcome. *Blood Purification, 21*(2), 170–175.

84. Van Den Berghe, G., Wouters, P., Weekers, F., et al. (2001). Intensive insulin therapy in critically ill patients. *New Engl J Med, 345*(19), 1359–1366.

85. Van Den Noortgate, N., Vogelaers, D., Afschrift, M., et al. (1999). Intensive care for very elderly patients: outcome and risk factors for in-hospital mortality. *Ageing, 28*(3), 253–256.

86. Von Korff, M., Wagner, E. H., Saunders, K. (1992). A chronic disease score from automated pharmacy data. *J Clin Epidemiol, 45*(2), 197–203.

87. Zimmerman, J. E., Wagner, D. P., & Seneff, M. G. (1996). Intensive care unit admissions with cirrhosis: risk-stratifying patient groups and predicting individual survival. *Hepatology, 23*(6), 1393–1401.

CHAPTER 4 Pain and Sedation

Sandra L. Siedlecki

Pain and discomfort are predictable consequences of injury, surgery, disease, and procedures common to critically ill patients. Yet pain and discomfort are frequently not anticipated, recognized, or managed well in the critical care population.[1,32,37] Common myths and misconceptions held by healthcare providers, both nurses and physicians, are often the cause of poor pain management (Box 4-1). Attempting to correct these misconceptions through education is essential for improving pain management and patient outcomes.[76–78a,b]

Pain impacts all aspects of a person's life, impairing physical, psychological, social, and spiritual well-being[26] (Table 4-1). Pain and discomfort are sources of physical and emotional stress. In response to stress, the autonomic nervous system (ANS) and hypothalamic-pituitary-adrenal (HPA) axis are activated. This activation results in the release of epinephrine and norepinephrine, increasing the work of the cardiovascular and respiratory systems, and at the same time releasing cortisol and various cytokines, altering immune function.[1,52,100] Prolonged stress, such as that experienced by critically ill patients, is associated with higher rates of mortality and morbidity.[1,47,52,106]

Nearly 4.5 million Americans will be admitted to critical care units this year;[106] nearly all will experience periods of discomfort and pain, and more than half will report their pain as moderate to severe.[76,77] Although knowledge by healthcare providers related to deleterious effects of uncontrolled pain has improved, nearly 64% of patients in critical care still receive no analgesia; this includes 61% of mechanically ventilated patients and 21% of paralyzed patients.[32] Identification and management of pain in critically ill patients is a challenge complicated by the presence of symptoms associated with major organ damage, system dysfunction or failure, altered mental status, and/or impaired communication. However, few nursing interventions have the potential to improve patient outcomes more than providing comfort, minimizing discomfort, and managing pain.

Box 4-1

Pain Myths

- Physical and behavioral symptoms are more reliable than self-report for assessing the presence of pain and its intensity.
- Pain rating scales are not reliable measures of pain in children, the elderly, or those with any cognitive impairment.
- Complaints of pain that occur in the absence of tissue damage are probably psychosomatic or psychogenic in origin.
- Pain intensity is directly related to size of wound or amount of tissue damage, suggesting a uniform pain threshold.
- The more frequent and severe the pain, the more tolerant patients become.
- Analgesics should be withheld until a definitive diagnosis is made, to prevent the masking of important symptoms.
- Cancer pain is more severe than non-cancer pain.
- Opioid abuse and addiction are common complications associated with the use of opioid analgesics to manage acute or chronic pain.
- Response to placebo analgesic is proof of malingering.
- Infants do not require analgesics, as their neurologic system is too immature to recognize and transmit nociceptive impulses.

Data from references 9, 28, 38, 39, 40, 67, 73.

PATIENTS AT RISK

All critically ill patients are at risk for pain; this risk is usually predictable. At increased risk are those who are aged, malnourished, confused, and nonresponsive, and those who have preexisting painful conditions (e.g., diabetic neuropathies or arthritis). Researchers found that more than half of patients were not medicated before or during painful procedures, and when analgesics were used, the amount was insufficient to adequately control pain.[1,32,37,72,76–78a,b] In a study of cancer patients in critical care, 55% to 75% reported moderate to severe pain as well as feelings of discomfort attributable to anxiety, fear, sleep disturbances, and

TABLE 4-1 Physiologic Consequences of Unrelieved Pain

SYSTEM	PHYSIOLOGIC EFFECT	CLINICAL MANIFESTATIONS
Endocrine/metabolic	Release of ADH, ACTH, cortisol, catecholamines (epinephrine and norepinephrine), and insulin	Weight loss, fever Increased respiratory and heart rates Fluid retention Shock
Cardiovascular	Sympathetic stimulation Increased vascular resistance Increased myocardial oxygen demand Hypercoagulation	Increased heart rate Increased blood pressure Unstable angina Myocardial ischemia Deep vein thrombosis
Respiratory	Decreased ventilatory effort	Atelectasis Pneumonia Acid-base disturbance
Gastrointestinal	Decreased gastric emptying Decreased gastric motility Hypermetabolic state	Anorexia Constipation/ileus Malnutrition
Musculoskeletal	Muscle spasm or cramping Muscle rigidity	Decreased range of motion Muscle weakness and/or fatigue
Genitourinary	Abnormal release of hormones (ADH, aldosterone) that affect urine output, fluid volume, and electrolyte balance	Decreased urine output Fluid retention Electrolyte disturbance Acid-base disturbance
Immune	Increased cortisol levels suppress inflammatory and immune response, decreasing number of circulating leukocytes and inhibiting their ability to migrate by decreasing capillary permeability Cortisol also inhibits release of histamine and prostaglandins, which depresses phagocyte activity High cortisol levels inhibit production of cytokines essential for mounting an immune response (interleukin-1)	Delayed wound healing Infection/sepsis

ACTH = Adrenocorticotropic hormone, ADH = antidiuretic hormone.

unsatisfied thirst or hunger.[72] Because pain and discomfort in critical care are often associated with predictable events, procedures, or conditions, they afford the nurse the opportunity to intervene preemptively (Table 4-2). Preemptive nursing interventions are those actions initiated by the nurse in an effort to prevent an anticipated and usually unpleasant situation or occurrence (i.e., pain or discomfort). Preemptive nursing interventions designed to promote comfort and to decrease pain should be initiated for all critically ill patients and continued throughout their hospitalization.

TABLE 4-2 Painful or Uncomfortable Conditions and Procedures

CONDITIONS	PROCEDURES
Environmental	**Line Placement**
Noise	Arterial lines
Odors	Central lines
Temperature	Peripheral lines

Table continues on page 46

Table 4-2 Painful or Uncomfortable Conditions and Procedures—cont'd

CONDITIONS	PROCEDURES
Musculoskeletal and/or Integument Trauma	**Tube or Drains (Insertion/Removal)**
Abrasions	Chest tubes
Burns	Indwelling urinary
Bruising	catheters
Fractures	Nasogastric tubes
Lacerations	
Thoracic and/or Abdominal Trauma	**Ventilation Support**
Blunt force injury	Intubation
Hemothorax	Mechanical ventilation
Pneumothorax	Suctioning
Rib fractures	Weaning
Disease	**Wound Care**
Arthritis	Dressing changes
Cancer	Sutures or suture
Neuropathies	removal
Sickle cell anemia	Wound irrigations
Side Effects of Treatment	**Surgery**
Constipation	Emergency
Ileus	Routine
Nausea/vomiting	
Physical	**Diagnostic Tests**
Hunger	Lab work
Shortness of breath	Hemodynamic tests
Hygiene	Radiologic tests
Immobility	
Positioning	
Thirst	

⬆ Case Study 4-1, Part A

Acute Versus Chronic Pain

While driving home from work late one night, M.T., a 52-year-old widowed female with no children, fell asleep at the wheel of her car. The car crossed the center line and collided head-on with a large truck. M.T. was found along the side of the road, having been ejected from the car during the crash. She was airlifted to the nearest trauma center, where her immediate life-threatening injuries were assessed and stabilized. She has sustained a subdural hematoma and fractures of several ribs, right shoulder, pelvis, and right femur. In addition, M.T. has multiple abrasions to her extremities and her back, and a large left cheek laceration. She arrives from the operating room after evacuation of the hematoma and stabilization of her pelvis. M.T. has no known allergies and no history of surgery or previous trauma; her only daily medications are aspirin 81 mg and a multivitamin. She is intubated and mechanically ventilated, but opens her eyes and is able to follow simple commands. Vital signs upon arrival include a BP of 150/96 mm Hg and a heart rate of 120 beats/min.

Decision point: What potential sources of *pain* can you anticipate during M.T.'s first 48 hours in the critical care unit?

Decision point: What potential sources of *discomfort* can you anticipate during M.T.'s first 48 hours in the critical care unit?

Case continues on page 63

ACUTE VERSUS CHRONIC PAIN

Pain is most frequently classified by duration. Acute pain is a symptom that alerts the body to a potential threat,[10] usually has an identifiable and treatable etiology, and diminishes with healing.[3,9] Critically ill patients often experience acute pain in several body locations simultaneously because of multiple injuries (e.g., trauma) or various insults (e.g., surgery, procedures) to the skin, bone, tissue, and/or organs. In addition, acute pain accompanies tissue injury that results in inflammation, complicating the nociceptive process and the body's response.[3,8,9,52,60a,b]

In contrast to acute pain, chronic pain is a syndrome rather than a symptom; it serves no useful purpose, persists for more than 6 months, and may or may not have a known cause.[4,82] Although the critically ill patient is most likely to experience acute pain during hospitalization, it should not be forgotten that many patients may have a preexisting chronic pain condition that also needs to be addressed. Of special concern are chronic pain patients who were using opioids for baseline pain management before admission and patients with a history of drug addiction or abuse. These patients may experience severe withdrawal symptoms if baseline levels of opioids are not maintained or if antagonists (e.g., naloxone hydrochloride [Narcan]) are administered (Chapter 53 contains more detail on withdrawal).[2,3] Collection of medical history information (from patient and/or family member) is essential to prevent this scenario. However, as prevention is not always possible, the nurse should be alert for symptoms of opioid withdrawal in all critically ill patients, because early recognition will prevent untoward complications (Box 4-2).

Box 4-2

Symptoms Associated With Opioid Withdrawal

MILD SYMPTOMS

- Restlessness
- Mydriasis (pupil dilation)
- Lacrimation
- Rhinorrhea
- Sneezing
- Piloerection
- Yawning
- Perspiration
- Restless sleep
- Aggressive behavior

SEVERE SYMPTOMS

- Muscle spasm
- Back pain
- Abdominal pain (cramping)
- Hot and cold flashes (chills alternating with diaphoresis)
- Insomnia
- Nausea and vomiting
- Diarrhea
- Tachypnea
- Hypertension or hypotension
- Tachycardia, bradycardia, or other cardiac dysrhythmias

Peripheral Versus Central Pain

Because there is a high concentration of nerve endings in cutaneous tissue, injury to the skin produces a well-defined and localized pain. In contrast, somatic pain occurs in response to injury of ligaments, tendons, bones, and blood vessels. With few nociceptors located in these areas, pain is usually dull and poorly localized. Visceral pain is the result of activation of nociceptors located in organs and body cavities. Because of the scarcity of nociceptors in these areas, the pain is diffuse and poorly localized, and is described as a persistent aching.*

Pain can be classified as either peripheral or central in origin. Trauma to peripheral nerves results in neurogenic pain, while damage to the central nervous system results in neuropathic pain. The main reason for distinguishing between origins of pain is to better understand the routes of transmission of painful stimuli. Nociceptive pain is a time-limited response to actual or potential tissue injury that serves as a protective

mechanism (Table 4-3). In contrast, neurogenic pain and neuropathic pain are the result of a nervous system malfunction related to disease or injury to the peripheral or central nervous system[21] (Table 4-4). Neurogenic or neuropathic pain can be caused by disorders such as diabetes, infiltration or compression of nerves by tumor or scar tissue, and inflammation attributable to infection.[7,9,58]

Pain Theory

The gate control theory (GCT), first described in 1968 by Melzack and Wall, identifies pain as a subjective experience composed of three components: (1) a sensory-discriminative component, described in terms of intensity, location, or quality of pain; (2) a motivational-affective component, characterized by feelings of anxiety, fear, or depression; and (3) a cognitive-evaluative component, responsive to thoughts about cause or meaning of the pain.[60b–62] This multidimensional conceptualization of pain emphasizes the broad range of factors that contribute to the experience of pain.

Pain perception is dependent on a system of sensory neurons (nociceptors) and neural afferent pathways that respond to noxious stimuli (Figure 4-1). In response to tissue damage, cells release neurochemical substances that stimulate nociceptors, causing them to discharge. Once discharged, the nociceptive impulse is transmitted by way of fast, myelinated A-delta fibers and slow, unmyelinated C-fibers to the dorsal horn of the spinal cord, where it is processed in the substantia gelatinosa (SG). In the SG, C-fibers release substance P, glutamate, aspartate, calcitonin gene-related peptide (CGRP), and nitric oxide, responsible for dorsal horn pain transmission. In the spinal cord, some impulses cross directly over to the anterior horn, where they stimulate sympathetic neurons and produce a reflex response (reflex arc). Other impulses cross the cord and ascend to the thalamus by way of the spinothalamic tract. The impulse is then transmitted to the cerebral cortex and the limbic system, where it is interpreted in light of physical, emotional, environmental, and personal factors that are unique to each person and each situation (Figure 4-2).*

Nociception and Inflammation

Nociceptors are nonspecific nerve endings that lie adjacent to blood vessels and mast cells. These structures create a functional unit that efficiently responds to tissue injury by initiation of an inflammatory response (Figure 4-3). In the presence of tissue damage,

---

*References 9, 15, 61, 71, 85, 94.

*References 7, 21, 58, 60b, 61, 94.

TABLE 4-3 Characteristics of Nociceptive Pain

	CUTANEOUS	SOMATIC	VISCERAL
Nociceptors	Superficial: skin and mucous membranes	Deep: muscles, joints, and bones	Visceral organs*
Stimulus	External: mechanical, chemical, or thermal	External mechanical or internal chemical	Internal mechanical or chemical
Localization	Very specific; related to point of tissue injury	Diffuse or radiating but generally associated with area of injury	Generalized and poorly localized
Quality	Sharp, pinching, or burning	Dull, aching, cramping	Sharp, stabbing, and deep aching
Signs and symptoms	Tenderness, erythema, or edema to specific area of injury	Tenderness, spasm, or edema in and around general area Tachycardia, hypertension, diaphoresis, muscle tension, nausea and vomiting	General malaise, fever, diaphoresis, nausea, vomiting, and generalized pain and tenderness
Etiology	Burns, abrasions, lacerations	Sprains, strains, tendinitis, fractures, arthritis	Organ or system inflammation, blockage, or pressure on organ because of lesions or tumors

Data from references 7, 9, 58, 67, 95.
*Visceral organs = Heart, lungs, liver, bowels, etc.

inflammation and physiologic changes occur that increase the sensation of pain.[87] The release of proinflammatory mediators (i.e., histamine, bradykinin, and prostaglandins) results in a lower sensory neuron threshold, leading to peripheral sensitization. Peripheral sensitization allows previously benign sensations, such as light touch, to cause pain (allodynia) by lowering the pain threshold. Inflammation also increases pain perception by altering properties and functions of neurons, through a process known as phenotypic switch or change, making more nociceptors available to transmit noxious stimuli.[7,57,61,62,87]

Central sensitization also affects pain impulse transmission. Central sensitization increases excitability and responsiveness of central nervous system neurons,[85] and has two major phases. The immediate nociceptive-dependent phase affects neurons in the dorsal horn, causing an effect similar to peripheral sensitization. In the delayed phase, inflammation results in hyperexcitability of central nervous system neurons, and blockage of descending inhibitory pain pathways. The combination of peripheral sensitization, phenotypic change, and central sensitization leads to a heightened response to painful stimuli, attributable to an increased response to stimuli (hyperalgesia) and a lowered pain threshold (allodynia).[85] Current research indicates that even a short period of persistent nociceptive activity can result in long-term changes in neural function that increase duration and intensity of pain.[94]

RESPONSE TO PAIN

The body responds to pain through production of neurochemicals (i.e., serotonin, norepinephrine, zinc, endorphins) in the brain and spinal tract that work by blocking release of substance P at the synapse, or by blocking substance P receptor sites. Gate control theory posits that at each synapse, there is a gate either opened by release of substance P or closed by inhibition of substance P.[5,12,21,60a,b–62,94] The mechanism of action for both pharmacologic and nonpharmacologic pain interventions is frequently explained through GCT. Because the perception of pain is influenced and directed by activity in the cerebral cortex and limbic system, interventions and environments that facilitate freedom from worry or stress, rest, and feelings of hope and control should close gates and raise the pain threshold.[27,33–35] In contrast, physical discomfort, fear, sadness, anxiety, isolation, and sleeplessness will lower the pain threshold, making patients more sensitive to pain and less sensitive to pain-inhibiting interventions.[11,43,52]

TABLE 4-4 Characteristics of Neuropathic Pain

| | PERIPHERAL NERVOUS SYSTEM | | | CENTRAL NERVOUS SYSTEM |
	NEUROPATHIES	DEAFFERENTATION	SYMPATHETIC	CENTRAL
Explanation	Pain caused by peripheral nerve damage	Loss of sensory input from a portion of the body, caused by interruption of peripheral sensory nerve fibers	Pain caused by sympathetic activity	Pain caused by primary CNS lesion or dysfunction
Pain quality	Cutaneous: deep burning, aching Paroxysmal: lancing	Burning, cramping, crushing, aching, stabbing, shooting	Burning, throbbing, shooting	Burning, numbing, shooting, tingling
Associated symptoms	Abnormal skin sensation	Hyperalgesia,* hyperpathia*	Allodynia,* ANS dysregulation	Sensory loss, allodynia,* hyperalgesia*
Etiology	Diabetes, alcohol abuse, herpetic disorder, repetitive motion injury	Damage to peripheral nerve or nerve plexus	Damage to peripheral nerve with stimulation by circulating catecholamines	CNS damage caused by ischemia, tumors, injury, or demyelinating* disorders
Disorder examples	Diabetic and alcoholic neuropathies,* postherpetic neuralgia,* carpal tunnel syndrome	Phantom limb pain, postmastectomy pain	Complex regional pain syndromes, phantom limb pain, postherpetic neuralgia	Poststroke syndrome, multiple sclerosis

*Hyperalgesia = Excessive sensitivity to pain, hyperpathia = a painful syndrome characterized by increased reaction to a stimulus, especially a repetitive stimulus, as well as an increased pain threshold, allodynia = condition in which normally non-painful stimuli evoke pain, demyelinating disorders = diseases in which the myelin sheath of nerves is destroyed, neuropathy = a general term denoting functional or pathologic changes in peripheral nervous system. Involvement of one nerve is mononeuropathy, involvement of several nerves is polyneuropathy.

The human body possesses its own analgesic system.[58] In response to stress or injury, specific endogenous opioids (i.e., enkephalins, beta-endorphins, and dynorphins) are released, modulating pain impulses at multiple locations.[52] Distributed in the dorsal horn and periaqueductal gray (PAG) in the midbrain and brain stem, enkephalins are the most widely distributed endogenous opioids in the human body.[60a,b–62] Of the three endogenous opioids, beta-endorphins produce the most morphine-like analgesic effect. The site of action and activation is the hypothalamus and pituitary gland. The most powerful of the endogenous opioids are dynorphins present in PAG and the spinal cord. These endogenous opioids moderate transmission of painful stimuli by altering release and activation of substance P.[23] To affect transmission of pain, endogenous opioids bind to opioid receptors. There are at least three types of receptor (i.e., mu, kappa, and delta) (Table 4-5).

Enkephalins bind with delta receptors, dynorphins bind with kappa receptors, and endorphins bind with mu and delta receptor sites. Mu receptors are located in laminae III and IV of the cortex, thalamus, periaqueductal gray, and substantia gelatinosa and when activated provide supraspinal analgesia. Kappa receptors, located in the hypothalamus, periaqueductal gray, and substantia gelatinosa, provide spinal analgesia; delta receptors, located in the amygdala, olfactory bulbs, and deep cortex, provide general analgesia.[23]

Stress Response Theory

A discussion of the pathophysiology of pain in critically ill patients would be incomplete without inclusion of the psychoneuroimmune (PNI) response to stress. Critically ill patients experience significant and prolonged exposure to stress from multiple sources

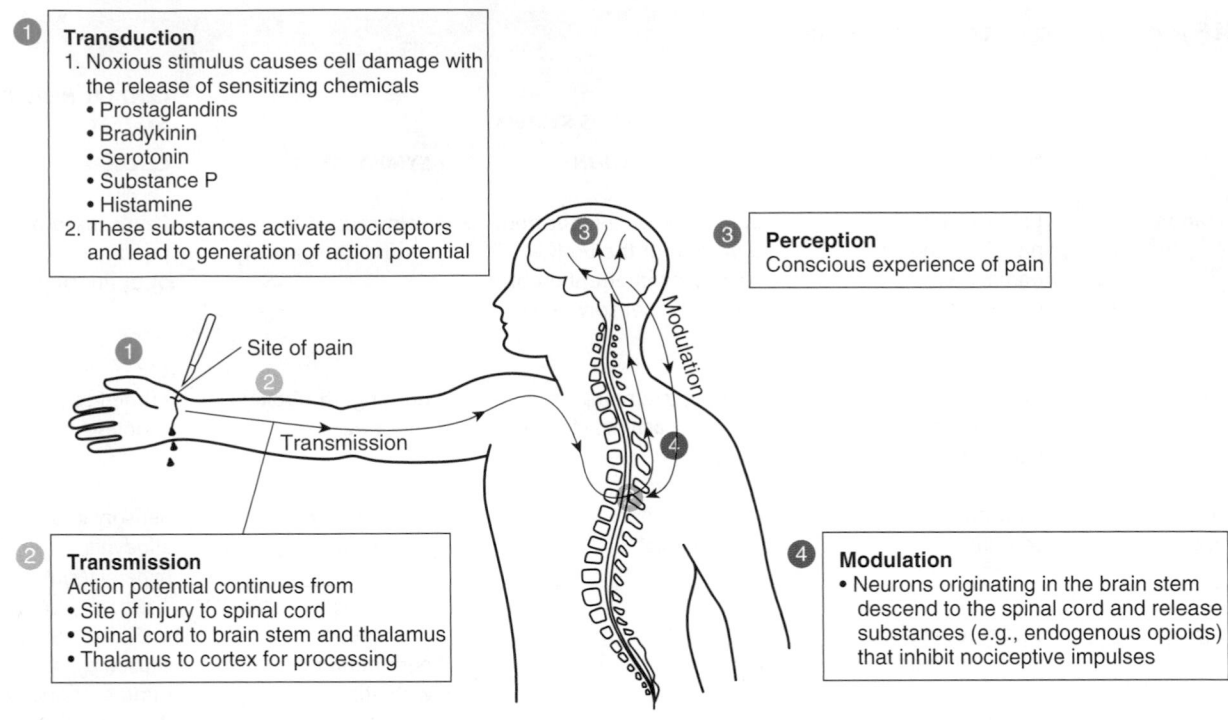

1 Transduction
1. Noxious stimulus causes cell damage with the release of sensitizing chemicals
   • Prostaglandins
   • Bradykinin
   • Serotonin
   • Substance P
   • Histamine
2. These substances activate nociceptors and lead to generation of action potential

Site of pain

Transmission

Modulation

3 Perception
Conscious experience of pain

2 Transmission
Action potential continues from
   • Site of injury to spinal cord
   • Spinal cord to brain stem and thalamus
   • Thalamus to cortex for processing

4 Modulation
   • Neurons originating in the brain stem descend to the spinal cord and release substances (e.g., endogenous opioids) that inhibit nociceptive impulses

⬥**FIGURE 4-1** Pain transmission.

related to injury and/or interventions. Stress produces a nonspecific response to a perceived threat. The body reacts to acute physical, emotional, and environmental stressors through activation of a complex series of PNI responses. These responses are essential for maintenance of homeostasis.[11,52]

The hypothalamic-pituitary-adrenal (HPA) axis and the autonomic nervous system (ANS) are responsible for modulation of the stress response. Physiologic responses occur when signals are transmitted from the limbic system to sympathetic neurons in the spinal cord, causing postganglionic nerves to release catecholamines (i.e., epinephrine and norepinephrine) to the heart, peripheral vessels, lungs, adrenal medulla, and liver. Catecholamine release activates the sympathetic nervous system (SNS), resulting in increased blood pressure and heart rate.[52]

Activation of the HPA axis begins with hypothalamic stimulation of the pituitary through corticotropin-releasing hormone (CRH), causing release of adrenocorticotropic hormone (ACTH). In response to release of ACTH, the adrenal cortex releases cortisol and dehydroepiandrosterone (DHEA). Activation of the HPA axis inhibits immune and inflammatory responses through the activity of glucocorticoids. Glucocorticoids directly affect leukocyte movement and function, and alter production of cytokines that mediate the inflammatory process. At the same time, ANS activation induces release of interleukin-6 (IL-6).

Interleukin-6 helps to control inflammation by further stimulating secretion of glucocorticoids and suppressing secretion of interleukin-1 and tumor necrosis factor-alpha. Finally, catecholamines, released by activation of the ANS, inhibit interleukin-12 and stimulate interleukin-10, resulting in suppression of cellular immunity.[11,27,47,52]

The stress response was intended to protect the body from effects of acute stress. However, a prolonged response, as seen in critically ill patients, can affect wound healing, fluid balance, metabolism, and cardiac and respiratory workload. Each of these potential complications can become additional stressors for the critically ill patient. The goal of nursing care for critically ill patients should be to minimize the number of stressors, moderate the severity of stressors, and provide interventions that can counteract negative effects of stress.

Guidelines Proposed by the Joint Commission on Accreditation of Healthcare Organizations

Recognizing that pain is a common component of nearly every patient's hospital experience and that unrelieved pain has negative physical and emotional consequences, in January, 2001 the Joint Commission on Accreditation of Healthcare Organizations (JCAHO)[43]

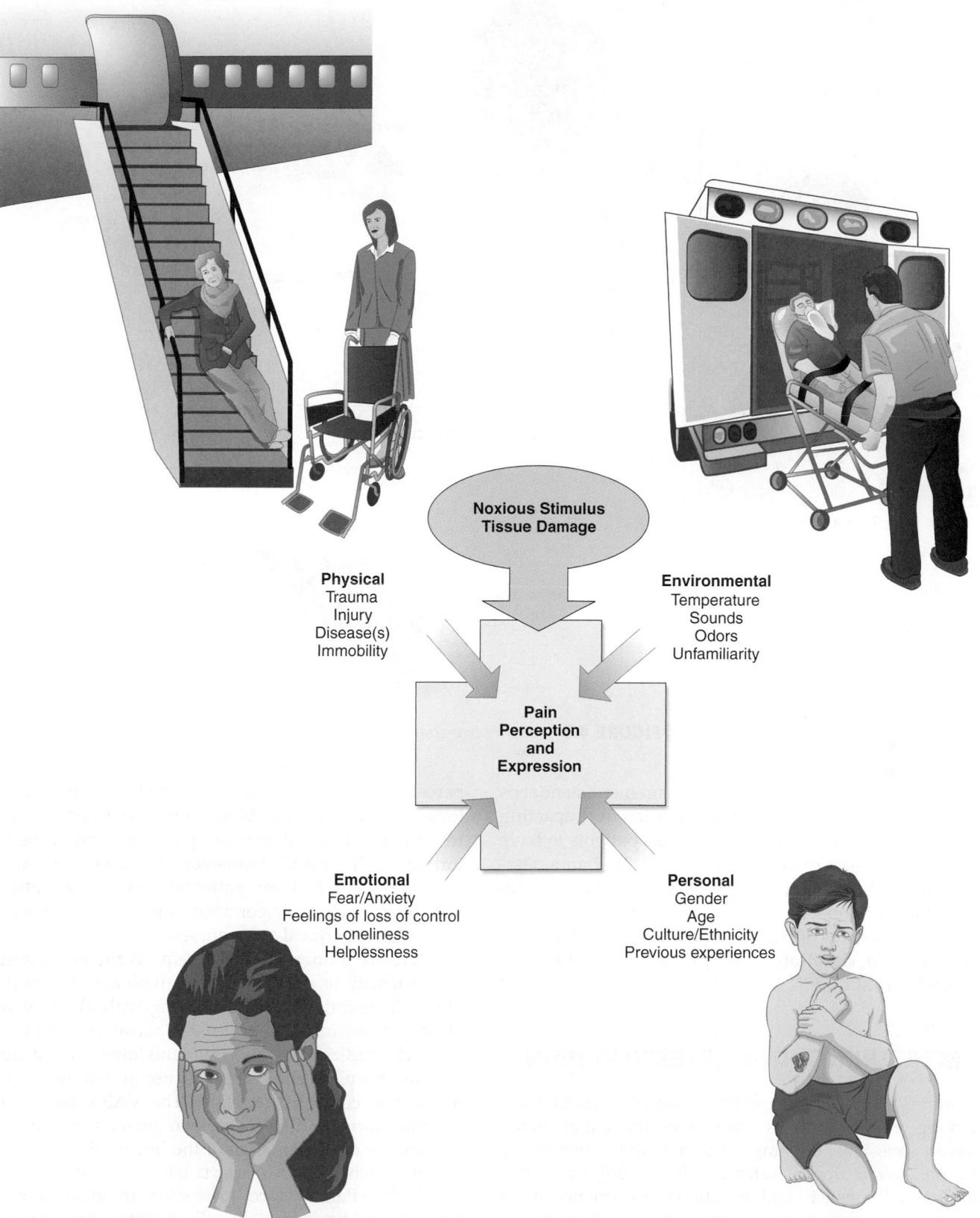

Noxious Stimulus Tissue Damage

Physical
Trauma
Injury
Disease(s)
Immobility

Environmental
Temperature
Sounds
Odors
Unfamiliarity

Pain Perception and Expression

Emotional
Fear/Anxiety
Feelings of loss of control
Loneliness
Helplessness

Personal
Gender
Age
Culture/Ethnicity
Previous experiences

◆**FIGURE 4-2**   Responses to noxious stimuli.

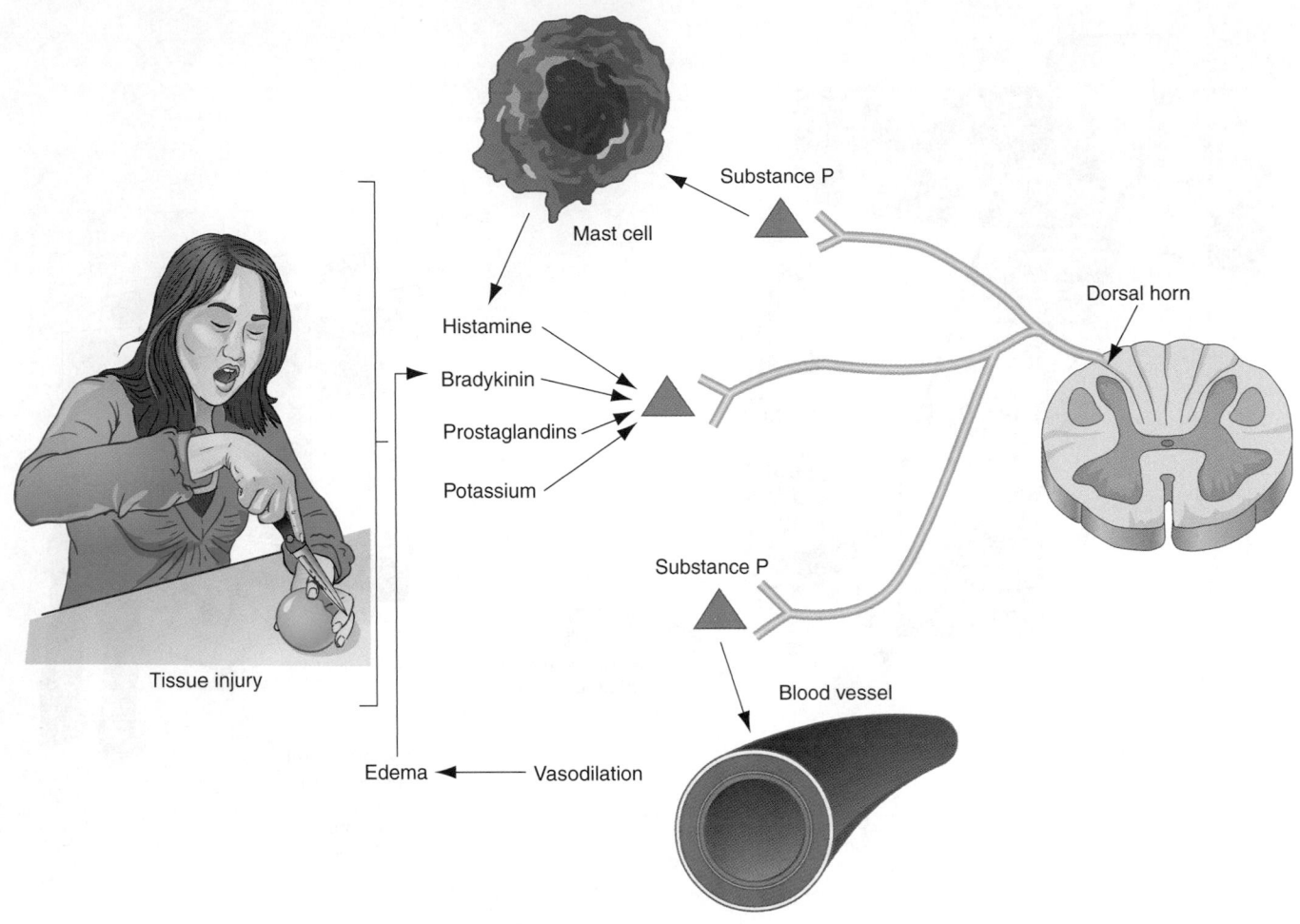

◆FIGURE 4-3 Nociceptive chemical mediation.

proposed pain assessment and management standards for hospitals. One of the standards directly impacting the critical care nurse is the right of all patients to have appropriate assessment of pain (Box 4-3). Pain assessment is used to evaluate the effectiveness of interventions, both pharmacologic and nonpharmacologic, and includes measures of pain intensity, quality, frequency, location, and duration, appropriate for the patient's age and condition.[43,44]

MEASURING AND ASSESSING PAIN

Pain is a subjective experience described as a hurt of varying intensity,[1,54] as "whatever the experiencing person says it is, existing whenever the experiencing person says it does" (reference 55, p. 86), or as "an unpleasant sensory and emotional experience associated with actual or potential tissue damage, or described as such" (reference 64, p. S217). As a subjective experience, there are no neurophysiologic or laboratory tests used to measure pain.[2] Research demonstrates

perceptions of pain are poorly correlated with physiologic measures such as blood pressure, heart rate, and respiratory rate; therefore pain is best assessed through self-report.* However, obtaining self-report measures of pain from patients who are critically ill and often unable to communicate presents a major challenge for critical care nurses.

There are numerous instruments available for assessing quantity of pain in patients who are able to provide self-report. The Visual Analog Scale (VAS) is one of the pain instruments used most frequently in research studies. However, patients often find it difficult to complete the VAS because it requires intact motor and cognitive function. The VAS consists of a 100-mm horizontal line with two anchors (Figure 4-4). The anchor on the left side of the line is labeled *no pain* and the anchor on the right is labeled *worst pain imagined*.[13–16,43] Patients are instructed to make a mark through the horizontal line that corresponds to their current level of pain. The scale is interpreted by

---

*References 2, 3, 9, 43, 44, 71.

TABLE 4-5 Opioid Receptor Responses to Activation

ACTIVATION RESPONSE	Receptor Sites		
	MU	KAPPA	DELTA
Analgesia	X	X	X
Respiratory depression	X	X	
Miosis	X	X	
Mydriasis			X
Decreased gastrointestinal motility	X		
Hypothermia	X		
Hallucinations			X
Dysphoria		X	X
Euphoria	X		
Psychomimetic effects		X	

Modified from reference 23.

placing a 100-mm rule along the bottom of the line and reading from left to right, recording in millimeters the place where the patient's mark crossed the horizontal line.[14] For patients who must complete this scale lying down, it has been suggested that converting the VAS to a 100-mm vertical line, with *no pain* at the bottom and *worst pain imagined* at the top, would make it easier for patients to use. However, in clinical practice the VAS is at best difficult for patients to use, and cumbersome for nurses to interpret.

The more useful clinical pain assessment instruments, for patients who are able to provide self-report, are verbal rating scales (VRS), numerical rating scales (NRS), and the FACES scale. Of the three, the VRS is used most often in clinical settings. To use the VRS, the nurse asks the patient to rate the current level of pain on a scale from 0 to 10, in which 0 is *no pain* and 10 is the *worst pain imagined,* and then the nurse records the patient's level of pain as the number (whole number and/or fraction) provided. In clinical practice, patients seem able to identify changes in pain halfway between two numbers, indicating that even small changes may be clinically significant.[14,40] Although 0 to 10 is the most frequently used VRS, some facilities use a 0 to 5 VRS. The 0 to 10 scale offers more variability and therefore is theoretically more sensitive to change; however, the most important factor when using either the 0 to 10 or the 0 to 5 scale is consistency. It is recommended that a single or limited set of pain assessment tools with similar variability and end points be used consistently within a facility.

The NRS is a written version of the VRS and requires intact motor and cognitive function. Patients are usually instructed to circle the number that corresponds to their current level of pain (Figure 4-5). The NRS score can vary from 0 to 5 or from 0 to 10. Anchor phrases that correspond to the numbers are no pain, mild pain, moderate pain, severe pain, and excruciating pain. Anchor phrases are labeled below a horizontal line or to the left of a vertical line, depending on the type of scale. Although instructed to circle a single number on the NRS, patients will often indicate a level of pain between pain categories. Since pain levels are recorded in whole numbers, the NRS may be less

---

Box 4-3

Principles of Pain Assessment and Management

- All patients have the right to appropriate assessment and management of their pain.
- Assess for pain in all patients at least with each set of vital signs and more often if indicated.
- Believe the patient's self-report. Pain is subjective and self-report is the most reliable indicator of pain.
- Do not rely on vital signs or behaviors. Physiologic signs (such as vital signs [e.g., tachycardia]) or behaviors (e.g., crying or grimacing) do not correlate well with pain and should not be used in place of self-report to assess pain.

- Assessment of pain should be appropriate to the patient population, taking into account language, culture, age, and cognitive and motor function.
- There are no neurophysiologic or laboratory tests that can be used to measure pain. Pain can exist even when no physiologic cause can be found.
- The same stimulus does not elicit the same response in different patients. There is no standard pain response.
- Chronic pain may make patients more sensitive to pain from other sources.
- Unrelieved pain has adverse physical and emotional consequences.

Data from references 2, 43, 71.

Visual Analog Scale (VAS) for Pain

On the line below, indicate how much pain you are currently
experiencing by placing a slash mark across the line.

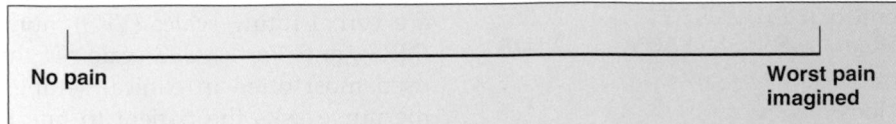

No pain   **Worst pain
                                                                    imagined**

⬍FIGURE 4-4 Visual Analog Scale.

Numerical Rating Scale (NRS) for Pain

On the line below, indicate how much pain you are currently experiencing
by circling the number that corresponds to your current pain experience.

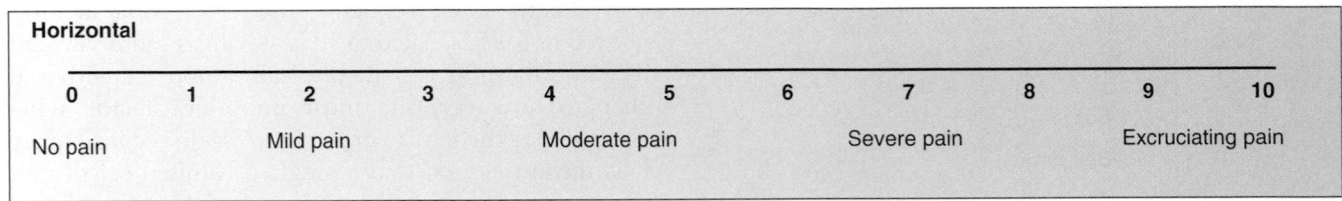

⬍FIGURE 4-5 Numerical pain rating scale.

sensitive than the VAS to small, though clinically significant, changes in pain.

The FACES scale has several variations, and is useful for individuals who are able to self-report but may have communication limitations (Figure 4-6). The FACES scale is often used with children, elderly, confused patients, or patients who speak a different language. Patients are presented a card with six faces that correspond to levels of pain, and asked to point to the face best describing their current level of pain.[40] For patients who are heavily sedated or for those with cognitive impairment, this scale may be the most useful. However, it is not as sensitive to small changes in pain as the VAS, VRS, and NRS.

In addition to assessing pain intensity, it is important to obtain a complete assessment including pain location, pain quality (e.g., sharp, dull, burning, and aching) at each location, pain duration, and factors that increase or decrease the pain. Quality and location of pain may provide information related to pathophysiology of the patient's injury or disease, and changes may indicate changes in the patient's condition. Assessing duration of pain and factors the patient perceives to increase or decrease pain provides information that can assist the nurse in developing individualized strategies to maximize comfort. There are several instruments available for assessing location and/or quality of pain. The McGill Pain Questionnaire (MPQ),

Brief word instructions: Point to each face using the words to describe the pain
intensity. Ask the patient to choose face that best describes own pain and record the
appropriate number.

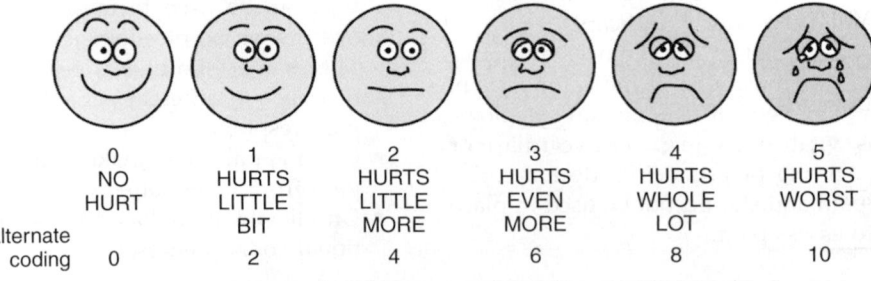

⬍FIGURE 4-6 FACES rating scale.

available in both long-form and short-form versions, can provide data on the sensory, affective, and evaluative nature of the pain experience[62] (Figure 4-7). Another instrument commonly used for initial pain assessment is the Brief Pain Inventory (BPI), available in both long-form and short-form versions (Figure 4-8).[13] The BPI is especially useful for recording baseline pain assessment data, and covers location, quality, quantity, and duration of pain. Drawbacks to use of MPQ and BPI are they require patients to have motor and cognitive function sufficient for providing self-report. In addition, unlike the VAS, VRS, and NRS, which take moments to complete and are sensitive to change over time, the MPQ and BPI take several minutes to complete and are less sensitive to small changes over brief periods.[13,14,16,62]

Short-Form McGill Pain Questionnaire
Ronald Melzack

Patient's name: _____   Date: _____

Pain Rating Index	None	Mild	Moderate	Severe
1. Throbbing	0) ____	1) ____	2) ____	3) ____
2. Shooting	0) ____	1) ____	2) ____	3) ____
3. Stabbing	0) ____	1) ____	2) ____	3) ____
4. Sharp	0) ____	1) ____	2) ____	3) ____
5. Cramping	0) ____	1) ____	2) ____	3) ____
6. Gnawing	0) ____	1) ____	2) ____	3) ____
7. Hot-burning	0) ____	1) ____	2) ____	3) ____
8. Aching	0) ____	1) ____	2) ____	3) ____
9. Heavy	0) ____	1) ____	2) ____	3) ____
10. Tender	0) ____	1) ____	2) ____	3) ____
11. Splitting	0) ____	1) ____	2) ____	3) ____
12. Tiring-exhausting	0) ____	1) ____	2) ____	3) ____
13. Sickening	0) ____	1) ____	2) ____	3) ____
14. Fearful	0) ____	1) ____	2) ____	3) ____
15. Punishing-cruel	0) ____	1) ____	2) ____	3) ____

Visual Analog Scale   No pain |——————————————————| Worst possible pain

Present Pain Index

0. No pain _____
1. Mild _____
2. Discomforting _____
3. Distressing _____
4. Horrible _____
5. Excruciating _____

> To complete the top of the questionnaire, the Pain Rating Index, the patient places a check mark in the column that represents the degree to which he or she feels each type of pain. Next, to indicate the overall pain experience, the patient places a tick mark on the Visual Analog Scale. The mark is interpreted as a number from 0 to 10. Finally, the patient selects the term on the Present Pain Index that best describes his or her current status. The clinician adds the numbers in each of the three sections to determine the patient's score.

◆FIGURE 4-7 McGill Pain Questionnaire.

STUDY ID #: _ _ _ _ _ _ _ _ _   DO NOT WRITE ABOVE THIS LINE   HOSPITAL #: _ _ _ _ _ _ _ _ _

Brief Pain Inventory (Short Form)

Date:_ _ _ _ /_ _ _ _ /_ _ _ _   Time: _ _ _ _ _ _ _

Name: _ _ _ _ _ _ _ _ _ _ _ _ _ _ _ _ _   _ _ _ _ _ _ _ _ _ _ _ _ _ _ _   _ _ _ _ _ _ _ _ _ _ _

               Last   First   Middle Initial

1. Throughout our lives, most of us have had pain from time to time (such as minor headaches, sprains, and toothaches). Have you had pain other than these everyday kinds of pain today?

           1.   Yes   2.   No

2. On the diagram, shade in the areas where you feel pain. Put an X on the area that hurts the most.

Front
Right   Left

Back
Left   Right

3. Please rate your pain by circling the one number that best describes your pain at its **worst** in the last 24 hours.

   0   1   2   3   4   5   6   7   8   9   10
   No   Pain as bad as
   Pain   you can imagine

4. Please rate your pain by circling the one number that best describes your pain at its **least** in the last 24 hours.

   0   1   2   3   4   5   6   7   8   9   10
   No   Pain as bad as
   Pain   you can imagine

5. Please rate your pain by circling the one number that best describes your pain on the **average**.

   0   1   2   3   4   5   6   7   8   9   10
   No   Pain as bad as
   Pain   you can imagine

6. Please rate your pain by circling the one number that tells how much pain you have **right now**.

   0   1   2   3   4   5   6   7   8   9   10
   No   Pain as bad as
   Pain   you can imagine

Page 1 of 2

⬍FIGURE 4-8   Brief Pain Inventory.

STUDY ID #:_____ DO NOT WRITE ABOVE THIS LINE HOSPITAL #:_____

Date:____/____/____   Time:_____

Name:_____ _____ _____
                    Last   First   Middle Initial

7. What treatments or medications are you receiving for your pain?

    _____

8. In the last 24 hours, how much relief have pain treatments or medications provided?
    Please circle the one percentage that most shows how much **relief** you have received.

    0%   10%   20%   30%   40%   50%   60%   70%   80%   90%   100%
    No   Complete
    Relief   Relief

9. Circle the one number that describes how, during the past 24 hours, pain has
    interfered with your:

    A. General Activity
    0   1   2   3   4   5   6   7   8   9   10
    Does not   Completely
    Interfere   Interferes

    B. Mood
    0   1   2   3   4   5   6   7   8   9   10
    Does not   Completely
    Interfere   Interferes

    C. Walking Ability
    0   1   2   3   4   5   6   7   8   9   10
    Does not   Completely
    Interfere   Interferes

    D. Normal Work (includes both work outside the home and housework)
    0   1   2   3   4   5   6   7   8   9   10
    Does not   Completely
    Interfere   Interferes

    E. Relations with other people
    0   1   2   3   4   5   6   7   8   9   10
    Does not   Completely
    Interfere   Interferes

    F. Sleep
    0   1   2   3   4   5   6   7   8   9   10
    Does not   Completely
    Interfere   Interferes

    G. Enjoyment of life
    0   1   2   3   4   5   6   7   8   9   10
    Does not   Completely
    Interfere   Interferes

Page 2 of 2

◆FIGURE 4-8, cont'd Brief Pain Inventory.

The real challenge for critical care nurses is monitoring and assessing pain in patients who are not able to self-report (Box 4-4). When patients are unable to provide self-report, the next consideration for the nurse is to assess the patient's risk for pain by considering that pain may be present because of pathologic conditions, disease, injury, equipment, positioning, or procedures. The nurse should be aware that because of altered levels of consciousness, sedation, and effects and side effects of many drugs used in critical care environments, critically ill patients may not exhibit physiologic indicators specific for pain (i.e., vital signs), nor will they be able to exhibit behaviors reflective of discomfort. The role of critical care nurses must be to anticipate and preempt pain whenever possible.

One of the most important variables associated with assessment of pain is appropriate timing of pain assessment. Pain should be assessed initially upon first contact with the patient; at intervals appropriate to the pharmacologic intervention, calculating onset and peak action of the drug; and at routine intervals based on knowledge of treatments or procedures scheduled for the patient.[2,43,44,71] For critically ill patients, who by virtue of their injury, disease, or treatment regimen are at significant risk for pain and discomfort, pain assessment should be carried out with at least the same frequency as measurement of vital signs and hemodynamic parameters.

Box 4-4

Guidelines for Assessing Pain in Patients Who Cannot Communicate

- Allow sufficient time to adequately assess patient's ability to respond to verbal or written communication.
- When in doubt, attempt use of rating scales appropriate for your population considering age, language, and functional ability.
- Follow the *Hierarchy of Indicators for Pain Assessment*, based on guidelines developed by the American Pain Society and recommended by JCAHO:[42,43]
  1. Patient self-report
  2. Exposure to pathologic conditions, injuries, or procedures known to be painful
  3. Reports from family members
  4. Pain-related behaviors, such as grimacing, restlessness, guarding, or crying out*
  5. Vital signs*

*Note that pain-related behaviors and vital signs are used as indicators of pain only when no other alternatives exist.

MANAGEMENT OF PAIN AND DISCOMFORT

All patients admitted to critical care have the potential to experience painful and uncomfortable events. Although often heavily sedated, as many as 54% of patients report pain and discomfort while in the intensive care unit.[101] Factors that affect comfort include presence of an endotracheal tube, medical procedures, pain, and noise.[101] As discussed earlier in this chapter, pain and discomfort are major stressors that ultimately affect the PNI system. Multiple stressors and prolonged periods of stress are common for critically ill patients and contribute to mortality and morbidity.[42] Interventions promoting comfort and decreasing discomfort and pain improve patient outcomes by decreasing the workload of the cardiovascular and respiratory systems and supporting immune system function.*

Nonpharmacologic Interventions

Pain and comfort measures for all patients, but especially for those who are critically ill, include both nonpharmacologic and pharmacologic interventions. Nonpharmacologic interventions should be started as soon as possible and continued throughout the duration of the patient's hospitalization. Both pharmacologic and nonpharmacologic interventions require continual assessment and reassessment to evaluate effectiveness. Treatment of pain, especially severe pain, is best accomplished through a multimodal approach that incorporates basic comfort measures, complementary therapies, and pharmacologic management[42] (Figure 4-9). This approach maximizes analgesia while minimizing the side effects of pharmacologic agents and the consequences of prolonged stress, resulting in better patient outcomes.

Comfort Measures. Comfort measures are often thought of as basic nursing care. Basic comfort measures are fundamental to nursing, often undervalued by nurses and other healthcare providers and frequently overlooked in favor of high-tech skills or administration of pharmacologic agents (Box 4-5). Yet to patients, these interventions are highly prized and welcomed ministrations providing comfort that minimize pain and suffering. Basic comfort measures include environment, hygiene, and positioning interventions.[42,89]

Complementary Therapies. Complementary therapies are nonpharmacologic interventions used to complement effects of traditional medical, surgical, or pharmacologic interventions. The list of complementary

---

*References 30, 42, 46, 52, 58, 68, 79.

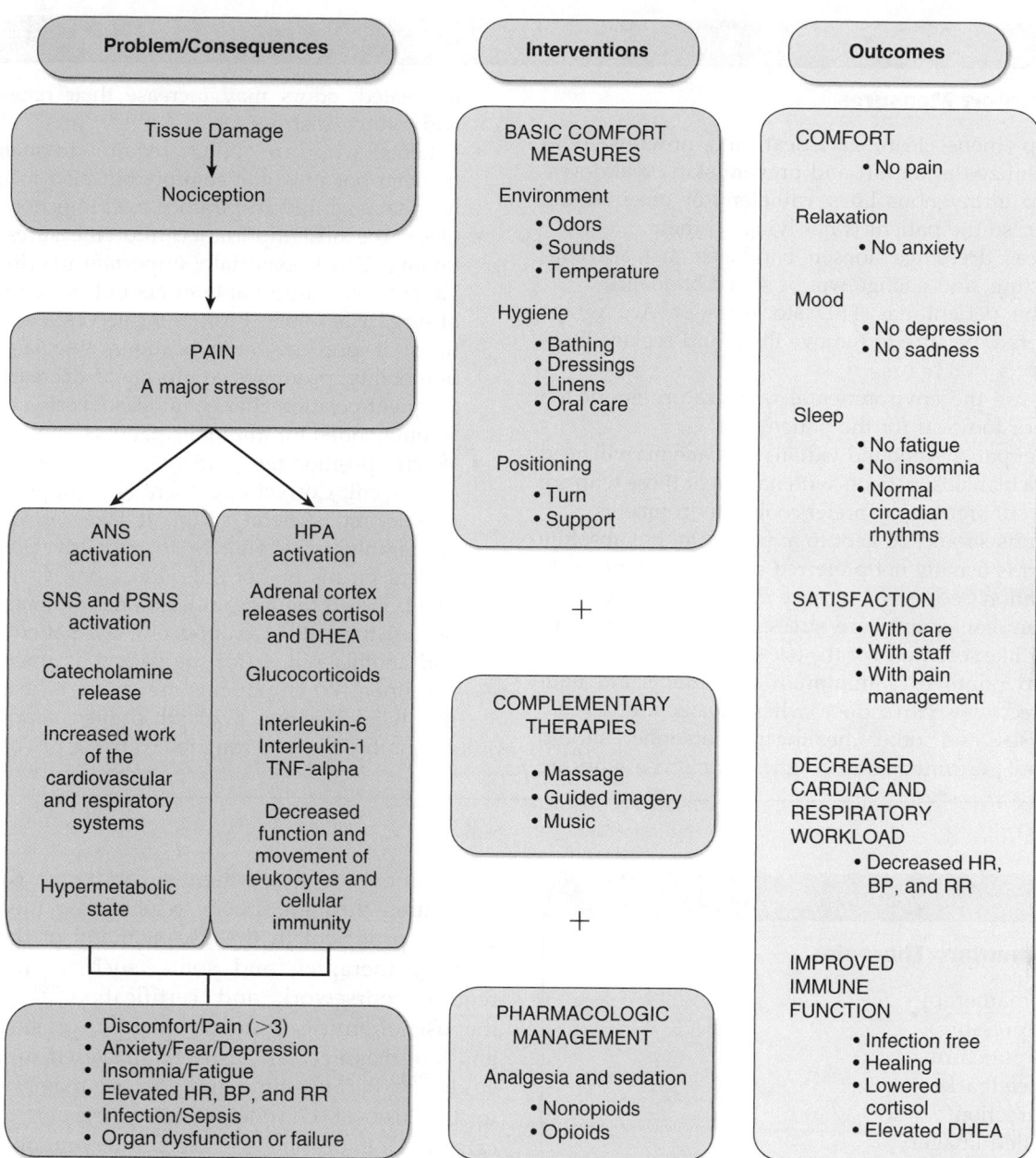

♦FIGURE 4-9 Multimodal pain management model. ANS = Autonomic nervous system, BP = blood pressure, DHEA = dehydro-epiandrosterone, HR = heart rate, PSNS = parasympathetic nervous system, RR = respiratory rate, TNF = tumor necrosis factor.

interventions is extensive (Box 4-6); however, for nurses in critical care, music, guided imagery, and massage are probably the easiest to use. Complementary therapies promote sleep and rest,[27,80] induce muscle relaxation,[34,35] strengthen immune function,[22,46] and decrease anxiety, depression, and pain.* The use of complementary therapies has been shown to be analgesic sparing, translating into fewer analgesic-related complications.[46] Complementary interventions should be started as soon

as possible, and thought of as first-line interventions for decreasing stress, pain, and discomfort[34,35,46] while promoting comfort, relaxation, and rest.[27] Pain perception and response to noxious stimuli are influenced by multiple physical, emotional, and cognitive factors unique to each individual. Stress, anxiety, fear, and fatigue decrease the threshold for pain, making perceptions of pain more intense. Interventions that decrease stress, anxiety, fear, and fatigue will increase the pain threshold and inhibit transmission of noxious impulses. At the same time, complementary interventions promote immune function, minimizing the potential for

*References 28–30, 33–35, 38, 39, 48, 53, 56, 63, 65–67, 73, 79, 88a,b, 91, 93, 96–99, 101, 103, 104, 108.

Box 4-5

Basic Comfort Measures

- Keep linens clean, dry, neat, and unwrinkled to minimize discomfort and prevent skin breakdown.
- Keep intravenous lines, catheters, or other tubing clear, so the patient is not lying on them.
- Assess dressings: loosen bandages that are constricting, and change wet or soiled bandages.
- If the patient has TED stockings or Ace wraps ordered, be sure to remove them and replace them every 4 to 8 hours.
- Be sure the environmental temperature is not too hot or too cold for the patient.
- Older patients and individuals with anemia will need extra blankets; patients with nausea or those who are short of breath may prefer cooler environments.
- Sounds should be kept to a minimum, but absolute quiet is usually not preferred and may contribute to agitation because of sensory deprivation. Loud and unfamiliar sounds are stressful; however, patients may like soft music or the television set left on.
- Keep odors to a minimum. If patients are nauseated, close the door when meals are served. Nurses and other healthcare personnel should avoid perfumes and colognes. For those who are

nauseated, odors may increase their nausea and add to their distress.
- Patients who are NPO require frequent oral hygiene not only for comfort but also to prevent hospital-acquired respiratory tract infection.
- One of the most important comfort measures is positioning. This is especially important to critically ill patients who are unable to get out of bed because of surgery or injury. Positioning serves several functions: it prevents complications associated with immobility; promotes comfort; and decreases pain. Frequent position change (at least every 2 hours) is recommended for immobile patients.
- When positioning patients, have appropriate equipment. Correct alignment and support reduce muscle and skeletal strain. It takes at least four (preferably five) pillows to properly position a patient on his or her side. Place one at the head, two between the legs, at least one (preferably two) behind the patient, supporting the patient's back, and another pillow for the patient's upper arm to rest upon. When patients are trying to maintain a side-lying position without proper support, the extremities become fatigued, causing discomfort.

Box 4-6

Complementary Therapies

- Aromatherapy
- Acupressure
- Acupuncture
- Biofeedback
- Distraction*
- Guided imagery*
- Massage therapy*
- Meditation
- Music therapy*
- Reiki
- Relaxation therapy
- Reflexology
- Therapeutic touch

Data from references 26, 44.

*Denotes those therapies that can be easily incorporated into critical care nursing practice.

iatrogenic complications of hospitalization (e.g., infection and poor wound healing).[11,22,47]

The selection of specific complementary nursing interventions should take into consideration the desires of the patient or family, knowledge of the nurse, and awareness of time constraints attributable to the

environment or the patient's condition. Knowledge acquisition through special education is necessary to become proficient in the use of many of the complementary therapies, and some, such as acupressure, require coursework and certification.[30,48] However, the use of music, guided imagery, or simple hand and foot massage can easily be mastered through self-study.[30,48] Because time and cost are major constraints to the use of complementary therapies in critical care, it is important to select interventions that are cost-effective, easy for the nurse to administer, and usually well received by patients and their families.

Music is an easy, inexpensive, and safe complementary intervention taking a minimal amount of time on the part of the nurse, but has a significant impact on perceptions of pain and discomfort for patients.[33–35,99,100] Music has been found to be effective as a complementary intervention for management of acute pain,[33–35,67] cancer pain,[108] and procedural pain.[46,63] Findings from previous music studies suggest that music facilitates relaxation,[33–35,93,103,104] decreases anxiety,[33–35,65,103,104] increases comfort and decreases perceptions of pain,[33–35,56,88a,b] and improves mood.[18,38,39,99]

Music interventions should be specific to patients' likes and dislikes; patient preference is the most important consideration. Ask the patient about his or her favorite music or have the family bring in a favorite compact disc (CD) or MP3 player. Many individuals will select calm, soothing, instrumental music to facilitate rest and relaxation, or to distract them from pain; however, some individuals will prefer more upbeat selections. Music can be fast or slow, loud or soft, or it may include the sounds of nature. To facilitate attention to music and to block out unpleasant environmental sounds, patients should be provided with personal headsets. Use music preemptively as you would pharmacologic interventions; and as with any intervention, pain and comfort should be assessed before and after the intervention; effectiveness should be documented in the patient's hospital record.

Like music, guided imagery is a mind-body intervention that can be provided in critical care settings to facilitate sleep, to promote relaxation, or to manage pain and discomfort. Guided imagery is a way to purposely focus a person's thoughts and divert attention away from unpleasant experiences.[96–98] There are essentially four types of guided imagery: pleasant imagery, physiologic focused imagery, mental rehearsal and reframing imagery, and receptive imagery.[101] For critical care patients, pleasant or physiologic focused imagery may be most useful. Research suggests that guided imagery can strengthen the immune system,[22] decrease feelings of anxiety[53] and pain,[29,96–98] and promote feelings of comfort.[96] In addition, guided imagery was found to be a cost-effective and opioid-sparing intervention for cardiac surgery patients, resulting in decreased length of stay and reduced postoperative pain and anxiety.[96–98] Finally, guided imagery was found to promote relaxation and facilitate sleep in critically ill adults.[80]

Although a personal one-on-one guided imagery session with a practitioner may be the most helpful, it is very impractical in the critical care setting. However, guided imagery audiotapes or CDs can be purchased and used by nurses in critical care. As with music, headsets should be provided to facilitate attention and increase the ability of the patient to focus. Headsets also serve to block out unfamiliar or frightening sounds in the critical care environment, thereby further decreasing anxiety and stress.

Massage is a complementary intervention that can promote relaxation, ease tension, and decrease fear.[42] Massage also promotes feelings of support and protection by the patient. Massage therapy refers to manual manipulation of soft tissue.[66] In critical care, nurses can incorporate hand massage, foot massage, or back massage into routine care and hygiene (Figure 4-10). However, caution is suggested if patients demonstrate evidence of peripheral or central sensitization, as even soft touch may be transmitted and interpreted as noxious stimuli.

Massage is thought to decrease perceptions of pain by providing competing stimuli that are conducted along faster neuronal networks, interfering with transmission and effectively closing pain gates before noxious stimuli can be processed.[66] Massage was found to decrease pain and distress in hospitalized cancer patients,[95] as well as patients with chronic and subacute pain.[79] In one study, massage was found to decrease release of substance P in patients with fibromyalgia.[27] Massage has also been associated with release of serotonin, which inhibits transmission of noxious signals to the brain,[28] and with release of endorphins, which modulate the transmission of pain.[73] Research in this area is discussed in the Research Utilization box below.

◆ RESEARCH UTILIZATION

Massage Therapy

CLINICAL ISSUE

Massage therapy is a relatively easy and cost-effective nursing intervention that can be incorporated into physical care. The purpose of this meta-analysis was to examine the evidence suggesting that massage is an effective and useful intervention that can be applied in a multitude of clinical settings and for a variety of clinical conditions.

SUMMARY

This meta-analysis evaluated 37 clinical trials that examined the effect or effectiveness of massage therapy (MT). Analysis found massage therapy was useful, with significant effects for both single-dose and multiple-dose treatments. Individuals in MT groups had 64% less anxiety than their counterparts in control groups. This reduction in anxiety corresponded to a reduction in blood pressure and heart rate. Multi-dose massage therapy was found to significantly reduce perceptions of pain; one study demonstrated a single 10-minute massage before cardiac catheterization reduced all measures of stress.

APPLICATION

Routine and preemptive use of massage therapy can have significant therapeutic effects, decreasing stress, anxiety, and pain; resulting in less strain on the cardiovascular and immune systems; and improving patient outcomes.

NEED FOR FURTHER STUDY

Future studies need to incorporate measurement of psychoneuroendocrine variables to determine the specific mechanisms of action associated with physical and emotional responses to MT. In addition, the effectiveness of preemptive and routine use of MT in critical care areas needs to be examined.

Moyer, C. A., Rounds, J., & Hannum, J. W. (2004). A meta-analysis of massage therapy research. *Psychol Bull, 130*(1), 3–18.

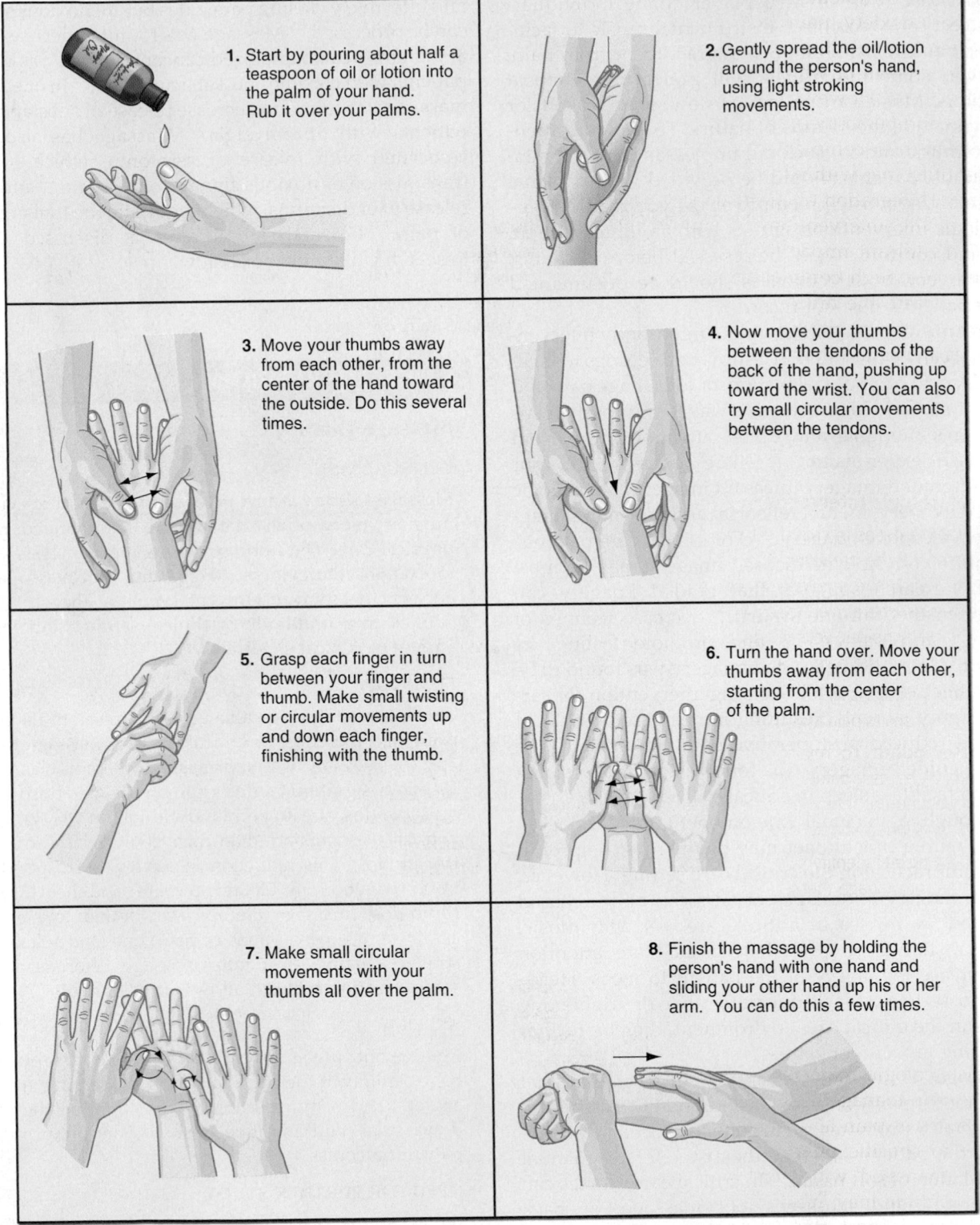

1. Start by pouring about half a teaspoon of oil or lotion into the palm of your hand. Rub it over your palms.

2. Gently spread the oil/lotion around the person's hand, using light stroking movements.

3. Move your thumbs away from each other, from the center of the hand toward the outside. Do this several times.

4. Now move your thumbs between the tendons of the back of the hand, pushing up toward the wrist. You can also try small circular movements between the tendons.

5. Grasp each finger in turn between your finger and thumb. Make small twisting or circular movements up and down each finger, finishing with the thumb.

6. Turn the hand over. Move your thumbs away from each other, starting from the center of the palm.

7. Make small circular movements with your thumbs all over the palm.

8. Finish the massage by holding the person's hand with one hand and sliding your other hand up his or her arm. You can do this a few times.

◆FIGURE 4-10 Hand massage technique.

In general, complementary interventions are thought to decrease anxiety, pain, and discomfort, improve or strengthen immune function, promote relaxation, and facilitate rest—all of which are important for the critically ill patient. However, because of limited resources (i.e., time and personnel), critical care nurses must identify and use those complementary therapies that provide the best outcomes within the constraints of their limited resources. Integration of complementary therapies and basic nursing interventions promoting comfort may have a significant impact on outcomes of critically ill patients. Although complementary therapies are usually welcomed, the nurse should always discuss their use with patients, providing options and explaining the rationale behind their use.

◆ Case Study 4-1, Part B

Pharmacologic Interventions

When M.T. arouses in critical care, she does not understand the reason for the breathing tube, restraints, or other equipment to which she is attached. She does not know where she is or how she arrived there. She is assaulted by unusual and unfamiliar noises, voices, and odors. She will be uncomfortable or in severe pain and unable to do anything about it.

Decision point: As M.T.'s nurse, what physiologic and emotional responses to pain and discomfort should you anticipate?

Decision point: To minimize physiologic and emotional consequences associated with pain and discomfort, what pain management interventions should you plan to initiate for M.T. and when should you start them?

Decision point: Identify potential side effects and methods to prevent or manage them.

Case continues on page 70

Pharmacologic Interventions

Pharmacologic management remains the mainstay of acute pain management (Figure 4-11). However, different types of pain and different people respond differently to specific pharmacologic agents. Mild pain may be managed with non-opioid analgesics, while moderate pain may require mild opioid analgesics. Severe pain is best managed by combining opioids and non-opioids to achieve the highest level of analgesia with fewest side effects.[2,5]

Non-Opioid Analgesics. Acetylsalicylic acid (aspirin), acetaminophen (Tylenol), and nonsteroidal anti-inflammatory drugs (NSAIDs) are useful and should be considered in management of patients with pain attributable to surgery, trauma, or cancer,[109] unless contraindicated by the patient's condition. Non-opioids are more effective anti-inflammatory agents than opioids. Aspirin (ASA), with its analgesic, anti-inflammatory, and antipyretic properties, is the oldest oral non-opioid analgesic agent. ASA acts in the periphery by inhibiting the production of prostaglandins. Because of its antiplatelet effect, gastrointestinal side effects, and association with Reye's syndrome, ASA has been largely replaced with acetaminophen and NSAIDs for management of pain and inflammation.[2]

Acetaminophen, another oral non-opioid analgesic, has analgesic and antipyretic properties similar to aspirin but lacks the anti-inflammatory potency of ASA. Acetaminophen does not have an antiplatelet effect nor does it cause irritation to gastrointestinal mucosa. However, excessive doses of acetaminophen can cause fatal liver damage; patients with poor liver function or a history of alcoholism can develop hepatotoxicity, even at therapeutic doses.[107] Acetaminophen has also been found to be a risk factor for excessive warfarin (Coumadin) anticoagulation.[41] The mechanism of action for acetaminophen remains unclear, but it appears to work at the level of the central nervous system (CNS).[2,92]

Nonsteroidal anti-inflammatory agents (NSAIDs) work specifically by blocking release of cyclooxygenase (COX) enzyme. Blocking COX inhibits production of prostaglandins. Prostaglandins produced by COX-1 enzymes protect the lining of the stomach, maintain normal platelet function, and maintain renal blood flow. Prostaglandins produced by COX-2 enzymes are inflammatory. The therapeutic effect of NSAIDs is a result of inhibition of COX-2, while side effects are attributable to inhibition of COX-1. Several new, COX-2–selective NSAIDs are currently on the market,[2,50,92,109] but recent problems related to side effects have limited their use.

All NSAIDs (selective and nonselective COX inhibitors) can cause renal insufficiency. Risk factors associated with serious renal side effects (i.e., acute renal failure [ARF]) include heart failure, chronic renal insufficiency, cirrhosis, ascites, lupus, dehydration, multiple myeloma, or atherosclerotic disease.[2] Symptoms of abrupt oliguria and sodium and water retention should be reported to the practitioner and NSAID treatment should be stopped. ARF secondary to NSAIDs usually reverses quickly once the drug is stopped.[2,92] Common non-opioid analgesics are listed in the Medication table on p. 64.

Opioid Analgesics. Opioid analgesics are the mainstay of pharmaceutical pain management.[37] Opioids act by

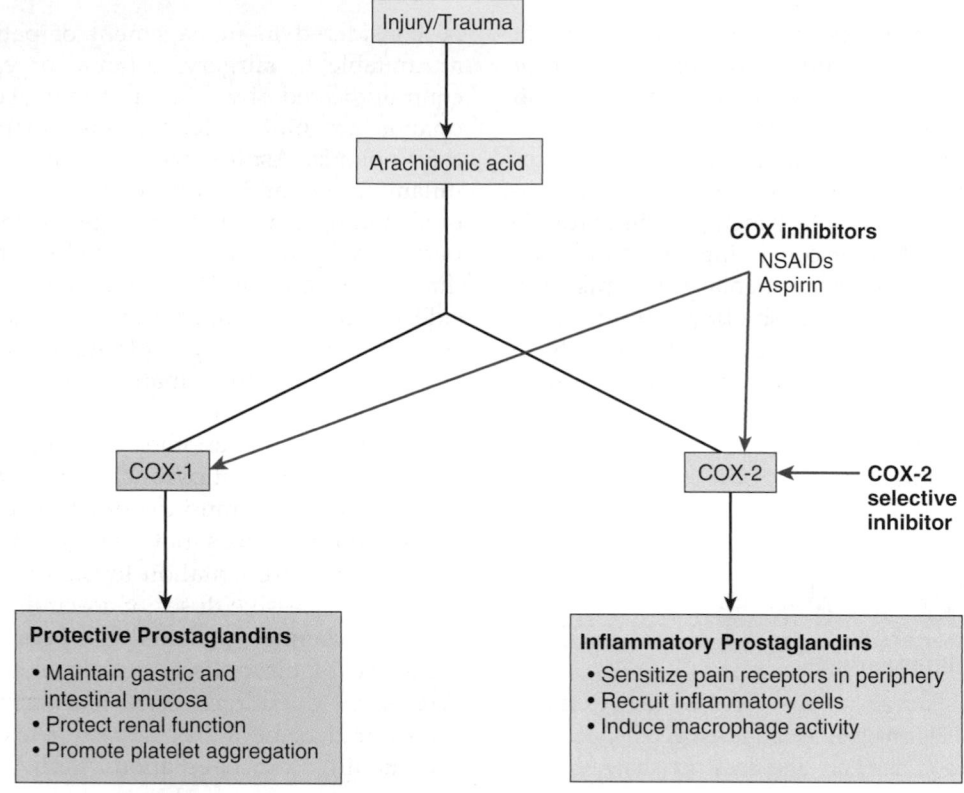

⇕FIGURE 4-11 Prostaglandins and action of aspirin and nonsteroidal antiinflammatory drugs (NSAIDs).

COMMON NON-OPIOID ANALGESICS

MEDICATION	INDICATIONS	DOSE	SPECIAL CONSIDERATIONS
Acetaminophen (Tylenol)	Mild to moderate pain Fever	650–975 mg every 4–6 hr PO or PRN	Total dose in 24 hours not to exceed 4000 mg. Use with caution in patients with renal or hepatic dysfunction.
Aspirin	Mild to moderate pain Fever Inflammation	650–975 mg every 4–6 hr PO or PRN	Monitor coagulation frequently; observe for signs of bleeding. Administer with food.
Ibuprofen (Motrin)	Mild to moderate pain Fever Inflammation	400 mg every 4–5 hr PO or PRN	Use with caution in patients with renal or hepatic dysfunction. Administer with food. Monitor renal and hepatic function frequently.
Ketorolac (Toradol)	Moderate to severe pain	60 mg IM or 30 IV as single dose or every 6 hr	Use with caution in patients with renal or hepatic dysfunction. Monitor renal and hepatic function frequently. Limit therapy to 5 days.
Naproxen (Naprosyn)	Mild to moderate pain caused by arthritis, tendinitis, or gout	500 mg (initial dose); 250 mg every 6–12 hr PO	Use with caution in patients with renal or hepatic dysfunction. Administer with food. Monitor renal and hepatic function frequently.

binding to specific receptors (mu, delta, and kappa) in the brain and spinal cord. The specific site(s) of action determine(s) the effect of the analgesic agent (see Table 4-5). Opioids do not alter the pain threshold of afferent nerve endings and they do not affect conduction of impulses along peripheral nerves. Opioid analgesia is mediated instead at the spinal cord and CNS through modulation of the release of substance P, gamma-aminobutyric acid (GABA), dopamine, acetylcholine, and noradrenaline. Opioids also modulate the endocrine and immune systems, alter emotional responses to pain, and inhibit release of vasopressin, insulin, and glucagon. Opioid analgesic agents are classified as agonists, partial agonists, or mixed agonist-antagonists[86] (Box 4-7). Common opioids are summarized in the Medication table on p. 66.

Agonists. Agonists are the most commonly used analgesic for critical care patients. The main effect of pure agonists occurs in the CNS, where agonists activate mu, delta, and kappa receptors located primarily in the limbic system, thalamus, midbrain, and spinal cord. Agonists have no ceiling effect, making side effects the dose-limiting factor in their administration.[12,23] Morphine,

first introduced more than 200 years ago, is a naturally occurring alkaloid derived from the poppy plant, and considered the preferred drug for opioid analgesia. Morphine is highly hydrophilic, so it crosses the blood-brain barrier poorly and diffuses slowly from the epidural space, increasing its general duration of action. Morphine, a potent agonist with both spinal and supraspinal actions, is available for oral, rectal, parenteral, and spinal administration.

Fentanyl (Sublimaze), a semisynthetic opioid, is more potent than morphine. Fentanyl is a lipophilic opioid that has a very limited duration of action (30 to 60 minutes) when administered by parenteral or intraspinal routes. Fentanyl is available for parenteral, transdermal, transmucosal, and spinal administration.[2,24,75,84]

Meperidine (Demerol), a synthetic opioid with analgesic properties similar to morphine, is primarily a kappa receptor agonist. Meperidine metabolizes into normeperidine (an active metabolite). Normeperidine is half as potent as meperidine but has nearly twice the side effects. In patients with impaired hepatic or renal function, the half-life of meperidine, normally 3 to 5 hours, is 7 to 11 hours; and the half life of normeperidine is even longer at 15 to 30 hours. The toxic effect of normeperidine causes anxiety, tremors, and seizures. Levels of normeperidine begin to accumulate with each dose. Patients with evidence of renal dysfunction, CNS disorders, and sickle cell disease; those receiving meperidine in doses greater than 600 mg in 24 hours; or those receiving meperidine for more than 48 hours are at risk for meperidine toxicity. Naloxone (Narcan) does not reverse the effects of normeperidine accumulation and is contraindicated because it may cause hyperexcitability.[2,43,45,71,92]

Partial Agonists. Partial agonists activate some but not all of the opioid receptor sites, have a ceiling effect, and produce less analgesia than full agonists, regardless of their concentration. Increasing doses of partial agonists beyond their ceiling would not increase the analgesic effect. When a partial agonist (buprenorphine [Buprenex]) is administered with a pure agonist (morphine), the partial agonist can displace the pure agonist at receptor sites, reducing analgesic action. If severe enough, this could cause opioid withdrawal. Therefore caution is required when using multiple analgesics or when switching patients from a pure to a partial agonist.[2,82]

Mixed Agonist-Antagonists. Mixed agonist-antagonists block some sites and activate others. For example, pentazocine (Talwin) has a weak antagonist effect on mu receptor sites and an agonist effect on kappa sites. Therefore in addition to analgesia, pentazocine is associated with psychotomimetic effects. Like partial

---

Box 4-7

General Opioid Classification

AGONISTS: ACTIVATE ALL OPIOID RECEPTOR SITES

- Morphine
- Codeine
- Oxycodone
- Dihydrocodeine
- Oxymorphone
- Meperidine
- Levorphanol
- Hydromorphone
- Methadone
- Fentanyl
- Dextropropoxyphene
- Tramadol
- Dextromoramide

PARTIAL AGONISTS: ACTIVATE SOME OPIOID RECEPTOR SITES

- Buprenorphine

AGONIST-ANTAGONISTS: ACTIVATE SOME AND BLOCK OTHER OPIOID RECEPTOR SITES

- Pentazocine (Talwin)
- Butorphanol (Stadol)
- Nalbuphine (Nubain)

DOSING DATA AND EXAMPLES OF COMMON OPIOID ANALGESICS

OPIOIDS	INDICATIONS	ROUTES OF ADMINISTRATION	APPROXIMATE EQUIANALGESIC ORAL DOSE*	APPROXIMATE EQUIANALGESIC PARENTERAL DOSE	RECOMMENDED ADULT STARTING ORAL DOSE	RECOMMENDED ADULT STARTING PARENTERAL DOSE	COMMENTS
Morphine	Severe pain caused by trauma, surgery, myocardial infarction, cancer, or chronic pain	Oral Intravenous bolus Infusion Intraspinal Subcutaneous Sublingual Rectal	30 mg every 3–4 hr (around-the-clock dosing) 60 mg every 3–4 hr (single dose or intermittent dosing)	10 mg every 3–4 hr	30 mg every 3–4 hr	4–10 mg every 3–4 hr	Gold standard against which all other opioids are measured
Fentanyl (Sublimaze)	Moderate to severe pain	Oral Intravenous bolus Infusion Intraspinal Transmucosal Transdermal	NA	NA	NA	Transdermal and intraspinal administration recommended	
Codeine	Mild to moderate pain	Oral	130 mg every 3–4 hr	NA	30–60 mg every 3–4 hr	NA	Doses higher than 65 mg increase constipation and other side effects without improving analgesic effect
Hydromorphone (Dilaudid)	Moderate to severe pain	Oral Intravenous Subcutaneous Rectal	7.5 mg every 3–4 hr	1.5 mg every 3–4 hr	6 mg every 3–4 hr	1.5 mg every 3–4 hr	Useful alternative to morphine
Meperidine (Demerol)†	Moderate to severe pain	Oral Intravenous Intramuscular Subcutaneous	300 mg every 2–3 hr	75–100 mg every 3 hr	Not recommended	100 mg every 3 hr	Normeperidine, a by-product of meperidine metabolism, is neurotoxic

Data from references 71, 90.
*Equianalgesic doses are compared to morphine. The equivalent of 30 mg of oral morphine is 130 mg of oral codeine.
†Meperidine is contraindicated for elderly patients, for individuals with renal or liver dysfunction, and for management of pain for more than 48 hours.

agonists, agonist-antagonists have a ceiling effect,[50,82] and when administered with a pure agonist can produce withdrawal symptoms.

Opioids are provided as individual or combination drugs. Caution should be taken when administering combination drugs, because their non-opioid component limits the dose. For example, agents such as oxycodone with codeine (Percocet) or acetaminophen with codeine (Tylenol with codeine) may cause hepatotoxicity if the acetaminophen dose exceeds 4000 mg per day. Note that in the presence of liver disease, hepatotoxicity occurs at an even lower dose.[2]

Routes of Administration. One advantage of opioids is they can be administered through a variety of routes. The oral route is preferred for long-term opioid treatment as it produces steady blood levels. The onset of action for oral morphine is usually 45 minutes with a peak effect in 1 to 2 hours.[2] Because oral opioids (e.g., morphine) are deactivated during their first pass through the liver, a larger oral dose compared to the usual parenteral dose is required. However, for patients with liver disease, dosage will need to be reduced to prevent overdose resulting from accumulation.

Intravenous Opioid Infusion. For rapid effect, intravenous (IV) bolus administration of opioids is recommended. Onset of action is nearly immediate, with a peak effect within 1 to 5 minutes for fentanyl, and 15 to 20 minutes for morphine. A second dose of opioid can be administered at expected peak times if severe pain persists and sedation level is within a safe range.[2] Managing continuous pain with repeated parenteral bolus is not recommended and may lead to a bolus effect, characterized by opioid toxicity at peak times and breakthrough pain at trough times.[42,43,92]

Continuous IV infusion of opioids avoids the "bolus effect," providing relatively stable blood levels. However, prolonged use may increase risk of adverse effects. This has implications for patient-controlled analgesia (PCA), as research has not demonstrated an advantage in maintaining a basal infusion and has found that it may lead to opioid overdose.[2,105]

Transdermal Opioid Administration. Some opioids, like fentanyl, are easily absorbed through the dermis. Fentanyl is available as a patch providing continuous opioid delivery without need for IV access.[75] Transdermal fentanyl is indicated for patients who require continuous opioid coverage; each patch provides a stable blood level for about 72 hours. This product is not indicated for acute procedural or postoperative pain, as onset of action is delayed by 12 to 18 hours, with a therapeutic lag time of up to 48 hours.[2,75]

It is important to note that skin integrity and heat can affect the rate of absorption from a fentanyl patch.[2,75] Patients with fever should be closely monitored for signs of excessive sedation or respiratory depression; use of warming blankets or heating pads should be avoided. Respiratory depression and excessive sedation may continue even after the patch has been removed; therefore patients will require close monitoring and/or periodic administration of naloxone hydrochloride (to reverse effects of oversedation).

Transmucosal Opioid Administration. Fentanyl is also available in a transmucosal formulation that comes as a sucker (a lozenge with a handle). Through this route, 25% of the drug is absorbed quickly via oral mucosa, providing immediate analgesia; the remainder is absorbed slowly through the gastrointestinal tract, providing prolonged analgesia. Levels peak in about 15 minutes.[24] Although developed for children, lozenge-style drug delivery can be used with any age-group and is especially useful for procedural analgesia.

Intramuscular and Subcutaneous Opioid Administration. Additional routes of administration for opioids include subcutaneous (subQ), intramuscular (IM), and rectal. Opioids can be given through continuous or intermittent subcutaneous infusion, but the amount of infusate must be limited.[2] The IM route, although commonly used, is the least effective. Intramuscular administration of pain medications is painful, and absorption rates are unpredictable at best, with a peak effect lag time of up to 60 minutes. In addition, the fall-off effect for IM opioids is rapid, resulting in levels of severe pain followed by periods of excessive sedation. Repeated IM administration should be avoided, as frequent injections may result in sterile abscesses and muscle or tissue fibrosis.[2]

Rectal Opioid Administration. Rectal administration of opioids is an acceptable alternative when patients are unable to take oral medications. Rectal opioids are rapidly absorbed,[16] and first-pass hepatic metabolism can be avoided if the suppository is inserted just past the rectal sphincter. If the suppository is inserted high into the rectum, there is danger of absorption into the superior renal vein, which empties into the portal vein, causing rapid hepatic metabolism.[2,17]

Intraspinal Opioid Administration. Opioid receptor sites are found in both the brain and dorsal horn of the spinal cord; thus it is possible to administer opioids directly to receptors in the spinal cord, minimizing supraspinal side effects and providing longer duration of analgesia with lower opioid doses than is possible with parenteral administration. Intraspinal routes of opioid administration are epidural and intrathecal.[84]

Epidural analgesia requires insertion of a catheter into the space just before the dura mater, and involves administration of an opioid or combination opioid and local anesthetic via a continuous infusion devise. The opioid works at opioid receptor sites in the spinal cord, while the local anesthetic blocks sensory nerve fibers.[84]

Intrathecal analgesia requires insertion of a catheter into the space where the cerebral spinal fluid (CSF) is located. Administration of opioids directly into the CSF allows rapid binding to opioid receptor sites in the spinal cord. This route requires less opioid than the epidural route. However, because of the location of the catheter, the opportunity for significant infection is high.[84]

Opioid analgesic doses vary significantly, with epidural doses approximately one tenth the parenteral dose, and intrathecal doses one tenth of epidural doses. For morphine, with a standard oral dose of 30 mg, the IV dose equivalent would be 10 mg, the epidural dose equivalent would be 1 mg, and the intrathecal dose equivalent would be 0.1 mg.[2,15,84]

Most often, morphine and fentanyl are the drugs chosen for intraspinal administration. It should be noted that morphine and fentanyl produce different levels of analgesia and side effects, due in part to variations in solubility.[84] Morphine, a hydrophilic opioid, diffuses poorly into capillaries and remains in cerebrospinal fluid for a longer time than fentanyl, a lipophilic opioid. Thus the duration of action for intraspinal morphine is longer than that of fentanyl, and intraspinal morphine is more likely to cause excess sedation and respiratory depression than fentanyl.[2,84]

Frequency and Titration of Opioids.

As needed (PRN) administration of opioids for patients known to be in pain or at probable risk for pain is inappropriate.[2] Opioid orders should include intermittent and continuous infusion orders, with specific provision for breakthrough pain.[2] Opioid dosing should begin small and be increased routinely until an acceptable level of analgesia is reached without unwanted side effects. Once the optimal dose for a 24-hour period has been determined, around-the-clock administration should be started. Effectiveness of opioid dosing should be reevaluated frequently and readjusted based on assessment of pain and sedation.

Recognizing and Managing Opioid Side Effects

Essential to management of pain with opioids is an understanding of side effects associated with their administration and knowledge of methods to minimize side effects (Table 4-6). The most common side effects are itching, constipation, nausea, vomiting, sedation, and respiratory depression.[12] When managing side effects, there are several options available: change dose, frequency, or route of administration; try a different opioid; consider addition of an opioid-sparing agent, such as an NSAID, to allow for a smaller dose of opioid; or add another drug that counteracts the troublesome side effects.[12,71] Changes in drug, dose, or route should be calculated using an equianalgesic table to determine starting doses (see the Medication table on p. 66). Equianalgesia refers to the relative potency of one opioid to another, using the parenteral dose of morphine (10 mg) as the standard for comparison. For example, to provide the same analgesia as 10 mg of parenterally administered morphine you would use the equianalgesic dose of 30 mg of oral morphine.

Respiratory Depression.

Adverse effects of most concern to healthcare providers are opioid toxicity and overdose. Overdose can lead to respiratory depression and/or respiratory arrest. To prevent this potentially fatal adverse effect, nurses should pay close attention to and frequently evaluate the patient's level of sedation, using a standard sedation scale. Because sedation precedes respiratory depression, monitoring sedation levels will allow the nurse to identify potential respiratory problems and prevent their occurrence. It is also important to recognize that respiratory depression or change in level of consciousness may be attributable to another problem (e.g., hypoxia or CNS insult). It is important to assess and treat the underlying condition appropriately. If respiratory depression (rate less than 6 to 8 respirations per minute) resulting from opioid toxicity occurs, an opioid antagonist (naloxone) may be administered in a dilute solution, made by mixing 0.4 mg of naloxone in 10 ml of saline. This solution can be administered at 0.5 ml every 2 minutes and titrated to response (increased rate and depth of respirations). Rapid administration of naloxone can precipitate withdrawal seizures, dysrhythmias, pulmonary edema, and severe pain.[2,43,71]

Tolerance and Dependence.

Potential for problems should be monitored on a regular basis, including development of tolerance and physical dependence. Tolerance is an adaptive process that occurs in response to a drug and leads to a decrease in the effect of the drug over time. Tolerance to analgesics usually occurs in the first weeks of therapy. Patients who experience increased pain on a dose of opioid that previously kept them comfortable should be evaluated for tolerance by ruling out other potential causes of

TABLE 4-6 Management of Analgesic Side Effects

SIDE EFFECT	RISK FACTORS	INTERVENTIONS
Sedation	Elderly Analgesics and sedatives	Assess sedation level frequently. Assess for nonpharmacologic causes, such as hypoxia or increased intracranial pressure. Eliminate unnecessary analgesics or sedatives. Provide frequent physical stimulation. Decrease dose or change drugs for excessive sedation. Consider reversal for emergent sedation.
Confusion (delirium)	Elderly Other CNS condition Head injury Electrolyte imbalance	Eliminate unnecessary medications. Identify and treat cause of delirium. Consider neuroleptics for persistent delirium.
Respiratory depression	Opioid-naïve patient Head injury Chest injury Respiratory disorder	Monitor sedation level and respiratory rate. Hold or reduce dose of opioid. Consider reversal for severe respiratory depression.
Itching		Apply cool compresses. Consider diphenhydramine.
Nausea/vomiting	May be dose or drug dependent	Control environmental odors. Assess cause; if caused by decreased gastric emptying, consider metoclopramide. Increase parenteral fluid intake. For chronic nausea, consider antiemetics.
Constipation	Elderly Immobility Dehydration	Maintain activity and encourage range-of-motion exercises. Monitor fluid balance; prevent dehydration. Administer stool softeners and stimulants as a preventive measure for all patients receiving opioids.
Ileus	Elderly Immobility Dehydration Constipation Surgery Analgesia and sedation	Maintain activity and encourage range-of-motion exercises. Monitor fluid balance; prevent dehydration. Administer stool softeners and stimulants as a preventive measure for all patients receiving opioids. Insert a nasogastric tube.
Altered hemodynamic status	Fluid imbalance Elderly Severity and length of illness Recurrent edema Sepsis CNS depression	Reduce analgesic. Administer parenteral fluids. Consider vasopressors. Administer antibiotics as indicated.

increased pain symptoms (e.g., new pathology, missed doses of pain medications). Increasing the dose, adding an opioid-sparing agent, or changing to another medication may be needed to treat increased pain caused by tolerance.[3,86]

Another potential problem is risk of physical dependence that can occur with many medications. Physical dependence is not addiction; it actually occurs to some degree with any medication (e.g., antihypertensive medications or steroids). Physical dependence is an adaptive state; withdrawal symptoms can occur with abrupt cessation of the drug or, in the case of opioids, with administration of an opioid antagonist such as naloxone.[86] Symptoms of withdrawal from opioids include anxiety, irritability, chills, excessive salivation, diaphoresis, nausea, abdominal cramps, and insomnia. Withdrawal symptoms are associated with drug half-life. Symptoms of morphine withdrawal may occur in as little as 6 to 12 hours and peak in 24 to 72 hours. Withdrawal symptoms from drugs with a longer half-life may not appear for several days. The role of the nurse is to anticipate and prevent withdrawal symptoms.[2,12,92] Patients treated with opioids for more than 2 weeks should have their medication gradually reduced before discontinuation. Reductions of 25% every day or two will generally prevent symptoms of withdrawal. If needed, clonidine (Catapres) can be used to treat withdrawal symptoms. The major drawback of clonidine therapy is the tendency towards hypotension.

◆ Case Study 4-1, Part C

Co-Analgesics

This patient (M.T.) is awake, but her cognitive ability is unclear, and she has a communication problem related to mechanical ventilation.

Decision point: What method of assessing pain and sedation will be most appropriate for this patient?

Co-Analgesics

In addition to non-opioid and opioid analgesics, a number of other drugs have the potential to improve analgesia or prevent side effects in special situations. Pharmacologic agents most commonly used as co-analgesics include tricyclic antidepressants, antiepileptic drugs, local anesthetics, skeletal muscle relaxants, antihistamines, benzodiazepines, and topical agents.[2]

Tricyclic antidepressants (TCAs) such as amitriptyline (Elavil), desipramine (Norpramin), imipramine (Tofranil), and nortriptyline (Pamelor) are useful for treatment of neuropathic pain related to surgery or trauma. Although studies have identified an analgesic effect for amitriptyline, occurring at relatively low doses (25 mg per day), anticholinergic side effects limit its tolerability. Sedation, hypotension, dry mouth, and urinary retention are common side effects associated with TCAs. In addition, TCAs may increase the incidence of ventricular dysrhythmias, making them risky for cardiovascular patients.[2,92]

Antiepileptic agents (e.g., gabapentin [Neurontin] and carbamazepine [Tegretol]) have been used to suppress the firing of sensory neurons. As with TCAs, these drugs are most often used to assist with management of neuropathic pain. The drawbacks to use of these drugs, especially gabapentin, are they require more than once a day dosing and must be used with caution and at reduced doses for individuals with renal insufficiency.[2]

Local anesthetic agents can be used for nerve blocks or topical anesthesia. Skeletal muscle relaxants provide temporary management of pain related to muscle injury or strain. However, muscle relaxants in the benzodiazepine, sedative, or antihistamine family of agents may cause dependence if used for prolonged periods. Antihistamines may be used to treat itching and nausea associated with opioid therapy[2] and because of their sedative effects they may be opioid sparing.[2,92]

Although phenothiazines, such as promethazine (Phenergan), have long been thought to potentiate analgesic effects of opioids, research demonstrates they only potentiate side effects, and prolonged use of phenothiazines can cause tardive dyskinesia, excessive sedation, and/or orthostatic hypotension. In addition, increased pain resulting from decreased analgesia can cause dysphoria, restlessness, and agitation (Box 4-8). Phenothiazines are contraindicated in patients receiving spinal or epidural anesthetics, and although they can be used to treat anxiety, benzodiazepines are recommended.[2,92]

ASSESSMENT AND MANAGEMENT OF SEDATION

Nearly 71% of patients in critical care experienced agitation as a result of sleep deprivation, anxiety, pain, immobility, or delirium,[31,42] making it the most common

---

Box 4-8

Tardive Dyskinesia

Tardive dyskinesia, a neurologic syndrome associated with prolonged use of neuroleptic drugs, is characterized by repetitive, involuntary, purposeless movements. Tardive dyskinesia is treated by stopping the offending drug. However, the symptoms may remain even after the drug has been discontinued. When assessing the patient, look for the following:
- Repetitive grimacing
- Tongue protrusion
- Lip smacking, puckering, and pursing
- Rapid eye blinking
- Rapid movements of the arms and legs

reason for sedating critical care patients. Both sedation and analgesia are essential tools for relieving pain, anxiety, fear, and stress in the critically ill patient and appear to have a synergistic effect.[5] A significant challenge for critical care nurses is to maintain balance between oversedation and undersedation. Oversedation is a dangerous event that leads to unnecessary tests, increased length of stay, and prolonged intubation and mechanical ventilation, whereas undersedation, costly in terms of human suffering (causing stress, anxiety, and agitation), has been associated with increased mortality and morbidity.[5,42,49] Using an algorithm for sedation and analgesia is important for safe and effective management of critically ill patients[52] (Figure 4-12).

Sedation may be indicated for patients who are mechanically ventilated and fighting the ventilator.

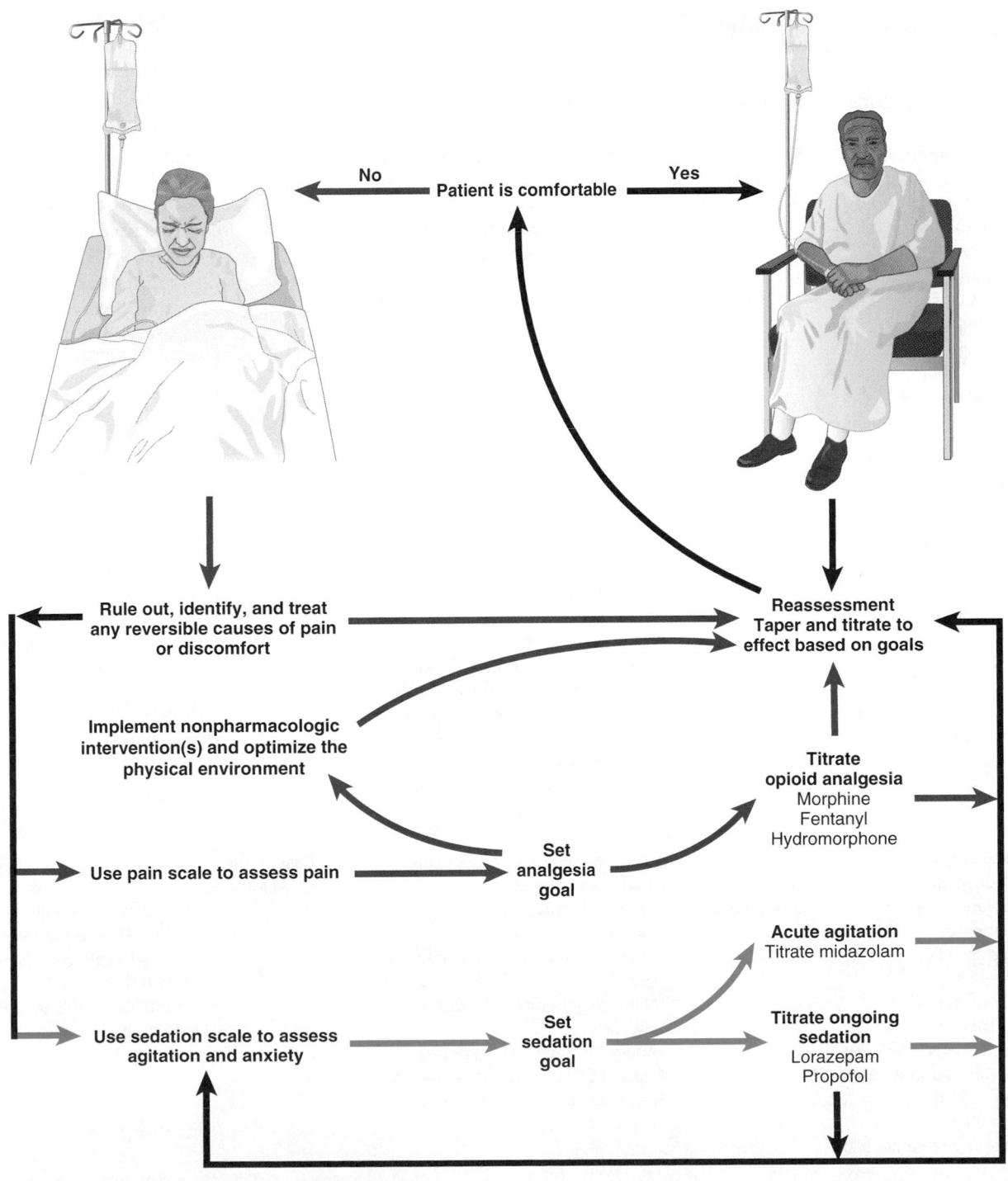

✦FIGURE 4-12 Sedation and analgesia algorithm.

Sedation for this purpose is appropriate only after attempting to manage the airway through adjustment of fraction of inspired oxygen (FiO_2) and ventilator modification to flow, tidal volume, rate, and synchrony. For patients who must be sedated in order to maintain a functional airway and adequate ventilation, it is desirable to administer both analgesic and sedating pharmacologic agents, as analgesics potentiate effects of sedating agents, requiring lower doses of sedating agents.[42,50,74,81,90]

There are four levels of sedation: minimal, moderate, deep, and general anesthesia.[43] For each level of sedation, there are indications and end points (Table 4-7). Sedation used in critical care fits into the moderate sedation category. With moderate sedation, the patient maintains protective reflexes and the ability

---

TABLE 4-7 Sedation End Points

ASSESSMENT FINDINGS	PROBLEM	INTERVENTIONS	END POINT	OUTCOME MEASURE
Chest movement that is poorly coordinated with ventilator cycling Extreme inspiratory or expiratory chest movement Frequent or sustained coughing Tightening of chest wall muscles during any phase of ventilator cycle Inadequate gas exchange Hemodynamic instability Increased peak airway pressure	Patient-ventilator dyssynchrony	Look for and correct any mechanical problems associated with ventilator or patient's airway. Look for and assess for metabolic, electrolyte, or cardiovascular cause of symptoms. Look for and correct any sources of discomfort. Assess sedation and pain levels. Titrate sedation and analgesia.	Patient-ventilator synchrony	Responds to ventilator breaths in coordinated manner Synchrony prevents excessive nonproductive muscle work Improved gas exchange Hemodynamic stability Normal peak airway pressure
Excessive restlessness Continuous non-purposeful physical activity: fidgeting, thrashing side to side, pulling at clothing, bedding, and tubes Disorientation/confusion Unable to follow commands	Agitation	Differentiate between delirium and agitation and treat appropriately. Look for, correct, and/or treat physical (pain, hypoxia, drug reaction, hyperglycemia, hypoglycemia), emotional (fear, anxiety), or environmental causes (loud unfamiliar noises, bright lights, odors, uncomfortable room temperatures). Assess sedation and pain levels. Titrate sedation and analgesia.	Calm, non-agitated	No excessive non-purposeful physical activity Orientation Ability to follow commands
Decreased level of consciousness Not aware of self or surroundings Unable to follow simple commands Stupor or coma Nonverbal Awake (opens eyes) but not aware (cannot carry out any cognitive functions) Persistent vegetative state	Altered level of consciousness	Look for, correct, and treat cause, which may include: Brain ischemia/lesions Metabolic disturbances Inflammatory conditions, infection, sepsis Neurodegenerative disorders Hypoxia Analgesic agents or sedatives Assess LOC and level of sedation. Titrate sedation and analgesia.	Baseline level of consciousness	Awake Aware of self and surroundings Able to follow simple commands Verbal Responds to verbal stimulus

Data from references 19 and 20.

to maintain a patent airway and respond to verbal stimuli. Critically ill patients usually require special care and consideration when receiving moderate sedation.[43]

The need for sedation will vary throughout the patient's stay. Typically, sedation and analgesic requirements are highest upon arrival, plateau, and decrease over time, depending on the patient's condition. Although the Task Force of the Society of Critical Care Medicine[36] recommended midazolam (Versed) and propofol (Diprivan) for short-term sedation and lorazepam (Ativan) for longer-term sedation, critical care sedation practices vary widely. A standard protocol is recommended to prevent under- and oversedation and polypharmacy problems.[5]

Once pharmacologic and nonpharmacologic interventions have been initiated, it is important to monitor effectiveness of treatment by assessing changes in pain and sedation. When a patient who was previously alert and/or awake becomes somnolent or has difficulty staying awake while in conversation, the patient's level of sedation may require action (e.g., frequent physical stimulation or opioid reversal) to prevent subsequent respiratory depression. Because sedation precedes respiratory depression, if the sedation level is assessed at appropriate time intervals, the nurse will be able to detect excessive sedation related to pharmacologic interventions and prevent untoward events (e.g., respiratory depression or respiratory arrest[20,42]).

Assessing sedation levels in critical care is an important skill. Sedation scales are tools available to the nurse in assessing a patient's response to physical, auditory, or verbal stimuli. The ideal scale would be easy to use and reliable, and able to distinguish between various degrees of sedation or agitation.[20,102] Several scales have been developed, with the most common being observational scales, where nurses rate level of sedation based on patients' response to various stimuli. Scales differ in their approach to assessing sedation or sedation and agitation. The Ramsay Sedation Scale (Box 4-9) assesses sedation on a six-point asleep-awake scale. Although simple to use, it does not provide an adequate measure of agitation, and is therefore less useful for monitoring sedation in critically ill patients.[20,36,42]

A more useful instrument for assessing sedation in critically ill patients is the Riker Sedation-Agitation Scale (SAS), which rates sedation and agitation on a continuum from 1 to 7 (Box 4-10). Similarly, the Motor Activity Assessment Scale (MAAS) evaluates both sedation and agitation. However, the MAAS uses a continuum from 0 to 6 and includes behavioral clarifiers that may make it easier for use in critical care (Box 4-11). A more extensive instrument is the Richmond Agitation-Sedation Scale (RASS). The RASS uses a 10-point scale and measures sedation on a continuum

---

Box 4-9

The Ramsay Sedation Scale

Response to Verbal Command	Numerical Score
Agitated	6
Responds readily to name in normal tone	5
Lethargic response to name in normal tone	4
Responds to name only if called loudly and repeatedly	3
Responds only after mild prodding or shaking	2
Does not respond to mild prodding or shaking	1
Does not respond to test stimulus	0

From reference 78b.

Box 4-10

Riker Sedation-Agitation Scale (SAS)

Score	Term	Descriptor
7	Dangerous agitation	Pulling at ET tube, trying to remove catheters, climbing over bed rail, striking at staff, thrashing side to side
6	Very agitated	Requiring restraint and frequent verbal reminding of limits, biting endotracheal tube
5	Agitated	Anxious or physically agitated, calms to verbal instructions
4	Calm and cooperative	Calm, easily arousable, follows commands
3	Sedated	Difficult to arouse but awakens to verbal stimuli or gentle shaking; follows simple commands but drifts off again
2	Very sedated	Arouses to physical stimuli but does not communicate or follow commands; may move spontaneously
1	Unarousable	Minimal or no response to noxious stimuli; does not communicate or follow commands

From reference 81.

Box 4-11

Motor Activity Assessment Scale (MAAS)

Score	Description	Definition
0	Unresponsive	Does not move with noxious stimulus*
1	Responsive only to noxious stimuli	Opens eyes OR raises eyebrows OR turns head toward stimulus OR moves limbs with noxious stimulus*
2	Responsive to touch or name	Opens eyes OR raises eyebrows OR turns head toward stimulus OR moves limbs when touched or name is loudly spoken
3	Calm and cooperative	No external stimulus is required to elicit movement AND patient is adjusting sheets or clothes purposefully and follows commands
4	Restless and cooperative	No external stimulus is required to elicit movement AND patient is picking at sheet or tubes OR uncovering self and follows commands
5	Agitated	No external stimulus is required to elicit movement AND attempting to sit up OR moves limbs out of bed AND does not consistently follow commands (e.g., will lie down when asked but soon reverts back to attempts to sit up or move limbs out of bed)
6	Dangerously agitated, uncooperative	No external stimulus is required to elicit movement AND patient is pulling at tubes or catheters OR thrashing side to side OR striking at staff OR trying to climb out of bed AND does not calm down when asked

From reference 49.
*Noxious stimulus, suctioning or 5 seconds of vigorous orbital, sternal, or nail bed pressure.

from −5 to 0 and agitation from 1 to 4 (Box 4-12). Like the MAAS, the RASS includes specific behavioral clarifiers, making it easy to use in critical care.[49,81]

Scales reviewed so far focus on a single domain. De Jong[19] recently described the development of the American Association of Critical-Care Nurses' Sedation Scale for Critically Ill Patients (Table 4-8). This scale consists of five domains: consciousness, agitation, anxiety, sleep, and patient-ventilator synchrony. Because the domains in this scale were designed to parallel the most common sedation therapy goals, it may offer advantages over scales that focus on a single domain. However, clinical testing is needed to determine if this scale is a valid and reliable tool for measuring sedation in the critically ill population.[19]

Of note is that observational scales are not useful for assessing patients who are receiving neuromuscular blockade, and although vital signs (e.g., blood pressure

Box 4-12

Richmond Agitation-Sedation Scale (RASS)

Score	Term	Description
+4	Combative	Overtly combative or violent: immediate danger to staff
+3	Very agitated	Pulls on or removes tube(s) or catheter(s) or has aggressive behavior toward staff
+2	Agitated	Frequent nonpurposeful movement or patient-ventilator dyssynchrony
+1	Restless	Anxious or apprehensive but movements not aggressive or vigorous
+0	Alert and calm	
−1	Drowsy	Not fully alert, but has sustained (more than 10 seconds) awakening, with eye contact to voice
−2	Light sedation	Briefly (less than 10 seconds) awakens with eye contact to voice
−3	Moderate sedation	Any movement (but no eye contact) to voice
−4	Deep sedation	No response to voice, but any movement to physical stimulation
−5	Unarousable	No response to voice or physical stimulation

From reference 88b.

TABLE 4-8 American Association of Critical-Care Nurses' Sedation Scale for Critically Ill Patients*

DOMAIN OR SUBSCALE	INDICATOR	BEST 1	2	3	4	WORST 5
Consciousness	Awake and aware of self and environment	Spontaneously opens eyes and initiates interaction with others	Wakens and responds after light verbal or tactile stimuli May return to sleep when stimuli stop	Wakens and responds after strong or noxious verbal or tactile stimuli Returns to sleep when stimuli stop	Displays localization or withdrawal behaviors to noxious stimuli	Displays posturing or no response to strong or noxious stimuli
Agitation	Body movement, patient/staff safety*	Calm body movements and tolerance of treatments and restrictions Movements do not pose a significant risk for safety of patient or staff		Body movements or noncompliance with treatments or restrictions does not pose a significant risk for safety of patient or staff		Body movements or noncompliance with treatments or restrictions poses a significant risk for safety of patient or staff
	Noises of patient	No noises		Frequent moaning or calling out		Shouting, screaming, or other disruptive vocalizations
	Patients' statements	Very calm				Very restless
Anxiety	Patient's perceived anxiety† (Faces Anxiety Scale)‡	No anxiety				Extreme anxiety

Table continues on page 76

Table 4-8 American Association of Critical-Care Nurses' Sedation Scale for Critically Ill Patients*—cont'd

DOMAIN OR SUBSCALE	INDICATOR	BEST 1	2	3	4	WORST 5
Sleep	Observed sleep	Looks asleep, calm, resting (eyes closed, calm face and body)	Looks asleep; periodically wakens and returns to sleep easily	Awake; naps occasionally for brief periods		Unable to sleep or nap
	Patient's perceived quality of sleep	I slept well		I slept fair		I slept poorly
Patient-ventilator synchrony	Breathing pattern relative to ventilator	Synchrony of ventilator and patient at all times, patient cooperative and accepting ventilation Coordinated, relaxed chest movements		Occasional resistance to ventilation or spontaneous breathing is out of synchrony with the ventilator Chest movement occasionally not coordinated with ventilator		Frequent resistance to ventilation or spontaneous breathing not synchronous with the ventilator Uncoordinated chest and ventilator movements

From reference 19. Used with permission.
*This component is assessed in all patients, regardless of the goal of sedation.
†Assumes the patient has the ability to understand directions and communicate his or her perceptions either verbally, in writing, or by pointing to words or pictures. If score is greater than 2 for this subscale, ask the patient if he or she needs something to help him or her relax.
‡Faces Anxiety Scale reprinted from McKinley, et al, with permission of Blackwell Publishing.

and heart rate) may be objective indicators of sedation, they may also be indicators of other variables. Vital signs are affected by the patient's underlying condition and pharmaceutical agents, making their usefulness as a measure of sedation suspect.[43,44]

Because sedation-agitation tools have limited usefulness in chemically paralyzed patients, objective instruments have been developed that use neurologic monitoring with electroencephalography (EEG) and auditory-evoked potentials (AEPs).[102] Bispectral index (BIS) uses a mathematical technique to analyze EEG wave data. This analysis provides a number between 0 and 100, with higher numbers indicating less sedation (100 = awake) and lower numbers (0 = isoelectric EEG) indicating increased sedation. Although currently used in many critical care units, some studies have demonstrated a poor correlation between BIS and subjective measures of sedation and agitation. Because muscle activity affects EEG data, the nurse needs to use BIS with caution in patients who exhibit either voluntary or involuntary muscle activity.[102] In contrast to BIS, AEP uses auditory stimulation through headphones to elicit and measure cortical response to sound, with a decreased response associated with increased levels of sedation. Auditory-evoked potentials (AEPs) have been correlated with subjective instruments such as the RASS.[102] However, these objective measures (BIS and AEP) are not yet universally used to assess levels of sedation and agitation; and because research is limited or conflicting related to their usefulness, they should be used only as adjuncts to subjective measures.[25,70,81,102]

Sedating Agents

Benzodiazepines, the most frequently used sedation agents, decrease anxiety and have amnesic and anticonvulsant properties. Benzodiazepines act by modulating GABA, an amino acid produced in the brain in response to stress.[42] GABA is our body's natural sedative. Unlike barbiturates, whose action mimics GABA, producing a pronounced CNS depressive effect, benzodiazepines potentiate the action of endogenous GABA, limiting the amount of CNS depression induced. As lipid-soluble agents, benzodiazepines cross the blood-brain barrier easily, and their effect (from decreasing anxiety to sedation to hypnosis) depends on the number of receptors occupied.[42,89] Benzodiazepines are easily absorbed and can be administered orally; however, the IV route is the most reliable. Benzodiazepines can be given intermittently (IV bolus) or by continuous infusion. Benzodiazepines should be used with caution in patients with signs of renal or hepatic dysfunction, and need for continuation should be evaluated at least daily.[42,82,89]

The most commonly used benzodiazepines are diazepam (Valium), lorazepam, and midazolam. Onset and duration of action for these agents varies by drug; side effects such as respiratory depression and hypotension are dose dependent. Sedation guidelines prepared by the Task Force of the American College of Critical Care Medicine[42] are shown in Box 4-13, and selected sedative agents are summarized in the Medication table on p. 78.

Although currently not recommended by the Task Force of the American College of Critical Care Medicine for reversal of prolonged benzodiazepine-induced sedation states,[42] flumazenil (Romazicon), a competitive agonist, can be administered intravenously to reverse the sedative effect of short-term benzodiazepine use. As a benzodiazepine antagonist, flumazenil's duration of action is short; so once reversed, sedation may reoccur from longer-acting benzodiazepines. The critical care nurse should assess for and anticipate the possibility of withdrawal seizures with flumazenil administration, especially if the patient has been receiving benzodiazepines for a prolonged time.[5,42]

Another agent frequently used for sedation, when rapid onset of action is required, is propofol. Propofol is a general anesthetic at high doses but has sedative and hypnotic properties at lower doses. With rapid onset and short duration of action, propofol is frequently used in critical care. Propofol, which can cause pain with peripheral administration, may also affect blood pressure and cause respiratory depression. These adverse effects are typically dose and rate

---

Box 4-13

Sedation Guidelines

- Midazolam and diazepam are useful for acutely agitated patients because of their rapid onset of action.
- When rapid awakening is essential for patient management, propofol is the preferred sedative.
- Midazolam is not recommended for prolonged use, and is associated with unpredictable waking times and prolonged intubation.
- Lorazepam, which can be given via continuous or intermittent infusion, is recommended for sedation in most patients.
- Sedative dosing should be titrated to a specific end point (using a sedation scale).
- Gradual tapering of sedative dose and daily drug interruption of sedation to assess underlying condition and reassess need for continued sedation are recommended for all sedating agents.

Data from reference 42.

SELECTED SEDATIVE AGENTS

MEDICATION	ACTIONS	DOSAGE	SPECIAL CONSIDERATIONS
Diazepam (Valium)	Depresses CNS at limbic and subcortical levels by increasing effects of GABA	Bolus 0.03–0.1 mg/kg IV	Contraindicated in patients who are hypersensitive to benzodiazepines or have a history of narrow-angle glaucoma, psychosis, coma, or respiratory depression
Lorazepam (Ativan)	Probably stimulates GABA receptors in ascending RAS	Bolus 0.02–0.06 mg/kg IV followed by infusion at 0.01–0.1 mg/kg/hr	Contraindicated in patients who are hypersensitive to benzodiazepines or have a history of narrow-angle glaucoma, psychosis, drug abuse, or chronic obstructive pulmonary disease
Midazolam (Versed)	Depresses CNS at limbic and subcortical levels by increasing effects of GABA	Bolus 0.02–0.08 mg/kg IV followed by infusion at 0.04–0.2 mg/kg/hr	Contraindicated in patients who are hypersensitive to benzodiazepines or have a history of narrow-angle glaucoma, coma, or alcohol intoxication
Propofol (Diprivan)	Inhibits sympathetic nervous system activity; decreases vascular resistance	Initially 5 mcg/kg/min IV over 5 minutes; may give 5–10 mcg/kg/min over 5–10 minutes until desired response. For maintenance: infusion at 0.1–0.2 mg/kg/min (6–12 mcg/kg/min)	Do not give to patients who have hypersensitivity to eggs or soybean oil Do not leave hanging longer than 6 hours Strict sterile technique Sedation may be prolonged in obese patients

dependent; the patient requires frequent monitoring of sedation level while receiving this agent. Propofol has a depressant effect on the cardiovascular system that can cause hypotension.[42,59] Of significant concern is the potential for patients receiving propofol for longer than 72 hours to develop pancreatitis. Monitoring of triglyceride levels is also critical, as hypertriglyceridemia is seen in patients with infusions longer than 3 days.[42,59] Another significant precaution related to continuous infusions of propofol is risk for microbial contamination of the infusion. Propofol is a lipid emulsion, a rich medium for many organisms.[42,59] Propofol infusions require a dedicated IV line to minimize incompatibility and infection problems. The infusion and setup should be replaced every 12 hours.[5,42,59] The Nutrition box at right contains more information about administration of propofol.

Although new as a sedating agent in critical care, dexmedetomidine (Precedex), a selective alpha agonist, has been approved for use as a sedative. Dexmedetomidine can be used as a short-term (less than 24 hours) sedative in mechanically ventilated patients. An advantage this agent offers is patients are sedated when left undisturbed, but arouse quickly with mild

▲ NUTRITION

Administration of Propofol

Propofol is available as an emulsion and provides calories from fat (1 kcal/ml) that should be included in dietary calculations. Prolonged use of propofol has been associated with hypertriglyceridemia, elevated pancreatic enzymes, and pancreatitis. Long-term use or administration of high doses of propofol has also been linked to lactic acidosis, bradycardia, and lipidemia in pediatric patients, and to dysrhythmias and increased risk of cardiac arrest in adult patients. Patients given propofol for prolonged periods should be routinely monitored for both metabolic acidosis and cardiac dysrhythmias.

stimulus. Dexmedetomidine is also analgesic sparing and has anxiolytic properties similar to benzodiazepines. Elevated blood pressure has been associated with rapid administration of dexmedetomidine; prolonged administration is associated with bradycardia and hypotension, especially in patients with intravascular volume depletion.[42]

A possible complication of sedation and analgesia is that it may cause or exacerbate episodes of delirium.[42] Delirium is a reversible condition characterized by sudden onset of confusion and agitation, and a change in level of consciousness.[3] All patients are at risk for development of delirium if they are extremely ill or taking medications that alter CNS function. However, sensory deprivation and sensory overload can also precipitate episodes of delirium. Factors that may contribute to delirium in critical care patients are social isolation, sedation, not wearing eyeglasses or hearing aids, sleep deprivation, and environmental noises and odors.[3,42] Just being admitted to the hospital, let alone critical care, contributes to delirium. Adverse effects of analgesics or sedatives are a frequent cause of delirium in critical care patients. However, abnormal levels of calcium, sodium, or magnesium can also cause delirium.[3,42] Before administering any drug to manage the symptoms of delirium, an attempt must be made to identify and treat the cause of delirium. Haloperidol (Haldol) is the drug most frequently used to treat critical care delirium. However, potential side effects require careful and critical monitoring to prevent untoward events. Patients should be monitored for prolonged Q-T intervals and cardiac dysrhythmias.[3]

NEUROMUSCULAR BLOCKADE

In addition to administration of sedating and analgesic medications, critically ill patients may also require neuromuscular blockade. Neuromuscular blocking (NMB) agents are used only when analgesia and sedation have not been effective, or when needed to facilitate treatment.[69] Neuromuscular blockade may be indicated for patients who are mechanically ventilated, for those with tetanus, or for patients with increased intracranial pressure (ICP). The goal of neuromuscular blockade is to maximize oxygenation and ventilation by control of ineffective breathing patterns that might be caused by either agitation or hyperdynamic states related to disease or trauma.[65] Neuromuscular blocking agents act by blocking the action of acetylcholine in postsynaptic receptor sites in neuromuscular junctions, causing muscle paralysis[51,69] (Figure 4-13).

Neuromuscular blocking agents reduce oxygen consumption, control intracranial pressure, and make intubation or procedures that require non-movement by the patient safer and easier.[51,69] Because of the potential for very serious side effects, NMB agents should always be used with extreme caution. When continuous NMB is indicated (more than 48 hours), the infusion should be stopped daily to assess for its continued need.[51] Basic nursing care for patients receiving NMB is essential as patients are at increased

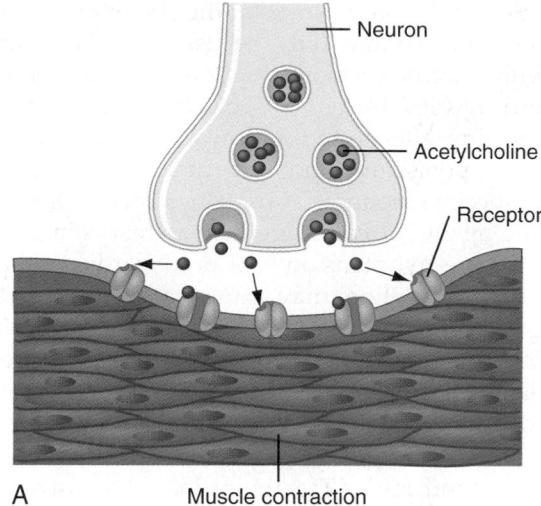

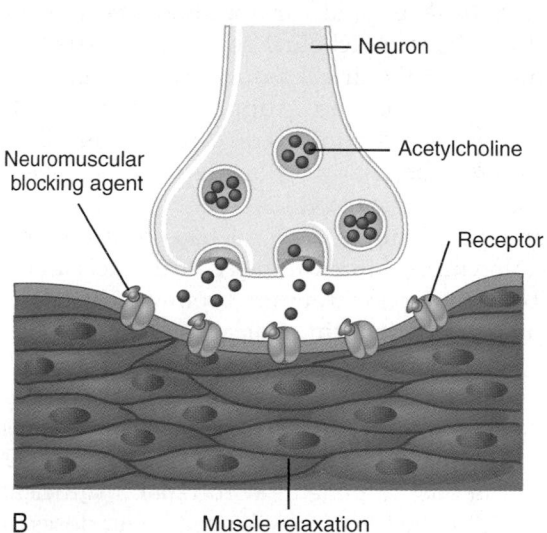

◆FIGURE 4-13   A, Normal muscle contraction. **B,** Neuromuscular blockade.

risk for problems associated with immobility. In addition, long-lasting weakness may occur after NMB, with patients demonstrating elevated serum creatine kinase levels, muscle fiber atrophy, and muscle fiber necrosis.[51,69] Prolonged weakness may be attributable to delayed clearing of the drug, or a synergistic effect that occurs when NMB agents are given with corticosteroids or aminoglycosides.[51,69] The actions of NMB agents are potentiated by aminoglycosides, antibiotics, hypothermia, hyperkalemia, and hypercalcemia.

Neuromuscular blocking agents are classified as either depolarizing or nondepolarizing.[51] Succinylcholine chloride (Anectine) is the only depolarizing agent. Succinylcholine chloride is given as a bolus (not as a continuous infusion) for rapid-sequence intubation. Because it can cause rapid elevation in serum potassium levels, risk of hyperkalemia and cardiac arrest is great. Succinylcholine works at the site of acetylcholine receptors and should only be used for short periods and with extreme caution.[2,52,92] Patients with acute spinal cord injuries, burns, and/or trauma are at highest risk for side effects and untoward events related to release of potassium and hyperkalemia. In addition, when succinylcholine is used in conjunction with sedating agents, it causes release of histamine, resulting in severe hypotension and bradycardia. Although rare, succinylcholine may cause a condition called malignant hyperthermia (Chapter 46).[51] Early recognition of malignant hyperthermia is essential to prevent muscle breakdown, acidosis, hyperthermia, and cardiac dysrhythmias. Warning symptoms include jaw spasms, muscle rigidity, increased heart and respiratory rates, and fever. Treatment includes discontinuation of the drug, correction of acid-base balance, treatment of fever, and cardiopulmonary support.[51,69] Overdose of succinylcholine chloride is treated by discontinuation of the drug, coupled with maintenance of airway and respiratory support. Anticholinesterase agents are not recommended to reverse NMB due to the action of depolarizing agents, and, if given, can increase the degree of NMB.[51,69]

Nondepolarizing agents, such as vecuronium bromide (Norcuron), atracurium (Tracrium), cisatracurium (Nimbex), and pancuronium bromide (Pavulon), are used most frequently in clinical practice and have an intermediate effect. Vecuronium, with an onset of action of 60 to 90 seconds (IV), peaks in 25 to 35 minutes and has few cardiovascular side effects. Thirty-five percent of vecuronium is excreted in the urine and 50% is excreted in bile, so patients with renal insufficiency or impaired hepatic function will need lower doses to prevent toxic accumulation. Because prolonged blockade has been noticed more frequently with vecuronium than with other NMB agents, it has fallen out of favor and the frequency of its use in critical care has decreased.[69]

An intermediate NMB agent with duration of action of 30 to 40 minutes, atracurium is used for patients with renal and hepatic failure because it degrades rapidly, making its clearance independent of liver and renal elimination. Atracurium has cardiovascular side effects associated with histamine release at high doses. The most common side effects are hypotension and tachycardia that can be prevented with administration of histamine blockers.[69] Atracurium, like other NMB agents, can cause persistent or prolonged neuromuscular blockade.[69]

Cisatracurium has greater NMB potency than atracurium, with similar elimination, primarily via degradation; unlike atracurium, cisatracurium has fewer cardiovascular side effects, is administered in smaller doses, and has a duration of 45 minutes, compared to 30 to 40 minutes for atracurium.

Pancuronium bromide, one of the first NMB agents used in critical care units, is long acting, with 1- to 2-hour duration of action. Pancuronium bromide can be used for continuous infusion. Because of its vagolytic effect on the sinoatrial node and blocking of norepinephrine, the most common side effects are hypertension and tachycardia.[5,51,69] Pancuronium bromide should not be used in patients who cannot tolerate an increased heart rate.

When monitoring patients who are receiving NMB, paralysis and sedation level should be assessed frequently. Paralysis can be monitored through assessment of clinical indicators and by using a peripheral nerve stimulator (Figure 4-14). Clinical indicators may be useful for detecting signs of inadequate sedation and paralysis. Clinical indicators include tachycardia, hypertension, diaphoresis, spontaneous breathing, and body movement.[51] However, these clinical indicators are not reliable indices of adequate sedation, nor can they be used to differentiate between adequate sedation and excessive sedation in patients with neuromuscular blockade.[51,69] In general, visual, tactile, and electronic methods can be employed to assess muscle tone and neuromuscular blockade. The mainstay of assessment is nursing observation of movement (musculoskeletal) and respiratory effort. However, electronic tools are available to assist the nurse in monitoring neuromuscular blockade.[6,69]

Perhaps one of the most promising methods of assessing paralysis is peripheral nerve stimulation (PNS). To assess paralysis, a stimulus is applied to either the ulnar nerve (Figure 4-15), the facial nerve (Figure 4-16), or the posterior tibial nerve (Figure 4-17). The same site should be used consistently, with the ulnar nerve being preferred because it is least affected by artifact. In the absence of NMB, twitching should occur four times in response to four electrical impulses. The goal of neuromuscular blockade is 90%, which corresponds to one twitch for every four electrical stimuli. When using the stimulator, if no twitches are elicited, the "tetanus mode," which delivers a 5-second stimulus, is used to generate a sustained twitch. This is followed by a repeat of the four stimuli. If no twitch occurs, the patient is overparalyzed and the NMB agent is stopped (intermittent dosing) or decreased (continuous dosing) until at least two twitches per four stimuli return. If the patient is receiving intermittent rather than continuous administration of neuromuscular blocking agents, then the four-sequence test should be performed every 30 to 60 minutes.*

Another tool that can be used to assess adequacy of neuromuscular blockade is continuous airway pressure

---

*References 2, 5, 6, 51, 69, 83.

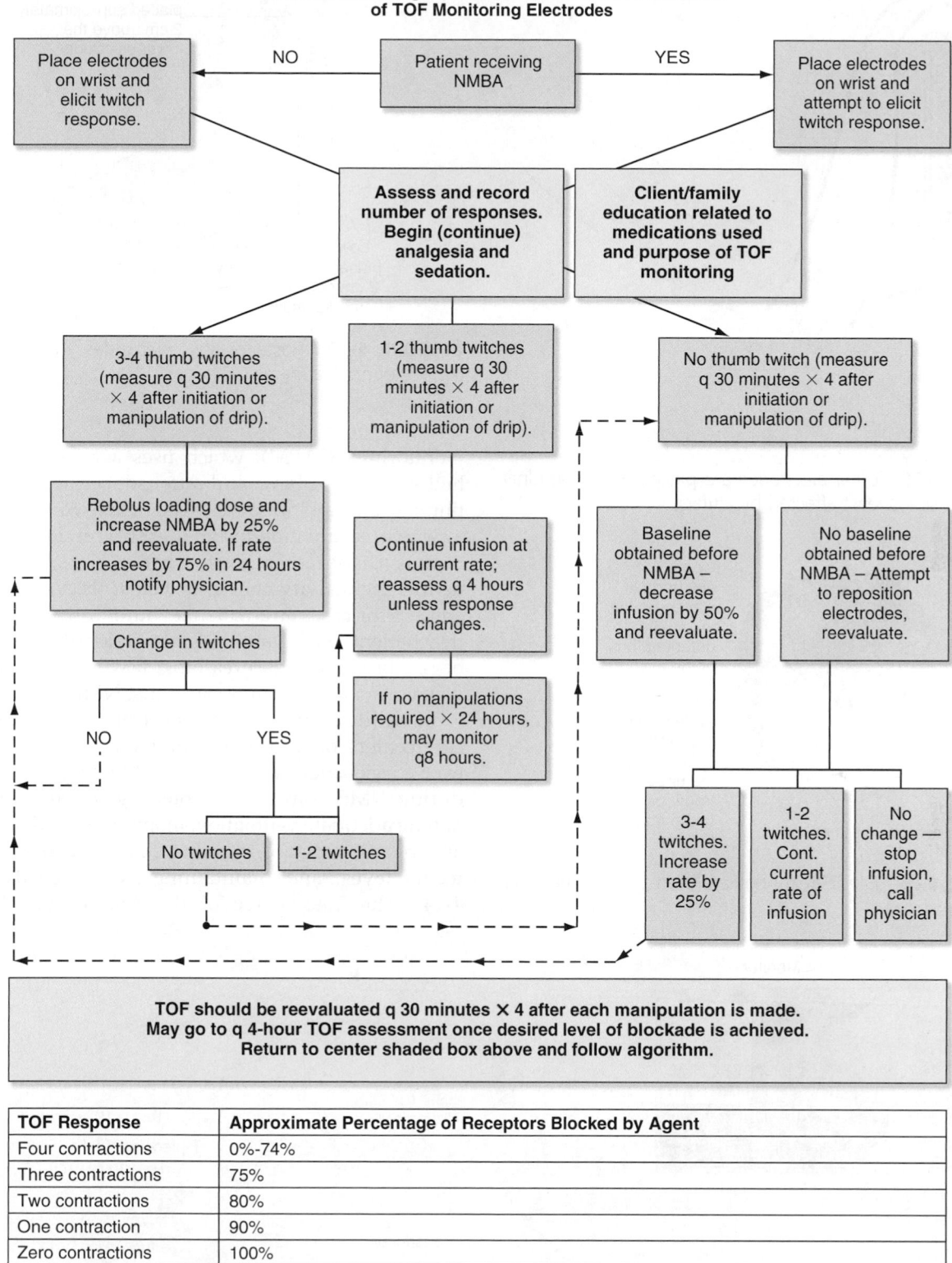

**Education/Training/Certification of Nurses in Placement
of TOF Monitoring Electrodes**

TOF Response	Approximate Percentage of Receptors Blocked by Agent
Four contractions	0%-74%
Three contractions	75%
Two contractions	80%
One contraction	90%
Zero contractions	100%

⬍FIGURE 4-14 Algorithm for assessing neuromuscular blockade.

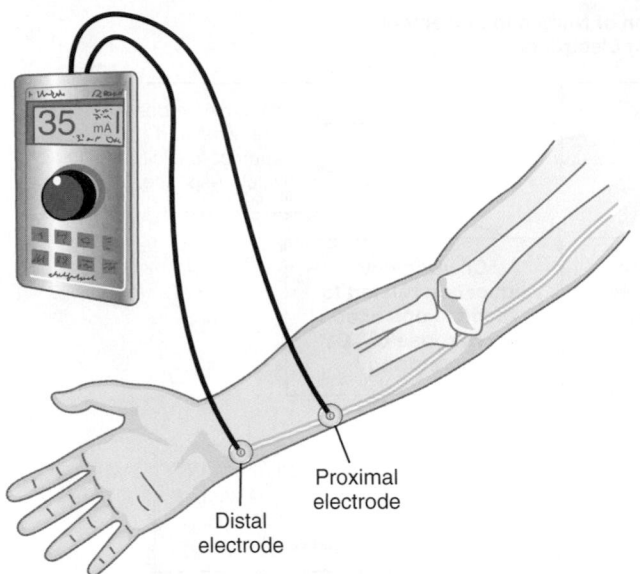

✦FIGURE 4-15 Ulnar electrodes are placed along the ulnar nerve. This site is least affected by artifact.

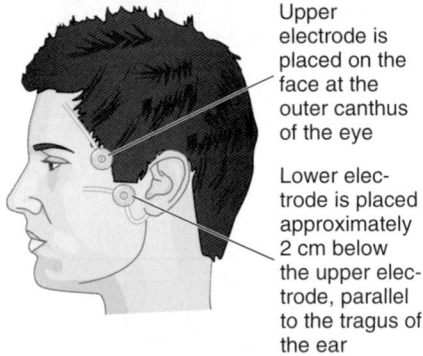

Upper electrode is placed on the face at the outer canthus of the eye

Lower electrode is placed approximately 2 cm below the upper electrode, parallel to the tragus of the ear

✦FIGURE 4-16 Facial electrodes are placed along the facial nerve.

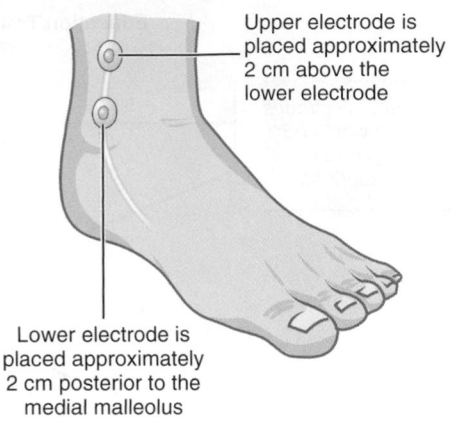

Upper electrode is placed approximately 2 cm above the lower electrode

Lower electrode is placed approximately 2 cm posterior to the medial malleolus

✦FIGURE 4-17 Posterior tibial electrodes are placed along the posterior tibial nerve.

monitoring (CAPM), which uses a transducer cable, high-pressure tubing, and a transducer to display continuous airway pressures[6] (Figure 4-18). Continuous airway pressure monitoring (CAPM) can identify spontaneous diaphragmatic effort before any other signs of neurologic activity can be detected; thus it is a useful adjunct for assessing patients with NMB. For example, if a patient on a ventilator set as assist-control (AC) begins breakthrough breathing, it will be noted on the waveform and the nurse can adjust NMB[6] (Figure 4-19).

In addition to assessing level of paralysis, nursing care centers on protecting the patient from untoward events associated with paralysis. Nursing management during NMB consists of protecting the airway, maintaining adequate ventilation, monitoring cardiac rhythm and blood pressure, treating pain and anxiety, protecting eyes, and maintaining skin integrity[51] (Box 4-14). The Task Force of the American College of

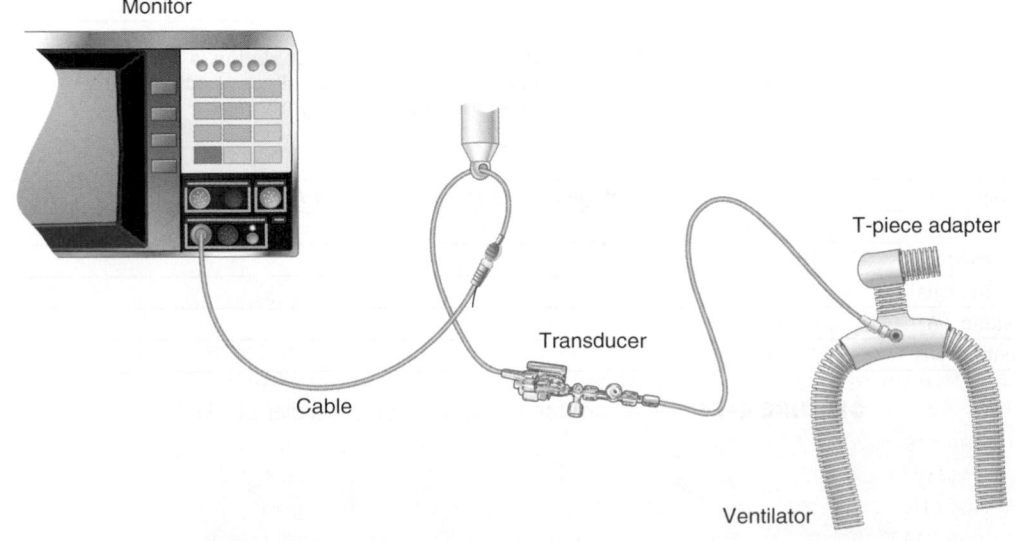

✦FIGURE 4-18 Continuous airway pressure monitoring.

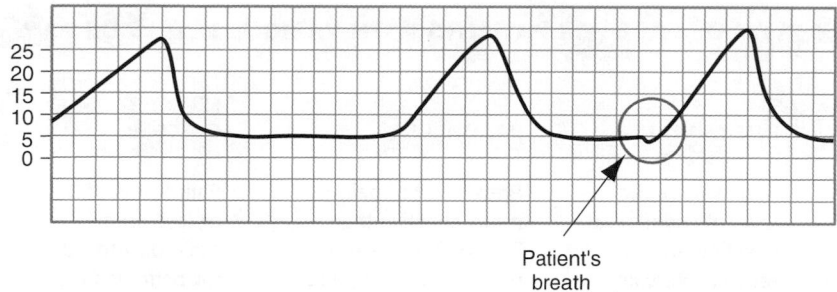

Patient's
breath

⬥FIGURE 4-19 Continuous airway pressure monitoring waveform in a patient on assist-control ventilation.

Box 4-14

Caring for Patients Receiving Neuromuscular Blockade

MANAGEMENT OF AIRWAY, BREATHING, AND CIRCULATION

- Establish and maintain a patent airway.
- Suction as indicated by patient's condition.
- Monitor ventilatory settings for accuracy.
- Evaluate oxygenation and ventilation through use of arterial blood gases and pulse oximetry.
- Maintain a manual resuscitation bag at the bedside at all times.
- Monitor for hemodynamic stability (blood pressure, heart rate and rhythm, temperature, peripheral pulses).
- Monitor and intervene as appropriate to maintain physiologic stability (acid-base status, electrolyte balance).
- Provide excellent physical assessment of cardiac and pulmonary systems to evaluate for effects of immobility.
- Observe skin for potential areas of breakdown.

- Reposition patient frequently.
- Consider use of a pressure-reducing mattress.
- Keep skin clean and dry. Consider use of massage to stimulate circulation as needed.
- Institute interventions to prevent deep vein thrombus.

MANAGEMENT OF EYE PROTECTION

- Close patient's eyes and cover with a soft eye pad.
- Use eye lubricants or artificial tears as ordered.

MANAGEMENT OF PAIN, SEDATION, AND LEVEL OF NEUROMUSCULAR BLOCKADE

- Institute monitoring to evaluate level of neuromuscular blockade with frequency established by patient's condition.
  - Peripheral nerve stimulation
  - Four-sequence testing
  - Continuous airway pressure monitoring
- Institute monitoring to evaluate patient's level of pain and sedation.
  - Administer adequate pain and sedation medications while patient is receiving neuromuscular blockade.

Critical Care Medicine recommends all patients receiving NMB also receive prophylactic eye care, physical therapy, and deep vein thrombosis (DVT) precautions.[69]

When excessive NMB has been identified or when there is no longer a need for NMB, chemically induced paralysis can be reversed by administering an anticholinesterase agent, such as physostigmine (Antilirium), pyridostigmine (Mestinon), or neostigmine (Prostigmin). Anticholinesterase agents work by increasing the availability of acetylcholine at receptor sites. While useful for reversing effects of nondepolarizing agents, use of anticholinesterase agents is contraindicated as

a method of reversing the effects of succinylcholine chloride.[69]

CONCLUSIONS

Pain is a common and usually predictable event for critically ill patients. Knowledge of and preemptive implementation of multimodal interventions that include basic comfort measures, the use of complementary therapies, and pharmacologic agents are essential to prevent the consequences of pain and to improve overall outcomes for critically ill patients. The

MULTIDISCIPLINARY PLAN OF CARE FOR PATIENTS WITH VARIOUS LEVELS OF PAIN AND ANXIETY

PROBLEM	INTERVENTION	RATIONALE	EXPECTED OUTCOME	COMMENTS
Acute pain related to: Surgery or trauma Procedures Immobility Inadequate pain management	Assess pain and level of sedation at baseline and at regular intervals. Anticipate pain and use preemptive pain management techniques.	Prevention of pain is more effective than PRN or "as needed" management of pain. Decreased stress results in improved immune function and reduced cardiorespiratory workload.	Pain levels of 3 or less on a scale of 0 to 10 for patients who can self-report	Include both pharmacologic and nonpharmacologic interventions to maximize analgesic effect and minimize side effects.
Anxiety/fear related to: Unfamiliar environment Confusion Lack of information Lack of control Pain/discomfort	Provide information. Provide touch. Provide options if possible. Assess orientation level and reorient as needed.	Communication and touch help patient differentiate self from surroundings and provide feelings of trust, allowing patient to sleep or rest.	Periods of uninterrupted sleep Oriented to time, place, person, and space Decreased pain levels Decreased anxiety	Anxiety and fear increase perceptions of pain, lower tolerance to pain, increase stress, and adversely affect immune system.
Discomfort related to: Temperature Positioning Odors Noise	Manage environment for patient's maximum comfort.	Discomfort is a stressor. By decreasing discomfort, stress is reduced.	Sleep/rest Pain levels of 3 or less Discomfort levels of 1 or less	Discomfort increases perceptions of pain, increases stress, and adversely affects immune system.
Potential for respiratory depression related to: Excessive sedation Side effects of pharmacologic agents	Provide frequent/ continuous sedation level monitoring (based on drug, dose, and route of administration).	Sedation *PRECEDES* respiratory depression.	Adequate management of pain (3 or less) with minimal side effects and adequate ventilation	Appropriate agent to reverse effects of drug administered should be readily available.

Multidisciplinary Plan of Care above outlines appropriate interventions for patients with varying levels of pain and anxiety. Nurses caring for critically ill patients must be aware of potential problems associated with pain management, sedation, and NMB that can impact patient outcomes. Research on management of pain and technology related to assessment of critically ill patients receiving sedative or neuromuscular blocking agents is rapidly changing the role of the nurse, requiring the acquisition of new knowledge and skills. Critical care nurses are in a unique position to monitor and assess the effectiveness of these innovations and provide important feedback on their usefulness for improving care of critically ill patients.

REFERENCES

1. Apfelbaum, J. L., et al. (2003). Postoperative pain experience: results from a national survey suggest postoperative pain continues to be undermanaged. *Anesth Analg, 97,* 534–540.
2. Ashburn, M. A., et al. (2003). *Principles of analgesic use in the treatment of acute pain and cancer pain* (5th ed.). Glenview, Ill: American Pain Society.
3. Beers, M. H., & Berkow, R. 1999–2005. *The Merck manual of diagnosis and therapy: internet edition.* www.merck.com/mrkshared/mmanual/home.jsp.

4. Bergman, S. (2003). A general practice approach to management of widespread musculoskeletal pain and fibromyalgia. *Rheumatic Disease: In Practice.* www.arc.org.uk/about_arth/med_reports/series4/ip/6510.htm.

5. Blanchard, A. R. (2002). Sedation and analgesia in intensive care: medications attenuate stress response in critical illness. *Postgrad Med, 111*(2), 59–74.

6. Burns, S. M. (2004). Continuous airway pressure monitoring. *Crit Care Nurs, 24*(6), 70–74.

7. Byers, M., & Bonica, J. J. (2001). Peripheral neural mechanisms of nociceptor plasticity. In J. D. Loeser, S. H. Butler, C. R. Chapman, et al. (Eds.), *Bonica's management of pain.* Philadelphia: Lippincott.

8. Cao, Y. Q., et al. (1998). Primary afferent tachykinins are required to experience moderate to intense pain. *Nature, 392,* 390–394.

9. Carr, D. B., et al. (2004). *The spectrum of pain.* New York: McMahon.

10. Carr, D., & Goudas, L. L. (1999). Acute pain. *Lancet, 353,* 2051–2058.

11. Charmandari, E., Tsigos, C., & Chrousos, G. (2005). Endocrinology of the stress response. *Annu Rev Physiol, 67,* 259–284.

12. Cherny, N., et al. (2001). Strategies to manage the adverse effects of oral morphine: an evidence-based report. *J Clin Oncol, 19,* 2542–2554.

13. Cleeland, C. S., & Ryan, K. M. (1995). Pain assessment: global use of the Brief Pain Inventory. *Ann Acad Med Singapore, 17,* 197–210.

14. Cork, R. C., et al. (2004). A comparison of the verbal rating scale and the visual analogue scale for pain assessment. *Internet J Anesthesiol, 8*(1), www.ispub.com/ostia/index.php?xmlFilePath=journals/ija/vol8n1/vrs.xml..

15. Cox, D. S. (2002). Definitions pertaining to pain management. In B. St. Marie (Ed.), *Core curriculum for pain management nursing.* Philadelphia: Saunders.

16. Crichton, N. (2001). Information point: visual analogue scale (VAS). *J Clin Nurs, 10*(5), 706.

17. Davis, M. P., et al. (2002). Symptom control in cancer patients: the clinical pharmacology and therapeutic role of suppositories and rectal suspensions. *Support Care Cancer, 10,* 117–138.

18. Davis-Rollans, C., & Cunningham, S. G. (1987). Physiological responses of coronary care patients to selected music. *Heart Lung, 16*(4), 369–378.

19. De Jong, M. J., et al. (2005). Development of the American Association of Critical-Care Nurses' sedation assessment scale for critically ill patients. *Am J Crit Care, 14*(6), 531–544.

20. Devlin, J. W., et al. (2001). Sedation assessment in critically ill adults. *Ann Pharmacother, 35,* 1624–1632.

21. Dickenson, A. H. (2002). Gate control theory of pain stands the test of time. *Brit J Anesthesia, 88,* 755–757.

22. Donaldson, V. W. (2000). A clinical study of visualization on depressed white blood cell count in medical patients. *Appl Psychophysiol Biofeedback, 25,* 117–128.

23. Doyle, D., Hanks, G. W. C.., & MacDonald, N. (Eds.). (1998). *Oxford textbook of palliative medicine* (2nd ed.). New York: Oxford University Press.

24. Egan, T. D., et al. (2000). Multiple dose pharmacokinetics of oral transmucosal fentanyl citrate in healthy volunteers. *Anesthesiology, 92,* 665–673.

25. Fatovich, D. M., Gope, M., & Paech, M. J. (2004). A pilot trial of BIS monitoring for procedural sedation in the emergency department. *Emerg Med Australasia, 16,* 103–107.

26. Ferrell, B. R. (1996). Humanizing the experience of pain and illness. In B. R. Ferrell (Ed.), *Suffering.* Boston: Jones and Bartlett.

27. Field, T. M., et al. (2002). Fibromyalgia pain and substance P decrease and sleep improve after massage therapy. *J Clin Rheumatol, 8,* 72–76.

28. Field, T., et al. (1996). Massage and relaxation therapies' effects on depressed adolescent mothers. *Adolescence, 31,* 903–911.

29. Fors, E. A., Sexton, H., & Gotestam, K. G. (2002). The effect of guided imagery and amitriptyline on daily fibromyalgia pain: a prospective, randomized controlled trial. *J Psychiatr Res, 36,* 179–187.

30. Fountaine, K. L. (2005). *Complementary and alternative therapies for nursing practice.* Upper Saddle River, NJ: Prentice Hall.

31. Fraser, G. L., Prato, S., Berthiaume, D., et al. (2000). Evaluation of agitation in ICU patients: incidence, severity, and treatment in the young versus the elderly. *Pharmacotherapy, 20,* 75–82.

32. Freire, A. X., et al. (2002). Characteristics associated with analgesia ordering in the intensive care unit and relationships with outcomes. *Crit Care Med, 30*(11), 2468–2472.

33. Good, M., & Chin, C. (1998). The effects of western music on postoperative pain in Taiwan. *Kaohsiung J Med Sci, 14,* 94–103.

34. Good, M., et al. (2001). Postoperative pain relief across activities and days with jaw relaxation, music, and their combination. *J Adv Nurs, 33*(2), 208–215.

35. Good, M., et al. (1999). Relief of postoperative pain with jaw relaxation, music, and their combination. *Pain, 81,* 163–172.

36. Habibi, C., & Coursin, D. B. (1996). Assessment of sedation, analgesia, and neuromuscular blockade in the perioperative period. *Int Anesthesiol Clin, 34*(3), 215–241.

37. Hamill-Ruth, R. J. (2002). Use of analgesics in the intensive care unit: who says it hurts? *Crit Care Med, 30*(11), 2597–2598.

38. Hanser, S. B. (1990). A music therapy strategy for depressed older adults in the community. *J Appl Geriatr, 9*(3), 283–298.

39. Hanser, S. B., & Thompson, L. W. (1994). Effects of music therapy strategy on depressed older adults. *J Gerontol, 49*(6), 265–269.

40. Hockenberry, M. J., Wilson, D., & Winklestein, M. L. (2005). *Wong's essentials of pediatric nursing* (7th ed.). St. Louis: Mosby.

41. Hylek, E., Heiman, H., Skates, S., et al. (1998). Acetaminophen and other risk factors for excessive warfarin over anticoagulation. *J Am Med Assoc (JAMA), 279,* 657–662.

42. Jacobi, J., et al. (2002). Clinical practice guidelines for the sustained use of sedatives and analgesics in the critically ill adult. *Crit Care Med, 30*(1), 119–141.

43. Joint Commission on Accreditation of Healthcare Organizations. (2001). *Pain management standards.* www.jcaho.org/standrads/pain_hap.html.

44. Joint Commission on Accreditation of Healthcare Organizations (JCAHO). (2001). Standards and intents of sedation and anesthesia. *Comprehensive accreditation manual for hospitals: the official handbook.* Chicago: Author.

45. Kaiko, R. F., et al. (1983). Central nervous system excitatory effects of meperidine in cancer patients. *Ann Neurol, 13,* 180–185.

46. Koch, M. E., et al. (1998). The sedative and analgesic sparing effects of music. *Anesthesiology, 89*(2), 300–306.

47. Kremer, M. J. (1999). Surgery, pain, and immune function. *CRNA: Clin Forum Nurse Anesthetists, 10*(3), 94–100.

48. Kuhn, M. A. (1999). *Complementary therapies for health care providers.* Philadelphia: Lippincott.

49. Lafleur, K. J. (2005). Will adequate sedation assessment include the use of actigraphy in the future? *Am J Crit Care, 14*(1), 61–62.

50. Lilley, L. L., Aucker, R. S., & Albanese, J. A. (Eds.). (1996). *Pharmacology and the nursing process.* St. Louis: Mosby.

51. Loyola, R., & Dreher, H. M. (2003). Management of pharmacologically induced neuromuscular blockade using peripheral nerve stimulation. *Dimensions Crit Care Nurs, 22*(4), 157–164.

52. Lusk, B., & Lash, A. A. (2005). The stress response, psychoneuroimmunology, and stress among ICU patients. *Dimensions Crit Care, 24*(1), 25–31.

53. Maguire, B. L. (1996). The effects of imagery on attitudes and mood in multiple sclerosis patients. *Altern Ther Health Med*, 2(5), 75–79.

54. Matas, K. E. (1997). Human patterning and chronic pain. *Nurs Sci Quart*, 10(2), 88–95.

55. McCaffery, M. (1968). *Nursing practice theories related to cognition, bodily pain, man-environment interactions*. Los Angeles: University of Los Angeles Student Store.

56. McCaffrey, R., & Freeman, E. (2003). Effect of music on chronic osteoarthritis pain in older adults. *J Adv Nurs*, 44(5), 517–524.

57. McCance, K.L., & Huether, S.E. (Eds.). (2006). *Pathophysiology: the biological basis for disease in adults and children*. St. Louis: Mosby.

58. McHugh, J., & McHugh, W. B. (2000). Pain: neuroanatomy, chemical mediators, and clinical implications. *AACN Clin Issues*, 11(2), 168–178.

59. McKeage, K., & Perry, C. M. (2003). Propofol: a review of its use in intensive care sedation of adults. *CNS Drugs*, 17(4), 235–272.

60a. Melzack, R. (1999). Pain—an overview. *Acta Anaesthesiol Scand*, 43, 880–884.

60b. Melzack, R. (1968). Neurophysiologic foundation of pain (pp. 1–12). In R. A. Sternbach (Ed.), *The psychology of pain* New York: Raven Press.

61. Melzack, R., & Casey, K. L. (1968). Sensory, motivational and central control determinants of pain: a new conceptual model (pp. 423–429). In D. Kenshalo (Ed.), *The skin senses*. Springfield, Ill: Charles C. Thomas.

62. Melzack, R., & Katz, J. (1992). The McGill pain questionnaire: appraisal and current status. In D. C. Turk & R. Melzack (Eds.), *Handbook of pain assessment*. New York: Guilford.

63. Menegazzi, J. J., et al. (1991). A randomized, controlled trial of the use of music during laceration repair. *Ann Emerg Med*, 20(4), 348–350.

64. Merskey, H. Classification of chronic pain: descriptions of chronic pain syndromes and definitions of pain terms. *In* Pain (Suppl 3, Pt II), pp. S215–S221).

65. Moss, V. A. (1988). Music and the surgical patient. *AORN J*, 48(1), 64–69.

66. Moyer, C. A., Rounds, J., & Hannum, J. W. (2004). A meta-analysis of massage therapy research. *Psychol Bull*, 130(1), 3–18.

67. Mullooly, A. M., Levin, R. F., & Feldman, H. R. (1988). Music for postoperative anxiety. *J NY State Nurses Assoc*, 19, 4–7.

68. Munro, C. L., & Grap, M. J. (2004). Oral health and care in the intensive care unit: state of the science. *Am J Crit Care*, 13(1), 25–34.

69. Murray, M. J., et al. (2002). Clinical practice guidelines for sustained neuromuscular blockade in the adult critically ill patient. *Crit Care Med*, 30(1), 142–156.

70. Nasraway, S. A., et al. (2002). How reliable is the bispectral index in critically ill patients? A prospective, comparative, single-blinded observer study. *Crit Care Med*, 30(7), 1483–1487.

71. National Pharmaceutical Councils and Joint Commission on Accreditation of Healthcare Organizations. (2001). *Pain: current understanding of assessment, management, and treatment (Monograph)*. Chicago: Author.

72. Nelson, J. E., et al. (2001). Self-reported symptom experience of critically ill cancer patients receiving intensive care. *Crit Care Med*, 29(2), 277–282.

73. Oumeish, O. Y. (1998). The philosophical, cultural, and historical aspects of complementary, alternative, unconventional, and integrative medicine in the old world. *Arch Dermatol*, 134, 1373–1386.

74. Park, G., Coursin, D., & Ely, E. W. (2001). Balancing sedation and analgesia in critical care. *Crit Care Clin*, 17, 1015–1027.

75. Payne, R., Chandler, S., & Einhaus, M. (1995). Guidelines for the clinical use of transdermal fentanyl. *Anticancer Drugs Suppl*, 3, 50–53.

76. Puntillo, K. (1990). The pain experience of intensive care patients. *Heart Lung*, 19, 526–533.

77. Puntillo, K. (2003). Pain assessment and management in the critically ill: wizardry or science? *Am J Crit Care*, 12(4), 310–316.

78a. Puntillo, K. A., et al. (2002). Practices and predictors of analgesic interventions for adults undergoing painful procedures. *Am J Crit Care*, 11(5), 415–432.

78b. Ramsay, M. A., et al. (1974). Controlled sedation with aphaxalone-alphadolone. *Brit Med J*, 2, 656–659.

79. Richards, K. C., Gibson, R., & Overton-McCoy, A. L. (2000). Effects of massage in acute and critical care. *AACN Clin Issues*, 11(1), 77–96.

80. Richardson, S. (2003). Effects of relaxation on the sleep of critically ill adults. *Dimensions Crit Care*, 22(4), 182–190.

81. Riker, R. R., et al. (1998). Assessing sedation levels in mechanically ventilated ICU patients with the bispectral index and the sedation agitation scale. *Crit Care Med*, 26(1S), 94A.

82. Rosner, H. L. (1996). The pharmacologic management of acute postoperative pain. In M. Lefkowitz & A. H. Lebovits (Eds.), *A practical approach to pain management*. Boston: Lippincott Williams & Wilkins.

83. Rudis, M. I., et al. (1997). A prospective, randomized, controlled evaluation of peripheral nerve stimulation versus standard clinical dosing of neuromuscular blocking agents in critically ill patients. *Crit Care Med*, 25(4), 575–583.

84. Sabbe, M. B., & Yaksh, T. L. (1990). Pharmacology of spinal opioids. *J Pain Symptom Manag*, 5, 191–203.

85. Samad, T. A. (2004). New understandings of the link between acute pain and chronic pain: can we prevent long-term sequelae? In D. B. Carr, G. Novak, J. P. Rathmell, et al. (Eds.), *The spectrum of pain* (pp. 16–27). New York: McMahon.

86. Savage, S., Covington, E., Heit, H., et al. (2001). *Definitions related to the use of opioids for the treatment of pain: a consensus document from the American Academy of Pain Medicine, the American Pain Society, and the American Society of Addiction Medicine*. Glenview, Ill.

87. Scholz, J., & Woolf, C. J. (2002). Can we conquer pain? *Nature Neurosci*, 5, 1062–1067.

88a. Schoor, J. A. (1993). Music and pattern change in chronic pain. *Adv Nurs Sci*, 15(4), 27–36.

88b. Sessler, C. N., et al. (2002). The Richmond agitation-sedation scale: validity and reliability in adult intensive care patients. *Am J Respir Crit Care Med*, 166, 1338–1344.

89. Siedlecki, S. L. (1996). *Pain management*. Torrance, Calif: Homestead Schools.

90. Skidmore-Roth, L. (2005). *2006 Mosby's nursing drug reference*. St Louis: Mosby.

91. Smith, M. C., Kemp, J., Hemphill, L., et al. (2002). Outcomes of therapeutic massage for hospitalized cancer patients. *J Nurs Scholarship*, 34(3), 257–262.

92. Springhouse. (2004). *Nurse's drug guide 2004* (5th ed.). Philadelphia: Lippincott.

93. Steelman, V. M. (1990). Intraoperative music therapy. *AORN J*, 52, 1026–1034.

94. Sufka, K. J., & Price, D. D. (2002). Gate control theory reconsidered. *Brain Mind*, 3, 277–290.

95. Swanson, R. W., & Klein, D. G. (2005). Comfort and sedation. In M. L. Sole, D. G. Klein, M. J. Moseley (Eds.), *Introduction to critical care nursing* (4th ed.). Philadelphia: Elsevier Saunders.

96. Tusek, D. L. (1999). Guided imagery: a powerful tool to decrease length of stay, pain, anxiety, and narcotic consumption. *J Invasive Cardiol*, 11(4), 265–267.

97. Tusek, D. L., & Cwynar, R. E. (2000). Strategies for implementing a guided imagery program to enhance patient experience. *AACN Clin Issues*, 11(1), 66–76.

98. Tusek, D. L., Cwynar, R., & Cosgrove, D. M. (1999). Effect of guided imagery on length of stay, pain, and anxiety in cardiac surgery patients. *J Cardiovasc Manag, 10*(20), 22–28.

99. Updike, P. (1990). Music therapy result for ICU patients. *Dimensions Crit Care Nurs, 9*, 39–45.

100. Van de Leur, J. P., et al. (2004). Discomfort and factual recollection in intensive care unit patients. *Crit Care, 8*(6), R467–R473.

101. Van Kuiken, D. (2004). A meta-analysis of the effect of guided imagery practice on outcomes. *J Holistic Nurs, 22*(2), 164–179.

102. Watson, B. D., & Kane-Gill, S. (2004). Sedation assessment in critically ill adults: 2001–2004 update. *Ann Pharmacol, 38*, 1898–1906.

103. White, J. M. (1992). Music therapy: an intervention to reduce anxiety in myocardial infarction patients. *Clin Nurse Specialist, 6*(2), 58–63.

104. White, J. M. (2000). State of the science of music interventions: critical care and peri operative practice. *Crit Care Nurs Clin, 12*(2), 219–225.

105. White, P. F., & Parker, R. K. (1992). Is the risk of using a ''basal'' infusion with patient-controlled analgesia therapy justified? *Anesthesiology, 76*, 489.

106. Young, M. P., & Birkmeyer, J. D. (2000). Potential reduction in mortality rates using an intensivist model to manage intensive care units. *Effective Clin Pract, 3*(6), 284–289.

107. Zimmerman, H., & Maddrey, W. (1995). Acetaminophen (paracetamol) hepatotoxicity with regular intake of alcohol: analysis of instances of therapeutic misadventure. *Hepatology, 22*, 767–773.

108. Zimmerman, L., Pozehi, B., Duncan, K., et al. (1989). Effects of music in patients who had chronic cancer pain. *West J Nurs Res, 11*(3), 298–309.

109. Zuckerman, L., & Ferrante, F. (1998). Nonopioid analgesics. In M. Ashburn & L. Rice (Eds.), *The management of pain*. Philadelphia: Churchill Livingstone.

Box 5-1

Common Etiologies of Nausea in Critical Care Patients

MEDICATIONS

Analgesics
  Aspirin
  Nonsteroidal antiinflammatory drugs

Cardiovascular medications
  Digoxin
  Antiarrhythmics
  Antihypertensives
  β-Blockers
  Calcium channel antagonists
  Diuretics

Antibiotics/antivirals
  Erythromycin
  Tetracycline
  Sulfonamides

Antituberculous drugs
  Acyclovir

Cancer chemotherapy
  Severe: cisplatin, dacarbazine, nitrogen mustard
  Moderate: etoposide, methotrexate, cytarabine
  Mild: fluorouracil, vinblastine, tamoxifen

Gastrointestinal medications
  Sulfasalazine
  Azathioprine
  Nicotine
  CNS active narcotics
  Antiparkinsonian drugs
  Anticonvulsants
  Antiasthmatics
  Theophylline

INFECTIOUS CAUSES

  Gastroenteritis
    Viral
      Bacterial
  Nongastrointestinal infections
  Otitis media

DISORDERS OF THE GUT AND PERITONEUM

  Mechanical obstruction
  Gastric outlet obstruction
  Small-bowel obstruction
  Functional gastrointestinal disorders
  Gastroparesis
  Chronic intestinal pseudo-obstruction
  Nonulcer dyspepsia
  Irritable bowel syndrome
  Organic gastrointestinal disorders
  Pancreatic adenocarcinoma
  Inflammatory intraperitoneal disease
  Peptic ulcer disease

  Cholecystitis
  Pancreatitis
  Hepatitis
  Crohn's disease
  Mesenteric ischemia
  Retroperitoneal fibrosis
  Mucosal metastases

CENTRAL NERVOUS SYSTEM CAUSES

  Migraine
  Increased intracranial pressure
  Malignancy
  Hemorrhage
  Infarction
  Abscess
  Meningitis
  Congenital malformation
  Hydrocephalus
  Pseudotumor cerebri
  Seizure disorders
  Demyelinating disorders
  Emotional responses
  Psychiatric disease
  Psychogenic vomiting
  Anxiety disorders
  Depression
  Pain
  Anorexia nervosa
  Bulimia nervosa
  Labyrinthine disorders
  Motion sickness
  Labyrinthitis
  Tumors
  Meniere's disease
  Iatrogenic
  Fluorescein angiography

ENDOCRINOLOGIC AND METABOLIC CAUSES

  Pregnancy
  Other endocrine and metabolic
  Uremia
  Diabetic ketoacidosis
  Hyperparathyroidism
  Hypoparathyroidism
  Hyperthyroidism
  Addison's disease
  Acute intermittent porphyria
  Postoperative nausea and vomiting
  Cyclic vomiting syndrome

MISCELLANEOUS CAUSES

  Cardiac disease
  Myocardial infarction
  Congestive heart failure
  Radiofrequency ablation

Modified from reference 41.

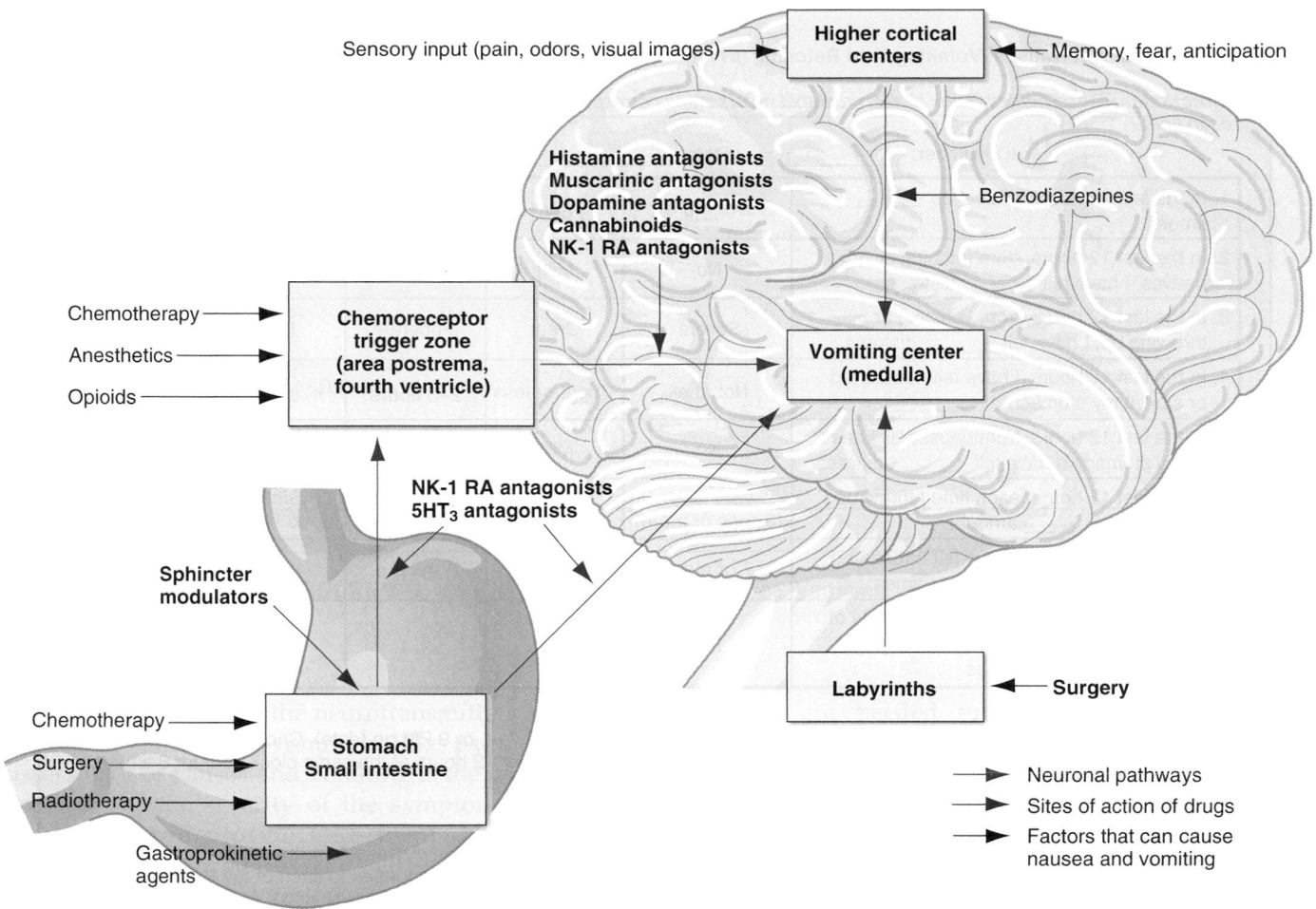

♦FIGURE 5-1 Mechanics of emesis. NK-1 = Neurokinin, 5HT₃ = serotonin.

Dehydration can precipitate nausea and vomiting, worsening the effects of anesthetic agents triggering the vomiting center.

Chemotherapy-induced nausea and vomiting (CINV) is among the most distressing and debilitating adverse effects of cancer treatment,[15,17,26,40] affecting as many as 50% of patients receiving chemotherapy. Patients may be admitted to critical care for management of the effects of nausea, vomiting, and associated complications such as aspiration pneumonia, severe dehydration, and electrolyte imbalances. CINV can be *anticipatory* (before chemotherapy), *acute* (within 24 hours of chemotherapy administration) or *delayed* (occurs 24 hours after chemotherapy administration). Treatment of CINV addresses identifying and treating the trigger. For anticipatory nausea and vomiting, anxiolytics may be beneficial. For acute and delayed nausea and vomiting, antiemetic agents are required for management.

Increased intracranial pressure can also trigger nausea and vomiting from increased pressure within the cranial vault. Patients experiencing increased intracranial pressure from traumatic injury, disease (e.g., hepatic encephalopathy, meningitis), or postoperative neurosurgical cerebral swelling are at significant risk of nausea and vomiting because of pressure changes within the cranial vault. Uncontrolled or unrelieved pain can also activate neurotransmitters that stimulate the CTZ and vomiting center (VC) in the brain and elicit a vomiting response.

ASSESSMENT AND TREATMENT

Treatment of nausea and vomiting requires a multifaceted approach, exploring the physical, emotional, chemical, and metabolic causative factors. Treatment of nausea and vomiting involves administration of

16. Gan, T. J. (2006). Risk factors for postoperative nausea and vomiting. *Anesth Analg, 102*(6), 1884–1898.

17. Garrett, K., et al. (2003). Managing nausea and vomiting: current strategies. *Crit Care Nurse, 23*(1), 31–50.

18. Grogan, T., & Kramer, D. (2002). The rectal trumpet: use of a nasopharyngeal airway to contain fecal incontinence in critically ill patients. *J Wound Ostomy Continence Nurs, 29*(4), 193–201.

19. Habib, A. S., et al. (2006). Postoperative nausea and vomiting following inpatient surgeries in a teaching hospital: a retrospective database analysis. *Curr Med Res Opin, 22*(6), 1093–1099.

20. Haynes, G. R., & Bailey, M. K. (1996). Postoperative nausea and vomiting: review and clinical approaches. *South Med J, 89*(10), 940–949.

21. Huether, S. (2002). Alterations of digestive function. In K. McCance & S. Huether (Eds.), *Pathophysiology: the biologic basis for disease in adults & children* (4th ed., pp. 1261–1284). St Louis: Mosby.

22. Hurley, B., & Nguyen, C. (2002). The spectrum of *Pseudomembranous enterocolitis* and antibiotic associated diarrhea. *Arch Intern Med, 162*, 2177–2184.

23. Insel, K., & Badger, T. (2002). Deciphering the 4 D's: cognitive decline, delirium, depression, and dementia. *J Adv Nurs, 38*(4), 360–368.

24. Jacobi, J., Fraser, G., Coursin, D., et al. (2002). Clinical practice guidelines for the sustained use of sedatives and analgesics in the critically ill adult. *Crit Care Med, 30*, 119–141.

25. Kazanowski, M. (2006). End-of-life care. In D. Ignatavicius & M. Workman (Eds.), *Medical-surgical nursing: critical thinking for collaborative care* (pp. 105–117). St Louis: Mosby.

26. King, C. (2001). Nausea and vomiting. In B. Ferrell & N. Coyle (Eds.), *Textbook of palliative nursing* (pp. 107–121). New York: Oxford University Press.

27. Kress, J., & Hall, J. (2004). Delirium and sedation. *Crit Care Clin, 20*(3), 419–433.

28. Kuebler, K., English, N., & Heidrich, D. (2001). Delirium, confusion, agitation, and restlessness. In B. Ferrell & N. Coyle (Eds.), *Textbook of palliative nursing* (pp. 290–308). New York: Oxford University Press.

29. Levy, J., & Turkish, A. (2002). Protective nutrients. *Curr Opin Gastroenterol, 18*, 717–722.

30. Maharaj, C., et al. (2005). Preoperative intravenous fluid therapy decreases postoperative nausea and pain in high risk patients. *Anesth Analg, 100*(3), 675–682.

31. Marcantonio, E., et al. (2003). Delirium symptoms in post acute care: prevalent, persistent, and associated with poor functional recovery. *JAGS, 51*, 4–9.

32. McGohan, L. (2005). Delirium. *J Continuing Educ Nurs, 36*(3), 102–103.

33. Micek, S., Anand, N., Laible, B., et al. (2005). Delirium as detected by the CAM-ICU predicts restraint use among mechanically ventilated medical patients. *Crit Care Med, 33*(6), 1260–1265.

34. Mirsa, S., & Ganzini, L. (2003). Delirium, depression, and anxiety. *Crit Care Clin, 19*(4), 771–787.

35. National Cancer Institute. (2005). Nausea and vomiting (PDQ) health professional version. www.cancer.gov/cancertopics/pdq/supportivecare/healthprofessional.

36. Nelson, J. (2002). Palliative care of the chronically critically ill patient. *Crit Care Clin, 18*, 659–681.

37. Newman, D., Fader, M., & Bliss, D. (2004). Managing incontinence using technology, devices, and products. *Nurs Res, 53*(6S), S42–S48.

38. Pan, C. (2000). Complementary and alternative medicine in the management of pain, dyspnea, and nausea and vomiting near the end of life. A systematic review. *J Pain Symptom Manag, 20*(5), 374–387.

39. Peterson, J., Pun, B., Dittus, R., et al. (2006). Delirium and its motoric subtypes: a study of 614 critically ill patients. *J Am Geriatr Soc, 54*(3), 479–484.

40. Polovich, M., White, J., Kelleher, L. (2005). *Chemotherapy and biotherapy guidelines and recommendations for practice* (pp. 109–118). Pittsburgh, Pa: Oncology Nursing Society Publishing Division.

41. Quigley, E. M. M., Hasler, W. L., & Parkman, H. P. (2001). American Gastroenterological Association technical review of nausea and vomiting. *Gastroenterology, 120*, 263–286.

42. Rhodes, V. A., & McDaniel, R. W. (1999). The index of nausea, vomiting, and retching: a new format of the index of nausea and vomiting. *Oncol Nurs Forum, 26*(5), 849–894.

43. Rhodes, V., & McDaniel, R. (2001). Nausea, vomiting, and retching: complex problems in palliative care. *Cancer J Clin, 51*(4), 232–248.

43a. Sabol, V., & Friedenberg, F. K. (1997). Diarrhea. *AACN Clin Issues, 8*(3), 425–436.

44. Truman, B., & Ely, E. (2003). Monitoring delirium in critically ill patients. *Crit Care Nurse, 23*(2), 25–37.

45. Wheeler, M. (2004). Palliative care is more than pain management. *Home Healthcare Nurse, 22*(4), 250–255.

46. Wickham, R. (2002). Dyspnea: recognizing and managing an invisible problem. *Oncol Nurs Forum, 29*(6), 925–933.

CHAPTER 6

Nutrition

Molly Clark

Nutritional support has become an essential feature in the care and treatment of the critically ill patient. The metabolic response to injury or stress is a highly variable process involving dramatic changes in the cardiovascular, respiratory, and central nervous systems (CNS). Over the years, the metabolic changes and malnutrition that occur with critical illness have been differentiated from those changes that occur with malnutrition associated with starvation. Additionally, the provision of timely and adequate nutritional support has been shown to be beneficial in improving the outcomes of critically ill patients. To address the varied components of managing the nutritional status of critically ill patients, practice guidelines for incorporating nutrition support have been published by several organizations.[5,16,20,36,80]

NORMAL AND ALTERED METABOLISM

The energy required for bodily functions is provided by the metabolism of carbohydrate, protein, and fat obtained from food. Carbohydrates, used for immediate or short-term energy needs, are stored in the liver and muscle as glycogen. Protein and amino acids are not stored and are metabolized immediately. If adequate protein is not available from dietary sources, muscle or body protein will be catabolized for energy and normal functions. The energy provided by the oxidation of muscle protein is less than the energy provided by exogenous sources.[51] Adipose tissue stores dietary fat for long-term energy needs.[51]

Carbohydrate Metabolism

Carbohydrates are metabolized to glucose and other simple sugars. Glucose is the preferred fuel for the CNS, bone marrow, red blood cells, and injured tissues.[55] Glucose can be supplied from the hydrolysis of carbohydrates, glycolysis (the breakdown of glycogen), and gluconeogenesis (the synthesis of glucose from noncarbohydrate sources in the liver).[51] In the metabolically stressed patient, half of the glucose oxidized can be through gluconeogenesis.[55] Substrates for gluconeogenesis are lactate from anaerobic metabolism in muscle tissue, glycerol from adipose tissue, and certain amino acids.[10] Hyperglycemia during the stress response is associated with increased hepatic glucose synthesis and insulin resistance in skeletal muscle and adipose tissue.[9] During starvation, the body uses glycogen reserves and protein stores for energy and gluconeogenesis. After glycogen stores are depleted, usually within 30 hours, fat and protein continue to be oxidized for energy.[10] With prolonged starvation, the basal metabolic rate decreases and energy expenditure is reduced. The metabolic advantage of this adaptation is that it allows the oxidation of ketones to provide energy so that the breakdown of protein is reduced.[4,51]

Protein Metabolism

Proteins consist of amino acid chains linked by peptide bonds. There are 20 amino acids that make up animal and plant proteins, 9 of which are essential. Essential amino acids are those that mammals are unable to synthesize in the body. Amino acids are needed for the synthesis of body proteins and other nitrogen-containing compounds, including creatine, peptide hormones, and neurotransmitters.[72] Protein and other nitrogen-containing compounds are constantly being synthesized and hydrolyzed. A greater amount of protein is recycled than consumed on an average basis. Protein is not stored in the body; rather, excess amino acids are degraded into nitrogen, which is excreted via the kidneys as urea, and into ketoacids, which are used for energy or converted to carbohydrate or fat. Proteins may contain carbohydrates (glycoproteins) or lipids (lipoproteins).[33]

During stress or critical illness, amino acids are shifted preferentially away from skeletal muscle to provide substrate for the liver, injured tissues, and cells involved in the inflammatory response for the synthesis of glucose, acute phase proteins, and enzymes.[42] With inadequate protein intake and the increase in energy expenditure during the metabolic response, the body catabolizes its own protein to provide amino acids for synthetic processes and energy. The longer this catabolic process occurs, the greater the loss of lean and visceral muscle mass, including muscles associated with the diaphragm and heart, leading to impaired immune response, difficulty with ventilatory weaning, organ dysfunction, and/or failure.

Lipid Metabolism

Dietary sources of fat consist mainly of triglycerides. A triglyceride is a compound formed by glycerol and three fatty acids; phospholipids and cholesterol are categorized as types of triglycerides. Lipid metabolism is characterized by digestion, emulsification, and absorption. In the body, fatty acids are oxidized to acetyl-coenzyme A (acetyl-CoA), which is used by the Krebs cycle—the enzyme-driven process that produces energy through the complete oxidation of carbohydrates, protein, and fat.[33] Acetyl-CoA can also be used to synthesize saturated and monounsaturated fatty acids and cholesterol. Like essential amino acids, there are essential polyunsaturated fatty acids required for the production of structural lipids and eicosanoids (prostaglandins, thromboxanes, and leukotrienes).[72] Fatty acids can be used for energy by almost all cells in the body, except by red blood cells and the CNS, which preferentially use glucose.

During starvation, the CNS can consume ketone bodies for energy when glucose is not readily available. As the liver and skeletal muscle store excess glucose as glycogen, adipose tissue stores excess lipids in the form of triglycerides. During the stress response, lipid metabolism is accelerated to provide energy substrate. As with protein metabolism, in the absence of adequate dietary intake, endogenous lipids are used. Triglycerides in the adipose tissue are hydrolyzed to fatty acids and glycerol. During starvation, glucagon (the major counter-regulatory hormone of insulin) causes glycogenolysis, gluconeogenesis, and the release of stored fatty acids for energy (lipolysis).[10]

THE METABOLIC RESPONSE

The metabolic changes brought on by stress or injury vary from those of starvation. Changes in arterial and venous blood pressure and flow, pain, and mediators released from wounds or infections trigger the hypothalamus, sympathetic nervous system, and adrenal medulla to initiate a response.[21] The metabolic response is characterized by the release of hormones, cytokines, and lipid mediators. These effects are attributed to the fight-or-flight response associated with an injurious event and are summarized in Box 6-1. The ultimate goal of the metabolic response is to restore homeostasis; otherwise, if the stress remains unmitigated, it can increase morbidity and mortality.[21]

The metabolic response increases blood flow to aid in the transfer of necessary substrates and removal of waste products, and to begin wound healing.[21] The amplified need for energy substrates to aid in inflammation, immune response, and wound healing increases energy expenditure. Alterations in macronutrient metabolism from the acute phase response are moderated by changes in hormones and cytokines.[4] These effects are outlined in Box 6-2. The physiologic changes associated with the metabolic response are summarized in Table 6-1. Protein breakdown is activated by the release of stress hormones and cytokines. Proteolysis leads to increased outflow of amino acids from the muscle to provide substrate to other areas of

---

Box 6-1

Effects of Hormones and Cytokines

Counter-regulatory hormones	Cytokines: peptide messengers secreted by macrophages
Glucagon: stimulates gluconeogenesis, glycogenolysis, and lipolysis	Tumor necrosis factor: mediates increased catabolism at specific tissues, produces anorexia, and activates hypothalamic-pituitary-adrenal axis
Cortisol: increases net protein catabolism	Interleukin-1: mediates acute phase response: increased body temperature, hypotension, inflammation, and accelerated protein catabolism
Catecholamines (epinephrine and norepinephrine): cause glucose intolerance	Interleukin-6: stimulates release of hepatic acute phase reactants (C-reactive protein, fibronectin, antitrypsin, ceruloplasmin, 1-acid glycoprotein); causes decreased levels of zinc, selenium, and iron and increased levels of copper

Data from reference 55.

Box 6-2

Alterations in Macronutrient Metabolism

Macronutrient	Catabolic	Anabolic
Protein	Cortisol	Insulin
	Glucagon	Growth hormone
	Catecholamines	Insulin-like growth factor-1
		Testosterone
		Catecholamines
Carbohydrate	Cortisol	Insulin
	Glucagon	
	Growth hormone	
	Catecholamines	
Fat	Catecholamines	Insulin

From reference 9.

the body that require protein synthesis.[94] The liver requires amino acids to synthesize acute phase proteins, while the rate of albumin synthesis decreases. Triglycerides are hydrolyzed to glycerol and free fatty acids from adipose tissue to provide energy to peripheral tissues and substrate for the liver to synthesize ketone bodies and triglycerides.[4]

Hyperglycemia in critically ill patients occurs as a result of insulin resistance by skeletal muscle, adipose tissue, and the liver as well as increased circulating glucose from the breakdown of glycogen.[4] The introduction of intensive insulin therapy for ventilated, critically ill surgical patients prompted widespread changes in their care to maintain blood sugar between 80 and 110 mg/dl.[92] Tight control of hyperglycemia is recommended to reduce the adverse effects of hyperglycemia, reduce infectious complications, and promote muscle protein synthesis.[92,94] The adverse effects of hyperglycemia are listed in Box 6-3. Improved glycemic control with intensive insulin

TABLE 6-1 Physiologic Changes Associated With the Metabolic Response

RESPONSE	BENEFIT	POTENTIAL RISK
Protein catabolism	Provision of adequate substrate for acute phase response, gluconeogenesis, wound healing, immune function	Hypoalbuminemia Tissue loss
Hyperglycemia	Substrate availability	Hyperglycemia Hyperosmolarity Immune dysfunction Osmotic diuresis Protein glycosylation
Sodium and water retention	Maintenance of intravascular volume	Congestive heart failure Hypervolemia Hypokalemia Hypomagnesemia Hyponatremia Pulmonary edema
Increased heart rate and cardiac output	Maintenance of organ perfusion	Dysrhythmias Increased cardiac work Increased myocardial ischemia
Hypercoagulability; increased platelet aggregation	Hemostasis	Deep venous thrombosis Microvascular thrombosis Pulmonary embolus
Increased sympathetic tone	Increased cardiac output Increased substrate availability (glycogenolysis, lipolysis)	Hyperglycemia Increased myocardial irritability Inhibition of insulin Shunting of blood flow to central organs, away from gut

From reference 55.

Box 6-3

Adverse Effects of Hyperglycemia

Decreased antibacterial function of polymorphonuclear
   leukocytes
       Adhesion capacity
       Chemotaxis
       Phagocytosis, superoxide radical production
Dehydration
Electrolyte and fluid imbalance
Impaired wound healing
Increased coagulability
   Platelet aggregation
   Coagulation factors
   Fibrinogen, plasminogen activator inhibitor, von
     Willebrand factor
   Increased susceptibility to infections

From reference 9.

therapy may benefit all critically ill patients with improved outcomes by lessening the inflammatory response, diminishing protein catabolism, and promoting wound healing.[9,13,94] Further studies are needed to evaluate the beneficial effects for other critically ill patient populations.[9,36] Chapter 34 provides more in-depth information about glycemic control.

NUTRITION SUPPORT

Numerous research studies have evaluated the timing and route of nutritional support in the critically ill patient. Nutrition support has become a routine component in the treatment of critical care patients to prevent malnutrition, correct macro- and micronutrient deficiencies, attenuate the catabolic response, improve wound healing, and improve outcomes.[5,16,31] In the 1960s total parenteral nutrition (TPN) was introduced as a means of providing macronutrients to the body in patients with nonfunctioning gastrointestinal (GI) tracts.[78] Original formulations contained only dextrose and protein hydrolysates because lipid emulsions were not available for intravenous infusion until the 1970s. The initial use of lipids was primarily for provision of essential fatty acids and, after FDA approval in the 1980s, as an energy source.[69] Despite advancements in formulations and infusion techniques to improve safety, parenteral nutrition can cause serious complications, including increased risk of infection and metabolic disorders. Enteral nutrition in various forms has been in existence for centuries, but did not

experience as rapid a technological advancement as parenteral nutrition.[18] In 2001 the American Society for Parenteral and Enteral Nutrition (ASPEN) established guidelines for patient selection and appropriate use of nutritional support.[2] Consensus statements from several physician groups have supported the use of enteral nutrition as the preferred route of nutrition support.[3,16,41] These recommendations and guidelines are outlined in Box 6-4.

Total Parenteral Nutrition

Intravenous nutrition typically includes carbohydrates (dextrose), proteins (crystalline amino acids), fats (lipid emulsion), electrolytes, vitamins, and trace elements. TPN formulations are hypertonic to body fluids and usually require central venous access to allow for dilution by the rapid rate of blood flow.[69] Lower osmolar concentrations (less than 900 mOsm/L) are required for peripheral venous access, which necessitates larger volumes of fluid and lower concentrations of dextrose, amino acids, and electrolytes. Consequently, peripheral parenteral nutrition provides less than the desired amount of calories and protein to meet patients' needs. Peripheral venous access may be difficult to maintain because of the common occurrence of thrombophlebitis, leading to frequent disruptions in nutrition support delivery.

Infectious complications associated with central venous access and TPN include skin flora at the site

---

Box 6-4

Indications for the Use of Nutritional Support

Total parenteral nutrition	Enteral nutrition
High-output proximal fistula	Adaptive phase of short bowel syndrome
Intractable emesis and diarrhea	Burns larger than 25% TBSA for children and adults; burns
Nonfunctioning GI tract	larger than 15% TBSA
Severe acute pancreatitis	for infants
Unable to meet nutritional requirements with enteral or oral intake	Malnourished patients after major surgery or severe trauma
Unobtainable enteral access	Normally nourished patients with expected non-oral intake or inadequate oral intake for more than 7–9 days

Data from references 2, 18, 58.
TBSA = Total body surface area.

of insertion, contamination of the catheter hub, infections from other parts of the body carried in the blood entering the line, and contamination of the infused solutions.[49] Other complications associated with access devices include thrombosis and occlusion.

TPN can also lead to metabolic disorders. Liver function can be altered and lead to changes in laboratory values, including increased serum levels of aspartate aminotransferase (AST), alanine aminotransferase (ALT), alkaline phosphatase, and bilirubin; however, this is not typically seen until TPN has been administered for 2 to 3 weeks. The rise in liver function assays may indicate hepatic steatosis from excess carbohydrate administration, which may present early in TPN therapy, yet is reversible.[43,57] Other complications of continued TPN therapy include intrahepatic cholestasis, cholelithiasis, and gallbladder sludge from the absence of enteral nutrients to stimulate bile flow. To reduce the risks of these complications, recommendations are to decrease the dextrose load (reduce the amount of carbohydrate), reduce the infusion period or "cycle," avoid overfeeding, and stimulate the GI tract by low-rate or "trickling" enteral support.[57]

The mucosa of the GI tract requires the flow of oxygen and nutrients to maintain function, cell integrity, and normal permeability. TPN, the metabolic response, starvation, opiates, and vasoactive drugs can disrupt the normal flow, leading to mucosal atrophy, decreased gastric function, altered permeability, and impaired immunity.[31,50,57] The mucosa facilitates the body's immune response against pathogens via gut-associated lymphoid tissue (GALT) by delivering primed beta cells through the lymphatic system to the gut and oropharyngeal mucosa to secrete antibodies.[52] The mucosa is coated by immunoglobulins, especially immunoglobulin A (IgA) and IgM, that prevent pathogenic organisms from entering the intestinal wall.[33] The enterocytes of the GI tract have a rapid turnover rate (replaced every 3 to 4 days) and are protected by various secretions, starting with saliva in the mouth and continuing throughout the intestinal tract.[5] There are more than 500 bacterial organisms that normally reside in the GI tract (mostly the colon), including enterococcus and pseudomonas.[5,95] Normal GI motility flushes pathogens out of the system before they have the opportunity to accumulate. Hypermotility and diarrhea may provide a defense mechanism against infectious substances.[52] During stress and lack of enteral nutrients, bacteria can attach to the mucosal cells and increase in concentration, leading to bacterial overgrowth.[52,95] With mucosal cell atrophy, there is a change in the permeability, allowing the passage of bacterial cells into the systemic circulation. Bacterial translocation has been shown to occur in humans and is believed to result in an inflammatory mediator response, systemic inflammatory response syndrome (SIRS), and single or multiple organ dysfunction.[23,31,74]

Other complications associated with TPN may be related to the composition of macronutrients (Box 6-5). Electrolyte abnormalities are also common secondary to fluid and electrolyte shifts between the extracellular and intracellular compartments. Evaluation of the components of other intravenous fluids provided to the patient is important to assess the intake of electrolytes. Daily evaluation of laboratory values and adjustments in the TPN prescription and other IV solutions are required until the patient is stable.

Vitamins, minerals, and trace elements may also be provided in the TPN prescription. Fat- and water-soluble vitamins are available in appropriate dosages to prevent deficiency. For patients with renal failure, adjustments to vitamin administration may be needed to reduce the risk of vitamin A toxicity. Trace elements can be provided individually or in a prepared mixture

---

Box 6-5

Complications Associated With TPN

Macronutrients	Complication
Amino acids	Prerenal azotemia: from excess protein administration, dehydration
	Hepatic encephalopathy (with liver disease)
Dextrose	Hyperglycemia: from stress-induced insulin resistance; excess carbohydrate administration; concurrent use of steroids
	Hypoglycemia: from excess insulin administration or if TPN discontinued abruptly
Energy	Overfeeding: hyperglycemia, hepatic disorders, increased CO_2 production
	Underfeeding: impaired immune function, increased infection risk, decreased respiratory muscle function
Lipids	Essential fatty acid deficiency: from omission of lipids and lack of linoleic and α-linolenic acids
	Hyperlipidemia: from excess or too rapid a rate of infusion
	Impaired immune response and vascular integrity

Data from reference 57.

and include zinc, copper, chromium, selenium, and manganese. Iron dextran is not compatible with lipid-containing TPN solutions.[47] Iron supplementation is usually not necessary for TPN therapy of short duration, except for patients with iron-deficiency anemia. For patients receiving TPN long-term or those with anemia, iron may be provided orally as ferrous sulfate or ferrous gluconate, or iron dextran can be administered intravenously (separately from lipid infusion) or intramuscularly.[47,57]

Enteral Nutrition

Numerous studies have determined that the enteral route for nutrition support is safe, provides a protective effect to maintaining splanchnic blood flow, moderates the metabolic response, maintains gut permeability, and prevents bacterial translocation.* The positive impact of early enteral nutrition in the postoperative period on improved immune function, improved wound healing, and decreased mortality has been demonstrated and has become a standard practice.† Previous concerns over lack of adequate bowel function in determining the ability to start enteral support have been evaluated and alleviated. Concerns for feeding the hypotensive patient include the risks for intestinal ischemia and small bowel necrosis.[7,8] The normal response to nutrient delivery is increased cardiac output, vasodilation of the mesenteric arteries, and decreased peripheral resistance, resulting in increased mucosal blood flow.[7,23] When cardiac output is reduced, oxygen delivery to the gut is decreased by poor vascular perfusion. Recommendations allow for the use of enteral nutrition for hypotensive patients after adequate fluid resuscitation and correction of electrolyte and acid-base disturbances.[23,31,41,89] Consideration should be given to a low initiation rate with slow progression to goal rate, feeding tube location, and close monitoring of tolerance (e.g., increased nasogastric tube output, new abdominal pain, sudden distention, or no bowel movements).[2,23,80] TPN should be considered for patients with continued poor tolerance of enteral support (greater than 5 to 7 days), inability to establish small bowel access, frequent surgical procedures, or intestinal obstruction.[17]

Surgery can lead to a stress response similar to the response trauma and burn injuries impose on the body. Gastric ileus is a common event in the postoperative period and is actually a multifactorial response to the fasted state, anesthesia, narcotic use, intestinal inflammation, abdominal distention, and hydration.[21,52,73] The

mechanisms associated with the development of postoperative ileus are listed in Table 6-2. The concerns for early enteral support in the postoperative period include poor tolerance, risk of ischemia, and bowel perforation. Studies have shown that enteral support provides protection from gastritis and improves blood flow and perfusion in the GI tract.[52] Evaluating gastric motility and intestinal function can be very difficult in critical care. The presence or absence of bowel sounds does not correlate to bowel function and may be difficult to assess because of trapped air from mechanical ventilation, abdominal dressings, the size of the patient, and other noises in the patient's room.[16,21,91]

An oral or nasal enteric tube can be positioned in the stomach or the small intestine for the provision of nutritional support. Gastric tubes are generally easier to place; verification of placement can be made at the bedside by portable radiograph, recognized as the most reliable method.[67] Other methods still commonly used to verify tube placement include aspiration of gastric contents and auscultation. The aspiration of gastric contents to check pH is not always a reliable indication of proper placement because of the large percentage of patients on proton pump inhibitors and acid-reducing medications.[67] Additionally, the appearance of the aspirated material may not be correctly identified in all cases.[67] Research has demonstrated that the auscultatory method, used to determine proper placement of gastric tubes, is ineffective.[67] Contraindications to gastric feeding include pancreatitis,

---

*References 4, 12, 31, 37, 41, 52, 73.

†References 3, 4, 12, 16, 21, 36, 52, 73, 80.

TABLE 6-2 Potential Etiologies of Postoperative Ileus

ETIOLOGY	COMPONENTS
Effects of anesthesia/ analgesia	Use of narcotic pain medications Use of general anesthetic Use of epidural anesthetic
Surgical stress	Decreased blood flow to the gut Sympathetic nervous system stimulation/inhibition
Release of systemic endocrine and/or inflammatory mediators	Increased macrophages Increased monocytes Increased T-cells Increased mast cells Increased cytokines Increased release of norepinephrine into the bowel

gastroparesis, or ileus; intolerance or inability to have head of bed elevated; and increased gastroesophageal reflux.[18] Small bowel feeding tubes *potentially* reduce the risk of aspiration or regurgitation of enteral formulas; there are limited supporting data available.[2,4,26,35] Placement of small bowel feeding tubes is more difficult to verify at the bedside and requires radiographic verification.[67] Small bowel feeding tubes are beneficial for patients with pancreatitis, where feeding beyond the ligament of Treitz limits pancreatic enzyme stimulation and secretion, and patients with low-output (less than 500 ml/day) enterocutaneous fistulas, where the feeding tube can be placed distal to the fistula.[16]

For enteral nutrition therapy of short duration, oral or nasal tubes are beneficial. Gastric or small bowel feeding tubes can be placed endoscopically or surgically for patients with dysphagia and demonstrated aspiration, or other patients who may require enteral nutrition support for longer duration. Complications of nasal feeding tubes include sinusitis, nasal necrosis, displacement, aspiration, and frequent occlusion.[68] Maintaining tube patency requires frequent flushing with water after medication administration, disruption of continuous formula infusion, or bolus delivery. If a feeding tube becomes occluded, the preferred method to dislodge the blockage is the instillation of warm water and application of light pressure or pancreatic enzyme treatments.[8,61] The use of carbonated soda or cranberry juice is not recommended because of the pH of these beverages.[59]

Complications associated with enteral support may be related to gastrointestinal disorders, mechanical disorders (e.g., displacement and occlusion), and metabolic disorders. Gastrointestinal intolerance includes aspiration, nausea and vomiting, abdominal distention, malabsorption, constipation, and diarrhea.[81]

Aspiration is a major concern for critically ill patients. Risk factors for aspiration are listed in Box 6-6. Patients can aspirate their own secretions regardless of whether enteral support is provided into the stomach or the small intestine. Gastric residuals remain an ongoing issue, with no clear definition of how much can be tolerated and when enteral feeding should be interrupted. Not including what is ingested orally, secretion volume in the stomach averages 2500 ml/day, whereas the intestinal tract is presented daily with 7000 ml of secretions from saliva, the stomach, bile, pancreas, and the intestinal tract itself.[33] With reabsorption, the GI tract is able to turn over greater than 95% of the volume; the remaining is excreted in the stool.[33] A consensus statement issued in 2002 from the Proceedings of the North American Summit in the Critically Ill Patient recommended guidelines for reducing the risk of aspiration (Box 6-7) and for the interpretation of gastric residual volumes (Table 6-3).

Box 6-6

Risk Factors for Aspiration

MAJOR RISK FACTORS

Decreased level of consciousness (sedation, increased intracranial pressure)
Documented previous episode of aspiration
Endotracheal intubation
Need for prolonged supine position
Neuromuscular disease and structural abnormalities of aerodigestive tract
Persistent high gastric residual volumes
Vomiting

ADDITIONAL RISK FACTORS

Abdominal/thoracic surgery or trauma
Age
Delayed gastric emptying (diabetes, hyperglycemia independent of diabetes, electrolyte abnormalities, medications known to reduce gastric emptying)
Inadequate nursing staff
Large size or diameter of feeding tube
Malpositioned feeding tube
Noncontinuous or intermittent feeding
Poor oral care
Presence of nasoenteric tube
Transport

Data from reference 63.

Box 6-7

Steps to Reduce the Risk of Aspiration

Elevate head of bed higher than 30–45 degrees (or reverse Trendelenburg at 30–45 degrees)
Good oral care
Regular assessment of tolerance and tube placement/position

FOR PATIENTS WITH ONE RISK FACTOR (see BOX 6-6)

Correct electrolyte abnormalities
Minimize narcotics
Maintain tight glycemic control
Use continuous enteral infusion

FOR PATIENTS WITH TWO OR MORE RISK FACTORS (see BOX 6-6)

Place small bowel feeding tube at or below ligament of Treitz
Use prokinetic agents

Data from reference 63.

TABLE 6-3 Recommended Practice for Gastric Residual Volumes

INDICATOR	ACTION
Obvious regurgitation/aspiration	Immediate discontinuation of tube feeding
Residuals larger than 500 ml	Hold tube feeding Reassess tolerance
Residuals 200–500 ml	Careful bedside evaluation
Residuals less than 200 ml	Continue tube feeding as no evidence of intolerance

Data from reference 60.

The use of motility drugs is strongly recommended to minimize the disruption of enteral nutrition and maximize the provision of calories and protein.[31,37,81] The use of blue dye to tint enteral formulas to detect pulmonary aspiration has been reviewed; current opinion is that blue dye is insensitive and unreliable as a marker and unsafe in critically ill patients because of potential mitochondrial toxicity with increased gut permeability.[45,54,62]

Diarrhea is also poorly defined and results from multiple causes (Box 6-8). Before discontinuing enteral support, consider changing the formula to one containing fiber, adding soluble fiber (e.g., banana flakes), or administering an antidiarrheal medication (if not contraindicated, e.g., *Clostridium difficile* infection).[81] Constipation may be related to multiple causes, including inadequate fluid to the GI tract, opioid use, lack of fiber, intolerance to fiber, or impaction.[81] Adequate fluid intake and administration of bowel medications are important to include with the initiation of enteral

support. Abdominal distention warrants further investigation for possible etiologies, including ascites, obstruction, and ileus.[81]

Metabolic disorders related to enteral support include fluid and electrolyte imbalances. Monitoring of laboratory values of critically ill patients is recommended to evaluate the nutrition support provided and to direct changes in enteral formula selection, where applicable, to correct abnormal electrolyte levels. Serum electrolytes should be monitored daily until stable.[2] Box 6-9 lists recommended laboratory values and frequency of monitoring.

Refeeding syndrome is a complication associated with the infusion of nutrition (either parenteral or enteral) to severely malnourished patients too quickly. Patients at risk for refeeding syndrome are listed in Box 6-10. Refeeding syndrome consists of hypokalemia, hypophosphatemia, and hypomagnesemia as a result

---

Box 6-9

Lab Monitoring Guidelines for Nutritional Support

Daily	Biweekly
Bicarbonate	C-reactive protein
BUN	Liver function tests:
Chloride	Alkaline phosphatase
Creatinine	AST
Glucose	ALT (primarily with TPN)
Hemoglobin	Prealbumin
Ionized calcium	Triglycerides (primarily with TPN)
Magnesium	
$Paco_2$	
Phosphorus	
Potassium	
Sodium	

Data from references 16, 55.

Box 6-8

Causes of Diarrhea

Bacterial overgrowth related to broad-spectrum antibiotics
Bolus feeding into small bowel
Impaction
Medication related (magnesium-containing antacids, sorbitol-containing liquids, stool softeners, laxatives, lactulose, theophylline, furosemide, metoclopramide)
Short bowel syndrome
Steatorrhea versus pancreatic insufficiency

Data from references 8, 48, 61.

Box 6-10

Conditions That May Place Patients at Risk for Refeeding Syndrome

Anorexia nervosa
Chronic alcoholism
Chemotherapy and/or radiation therapy
Kwashiorkor or marasmus
HIV
Morbid obesity with rapid weight loss
NPO/fasting greater than 7–10 days

Data from references 2, 18, 29, 64, 81.

TABLE 6-4 Effects of Hypokalemia, Hypophosphatemia, and Hypomagnesemia

	HYPOKALEMIA	HYPOPHOSPHATEMIA	HYPOMAGNESEMIA
Cardiac	Dysrhythmias Arrest Digoxin toxicity	Dysrhythmias Congestive heart failure Cardiomyopathy Decreased cardiac contractility Hypotension	Dysrhythmias Tachycardia
Neurologic	Weakness Paralysis Rhabdomyolysis Lethargy Confusion	Rhabdomyolysis Weakness Altered mental status Paralysis Seizures	Altered mental status Tetany Paresthesias Seizures Paralysis
Metabolic	Metabolic acidosis	Insulin resistance Osteomalacia	
Gastrointestinal	Paralytic ileus Constipation		Abdominal pain Anorexia Diarrhea Constipation
Hematologic		Thrombocytopenia Platelet dysfunction Hemolytic anemia RBC morphology changes	

From reference 88.

of insulin release in response to carbohydrate infusion. Insulin secretion causes the intracellular shift of potassium, phosphorus, and magnesium from the serum levels.[29,64] In addition, insulin secretion leads to sodium retention and increased extracellular fluid retention.[13] The effects of decreased serum levels of potassium, phosphorus, and magnesium are listed in Table 6-4. Thiamine deficiency may also be associated with refeeding syndrome due to depletion of stores from weight loss and malnutrition.[29,64,81] Thiamine, or vitamin B_1, is an essential cofactor for carbohydrate metabolism. Thiamine supplementation may be of benefit to patients at risk for refeeding syndrome, but there are insufficient data to define the amount or length of time to replenish thiamine stores. Guidelines for the administration of nutritional support to at-risk patients are listed in Box 6-11.

Box 6-11

Nutritional Support Guidelines for Patients at Risk for Refeeding Syndrome

Advance nutrition support only when electrolytes are stable. Advancement should be slow and gradual over several days (some references suggest over 5 days).[46]

Correct electrolyte abnormalities before initiation of nutrition support.

Monitor electrolytes frequently (may require multiple draws per 24-hour period if patient requires replacement).

Provide maximum of 20 kcal/kg actual body weight per day.

Data from references 29, 46, 64.

NUTRITION ASSESSMENT

Energy expenditure, or metabolic rate, is the amount of calories used to support bodily functions, including catabolism and anabolism. Factors that affect the metabolic rate are listed in Box 6-12. Critical illness increases energy expenditure by escalating levels of catecholamines, cytokines, and insulin.[87] To prevent the devastating effects of malnutrition in the critically ill, adequate nutrition support is required; however, determining the appropriate amount of calories and protein is difficult. There are risks associated with

---

Box 6-12

Effects Contributing to Metabolic Rate

Age
Ambient temperature
Anxiety
Body mass
Body temperature
Digestion (thermic effect of food)
Exercise or activity
Gender
Mechanical ventilation
Paralytics
Regulatory and counter-regulatory hormones
Sedatives
Thyroid levels

Data from reference 33.

Box 6-13

Complications of Overfeeding and Underfeeding

Overfeeding	Underfeeding (inadequate calories and protein to meet needs)
Azotemia (uremia)	Impaired immune response
Lipogenesis	Loss of visceral protein
Hepatic steatosis	Hypercapnia
Hypercapnia	Poor wound healing
Hyperglycemia	
Hypertriglyceridemia	

Box 6-14

Criteria to Improve Reliability of Indirect Calorimetry

Ventilatory support of fraction of inspired oxygen (FiO_2) less than 0.60
Chest tubes to water seal
Tracheal cuffs without leaks
At least 60 minutes since physical therapy, ventilator setting changes, dressing changes
Either continuous nutrition support or 2 hours after a meal or tube-feeding bolus

Data from reference 40.

---

overfeeding and underfeeding patients (Box 6-13). The measurement of energy expenditure can be either by indirect calorimetry or by predictive equations.

Indirect Calorimetry

Indirect calorimetry, considered the gold standard, involves the measurement of oxygen consumed and carbon dioxide produced over a steady, or resting, state.[2,28,41] The equipment required for indirect calorimetry is expensive, and trained personnel are required to administer the test. Some indirect calorimeters are able to measure energy expenditure on spontaneously breathing patients, while others are only able to measure during mechanical ventilation. For mechanically ventilated patients, recommended selection criteria to improve the reliability of measurement are listed in Box 6-14. The measured energy expenditure extrapolates the calories used during the testing period for a 24-hour period as well as the respiratory quotient (RQ)—the ratio of carbon dioxide produced to oxygen consumed. The RQ can provide information about substrate utilization (the oxidation of carbohydrate, protein, and fat); established RQ values are 0.95–1.0 for glucose, 0.8 for protein, 0.7 for fat, and 0.85 for mixed substrate.[40] Values greater than 1.0 may indicate overfeeding of total calories or excessive carbohydrate infusion, while values less than 0.6 may indicate ketosis. Although indirect calorimetry provides the most accurate measurement of energy expenditure, it may not account for additional energy expenditure related to activity from agitation, physical therapy, and dressing changes. Indirect calorimetry is beneficial for determining caloric needs for difficult patient populations, including obese patients,

brain-injured patients, and those not responding to current nutritional support with improved nutritional parameters.

Predictive Equations

The Harris-Benedict equation, published in 1919, was one of the original equations developed to determine metabolic rates of healthy people. The original data set included gender, age, height, weight, and body mass index of participants. Indirect calorimetry was performed to measure gas exchange; energy expenditures were calculated for the study population.[30,77] Additional studies were completed between 1928 and 1935 to expand the age and body mass index range of participants.[30] Despite the data set including primarily healthy individuals, the Harris-Benedict equation is still commonly used in the clinical setting as a means of estimating the basal energy expenditure of patients. Adjustments for stress or activity factors are added to compensate for changes in energy expenditure from trauma, illness, and surgical procedures. Research continues on malnutrition in critically ill patients and ways to provide appropriate amounts of calories and protein to lessen the effects of the metabolic response, yet avoid the deleterious effects of over- or underfeeding. Various predictive equations have been generated in an attempt to provide practical, improved means of estimating energy needs when indirect calorimetry is not available. The development of predictive equations is typically based on the comparison of results from the equations to those results determined by indirect calorimetry. Examples of predictive equations are listed in Box 6-15. While some of the equations account for changes in energy expenditure as a result of a condition, others are used to estimate basal energy needs. The factors used to correct or adjust basal energy expenditure to account for activity, illness, or injury are summarized in Table 6-5. Age, sedation, body mass, anabolism, and state of illness contribute to energy expenditure.[70,77] Because of the variety of means available to determine energy expenditure with predictive equations and indirect calorimetry, healthcare institutions will identify a standard of practice for determining which method will be used to calculate energy expenditure for their patient populations.

The American College of Chest Physicians, the American Society for Parenteral and Enteral Nutrition, and the *Journal of Trauma* have published guidelines for nutrition support, outlined in Table 6-6.

Obesity

With the increasing rate of obesity in the United States, this group of patients presents a special challenge in determining energy expenditure. Body mass index (BMI) is commonly used to grade and/or diagnose the severity of obesity by comparing the ratio of weight to height versus an accepted standard. The equation used to calculate BMI is shown in Box 6-16. The U.S. National Health and Nutrition Examination Surveys (NHANES) define overweight as a BMI greater than 25, obesity as a BMI greater than 30, and extreme obesity as a BMI greater than 40. Comorbid conditions associated with obesity are listed in

---

Box 6-15

Commonly Used Predictive Equations

HARRIS-BENEDICT

Male:

$$66 + 13.75(\text{weight [wt] in kg}) + 5(\text{height [ht] in cm}) - 6.8(\text{age in years})$$

Female:
$$655 + 9.6(\text{wt in kg}) + 1.8(\text{ht in cm}) - 4.7(\text{age in years})$$

IRETON-JONES

$$EEE(V) = 1784 - 11(A) + 5(W) + 244(S) + 239(T) + 804(B)$$

$$EEE(S) = 629 - 11(A) + 25(W) - 609(O)$$

EEE = kcal/day
S = spontaneously breathing
V = ventilator-dependent
A = age in years
W = body weight in kg
S = sex (male = 1, female = 0)
T = trauma
B = burn
O = obesity (present = 1, absent = 0)

FICK

$$REE = CO \times Hb(SaO_2 - SvO_2)95.18$$

REE = resting energy expenditure
CO = cardiac output in L/min
Hb = hemoglobin concentration in mg/L
SaO_2 = oxygen saturation of arterial blood
SvO_2 = oxygen saturation of mixed venous blood

OWEN

Male:
$$EE = 879 + 10.2(\text{wt in kg})$$

Female:
$$EE = 795 + 7.18(\text{wt in kg})$$

EE = energy expenditure

MIFFLIN-ST. JEOR

Male:

$$EE = 5 + 10(\text{wt in kg}) + 6.25(\text{ht in cm}) - 5(\text{age in years})$$

Female:
$$EE = -161 + 10(\text{wt in kg}) + 6.25(\text{ht in cm}) - 5(\text{age in years})$$

EE = energy expenditure

Data from references 28, 87.

TABLE 6-5 Factors Used to Adjust Basal Energy Expenditure or Basal Metabolic Rate

FACTOR	RELATED VARIABLES	EFFECT ON BASAL ENERGY EXPENDITURE OR BASAL METABOLIC RATE
Activity	Bed rest	1.2
	Out of bed	1.3
Burns	Less than 20% body surface area (BSA)	1.0–1.5
	40% BSA	1.5–1.85
	Greater than 45% BSA	1.5–2.0
Infection	Fever	1.0 ± 0.13 per °C
	Peritonitis	1.2–1.37
	Sepsis	1.4–1.8
Trauma	Soft tissue trauma	1.14–1.37
	Closed head injury	1.4–1.6
	Skeletal trauma	1.2–1.37

Data from references 53, 87.

Box 6-17. The provision of hypocaloric nutritional support has become an area of research in critically ill patients as a means of restricting calories below requirements (primarily from glucose), yet providing adequate protein to stimulate the use of fat stores to meet energy needs.[86] Because of the increased risk of insulin resistance with obesity, the reduction of glucose may avoid or reduce the complications associated with hyperglycemia (i.e., impaired wound healing, increased risk of infection, lipogenesis, increased respiratory effort). The potential error in overestimating energy needs with predictive equations is enhanced with obese patients because of differences in body composition. Obesity results in larger fat free mass, larger organs, increased skeletal mass, and increased skeletal weight.[86] Debate continues over what weight should be used to estimate energy needs: an adjusted body weight, ideal body weight based on height, or actual weight. Adjusted body weight formulas vary from 25% to 50% of ideal without strong evidence supporting any particular formula.[25,27,70,77] Indirect calorimetry to measure actual energy expenditure remains the most accurate method to determine the caloric needs of the obese critically ill patient.

Overfeeding

Despite multiple ways of estimating energy needs, there are risks associated with overestimating a patient's calorie needs. Overfeeding, the provision of calories in excess of metabolic needs, can lead to hyperglycemia, lipogenesis, increased carbon dioxide production, increased minute ventilation, and respiratory acidosis, taxing a metabolic system already burdened with injury, inflammation, and stress. Studies comparing the ability of predictive equations to estimate energy needs compared to needs measured by indirect calorimetry have yielded mixed results because of the heterogeneity of the critically ill patient population. While the consensus remains that indirect calorimetry provides the most accurate measurement, predictive equations remain a useful, practical, readily available, and inexpensive tool.[27,28,70,77]

Protein Needs

The assessment of protein status and the estimation of protein requirements are difficult to measure in the critically ill patient. Normal, healthy adults experience obligatory nitrogen losses via urine, feces, sweat, and sloughed skin, hair, and nails. The recommended dietary allowance of protein intake for healthy adults is 0.75 g/kg/day.[12] Nitrogen balance studies are the classic method of measuring the difference between intake and output. Nitrogen loss is calculated by measuring urinary losses and urea nitrogen levels along with the addition of an estimate of insensible losses from skin, secretions, feces, etc. Nitrogen balance can be used to measure the adequacy of nutritional support with limited interpretation of the results to indicate current net protein metabolism.[9,46] The equations involved are listed in Box 6-18. For patients with open wounds or burn injuries, additional nitrogen loss should be estimated and added to the balance equation (Box 6-19). Nitrogen balance studies will be rendered less valid by renal failure (creatinine clearance less than 50 ml/min), severe hepatic failure, large volume diuresis, diarrhea, and inaccurate urine collection.[22]

Serum Proteins

Nitrogen balance studies in the clinical setting are imperfect means of measuring nutritional status. Serum proteins, synthesized in the liver, are commonly used to indicate nutritional status with the belief that low levels result from malnutrition.[22] Serum proteins also function as transport proteins and require adequate amino acids and hepatic function for their synthesis.[22] The metabolic response initially changes the priority of hepatic protein synthesis to increase the production of acute phase reactants (i.e., C-reactive protein [CRP], fibrinogen, ceruloplasmin, and α_1-antitrypsin) and decrease the production of transport proteins.[16,22,41,87,91] Serum albumin has traditionally

TABLE 6-6 General Guidelines for Nutrition Support

	AMERICAN COLLEGE OF CHEST PHYSICIANS	AMERICAN SOCIETY OF PARENTERAL AND ENTERAL NUTRITION	THE JOURNAL OF TRAUMA INJURY, INFECTION, AND CRITICAL CARE[41]
Calorie needs	25 kcal/kg usual body weight	20–25 kcal/kg	25–30 kcal/kg or 120%–140% of BEE calculated by H-B Severe head injury (GCS score less than 8) 30 kcal/kg or 140% of MEE for nonpharmacologically paralyzed; 25 kcal/kg or 100% MEE for paralyzed
Carbohydrates	30%–70% of total calories from glucose (2–5 g/kg/min)	Not to exceed 7 g/kg/min	Not to exceed 5 mg/kg/min or 25 kcal/kg/day
Protein	15%–20% of total calories or 1.2–1.5 g/kg/day	0.8–2 g/kg/day depending on metabolic needs	1.25 g/kg and up to 2.0 g/kg for severely burned
Fat	15%–30% of total calories (at least 7% from omega-6 polyunsaturated fatty acids to prevent EFAD)	Not to exceed 2.5 g/kg/day (1%–2% of total kcal from omega-6 and 0.5% from omega-3 fatty acids to prevent EFAD)	Less than 30% of total calories
Micronutrients	Doses to maintain normal serum levels	Based on RDAs	Not specified
Fluid	1 ml/kcal administered	30–40 ml/kg for adults or 1–1.5 ml/kcal	Not specified

BEE = Basal energy expenditure, H-B = Harris-Benedict equation, GCS = Glasgow Coma Scale, MEE = measured energy expenditure, EFAD = essential fatty acid deficiency, RDA = recommended dietary allowance.

Box 6-16

Calculation of Body Mass Index

$$BMI = Weight\ (kg) \div Height\ (m^2)$$
1 kg = 2.2 lb
1 inch = 2.54 cm
1 meter = 100 cm

---

been a preoperative indicator of morbidity and mortality following surgery and an indicator of long-term nutritional status because of its extended half-life over other serum proteins. However, its half-life and the influence of fluid volumes, catabolism, and hepatic synthesis on serum levels make albumin a poor marker in the critically ill patient. Other serum proteins commonly used in the assessment of critically ill patients are listed in Table 6-7. Early in the inflammatory response, the low levels of these hepatic serum proteins are more indicative of the severity of illness, not nutritional status.[32,55] Transport protein synthesis

---

Box 6-17

Comorbid Conditions Associated With Obesity

Cardiomyopathy
Cerebrovascular disease
Chronic back pain
Coronary artery disease
Degenerative joint disease
Depression
Diabetes mellitus
Endocrine abnormalities
Gallstones
Gastroesophageal reflux
Hepatic steatosis
Hepatobiliary disease
Hypertension
Infertility
Malignancies
Respiratory abnormalities
Sudden death

From reference 86.

Box 6-18

Nitrogen Loss and Balance Equations

NITROGEN LOSS EQUATIONS:

24-hr urine urea nitrogen (UUN)(g/day)

$$= UUN(mg/day) \times urine\ output(ml/day)$$

$$\times 1\,g/1000\,mg \times 1\,dl/100\,ml$$

Total nitrogen loss (g/day)
$$= 24\text{-hour UUN (g/day)} + (0.02$$
$$\times 24\text{-hr UUN g/day)} + 2\,g/day$$

NITROGEN BALANCE EQUATION:

24-hr protein intake (g)
$$\div 6.25 - urinary\ nitrogen\ (g/day) = N/day$$

From reference 87.

Box 6-19

Additional Nitrogen Loss From Wounds

**NITROGEN (N) LOSSES FOR BURNS OR OPEN
WOUNDS (BASED ON BODY SURFACE AREA)**

Less than 10% = 0.02 g of N/kg/day
11%–30% = 0.05 g of N/kg/day
Greater than 31% = 0.12 g of N/kg/day

Data from reference 44.

---

should return to normal within several days unless sepsis or additional complications arise.[55] Continued monitoring of serum hepatic protein levels may provide data to support the persistence of the inflammatory response and continued catabolism.[32] Recommendations are to measure serum proteins and acute phase reactants (CRP, fibrinogen, α_1-glycoprotein) on a regular basis to trend changes that occur throughout the metabolic response, from initial onset through anabolism, to monitor the efficacy of nutritional support.[16,41,46]

MICRONUTRIENTS

Micronutrients include vitamins, minerals, and trace elements that are necessary for normal metabolism and physiologic function in addition to the energy and metabolites provided by macronutrients. The stress response affects body stores of micronutrients by changing the concentrations found in serum, plasma, tissue, breast milk, and enzyme activity.[91] Measuring

micronutrient levels cannot always differentiate true deficiencies from reduced levels caused by the inflammatory response because of fluid shifts, dilutional effects, increased utilization, and redistribution in the body. CRP, an acute phase protein, is stimulated by the inflammatory response to protect against the damaging effects of cytokines. With the upregulation of CRP synthesis in the liver, there is a downregulation in the synthesis of retinol-binding protein. Retinol-binding protein is necessary to deliver retinol to dependent tissues like the eye, epithelial surfaces, and immune cells, but the decreased serum levels of retinol may not indicate a deficiency.[91] There is an increase in free radical formation during the inflammatory response, with increased utilization of antioxidants, including vitamins C and E, selenium, and carotenoids.[56] The increased use of antioxidants yields lower plasma concentrations of these micronutrients. Plasma zinc levels will also be decreased during the inflammatory response, with additional losses in urine, prolonged diarrhea, high-output fistulas, and large open wounds.[56,91] Research has indicated that propofol (Diprivan) increases urinary excretion of zinc and iron because of ethylenediaminetetraacetic acid (EDTA), a chelating agent found in propofol.[39] Diagnosing iron deficiency is difficult in critical illness as free iron decreases iron-binding proteins (e.g., ferritin) in response to stress.[39,56] Although many studies have reported on the effects of the inflammatory response on micronutrient status, clear guidelines do not exist for the interpretation of the results and the role of individual micronutrient supplementation during critical illness.

Antioxidants and Critical Illness

Free radicals are unstable atoms or molecules with unpaired electrons.[6] In the body, oxygen takes electrons from other molecules during aerobic metabolism and forms reactive oxygen species, and nitric oxide metabolism forms reactive nitrogen-oxygen species.[6,82] Reactive oxygen species' harmful effects include DNA damage, lipid peroxidation in cell membranes, enzyme alterations leading to protein damage, and changes in reduction-oxidation signals affecting cellular activities.[6,34,38,79,82] To defend against free radical damage, the body uses intracellular enzymatic and nonenzymatic antioxidants. The primary intracellular antioxidants are superoxide dismutase, catalase, glutathione peroxidase, and lipid peroxidases.* Nonenzymatic antioxidants include the micronutrients—vitamins C and E, β-carotenes, zinc, selenium, copper, iron, and manganese.* The intracellular antioxidants remove

---

*References 6, 34, 38, 44, 75, 79, 82.

TABLE 6-7 Serum Hepatic Proteins

PROTEIN	HALF-LIFE	ROLE	AFFECTED BY
Albumin	20–21 days	Maintains plasma oncotic pressure, transports amino acids, zinc, magnesium, calcium, free fatty acids, drugs	Increased by: dehydration, insulin, infection, anabolic steroids
			Decreased by: heart failure, edema, cirrhosis, renal failure, overhydration, burns
Retinol-binding protein	12–24 hours	Transports vitamin A in plasma, binds to prealbumin	Increased by: renal failure
			Decreased by: cirrhosis, stress, vitamin A and zinc deficiency, hyperthyroidism
Transferrin	8–10 days	Binds iron in plasma, transports to bone	Increased by: iron deficiency, chronic blood loss, pregnancy, estrogens, hepatitis
			Decreased by: renal failure, cirrhosis, cancer, aminoglycosides, tetracycline
Transthyretin or prealbumin	2–3 days	Binds thyroxin, carrier of retinol-binding protein	Increased by: renal failure
			Decreased by: cirrhosis, hepatitis, inflammation, stress

From reference 22.

the reactive oxygen species and form hydrogen peroxide, which is further reduced to water and oxygen.[6,34,82] Nonenzymatic antioxidants are primarily extracellular and function to neutralize free radicals by donating an electron, decrease peroxide concentrations, repair cellular membranes, and sequester iron.[6,34,75,82]

Oxidative stress results from excess free radicals and insufficient antioxidants to maintain homeostasis. Excess free radicals can result from hypoxia, wounds, the immune response to pathogens, pollution, smoking, ischemia, and the inflammatory response.* Acute and chronic diseases are also associated with excess free radicals or oxidative stress, including asthma, coronary artery disease, diabetes, myocardial infarction, cerebral vascular accident, hypertension, pneumonia, congestive heart failure, multisystem organ failure, cancer, and acute respiratory distress syndrome (ARDS).*

Research has investigated the supplementation of antioxidants in critically ill patients to determine their effect on diminishing oxidative stress and mortality. The antioxidants most commonly studied include vitamins C and E, selenium, copper, and zinc. Meta-analysis

of the studies revealed differences in doses, timing, and route of administration, and varied combinations of antioxidants were present, leading to inconclusive recommendations for the heterogeneous population of critically ill patients.[6,38,75] General recommendations indicate early administration is more beneficial and doses exceeding the RDA are relatively safe.[6,38,71,79] In critically ill surgery patients, vitamins E and C were shown to be effective in reducing the incidence of organ failure and ICU length of stay.[71] Selenium may reduce mortality, but it remains unclear if its benefits are from supplementation by itself or in combination with other antioxidants.[38]

Wound Healing

Thermal injuries, necrotizing fasciitis, and pressure ulcers increase critically ill patients' metabolic requirements for wound healing. The properties and functions of vitamins and minerals have been studied to evaluate their role in the promotion of wound healing and enhanced skin integrity. Vitamins A and C and zinc are most commonly recommended for supplementation to shorten the duration of wound healing. Common dosing regimens are listed in Table 6-8. The general practice is to provide these additional micronutrients with a daily multivitamin.

*References 6, 34, 38, 44, 75, 79, 82.

TABLE 6-8 Micronutrients Provided for Wound Healing

MICRONUTRIENT	ENTERAL DOSAGE	PARENTERAL DOSAGE
Vitamin A	5000–10,000 units per day	
Vitamin C	500 g twice per day	100–200 mcg per day
Zinc	50–100 mg elemental (220 mg zinc sulfate) per day	5–10 mg per day

Data from references 58, 65.

Immunonutrition

Immune-enhancing nutrients are continually studied to determine their role in modulating the inflammatory and immune responses to stress and illness. Many immune-enhancing nutrients are common to typical dietary intakes, but in amounts not found to have a modulating or stimulating effect. The provision of these nutrients in greater quantities, sometimes pharmacologic dosages, can be beneficial to the immune system.[1,9,15,83,85] Several immune-enhancing enteral formulas are available with these nutrients included individually or in various combinations. The most common nutrients referred to as immune-enhancing are arginine, glutamine, nucleotides, and the n-3 long-chain polyunsaturated fatty acids eicosapentaenoic acid and docosahexaenoic acid (commonly known as omega-3 fatty acids).[1,9,15,83,85] Arginine is a conditionally-essential amino acid, where under normal circumstances the diet provides adequate protein for endogenous synthesis to meet the body's needs. With stress from growth, illness, or the inflammatory response, the body is unable to meet its needs and exogenous arginine is required.[83] Glutamine, another conditionally-essential amino acid, is the most abundant amino acid in plasma and is rapidly depleted during the early stages of the inflammatory response.* Nucleotides form the foundations of deoxyribonucleic acid (DNA) and ribonucleic acid (RNA), and mediate cellular energy transfer and hormone signals.[1,83] Dietary sources of nucleotides include milk, meat, beans, peas, and yeast.[83] The omega-3 fatty acids together with omega-6 fatty acids (precursors of arachidonic

acid) are known as essential fatty acids because the body cannot synthesize them and dietary intake is required. The omega-6 fatty acids function as structural elements of cell membranes and as precursors for prostaglandins and leukotrienes, the localized hormones that mediate the inflammatory response.[1,83] High levels of omega-6 fatty acids are proinflammatory and immunosuppressive. Omega-3 fatty acids, commonly found in fish and canola oils, function to decrease platelet aggregation and increase bleeding time and are antiinflammatory.[1,83] Table 6-9 lists the effects of these nutrients on the immune and inflammatory responses. There is generalized support for the use of arginine and glutamine in patients with the greatest metabolic stress, such as burn and postsurgical trauma patients.[9,16,20,83] Despite the numerous studies available on immune-enhancing nutrition and its potential

TABLE 6-9 Beneficial Effects of Immune-Enhancing Nutrients

NUTRIENT	EFFECTS
Arginine	Improves T-cell function Wound healing Detoxification of ammonia Antihypertensive Improves myocardial, cerebral, and ischemic reperfusion Increases secretion of insulin-like growth factor, insulin, vasopressin, adrenal catecholamines, somatostatin Inhibits lipid peroxidation
Glutamine	Cell proliferation (immune cells, enterocytes) Glutathione synthesis (antioxidant) Protein synthesis, gluconeogenesis, precursor for nucleotides Immunoglobulin synthesis Maintenance of gut-associated lymphoid tissue
Nucleotides	Exogenous supplementation decreases energy-wasting endogenous synthesis to maximize proliferation of gastrointestinal enterocytes and immune cells (no human trials)
Omega-3 fatty acids	Favor antiinflammatory prostaglandin and leukotriene synthesis

Data from references 1, 9, 15, 20, 83, 85, 93.

*References 1, 9, 20, 76, 83, 85, 93.

◆ RESEARCH UTILIZATION

Outcomes in Critically Ill Patients Before and After the Implementation of an Evidence-Based Nutritional Management Protocol

CLINICAL ISSUE

It is widely accepted that many critically ill patients are malnourished. As well, it is known that any type of acute illness has the potential to increase the patient's metabolic rate and may impair the body's ability to use nutritional substrates. While there is a growing awareness of the importance of nutrition on outcomes in the critically ill, there is no evidence-based approach for delivering early, appropriate nutrition.

SUMMARY

This study did a prospective evaluation of patients before and following the introduction of evidence-based guidelines for providing nutritional support in critical care. Two hundred critically ill adults, all NPO for more than 48 hours, were enrolled; 100 patients in the pre-implementation group and 100 patients in the post-implementation group. Both nutritional and clinical outcomes were measured. Nutritional outcomes evaluated included number of patients who received enteral nutrition, the time to initiation of support, and the percent caloric target administered on day 4 of support. Clinical outcomes included duration of mechanical ventilation, critical care and hospital length of stay, and in-hospital mortality rates. Implementation of the evidence-based nutritional protocol increased the likelihood that critical care patients would receive enteral nutrition and shortened the duration of mechanical ventilation. The introduction of enteral feedings was also associated with a reduced in-hospital mortality.

APPLICATION

Introduction of an evidence-based nutritional protocol has the potential to improve outcomes and decrease costs. Early attention to meeting the nutritional needs of critically ill patients has the potential to shorten days on mechanical ventilation and decrease in-hospital mortality, resulting in better outcomes for patients.

NEED FOR FURTHER STUDY

Use of this evidence-based nutritional protocol should be studied in a variety of critically ill patients, including the critically ill surgical population. As well, studies to increase compliance with use of such a protocol should be undertaken.

Barr, J., et al. (2004). Outcomes in critically ill patients before and after the implementation of an evidence-based nutritional management protocol. *Chest, 125*(4), 1446–1458.

benefit to reduce the rate of infection and attenuate the inflammatory response, there remains limited evidence to support widespread supplementation to all critically ill patients.[9,16,36,41]

MULTIDISCIPLINARY CARE

The care and management of critically ill patients have been improved with the direction of a multidisciplinary team consisting of physicians, nurses, pharmacists, clinical nutritionists, respiratory therapists, and physical and occupational therapists. Ongoing research, of course, is inextricably linked with practice advances in this area (see the Research Utilization box at left). The clinical nutritionist, or nutrition support–certified pharmacist or nurse, is able to provide recommendations for the route and timing of nutritional support, the selection of enteral formulas, the calculation of parenteral formulations, assessment of patients' calorie and protein requirements, and monitoring the response to nutritional support. A nutrition care plan will be developed and monitored by the nutritionist for necessary adjustments based on medical status and clinical improvement throughout the patient's hospitalization.

CONCLUSIONS

Nutrition plays a vital role in improving the outcomes of critically ill patients. The inflammatory response to stress or injury can be attenuated by the timely introduction of nutrition support to provide energy and nutrients to diminish catabolism and promote anabolism and wound healing. The type and route of nutrition support are important considerations, with established guidelines available to determine the most advantageous means of providing calories and protein to the critically ill patient. Monitoring the adequacy and tolerance of nutrition support ensures patients receive appropriate nutrition to improve their health and outcome from illness.

REFERENCES

1. Alexander, J. W. (2002). Nutritional pharmacology in surgical patients. *Am J Surg, 183*(4), 349–352.
2. August, D., et al. (2002). Guidelines for the use of parenteral and enteral nutrition in adult and pediatric patients. *JPEN, 26*(1 suppl), 1SA–138SA.
3. Barr, J., et al. (2004). Outcomes in critically ill patients before and after the implementation of an evidence-based nutritional management protocol. *Chest, 125*(4), 1446–1458.

4. Baudouin, S. V., & Evans, T. W. (2003). Nutritional support in critical care. *Clin Chest Med, 24*, 633–644.

5. Bengmark, S. (1998). Ecological control of the gastrointestinal tract. The role of probiotic flora. *Gut, 42*, 2–7.

6. Berger, M. M. (2005). Can oxidative damage be treated nutritionally? *Clin Nutr, 24*(2), 172–183.

7. Berger, M. M., Revelly, J.-P., & Cayeux, M.-C. (2005). Enteral nutrition in critically ill patients with severe hemodynamic failure after cardiopulmonary bypass. *Clin Nutr, 24*, 124–132.

8. Bernard, A. C., et al. (2004). Defining and assessing tolerance in enteral nutrition. *Nutr Clin Pract, 19*(5), 481–486.

9. Biolo, G., et al. (2002). Position paper of the ESICM Working Group on Nutrition and Metabolism. Metabolic basis of nutrition in intensive care patients: ten critical questions. *Intensive Care Med, 28*, 1512–1520.

10. Borum, P. R. (2001). Nutrient metabolism. In M. M. Gottschlich, et al. (Eds.), *The science and practice of nutrition support: a core-based curriculum*. Dubuque, Iowa: Kendall/Hunt.

11. Boosalis, M. G. (2001). Micronutrients. In M. M. Gottschlich, et al. (Eds.), *The science and practice of nutrition support: a core-based curriculum*. Dubuque, Iowa: Kendall/Hunt.

12. Braga, M., et al. (2002). Feeding the gut early after digestive surgery: results of a nine-year experience. *Clin Nutr, 21*(1), 59–65.

13. Btaiche, I. F., & Khalidi, N. (2004). Metabolic complications of parenteral nutrition in adults, part 1. *Am J Health Syst, 61*, 1938–1949.

14. Btaiche, I. F., & Khalidi, N. (2004). Metabolic complications of parenteral nutrition in adults, part 2. *Am J Health Syst, 61*, 2050–2057.

15. Calder, P. C. (2004). n-3 fatty acids, inflammation, and immunity—relevance to postsurgical and critically ill patients. *Lipids, 39*, 1147–1161.

16. Cerra, F. B., et al. (1997). Applied nutrition in ICU patients: a consensus statement of the American College of Chest Physicians. *Chest, 111*(3), 769–778.

17. Chang, V. H., & Peck, M. D. (2001). Nutrition in sepsis and infection. In M. M. Gottschlich, et al. (Eds.), *The science and practice of nutrition support: a core-based curriculum*. Dubuque, Iowa: Kendall/Hunt.

18. Charney, P. (2001). Enteral nutrition: indications, options, and formulations. In M. M. Gottschlich, et al. (Eds.), *The science and practice of nutrition support: a core-based curriculum*. Dubuque, Iowa: Kendall/Hunt.

19. Chiolero, R. L., & Kudsk, K. (2004). Current concepts in nutrition delivery in critically ill patients: route, insulin, and economics. *Curr Opin Clin Nutr Metabolic Care, 7*, 157–159.

20. Coeffier, M., & Dechelotte, P. (2005). The role of glutamine in intensive care unit patients: mechanisms of action and clinical outcome. *Nutr Rev, 63*(2), 65–69.

21. Correia, M. I. T. D., & da Silva, R. G. (2004). The impact of early nutrition on metabolic response and postoperative ileus. *Curr Opin Clin Nutr Metabolic Care, 7*, 577–583.

22. Cresci, G. A. (2002). Nutrition assessment and monitoring. In S. A. Shikora, et al. (Eds.), *Nutritional considerations in the intensive care unit: science, rationale and practice*. Dubuque, Iowa: Kendall/Hunt.

23. Cresci, G. A., & Martindale, R. G. (2001). Nutrition support in trauma. In M. M. Gottschlich, et al. (Eds.), *The science and practice of nutrition support: a core-based curriculum*. Dubuque, Iowa: Kendall/Hunt.

24. DeLegge, M. H. (2002). Aspiration pneumonia: incidence, mortality, and at-risk populations. *JPEN, 26*(6), 519–525.

25. Dickerson, R. N. (2005). Hypocaloric feeding of obese patients in the intensive care unit. *Curr Opin Clin Nutr Metabolic Care, 8*, 189–196.

26. DiSario, J. A. (2002). Future considerations in aspiration pneumonia in the critically ill patients: what is not known, areas for future research and experimental methods. *JPEN, 26*(6), S75–S79.

27. Faisy, C., et al. (2003). Assessment of resting energy expenditure in mechanically ventilated patients. *Am J Clin Nutr, 78*, 241–249.

28. Flancbaum, L., et al. (1999). Comparison of indirect calorimetry, the Fick method, and prediction equations in estimating the energy requirements of critically ill patients. *Am J Clin Nutr, 69*, 461–466.

29. Flesher, M. E., et al. (2005). Assessing the metabolic and clinical consequences of early enteral feeding in the malnourished patient. *JPEN, 29*(2), 108–117.

30. Frankenfield, D. C., Muth, E. R., & Rowe, W. A. (1998). The Harris-Benedict studies of human basal metabolism: history and limitations. *J Am Diet Assoc, 98*(4), 439–445.

31. Frost, P., & Bihari, D. (1997). The route of nutritional support in the critically ill: physiological and economical considerations. *Nutrition, 13*(suppl), 58S–63S.

32. Fuhrman, M. P., Charney, P., & Mueller, C. M. (2004). Hepatic proteins and nutrition assessment. *JADA, 104*(8), 1258–1264.

33. Ganong, W. F. (Ed.). (1991). *Review of medical physiology* (15th ed.). Norwalk, Conn: Appleton & Lange.

34. Goodyear-Bruch, C., & Pierce, J. D. (2002). Oxidative stress in critically ill patients. *Am J Crit Care, 11*(6), 543–551.

35. Heyland, D. K., et al. (2002). Optimizing the benefits and minimizing the risks of enteral nutrition in the critically ill: role of small bowel feeding. *JPEN, 26*(6), S51–S57.

36. Heyland, D. K., et al. (2003). Canadian clinical practice guidelines for nutrition support in mechanically ventilated, critically ill adult patients. *JPEN, 27*(5), 355–373.

37. Heyland, D. K., et al. (2004). Validation of the Canadian clinical practice guidelines for nutrition support in mechanically ventilated, critically ill adult patients: results of a prospective observational study. *Crit Care Med, 32*(11), 2260–2266.

38. Heyland, D. K., et al. (2004). Antioxidant nutrients: a systematic review of trace elements and vitamins in the critically ill patient. *Intensive Care Med, 31*, 327–337.

39. Higgins, T. L., et al. (2000). Trace element homeostasis during continuous sedation with propofol containing EDTA versus other sedatives in critically ill patients. *Intensive Care Med, 26*, S413–S421.

40. Ireton-Jones, C. S. (2002). Estimating energy requirements. In S. A. Shikora, et al. (Eds.), *Nutritional considerations in the intensive care unit: science, rationale and practice*. Dubuque, Iowa: Kendall/Hunt.

41. Jacobs, D. G., et al. (2004). Practice management guidelines for nutritional support of the trauma patient. *J Trauma, 57*, 660–679.

42. Jaksic, T. (2002). Effective and efficient nutritional support for the injured child. *Surg Clin North Am, 82*(2), 379–391.

43. Jeejeebhoy, K. N. (2005). Management of PN-induced cholestasis. *Practical Gastroenterol, 24*, 62–68.

44. Kien, C. L., et al. (1978). Increased rates of whole body protein synthesis and breakdown in children recovering from burns. *Ann Surg, 187*, 383–391.

45. Klein, L. (2004). Is blue dye safe as a method of detection for pulmonary aspiration? *JADA, 104*(11), 1651–1652.

46. Kozar, R. A., McQuiggan, M. M., & Moore, F. A. (2002). Nutritional support of trauma patients. In S. A. Shikora, et al. (Eds.), *Nutritional considerations in the intensive care unit: science, rationale and practice*. Dubuque, Iowa: Kendall/Hunt.

47. Krumpf, V. J. (2003). Update on parenteral iron therapy. *Nutr Clin Pract, 18*(4), 318–326.

48. Krumpf, V. J., & Gervasio, J. (2001). Pharmacotherapeutics. In M. M. Gottschlich, et al. (Eds.), *The science and practice of nutrition support: a core-based curriculum*. Dubuque, Iowa: Kendall/Hunt.

49. Krzywda, E. A., et al. (2001). Parenteral access devices. In M. M. Gottschlich, et al. (Eds.), *The science and practice of nutrition support: a core-based curriculum*. Dubuque, Iowa: Kendall/Hunt.

50. Kudsk, K. A. (2002). Parenteral vs. enteral nutrition. In S. A. Shikora, et al. (Eds.), *Nutritional considerations in the intensive care unit: science, rationale and practice.* Dubuque, Iowa: Kendall/Hunt.

51. Lafrance, J. P., & Leblanc, M. (2005). Metabolic, electrolytes, and nutritional concerns in critical illness. *Crit Care Clin, 21,* 305–327.

52. Lin, L., & Cohen, N. H. (2005). Early nutritional support for the ICU patient: does it matter? *Contemp Crit Care,* (9), 1–10.

53. Long, C. L., et al. (1979). Metabolic response to injury and illness: estimation of energy and protein needs from indirect calorimetry and nitrogen balance. *JPEN, 3,* 452–456.

54. Maloney, J. P., & Ryan, T. A. (2002). Detection of aspiration in enterally fed patients: a requiem for bedside monitors of aspiration. *JPEN, 26*(6), S34–S42.

55. Martindale, R. G., et al. (2002). The metabolic response to stress and alterations in nutrient metabolism. In S. A. Shikora, et al. (Eds.), *Nutritional considerations in the intensive care unit: science, rationale and practice.* Dubuque, Iowa: Kendall/Hunt.

56. Mason, J. B. (2002). Vitamins and trace elements in the critically ill patient. In S. A. Shikora, et al. (Eds.), *Nutritional considerations in the intensive care unit: science, rationale and practice.* Dubuque, Iowa: Kendall/Hunt.

57. Matarese, L. E. (2001). Metabolic complications of parenteral nutrition therapy. In M. M. Gottschlich, et al. (Eds.), *The science and practice of nutrition support: a core-based curriculum.* Dubuque, Iowa: Kendall/Hunt.

58. Mayes, T., & Gottschlich, M. M. (2001). Burns in wound healing. In M. M. Gottschlich, et al. (Eds.), *The science and practice of nutrition support: a core-based curriculum.* Dubuque, Iowa: Kendall/Hunt.

59. McCarthy, M. S., Fabling, J. C., & Bell, D. E. (2002). Drug-nutrient interactions. In S. A. Shikora, et al. (Eds.), *Nutritional considerations in the intensive care unit: science, rationale and practice.* Dubuque, Iowa: Kendall/Hunt.

60. McClave, S. A., & Snider, H. L. (2002). Clinical use of gastric residual volumes as a monitor for patients on enteral tube feeding. *JPEN, 26*(6), S43–S50.

61. McClave, S. A., & Chang, W.-K. (2003). Complications of enteral access. *Gastrointestinal Endoscopy, 58*(5), 739–775.

62. McClave, S. A., et al. (2005). Poor validity of residual volumes as a marker for risk of aspiration in critically ill patients. *Crit Care Med, 33*(2), 324–330.

63. McClave, S. A., et al. (2002). North American summit on aspiration in the critically ill patient: consensus statement. *JPEN, 26*(6), S80–S85.

64. McCray, S., Walker, S., & Parrish, C. R. (2005). Much ado about refeeding. *Practical Gastroenterol, 23,* 26–44.

65. Mechanick, J. I., & Brett, E. M. (2002). Nutrition support of the chronically critically ill patient. *Crit Care Clin, 18,* 597–618.

66. Mechanick, J. I. (2004). Practical aspects of nutritional support for wound-healing patients. *Am J Surg, 188*(Suppl to July 2004), 52S–56S.

67. Metheny, N. A., & Meert, K. L. (2004). Monitoring feeding tube placement. *Nutr Clin Pract, 19*(5), 487–495.

68. Minard, G., & Lysen, L. K. (2001). Enteral access devices. In M. M. Gottschlich, et al. (Eds.), *The science and practice of nutrition support: a core-based curriculum.* Dubuque, Iowa: Kendall/Hunt.

69. Mirtallo, J. M. (2001). Introduction to parenteral nutrition. In M. M. Gottschlich, et al. (Eds.), *The science and practice of nutrition support: a core-based curriculum.* Dubuque, Iowa: Kendall/Hunt.

70. Moreira da Rocha, E. E., et al. (2005). Can measured resting energy expenditure be estimated by formulae in daily clinical nutrition practice? *Curr Opin Clin Nutr Metabolic Care, 8,* 319–328.

71. Nathens, A. B., et al. (2002). Randomized, prospective trial of antioxidant supplementation in critically ill surgical patients. *Ann Surg, 236*(6), 814–822.

72. National Research Council. (1989). *Recommended dietary allowances* (10th ed.). Washington, DC: National Academy Press.

73. Nelligan, P., Deutschman, C. S., & Maccioli, G. A. (2005). Early enteral nutrition. *Contemp Crit Care, 2*(12), 1–10.

74. O'Boyle, C. J., et al. (1998). Microbiology of bacterial translocation in humans. *Gut, 42,* 29–35.

75. Oldham, K. M., & Bowen, P. E. (1998). Oxidative stress in critical care: is antioxidant supplementation beneficial? *J Am Diet Assoc, 98,* 1001–1008.

76. Preiser, J. C., & Wernerman, J. (2003). Glutamine, a life-saving nutrient, but why? *Crit Care Med, 31*(10), 2555–2556.

77. Reeves, M. M., & Capra, S. (2003). Predicting energy requirements in the clinical setting: are current methods evidence based? *Nutr Rev, 61*(4), 143–151.

78. Rhoads, J. E., & Dudrick, S. J. (1993). History of intravenous nutrition. In J. L. Rombeau & M. D. Caldwell (Eds.), *Clinical nutrition, parenteral nutrition* (2nd ed.). Philadelphia: Saunders.

79. Richards, G. A. (2004). Nutrition and antioxidants in the critically ill patient. *Clin Pulm Med, 11,* 183–187.

80. Roberts, S. R., et al. (2003). Nutrition support in the intensive care unit: adequacy, timeliness, and outcomes. *Crit Care Nurse, 23*(6), 49–57.

81. Russell, M., et al. (2001). Complications of enteral nutrition therapy. In M. M. Gottschlich, et al. (Eds.), *The science and practice of nutrition support: a core-based curriculum.* Dubuque, Iowa: Kendall/Hunt.

82. Scheibmeir, H. D., et al. (2005). A review of free radicals and antioxidants for critical care nurses. *Intensive Criti Care Nurs, 21*(1), 24–28.

83. Schloerb, P. R. (2001). Immune-enhancing diets: products, components, and their rationales. *JPEN, 25*(2), S3–S7.

84. Sedman, P. C., et al. (1995). The prevalence of gut translocation in humans. *Gastroenterology, 107*(3), 643–649.

85. Sentengo, T., & Mascarenhas, M. R. (2002). Newer components of enteral formulas. *Pediatr Clin North Am, 49*(1), 113–125.

86. Shikora, S. A., & Naylor, M. J. (2002). Nutritional support for the obese patient. In S. A. Shikora, et al. (Eds.), *Nutritional considerations in the intensive care unit: science, rationale and practice.* Dubuque, Iowa: Kendall/Hunt.

87. Sloane, D. S. (2004). Nutritional support of the critically ill and injured patient. *Crit Care Clin, 20,* 135–157.

88. Soloman, S. M., & Kirby, D. F. (1990). The refeeding syndrome: a review. *JPEN, 14,* 90–97.

89. Spain, D. A. (2002). When is the seriously ill patient ready to be fed? *JPEN, 26*(6), S62–S68.

90. Swanson, R. W., & Winkelman, C. (2002). Special feature: exploring the benefits and myths of enteral feeding in the critically ill. *Crit Care Nurse Quart, 24*(4), 67–74.

90. Swanson, R. W., & Winkelman, C. (2002). Special feature: exploring the benefits and myths of enteral feeding in the critically ill. *Crit Care Nurse Quart, 24*(4), 67–74.

91. Tomkins, A. (2003). Assessing micronutrient status in the presence of inflammation. *J Nutr, 133,* 1649S–1655S.

92. Van den Berghe, G., et al. (2001). Intensive insulin therapy in critically ill patients. *New Engl J Med, 345*(19), 1359–1368.

93. Wischmeyer, P. E. (2003). Clinical applications of L-glutamine: past, present, and future. *Nutr Clin Pract, 18,* 377–385.

94. Wolfe, R. R. (2005). Regulation of skeletal muscle protein metabolism in catabolic states. *Curr Opin Clin Nutr Metabolic Care, 8,* 61–65.

95. Zaidel, O., & Lin, H. C. (2003). Uninvited guests: the impact of small intestinal bacterial overgrowth on nutritional status. *Practical Gastroenterol, 7,* 27–34.

CHAPTER 7

Thermoregulation

Richard Henker

Thermoregulation in the critically ill is affected by underlying pathophysiology and treatment of patients. Fever can be generated from infection or inflammation, and hypothermia can occur in the postoperative patient admitted to critical care. Examples of consequences of altered thermoregulation include a hypermetabolic state in the febrile septic patient and problems with clotting in the hypothermic trauma patient. Although temperature measurement and thermoregulation are often considered in terms of the priorities in the management of a critically ill patient, consequences associated with a hyperthermic or hypothermic state can be dire.

It should be mentioned that although decreased core body temperature has often been viewed as detrimental, one condition treated with hypothermia is hypoxic injury.[29] In other conditions, such as traumatic brain injury, the benefits of hypothermia are less conclusive. Results from animal studies suggest that decreased core body temperature is helpful in patients with neurologic injury, but human studies have been inconclusive.[9,13,52,55]

PHYSIOLOGY OF THERMOREGULATION

The ability to thermoregulate involves a system that includes a sensory component, an integrator, and effector mechanisms. The sensory component of thermoregulation consists of thermoreceptors existing mostly in the skin but also residing in the central nervous system in areas such as the hypothalamus, and in other organs, such as the gut. Signals sent from thermoreceptors travel via the spinothalamic tracts to integrators in the central nervous system. The hypothalamus is often thought to be the main site of integration of signals, but other portions of the brain such as the brain stem and spinal cord are also involved in receiving and sending signals associated with thermoregulation. Effector mechanisms that help to maintain a constant core body temperature include skin blood flow, sweating, and shivering. Changes in skin blood flow help to regulate the amount of heat lost to the environment. Increases in core body temperature lead to vasodilation of the vessels of the skin and thus greater heat loss. Cooling leads to a decrease of the skin blood flow and thus less heat loss to the environment. Shivering is an inefficient effector mechanism that increases core body temperature by increasing the metabolic rate.[28] Sweating leads to heat loss via evaporation.

Control of effector mechanisms is maintained by the motor system and the sympathetic component of the autonomic nervous system. Shivering is controlled by the motor component of the central nervous system. Skin blood flow and sweating are controlled by the sympathetic component of the autonomic nervous system. Although sympathetic tone controls sweating, the neurotransmitter that is associated with sweating is acetylcholine. These effector mechanisms help to tightly control core body temperature within what is often referred to as a thermoneutral zone.

The thermoneutral zone is the term used when temperature levels do not stimulate shivering or sweating. Temperature is maintained in the thermoneutral zone by changes in skin blood flow. Increased skin blood flow leads to greater heat loss, and decreased skin blood flow results in less heat loss. Therefore vasoconstriction of vessels that may occur with the use of vasopressors will decrease heat loss. Elevations in core body temperature pushing the upper limits of the thermoneutral zone lead to sweating, and decreases in core body temperature lead to shivering; these two mechanisms help maintain tight regulation of core body temperature.

Mechanisms of heat loss include radiant, evaporative, conductive, and convective (Figure 7-1). Radiant heat loss is attributed to 60% of the total heat loss by an individual and occurs by loss of electromagnetic radiation that moves from individuals to objects in the environment. An example of this type of heating is the electromagnetic radiation from the sun. A sunny day seems warmer than a cloudy day even though the air temperature is the same on both days. Evaporative heat loss can occur via the skin by sweating or through the lungs. Evaporative heat loss can be a

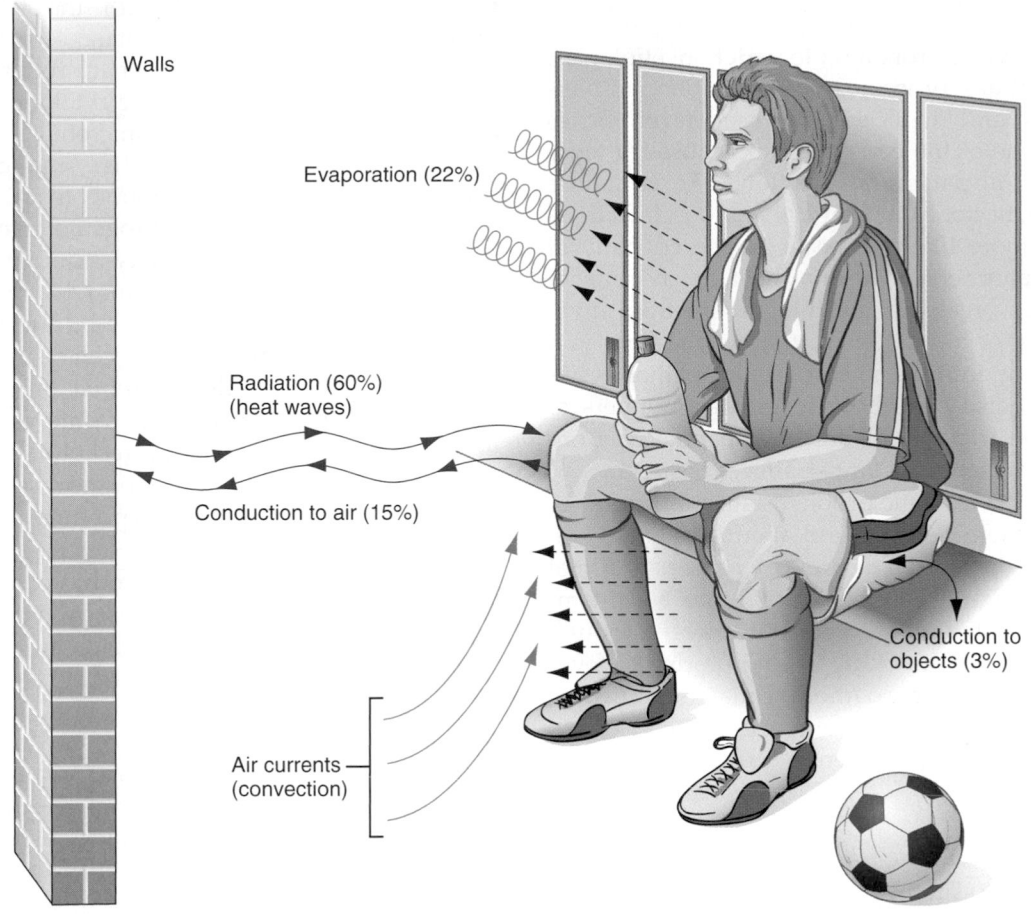

Walls

Evaporation (22%)

Radiation (60%)
(heat waves)

Conduction to air (15%)

Conduction to objects (3%)

Air currents
(convection)

⬍FIGURE 7-1 Mechanisms of heat loss.

very effective method of heat loss in environments that are dry. Greater heat loss occurs in the patient who has a greater respiratory rate. Conductive heat loss occurs with direct contact with the skin. For example, transfer of a patient onto a cold bed will increase heat loss until heat transferred from the patient warms the bed. Convective heat loss is greater in areas that have frequent exchange of air. In the operating room, for example, increased airflow passing over the patient's skin increases convective heat loss.

There are a variety of pathophysiologic processes associated with critically ill patients. Primary thermoregulatory problems include hypothermia resulting from environmental exposure or hyperthermia caused by heatstroke, malignant hyperthermia, neuroleptic malignant syndrome, or recreational drug use. More frequent problems associated with thermoregulation in the critically ill are secondary problems such as fever resulting from infection and hypothermia attributable to surgery or medications that inhibit thermoregulation in patients.

FEVER

Definition

Fever is a regulated rise in core body temperature that is a component of the host defense response. Providing a particular level of core body temperature as an indicator of fever is difficult because of the many factors that impact core body temperature. Circadian rhythm alters core body temperature approximately 0.5°C each day.[38] In an individual who has a typical sleep-wake cycle, the highest temperature is usually in the evening and the lowest temperature is in the morning. Most critically ill patients do not have normal sleep-wake cycles; therefore they have altered temperature circadian rhythms.[54] Another factor that impacts temperature circadian rhythm is the menstrual cycle. According to the Society of Critical Care Medicine and the Infectious Disease Society of America, fever requiring attention is defined as a core body temperature greater than 38.3°C (100.9°F).[43]

Patients at Risk

Fever may develop from a wide variety of etiologies, including infectious processes, inflammation, autoimmune diseases, and medication-induced fever (Boxes 7-1 and 7-2). One of the most common causes of fever in the critically ill patient is infection.[43] Fever can be caused by viral, bacterial, or fungal infections. Infectious processes are more likely to occur in the critically ill because of impairment of normal host defense mechanisms, such as breaks in the integument from invasive monitoring or alterations in the normal flora in a patient receiving antibiotics. Underlying pathophysiologic processes also contribute to greater numbers of infections in the critically ill, and the hospital environment harbors virulent resistant strains of bacteria.

Patients with neurologic problems such as traumatic brain injury, ischemic stroke, and aneurysm have been identified as having a high incidence of fever.[33] Animal studies have suggested that elevated core body temperature is associated with poorer outcomes. Although clinical trials are still not clear,[52,55] monitoring of fever in patients with neurologic pathology may require more vigilance. Early treatment is thought to be beneficial to improve outcomes in this patient population.

Pathophysiology

Fever in the critically ill is often caused by infectious processes that stimulate an elevation in temperature set-point in the hypothalamus.[16] Identification of the first mediators associated with the febrile process started in 1948.[1] Dinarello[16] suggests that fever is generated by stimulation of what are termed toll-like receptors (TLRs) and pyrogenic cytokines.[16] The TLRs are sensitive to a variety of microbial products such as cell walls from gram-negative and gram-positive bacteria. TLRs have been found to stimulate fever without the generation of pyrogenic cytokines. These microbial products can directly stimulate endothelial cells in the organum vasculosum laminae terminalis (OVLT) of the hypothalamus. In addition, TLRs have been found on host defense cells such as macrophages and neutrophils. Microbial products bind to the TLRs on these cells and generate pyrogenic cytokines that stimulate cytokine receptors in the OVLT. Stimulation of the TLRs and cytokine receptors activates the arachidonic acid cascade to produce prostaglandins via the cyclooxygenase II pathway.

Prostaglandin E_2 (PGE_2), produced as part of the cyclooxygenase II pathway, has been found to alter thermoregulation in the hypothalamus. The changes that occur in thermoregulation are often referred to as a change in temperature set-point. The thermostat that controls temperature in the central nervous system is shifted to a higher temperature. As part of this shift, PGE_2 decreases the activity of warm-sensing neurons and increases the activity of cold-sensing neurons in the hypothalamus.[8] The set-point in the human body is comparable to the thermostat in a house. Turning up the thermostat leads to a greater temperature by turning on the furnace in the house. During fever,

---

Box 7-1

Etiology of Fever

INFECTIOUS

Bacterial
Fungal
    Candidiasis
    Cryptococcosis
    Histoplasmosis
Parasitic
    Amebiasis
    Malaria
    Pneumocystis jiroveci infection
    Toxoplasmosis
    Trichinosis
Viral
    Coxsackie B
    Cytomegalovirus
    Hanta
    Hepatitis A
    Hepatitis B

Human immunodeficiency virus
SARS-associated coronavirus
West Nile virus

INFLAMMATORY

Burns
Collagen vascular diseases
Diverticulitis
Gout
Rheumatic fever
Rheumatoid arthritis
Sarcoidosis
Systemic lupus erythematosus
Thrombophlebitis
Thyroiditis
Trauma

VASCULAR OCCLUSION

Myocardial infarction
Pulmonary embolism

Box 7-2

Noninfectious Processes Associated With Elevated Core Body Temperature

CENTRAL NERVOUS SYSTEM

Head injury
Heat exhaustion
Heatstroke
Stroke
Subarachnoid hemorrhage
Seizures

DRUG FEVER

Anesthetic agents
Enflurane
Halothane
Succinylcholine

ANTIMICROBIAL AGENTS

Aminoglycosides
Gentamicin
Amphotericin

BETA-LACTAM ANTIBIOTICS

Cephalosporins
Isoniazid
Macrolides
   Penicillin G
   Second-generation penicillins
Amoxicillin
Ampicillin
Nafcillin
Piperacillin
Streptomycin
Sulfonamides
Trimethoprim-sulfamethoxazole
Vancomycin

ANTINEOPLASTIC AGENTS

5-Fluorouracil
Bleomycin
Chlorambucil
Cisplatin
Doxorubicin
Hydroxyurea

Methotrexate
Procarbazine

BIOLOGIC AGENTS

Interferon
Interleukin-2

CARDIOVASCULAR AGENTS

α-Methyldopa
Captopril
Catecholamines
Hydralazine
Nifedipine
Procainamide
Quinidine
Triamterene

CENTRAL NERVOUS SYSTEM AGENTS

Amphetamines
Anticholinergic agents
Barbiturates
Cocaine
Ecstasy (MDMA)
Methyldopa
Monoamine oxidase inhibitors
Phenothiazides
Phenytoin

OTHER

Allopurinol
Aspirin
Cimetidine
Folic acid
Ibuprofen
Iodides
Propylthiouracil

NEOPLASMS

Atrial myxomas
Hodgkin's disease
Hyperthyroidism
Leukemia
Metastatic cancer
Non-Hodgkin's lymphoma

---

there is an increase in the activity of cold-sensing neurons that leads to the chills. In addition to chills, cutaneous vasoconstriction and shivering occur to increase core body temperature. Cutaneous vasoconstriction decreases heat loss to help raise the core body temperature to meet the new elevated set-point that occurs with fever. Shivering is an inefficient mechanism that increases heat generated by the body to attain the new, elevated temperature set-point.

Considerable controversy exists regarding whether fever should be treated in the critically ill. Animal studies by Kluger et al.[34] suggest that fever is a host defense response. Interference in the ability to generate febrile response in animals has been associated with greater mortality. There are no randomized controlled trials in humans evaluating the effectiveness of fever as a host defense response. The second controversy regarding fever involves the treatment of fever. Fever is often treated in the critically ill with antipyretics and cooling blankets. If fever is treated based upon the set-point theory, then cooling will lead to shivering.[27] In critical care, however, cooling is often used to treat fever.[42] Despite the high frequency of fever in the critically ill, there are very few studies evaluating the effectiveness of treatments. Antipyretics used to treat fever block the production of eicosanoids via the arachidonic acid cascade. In particular, the eicosanoid that is closely associated with the generation of fever is PGE_2.[14] Changes in thermoregulation in the hypothalamus have been associated with the administration of PGE_2 in animals.[8] Medications such as aspirin, nonsteroidal antiinflammatory drugs, and cyclooxygenase II inhibitors prevent the production of PGE_2 via the cyclooxygenase II pathway, thereby inhibiting the generation of fever.[14] Acetaminophen (Tylenol) is another antipyretic proposed to have more central effects than the antiinflammatory medications mentioned. Although it is thought that acetaminophen blocks the production of PGE_2, the exact mechanism of action of acetaminophen is not well understood.

Fever Management

Fever is most typically viewed as an indicator of infection. Therefore once a patient has a fever it leads to evaluating a variety of other signs and symptoms to determine the underlying cause. Fever can be attributed to a variety of causes, including but not limited to viral or bacterial infection, inflammatory processes, neoplasia, and autoimmune processes (see Box 7-2).

Temperature greater than 38.3°C (100.9°F) is recommended as the threshold for the collection of blood cultures to determine if the cause is bacterial infection.[43] Bacteremia in blood cultures collected is typically in the 10% range or less.[23] This may be a result of the fact that fever is often generated well after the stimulus for the fever has occurred, or local infection could be the stimulus for the production of pyrogenic cytokines. The cause of the fever could be from viral or other nonbacterial infectious agents or an inflammatory response.

Although 38.5°C (101.3°F) is often the threshold for collecting blood cultures, there are many factors that impact the ability to generate fever in the critically ill. The elderly are less likely to generate fever and are at risk for a phenomenon termed afebrile bacteremia.[43] Septic patients may be unable to generate a fever because of cutaneous vasodilation, leading to a decrease in core body temperature. Patients who have autonomic neuropathy such as those with diabetes mellitus may be unable to conserve heat because of lack of cutaneous vasoconstriction. Immunosuppressed patients are less likely to generate fever. Patients who

are receiving continuous renal replacement therapy lose heat from convective heat loss from the extracorporeal circuit to the air. Lowering of the temperature threshold for collection of blood cultures in the these patients may be considered. In addition, other signs of bacteremia should be considered, such as changes in mental status, heart rate, or blood pressure.

Considerations when treating fever in the critically ill include host defense and cardiopulmonary responses. In a landmark study, Kluger et al.[34] discovered the beneficial effects of fever in animals. Additional animal studies have supported the beneficial host defense responses associated with fever. There are few human studies that have considered the host defense benefits of fever.[3,12,56] Because of the many factors that impact outcome in febrile hospitalized patients, these studies are not conclusive. Cardiopulmonary response is also a consideration in the treatment of fever. Fever is known to increase heart rate[22] and oxygen consumption[38]; therefore patients who have a history of cardiac disease or have many of the risk factors for heart disease may benefit from treatment of fever to decrease myocardial oxygen consumption. This is discussed further in the Research Utilization box below. Patients with respiratory disease may have difficulty increasing the oxygen delivery needed for the increased oxygen consumption associated with fever.

◆ RESEARCH UTILIZATION

Hypothermia as a Treatment After Cardiac Arrest

CLINICAL ISSUE

The use of hypothermia has been studied as a treatment of neurologic injury since the 1950s. Hypothermia decreases the metabolic requirements of brain tissue and retards the production of reactive oxygen species concomitant with other suggested mechanisms. Although there is controversy regarding the benefits of hypothermia for head injury, this study suggests that hypothermia has a place in the treatment of patients after cardiac arrest.

SUMMARY

In this comparison of cardiac arrest patients treated with normothermia (n = 138) vs. hypothermia (n = 137), patients receiving hypothermia (32° to 34°C for 24 hours) were more likely to have a favorable neurologic outcome (risk ratio 1.4; 95% confidence interval 1.08 to 1.81). A favorable neurologic outcome was defined as good recovery or moderate disability. Favorable outcome for the hypothermia group was 55% vs. 39% for the normothermia group.

(Continued)

APPLICATION

The use of hypothermia after cardiac arrest is becoming a standard of care. Although there were no statistically significant differences in complications between groups, there is the potential for cardiac dysrhythmias, coagulopathies, and infection in patients receiving hypothermia.

NEED FOR FURTHER STUDY

There are no studies in neurologically injured patients that have compared various temperature levels or lengths of time of hypothermia on outcomes.

Hypothermia after Cardiac Arrest Study Group. (2002). Mild therapeutic hypothermia to improve the neurologic outcome after cardiac arrest. *N Engl J Med, 346*(8), 549–556.

Although fever may be considered beneficial in most patient populations, there is growing evidence the treatment of fever should be more aggressive in patients with neurologic injury. Kilpatrick and colleagues[33] found that 47% of patients admitted to a neurology critical care unit would have a fever during their stay and 93% of patients would develop a fever if their stay was greater than 14 days. Outcomes in patients with ischemic stroke were significantly improved in patients who were hypothermic on admission compared to those who were febrile.[55] Although more clinical studies evaluating temperature and neurologic problems are needed, early treatment of fever in patients with neurologic injury seems appropriate.

Treatments for fever include the administration of antipyretics and physical cooling. The Medication table below describes the medications most commonly

MEDICATIONS USED TO TREAT PROBLEMS OF THERMOREGULATION

MEDICATION	ACTIONS	DOSAGE	SPECIAL CONSIDERATIONS
Acetaminophen (Tylenol)	Antipyretic and analgesic that blocks production of prostaglandins in central nervous system	Adults: 325–650 mg every 4–6 hr PO or PR	Greater than 4 g of acetaminophen a day can lead to hepatic toxicity.
Acetylsalicylic acid (aspirin)	Antipyretic, antiinflammatory, and analgesic that blocks production of prostaglandins and thromboxanes	Adults: 325–650 mg every 4–6 hr PO or PR	Aspirin will inhibit platelet clotting by preventing production of thromboxane A_2 for life of platelet, approximately 10 days.
Bromocriptine mesylate (Parlodel)	Dopamine agonist that can decrease muscle rigidity	For treatment of neuroleptic malignant syndrome: adults, 2.5–5 mg, 3 times per day PO	Not FDA approved for neuroleptic malignant syndrome due to insufficient evidence of efficacy.
Dantrolene sodium (Dantrium)	Skeletal muscle relaxant that interferes with release of calcium; drug of choice for treatment of malignant hyperthermia	As an emergent treatment for malignant hyperthermia, 2 mg/kg every 5 minutes up to 10 mg/kg IV	Treatment with dantrolene after malignant hyperthermia crisis should continue for at least 24 hr.
Rofecoxib (Vioxx)	Nonsteroidal antiinflammatory drug (NSAID) that inhibits production of prostaglandins by blocking cyclooxygenase II in arachidonic acid cascade		Voluntarily removed from market by manufacturer because of association with increased incidence of myocardial infarction and stroke.
Ibuprofen (Motrin, Advil)	NSAID that inhibits production of prostaglandins by blocking cyclooxygenases I and II in arachidonic acid cascade	Adults: 200–400 mg every 4–6 hr PO	May decrease effectiveness of angiotensin-converting enzyme (ACE) inhibitors that can lead to hypertension. Increased bleeding is associated with NSAIDs. NSAIDs can also affect kidney function by interfering with prostaglandin release.

used to treat problems of thermoregulation. Antipyretics such as aspirin, nonsteroidal antiinflammatory drugs (NSAIDs), cyclooxygenase II inhibitors, and acetaminophen block the production of eicosanoids such as prostaglandin E_2. Prostaglandin E_2 alters thermoregulation in the hypothalamus, leading to the development of fever.[8] Methods of physical cooling promote heat loss, thus decreasing core body temperature.

A variety of antipyretics can be used to treat fever, but there are considerations when choosing an appropriate antipyretic. Although aspirin is an effective antipyretic, analgesic, and antiinflammatory medication, aspirin permanently binds to cyclooxygenase, inhibiting the release of thromboxane A_2, an inducer of platelet aggregation.[46] In addition, aspirin blocks the production of prostaglandins required for the development of mucus in the stomach, leading to gastric irritation. Nonsteroidal antiinflammatory medications have similar actions, although the effects on cyclooxygenase in platelets are reversible.[45] One other consideration in trauma patients with using NSAIDs is the decrease in bone healing that occurs with use of NSAIDs.[15] One of the more frequently used antipyretics for the treatment of fever is acetaminophen. Although acetaminophen does not have any antiinflammatory capabilities, it has been found to be effective in treating fever with no platelet effects and no gastric irritation.[2] One of the considerations when using any of these antipyretics in the critically ill is the variability in absorption from the stomach.[50]

Fever is also frequently treated with physical cooling in the critically ill to promote heat loss and decrease core body temperature.[42] One of the frequent comments regarding the use of physical cooling is the lack of regard for thermoregulatory mechanisms generating fever.[27] Physical cooling can generate shivering in the critically ill, leading to an increase in oxygen consumption. More conventional physical cooling therapies include water-filled cooling blankets, convective cooling, ice packs, and iced gastric lavage. One of the problems with cooling the skin is the resultant cutaneous vasoconstriction leads to a decrease in heat loss. A recent method that has been used to control fever in patients with head injuries is a central venous catheter with a closed-loop internal cooling circuit.[47] This more invasive method avoids the problem of cutaneous vasoconstriction that decreases heat loss with fever.

Comparisons between antipyretic and physical cooling methods have been somewhat inconclusive. The differences in decreasing the core body temperature between antipyretics and physical cooling have not been found to be significant in most studies, but there were differences in metabolic activity.[19,25,41] Oxygen consumption decreased with antipyretic administration but increased in the patients treated with physical cooling.[19] Additional studies evaluating metabolic effects of cooling would be helpful for clinical decision making regarding the treatment of fever.

◆ Case Study 7-1

Thermoregulation After Trauma

R.A. is a 25-year-old trauma patient who lost control of his all-terrain vehicle (ATV) and hit a tree. He was riding with a helmet and upon admission to the emergency department was diagnosed with the following injuries: hemothorax and pulmonary contusion of the right lung; three rib fractures on the right side; fracture of the right femur; fractures of the right tibia and fibula. After surgery for the hemothorax, R.A. was admitted to the surgical intensive care unit (SICU) and intubated with an arterial line and right internal jugular central line. Vital signs on admission to the SICU were a bladder temperature of 35.9°C (96.6°F), heart rate of 96 beats/min, and blood pressure of 100/56 mm Hg. On day 5 of his stay in the SICU, he continued to be intubated and had the following vital signs: bladder temperature 38.8°C (101.8°F), heart rate 110 beats/min, blood pressure 104/64 mm Hg. Antibiotic therapy was reinitiated and R.A. was given 650 mg of acetaminophen per rectum. Two hours later his temperature continued to rise to 39°C and his heart rate increased to 116 beats/min. He was cooled using a convective cooling system. Six hours after starting convective cooling, his heart rate decreased to 96 beats/min and his temperature decreased to 37.9°C (100.2°F).

Decision point: What are the benefits of fever in R.A.?

Decision point: What are the consequences of fever?

HYPOTHERMIA

Patients at Risk

Hypothermia in patients admitted to critical care is often seen in trauma patients or postoperative patients who have required considerable fluid resuscitation. Trauma patients can be at risk for hypothermia because of long extraction time before entry into the healthcare delivery system, fluid resuscitation, or administration of medications that may contribute to inability to thermoregulate normally. Fluid resuscitation is known to decrease core body temperature.[49] Patients undergoing surgical procedures receive medications such as thiopental, propofol (Diprivan), opioids, and anesthetic gases that are known to decrease the temperature threshold for shivering and cause heat loss through cutaneous vasodilation.[14] Patients who have large surface areas exposed during surgical procedures or open intra-abdominal procedures are at risk for the development of hypothermia. Skin prep for surgical procedures promotes evaporative heat loss. In addition, the amplified air exchange present in the operating room promotes convective heat loss. Therefore the environment and many of the medications used in critical care, such as propofol, contribute to increased heat loss in patients.

Accidental hypothermia is seen in patients as a result of exposure to cold environmental temperatures. Individuals at risk for hypothermia include children because of their high body surface to mass ratio and the elderly because of their decreased ability to generate heat.[5] Decreased body mass index is associated with increased heat loss. Other factors that increase risk for accidental hypothermia include alcohol use, medications that block serotonin receptors, psychiatric illness, and homelessness.[36]

Extracorporeal circuits can induce cooling. Patients receiving continuous renal replacement therapy are at risk for a decrease in core body temperature resulting from heat loss through the dialysate and tubing of the continuous renal replacement system. In a study by Jones,[31] the average temperature drop during the first 12 hours of continuous renal replacement therapy was 1.9°C (3.4°F), and 64% of patients started to shiver. Therefore these patients are at risk for the development of hypothermia.

Patients with autonomic neuropathies attributable to diabetes mellitus or spinal cord injury have been reported to be at risk for hypothermia.[48] The inability to vasoconstrict and vasodilate places these patients at risk not only for hypothermia but also for hyperthermia. Altered ability to thermoregulate in patients with spinal cord injury is termed poikilothermia.

Definition

Hypothermia caused by exposure is classified as mild hypothermia (greater than 32°C; 89.6°F), moderate hypothermia (28° to 32°C; 82.4° to 89.6°F), and severe hypothermia (less than 28°C; 82.4°F).[5] Shivering is intact in patients with mild hypothermia but absent in patients suffering from moderate or severe hypothermia.

Pathophysiology

Although hypothermia can occur from a variety of causes (e.g., accidental, trauma), physiologic and pathophysiologic responses are somewhat similar and include many body systems. As core body temperature decreases, the initial thermoregulatory response is for shivering to occur. Subsequently, shivering increases oxygen consumption.[28] As core body temperature continues to decrease, shivering slows and oxygen consumption will decrease.[53]

Pathophysiologic manifestations that occur with hypothermia include central nervous system changes such as impaired judgment, apathy, ataxia, and confusion (Table 7-1). As temperature continues to decrease, coma will occur. Initial cardiovascular changes that occur include vasoconstriction that leads to shifts in fluid from the peripheral vasculature to the central vasculature. Because of this fluid shift, there is what is termed a cold diuresis and subsequent hypovolemia. The hypovolemia becomes a concern as the patient is rewarmed. Severe hypothermia leads to depressed cardiac function and decreased cardiac output. Bradycardia and atrial fibrillation will start to occur during moderate hypothermia, and ventricular fibrillation and asystole will occur during severe hypothermia.[53] The development of a J wave is a classic sign of hypothermia (Figure 7-2). Respiratory rate and oxygen consumption decrease with moderate and severe hypothermia. Metabolism is slowed during hypothermia because of the slowing of many enzymatic reactions. The clotting cascade is dependent upon enzymatic reactions. During hypothermia at 33°C, coagulation is at less than 50% of normal activity.[30] The coagulation profile typically looks normal in the patient with hypothermia because the specimens are usually warmed to 37°C for analysis.[53]

Decreased enzymatic activity not only affects the clotting cascade but also will decrease the metabolism of some medications. The duration of action of medications such as muscle relaxants and benzodiazepines can be prolonged by as much as 40% to 50%.[53]

Multidisciplinary Plan of Care

Temperature monitoring is a priority in patients with accidental hypothermia but often other clinical issues are prioritized above temperature measurement. There are significant implications associated with hypothermia for processes such as coagulation, acid-base balance, and cardiac rhythms. Of the various clinical sources available for core body temperature measurement, the best are esophageal, pulmonary artery, or urinary bladder. Moderately accurate sites of core body temperature are oral and rectal temperature measures, and the least accurate are tympanic and axillary measurements.[17,24,26] Monitoring trends is important to evaluate in terms of temperature measurement; therefore switching monitoring sites during the care of a patient will adversely affect the ability to trend temperature alterations. Of note, when monitoring temperature in hypothermic patients, many clinical thermometers do not measure temperatures less than 34.4°C (93.9°F).[40]

In addition to temperature monitoring, changes in acid-base balance, oxygenation, and coagulation should

TABLE 7-1 Manifestations of Hypothermia

CLASSIFICATION OF HYPOTHERMIA	PHYSIOLOGIC CHANGES	SIGNS AND SYMPTOMS
Mild hypothermia, 32°–35°C (90–95°F)	Increased basal metabolic rate Increased oxygen consumption Vasoconstriction Inability to concentrate urine Decreased intestinal motility Decreased liver function	Shivering: tachycardia, increased stroke volume, increased cardiac output, increased blood pressure Tachypnea, decreased tidal volume, cyanosis, pallor Diuresis Ileus Decreased clearance time for medications
Moderate hypothermia, 28°–32°C (83°–90°F)	Decreased basal metabolic rate Inability to spontaneously rewarm Decreased oxygen consumption Decreased cerebral blood flow Coagulopathies Acidosis or alkalosis	Bradycardia, decreased blood pressure Shivering stops Bradypnea, decreased cough reflex Confusion, uncoordination, decreased level of consciousness Increased PT and PTT, platelet dysfunction Muscle rigidity
Severe hypothermia, 25°–28°C (77°–83°F)	Decreased systematic vascular resistance Decreased cardiac conduction Increased cardiac irritability Decreased nerve conduction Lack of central nervous system activity	Decreased heart rate, decreased stroke volume, decreased cardiac output, decreased blood pressure Dysrhythmias, ECG changes, J (Osborne) wave, decreased sinus rate, T wave inversions and interval prolongation Ventricular fibrillation Hyporeflexia or areflexia Fixed, dilated pupils; unconsciousness

Modified from reference 4.
PT = Prothrombin time, PTT = partial thromboplastin time, ECG = electrocardiogram.

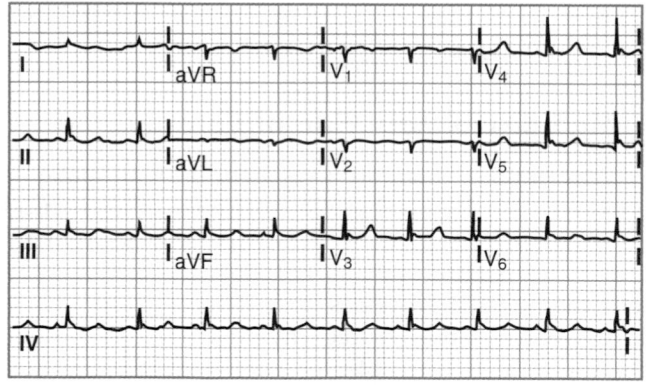

⬥**FIGURE 7-2** Patient showing J waves during hypothermia.

be monitored in patients with hypothermia. Changes in potassium levels will be associated with acid-base alterations, and sodium concentrations will change with fluid shifts. Thus electrolytes should also be evaluated frequently.[40] Reversal of coagulopathies will occur with warming of the patient.[40]

There are a variety of methods for warming patients; some are more invasive than others. The most important consideration in warming patients is that the patient should be kept dry. Wet clothing is a factor in decreasing core body temperature, and should be removed as soon as possible. Passive warming methods such as warm blankets or any protective covering will help prevent heat loss. More active warming methods include conductive warming with a circulating water mattress and convective blankets. Of the noninvasive methods for treating hypothermia, convective warming has been shown to be most effective.[49] Other methods of active core warming include administration of warmed intravenous (IV) fluids and lavage of body cavities such as the stomach, colon, or bladder. An example is the use of a peritoneal dialysis catheter to warm the peritoneum with fluids. More invasive methods have emerged to warm hypothermic patients using extracorporeal systems such as hemodialysis, cardiopulmonary bypass, arteriovenous warming, and venovenous warming.[40]

One of the concerns when warming patients with hypothermia is the development of afterdrop.[35] Afterdrop, a decrease in core body temperature, occurs when warming a patient who is cold. Application of warming blankets or other types of warming causes changes in blood flow that cause more blood to move through cold tissues. This subsequently decreases the core body temperature. The Multidisciplinary Plan of Care on pp. 139-140 summarizes the care of patients with disorders of thermoregulation.

MULTIDISCIPLINARY PLAN OF CARE FOR PATIENTS WITH DISORDERS OF THERMOREGULATION

PROBLEM	INTERVENTION	RATIONALE	EXPECTED OUTCOME	COMMENTS
Fever	Collect blood cultures; identify underlying cause of infection. Consider other appropriate diagnostic procedures to identify underlying cause of fever.	Fever is often a sign of infection but is also associated with many other etiologies.	Early identification of underlying cause of fever	Fever may not be present in some patients who have infectious processes. The elderly may have subtle changes in mentation that are associated with development of infection.[18]
Fever	Administer antipyretics if patient cannot tolerate increased metabolic demands associated with fever.	Although fever is thought to be beneficial as a host defense mechanism, some patients will benefit from treatment of fever, such as patients with a history of cardiac disease, pulmonary disease, or neurologic disease. The demands of fever in the elderly may provide considerable stress; therefore treatment of fever should be considered.	Decreased core body temperature, decreased heart rate, decreased respiratory rate, and decreased fluid loss	
Fever	Use physical cooling with excessive elevation in core body temperature.	Application of physical cooling is somewhat controversial as a treatment for fever. Shivering can occur with application of a cooling blanket, leading to increased oxygen consumption. In a study by O'Donnell et al.,[42] the investigators found that critical care nurses most frequently used cooling blankets when core body temperatures reached 39.7°C (103.5°F).	Decreased core body temperature, decreased heart rate, decreased respiratory rate, and decreased fluid loss	If patients shiver with application of cooling, oxygen consumption will increase.
Hypothermia	Measure core body temperature. Monitor assessments that typically change with hypothermia.	Core body temperature assessment is often not considered a priority in critically ill patients. Decreased core body temperature can increase blood loss in patients at risk for hemorrhage.	Assess for decreased core body temperature; assess for dysrhythmias, acid-base abnormalities, changes in cognitive function	
Hypothermia	Increase insulation and remove any wet clothing. Actively apply external warming methods such as convective warming or fluid-filled warming blankets.	Decreasing gradient between core body temperature and ambient temperature will decrease heat loss, increasing patient's core body temperature.	Normal core body temperature, absence of shivering	

Table continues on page 140

MULTIDISCIPLINARY PLAN OF CARE FOR PATIENTS WITH DISORDERS OF THERMOREGULATION—CONT'D

PROBLEM	INTERVENTION	RATIONALE	EXPECTED OUTCOME	COMMENTS
Hypothermia	Infuse warmed intravenous fluids. Consider other invasive active methods of warming such as peritoneal lavage or extracorporeal circuits.	A heat load can be provided to patient with warmed intravenous fluids or other types of active invasive methods of warming.[53]	Normal core body temperature, absence of shivering	
Hyperthermia	Accurately measure core body temperature.	Thermometers may not be accurate at temperatures higher than 40°C.	Determination of core body temperature	
Hyperthermia	Interventions used for each type of hyperthermia are dependent upon etiology. In general the key is to decrease heat production and promote heat loss by using medications or physical cooling.	Examples: Priority for treatment of heatstroke is a decrease in core body temperature using physical cooling (iced gastric lavage, ice packs, cooling blankets, cold water immersion, continuous fanning).[7]	Normal core body temperature	Priority for treatment of malignant hyperthermia is administration of dantrolene.
Hyperthermia	Consider administration of sodium bicarbonate.	Treat metabolic acidosis associated with hyperthermia and rhabdomyolysis.	pH 7.35–7.45	
Hyperthermia	Consider administration of benzodiazepines.	Treat or prevent seizure activity.	Absence of seizures	
Hyperthermia	Infuse isotonic fluids for hypovolemia and consider monitoring central venous pressure.	Vasodilation during hyperthermia causes hypotension.	Systolic blood pressure higher than 100 mm Hg and mean blood pressure higher than 70 mm Hg	
Hyperthermia	Administer oxygen and consider intubation.	Administer oxygen for increased metabolic rate. Provide airway if patient has decreased neuro status or respiratory failure.		

HYPERTHERMIA

Patients at Risk

Elevated core body temperature can occur from environmental heat exposure, malignant hyperthermia, neuroleptic malignant syndrome, or recreational drug use. Heatstroke is considered a core body temperature of greater than 40.0° C and is classified as either classic heatstroke or exertional heatstroke.[7] Classic heatstroke is more likely to occur in children or the elderly. Children left in cars during summer months are at risk for the development of heatstroke.[21] Elderly that do not have air-conditioned living quarters are at risk for heatstroke during heat waves. Heat stress is known to occur more frequently in states that have warmer climates, such as Arizona.[9] Exertional heatstroke is more likely to occur in marathon runners, football players, and military recruits.[7]

Recreational drugs such as cocaine and ecstasy, also known as MDMA (3,4-methylenedioxymethamphetamine), increase the risk for hyperthermia. Although both drugs increase metabolic rate, it is usually the combination of a warm environment in addition to use of these drugs that leads to heatstroke.[20] The use of ecstasy in combination with increased physical activity such as dancing increases metabolic rate. In addition, the environments where ecstasy is used often are hot, crowded dance clubs with poor ventilation.[20]

Ephedra, an herbal supplement, has been associated with heatstroke-related deaths in athletes and also army recruits.[57] The mechanism associated with death caused by hyperthermia in individuals taking ephedra is thought to be associated with the peripheral vasoconstriction that occurs. This cutaneous vasoconstriction decreases the ability to lose heat, therefore causing a rise in core body temperature.

Genotype may also play a role in the development of heatstroke. Heat shock proteins have been identified as having a beneficial effect by allowing cells to survive in times of heat stress. Some individuals do not have the genetic capabilities to transcribe heat shock proteins and are thought to be at particular risk for the development of heatstroke.[7]

Malignant hyperthermia (MH) is associated with a genetic mutation in the ryanodine receptor that leads to a hyperthermic state when patients are exposed to particular medications.[11] The most frequent mutation associated with MH is located on chromosome 19q13.1 and is inherited via autosomal dominant transmission, although other genes are associated with MH. Anesthetic agents that trigger malignant hyperthermia include halothane, isoflurane, sevoflurane, and desflurane. Succinylcholine is also known to trigger malignant hyperthermia. Before surgery, patients should be asked if any family members have had problems with previous surgeries. In addition to these more common triggers of MH, other triggers of MH include exercise in hot conditions, infection, alcohol, and neuroleptic medications.[11]

Neuroleptic malignant syndrome (NMS) is associated with an increase in core body temperature in patients that are taking neuroleptic medications. Medications that are reported to be associated with NMS include haloperidol (Haldol), chlorpromazine (Thorazine), fluphenazine (Prolixin, Decanoate), loxapine (Loxitane), aripiprazole (Abilify), ziprasidone (Geodone), clozapine (Clozaril), olanzapine (Zyprexa), quetiapine (Seroquel), and risperidone (Risperdal).[10] Dopamine is thought to have an inhibitory effect on the heat-

generating capabilities of serotonin; therefore if the production of dopamine is blocked, as occurs with many of the previously listed medications, there is an elevation in core body temperature.[10] Additional support for this theory comes from reported cases of patients with Parkinson's disease having elevation in core body temperature. Other factors that contribute to the development of NMS include dehydration, malnutrition, exhaustion, and infection.[32] A genetic polymorphism (Taq I A) has also been suggested to be associated with the development of NMS.[32]

Definition

Hyperthermic states caused by environmental heat exposure are classified as heat stress, heat exhaustion, and heatstroke. Heat stress is the development of discomfort, cramps, and possibly syncope. Heat exhaustion is a body temperature greater than 37°C and less than 40°C. Heatstroke is defined as a core body temperature that is greater than 40.0°C with central nervous system dysfunction.[7]

Pathophysiology

Mechanisms related to the generation of heatstroke are associated with the particular cause. Environmental conditions such as a heat wave (3 days greater than 90°F) contribute to heatstroke in the very young, the elderly, and those that do not have access to air conditioning. The very young have difficulty with thermoregulation because of their surface area to mass ratio and the very old are often unable to lose heat as effectively as healthy adults. The elderly often have diseases that impair heat loss, such as diabetes or neurologic problems.

Heatstroke, a core body temperature greater than 40°C, leads to pathophysiologic changes in many body systems, resulting in increased mortality in the critically ill patient. Some of the consequences of heatstroke include a systemic inflammatory response with increased production of proinflammatory and antiinflammatory cytokines.[7] In addition, coagulation abnormalities similar to disseminated intravascular coagulation occur with heatstroke. These include increased clotting and increased fibrinolytic activity. Additionally, there is a hyperpermeability that occurs in the gut, leading to endotoxin entry into the circulation. Endotoxemia that occurs from this hyperpermeability is associated with hemodynamic instability.

Clinical manifestations associated with heatstroke affect multiple body systems. Central nervous system manifestations may be as subtle as changes in judgment or inappropriate behavior although manifestations can be as severe as coma with seizures that occur during cooling.[7] Cardiovascular manifestations that occur in these patients include increased heart rate with a decrease in blood pressure. Acid-base abnormalities that occur include lactic acidosis and respiratory alkalosis. Carbon dioxide levels are usually decreased in these patients because of hyperventilation.[6,7] If the cause of heatstroke in patients is exertional, there is more likely to be a metabolic acidosis that is often associated with rhabdomyolysis.[6] Patients may go on to develop multisystem failure including encephalopathy, renal failure, acute respiratory distress syndrome, myocardial injury, hepatic injury, intestinal ischemia, pancreatic injury, and hemorrhagic problems.

MH is a rise in core body temperature from increased muscle activity caused by exposure to halogenated anesthetic agents and depolarizing muscle relaxants.[38] Cases in the literature have also cited exercise and heat stress as triggers that may lead to the development of MH.[51] A genetic mutation of the ryanodine receptor is associated with increased intracellular calcium levels. This increase in calcium released from the sarcoplasmic reticulum stimulates vigorous contraction of the muscle, leading to increased heat production.

In addition to the rise in core body temperature that occurs with MH, other body systems are also affected.[39] Acid-base abnormalities that occur include acidosis resulting from increased production of carbon dioxide. Muscle rigidity occurs despite the administration of muscle relaxants. If the patient is not intubated before the onset of MH, contraction of the jaw may make oral intubation difficult. Potassium levels rise and patients will have elevated creatine kinase levels. Patients become tachycardic, increasing myocardial consumption, and they often have dysrhythmias. Rhadomyolysis and subsequent myoglobinuria can lead to renal failure.

There are some theories regarding the generation of NMS.[10] One of the theories suggests that dopamine inhibits increases in core body temperature and that serotonin increases core body temperature. Inhibition of dopamine production leads to an increase in core body temperature. Patients with Parkinson's disease sometimes have elevations in core body temperature with cessation of levodopa-carbidopa therapy, thus supporting this theory. A second theory suggests that patients with NMS are similar to patients with MH.[10] Patients with NMS have alterations in muscle contraction that suggest release of calcium from the sarcoplasmic reticulum at lower thresholds.

◆ Case Study 7-2

Malignant Hyperthermia

P.P is a 25-year-old female weighing 55 kg who presented to the emergency department with right lower quadrant pain (pain rating: 8/10) and a core body temperature of 38.1°C. She had no previous surgeries and there was no family history of problems with surgery. The patient was taken to the operating theater for an appendectomy. Preoperative medications administered include 2 mg of midazolam (Versed) and 100 mcg of fentanyl (Duragesic). Induction during the case included sodium thiopental and succinylcholine chloride (Anectine). The patient was kept anesthetized during the case with isoflurane, and rocuronium (Zemuron) was administered to provide paralysis. Toward the end of the case the surgeon asked that the patient receive more paralytic because the patient's abdomen was very rigid. The heart rate at this time was 110 beats/min. The patient's end tidal CO_2 level had risen from a baseline of 33 to 55 mm Hg and the core body temperature was now 38.9°C. An arterial blood gas was drawn; results were a pH of 7.21 and a pco_2 of 60 mm Hg. The isoflurane was discontinued. Dantrolene (Dantrium) 2.5 mg/kg was administered IV. The patient was cooled using ice bags to the thorax, head, arms, and legs, and the patient was placed on a Fio_2 of 1.0. Postoperatively the patient was admitted to critical care. The patient received 1 mg/kg dantrolene every 6 hours for 24 hours to prevent the redevelopment of MH.

Decision point: What is the cause of P.P.'s MH?

Decision point: What is the mechanism for the rise of her core body temperature?

Decision point: What manifestations of malignant hyperthermia did P.P. display?

Multidisciplinary Plan of Care

Although the goal for treatment of the patient with hyperthermia is a normal core body temperature, management of patient will vary depending upon the underlying cause of the hyperthermia. For example, the management of the patient with hyperthermia caused by environmental exposure will differ compared to that for the patient with malignant hyperthermia. One of the considerations with hyperthermia is accurate measurement of core body temperature. Thermometers normally used to measure core body temperature may not be accurate above 40°C.[7]

The goal when treating hyperthermia is to decrease the core body temperature. This can be accomplished by conductive cooling, that is, decreasing skin temperature and promoting heat loss by increasing the gradient between core and skin temperatures. This could be accomplished by use of ice packs or water-filled cooling blankets. One of the problems with conductive cooling of the skin is the subsequent vasoconstriction that decreases heat loss. Other methods of cooling include the use of warm air spray, similar to the devices seen on the sidelines of football games in warm environments. The warm air spray promotes heat loss by evaporation of the mist and convective heat loss by the air movement of the fan. The warmth of the mist promotes cutaneous vasodilation and thus greater heat loss. In a study by Plattner et al.,[44] the most effective method to decrease core body temperature is placing the patient in a water and ice mixture.

In addition to cooling, treatments for heatstroke include fluid resuscitation with an isotonic crystalloid solution or administration of vasopressors if the patient is hypotensive. Patients will require administration of oxygen and possibly intubation if they are unable to adequately protect their airway or have respiratory failure. Seizure activity with heatstroke is treated with benzodiazepines. If rhabdomyolysis is suspected, patients are treated with an infusion of saline in addition to mannitol, furosemide (Lasix), and sodium bicarbonate.[7] Administration of sodium bicarbonate is dependent upon acid-base balance. In addition to monitoring acid-base balance by measurement of arterial blood gases, potassium level is monitored to detect hyperkalemia. Additional measures may be required to treat hyperkalemia.

MH is another possible cause of hyperthermia that is treated differently because of the intense generation of heat from muscle contraction. Treatments include removing the triggering agent and placing the patient on a fraction of inspired oxygen (Fio_2) of 1.0 because of the increased metabolic rate.[44] Dantrolene (Dantrium) 2 mg/kg up to 10 mg/kg is the drug of choice for treatment of MH. Dantrolene decreases the release of calcium from the sarcoplasmic reticulum and relaxes muscle contraction. Once MH occurs, treatment with dantrolene must be repeated during the following 24 hours. Monitoring and treatment of acid-base and electrolyte abnormalities can help to prevent complications of MH such as renal failure from rhabdomyolysis.[45] Evaluation of MH includes muscle contracture biopsy studies in response to halothane and caffeine.[45] If the contracture study is positive, subsequently there is a search for genetic mutations. Family members can be evaluated for similar genetic mutations to identify risk for MH.[45]

Treatment of NMS is similar to that for MH. Dantrolene is administered to decrease the muscle rigidity that occurs with NMS.[10] Fluids are administered, and rhabdomyolysis similar to that seen in MH is also a concern. The other medication that may be administered specifically for NMS is bromocriptine (Parlodel). Bromocriptine is used to facilitate dopamine production to help with muscle relaxation. One of the concerns with holding medications that cause NMS is the increase in psychotic symptoms experienced by patients.[10] See the Multidisciplinary Plan of Care on pp. 139-140.

CONCLUSIONS

Although temperature monitoring and thermoregulation are not always priorities in care of the critically ill patient, the effects of core body temperature alter the physiologic responses of other body systems. Early treatment of extremes of core body temperature can prevent problems such as bleeding, infection, and increased oxygen consumption. Fever, although typically viewed as an indicator of infection, should also be considered an adaptive response that may benefit the host. Other extremes in core body temperature are not adaptive responses and contribute to patient mortality and morbidity. Hypothermia during surgery has been associated with increased infection rates; therefore it is important to prevent decreases in core body temperature.

REFERENCES

1. Atkins, E. (1985). Fever: the old and new. *J Infect Dis, 151*(3), 570.
2. Benson, G. D., Koff, R. S., & Tolman, K. G. (2005). The therapeutic use of acetaminophen in patients with liver disease. *Am J Therapeutics, 12*(2), 133–141.
3. Bernard, G. R., Wheeler, A. P., Russell, J. A., et al. (1997). The effects of ibuprofen on the physiology and survival of patients with sepsis. The Ibuprofen in Sepsis Study Group. *New Engl J Med, 336*(13), 912–918.
4. Bernardo, L. M., & Henker, R. (1999). Thermoregulation in pediatric trauma: an overview. *Int J Trauma Nurs, 5*(3), 101–105.
5. Biem, J., Koehncke, N., Classen, D., et al. (2003). Out of the cold: management of hypothermia and frostbite. *CMAJ Can Med Assoc J, 168*(3), 305–311.
6. Bouchama, A., & De Vol, E. B. (2001). Acid-base alterations in heatstroke. *Intensive Care Med, 27*(4), 680–685.
7. Bouchama, A., & Knochel, J. P. (2002). Heat stroke. *New Engl J Med, 346*(25), 1978–1988.
8. Boulant, J. A. (1998). Hypothalamic neurons. Mechanisms of sensitivity to temperature. *Ann NY Acad Sci, 856*, 108–115.
9. Centers for Disease Control and Prevention. (2005). Heat-related mortality—Arizona, 1993–2002, and United States, 1979–2002. *MMWR Morbidity Mortality Weekly Rep, 54*(25), 628–630.
10. Chandran, G. J., Mikler, J. R., & Keegan, D. L. (2003). Neuroleptic malignant syndrome: case report and discussion. *CMAJ Can Med Assoc J, 169*(5), 439–442.
11. Christiansen, L. R., & Collins, K. A. (2004). Pathologic findings in malignant hyperthermia: a case report and review of literature. *Am J Forensic Med Pathol, 25*(4), 327–333.
12. Clemmer, T. P., Fisher, C. J., Jr., Bone, R. C., et al. (1992). Hypothermia in the sepsis syndrome and clinical outcome. The Methylprednisolone Severe Sepsis Study Group. *Crit Care Med, 20*(10), 1395–1401.

13. Clifton, G. L., Miller, E. R., Choi, S. C., et al. (2001). Lack of effect of induction of hypothermia after acute brain injury. *New Engl J Med*, 344(8), 556–563.

14. Cuddy, M. L. (2004). The effects of drugs on thermoregulation. *AACN Clin Issues*, 15(2), 238–253.

15. Dahners, L. E., & Mullis, B. H. (2004). Effects of nonsteroidal anti-inflammatory drugs on bone formation and soft-tissue healing. *J Am Acad Orthopaedic Surgeons*, 12(3), 139–143.

16. Dinarello, C. A. (2004). Infection, fever, and exogenous and endogenous pyrogens: some concepts have changed. *J Endotoxin Res*, 10(4), 201–222.

17. Erickson, R. S. (1999). The continuing question of how best to measure body temperature. *Crit Care Med*, 27(10), 2307–2310.

18. Gleckman, R., & Hibert, D. (1982). Afebrile bacteremia. A phenomenon in geriatric patients. *JAMA*, 248(12), 1478–1481.

19. Gozzoli, V., Treggiari, M. M., Kleger, G. R., et al. (2004). Randomized trial of the effect of antipyresis by metamizol, propacetamol or external cooling on metabolism, hemodynamics and inflammatory response. *Intensive Care Med*, 30(3), 401–407.

20. Green, A. R., O'Shea, E., & Colado, M. I. (2004). A review of the mechanisms involved in the acute MDMA (ecstasy)-induced hyperthermic response. *Eur J Pharmacol*, 500(1–3), 3–13.

21. Guard, A., & Gallagher, S. S. (2005). Heat related deaths to young children in parked cars: an analysis of 171 fatalities in the United States, 1995–2002. *Injury Prevention*, 11(1), 33–37.

22. Haupt, M. T., & Rackow, E. C. (1983). Adverse effects of febrile state on cardiac performance. *Am Heart J*, 105(5), 763–768.

23. Henker, R. (2000). Infection control. Use of blood cultures in critically ill patients. *Crit Care Nurse*, 20(1), 45–50.

24. Henker, R., & Coyne, C. (1995). Comparison of peripheral temperature measurements with core temperature. *AACN Clin Issues*, 6(1), 21–30.

25. Henker, R., Rogers, S., Kramer, D. J., et al. (2001). Comparison of fever treatments in the critically ill: a pilot study. *Am J Crit Care*, 10(4), 276–280.

26. Henker, R. A., Brown, S. D., & Marion, D. W. (1998). Comparison of brain temperature with bladder and rectal temperatures in adults with severe head injury. *Neurosurgery*, 42(5), 1071–1075.

27. Holtzclaw, B. J. (2004). Shivering in acutely ill vulnerable populations. *AACN Clin Issues*, 15(2), 267–279.

28. Horvath, S. M., Spurr, G. B., Hutt, B. K., et al. (1956). Metabolic cost of shivering. *J Appl Physiol*, 8(6), 595–602.

29. Hypothermia after Cardiac Arrest Study Group. (2002). Mild therapeutic hypothermia to improve the neurologic outcome after cardiac arrest. [see comment] [erratum appears in *N Engl J Med*, (2002). 346(22), 1756]. *New Engl J Med*, 346(8), 549–556.

30. Johnston, T. D., Chen, Y., & Reed, R. L., 2nd. (1994). Functional equivalence of hypothermia to specific clotting factor deficiencies. *J Trauma Injury Infection Crit Care*, 37(3), 413–417.

31. Jones, S. (2004). Heat loss and continuous renal replacement therapy. *AACN Clin Issues*, 15(2), 223–230.

32. Kawanishi, C. (2003). Genetic predisposition to neuroleptic malignant syndrome: implications for antipsychotic therapy. *Am J Pharmaco Genomics*, 3(2), 89–95.

33. Kilpatrick, M. M., Lowry, D. W., Firlik, A. D., et al. (2000). Hyperthermia in the neurosurgical intensive care unit. *Neurosurgery*, 47(4), 850–855; discussion 855–856.

34. Kluger, M. J., Ringler, D. H., & Anver, M. R. (1975). Fever and survival. *Science*, 188(4184), 166–168.

35. Koller, R., Schnider, T. W., & Neidhart, P. (1997). Deep accidental hypothermia and cardiac arrest—rewarming with forced air. *Acta Anaesthesiol Scand*, 41(10), 1359–1364.

36. Koutsavlis, A. T., & Kosatsky, T. (2003). Environmental-temperature injury in a Canadian metropolis. *J Environ Health*, 66(5), 40–45.

37. Mackowiak, P. A., Wasserman, S. S., & Levine, M. M. (1992). A critical appraisal of 98.6 degrees F, the upper limit of the normal body temperature, and other legacies of Carl Reinhold August Wunderlich. *JAMA*, 268(12), 1578–1580.

38. Manthous, C. A., Hall, J. B., Olson, D., et al. (1995). Effect of cooling on oxygen consumption in febrile critically ill patients. *Am J Respiratory Crit Care Med*, 151(1), 10–14.

39. McCarthy, E. J. (2004). Malignant hyperthermia: pathophysiology, clinical presentation, and treatment. *AACN Clin Issues*, 15(2), 231–237.

40. McCullough, L., & Arora, S. (2004). Diagnosis and treatment of hypothermia. *Am Fam Physician*, 70(12), 2325–2332.

41. Morgan, S. P. (1990). A comparison of three methods of managing fever in the neurologic patient. *J Neurosci Nurs*, 22(1), 19–24.

42. O'Donnell, J., Axelrod, P., Fisher, C., et al. (1997). Use and effectiveness of hypothermia blankets for febrile patients in the intensive care unit. *Clin Infect Dis*, 24(6), 1208–1213.

43. O'Grady, N. P., Barie, P. S., Bartlett, J., et al. (1998). Practice parameters for evaluating new fever in critically ill adult patients. Task Force of the American College of Critical Care Medicine of the Society of Critical Care Medicine in collaboration with the Infectious Disease Society of America. *Crit Care Med*, 26(2), 392–408.

44. Plattner, O., Kurz, A., Sessler, D. I., et al. (1997). Efficacy of intraoperative cooling methods. *Anesthesiology*, 87(5), 1089–1095.

45. Rosenberg, H., Brandom, B. W., Sambuughin, N., et al. (2006). Malignant hyperthermia and other pharmacogenetic disorders. In B. F. Cullen, P. G. Barash & R. K. Stoelting (Eds.), *Clinical anesthesia* (5th ed., pp 529–556). Philadelphia: Lippincott Williams & Wilkins.

46. Schafer, A. I. (1999). Effects of nonsteroidal anti-inflammatory therapy on platelets. *Am J Med*, 106(5B), 31.

47. Schmutzhard, E., Engelhardt, K., Beer, R., et al. (2002). Safety and efficacy of a novel intravascular cooling device to control body temperature in neurologic intensive care patients: a prospective pilot study. *Crit Care Med*, 30(11), 2481–2488.

48. Scott, A. R., Bennett, T., & Macdonald, I. A. (1987). Diabetes mellitus and thermoregulation. *Can J Physiol Pharmacol*, 65(6), 1365–1376.

49. Sessler, D. I. (1997). Mild perioperative hypothermia. *New Engl J Med*, 336(24), 1730–1737.

50. Tarling, M. M., Toner, C. C., Withington, P. S., et al. (1997). A model of gastric emptying using paracetamol absorption in intensive care patients. *Intensive Care Med*, 23(3), 256–260.

51. Tobin, J. R., Jason, D. R., Challa, V. R., et al. (2001). Malignant hyperthermia and apparent heat stroke. *JAMA*, 286(2), 168–169.

52. Todd, M. M., & Hindman, B. J., Intraoperative Hypothermia for Aneurysm Surgery Trial. (2005). Mild intraoperative hypothermia during surgery for intracranial aneurysm [see comment]. *New Engl J Med*, 352(2), 135–145.

53. Tsuei, B. J., & Kearney, P. A. (2004). Hypothermia in the trauma patient. *Injury*, 35(1), 7–15.

54. Tweedie, I. E., Bell, C. F., Clegg, A., et al. (1989). Retrospective study of temperature rhythms of intensive care patients. *Crit Care Med*, 17(11), 1159–1165.

55. Wang, Y., Lim, L. L., Levi, C., et al. (2000). Influence of admission body temperature on stroke mortality. *Stroke*, 31(2), 404–409.

56. Weinstein, M. P., Murphy, J. R., Reller, L. B., et al. (1983). The clinical significance of positive blood cultures: a comprehensive analysis of 500 episodes of bacteremia and fungemia in adults. II. Clinical observations, with special reference to factors influencing prognosis. *Rev Infect Dis*, 5(1), 54–70.

57. Yeo, T. P. (2004). Heat stroke: a comprehensive review. *AACN Clin Issues*, 15(2), 280–293.

CHAPTER 8   Families in Critical Care

Nancy C. Molter

Do family members of critically ill patients consider themselves healers or visitors during the critical care experience? What role do they perceive they have in helping the critically ill patient heal? What do nurses need to know to create healing, family-centered environments for the critically ill? What is already known? What else needs to be explored? To answer these questions, this chapter will explore the interface of theory, clinical research, and practice to establish the boundaries of knowledge related to family-centered care (FCC) in the critical care environment.

Defining the key elements of FCC is germane to the exploration of the other questions. FCC is a concept originally developed by healthcare practitioners working with children.[17] It is a synthesis of philosophies, attitudes, and approaches to care; it is a concept translated from caring for children to caring for all patients and their families in healthcare delivery systems. The key elements of FCC, summarized in Box 8-1, reflect the consideration of an individual as a member of a self-defined family unit and directly support the rights and responsibilities of patients and families espoused by healthcare delivery systems. Recently, FCC has been further refined to include the concept of *family-sensitive care*. This term refers specifically to the nurse-family interface reflective of the receptivity of the nurse to the family's experience, and the use of these perceptions to be responsive to the developing family needs.[48] Patients define their "family," whether or not a blood relative; the members of this "family" become the primary support system for the patient. As a support system, they often complement nurses in creating a healthy, healing environment for the patient.

The complexity of working with families of critical care patients is often daunting to the critical care staff.[11,24,25,33] Practice based on a variety of theoretical foundations is needed to assist families during the critical care experience. Therefore an understanding of concepts including complexity, family systems, relatedness, role, crisis, and hierarchical needs theories can assist nurses in developing skills to work with families in crisis. A brief review of the premises of these theories lays the foundation for evidence-based

Box 8-1

Eight Elements of Family-Centered Care

1. Incorporating into policy and practice the recognition that the family is the constant in a person's life, while the service systems and support personnel within those systems fluctuate.
2. Facilitating family/professional collaboration at all levels of hospital, home, and community care.
3. Exchanging complete and unbiased information between families and professionals in a supportive manner at all times.
4. Incorporating into policy and practice the recognition and honoring of cultural diversity, strengths, and individuality within and across all families.
5. Recognizing and respecting different methods of coping and implementing comprehensive policies and programs that provide developmental, educational, emotional, environmental, and financial supports to meet the diverse needs of families.
6. Encouraging and facilitating family-to-family support and networking.
7. Ensuring that hospital, home, and community service and support systems for individuals and their families needing specialized health and development care are flexible, accessible, and comprehensive in responding to diverse family-identified needs.
8. Appreciating families as families and individuals as individuals, recognizing that they possess a wide range of strengths, concerns, emotions, and aspirations beyond their need for specialized health services and support.

Data from reference 17.

care for families of critically ill patients. This will be followed by a review of the evidence for practice related to family needs, the role of family presence, and FCC interventions and outcomes.

145

The chapter will close with suggestions about implementing FCC. It will include strategies, tools, and outcome evaluation information that can assist critical care staff in establishing FCC programs. Evidence exists to support the positive outcomes of FCC. The goal of this chapter is to help critical care nurses meet the challenge of making FCC a reality.

THEORETICAL FOUNDATIONS FOR FAMILY-CENTERED CRITICAL CARE

There are many theories related to ensuring family-friendly environments that promote FCC to ensure healthy, healing environments for the patient and family. Figure 8-1 depicts six theories with direct relevance to nursing practice for implementing FCC principles. Each theory provides insight into the importance of a holistic, comprehensive model of critical care practice that establishes the patient and family as a unit central to the care provided. The patient/family unit must be considered holistically to achieve optimal FCC outcomes.

Chaos/Complexity Theory

An overview of chaos/complexity theory is helpful because this theory challenges the traditional thinking of the scientific community in Western civilization. For the most part, science follows the scientific method or a model of reductionism. This scientific method requires detached objectivity, a philosophy that is slowly changing based on the knowledge acquired from emerging new sciences.[51] Chaos/complexity theory is the study of dynamic nonlinear systems evolving from mathematical and physical sciences, humanistic behavior, and social sciences, as well as the humanities.[14,34,51] Complexity theory lends rationality to the "serendipitous" findings that were so difficult to explain with linear science.

Complexity is the reaction of a system away from maximal entropy (a measure of the disorder in systems) that leads to deterioration of a system. The edge of chaos is where mutation and innovation occur. As a system passes through this phase, it can transform to more adaptive functioning for the environment. Critical moments force an existing system to the edge of chaos. The outcome is unpredictable because of the sensitivity of the system to initial conditions. James York gave chaos (now termed "complexity") theory its name, but Edward Lorenz is the meteorologist who initially described the effects of nonlinear dynamic interactions. As he made a slight change in the number of a formula he was using to predict the weather, he observed significant, unpredictable changes in the outcome of his program. The "sensitivity to initial conditions" he observed is termed the "butterfly effect" to describe the phenomena of a butterfly flapping its wings in one part of the world and causing a significant change in weather in another part.[34,51] His discovery showed the apparently irregular, unpredictable behavior of nonlinear systems.

Butz et al.[9] applied chaos/complexity theory concepts to family systems. Family members in crisis will exhibit behavior that they believe will protect the family system. However, the critical care environment can pose "initial conditions" that can affect how the family adapts to a new level of functioning. Based on complexity theory, there is evidence that the interaction between families in crisis and the critical care healthcare delivery system could benefit from reframing the healthcare system as a nonlinear system. As critical care staff work with families in crisis, they will experience the importance of how they relate to the patient's family as a key element of the family's "initial sensitivity to conditions" as they enter the critical care system.

Theory of Human Relatedness

An emerging theory in nursing, called the theory of human relatedness, has as its core construct "an individual's level of involvement with persons, objects, groups or natural environments and the concurrent level of comfort or discomfort with that involvement."[20] Hartrick also writes about the importance of having relational capacity in nursing practice.[22] The implications for nursing of a theory of human relatedness

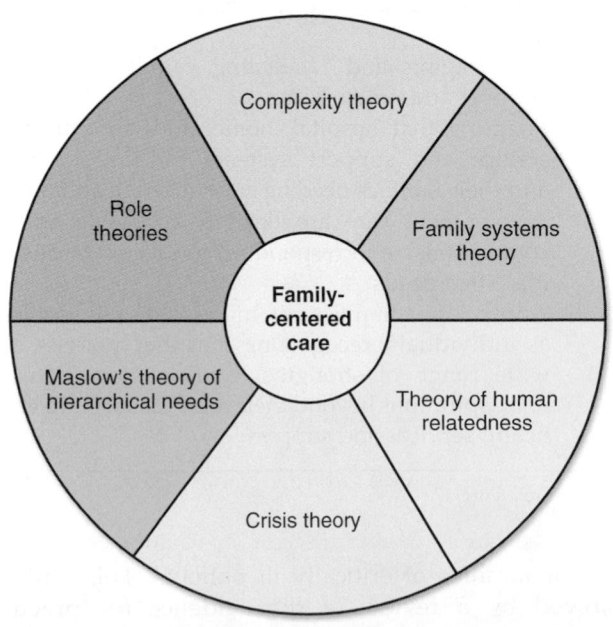

♦ FIGURE 8-1 Theoretical foundations of family-centered care.

are based on the four major processes or social competencies involved in promoting relatedness states: sense of belonging, reciprocity, mutuality, and synchrony. Promoting a *sense of belonging* in relation to an environment can reduce anxiety. For example, if family members are oriented to the critical care environment and are aware how they will function within the environment, anxiety can be reduced. *Reciprocity* relates to an equitable quality and intensity of interchange. Families expect to be kept informed of the patient's condition, and as trust develops they in turn will be able to contribute more intensely to the plan of care. *Mutuality* is defined as the experience of shared commonalities of goals, visions, characteristics, or sentiments, including shared acceptance of differences. When interactions with family members are open, and based on respect and trust, care becomes more individualized for the patient. *Synchrony* describes rhythmic patterns and the congruence the person has with internal patterns and external environments. Over time, the staff/family interactions become synchronized, just as a fine orchestra of expert individual musicians becomes synchronized. The outcome to the patient is greater than the contributions of any single player.

These four processes are also foundational for the Synergy Model of care developed by the American Association of Critical-Care Nurses (AACN).[2] Within this model are nursing competencies that should be matched to patient/family requirements for care. Two key competencies are *caring practices* and *systems thinking*. *Caring practices* are defined as "nursing activities that create a compassionate, supportive, and therapeutic environment for patients and staff, with the aim of promoting comfort and healing and preventing unnecessary suffering. These caring behaviors include but are not limited to vigilance, engagement, and responsiveness of caregivers." *Systems thinking* is described as a "body of knowledge and tools that allow the nurse to manage whatever environmental and system resources exist for the patient and family, within or across healthcare systems." The competencies involve a collaborative sharing of mutual goals that implies reciprocity in nurse/family interactions. When a nurse's competencies for practice match the required needs of the patient/family unit, synergy results and better outcomes can occur (see Figure 1-2). This match could also lead to synchrony between how the family internalizes the critical care experience and the reality of the critical care environment.

Family Systems Theory

Another key theoretical foundation for incorporating family into critical care is family systems theory. This theory emerged from the concept of *cybernetics*,

focusing on the science of communication and control in man as well as machines. Gregory Bateson, an anthropologist and ethnologist, became interested in applying the concept of cybernetics to human communication and introduced viewing the family as a cybernetic system. In 1952 he and his group developed the field of family therapy. Family was construed as a group of individual members each with their own sense of family. Thus families are viewed as complex emotional systems comprising three or four generations. Families are no longer traditional in that there are several permutations (e.g., stepfamilies, single-parent families) of "family" in today's world.[9] In addition, evidence also suggests that individuals consider pets as "family" and that pet visitation assists in healing.[13]

Family systems theory views family as an interdependent whole greater than the sum of its parts.[18] Although many nursing theories define "client" as an individual, family, or community, they do not differentiate between working with individuals and working with family units. One major model for family systems nursing, the Calgary Family Assessment and Intervention model, does make this distinction. The client is the family. Some of the basic tenets of the Calgary model are outlined in Box 8-2.[52]

Role Theories

Despite the extensive body of literature about family needs, very little is known about what the family's role is or should be during the critical care experience. Thus role theories (sometimes called symbolic interaction theories) may provide useful knowledge related to working with families in the critical care environment. Although not new theories, they provide provocative assumptions and well-researched concepts that can assist in defining the role of family members during a critical illness. "Role" is defined as an integrated set "of social norms that [is] distinguishable from other sets

---

Box 8-2

Principles of the Calgary Family Assessment and Intervention Model

- The family as a whole is greater than the sum of its parts.
- A change in one family member affects all family members.
- The family is able to create a balance between change and stability.
- Family members' behaviors are best understood from a view of circular rather than linear causality.

Modified from reference 52.

of norms that constitute other roles."[8] Table 8-1 summarizes some of the middle-range role theories of symbolic interactionism. Only a few studies have explored the "role" of family members of critically ill patients.

One of the first to write about family roles was Gerald Caplan,[10] describing the family "role" in terms of support functions. Simpson[44] explored the supportive functions of families during a critical illness from the perspective of the critically ill patients. She found similarities with Caplan's conceptual framework (Table 8-2). In Simpson's descriptive survey of 100 patients in a surgical ICU (50) or coronary care unit (50), the categories of supportive functions were validated. She outlines the following principles that have implications for practice:

- Family interaction patterns before the critical illness episode may influence how patients will perceive visits as supportive.
- What actually occurs during visits is not as important as the patient's perception of what occurs.

- What may be helpful to one patient may be upsetting to another.
- Families provide a positive outlook for patients.
- Families should be included in patients' interactions with healthcare personnel.
- Critically ill patients are concerned about family welfare.

The experience of relatives of critically ill patients was explored in a qualitative study by Walters.[49] Four themes were identified as important to the relatives: *being with, seeing, plain talk,* and *making sense. Being with* involves genuine feelings of respect and love. It is the physical and emotional presence of the family that could involve just holding the patient's hand or providing companionship to relieve loneliness. *Seeing* and having access to the patient in the critical care unit were important for family members. Family members focus on all aspects of the patient and relate their observations to their knowledge of the patient's normal state. This focus may relieve or increase the anxiety

TABLE 8-1 Middle-Range Role Theories of Symbolic Interactionism	
MIDDLE-RANGE ROLE THEORY	**DESCRIPTION**
Theory of interpersonal competence	Ability to function effectively in long-term and fairly complex human relationships. Four mental phenomena related to interpersonal competence are defined: number of cultural symbols; role-taking ability; repertory of role skills; complexity of self-conceptions.
Situation theory	Situations that are defined as real, are real in their consequences. A "situation" is what or how an individual perceives something to be. The meaning is the essential element.
Theory of satisfaction	Central concept of "satisfaction" is defined as an individual's affective response varying in amount of gratification with something.

A theory of role enactment	Central concept is quality of role enactment, which is related to:
	  Number of roles, and role strain
	  Ease of role transitions or moving in and out of roles and perceived accuracy of contextual alignment of role with circumstances
	Self-role congruence (degree of alignment of role requirements and qualities of self)
	  Consensus on role expectations among parties
	  Sensitivity to role demands by others
	  Audience sanctions (rewards or punishments for complying with role expectations)

Role transition theory	Ease of role transition is a concept that is concerned with difficulty in beginning or ending a role and depends on availability of resources to begin or exit from a role. Variables affecting ease of role transition include anticipatory socialization (process of learning the norms, values, attitudes, and dimensions of the role); role strain; transition procedures; amount of normative change; and facilitation of goal attainment.
A theory of role strain	Role strain is defined as perceived difficulty in fulfilling role obligations. Four variables affect role strain: consensus of expectations; clarity of expectations; diversification or requirement to maintain working relationships with a wide variety of complementary roles; and amount of activity related to role, role accumulation, and role incompatibility.

TABLE 8-2 Comparison of General Family Role Functions Versus Those During Hospitalization of a Family Member for Critical Care

CAPLAN*	SIMPSON†
Includes family members in general.	Includes family members during hospitalization experience.
Collect and disseminate information about the world for its members.	Foster a link between patient and environment external to critical care unit.
Filter, interpret, and make assessments for each other about feedback cues in environment.	
Provide each other with feedback about behavior in terms of family value system. (Families are major source of belief systems for their members.)	Assist patients to cognitively process concerns about health by helping them to solve problems or providing anticipatory guidance.
Guide each other in problem solving or assume this function for an individual member if needed.	
Give practical assistance to each other and serve as a haven for rest and recuperation.	Assist patients with daily functions they cannot perform, such as feeding, comfort, sleep/rest needs, grooming/hygiene, mobility, and elimination (in order of frequency).
	Further positive relationships by offering love and comfort and reinforcing positive self-esteem.

*Reference 10.
†Reference 44.

of the family. Communication with the patient often is increased because of shared intimacy. *Plain talk* refers to eliminating hospital jargon and explaining the situation in terms the family member can understand. If the family does not understand what is happening, they cannot interpret accurately for the patients. *Making sense* relates to the reflection of family members on what the experience means to them and the family. *Making sense* involves maintaining a positive attitude of hope. Although this study provides some insight into how family members perceive the critical care experience, it is up to the reader to infer specific roles that family members perceive as important in helping the patient.

Confusion about the role of the family during critical illness is illustrated in a comparative study of hospital staff (lawyers and medical staff) and family members.[33] Respondents were asked in interviews what created the most difficulty in end-of-life situations. The staff perceived that conflicts arose most often in acute care situations when family members failed to conform to behaviors expected by the staff. When family members disagreed with staff, they were labeled as "dysfunctional." A significant source of tension between staff and families was the differing perceptions of the roles that family members should

have. Sixty family members reported severe stress with the hospitalization of a family member. Family members felt that they had to be an advocate for the patient. If the patient had a chronic disease, the advocacy role was especially stressful because of the perception that the hospital staff did not respect the family's expertise in caring for the patient. Other roles the family members assumed, or were expected by staff to fulfill, included caregiver, trusted companion and link to identity beyond the illness, and surrogate decision maker. The findings reinforced those in Simpson's study and Caplan's framework but also highlighted the differences between staff and families concerning the perceptions of role functions.

Role conflict was also a major theme identified by spouses of critically ill patients in a study conducted by Johnson and colleagues.[27] The conflict resulted from trying to balance many roles as spouse, parent, employee, and support person to the patient and other family members. Family-sensitive care would incorporate the impact of the changing roles of family members and provide assistance or guide family members to resources to assist with new roles they may have to assume. Role theory may assist in helping nurses understand the changing roles of family members and what role they should have in helping the critically ill patient heal. Much more research is needed in this area.

Crisis Theory

The life-threatening nature of a critical illness often propels the family into a crisis state. Contemporary crisis theory is organized around efforts to stabilize families in crisis and/or to use family to stabilize individuals in crisis. A very functional model for crisis intervention is the double ABCX model, by McCubbin and Patterson (Figure 8-2).[38] In this model there is a precrisis (or adjustment) phase and a postcrisis (or adaptation) phase. The meaning of the situation to an individual determines whether the demands are perceived as a threat. The same variables interacting to produce a crisis also produce crisis adaptation. The accumulation of demands (or stressors) produces tension until the demands are met.

McCown and Johnson[37] describe two dimensions of family crisis: instrumental and perceptual. An instrumental crisis occurs when there is a loss of resources because of stressors such as an accident, illness, or sudden financial loss. The family perceives a threat to its physical existence or the existence of a member of the family. This type of crisis occurs suddenly. A perceptual crisis occurs when members perceive that they cannot function as a family unit, or as they previously functioned. There is a sudden behavior shift directed toward a condition that is not changing or is changing very slowly. There is often no clear precipitant of the crisis.

In the instrumental crisis there is reliance on external resources to help the family adapt. The perceptual crisis relies on the family's internal resources to help the system evolve through self-organization to a new level of functioning. Individual family member resources can be knowledge, intelligence, and self-esteem. Family resources include cohesion, adaptability, or communication skills. Chaos theory is most helpful in explaining the dynamics of perceptual crises. The unpredictability of the crisis may assist in helping the family to evolve to a higher level. Instrumental crises respond well to interventions based on crisis theory.[9,37] However, these types of crises can also instigate factors that will surface a perceptual crisis.

Although a person can grow and develop new coping strategies from a crisis, the goals of crisis intervention are to prevent further dysfunction and to return the person (or family) to the precrisis condition. In a study done by Reeder,[43] the family's perception of the critical illness was the key to finding effective interventions to assist the family to adapt positively to the situation.

Critical care nurses work with families in crisis every day. Often the crisis is instrumental, but frequently there is an underlying perceptual crisis further complicating interventions. The primary goal in delivering critical care nursing is to prevent crises from occurring or to minimize the effects of those that do occur. This holds true for emotional as well as physiologic crises. If it is true, as most family therapists believe, that what happens to one family member affects the entire family system, then it is crucial that nurses interact with the family members to prevent or minimize the effects of an acute illness on the family system, or to help the family adapt functionally to the crisis. The support such interventions can provide may allow the family members to better support the critically ill member in healing.[10,38,44]

Maslow's Theory of the Hierarchy of Needs

Another theory that works in concert with crisis theory is Maslow's theory of the hierarchy of needs.[35] Most people want to be the best they can be, but unmet needs may interfere with growth. Maslow defines five basic needs that need to be met in a certain order. From the lowest level to the highest, these needs are physiologic, safety, belongingness or social needs, esteem, and self-actualization. During a crisis, individuals often regress to the lowest level needs of this hierarchy. An understanding of this movement assists

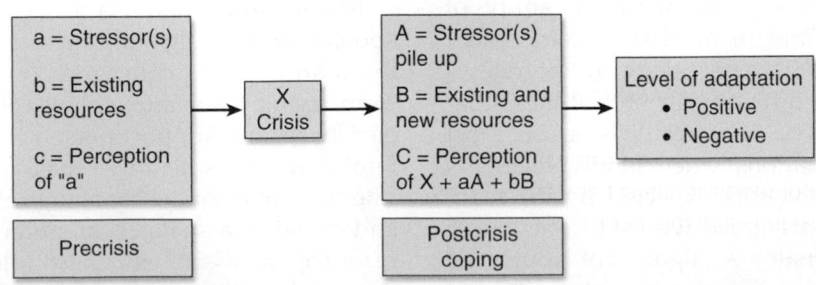

◆FIGURE 8-2 The double ABCX model of stress and adaptation.

in understanding behaviors observed and provides a framework to provide interventions to meet such needs. Thus this theory provides a theoretical foundation for understanding and supporting the needs of family members during a critical illness.

In summary, there are a variety of theoretical foundations to providing FCC in the critical care environment. A better understanding of the theories discussed can assist the expert nurse in choosing the most appropriate interventions to meet the needs of an individual patient/family unit. Critical care nurses must be competent in relating to families in crisis and must work with a team of healthcare providers in meeting the challenges of families in crisis.

Small changes in how the staff approaches care (systems thinking) and implements caring practices ("initial conditions") can have significant effects on the outcomes of care. The more difficult the crisis is for a family, the more important it is to match the competencies of the critical care nurse to the patient/family's needs at the various stages of the critical illness. The critical care environment is a complex system within a greater complex system of healthcare. Care delivered in this environment must be holistic, and nurses must view their organizations as social systems in which humans relate to each other. Implementing a FCC environment requires support from the entire system.

Case Study 8-1, Part A

Matching the Patient and Family's Needs

Mr. B. recently underwent a Whipple procedure for pancreatic cancer. Because this procedure involved removal of the head of the pancreas, the attached duodenum, a portion of the bile duct, the gallbladder, and a portion of his stomach, he remained in critical care for an extensive period. Mrs. B. was overwhelmed by the situation and began to display behaviors difficult for the nursing staff to manage. She had a belligerent and challenging tone when questioning staff about Mr. B.'s care. She wanted a complete review of his blood glucose values and the doses of insulin he received daily. She often would receive information about his pain medication and then turn to another staff member immediately and ask if the information was correct. The staff dealt with these behaviors by limiting her time in critical care and distancing themselves from her when she was in the unit. Unfortunately, this behavior had a negative effect on Mr. B. One day, when Mrs. B. was exhibiting this type of behavior during her visit, Mr. B. pulled out his endotracheal tube and told her to "shut up."

Decision point: How does theory help us explain what happened and how we could prevent such a situation?

Case continues on page 153

EVIDENCE-BASED CARE FOR FAMILIES OF THE CRITICALLY ILL

Paradoxically, the very complex nature of family systems may be the underlying reason why nurses find it difficult to work with families in critical care. It is much easier to focus on the patient and attempt to eliminate as much of the chaos or turmoil that occurs in delivering care when family members are present. In a qualitative study describing the breakdown in nursing care of families in the critical care environment, the following five approaches by nurses were identified as constraining forces to family members providing supportive functions for the patient[11]:

1. Distancing the family physically from the patient and the patient's bedside
2. Distancing themselves from the patient and the patient's family
3. Characterizing the family's perspective as pathologic
4. Dissipating responsibility for family care
5. Taking an elemental rather than a systemic perspective in providing care

In seeking solutions to reduce such barriers, extensive research was conducted to identify the perceived needs family members have while experiencing a critical illness in the family.[31,32,47] Despite knowing the needs, studies evaluating effective interventions to support family members during critical illness have not been conclusive.[31,46] If nurses do not know how family members perceive their role in the healing of a critically ill family member, it is difficult to develop systems and interventions to support the family in such a role. The complex nature of the interactions of the patient/family/nurse system may not be amenable to the quantitative evaluations of specific interventions. More qualitative research may assist in evaluating specific interventions.

Family Needs

Molter[40] first identified and quantified needs of family members of critically ill patients. Leske,[30,32] through psychometric evaluation, refined the Critical Care Family Needs Inventory (CCFNI) and grouped the 45 items into 5 concept areas: proximity, assurance, information, support, and comfort needs (Box 8-3). These needs are universally experienced by most families with a critically ill family member. There is a universal need for hope followed by the need for honest information about the patient's condition and the need to feel that staff care about the patient, to have a waiting room near the patient, and to be informed about changes in the patient's condition. The CCFNI has been translated into a number of languages and modified or adapted to a variety of environments, most recently for the emergency department.[37] There is

Box 8-3

Five Categories of Needs Based on the Critical Care Family Needs Inventory

1. **Receiving assurance.** The need for assurance reflects the family's need for reinforcing hope about the patient's outcome. Meeting this need promotes confidence, security, and freedom from doubt about the healthcare team and system.
2. **Remaining near the patient.** The need to be present with the critically ill patient reflects linking and maintaining familial relationships. Meeting this need helps family members remain emotionally close and provide support to the patient.
3. **Receiving information.** The need for information reflects the goal of understanding the patient's condition. Meeting this need lays the foundation for family members' decision making and coaching of the patient. Anxiety is reduced, and sense of control is promoted.
4. **Being comfortable.** The need for comfort reflects reducing distress. When a person is comfortable, energy is conserved, and less stress and anxiety occur.
5. **Having support available.** The need for support reflects seeking or accepting expert help, assistance, or aid. Meeting this need assists with coping with stress, augmenting family resources, and maintaining strength to support the patient.

From reference 32.

no evidence that the needs vary significantly from cultural factors.[29,32]

There is evidence that the needs for information and proximity to the patient are often met; however, the needs for assurance, comfort, and support were frequently not met.[18,31,32] This may be related to the fact that nurses and families rarely agree on such needs as to feel accepted by hospital staff, to help with physical care, to be informed about transfers, or to visit the patient frequently.[28] There also is evidence that nurses and families have different perceptions of the role of the family in critical care.[25] Families feel they have an important role while nurses need to maintain control of the environment and their perception of the patient's needs. Although nurses do feel it is important for them to comfort the family, they find it challenging to communicate with families in crisis.[29] While family needs are well identified, the family's role in critical care needs further exploration; nurses need to develop competencies to manage complex family dynamics during the critical illness of a family member.

Family Presence

In extensive reviews of the literature related to visiting in adult critical care,[32,47] as well as presence during resuscitation procedures,[22] movement toward less restricted, more liberal policies to allow family presence in critical care is recommended. There is, however, no consensus on an ideal visiting policy; some do not perceive family as "visitors."[36,41] However, evidence shows that having the family present with the patient in critical care is not detrimental to the patient, may actually help the patient heal, and is definitely helpful to the family in coping with the trauma of critical illness.[21] This holds true for children visiting in adult critical care.[12] There is no evidence of increased litigation related to the family's presence during emergency life-saving procedures.[21] Families want and expect to be near a critically ill member during hospitalization.[19] There should not be a "one policy fits all" approach.[45] Each family unit should be evaluated and a schedule for being with the patient negotiated. "Visiting hours" is a tradition that must go the way of other traditions shown by research to be detrimental to patients.[36,40,41] Families need help in determining what role they should play in helping the patient heal. Often they are the "expert" in terms of how the patient is responding. Therefore they need to be an important part of the team.

Family-Centered Interventions and Outcomes

The essence of nursing is caring. The Synergy Model addresses the caring practices required for healing as they are integrated with other interventions driven by the patient's needs. Exploring the essence of nursing related to families of critical care patients, Warren[50] used a grounded theory methodology to elicit the meaning of caring behaviors used by the nurses in the critical care waiting room. The guided interviews explored nurses' behaviors perceived as caring, the personal importance of engaging in caring transactions, the role of reciprocity, and any other information the family believed was important.

Four categories emerged from the data. *Informing* is the behavior of providing information about the patient's condition and treatment. Dialogue is an essential element of this behavior to ensure that the family is oriented to the situation; the family should be encouraged to share their stories. *Enhancing* is defined as behaviors that intensify and magnify the spirit of the family group. Open, honest communication promotes trust and confidence in the nurses and their care. Eye contact and facial expressions are nonverbal cues perceived by the family as reassurance from the nurse. Understanding messages of encouragement gives hope. Factual information provides family members realistic appraisal of the patient's progress. *Touching* is perceived as one of the most important behaviors exhibited by nurses. It conveys nurturing and compassion that are perceived by family members as helping with their healing process. *Spiriting* relates to the behaviors of a nurse in terms of healing powers and being guided by a higher power. Spiriting enhances the ability of the nurse to detect changes in the status of the patient.

Because a critical illness of a family member is a crisis for the family, how the healthcare team involves the family has significant impact on how the family will respond to the crisis and adapt to the changes occurring in the family.[4,31,46] Most recently, the effects of having family members present during life-saving and invasive procedures and improving communications with families at the end of life have indicated that such interventions can assist families to adapt functionally to the crisis and lead to reduced length of stays and resource utilization.[1,3,21] Family presence during critical illness or end of life should not be dependent on a particular nurse being on duty. It should be a right that all families have. The healthcare team should develop expertise in planning the methods that will be the most effective for an individual family situation.

◆ Case Study 8-1, Part B

Matching the Patient and Family's Needs

Both staff and Mrs. B. need assistance in developing insight into the reasons behind Mrs. B.'s behavior. Clearly, without the help of Mrs. B., Mr. B. will continue to suffer and healing will be delayed. Mrs. B. needs to be with her husband and he needs her to be there for support. However, without a plan to meet Mrs. B.'s specific needs, her presence was detrimental to Mr. B. With some specific interventions negotiated with Mrs. B., the staff was able to meet her needs and those of her husband, and achieve mutual goals for the rapid healing of Mr. B. Assistance for this family required involvement of all disciplines and a systems approach to providing care.

The surgical intensive care staff caring for Mr. B. asked for help from the clinical nurse specialist in evaluating Mrs. B.'s needs and assisting staff in developing an effective plan of care to meet the needs of Mr. and Mrs. B. and the staff. The CNS spoke with Mrs. B. and learned she was very fearful that her husband would die. The only information Mrs. B. received from the staff that she understood was the need to monitor glucose and provide insulin as needed. Mrs. B. also was very upset when she saw Mr. B. in pain. She wanted to be with him as much as possible but had to care for her teenage children. Visiting hours were very restricted and inconvenient for Mrs. B. After Mr. B. extubated himself, Mrs. B. understood that her behavior was hurting her husband.

Decision point: What evidence is available to formulate an effective plan of care to help this family?

Case continues on page 156

IMPLEMENTING FAMILY-CENTERED CRITICAL CARE

It is unclear which nurse behaviors help family members improve their role as healers. More research is needed to answer this question fully. However, the implementation of FCC appears to be a step forward in achieving collaboration with families so that their energy can be used to help a family member heal. Once such programs are established, they can be studied for their effectiveness. FCC is not a new concept; pediatric and obstetric units have been providing such care for a long time. It may be difficult to establish a FCC program in a unit with a history of patient-focused care; most adult critical care units are patient focused. With some practical planning, it can happen.[15,23,26,29] The Chest Foundation, in conjunction with Eli Lilly and Company Foundation, developed a Critical Care Family Assistance Program (CCFAP) to respond to the unmet needs of family of critically ill patients.[29] The program model is based on five principles emphasizing the importance of a systemic approach to providing resources and support to families during the period of critical care (Box 8-4). The program was piloted in several facilities; a replication tool kit can be obtained through AACN or the Chest Foundation. The CCFAP is also in agreement with the *AACN Standards for Establishing and Sustaining Healthy Work Environments*[5] that promotes the necessity of excellent communication and true collaboration for safe and effective critical care.

Unit and Organizational Assessment

A necessary first step is to obtain commitment for FCC from all stakeholders, including administration, physicians, nursing staff, families, and patients. Clarification of what FCC is for all involved should begin the process. Box 8-5 summarizes key points to remember in this clarification process. To obtain the input from patients and families, the use of focus groups to validate that this is a welcomed direction in care may be helpful. Having direct input from patients and families may be the impetus for staff to embrace the need to adopt the FCC approach to care. Using a survey to identify staff attitudes toward family presence and visitation policies[15] will provide necessary information useful to both making change and evaluating the impact of the change. The focus groups and staff survey can serve as a baseline measurement for performance improvement once FCC is implemented. Without the commitment of all stakeholders, it will be difficult to truly adopt FCC. Henneman and colleagues[23] also suggest including security personnel in planning and education so that family issues are not confused with security or confidentiality issues. The potential for violence can be significant in

Box 8-4

Principles of the Critical Care Family Assistance Program Model

1. Healthcare organizations have a responsibility to foster an environment that protects the physical and emotional health of severely stressed family members who assemble in their facilities to participate in the treatment of a relative.
2. Any family-friendly or patient-friendly program must ultimately justify its presence in a hospital by demonstrating over time that it can have a positive impact on key issues, such as the health of the patient, length of stay in the hospital, satisfaction of family members, and cost-effectiveness.
3. Nothing is as effective in meeting needs and promoting satisfaction, not only with the families but also with the hospital staff, as improved and consistent communication. All members of the staff must be able to depend on every other team member to be faithful to communication responsibilities.
4. The implementation of a program, such as the CCFAP, requires a staff that is able to think and act in nontraditional ways. This ability to work constructively "outside the box" becomes a hallmark of a family-friendly program.
5. While the ICU is the contact point for family members, the unit itself only exists as a part of the larger whole—the hospital. The CCFAP can only succeed when the goals and objectives of the program are in harmony with the priorities of the hospital. The changes made in the ICU must be integrated into the goals and objectives of the hospital and at other points in the care of critically ill patients.

Data from reference 29.

Box 8-5

Family-Centered Critical Care: What It Is and Is Not

WHAT IT *IS*

Family-centered care is a philosophical approach for providing care to patients and their families. The basic premise of this philosophy is that patients are part of a larger "whole" of which we must be aware if we are to provide the best possible care.

Family-centered care is care that demands a collaborative approach to care in which *all* members of the team support and value this philosophy.

Providing care that is family centered means that we recognize our responsibility to help the family as well as the patient survive the crisis of an illness. It means we have an obligation to meet the three basic needs of the family:

1. The need for information
2. The need for reassurance/support
3. The need to be near the patient

WHAT IT IS *NOT*

Family-centered care is *not* new. Many clinicians (such as in pediatrics) have been practicing family-centered care for a long time with much success.

Family-centered care does *not* mean that staff must relinquish all decision making to patients' family members. Patients' families need and appreciate structure and guidance during a time of crisis.

Family-centered care does *not* mean that the patients' families have the right to be rude or abusive to staff.

Family-centered care is *not* difficult, but it requires a thoughtful and caring appreciation of the needs of the patients and their families.

Data from reference 23.

critical care but it should not prevent patients and families from being together.

When everyone is clearly oriented to FCC, a multidisciplinary team needs to be developed to design a basic policy statement and an implementation plan. A unit policy statement clearly states the unit has adopted the principles of FCC. Supporting policies may also be needed, especially a policy defining when family can be in the unit. Having all staff members sign the policy documents may help in ensuring that individual staff members understand what FCC is and are committed to its implementation. One of the biggest frustrations for families is inconsistency among staff in interpreting unit rules.

The implementation plan should be constructed to ensure that there are strategies and tools in place to educate staff and families, and to evaluate patient/family and staff satisfaction. Designing outcome measures of implementing FCC care is important at the beginning of the process. The CCFAP tool kit can provide assistance with these processes.

Strategies and Tools for Implementing Family-Centered Care

An understanding of the needs of the population of families coming to the unit is foundational to implementing FCC. Use of a tool like the CCFNI may assist in focusing on what types of needs are most important. It is also an opportunity to gather evidence of how well the needs are perceived as being met. From this assessment, educational tools for the staff can be structured to focus on strategies to meet the unmet needs. For example, if the need to be with the patient is of high priority, what does your unit do to facilitate this need? What messages or signs are posted outside your unit describing access to the unit? How does staff feel about having families in the unit based on a family's need rather than the staff's need? How do physicians feel about family being at the bedside? From experience, eliminating set visiting hours will be one of the most difficult "traditions" to change! Videotaping your family focus groups or having family members and past patients speak with the staff provide powerful messages to staff about how important FCC is to the family. Documentation templates that assist staff in assessing family-focused needs will be useful. Box 8-6 outlines elements that should be addressed in these tools.

It is also important to develop educational resources for the family. The family may have past experiences with critical illness and have preconceived ideas of how they will be treated. Written and oral educational tools are helpful. Types of care that family members can assist with, such as bathing, oral care, or simple range of motion, should be included. Develop some way to communicate to other staff members what types of care family members are providing for the patient. Remember, inconsistency among staff approaches to family causes frustration.

FCC is a team effort that needs to include a variety of disciplines. Nurses are not the only staff that need to work with families. In a recent study, physicians were identified by families as being more controlling than bedside nurses, with physicians' refusal to share information being the biggest complaint for families interacting with physicians.[4] The creation of referral guidelines for chaplains, social workers, and clinical specialists may help promote more consistent FCC among all healthcare personnel. Education about FCC for other staff working with the patient at the bedside (e.g., physical and respiratory therapists, dietitians) should be developed, using those specialists to assist in providing education related to working with families under stress. Satisfaction with care is often based on interactions with all staff members, not just nurses.

A method to formally evaluate satisfaction with care should be implemented and incorporated into the unit performance improvement plan. Staff should be involved in the development of a unit-based satisfaction survey administered after discharge from critical care to another unit in the hospital. This should be an anonymous survey reflective of recent recall of events. Such a survey provides staff a way to evaluate the perception of the care provided to families and patients. Eventually, there can be predictors of satisfaction based on a model of FCC.[16]

Once the FCC program is implemented, it needs to be sustained and supported. Management should consider hiring staff that will support FCC. Ongoing continuing education is needed to help staff deal with difficult family situations and issues. Consultants such as advance practice nurses, chaplains, and psychology staff can assist in providing education to other staff or with debriefing critical incidents related to family.[7] It is helpful to use performance improvement methods to tackle specific issues identified through staff meetings or family satisfaction surveys.

EVALUATION OF OUTCOMES

Before implementing FCC, strategies must be designed to measure current outcomes of care. Both family needs and the degree to which those needs are being met need to be evaluated. Data reflecting the average length of stay adjusted for the severity of illness will be helpful. Assessment of staff turnover rate and satisfaction with unit policies related to families should be included in this initial data collection. Assessment of the patient/family level of satisfaction with care as currently delivered is vital. After implementation of the FCC approach, the same outcomes should be evaluated 4, 6, and 12 months later.

Box 8-6

Elements of an Effective Documentation Template for Assessing Family Structure

- Who will be staying with the patient on a regular basis?
- Who is the family spokesperson to be contacted for vital updates?
- Who usually supports the family in times of crisis? Does the patient have other family, church members, or support groups?
- When is the best time for the family to communicate with the healthcare team? Who should the family contact for information about sudden changes in condition?
- Would the family like to be present during morning rounds when the patient's condition and plan of care are reviewed?
- What else does the staff need to know about the family to help them during this stressful time?

▲ Case Study 8-1, Part C

Matching the Patient and Family's Needs

Mrs. B. stayed at Mr. B.'s bedside during times that she easily could be away from home responsibilities. She was able to stay quietly at the bedside and perform small comfort measures for Mr. B. He visibly relaxed when she was there. She was more relaxed because she trusted the staff to call her if there were major changes in Mr. B.'s condition when she was not at the hospital. Staff recognized the need and right of Mr. and Mrs. B. to be together during this difficult time for their family. Mrs. B.'s presence was very important for Mr. B. She provided reassurance and support for him. Plans were made for the children to visit on a regular basis.

Decision point: What outcomes might be expected as a result of this new plan of care?

CONCLUSIONS

This chapter has introduced the need for FCC and reviewed the theoretical foundations for such an approach. A review of evidence-based practice related to family needs, family presence, and family-centered interventions and outcomes was presented. Finally, strategies and tools for implementing FCC were discussed and suggested measures of satisfaction and outcome were presented. In our complex and mobile society, the stress of a critical illness poses a significant burden on the entire family. The Research Utilization box below discusses this issue further. Now is the time to challenge and change our approach to caring for the critically ill. Providing care to the patient and family as a unit of care is critical to long-term outcomes for the family. Using the research related to FCC is essential in developing cost-effective programs.

▲ RESEARCH UTILIZATION

Categories of Needs Among Families of Critically Ill Patients

CLINICAL ISSUE

Research indicates that families of critically ill patients have five general categories of needs: need for information, proximity, comfort, reassurance, and support. The need for clear and honest information is of the highest priority and often is not met. Family members also experience significant stress with critical care hospitalization of a family member. What is the relationship between satisfaction of needs met, signs and symptoms of acute stress disorder, interpersonal perception of healthcare staff, and the level of optimism of the family member?

SUMMARY

This study assessed 1 family representative for each of 40 patients admitted to a surgical trauma ICU in one East Coast level I trauma center. Assessment tools included a 14-item modified version of the Critical Care Family Needs Inventory, the Acute Stress Disorder Scale, the Brief Symptom Inventory, the Impact Message Inventory, and the Life Orientation Test administered at time of admission (mean = 3 days) and at time of discharge (mean = 30 days). Unmet needs involved lack of information about the patient's condition and why actions/procedures were being done. The Acute Stress Disorder scores were approximately the same as those for patients admitted to a psychiatric hospital for posttraumatic stress disorder. However, the scores decreased to normal once the patient was discharged. Family representatives perceived physicians as more controlling than nurses, and this affected satisfaction with needs met. The more optimistic the family representatives were, the more they were satisfied that their needs were met.

APPLICATION

Family members of critically ill patients will likely be stressed and require interpersonal contact to determine their needs. Other disciplines (e.g., chaplains and social workers) can assist with reducing anxiety. However, information needs are significant early in the hospitalization and should be provided by both physicians and nurses. Family members will adapt to stress and staff should help them be optimistic about coping with the stress of the critical illness. It requires diligence on the part of the critical care team and planning with the family to assist them during this stressful period.

NEED FOR FURTHER STUDY

Healthcare organizations want their customers to be happy, and meeting the needs of critically ill family members is important for the patient and family dynamics. More research will be needed to validate the effectiveness of FCC programs.

Auerbach, S. M., et al. (2005). Optimism, satisfaction with needs met, interpersonal perceptions of the healthcare team, and emotional distress in patients' family members during critical care hospitalization. *Am J Crit Care*, 14(3), 202–210.

REFERENCES

1. Ahrens, T., Yancey, V., & Kollef, M. (2003). Improving family communications at the end-of-life: implications for length of stay in the intensive care unit and resource use. *Am J Crit Care, 12,* 317–324.

2. American Association of Critical-Care Nurses Certification Corp. (2003). *The synergy model of certified practice.* Available at www.aacn.org/certcorp.

3. American Association of Critical-Care Nurses (AACN). (2004). *Practice alert: family presence during CPR and invasive procedures.* Available at www.aacn.org.

4. Auerbach, S. M., et al. (2005). Optimism, satisfaction with needs met, interpersonal perceptions of the healthcare team, and emotional distress in patients' family members during critical care hospitalization. *Am J Crit Care, 14*(3), 202–210.

5. Barden, C. (Ed.) (2005). *AACN standards for establishing and sustaining healthy work environments: a journey to excellence.* Aliso Viejo, Calif: American Association of Critical-Care Nurses.

6. Berwick, D., & Kotagel, M. (2004). Restricted visiting hours in ICUs. Time to change. *JAMA, 292*(6), 736–737.

7. Bradley, C. P. (1992). Turning anecdotes into data—the critical incident technique. *Family Practice, 9*(1), 98–103.

8. Burr, W. R., et al. (1979). Symbolic interaction and the family. In W. R. Burr, R. Hill, F. I. Nye, et al. (Eds.), *Contemporary theories about the family* (Vol 2, pp 42–111). New York: The Free Press.

9. Butz, M. R., Chamberlain, L. L., & McCown, W. G. (1997). *Strange attractors, chaos, complexity, and the art of family therapy.* New York: Wiley & Sons.

10. Caplan, G. (1982). The family as a support system. In H. McCubbin, A. Cauble & J. Patterson (Eds.), *Family stress, coping, and social support.* Springfield, Ill: Charles C. Thomas.

11. Chesla, C. A., & Stannard, D. (1997). Breakdown in the nursing care of families in the ICU. *Am J Crit Care, 6*(1), 64–71.

12. Clark, C., & Harrison, D. (2001). The needs of children visiting on adult intensive care units: a review of the literature and recommendations for practice. *J Adv Nurs, 34*(1), 61–68.

13. Cullen, L., Titler, M., & Drahozal, R. (2003). Family and pet visitation in the critical care unit. *Crit Care Nurs, 23*(5), 62–66.

14. Coppa, D. F. (1993). Chaos theory suggests a new paradigm for nursing science. *J Adv Nurs, 18*(6), 985–991.

15. Damboise, C., & Cardin, S. (2003). Family-centered critical care. *AJN, 103*(6), 56AA–56EE.

16. Dowling, J., et al. (2005). A model of family-centered care and satisfaction predictors: the critical care family assistance program. *Chest, 128,* 81S–92S.

17. Edelman, L. (Ed.) (1995). *Getting on board: training activities to promote the practice of family-centered care* (2nd ed.). Bethesda, Md: Association for the Care of Children's Health.

18. Gavaghan, S. R., & Carroll, D. L. (2002). Families of critically ill patients and the effect of nursing interventions. *Dimensions Crit Care Nurs, 21*(2), 64–71.

19. Gonzales, C. E., et al. (2004). Visiting preferences of patients in the intensive care unit and in a complex care medical unit. *Am J Crit Care, 13*(3), 194–198.

20. Hagerty, B. M. K., et al. (1993). An emerging theory of human relatedness. *Image: J Nurs Scholar, 25*(4), 291–296.

21. Halm, M. A. (2005). Family presence during resuscitation: a critical review of the literature. *Am J Crit Care, 14*(6), 494–511.

22. Hartrick, G. (1997). Relational capacity: the foundation for interpersonal nursing practice. *J Adv Nurs, 26,* 523–528.

23. Henneman, E., & Cardin, S. (2002). Family-centered critical care: a practical approach to making it happen. *Crit Care Nurse, 22,* 12–19.

24. Holden, J., Harrison, L., & Johnson, M. (2002). Families, nurse and intensive care patients: a review of the literature. *J Clin Nurs, 11,* 140–148.

25. Hupcey, J. E. (1999). Looking out for the patient and ourselves—the process of family integration into the ICU. *J Clin Nurs, 8,* 253–262.

26. Jansen, M., & Schmitt, N. A. (2003). Family-focused interventions. *Crit Care Nurs Clin North Am, 15,* 347–354.

27. Johnson, S. K., et al. (1995). Perceived changes in adult family members' roles and responsibilities during critical illness. *Image: J Nurs Scholar, 27*(3), 238–243.

28. Kosco, M., & Warren, N. (2000). Critical care nurses' perceptions of family needs met. *Crit Care Nurs Q, 23,* 60–72.

29. Lederer, M. A., Goode, T., & Dowling, J. (2005). Origins and development: the critical care family assistance program. *Chest, 128,* 65S–75S.

30. Leske, J. S. (1991). Internal psychometric properties of the Critical Care Family Needs Inventory. *Heart Lung, 20,* 236–244.

31. Leske, J. S., & Jiricka, M. K. (1998). Impact of family demands and family strengths and capabilities on family well-being and adaptation after critical injury. *Am J Crit Care, 7*(5), 383–392.

32. Leske, J. S., & Pasquale, M. A. (2007). Family needs, interventions, and presence. In: Molter NC, ed. *AACN Protocols for Practice: Creating Healing Environments* (2nd ed.). Sudbury, MA: Jones and Bartlett.

33. Levine, C., & Zuckerman, C. (1999). The trouble with families: toward an ethic of accommodation. *Ann Intern Med, 130,* 148–152.

34. Lewin, R. (1993). *Life at the edge of chaos.* London: Dent.

35. Maslow, A. H. (1970). *Motivation and personality* (2nd ed.). New York: Harper Collins.

36. Mason, D. J. (2000). Families: in the way? *AJN, 100*(2), 7.

37. McCown, W. G., & Johnson, J. (1993). *Therapy with treatment resistant families, a consultation-crisis intervention model.* New York: Hayworth.

38. McCubbin, H., & Patterson, J. (1983). The family stress process: the double ABCX model of family adjustment and adaptation. In H. McCubbin, M. Sussman & J. Patterson (Eds.), *Social stress and the family: advances and developments in family stress theory and research.* New York: Haworth Press.

39. Medina, J. (2005). A natural synergy in creating a patient-focused care environment: the critical care family assistance program and critical care nursing. *Chest, 128,* 99S–102S.

40. Molter, N. C. (1979). Needs of relatives of critically ill patients: a descriptive study. *Heart Lung, 20,* 229–235.

41. Molter, N. C. (1994). Families are not visitors in the critical care unit. *Dimensions Crit Care Nurs, 13,* 2–3.

42. Redley, B., & Beanland, C. (2004). Revising the Critical Care Family Needs Inventory for the emergency department. *J Adv Nurs, 45*(1), 95–104.

43. Reeder, J. M. (1991). Family perception: a key to intervention. *AACN Clin Issues, 2*(2), 188–194.

44. Simpson, T. (1991). The family as a source of support for the critically ill adult. *AACN Clin Issues, 2*(2), 229–235.

45. Slota, M., et al. (2003). Perspectives on family-centered, flexible visitation in the intensive care setting. *Crit Care Med, 31*(5), S262–S266.

46. Swoboda, S. M., & Lipsett, P. A. (2002). Impact of a prolonged surgical critical illness on patients' families. *Am J Crit Care, 11,* 459–466.

47. Titler, M. G. (1998). Family visitation and partnership in the critical care unit. In M. Chulay & N. C. Molter (Eds.), *Protocols for practice: creating a healing environment series.* Aliso Viejo, Calif: American Association of Critical-Care Nurses.

48. Tomlinson, P. S., et al. (2002). Clinical innovation for promoting family care in paediatric intensive care: demonstration, role modeling and reflective practice. *J Adv Nurs, 38*(2), 161–170.

49. Walters, A. J. (1995). A hermeneutic study of the experiences of relatives of critically ill patients. *J Adv Nurs, 22,* 998–1005.

50. Warren, N. A. (1994). The phenomena of nurses' caring behaviors as perceived by the critical care family. *Crit Care Nurs Q, 17*(3), 67–72.

51. Wheatley, M. J. (2002). *Leadership and the new science. Discovering order in a chaotic world* (2nd ed.) San Francisco: Berrett-Koehler.

52. Wright, L. M., & Leahey, M. (2002). *Nurses and families. A guide to family assessment and intervention* (3rd ed.). Philadelphia: F. A. Davis.

CHAPTER 9

Improving Outcomes Through Prophylaxis

Denise M. Lawrence, Vicki S. Good, and Karen K. Carlson

Critical care units are considered some of the most complex and hazardous environments in acute care. Annually, between 4 and 5 million patients are admitted to critical care across the United States.[51] Many patients suffer potentially preventable morbidity and mortality during their hospitalizations; mortality rates have been estimated between 10% and 25%, depending on the complexity of the critical care unit.[2,51,69] Improvements in care processes have been shown to yield improvements in both clinical and financial outcomes for the critically ill patient.*

Historically, hospitals initiated critical care units to "concentrate" the sickest patients into one location. By the late 1970s the clinical effectiveness of critical care units began to be explored. Efforts to improve care focused on structure and peer review, along with written documentation of policies, procedures, and patient care. The 1980s brought explosive increases in technologies and therapies; however, little attention was paid to assessing clinical outcomes associated with these advances.[4] During the 1990s quality improvement activities focused on process tools and scales to assess and compare morbidity and mortality. By the end of the 1990s and into this century, clinical practice became driven by evidence-based outcomes. Continuous quality improvement efforts are focused on systems and processes of care versus attention to individual clinicians.[10]

This chapter will describe implementable preventive strategies that may improve the outcomes of critically ill patients. Rapid response teams will be discussed along with prophylactic strategies for prevention of venous thromboembolism (VTE), stress ulcer, central line infection, and ventilator-associated pneumonia (VAP).

Prophylactic interventions, with a focus on improving outcomes, should be an ongoing initiative. As new treatment recommendations and protocols become available, they should be used to guide clinicians in caring for patients, using the latest clinical evidence.

*References 2, 10, 11, 23, 39, 41, 45, 50, 53, 66, 68.

RAPID RESPONSE TEAMS

As part of the Institute for Healthcare Improvement's (IHI) 100K Lives campaign, the concept of a rapid response team (RRT) (also known as a medical emergency team [MET]) was introduced as a way to improve overall mortality in the acute care setting.[37] Foundational to the development of RRTs was the revelation that patients were dying unnecessarily in hospitals on a daily basis.[17,37] Therefore, challenged to explore opportunities to address this issue, RRTs were introduced into many healthcare institutions throughout the United States.

The goal of assessment and intervention by an RRT is to respond to patients as their clinical condition is deteriorating before they suffer cardiopulmonary arrest.[25,30,31,55] Studies have confirmed that between 60% and 70% of patients demonstrate clinical signs of physiologic instability before cardiopulmonary arrest (Box 9-1).* The RRT should be activated anytime serious physiologic changes occur in the patient's status or whenever the clinician is uncomfortable with symptoms the patient is displaying. Many RRT programs use the criteria listed in Box 9-1 to determine trigger

*References 6, 7, 25, 31, 33, 55.

Box 9-1

Clinical Warning Signs of Cardiopulmonary Arrest

- Mean arterial pressure less than 70 or greater than 130 mm Hg
- Heart rate less than 40 or greater than 130 beats per minute
- Respiratory rate less than 8 or greater than 30 breaths per minute
- Acute changes in pulse oximetry saturation to less than 90% despite oxygen administration
- Acute changes in urine output to less than 50 ml in 4 hours
- Chest pain
- Altered mental status

points for activation of the team. The overall goal of the RRT is to use the clinical expertise and skills of critical care personnel at the bedside of a patient becoming ill no matter the patient's location within an acute care facility. Therefore the RRT represents a proactive model of prophylaxis for acutely ill patients.

The role of the RRT is multifunctional and includes assessment and stabilization of the patient, assistance with the communication among all team members, education and support of the staff who activated the team, and lastly, assistance with the proper placement of the patient after intervention (patients may stay on the unit where they were previously located or be transferred to a higher level of care). The team often uses standardized delegated medical orders to guide the care provided to the patient. These orders (Figure 9-1) include diagnostic testing and medical interventions to assist with stabilization of the patient.

The composition of an RRT varies from facility to facility. Each facility determines the best model for their team on the basis of the availability of clinical resources. Some examples of types of team composition include a critical care registered nurse and respiratory therapist (RT); or a critical care registered nurse, respiratory therapist, and medical resident, intensivist, hospitalist, or physician assistant.[37,45] No model has demonstrated superiority over other models.[37]

The clinical outcomes of the RRT model are somewhat controversial. The original goal of the RRT program was to decrease hospital cardiopulmonary arrests.[3,7,28,32,56] While researchers have successfully proven this goal, others have questioned the methodologies used to measure such success.[68] Some patients have benefited from earlier implementation of "do not resuscitate" (DNR) interventions when the patient displayed signs and symptoms of deterioration versus addressing DNR status during a cardiopulmonary arrest situation.[20,39] Other possible benefits of RRTs include improved teamwork and communications among caregivers; improved nurse, physician, and patient satisfaction; increased nursing retention; and financial benefits.[17,32] All of these benefits require further research before their clinical significance can be demonstrated.

VENOUS THROMBOEMBOLISM

Thromboembolic disease is a significant source of morbidity and mortality for the critical care patient. Many patients in the critical care unit have associated risk factors for the development of a VTE (Box 9-2). The many risk factors for VTE before critical care admission (including age, previous thromboembolic event, heredity, immobility, malignancy, obesity, and myocardial infarction) are complicated once in critical care because of common sedation and paralysis, central venous line catheters, and mechanical ventilation, which heighten the risk for VTE. In fact, 10% to 30% of medical and surgical critical care unit patients develop a VTE within the first week of critical care unit admission.[26] All critically ill patients are at risk for VTE. There is no best treatment for prevention, but data have supported that the use of some form of prophylaxis decreases the incidence of VTE and improves patient outcomes. These interventions may include early ambulation, use of elastic stockings or sequential compression devices, or pharmacologic intervention such as warfarin (Coumadin) or enoxaparin (Lovenox).[26,61] Prevention of VTE is the key in the critically ill patient population, because diagnosis and treatment are complicated once a VTE develops (Box 9-3).

Thromboprophylaxis in the critically ill patient is effective in preventing the development of VTEs. However, the methods of prophylaxis proven in one patient population cannot be generalized to another. Many forms of deep venous prophylaxis are available. Mobility is a simple and highly effective tool to fight thrombus formation. Ambulation prevents venous stasis through position change and muscle contraction. If patients are unable to ambulate, active range of motion should be encouraged. Passive range of motion does help to prevent venous stasis, but does not have the benefit of muscle contraction. Mobility is something that can be taught to the patient and family and is a way of involving them in the care.

Elastic stockings have been shown to be effective in preventing a VTE in some populations. Although the exact mechanism for preventing a VTE is unclear, it is hypothesized that stockings prevent venous pooling by compressing the diameter of the veins. Elastic stockings have been shown to be an effective method of preventing a VTE. There is no conclusive evidence that favors thigh-high over knee-high stockings. Proper fitting of the stocking is essential to provide the appropriate compression without causing overcompression. Patients should be fitted according to manufacturers' recommendations in order to achieve the benefits of this therapy.

Sequential compression devices (SCDs) are often used to prevent venous stasis through compression and relaxation of the calf muscles, similar to the effect of muscle contraction. Sequential compression devices have been proven to effectively reduce the risk of a VTE and have been shown to be an effective primary therapy for patients who are unable to receive anticoagulation therapy. There are several types of SCDs including foot, calf, and thigh-high compression as well as graduated, asymmetric, and circumferential

Date	Hour	Nurse Initials	Authorization is granted to supply drugs by nonproprietary name unless the physician writes words "This brand only" after the drug name.
			STANDING DELEGATED MEDICAL ORDER
			Medical Emergency Response Team (MERT)
			MERT to assess patient and initiate the appropriate orders
			☐ Normal saline IV to keep open rate
			☐ Continuous electrocardiogram monitoring
			☐ Insert Foley catheter if urine output < 250 mL in last 8 hr
			☐ Check oxygen saturation
			☐ Oxygen protocol per Respiratory Therapy
			☐ Stat 12-lead ECG
			☐ Stat portable chest x-ray
			Stat labs: • ISTAT (Cg8 cartridge) • Arterial blood gas
			Medications: ☐ Naloxone 0.4 mg IV push times one dose; may repeat one time in 5 min if no response ☐ Flumazenil 0.2 mg IV push times one dose; may repeat one time in 5 min if no response ☐ Acetominophen (Tylenol Extra Strength) 500 mg times two by mouth for a temperature greater than 101.9 °F ☐ Acetominophen (Tylenol Extra Strength) 500 mg by rectum for temperature greater than 101.9 °F if unable to take medications ☐ D50 one ampule IV push times one dose ☐ Albuterol 0.5 mL hand-held nebulizer now times one dose ☐ Xoponex 1.25 mg hand-held nebulizer now times one dose ☐ Atrovent 2.5 mg hand-held nebulizer now times one dose
			☐ Notify patient's physician

Patient Label	**Baylor All Saints Medical Center** **Medical Emergency Response Team** **Orders**

⬍FIGURE 9-1 Sample of rapid response team physician orders.

compression. Studies comparing foot, calf, and thigh-high compression found little difference in effectiveness. However, to achieve adequate compression, foot compression devices required pressures of 130 mm Hg compared with 40 mm Hg necessary for calf compres-sion. There is little evidence favoring the type of compression used. During graduated compression, the air moves sequentially up the leg and then relaxes. The advantage of this therapy has been the extended length of time of compression compared with standard

Box 9-2

Risk Factors for Venous Thromboembolism

Surgery
Trauma (major or lower extremity)
Immobility, paresis
Malignancy
Cancer therapy (hormonal, chemotherapy, or radiotherapy)
Previous VTE
Increasing age
Pregnancy and the postpartum period
Estrogen-containing oral contraception or hormone replacement therapy
Selective estrogen receptor modulators
Acute medical illness
Heart or respiratory failure
Inflammatory bowel disease
Nephrotic syndrome
Myeloproliferative disorders
Paroxysmal nocturnal hemoglobinuria
Obesity
Smoking
Varicose veins
Central venous catheterization
Inherited or acquired thrombophilia

Box 9-3

Interventions for Prevention of VTE

Assessment of clinical risk factors
Selective screening with Doppler
Nonpharmacologic measures (early ambulation, pneumatic compression boots)
Inferior vena cava filter for proximal VTE in presence of contraindication to therapeutic anticoagulation

Data from reference 26.

inflation. Asymmetric compression involves only inflating the area on the back of the leg or foot. Lastly, circumferential devices compress the circumference of the leg or foot evenly.

In 2003 the American College of Chest Physicians published recommendations for VTE prophylaxis in many patient populations.[26,27,35] These guidelines address the concerns about balancing the risk of bleeding against the need for prophylaxis. When determining the appropriate intervention for the prevention of VTE, clinical parameters should be reviewed before initiating any treatment. These recommendations,

TABLE 9-1 Bleeding Risk/Recommendations for Treatment of Venous Thromboembolism

BLEEDING RISK	VTE RISK	RECOMMENDATIONS
Low	Moderate	Low-dose unfractionated heparin
Low	High	Low molecular weight heparin
High	Moderate	Graduated compression stockings or intermittent pneumatic compression; low-dose unfractionated heparin when risk decreases
High	High	Graduated compression stockings or intermittent pneumatic compression, low molecular weight heparin when risk decreases

Data from reference 26.

given in Table 9-1, stratify patients by both their risk for bleeding and their risk for VTE.[26]

All critically ill patients are at risk for VTE. There is no best treatment for prevention, but data have supported that the use of some form of prophylaxis decreases the incidence of VTE and improves patient outcomes. Prevention of VTE is the key in the critically ill patient population because diagnosis is difficult and treatment is hindered due to the high risk for bleeding associated with anticoagulation.

STRESS-RELATED EROSIVE SYNDROME

Knowledge regarding stress-related erosive syndrome (SRES) and stress ulcer prophylaxis has evolved throughout the years and is supported by clinical research and recommendations. This section will discuss the pathophysiology of SRES, risk factors for development, and recommended patient populations for prophylaxis and then conclude with the medication regimen.

The primary function of the upper gastrointestinal tract includes the maintenance of mucosal integrity, acid secretion, and motility.[24] Critical care disease–related physiologic stress places undue strain on these functions, leading to the development of gastrointestinal ulcerations. While there is a strong association between physiologic stress and the development of SRES, the pathophysiology is not entirely understood.[1,24,53]

Patients who undergo a stressful event such as trauma, mechanical ventilation, sepsis, or burns are at risk for developing a hemorrhagic gastritis from stress ulcerations. Stress ulcerations result from multiple factors, including acid hypersecretion, alteration of normal protective mechanisms, reduced mucosal blood flow leading to ischemia, and degeneration of the mucosal lining. These lesions are typically highly vascular and involve multiple sites within the upper gastrointestinal tract, and therefore place the patient at high risk for developing gastrointestinal bleeding.[1]

The pathogenesis of SRES is multifactorial; there is no evidence to support one pathologic finding over another.[1,8,18,24] One of the first pathologic findings implicated is acid hypersecretion. Acid hypersecretion has not been found consistently in patients who develop SRES, nor does a higher pH value (greater than 4.5) prevent the development of SRES.[1,29,48] A second pathologic finding is reduction in mucosal blood flow. The decrease in blood flow leaves the mucosal layer vulnerable to the development of erosions, which may lead to ulcerations or bleeding.[1] The last pathologic finding consistently implicated in SRES development is the alteration of the normal protective mechanisms of the mucosal layer of the gastrointestinal tract. During stress a variety of mediators are released, leading to erosions that may cause ulcerations or bleeding.[1]

There are three different types of gastrointestinal bleeding found in the critically ill patient. Occult bleeding is defined as guaiac-positive gastric aspirate or stool. Overt bleeding is defined as hematemesis, hematochezia, or melena. When a patient with overt bleeding develops hemodynamic instability, need for transfusion, or a drop in hemoglobin level of greater than 2 g/dl, the patient is considered to have clinically important bleeding.[1,24] The incidence of clinically important bleeding has been estimated between 1% and 4% of critically ill patients across the United States.[1,13–15,24,53]

SRES prophylaxis has evolved over the recent past and moved from treating each individual admitted to the critical care unit to judicious use of prophylaxis based on selection of patients with significant predictors.[50] Prophylactic treatment should focus on the individual patient. Two risk factors have been identified as the primary risks for developing clinically significant bleeding: (1) the patient with respiratory failure requiring mechanical ventilation for at least 48 hours; and (2) the patient with a coagulopathy.[1,8,15,18,43] Other contributing risk factors implicated in the development of SRES include sepsis,[1,8,18] prolonged critical care length of stay,[18,57] and high-dose corticosteroids (greater than 250 mg/day).[1,8,18] As the number of risk factors increases, the probability of the patient developing clinically important bleeding increases.[1]

As shown in the Medication table on p. 163, pharmacologic prophylactic treatment of critical care patients is recommended only for those with high risk of clinically important bleeding. It has been estimated that prophylaxis treatment would need to be given to greater than 900 low-risk patients to prevent one episode of bleeding.[1,8,18] The two medication classifications primarily used for pharmacologic prophylaxis include histamine-2 receptor antagonists (H_2RAs) and proton pump inhibitors (PPIs). There is no evidence that one medication regimen is more effective than the other. Therefore there are no specific recommendations for use of one medication regimen rather than the other, nor is there support for combining therapies.[1,18,19,24,43]

The use of sucralfate (Carafate) is somewhat controversial in the literature. The medication is not labeled for the indication of gastrointestinal bleeding prophylaxis despite the strong usage of the medication for this purpose. Sucralfate exerts its effects locally; therefore it must be given orally, which provides limitations in several critical care patients.[1]

As the risk factors of critical care patients are treated or eliminated, the risk for development of SRES decreases. Therefore the current recommendation is discontinuation of pharmacologic prophylaxis upon extubation or with discharge from critical care.[1,43]

BLOODSTREAM INFECTION RELATED TO CENTRAL LINES

The use of intravascular catheters for medication, blood, and fluid administration as well as blood sampling is indispensable in critical care units. However, there is no doubt that the presence of these catheters increases the patient's risk of complications, including catheter-related bloodstream infection (CRBSI).

Patients in the critical care unit have a higher risk of acquiring hospital-associated infections than those in noncritical care areas. Central lines are more commonly inserted in an urgent setting, are in use for a longer period of time, require frequent manipulation, and may be placed in patients who have already become colonized with hospital-acquired organisms. CRBSIs are associated with significant mortality, morbidity, and costs. Patients in critical care are at increased risk for CRBSIs because 48% to 50% of them

MEDICATIONS FOR STRESS-RELATED EROSIVE SYNDROME (SRES)

MEDICATION	ACTIONS	DOSAGE	SPECIAL CONSIDERATIONS
Histamine-2 Receptor Antagonists			
Ranitidine (Zantac)	Inhibits histamine action at H_2 receptors of gastric parietal cells.	150 mg twice daily PO or by nasogastric tube; can also be prepared in a suspension	If creatinine clearance is less than 50 ml/min, reduce dose to 150 mg once daily PO or by nasogastric tube
		or 50 mg every 6–8 hr IV	or 50 mg every 12–24 hr IV; may dose every 12 hours with careful renal monitoring
		or 6.25 mg/hr by continuous IV infusion	
Famotidine (Pepcid)	Inhibits histamine action at H_2 receptors of gastric parietal cells.	20 mg twice daily PO, IV, or by nasogastric tube	If creatinine clearance is less than 30 ml/min, 20 mg once daily PO, IV, or by nasogastric tube
		or 1.7 mg/hr by continuous IV infusion	
Cimetidine (Tagamet)	Inhibits histamine action at H_2 receptors of gastric parietal cells.	300 mg 4 times a day by mouth, nasogastric tube, or intravenously	If creatinine clearance is less than 30 ml/min, 300 mg twice a day by mouth, nasogastric tube, or intravenously
		or 50 mg/hr by continuous intravenous infusion	or 25 mg/hr by continuous intravenous infusion
Proton Pump Inhibitors			
Omeprazole (Prilosec)	Converted to active metabolites that irreversibly bind to and inhibit H^+, K^+, and ATPase. Inhibits hydrogen ion transport into gastric lumen.	40 mg loading dose, then 20–40 mg daily by mouth or nasogastric tube	No dosage adjustments needed for impaired renal function Capsules should be swallowed whole; do not chew or crush
Others			
Sucralfate (Carafate)	Forms a viscous, adhesive barrier on surface of intact mucosa of stomach/duodenum.	1 g 4 times a day PO or by nasogastric tube	Avoid meals and antacids for 30 min to 1 hr before administration of sucralfate No dosage adjustment needed for patients with impaired renal function; however, risk of toxicity may be increased due to accumulation of aluminum

have central venous catheters; an estimated 28,000 patients die of CRBSIs each year.[5]

A catheter-related infection (CRI) is defined as greater than 15 colony-forming units and is identified as colonization (all other cultures negative and no clinical symptoms), local or exit site infection (erythematic, cellulitis, purulence), catheter-related bacteremia (systemic blood cultures positive for identical organism on catheter segment and no other source), or catheter-related sepsis or septic shock.[59] Catheters can become infected from four potential sources: the skin insertion site, the catheter hub(s), hematogenous seeding, and infusate contamination. Care of the catheter after insertion is extremely important in minimizing infection; all medical personnel should follow standardized protocols.

Specific prevention strategies and improved guidelines for the use of intravascular catheter devices can decrease the rate of infection. A number of studies have investigated interventions aimed at decreasing bloodstream infections (BSIs) in critical care and have demonstrated that certain interventions are linked with a statistically significant decrease in infections.[5,16,22,47,66] In 2002 the Centers for Disease Control and Prevention (CDC) published guidelines for the prevention of intravascular catheter-related infections. Each recommendation was made on the basis of the existing science, theoretical rationale, applicability, and economic impact.[9] A summary of those recommendations receiving the strongest level of recommendation (1A: strongly recommended for implementation and strongly supported by well-designed experimental, clinical, or epidemiologic studies, and a strong theoretical rationale) is shown in Box 9-4. Other strategies suggested by the literature include creating a line insertion cart, asking daily whether the catheter can be removed, implementing a checklist to be completed by the nurse or supervising physician before insertion, and empowering nurses to stop procedures if guidelines are not followed.

Catheter-related bloodstream infections are a preventable cause of morbidity and mortality in the critically ill patient. By instituting a quality improvement model with infection control strategies, an education program to increase awareness, a checklist reminder, and empowerment of nurses, a substantial decrease in morbidity and mortality and costs has been shown.

VENTILATOR-ASSOCIATED PNEUMONIA

Ventilator-associated pneumonia (VAP) continues to pose many challenges for the critically ill patient. While the economic burden and clinical outcomes of VAP are unambiguous, ambiguity does exist over strategies for diagnosis, prevention, and management of VAP (Box 9-5).[36,60] Among the hospital-acquired infections, VAP causes the greatest number of deaths, exceeding those resulting from central line infections, severe sepsis, and respiratory tract infections in nonintubated patients.[34,36] In addition to the physiologic toll, there is also an economic toll. It has been estimated the VAP adds an estimated $40,000 to the hospital admission.[63] This section of the chapter will discuss the recommended prevention strategies for VAP.

Box 9-4

Level 1A Recommendations for the Prevention of Intravascular Catheter–Related Infections

- Develop and implement an education program on the insertion and care of central venous catheters for nurses, physicians, and residents. Program should include indications for use, proper insertion procedures, maintenance of catheters, and appropriate infection control strategies.
- Use appropriate hand hygiene before and after palpation of insertion site as well as before and after inserting, replacing, accessing, repairing, or dressing an intravascular catheter.
- Use the catheter, insertion technique, and insertion site with the lowest risk of complications for the anticipated type and duration of the therapy.
- Maintain aseptic technique for the insertion and care of intravascular catheters.
- Use maximal barrier precautions during central venous catheter insertion (cap, mask, sterile gown, sterile gloves, sterile drape).
- Use 2% chlorhexidine preparation for skin antisepsis before insertion and with dressing changes.
- Use sterile gauze or sterile, transparent semipermeable dressing to cover catheter site.
- Do not use topical antibiotic ointments on insertion sites.
- Do not apply organic solvents to the skin before insertion of catheters or during dressing changes.
- Use the subclavian vein as the preferred site for insertion, rather than the jugular or femoral vein.
- Remove any nonessential intravascular catheter.

Data from reference 9.

Definition

One of the challenges in addressing VAP is the lack of consensus on a definition or determination of VAP.[36,62] A patient is deemed to have VAP when he or she has been on a mechanical ventilator for longer than 48 hours and develops new or progressive pulmonary infiltrates with fever, leukocytosis, and purulent tracheobronchial secretions.[7,8]

The incidence of VAP is defined as the number of ventilator-associated pneumonias per 1000 ventilator days.[36] Rello et al. used a multicenter U.S. database to evaluate the epidemiology and outcomes of patients with VAP.[54] These data demonstrated that 9.3% of

Box 9-5

Evidence-Based Practice Guidelines for the Prevention of Ventilator-Associated Pneumonia (VAP)

GASTRIC REFLUX PREVENTION

1. All mechanically ventilated patients, as well as those at high risk for aspiration (e.g., decreased level of consciousness, enteral tube in place), should have the head of the bed elevated at an angle of 30 to 45 degrees unless medically contraindicated.
2. Routinely verify appropriate placement of the feeding tube.

AIRWAY MANAGEMENT

1. If feasible, use an endotracheal tube with a dorsal lumen above the endotracheal cuff to allow drainage (by continuous or intermittent suctioning) of tracheal secretions that accumulate in the patient's subglottic area.
2. Unless contraindicated by the patient's condition, perform orotracheal rather than nasotracheal intubation.
3. Endotracheal tube (ETT) cuff management: Before deflating the cuff of an ETT in preparation for tube removal, or before moving the tube, ensure that secretions are cleared from above the tube cuff.
4. Use only sterile fluid to remove secretions from the suction catheter if the catheter is to be used for reentry into the patient's lower respiratory tract.
5. Perform tracheostomy under aseptic conditions.

ORAL CARE

1. Develop and implement a comprehensive hygiene program.
2. Use an oral chlorhexidine gluconate (0.12%) rinse during the perioperative period on patients who undergo cardiac surgery.

CROSS-CONTAMINATION PREVENTION

1. Hand washing: Decontaminate hands with soap and water or a waterless antiseptic agent after contact with mucous membranes, respiratory secretions, or objects contaminated with respiratory secretions, whether or not gloves are worn.
2. Decontaminate hands with soap and water or a waterless antiseptic agent before and after contact with a patient who has an endotracheal or tracheostomy tube, and before and after contact with any respiratory device that is used on the patient, whether or not gloves are worn.
3. Wear gloves for handling respiratory secretions or objects contaminated with respiratory secretions of any patient.
4. When soiling with respiratory secretions is anticipated, wear a gown and change it after soiling and before providing care to another patient.
5. Room-air humidifiers: Do not use large-volume room-air humidifiers that create aerosols (nebulizers) unless they can be sterilized or subjected to high-level disinfection at least daily and filled only with sterile water.

MOBILIZATION

1. Ambulate as soon as medically indicated in the postoperative period.

EQUIPMENT CHANGES

1. Do not change routinely, on the basis of duration of use, the patient's ventilator circuit. Change the circuit when it is visibly soiled or mechanically malfunctioning. Periodically drain or discard any condensate that collects in the tubing. Do not allow condensate to drain toward the patient.
2. Between use on different patients, sterilize or subject to high-level disinfection all manual resuscitation bags.

From reference 9a.

patients requiring mechanical ventilation for greater than 24 hours developed VAP. Stephan et al. disclosed a VAP rate in the trauma patient population of 44%.[62] Because of the variability of the definition of VAP, it is difficult to determine a true "incidence" of VAP.[36] Efforts of critical care clinicians should be to bring the incidence of VAP to zero.

PATIENT OUTCOMES OF VAP

Despite the disagreement on the incidence, there is agreement that VAP increases the risk of mortality and length of stay in the critical care unit, and increases the length of time on the mechanical ventilator.[34,36,54,62] Rello et al. found an increase of 9.6 additional days of mechanical ventilation, 6.1 additional days in the critical care unit, and 11.5 additional days in the hospital.[54] Patients who develop VAP have an associated mortality risk of 46% compared with 32% for those patients who do not develop VAP.[34]

Ventilator Bundle of Care

During the work by the IHI to decrease mortality of hospitalized patients, "bundles of care" were defined.

A bundle of care is individual interventions or best practices for a specific disease process that when grouped together have an even greater positive impact on the patient outcome. Interventions are placed on a bundle on the basis of multiple factors, including demonstrated patient outcomes, cost, ease of implementation, and basic fundamentals of care. Therefore each and every possible intervention has not been placed on the ventilator bundle, but only those interventions proven most effective and reliable. To obtain the maximum effect of the bundle, all interventions should be used together, an "all-or-none" strategy.[36]

According to the IHI, the interventions bundled together for the prevention of VAP include elevation of the head of the bed (between 30 and 45 degrees), daily "sedative interruption" with daily assessment of readiness to extubate, peptic ulcer disease (PUD) prophylaxis, and VTE prophylaxis (unless contraindicated).[36]

To ensure compliance with the bundled interventions, the IHI recommends that facilities use a multidisciplinary team to implement all strategies to improve patient care. The ventilator bundle interventions should be integrated into a standardized order set for all patients on a mechanical ventilator.[36] It is important for the critical care practitioner to remember that despite the fact that this section does not address hand hygiene, hand hygiene remains of utmost importance in preventing nosocomial infections.[41]

Elevation of Head of Bed.

The elevation of the head of the bed of the mechanically ventilated patient is one of the core strategies of the VAP bundle. Drakulovic et al. demonstrated that patients maintained with the head of the bed elevated experienced an 8% incidence of VAP, whereas those patients kept supine experienced an incidence of VAP at 34%.[21]

The recommended elevation of the head of the bed is between 30 and 45 degrees.[29,36,64] Researchers have demonstrated that elevating the head of the bed at 30 degrees is more feasible than the 45-degree level.[64] When the head of the bed is elevated to 45 degrees, direct nursing care tasks become a challenge and there is fear that shearing of skin may occur because the patient is at increased risk for sliding down the bed.[36,64]

There are two demonstrable benefits to elevating the head of the bed for the mechanically ventilated patient. First, by elevating the head of the bed, there is a decreased chance of aspirating gastric contents or nasopharyngeal or oropharyngeal secretions.[18,64] Second, the patient's tidal volume may be increased when the head of the bed is elevated compared to the patient in the supine position. This increase in ventilatory volume may augment ventilatory efforts and decrease atelectasis.[18,29,36]

Despite the evidence, challenges exist in maintaining this practice as a standard of care. The IHI recommends that head of bed elevation be an intervention included on the critical care nursing flow sheet and that it be discussed in multidisciplinary rounds. The elevation of the head of the bed must be an integrated multidisciplinary responsibility; for example, if the respiratory therapist notes that the patient's head of bed is not elevated, the therapist should be empowered to elevate the head of the bed. By increasing the number of triggers in the critical care environment, greater compliance will be obtained on the bundle.[36]

Daily Sedative Interruption.

The provision of continuous sedation infusions has been very beneficial for mechanically ventilated patients in recent years, allowing patients to undergo ventilatory interventions not tolerated without the sedation.[5] Despite the advantages provided by continuous sedation infusion, the disadvantage has been the increased amount of time these patients spend on the mechanical ventilator, thereby prohibiting neurologic assessments.[42,58]

Researchers have demonstrated that by removing the sedation infusion daily from patients, the patient's time on the mechanical ventilator can be decreased. Kress et al. found that patients experienced a reduction in mechanical ventilation time of 2.4 days (P value = 0.004) when a daily sedation interruption was implemented.[42] Similarly, Schweickert et al. demonstrated a decrease of 2.5 days (P value = 0.003) on the mechanical ventilator and a decrease of 3.7 days (P value = 0.01) in critical care.[58] In both studies, patients were removed from the sedation infusion until awake and able to follow commands or until they became uncomfortable or agitated. If the patient needs to be returned to the sedation infusion, the rate of infusion should be decreased by half of the previous dosage. By reducing the dosage, weaning of the infusion is more successful during the next sedation interruption.[36]

During the interruption of sedation, two important assessment parameters are monitored. The first, a neurologic assessment, benefits the patient by identifying early neurologic changes. By identifying changes early, interventions can be implemented, resulting in improved outcomes and a decrease in further testing.[36,42] The second assessment, readiness to wean, benefits the patient by identifying patient readiness to wean from mechanical ventilation. During interrupted sedation, practitioners are able to assess overall lung function of the patient, thus determining when the patient is physiologically ready to begin the weaning process.[36]

When using sedation interruption, the significance of decreased length of time both on the mechanical ventilator and in critical care is insignificant compared to the impact on the complication rate of the critical care patient. By decreasing the time spent on the mechanical ventilator, the number of complications the patient experiences may also be reduced. Complication rates when sedation interruption is used decrease by approximately 50%, thus leading to a decreased rate of VAP development.[40]

The IHI recommends key strategies to ensure sedation interruption is performed on all patients being maintained on a continuous infusion of sedative agents. Facilities should implement a protocol for the sedation interruption. Compliance with the protocol should be assessed during multidisciplinary rounds and overall compliance should be posted to increase staff engagement in the process. If the facility uses a weaning protocol or standing order sets, the sedation interruption should be included in these protocols or order sets. Lastly, there should be agreement between all disciplines on the utilization of a sedation scale to avoid oversedation.[36]

Stress Ulcer Prophylaxis in Mechanically Ventilated Patients. In the previous section of this chapter, the importance of stress ulcer prophylaxis was discussed in relation to the prevention of gastrointestinal bleeding. Therefore it is a necessary intervention for critically ill patients, despite the controversy surrounding stress ulcer prophylaxis and the development of pneumonia.

Early research studies demonstrated that aspiration of gastric contents with a higher pH may lead to the development of pneumonia.[1,15,46] One of the key mechanisms of action of the medications used for the prevention of stress ulceration development is raising the pH of gastric contents.[1] Critical care patients are at high risk for aspiration of gastric contents; therefore practitioners have been hesitant to place patients on stress ulcer prophylaxis.

In 1991 Cook et al. completed a randomized controlled trial demonstrating no increased incidence of hospital-acquired pneumonia when the gastric pH was elevated.[12] Contrarily, the researchers found a trend toward a reduction in hospital-acquired pneumonia when sucralfate was used.[12] Unfortunately, there is a slight increase in the number of patients who develop gastric bleeding when taking sucralfate, compared to other histamine blocking agents.[1]

In light of the controversies surrounding gastric prophylaxis and the development of hospital-acquired pneumonia, the risk of developing a gastric bleed is greater; therefore current recommendations are that all mechanically ventilated patients should receive stress ulcer prophylaxis as an element in the VAP prevention bundle of care.[36]

Venous Thromboembolism Prophylaxis in Mechanically Ventilated Patients. It is uncertain that there is any relationship between VTE prophylaxis and the prevention of VAP. What is certain is that mechanically ventilated patients are sedentary and have a high acuity, both placing the patient at high risk of developing a VTE. Therefore the IHI recommends VTE prophylaxis for all mechanically ventilated patients as a part of the ventilator bundle of care. For details of VTE prophylaxis, please refer to the section on VTE prophylaxis within this chapter.[36]

VAP prophylaxis must take priority with all mechanically ventilated patients. The negative financial and clinical outcomes of this disease necessitate diligence on the part of critical care practitioners. By use of the ventilator bundle of care, VAP prevention can be made a reality in the critical care environment.

CONCLUSIONS

Care provided to patients in the critical care environment is complex. The key to improving outcomes is through prevention. As discussed in this chapter, there are many ways critical care nurses can assume the lead role in implementing prevention strategies. These evidence-based interventions can decrease cost and length of stay, and improve patient and family satisfaction. There are many new thoughts on improving patient care focusing on instituting guidelines, initiation of bundles, and checklists to prevent complications and provide a safe environment for patients.

Prophylactic interventions, with a focus on improving outcomes, should be an ongoing initiative. As new treatment recommendations and protocols become available, they should be used to guide clinicians in caring for patients, utilizing the latest clinical evidence.

REFERENCES

1. American Society of Health System Pharmacists. (1999). ASHP therapeutic guidelines on stress ulcer prophylaxis. *Am J Health-System Pharmacy, 56*(4), 347–379.
2. Angus, D., & Black, N. (2004). Improving care of the critically ill: institutional and health-care system approaches. *Lancet, 363* (9417), 1314–1320.

3. Bellomo, R. D., et al. (2003). A prospective before-and-after trial of a medical emergency team. *Med J Aust, 179*(6), 283–287.

4. Berenholtz, S. M., et al. (2002). Qualitative review of critical care unit quality indicators. *J Crit Care, 17*, 1–12.

5. Berenholtz, S. M., et al. (2004). Eliminating catheter related bloodstream infections in the CCU. *Crit Care Med, 32*(10), 2014–2020.

6. Braithwaite, R. S., et al. (2004). Use of medical emergency team (MET) responses to detect medical errors. *Qual Saf Health Care, 13*(4), 255–259.

7. Buist, M. D., et al. (1999). Recognising clinical instability in hospital patients before cardiac arrest or unplanned admission to intensive care. A pilot study in a tertiary-care hospital. *Med J Aust, 171*(1), 22–25.

8. Cash, B. D. (2002). Evidence-based medicine as it applies to acid suppression in the hospitalized patient. *Crit Care Med, 30*(6), S373–S378.

9. Centers for Disease Control and Prevention. (2002). Guidelines for the prevention of intravascular catheter-related infections. *MMWR, 51*(RR-10).

9a. Chulay, M. (2006). Respiratory System. In M. Chulay & S. Burns (Eds.), *AACN Essentials of Critical Care Nursing*, New York: McGraw-Hill.

10. Clemmer, T., et al. (1999). Results of a collaborative quality improvement program on outcomes and costs in a tertiary critical care unit. *Crit Care Med, 27*(9), 1768–1774.

11. Clemmer, T. (2004). Monitoring outcomes with relational databases: does it improve quality of care? *J Crit Care, 19*(4), 243–247.

12. Cook, D., et al. (1991). Nosocomial pneumonia and the role of gastric pH—a meta-analysis. *Chest, 100*(1), 7–13.

13. Cook, D., et al. (1996). Stress ulcer prophylaxis in critically ill patients: resolving discordant meta-analyses. *JAMA, 275*(4), 308–314.

14. Cook, D., et al. (1998). A comparison of sucralfate and ranitidine for the prevention of upper gastrointestinal bleeding in patients requiring mechanical ventilation. *New Engl J Med, 338*, 791–797.

15. Cook, D., et al. (1999). Risk factors for clinically important upper gastrointestinal bleeding in patients requiring mechanical ventilation. *Crit Care Med, 27*, 2812–2817.

16. Coopersmith, C. M., et al. (2002). Effect of an education program on decreasing catheter related bloodstream infections in the surgical critical care unit. *Crit Care Med, 30*(1), 59–64.

17. Cretikos, M., & Hillman, K. (2003). The medical emergency team: does it really make a difference? *Intern Med J, 33*(11), 511–514.

18. Daley, R. J., et al. (2004). Prevention of stress ulceration: current trends in critical care. *Crit Care Med, 32*(10), 2008–2013.

19. Dellinger, R., et al. (2004). Surviving sepsis campaign guidelines for management of severe sepsis and septic shock. *Crit Care Med, 32*(3), 858–873.

20. DeVita, M. A., et al. (2004). Use of medical emergency team responses to reduce hospital cardiopulmonary arrests. *Qual Saf Health Care, 13*(4), 251–254.

21. Drakulovic, M., et al. (1999). Supine body position as a risk factor for nosocomial pneumonia in mechanically ventilated patients: a randomised trial. *Lancet, 354*(9193), 1851–1858.

22. Eggimann, P., et al. (2000). Impact of a prevention strategy targeted at vascular access care on incidence of infection acquired in the critical care. *Lancet, 355*(9218), 1864–1868.

23. Eisenberg, J. (2003). The leapfrog group for patient safety: rewarding high standards. *Jt Commission J Qual Patient Saf, 29*(12), 634–639.

24. Fennerty, M. B. (2002). Pathophysiology of the upper gastrointestinal tract in the critically ill patient: rationale for the therapeutic benefits of acid suppression. *Crit Care Med, 30*(6 suppl), S351–S355.

25. Franklin, C., & Mathew, J. (1994). Developing strategies to prevent in-hospital cardiac arrest: analyzing responses of physicians and nurses in the hours before the event. *Crit Care Med, 22*(2), 244–247.

26. Geerts, W., et al. (2004). Prevention of venous thromboembolism: the Seventh ACCP Conference on Antithrombotic and Thrombolytic Therapy. *Chest, 126*(3 suppl), 338S–400S.

27. Goldhaber, S., & Turpie, A. (2005). Prevention of venous thromboembolism among hospitalized medical patients. *Circulation, 111*, e1–e3.

28. Goldhill, D., et al. (1999). The patient-at-risk team: identifying and managing seriously ill ward patients. *Anesthesia, 54*(9), 853–860.

29. Gudeman, S., et al. (1983). Gastric secretory and mucosal injury response to severe head trauma. *Neurosurgery, 12*, 175–179.

30. Hillman, K., et al. (2001a). Redefining in-hospital resuscitation: the concept of the medical emergency team. *Resuscitation, 48*(2), 105–110.

31. Hillman, K. M., et al. (2001b). Antecedents to hospital deaths. *Intern Med J, 31*(6), 343–348.

32. Hillman, K., et al. (2005). Introduction of the medical emergency team (MET) system: a cluster-randomised controlled trial. *Lancet, 365*(9477), 2091–2097.

33. Hodgetts, T. J., et al. (2002). The identification of risk factors for cardiac arrest and formulation of activation criteria to alert a medical emergency team. *Resuscitation, 54*(2), 125–131.

34. Ibrahim, E., et al. (2001). The occurrence of ventilator-associated pneumonia in a community hospital: risk factors and clinical outcomes. *Chest, 120*(2), 555–561.

35. Institute for Clinical Systems Improvement (ICSI). (2006). *Venous thromboembolism prophylaxis*. Institute for Clinical Systems Improvement (ICSI). Available at www.icsi.org/knowledge.

36. Institute for Healthcare Improvement. (2006a). *Getting started kit: prevent ventilator-associated pneumonia: how-to guide*. Available at www.ihi.org/IHI/Programs/Campaign.

37. Institute for Healthcare Improvement. (2006b). *Getting started kit: rapid response teams: how-to guide*. Available at www.ihi.org/IHI/Programs/Campaign.

38. Irwin, R., Marcus, L., & Lever, A. (2004). The critical care professional societies address the critical care crisis in the United States. *Chest, 125*(4), 1512–1513.

39. Kenward, G., et al. (2004). Evaluation of a medical emergency team one year after implementation. *Resuscitation, 61*(3), 257–263.

40. Knaus, W., et al. (1986). An evaluation of outcome from intensive care in major medical centers. *Ann Intern Med, 104*(3), 410–418.

41. Kollef, M. H. (2004). Prevention of hospital-associated pneumonia and ventilator-associated pneumonia. *Crit Care Med, 32*(6), 1396–1405.

42. Kress, J. P., et al. (2000). Daily interruption of sedative infusions in critically ill patients undergoing mechanical ventilation. *New Engl J Med, 342*(20), 1471–1477.

43. Lam, N., et al. (1999). National survey of stress ulcer prophylaxis. *Crit Care Med, 27*(1), 98–103.

44. Metnitz, P., et al. (2004). More interventions do not necessarily improve outcome in critically ill patients. *Intensive Care Med, 30*(8), 2154–2158.

45. Morse, K. J., et al. (2006). A new role for the ACNP: the rapid response team leader. *Crit Care Nurs Q, 29*(2), 137–146.

46. Navab, F., & Steingrub, J. (1990). Stress ulcer: is routine prophylaxis necessary? *Am J Gastroenterol, 90*, 708–712.

47. O'Grady, N. P. (2002). Applying the science to the prevention of catheter related infections. *J Crit Care, 17*(2), 114–121.

48. O'Neill, J. (1970). The influence of thermal burns on gastric acid secretion. *Surgery, 67*, 267–271.

49. Ottolini, M., & Pollack, M. (2003). Pediatric hospitals improve critical care outcomes. *Crit Care Med, 31*(3), 986–987.

50. Peura, D. (1990). Prophylactic therapy of stress-related mucosal damage: why, which, who, and so what? *Am J Gastroenterol, 85*, 935–937.

51. Pronovost, P., et al. (2004). Interventions to reduce mortality among patients treated in intensive care units. *J Crit Care, 19*(3), 158–164.

52. Pronovost, P., et al. (2006). A practical tool to learn from defects in patient care. *J Qual Patient Saf, 32*(2), 102–108.

53. Reilly, J., & Fennerty, M. B. (1998). The prevention of gastrointestinal bleeding and the development of nosocomial infections in critically ill patients. *J Pharm Prac, 11*, 418–432.

54. Rello, J., et al. (2002). Epidemiology and outcomes of ventilator-associated pneumonia in a large U.S. database. *Chest, 122*(6), 2115–2121.

55. Schein, R. M., et al. (1990). Clinical antecedents to in-hospital cardiopulmonary arrest. *Chest, 98*(6), 1388–1392.

56. Scholle, C. C., & Mininni, N. C. (2006). Best-practice interventions: how a rapid response team saves lives. *Nursing, 36*(1), 36–40.

57. Schuster, D., et al. (1984). Prospective evaluation of the risk of upper gastrointestinal bleeding after admission to a medical intensive care unit. *Am J Med, 76*, 623–630.

58. Schweickert, W. D., et al. (2004). Daily interruption of sedative infusions and complications of critical illness in mechanically ventilated patients. *Crit Care Med, 32*(6), 1272–1276.

59. Seneff, M. G. (2003). Central venous catheters. In J. M. Rippe & R. S. Irwin (Eds.), *Critical care medicine*. Philadelphia: Lippincott Williams & Wilkins.

60. Shorr, A. F., & Kollef, M. H. (2005). Ventilator-associated pneumonia: insights from recent clinical trials. *Chest, 128*(5), 583S–591S.

61. Spyropoulos, A. (2005). Emerging strategies in the prevention of venous thromboembolism in hospitalized medical patients. *Chest, 128*(2), 958–969.

62. Stephan, F., et al. (2006). Ventilator-associated pneumonia leading to acute lung injury after trauma: importance of *Haemophilus influenzae*. *Anesthesiology, 104*(2), 235–241.

63. Tablan, O., et al. (2004). Guidelines for preventing health-care-associated pneumonia, 2003 recommendations of CDC and the Healthcare Infection Control Practices Advisory Committee. *MMWR, 53*(RR-3), 1–36.

64. van Nieuwenhoven, C., et al. (2006). Feasibility and effects of the semirecumbent position to prevent ventilator-associated pneumonia: a randomized study. *Crit Care Med, 34*(2), 396–402.

65. Wall, R., et al. (2005). Using real time process measurements to reduce catheter related bloodstream infections in the intensive care unit. *Qual Saf Health Care, 14*(4), 295–302.

66. Warren, D. K., et al. (2004). The effect of an education program on the incidence of central venous catheter-associated bloodstream infections in a medical CCU. *Chest, 126*(5), 1612–1618.

67. Willeumier, D. (2004). Advocate health care: a system wide approach to quality and safety. *Jt Commission J Qual Patient Saf, 30*(10), 559–566.

68. Winters, B., et al. (2006). Rapid response teams—walk, don't run. *JAMA, 296*(13), 1645–1647.

69. Young, M., & Birkmeyer, J. (2000). Potential reduction in mortality rates using an intensivist model to manage intensive care units. *Effect Clin Pract, 3*(6), 284–289.

Kristine J. Peterson

Observation of a patient's cardiac rhythm is one of the most important aspects of critical care nursing. Early detection and accurate diagnosis of dysrhythmias or ST-T wave changes may prevent adverse consequences for the patient. The goal of this chapter is to provide information on select cardiac dysrhythmias that have important implications for patient care. Understanding of basic electrocardiography is required.

THE CARDIAC ACTION POTENTIAL

Normal Cardiac Cell Function

The cardiac *action potential* is the electrical activity occurring in individual cardiac cells during one cardiac cycle. It is the result of movement of charged ions across the cell membrane (*sarcolemma*). All cardiac muscle cells are electrically active; however, the morphology of their action potential depends on their unique characteristics. The arrangement and balance of positively and negatively charged ions on both sides of the sarcolemma create a net charge on each side of the membrane. When ready to conduct an impulse, the net charge inside the cell is called the *resting membrane potential* (−90 mV). This is a period of electrical stability also known as *electrical diastole*. The electrical potential at which the cell discharges and conducts an electrical impulse is called the *threshold potential* (−70 mV). Most atrial and ventricular muscle cells (as well as other muscle cells) cannot conduct an impulse without an outside stimulus. That is, when they are at their resting membrane potential, they require an electrical impulse to allow ionic movement to drive the charge inside the cell to threshold. Cardiac pacemaker cells, on the other hand, have a unique characteristic called *automaticity*. Automaticity is the capability of a cell to depolarize spontaneously and propagate an impulse. Although primarily found in the cells of the sinoatrial (sinus or SA) node, the atrioventricular (AV) node and His-Purkinje cells also possess this characteristic. The SA node and conduction system and the phases of the action potentials of ventricular muscle cells are illustrated in Figure 10-1.

Action Potential of Ventricular Muscle Cells

Phase 0: Rapid Depolarization. In the normal heart, an electrical impulse is initiated at the SA node and is propagated through the entire muscle via the conduction system. Once it reaches a muscle cell, it causes an influx of sodium (Na^+) that drives the net charge to threshold. Because Na^+ is a positively charged ion, when Na^+ ions move into the cell the net charge inside the cell increases (changes from −90 mV to −70 mV). At threshold, there is a brief (1 to 2 milliseconds) opening of the Na^+ channels, allowing a further rapid influx of Na^+. The charge inside the cell rapidly increases to about +30 to +40 mV. The speed of conduction is directly related to the amount of negativity at activation and the number of Na^+ channels that open. In addition, calcium (Ca^{++}) channels begin opening in clustered bursts, which allows the influx of Ca^{++} and also causes the sarcoplasmic reticulum to release Ca^{++} for muscle contraction.

Phase 1: Early Repolarization. Phase 1 is the beginning of repolarization and is caused chiefly by the closing of inward Na^+ and Ca^{++} channels. An outward potassium (K^+) channel opens, allowing K^+ to exit the cell. This results in a slight decrease in charge (repolarization) of the cell to about +10 mV.

Phase 2: Plateau. During phase 2, inward and outward ion flows are in balance so the charge stays relatively stable. Ca^{++} and Na^+ continue to flow into the cell while K^+ flows out of the cell. The flow of K^+ builds until the outward flow of K^+ exceeds the inward flow of Na^+ and Ca^{++}. At this point, contraction ends and repolarization begins. During phase 2, the cell is refractory or unable to respond to another stimulus. The property of cardiac *refractoriness* prevents tetany. The plateau phase does not occur in skeletal muscle action potentials.

Phase 3: Rapid Repolarization. Slow Ca^{++} channels close while outward movement of K^+ continues,

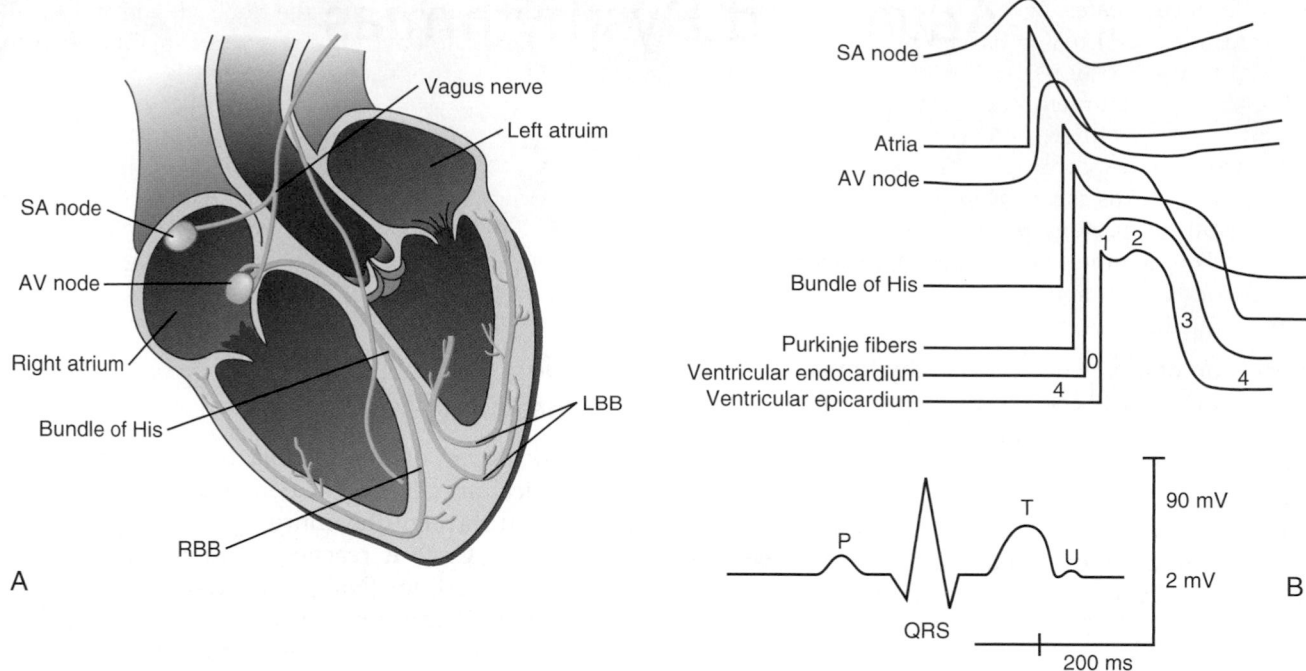

⬍FIGURE 10-1 A, Sinus node and conduction system. **B,** Action potentials. AV = Atrioventricular, LBB = left bundle branch, RBB = right bundle branch, SA = sinoatrial (sinus).

making the inside charge increasingly negative. Na⁺ channels are readied to respond to another impulse.

Phase 4: Electrical Diastole. During phase 4, muscle cells are permeable to K^+. The K^+ rectifier current returns K^+ and Na^+ to normal proportions and the charge reaches its resting potential, ready to receive another impulse. Outward K^+ movement and inward Na^+ movement continue during phase 4. If not depolarized by an impulse from a higher pacemaker, a muscle cell could conceivably reach threshold potential through this influx of Na^+ ions.

Action Potential of Pacemaker Cells

The action potential in the SA node, AV node, and His-Purkinje cells differs in many respects from the action potential of a working myocardial cell. The action potential here begins in phase 4.

Phase 4: Slow Diastolic Depolarization. As noted earlier, pacemaker cells have the property of automaticity, meaning that they do not require an outside stimulus to bring them to threshold potential. At the end of phase 3, the charge inside the pacemaker cell reaches its most negative (*maximum diastolic potential*). At this point, outward K^+ flow slows and there is a slow inward flux of Na^+ and then Ca^{++}. This inward flow slowly raises the charge inside the cell to

threshold potential, which initiates phase 0. The slope of phase 4 is steeper in pacemaker cells, meaning that threshold potential is reached sooner here than in other cells. Under normal conditions, the SA node controls the heart rate because the SA node cells generate threshold potential faster than other conductive tissue.

Phases 0–4. In pacemaker cells, phase 0 is the result of Ca^{++} influx rather than Na^+, and the change in potential between phase 4 and phase 0 is not as abrupt. The upstroke is shorter and not as steep. Phase 1 is absent in pacemaker cells. After maximum positive voltage is reached, a slow outward K^+ current begins repolarization. Phases 2 and 3 are present but brief. The rate of phase 3 repolarization is slower and results in a maximum diastolic potential that is less negative than in muscle cells. At the maximum diastolic potential, phase 4 begins.

Ionic Channels and Pumps

Ions move across the cell membrane according to the permeability to that ion as well as the electrical and diffusion forces on that ion. Equilibrium is a state of no net movement of ions, although transmembrane movement can still occur. The electrical difference between areas, such as the inside and outside of a cell membrane, is called the *potential difference.*

This difference creates an electromotive force that is measured in volts (1 mV = 0.001 V).

The movement of ions is closely regulated via permeability of the cell membrane and molecular pumps. Ion movement is either passive or active. Cell membranes are able to control which ions move across the membrane. This is called *selective permeability* and is the result of protein pores in the membrane, or channels. The channels are composed of several proteins encoded by specific genes. One membrane protein traverses the membrane while others act as gates. These channels open and close like gates via electrical or chemical signals. When a channel is open, specific ions are permitted to cross according to the electrical and concentration gradients. When the channel closes, movement of those ions stops. Effective cardiac conduction depends on the correct timing, sequence, and voltage activation of the membrane channels. A more detailed description of ion movement and channels may be found in other sources.[66,106]

Ionic Channels. I_{Na} is the fast inward Na^+ channel responsible for phase 0. It opens at threshold potential (−70 mV) for 1 to 2 msec. There are many Na^+ channels that open sequentially, producing a large, rapid influx of Na^+. The more Na^+ channels open, the faster the speed of conduction. The Na^+ channel is inactivated by the positive voltage caused by the Na^+ influx. It cannot be reactivated again until the cell repolarizes. I_{Na} channels are not present in pacemaker cells of the SA and AV nodes.

I_{Ca} produces a slow influx of Ca^{++} during slow diastolic depolarization and during phase 2 plateau. The inward Ca^{++} channel activates Ca^{++} release from the sarcoplasmic reticulum as well. I_{Ca} opens at positive potentials and inactivates at negative potentials.

K^+ currents generally produce the opposite effects of Na^+ channels. The timing of activation and inactivation of I_K directly influences the length of the refractory period. Opening early predisposes the cell to premature excitation while late activation shortens repolarization. The outward K^+ current increases with time during phase 2 until it is inactivated. This terminates the plateau phase. Furthermore, outward K^+ channels can be activated by acetylcholine. This outward K^+ current creates a more negative maximum diastolic potential than would be present without the influence of acetylcholine. From this voltage it takes longer to reach threshold potential, which accounts for the parasympathetic effect of slowing the heart rate. Some K^+ channels are sensitive to adenosine triphosphate (ATP) and are activated by ischemia, anoxia, or contractile failure.

The pacemaker current (I_f) is actually a combination of several effects. This current is present in SA and AV node cells and in Purkinje fibers. I_f activates at the end of phase 3 at maximum negative diastolic potential and produces a net inward positive current via movement of Na^+ and K^+. Inward Na^+ and Ca^{++} currents activating at specific voltages are also involved.

Ionic Pumps. While ion movement through channels is passive, not requiring energy, pumps move ions against electrochemical gradients and are dependent upon the presence of ATP. Two pumps have direct effects on the action potential.

Na^+-K^+-ATPase Pump. The Na^+-K^+-ATPase pump moves Na^+ ions outside of the cell in exchange for K^+ ions moved into the cell at a ratio of 3:2. This pump maintains the negative resting potential by returning the concentrations of Na^+ and K^+ to the resting state. The pump continually moves K^+ to the inside of the cell, creating a large K^+ gradient, and removes the Na^+ that enters during depolarization, thus ensuring that the cell is excitable.

Sodium-Calcium Exchange Pump. The purpose of the Na^+-Ca^{++} exchange pump is to remove the free Ca^{++} transported into the cell to activate contraction. Na^+ is pumped down the concentration gradient, which produces energy to move Ca^{++} out of the cell against the concentration gradient.

Implications for Patient Care

Classifications and Actions of Antidysrhythmic Agents. The Vaughn Williams classification lists antidysrhythmic agents according to the types of effects (Table 10-1). The Medication table on pp. 177–181 lists common antidysrhythmic agents and their points of action.

Prodysrhythmia. Antidysrhythmic medications affect specific points in the action potential. In addition, antidysrhythmics may be negative inotropes and prodysrhythmic. *Prodysrhythmia* is defined as "the aggravation of an existing dysrhythmia or the development of a new dysrhythmia during antidysrhythmic drug therapy."[75] The paradox of most antidysrhythmic agents is that instead of suppressing dysrhythmias, these agents may actually worsen the dysrhythmia or precipitate a new one. Prodysrhythmic effects have been noted for many years; however, it was not until 1989 that the lethal consequences of these effects were fully realized and demonstrated. The Cardiac Arrhythmia Suppression Trial (CAST), published in 1989, tested class I antidysrhythmic agents in patients with prior myocardial infarction (MI).[30] The study was terminated at the 10-month follow-up because of a significant increase in lethal

TABLE 10-1 The Vaughn Williams Classification of Antidysrhythmic Agents

CLASS	ACTIONS	EXAMPLES*
Ia	Moderate fast Na$^+$ channel blockade Decreased conduction velocity Prolonged refractory period (QT) Prolonged vulnerable period	Disopyramide Procainamide Quinidine
Ib	Mild fast Na$^+$ channel blockade Decreased conduction velocity Shortened repolarization Prolonged vulnerable period	Lidocaine Mexiletine Phenytoin Tocainide
Ic	Potent fast Na$^+$ channel blockade Decreased conduction velocity Prolonged vulnerable period	Encainide Flecainide Moricizine Propafenone
II	Beta receptor blockade Decreased conduction velocity Decreased heart rate Negative inotrope	Atenolol Carvedilol Esmolol Metoprolol Propranolol
III	K$^+$ channel blockade (I_{Kf}) Prolonged repolarization Prolonged QT	Amiodarone Azimilide Dofetilide Dronedarone Ibutilide Sotalol Tedisamil Trecetilide
IV	Calcium slow channel blockade Decreased AV conduction	Bepridil Diltiazem Nifedipine Verapamil

Data from references 17, 33, 62.
*Adenosine and digitalis are not classified.

dysrhythmias and cardiac arrest in the patients taking encainide (Enkaid) and flecainide (Tambocor). CAST-II, studying moricizine, was also terminated early because of lack of benefit and a trend toward harm.[44] Lethal prodysrhythmic effects occurred in patients with prior MI despite successful premature ventricular contraction (PVC) suppression by these medications. Examples of prodysrhythmic effects include new onset of bradycardia or other bradydysrhythmias, supraventricular premature beats and tachycardias, PVCs, and various types of ventricular tachycardia including torsades de pointes (TdP) and ventricular fibrillation.[75]

Prodysrhythmic effects are produced through several electrical and chemical mechanisms. The result of these mechanisms is that tissue that can conduct normally is changed into areas of depressed conduction. Such areas are then subject to dysrhythmogenic mechanisms such as triggered activity or reentry. Medications that slow conduction and suppress lethal dysrhythmias are not selective to only ischemic or depressed tissue. Therefore, while eliminating abnormal conduction in abnormal tissue, the same effects can turn normal tissue into areas of slowed conduction capable of sustaining dysrhythmias. Medications that prolong refractory periods and vulnerable periods make the same tissue susceptible to afterdepolarizations or reentry circuits. In addition, acid pH states can change the binding of agents to channels and alter their effects. In particular, binding and dissociation of medications to the Na$^+$ channel may be involved.[75]

Research to date has not identified reliable clinical predictors of prodysrhythmia. Occurrence of prodysrhythmia with one agent does not predict that use of another agent, even within the same class, will cause prodysrhythmia although class Ia, Ic, and III drugs seem to carry some risk.[75] Prodysrhythmia can occur at normal therapeutic drug levels. Individuals with heart failure, those with a history of sustained ventricular dysrhythmias, and those with ischemia are at high risk for dysrhythmias, and those same conditions predispose to prodysrhythmic effects.

DYSRHYTHMOGENIC MECHANISMS

Dysrhythmias fall into two categories: abnormalities of impulse formation and abnormalities of impulse conduction. Abnormal impulse formation can result from alterations in automaticity or from triggered activity, while abnormal impulse conduction can result from reentry or ischemia.

Alterations in Impulse Formation

Altered Automaticity

Enhanced Normal Automaticity. As discussed, automaticity is the ability of a cardiac cell to depolarize spontaneously and propagate an impulse. Automaticity is due to slow diastolic depolarization during

EFFECTS OF ANTIDYSRHYTHMIC MEDICATIONS

DRUG	CLASS	EFFECT ON ACTION POTENTIAL	CLINICAL EFFECTS	USUAL DOSE RANGE	INDICATIONS	ADVERSE EFFECTS
Adenosine (Adenocard)		Opens ATP-dependent K$^+$ channel I_{KAdo} Inhibits I_f pacemaker current in SA and AV nodal cells	Slows SA node Shortens atrial action potential Slows heart rate Slows AV conduction	6 mg rapid IV push, followed by 12 mg and 12 mg at 2-min intervals PRN Maximum total dose is 30 mg	PSVT, including accessory pathways and WPW Not effective for atrial fibrillation, flutter, or VT	Flushing, chest pain, hypotension, headache, dyspnea Long sinus pauses or increased conduction block possible Bronchoconstriction if asthma Effects may be antagonized by methylxanthines such as caffeine and theophylline.
Amiodarone (Cordarone)	III	Blocks K$^+$ channel I_K Blocks I_{Na} and I_{Ca} Potent alpha and beta blockade	Prolongs action potential Prolongs refractory period Decreases AV conduction	Pulseless VT or VF: 300 mg IV push, 150 mg IV push if needed, follow with infusion Breakthrough VF or VT: 150 mg IV over 10 min Infusion: 1 mg/min for 6 hr, then 0.5 mg/min	Treatment and prophylaxis for unstable VT and VF Supraventricular tachycardias	Hypotension, bradycardia, dysrhythmias Many drug interactions Can increase AV block Liver toxicity Lengthening QT interval
Azimilide	III	Blocks K$^+$ channel I_{Ks}	Prolongs refractory period, QT interval	Investigational	Atrial fibrillation, flutter, PSVT Investigational for reducing ICD discharges in patients with dysrhythmias post AMI	Prolonged QT, headache, nausea
Diltiazem (Cardizem)	IV	Inhibits slow inward L-type Ca^{++} channels	Slows AV conduction Shortens action potential	0.25 IV mg/kg/actual body weight, given over 2 min Infusion at 5–15 mg/hr for 24 hr	Atrial fibrillation or flutter PSVT **NOT for tachycardias of WPW**	Dizziness, hypotension, edema, AV block

Table continues on page 178

DRUG	CLASS	EFFECT ON ACTION POTENTIAL	CLINICAL EFFECTS	USUAL DOSE RANGE	INDICATIONS	ADVERSE EFFECTS
Disopyramide (Norpace)	Ia	Blocks fast Na$^+$ channels Blocks K$^+$ channels	Decreases excitability Decreases conduction velocity Prolongs vulnerable period	150 mg PO every 6 hr (immediate release form) or 300 mg PO every 12 hr (controlled release form)	Ventricular ectopy, atrial fibrillation and flutter, PAT	Prolonged QT, anticholinergic effects, hypotension, CHF
Dofetilide (Tikosyn)	III	Blocks K$^+$ channel I$_K$	Prolongs refractory period (QT)	Inpatient initiation of therapy 125–500 mcg PO daily with QTc monitoring during first 3 days	Symptomatic atrial fibrillation or flutter	Prolonged QT, AV blocks, torsadesde pointes Dose must be adjusted for renal impairment
Dronedarone	III	Blocks K$^+$ channels	Prolongs action potential, refractory period, QTc Prolongs AV conduction	Investigational	Atrial fibrillation, ICD patients	Prolonged QT
Esmolol (Brevibloc)	II	Blocks beta receptors (more beta$_1$ than beta$_2$ activity)	Slows SA rate Slows AV conduction Negative inotrope	Loading: 500 mcg/kg/min IV for 1 min, then 50 mcg/kg/min IV for 4 min Increase infusion by 50 mcg/kg/min up to 200 mcg/kg/min until desired effect May repeat loading dose with each increase PRN	SVT Atrial fibrillation or flutter	Hypotension, dizziness, CHF, bradycardia, bronchospasm, nausea
Flecainide (Tambocor)	Ic	Blocks fast Na$^+$ channels	Slows AV conduction Prolongs refractory period Negative inotrope	100 mg PO every 12 hr, maximum dose 400–600 mg/day	Life-threatening ventricular dysrhythmias SVT when other agents failed and no structural heart disease	Exacerbation of CHF, prolonged QT, visual disturbances, dyspnea

Drug	Class	Mechanism	Action	Indication	Dose	Side effects
Ibutilide (Corvert)	III	Blocks K$^+$ channel I$_K$, Increases inward Na$^+$ channel	Prolongs action potential, Prolongs refractory period	Conversion of new or recent onset AF or atrial flutter to sinus rhythm	For patients ≥60 kg, 1 mg IV given over 10 min, may repeat dose in 10 min PRN. For patients <60 kg, 0.01 mg/kg given over 10 min	AV blocks, bradycardia, torsades de pointes, prolonged QT, ventricular dysrhythmias
Lidocaine (Xylocaine)	Ib	Blocks fast Na$^+$ channels, Increases electrical threshold	Slows conduction, Slows AV conduction, Local anesthetic	Ventricular dysrhythmias	1.0–1.5 mg/kg IV over 2 min, repeat 0.5–0.75 mg/kg every 5–10 min up to total dose of 3 mg/kg. Continuous infusion of 1–4 mg/min	Heart blocks, confusion (especially in elderly patients), agitation, anxiety
Metoprolol (Lopressor)	II	Blocks beta receptors (more beta$_1$ than beta$_2$ activity)	Slows SA rate, Slows AV conduction, Negative inotrope	Atrial fibrillation and flutter	100–450 mg/day IV divided into 2–3 doses	Bradycardia, CHF, insomnia, impotence, bronchospasm
Mexiletine (Mexitil)	Ib	Blocks fast inward Na$^+$ channel, Slows rate of rise of phase 0	Prolongs refractory period	Ventricular dysrhythmias, suppression of PVCs	200–300 mg PO every 8 hr, maximum dose 1.2 g/day	AV blocks, dizziness, GI distress, nausea/vomiting, tremor. Prodysrhythmic agent. Give with food
Nifedipine (Procardia)	IV	Inhibits slow inward Ca^{++} channels	Antianginal	Hypertension, angina	10–30 mg PO 3 times per day, maximum of 120–180 mg/day	Flushing, dizziness, headache, nausea, heartburn, weakness
Phenytoin (Dilantin)	Ib	Blocks outward Na$^+$ channels, Activates inward Na$^+$ channels	Prolongs refractory period, Shortens action potential, Suppresses automaticity	Old indication for ventricular dysrhythmias	20–50 mg/min IV with filter	Hypotension, bradycardia, prodysrhythmic agent, Vesicant, Prolonged QT

Table continues on page 180

DRUG	CLASS	EFFECT ON ACTION POTENTIAL	CLINICAL EFFECTS	USUAL DOSE RANGE	INDICATIONS	ADVERSE EFFECTS
Procainamide (Pronestyl)	Ia	Blocks fast Na$^+$ channels Blocks K$^+$ channels	Prolongs refractory period Decreases conduction velocity Negative inotrope	15–18 mg/kg IV over 30 min or 100–200 mg IV, repeated every 5 min to total dose of 1 g Follow by infusion of 1–4 mg/min	VT, PVCs, PSVT, atrial fibrillation	Hypotension, prolonged QT, prodysrhythmic agent, lupus-like syndrome, blood dyscrasias, nausea, vomiting, diarrhea, taste disturbances
Propafenone (Rythmol)	Ic	Blocks fast inward Na$^+$ current Mild beta blockade	Slows conduction velocity Prolongs vulnerable period Decreases automaticity	150–300 mg PO every 8 hr	Life-threatening ventricular dysrhythmias	Prodysrhythmic agent, CHF, AV blocks, syncope, prolonged QT, dizziness, headache, GI complaints
Quinidine (Quinidex, Quinaglute)	Ia	Blocks fast Na$^+$ channels Blocks K$^+$ channels Blocks Ca^{++} influx	Depresses phase 0 Decreases excitability Decreases conduction velocity Decreases contractility Prolongs vulnerable period	Depends on formulation • Quinidine sulfate 200–400 mg PO every 4–6 hr • Quinidine gluconate 324–648 mg PO every 8–12 hr • Quinidine polygalacturonate 275 mg PO every 6–8 hr Must adjust doses when switching from one form to another	Prophylaxis after conversion of atrial fibrillation or flutter, PSVT, VT	Prolonged QT, hypotension, syncope, prodysrhythmic agent, dizziness, diarrhea, taste disturbance, nausea, vomiting, anorexia, heartburn, cramping

Drug	Class	Mechanism	Action	Dose	Indication	Side Effects/Comments
Sotalol (Betapace)	II, III	Beta blocker, Blocks K⁺ channels	Slows heart rate, Decreases AV conduction velocity, Increases AV refractory period, Prolongs action potential, Prolongs refractory period	80 mg PO 2 times per day, maximum of 240–320 mg/day	Ventricular dysrhythmias, maintenance of sinus rhythm after conversion of atrial fibrillation or flutter	Prolonged QT, bradycardia, palpitations, fatigue, dizziness, weakness, respiratory distress. Dose must be adjusted for renal impairment
Tedisamil	III	Blocks K⁺ channel **I**$_K$	Prolongs refractory period (QT), Slows heart rate	Investigational	Bradycardia, anti-ischemic ventricular dysrhythmias, Atrial fibrillation, flutter	Investigational
Tocainide (Tonocard)	Ib	Blocks fast Na⁺ channels	Suppresses automaticity, Increases diastolic depolarization threshold, Blocks AV conduction	1200–1800 mg/day PO divided into 3 doses, maximum dose 2400 mg/day	Life-threatening ventricular dysrhythmias	Prodysrhythmic agent, dizziness, nausea, hypotension, diarrhea, paresthesias, tremor
Trecetilide	III	Blocks K⁺ channel **I**$_K$	Prolongs refractory period, QTc, action potential	Investigational	Atrial fibrillation/flutter	Investigational
Verapamil (Calan)	IV	Blocks slow Ca⁺⁺ channels, Deceases automaticity	Slows heart rate, Slows AV conduction, Relaxation of coronary vascular smooth muscle	2.5–5 mg IV over 2 min, followed by 5–10 mg in 15–30 minutes, maximum total dose of 20 mg	PSVT, atrial fibrillation, flutter, angina. Not for use in rhythms with accessory pathway	AV blocks, bradycardia, hypotension, gingival hyperplasia, constipation

Data from references 33 and 62.
AF = Atrial fibrillation, AMI = acute myocardial infarction, ATP = adenosine triphosphate, AV = atrioventricular, CHF = congestive heart failure, GI = gastrointestinal, ICD = implantable cardioverter-defibrillator, K⁺ = potassium, Na⁺ = sodium, PAT = paroxysmal atrial tachycardia, PRN = as needed, PSVT = paroxysmal supraventricular tachycardia, PVC = premature ventricular contraction, QTc = QT interval corrected, SA = sinoatrial, SVT = supraventricular tachycardia, VF = ventricular fibrillation, VT = ventricular tachycardia, WPW = Wolff-Parkinson-White.

phase 4. In cells other than the SA and AV nodes, it is the result of an inward positive current through the fast Na^+ channel during phase 4. This inward movement of Na^+ stimulates the Na^+-K^+-ATPase pump. Na^+ is rapidly moved out of the cell, which causes a brief hyperpolarization (very negative charge) of the cell. In pacemaker cells, automaticity is the result of an inward Na^+ movement, I_f, and a slow influx of Ca^{++}. Normal automaticity responds to physiologic need, increasing with increased oxygen demand and decreasing with lower oxygen demand.

All pacemaker cells, such as those in the SA node, AV node, and His-Purkinje system, have automaticity. The SA node has the fastest rate of automaticity and therefore normally controls the heart rate. Pacemaker cells located farther down the conduction system are depolarized by the sinus impulse before they can reach threshold. This is known as *overdrive suppression*. Sites usually suppressed by the SA impulse are known as *subsidiary* or *latent pacemakers*. Figure 10-2 illustrates the action potential of altered automaticity.

Enhanced normal automaticity is the result of accelerated generation of action potentials by normal pacemaker tissue.[80] The slope of phase 4 becomes steeper, meaning that it takes less time for the cell to reach threshold potential. The action potential produced is otherwise normal. Enhanced normal automaticity can be caused either by an increase or decrease in the sinus rate or by an increase in another pacemaker cell's automatic rate. A major cause of enhanced normal automaticity is increased sympathetic activity that increases the sinus rate. Other conditions that increase subsidiary pacemaker cell automaticity include sympathomimetic agents, digitalis, chronic pulmonary disease, coronary artery disease, and hormones such as aldosterone, angiotensin, thyroid hormone, and insulin.[80]

Conditions that may depress normal sinus automaticity include increased vagal (parasympathetic) stimulation, drug levels, abnormal electrolyte levels, and disease of the sinus node.[80] In these situations, overdrive suppression of latent pacemakers does not occur, so a subsidiary pacemaker cell reaches threshold potential and usurps control of the heart rate. This can be protective, as happens in escape rhythms.

Rates produced from altered normal automaticity are seldom much higher than low 100s. Dysrhythmias resulting from enhanced normal automaticity include inappropriate sinus tachycardia, atrial tachycardias, wandering atrial pacemaker, junctional tachycardia, and accelerated idioventricular rhythms.[66]

Abnormal Automaticity. Abnormal automaticity is the accelerated generation of action potentials in abnormal myocardial tissue.[80] In depressed tissue, such as ischemic areas, the resting membrane potential is reduced (it is less negative than normal). The less negative the membrane potential becomes, the fewer fast Na^+ channels are available because they are voltage-dependent. Depressed cells will not have enough Na^+ channels available to create the conditions described to hyperpolarize.[66] In such situations, any atrial or ventricular cell may reach threshold and fire spontaneously via the normally occurring slow calcium influx during phase 4. The action potential produced is abnormal (Figure 10-2).

Abnormal automaticity may be caused by anything that makes the inside of the cell more positive or that impairs the Na^+-K^+-ATPase pump, such as decreased permeability to K^+ or increased permeability to Na^+

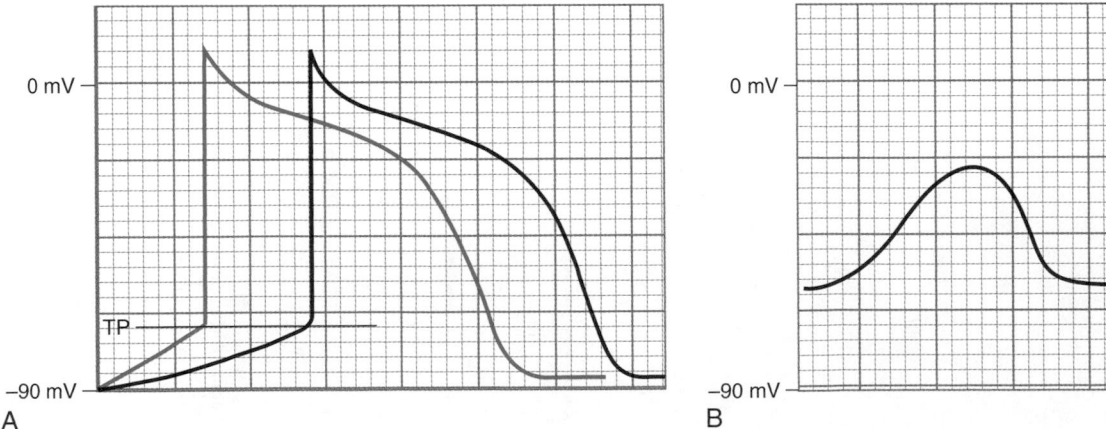

♦FIGURE 10-2 Two types of altered automaticity. **A,** Enhanced normal automaticity (caused by catecholamines) occurs in pacemaker cells such as His-Purkinje cells. Note that the phase 4 slope is steeper in enhanced automaticity. **B,** Abnormal automaticity resulting from ischemia or injury may occur anywhere in the heart. The membrane potential is only −60mV. TP=Threshold potential.

or Ca^{++}. Factors that lead to abnormal automaticity include hypoxia, ischemia, infarction, hyperkalemia, hypocalcemia, abnormal myocardial stretch, increased catecholamines, decreased parasympathetic tone, or digitalis. Atrial tachycardias, accelerated idioventricular rhythms, ventricular tachycardia associated with acute MI, and junctional tachycardias may all be the result of abnormal automaticity.[66] Tachycardias produced by abnormal automaticity typically are faster than those produced by normal automaticity. The less negative the resting potential, the faster the resulting rate. Abnormal automaticity produces rates between 100 and 200 beats per minute.

Triggered Activity. Triggered activity is a result of *afterdepolarizations*. Afterdepolarizations are fluctuations in the membrane potential that occur in late repolarization or just after repolarization. If these fluctuations reach threshold, a new action potential is "triggered."

Early Afterdepolarizations. Early afterdepolarizations (EAD) occur during phase 3 repolarization and result from a change in the inward positive current, probably because of activation of one type of slow Ca^{++} channel. If an EAD reaches threshold, it causes a new upstroke depolarization and an early beat. EAD differs from abnormal automaticity in that it is dependent on (triggered by) the previous action potential (Figure 10-3). EAD activity is associated with long QT intervals, bradycardia, sinus pauses, or anything that prolongs repolarization. Such conditions include hypoxia, acidosis, hypokalemia, hypomagnesemia, hypothermia, hypercapnia, and increased catecholamines. TdP and reperfusion dysrhythmias are the result of EAD activity.

Delayed Afterdepolarizations. Delayed afterdepolarizations (DAD) are fluctuations in the membrane potential that occur after complete repolarization. Again, should this activity reach threshold, another action potential will be triggered (Figure 10-4). Increased intracellular calcium levels predispose to DAD. Fast heart rates, hypercalcemia, digitalis toxicity, and increased catecholamines can result in DAD.

Alterations in Impulse Conduction

Reentry. Reentry means that an impulse repeatedly depolarizes the same area of tissue (Figure 10-5). Several conditions are required for reentry to occur: an area with unidirectional conduction block; an area of delayed conduction; and an area of inexcitable tissue. Essentially, the impulse travels down one branch of tissue while being blocked in another branch. Tissue beyond the area of unidirectional block is not depolarized, which allows the impulse to activate that tissue from the opposite direction and conduct slowly through it. By the time the impulse reaches the previously depolarized area, the tissue has repolarized, which allows the original impulse to reenter and stimulate it again. As long as the refractory period is short enough and the conduction is slow enough to allow the depolarized area to recover, the impulse can continue to traverse the circuit. If the refractory period lengthens or the conduction velocity increases, the impulse will reach refractory tissue and die out.

Reentry has been variously termed circus movement, reciprocal tachycardia, echo beats, and reentrant tachycardia. Dysrhythmias seen as a result of reentry include the tachycardia of Wolff-Parkinson-White syndrome, paroxysmal supraventricular tachycardia,

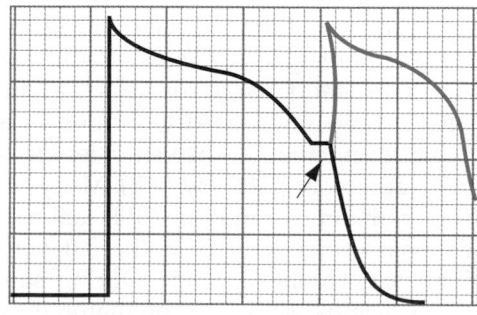

Early afterdepolarization

⬧**FIGURE 10-3** Early afterdepolarization distorts the action potential during phase 3, reaches the threshold potential, and produces a triggered beat.

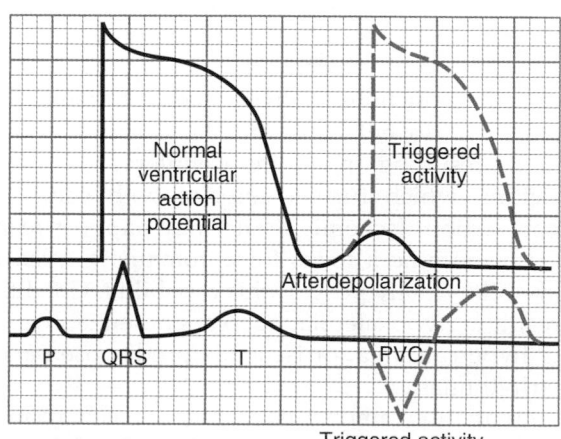

Triggered activity

⬧**FIGURE 10-4** Delayed afterdepolarization shown following the action potential. When the threshold potential is reached, a triggered beat is produced.

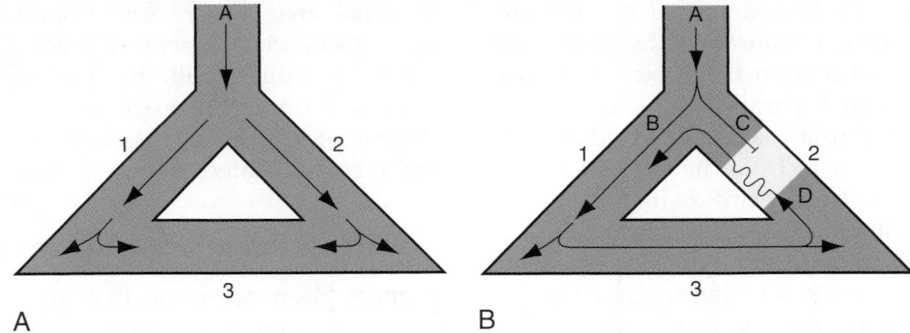

FIGURE 10-5 A, Normal conduction of an impulse through cardiac muscle with limbs 1 and 2 being depolarized simultaneously. **B,** Shaded area demonstrates unidirectional block. Impulse begins at point A and depolarizes limb 1 but is blocked in limb 2 at point C. The impulse continues from limb 1 to depolarize limb 3 and enters limb 2 at D. At point D, the impulse is able to conduct backward through the depressed segment and reenter limb 1 at point B.

scar-related ventricular tachycardia, intraatrial reentrant tachycardia, and atrial flutter.[18]

Ischemia. Cardiac ischemia alters the action potential in several ways. The resting membrane potential becomes less negative; then the upstroke and amplitude of phase 0 decrease, phases 2 and 3 are shortened, and fast Na^+ channels are inactivated. Because of these changes, the cell never reaches the normal resting membrane potential. The result is a slow-response action potential and an area of depressed conduction. Within minutes, cells become inexcitable. Ischemia inactivates the Na^+-K^+ pumps, cell membranes are damaged, and K^+ leaves the cell.

Because sympathetic activity is increased during ischemia, norepinephrine accumulates. During ischemia the effect of norepinephrine is to prolong both the action potential and the vulnerable period. Normally the cardiac muscle contracts in an all-or-nothing manner because the junctions between cells are low resistance and enhance conduction between fibers. During ischemia "electrical uncoupling" occurs because the junctions between cells become more resistant and do not conduct. The calcium pump is impaired, resulting in an intracellular accumulation of calcium, which further impairs both conduction and contraction. Ischemic tissue may support reentry circuits or become a focus for automaticity, even if it would not normally possess this capability. Conditions that result in hypokalemia, hypomagnesemia, hypocalcemia, hypercalcemia, or ischemia predispose patients to dysrhythmias.

Differentiation among the various mechanisms of dysrhythmias via the surface ECG is difficult. Management depends to a large extent on how well the patient tolerates the tachycardia. Most of the tachycardias resulting from these mechanisms respond to vagal maneuvers, overdrive pacing, medications that block AV conduction, or cardioversion.

SUPRAVENTRICULAR TACHYCARDIAS

Supraventricular tachycardia (SVT) is defined as any tachycardia that originates above the bifurcation of the bundle of His. Atrial tachycardias, atrial flutter, atrial fibrillation, junctional tachycardia, sinus tachycardia, atrioventricular nodal reentry tachycardia (AVNRT), and atrioventricular reciprocating tachycardia (AVRT or circus movement tachycardia) can all be termed SVT. Most often, SVT has a narrow QRS complex; however, aberrant conduction of a supraventricular rhythm may cause a wide QRS. The term paroxysmal supraventricular tachycardia (PSVT) is used when the rhythm begins and ends abruptly. AVNRT and AVRT are the two most common mechanisms of PSVT.[18]

Wolff-Parkinson-White Syndrome

Wolff-Parkinson-White (WPW) syndrome is a specific ECG pattern found in persons with repeated episodes of symptomatic PSVT. These findings indicate ventricular preexcitation and consist of a short P-R interval, delta wave, and broad QRS. Preexcitation is defined as early activation of the ventricles via conduction down an accessory pathway (AP). Many such APs exist; however, the most common AP location in WPW is an AV bypass tract located in the left ventricular free wall or posteroseptal region. During sinus rhythm the ventricle is activated prematurely via the AP while the impulse is simultaneously conducted down the AV-His-Purkinje system. The AP conduction time is faster than the AV node and because there is no AV delay, like that which occurs in the AV node, the AP impulse reaches the ventricle first. The AP impulse produces a characteristic slurring of the upstroke of the QRS, known as a delta wave. The ventricle is then activated by two simultaneous impulses, resulting in a fusion beat. Figure 10-6 illustrates the characteristic features of WPW. WPW is thought to be caused by a genetic defect that leads to abnormal fetal development of the fibrous ring (annulus fibrosus) that keeps the atria and ventricles electrically separate. Bridging strands of myocardium present after birth. There is a familial tendency to develop WPW.

ECG Characteristics. In sinus rhythm of a patient with WPW the P-R interval is usually less than 120 msec, and a delta wave is present, resulting in a QRS slightly broader than normal. The size of the delta wave varies depending on the speed of conduction down the AP and the location of the AP. Because of the abnormality in conduction, abnormal repolarization represented by inverted T waves is often present as well. Sinus rhythm and the tachycardias can be present without the characteristic ECG findings when the AP is not used for anterograde conduction. This is called *latent* or *concealed accessory pathway*. Most WPW patients seen clinically have a history of PSVT.

There are different degrees of preexcitation, depending on the conduction time of the atria, AV node, and the AP. This manifests in differing widths and degrees of visibility of the delta waves. Similarly, depending on the location of the AP, sinus rhythm in WPW may resemble hypertrophy, bundle branch block (BBB), or an acute MI. WPW may be asymptomatic or, rarely, the first symptom may be sudden cardiac death. The most frequent dysrhythmia associated with WPW is orthodromic AV reciprocating tachycardia (AVRT), although atrial fibrillation may be seen as well.[18,81]

Episodes may be so frequent as to be disabling. Severity depends on the duration and rate of the tachycardia.

Atrial flutter and fibrillation that occur in the presence of an AP can result in a ventricular rate as fast as 250 to 300 beats per minute and can potentially degenerate into ventricular fibrillation. The precise mechanism for the development of atrial fibrillation in WPW is unknown. Atrial fibrillation with antegrade conduction over an AP manifests as an irregular, rapid, wide complex tachycardia with varying degrees of preexcitation.

Atrioventricular Nodal Reentry Tachycardia

Atrioventricular nodal reentry tachycardia (AVNRT) is a tachycardia resulting from a reentry circuit using two separate pathways into the AV node. Multiple pathways into the AV node are possible, although abnormal. These include the fast and slow pathways, accessory pathways, and others. Any combination of pathways with differing conduction velocities and refractory periods can maintain a reentry circuit. AVNRT tachycardia involves the "fast pathway," which conducts rapidly but has a long refractory period, and the "slow pathway," which conducts more slowly but has a shorter refractory period. AVNRT is most commonly initiated by a premature atrial complex that is blocked at the fast pathway and conducted through the AV node via the slow pathway. The delay in conduction through the slow pathway allows the impulse to traverse the AV node through to the ventricle and simultaneously back to the atria retrograde through the fast pathway. The impulse can then reactivate the slow pathway and initiate a tachycardia.[64]

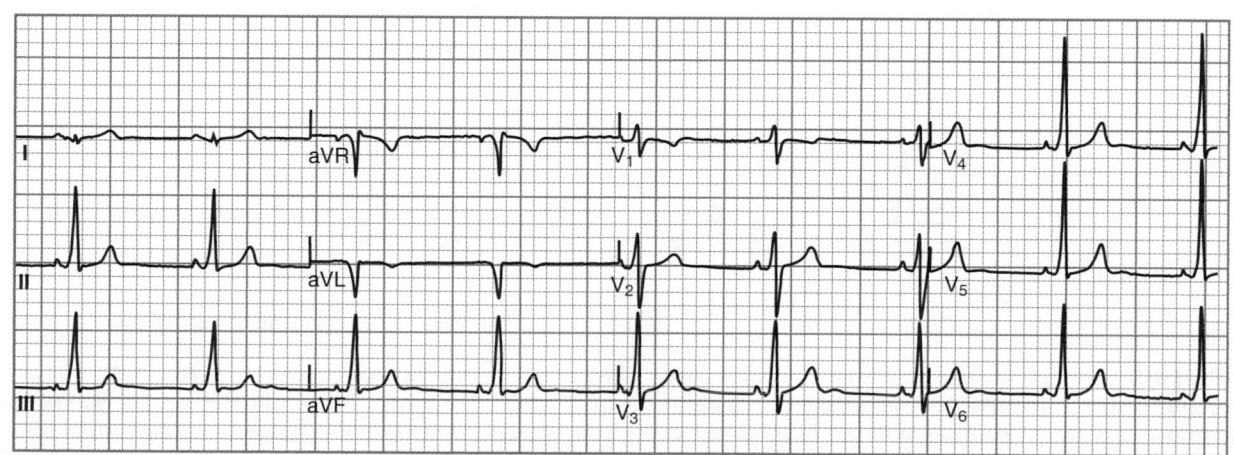

⇕FIGURE 10-6 Wolff-Parkinson-White pattern. Note the short P-R interval and delta wave in leads II, III, aVF, and V₃-V₆.

There are two distinguishing ECG features for AVNRT. First, because conduction is delayed in the slow pathway, the interval from the premature P wave to the corresponding R wave is usually greatly prolonged to longer than 300 msec.[18] Additionally, because the atria and ventricles are activated simultaneously, the retrograde P (P') occurs at the end of the QRS complex, which often distorts the final portion and creates a pseudo right bundle branch block (RBBB) pattern in lead V_1. Best seen as a small, late positive deflection in V_1 and a small terminal negative component in the inferior leads, this distortion can often be mistaken for part of the QRS (Figure 10-7).[64] Figure 10-8 illustrates the development of AVNRT. Sometimes, detection of a retrograde P wave is recognized only upon careful comparison of the sinus rhythm ECG with the SVT ECG.

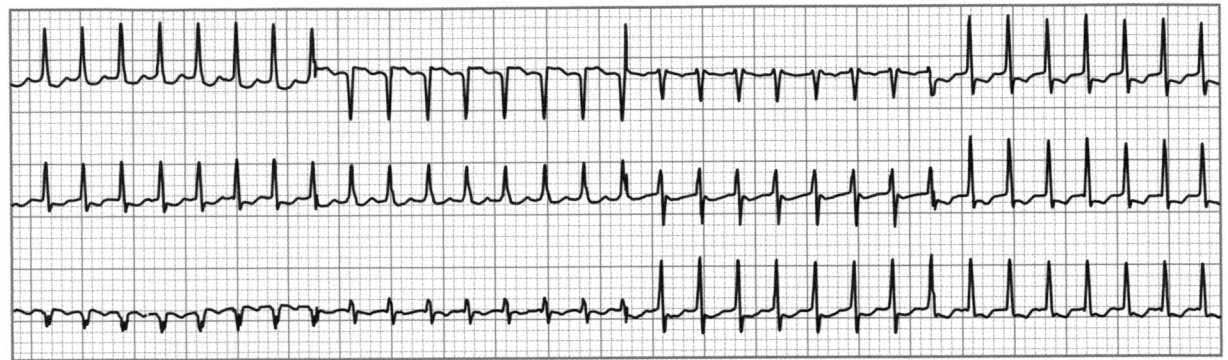

♦FIGURE 10-7   AV nodal reentry tachycardia. Note the pseudo right bundle branch block pattern in V_1 that was not present during normal sinus rhythm, representing the P wave at the end of the QRS complex.

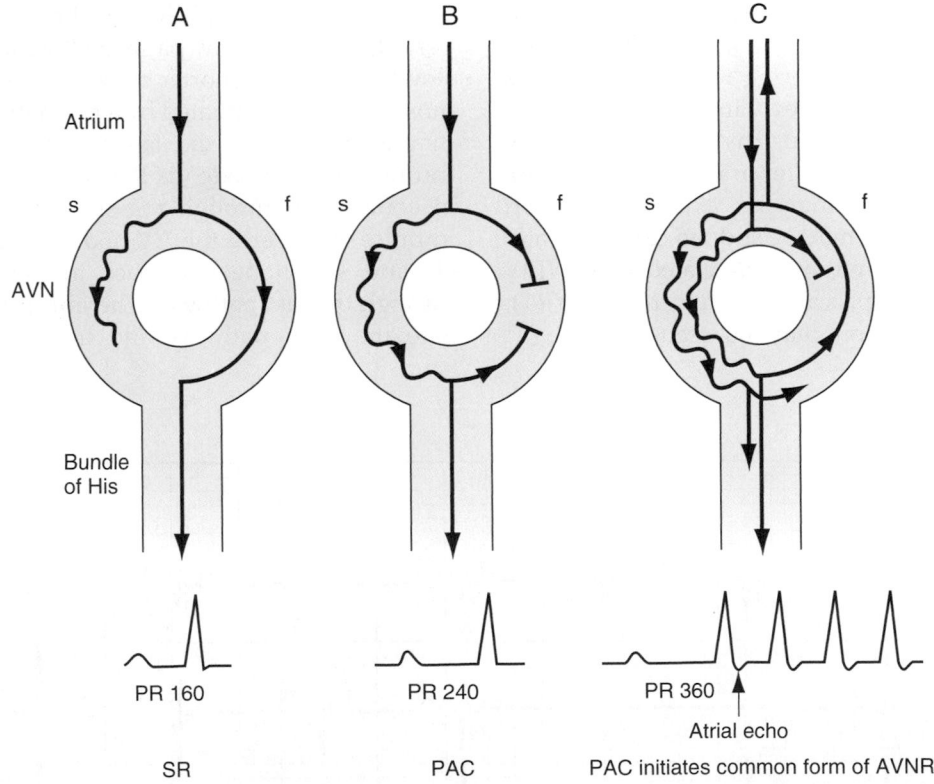

♦FIGURE 10-8   Premature atrial contraction (PAC) initiation of AV nodal reentry tachycardia (AVNRT). **A,** Sinus rhythm (SR): atrial impulse reaches the bundle of His via the fast (f) pathway, resulting in a normal P-R interval. **B,** PAC is conducted over a slow (s) pathway because of the block in the fast pathway, resulting in the sudden prolongation of the P-R interval. **C,** A PAC with slower conduction reenters the fast pathway and initiates AV nodal reentry tachycardia. Atrial echo represents the retrograde atrial conduction; also called a retrograde P wave.

ECG Characteristics. Heart rate is 130 to 250 beats per minute. Rhythm is most often regular. P′ waves are, if seen, within the terminal portion of the QRS and are negative in inferior leads (leads II, III, and aVF) because of retrograde conduction into the atria. The initiating P′-R interval is prolonged and the QRS is of normal duration unless aberrant conduction is also present. Often the P′ distorts the terminal portion of the QRS. This resembles a terminal s wave in the inferior leads and a terminal r wave in V_1. AVNRT is benign and paroxysmal and represents about two thirds of cases of PSVT in adults.[6] It is more common in adult women than in men. AVNRT can be terminated by inducing a temporary block in the AV node through a vagal maneuver or antidysrhythmics. Once normal rhythm is restored, a definitive diagnosis can sometimes be made by comparing the 12-lead ECG of the tachycardia to the 12-lead ECG of the patient's normal rhythm. An electrophysiology study is often needed to determine the exact mechanism of the tachycardia. AVNRT may also be termed *AV junctional reentrant tachycardia* or *reciprocating AV nodal reentrant tachycardia.*

AV Reciprocating Tachycardia

AV reciprocating tachycardia or circus movement tachycardia (CMT) is a reentry circuit that uses both the normal AV node pathways and an AP. An AP, sometimes termed a *bypass tract*, is an extra bundle of muscle fibers connecting the atria to the ventricles. Since the atria and ventricles are normally electrically isolated, an AP forms an abnormal connection between them and can support dysrhythmias. APs are most commonly located at the intraventricular septum or the left ventricle free wall; however, an electrophysiology study is required to precisely locate an accessory pathway.

If anterograde conduction is through the AV node and retrograde conduction uses the accessory pathway, the tachycardia is termed *orthodromic reciprocating tachycardia* (ORT). This is the most common form of AVRT.[53] Less common is *antidromic* AVRT, in which where conduction occurs in the opposite direction. AVRT is the most common mechanism for the tachycardias of WPW.

In ORT the reentry circuit is usually initiated by a premature atrial contraction (PAC) or a PVC. The premature impulse is blocked by the accessory pathway, but is conducted through the AV node to the ventricles. The accessory pathway is now nonrefractory and the impulse uses it to travel retrograde back to the atria. Thus an orthodromic reentry circuit is formed with the impulse activating the ventricles through normal conduction pathways and traveling backward up the accessory pathway to activate the atria (Figure 10-9). Because the atria and ventricles are activated in sequence, P′ will be after the QRS, rather than connected to it as in AVNRT. The faster the conduction up the accessory pathway, the closer P′ will be to the QRS. A characteristic ECG finding is *ventricular preexcitation*—premature activation of the ventricles through an accessory pathway. This can be seen during sinus rhythm and is considered evidence

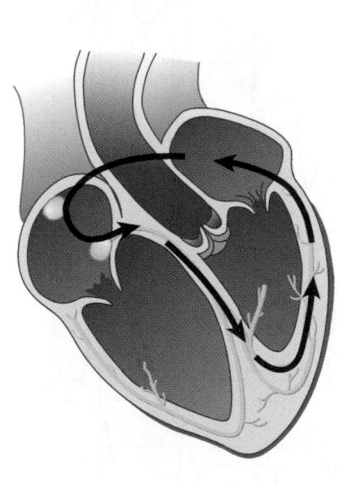
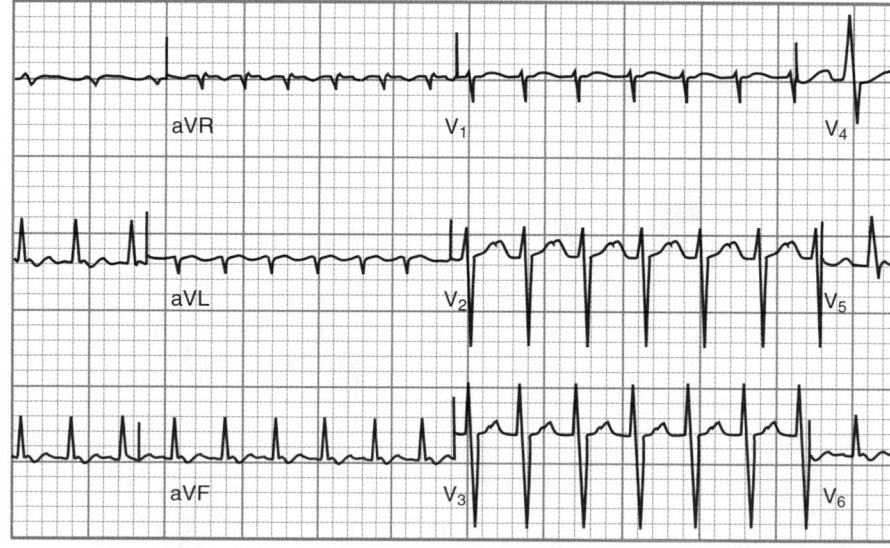

⬍FIGURE 10-9 Conduction and ECG in orthodromic AV reentry tachycardia. P waves are visible in the ST segment, especially in V_2 and V_3, and are inverted in leads I, III, and aVF.

of the presence of an accessory pathway.[53] Another distinguishing factor between AVNRT and AVRT is that the P-R interval initiating the tachycardia is normal in AVRT while it is prolonged in AVNRT.[18] Figure 10-9 illustrates an orthodromic AVRT, and Figure 10-10 shows an antidromic AVRT.

ECG Characteristics. The rate of AVRT is typically 130 to 250 beats per minute with a regular rhythm. The rate can be faster than 200 beats per minute, and as the rate becomes faster, AV node conduction may vary, producing an irregular rhythm and possible aberrant conduction. The initiating P-R interval is normal and P′ is always separate from the QRS. The polarity of P′ waves varies depending on the location of the accessory pathway.

Clinical Presentation of AVNRT and AVRT

Most types of PSVT occur intermittently. Symptoms depend on the rate and duration of the rhythm. Patients may experience palpitations, anxiety, angina, syncope, heart failure, or shock. Changes in atrial pressure during the tachycardia are thought to cause release of atrial natriuretic factor (ANF), causing polyuria.[18] A classic sign of PSVT is "cannon" atrial waves in the jugular pulse. Because atrial and ventricular contractions occur simultaneously rather than in sequence, the atria contract against closed tricuspid and mitral valves. This causes a rise in atrial pressure that is reflected back into the central venous circulation and is seen as regular, visible pulsations in the jugular veins.

Management of AVNRT and AVRT

Management of Tachycardias of WPW. The most effective pharmacologic agents slow conduction and lengthen the refractory period in the accessory pathway. Amiodarone (Cordarone), procainamide (Pronestyl), propafenone (Rythmol), sotalol (Betapace), flecainide, and quinidine may be used.[18,39,90] Intravenous procainamide or ibutilide (Corvert) are effective agents for atrial fibrillation induced by WPW.[39] Agents that shorten refractory periods, such as digoxin (Lanoxin) and calcium channel blockers, are contraindicated during atrial fibrillation because they can accelerate conduction through the AP. Because diltiazem (Cardizem) and digoxin may be used to treat atrial fibrillation, WPW must be ruled out before using them.[18] When a patient presents with a very fast, very broad, and irregular (FBI[18]) tachycardia, the 12-lead

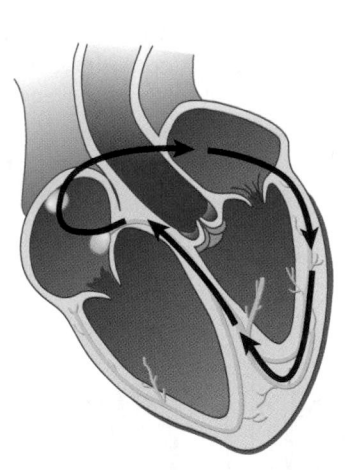
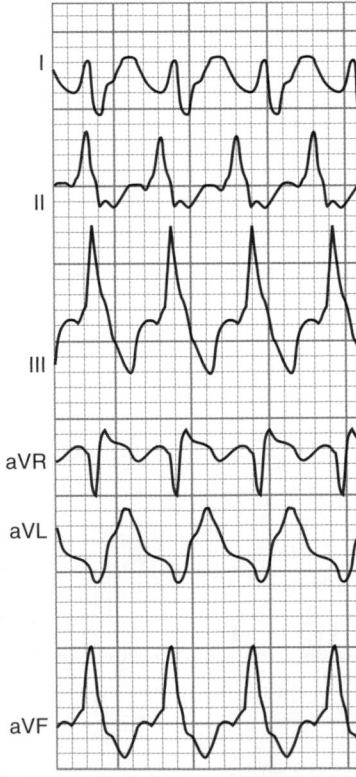
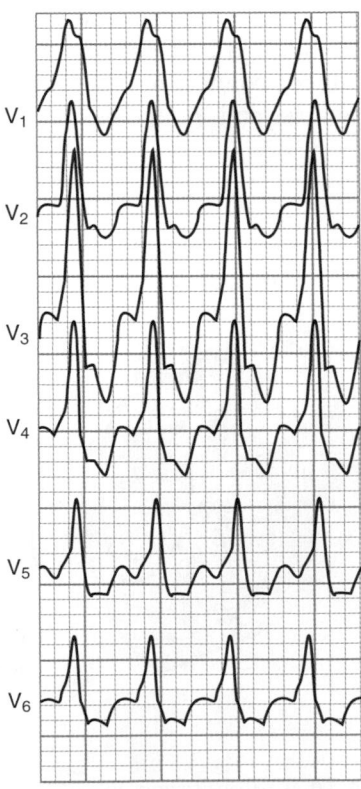

✦FIGURE 10-10 Conduction and ECG in antidromic circus movement tachycardia with AV conduction over a left posterior accessory pathway.

ECGs should be carefully checked for the presence of preexcitation. Treatment options range from none, to pharmacologic agents, to ablation. Radiofrequency ablation of the accessory pathway is very successful in eliminating the tachycardias and is the treatment of choice for symptomatic WPW.[32,86]

Management of AVNRT and AVRT. Because the AV node is actively involved in the reentry circuit of AVNRT, blocking the AV node will usually terminate the tachycardia. Acute use of vagal maneuvers is particularly effective for these rhythms.[6,18] Vagal stimulation causes a release of acetylcholine, which prolongs the refractory period of the AV node, terminating the rhythm. The vagus nerve also affects the sinus node, so a possible adverse effect of vagal stimulation is sinus bradycardia or sinus pauses. Examples of vagal maneuvers that patients can use include coughing, blowing out against a closed glottis, gagging, or squatting. Most patients should be taught several vagal maneuvers so that they are likely to find an effective one when the tachycardia occurs. Carotid sinus massage should be reserved for patients with no symptoms of transient ischemic attacks and no carotid bruits. Eyeball pressure should never be used.[18]

Any drug that blocks the AV node fast or slow pathways, increases the refractory period of the AV node, or slows conduction through the AP would be effective. Adenosine (Adenocard) is the drug of choice for narrow-complex tachycardia. It acts by blocking conduction through the slow pathway into the AV node. Flushing, headache, chest pain, and long sinus pauses may occur. Because of the very short action of adenosine, these effects are brief and well tolerated.

Beta blockers, diltiazem, and verapamil (Calan) slow conduction through the AV node, and sotalol blocks the slow pathways. Class Ic agents such as propafenone may work on both fast and slow pathways. Amiodarone's effects include slowing AV conduction by slowing both the fast and slow pathways, and it is useful for most narrow-complex tachycardias. Procainamide can interrupt either an AVNRT or an AVRT by lengthening the refractory period of both the fast AV pathway and accessory pathways. Both amiodarone and procainamide have toxicity issues and therefore are infrequent first-line agents. If the QRS is wide, digitalis, diltiazem, and verapamil are contraindicated because they can shorten the refractory period in the accessory pathway.

Dysrhythmias that use an AP for antegrade conduction (such as atrial fibrillation with rapid ventricular response using the AP) should be terminated as soon as possible because they may deteriorate into ventricular fibrillation. AVNRT seldom requires synchronized cardioversion, but if the patient is unstable, it is the recommended therapy. AVNRT and AVRT are the most common forms of PSVT, but there are variants of PSVT that use multiple pathways into the AV node or accessory pathways. These are difficult to distinguish outside of the electrophysiology laboratory. In any case, synchronized cardioversion is the therapy of choice for emergency management of an unstable patient with PSVT. In practice, cardioversion is rarely required because pharmacologic agents today are rapidly effective for most patients.

Radiofrequency modification or ablation is the preferred treatment.[6] For AVNRT, Scheinman et al.[86] reported a 96% rate of permanent elimination of the tachycardia after ablation of the slow pathway. This carries a very low risk of AV block (0.1% of patients). Radiofrequency ablation of the accessory pathway is effective in 94% of patients with symptomatic AVRT and carries a similarly very low risk of complications.[53,86]

When there is time, obtaining a 12-lead ECG of the tachycardia is very helpful. Many patients experience these rhythms only sporadically so there may be few opportunities to record the rhythm in many leads. If the patient does not have the overt markers of WPW, the diagnosis may only be possible during the tachycardia. During an electrophysiology study, a number of dysrhythmias may be elicited. Accurate identification of the clinically significant rhythm is essential to eliminating the correct focus.

VENTRICULAR TACHYCARDIAS

Ventricular tachycardia (VT) is defined as at least three consecutive ventricular complexes at a rate of faster than 100 per minute. There are two types of ventricular tachycardia—monomorphic and polymorphic. TdP is a specific variant of polymorphic VT.

Monomorphic Ventricular Tachycardia

Monomorphic ventricular tachycardia arises from one reentrant circuit or pathway in the ventricle; therefore all QRS complexes have the same morphology (Figure 10-11). It is the most common type of VT. The rhythm is regular with a broad QRS. P waves, if present, are dissociated from the ventricular rhythm. In a wide-complex tachycardia, AV dissociation is highly suggestive of VT.

The mechanism of monomorphic VT is reentry, altered automaticity of a ventricular fiber, or it may be triggered by delayed afterdepolarizations. Acute MI is the most common precipitant for monomorphic VT. Dilated cardiomyopathy, hypokalemia, hypomagnesemia, hypoxia, and ischemia may all predispose to

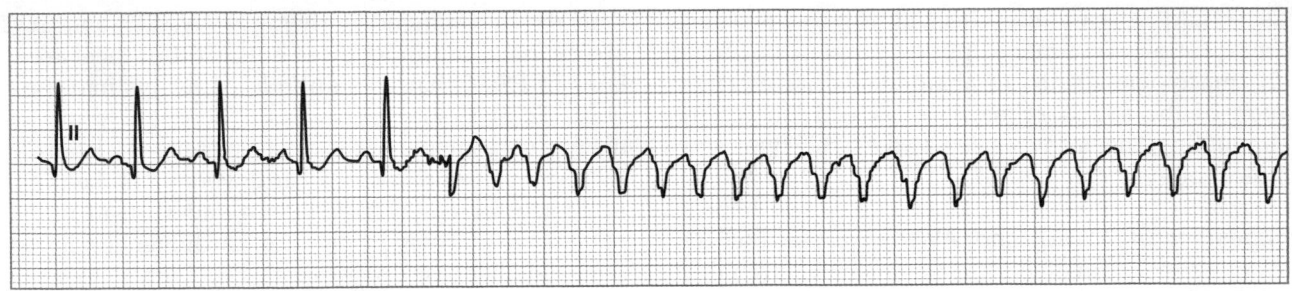

✦FIGURE 10-11 Monomorphic ventricular tachycardia.

this dysrhythmia. Sustained monomorphic VT usually requires treatment to prevent hemodynamic compromise and deterioration into ventricular fibrillation. Amiodarone is the first-line therapy for acute monomorphic VT. Lidocaine or procainamide may be used as well. For long-term management of ischemic VT, amiodarone or sotalol may be used. Implantable antitachycardia device therapy and surgical ablation may be necessary for recurrent, refractory VT.

Alternative Forms of Monomorphic VT. One form of monomorphic VT originates in the right ventricular outflow tract (RVOT VT). The morphology is that of left bundle branch block (LBBB) with an inferior axis. It is thought that this type of VT is the result of a triggered or automatic focus and is characterized by repetitive short bursts of VT. It is more common in males.[70] This VT may be the result of dysrhythmogenic right ventricular dysplasia.[70] Treatment is administration of antidysrhythmic agents, including beta blockers, adenosine, or verapamil; radiofrequency ablation; or, rarely, an implantable cardioverter-defibrillator. Monomorphic VT may arise from either the right or the left ventricle and may occur with or without structural heart disease. Many of these dysrhythmias occur in overtly structurally normal hearts. Magnetic resonance imaging may reveal mild abnormalities such as fatty infiltration and wall motion abnormalities. The significance of these is not well understood. It is important to distinguish VT that occurs in the absence of a definable cause (idiopathic) from VT that occurs in patients with dysrhythmogenic right ventricular dysplasia or Brugada syndrome, because these syndromes carry a higher risk of sudden cardiac death.

Polymorphic Ventricular Tachycardia

This type of VT has an irregular and varying morphology. Polymorphic VT may be associated with a normal QT or prolonged QT interval. The changing morphology is due to differing foci and reentry circuits. Acute myocardial ischemia is the most common cause of polymorphic VT. Polymorphic VT with a normal QT interval is probably caused by reentry and is treated the same as monomorphic VT. Figure 10-12 illustrates polymorphic VT.

Torsades de Pointes. Polymorphic VT associated with a prolonged QT interval is known as TdP. It has a continuously varying QRS that appears to rotate around a central line. The mechanism of TdP is a prolonged QT interval and early afterdepolarizations.[31,101] ECG manifestations include a prolonged QT interval, merging of the T and U waves, initiation by an R-on-T PVC with a long coupling interval, and irregular, wide, bizarre QRS complexes with continuously changing morphology that are often notched. It may resemble coarse ventricular fibrillation. The short-long-short cycle initiating sequence is classic for TdP. The initiating PVC comes on the T wave of a beat after a long cycle. The varying cycle lengths set up differing refractory periods and predispose to TdP.[66] The rate is usually 200 to 250 beats per minute and occurs in paroxysmal, repeating episodes (Figure 10-13).

Identifying TdP via the ECG clues is important because it does not respond to the usual VT therapies. The medications used to treat ordinary VT will often exacerbate TdP. Amiodarone, procainamide, and sotalol are contraindicated because they prolong

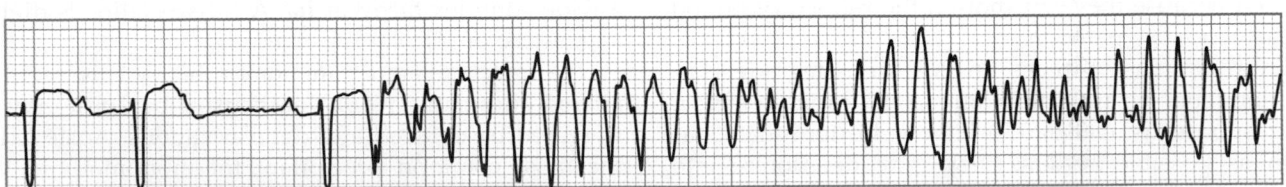

✦FIGURE 10-12 Polymorphic ventricular tachycardia. The QT interval is normal (400 msec).

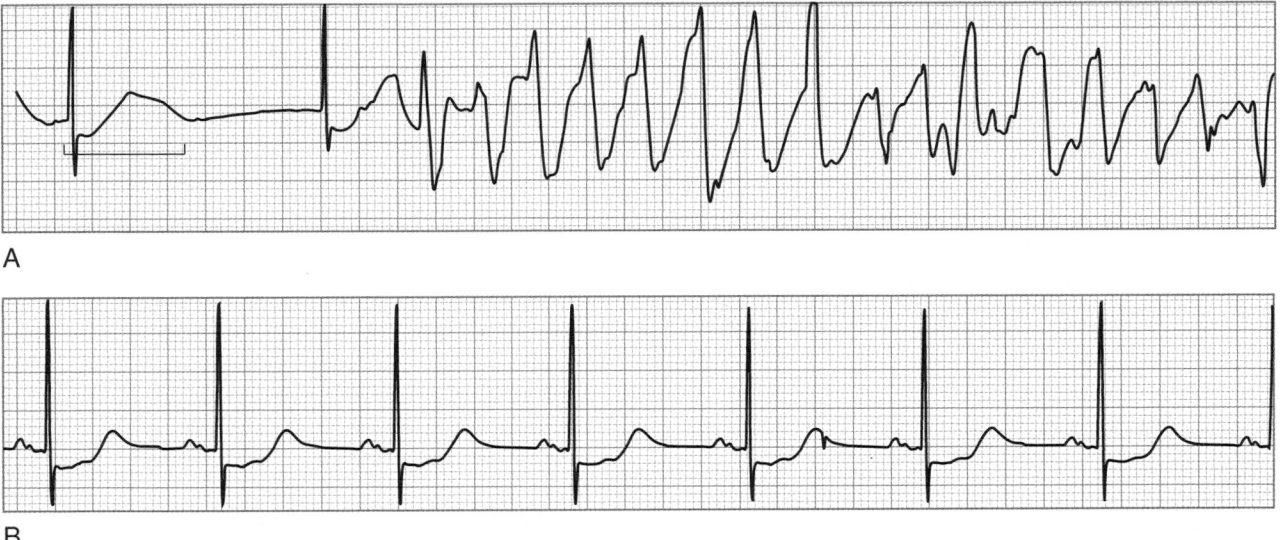

⬍FIGURE 10-13 A, Torsades de pointes. Note the longer QT interval of 800 msec at the beginning of the strip. **B,** Same patient in normal sinus rhythm. QT interval is about 560 msec.

refractory periods. Treatment must be aimed at shortening the refractory period, increasing the heart rate, and correcting underlying causes. The two most effective acute therapies are overdrive pacing and IV magnesium.[31]

Although a role remains for antidysrhythmic agents in helping to control frequent dysrhythmias, the implantable cardioverter-defibrillator (ICD) is very effective for long-term therapy. Data from multiple clinical trials now indicate there is a significant mortality reduction in patients who have survived sudden cardiac death, in patients at risk for sudden cardiac death, and in patients with heart failure with ICD implantation as compared with pharmacologic therapy.[8,9,11,84] The Research Utilization box below discusses some implications of longer survival with ICDs.

⬍ RESEARCH UTILIZATION

Use of the Implantable Cardioverter-Defibrillator

CLINICAL ISSUE

The use of the implantable cardioverter-defibrillator (ICD) is increasing. More than 100,000 ICDs were implanted in 2004 at a cost of $2 billion. In a review of 1280 patients who received ICDs since 1987 at one institution, 40% of patients survived 10 years post implantation. Battery life, on average, was 4.0 ± 1 years. Battery depletion accounts for 90% of ICD pulse generator failures.

SUMMARY AND APPLICATION

Over the next decade, the number of ICD implants is expected to increase dramatically as a result of the aging population, the increasing life span of patients with cardiovascular disease, the expanding indications for ICD implantation, and the increasing combination of ICD with cardiac resynchronization therapy. The economic and clinical impact will be substantial. Clinicians will be increasingly challenged to assist ICD patients with planning for follow-up and reimplantation.

NEED FOR FURTHER STUDY

How does patient quality of life relate to length of survival post implantation? What are the psychological, clinical, and economic implications of multiple implants? How will patient perspectives affect the development of ICD technology? What are the technological and clinical implications of increasing battery life? What is the role of rechargeable ICD batteries? What effect will increasing survival length have on reimbursement, utilization, and access to healthcare services? What are the ethical implications of multiple implants? How do we align incentives for industry, clinicians, providers, and patients to optimize battery life and ICD function?

Hauser, R. G. (2005). The growing mismatch between patient longevity and the service life of implantable cardioverter-defibrillators. *J Am Coll Cardiol, 45*(12), 2022-2025.

DISORDERS OF REPOLARIZATION

The QT Interval

The QT interval represents the time of ventricular depolarization and repolarization, including the refractory period. The QT interval is measured from the time the QRS complex leaves the isoelectric line to the time the T wave returns to the isoelectric line. Its duration varies with gender, age, autonomic activity, and time of day; and it varies inversely with heart rate.[18] The QT interval should be measured in lead II.[54,58,105]

Because of the variation in QT, it is customary to correct for the heart rate (QTc) to give a more precise measure of refractoriness. Bazett's formula, first introduced in 1920,[58] is the most commonly used formula for this purpose:

$$QTc = QT(ms) \div \sqrt{preceding\ R\text{-}R\ interval(msec)}$$

There is considerable variation in the length of the QT interval in individuals with and without structural heart disease. An interval of 460 msec or greater is generally considered abnormal, although the exact limits of normal remain unknown. Because of this, a long-standing undocumented rule-of-thumb has been commonly used to evaluate the QT interval. This rule states that the QT interval should be no longer than half the preceding R-R interval. This rule applies to heart rates of 60 to 100 beats per minute. The rule was first described by Marriott[66] and has since been mathematically validated. It is widely accepted as a clinically useful tool to quickly determine if the QT interval is normal.[18]

Long QT Syndrome

Long QT syndrome (LQTS) is divided into two types—acquired and congenital. Acquired or iatrogenic long QT syndrome is more common and may be caused by any factor that prolongs the QT interval, such as bradycardia, hypomagnesemia, hypokalemia, heart failure, cardiac hypertrophy, hypocalcemia, thyroid disorders, liver disease, renal disease, and subarachnoid hemorrhage.[18,58] It may be induced by drugs such as class Ia and III antidysrhythmics, antibiotics, psychotropic drugs, antihistamines, and many others. Box 10-1 lists selected drugs that can prolong the QT interval.

Congenital LQTS is an inherited disorder of the ion channels controlling cell permeability, specifically the I_K and I_{Na} channels that are responsible for repolarization.[18,88] These disorders cause prolonged refractory

---

Box 10-1

Selected Drugs That Prolong the QT Interval

Acrivastine	Diphenhydramine	Moricizine
Almokalant	Disopyramide	N-Acetylprocainamide
Amantadine	Dofetilide	Nortriptyline
Amiodarone	Doxepin	Papaverine, intracoronary
Amitriptyline	Droperidol	Pentamidine
Amoxapine	Erythromycin	Phenothiazines
Ampicillin	Flecainide	Procainamide
Aprindine	Fludrocortisone	Prochlorperazine
Astemizole	Fluoroquinolones	Propafenone
Azimilide	Fluphenazine	Protriptyline
Bepridil	Haloperidol	Quetiapine
Chloral hydrate	Hydroxyzine	Quinidine
Chloroquine	Ibutilide	Quinine
Chlorpromazine	Imidazole	Risperidone
Cisapride	Imipramine	Sotalol
Citalopram	Ipecac	Tamoxifen
Clemastine	Itraconazole	Terfenadine
Clomipramine	Ketoconazole	Thioridazine
Cocaine	Lithium	Thiothixene
Co-trimoxazole	Loratadine	Trifluoperazine
Desipramine	Milrinone	Trimethoprim sulfamethoxazole

From reference 18.

periods and abnormal T-U waves, which predispose the patient to reentry and triggered activity.

Prolonged repolarization equals prolonged refractoriness. Repolarization rate is related to heart rate, and sets up the refractory period for the next beat. A long beat-to-beat interval results in the next beat having a longer refractory time. The repolarization rate normally varies somewhat from cell to cell. Prolonged repolarization increases the disparity of refractoriness within the ventricular muscle cells. This is called *dispersion of repolarization*. The greater the disparity of refractoriness, the more dysrhythmogenic the situation.[66] Thus increased disparity in refractory times among ventricular cells is one adverse consequence of prolonged refractory periods, represented on the ECG by a prolonged QT interval. The second consequence of prolonged refractory periods is the potential for early afterdepolarizations. EADs occurring during the vulnerable period can result in triggered activity and reentrant tachycardias. It is the combination of EADs and dispersion of refractoriness that is dysrhythmogenic.

Clinical Significance. Individuals with LQTS are susceptible to torsades de pointes, ventricular fibrillation, and sudden cardiac death. In some patients, the first symptom is sudden cardiac death. In about 33% of patients, it is diagnosed during investigation of signs and symptoms such as palpitations, syncope, chest pain, or seizures.[58] Genetic studies have identified genes responsible for congenital LQTS and specific subtypes of the disorder; however, genetic testing for congenital LQTS is available only in research settings. It is estimated that a specific gene mutation will be identifiable in only about 50% of the cases.[106] As yet, genetic testing has little practical applicability. LQTS is diagnosed based on ECG findings as well as medical and family history. A family history of sudden, unexplained death should raise the index of suspicion.

Intravenous haloperidol (Haldol) is increasingly used to manage acute confusion in acutely and critically ill patients. Intravenous haloperidol has been associated with prolongation of the QT interval and TdP. Haloperidol blocks the K^+ channel, I_K, and therefore prolongs repolarization and QT. This effect is dose-related.[21] The incidence of TdP in patients who receive IV haloperidol is greater in those who have a prolonged QT interval than in those patients who do not. QT dispersion is increased in patients who develop TdP as well.[96] The new generation antipsychotic drugs such as ziprasidone (Geodon), risperidone (Risperdal), olanzapine (Zyprexa), and quetiapine (Seroquel), may cause QT prolongation as well; however, no cases of drug-induced TdP have been reported.[99]

Patients who receive IV haloperidol should have a baseline and daily ECGs for measurement of the QTc. K^+ and magnesium levels should be closely monitored. Zareba and Lin[105] recommend categorizing patients on antipsychotics into three groups: those with QTc of 410 msec or less, who are unlikely to develop prodysrhythmia; those with borderline risk at QTc of 420 to 440 msec; and those with a QTc of 450 msec or greater. Those patients at low risk should have a baseline ECG with further ECGs required only if other QT-prolonging drugs are added. Borderline patients are at low risk, and a regular ECG for monitoring QTc is sufficient. Those with prolonged QTc intervals need regular 12-lead ECGs for monitoring the QTc and close monitoring of serum K^+ and magnesium levels. Because a QTc of greater than 500 ms is associated with the greatest risk of TdP, haloperidol should be discontinued if the QTc reaches 500 msec or if multiple QTc-prolonging drugs are needed.[96,105]

Because so many drugs and medical conditions can affect the QT interval, clinicians must be very alert to possible drug interactions. Of special interest are interactions involving drugs that inhibit the cytochrome P-450 system (for example, diltiazem, erythromycin, fluconazole [Diflucan], and methylprednisolone) given concurrently with cisapride (Propulsid) or pimozide (Orap).* The cytochrome P-450 system is an enzymatic drug metabolism system expressed in the liver and in the intestinal endothelium. In this system, drugs are metabolized by binding to receptors for the system enzymes. If two or more P-450 drugs are given concurrently, they compete for the receptors; some will bind more than others. This will result in increased plasma concentrations of the drugs that bind less, which can lead to adverse effects from those drugs.

Grapefruit interacts with many cardiac drugs (such as calcium channel blockers and statins), tranquilizers, and sertraline (Zoloft) through the P-450 system expressed in the intestinal wall.[7,36] Grapefruit juice inhibits this enzyme system and can lead to increased serum concentrations of drugs metabolized through this system. This effect is highly variable among individuals. To date the data on grapefruit juice-drug interactions are based on small studies of healthy volunteers. No studies have addressed adverse effects of these interactions.[36] Because of the popularity of grapefruit juice, the clinician is well advised to be aware of and monitor for food-drug interactions when cytochrome P-450 drugs are prescribed. Avoiding concomitant administration of drugs that prolong QT intervals, monitoring electrolyte levels, and

---

*References 18, 24, 51, 57, 63, 104.

decreasing dosage in individuals with multiple risk factors are all important for prevention of adverse effects related to the QT interval. It is also important to teach patients with known LQTS about risk factors, potential drug interactions, and symptoms of tachycardias. Events that cause sudden arousal are likely triggers of dysrhythmias in patients with some specific subtypes of congenial LQTS. Such events might include exercise, emotion, alarm clocks, or telephones.[89] Patient counseling should include avoidance of vigorous sporting activities and other situations that evoke adrenergic surges, even including doorbells, alarm clocks, and loud concerts. Fainting spells require a prompt medical evaluation.[73]

There is preliminary evidence that cranberry juice and pomegranate juice may also inhibit some of the hepatic enzymes. Although there have been no reports of QT interval prolongation associated with use of herbal products, they may interact with cardiac medications via the cytochrome P-450 system.

Treatment. For symptomatic individuals, the risk of abrupt syncopal events is 5% per year and mortality is nearly 50% without treatment.[58] Beta blockers, such as atenolol (Tenormin), metoprolol (Lopressor), propranolol (Inderal), and nadolol (Corgard), are the first-line treatment. Other possible therapies include pacing, ICD, and cardiothoracic sympathectomy. Gene therapy is still evolving.[58,73]

Brugada Syndrome

Brugada syndrome is an inherited genetic disorder of the Na^+ channels that leads to shortened repolarization in the right ventricle. First described in 1992, it is diagnosed by a characteristic cluster of ECG signs in otherwise healthy young adults with no structural heart disease.[10] Brugada syndrome leads to a propensity for sudden cardiac death, which is often the first symptom.

In Brugada syndrome, the inward Na^+ current in the right ventricle is reduced, shortening repolarization. This increases the dispersion of refractoriness over the myocardium, which is dysrhythmogenic. The characteristic ECG signs (Figure 10-14) occur most prominently in V_1 to V_3 and include the following:

- J point elevation
- RBBB pattern in V_1 to V_3 with terminal R waves (epsilon waves) and absence of wide S wave in I, V_5, and V_6
- ST elevation unrelated to ischemia or other abnormalities
- Normal QT

Individuals with Brugada syndrome are prone to syncope and life-threatening dysrhythmias that appear to be vagally mediated. Most deaths occur during sleep. It occurs more frequently in males of Southeast Asian and Japanese descent. Amiodarone and beta blockers have not proven beneficial. ICD implantation is the current treatment of choice.[58]

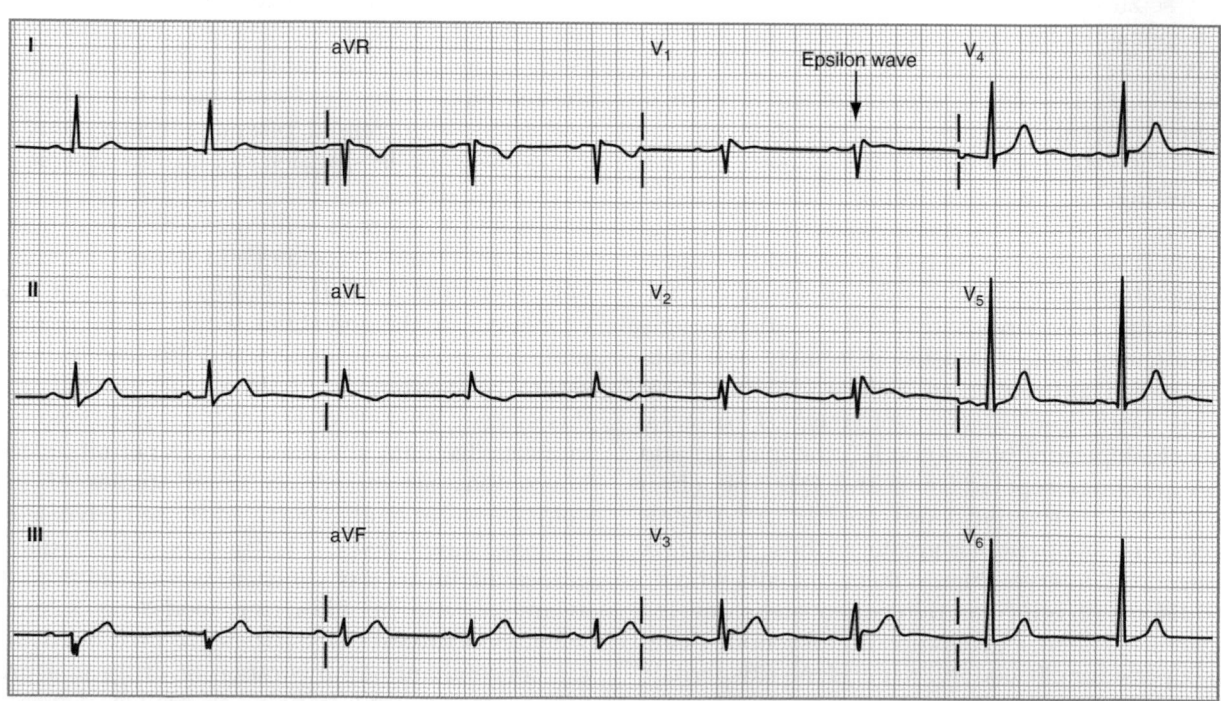

♦**FIGURE 10-14** Brugada syndrome. Note the epsilon waves in V_1-V_3 and the absence of S waves in leads I, aVL, and V_6.

ABERRANCY VERSUS ECTOPY

Mechanisms of Aberrancy

Aberrancy is defined by *Stedman's Medical Dictionary* as "deviating from the normal course or pattern."[93] In cardiac terms, when a supraventricular impulse is conducted abnormally through the ventricles, it is termed aberrant. Aberrrant conduction will take longer to activate the ventricle, resulting in a wide QRS. Situations that result in wide QRS complexes include beats of ventricular origin, preexcitation through an AP, and temporary or permanent BBB. The term *aberration* is usually reserved for temporary conditions. Therefore both supraventricular and ventricular impulses may result in a wide QRS complex. Distinguishing between the two is one of the most common clinical problems in cardiac nursing. Accurate diagnosis is important both for effective management of the acute event and for long-term therapy. Aberrant conduction occurs when an impulse arrives at the His-Purkinje system during phase 3 of the action potential and finds it partially or completely refractory. As discussed earlier, refractory period length is directly related to the preceding cycle length so that a long cycle (slow heart rate) is followed by a long refractory period and a short cycle (fast heart rate) is followed by a short refractory period. If the cycle length suddenly changes or is constantly fluctuating, aberrancy is likely. Situations prone to aberrancy include premature supraventricular beats, which arrive too early; rapid heart rates, which may not allow enough time for the bundle branches to completely repolarize; and atrial fibrillation or other irregular rhythms, where cycle length continually changes. If the aberrancy only occurs at rapid heart rates, the term rate-dependent BBB is used. The right bundle branch conducts more slowly and has a longer refractory period than the left bundle so aberrant beats most often have an RBBB morphology.

General Principles of Diagnosis

Contrary to commonly held myths, the most reliable clues to distinguishing aberrancy from ectopy are ECG clues. VT is much more common than SVT with aberration. In addition, hemodynamic stability is not reliably associated with one or the other. Patients may remain stable for some time with either VT or SVT and, similarly, may deteriorate quickly with either rhythm. If available, the patient's history is helpful. Known structural heart disease or history of MI suggests VT. Because very rapid rates may occur in both supraventricular and ventricular rhythms, heart rate is not a useful clue (Table 10-2).[45] VT is most often regular. An irregular wide-complex tachycardia with a rate greater than 220 beats per minute is likely to be atrial fibrillation with aberrant conduction.[45]

Physical Signs. The neck veins provide useful clues to the diagnosis. Atrial contraction against closed AV valves results in a reflux of blood back through the jugular veins. In PSVT, this results in regular venous pulsations while in VT there may be irregular jugular venous pulsations if the atrial and ventricular rhythms are dissociated. Retrograde conduction into the atria during VT may result in regular cannon waves. The intensity of the first heart sound (S_1) varies when there is AV dissociation. This occurs because the first heart sound is produced by the closure of the AV valves. The intensity of S_1 depends on the proximity of the AV leaflets to one another when the ventricles contract. In AV dissociation, the ventricles contract at varying intervals related to the atrial cycle. Thus the leaflets may be closer together or farther apart beat to beat, and the intensity of the closing sound varies. PSVT may be associated with polyuria, which is likely related to release of atrial natriuretic factor.[18] VT usually does not respond to carotid sinus massage, whereas supraventricular rhythms may either be converted to sinus rhythm or be slowed enough to diagnose the atrial mechanism.

ECG Clues. AV dissociation is an important ECG clue. The presence of P waves dissociated from the ventricular rhythm is considered diagnostic for VT.[18] Be careful when looking for P waves because it is easy to mistake irregularities in the QRS for P waves. The most reliable approach is to look for distortions in QRS complexes that are not present in every cycle, rather than looking for P wave presence in every cycle. Extreme right electrical axis (no-man's land, suggesting that the electrical location of axes lying within this quadrant is imprecise) suggests VT. Concordance of the precordial leads means that all six precordial leads have the same deflection direction. Negative precordial concordance is diagnostic for VT.[18] Positive concordance, while not as diagnostic, is strongly suggestive of VT.[18,45] In addition, a QRS width 0.16 second or greater suggests VT, as does QRS morphology similar to that of previous PVCs. Other axis conditions that suggest VT include a left axis ($-60°$ to $-90°$) with an RBBB morphology and a right axis ($+120°$ to $+180°$) LBBB morphology.[29] Capture beats happen when the sinus impulse randomly arrives at nonrefractory bundle branches, is conducted through the ventricles, and produces a narrow QRS during a wide-complex tachycardia. If a second ventricular ectopic focus fires in concert with the primary ectopic focus, ventricular fusion may occur. In fusion, the ventricle is depolarized by both a supraventricular impulse and a ventricular impulse, producing a QRS of different morphology than either. Although uncommon, capture and fusion beats are diagnostic for VT.[18] In order to

TABLE 10-2 Differential Diagnosis of Aberrancy Versus Ectopy According to V_1 Polarity

	V_1—POSITIVE	V_1—NEGATIVE
Suggests VT	Monophasic R in V_1 Biphasic V_1 R or qR in V_1 with taller left rabbit ear QRS >0.14 sec R:S ratio >1 in V_6 if left axis QS or rS in V_6 R-S interval >100 ms in any precordial lead Onset of QRS to tallest peak >70 msec	Broad R (>0.03 sec) V_1 or V_2 Slurred downstroke V_1 or V_2 Delayed S nadir (>0.06 sec) V_1 or V_2 Any Q in V_6 Right axis deviation QRS >0.16 sec R-S interval >100 msec in any precordial lead
Suggests SVT	Triphasic V_1 (rSR') Triphasic V_6 (qRs) ONLY if V_1 positive QRS ≤0.14 sec Onset of QRS to tallest peak <50 msec	Narrow initial r wave V_1 or V_2 Smooth downstroke V_1 or V_2 No Q in V_6 Onset of QRS to nadir <50 msec

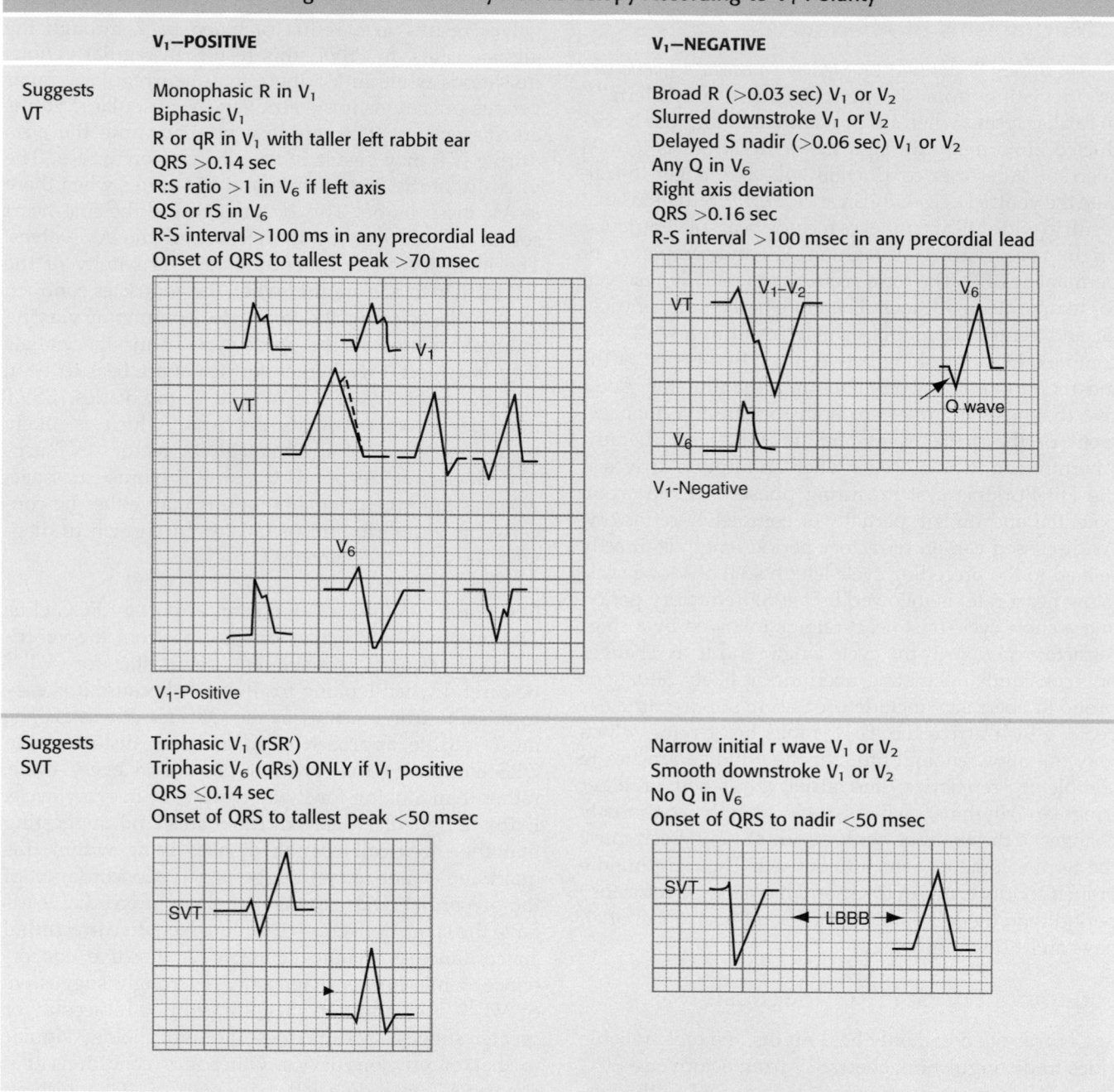

use QRS morphology to distinguish aberrancy from ectopy, it is helpful to sort the clues into V_1-positive and V_1-negative complexes (see Table 10-2). Figure 10-15 demonstrates sinus tachycardia with RBBB (V_1 positive) aberration. Figure 10-16 demonstrates VT with RBBB (V_1 positive) morphology. Figure 10-17 illustrates SVT with LBBB aberration (V_1 negative). Figure 10-18 illustrates VT with LBBB morphology (V_1 negative).

DIGITALIS TOXICITY

Digitalis Dysrhythmias

Because digitalis has a narrow therapeutic range, toxicity is not uncommon and can be a source of significant dysrhythmias. Digitalis can produce a great variety of dysrhythmias; however, profound bradycardia, junctional tachycardia, atrial tachycardia, and fascicular

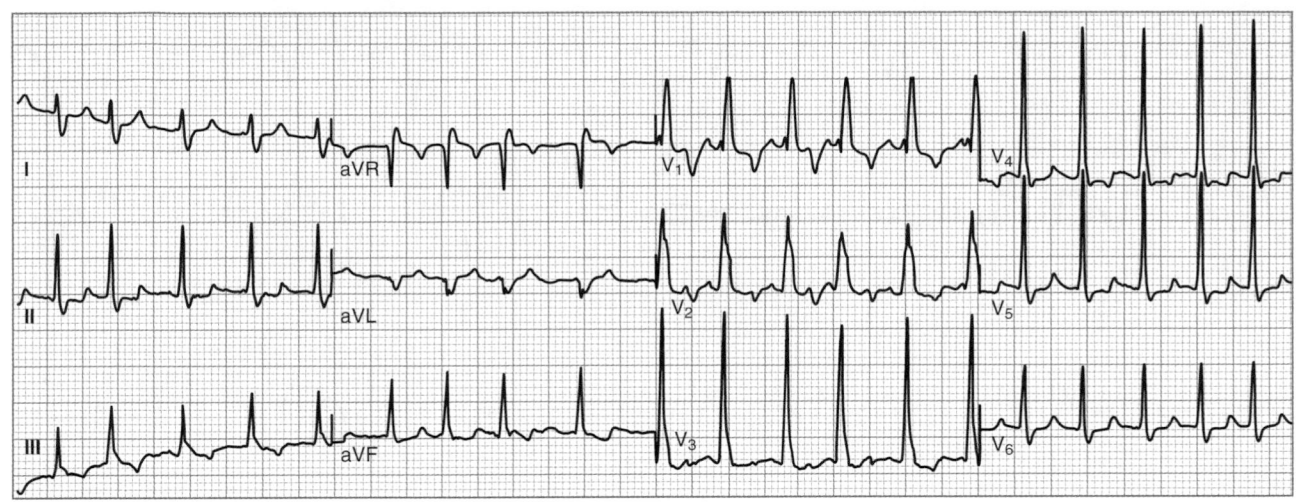

✦FIGURE 10-15 Sinus tachycardia with right bundle branch block aberration. Features favoring a diagnosis of SVT include typical rsR′ pattern in V_1 and wide S waves in leads I, aVL, and V_6. P waves are best seen preceding QRS complexes in V_1 and the early beats are most likely PACs.

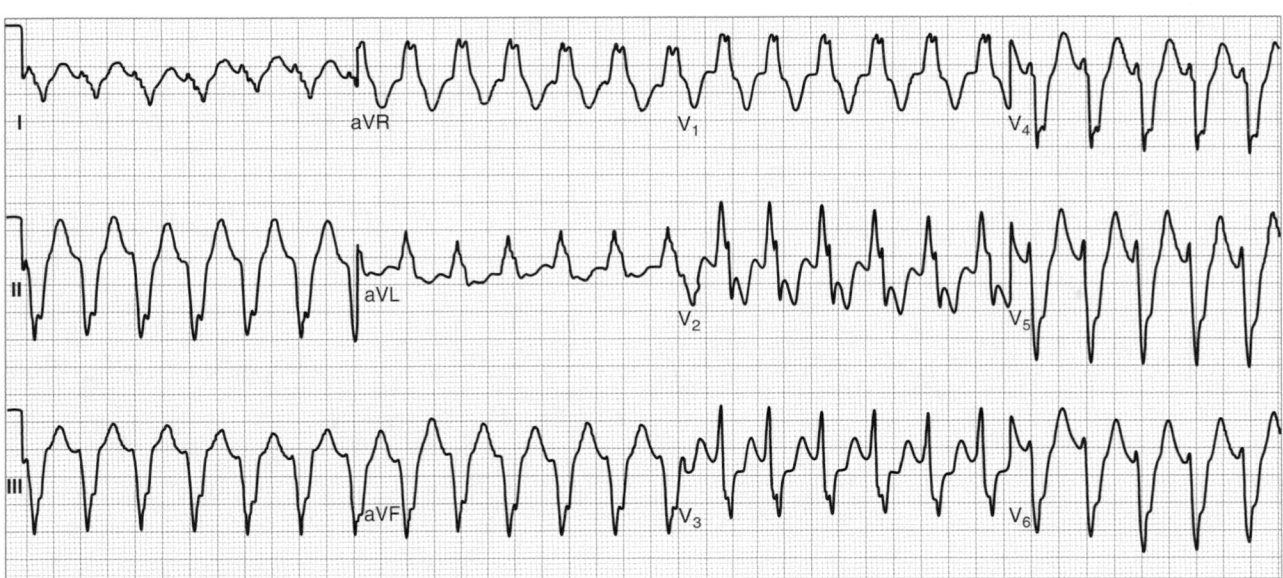

✦FIGURE 10-16 Ventricular tachycardia with right bundle branch block morphology. Features favoring the diagnosis of ventricular tachycardia include the following: taller left peak in V_1, rS in V_6, indeterminate axis, and QRS width of 0.16 sec.

ventricular tachycardia are of particular interest because they can be life threatening. Monitor ECGs of digitalized patients and systematically review rhythm strips for the following characteristics[18]:

- New bradycardias
- AV blocks
- New tachycardias
- Junctional tachycardia (rate greater than 70 beats per minute)
- Fascicular ventricular tachycardia

- Unexpected regularity of atrial fibrillation
- Group beating in atrial fibrillation (escape rhythm is junctional tachycardia with Wenckebach conduction)
- Group beating in sinus rhythm (bigeminy, AV Wenckebach)

Bradycardia. The sinus node rate can be slowed by the direct actions of digitalis in combination with vagal activity. In digitalis toxicity, bradycardia is often

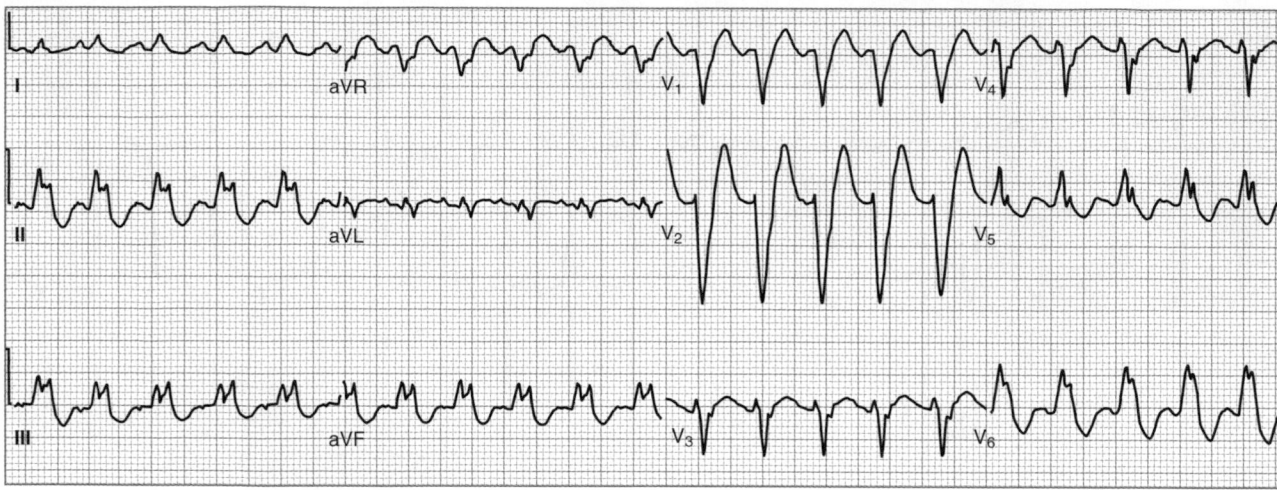

♣FIGURE 10-17 SVT with left bundle branch block morphology. Features favoring diagnosis include the following: narrow r wave and straight downstroke of QRS in V_2; measurement from onset of QRS to nadir of S wave in V_1 and V_2 is not greater than 0.06 sec; no q wave in V_6; P waves are best seen preceding each QRS in aVL, and they appear inverted in lead III.

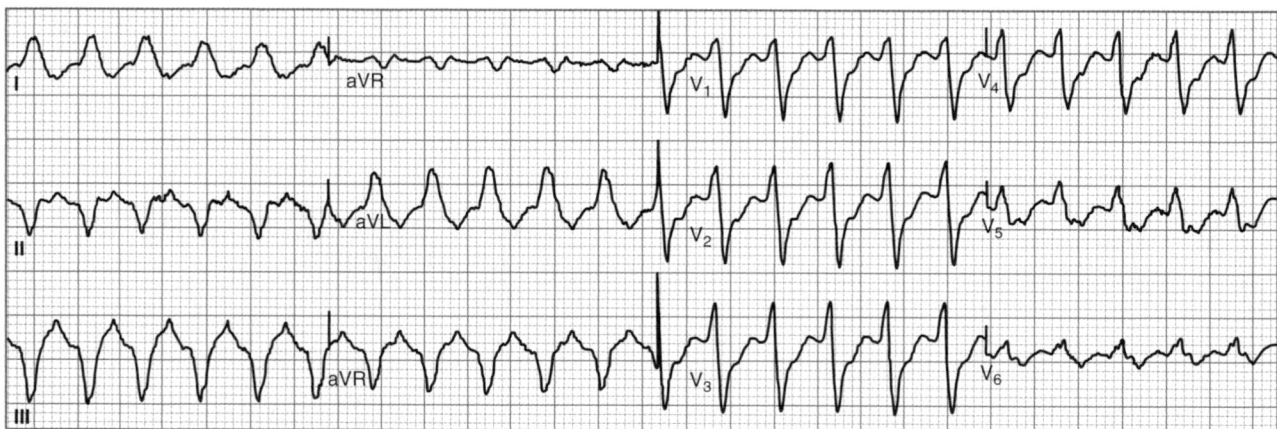

♣FIGURE 10-18 VT with left bundle branch block morphology. Features favoring the diagnosis of ventricular tachycardia include the following: wide r wave (0.08 sec) in V_1 and V_2; delay from onset of QRS to nadir of S wave of 0.14 sec in V_1 and V_2.

associated with junctional escape beats. Either SA Wenckebach, AV Wenckebach, or both can occur with digitalis toxicity. They would be indicated by the classic Wenckebach signs of group beating, shortening R-R intervals, lengthening P-R intervals (AV Wenckebach only), and pauses less than twice the shortest interval. Prolongation of the P-R interval during sinus bradycardia in a digitalized patient is a sign of toxicity as well.

Atrial Tachycardia. Digitalis toxicity can produce atrial tachycardias of rates 130 to 250 beats per minute. AV block of varying degrees is often associated with these tachycardias. Atrial fibrillation may convert to a rapid

atrial tachycardia with a high degree of block in the setting of digitalis toxicity.

Junctional Tachycardia. Junctional tachycardia is one of the most alarming digitalis-induced dysrhythmias. The junctional rate will be 70 to 140 beats per minute. It is a regular rhythm with a gradual onset, best seen in V_1. P waves may or may not be seen, but retrograde P waves will not be seen because of the AV block from the digitalis. Again, conduction variations between the junctional tissue and the ventricles can occur and a Wenckebach pattern of group beating will be noted. Junctional tachycardia during atrial fibrillation may occur and can be recognized by a change to a regular ventricular rhythm. When junctional tachycardia occurs with atrial flutter, the flutter waves have no constant relationship to the QRS, indicating AV dissociation. Junctional tachycardia in the presence of digitalis toxicity indicates severe AV block and should be immediately treated.

Fascicular Ventricular Tachycardia. Fascicular ventricular tachycardia of digitalis toxicity occurs when the tachycardia originates in one of the left bundle fascicles. Its rate is 90 to 160 beats per minute, and produces an RBBB morphology. Axis deviation occurs and may alternate between right and left deviation if the rhythm alternates between fascicles. The characteristic down-sloping ST segment known as the "digitalis effect" may be very noticeable in fascicular VT. The tachycardia is actually multifocal, indicated by changing morphology between the precordial leads, and is a result of changing conduction pathways through the Purkinje fibers.[18] Unlike other VTs, fascicular VT may respond to verapamil.

Management of Digitalis Dysrhythmias

The key to management is early recognition. The manifestations can be gradual and very subtle; therefore the rhythm strips of digitalized patients should be analyzed carefully for signs. In addition, watch patients carefully for physical symptoms of digitalis toxicity, especially if the patient is not monitored. Symptoms include nausea, vomiting, anorexia, headaches, malaise, disorientation, memory problems, hallucinations, nightmares, and insomnia. Visual changes are classic symptoms of digitalis toxicity and include halos and spots. In addition, unexpected difficulty with red-green contrast of color monitors may indicate digitalis toxicity.[18] Serum digitalis levels are helpful but not sufficient indicators of toxicity. Patients may manifest symptoms of toxicity in the presence of a normal level and, conversely, may be asymptomatic in the presence of an elevated digitalis level. Physical symptoms and ECG changes are the most reliable indication of toxicity.

Once diagnosed, the digitalis should be immediately stopped. Bed rest is helpful to avoid catecholamine surges and syncope. Cardiac monitoring is recommended. Because both hypokalemia and hypomagnesemia potentiate digitalis, these abnormalities should be corrected as soon as possible. Treat tachycardias as indicated by hemodynamic status. For bradycardia, temporary pacing may be necessary. Digoxin immune Fab (Digibind), which binds to free digoxin, is used if the patient shows signs of hemodynamic instability or hyperkalemia. Underlying exacerbating conditions such as acute ischemia or acute heart failure should be eliminated or controlled.

ATRIAL FIBRILLATION

Electrophysiologic Features

It is estimated that 4% of the U.S. population older than age 60, about 2 million people, have atrial fibrillation (AF). It is the most common sustained clinical dysrhythmia seen.[42] AF is a rhythm characterized by rapid and disorganized depolarization in the atria resulting in the replacement of P waves on the ECG with irregular fibrillatory (F) waves at rates of 350 to 600 impulses per minute with an irregularly irregular ventricular response. The electrical activity is characterized by "multiple wandering wavelets"[5] that do not reenter their own pathway but can randomly reexcite other pathways that have been previously excited by another wavelet.

This is termed *microreentry*.[5] Resulting circuits are unstable, disappearing and re-forming at random. There also appears to be short and variable cycle lengths and increased dispersion of refractoriness.[5] The AV node allows only a certain number of the fibrillation impulses to be conducted to the ventricle, which results in an irregular and often rapid ventricular response. The number of impulses that reach the ventricles is dependent on a number of factors, including the amount of sympathetic stimulation and electrophysiologic properties of the AV node.[5,35,76] AF is associated with significant morbidity and hospitalization; major risks associated with AF include substantial threat of thromboembolism because of stasis of blood in the fibrillating atria, development of congestive heart failure, increased hospitalizations, and death.[13,19,42] Costs attributed to AF are estimated at $1 billion in the United States alone.[13]

The most common cause of AF is initiation by atrial premature beats. Studies have demonstrated that areas around the pulmonary vein, superior vena cava, and coronary sinus are common sites for these premature beats.[5,49,50] There is evidence that the presence of AF can alter the atrial electrophysiology and structure in ways that perpetuate AF. This is termed *atrial remodeling* and contributes to the difficulty seen in abolishing established AF.[76]

The American Heart Association recommends classifying new AF that is unassociated with a reversible cause (not secondary to cardiac surgery or pericarditis, for example) into one of four types: (1) paroxysmal, in which episodes last 7 days or less; (2) persistent, in which episodes last longer than 7 days; (3) permanent, in which AF lasts more than 1 year; and (4) lone AF for any of the above types that occur without structural heart disease.[35]

Management of Atrial Fibrillation

Goals of management of AF are symptom alleviation and prevention of stroke. A great deal of study has been devoted to the question of whether to restore sinus rhythm (rhythm control) or to control the ventricular response but allow the AF to continue (rate control). Rate control with chronic anticoagulation is currently recommended for most patients.[69,92,103] To achieve rate control via pharmacologic means, the strongest efficacy and safety evidence is for atenolol, metoprolol, diltiazem, and verapamil.[69] For conversion to sinus rhythm, the best evidence exists for amiodarone, dofetilide (Tikosyn), ibutilide, propafenone, and flecainide.[102]

Nonpharmacologic Approaches to Management of Atrial Fibrillation. There are significant disadvantages to pharmacologic options for conversion of AF to sinus rhythm, notably recurrence of AF and side effect profiles. Because of this, there is growing interest in nonpharmacologic approaches to restoring sinus rhythm. Sinus rhythm offers several advantages such as symptom alleviation and decreased risk of thromboembolism. Nonpharmacologic techniques offer the additional advantage of avoiding drug side effects. There are four currently available options: surgical techniques, radiofrequency catheter ablation, pacing, and implantable atrial defibrillators. The ideal operative procedure for AF would abolish AF and restore sinus rhythm, maintain atrioventricular synchrony, maintain atrial function, and reduce the risk of thromboembolism.[14]

Surgery for Atrial Fibrillation. Cox[20] developed the Maze procedure in the 1980s. In this procedure, incisions in the atria isolate parts of the atria and interrupt the reentry circuits. The radial modification uses the same principle; however, the incisions are made in such a way as to preserve more of the natural atrial activation, and thus improve atrial contractility.[5,14] The procedure has since evolved into the Maze III procedure in which incisions are made in the right atrial free wall, cryoablation is used to create conduction block at the tricuspid valve, the orifices of the pulmonary veins are electrically isolated with an encircling incision, and both atrial appendages are resected.[78] Successful cure of AF has been achieved in 81% to 99% patients who have received Maze procedures since 1987; operative mortality is 2% to 3%.[67,78,85] At 10-year follow-up of 197 patients who underwent the procedure, one study reported 89.3% patients had no recurrence of AF.[37] Stroke rate is also substantially reduced.[3] Because the pulmonary veins were noted to be initiating sites for AF, surgical isolation of the orifices has been used as a strategy for preventing AF. Initial success with this approach led to its incorporation into the Maze III procedure.[78]

The surgery requires a median sternotomy, cardiopulmonary bypass, and cold circulatory arrest for a portion of the procedure. Postulated complications include sinus node dysfunction and disrupted atrial contractility. These complications remain rare. Left atrial function is intact in 93% of patients and right atrial function in 99% of patients, with no long-term damage to the sinus node.[78]

Ablative Procedures. Ablation for AF evolved from surgical techniques. Advantages of ablative techniques over the classic Maze surgery include eliminating surgical incisions (replacing them with tissue ablation lesions) and making fewer incision in the right atrium, focusing on the pulmonary vein orifices (which allows for better left atrial function), and using a less invasive and more patient-specific approach.[78] Several technologies have been utilized including radiofrequency energy (monopolar and bipolar), cryoablation, microwave energy, and laser energy. All of these technologies have been used with success.[78] Ablative approaches include focal ablation of ectopic foci, pulmonary vein isolation, catheter-based electroanatomic mapping system (CARTO, which allows for detailed mapping of the atria and focused pulmonary vein isolation), focal ablation of reentry sites using complex fractionated atrial electrocardiograms, and ablation of cardiac autonomic nerves. The techniques are still evolving; however, results to date are encouraging. Absence of atrial fibrillation at 1 year ranges from 50% to 85%, and absence of thromboembolic events is also high.[78] In a study of 181 centers worldwide, reporting on 8745 patients, Cappato et al.[12] found an average of 52% reported the absence of AF without antidysrhythmic agents, and an additional 23.9% were free of AF with the addition of antidysrhythmic agents. Two procedures were required in 24.3% of the patients and three procedures were required in 3.1% of patients. Major complications were reported in 6% of patients. An additional finding is that outcomes were better in higher-volume centers. These data indicate that the use of ablative techniques is rapidly expanding but still evolving. Although success is achieved in significant numbers of patients, complication rates appear higher than with surgical techniques and success is related to operator experience.[5,14]

Pacing Therapies. Pacing in atrial fibrillation has largely been used to maintain acceptable ventricular rates in patients with slow ventricular response. There is substantial evidence that, especially in patients with sinus node dysfunction, physiologic pacing using atrial or dual-chamber pacing modes also decreases the occurrence of atrial fibrillation.[17,42,47,56]

In patients with a history of AF, alternative pacing modalities have been used to prevent recurrences of AF with some success. Dual-site atrial pacing, in which a lead is placed in the right atrial appendage and one in the coronary sinus, paces both atria simultaneously. The proposed advantage is that greater synchronization of atrial activity reduces the occurrence of AF.[19] Several studies investigated this technique to prevent postoperative AF in cardiac surgery patients. Three randomized studies found a significant reduction in postoperative AF with dual-site simultaneous pacing as opposed to single-site pacing.[22,34,61]

The Dual-Site Atrial Pacing to Prevent Atrial Fibrillation (DAPPAF) trial randomized 118 patients to high right atrial (RA) pacing, dual-site RA pacing, or support pacing (DDI or VDI). Time to recurrence of AF was longer with dual-site RA pacing, and in patients treated with both an antidysrhythmic and pacing, dual-site RA pacing reduced AF recurrence by 34%.[19,82] Proposed advantages of this technique include a shortened P wave, which could be useful in patients with delayed interatrial conduction. Disadvantages include the difficulty in placing the second atrial lead and other technical issues.[19]

Another application for pacemakers in the setting of AF is the use of overdrive atrial pacing. In demand pacing, the faster the pacemaker's programmed rate, the more paced beats that occur. Atrial pacing affects the dynamics of atrial contraction and appears to suppress premature atrial beats.[15,19] Early results from studies of fixed-rate atrial pacing at faster rates for prevention of AF were mixed. Since then, work has focused on developing devices with algorithms that provide overdrive suppression of premature atrial beats, maintain a high percentage of paced beats, minimize sudden rate changes, prevent excessively high paced rates, and maintain the normal circadian variations in heart rate.[13,15] The Atrial Dynamic Overdrive Pacing Trial (ADOPT) tested the efficacy of one such algorithm— the AF Suppression Algorithm (St. Jude Medical Cardiac Rhythm Management Division, Sylmar, California). Results showed a small but significant reduction in number of days when AF occurred but showed no differences in mean number of AF episodes, hospitalizations, complications, adverse events, and death.[13] This algorithm has since been approved for use by the FDA.

In patients with antibradycardia dual-chamber pacing who have recurrent AF, a function termed *mode-switching* is used to prevent inappropriate tracking of the rapid atrial rate. When a rapid atrial rate is sensed, the pacemaker switches from the dual-chamber pacing mode into an atrial sensing, but not atrial tracking, mode. This feature allows for physiologic pacing but prevents pacing at a fast atrial rate. This is particularly useful in patients who have radiofrequency ablation of the AV node for rate control.[15]

The American Heart Association published a *Science Advisory* in 2005 making the following recommendations:[52]

1. Patents who have a history of AF and who need a pacemaker for bradycardia should receive a physiologic pacemaker (dual chamber or atrial) rather than a single-chamber ventricular pacemaker.
2. For patients who need a pacemaker for bradycardia and also have AF, there are no consistent data to support alternative single-site atrial pacing, multisite RA pacing, biatrial pacing, overdrive pacing, or antitachycardia atrial pacing.
3. Currently, pacing to prevent AF in patients without a bradycardia indication for pacing is not indicated.

Electrical Cardioversion. The Metrix (InControl) was the first atrial defibrillator with successful clinical use. This device had both automatic shock and patient-activated shock modes and was found to be feasible and safe; however, it is no longer on the market.[38,59] Subsequently, several devices capable of terminating both atrial and ventricular dysrhythmias have been approved for use. The Jewel AF device (Medtronic) provides antitachycardia pacing and defibrillation for both atrial and ventricular dysrhythmias, as well as dual-chamber pacing and patient-activated therapy. It successfully terminated drug-refractory AF with high-frequency burst pacing in 16.8% of episodes and in 76% of episodes with atrial defibrillation. Six-month complication-free survival was 88% for burst pacing and 94% with atrial defibrillation.[87] In a second study, termination of AF with burst pacing occurred in 30% of episodes.[4] A number of small studies have demonstrated feasibility of this therapy, good tolerance by patients, decreased resource utilization, and maintained or improved quality of life.[72,77,82] A newer model of this same therapy, the GEM III AT (Medtronic), is now on the market as are other models. Gillis et al.[40] reported 26% termination of AF episodes via antitachycardia pacing and 26% success with burst pacing without evidence of inducing ventricular dysrhythmias with the GEM III device. Two important limitations to use of these devices remain. Cost remains problematic. In addition, the exact group of patients who will most benefit from this therapy is not yet established.[60]

HEART RATE VARIABILITY

Measurement

Both the sympathetic and parasympathetic nervous systems have significant influence on cardiac function.[43] Heart rate variability (HRV) measurement has emerged as a valid tool with which to measure the balance of autonomic influences. The heart rate is based chiefly on the amount of sympathetic or parasympathetic influence on the SA intrinsic rate. Normally, the parasympathetic system has the most influence. Periods of sympathetic predominance occur intermittently over 24 hours; however, sustained sympathetic dominance is abnormal. Sympathetic nervous system (SNS) activity alters the ability of the heart to modulate rate and enhances electrical instability.[65] Normal heart rates vary even at rest, and this variability has been referred to as *respiratory variation*. Sleep-wake state, age, gender, body position, activity level, pain, and sleep apnea influence HRV.[68]

HRV is a measure of the beat-to-beat variability between cardiac cycles in normal sinus rhythm. The common unit of measurement is the R-to-R interval between normal beats, or the NN interval. HRV measurement is performed through a normal ECG recording analyzed through software programs. The various programs use complex statistical analyses called *time domain analysis* and *frequency domain analysis* as well as various techniques of nonlinear analysis. Time domain analysis is based on the time of NN intervals whereas frequency domain or spectral analysis provides information on how variance in rhythm is distributed as a function of rate.[65] Only sinus rhythm beats are used for HRV analysis.

Clinical Significance

Depressed HRV (less variability than expected) is associated with increased sympathetic activity. Research to date indicates that depressed HRV over 24 hours is an independent predictor of mortality and risk of sustained ventricular tachycardia after MI. Combined with other risk factors, HRV is a powerful predictor of mortality. Chronic activation of the sympathetic system is seen in patients with heart failure, and depressed HRV is associated with worse LV function and peak oxygen consumption, and is an independent predictor of survival in heart failure.[46,65]

Several studies have shown that the combination of increased age, insulin-dependent diabetes, and depressed HRV predicts increased length of stay after cardiovascular surgery.[55,95,97] In patients with hypertension, HRV patterns are abnormal, and reduced HRV in men is a strong predictor for the development of hypertension.[68] Studies of beta blockade on HRV have indicated that these agents increase the vagal effect on HR and decrease sympathetic effects.[94] Finally, HRV is a marker of the extent of diabetic neuropathy. The metabolic syndrome (diabetes, dyslipidemia, and hypertension) is associated with depressed HRV patterns.[68] Given the clinical usefulness of HRV measurement for diagnosis, prognosis, and risk stratification, critical care nurses can expect to see it with increasing frequency and are well advised to become familiar with its use.

MONITORING IN CRITICAL CARE

Accurate Lead Placement

Precise placement of the ECG electrodes is critical for accurate rhythm monitoring. Studies indicate that misplacement by as little as one intercostal space can alter the morphology of the QRS enough to change a diagnosis.[27] Misplacement of precordial electrodes can mimic anterior MI or RBBB.[71] Skin preparation is important both for accuracy and for prevention of erroneous alarms. Skin preparation strategies include cleaning the skin with alcohol to remove skin oils and clipping hair from areas where electrodes are to be placed. In addition, leads should be checked for proper placement and dryness and electrodes changed at regular intervals. Alarms should be individualized to the patient's baseline and clinical condition.

Choosing a Monitoring Lead

Ischemia. Because of the localized nature of ischemia, multiple leads are necessary to monitor for ischemia across a variety of areas. Thus studies have focused on associating coronary arteries with specific leads that are best at detecting ischemia in that area. The monitoring lead should be chosen to correlate with the area at risk. For the right coronary artery, lead III is recommended; for the left anterior descending artery, V_3; and for the circumflex, V_3.[18,27] Interestingly, common monitoring leads, leads II and V_1, are not sensitive for detecting ischemia. Therefore if the goal is to detect acute ischemia, the combination of leads III and V_3 would be recommended.

Reduced-lead configuration methods, such as the EASI 12-Lead system (Philips Medical Systems, Andover, Massachusetts), have been developed that may be used for ischemia monitoring. Technology such as this enables the clinician to obtain 12 ECG leads from a smaller number of electrodes. This creates a practical means of continuously monitoring 12 leads. The EASI configuration is a *derived ECG* and was developed by

Dower et al.[23] This system has been systematically studied and is considered diagnostically comparable to a standard 12-lead ECG for several purposes. These include analysis of wide-complex tachycardias, acute MI, angioplasty-induced ischemia, transient ischemia, and dysrhythmias.[26,28,48]

ST Segment Monitoring. ST segment monitoring is increasingly popular for detecting episodes of transient ischemia. Again, the leads best for detecting ischemia (III and V_3) are recommended.

Set the measuring point at J point + 60 ms because this will avoid the upslope of the T wave. Establish the patient's baseline and set the alarm 100 to 200 microvolts above this baseline, even if abnormal.[18] In a study of 237 telemetry patients admitted for acute coronary syndromes, Pelter et al. found that those with episodes of transient ischemia via continuous 12 lead ST segment monitoring were 8.5 times more likely to have in-hospital complications.[79]

ST segment monitoring has several limitations, including a propensity for false-positive alarms. Patients with intermittent BBB, permanent LBBB, ventricular pacemaker, or excessive restlessness are not good candidates for ST segment monitoring because of interference with the ST-T wave configuration.

Dysrhythmia Detection. Lead II is a good diagnostic lead for a variety of atrial dysrhythmias since P waves are easily visible. Leads I, III, and V_1 or V_6 are also very good general monitoring leads. To detect Wellens' syndrome, a marker of critical proximal left anterior descending coronary artery stenosis, V_2 or V_3 should be used. Therefore these leads are also useful for monitoring unstable angina. For wide complex tachycardia, V_1 should be used, with findings confirmed using V_2, and V_6.

Given the variety of patients and conditions that require monitoring, using a standard monitoring lead is illogical. It may be dangerous if incorrect monitoring results in delay of detection or diagnosis of changes. Choice of a monitoring lead should be based on the patient's clinical condition and the goals of monitoring. More information on clinical monitoring can be found in the AACN *Protocols for Practice.*[1,2]

CONCLUSIONS

Diagnosis and management of dysrhythmias require understanding of normal cardiac electrophysiology and dysrhythmogenic mechanisms, and knowledge of pharmacologic effects on cardiac electrophysiology.

Given the adverse effects possible if a dysrhythmia is misdiagnosed or missed, and given that the nurse is the constant presence at the bedside, the critical care nurse must have extensive knowledge of all these areas in order to ensure safe passage of dysrhythmia patients through their critical care stay.

REFERENCES

1. AACN. (Aug 2004). *Practice alert: ST segment monitoring.* Accessed at www.aacn.org.
2. AACN. (2006). *Protocols for practice: noninvasive monitoring* (2nd ed.). Sudbury, Mass: Jones & Bartlett.
3. Ad, N., & Cox, J. L. (2000). Stroke prevention as an indication for the Maze procedure in the treatment of atrial fibrillation. *Semin Thorac Cardiovasc Surg, 12,* 56–62.
4. Adler, S. W., et al. (2001). Efficacy of pacing therapies for treating atrial tachyarrhythmias in patients with ventricular arrhythmias receiving a dual-chamber implantable cardioverter defibrillator. *Circulation, 104,* 887–892.
5. Arnsdorf, M. F. (2006). *Electrocardiographic and electrophysiologic features of atrial fibrillation.* Accessed at www.uptodate.com.
6. Arnsdorf, M. F., & Wilber, D. (2006). *Atrioventricular nodal reentrant tachycardia (junctional reciprocating tachycardia).* Accessed at www.uptodate.com.
7. Bailey, D. G., et al. (1998). Grapefruit juice-drug interactions. *Brit J Clin Pharmacol, 46,* 101–110.
8. Bardy, G. H., et al., for the Sudden Cardiac Death in Heart Failure Trial (SCD-HeFT) investigators. (2005). Amiodarone or an implantable cardioverter-defibrillator for congestive heart failure. *New Engl J Med, 352*(3), 225–237.
9. Brennan, T. D., & Haas, G. J. (2005). The role of prophylactic implantable cardioverter defibrillators in heart failure: recent trials usher in a new era of device therapy. *Curr Heart Fail Rep, 2*(1), 40–45.
10. Brugada, P., & Brugada, J. (1992). Right bundle branch block, persistent ST segment elevation and sudden cardiac death: a distinct clinical and electrocardiographic syndrome. A multicenter report. *J Am Coll Cardiol, 20,* 1391–1396.
11. Buxton, A. E. (2004). Results of clinical trials of automatic external defibrillators and implantable cardioverter-defibrillators in patients at risk for sudden death. In D. P. Zipes & J. Jalife (Eds.), *Cardiac electrophysiology: from cell to bedside* (4th ed.). Philadelphia: Saunders.
12. Cappato, R., et al. (2005). Worldwide survey on the methods, efficacy, and safety of catheter ablation for human atrial fibrillation. *Circulation, 111*(9), 1100–1105.
13. Carlson, M. D., et al. (2003). A new pacemaker algorithm for the treatment of atrial fibrillation. Results of the atrial dynamic overdrive pacing trial (ADOPT). *J Am Coll Cardiol, 42*(4), 627–633.
14. Cheng, J., & Arnsdorf, M. F. (2006). *Surgical approaches to prevent recurrent atrial fibrillation.* Accessed at www.uptodate.com.
15. Cheng, J., & Arnsdorf, M. F. (2006). *The role of pacemakers in the prevention of atrial fibrillation.* Accessed at www.uptodate.com.
16. Cheng, J., & Arnsdorf, M. F. (2006). *Radiofrequency catheter ablation to prevent recurrent atrial fibrillation.* Accessed at www.uptodate.com.
17. Connolly, S. J., et al. (2000). Effects of physiologic pacing versus ventricular pacing on the risk of stroke and death due to cardiovascular causes. *New Engl J Med, 342,* 1385–1391.
18. Conover, M. B. (2003). Mechanisms of arrhythmias. In *Understanding electrocardiography* (8th ed.). St. Louis: Mosby.

19. Cooper, J. M., Katcher, M. S., & Orlov, M. V. (2002). Implantable devices for the treatment of atrial fibrillation. *New Engl J Med, 346*, 2062–2068.

20. Cox, D. L. (1991). The surgical treatment of atrial fibrillation. IV. Surgical technique. *J Thorac Cardiovasc Surg, 101*(4), 584–592.

21. Crouch, M. A., et al. (2003). Clinical relevance and management of drug-related QT interval prolongation. *Pharmacotherapy, 23*(7), 881–908.

22. Daoud, E. G., et al. (2000). Randomized, double-blind trial of simultaneous right and left atrial epicardial pacing for prevention of post-open heart surgery atrial fibrillation. *Circulation, 102*, 761–765.

23. Dower, G. E., Machado, H. B., & Osborne, J. A. (1980). On deriving the electrocardiogram from vectorcardiographic leads. *Clin Cardiol, 3*, 87–95.

24. Dresser, G. K., et al. (2000). Pharmacokinetic-pharmacodynamic consequences and clinical relevance of cytochrome P450 3A4 inhibition. *Clin Pharmacokinet, 38*, 41–57.

25. Drew, B. J., et al. (2005). Practice standards for electrocardiographic monitoring in hospital settings. An American Heart Association scientific statement from the councils on cardiovascular nursing, clinical cardiology, and cardiovascular disease in the young: Endorsed by the International Society of Computerized Electrocardiology and the American Association of Critical-Care Nurses. *J Cardiovasc Nurs, 20*(2), 76–106.

26. Drew, B. J., et al. (2002). Comparison of a new reduced lead set ECG with the standard ECG for diagnosing cardiac arrhythmias and myocardial ischemia. *J Electrocardiol, 35*(suppl), 13–21.

27. Drew, B. J. (2002). Celebrating the 100th birthday of the electrocardiogram: lessons learned from research in cardiac monitoring. *Am J Crit Care, 11*(4), 378–388.

28. Drew, B. J., et al. (1999). Accuracy of the EASI 12-lead electrocardiogram compared to the standard 12-lead electrocardiogram for diagnosing multiple cardiac abnormalities. *J Electrocardiol, 32*(suppl), 38–47.

29. Drew, B. J., & Scheinman, M. M. (1995). ECG criteria to distinguish between aberrantly conducted supraventricular tachycardia and ventricular tachycardia: practical aspects for the immediate care setting. *PACE, 18*, 2194–2208.

30. Echt, D. S., et al. (1991). Mortality and morbidity in patients receiving encainide, flecainide or placebo: the cardiac arrhythmia suppression trial. *New Engl J Med, 324*, 781.

31. El-Sherif, N., & Turrito, G. (2004). Torsades de pointes. In D. P. Zipes & J. Jalife (Eds.), *Cardiac electrophysiology: from cell to bedside* (4th ed.). Philadelphia: Saunders.

32. Ernst, S., et al. (2004). Catheter ablation of atrioventricular reentry. In D. P. Zipes & J. Jalife (Eds.), *Cardiac electrophysiology: from cell to bedside*. Philadelphia: Saunders.

33. Estes, N. A. M. (2004). New antiarrhythmic drugs. In D. P. Zipes & J. Jalife (Eds.), *Cardiac electrophysiology: from cell to bedside*. Philadelphia: Saunders.

34. Fan, K., et al. (2000). Effects of biatrial pacing in prevention of postoperative atrial fibrillation after coronary artery bypass surgery. *Circulation, 102*, 755–760.

35. Fuster, V., et al. (2001). ACC/AHA/ESC guidelines for the management of patients with atrial fibrillation: executive summary. A report of the American College of Cardiology/American Heart Association Task Force on Practice Guidelines and the European Society Cardiology Committee for Practice Guidelines and Policy Conferences (Committee to Develop Guidelines for the Management of Patients with Atrial Fibrillation) developed in collaboration with the North American Society of Pacing and Electrophysiology. *Circulation, 104*(17), 2118–2150.

36. Garvan, C. K., & Lipsky, J. J. (2000). Drug-grapefruit juice interactions. *Mayo Clin Proc, 75*, 933–942.

37. Gaynor, S. L., et al. (2005). Surgical treatment of atrial fibrillation: predictors of late recurrence. *J Thorac Cardiovasc Surg, 129*(1), 104–111.

38. Geller, J. C., et al. (2003). Treatment of atrial fibrillation with an implantable atrial defibrillator—long term results. *Eur Heart J, 24*, 2083–2098.

39. Gillis, A. M., et al. (2004). Class I antiarrhythmic drugs: quinidine, procainamide, disopyramide, lidocaine, mexiletine, flecainide, and propafenone. In D. P. Zipes & J. Jalife (Eds.), *Cardiac electrophysiology: from cell to bedside*. Philadelphia: Saunders.

40. Gillis, A. M. (2002). Safety and efficacy of advanced atrial pacing therapies for atrial tachyarrhythmias in patients with a new implantable dual chamber cardioverter-defibrillator. *J Am Coll Caridiol, 40*(9), 1653–1659.

41. Glitsch, H. G. (2001). Electrophysiology of the sodium-potassium-ATPase in cardiac cells. *Physiol Rev, 81*, 1791–1826.

42. Gold, M. R., & Peters, R. W. (2004). Newer applications of pacemakers. In D. P. Zipes & J. Jalife (Eds.), *Cardiac electrophysiology: from cell to bedside*. Philadelphia: Saunders.

43. Goldberger, A. L., Mietus, J. E., & Stein, P. K. (2006). *Heart rate variability: technical aspects.* Accessed at www.uptodate.com.

44. Greene, H. L., et al. (1992). The cardiac arrhythmia suppression trial: first CAST . . . then CAST II. *JACC, 19*(5), 894–898.

45. Gupta, A. K., & Thakur, R. K. (2001). Wide QRS complex tachycardias. *Med Clin North Am, 85*(2), 245–266.

46. Hallstrom, A. P., et al. (2005). Characteristics of heart beat intervals and prediction of death. *Int J Cardiol, 100*, 37–45.

47. Hayes, D. L. (2004). Implantable pacemakers. In D. P. Zipes & J. Jalife (Eds.), *Cardiac electrophysiology: from cell to bedside*. Philadelphia: Saunders.

48. Horacek, B. M., et al. (2000). Diagnostic accuracy of derived versus standard 12-lead electrocardiograms. *J Electrocardiol, 33*(suppl), 155–160.

49. Hsieh, M. H., et al. (2001). Mechanism of spontaneous transition from typical atrial flutter to atrial fibrillation: role of ectopic atrial fibrillation foci. *Pacing Clin Electrophysiol, 24*, 46–52.

50. Jensen, T. J., et al. (2004). Impact of premature atrial contractions in atrial fibrillation. *Pacing Clin Electrophysiol, 27*, 447–452.

51. Kivisto, K. T., et al. (1999). Repeated consumption of grapefruit juice considerably increases plasma concentrations of cisapride. *Clin Pharmacol Ther, 66*, 448–453.

52. Knight, B. P., et al. (2005). Role of permanent pacing to prevent atrial fibrillation: science advisory from the American Heart Association Council on Clinical Cardiology (Subcommittee on Electrocardiography and Arrhythmias) and the Quality of Care and Outcomes Research Interdisciplinary Working Group, in collaboration with the Heart Rhythm Society. *Circulation, 111*(2), 240–243.

53. Knight, B. P., & Morady, F. (2004). Atrioventricular reentry and variants. In D. P. Zipes & J. Jalife (Eds.), *Cardiac electrophysiology: from cell to bedside*. Philadelphia: Saunders.

54. Kunkler, K. (2002). Acquired long QT syndrome: risk assessment, prudent prescribing and monitoring, and patient education. *J Am Acad Nurse Pract, 14*(9), 382–389.

55. Laitio, T. T., et al. (2002). Relation of heart rate dynamics to the occurrence of myocardial ischemia after coronary artery bypass grafting. *Am J Cardiol, 89*, 1176–1181.

56. Lamas, G. A., et al. (2002). Ventricular pacing or dual-chamber pacing for sinus-node dysfunction. The Mode Selection Trial in Sinus-Node Dysfunction. *New Engl J Med, 346*, 1854–1862.

57. Lee, A. J., et al. (1999). The effects of grapefruit juice on sertraline metabolism: an in vitro and in vivo study. *Clin Ther, 21*, 1890–1899.

58. LeRoy, S. S., & Russell, M. (2004). Long QT syndrome and other repolarization-related dysrhythmias. *AACN Clin Issues, 15*(3), 419–431.

59. Levy, S., & Camm, A. J. (2006). *Implantable atrial defibrillators for the treatment of atrial fibrillation.* Accessed at www.uptodate.com.

60. Levy, S. (2004). Implantable atrial defibrillators for atrial fibrillation. In D. P. Zipes & J. Jalife (Eds.), *Cardiac electrophysiology: from cell to bedside.* Philadelphia: Saunders.

61. Levy, T., et al. (2000). Randomized controlled study investigating the effect of biatrial pacing in prevention of atrial fibrillation after coronary after bypass grafting. *Circulation, 102,* 1382–1387.

62. Lexi-Drugs (Comp + Specialties). (2006).

63. Lilja, J. J., et al. (2000). Duration of effect of grapefruit juice on the pharmacokinetics of the CYP3A4 substrate simvastatin. *Clin Pharmacol Ther, 68,* 384–390.

64. Lockwood, D., et al. (2004). Electrophysiologic characteristics of atrioventricular nodal reentrant tachycardia: implications for the reentrant circuits. In D. P. Zipes & J. Jalife (Eds.), *Cardiac electrophysiology: from cell to bedside.* Philadelphia: Saunders.

65. Malik, M. (2004). Heart rate variability and baroreflex sensitivity. In D. P. Zipes & J. Jalife (Eds.), *Cardiac electrophysiology: from cell to bedside* (4th ed.). Philadelphia: Saunders.

66. Marriott, H. J. L., & Conover, M. B. (1998). Chapter 2: Membrane channels; and Chapter 5: Arrhythmogenic mechanisms and their modulation. In *Advanced concepts in arrhythmias* (3rd ed.). St. Louis: Mosby.

67. McCarthy, P. M., et al. (2000). The Cox-Maze procedure: the Cleveland Clinic experience. *Semin Thorac Cardiovasc Surg, 12,* 25–29.

68. McMillan, D. E. (2002). Interpreting heart rate variability sleep/wake patterns in cardiac patients. *J Cardiovasc Nurs, 17*(1), 69–81.

69. McNamara, R. L., et al. (2003). Management of atrial fibrillation: review of the evidence for the role of pharmacologic therapy, electrical cardioversion, and echocardiography. *Ann Intern Med, 139,* 1018–1033.

70. McRae, A. T. III, Chung, M. K., & Asher, C. R. (2001). Arrhythmogenic right ventricular cardiomyopathy: a cause of sudden death in young people. *Cleveland Clinic J Med, 69,* 459–467.

71. Mieghem, C. V., et al. (2004). The clinical value of the ECG in noncardiac conditions. *Chest, 125,* 1561–1576.

72. Mitchell, A. R., et al. (2003). Psychosocial aspects of patient-activated atrial defibrillation. *J Cardiovasc Electrophysiol, 14*(8), 812–816.

73. Moss, A. J., & Zareba, W. (2004). Long QT syndrome: therapeutic considerations. In D. P. Zipes & J. Jalife (Eds.), *Cardiac electrophysiology: from cell to bedside.* Philadelphia: Saunders.

74. Moss, A. J., et al. (2002). Prophylactic implantation of a defibrillator in patients with myocardial infarction and reduced ejection fraction. *New Engl J Med, 346,* 877–883.

75. Naccarelli, G. V., Wolbrette, D. L., & Luck, J. C. (2001). Proarrhythmia. *Med Clin North Am, 85*(2), 503–526.

76. Nattel, S., & Ehrlich, J. R. (2004). Atrial fibrillation. In D. P. Zipes & J. Jalife (Eds.), *Cardiac electrophysiology: from cell to bedside.* Philadelphia: Saunders.

77. Newman, D. M., et al. (2003). Effect of an implantable cardioverter defibrillator with atrial detection and shock therapies on patient-perceived, health-related quality of life. *Am Heart J, 145*(5), 841–846.

78. Page, P. L. (2004). Surgery for cardiac arrhythmias. In D. P. Zipes & J. Jalife (Eds.), *Cardiac electrophysiology: from cell to bedside.* Philadelphia: Saunders.

79. Pelter, M. M., et al. (2003). Transient myocardial ischemia is an independent predictor of adverse in-hospital outcomes in patients with acute coronary syndromes treated in the telemetry unit. *Heart Lung, 32*(2), 71–78.

80. Podrid, P. J. (2006). *Enhanced cardiac automaticity.* Accessed at www.uptodate.com.

81. Prystowsky, E., et al. (2004). Wolff-Parkinson-White syndrome. In D. P. Zipes & J. Jalife (Eds.), *Cardiac electrophysiology: from cell to bedside.* Philadelphia: Saunders.

82. Ricci, R., et al. (2004). Dual defibrillator improves quality of life and decreases hospitalizations in patients with drug refractory atrial fibrillation. *J Interv Cardiol Electrophysiol, 10*(1), 85–92.

83. Saksena, S., et al. (2002). Improved suppression of recurrent atrial fibrillation with dual-site right atrial pacing and antiarrhythmic therapy. *J Am Coll Cardiol, 40*(6), 1140–1150.

84. Sanders, G. D., Hlatky, M. A., & Owens, D. K. (2005). Cost-effectiveness of implantable cardioverter-defibrillators. *New Engl J Med, 353*(14), 1471–1480.

85. Schaff, H. V., et al. (2000). The Cox-Maze procedure for atrial fibrillation: the Mayo Clinic experience. *Semin Thorac Cardiovasc Surg, 12,* 30–37.

86. Scheinman, M. M., & Huang, S. (2000). The 1998 NASPE prospective catheter ablation registry. *Pacing Clin Electrophysiol, 23*(6), 1020.

87. Schoels, W., et al. (2001). Worldwide clinical experience with a new dual-chamber implantable cardioverter defibrillator system. *Worldwide Jewel AF Investigators, 12*(5), 521–528.

88. Schwartz, P. J., & Priori, S. G. (2004). Long QT syndrome: genotype-phenotype correlations. In D. P. Zipes & J. Jalife (Eds.), *Cardiac electrophysiology: from cell to bedside.* Philadelphia: Saunders.

89. Seslar, S. P., et al. (2006). *Clinical features of congenital long QT syndrome.* Accessed at www.uptodate.com.

90. Siddoway, L. A. (2003). Amiodarone: guidelines for use and monitoring. *Am Family Physician, 68*(11), 2189–2196.

91. Smith, T. W., & Cain, M. E. (2004). Class III antiarrhythmic drugs: Amiodarone, ibutilide, and sotalol. In D. P. Zipes & J. Jalife (Eds.), *Cardiac electrophysiology: from cell to bedside.* Philadelphia: Saunders.

92. Snow, V., et al. (2003). Management of newly detected atrial fibrillation: a clinical practice guideline from the American Academy of Family Practice Physicians and the American College of Physicians. *Ann Intern Med, 139,* 1009–1017.

93. *Stedman's Medical Dictionary.* (2004). Philadelphia: Lippincott Williams & Wilkins.

94. Stein, P. K., Mietus, J. E., & Goldberger, A. L. (2006). *Heart rate variability: uses other than after myocardial infarction.* Accessed at www.uptodate.com.

95. Stein, P. K., et al. (2001). Association between heart rate variability recorded on postoperative day 1 and length of stay in abdominal aortic surgery patients. *Crit Care Med, 29,* 1738–1743.

96. Tisdale, J. E., et al. (2001). The effect of intravenous haloperidol on QT interval dispersion in critically ill patients: comparison with QT interval prolongation for assessment of risk of torsades de pointes. *J Clin Pharmacol, 41,* 1310–1318.

97. Towbin, J. A., & Vatta, M. (2001). Molecular biology and the prolonged QT syndromes. *Am J Med, 110,* 385–389.

98. van De Borne, P., et al. (2001). Differential characteristics of neural circulatory control: early versus late after cardiac transplantation. *Circulation, 104,* 1809–1813.

99. Vieweg, W. V. R. (2003). New generation antipsychotic drugs and QTc interval prolongation. *Primary Care Companion J, 5*(5), 205–215.

100. Viskin, S. (1999). Torsades de pointes. *Curr Treat Options Cardiovasc Med, 1,* 187–195.

101. Volders, P. G., et al. (2000). Progress in the understanding of cardiac early afterdepolarizations and torsades de pointes: time to revise current concepts. *Cardiovasc Res, 46,* 376–392.

102. Wyse, D. G. (2004). Results of clinical trials on atrial fibrillation. In D. P. Zipes & J. Jalife (Eds.), *Cardiac electrophysiology: from cell to bedside.* Philadelphia: Saunders.

103. Wyse, D. G., et al. (2002). Atrial fibrillation follow-up investigation of rhythm management (AFFIRM) investigators: a comparison of rate control and rhythm control in patients with atrial fibrillation. *New Engl J Med, 347,* 1825–1833.

104. Yap, Y. G., & Camm, J. (2000). Risk of torsades de pointes with non-cardiac drugs. Doctors need to be aware that many drugs can cause QT prolongation. *BMJ, 320,* 1158–1159.

105. Zareba, W., & Lin, D. A. (2003). Antipsychotic drugs and QT interval prolongation. *Psychiatric Quart, 74*(3), 291–306.

106. Zimetbaum, P., & Josephson, M. E. (2006). *Genetics of congenital and acquired long QT syndrome.* Accessed at www.uptodate.com.

107. Zipes, D. P., & Jalife, J. (2004). *Cardiac electrophysiology: from cell to bedside* (4th ed.). Philadelphia: Saunders.

CHAPTER *11* Acute Coronary Syndromes

Nancy Munro

Acute coronary syndrome is an evolving term, found in the literature as early as 1972.[52] It began to be used more commonly in the late 1980s, when it was used to describe the presentation of an acute myocardial infarction (MI), accompanied by hypotension and dysrhythmias.[3] *Acute MI* and *unstable angina* are terms that have been used in the past. However, terminology is changing as scientific information about ruptured or eroded atheromatous plaque increases. Acute coronary syndrome (ACS) represents an entire spectrum of events (ischemia to infarction) that occur at the cellular and muscular levels. The conditions included in this syndrome are categorized according to 12 lead electrocardiogram (ECG) findings, including non–ST elevation myocardial infarction (NSTEMI), ST segment elevation myocardial infarction (STEMI), ST segment depression, and nondiagnostic ST segment and T wave abnormalities.[2]

In 2002 the American College of Cardiology (ACC) and the American Heart Association (AHA) published guidelines describing ACS as a condition resulting in an imbalance between myocardial oxygen supply and demand. This imbalance can be the consequence of (1) coronary artery narrowing from nonocclusive thrombus, (2) intense focal coronary artery spasm, (3) severe narrowing without spasm or thrombus, (4) arterial inflammation, or (5) secondary unstable angina (UA).[2a] If the imbalance of supply and demand persists, cell death or MI occurs. The term *angina* is still used but may disappear as the guidelines continue to evolve. The development of the term *ACS* reflects the rapid and significant growth of scientific knowledge involving atherogenesis, thrombus formation, and arterial inflammation now associated with cardiovascular disease.

The extent of this disease in the United States is staggering. Seventy million Americans (25% of men and women) have one or more types of cardiovascular disease.[1] Coronary artery disease (CAD) is the leading cause of death in the United States and is commonly manifested as UA or NSTEMI.[2a] The prevalence of angina is higher in women, while men have a higher occurrence of MI.[1] Chapter 13 provides more comprehensive information about women and heart disease.

Race and gender are influential factors when studying CAD. African Americans and American Indians have higher incidence rates of CAD than do Caucasians.[1] CAD had a significant impact on healthcare costs in 2005, with the direct and indirect costs estimated to be $142.1 billion.[1]

PATHOPHYSIOLOGY

As the science of vascular biology and cellular functions advances, the understanding of the pathophysiology of CAD has evolved. The concept of "hardened arteries" of atherosclerosis is now known to be more complicated and encompasses the hematologic, immunologic, and inflammatory responses of the body. A review of the inflammatory process enhances the understanding of the cellular activity in the arteries.

The inflammatory response is a nonspecific, protective response to tissue damage elicited by various triggers such as pathogens, chemical irritations, or disturbance of cellular homeostasis.[61] After damage has occurred, return of homeostasis is achieved in three phases. Initially, vasodilation and increased permeability of the local vessels provide increased blood flow, allowing mediators, cells, and other substances to infiltrate the damaged area. Phagocytes (white blood cells migrating to the area following signaling of cellular mediators) employ chemotactic maneuvers to access the damaged cell material, thereby becoming tissue macrophages. Once in the tissue, the macrophages initiate the process of cellular repair.[61]

Inflammation has been identified as a pivotal component of the atherosclerotic process (Figure 11-1). The theory of atherosclerosis proposes that the initiation of this process may start asymptomatically as early as the teenage years.[63] Diets high in saturated fats and cholesterol contribute to the collection of lipids in the arterial wall.[37] With high levels of lipoproteins circulating, they begin to accumulate in the intricate collagen fibers of the intima of the arterial wall, developing into an atheroma. This insidious process reflects the "chronic" component of ACS, as it may take years to develop and even longer

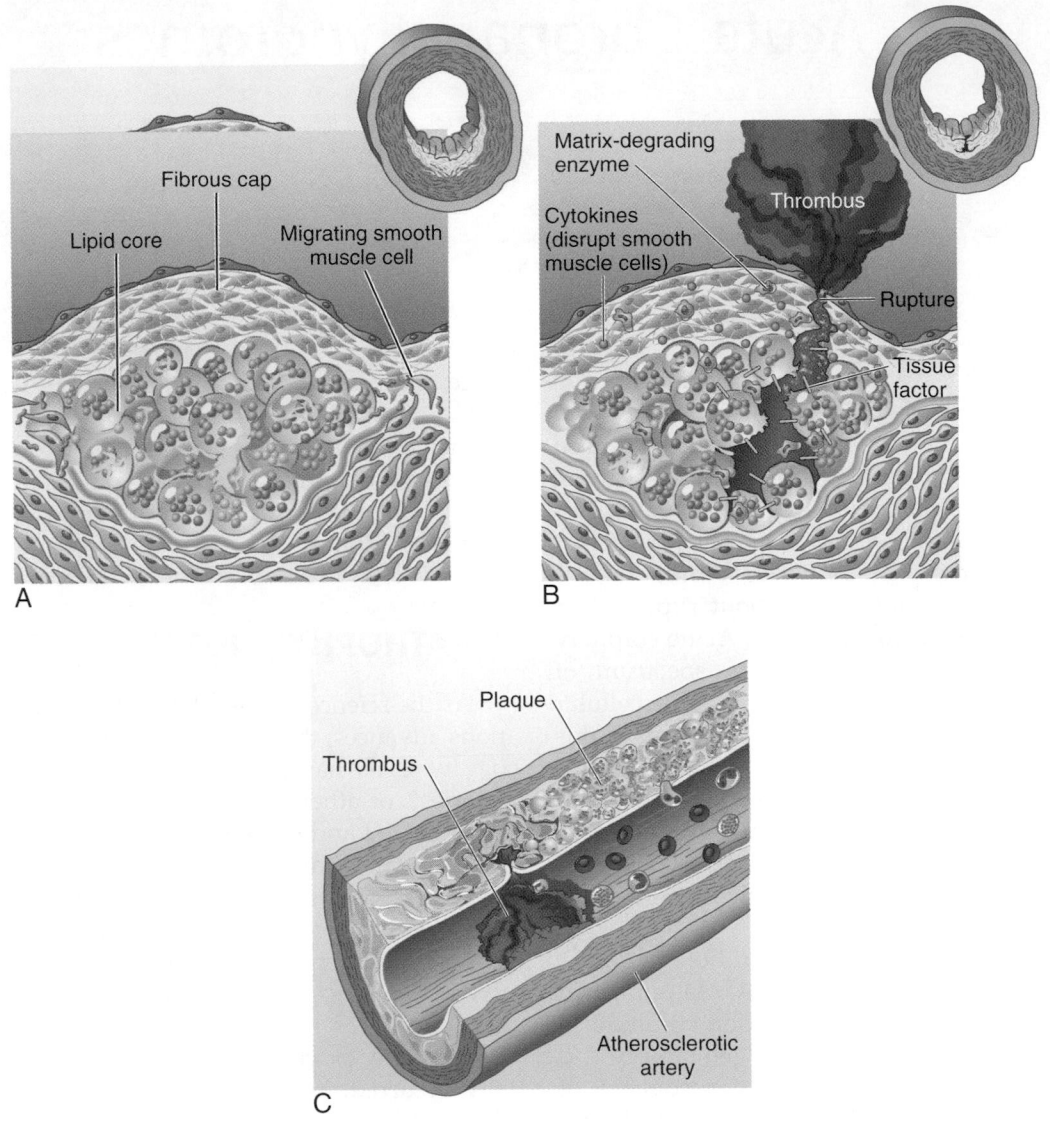

⬍FIGURE 11-1   Role of inflammation in CAD. A, Inflammation encourages growth of plaque, which becomes covered by a fibrous cap when smooth muscle cells move into the intima. The cap enlarges the size of the plaque deposit. **B,** Over time, inflammatory substances weaken the cap and damage smooth muscle. If the weakened plaque ruptures, a thrombus may form and block blood flow to the heart. **C,** Narrowing of an artery by plaque and thrombus.

before symptoms occur.[37] Once the low-density lipoproteins (LDLs) are bound to the proteoglycan of the intima, they become more susceptible to oxidation (loss of electrons) and other chemical modifications, such as glycation (binding by glucose). The chemical alteration of the LDLs entrapped in the intimal wall is thought to be an important component of atherosclerosis.[12] The cellular changes of the LDLs are recognized as abnormalities by the endothelial cells, which respond by defending the damaged cells. The endothelial cells release adhesion molecules (vascular cell adhesion molecule-1 [VCAM-1] and intercellular adhesion molecule-1 [ICAM-1]) at their surface, which attract monocytes that adhere to the endothelial cell surface.[46] The monocytes receive a signal from the endothelial cell in the form of protein molecules called *chemokines* that direct their migration.[40]

They will diapedese between the endothelial cell junctions and enter the intima, beginning to ingest lipoproteins. To attract more abnormal LDL cells, these macrophages display scavenger receptors on their cell walls, successfully engaging more abnormal lipoproteins. Microscopically, these macrophages surrounded by LDL cells appear to have a foamy nature and are appropriately named "foam cells."[35]

Plaque formation continues to progress as the foam cells replicate in response to macrophage-colony stimulating factor. The foam cells also are a source of proinflammatory mediators such as chemokines and superoxides.[26] Plaque formation is enhanced by the inflammatory process. Other phagocytes gather in the intima, attracting T cells to the site by presenting antigens. When the T cells interact with the antigens, they become activated and release large amounts of cytokines, again encouraging atherogenesis.[37] Smooth muscle cells migrate from the media to the atherosclerotic intima but are not like the normal smooth muscle cell. They have fewer contractile fibers and more rough endoplasmic recticulum.[37] These cells eventually form a tough fibrous cap, protecting the foam cells from exposure to blood. However, the cells continue through their life cycle and eventually experience apoptosis (programmed cell death), perhaps enhanced by the inflammatory cytokines.[37]

The atherosclerotic process described is considered the chronic phase of atheroma development, occurring over many years. The acute phase of atherosclerosis involves the formation of a thrombus, actually occluding arterial blood flow. The fibrous cap protects the inner endothelial cell content but is not impervious to damage itself. The T cells and macrophages accumulated in the collagen fibers release cytokines and matrix metalloproteinases, respectively, decreasing synthesis and degrading the collagen fibers, thereby thinning the cap.[57] This interaction links the inflammatory response with the development of the atheroma at the cellular level. As the fibrous cap becomes thinner, it eventually ruptures and exposes the foam cells. These cells display tissue factor, a potent procoagulant, initiating the activation of the extrinsic pathway of the coagulation cascade. Once exposed, tissue factor binds with factor VII, creating its activated form, factor VIIa. Factor VIIa is a potent enzyme that activates factor X to Xa. This chemical step initiates the common pathway of the coagulation cascade and the release of platelet activating factor. The platelets become sticky and adhere to each other. Arachidonic acid from the phospholipids in the platelet membrane assists in the formation of thromboxane A_2, further encouraging platelet aggregation. Glycoprotein IIb/IIIa, a receptor on the platelet surface, experiences conformational changes caused by thromboxane A_2, exposing fibrinogen binding sites. Fibrinogen builds bridges to adjacent platelets and advances platelet aggregation. Fibrin reinforces these aggregates; a thrombus is formed.[62] The thrombus eventually obstructs blood flow in the area of the affected coronary artery, resulting in an acute coronary syndrome. A more detailed review of coagulation is discussed in Chapter 37, and Figure 37–2 illustrates the clotting cascades.

The cellular changes discussed initiate a chain reaction once a thrombus is formed. The precarious balance between supply and demand of oxygen at the cellular level is easily disrupted. If blood flow to myocardial cells is diminished for even 10 seconds, myocardial ischemia can occur because of oxygen deprivation.[34] Anaerobic metabolism ensues, inhibiting the ion pumps, altering membrane potential, and causing cellular edema. Intracellular hydrogen ions and lactic acid accumulate, which quickly depress left ventricular function. Ventricular performance deteriorates and triggers compensatory mechanisms, causing oxygen delivery to tissues to decrease because of a decrease in cardiac output (CO). Cardiogenic shock is discussed in Chapter 40. Not only do other organs of the body suffer when cardiac performance is compromised, but the myocardial muscle continues to be negatively affected as well. Coronary artery blood flow is regulated by the driving pressure in the vascular system, requiring at least a mean arterial pressure of 60 mm Hg to maintain flow. The endothelial cells attempt to control flow by maintaining vascular tone. There are many mediators that influence vascular tone, either causing coronary artery vasodilation or causing constriction, depending on the surrounding environment. Once ischemia has occurred, various mediators including prostacyclin, endothelial-derived relaxing factor (nitric oxide), and others will be released, causing vasodilation in an attempt to reestablish homeostasis.[34] In addition, there are mediators such as endothelin-1 that not only cause vasoconstriction but also reduce adenosinetriphosphatase (ATPase), leading to the production of hydrogen peroxide and superoxides and causing cell injury.[34] Ideally blood flow can be quickly restored by various interventions so that cellular activity can be returned to normal. Many outside factors influence and enhance these abnormal cellular disruptions and are considered risk factors in CAD.

PATIENTS AT RISK

Understanding the newer perspectives of cardiac heart disease (CHD) involving the inflammatory process adds new dimensions when considering risk factors for CHD. Hyperlipidemia is commonly recognized as a major contributor to CHD.[1] The insidious process of accumulating lipoproteins in the intima of the arterial wall is postulated to occur over many years. If hyperlipidemia is recognized and controlled in the early stages, CHD could be decreased. Diabetes mellitus results in an elevation of blood glucose levels, enhancing the glycation of LDLs and triggering the initial stages of the inflammatory response. Cigarette smoking is also thought to elicit the early inflammatory process by facilitating the formation of oxidants that increase oxidation of LDLs.[35,36] Tighter glucose control and prevention or early cessation of smoking should be clinical goals when dealing with CHD.

Obesity is another contributor to both diabetes and intravascular inflammation.[35] Hypertension can lead to chronic heart failure, and may also involve the inflammatory process. Angiotensin II, a potent vasoconstrictor and factor in hypertension, may have some role in inflammation as well.[35]

Hormone manipulation, as in the use of oral contraceptives and postmenopausal replacement, is thought to increase risk of CHD. Oral contraceptives may promote atherogenesis by affecting blood pressure (BP) and concentrations of lipids and glucose.[54] Hormone replacement therapy (HRT) has similar mechanisms and is discussed in Chapter 13.

Metabolic factors such as homocysteine levels may be a risk factor for CHD, although the evidence is not clear currently. Homocysteine is an amino acid byproduct of methionine metabolism. It has been associated with endothelial dysfunction, intimal thickening, and procoagulant activity that may stimulate and aggravate atherogensis.[41]

Other classic, nonmodifiable risk factors such as age, gender, race, and familial history should not be forgotten. CHD increases with age for both men and women.[1] African Americans, especially men, are at greater risk than other races, and family history remains a strong predictor of CHD.[1]

A more atypical but important risk factor is recent cocaine use. The drug is thought to cause coronary artery spasm. These risk factors and preventive interventions are discussed later in the chapter.

CLASSIC (STABLE) ANGINA

Physical Assessment

Although stable angina is not included in the definition of ACS, it is important to understand the difference in presentation of various types of chest pain. Angina pectoris is a clinical syndrome composed of transient episodes of substernal chest pain or discomfort caused by myocardial ischemia.[21] There are many variables of this discomfort, including nausea, vomiting, diaphoresis, jaw pain, back pain, and dyspnea. Chest pain is the classic symptom assumed to be the major presentation; however, there are anginal equivalents that should be integrated into the diagnostic process. This type of presentation includes sensation of dyspnea, excessive fatigue or weakness, or isolated arm or jaw pain.[21] Women and patients with diabetes are two patient populations that do not usually have classic chest pain. Women present with nonspecific chest pain syndromes (Chapter 13). Additionally, chest pain in women does not have the same prognostic value as it does in men. When women with classic chest pain were studied angiographically, they did not have significant occlusions as frequently as men.[45] Diabetic patients may not experience pain because of neuropathy associated with the disease. It becomes important to recognize these variances and understand the differential diagnosis. Table 11-1 summarizes chest pain syndromes.

Anginal chest pain may last from 2 to 30 minutes and generally occurs with physical exertion or after eating a heavy meal. It is often relieved with rest. Nitroglycerin (NTG) may be used to treat the chest pain as well as esophageal spasm. Location of chest pain is variable. Eslick[23] developed a schematic diagram using a cluster analysis technique to help the clinician determine the origin of chest pain (Figure 11-2). It is very important to remember that there is no absolute chest pain description; the clinician should maintain a high index of suspicion with any type of chest pain. Other testing is necessary to ascertain the source of the pain. A focused physical exam should also include assessment for signs of heart failure, including pulmonary crackles, jugular vein distention, peripheral edema, and other signs of right or left ventricular failure. The focused exam enables faster implementation of interventions during this important period. Treatment should not be delayed to follow-up on noncritical assessment findings until after the immediate conditions have been treated. However, any abnormal data should be pursued when the immediate threat has been treated.

Laboratory Tests

Measurement of serum cardiac biomarkers is useful in the diagnosis of ACS. The most common laboratory tests used are creatine kinase (CK) and troponin. These markers are proteins released into the blood as a result of muscle destruction. CK is the older marker and is found in skeletal muscle, heart muscle, and brain tissue. Isoenzymes of CK reflect tissue origins: CK-MB is predominantly cardiac muscle, CK-MM is skeletal muscle, and CK-BB is brain and kidney. Even though there is a small skeletal muscle component of the isoenzyme, lowering its specificity, CK-MB has been the gold standard used to assist with the diagnosis of MI. It is important to recognize when biomarkers begin to rise and when they peak so that diagnostic goals can be set. CK-MB starts to rise in 4 to 8 hours and peaks in 12 to 24 hours.[14] While this biomarker continues to be used in the diagnosis of ACS, there are newer, more specific markers.

Troponin is a protein found in cardiac and skeletal muscle that covers the binding site for the actin and myosin filaments. There are two troponin components specific for cardiac muscle: troponin I and troponin T. Cardiac troponin I (cTnI) inhibits muscle contraction, and cardiac troponin T (cTnT) connects the troponin complex to tropomyosin.[14] Both of these biomarkers rise in 3 to 4 hours, peak in 10 to 24 hours, and remain elevated up to 10 days after an event; this is helpful if a patient presents long after the chest discomfort occurred. This is the preferred marker as recommended by the ACC/AHA 2007 guidelines.[2a]

TABLE 11-1 Differential Diagnosis of Episodic Chest Pain

DIAGNOSIS	DURATION	QUALITY	PROVOCATION	RELIEF	LOCATION	COMMENT
Effort angina	5–15 min	Visceral (pressure)	During effort or motion	Rest, nitroglycerin (NTG)	Substernal, radiates	First episode vivid
Rest angina	5–15 min	Visceral (pressure)	Spontaneous	NTG	Substernal, radiates	Usually nocturnal
Mitral prolapse	Minutes to hours	Superficial	Spontaneous	Time	Left anterior	No pattern, variable character
Esophageal reflux	10–60 min	Visceral	Recumbency, lack of food	Food, antacids	Substernal, epigastric	Rarely radiates
Esophageal spasm	50–60 min	Visceral	Spontaneous, cold liquids, exercise	NTG	Substernal, radiates	Mimics angina
Peptic ulcer	Hours	Visceral (burning)	Lack of food, "acid food"	Food, antacids	Epigastric, substernal	
Biliary disease	Hours	Visceral (wax and wane)	Spontaneous, food	Time, analgesia	Epigastric, radiates	Colic
Cervical disk	Variable (gradually subsides)	Superficial	Head and neck movement, palpation	Time, analgesia	Arm, neck	Not relieved by rest
Hyperventilation	2–30 min	Visceral	Emotion, tachypnea	Stimulus removed	Substernal	Facial paresthesia
Musculoskeletal	Variable	Superficial	Movement, palpation	Time, analgesia	Multiple	Tenderness
Pulmonary	30 min+	Visceral (pressure)	Often spontaneous	Rest, time, bronchodilator	Substernal	Dyspneic

Modified from reference 16a.

Other biomarkers have a role in the detection of ACS. Myoglobin, a heme protein found in cardiac and skeletal muscle, is rapidly released from damaged tissue. Found in skeletal muscle, its use is limited because it is not specific to cardiac muscle. It is also cleared by the kidney, so patients with renal disease may have false-positive findings. Another screening marker is C-reactive protein (CRP), which is developing a role in the prediction of ACS. CRP is a peptide produced by the liver in response to inflammation, infection, or tissue damage. Highly elevated levels may be more predictive of CAD than LDL levels.[35] CRP levels should be used in conjunction with other data, such as risk factors and family history, because specificity with this marker can be an issue. Levels could be high with an infection or other tissue damage. Table 11-2 summarizes the biomarkers used in the diagnosis of ACS.

Other Diagnostic Tests

The electrocardiogram (ECG) is the other classic diagnostic tool used in ACS. The ECG should be performed and interpreted by an experienced healthcare provider within 10 minutes of the start of chest discomfort.[2a] The ECG is most helpful for diagnosis of ischemia or infarction when the ST segment and T wave are evaluated and the presence of a Q wave determined. With stable angina, there may be no ECG changes, or nonspecific ST-T wave findings. Another helpful evaluation tool, useful in the differential

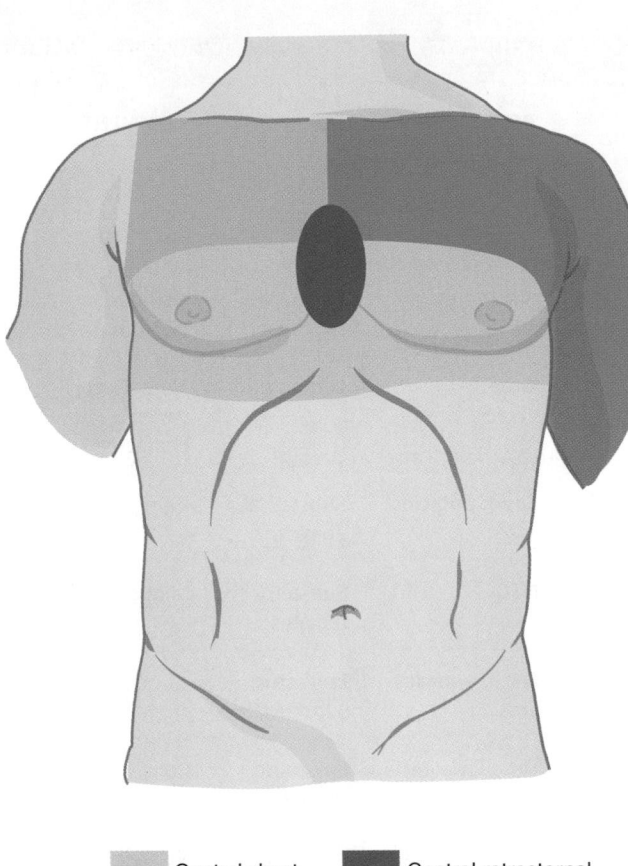

- Central chest
- Central retrosternal
- Upper chest
- Left chest and arm

⬥FIGURE 11-2 Cluster locations of acute chest pain.

TABLE 11-2 Diagnostic Biomarkers of Acute Coronary Syndrome

BIOMARKER	INITIAL RISE	PEAK	ABNORMAL VALUES
Troponin cTnI and cTnT	3–4 hr	10–24 hr	cTnI greater than 1.5 mcg/L cTnT greater than 0.1 mcg/ml
CK-MB	4–8 hr	12–24 hr	Greater than 10 mcg/ml or greater than 3% total
Myoglobin	1–3 hr	NA	Males 20–90 ng/ml Females 10–75 ng/ml

Modified from reference 14.

diagnosis of chest pain, is the chest radiograph. It shows the heart and aorta size. If the chest pain is the result of an aortic dissection, the aortic size could be notably increased. Standard laboratory testing including electrolytes, blood urea nitrogen (BUN), creatinine, hematocrit, lipid profile, and glucose should also be obtained to establish a baseline for the patient.

Further evaluation of chest pain can be done using stress testing. Under controlled conditions, the workload of the heart is increased, while heart rate (HR), BP, and the ECG are monitored for any changes in the ST segment, T waves, or the development of dysrhythmias or angina. The workload of the heart can be increased by exercise, or if the patient is unable to exercise, pharmacologic agents such as dobutamine (Dobutrex), dipyridamole (Persantine), or adenosine (Adenocard) can be administered while the patient remains stationary. Stress testing combined with cardiac imaging assists in the diagnosis of ischemic heart disease. Radionuclides (e.g., thallium-201 or technetium-99m sestamibi) are injected during maximal stress and traced to determine how myocardial blood flow is distributed for that patient. These tests are very sensitive and accurate. Cardiac positron emission tomography (PET) uses radiolabeled glucose to differentiate between ischemic and infarcted myocardium.[21] Computed tomography (CT) and magnetic resonance imaging (MRI) are also being adapted as diagnostic tools for ACS. Two-dimensional cardiac echocardiography is less invasive and can evaluate for abnormal cardiac wall motion, ejection fraction, and valvular motion, and can also be performed with stress testing technology. However, the gold standard for evaluation of coronary artery anatomy and obstructive atherosclerosis is coronary angiography.

UNSTABLE ANGINA AND NON–ST SEGMENT ELEVATION MYOCARDIAL INFARCTION

The difference between stable and UA is in the changing pattern of the chest pain. There are three presentations of UA: (1) rest angina; (2) new-onset severe angina; and (3) increasing angina, which is more frequent, of longer duration, and lower in threshold.[2a] Threshold refers to the Canadian Cardiovascular Society (CCS) classification system established in 1976, which is used to describe UA (Table 11-3).[13] UA can result from the prolonged imbalance of oxygen supply and demand of the myocardial muscle attributable to one or more of the following reasons: (1) coronary artery narrowing from nonocclusive thrombus; (2) intense focal coronary artery spasm; (3) severe narrowing without spasm or

TABLE 11-3   Grading of Angina

Class I	In this stage, angina is not caused by ordinary physical activity (e.g., stair climbing, walking). Angina is caused by demanding, rapid, or extended exertion at either work or recreation.
Class II	In this stage, ordinary activities must be limited slightly. Angina occurs when walking or climbing stairs quickly or after a meal; when walking uphill; in cold or wind; under emotional duress; and during the first few hours after waking up. Angina also occurs when walking more than two blocks on level terrain and when climbing more than one flight of ordinary stairs at a normal pace, under normal conditions.
Class III	This stage is characterized by marked limitations in ordinary physical activity. Angina occurs when walking one to two blocks on level terrain and when climbing only one flight of stairs at a normal pace, under normal conditions.
Class IV	This stage is characterized by a complete inability to perform any type of physical activity without discomfort. Symptoms of angina may also occur while at rest.

Data from the Canadian Cardiovascular Society Classification.

thrombus; (4) arterial inflammation; or (5) secondary UA.[2a] UA and NSTEMI are closely related conditions whose presentations and pathogenesis are very similar, differing only in severity.[2a] With NSTEMI, the ischemia is severe enough to cause sufficient myocardial damage for detectable levels of biomarkers to be released. This condition was previously referred to as a "non Q wave MI" because there were ST-T wave abnormalities with elevated biomarker levels but no Q wave development. UA can have ST-T wave changes, but they are usually transient.[2a] When a patient has any type of chest discomfort, it is important to consider these diagnoses immediately and to initiate an evidence-based plan of care. Fast, appropriate interventions can save myocardial muscle and improve functional outcomes.

MULTIDISCIPLINARY PLAN OF CARE

Once ACS is recognized, timing of interventions is crucial. Education of the public focuses on entering the healthcare system as soon as possible by calling the emergency medical services (EMS). Initial contact with a patient with chest pain commonly occurs over the telephone. Telephone triage quickly assesses the patient's symptoms and refers the patient to a facility with a physician and 12 lead ECG capabilities.[2a] While waiting for the ambulance, the patient should chew an adult, nonenteric coated aspirin if there is no allergy or recent gastrointestinal bleeding history. Once the patient has arrived in the facility (usually an emergency department or chest pain unit), the triage nurse should explore the nature of the chest discomfort and ask about associated symptoms (i.e., nausea, vomiting, dyspnea, diaphoresis). Medical history including CAD, angina, MI, or coronary artery bypass graft (CABG) as well as the presence of any risk factors should be established. Special consideration should be given to women, diabetic patients, and older adults because their chest pain presentation is usually atypical. Important questions to be considered are the following: (1) What is the possibility that the signs and symptoms represent ACS secondary to obstructive CAD? (2) What is the likelihood of an adverse clinical outcome?[2a]

Immediate cardiac assessment begins with a 12 lead ECG. The ST segment is examined for elevation or depression. Depending on 12 lead ECG findings, anticoagulation interventions that begin with aspirin are augmented with heparin therapy, clopidogrel (Plavix), and possible administration of glycoprotein IIb/IIIa inhibitors.[2] These interventions disable the coagulation cascade in an effort to increase blood flow to the compromised cardiac muscle. Additional therapies to decrease cardiac workload and myocardial oxygen consumption include beta blockers to decrease HR and contractility and NTG to decrease preload. Data collected through history, physical examination, 12 lead ECG, and biomarker levels will help the healthcare team estimate the level of risk for a patient.

Risk stratification will assist in decision making about appropriate patient interventions. The categories for risk include low, intermediate, or high likelihood of death or nonfatal cardiac ischemic events. Table 11-4 summarizes these risk categories. Reperfusion therapy includes percutaneous coronary intervention (PCI) or fibrinolysis (clot lysis). Additional adjunctive therapies initiated after reperfusion therapy include angiotensin-converting enzyme (ACE) inhibitors, angiotensin receptor blockers (ARBs), and statin therapy.[2a] Each of these interventions is discussed in more detail in the following sections.

Anti-Ischemic Nursing Interventions and Bedside Monitoring

Bedrest is a simple and effective intervention that helps decrease myocardial ischemia, especially in patients with ongoing pain at rest. If there is ischemia, decreasing myocardial work decreases the muscle's

TABLE 11-4 Risk Stratification for Acute Coronary Syndrome

FEATURE	HIGH LIKELIHOOD	INTERMEDIATE LIKELIHOOD	LOW LIKELIHOOD
History	Chest or left arm pain or discomfort as chief symptom with known history of CAD including MI	Chest or left arm pain or discomfort as chief symptom; age greater than 70 years; male sex and diabetes mellitus	Probable ischemic symptoms in absence of any of intermediate likelihood characteristics; recent cocaine use
Exam	Transient mitral regurgitation, hypotension, diaphoresis, pulmonary edema or rales	Extracardiac vascular disease	Chest discomfort reproduced by palpation
ECG	New or presumed new transient ST segment elevation (greater than 0.05 mV) or T wave inversion (0.2 mV) with symptoms	Fixed Q waves; abnormal ST segments or T waves not documented to be new	T wave flattening or inversion in leads with dominant R waves or normal ECG
Cardiac markers	Elevated cardiac TnI, TnT, or CK-MB	Normal	Normal

Modified from reference 11a.
CAD = Coronary artery disease, CK-MB = creatine kinase-MB, MI = myocardial infarction, TnI = troponin I, TnT = troponin T.

demand for oxygen. This is a simple initial intervention implemented while the results of the ECG, serum markers, and the history and physical are collected. Ambulation and return to regular activity should be promoted as soon as the patient's condition is stabilized. Supplemental oxygen should be administered in the presence of arterial saturation less than 90% or overt pulmonary edema.[2] The clinical goal should be to keep the oxygen saturation to greater than 90% and wean oxygen as symptoms improve.[2]

Cardiac monitoring is also required for this patient population. Evidence-based practice using bedside monitoring facilitates proper recognition of changes in patients' status and may improve outcomes. The preferred cardiac monitoring using five electrodes allows the clinician to obtain a true V_1 lead, whereas a three-electrode system produces a modified chest lead (MCL_1). Lead V_1 is the optimal lead for diagnosing bundle branch blocks and confirming proper right ventricular pacemaker location when using temporary pacing, and can be used to distinguish supraventricular tachycardia versus ventricular tachycardia.[22] However, monitoring can only provide valid data if used appropriately. Skin preparation and lead placement are vital steps and, when properly performed, optimize the monitoring data and lessen the likelihood of false alarms. Skin preparation includes shaving electrode sites and removing skin oils and debris with alcohol or a rough washcloth.[22] Once the skin is prepared, proper lead placement has been shown to assist in the differentiation of rhythms. Figure 11-3 shows the

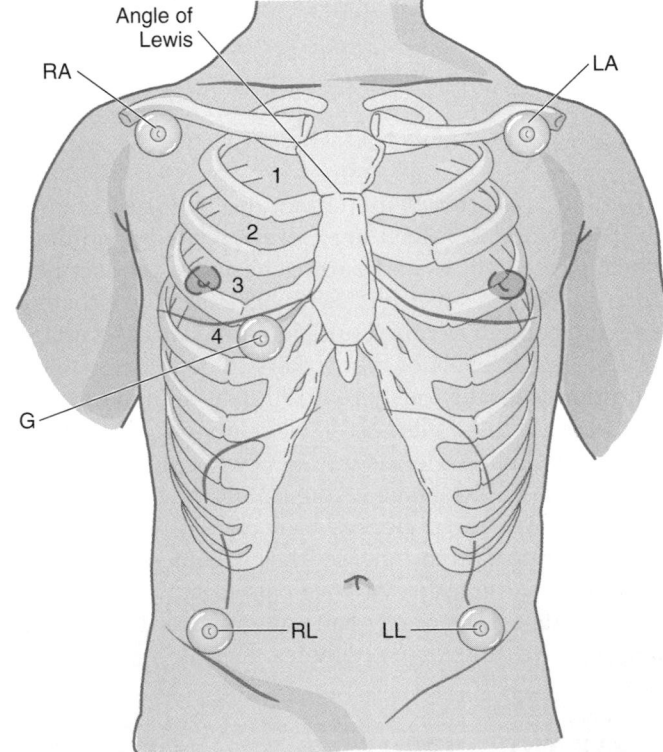

FIGURE 11-3 Correct five-electrode lead placement. Commonly used five-electrode lead system that allows for recording any of the six limb leads plus one precordial (V) lead. Shown here is lead placement for recording V_1. A limitation of this system is that only one precordial lead can be recorded. RA = Right arm, LA = left arm, RL = right leg, LL = left leg, G = ground.

correct five-electrode lead placement. It is important to emphasize that the right and left leg leads should be placed *below* the rib cage.[22] Consistency of lead placement improves the information gained from bedside monitoring as well as when obtaining a 12 lead ECG. Indelible ink or other permanent method should be employed to ensure consistent placement of the precordial leads. These evidence-based practices facilitate accurate, efficient nursing practice.

The critical care nurse should have the basic knowledge required for interpreting a 12 lead ECG. There are many books available to assist with this instruction.[22a] Initial interpretation of a 12 lead ECG helps the nurse anticipate possible interventions. Knowledge of the anatomy of the coronary arteries is needed to understand the relationship between the leads and the anatomic area of the heart represented. Table 11-5 describes the coronary artery system, regions of blood supply, and their corresponding leads. Lesions involving the left anterior descending artery (LAD) usually include the anterior wall of the left ventricle and can lead to pump failure and, if extensive damage occurs, cardiogenic shock. The right coronary artery (RCA) supplies the inferior and posterior wall of the left ventricle and the conduction system in the majority of the population. Lesions in this artery can lead to conduction disorders and possible right ventricular dysfunction. Right ventricular dysfunction can be detected by evaluating right-sided chest leads. The lateral wall is usually supplied by the left circumflex artery (LCA). Depending on the individual's coronary anatomy, lateral wall damage rarely occurs alone; it is typically found in conjunction with any of the other types of wall damage. Lateral wall damage can be associated with sinus node dysrhythmias. This baseline knowledge allows the nurse to anticipate patient presentation and clinical needs.

The ECG changes seen with myocardial damage are a component of the objective data that assist in the diagnostic process. Because the ventricle is the muscle mass experiencing ischemia, ventricular depolarization and repolarization are altered. The QRS complex, ST segment, and T wave are the ECG elements that will be affected. Development of a pathologic Q wave was once considered a hallmark of a myocardial infarction. However, the development of more sensitive and specific biomarkers (i.e., troponin I and troponin T) identifies approximately 25% of patients who had elevation in troponin levels along with ST elevation but did not develop pathologic Q waves.[4,5,27] Q waves are considered pathologic if (1) the width is greater than 30 milliseconds (ms) or (2) the width is greater than or equal to 25% of the height of the subsequent R wave.[44] The presence of pathologic Q waves in contiguous leads indicates necrosis, because dead cells cannot conduct action potentials or electric current. It was thought that Q wave MIs were indicative of a transmural MI and carried a higher mortality.[48] However, investigators have shown that there is no difference in total mortality between Q wave and non–Q wave MIs.[6,49]

Bundle branch blocks (BBBs) seen in the CAD patient are another distortion of the QRS complex with potential clinical significance. A new left BBB makes the identification of an MI difficult because it alters

TABLE 11-5 Anatomic Regions of the Myocardium and Their Corresponding Leads

ANATOMIC REGION	AFFECTED CORONARY ARTERY	CORRESPONDING ECG LEADS	CLINICAL IMPLICATIONS
Anteroseptal wall	LAD	V_1, V_2, V_3, V_4	Potential for failure, cardiogenic shock, conduction defects
Left lateral wall	LCX	I, aV_L, V_5, V_6	Potential for dysrhythmias
Inferior wall	RCA, LCX, PDCA	II, III, aV_F	Potential for conduction defects
Posterior wall	RCA	Tall R wave and ST depression in right precordial leads V_1, V_2	May occur with inferior MI; SA and AV node dysfunction
Right ventricular infarction	RCA	V_{4R}, ST elevation in V_1, II, III, aV_F	Potential for right-sided heart failure; dependent on preload

Modified from reference 44a.
LAD = Left anterior descending coronary artery, LCX = left circumflex coronary artery, PDCA = posterior descending coronary artery, RCA = right coronary artery.

the early and late phases of ventricular depolarization and is associated with increased risk of poor outcomes.[19] A new right BBB has less clinical significance but has been associated with heart failure or may indicate need for a pacemaker.[43]

The ST segment has been the focus of intense study over the past 15 to 20 years.[2a,48] The S wave is the first negative deflection after the QRS complex and ends with the J point—the beginning of the ST segment. It is important to identify the J point to help analyze injury patterns. Changes in the ST segment along with biomarker serial elevations are indications of an MI. Again, obstruction of blood flow to myocardial cells because of thrombosis will ultimately lead to a change in electrical current. These changes in current are reflected in abnormal findings in the ST segment and T wave (ventricular repolarization). Hyperacute T waves, ST elevation, T wave inversion, and ST depression are all referred to as "currents of injury."[15] Ischemic changes are usually represented by ST depression and deep T wave inversion (greater than 0.1 mV).[15] ST segment depression is positive for ischemia when it is *greater than or equal to* 1 mm below the baseline of two contiguous leads.[2a,18] Inversely, ST elevation *greater than or equal to* 0.1 mV (1 mm) in two contiguous leads can indicate an acute MI.[6] It is important to recognize that ECG findings need to be present in *at least* two contiguous leads in order for the finding to be diagnostic.[15] Figure 11-4 summarizes ECG changes for ischemia and infarction.

Because ST segment changes are so important, continuous ST segment monitoring is now recommended by the AHA.[22] There are no randomized clinical trials documenting improved outcomes, but this technology does enable (1) monitoring of the impacted artery, (2) detection of abrupt closure after a primary PCI, (3) detection of ongoing ischemia, and (4) detection of transient myocardial ischemia.[22] Unfortunately, ST segment monitoring is widely underused in hospitals, even if the system is available. One reason this tool is not widely used is the high rate of false alarms as well as lack of understanding about how to properly use this technology. Many of the strategies for improving bedside cardiac monitoring apply to improving the accuracy of ST monitoring. Some of the strategies recommended by the AHA are the following: (1) understand that body position changes can cause ST fluctuations; (2) follow careful skin preparation techniques; (3) maintain consistent lead placement; (4) tailor alarm parameters to the patient's baseline ST level; (5) understand the goals of monitoring; and (6) analyze ECG printout rather than just graphic trends.[22] Using this technology effectively may help improve patient care.

Anti-Ischemic Medication Therapy

Nitrates are one of the first medications given to reduce myocardial oxygen demand. NTG is a potent vasodilator of the capacitance vessels, reducing preload, ventricular wall tension, and myocardial oxygen consumption. It also dilates large coronary arteries and increases collateral flow to ischemic areas. In critical care, NTG can be administered sublingually, but when the patient has marginal hemodynamic parameters, intravenous administration may be preferred to better control patient response. Hypotension can occur as a result of hypovolemia, poor myocardial function, or the combination of pharmacologic agents given quickly. The 2007 AHA guidelines[2a] include morphine sulfate in this category as an adjunct therapy. Morphine sulfate is a potent analgesic and anxiolytic that may be given concurrently with NTG to control chest pain or acute pulmonary congestion. Morphine causes venodilation, decreasing preload and the workload of the compromised myocardium, indirectly assisting with anti-ischemic effects of other drugs. The patient's home medications should be reviewed carefully for other drugs that may exacerbate hypotension. Alpha agonists for erectile dysfunction, such as sildenafil (Viagra), are commonly prescribed and can have vasodilatory effects up to 24 hours after a dose.[2a] Combination of various drugs can produce pharmacologic-induced hypotension, which can cause further myocardial ischemia; BP needs to be carefully monitored.

Beta blockers can also combat myocardial ischemia. These drugs block the effects of catecholamines at beta-receptor sites on cell membranes. In the myocardium,

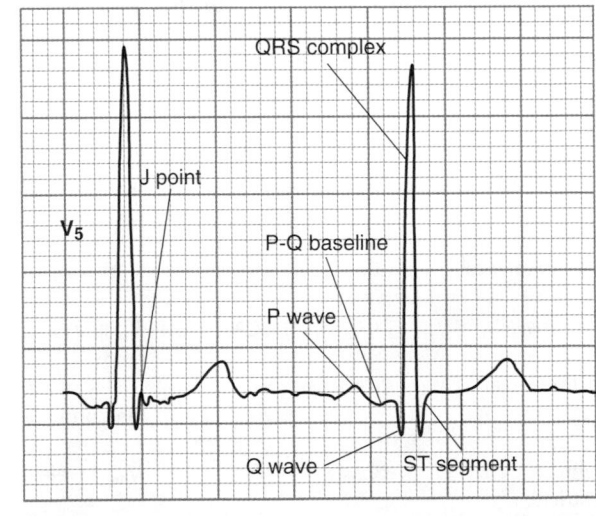

A

♦**FIGURE 11-4** Summary of ECG changes for ischemia and infarction. **A,** Normal ECG.

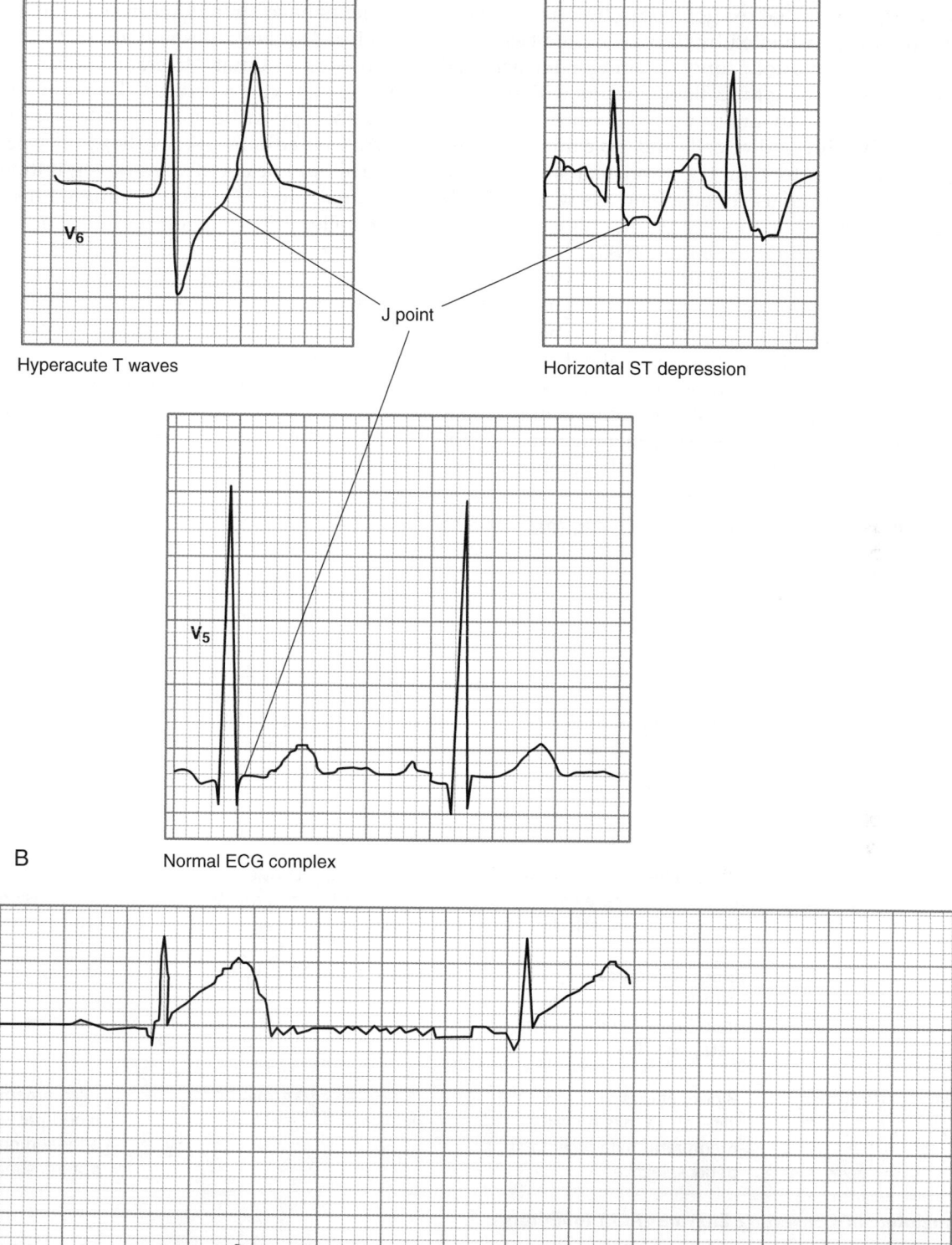

FIGURE 11-4, cont'd   B, ST depression and hyperacute T waves. **C,** ST elevation.

this action decreases HR and contractility, thereby decreasing myocardial oxygen consumption. Adequate beta blockade is achieved by decreasing the heart rate, which increases diastolic time, resulting in an increased coronary artery filling time. Beta blockers with selective beta₁ receptor activity are preferred because they interact primarily with cardiac cells and have minimal activity on beta receptors in the bronchial airways and pancreatic cells. The use of beta blockers was originally shown to decrease morbidity or mortality in patients with MIs and heart failure in the 1980s,[69] and remains an important intervention in the 2007 AHA guidelines.[2a] Initial doses of beta blockers are usually given intravenously for more immediate effect and can be converted to an oral equivalent dose once the patient is stable.

Calcium antagonists can decrease myocardial ischemia by inhibiting myocardial contractility and slowing atrioventricular (AV) node conduction, reducing the inward calcium flux across the cell membrane. This action decreases myocardial oxygen consumption. If patients have already received nitrates and beta blockers in adequate doses and are still experiencing symptoms or cannot tolerate those drugs, calcium antagonists can be added. They are also good adjunctive therapy in treating hypertension in patients with UA.[2a] Nifedipine (Procardia) is a calcium antagonist that should be avoided, however, if there is not already adequate beta blockade (controlled heart rate) because controlled trials suggest increased adverse effects.[24]

Another medication classification associated with decreased mortality in patients with recent MI, left ventricular (LV) systolic dysfunction, or normal LV function is the ACE inhibitors.[2a] If the patient does not tolerate ACEIs, ARBs can be used. Combinations of these medication classifications can be used to control symptoms and limit ischemia. The Medication table below summarizes information on the anti-ischemic drugs.

MEDICATIONS USED FOR ANTI-ISCHEMIC THERAPY

MEDICATION	ACTIONS	DOSAGE	SPECIAL CONSIDERATIONS
Nitrates			
Nitroglycerin (NTG)	Potent vasodilator of capacitance vessels; reduces preload, thereby reducing ventricular wall tension and myocardial oxygen consumption	0.3–0.6 mg up to 1.5 mg; 0.4 mg sublingual or spray as needed; 10 mcg/min IV infusion and increase 10 mcg q 3–5 min	Monitor for hypotension
Beta Blockers			
Metoprolol (Lopressor)	Blocks effects of catecholamines on cell membrane beta receptors; beta₁ selective	50–200 mg PO twice daily; IV with chest pain, 5 mg IV q 5 min × 3	Monitor for bradycardia; hypotension; bronchospasm less likely
Atenolol (Tenormin)	Blocks effects of catecholamines on cell membrane beta receptors; beta₁ selective	50–200 mg PO daily	Monitor for bradycardia; hypotension; bronchospasm less likely
Esmolol (Brevibloc)	Blocks effects of catecholamines on cell membrane beta receptors; beta₁ selective	50–300 mcg/kg/min IV infusion	Recommend monitoring blood pressure with intra-arterial monitoring; potent, short acting
Angiotensin-Converting Enzyme (ACE) Inhibitors			
Captopril (Capoten)	Inhibits formation of converting enzyme, thus formation of aldosterone	25–100 mg PO q day to three times daily Max dose is 450 mg per day	Cough is side effect, not allergy; monitor for hyperkalemia and decreased renal function
Enalapril maleate (Vasotec)	Inhibits formation of converting enzyme, thus formation of aldosterone	2.5–40 mg PO once or twice daily	Cough is side effect, not allergy; monitor for hyperkalemia and decreased renal function

MEDICATION	ACTIONS	DOSAGE	SPECIAL CONSIDERATIONS
Lisinopril (Prinivil, Zestril)	Inhibits formation of converting enzyme, thus formation of aldosterone	10–40 mg PO once daily	Cough is side effect, not allergy; monitor for hyperkalemia and decreased renal function
Calcium Channel Blockers			
Amlodipine (Norvasc)	Reduces influx of transmembrane calcium influx, thus decreasing vascular wall contraction	5–10 mg PO once daily	Monitor for hypotension
Nifedipine (Procardia)	Reduces influx of transmembrane calcium influx, thus decreasing vascular wall contraction	30–90 mg PO once daily	Not recommended in this patient population

Data from references 11 and 29.

Antiplatelet and Anticoagulation Therapy

Disabling platelet activity has been shown to be an effective treatment for UA/NSTEMI and should be initiated immediately.[2a] Once the plaque is disrupted, platelets are one of the major participants in thrombus formation. Aspirin (ASA) irreversibly inhibits the cyclooxygenase-1 within platelets, thereby preventing the formation of thromboxane A_2, disabling platelet aggregation. ASA should be administered as soon as possible after patient presentation and continued on a daily basis indefinitely.[2a] It also is thought to alter the inflammatory process at the cell level. However, some patients may not tolerate ASA because of hypersensitivity, gastric intolerance, or bleeding.

Thienopyridines are another type of medication that disables platelets by interacting with platelet glycoprotein IIb/IIIa to prevent fibrinogen binding to activated platelets.[29] Clopidogrel (Plavix) is a thienopyridine used when ASA intolerance is an issue and as adjunctive therapy with ASA in the hospitalized patient where a noninterventional approach is planned.[8,2a] Because thienopyridines and ASA prevent platelet aggregation by different mechanisms, there can be an additive effect when using both medications. Clopidogrel should be given when there is serious suspicion of myocardial injury.[2] The findings of the Clopidogrel in Unstable Angina to Prevent Recurrent Events (CURE) trial demonstrated a 20% decrease in the combined end point of cardiovascular death, nonfatal MI, and stroke when using a loading dose of 300 mg followed by 75 mg daily in NSTEMI patients.[25] Of note, these results were achieved with an increased risk of bleeding; therefore this consequence must be considered in centers using aggressive interventional strategies.

Ticlopidine (Ticlid), another available thienopyridine, can be used; however, Urban et al.[64] demonstrated clopidogrel was tolerated better. If coronary artery bypass graft (CABG) surgery is being considered, the current recommendation is that clopidogrel be discontinued 5 to 7 days before surgery to help limit postoperative bleeding.[2a] There are ongoing studies examining the risk-benefit issues of this practice.

If more immediate action against platelet aggregation is needed, intravenous glycoprotein IIb/IIIa (GP IIb/IIIa) receptor antagonists are recommended when myocardial injury is suspected and a catheterization or PCI is planned.[2a] Since the PCI will cause further endothelial disruption, a GP IIb/IIIa inhibitor should be administered just before the procedure to achieve optimal platelet aggregation antagonism. There are three commonly used GP IIb/IIIa inhibitors in clinical practice: abciximab (ReoPro), eptifibatide (Integrilin), and tirofiban (Aggrastat). Although the final action of these drugs is similar, the pharmacokinetics and pharmacodynamic properties are different. The GP IIb/IIIa antagonists occupy receptors, preventing fibrinogen binding and thereby preventing platelet aggregation. Abciximab has a strong affinity for the receptor sites but is less specific and inhibits the vitronectin receptors on the endothelial cell.[17] Eptifibatide and tirofiban affect different peptide sequences of fibrinogen and are highly specific for the GP IIb/IIIa receptors.[2a]

Because the mechanism of acute myocardial injury is thrombus formation, pharmacologic interventions are aimed at decreasing thrombus formation at various levels in the clotting cascade. Antithrombotic interventions include antiplatelet and anticoagulation therapy. Unfractionated heparin (UFH) and low molecular weight heparins (LMWHs) are the most commonly used anticoagulation agents. Heparin accelerates the action of antithrombin, which inactivates factor IIa (thrombin), whereas LMWH inactivates both thrombin and factor Xa.[29] Heparin activity requires partial prothrombin time (PTT) monitoring while LMWHs do not require laboratory monitoring. It is important to remember that heparins prevent thrombi formation but do not lyse existing thrombi.

With the increased use of heparins, heparin-induced thrombocytopenia (HIT) has become a more common clinical syndrome. HIT, a platelet disorder associated with development of a drug-induced thrombocytopenia, can be frequently complicated by life-threatening thrombotic events.[67] HIT may be seen in patients who receive heparin, and should be an early consideration in the cardiac patient with new thrombocytopenia that develops 5 to 8 days after the initiation of heparin therapy.[67] An in-depth discussion of HIT can be found in Chapter 37. If HIT is suspected, lepirudin (Refludan), a direct thrombin inhibitor, can be substituted for heparin. Another direct thrombin inhibitor, bivalirudin (Angiomax), has been used in recent studies during percutaneous coronary revascularization. Patients randomly received either bivalirudin with provisional (if necessary during the procedure) GP IIb/IIIa blockade or heparin with planned GP IIb/IIIa blockade.[38] The long-term outcomes are comparable to those of heparin, but further study is required before including bivalirudin in national guidelines.[38]

The antiplatelet and anticoagulation medications discussed are summarized in the Medication table below. Once the patient's condition stabilizes, long-term therapy can be implemented. It is important to note that even though the cause of myocardial injury in UA/NSTEMI may be a nonocclusive thrombus, thrombolysis has not been shown to improve outcomes and is not recommended.[2a]

MEDICATIONS USED FOR ANTIPLATELET AND ANTICOAGULATION THERAPY

MEDICATION	ACTIONS	DOSAGE	SPECIAL CONSIDERATIONS
Oral Antiplatelet Therapy			
Aspirin (ASA)	Blocks production of thromboxane A_2, which induces platelet aggregation	Initial dose 162–325 mg PO nonenteric followed by 75–160 mg PO daily	Important for first dose to be nonenteric for better absorption
Clopidogrel (Plavix)	Adenosine diphosphate antagonist	75 mg PO daily; loading can be 4–8 tablets (300–600 mg)	Loading for more rapid onset
Ticlopidine (Ticlid)	Interacts with platelet glycoprotein IIb/IIIa to inhibit fibrinogen binding to activated platelets	250 mg PO twice daily; loading can be 500 mg	Loading for more rapid onset
Heparins			
Dalteparin (Fragmin)	Increases action of antithrombin, inactivating thrombin, but more potent on inhibition of factor Xa	120 units/kg subcutaneously q 12 hr	Maximum is 10,000 units twice daily. Has not been approved for post-MI use.
Enoxaparin (Lovenox)	Increases action of antithrombin, inactivating thrombin, but more potent on inhibition of factor Xa	1 mg/kg subcutaneously q 12 hr; may use loading dose 30 mg IV bolus	No lab parameter to measure effects (can check anti-Xa levels if using long-term) Dose should be adjusted for renal impairment Monitor platelet count
Heparin (UFH)	Increases action of antithrombin, inactivating thrombin	Bolus 60–70 units/kg IV (max is 5000 units) followed by 12–15 units/kg/hr (max is 1000 units/hr)	Goal is a PTT 1.5–2.5 times control Monitor platelet count

MEDICATION	ACTIONS	DOSAGE	SPECIAL CONSIDERATIONS
Direct Thrombin Inhibitor			
Bivalirudin (Angiomax)	Direct thrombin inhibitor	Bolus 0.75 mg/kg IV at start of intervention and infusion of 1.75 mg/kg/hr during intervention	
Intravenous Antiplatelet Therapy			
Abciximab (ReoPro)	Prevents platelet aggregation by preventing fibrinogen binding	0.25 mg/kg IV followed by 0.125 mcg/kg/min infusion (max is 10 mcg/min) for 12–24 hr	Monitor for occult bleeding (retroperitoneal or groin) Monitor platelet count
Eptifibatide (Integrilin)	Prevents platelet aggregation by preventing fibrinogen binding	180 mcg/kg IV bolus followed by 2 mcg/kg/min infusion for 72–96 hr Can give second bolus 10 minutes after first bolus if needed	Monitor for occult bleeding (retroperitoneal or groin) Monitor platelet count
Tirofiban (Aggrastat)	Prevents platelet aggregation by preventing fibrinogen binding	0.4 mcg/kg/min IV for 30 min followed by 0.1 mcg/kg/min for 48–96 hr	Monitor for occult bleeding (retroperitoneal or groin) Monitor platelet count

Data from references 11 and 29.

Preventive Nursing Interventions

The obvious complication that can occur with antithrombotic therapy is bleeding. A high index of suspicion should be the driving force for nursing interventions. Complications can be avoided by close monitoring of all disruptions in skin integrity, including mucous membranes, wounds, and vascular access sites. Monitoring for adequate tissue perfusion should include specific attention to certain body systems. Hypovolemia and hypotension can exacerbate myocardial perfusion issues and can lead to increased frequency or intensity of chest pain, ECG changes, or associated respiratory distress. Cerebral hemorrhage can be another devastating complication of anticoagulation. Neurologic assessment skills should be refined to detect more subtle changes in level of consciousness. Change in cognitive processes, subtle changes in speech, or minor motor deficits may be early signs of cerebral bleeding. Renal perfusion may also be compromised because of hypoperfusion or myocardial dysfunction. Careful monitoring of urine output and renal function, including trending BUN, creatinine, and calculated creatinine clearance values, should be integrated into nursing care. Testing all body secretions for blood, measuring and accurately recording blood loss, and participating in interventions to prevent injury, such as use of soft mouth care utensils, minimal blood sampling, and avoidance of invasive procedures (e.g., nasogastric tubes, rectal tubes), are all standard nursing interventions.

◆ Case Study 11-1, Part A

Acute Coronary Syndrome

Mr. C. is a 55-year-old male experiencing severe chest pain radiating down his left arm. He has a past medical history of hypertension and obesity and is unsure about his cholesterol levels. His family history is significant: both his father and his brother have a history of heart attacks, and his mother has type 2 diabetes. He also complains of shortness of breath and is diaphoretic. He states the pain started this evening after dinner (about 3 hours earlier). He initially thought it was indigestion, for which he took an antacid. When the discomfort persisted, his wife convinced him to go to the hospital. The emergency medical services personnel recognized the symptoms of ACS and advised him to chew an aspirin (160 to 325 mg) while waiting for the ambulance to arrive (after assessment for any aspirin allergy and recent history of gastrointestinal bleeding).

Once in the emergency department (ED), Mr. C. was immediately triaged.

Decision point: What interventions should be instituted immediately?

Decision point: Should fibrinolytic therapy also have been initiated to help improve Mr. C.'s outcome?

Case continues on page 229

Revascularization Therapy

If UA persists despite medical therapy or if the patient has any of the high-risk indicators, an early invasive strategy is suggested (Box 11-1).[2a] Invasive strategies include coronary angiography with PCI or CABG. Coronary angiography is the gold standard in studying coronary artery anatomy and flow. Once the anatomy is visualized, treatment options can be considered. This study usually includes a left-sided heart catheterization consisting of a ventriculogram that can determine ventricular anatomy and function (ejection fraction) as well as visualize valve structure and function. The usual access site for any angiographic intervention is the right common femoral artery, but the left femoral artery can also be used. If needed, alternative sites are the radial and brachial arteries. A right-sided heart catheterization can be performed by accessing either the femoral, internal jugular, or subclavian veins. This study is obtained to evaluate the right heart performance, pressures, and valve function as well as to detect the presence of a pathologic left to right shunt by measuring progressive oxygen saturation in the vessels, right atrium, and right ventricle.

If the information obtained in the catheterization indicates a need for further intervention, a PCI can be performed at that time. The expertise of the operator plays an important role. The ACC/AHA guidelines for PCI, revised in 2005,[56] recommend that the operator maintain an acceptable volume of interventions (greater than 75 procedures per year) in a center with cardiac surgery capability. The procedures currently available are (1) percutaneous transluminal coronary angioplasty (PTCA), (2) coronary atherectomy, (3) coronary stent placement, and (4) brachytherapy. The more common procedures are the PTCA and coronary stent placement.

PTCA is an intervention often transitioned to during the catheterization. A guide catheter is placed with a wire across the lesion. A prepared balloon is inserted over the wire, placed across the lesion, and inflated multiple times at various pressures, depending on the physician's preference (Figure 11-5). Because early outcomes of PTCA initially included acute or delayed restenosis (5% to 10%), the coronary stent was introduced to counteract the elastic recoil that occurred in the coronary artery after PTCA[20] (Figure 11-6). These metal devices were designed to be mounted on a balloon that, when expanded, would deploy the device and implant it into the lesion of the coronary artery. They have various designs (e.g., mesh, coil, slotted tube, ring) and are composed of various materials (e.g., stainless steel, cobalt alloy, tantalum).[20] Initial stenting procedures also had variable outcomes. The stent actually produces injury to the endothelium of the artery and can initiate or worsen the inflammatory process, leading to hyperplasia, restenosis, or thrombosis. To counteract the complications of the bare-metal stent, the drug-eluting stent was developed. These stents are coated with a drug or material with antiproliferative properties to prevent or lessen the insult to the arterial endothelium and maintain blood flow through the lumen. One such stent is the BX VELOCITY stent, which has a polymer coating and is impregnated with the drug sirolimus. Sirolimus is an immunosuppressant that allows normal growth of the endothelium; the polymer coating decreases the cytokine response of the smooth muscle cell.[20,50] These two actions decrease the restenosis rate associated with this intervention.[20,50]

Coronary atherectomy is a technique in which the atheromatous plaque is removed by either a cutter or a burr rotating at a high speed. Because the technique also causes damage to the endothelial wall, cell hyperplasia and restenosis can occur. This is another intervention that may be accompanied by a stent placement to enhance the likelihood that the lumen remains patent.

Because restenosis is a major complication of any PCI, other interventions have been developed to treat the complication. Laser angioplasty has been revisited. It was originally used to remove atherosclerotic lesions but had poor outcomes. Tissue ablation is thought to be achieved using a combination of photochemical, localized thermal, and mechanical effects.[20]

Another technique to deal with restenosis is brachytherapy—local radiation treatment to the coronary artery wall to decrease the formation of hyperplastic

---

Box 11-1

Indicators of High Risk for Unstable Angina/ Non–ST Elevation Myocardial Infarction

- Recurrent angina/ischemia at rest or with low-level activities despite intensive anti-ischemic therapy
- Elevated TnT or TnI
- New or presumably new ST segment depression
- Recurrent angina/ischemia with CHF symptoms, S_3 gallop, pulmonary edema, worsening rales, or new or worsening mitral regurgitation
- High-risk findings on noninvasive stress testing
- Depressed left ventricular systolic function (ejection fraction <40%)
- Hemodynamic instability
- Percutaneous coronary intervention within 6 months
- Prior CABG

From reference 11.

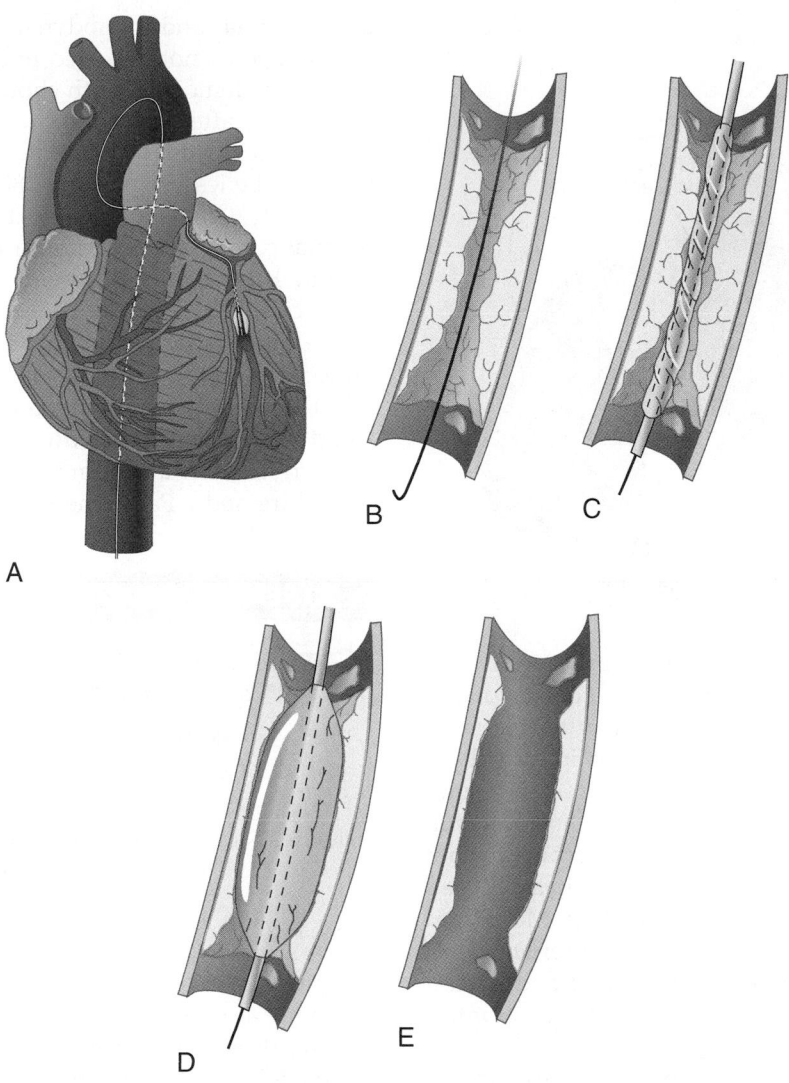

✦FIGURE 11-5 Percutaneous transluminal coronary angioplasty (PTCA). Mechanism of intracoronary balloon angioplasty. **A,** The balloon catheter is introduced into the coronary artery via the catheter in the aorta. **B,** A guidewire is advanced across the area of narrowing. **C,** The balloon catheter is advanced over the wire across the lesion. **D,** The balloon is inflated. **E,** The opened coronary artery as it appears after the PTCA.

cells. Any of these techniques can have complications, including perforation or late thrombosis. Other complications associated with these interventions are recurrent chest pain, abrupt closure, vascular spasm, stroke, transient ischemic attack (TIA), NSTEMI, STEMI, dysrhythmias or conduction disorders, and contrast-related complications.

Revascularization of the coronary arteries can also be achieved surgically. CABG surgery has been used for revascularization for many years and continues to be a viable option even with the development of PCIs. These grafts can also be subject to restenosis that may be amenable to some of the previously mentioned interventions. A more complete discussion of cardiac surgery can be found in Chapter 14.

Nursing Interventions for Patients Treated With Percutaneous Coronary Interventions

The preparation for, observation period during, and follow-up after a PCI can be pivotal periods of time for the cardiac patient. It is imperative the nurse have proper education in caring for these patients to help avoid complications and properly educate the patients. Before the study, the nurse should ensure baseline laboratory tests are obtained, including electrolytes, BUN and creatinine, glucose, a complete blood count (CBC), and, if the patient has been prescribed anticoagulation therapy, coagulation studies. A baseline 12-lead ECG should also be available. If there is a suspicion of

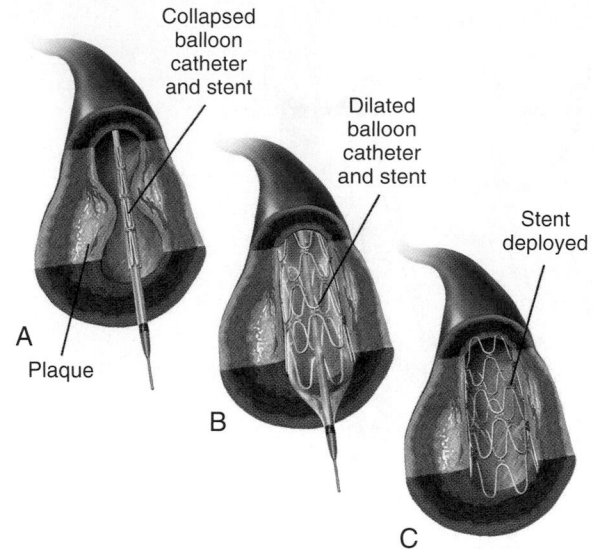

Collapsed balloon catheter and stent

Dilated balloon catheter and stent

Stent deployed

A

Plaque

B

C

⬍**FIGURE 11-6** Cardiac stent.

ongoing ischemic events, cardiac biomarkers may also be measured. Evaluation of the intravascular volume status of these patients is critical to maintaining adequate renal function. Because the patient will be NPO, intravenous fluids should be ordered. Diuretics may be held, depending on the patient's volume status. Oral hypoglycemic agents, especially metformin (Glucophage), are held because their use is associated with an increased risk of renal dysfunction. Metformin should also be held 48 hours after the intervention.[30] Blood glucose levels should be monitored and insulin ordered to maintain good blood glucose control (Chapter 34).

Renal function is an important parameter that can be compromised, especially with the contrast administered during a PCI. Adequate intravascular volume must be maintained to protect renal function. Assessment of intravascular volume includes HR, BP, and other hemodynamic parameters as available. HR may not be a reliable parameter if beta blockade is used. There are three types of contrast available for these procedures: (1) high osmolar ionic agents, (2) low osmolar ionic agents, and (3) low osmolar nonionic agents. The low osmolar nonionic agents are most commonly used to lessen intravascular depletion from the contrast. As well, more recent literature suggests that the most effective intervention is adequate hydration before and after the procedure.[66] Chapter 33 provides more comprehensive information about the prevention of renal failure. If the patient has a contrast or iodine allergy, premedication with an antihistamine and steroids can be used.

After the PCI, the same laboratory values (electrolytes, CBC, BUN, and creatinine) that were measured as a baseline are obtained concomitant with a 12 lead ECG. Close observation for chest pain, any type of

dysrhythmia, and hemodynamic instability should be maintained. If not removed in the catheterization laboratory, the femoral sheath should be removed within 4 to 6 hours after the procedure. An activated clotting time (ACT) is used to monitor anticoagulation status; it should be less than 150 to 180 seconds before pulling the sheath. The sheath can be discontinued using either manual compression or a compression device. Pressure should be maintained for 20 minutes, observing for distal circulation, hemodynamic stability, and bleeding at the site. Visualization of the insertion site is very important. Equipment obscuring the site (such as sandbags) can limit the ability to detect bleeding. To help avoid a vagal reaction during sheath removal, adequate hydration and femoral site pain control should be addressed. Pain medication can decrease the

▲ RESEARCH UTILIZATION

Complications Occurring After Percutaneous Coronary Intervention

CLINICAL ISSUE

There are many complications that can occur after a PCI related to the sheath removal. Newer closure devices such as an implantable collagen plug and a percutaneous suture device have decreased the incidence of complications. However, identification of risk factors and predictors of complications is needed.

SUMMARY

The nurse researchers conducted a descriptive correlation design with comparative procedures for subgroups to compare the variables of patients who experienced complications when using the two closure devices.

APPLICATION

The following variables were found to be predictive of complications with closure devices:
1. Low preprocedural hematocrit
2. Bleeding disorder
3. Previous use of a closure device (strongest predictor variable)

Because of the results, previous placement of a closure device should be included in the admission process and in screening tools.

NEED FOR FURTHER STUDY

This study demonstrated that more studies with similar design are needed to identify variables that may predict complications with closure devices.

Hammer, J. B., Dubois, J. E., & Rice, T. P. (2005). Predictors of complications associated with closure devices after transfemoral percutaneous coronary procedures. *Crit Care Nurse, 25,* 30–37.

tendency of the patient to "bear down," which increases vagal tone. The head of the bed should be at 30 degrees to ensure comfort. Once the sheath is removed, frequent neurovascular checks of the affected extremity and puncture site should be performed as per institutional protocol.[33] Initial checks every 15 minutes for 1 hour would commonly be included in observation guidelines. Newer vascular closure devices (e.g., implantable collagen plugs or percutaneous suture devices) are now used to achieve rapid hemostasis, improve patient comfort, and allow early ambulation (see the Research Utilization box on p. 224).[28] Proper management of the puncture site can allow faster mobilization of this patient population.

Complications of the groin include hematoma, retroperitoneal bleeding, arterial thrombosis, pseudo-aneurysm, and arteriovenous fistula. A high index of suspicion should be maintained when observing these patients. Gentle palpation of the groin puncture site may assist with hematoma detection. Auscultation over the site for a vascular bruit can help with early detection of an arteriovenous fistula. Monitoring hemoglobin and hematocrit provides trends indicating increased bleeding. Monitoring of flank areas near the sheath site should be done to evaluate for retroperitoneal bleeding. Subtle changes, such as increased numbness and tingling of the effected extremity, may indicate pressure from an expanding hematoma on nerves in the groin. Astute observations may help detect issues earlier, leading to interventions that may lessen devastating complications. The Multidisciplinary Plan of Care is outlined below. Use of a multidisciplinary team is essential.

MULTIDISCIPLINARY PLAN OF CARE FOR PATIENTS WITH ACUTE CORONARY SYNDROMES

PROBLEM	INTERVENTION	RATIONALE	EXPECTED OUTCOMES
Risk of patient developing heart failure or cardiogenic shock	Early identification of possible ACS patients.	Early identification of ACS patients will enable early treatment.	No cardiac muscle dysfunction or minimal muscle dysfunction
	Administer ASA. Support with oxygen. NTG and morphine for pain control.	ASA disables platelets. NTG and morphine will decrease preload and decrease myocardial oxygen consumption.	
	Entrance into healthcare system to start assessment with 12 lead ECG and cardiac biomarkers.	ECG and cardiac biomarkers are best initial assessment methods.	
	Determine if there is injury (STEMI), ischemia (UA/NSTEMI).	Type of muscle damage will determine type of intervention.	
	If STEMI, start beta blockers, clopidogrel, and heparin. Consider reperfusion therapy, either PCI or fibrinolysis.	Beta blockers decrease myocardial oxygen consumption. Clopidogrel disables platelets, and heparin decreases further clot formation. PCI will mechanically relieve obstruction whereas fibrinolysis will lyse clot.	
	If UA/NSTEMI, start NTG, beta blockers, clopidogrel, heparin, and glycoprotein IIb/IIIa inhibitors. Admit, monitor, and assess risk status.	Addition of glycoprotein IIb/IIIa inhibitors will provide additive antiplatelet activity.	
	Continue therapies and start ACE inhibitor/ARB and statin therapy for both STEMI and UA/NSTEMI patients.	ACE inhibitor and statin therapy will decrease mortality in this patient population.	
Risk of patient developing groin complication	Provide close monitoring of femoral site of PCI, including frequent visual inspection of site as well as neurovascular assessment of affected extremity.	Permits early detection of femoral hematoma or neurovascular injury.	No or minimal femoral bleeding or focal deficit from neurovascular injury

ST SEGMENT ELEVATION MYOCARDIAL INFARCTION

When there is acute ST segment elevation, an acute MI is occurring. Cell death is not recoverable, as may be the case with cell ischemia. Therefore urgency in implementing interventions becomes the focus. The plan of care is similar to that discussed for UA/NSTEMI. However, the one major difference is urgent reperfusion therapy becomes the priority, as it is presumed that the atheromatic plaque has ruptured and initiated the coagulation cascade, forming a thrombus large enough to completely obstruct blood flow in one or several coronary arteries. Fibrinolytic therapy may be considered, but is not without risks that must be evaluated before administration of any drug.[4] The risk of bleeding is a major concern, and evaluation for that risk needs to be efficient in order to avoid major complications. Because of this risk, PCI is considered the preferred intervention in this patient population.[56]

Physical and Laboratory Assessment

Assessment of patients with a STEMI focuses on evaluation of chest pain and medical history, as well as the presence of heart failure or renal dysfunction, similar to recommendations for UA/NSTEMI patients. Because the STEMI patient may be considered immediately for fibrinolytic therapy, a brief, focused neurologic exam should be performed to detect evidence of prior stroke or cognitive defects.[4] This information will assist with risk stratification as well as establish a neurologic baseline for future assessment. A 12 lead ECG should be performed and evaluated immediately to help determine the extent and location of the STEMI. Laboratory data should be collected, but should not delay implementation of reperfusion therapy.[4] The optimal biomarkers are the cardiac-specific troponins that should be drawn before and within 24 hours after fibrinolytic therapy, especially in patients not undergoing angiography.[4] Trends in the levels of these biomarkers will provide supportive, noninvasive evidence about the effectiveness of reperfusion of the infarct artery. A qualitative assessment of these biomarkers can be performed using handheld bedside (point-of-care) assays that are especially helpful in emergency departments or chest pain units. However, subsequent assessments should be performed with a quantitative test or standard laboratory testing to ensure valid measurement.[4]

Other Diagnostic Tests

A chest x-ray is an important test to assist with a differential diagnosis. Suspicion of aortic dissection should be pursued because it is one of the contraindications for the use of fibrinolytic therapy. A high-quality chest x-ray will give some helpful information about the size of the aorta, as can a transthoracic or transesophageal echocardiogram.[2] A portable echocardiogram can also assist with risk stratification, especially if the possible STEMI patient has a new left BBB.[4]

REPERFUSION THERAPY

As the decision about reperfusion therapy is being considered, routine management of the STEMI patient should be continued. Oxygen should be administered if the oxygen saturation of arterial blood is less than 90%.[2] NTG should be administered in the presence of chest pain if the patient is hemodynamically stable. However, nitrates should not be given if (1) the systolic blood pressure (SBP) is less than 90 mm Hg; (2) the SBP is greater than or equal to 30 mm Hg below baseline; (3) there is severe bradycardia (less than 50 beats per minute) or tachycardia (greater than 100 beats per minute); (4) a right ventricular infarction is suspected; or (5) the patient has taken a phosphodiesterase inhibitor for erectile dysfunction (e.g., Viagra) within the last 24 hours.[4] Because STEMI patients may have experienced significant myocardial muscle damage, they may be prone to cardiogenic shock and preload reduction with nitrates could exacerbate that situation.

The major decision in therapy is centered on reperfusion therapy. Evidence supports expeditious restoration of blood flow to the affected artery. Short- and long-term outcomes are improved regardless of whether reperfusion was achieved via fibrinolytic therapy or PCI.[4] The emphasis is on rapid recognition and treatment. If the patient enters the healthcare system through an emergency department, the timeline goal is a door-to-needle time of 30 minutes for initiation of fibrinolytic therapy. If the patient does not qualify for fibrinolytic therapy or if the institution has 24-hour access to the catheterization lab, PCI is the other treatment consideration and the timeline goal is a door-to-balloon time of 90 minutes for initiation of a PCI.[4] These timeline goals are guidelines to help organize and direct care but may not be achieved because of various unavoidable circumstances.

Selection of a reperfusion strategy is influenced by several factors. The time from onset of symptoms to presentation to a medical system is a pivotal factor to consider. The longer the time between onset of symptoms and presentation, the less likely fibrinolytic therapy will be successful. Ideally, fibrinolytic therapy should be administered within the first 2 hours of onset of chest pain.[9] The risk of mortality with a STEMI can be estimated and considered in making the decision about the type of reperfusion therapy. If the patient is in cardiogenic shock, PCI may be the better intervention.[4] Another factor influencing this decision is the time required for transport to a skilled PCI laboratory. The decision will be dependent on how long the trip will take and how quickly the skilled laboratory can mobilize into a functional state. The clinician must consider many factors to make the most efficacious decision about which intervention to pursue.

Pharmacologic Reperfusion Therapy

Restoration of blood flow is the top priority for patient management. Pharmacologic therapy to "dissolve" a thrombus is referred to as fibrinolytic therapy. The goal is early clot lysis by attacking the fibrin component of the clot, hence the term *fibrinolysis*. According to the classic work by Topol,[60] this pharmacologic intervention is achieved using thrombolytic agents that can be divided into two categories: (1) fibrin selective, which activate the fibrin-bound plasminogen and lyse clots quickly; and (2) nonselective agents, which provide more systemic plasminogenolysis and fibrinogenolysis at a slower rate and a more prolonged systemic lytic state. The optimum goal time for implementation of fibrinolytic therapy for the STEMI patient is 30 minutes "door to needle."[4] If the diagnostic process is prolonged, initiation of therapy can be postponed up to 12 hours to ensure a correct diagnosis.[4] Before choosing a thrombolytic agent, it is imperative that a risk assessment for bleeding be completed. Absolute and relative contraindications are summarized in Box 11-2. A complete focused assessment, including neurologic history, becomes essential to establish a baseline and provide clues to possible contraindications for fibrinolysis. A summary of the more commonly used thrombolytics can be found in the Medication table on p. 228. In the past, nonselective thrombolytics were used, but patients were found to have prolonged bleeding tendencies. Streptokinase (SK) is a nonenzymatic protein product of hemolytic streptococci that combines with circulating plasminogen to form complexes that catalyze plasmin formation. The excessive plasmin levels dissolve all recent thrombi in the body, thereby depleting circulating fibrinogen, plasminogen, factor

---

Box 11-2

Contraindications and Cautions for Fibrinolysis

ABSOLUTE CONTRAINDICATIONS

- Any prior intracranial hemorrhage
- Known structural cerebral vascular lesion
- Known malignant intracranial neoplasm (primary or metastatic)
- Ischemic stroke within 3 months EXCEPT acute ischemic stroke within 3 hours
- Suspected aortic dissection
- Active bleeding or bleeding diathesis (excluding menses)
- Significant closed head or facial trauma within 3 months

RELATIVE CONTRAINDICATIONS

- History of chronic, severe, poorly tolerated hypertension
- Severe uncontrolled hypertension on presentation (SBP greater than 180 mm Hg or DBP greater than 110 mm Hg)
- History of prior ischemic stroke greater than 3 months, dementia, or known intracranial pathology not covered in contraindications
- Traumatic or prolonged (greater than 10 min) CPR or major surgery (less than 3 weeks)
- Recent (within 2–4 weeks) internal bleeding
- Noncompressible vascular punctures
- For streptokinase: prior exposure (more than 5 days ago) or prior allergic reaction to these agents
- Pregnancy
- Active peptic ulcer
- Current use of anticoagulants

Modified from reference 4.

V, and factor VIII and increasing accumulation of fibrin split or degradation products.[21] These increased levels also have anticoagulation activity. Another issue with SK is a possible allergic reaction if the patient has had a recent known streptococcal infection or has received SK in the previous 6 months. Hypotension resulting from an activation of plasmin-mediated kinins can occur, which may exacerbate hypotension already present from myocardial dysfunction.[60] Anisoylated plasminogen streptokinase activator complex (APSAC) is a chemically altered form of SK that converts circulating and fibrin-bound plasminogen into plasmin. Because this drug has a prolonged half-life and fibrinolysis activity as well as allergic reactions similar to SK, it is not used frequently in the clinical setting.

MEDICATIONS USED AS THROMBOLYTIC AGENTS

MEDICATION	ACTION	DOSAGE	SPECIAL CONSIDERATIONS
Fibrin Selective			
Alteplase (rt-PA)	Increased affinity to fibrin, which activates fibrin-bound plasminogen	Accelerated dose: Patients over 67 kg: total dose 100 mg. Give 15 mg IV bolus, 50 mg over 30 minutes, and then 35 mg over 60 minutes. Patients 67 kg or less: give 15 mg IV bolus, then 0.75 mg/kg over 30 min, then 0.5 mg/kg over 60 min. Total dose not to exceed 100 mg. 3-hour infusion: Patients 65 kg or more: 60 mg in the first hour (6 to 10 mg of which is to be given as a bouls), 20 mg over the second hour, and 20 mg the third hour. Patients less than 65 kg: 1.25 mg/kg IV administered over 3 hours. Give 60% the first hour (10% of which to be given as a bolus); give remaining 40% over next 2 hours	Monitor for occult bleeding (retroperitoneal or groin)
Reteplase (r-PA)	Increased affinity to fibrin, which activates fibrin-bound plasminogen	Two 10-megaunit IV boluses 30 min apart	Monitor for occult bleeding (retroperitoneal or groin)
Tenecteplase (TNKase)	Increased affinity to fibrin, which activates fibrin-bound plasminogen; very fibrin specific	Weight based in 5-sec bolus: <60 kg = 30 mg; ≥60 to <70 kg = 35 mg; ≥70 to <80 kg = 40 mg; ≥80 to <90 kg = 45 mg; ≥90 kg = 50 mg, which is highest recommended dose	Monitor for occult bleeding (retroperitoneal or groin)
Nonselective			
Streptokinase (SK)	Combines with circulating plasminogen, forming complexes that catalyze plasmin formation	1.5 million units infused over 30–60 min	Monitor for occult bleeding (retroperitoneal or groin); monitor for allergic reaction
Anisoylated plasminogen streptokinase activator complex (APSAC)	Combines with circulating plasminogen, forming complexes that catalyze plasmin formation	30-unit IV bolus over 2–5 min	Monitor for occult bleeding (retroperitoneal or groin); monitor for allergic reaction

Data from reference 58.

One of the more common thrombolytic agents is alteplase (recombinant tissue plasminogen activator [rt-PA]). Alteplase is a drug produced by recombinant DNA techniques and has similar actions to tissue plasminogen activator (t-PA). A protease produced by the vascular endothelial cell, t-PA has an increased affinity for fibrin, which activates fibrin-bound plasminogen. Reteplase (r-PA) is derived from t-PA and also has similar actions but is dosed differently. Tenecteplase is also derived from native t-PA and is designed to have a very fibrin-specific affinity, thus allowing selective clot lysis, attempting to decrease intracranial bleeding.[21] Combinations of pharmacologic therapies have been tested to help maintain arterial flow. Because alteplase has a short half-life, continuous IV heparin is recommended to maintain arterial patency.

Intravenous antiplatelet therapy with abciximab can be combined with pharmacologic reperfusion therapy with reteplase or tenecteplase to prevent reinfarction.[4]

Obvious complications can occur with fibrinolytic therapy. One of the most devastating consequences can be intracranial hemorrhage (ICH). If there is any suspicion of ICH, the stroke team institutional protocol should be initiated including neurology or neurosurgery consults while any type of anticoagulation or fibrinolytic therapy is discontinued until there is radiologic evidence of the absence of ICH.[4] Further in-depth discussion about the management of ICH can be found in Chapter 23. Gastrointestinal bleeding (Chapter 26) may also become an issue because related hypotension can aggravate myocardial dysfunction.

Other pharmacologic interventions for the STEMI patient are similar to those discussed concerning the UA/NSTEMI patients. Interventions are aimed at disrupting the coagulation cascade at all levels so thrombi cannot develop. Antiplatelet and antithrombin drugs are aggressively initiated once the diagnosis of UA is made. Medications to decrease myocardial workload, including beta blockers and ACE inhibitors, should also be considered as soon as BP and cardiac function are within normal parameters.

Interventional Reperfusion Therapy

If immediately available, primary PCI should be performed on STEMI patients within 12 hours of onset of symptoms.[4] The optimum timeline goal is 90 minutes from "door to balloon" or as quickly as possible, especially if congestive heart failure, pulmonary edema, or cardiogenic shock is present.[4] These high-risk patients experience the greatest mortality benefit from primary PCI.[31] PCI can also be used with fibrinolysis. "Rescue PCI" refers to PCI within 12 hours after failed fibrinolysis and is used in patients who continue to have myocardial ischemia. This strategy should be implemented if shock develops within 36 hours of pharmacologic reperfusion therapy.[4] Support systems of a hospital are important factors that can influence the decision to perform a PCI, as it is best supported in hospitals that have on-site cardiac surgery. PCI can be performed in hospitals without cardiac surgery options, but a plan should be in place to expedite rapid transport to an appropriately equipped institution.

Surgical revascularization is also an option, particularly in the following circumstances: (1) failure of PCI; (2) persistent or recurrent myocardial ischemia; (3) severe mitral valve insufficiency; (4) cardiogenic shock; (5) life-threatening ventricular dysrhythmias with 50% left main stenosis or triple vessel disease; (6) patient

is not a candidate for PCI or fibrinolysis.[4] Patients who have received fibrinolytic therapy may also be candidates for surgical intervention, but present a challenge for postsurgical care because of the tendency to bleed.

Complications of STEMI

If myocardial muscle is deprived of blood flow, cardiac function will deteriorate and cardiogenic shock occurs (Chapter 40). The degree of dysfunction is somewhat dependent on the amount of muscle lost and the anatomic region of the damage. Anterior wall damage can result in major pump failure and cardiogenic shock. Recommended interventions for shock are (1) volume management using a pulmonary artery catheter (PAC) and (2) inotropic support, if needed, with sympathomimetic drugs such as dobutamine (Dobutrex) or milrinone (Primacor). These agents have $beta_1$ and $beta_2$ activity that improve myocardial contractility as well as decrease afterload. If shock is severe, alpha agonists such as norepinephrine (Levophed)

◆ Case Study 11–1, Part B

Acute Coronary Syndrome

Mr. C. was transported to the cardiac catheterization laboratory and the intervention initiated within the 90-min "door to balloon inflation" goal. The findings of the coronary angiogram revealed 80% occlusion of the RCA and the LCX with some diffuse distal lesions (less than 50%) in the remaining left coronary system. The decision was made to balloon and stent the RCA and LCX lesions; other lesions were not amenable to interventions. The procedure was successful but Mr. C. remained hypotensive (BP = 80/50 mm Hg) in the recovery room. His initial troponin level was 8 mcg/L, and an additional 12 lead ECG with right chest leads demonstrated a significant Q wave in V_{4R}, indicating a right ventricular infarct. Previous ECGs for Mr. C. also showed an inferior wall MI. A 2D echocardiogram confirmed abnormal wall motion and decreased ejection fraction of the right ventricle. Volume resuscitation was given, which improved the patient's BP. GP IIb/IIIa inhibitor was not used because there is not enough evidence to support use in STEMI.[2]

Mr. C. continued to improve over the next 12 hours and his BP stabilized. Initiation of beta blockers was a goal of therapy, but had to be cautiously considered with the inferior wall MI. Mr. C.'s rhythm has been sinus bradycardia with a ventricular response of approximately 50 to 55 beats/min.

Decision point: Should Mr. C. have had a temporary pacemaker placed?

Case continues on page 234

and phenylephrine (Neo-Synephrine) are used to maintain adequate perfusion. Patients with inferior wall STEMI should be assessed for right ventricular infarction using right precordial chest leads as well as echocardiography. STEMI patients with right ventricular infarctions are dependent on adequate preload and atrial-ventricular synchrony for optimal function.

Mechanical interventions can also support myocardial muscle as it recovers from significant insult. The intra-aortic balloon pump (IABP) is a device that employs the concept of counterpulsation to improve myocardial performance. Counterpulsation is inflation during ventricular diastole and deflation during isometric ventricular contraction—"counter" balloon movement in relation to ventricular activity.[50] The balloon is placed in the aorta just below the left subclavian artery and above the renal artery via percutaneous insertion in the femoral artery. The device actually displaces volume while moving in the aorta. With balloon inflation, volume is displaced proximally, which increases aortic root pressure while the aortic valve is closed. This action improves the perfusion of the coronary arteries, increasing oxygen delivery to the myocardial muscle. Blood volume is also displaced distally during balloon inflation, which can improve renal perfusion. Deflation of the balloon causes a decrease in intra-aortic blood volume, thereby decreasing impedance of blood flow out of the ventricle or

reducing afterload of the left ventricle (Figure 11-7).[50] Increasing oxygen delivery to compromised myocardial muscle improves contractility and CO. With increased CO, intraventricular pressures (estimated by the PAC) decrease, thereby decreasing preload. Afterload reduction also improves CO and function. It is the mechanical equivalent of pharmacologic inotropic support and arterial vasodilation and is used alone or in conjunction with pharmacologic agents if the myocardium is severely compromised.

Proper function of the IABP is evaluated by several methods. Hemodynamic parameter trends are monitored, especially the pulmonary artery diastolic (PAD) pressure, the pulmonary artery wedge pressure (PAWP), and the CO. Pulmonary artery pressures (PAPs) decrease and the CO increases when the IABP is properly positioned. Another method used to evaluate proper IABP function is the observation and analysis of the arterial line waveform. There are expected "abnormalities" of the arterial line waveform when using the IABP. Figure 11-8 displays the proper arterial line waveform when using the IABP. Diastolic augmentation is apparent and afterload reduction is demonstrated with the reduction of end-diastolic pressure. The critical care nurse needs to be familiar with the IABP and appropriate monitoring techniques. However, an in-depth discussion of IABP is beyond the scope of this chapter.

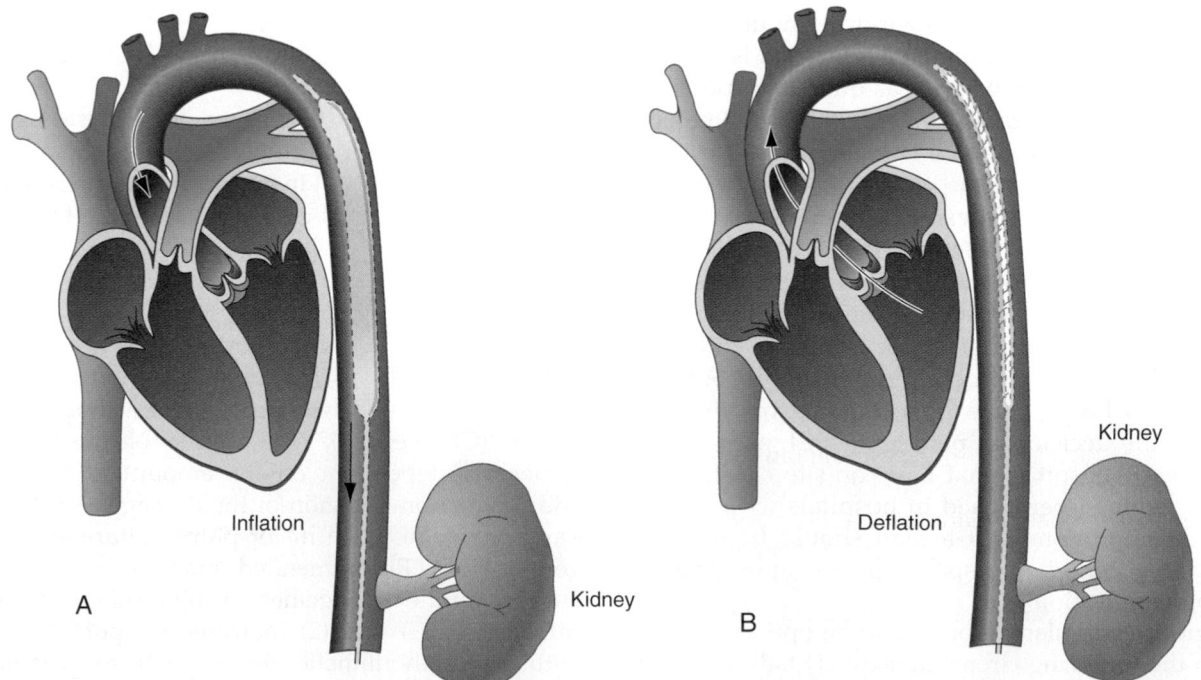

◆**FIGURE 11-7** Intra-aortic balloon pump movement. **A,** Inflation during diastole moves blood toward the heart. **B,** Deflation during systole moves blood away from the heart.

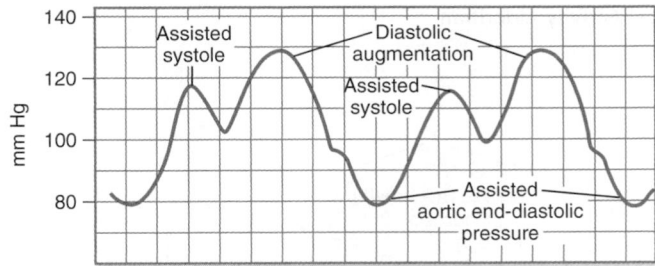

◆FIGURE 11-8 Intra-aortic balloon pump arterial waveform.

Dysrhythmias are another complication of the STEMI patient. Serious ventricular dysrhythmias, such as ventricular tachycardia and fibrillation, can be treated using various methods. Emergent deterioration resulting in ventricular fibrillation or pulseless ventricular tachycardia requires immediate, unsynchronized electric shock following advanced cardiac life support (ACLS) algorithms.[2] Amiodarone (Cordarone) (used after epinephrine in arrest situations) is a drug recommended to control these life-threatening rhythms. If the patient continues to experience ventricular fibrillation or sustained pulseless ventricular tachycardia for more than 2 days after the STEMI or has an ejection fraction of 30% or less, the placement of an implantable cardioverter-defibrillator (ICD) is recommended.[4]

Atrial fibrillation is another rhythm that can complicate the post-STEMI course. Treatment priorities are to control the heart rate and convert to sinus rhythm. Lifelong anticoagulation to decrease the risk of stroke may be indicated if the patient remains in atrial fibrillation. Bradycardia and conduction defects are complications of inferior and anterior MIs. Depending on the severity of the disorder, a permanent pacemaker can be inserted to maintain adequate atrial-ventricular synchrony. A complete discussion of dysrhythmias and associated interventions can be found in Chapter 10.

Other complications of a STEMI include the following:

1. Pericarditis (inflammation of the pericardium), which can be treated with antiinflammatory medications (aspirin or nonsteroidal antiinflammatory drugs [NSAIDs]). If a pericardial effusion develops, anticoagulation should be discontinued immediately to avoid cardiac tamponade.[4]
2. Ischemic stroke, in which treatment focuses on finding the source of the embolism (i.e., mural thrombus, akinetic segment, or atrial fibrillation)[4] and immediately consulting the stroke team.

The critical care nurse should always be alert for signs of these complications and initiate institutional protocols early.

Emergency Interventions

If the myocardium sustains significant damage, function is severely compromised and the patient may become hemodynamically unstable or experience cardiac arrest. In 2005 the AHA published updated guidelines for cardiopulmonary resuscitation (CPR) and emergency cardiovascular care (ECC).[2] The guidelines have been updated in an attempt to reflect the most recent scientific evidence and expert consensus opinion when evidence is limited. A new algorithm for cardiac arrest, *pulseless arrest*, has combined content from the ventricular fibrillation/pulseless ventricular tachycardia (VF/VT) algorithm with content from the asystole and pulseless electrical activity (PEA) algorithms (Figure 11-9). A major theme in the update emphasizes minimal interruption of CPR especially after defibrillation, in order to enhance coronary perfusion pressure.[70] The most critical intervention when a pulseless arrest is recognized is to initiate CPR and prepare for defibrillation. The three successive ("stacked") shocks have been replaced with one shock because first-shock success rate has improved, especially with biphasic defibrillators.[42] When stacked shocks were used, researchers found that seconds were lost (up to 37 seconds) in charging the defibrillator, releasing the shock, and checking a pulse.[70] Evidence suggests that one shock immediately followed by effective CPR may improve patient outcomes.[2]

Energy levels for shocks were also addressed in the 2005 revision. The amount of energy used depends on the type of defibrillator. Biphasic devices have individual effective joule levels ranging from 120 to 200 joules, but if the provider is unsure of the appropriate machine level, 200 joules is an acceptable dose.[2] If a monophasic machine is used, 360 joules is the appropriate dose. If VF reoccurs, the previously successful energy level is delivered. Automated electrical defibrillators (AEDs) are now being used more frequently and are preset to deliver a set electrical dose. Once the shock is delivered, CPR is resumed for 5 cycles, although that time period may be altered in a hospital-monitored situation at the discretion of a physician.[2]

If VF/VT persists after 2 shock and CPR cycles, administration of a vasopressor is suggested. Epinephrine is the drug of choice at the dose of 1 mg IV/IO (intraosseous) every 3 to 5 minutes. Vasopressin 40 units IV/IO can be given once to replace the first or second dose of epinephrine.[2] It is important not to interrupt CPR when administering any drug. Antidysrhythmics may be needed if electrical therapy is not successful in converting VF. Amiodarone should be administered as a bolus (first dose of 300 mg IV/IO and 150 mg IV/IO if an additional dose is required).[2] Lidocaine can be considered if amiodarone is not available. The dose of lidocaine is 1 to 1.5 mg/kg IV/IO initially and then 0.5 to

Asystole/Pulseless Electrical Activity Algorithm

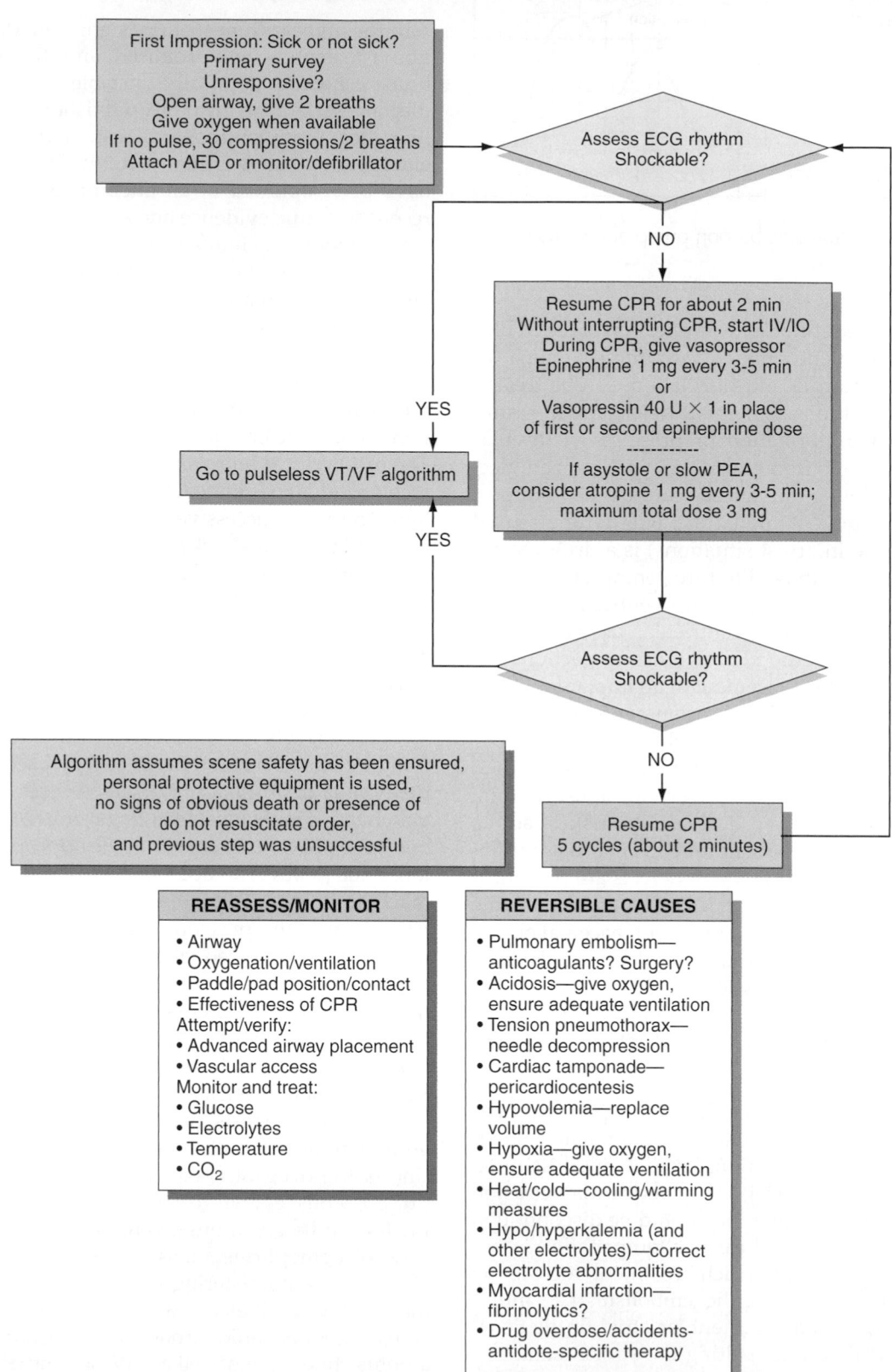

First Impression: Sick or not sick?
Primary survey
Unresponsive?
Open airway, give 2 breaths
Give oxygen when available
If no pulse, 30 compressions/2 breaths
Attach AED or monitor/defibrillator

Assess ECG rhythm
Shockable?

NO

Resume CPR for about 2 min
Without interrupting CPR, start IV/IO
During CPR, give vasopressor
Epinephrine 1 mg every 3-5 min
or
Vasopressin 40 U × 1 in place
of first or second epinephrine dose

If asystole or slow PEA,
consider atropine 1 mg every 3-5 min;
maximum total dose 3 mg

YES

Go to pulseless VT/VF algorithm

YES

Assess ECG rhythm
Shockable?

Algorithm assumes scene safety has been ensured,
personal protective equipment is used,
no signs of obvious death or presence of
do not resuscitate order,
and previous step was unsuccessful

NO

Resume CPR
5 cycles (about 2 minutes)

REASSESS/MONITOR

- Airway
- Oxygenation/ventilation
- Paddle/pad position/contact
- Effectiveness of CPR
Attempt/verify:
- Advanced airway placement
- Vascular access
Monitor and treat:
- Glucose
- Electrolytes
- Temperature
- CO_2

REVERSIBLE CAUSES

- Pulmonary embolism—
anticoagulants? Surgery?
- Acidosis—give oxygen,
ensure adequate ventilation
- Tension pneumothorax—
needle decompression
- Cardiac tamponade—
pericardiocentesis
- Hypovolemia—replace
volume
- Hypoxia—give oxygen,
ensure adequate ventilation
- Heat/cold—cooling/warming
measures
- Hypo/hyperkalemia (and
other electrolytes)—correct
electrolyte abnormalities
- Myocardial infarction—
fibrinolytics?
- Drug overdose/accidents-
antidote-specific therapy

✦**FIGURE 11-9** Pulseless arrest algorithm.

TABLE 11-6 Causes of Asystole and Pulseless Electrical Activity

H'S	T'S
Hypovolemia	Toxins
Hypoxia	Tamponade (cardiac)
Hydrogen ion (acidosis)	Tension pneumothorax
Hypo/hyperkalemia	Thrombosis (coronary or
Hypoglycemia	pulmonary)
Hypothermia	Trauma

Modified from reference 2.

♦ NUTRITION

Recommended Dietary Intake to Prevent and Treat High Blood Cholesterol

Nutrient	Recommended Intake
Calories	Balance energy intake and expenditure to maintain desirable body weight and prevent weight gain
Physical activity	Include enough moderate exercise to expend at least 200 kcal per day
Total fat	25%-35% of total calories
Saturated	Less than 7% of total calories
Polyunsaturated	Up to 10% of total calories
Monounsaturated	Up to 20% of total calories
Cholesterol	Less than 200 mg/day
Protein	Approximately 15% of total calories
Carbohydrate	50%-60% of total calories
Soluble fiber	10–25 g per day
Plant stanols/ sterols	2 g per day

Data from reference 37a.

0.75 mg/kg IV/IO for a total of 3 mg/kg maximum dose.[2] If torsades de pointes is observed, magnesium sulfate 1 to 2 grams IV/IO over 5 to 20 minutes is recommended.[2]

Asystole and PEA are rhythms that display electrical activity, but the mechanical activity associated with these rhythms is too weak to detect a palpable pulse.[2] The sequence of interventions is as described previously except without electrical therapy, which is not effective with these rhythms. The focus in reversing these rhythms is to determine the underlying cause of the rhythm (Table 11-6).

PREVENTION OF CORONARY ARTERY DISEASE

Lipid Management

Because excess LDLs contribute to the formation of plaque, more stringent goals for controlling cholesterol have been set. An LDL level less than 100 mg/dl is now the general goal.[47] The first-line intervention to control hypercholesterolemia is to maintain a diet that is low in saturated fat and cholesterol (less than 7% of total calories as saturated fat and less than 200 mg/dl cholesterol). Foods high in omega-3 fatty acids and high in fiber, fruits, vegetables, and whole grains should be part of the daily intake.[47] A balanced diet combined with an exercise regimen can also help control cholesterol levels. An example of a recommended diet is shown in the Nutrition box above, right.[59] If the patient has multiple risk factors and has an LDL level of 130 mg/dl or greater, drug intervention should be considered.[47] The STEMI patient should have a lipid assessment profile performed within 24 hours of the acute event.[4] If drug intervention is indicated, a statin is the preferred medication.[39] There is evidence that statin medications will not only lower cholesterol but also may assist in

decreasing the inflammatory response.[55] The medication should be initiated immediately, and liver function tests should be followed at 3- and 6-month intervals.

Smoking Cessation

It is postulated that cigarette smoking accelerates atherosclerosis by several mechanisms: (1) adverse effects on lipid profiles; (2) endothelial damage or dysfunction; (3) hemodynamic stress; (4) oxidant injury; (5) neutrophil activation; (6) enhanced thrombosis; and (7) increased blood viscosity.[7] Smoking cessation education is an integral part of the ACS patient education. In 2000 the Department of Health and Human Services published an evidence-based guideline to treat tobacco use.[65] This guideline promotes a systematic approach to assess for tobacco use. The first step is to ask every patient if they use tobacco products. If tobacco use is present, the second step should be to strongly urge the patient to quit. The third step recommended is to assess the willingness of the smoker to attempt to quit. If the patient indicates a resolve to quit, the healthcare provider should aid the patient in quitting smoking. Nicotine replacement therapy using gum or a patch can be used to aid this process. The final step should be to schedule a follow-up appointment to monitor progress. There are multiple sources of educational literature available that can supplement patient counseling.[58]

Blood Pressure Control

The most recent recommendations for BP control were published in 2003 by the Joint National Committee of the National High Blood Pressure Education Program and the Guidelines Subcommittee of the World Health Organization and the International Society of Hypertension.[16] The general preemptive goal is an SBP less than 120 mm Hg and a diastolic BP less than 80 mm Hg for the average patient. For the STEMI patient, the recommended target BP is less than 140/90 mm Hg, or less than 130/80 mm Hg for those with chronic kidney disease or diabetes.[4,16] BP should be controlled with beta blockers, ACE inhibitors, and, if needed, aldosterone antagonists. Angiotensin II, a potent vasoconstrictor of the renin-aldosterone-angiotensin axis, plays a major role in hypertension. It is also thought to have inflammatory effects that contribute to the long-term process.[36] In general, hypertension may contribute to the atherosclerotic process of vessels, especially at bifurcations, because of damage to the endothelial cells.[36] Two or three types of drugs may be needed to attain BP goals, with the emphasis placed on optimizing the dosing of beta blockers and ACE inhibitors.[16] Short-term calcium channel blocking agents (e.g., verapamil) should not be used to control hypertension.[4] Weight management, if appropriate, should automatically be included in an antihypertensive regimen.

General Preventive Interventions

Obesity has been recognized as a major contributor to cardiovascular disease in the United States.[10] The recommended body mass index (BMI) is 18.5 to 24.9 kg/m^2.[4] Waist circumference is another parameter that may be easier to use when counseling patients. Women should have a waist circumference less than 35 inches, and men's waist circumference should be less than 40 inches.[4] A combination of diet control and an increase of physical activity is the first level of intervention. Physical activity goals should be 30 minutes at least 5 times per week. Another parameter is optimal glucose control. Diabetic management is guided by measuring the HbA$_{1c}$ level. The recommended goal for HbA$_{1c}$ is less than 7%.[4] There is a detailed discussion of glycemic control in Chapter 34.

◆ Case Study 11-1, Part C

Acute Coronary Syndrome

After several days of hospitalization for continual monitoring, Mr. C. was ready to be discharged home. His medications include aspirin, clopidogrel (Plavix), metoprolol (Toprol), and atorvastatin (Lipitor). Mr. C.'s heart rate is now 65 beats/min and his BP is 110/60 mm Hg, thereby allowing a beta blocker to be added.

Additional counseling has been provided about exercise, weight reduction, cholesterol monitoring, and diabetes prevention. His HbA$_{1c}$ level was 4%; therefore medication was not indicated at present. The focus of therapy for now was to lose 10 pounds in the next 2 months and to start exercising two or three times per week.

Decision point: How soon after initiation of atorvastatin therapy should Mr. C. have liver function tests performed?

CONCLUSIONS

The concepts of the pathophysiology and treatment of CAD are rapidly evolving. Discovery of new cellular processes of atherosclerosis continues to affect the treatment and prevention of the disease. Atherosclerosis is no longer considered a disease of lipid accumulation, but instead a disorder characterized by low-grade vascular inflammation.[36] The focus of treatment is centered on disabling the coagulation system at all levels, reestablishing blood flow, and maintaining adequate blood flow long term. PCIs are coupled with anticoagulation and implemented as early as possible. With earlier interventions, less myocardial muscle damage is incurred and better outcomes are achieved. These efforts, along with preventive interventions and aggressive patient education, will hopefully contribute to the eventual demise of CAD.

REFERENCES

1. American Heart Association. (2005). *Heart disease and stroke statistics—2005 update.* Dallas, Tex: AHA.
2. American Heart Association Guidelines for Cardiopulmonary Resuscitation and Emergency Cardiovascular Care. (2005). *Circulation, 112*(suppl IV), IV-58–IV-66.
2a. Anderson, J. L., et al. (2007). ACC/AHA 2007 guideline update for the management of patients with unstable angina and non-ST-segment elevation myocardial infarction. *Circulation, 116,* e148–e304.
3. Angelini, P., Leachman, R., & Heibig, J. (1986). Flow characteristics of coronary balloon catheters. *Tex Heart Inst J, 13,* 213–215.
4. Antman, E. M., et al. (2004). ACC/AHA guidelines for the management of patients with ST-elevation myocardial infarction: executive summary. *J Am College Cardiol, 44,* 671–719.

5. Antman, E. M., et al. (2004). Cardiac specific troponin I levels to predict the risk of mortality in patients with acute coronary syndrome. *N Engl J Med, 355,* 1342–1349.

6. Benhorin, J., et al. (1990). The prognostic significance of first myocardial infarction type (Q wave versus non-Q wave) and Q wave location. The Multicenter Diltiazem Post-Infarction Research Group. *J Am College Cardiol, 15,* 1201–1207.

7. Benowitz, N., & Gourlay, S. (1997). Cardiovascular toxicity of nicotine: implications for nicotine replacement therapy. *J Am College Cardiol, 29,* 1422–1431.

8. Bertrand, M. E., et al. (1999). Double-blind study of the safety of clopidogrel with and without a loading dose in combination with aspirin compared with ticlopidine in combination with aspirin after coronary stenting. *Circulation, 103,* 624–629.

9. Boersma, E., et al. (1996). Early thrombolytic treatment in acute myocardial infarction: reappraisal of the golden hour. *Lancet, 348,* 771–775.

10. Bonow, R. O., & Eckel, R. H. (2003). Diet, obesity and cardiovascular risk. *N Engl J Med, 348,* 2057–2058.

11. Deleted in proofs.

11a. Braunwald, E., Jones, R. H., et al. (1994). *Unstable angina: diagnosis and management.* AHCPR Publication No. 94–060, Rockville, Md: Agency for Health Care Policy and Research and the National Heart, Lung and Blood Institute, U.S. Public Health and Human Services.

12. Camejo, G., et al. (1998). Association of apo B lipoproteins with arterial proteoglycans: pathological significance and molecular basis. *Atherosclerosis, 139,* 205–222.

13. Campeau, L. (1976). Grading of angina pectoris (letter). *Circulation, 54,* 522–523.

14. Casey, P. (2004). Markers of myocardial injury and dysfunction. *AACN Clin Issues, 15,* 547–557.

15. Channer, K., & Morris, F. (2002). ABC of clinical electrocardiography: myocardial ischemia. *BMJ, 324,* 1023–1026.

16. Chobanian, A. V., et al. (2003). The seventh report of the Joint National Committee of Prevention, Detection, Evaluation and Treatment of High Blood Pressure: the JNC-7 report. *JAMA, 290,* 2560–2572.

16a. Christie, L. G., & Conti, C. R. (1981). Systematic approach to the evaluation of angina-like chest pain. *Am Heart J, 102,* 899.

17. Coller, B. S. (1999). Potential non-glycoprotein IIb/IIIa effects of abciximab. *Am Heart J, 138,* 1085–1091.

18. Committee for the Redefinition of Myocardial Infarction. (2000). Myocardial infarction redefined—a consensus document of the Joint European Society of Cardiology/American College of Cardiology. *J Am College Cardiol, 36,* 959–969.

19. Consensus Panel Statements for Outcomes—Effective and Evidence-Based Patient Management. (2001). *Acute myocardial infarction and ischemic coronary syndromes: optimizing selection of reperfusion and revascularization therapies in the coronary care unit and emergency department.* Atlanta, Ga: American Health Consultants.

20. Deelstra, M. H. (2005). Interventional cardiology techniques. In *Cardiac nursing* (5th ed.). Philadelphia: Lippincott, Williams & Wilkins.

21. Del Bene, S., & Vaughan, A. (2005). Acute coronary syndromes. In *Cardiac nursing* (5th ed.). Philadelphia: Lippincott, Williams & Wilkins.

22. Drew, B. J., et al. (2004). Practice standards for electrocardiographic monitoring in hospital settings. *Circulation, 110,* 2721–2746.

22a. Dubin, D. (2000). *Rapid interpretation of EKGs: An interactive course* (6th ed.). Tampa: Cover Publishing.

23. Eslick, G. D. (2005). Usefulness of chest pain character and location as diagnosis indicators of an acute coronary syndrome. *Am J Cardiol, 95,* 1228–1231.

24. Furberg, C. D., Psaty, B. M., & Meyer, J. V. (1995). Nifedipine dose-related increase in mortality in patients with coronary heart disease. *Circulation, 92,* 1326–1331.

25. Gerschutz, G. P., & Bhatt, D. L. (2002). The CURE trial: using clopidogrel in acute coronary syndromes without ST-segment elevation. *Cleveland Clinic J Med, 69,* 377–385.

26. Griendling, K. K., & Harrison, D. G. (2001). Out, damned dot: studies of the NADPH oxidase in atherosclerosis. *J Clin Invest, 108,* 1423–1424.

27. Ham, C. W., et al. (2004). Emergency room triage of patients with acute chest pain by means of rapid testing for cardiac troponin T or troponin I. *N Engl J Med, 337,* 1648–1653.

28. Hamner, J. B., Dubois, E. J., & Rice, T. P. (2005). Predictors of complications associated with closure devices after transfemoral percutaneous coronary procedures. *Crit Care Nurse, 25,* 30–37.

29. Hardman, J., & Limbird, L. (2000). *Goodman and Gillman's the pharmacological basis of therapeutics* (10th ed.). New York: McGraw-Hill Medical Publishing Division.

30. Heupler, F. A. (1998). Guidelines for performing angiography in patients taking metformin. Members of the Laboratory Performance Standards Committee of the Society for Cardiac Angiography and Interventions. *Cathet Cardiovasc Diagn, 43,* 121–123.

31. Hochman, J. S., et al. (1999). Should we emergently revascularize occluded coronaries for cardiogenic shock (SHOCK) investigators. Early revascularization in acute myocardial infarction complicated by cardiogenic shock. *N Engl J Med, 341,* 625–634.

32. Dubin, D. (2000). *Rapid interpretation of EKGs: An interactive course* (6th ed.). Tampa, Fla: Cover Publishing Company.

33. Juran, N. B., et al. (1999). Nursing interventions to decrease bleeding at the femoral access site after percutaneous coronary intervention. *Am J Crit Care, 8,* 303–313.

34. Libby, P. (1995). Molecular basis of the acute coronary syndromes. *Circulation, 91,* 2844–2850.

35. Libby, P. (2002). Atherosclerosis: the new view. *Scientific Am, 286,* 48–55.

36. Libby, P., Ridker, P., & Maseri, A. (2002). Inflammation and atherosclerosis. *Circulation, 105,* 1135–1143.

37. Libby, P. (2005). The vascular biology of atherosclerosis. In *Braunwald's heart disease: a textbook of cardiovascular medicine* (7th ed.). Philadelphia: Elsevier.

38. Lincoff, A. M., et al. (2005). Long-term efficacy of bivalirudin and provisional glycoprotein IIb/IIIa blockade vs heparin and planned glycoprotein IIb/IIIa blockade during percutaneous coronary revascularization (REPLACE-2 randomized trial). *JAMA, 292,* 696–703.

39. Long-Term Intervention with Pravastatin in Ischaemic Disease (LIPID) study group. (1998). Prevention of cardiovascular events and death with pravastatin in patients with coronary heart disease and a broad range of initial cholesterol levels. *N Engl J Med, 339(19),* 1349–1357.

40. Luster, A. D. (1998). Chemokines: chemotactic cytokines that mediate inflammation. *N Engl J Med, 338,* 436–445.

41. Mangoni, A. A., & Jackson, S. H. (2002). Homocysteine and cardiovascular disease: current evidence and future prospects. *Am J Med, 112,* 556–565.

42. Martens, P. R., Russell, J. K., Wolcke, B., et al. (2001). Optimal response to cardiac arrest study: defibrillation waveform effects. *Resuscitation, 49,* 233–243.

43. Melfarejo, A. M., et al. (1997). Incidence, clinical characteristics and prognostic significance of right bundle-branch block in acute myocardial infarction: a study in the thrombolytic era. *Circulation, 96,* 1139–1144.

44. Morris, F., & Brady, W. J. (2002). ABC of clinical electrocardiography: acute myocardial infarction—part I. *BMJ, 324,* 831–834.

44a. Morton, P. G. (1996). Using the 12-lead ECG to detect ischemia, injury and infarction. *Crit Care Nurse, 16,* 85–95.

45. Mosca, L., et al. (1997). Cardiovascular disease in women: a statement for healthcare professionals from the American Heart Association Writing Group. *Circulation, 96*, 2468–2482.

46. Nakashima, Y., et al. (1998). Upregulation of VACM-1 and ICAM-1 at atherosclerosis-prone sites on the endothelium in the apoE-deficient mouse. *Arterioscler Thromb Vasc Biol, 18,* 842–851.

47. National Cholesterol Education Program. (2001). *Expert Panel on Detection, Evaluation and Treatment of High Blood Cholesterol in Adults (Adult treatment panel III).* National Institutes of Health, Publication No. 01–3670, Bethesda, Md: U.S. Department of Health and Human Services.

47a. National Cholesterol Education Program. (2002). Third Report of the NCEP Expert Panel on Detection, Evaluation, and Treatment of High Blood Cholesterol in Adults (Adult Treatment Panel III). *Circulation, 106*, 3143–3421.

48. Payne, C. (2004). Classification of acute coronary syndromes using 12-lead electrocardiogram as a guide. *AACN Clin Issues, 15*, 558–567.

49. Phibbs, R., et al. (1999). Q-wave versus non-Q wave myocardial infarction: a meaningless distinction. *J Am College Cardiol, 33*, 576–582.

50. Quaal, S. (1993). *Comprehensive intraaortic balloon counterpulsation.* (2nd ed.). St. Louis: Mosby.

51. Regar, E., et al. (2002). Angiographic findings of the multicenter Randomized Study With the Sirolimus-Eluting Bx Velocity Balloon-Expandable Stent (RAVEL): sirolimus-eluting stents inhibit restenosis irrespective of the vessel size. *Circulation, 106*, 1949–1956.

52. Rogers, W. R. (1972). Maximal QS 2-interval shortening in acute coronary syndromes: experience with a simple method in fifty patients. *Northwest Med, 71*, 605–608.

53. Rong, J. X., et al. (1998). Arterial injury by cholesterol oxidation products causes endothelial dysfunction and arterial wall cholesterol accumulation. *Arterioscler Thromb Vasc Biol, 18*, 1885–1894.

54. Rosenberg, L., Palmer, J. R., & Shapiro, S. (1990). Oral contraceptive use and the risk of myocardial infarction. *Am J Epidemiol, 131*, 1009–1016.

55. Schwartz, G. G., & Olsson, A. G. (2005). The case for intensive statin therapy after acute coronary syndrome. *Am J Cardiol, 96*, 45–53.

56. Smith, S. C., et al. (2006). ACC/AHA/SCAI 2005 guideline update for percutaneous coronary intervention. *Circulation, 113*, 156–175.

57. Sukhova, G. K., et al. (1999). Evidence for increased collagenolysis by interstitial collagenases-1 and -3 in vulnerable human atheromatous plaques. *Circulation, 99*, 2503–2509.

58. Surgeon General Report. U.S. Department of Health and Human Services. (2004). *The health consequences of smoking: a report of the surgeon general.* U.S. Department of Health and Human Services, Centers for Disease Control and Prevention, National Center for Chronic Disease Prevention and Health Promotion, Office on Smoking and Health.

59. Third Report of the NCEP Expert Panel on Detection, Evaluation, and Treatment of High Blood Cholesterol in Adults (Adult Treatment Panel III). (2002). *Circulation, 106*, 3143–3421.

60. Topol, E. J. (1990). Thrombolytic intervention. In *Textbook of interventional cardiology.* Philadelphia: Saunders.

61. Tortora, G., & Grabowski, S. (2003). *Principles of anatomy and physiology* (10th ed.). New York: John Wiley & Sons.

62. Turgeon, M. (1999). *Clinical hematology: theory and procedures.* Philadelphia: Lippincott, Williams & Wilkins.

63. Tuzcu, E. M., et al. (2001). High prevalence of coronary atherosclerosis in asymptomatic teenagers and young adults: evidence from intravascular ultrasound. *Circulation, 103*, 2705–2710.

64. Urban, P., et al. (1999). *The clopidogrel aspirin stent international cooperative study,* oral presentation, Atlanta, Ga: AHA Scientific Sessions.

65. U.S. Department of Health and Human Services. (2000b). *Treating tobacco use and dependence: clinical practice guideline.* Washington, DC: Government Printing Office.

66. Van den Berk, G., et al. (2005). Bench-to-bedside review: preventive measures for contrast-induced nephropathy in critically ill patients. *Crit Care, 9*, 361–370.

67. Warkentin, T., Chong, B., & Grienacher, A. (1998). Heparin-induced thrombocytopenia: towards consensus. *Thrombosis Haemostasis, 79*, 1–7.

68. Woods, S. L., Froelicher, E. S., Motzer, S, & Bridges, E. J. (2005). *Cardiac Nursing* (5th ed.). Philadelphia: Lippincott Williams & Wilkins.

69. Yusuf, S., Wittes, J., & Friedman, L. (1988). Overview of results of randomized clinical trials in heart disease, II: unstable angina, heart failure, primary prevention with aspirin and risk factor modification. *JAMA, 260*, 2259–2263.

70. Yu, T., et al. (2002). Adverse outcomes of interrupted precordial compression during automated defibrillation. *Circulation, 106*, 368–372.

CHAPTER 12

Heart Failure

Debra K. Moser, Barbara Riegel, Sara Paul, Terry A. Lennie, and Peggy L. Kirkwood

Heart failure is a clinical syndrome that commonly is the final manifestation of cardiac risk factors (e.g., untreated hypertension) and cardiac diseases or events (e.g., acute myocardial infarction [MI]). The prevalence of heart failure is high in the United States and worldwide; at least 5 million people in the United States suffer from heart failure,[150] while more than 15 million individuals worldwide have heart failure.[188] In the United States alone, approximately 500,000 new cases are diagnosed each year, and the incidence is not declining[148,150] despite apparent improvements in survival.[93,148,172] Survival rates have not improved as much among women as they have among men, nor among elderly individuals.[148] The aging of the population will only increase the incidence and prevalence of heart failure, and the survival disparity.

The steep price of caring for patients with heart failure is largely attributable to hospitalizations for exacerbations of chronic heart failure. The number of hospital discharges for heart failure rose 157% from 1979 to 2002.[150] Three-month readmission rates are as high as 20% to 30%, while 6-month readmission rates among symptomatic patients are about 50%.[188] Hospitalization for heart failure is thought to be the largest and most expensive Medicare diagnosis-related group.

Concentration on statistics can obscure the immense personal burden of heart failure. Patients with heart failure commonly report very poor quality of life because heart failure has a negative impact on all aspects of life, particularly symptom burden and ability to perform usual activities.[7,190] Heart failure has an impact on quality of life comparable to, or worse than, that seen in other serious chronic conditions.[29]

Given the enormous personal, social, and economic burdens of heart failure, preventing it from occurring in the first place is a major priority that all healthcare providers must embrace. Once heart failure develops, prevention of both rehospitalization and progression of heart failure becomes a major priority. The emphasis of this chapter is to provide nurses with the knowledge and skills to manage patients with acute decompensated heart failure (ADHF) so that rehospitalizations are prevented, quality of life is improved, and further progression of heart failure is halted. Achieving these outcomes requires delivery of care emphasizing resolution of the acute problem, ensuring patients have optimal chronic care delivery once discharged, and preparing the patient and family to assume self-care responsibilities.

PREVENTION OF ACUTE DECOMPENSATED HEART FAILURE

Heart failure is an obviously chronic condition. Yet the acute care focus taken by the vast majority of healthcare providers in the management of heart failure belies this fact and contributes to the high rate of rehospitalizations seen in this condition.[111] It is imperative that critical care nurses extend their viewpoint beyond the acute, critical care environment and embrace the totality of chronic care strategies necessary for optimizing heart failure patient outcomes. Attention to only the acute problems without attending to patient needs engendered by the chronicity of heart failure leaves patients without the solutions they need to manage their condition on a daily basis. Critical care nurses must understand both acute and chronic care. They must know how to promote patient self-care, and they need to advocate for appropriate pharmacologic and nonpharmacologic chronic care.

Definition

Heart failure is not a specific disease, but a clinical syndrome characterized by dyspnea, activity intolerance, and fluid overload adversely affecting patients' functional status and quality of life.[76] Dyspnea and activity intolerance are the two most common symptoms of heart failure, while manifestations of fluid overload, such as edema and jugular venous distention, are the most common signs. This clinical syndrome occurs as a consequence of structural or functional (or both) cardiac abnormalities that impair cardiac pumping or filling.[76]

ADHF is the appearance of signs and symptoms of heart failure that are not self-limiting, that escalate, and that need intervention.[119] ADHF most commonly occurs in the setting of existing chronic heart failure, but can be the first manifestation of emergent heart failure. Acute decompensated heart failure can occur in patients with systolic or diastolic dysfunction and requires urgent treatment. Although usually (about 75% of the time[5]) a consequence of chronic heart failure, patients with ADHF can present with one of the six clinical manifestations outlined in Box 12-1.[119]

Pathophysiology of Heart Failure

ADHF most often occurs in the context of chronic heart failure. A full understanding of the pathophysiology of chronic heart failure is necessary to appreciate the rationale for using the various drug classes recommended in the management of heart failure. The pathophysiology of chronic heart failure will be described, followed by the pathophysiologic events that culminate in ADHF.

Clinical heart failure usually develops after sufficient myocardial cell damage has occurred to impair ventricular contractility. In response to impaired contractility, and in order to maintain tissue and organ perfusion, several components of the neurohumoral axis are activated. Neurohumoral activation initially is adaptive and serves to support circulation and blood pressure.[122] However, with time, sustained neurohumoral activation produces symptomatic heart failure, and progression of heart failure. Recent advances in heart failure treatment can be traced to better understanding of the role of neurohumoral activation in the pathophysiology of heart failure.

Initial Adaptation to Depressed Contractility: The Role of Neurohumoral Activation. Two responses, both of which improve contractility, characterize the early phase of adaptation to depressed contractility (Figure 12-1). Both of these responses occur in any condition characterized by reduced cardiac output (CO) and tissue perfusion when relative or absolute fluid volume is decreased. Their purpose is maintenance of ventricular filling pressure, CO, and tissue perfusion. One response is immediate augmentation of cardiac inotropy by the Frank-Starling mechanism. The Frank-Starling mechanism results in enhanced inotropy from fluid retention that increases ventricular filling pressures and end-diastolic volume, both of which stretch cardiomyocytes (a fundamental mechanism for enhancing inotropy). The end result of increased cardiac myocyte stretch is an increase in contractility owing to augmented sarcomere sensitivity to calcium.

The second response is activation of the sympathetic nervous system, which also increases inotropy through a different calcium-dependent mechanism. Sympathetic nervous system activation stimulates contractility and heart rate (HR) to improve CO directly through beta$_1$-receptor activation and indirectly through venous and arteriolar vasoconstriction. By recruiting volume from the capacitance vessels, venoconstriction enhances venous return to the ventricles, thereby increasing preload. These responses initially maintain perfusion by improving CO, but at a cost. Ultimately, prolonged neurohumoral activation produces abnormalities that contribute to ventricular remodeling, alterations in local vascular control that produce vasoconstriction, progression of ventricular dysfunction, and expression of symptomatic heart failure.

Both internal wall tension and external wall tension are increased in heart failure (see Figure 12-1). Internal wall stress increases as a result of increased end-diastolic volume dilating the ventricle. Increased external

---

Box 12-1

Clinical Manifestations of Acute Decompensated Heart Failure

1. Mild acute decompensated heart failure, either new or exacerbation of chronic heart failure, with mild signs and symptoms of acute heart failure.
2. Hypertensive ADHF with signs and symptoms of heart failure along with hypertension, relatively preserved left ventricular function, and pulmonary edema on chest x-ray.
3. Pulmonary edema on chest x-ray with severe dyspnea and orthopnea, rales, and oxygen saturation less than 90%.
4. Cardiogenic shock with tissue hypoperfusion induced by heart failure after correction of preload; systolic BP less than 90 mm Hg, or a drop of mean arterial pressure greater than 30 mm Hg, or low urine output (less than 0.5 ml/kg/hr), with a pulse rate greater than 60 beats/min with or without evidence of organ congestion.
5. High-output heart failure with elevated cardiac output, tachycardia, warm periphery, and pulmonary congestion (e.g., dysrhythmias, thyrotoxicosis, and anemia). Hypotension may be present with septic shock.
6. Right ventricular heart failure, which is manifested by low-output syndrome, increased jugular venous pressure, increased liver size, and hypotension.

ADHF = Acute decompensated heart failure,
BP = blood pressure.

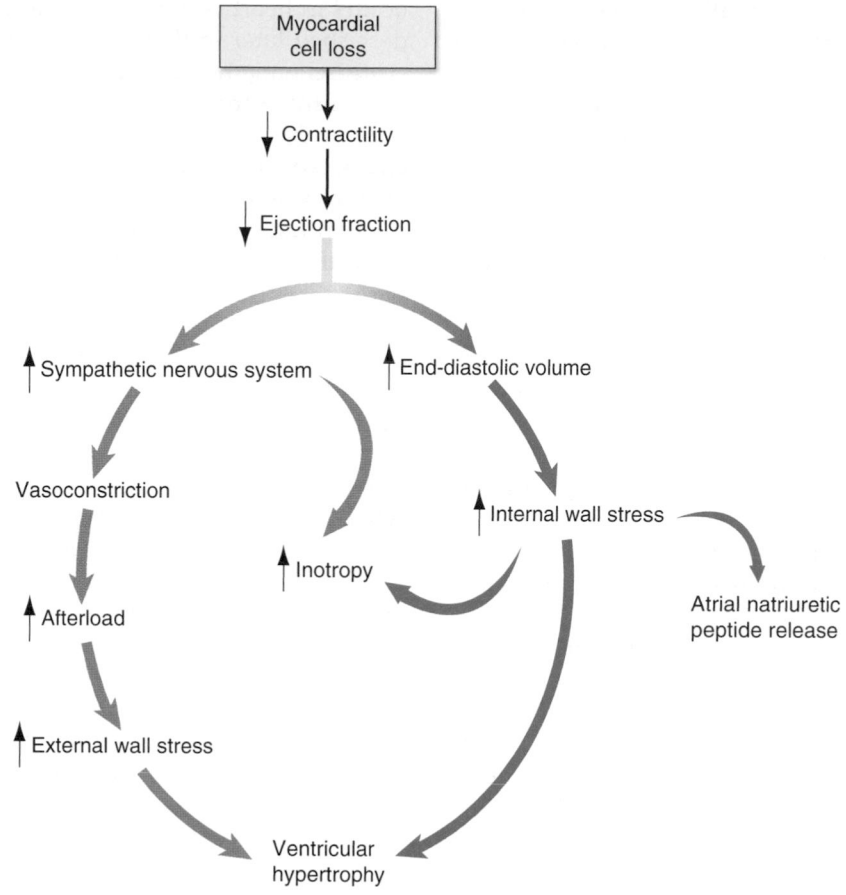

♦FIGURE 12-1 Early compensatory responses to impaired contractility.

wall stress is a result of increased afterload against which the heart must eject blood. Increased afterload is a function of marked vasoconstriction secondary to sympathetic nervous system activation with adrenergic stimulation of alpha receptors in the vasculature.

Early in heart failure, three adaptive forces compensate for increasing wall tension: myocardial hypertrophy, attenuation of sympathetic nervous system activation, and release of atrial natriuretic peptide.[125] Elevated wall tension triggers hypertrophy and subsequently wall tension is reduced. Hypertrophy of healthy myocardium reduces wall tension because the stress induced by ventricular dilation is distributed across a larger mass of myocardium. Sympathetic nervous system activity is attenuated by atrial stretch and stimulation of baroreceptors. Atrial natriuretic peptide is released in response to atrial stretch. Atrial natriuretic peptide has both vasodilator and natriuretic properties that reduce wall stress.

Early in heart failure, the vasoconstrictor and vasodilator systems, and the forces that produce ventricular dilation and hypertrophy, maintain perfusion with no or few symptoms. Protracted activation of these compensatory mechanisms eventually results in progression of ventricular dysfunction and the expression of symptomatic heart failure.

Progression of Ventricular Dysfunction and Expression of Symptomatic Heart Failure.
Ventricular remodeling, neurohumoral activation, inflammation, and alterations in local vascular and hormonal control all contribute to the pathophysiologic changes seen in overt heart failure. None of these systems acts in isolation.

Ventricular Remodeling. Ventricular remodeling occurs in response to injury, for example, infarction or long-standing pressure overload such as occurs in hypertension. Ventricular remodeling refers to changes in size, shape, and structure of the myocardium. Ventricular remodeling is an early adaptive response to loss of healthy contractile units in the myocardium, and is characterized in the early stages by ventricular dilation and wall thinning.[133] Ventricular dilation initially preserves stroke volume through the Frank-Starling mechanism. Dilation increases wall stress because, by Laplace's law, wall stress increases when ventricular pressure or radius increases and wall stress is reduced when wall thickness increases. Thus ventricular hypertrophy is initially compensatory, and hypertrophy compensates for increased ventricular cavity size (increased radius). Ventricular dilation progresses even in this initial compensated state; ultimately hypertrophy is not adequate to reduce wall stress.[133]

The structural changes seen in ventricular remodeling are thought to be produced by several mechanisms.[123] Ventricular remodeling occurs in heart failure from many causes, but is most thoroughly described after MI.[177] After an MI, "infarct expansion"—dilation and thinning of the infarcted area—occurs and appears to be the result of "cell slippage" produced by activation of collagenase. Collagenase disrupts the collagen myocyte support network. Despite the presence of collagenase, new collagen is deposited and existing collagen expands in response to myocardial damage. Collagen deposition and expansion result in hypertrophy. Collagen overgrowth reduces ventricular distensibility and compliance.

The remodeling changes described are initially compensatory, but ultimately they alter myocardial structure such that pumping efficiency is further impaired. Identification of triggers of the onset of ventricular remodeling and of the progression from compensatory hypertrophy to failure could provide important targets for intervention.

Triggers of Ventricular Remodeling. More than one factor triggers the process of hypertrophy; it is likely several triggers interact.[123] Likely triggers of remodeling include mechanical (i.e., cardiac myocyte stretch) and biochemical factors. The biochemical factors include neurohormones acting both as hormones and as paracrine substances, intracellular second messengers, and other trophic (e.g., fibroblast growth) factors.[123] The most likely neurohormones implicated in triggering hypertrophy are norepinephrine, angiotensin II, and arginine vasopressin, all of which stimulate cell proliferation. Norepinephrine also induces hypertrophy and myocardial cell remodeling through the promotion of proto-oncogene expression. Angiotensin II promotes gene expression responsible for protein synthesis leading to hypertrophy. Growth factors normally found in the heart initiate cardiac cell growth and synthesis of fetal cardiac muscle proteins. Various intracellular second messengers, including cyclic AMP and calcium, initiate cardiac cell growth and are potentially important in hypertrophy.

Progression From Hypertrophy to Overt Heart Failure. Compensated hypertrophy frequently progresses to produce deterioration of cardiac function. It has been hypothesized that the failing heart is "energy-starved," contributing to heart failure by allowing progressive myocardial cell death.[84] Myocardial cell loss occurs in heart failure as a result of a variety of causes, described later in this chapter, and not just in patients with ischemic heart failure (Figure 12-2).[106]

The hypertrophied heart has abnormalities of coronary artery flow, capillary morphology, mitochondrial characteristics, and high-energy phosphate delivery that appear to alter the balance between energy production and utilization.[84] Perfusion is impaired in the hypertrophied heart; angina with exertion occurs in patients with hypertrophy, even in the absence of coronary artery disease (CAD). Capillary supply to the hypertrophied myocardium does not increase at the same rate as does growth of muscle tissue. The consequence of inadequate myocardial perfusion is regional necrosis and subsequent fibrosis. Mitochondrial function and oxidative phosphorylation, the process whereby energy is produced, are abnormal in the hypertrophied heart. Together these abnormalities result in loss of functioning myocardial tissue and progression of heart failure.

Other factors that may contribute to the progression of heart failure include processes that promote subendocardial ischemia. Increased end-diastolic volume seen in heart failure produces elevated intraventricular pressures. Elevated pressures promote subendocardial ischemia even in the absence of CAD. The elevated circulating levels of norepinephrine and angiotensin II seen in heart failure can cause subendocardial and coronary artery vasoconstriction that produce subendocardial ischemia. Both of these processes can cause myocardial cell loss that stimulates fibrosis, which further impairs cardiac function. The process of remodeling results in a reduction in myocardial compliance that promotes cell death and fibrosis, because decreased compliance leads to increased wall stress that increases myocardial oxygen demand. Together, these processes lead to heart failure progression by decreasing the number of functional contractile units.

Inflammation (discussed at greater length later in this chapter), wall stress, and reduced coronary blood flow promote apoptosis in heart failure. Apoptosis is programmed cell death or "cellular suicide" and is thought to be important in the development of ventricular hypertrophy. Apoptosis may be modulated by expression of the proto-oncogenes BCL2 and BAX.[121] BCL2 protects cells against apoptosis, while BAX promotes apoptosis by countering BCL2. Cell death in patients with ischemic and idiopathic heart failure is caused by both necrosis and apoptosis.[121] Rates of apoptosis are increased more than 200-fold in heart failure compared to normal hearts.

Neurohumoral Activation. Neurohumoral activation results in vasoconstrictor and vasodilator responses as well as in volume retention and diuretic responses

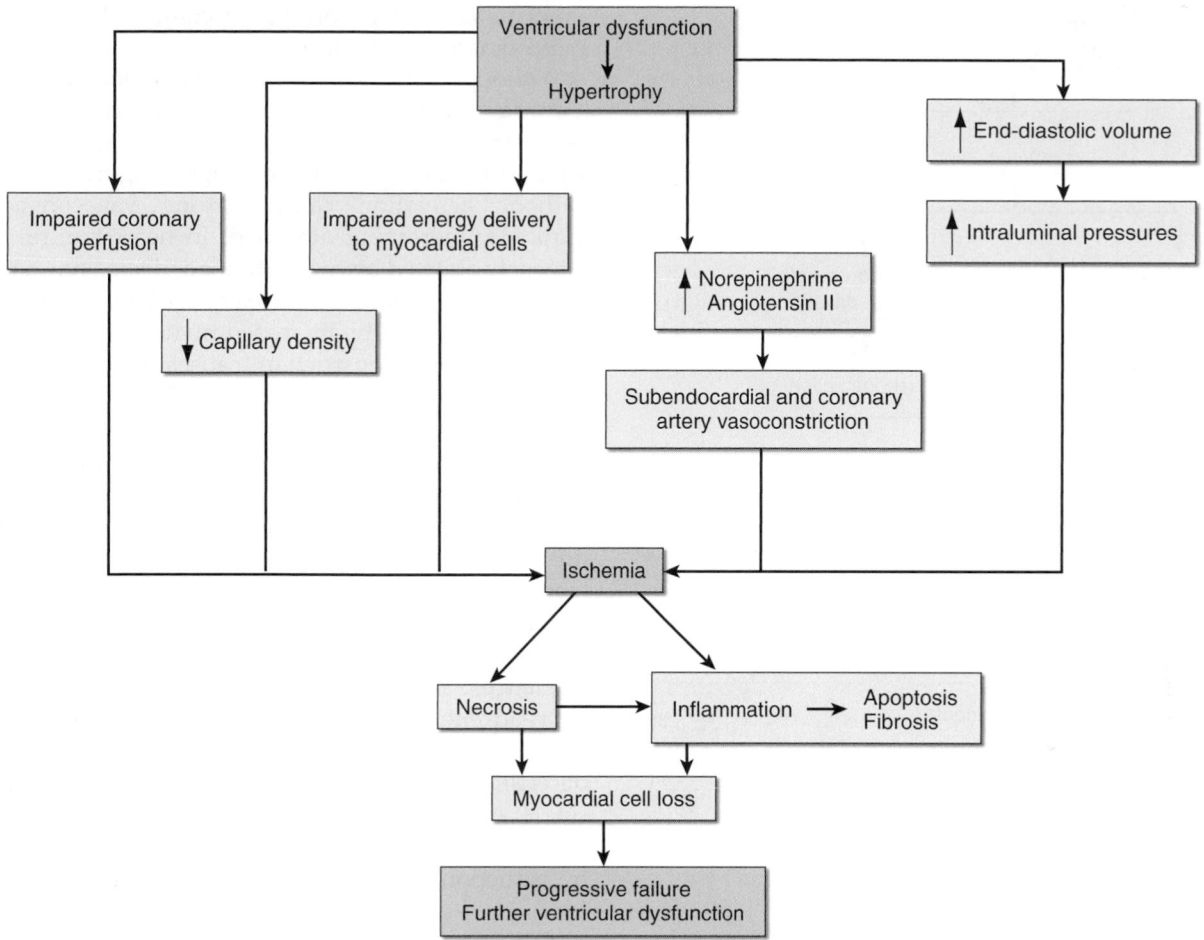

♦FIGURE 12-2 Factors contributing to the progression from hypertrophy to overt heart failure.

(Box 12-2). Early in heart failure these forces balance each other to maintain homeostasis. With time, the vasoconstrictor and volume retention systems overwhelm the vasodilator forces to produce symptomatic heart failure.

Sympathetic Nervous System Activation. Activation of the sympathetic nervous system initially compensates for impairment of stroke volume/CO. Heightened adrenergic activity improves CO directly and indirectly (Figure 12-3). Direct effects include beta$_1$-receptor activation that stimulates contractility and HR. Indirect effects include enhanced CO as a product of norepinephrine interacting with alpha$_1$ receptors in the vasculature to produce arteriolar vasoconstriction and venoconstriction. When volume is recruited from the capacitance vessels during venoconstriction, venous return to the ventricles is increased, increasing preload and CO. Arterial vasoconstriction maintains blood pressure and tissue perfusion. Sympathetic nervous system activation is sustained inappropriately because of

---

Box 12-2

Vasoconstrictor and Vasodilator Neurohormonal Activation Participating in Heart Failure

VASOCONSTRICTION AND VOLUME RETENTION FACTORS

- Sympathetic nervous system
- Renin-angiotensin-aldosterone system (both systemic and local tissue systems)
- Arginine vasopressin
- Neuropeptide Y

VASODILATION AND NATRIURESIS FACTORS

- Atrial natriuretic peptide
- Bradykinin
- Prostaglandins
- Vasoactive intestinal peptide

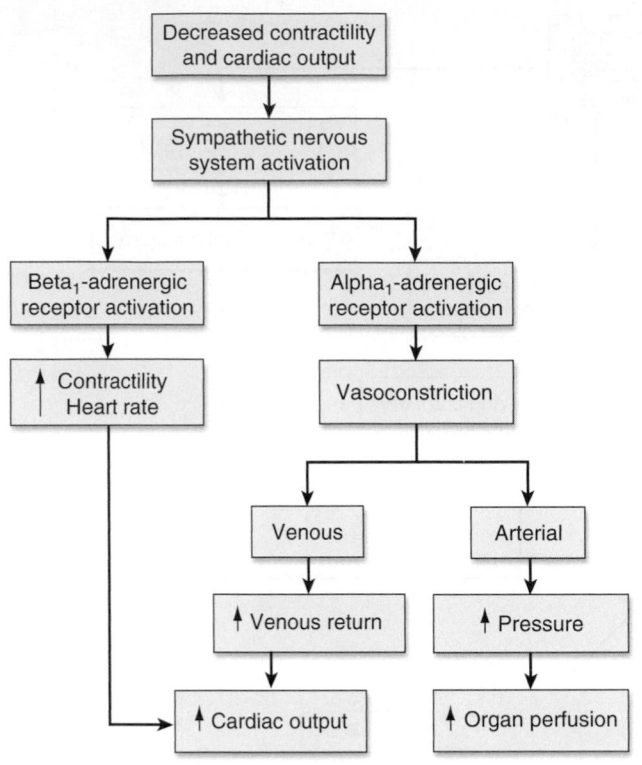

⇕FIGURE 12-3 Initial response of the sympathetic nervous system to decreased cardiac output. Cardiac output improves through beta₁-adrenergic and alpha₁-adrenergic receptor activation.

abnormalities of baroreceptor control;[103] as a result, symptomatic heart failure occurs.

Although activation of the sympathetic nervous system may have beneficial effects early in the course of heart failure, ultimately ventricular performance is affected adversely by this response (Figure 12-4). Sympathetic activation causes strong vasoconstriction, markedly increasing afterload. In heart failure, CO is intensely affected by high afterload, decreasing as a consequence of increasing afterload. Cardiac performance is adversely affected by increased myocardial oxygen consumption. Venoconstriction causes increased venous return, which elevates ventricular filling pressures leading to increased wall stress. Tachycardia from beta-adrenergic stimulation increases myocardial oxygen consumption while decreasing diastolic filling time and coronary artery perfusion, all of which can promote ischemia. Diastolic function is also adversely affected by increased HR because it reduces ventricular filling time.

Excessive adrenergic stimulation affects myocardial beta-adrenergic receptors with clinically important consequences. In heart failure, beta₁-adrenergic, but not beta₂-adrenergic, receptors undergo downregulation in that there is decreased density of beta₁ receptors and desensitization of remaining receptors to norepinephrine.[25] Additionally, in clinical heart failure beta receptors are uncoupled from adenylate cyclase, their signal transduction pathway. The overall effect is a depressed

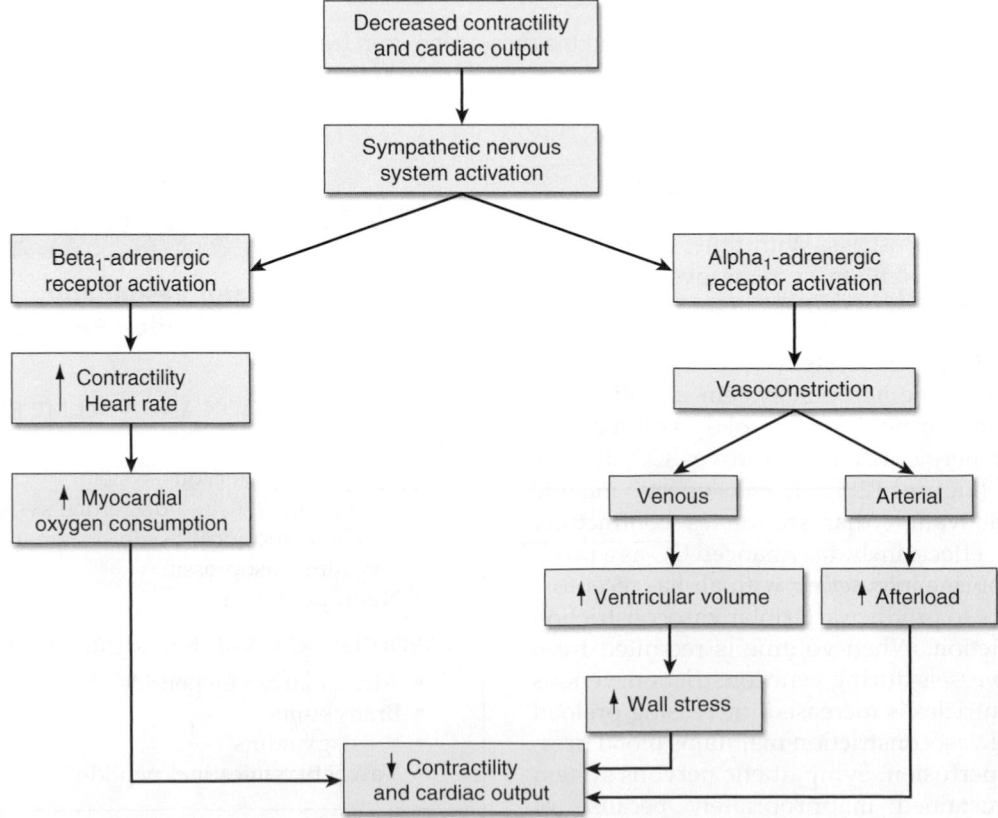

⇕FIGURE 12-4 Continued activation of the sympathetic nervous system leads to progression of ventricular dysfunction through several mechanisms.

response to beta-adrenergic stimulation, an adaptive response to sustained sympathetic stimulation.

Atrial Natriuretic Factor. Atrial natriuretic factor is a peptide released early in the course of heart failure in response to atrial stretch. Atrial natriuretic factor has vasodilator, diuretic, and natriuretic properties that attempt to maintain homeostasis by counteracting vasoconstriction and fluid retention. Atrial natriuretic factor opposes the renin-angiotensin system, suppresses aldosterone and vasopressin arginine release, and prevents norepinephrine release. The beneficial effects of atrial natriuretic factor are attenuated in advanced heart failure and appear to be overwhelmed by the other neurohumoral systems activated.

Renin-Angiotensin-Aldosterone System Activation. The renin-angiotensin-aldosterone (RAA) system is activated early in heart failure. A number of factors can stimulate activation of the renin-angiotensin system (Figure 12-5). In response, renin is released from the juxtaglomerular apparatus. Angiotensinogen (formed in the liver) and renin interact to produce angiotensin I. Angiotensin I is converted to angiotensin II by converting enzyme. Compensatory actions of angiotensin II are arteriolar vasoconstriction, aldosterone release from the adrenal cortex, vasopressin arginine release, stimulation of thirst, and sodium retention. Aldosterone release promotes additional sodium and water

retention. Arginine vasopressin release augments water retention. Angiotensin II also potentiates sympathetic system activity.

Vasoconstriction, sodium and water retention, and added sympathetic activity place the failing myocardium in further jeopardy by further increasing preload and afterload and by promoting ventricular dysrhythmias, subendocardial ischemia, hyponatremia, and hypokalemia. There are circulating and local or tissue renin-angiotensin systems that appear to act independently. Locally produced angiotensin II influences vascular tone, cardiac contractility, myocardial hypertrophy, and sodium level.

Arginine Vasopressin Release. Arginine vasopressin (or antidiuretic hormone) is a vasoconstrictor that promotes water retention. Dilutional hyponatremia seen in advanced heart failure is related to the activity of arginine vasopressin on the kidneys. Although a potent vasoconstrictor, vasopressin is thought to make the smallest contribution to the vasoconstriction seen in heart failure.

Eicosanoids. In addition to renin, vasodilator renal hormones are active in heart failure, including prostaglandins from the arachidonic acid cascade and bradykinin from the kallikrein-kinin system (Figure 12-6). Prostaglandins are released in response to hyponatremia, norepinephrine, and angiotensin II in order to

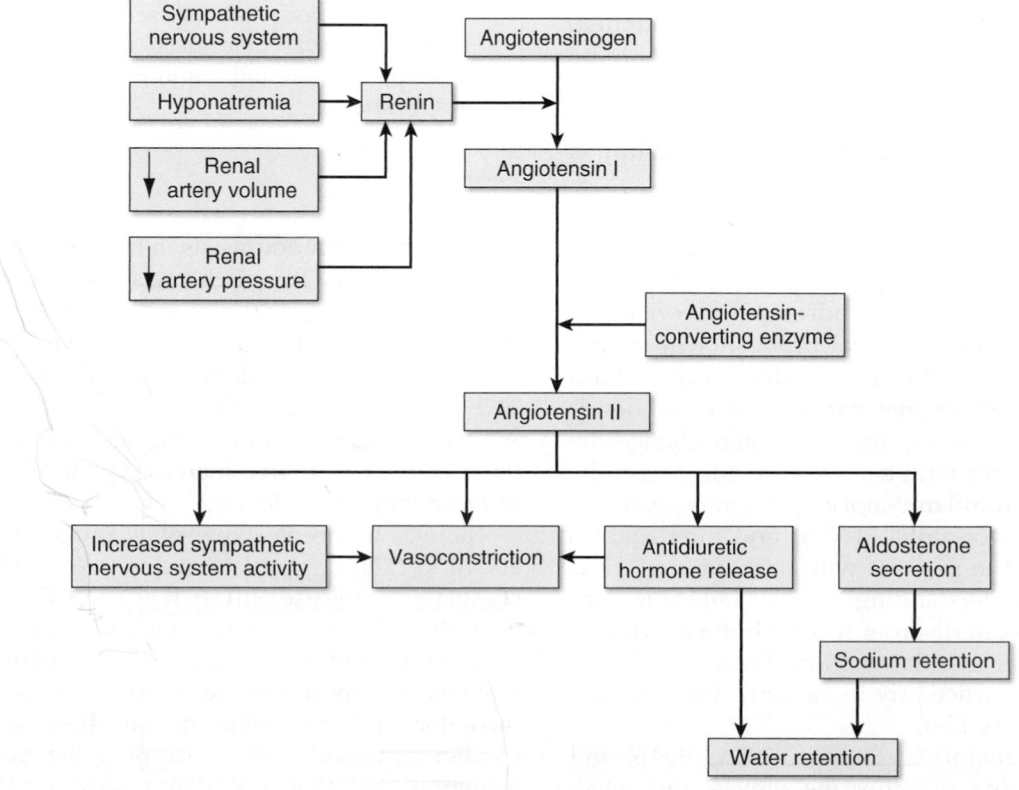

✦FIGURE 12-5 Activation of the renin-angiotensin-aldosterone system leading to vasoconstriction and volume retention.

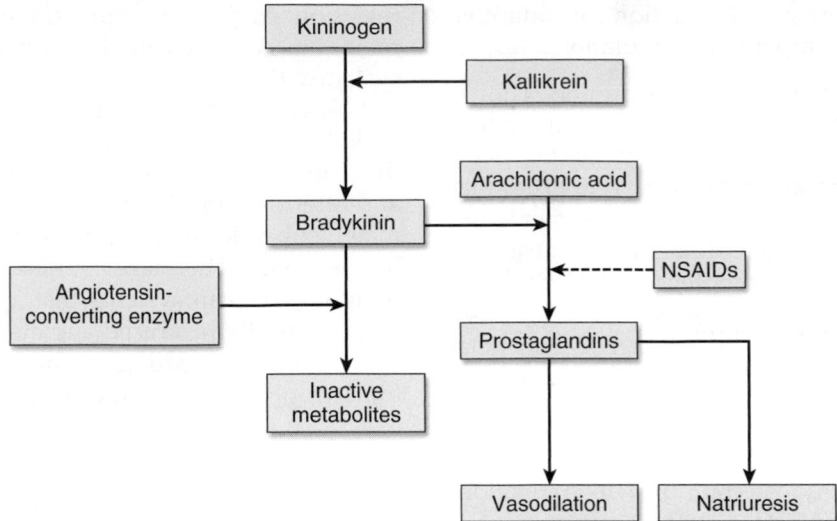

♣FIGURE 12-6 Other renal hormones released in heart failure include bradykinin and prostaglandins. Angiotensin-converting enzyme, which is responsible for the production of angiotensin II, also degrades bradykinin. NSAIDs can antagonize prostaglandin production. Dashed arrow indicates antagonized response; solid arrows indicate promoted response. NSAIDs, Nonsteroidal antiinflammatory drugs.

attenuate vasoconstriction and fluid retention. These potentially beneficial effects are overcome by the vasoconstrictor systems activated in heart failure. However, prostaglandins may maintain renal blood flow despite decreased CO. Both renal and ventricular function may worsen when nonsteroidal antiinflammatory agents that antagonize prostaglandins are used in patients with severe heart failure and hyponatremia. Thus although their vasodilator activity appears to be overwhelmed, prostaglandins still may play a protective role in the prevention of rapid deterioration in heart failure. The role of bradykinin in heart failure is not known.

Inflammation. The conceptualization of heart failure pathophysiology has undergone a number of changes in the past 5 decades. The syndrome was originally considered simply a cardiorenal problem with hemodynamic consequences to be corrected. Appreciation of the role of neurohormonal activation allowed development of medication therapy that could change the prognosis for patients with heart failure. Most recently, evidence that proinflammatory cytokines such as tumor necrosis factor-alpha (TNFα) and interleukin 6 (IL-6) are elevated in patients with heart failure[155] has progressed our understanding of heart failure toward that of a multisystem disorder in which the overriding pathologic process is inflammation. Potential triggers of inflammation, particularly in ischemic heart failure, are indicated in Box 12-3.

The proinflammatory cytokines TNFα, IL-1β, and IL-6 exert paracrine or autocrine effects, but when

---

Box 12-3

Potential Triggers of Inflammation in Heart Failure

- **C-reactive protein:** acute phase protein
- **Infectious agents:** chronic nonvascular infections such as periodontal disease, prostatitis, and bronchitis; also vascular infections
- **Hypertension and angiotensin II**
- **Obesity**

---

secreted in large amounts, as in heart failure, they exert endocrine effects. Elevated levels of these cytokines are seen in patients with heart failure.[155] At high levels, these cytokines can cause left ventricular dysfunction and ventricular remodeling and promote apoptosis. TNFα and IL-6 levels correlate with New York Heart Association (NYHA) functional class, and patients with the highest levels have increased mortality compared to those with lower levels.[178]

There is a complex interplay among TNFα, IL-1β, and IL-6. TNFα stimulates release of IL-1β; both can stimulate the release of IL-6. IL-1β and TNFα act synergistically in autocrine and paracrine manners to induce many of the metabolic alterations that occur during the systemic inflammatory response. IL-6 is a systemic mediator of local inflammation. IL-6 may serve a counter-regulatory role of capping the magnitude of activity of the other proinflammatory cytokines.

The origin of proinflammatory cytokines found in the blood of patients with heart failure is unknown, but there are several potential sources. One source may be the proinflammatory cytokines synthesized in the myocardium that leak out into circulation. A second source is thought to be cytokines produced by immune and other cells in ischemic tissues. Ischemic injury initiates a cascade of events that simulate immune, epithelial, and other cells in the ischemic tissue to produce proinflammatory cytokines. A third source may be stimulation of immune cells by lipopolysaccharide (LPS) from the cell wall of gram-negative bacteria. Gram-negative bacteria translocate across the ischemic gut into the blood, where LPS binds to immune cells. LPS is a potent stimulator of tumor necrosis factor-alpha production in immune cells. Patients with heart failure, particularly those with edema, have been reported to have elevated blood levels of LPS associated with higher circulating TNFα levels. Once edema in these patients was treated, LPS levels decreased.[118]

The most prominent consequence of systemic inflammation associated with heart failure is the development of cardiac cachexia. Researchers have established a positive relationship between proinflammatory cytokine levels and severity of cardiac cachexia.[8–11] Proinflammatory cytokines have direct and indirect actions on peripheral tissues and the brain. The combined effects of cytokine activity in these areas include decreased food intake, catabolism of muscle and adipose tissue, stimulation of catabolic hormones, such as epinephrine and cortisol, increased metabolism, and fatigue.

Counter-Regulation of Proinflammatory Cytokines. To maintain homeostasis, proinflammatory cytokines are opposed by antiinflammatory cytokines, including IL-4, IL-10, and IL-12. IL-10 in particular has potent antiinflammatory properties, including downregulation of TNFα, IL-1β, and IL-6 production.[14] Patients with heart failure do not produce enough IL-10 to counter proinflammatory cytokine activity. Activation of the hypothalamic-pituitary-adrenal axis is the second major counter-regulatory mechanism to control proinflammatory cytokine activity. Proinflammatory cytokines stimulate the hypothalamic-pituitary-adrenal axis, resulting in release of glucocorticoids, primarily cortisol. Antiinflammatory properties of cortisol include suppression of proinflammatory cytokine and stimulation of IL-10.

Peripheral Changes

Endothelial-Derived Factors. In addition to activation of the sympathetic and renin-angiotensin systems, vasoconstriction in heart failure is mediated by peripheral mechanisms. These mechanisms include vascular remodeling with inhibition of vasodilation, increased vascular stiffness secondary to elevated sodium and water content in the vascular wall, and alterations in endothelial-derived factors.[42,44]

The vascular endothelium produces vasoactive substances that locally promote smooth muscle relaxation and contraction. These substances include the vasodilator endothelium-derived relaxing factor (i.e., EDRF, nitric oxide) and the potent vasoconstrictor endothelin. Abnormalities of EDRF and endothelin contribute to the vasoconstriction seen in heart failure.[42,43] Endothelial-dependent vasodilation in heart failure is decreased, possibly because of abnormalities in the formation or release of EDRF, and abnormalities in smooth muscle response. Endothelin levels are markedly increased in heart failure patients. Increased cytokine expression has been implicated in endothelial dysfunction. Increased levels of free oxygen radicals seen in heart failure can impair vasodilation by inactivating EDRF.

PATHOPHYSIOLOGY OF ACUTE DECOMPENSATION IN THE SETTING OF CHRONIC HEART FAILURE

The pathophysiologic chain of events converting compensated to decompensated heart failure has been the subject of considerable controversy and is not yet clear. For decades, it has been believed that ADHF occurred because systemic fluid overload and impairment in contractility produced fluid buildup in the lungs.[54] Evidence that ADHF occurs in the setting of normal CO and ejection fraction (EF) led to the observation that ADHF is most commonly manifested by marked elevations in systemic vascular resistance and ventricular filling pressures. Together these changes produce a shift in fluid to the lungs, with resulting symptoms of dyspnea. Thus many cases of ADHF are the result of markedly increased afterload and not simply increased preload alone.

Stages and Types of Heart Failure

Stages of Heart Failure. The American College of Cardiology/American Heart Association (ACC/AHA) guideline for the management of heart failure emphasizes prevention at several levels in the development and progression of heart failure by conceptualizing heart failure in four progressive stages (Figure 12-7). Those patients in stage A are considered to be in "pre-heart failure," meaning they do not yet have heart failure or structural heart disease, but are at risk for the

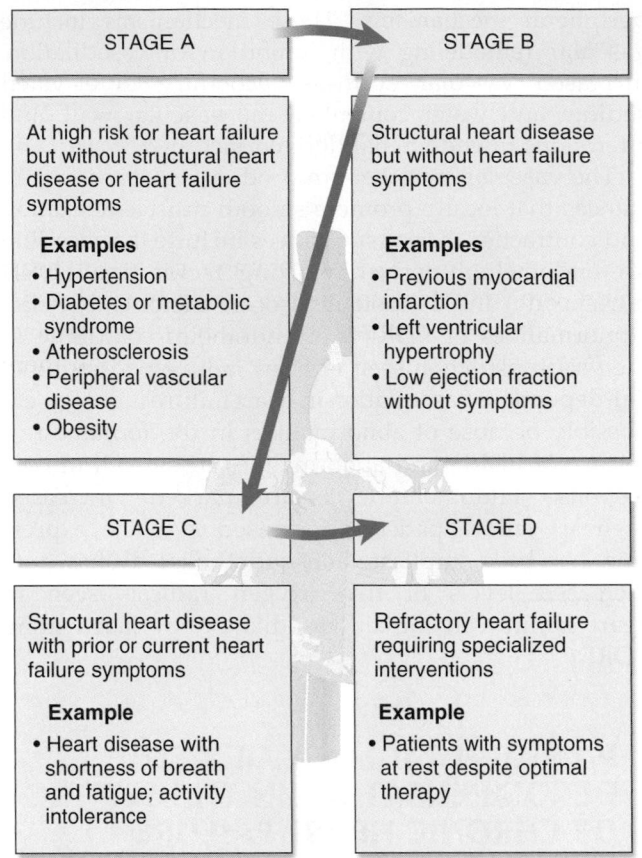

STAGE A	STAGE B
At high risk for heart failure but without structural heart disease or heart failure symptoms **Examples** • Hypertension • Diabetes or metabolic syndrome • Atherosclerosis • Peripheral vascular disease • Obesity	Structural heart disease but without heart failure symptoms **Examples** • Previous myocardial infarction • Left ventricular hypertrophy • Low ejection fraction without symptoms

STAGE C	STAGE D
Structural heart disease with prior or current heart failure symptoms **Example** • Heart disease with shortness of breath and fatigue; activity intolerance	Refractory heart failure requiring specialized interventions **Example** • Patients with symptoms at rest despite optimal therapy

◆FIGURE 12-7 The four stages in the development of heart failure as described by the American College of Cardiology/ American Heart Association.

development of such. The goal of therapy for patients in this stage is the prevention of heart failure. Individuals with stage B heart failure have developed structural heart disease, but do not have symptoms of heart failure. Stage C heart failure is heralded by the development of overt symptomatic heart failure. Stage D heart failure is refractory heart failure in which specialized interventions are needed. Therapy for each stage is outlined in Box 12-4.[76]

Types of Heart Failure. Heart failure can result from impairment of left ventricular systolic function, from diastolic dysfunction where systolic function is relatively preserved, or from a combination of these.

Systolic Dysfunction. Heart failure with systolic dysfunction is the occurrence of specific signs and symptoms in the setting of impaired systolic function as evidenced by a left ventricular EF below 40% (Box 12-5).

Preserved Systolic Function or Diastolic Heart Failure. Increasingly it is clear that 40% to 50% of cases

Box 12-4

Management of Stages of Heart Failure From the American College of Cardiology/American Heart Association Heart Failure Guidelines

STAGE A THERAPY: TREAT RISK FACTORS FOR HEART FAILURE AND ITS PRECURSORS
• Treat hypertension aggressively
• Treat dyslipidemias
• Control diabetes and metabolic syndrome
• Smoking cessation
• Promote regular exercise
• Obesity control
• Other measures to prevent atherosclerosis and coronary artery disease
• Discourage excess alcohol intake, illicit drug use
• Angiotensin-converting enzyme inhibitors or angiotensin receptor blockers in at-risk patients

STAGE B THERAPY: TREAT STRUCTURAL HEART DISEASE
• All measures in stage A
• Beta blockers in appropriate patients

STAGE C THERAPY: TREAT HEART FAILURE
• All stage A and stage B lifestyle measures
• Dietary sodium restriction
• Angiotensin-converting enzyme inhibitors or angiotensin receptor blockers in at-risk patients
• Beta-adrenergic receptor blockers
• Diuretics
• Digoxin
• Aldosterone antagonists
• Hydralazine/nitrates
• Biventricular pacing or implantable defibrillators in select patients

STAGE D THERAPY: TREAT REFRACTORY HEART FAILURE REQUIRING SPECIALIZED INTERVENTIONS
• All measures under stages A, B, C
• Mechanical assist devices
• Heart transplantation
• Palliative/hospice care

of heart failure occur in the presence of preserved systolic function, whereas approximately 10% have a combination of systolic and diastolic dysfunction.[191] Diastolic heart failure is defined as the occurrence of signs and symptoms of heart failure in the setting of unimpaired (or only slightly impaired) left ventricular systolic function and diastolic dysfunction (see Box 12-5).[119] Although mortality rates among those with diastolic

Box 12-5

Signs and Symptoms of Heart Failure

SIGNS

- Edema (peripheral, sacral)
- Jugular venous distention or elevated venous pressure (>16 mm Hg)
- Rales (although can be absent in most patients with heart failure because of compensation by pulmonary lymphatic system)
- Cardiomegaly
- Hepatojugular reflex
- Displaced apical pulse
- Ascites
- Third heart sound

SYMPTOMS

- Dyspnea or orthopnea
- Paroxysmal nocturnal dyspnea
- Nocturnal cough
- Activity intolerance, fatigue
- Anorexia or other gastrointestinal symptoms

failure are lower than those seen in patients with systolic dysfunction, hospitalizations rates are similar. There are few existing clinical studies to guide clinicians in the management of patients with diastolic heart failure and preserved systolic function, but several ongoing studies will soon provide important evidence and consensus guidelines are beginning to address it.

Diastolic Heart Failure. Diastolic heart failure is the result of the heart's inability to accept an adequate blood volume. This inability is caused by abnormal ventricular relaxation or by loss of ventricular compliance (i.e., increased ventricular stiffness).

Patients at Risk

Given the high morbidity and mortality associated with heart failure, knowledge of at least three groups of risk factors could help healthcare providers use risk profiles to target the most at-risk patients. Individuals have varying degrees of risk for (1) the development of heart failure and (2) an exacerbation of heart failure.

At Risk for Development of Heart Failure. There is a difference between a cause of heart failure and a risk factor for heart failure. A cause is a factor that has a strong association with heart failure, is consistent among studies, and has an appropriate temporal sequence and a biologically plausible dose-response relationship.[58] A risk factor is a characteristic suspected

of being associated with heart failure, but it is not sufficient or necessary to cause heart failure (Box 12-6).[58]

Based on data from the Framingham study, the lifetime risk for the development of heart failure in both men and women is thought to be 1 in 5.[95] This risk increases substantially with age. For example, the prevalence of heart failure in men ages 50 to 59 years is 3 in 1000, while the prevalence in those ages 80 to 89 years is 27 in 1000.[188] The most common causes of heart failure are hypertension and ischemic heart disease, particularly antecedent MI.[95] Other causes and risk factors are outlined in Box 12-6. Of note, although there

Box 12-6

Causes of, and Risk Factors for, Heart Failure

CAUSES

1. Myocardial
   - Ischemic (coronary artery disease)
   - Chamber dilation (idiopathic, viral, toxins, inflammatory, peripartum)
2. Volume
   - Aortic and mitral regurgitation
   - Anemia
   - Pressure loading
   - Hypertension
   - Aortic stenosis
   - Restrictive
   - Constrictive pericarditis
   - Amyloidosis
   - Sarcoidosis
   - Thyroid abnormality
   - Renal insufficiency

RISK FACTORS

1. Modifiable
   - Diabetes
   - Valve disease
   - Obesity
   - Left ventricular hypertrophy
   - Smoking
   - Physical inactivity
   - Achieved less than a high school education
2. Nonmodifiable
   - African-American race
   - Older age
3. Novel/Potential
   - Toxins
   - Metabolic syndrome
   - Sleep-disordered breathing
   - Depression
   - Alcohol

Modified from reference 58.

are no gender differences in risk of developing heart failure, there are gender differences in the risk profile. For example, men are more likely to have CAD as a precursor to heart failure, while women more often have hypertension as a precursor. Among the nine predictors of incident heart failure in women identified by the Heart and Estrogen/Progestin Replacement Study (HERS), diabetes was the strongest risk factor, especially when it was not well controlled or when it was coupled with obesity or renal insufficiency (Box 12-7).[19]

At Risk for Exacerbation of Chronic Heart Failure.

A number of medical and nonmedical factors can precipitate an exacerbation of chronic heart failure, the most common cause of readmission to the hospital with ADHF. Although determining the most common causes or risk factors for rehospitalization is difficult because investigators only test a selected number of potential predictors in each study, comparison of studies indicates important trends. Two of the most common reasons for disease exacerbation leading to rehospitalization are patient nonadherence and failure to report deteriorating symptoms in a timely fashion.* Failure to take medications as prescribed or to follow the low-sodium diet are the most frequent types of nonadherence.[102,116,169,181] Reasons for patients' apparent inability to recognize escalating symptoms until they have seriously deteriorated are unclear, but may include the variable, and sometimes subtle, nature of symptom fluctuation. Another factor contributing to readmission is discharge of patients before they are clinically stable. Patients can be discharged before they are stable and with a variety of risk factors for rehospitalization,[108,167] all of which can place them at risk for

---

*References 48, 49, 102, 116, 169, 181.

---

early rehospitalization. The full variety of factors that place patients at risk for rehospitalization for ADHF is outlined in Box 12-8.

Profile of Patients Admitted With Acute Decompensated Heart Failure. The Acute Decompensated Heart Failure National Registry (ADHERE) has provided a snapshot of the typical ADHF patient.[1,5,187] The mean age of patients admitted to the hospital for ADHF in the most recent report, which includes 105,388 patients, is 72 years; 52% were women. A total of 72% of patients were Caucasian and 20% African American. Medicare and Medicaid were the predominant insurers, covering 78% of patients. Common comorbidities included hypertension (73%), CAD (57%), diabetes (44%), atrial fibrillation (31%), obstructive pulmonary disease or asthma (31%), and renal insufficiency (30%), with 21% of patients having a serum creatinine level greater than 2 mg/dl. Of the patients admitted, 46% had heart failure with preserved or only mildly impaired left ventricular function (left ventricular ejection fraction [LVEF] greater than 40%).

In 75% of patients, the ADHF was a result of exacerbation of chronic heart failure.[5] A total of 33% of patients from this report had been admitted for heart failure in the prior 6 months. The most common symptom present on admission was dyspnea (89%). Rales

---

Box 12-7

Predictors of Development of Heart Failure in Postmenopausal Women With Coronary Artery Disease Enrolled in the Heart and Estrogen/Progestin Replacement Study (HERS)

- Diabetes
- Atrial fibrillation
- Myocardial infarction
- Renal insufficiency
- Hypertension
- Obesity
- Current smoking
- Left bundle branch block
- Left ventricular hypertrophy

Box 12-8

Factors Placing Patients at Risk for Hospitalization for Exacerbation of Heart Failure

MODIFIABLE

- Poor medication and dietary adherence
- Lack of or inadequate patient and family education and counseling
- Inadequate follow-up
- Inadequate or inappropriate medical therapy
- Depression
- Social isolation
- Failure to respond to escalating symptoms in a timely manner
- Ischemia
- Dysrhythmias (including atrial fibrillation)
- Uncontrolled hypertension
- Infections

NONMODIFIABLE

- Older age
- Presence of comorbidities
- Renal dysfunction
- Previous admission

and peripheral edema occurred in 68% and 66% of the cases, respectively. Patients commonly received aggressive treatment, especially the approximately 14% admitted to critical care. Mechanical ventilation was required in 23% of these patients. The median hospital length of stay for all hospitalized patients was 4.3 days. Overall the hospital mortality rate was 4%; mortality was 10.6% for the subset of patients who received care in critical care.

Assessment

Patients presenting to the emergency department (ED) with ADHF are usually in significant distress from dyspnea and other symptoms of fluid overload, occurring rapidly (within minutes to hours), or developing over the course of several days. Patients' difficulty assessing their own escalating symptoms over the course of several days is a target for intervention. Many patients delay days before seeking treatment, when earlier recognition of symptoms might have prevented hospitalization.[49]

Based on the Forrester classification,[56] clinicians can employ the clinical severity classification to classify patients presenting with ADHF so that therapy can be guided appropriately (Figure 12-8).[120] This classification system uses data derived from bedside examination to assess whether clinical symptoms of elevated filling pressure and inadequate perfusion are present. The profile is predictive of post-discharge mortality.[120]

Using the system, patients are classified as group A (warm and dry), group B (warm and wet), group L (cold and dry), or group C (cold and wet). With regard to congestion, patients can present as "dry" (without fluid overload) or "wet" (with fluid overload). Those who present "wet" have fluid overload with elevated ventricular filling pressure, and signs and symptoms of congestion including orthopnea, peripheral edema, jugular venous congestion, hepatojugular reflux, or ascites. If a pulmonary artery catheter (PAC) was inserted, pulmonary artery wedge pressure (PAWP) would be elevated. With regard to perfusion, patients can present as "warm" (adequate perfusion) or "cold" (poor perfusion). Patients who present "cold" can have the following signs and symptoms: narrow proportional pulse pressure (systolic minus diastolic blood pressure divided by systolic blood pressure less than 25%); symptomatic hypotension; cool extremities; pulsus alternans; and obtunded mentation. Patients in the wet and cold category have the worst prognosis (40% mortality at 6 months) while those in the dry and warm category have the best prognosis (11% mortality at 6 months).[120]

Of the four profiles, "warm and wet" is the most commonly seen in hospitalized patients. The warm and wet profile means that the patient has adequate perfusion but fluid volume excess. Patients who present "cold and wet" have a combination of elevated filling pressures and low CO. Patients who present as "cold and dry" have normal filling pressures and low CO; it is thought that many of these patients have fluid overload that has not been assessed adequately.[54,164] Finally, patients who have the "warm and dry" presentation often do not actually have ADHF, but rather have escalating symptoms similar to those of ADHF from another cause such as pulmonary disease. However, a "warm and dry" ADHF presentation is possible and occurs in patients with heart failure and anemia, for example.

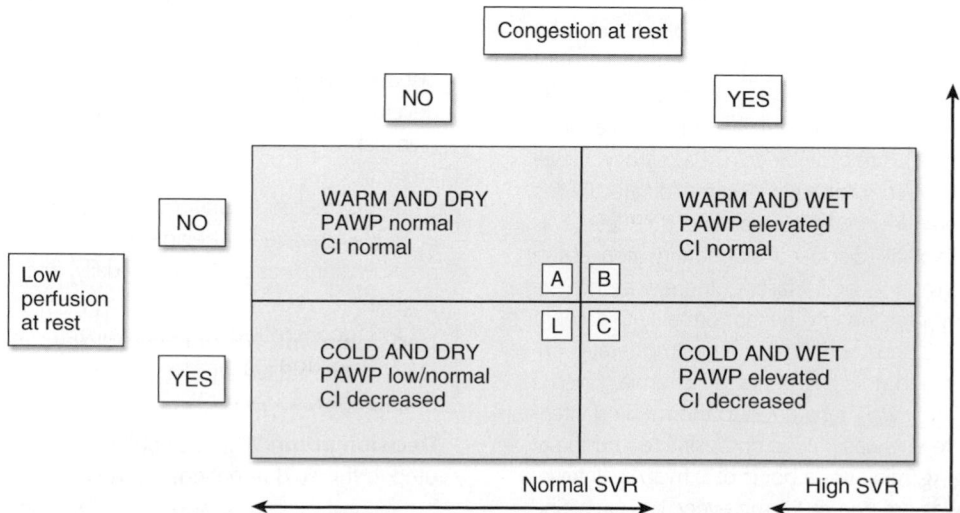

♦**FIGURE 12-8** Clinical assessment of patient hemodynamic profiles that occur in acute decompensated heart failure. CI = Cardiac index, PAWP = pulmonary artery wedge pressure, SVR = systemic vascular resistance.

Case Study 12-1, Part A

Etiology of Heart Failure

R.S. is a 56-year-old African-American woman with a history of prior acute, long-standing hypertension, type 2 diabetes, and "a little congestive heart failure." She is a widow and lives alone. Each member of her family (two married daughters and two married sons) has asked her to live with them because they are concerned about her steadily worsening medical condition. R.S. has resisted because she values her independence and does not want to be a burden to her family. She was brought to the ED by her daughters, who went to R.S.'s home to pick her up for a family celebration and found her struggling to breathe while sitting up in a chair.

R.S. has a long medical history of poorly controlled hypertension, partially related to her own nonadherence to prescribed medical therapy, and partially related to failure of her primary care provider to aggressively treat her hypertension. Her diabetes similarly is poorly controlled as she "loves to eat the sweet stuff and cook for my family." She has resisted following a low-salt diet because she loves family dinners and does not want to impose her diet on anyone else and because it is "too much trouble and bad tasting to go low salt." Her body mass index (BMI) is 32 kg/m². Medications before admission were furosemide 20 mg twice per day, digoxin 0.125 mg once per day, and metformin (Glucophage) 500 mg once per day.

In the ED, she is observed to be anxious and in moderate, escalating respiratory distress. Heart rate is 126 beats/min, respiratory rate is 32 breaths/min, and blood pressure is 160/96 mm Hg. Pulse oximetry reveals an oxygen saturation of 82%. She has distended neck veins with elevated venous jugular pressure, an S_3 gallop with a systolic ejection murmur, and 4+ pedal edema. R.S. does not know if she has gained weight in the past few days because she does not weigh herself daily because "it's not good to be obsessed with your weight." Lung sounds include crackles at both bases. She was placed on oxygen and given 80 mg of intravenous furosemide. Laboratory studies, chest x-ray, and 12 lead ECG were obtained. Her complete blood cell count revealed anemia, creatinine level 1.8 mg/dl, blood urea nitrogen level 42 mg/dl, and glucose concentration 350 mg/dl; electrolytes were normal, troponin level was normal, and BNP level was 1325 pg/ml. Chest x-ray disclosed pulmonary congestion consistent with congestive heart failure; there was no evidence of pulmonary infection or other abnormality to account for dyspnea. The ECG showed her old infarct, moderate ventricular hypertrophy, and no signs of acute ischemia. Given a diagnosis of ADHF, R.S. was transferred to the medical intensive care unit, where she was placed on nesiritide infusion at a rate of 0.01 mcg/kg/min after a bolus of 2 mcg/kg. Intravenous furosemide was ordered at 40 mg every 12 hours. She was started on lisinopril (Zestril) 10 mg daily with plans to start carvedilol (Coreg) 3.125 mg twice daily and titrate once her condition stabilizes. Sliding-scale insulin was used to control blood glucose level.

Decision point: What signs and symptoms of heart failure was R.S. exhibiting?

Decision point: What causes, risk factors, and lifestyle choices does R.S. have for heart failure?

Case Study 12-1, Part B

Etiology of Heart Failure

R.S. met criteria for the "warm and wet" profile of ADHF. After 24 hours she had diuresed 3 liters of urine; her blood pressure was 126/66 mm Hg, her respiratory rate was 20 breaths/min with no complaints of dyspnea, and her heart rate was 80 beats/min. She no longer had evident jugular venous distention, and her lungs were clear. Oxygen was discontinued. Echocardiography revealed left ventricular dysfunction with an ejection fraction of 30% and left ventricular hypertrophy.

Patient and family education and counseling were begun to assist the patient to assume greater self-care responsibility. The fundamentals of daily weighing along with the rationale (and the differences between weighing for fat and weighing to monitor for fluid gain) were explained. Instruction on monitoring for symptoms of worsening heart failure was also given. The patient was asked to return demonstrate each of these skills. Social services were consulted to begin discharge planning. Arrangements were made for a dietitian consult for the patient and family to begin teaching R.S. to make low-sodium diet choices. Each day of the 4-day admission, the information was reinforced. Strategies for medication adherence were also taught. Because there was no heart failure disease management program, critical care unit nurses had developed a phone follow-up program for patients with a high risk of rehospitalization, and R.S. was referred to this program.

After consultation with a cardiologist, R.S.'s medication regimen was changed to begin optimizing her drug therapy. Lisinopril was increased to 20 mg daily, and the carvedilol was begun.

Decision point: What pathophysiologic mechanism contributed to the left ventricular hypertrophy and left ventricular dysfunction?

Decision point: What pathophysiologic mechanism contributed to the fluid retention?

Case continues on page 266

Diagnostic Evaluation. There is no single test that definitely diagnoses ADHF; rather the diagnosis is made based on clinical judgment after consideration of a number of factors. The following diagnostic tests may be employed to assist in the decision-making process.

B-Type Natriuretic Peptide. The natriuretic peptides have diverse cardiovascular, renal, and endocrine system effects. B-type natriuretic peptide (BNP) is released from the ventricles as a result of increased myocardial pressure and stretch. Thus BNP is released in heart failure as a protective response to fluid overload. Endogenous BNP causes natriuresis (i.e., urinary loss of sodium and water) and vasodilation. These effects are not adequate to overcome the adverse effects of the counter-regulatory hormones of the neurohormonal system activated in heart failure. BNP is a biomarker of heart failure, and is used as a diagnostic and prognostic tool, as well as a therapeutic agent in the management of ADHF.

The Breathing Not Properly study was the first large multinational prospective study using BNP levels to evaluate the causes of dyspnea.[97] In this study, BNP levels were found to be better at accurately predicting presence of heart failure than history, physical findings, or laboratory values. A BNP level greater than 100 pg/ml had a 90% sensitivity and 76% specificity for differentiating heart failure from other causes of dyspnea.[97] As a result of this and other studies, BNP levels are now commonly used in the ED to determine whether heart failure is the cause of dyspnea.

A BNP level is usually measured when the patient first presents to the hospital with symptoms of ADHF and again before discharge. If BNP levels do not fall after 24 hours of therapy, this may indicate that the patient needs more aggressive treatment. Failure of BNP to improve with treatment is a poor prognostic sign.[183] The frequency of BNP evaluation throughout the hospitalization depends on the provider's clinical judgment. Although BNP levels are associated with disease severity and prognosis in patients with heart failure, there are as yet no definitive data demonstrating that BNP levels can be used for determining optimization of therapy. Ongoing studies will provide these data in the future.[183]

The level of BNP can be determined from serum assays of BNP or of NT-proBNP, the biologically inactive N-terminal fragment of proBNP cleavage that produces the biologically active BNP. Both BNP and NT-proBNP assays perform equally well in clinical situations. The cut-point for BNP for the best negative predictive value is 100 pg/ml, while the similar cut-point for NT-proBNP is 300 pg/ml. NT-proBNP and BNP values are not comparable and there is no conversion factor for one to the other.[183] There is marked interindividual variation in repeat BNP and NT-proBNP levels, and BNP and NT-proBNP are affected by age (higher at older ages), gender (women have higher levels), renal failure (higher levels seen with worse renal function), body weight, and the presence of other comorbidities (e.g., diabetes and hypertension). BNP levels may not be elevated in cases of "flash pulmonary edema" from ADHF, and BNP levels are most predictive in ADHF patients with new symptoms. More research is needed to clarify level norms in various subgroups.

Other Laboratory Testing. Laboratory testing in patients who present with ADHF includes a complete blood count, panel of electrolytes, and blood urea nitrogen (BUN) and serum creatinine levels. Patients should be tested for diabetes mellitus, or if already diagnosed with diabetes, a hemoglobin A_{1c} level should be obtained. A fasting lipid panel and thyroid panel should also be evaluated. These laboratory tests are helpful to evaluate comorbidities that contribute to worsening HF (i.e., anemia, diabetes, renal insufficiency, hyperlipidemia, and thyroid abnormalities).

Chest Radiograph. The chest x-ray is an important part of the assessment of ADHF. Despite the absence of rales on physical exam, findings of pulmonary congestion may be seen on x-ray.[82] An early sign of fluid accumulation in the interstitium is the presence of Kerley B lines, which represent fluid accumulation in the interlobular septa. The findings of cardiomegaly, pulmonary edema, or pleural effusion on the chest x-ray are indicative of heart failure, but these findings alone do not confirm the diagnosis.

Electrocardiogram. The electrocardiogram (ECG) is of limited use in establishing a diagnosis of heart failure; however, it is helpful in determining the onset of new dysrhythmias that may precipitate or exacerbate ADHF. In addition, the ECG can provide evidence of myocardial ischemia or infarction, and conduction abnormalities such as bundle branch block.[82]

Echocardiogram. Echocardiography with identification of the left ventricular EF is a fundamental aspect in the evaluation of heart failure. However, repeated assessment of left ventricular function in patients with heart failure does not affect or alter the treatment plan unless significant changes in the patient's cardiac function or clinical status have occurred. Thus echocardiography is indicated in ADHF only when there is evidence that changes in patients' myocardial performance or valvular integrity may have precipitated ADHF. It may also provide information about the presence of an acute ischemic syndrome and the status of the pericardium.

Coronary Angiography. Coronary angiography may be appropriate in the evaluation of ADHF if it appears that acute MI or unstable acute coronary syndrome amenable to intervention precipitated the patient's ADHF. However, it is important to speak with the patient and outline possible interventions before proceeding to the catheterization lab, to determine the patient's wishes for future therapy.

Pulmonary Artery Catheterization. Until concerns emerged about the possibility that use of the PAC might increase mortality, it was commonly used to guide therapy for patients with severe ADHF. Tailored therapy, or therapy guided to specific hemodynamic goals, was shown to improve outcomes in some clinicians' hands.[165] However, the results of a recent randomized controlled trial of ADHF therapy in patients with severe heart failure guided by PAC data versus clinical judgment revealed no difference in outcomes between the two groups.[20] These data, combined with the results of a meta-analysis of randomized controlled trials,[156] suggest that although there is no excess harm from using PAC to guide therapy during ADHF, neither is there a survival benefit. However, it may be that the lack of evidence-based guidelines for management of ADHF has prevented demonstration of an advantage. Further research on PAC is warranted as evidence-based guidelines for the care of ADHF develop. Until such time, use of the PAC to guide therapy in ADHF should be reserved for those situations in which fluid status is difficult to determine or medication needs are complex (e. g., balancing inotropes and vasodilators when blood pressure is extremely low or very labile).

Multidisciplinary Plan of Care

Achieving the goals of therapy in ADHF involves the commitment of multiple disciplines. As such, an integrated Multidisciplinary Plan of Care as shown below is essential. The plan must address each of the following goals[54]:

- Prompt relief of respiratory distress and treatment of other symptoms
- Prompt treatment of acute hemodynamic abnormalities
- Optimization of pharmacologic and nonpharmacologic therapies to improve quality of life and survival, prevent future hospitalizations, and slow progression of heart failure

MULTIDISCIPLINARY PLAN OF CARE FOR PATIENTS WITH ACUTE DECOMPENSATED HEART FAILURE

PROBLEM	INTERVENTION	RATIONALE	EXPECTED OUTCOME
Presentation with ADHF	Assess clinical severity based on fluid status and perfusion. Assign patient to one of four quadrants: warm and dry, warm and wet, cold and dry, or cold and wet.	Choice of therapy guided by assignment of patient to one of four clinical severity quadrants is associated with improved outcomes.	Appropriate therapy is chosen and implemented with rapid relief of symptoms.
Warm and dry presentation	Assess for other causes of escalating symptoms, such as anemia or pulmonary disease. Ensure chronic outpatient heart failure therapy is optimal.	Warm and dry presentation unusual for ADHF, so search for other causes of symptoms is warranted. Any hospitalization is a good time to check for optimal heart failure therapy.	Patient is appropriately treated and symptoms resolve.
Warm and wet presentation	Administer intravenous diuretic therapy to reduce or redistribute volume to meet following goals: (1) relief from congestion (i.e., absence of dyspnea/orthopnea, achievement of dry weight, none to minimal edema or ascites); (2) absence of electrolyte abnormalities (i.e., potassium level >4 mEq/L and magnesium level >1.8 mEq/L).	Volume overload or inappropriate distribution of blood volume in pulmonary and systemic vessels is a fundamental alteration in ADHF. Intravenous administration is recommended for optimum speed of action and greatest drug concentration because gastrointestinal absorption is affected by gut edema.	Patient has relief of congestion with maintenance of adequate blood pressure.

PROBLEM	INTERVENTION	RATIONALE	EXPECTED OUTCOME
Warm and wet presentation—Cont'd	Administer vasodilators if diuretics insufficient to meet following goals: (1) relief from congestion (i.e., absence of dyspnea/orthopnea, absence of adventitious breath sounds); (2) adequate arterial blood pressure (i.e., absence of symptomatic hypotension).	Vasodilation induces redistribution of blood volume to capacitance vessels, reduces venous return to right atrium, decreases vascular pressures, and optimizes cardiac function by moving heart to a more normal Frank-Starling curve. Vasodilators also reduce afterload and improve systolic function by decreasing systemic vascular resistance and reducing resistance to ventricular ejection and forward blood flow.	
Cold and wet presentation	Use diuretics and vasodilators as above. Administer intravenous inotropic therapy in doses as small as possible to improve systolic function to meet following goals: (1) augmentation of stroke volume and cardiac output; (2) direct and indirect vasodilation; (3) no significant increase in myocardial oxygen consumption.	See above. Inotropic agents improve myocardial contractility by enhanced release and use of myocardial intracellular calcium. Augmented contractility enhances ventricular ejection of blood and reduces pulmonary congestion.	Patient shows symptom relief and return to compensated state.
Cold and dry presentation	Reassess fluid status. Follow inotropic therapy as above.	Fluid overload is often present yet not adequately assessed. See above.	
High risk for early rehospitalization for ADHF after discharge	Assess for and treat modifiable factors contributing to ADHF. Ensure chronic outpatient heart failure therapy is optimal. Assess for criteria for stability before discharge and for factors increasing risk for rehospitalization and intervene as appropriate.	Attention to modifiable risk factors decreases future rehospitalizations. Any hospitalization is a good time to check for optimal heart failure therapy. Premature discharge before clinical stability is reached or failure to intervene with other risk factors are two major causes of early rehospitalization.	There is no early rehospitalization for patient.
High risk for any heart failure rehospitalization	Refer any patient who has been hospitalized for an exacerbation of heart failure; who has problems with adherence, multiple comorbidities, renal insufficiency or failure; or who is an older adult and living alone to a heart failure disease management program or to a practitioner who employs disease management principles. Promotion of self-care.	Hospitalization for heart failure is one major risk factor for subsequent rehospitalization. Heart failure disease management is an effective model of care for decreasing rehospitalizations and costs and increasing quality of life. Self-care strategies are fundamental to maintaining heart failure stability.	Patient is not hospitalized for ADHF.

ADHF = Acute decompensated heart failure.

Both pharmacologic and nonpharmacologic therapies are essential to improving outcomes in patients with heart failure.

Pharmacologic Therapy: Acute Management

Although it is now known that heart failure is not simply the result of hemodynamic abnormalities, correcting derangements in hemodynamics continues to remain a goal of acute treatment of ADHF because it is these derangements that produce the symptomatic presentation in ADHF.[164] Intravenous diuretics, vasodilators, inotropic agents, and natriuretic peptides are the drugs useful in ADHF treatment.

Correcting Clinical Severity Profile. Intravenous vasodilators decrease filling pressures and increase CO in most patients with ADHF. Vasodilator therapy with nitroprusside (Nipride), nitroglycerin, or nesiritide (Natrecor) decreases afterload, thus increasing CO. These agents and intravenous diuretic therapy decrease filling pressures.[81] If diuretic therapy is used without vasodilators, the reduction in intravascular volume

could decrease CO and increase RAA system activation. Excessive diuresis leads to hypotension and worsening azotemia, which make initiation and titration of afterload-reducing agents such as angiotensin-converting enzyme (ACE) inhibitors difficult. Initiation of vasodilator therapy augmented with modest doses of diuretics can quickly stabilize most patients with ADHF.[81]

For patients who need added support to improve CO, small doses of a positive inotropic agent (such as inamrinone [Inocor], dobutamine [Dobutrex], or milrinone [Primacor]) may be used.[164] These drugs must only be used in the short-term, as use of inotropic drugs in patients with heart failure increases the incidence of dysrhythmias and increases mortality. The Medication table on pp. 1116-1121 of Chapter 41 describes the most common vasoactive drugs used in the management of ADHF.

Overall, therapy can be guided according to the patient's hemodynamic profile on admission (Figure 12-9). Patients who present "warm and wet" usually do well after diuresis induced by intravenous diuretics. Occasionally, vasodilator therapy may be needed to enhance symptom relief by reducing afterload. The average diuresis for patients hospitalized with ADHF is 4 L.

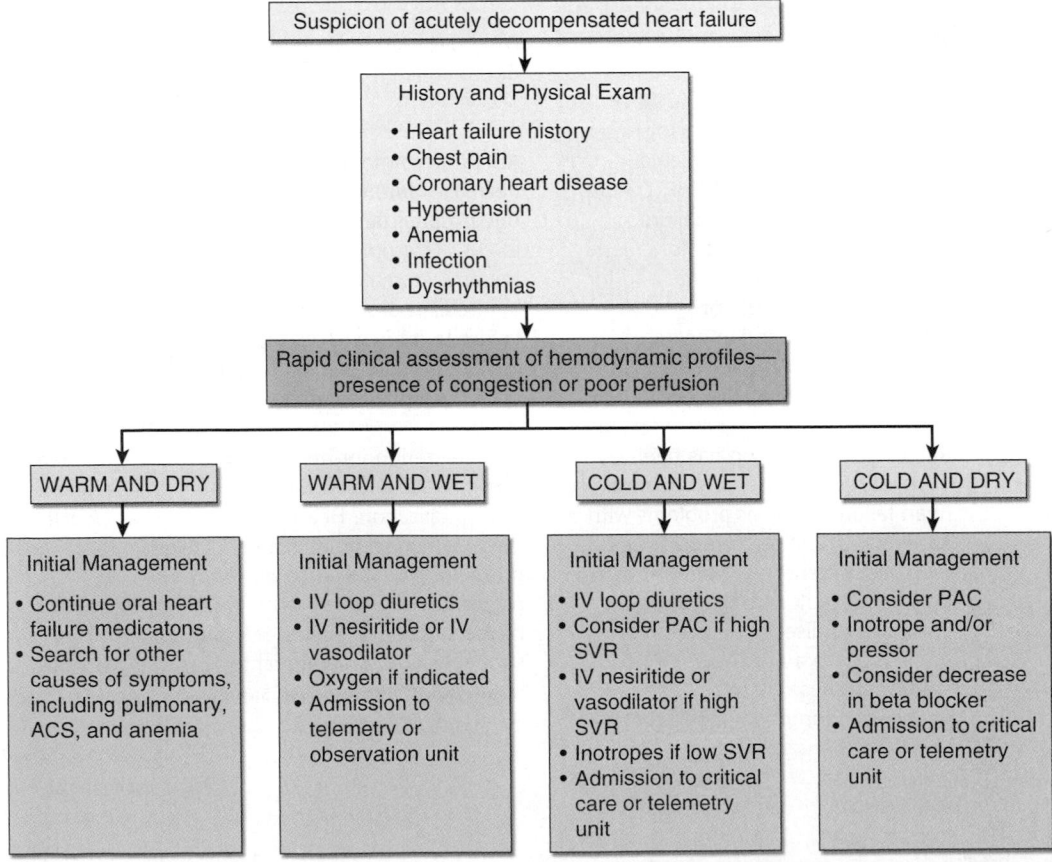

♦FIGURE 12-9 Management algorithm based on clinical severity classification for acute decompensated heart failure. ACS = Acute coronary syndrome, IV = intravenous, PAC = pulmonary artery catheterization, SVR = systemic vascular resistance.

MEDICATIONS FOR CHRONIC OUTPATIENT DRUG THERAPY

DRUG	INITIAL DOSE	MAXIMUM DOSE	SIDE EFFECTS	SPECIAL CONSIDERATIONS
Angiotensin-Converting Enzyme Inhibitor Therapy				
Captopril (Capoten)	6.25 mg tid	50 mg tid	Hypotension, hyperkalemia, renal insufficiency, cough, angioedema	Efforts to avoid sodium retention or depletion should be made, because volume imbalance affects effectiveness of ACE inhibitor therapy; fluid retention decreases benefits and fluid depletion increases potential for hypotension or renal insufficiency. NSAIDs adversely affect ACE inhibitor effectiveness and should be avoided.
Enalapril (Vasotec)	2.5 mg bid	10–20 mg bid		
Lisinopril (Zestril)	2.5–5 mg daily	20–40 mg daily		
Quinapril (Accupril)	5 mg bid	20 mg bid		
Ramipril (Altace)	1.25–2.5 mg daily	10 mg daily		
Angiotensin Receptor Blocking Agents				
Candesartan (Atacand)	4–8 mg daily	32 mg daily	Hypotension, hyperkalemia, worsening renal function, angioedema (less often than ACE inhibitors, but still occurs)	ACE inhibitors are first choice renin-angiotensin system antagonism. ARBs are an alternative in patients intolerant to ACE inhibitors because of refractory cough. ARBs appear to cause hypotension, worsening renal function, and hyperkalemia as often as ACE inhibitors.
Losartan (Cozaar)	25–50 mg daily	50–100 mg daily		
Valsartan (Diovan)	20–40 mg bid	160 mg bid		
Beta-Adrenergic Blocking Agents				
Bisoprolol (Zebeta)	1.25 mg daily	10 mg	Hypotension, bradycardia and heart block, fatigue, fluid retention, and worsening heart failure	Use with ACE inhibitors, but if hypotension a problem consider giving ACE inhibitors and beta blocker at different times of day. In patients with fluid overload, diuretics improve action of beta blockers by maintaining fluid and sodium balance. May increase fluid retention during initiation of therapy; close monitoring of fluid status by patient with daily weights is necessary. May take weeks to months for symptoms to improve, and beta blockers should be continued even if symptom status is unchanged because they protect against future adverse cardiac events.
Carvedilol (Coreg)	3.125 mg bid	25 mg bid or 50 mg bid for patients >85 kg; 50 mg bid for patients ≥85 kg		
Carvedilol CR (Coreg CR)	10 mg daily	80 mg daily		
Metoprolol CR/XL (Toprol XL)	12.5–25 mg daily	200 mg		
Diuretic Therapy				
Loop Diuretics				
Bumetanide (Bumex)	0.5–1 mg daily or bid	10 mg	Electrolyte depletion, hypotension, azotemia	Diuretics cannot be used alone for management of heart failure. By promoting fluid and sodium balance, diuretics enhance effectiveness of other heart failure medications. Care should be taken to avoid over- and underdiuresis. Diuretic equivalencies: bumetanide 1 mg = furosemide 40 mg = torsemide 10–20 mg
Furosemide (Lasix)	20–40 mg daily or bid	600 mg		
Torsemide (Demadex)	10–20 mg daily	200 mg		

Table continues on page 256

DRUG	INITIAL DOSE	MAXIMUM DOSE	SIDE EFFECTS	SPECIAL CONSIDERATIONS
Thiazides				
Chlorothiazide (Diuril)	250–500 mg daily or bid	1000 mg	Electrolyte depletion, hypotension, azotemia, photosensitivity	
Chlorthalidone (Hygroton)	25–50 mg daily	200 mg		
Hydrochlorothiazide (Microzide)	25 mg daily or bid	100 mg		
Indapamide (Lozol)	2.5 mg daily	5 mg		
Metolazone (Zaroxolyn)	5 mg daily	20 mg		
Potassium-Sparing Diuretics				
Amiloride (Midamor)	5–10 mg daily	20 mg	Hyperkalemia, volume depletion (particularly when taken with other diuretics)	Risk of hyperkalemia is increased by concomitant administration of ACE inhibitors.
Spironolactone (Aldactone)	12.5–25 mg daily	50 mg		
Triamterene (Dyrenium)	100 mg bid	300 mg		
Sequential Nephron Blockade				
Metolazone (Zaroxolyn)	2.5–10 mg once plus loop diuretic			
Hydrochlorothiazide (Microzide)	25–100 mg once or twice plus loop diuretic			
Chlorothiazide (IV)	500–1000 mg once plus loop diuretic			
Aldosterone Antagonist Therapy				
Eplerenone (Inspra)	25 mg daily	50 mg	Hyperkalemia, volume depletion (particularly when taken with other diuretics)	Used with other diuretics for management of severe symptomatic heart failure. Monitor renal function and potassium levels closely during therapy; monthly for first 3 months, then every 3 months.
Spironolactone (Aldactone)	12.5–25 mg daily	25–50 mg		

Modified from reference 135a.

ACE = Angiotensin-converting enzyme, ARB = angiotensin receptor blocker, bid = twice per day, NSAIDs = nonsteroidal antiinflammatory drugs, tid = three times per day.

Patients who present as "cold and wet" usually need vasodilation in order to increase CO and decrease filling pressures before initiating diuretic therapy. The mitral regurgitant flow that is increased in the presence of elevated afterload may consume up to 75% of total stroke volume. By unloading the ventricle and improving CO, mitral regurgitant flow may be markedly reduced.[166] Low doses of dopamine (Intropin), dobutamine, or milrinone may help improve contractility in these patients, but at the expense of increasing risk of dysrhythmias or ischemia.[164] Thus if therapy with these agents is chosen, vigilance is needed to detect these complications.

Patients who present "cold and dry" are the most difficult to manage. They should be carefully evaluated to make sure that filling pressures are not actually elevated. If filling pressures are truly reduced in these patients, a very cautious trial of fluid replacement may be attempted.[164] Treatment depends on the patient's clinical situation. Inotropic support may temporarily benefit the patient, but may lead to further deterioration. Additional afterload reduction with vasodilators may exacerbate hypotension.

Diuretics

Diuretics have never been subjected to randomized controlled trials. Yet they remain the most commonly used drugs in heart failure because of their ability to effectively treat volume overload and improve symptoms. Loop diuretics, such as furosemide (Lasix), bumetanide (Bumex), and torsemide (Demadex), are the most commonly used. Diuretics are initially given intravenously, resulting in a reduction in filling pressures and intravascular pressure. Consequently, fluid is mobilized from the interstitium back into the intravascular space, where it can be filtered by the kidney and excreted.

Loop diuretics are short-acting, lasting about 6 hours. After the drug effect wears off, the RAA system will become activated because of a sudden decrease in sodium excretion. This will make subsequent daily doses of diuretic become less effective. Concomitant use of neurohormonal blocking agents, such as ACE inhibitors, will decrease this effect. Patients who do not respond to diuretic therapy may have "diuretic resistance," which occurs in 20% to 30% of patients with severe left ventricular dysfunction.[45a] Suggestions to improve diuretic effectiveness in patients with diuretic resistance include doubling the dose of diuretic, using a continuous infusion of the diuretic rather than bolus dosing, or adding a thiazide or thiazide-like diuretic, such as metolazone (Zaroxolyn), to the patient's medication regimen. The combination of a thiazide diuretic and a loop diuretic may result in electrolyte wasting, particularly potassium and sodium. Patients receiving these medications must be carefully monitored for electrolyte disturbances, and any resulting deficiencies should be corrected.

The term "cardiorenal syndrome" has been coined to describe those patients in whom renal function declines progressively while diuresis relieves symptoms of ADHF. About 25% of patients hospitalized with heart failure have aggravated renal dysfunction, which can lead to prolonged hospitalization and increased mortality.[91] Preexisting renal insufficiency can be aggravated with diuretic therapy, use of ACE inhibitors or angiotensin receptor blockers (ARBs), and infusion of nesiritide.[152] The main components of cardiorenal syndrome include an increase in serum creatinine level, diuretic resistance, anemia, hyperkalemia, and decreased systolic blood pressure.

Parameters to identify patients at risk for the development and progression of renal dysfunction include admission BUN level greater than or equal to 43 mg/dl and serum creatinine level greater than or equal to 2.75 mg/dl.[50] Temporary inotropic support may improve CO and attenuate the cardiorenal syndrome, but renal function often declines once again after inotropic support has been removed.[164] Renal function may improve over several weeks if the patient maintains a lower volume status. Discontinuation of ACE inhibitors or ARB therapy may be required with transition to hydralazine (Apresoline) and nitrate combination if the serum creatinine level rises by greater than 25% of baseline during acute exacerbation treatment and fails to fall back to baseline, or if the BUN level remains above 80 to 100 mg/dl.[164]

Generally, patients should respond to diuretic therapy within 2 to 3 hours. Fluid-overloaded patients who are refractory to maximal medical therapy (i.e., diuretics, vasodilators, and inotropic agents) may require hemofiltration to relieve fluid overload. This procedure is similar to hemodialysis, except that only water is extracted; the large fluctuations in electrolyte levels or acid-base balance are avoided. As short-term therapy for diuretic-refractory ADHF, hemofiltration relieves symptoms of pulmonary edema, reduces ascites and peripheral edema, and enhances the subsequent response to diuretics.[21] Though shown to be effective in a subset of patients, hemofiltration has not been a widely used treatment in ADHF. One reason is the need for central line access and the inherent risks involved with invasive lines and anticoagulation.

Vasodilators

When used, vasodilator therapy should be initiated early in patients with ADHF. Vasodilating drugs do not directly improve cardiac function but rather they reduce preload and afterload, which increases forward flow. Together with diuretic therapy, vasodilators improve CO by unloading the heart and reducing mitral regurgitation, while decreasing neurohormone levels.

Nitroprusside. Nitroprusside was the first intravenous vasodilator shown to improve CO in heart failure. With a half-life of approximately 2 minutes, nitroprusside has a very rapid onset and offset and is easily titrated or weaned. Nitroprusside is titrated up by 10 to 20 mcg/min every 10 to 20 minutes, with a goal of lowering the PAWP to 16 mm Hg without causing the systolic blood pressure to fall below 80 mm Hg. Dosages are usually measured as absolute doses, but may also be defined as micrograms per kilogram per minute, ranging from 0.5 mcg/kg/min to 10 mcg/kg/min. Dosage requirements will vary from patient to patient. Some patients may have improved filling pressures at 50 mcg/min, whereas others require up to 400 mcg/min.

Side effects from nitroprusside include nausea, vomiting, and disorientation, particularly if the infusion continues for more than 48 hours.[124] The most serious danger of nitroprusside is cyanide toxicity, which is most likely to occur in patients with reduced hepatic or renal function. If cyanide toxicity is suspected, the infusion should be discontinued and no further treatment is usually required.

Nitroglycerin. Nitroglycerin is predominantly a venodilator with mild arteriolar vasodilating effects. It has a rapid onset of action, usually within 3 to 5 minutes, and may be rapidly titrated to hemodynamic goals. It is most effective in pulmonary edema related to myocardial ischemia, but is an effective vasodilator in ADHF as well. The tubing used for administration may affect the dose because of adsorption of drug. If polyvinyl chloride (PVC) tubing is used, dosing is usually initiated at 20 mcg/min and increased by 20-mcg increments until the hemodynamic goals are achieved.[164] If a non-PVC set is used, the dose should be initiated at 5 mcg/min with titration every 3 to 5 minutes. Larger dosing increments of 10 to 20 mcg/min may be used if no response is seen at 20 mcg/min. The most common side effect of nitroglycerin is headache, which can be treated with analgesics. Nitrate tolerance may occur after 4 to 8 hours of infusion but is usually overcome by increasing the dose. As with nitroprusside, hypotension may occur and the patient's blood pressure should be monitored frequently.

Nesiritide. Nesiritide is an intravenous vasodilator for the treatment of patients with ADHF that lowers preload and afterload. It is a recombinant form of BNP. Clinical response to nesiritide is usually rapid, with significant reduction in filling pressures and symptoms of dyspnea in 15 minutes.[134] Nesiritide potentiates diuretics, such that lower doses of diuretics may be used to reduce filling pressures. It also inhibits the RAA system, leading to a reduction in levels of plasma aldosterone and norepinephrine.[3] Nesiritide has a renal effect as an efferent arteriolar vasoconstrictor that augments the glomerular filtration rate and urine output and promotes sodium excretion.[79] Unlike nitroprusside or nitroglycerin, nesiritide may be infused safely in an intermediate care unit, emergency department, or observation unit and does not require critical care admission.

The recommended starting dose of nesiritide is a 2 mcg/kg bolus followed by an infusion of 0.01 mcg/kg/min until the desired hemodynamic profile is achieved. Many clinicians opt to start the infusion without a loading bolus for a more gradual onset of vasodilation.[188] Hypotension is rare, but may occur with nesiritide; thus close blood pressure monitoring is required. The half-life is about 20 minutes. If the patient becomes hypotensive, the infusion should be stopped until an adequate blood pressure is obtained. Once the blood pressure is stabilized, the nesiritide infusion may be restarted at a dose that is reduced by 30%. Nesiritide should not be infused through heparin-coated catheters or through the same intravenous tubing as heparin or furosemide.[188]

Inotropic Agents

The use of nesiritide and other vasodilators in ADHF is associated with better outcomes than the use of inotropic agents.[1] However, patients with end-stage heart failure resulting from contractile dysfunction may not benefit from receiving vasodilating agents. These patients with refractory hypoperfusion may require pharmacologic inotropic support or the use of an intra-aortic balloon pump or other cardiac support device.

Dobutamine. Dobutamine is a beta-adrenergic stimulating agent that exerts a potent inotropic effect, and a peripheral and pulmonary vasodilating effect. Inotropic therapy should only be used in situations in which improved contractility is the desired end point, and should be used for as short duration as possible because of the increased risk of tachydysrhythmias and increased ischemia. Situations that may require inotropic support include profound hypotension, inadequate renal perfusion, and multiorgan dysfunction until cardiac transplantation or left ventricular assist device insertion can be performed. It may also be used short-term following surgery or myocardial infarction.[164] Occasionally patients may become dependent on inotropic infusion for palliative support in end-stage heart failure and may be discharged from the hospital with a permanent intravenous catheter for home infusion.

Dosages usually start at 2 mcg/kg/min, titrating to the desired hemodynamic profile. Patients who are taking beta-adrenergic blocking agents may require slightly higher doses of dobutamine; however, dosage should not exceed 10 to 15 mcg/kg/min because of the possibility of inducing dysrhythmias.

Dopamine. Dopamine stimulates both alpha and beta receptors in the heart, as well as dopaminergic receptors that cause vasodilation in the renal and peripheral vasculature. At low doses, dopamine increases blood flow to the renal, mesenteric, coronary, and cerebral beds; however, at high doses it causes alpha-receptor stimulation and peripheral vasoconstriction.[124] By increasing renal blood flow, dopamine may improve diuresis by augmenting the effects of loop diuretics. The starting dosage of dopamine is 0.5 to 1 mcg/kg/min and is increased until the desired effect is achieved, such as increased urine output or improved blood pressure. Up to 3 mcg/kg/min, dopamine is predominantly vasodilatory; however, when a dosage of 5 mcg/kg/min is reached, alpha receptors are stimulated and it becomes a vasoconstrictor.[164] When dopamine is used as a vasoconstricting agent, weaning may have to be discontinued at 3 mcg/kg/min, because lower doses may promote vasodilation and will lower blood pressure. Like dobutamine, dopamine may promote tachydysrhythmias and ischemia.

Milrinone. Milrinone is a phosphodiesterase inhibitor that increases contractility by improving sarcolemma calcium uptake. It produces positive inotropic effects in the myocardium and promotes peripheral and pulmonary vasodilation through smooth muscle relaxation.[63] In contrast to dobutamine, milrinone does not compete for receptor sites in patients taking beta blockers. Hypotension may be a problem, so the patient's blood pressure should be monitored closely. If hypotension is the reason for inotropic support in a patient with ADHF, milrinone would not be the appropriate agent to use. Similar to other inotropic agents, milrinone may increase the frequency of tachydysrhythmias and ischemic events. The elimination half-life of milrinone is quite long, and is increased even further in the presence of renal failure. After weaning off milrinone, patients should be carefully observed for 48 hours.

The recent Outcomes of a Prospective Trial of Intravenous Milrinone for Exacerbations of Chronic Heart Failure (OPTIME-CHF) trial divulged that treatment with intravenous milrinone as an adjunct to standard medical care did not reduce the average length of hospital stay or mortality rate when compared with placebo. Furthermore, an increase in adverse events was seen in the patients receiving milrinone.[36a] Milrinone is excreted via the kidneys, so the dose should be reduced in patients with renal insufficiency. Milrinone may be used to support patients awaiting cardiac transplantation and can be infused either alone or in combination with dobutamine. It is also used as palliative care to improve symptoms and quality of life in end-stage patients with heart failure.

Other Vasoactive Agents

Occasionally, patients with ADHF require additional vasoconstricting agents. In patients with worsening circulatory status and life-threatening hypoperfusion, dopamine is the initial agent for blood pressure support. If dopamine fails to improve the patient's clinical status, intravenous epinephrine infusion may be necessary for short-term therapy. It provides profound vasoconstriction for stabilization of blood pressure until more definitive action may be taken, such as surgical intervention or insertion of a ventricular assist device. Epinephrine is given at a starting dose of 1 mcg/min and titrated until the patient's hemodynamics have been stabilized. Vasopressin (Pitressin) may be used in patients who maintain a systolic blood pressure of less than 70 mm Hg, despite maximum vasopressor therapy. It may be used for short periods at doses of 0.05 to 0.1 unit/min.[164] Powerful vasoconstricting agents can contribute to dysrhythmias and worsening ischemia, as well as necrosis of organs and extremities.[164]

Device Therapy

Many patients with heart failure who have low EF and are symptomatic also have a ventricular conduction delay with a prolonged QRS (greater than 0.12 ms) on ECG.[66] This conduction delay (left bundle branch block [LBBB]) produces ventricular dyssynchrony, which causes suboptimal ventricular filling because of shortened diastolic filling time. In addition, the LBBB causes septal contraction before activation of the lateral wall of the left ventricle, creating paradoxical septal wall motion. The prolonged QRS causes a more severe mitral regurgitation,[57] resulting in greater impairment of LV contractility.[63a] The hemodynamic consequences of the left atrioventricular mechanical delay are a decreased stroke volume and increased left atrial pressure as a result of the mitral regurgitation.[61a] Ventricular dyssynchrony has also been associated with an increased mortality and sudden death in heart failure patients.[15,190a]

Cardiac resynchronization therapy (CRT), or biventricular (BiV) pacing, coordinates the right and left ventricular contractions to resynchronize the ventricles, thus enhancing ventricular contraction and reducing the degree of mitral regurgitation.[116a,179] The pulse generator device used is approximately the same size as a standard pacemaker, but it allows for three lead connections to the right atrial lead, right ventricular lead, and left ventricular lead. The leads are placed transvenously, similar to a traditional pacemaker, with the addition of the left ventricular lead inserted through the coronary sinus into the coronary vein (Figure 12-10). Other than standard pacemaker insertion risks, specific risks of this implant procedure are that the left ventricular lead implant is unsuccessful about 8% of the time and that dissection or perforation of the coronary sinus occurs about 6% of the time.[2] Patients with BiV pacemakers should be afforded the same cautions as those with standard pacemakers: avoid magnetic resonance imaging, diathermy, high sources of radiation, electrosurgical cautery, lithotripsy, and radiofrequency ablation. External defibrillation pads should not be placed directly over the device.[6] The patient's ECG after CRT will depend on the conduction delay before implantation and device settings (Figure 12-11). The device should capture both the right and left ventricles, which will produce a smaller and narrower QRS, ST segment, and T wave.[6]

It has been shown that when added to optimal medical therapy in persistently symptomatic patients, CRT results in significant improvements in quality of life, functional class, exercise capacity, CO, and EF[2,26,189] as well as decreased hospitalizations.[34] Therefore the current recommendations are that symptomatic patients who have an EF less than or equal to 35%, are in sinus rhythm, have a QRS greater than 0.12 ms, and are NYHA functional class III or IV despite optimal medical therapy should receive CRT.[76]

Mortality is high in patients with heart failure with left ventricular dilation and reduced EF.[16,24] Patients frequently manifest ventricular tachydysrhythmias, both nonsustained and sustained. Implantable

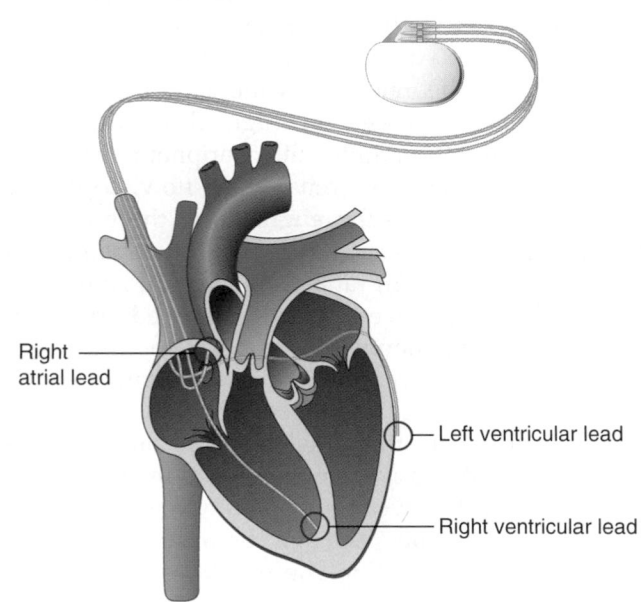

⬧FIGURE 12-10 Biventricular pacemaker with lead placement.

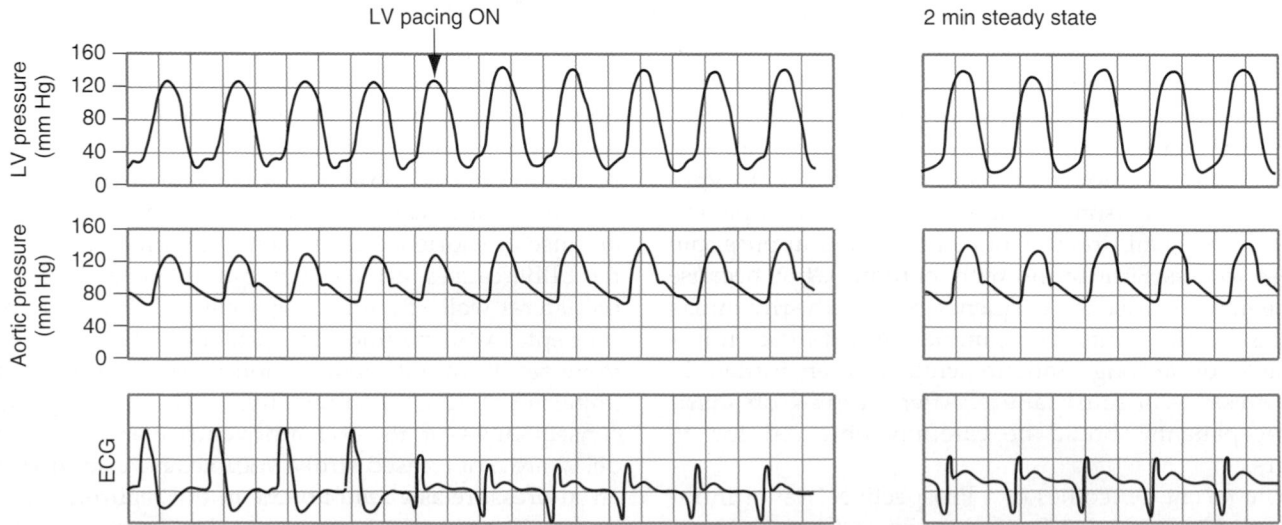

⬧FIGURE 12-11 Raw data tracings before, immediately on initiation of biventricular pacing, and after 2 minutes of steady-state left ventricular stimulation in patient with LBBB. ECG = Electrocardiogram, LV = left ventricle.

cardioverter-defibrillators (ICDs) have been found to reduce the risk of sudden death in patients with marked left ventricular dysfunction, regardless of etiology.[60,113] ICDs are now the treatment of choice in patients with left ventricular dysfunction who have survived sudden cardiac death; have symptomatic sustained ventricular tachycardia; have asymptomatic nonsustained but inducible ventricular tachycardia; or have an ischemic cardiomyopathy with an LVEF less than 30%.[75]

Managing Comorbidities

Most patients with heart failure have at least one comorbid condition complicating their treatment plan and negatively impacting outcomes. In those older than age 65, about 40% of people with heart failure have five or more noncardiac comorbid conditions.[23] Older adults hospitalized for heart failure have a high incidence of diabetes (38%), chronic lung disease (33%), atrial fibrillation (30%), and prior stroke (18%).[66] Those with multiple comorbid conditions have more frequent hospitalizations and a relatively higher mortality rate.

Chronic Lung Disease. Chronic lung disease, including chronic obstructive lung disease (OLD), asthma, and other lower respiratory tract diseases, is the most common comorbid condition found in patients with heart failure.[23] Refining the drug regimen in patients with these conditions can be challenging. Most problematic are bronchodilators, corticosteroids, loop diuretics, and digitalis. Beta blockers, important in heart failure therapy, are thought to be traditionally contraindicated in those with chronic lung disease. However, newer evidence demonstrates that these drugs can be used in persons with mild-to-moderate chronic lung disease.[13] Bronchodilators are important in chronic lung disease, but may increase mortality in patients with heart failure.[174,175] Corticosteroids used in chronic lung disease cause fluid retention, which makes fluid management more difficult in heart failure. Digoxin (Lanoxin) can cause pulmonary vasoconstriction, dysrhythmias secondary to hypoxia, and acidosis in persons with chronic lung disease. Loop diuretics can cause acidosis in those with chronic OLD because patients have increased minute ventilation, which can decrease respiratory drive and accentuate the risk of metabolic acidosis. Patients with both heart failure and chronic lung disease should be taught to seek care immediately with escalating dyspnea not relieved by their usual measures.

Renal Failure. Renal dysfunction is a common comorbidity and is one of the strongest predictors of mortality in patients with heart failure.[158] Chronic renal insufficiency, anemia, and heart failure commonly occur together as part of the cardio-renal syndrome. Anemia is present in 15% to 55% of patients with heart failure.[129] Anemia is associated with worse functional status, malnutrition, and increased morbidity and mortality. Even appropriate drug therapy can fail to improve heart failure if anemia is untreated. When anemia is corrected with erythropoietin and iron therapy, LVEF, symptoms, and exercise capacity improve.[129]

Diabetes Mellitus. Diabetes is present in about 20% to 25% of patients with heart failure.[64] The metabolic consequences of diabetes (i.e., elevated proinsulin level, hyperinsulinemia, and hyperglycemia) adversely affect the vascular endothelium to cause accelerated atherosclerosis. Insulin resistance has been linked with cardiovascular remodeling.[59] When diabetes and heart failure coexist, morbidity and mortality are significantly increased,[64] especially in heart failure patients with an ischemic etiology.[39]

ACE inhibitors, the first line of drug therapy for heart failure, have additional benefits for patients with diabetes because they improve glucose handling. Another important component of drug therapy in heart failure, beta-adrenergic blockade, was formerly thought to be contraindicated in diabetic patients. Nonetheless, many clinicians carefully monitored their patients and used beta blockers without problem. Recently, BEST (Beta-Blocker Evaluation of Survival Trial) demonstrated in heart failure patients with diabetes that bisoprolol (Zebeta) therapy reduced death, heart failure hospitalizations, total hospitalizations, and the incidence of acute myocardial infarction.[39] A meta-analysis subsequently confirmed the finding of a mortality benefit in patients with diabetes and heart failure.[64] Thiazolidinediones (TZDs) are likely to be of cardiovascular benefit in patients with diabetes and heart failure because they improve insulin sensitivity.[59] TZDs can cause edema or weight gain as a result of fluid retention, and monitoring is required.

Anxiety and Depression. Anxiety and depression are the most common expression of emotional distress, and are common in heart failure. Approximately 11% to 25% of heart failure outpatients and 35% to 70% of those hospitalized are depressed.[83] Heart failure patients with depression have a substantially greater risk of functional decline, rehospitalization, and death than those who are not depressed.[176]

Although anxiety is an important, debilitating symptom of heart failure, few investigators have studied this response. A recent comparison of heart failure patients, acute myocardial infarction patients, coronary artery bypass patients, and healthy older adults revealed that although patients with heart failure have anxiety levels similar to the other cardiac groups, they have substantially more anxiety than healthy older adults.[109]

Dracup and colleagues[41] studied the relationship between perceived control and anxiety, depression, and hostility and demonstrated that heart failure patients with low perceived control were more anxious, more depressed, and more hostile than those with perceptions of greater control. Perceived control can be increased by promoting self-care, and with comprehensive education and counseling.

Assessing Stability for Hospital Discharge

Persistently high rates of readmission, especially within the first month of discharge, continue to be a problem in persons with heart failure. Recent data demonstrating that many patients with heart failure are discharged with multiple unaddressed risk factors for rehospitalization[132] highlight the need to ensure true readiness for discharge. Patients should be assessed and should meet specific criteria before they are discharged (Box 12-9).[54,62,108,164]

Box 12-9

Criteria for Discharge After Hospitalization for Acute Decompensated Heart Failure

- Reversible causes of heart failure are treated.
- Exacerbating causes of heart failure are corrected, if possible.
- Congestion is relieved (i.e., definition of and achievement of dry weight, absence of orthopnea, absence of or minimal edema).
- Oral drug regimen is established (i.e., oral diuretic, potassium replacement, and ACE inhibitor doses stable for 24 hours; no intravenous inotropes for 48 hours).
- Stability of noncardiac illnesses, including vital signs and laboratory values (e.g., sodium, potassium, creatinine), is achieved.
- Plans for home care are made, if needed (i.e., scale at home, arrangement of visiting nurse or phone follow-up within 3 days).
- Written information is prepared for patients (i.e., medication schedule, scheduled cardiologist follow-up information, indications for urgent call to healthcare provider, 24-hour phone number of clinician familiar with prescribed regimen).
- Determination is made of social or financial barriers to adherence with prescribed regimen or safe return to home.
- Patient and family/caregiver education has begun and plans for its continuation after discharge are made.

Pressures to decrease the length of hospital stay have resulted in earlier discharges. A common reason for early rehospitalization is that patients are discharged before they are able to meet criteria that indicate readiness. One team of investigators tested the effect of adherence to clinical stability criteria plus receipt of a target dose of ACE inhibitor before hospital discharge.[101] Before using this approach, 20% of heart failure patients were readmitted within 30 days. After implementing this approach, the problem with early hospital readmissions was totally eliminated. This trial dramatically illustrates the potential effects of adherence to clinical guidelines and a sensible approach to ensuring clinical stability before discharging patients.

Pharmacologic Therapy: Chronic Management

Once patients with ADHF are stabilized, it is important to assess their current chronic drug therapy, begin to take steps to optimize therapy using current guidelines, and ensure that inappropriate drugs are discontinued to avoid further episodes of decompensation. Starting appropriate drugs during hospitalization or making sure that they are continued after discharge is one method of ensuring optimal outpatient drug therapy.[126]

It is essential that critical care nurses advocate for use of evidence-based pharmacologic therapy in their patients. The appropriate therapy improves symptoms, enhances functional status, reduces the risk of hospitalization, and increases survival,[68,75] yet too many patients still do not receive appropriate therapy.[55] Routine pharmacologic therapy for patients with heart failure with nonpreserved left ventricular function consists of an ACE inhibitor (or ARB if patient is truly unable to take an ACE inhibitor), a beta-adrenergic blocking agent, and diuretics. Aldosterone antagonists, digoxin, and hydralazine/nitrates are added in appropriate patients. Details of outpatient drug therapy are outlined in the Medication table on pp. 255-256. The importance of neurohumoral activation to the pathophysiology of heart failure is demonstrated by the finding that only neurohumoral blocking drugs (i.e., ACE inhibitors, beta-adrenergic blockers, and aldosterone antagonists) increase survival. Thus their use is essential in the management of heart failure.[75]

Calcium channel blockers, even newer generation formulations, should be avoided in heart failure because they stimulate neurohumoral activation.[68] Two recent trials of newer generation calcium channel blockers, amlodipine (Norvasc) (the prospective randomized amlodipine survival evaluation [PRAISE] trial) and felodipine (Plendil) (V-HeFT III), in patients with heart failure suggest that these drugs may have beneficial effects, although further studies are needed. Also to be avoided in heart failure are antidysrhythmic agents (with the exception of amiodarone [Cordarone]) because they have cardiodepressant and prodysrhythmic effects that negatively affect survival. Nonsteroidal antiinflammatory agents should be avoided because they can cause sodium retention and decrease the efficacy of ACE inhibitors.

Underuse of Optimal Therapy. Several investigative teams have demonstrated a consistent failure of providers to use clinical guidelines.[33,90] In a recent study, only 55% of a cohort of 960 patients hospitalized with heart failure were discharged on an ACE inhibitor.[27] Of these, only 77.1% had filled the prescription within 30 days after discharge and only 63.3% were current users at 1 year. An important additional finding was that patients who were not started on an ACE inhibitor during hospitalization were unlikely to have started the medication after discharge. A recent study of 30,228 Medicare patients hospitalized with heart failure disclosed regional differences in the pattern of ACE inhibitor prescriptions, with prescribing rates varying from 56% to 87%.[67] Adherence to guidelines is a predictor of better outcomes in patients with heart failure.[87]

Nonpharmacologic Therapy

Nonpharmacologic therapy assumes its greatest importance after the initial acute phase has passed. Nonpharmacologic therapies are essential to slowing heart failure progression, improving quality of life, and preventing rehospitalization. There is also evidence that comprehensive education and counseling, the cornerstone of nonpharmacologic therapy, improves survival.[89] Improving these outcomes depends in large part on adoption of good self-care practices by patients and their families. Although critical care nurses may feel that they have only cursory responsibility for promoting self-care as it is largely an outpatient activity, all nurses must understand the complexity of self-care before they can adequately teach patients to adopt it. Education and counseling, along with reinforcement of what has already been learned, needs to begin as soon as possible. Thus it is essential that critical care nurses have a comprehensive understanding of the self-care process.

Self-Care. Self-care consists of two processes: self-care maintenance (i.e., behaviors that maintain physiologic stability, including treatment adherence) and self-care management (i.e., recognizing and managing escalating symptoms).[145]

Self-Care Maintenance. The healthy behaviors that keep the patient with heart failure physiologically stable and that must be taught to each patient or his or her family caregivers include the following:

- Monitor daily weights and take action (call healthcare provider or take extra diuretic doses if prescribed by provider) for any 2-day 3-pound weight gain or 1-week 3- to 5-pound weight gain.
- Follow a low-sodium diet.
- Take medications as prescribed.
- Prevent infections (including obtaining annual flu vaccination and Pneumovax every 5 years).
- Modify unhealthy lifestyle behaviors, such as smoking, inactivity, or excess alcohol intake.

Adherence is a fundamental element of self-care, but one that is very difficult for patients. The difficulties with adherence faced by many patients are illustrated in Table 12-1, which shows results of a study describing self-care practices followed early after discharge by 202 patients with chronic heart failure.[108]

Daily Weighing. Daily weighing is useful for monitoring fluid status, yet fewer than half of all patients weigh themselves daily,[71] even when newly discharged from a hospitalization for ADHF.[108] One reason may be failure of providers to recommend daily weighing[51] or failure to teach patients the rationale behind daily weighing.[73] Patients should be taught the fundamentals of daily weighing at each hospitalization: weigh every day under similar conditions, log weight, and call provider with increases in weight.

Dietary Sodium Restriction. Fluid overload secondary to excess dietary sodium intake is one of the most common proximate causes of ADHF.[180] Less than half of patients adequately limit dietary sodium,[180] and this number does not improve even after a recent hospitalization for ADHF.[108] Patients have difficulty adhering for a number of reasons including the following: (1) inadequate knowledge about how to follow a low-sodium diet; (2) lack of helpful instructions from providers; (3) lack of skill in applying knowledge gained; (4) difficulties eating with family and friends, or eating out; (5) age-related changes in smell and taste that add to the unpalatability of salt restriction; and (6) lack of motivation.[17,72,117] The Nutrition box on p. 264 provides more information on prescribing a low-sodium diet.

Medication Adherence. Medication nonadherence is common and has been demonstrated in more than half of heart failure patients.[117,180] Poor medication adherence is associated with increased rates of hospitalization, longer lengths of hospital stay, and higher

TABLE 12-1   Percentage of Chronic Heart Failure Patients Adhering to Selected Discharge Recommendations*

WEIGHING BEHAVIOR, %	
Daily	14
Weekly	17
Monthly	22
Never	47

Knowledge of Symptoms of Worsening Heart Failure, %	
Knew greater than two symptoms	16
Knew at least one symptom	53
Did not know any symptoms	31

Monitored for Symptoms of Worsening Heart Failure, %	9

Medication Adherence, %	
Taking all medications as prescribed and not taking unprescribed medications	34
Taking all prescribed medications plus greater than one not prescribed	12
Not taking all prescribed medications and not taking unprescribed medications	28
Not taking all prescribed medications and taking medications not prescribed	26

Low-Sodium Diet Adherence, %	
Stated their physician did not prescribe a low-sodium diet	20
Followed a low-sodium diet and could calculate sodium content	8
Followed a low-sodium diet, but could not calculate sodium content	5
Did not follow a low-salt diet, but could calculate sodium content	12
Did not follow a low-salt diet and could not calculate sodium content	55

*N = 202 patients newly discharged from a hospitalization for exacerbation of chronic heart failure.[108]

mortality.[31] Patients who should be screened carefully for medication nonadherence are those who are unmarried or unsupported, taking multiple medications, and low in self-efficacy.[47,117] Box 12-10 describes ways to improve medication adherence.

Preventing Infection. All patients with heart failure should receive an annual influenza vaccination, and anyone older than age 2 with heart failure should receive a pneumonia vaccination every 5 years. Vaccination for pneumonia is particularly important for any heart failure patient who is exposed to cigarette smoke.[161]

▲ NUTRITION

Nutrition: Prescribing a Low-Sodium Diet

- Restricting sodium to about 2 to 3 g per day improves clinical presentation and increases sensitivity to diuretics.
  - For patients with mild heart failure, a 3-gram sodium diet is usually sufficient.
  - For most patients with more advanced heart failure, especially those who require large doses of diuretics, prescribe a 2-g sodium diet.
- Begin with a thorough assessment of the patient's current sodium intake and eating habits: "What did you eat for each meal and snack for the past few days?"
- Assess the patient's knowledge of the sodium content of foods.
- To assess skill in choosing low-sodium foods, keep a supply of food containers and ask patients to sort them into low-, medium-, and high-sodium foods.
- Include both the patient and the family/caregiver in all dietary education and counseling sessions, particularly when the family/caregiver buys the food and cooks meals.
- Remember that eating is a social endeavor and include instructions for patient and family about eating out in restaurants and choosing foods at social gatherings.
- Provide specific instructions about how to achieve the prescribed sodium restriction, with provision of carefully chosen resource materials (e.g., the Heart Failure Society of America's educational module *How to Follow a Low-Sodium Diet,* available free at www.hfsa.org/hf_modules.asp).
- Suggest substitutions for high-sodium foods and medicines.
- Consider referral to a registered dietitian or advanced practice nurse with expertise in diet counseling.
- Referral for dietary counseling is particularly important for patients from diverse cultural backgrounds and for those having difficulty adapting their preferences to a low-salt diet.

Modified from reference 135a.

Alcohol Restriction. Because there are no prospective studies of the impact of alcohol consumption on heart failure, there is controversy about what to tell patients, and providers differ in their advice.[146] Patients with heart failure commonly are asked to abstain totally from drinking alcohol because of its

Box 12-10

Techniques for Improving Medication Adherence

- Remember that knowledge is necessary but not sufficient to achieve medication compliance.
- Engage the patient to undertake a greater personal role (self-care) in managing heart failure.
- Identify patients able to self-dose and teach these patients how to medicate with diuretics and potassium based on changes in body weight.
- Use once-a-day dosing whenever possible.
- Consider providing pre-prepared pill dispensers, particularly for patients having visual or cognitive difficulties and without a source of social support.
- Assess potential barriers to medication adherence such as lack of knowledge, memory problems, illiteracy, depression, financial difficulty.
- Make sure that all pill bottles are labeled in large print with the drug name and dosing regimen.
- Provide patients with an updated medication list at each visit.
- Carefully educate patients about taking only medications prescribed and clarify prescriptions, particularly when there is more than one provider.
- Do not assume that patients are taking all of their medicines all of the time. Be open to hearing about problems and working through solutions: "Lots of patients have trouble taking their water pills on a regular basis. Are you having this problem? Other problems?"

Modified from reference 135a.

TABLE 12-2 Alcohol Recommendations for Persons With Heart Failure

RECOMMENDATION	RATIONALE
Carefully consider cause of heart failure before advising patients about use of alcohol. Someone with ischemic left ventricular dysfunction can probably consume one standard (12 g of alcohol) drink on an occasional basis if taken with a meal.	Evidence is accumulating that small amounts of alcohol provide some physiologic benefit for persons with ischemic heart disease. Food slows absorption of alcohol and moderates physiologic effects.
Avoid alcohol if heart failure is a result of nonischemic causes or alcoholic cardiomyopathy.	There are no data to support benefit of alcohol in someone without ischemic heart disease. There is some indication that alcohol consumption may increase hospitalization rates. Alcoholic cardiomyopathy responds favorably to alcohol abstinence.
Avoid alcohol in persons with major depression, anxiety disorder, behavioral disorder, sleep disorders.	Alcohol can interfere with effectiveness of some antidepressants, complicate a psychiatric condition, and interfere with sleep.
Avoid alcohol in persons with recurrent dysrhythmias, a history of hypertension, and diabetes.	Dysrhythmias and high blood pressure could be accentuated. The sugar content of alcohol could complicate control of diabetes.
Women should drink less alcohol than men.	Alcohol is metabolized differently in men and women.
Always avoid intoxication, drinks high in alcohol content (greater than 60%), and those with additives.	Hemodynamic effects of alcohol are accentuated at higher doses.

From reference 135a.

presumed myocardial depressant effects, although these effects have not been demonstrated in heart failure and are thought to be minor and transient.[131] Recommendations for alcohol intake in heart failure patients based on current data are summarized in Table 12-2.

Exercise. An important goal for patients with heart failure is maintenance of functional capacity and quality of life. A meta-analysis of 9 studies with 801 patients revealed a survival advantage in the 395 persons randomized to exercise training.[132] A Cochrane review concluded that exercise training improved short-term aerobic capacity and quality of life in persons with mild to moderate heart failure.[135] Exercise is beneficial for those with mild to moderate heart failure, and ongoing studies are defining its role in patients with severe heart failure. Although questions may remain about the specifics of prescribing activity for patients with heart failure, it is clear that inactivity is damaging and activity should be encouraged.

Self-Care Management. In addition to self-care *mainte-nance* behaviors, individuals with heart failure also must engage in self-care *management*. Self-care management is the use of problem-solving skills, decision making, and rapid assessment of new signs and symptoms. One key to self-care management is symptom recognition;[30,142] thus critical care nurses can play an important role in preparing patients to assume self-care by teaching them how to monitor for and recognize escalating symptoms.

Patients with heart failure encounter considerable difficulty recognizing their own worsening symptoms.[30,142] The reasons for this are unclear, but likely include failure of nurses to teach patients in an understandable way which symptoms to watch for and how to recognize worsening symptoms[51,73] as well as failure of patients to follow recommendations once they are given.[108] Patients commonly wait hours to days before responding to escalating dyspnea, something that is quite hard for clinicians to understand. Yet, for patients with heart failure who have never been taught how to gauge worsening dyspnea, who may have experienced worsening and then spontaneously improving dyspnea, and who encounter system difficulties whenever they try to contact their healthcare provider, waiting until symptoms are unbearably severe may seem appropriate.[110]

Individuals most likely to master heart failure self-care are those who are more highly educated,[47] have experience with the diagnosis,[145] have received patient education,[128] and have support from others.[128] Factors that impair self-care include financial hardship, low health literacy, impaired cognition, poor functional status, and sensory impairments.[142]

◆ Case Study 12-1, Part C

Etiology of Heart Failure

R.S. continued to improve during her hospitalization. She demonstrated skills taught to her and verbalized new appreciation for why symptom and weight monitoring was important. Because she had trouble seeing the number on the scale, her children bought her a new scale with large digital numbers, and a diary for recording her weights and symptoms. Additional teaching was done to try to avoid confusion regarding diabetes and heart failure requirements. Workup of anemia revealed no apparent bleeding sources, and her anemia was attributed to chronic heart failure. She was referred for consideration for iron erythropoietin therapy. Her children worked out a schedule where they could check on her more frequently and provide greater support for her as she assumed self-care for her heart failure.

Decision point: What nonpharmacologic therapies are essential for R.S. after discharge?

Heart Failure Disease Management

Although most critical care nurses are not involved directly in heart failure disease management, they should understand its usefulness and advocate for its use in patients at risk for rehospitalization. In addition, the principles of successful heart failure disease management can be adopted and used by critical care nurses. Disease management involves practice redesign with increased availability of experts, use of evidence-based guidelines, improved education and counseling, and use of monitored outcomes to improve care processes.[46,192] Although a few reports have demonstrated a neutral or negative impact of heart failure disease management,[45,78,143,184] the majority of heart failure disease management programs, regardless of type, have demonstrated positive outcomes. Disease management has been shown to (1) improve patients' heart failure knowledge,[71,94] (2) facilitate health behavior change that improves self-care,[78] including treatment adherence and symptom management, (3) improve symptoms and functional status, and (4) improve clinical outcomes such as rehospitalization rates, hospitalization costs, and mortality.* Stewart and Horowitz, among others, demonstrated a survival advantage on long-term follow-up for patients who participated in a home-based disease management intervention.[170] This body of literature now provides compelling evidence for the superiority of heart failure disease management over usual care.[111,171]

Applying Heart Failure Disease Management Principles. Despite the superiority of heart failure disease management for outpatient management, only a minority of heart failure patients are cared for using these care delivery models. Assuming that non-adherence is the result of patient, provider, and healthcare system factors, a concerted effort to influence each of these components will have the best chance of improving outcomes in this challenging patient population, as explained in the Research Utilization box on p. 267. Thus appropriate patients should be referred to heart failure disease management programs when possible.[68] However, heart failure disease management programs are not available to the majority of patients and providers. In such cases, it is possible for providers to employ the principles of heart failure disease management in their practice (Box 12-11).[112]

---

*References 22, 32, 35, 40, 53, 65, 69, 71, 78, 89, 99, 107, 115, 128, 136–141, 144, 149, 154, 157, 162, 168, 170, 173–175, 185.

RESEARCH UTILIZATION

Effectiveness of Comprehensive Disease Management in Improving Clinical Outcomes in Heart Failure Patients

CLINICAL ISSUE

Heart failure rehospitalization rates are extremely high, and most hospitalizations are thought to be preventable with better care delivery. Heart failure disease management enhances patient adherence and provider adherence to treatment guidelines. Randomized controlled trials of heart failure disease management have included relatively small numbers of subjects to date, and the impact on mortality is unclear.

SUMMARY

This meta-analysis included studies located through a systematic literature search. Only randomized controlled trials of heart failure patients who were allocated to disease management or usual care were included. A study quality assessment was performed. The main clinical outcomes assessed were all-cause mortality and rehospitalizations, and heart failure rehospitalizations and mortality. Thirty-three trials were included. Mortality was significantly reduced by disease management compared with usual care: OR = 0.80 (CI 0.69–0.93, $p = 0.003$). All-cause and heart failure–related hospitalization rates were also reduced: OR = 0.76 (CI 0.69–0.94, $p < 0.00001$) and OR = 0.58 (CI 0.50–0.67, $P < 0.00001$), respectively. Different disease management approaches appeared to be equally effective.

APPLICATION

Patients at risk for hospitalizations for ADHF should be referred to a heart failure disease management program to reduce mortality and hospitalizations. Various types of disease management appear to be equally effective, so the choice of a specific program depends on characteristics of local health services, patient population, and resources available.

NEED FOR FURTHER STUDY

Future investigations should seek to uncover the components of disease management programs necessary for improved outcomes and how to promote widespread use of heart failure disease management.

Roccaforte, R., et al. (2005). Effectiveness of comprehensive disease management programmes in improving clinical outcomes in heart failure patients. A meta-analysis. *Eur J Heart Fail, 7*, 1133–1144.

Nutrition Management. Ignored for years, there is now increased interest in the role of nutrition in the management of patients with heart failure. Table 12-3 provides a list of nutrients known to be important in the

Box 12-11

Components of Successful Heart Failure Disease Management Programs

- Promote patient self-care.
- Assess and address patient factors that affect adherence and ability to engage in self-care.
- Include family members and other informal caregivers.
- Identify and target patients who are at high risk for rehospitalization.
- Employ components of heart failure disease management programs that improve outcomes.
- Use behavioral strategies to increase adherence.
- Provide individualized, comprehensive patient and family or caregiver education and counseling on an outpatient basis that includes the following:
  - Optimization of medical therapy
  - Vigilant follow-up
  - Increased access to healthcare professionals
  - Early attention to fluid overload
  - Coordination with other agencies as appropriate
  - Physician-directed care with assistance from nurse coordinators or nurse-managed care by experienced advanced practice cardiovascular nurses with access to a cardiologist

Modified from reference 135a.

management of heart failure.[18,159] Heart failure is viewed as a complex disorder with a major systemic inflammatory component.[36,85,96,98,104]

Proinflammatory cytokines, including TNFα and IL-6, in conjunction with other inflammatory mediators, directly or indirectly elicit catabolism of protein-based tissues, fluid and sodium retention, and altered nutritional intake and metabolism.[98] In addition, body fat may affect the underlying inflammatory processes in heart failure, and thus it is important to address recent data suggesting that increased body fat improves outcomes.

Nutrient deficiencies have been identified even in the normal or high body weight patients. In one study,[12] the majority of patients had a negative caloric balance, negative nitrogen balance, and malnutrition. Others have found deficiencies in calcium, folic acid, manganese, riboflavin, thiamine, and zinc in hospitalized patients.[61] Dietary deficiency in magnesium appears common in patients with heart failure. Diuretics increase magnesium loss as well as the loss of many other water-soluble micronutrients such as thiamine, calcium, and vitamin C.[186] These data suggest that poor nutritional intake may be present in a large number of patients who do not appear cachectic. Thus nutritional intake should be assessed in all patients with heart failure, regardless of whether they appear malnourished.

TABLE 12-3 Nutrients Important in Managing Heart Failure

NUTRIENT	ROLES	RECOMMENDED DAILY INTAKE
Protein*	Major component of lean body mass and all biologically active molecules in body	1 g/kg
Calories	Provide energy for all metabolic processes	Underweight: 32 kcal/kg Normal weight: 28 kcal/kg
Fat	Provides energy and essential substrates for cell membranes	Saturated <10% of kcal Trans <2% of kcal Omega-3 fatty acids 1.3 g
Calcium*	Necessary for bone metabolism and muscle contraction	1200 mg Note: requirement may be higher for patients taking loop diuretics
Folate Vitamin B$_{12}$	Folate converts homocysteine to harmless compound; B$_{12}$ is a cofactor in this conversion pathway	Folate: 400 mcg B$_{12}$: 2.4 mcg
Iron	Important element in a number of proteins, enzymes, and oxygen-carrying component of hemoglobin	Males: 8 mg Postmenopausal females: 8 mg Premenopausal females: 18 mg
Magnesium*	Activation of cellular sodium-potassium pumps; endogenous calcium channel blocker	Males: 420 mg Females: 320 mg Note: requirement may be higher for patients taking loop or thiazide diuretics
Vitamin C	Antioxidant properties, plus maintains tissue levels of vitamins A and E	Males: 90 mg Females: 75 mg
Vitamin D*	Essential for intestinal absorption of calcium	<70 yr: 10 mcg ≥70 yr: 15 mcg
Vitamin E	Antioxidant properties	15 mg[95] Note: intake >400 mg may be associated with an increase in all-cause mortality
Potassium	Maintains necessary electrical voltage difference across cell membranes to generate electrical impulse for nerve conduction and cardiac muscle contraction	4.7 g Note: requirement may be higher for patients prescribed loop and thiazide diuretics and lower for patients taking ACE inhibitors, angiotensin receptor blockers, and aldosterone inhibitors
Selenium	Incorporated into several antioxidant proteins essential to prevent cellular free radical damage	55 mcg
Sodium	Primary component of osmotic fluid pressure; generation of nerve impulses and muscle contraction	<2300 mg Advanced heart failure: ≤2000 mg
Thiamine*	Coenzyme in many physiologic functions, including carbohydrate metabolism and maintenance of myelin necessary for proper nerve and muscle function	Males: 1.2 mg Females: 1.1 mg Note: requirement may be higher for patients prescribed loop diuretics
Water	Largest component of human body; essential for cellular homeostasis	Advanced heart failure with hyponatremia: ≤2 liters

Modified from reference 92a.
*Nutrients with the greatest likelihood of being deficient in patients with heart failure.

Of the three macronutrients—protein, carbohydrates, and fats—protein is the only nutrient capable of being transformed into all of the other macronutrients.[127] Protein is essential for maintaining lean body mass and is the major component of all biologically active molecules in the body. Protein depletion can impair metabolism, adversely affect immune function, lead to muscle (including organ muscle) wasting, and, in severe cases, cause death.[38] Despite the fact that the protein intake of patients was comparable to that of similarly healthy controls, most patients with heart failure in a recent study presented with negative nitrogen balance.[12] This finding suggests that patients with heart failure need more protein than healthy adults to meet their metabolic demands. Thus the dietary reference intake for protein of 0.8 g/kg body weight[77] may be too low to meet the needs of most patients with heart failure.

Typically, nutritional interventions have been reserved for patients who are markedly underweight. The data suggest that all patients with heart failure are at risk for malnutrition and therefore should have nutritional intake assessed. Routine referral of patients to a dietitian would be helpful in determining the adequacy of patients' diets. At the minimum, nutritional intake should meet the current dietary reference intake levels for each micronutrient. All patients, but especially for those prescribed diuretics, may benefit from a daily multivitamin with minerals to decrease the risk of developing micronutrient deficiencies. In addition, ensuring protein intake of at least 1 g/kg could help offset the catabolic effects of inflammation and decrease the risks associated with body protein depletion.

Omega-3 fatty acids may play a role in heart failure for the following reasons. When the proportion of omega-3 fatty acids in the diet increases to about one third the amount of omega-6 fatty acids, they replace omega-6 fatty acids in cell membranes. In response to inflammatory stimuli, these cells produce mediators that are less inflammatory than those derived from omega-6 fatty acids.[70] This, in turn, may decrease release of proinflammatory cytokines.[28,70,160] Additional positive effects attributed to omega-3 fatty acids in patients with heart failure include antivasopressor, antihypertension, and antidysrhythmic activities; decreased blood viscosity; and slowed progression of atherosclerosis.[100] Western diets typically contain a much greater proportion of omega-6 fatty acids than is thought to be beneficial.[160] The primary dietary sources of omega-3 fatty acids are limited to oily fish such as sardines, mackerel, herring, trout, and salmon.[70] Other sources include flaxseed, soy, and canola oils, but the process of converting these to omega-3 fatty acids is inefficient in humans, thereby limiting the use of these oils as good sources of omega-3 fatty acids.

There are no clinical trials demonstrating the benefit of omega-3 fatty acid supplementation in patients with heart failure. However, the omega-3 fatty acids eicosapentaenoic acid (EPA) and docosahexaenoic acid (DHA) are essential nutrients, and ensuring adequate intake is necessary to meet nutritional requirements. For patients who cannot obtain the recommended daily intake of 1 g of EPA plus DHA[77] from dietary sources, daily fish or flaxseed oil supplements will assist in reaching this goal.[88]

Dietary Supplements. The supplements coenzyme Q_{10} (coQ10), carnitine, creatine, and taurine have been suggested as useful for patients with heart failure.[163,186] coQ10 is an antioxidant, and supplementation with it has been reported in small, uncontrolled studies to improve EF, exercise tolerance, and quality of life in patients with heart failure.[151,186] However, clinical trials to date have been too small to draw definitive conclusions about its efficacy.[151,163]

Carnitine is involved in the transport of long-chain fatty acids to the mitochondria, an important component of muscle metabolism.[163] Studies suggest that supplementation improves exercise tolerance.[130] Although promising, there are no large, controlled clinical trials that demonstrate the efficacy of carnitine in patients with heart failure.

Creatine phosphate serves as a donor of high-energy phosphate in the formation of adenosine triphosphate, the primary source of cellular energy. Supplementation appears to benefit skeletal muscle much more than myocardial muscle.[163] Functional capacity has not consistently been shown to improve, nor has the long-term safety and efficacy of creatine been studied.[186]

Taurine, a nonessential amino acid, assists in the control of cellular calcium levels. It may also promote diuresis and interfere with angiotensin II signaling.[153]

Taurine is found in high concentrations in normal myocardium, but is reduced by ischemia.[163] There are no well-controlled studies that demonstrate taurine is effective in improving myocardial function in patients with heart failure.

There are no definitive data establishing the safety or efficacy of coQ10, carnitine, creatine, or taurine in the management of heart failure. Thus the use of these supplements in the management of heart failure is not recommended at this time.

Impact of Excess Body Fat. In theory, patients with heart failure who have either abnormally low fat mass (BMI less than 19 kg/m^2) or abnormally high fat mass (BMI greater than 25 kg/m^2) should have poorer outcomes than patients with BMIs in the normal range (20 to 25 kg/m^2).[182] Indeed, patients with below-normal BMIs do have increased morbidity and mortality.[9,10]

However, patients who meet criteria for overweight and even obesity have recently been shown to have better outcomes than those in all other weight groups, including normal-weight patients.[37,74,92,114] The negative outcomes reported for patients with low BMIs are consistent with our current understanding of the consequences of cardiac cachexia and with current recommendations to promote nutritional intake and weight gain in this population.[127] In contrast, the positive outcomes reported for patients with increased BMIs are inconsistent with our understanding of the cardiovascular risk factors associated with overweight/obesity and contradict current recommendations to promote weight loss in this population.[52,92]

A number of mechanisms have been suggested for the apparent paradox that overweight and obesity appear to improve outcomes in patients with heart failure. It may be that increased body fat provides a metabolic reserve that allows overweight and obese patients to tolerate the metabolic/catabolic stress of heart failure for a longer period of time.[37] A second potential mechanism lies in possible differences in proinflammatory cytokine activity between underweight and overweight/obese individuals.[74] Adipose tissue releases both proinflammatory and antiinflammatory cytokines, and higher levels of circulating antiinflammatory cytokines are present in overweight and obese patients. These higher levels may attenuate proinflammatory activity.[105]

There are several issues that need to be addressed before it can be definitely stated that obesity is protective in heart failure. First, BMI is a useful, but rather simple, estimate of body fat mass. It does not capture the impact of body fat distribution on health. Central body fat, particularly visceral fat, is associated with several negative health effects, including hypertension, diabetes, dyslipidemia, and premature coronary death.[80] It is unknown whether the potential positive effects of excess body fat vary depending on body fat distribution. Second, obesity is associated with a number of cardiac structural and hemodynamic alterations that can decrease survival.[86] It is not known whether there is an upper limit above which additional body fat may worsen prognosis.

The risks versus benefits of encouraging voluntary weight loss in heart failure patients who are overweight or obese have not been clearly defined. Although excess body fat is associated with cardiac structural and hemodynamic alterations that can decrease survival, the data demonstrating improved outcomes in obese patients are sufficiently compelling to merit careful consideration. Given the current evidence, the most prudent recommendation for overweight and obese patients is to maintain current body weight (i.e., no weight gain or loss) unless there is clinical evidence that excess body fat is impairing myocardial function or limiting functional staus.

CONCLUSIONS

The care of patients with ADHF is complex, and ensuring optimal patient outcomes demands that nurses who care for these patients have a full grasp of appropriate care. Optimal short- and long-term outcomes can be achieved only when attention is given to optimizing both pharmacologic and nonpharmacologic therapies. Ultimately an integrated multidisciplinary approach is needed to deliver such care to these patients and prevent further exacerbations from occurring.

REFERENCES

1. Abraham, W. T., et al. (2005). In-hospital mortality in patients with acute decompensated heart failure requiring intravenous vasoactive medications: an analysis from the Acute Decompensated Heart Failure National Registry (ADHERE). *J Am Coll Cardiol, 46,* 57–64.
2. Abraham, W. T., et al. (2002). Cardiac resynchronization in chronic heart failure. *N Engl J Med, 346,* 1845–1853.
3. Abraham, W., et al. (1998). Systemic hemodynamic, neurohormonal, and renal effects of a steady-state infusion of human brain natriuretic peptide in patients with hemodynamically decompensated heart failure. *J Card Fail, 4,* 37–44.
4. Abraham, W. T., Port, J. D., & Bristow, M. R. (1997). *Neurohormonal receptors in the failing heart.* New York: Churchill Livingstone.
5. Adams, K. F., Jr., et al. (2005). Characteristics and outcomes of patients hospitalized for heart failure in the United States: rationale, design, and preliminary observations from the first 100,000 cases in the Acute Decompensated Heart Failure National Registry (ADHERE). *Am Heart J, 149,* 209–216.
6. Albert, N. M. (2003). Cardiac resynchronization therapy through biventricular pacing in patients with heart failure and ventricular dyssynchrony. *Crit Care Nurse, 23,* (3 Suppl), 2–13.
7. Alla, F., et al. (2002). Self-rating of quality of life provides additional prognostic information in heart failure. Insights into the EPICAL study. *Eur J Heart Fail, 4,* 337–343.
8. Anker, S. D., et al. (1997). Hormonal changes and catabolic/anabolic imbalance in chronic heart failure and their importance for cardiac cachexia. *Circulation, 96,* 526–534.
9. Anker, S. D., & Coats, A. J. (1999). Cardiac cachexia: a syndrome with impaired survival and immune and neuroendocrine activation. *Chest, 115,* 836–847.
10. Anker, S. D., et al. (1997). Wasting as independent risk factor for mortality in chronic heart failure. *Lancet, 349,* 1050–1053.
11. Anker, S. D., & Sharma, R. (2002). The syndrome of cardiac cachexia. *Int J Cardiol, 85,* 51–66.
12. Aquilani, R., et al. (2003). Is nutritional intake adequate in chronic heart failure patients? *J Am Coll Cardiol, 42,* 1218–1223.
13. Aronow, W. S. (2003). Treatment of heart failure in older persons. Dilemmas with coexisting conditions: diabetes mellitus, chronic obstructive pulmonary disease, and arthritis. *Congest Heart Fail, 9,* 142–147.
14. Asadullah, K., Sterry, W., & Volk, H. D. (2003). Interleukin-10 therapy—review of a new approach. *Pharmacol Rev, 55,* 241–269.
15. Baldasseroni, A., et al. (2002). Left bundle-branch block is associated with increased 1-year sudden and total mortality rate in 5517 outpatients with congestive heart failure: a report from the Italian Network on Congestive Heart Failure. *Am Heart J, 143,* 398–405.

16. Bardy, G. H., et al. for the Sudden Cardiac Death in Heart Failure Trial (SCD-HeFT) investigators. (2005). Amiodarone or an implantable cardioverter-defibrillator for congestive heart failure. *N Engl J Med*, *352*, 225–237.

17. Bentley, B., et al. (2005). Factors related to nonadherence to a low sodium diet in heart failure patients. *Eur J Cardiovasc Nur*, *4*, 331–336.

18. Berry, C., & Clark, A. L. (2000). Catabolism in chronic heart failure. *Eur Heart J*, *21*, 521–532.

19. Bibbins-Domingo, K., et al. (2004). Predictors of heart failure among women with coronary disease. *Circulation*, *110*, 1424–1430.

20. Binanay, C., et al. (2005). Evaluation study of congestive heart failure and pulmonary artery catheterization effectiveness: the ESCAPE trial. *JAMA*, *294*, 1625–1633.

21. Blake, P., & Paganini, E. (1997). Refractory congestive heart failure: overview and application of extracorporeal ultrafiltration. *Adv Renal Replacement Therapy*, *3*, 166–173.

22. Blue, L., et al. (2001). Randomised controlled trial of specialist nurse intervention in heart failure. *BMJ*, *323*, 715–718.

23. Braunstein, J. B., et al. (2003). Noncardiac comorbidity increases preventable hospitalizations and mortality among Medicare beneficiaries with chronic heart failure. *J Am Coll Cardiol*, *42*, 1226–1233.

24. Brennan, T. D., & Haas, G. J. (2005). The role of prophylactic implantable cardioverter defibrillators in heart failure: recent trials usher in a new era of device therapy. *Curr Heart Fail Rep*, *2*, 40–45.

25. Bristow, M. R. (1993). Pathophysiologic and pharmacologic rationales for clinical management of chronic heart failure with beta-blocking agents. *Am J Cardiol*, *71*, 12C–22C.

26. Bristow, M. R., et al. (2004). Cardiac-resynchronization therapy with or without an implantable defibrillator in advanced chronic heart failure. *N Engl J Med*, *350*, 2140–2150.

27. Butler, J., et al. (2004). Outpatient utilization of angiotensin-converting enzyme inhibitors among heart failure patients after hospital discharge. *J Am Coll Cardiol*, *43*, 2036–2043.

28. Calder, P. C. (1998). Immunoregulatory and anti-inflammatory effects of n-3 polyunsaturated fatty acids. *Braz J Med Biol Res*, *31*, 467–490.

29. Calvert, M. J., Freemantle, N., & Cleland, J. G. (2005). The impact of chronic heart failure on health-related quality of life data acquired in the baseline phase of the CARE-HF study. *Eur J Heart Fail*, *7*, 243–251.

30. Carlson, B., Riegel, B., & Moser, D. K. (2001). Self-care abilities of patients with heart failure. *Heart Lung*, *30*, 351–359.

31. Chui, M. A., et al. (2003). Association between adherence to diuretic therapy and health care utilization in patients with heart failure. *Pharmacotherapy*, *23*, 326–332.

32. Cintron, G., et al. (1983). Nurse practitioner role in a chronic congestive heart failure clinic: in-hospital time, costs, and patient satisfaction. *Heart Lung*, *12*, 237–240.

33. Cleland, J. G., et al. (2002). Management of heart failure in primary care (the IMPROVEMENT of Heart Failure Programme): an international survey. *Lancet*, *360*, 1631–1639.

34. Cleland, J. G., et al. (2005). The effect of cardiac resynchronization on morbidity and mortality in heart failure. *N Engl J Med*, *352*, 1539–1549.

35. Cline, C. M., et al. (1998). Cost effective management programme for heart failure reduces hospitalisation. *Heart*, *80*, 442–446.

36. Conraads, V. M., Bosmans, J. M., & Vrints, C. J. (2002). Chronic heart failure: an example of a systemic chronic inflammatory disease resulting in cachexia. *Int J Cardiol*, *85*, 33–49.

36a. Cuffe, M., et al. (2002). Short term intravenous milrinone for acute exacerbation of chronic heart failure: a randomized controlled trial. *JAMA*, *287*, 1541–1547.

37. Davos, C. H., et al. (2003). Body mass and survival in patients with chronic heart failure without cachexia: the importance of obesity. *J Card Fail*, *9*, 29–35.

38. Demling, R. H., & DeSanti, L. (2001). *Involuntary weight loss and protein-energy malnutrition: diagnosis and treatment.* Accessed at Medscape:www.medscape.com/viewprogram/713_pnt.

39. Domanski, M., et al. (2003). The effect of diabetes on outcomes of patients with advanced heart failure in the BEST trial. *J Am Coll Cardiol*, *42*, 914–922.

40. Doughty, R. N., et al. (2002). Randomized, controlled trial of integrated heart failure management: the Auckland Heart Failure Management Study. *Eur Heart J*, *23*, 139–146.

41. Dracup, K., et al. (2003). Perceived control reduces emotional stress in patients with heart failure. *J Heart Lung Transplant*, *22*, 90–93.

42. Drexler, H. (1996). Endothelial function in heart failure: some unsolved issues. *Eur Heart J*, *17*, 1775–1777.

43. Drexler, H. (1998). Factors involved in the maintenance of endothelial function. *Am J Cardiol*, *82*, 3S–4S.

44. Drexler, H., & Horing, B. (1996). Importance of endothelial function in chronic heart failure. *J Cardiovasc Pharmacol*, *27*(Suppl 2), S9–S12.

45. Ekman, I., et al. (1998). Feasibility of a nurse-monitored, outpatient-care programme for elderly patients with moderate-to-severe, chronic heart failure. *Eur Heart J*, *19*, 1254–1260.

45a. Ellison, D. (1994). Diuretic drugs and the treatment of edema: from clinic to bench and back again. *Am J Kidney Dis*, *23*, 623–643.

46. Ellrodt, G., et al. (1997). Evidence-based disease management. *JAMA*, *278*, 1687–1692.

47. Evangelista, L. S., & Dracup, K. (2000). A closer look at compliance research in heart failure patients in the last decade. *Prog Cardiovasc Nurs*, *15*, 97–103.

48. Evangelista, L. S., Dracup, K., & Doering, L. V. (2000). Treatment-seeking delays in heart failure patients. *J Heart Lung Transplant*, *19*, 932–938.

49. Evangelista, L. S., Dracup, K., & Doering, L. V. (2002). Racial differences in treatment-seeking delays among heart failure patients. *J Card Fail*, *8*, 381–386.

50. Fonarow, G. C., et al. (2005). Risk stratification for in-hospital mortality in acutely decompensated heart failure: classification and regression tree analysis. *JAMA*, *298*, 572–580.

51. Fonarow, G. C., & Corday, E. (2004). Overview of acutely decompensated congestive heart failure (ADHF): a report from the ADHERE registry. *Heart Fail Rev*, *9*, 179–185.

52. Fonarow, G. C., & Horwich, T. B. (2002). Obesity, weight reduction and survival in heart failure: reply. *J Am Coll Cardiol*, *39*, 1563–1564.

53. Fonarow, G. C., et al. (1997). Impact of a comprehensive heart failure management program on hospital readmission and functional status of patients with advanced heart failure. *J Am Coll Cardiol*, *30*, 725–732.

54. Fonarow, G. C., & Weber, J. E. (2004). Rapid clinical assessment of hemodynamic profiles and targeted treatment of patients with acutely decompensated heart failure. *Clin Cardiol*, *27*(suppl V), V1–V9.

55. Fonarow, G. C., Yancy, C. W., & Heywood, J. T. (2005). Adherence to heart failure quality-of-care indicators in US hospitals: analysis of the ADHERE Registry. *Arch Intern Med*, *165*, 1469–1477.

56. Forrester, J. S., et al. (1976). Medical therapy of acute myocardial infarction by application of hemodynamic subsets (second of two parts). *N Engl J Med*, *295*, 1404–1413.

57. Fried, J. S., et al. (1999). Electrical and hemodynamic correlates of the maximal rate of pressure increase in the human left ventricle. *J Cardiac Failure*, *5*, 8–16.

58. Funk, M., & Winkler, C. G. (2007). Epidemiology of heart failure. In D. K. Moser & B. Riegel (Eds.), *Cardiac nursing: a companion to Braunwald's heart disease*. Philadelphia: Elsevier.

59. Giles, T. D. (2003). The patient with diabetes mellitus and heart failure: at-risk issues. *Am J Med*, *115*(suppl 8A), 107S–110S.

60. Goldberger, Z., & Lampert, R. (2006). Implantable cardioverter-defibrillators; expanding indications and technologies. *JAMA*, *295*, 809–818.

61. Gorelik, O., et al. (2003). Dietary intake of various nutrients in older patients with congestive heart failure. *Cardiology*, *99*, 177–181.

61a. Gottlieb, S. S. (1998). The use of pacemakers as treatment for systolic dysfunction. *J Cardiac Failure*, *4*, 145–150.

62. Grady, K. L., et al. (2000). Team management of patients with heart failure: a statement for healthcare professionals from The Cardiovascular Nursing Council of the American Heart Association. *Circulation*, *102*, 2443–2456.

63. Greenberg, B., & Hermann, D. (2002). *Contemporary diagnosis and management of heart failure*. Newton, Pa: Handbooks in Health Care.

63a. Gura, M. T., & Foreman, L. (2004). Cardiac resynchronization therapy for heart failure management. *AACN Clin Issues*, *15*, 326–339.

64. Haas, S. J., et al. (2003). Are beta-blockers as efficacious in patients with diabetes mellitus as in patients without diabetes mellitus who have chronic heart failure? A meta-analysis of large-scale clinical trials. *Am Heart J*, *146*, 848–853.

65. Hanumanthu, S., et al. (1997). Effect of a heart failure program on hospitalization frequency and exercise tolerance. *Circulation*, *96*, 2842–2848.

66. Havranek, E. P., et al. (2002). Spectrum of heart failure in older patients: results from the National Heart Failure project. *Am Heart J*, *143*, 412–417.

67. Havranek, E. P., et al. (2004). Provider and hospital characteristics associated with geographic variation in the evaluation and management of elderly patients with heart failure. *Arch Intern Med*, *164*, 1186–1191.

68. Heart Failure Society of America. (2006). HFSA 2006 comprehensive heart failure practice guideline. *J Card Fail*, *12*, e86–e103.

69. Heidenreich, P. A., Ruggerio, C. M., & Massie, B. M. (1999). Effect of a home monitoring system on hospitalization and resource use for patients with heart failure. *Am Heart J*, *138*, 633–640.

70. Heller, A. R., Theilen, H. J., & Koch, T. (2003). Fish or chips? *News Physiol Sci*, *18*, 50–54.

71. Hershberger, R. E., et al. (2001). Prospective evaluation of an outpatient heart failure management program. *J Card Fail*, *7*, 64–74.

72. Horan, M., et al. (2000). The basics of heart failure management: are they being ignored? *Eur J Heart Fail*, *2*, 101–105.

73. Horowitz, C. R., Rein, S. B., & Leventhal, H. (2004). A story of maladies, misconceptions, and mishaps: effective management of heart failure. *Social Sci Med*, *58*, 631–643.

74. Horwich, T. B., et al. (2001). The relationship between obesity and mortality in patients with heart failure. *J Am Coll Cardiol*, *38*, 789–795.

75. Hunt, S. A., et al. (2005). ACC/AHA 2005 guideline update for the diagnosis and management of chronic heart failure in the adult—summary article: a report of the American College of Cardiology/American Heart Association task force on practice guidelines (writing committee to update the 2001 guidelines for the evaluation and management of heart failure). *J Am Coll Cardiol*, *46*, 1116–1143.

76. Hunt, S. A., et al. (2005). ACC/AHA 2005 guideline update for the diagnosis and management of chronic heart failure in the adult: a report of the American College of Cardiology/American Heart Association task force on practice guidelines (writing committee to update the 2001 guidelines for the evaluation and management of heart failure): developed in collaboration with the American College of Chest Physicians and the International Society for Heart and Lung Transplantation: endorsed by the Heart Rhythm Society. *Circulation*, *112*, e154–e235.

77. Institute of Medicine. (2000). *Dietary reference intakes. Applications in dietary assessment*. Washington, DC: National Academies Press.

78. Jaarsma, T., et al. (1999). Effects of education and support on self-care and resource utilization in patients with heart failure. *Eur Heart J*, *20*, 673–682.

79. Jensen, K. T., et al. (1999). Renal effects of brain natriuretic peptide in patients with congestive heart failure. *Clin Sci*, *96*, 5–15.

80. Jensen, M. D. (1997). Health consequences of fat distribution. *Horm Res*, *48*(suppl 5), 88–92.

81. Johnson, W., et al. (2002). Neurohormonal activation rapidly decreases after intravenous therapy with diuretics and vasodilators for class IV heart failure. *J Am Coll Cardiol*, *39*, 1623–1629.

82. Jones, R. C., Francis, G. S., & Lauer, M. S. (2004). Predictors of mortality in patients with heart failure and preserved systolic function in the Digitalis Investigation Group trial. *J Am Coll Cardiol*, *44*, 1025–1029.

83. Joynt, K. E., Whellan, D. J., & O'Connor, C. M. (2004). Why is depression bad for the failing heart? A review of the mechanistic relationship between depression and heart failure. *J Card Fail*, *10*, 258–271.

84. Katz, A. M. (1996). Is the failing heart an energy-starved organ? *J Card Fail*, *2*, 267–272.

85. Katz, S. D., et al. (1994). Pathophysiological correlates of increased serum tumor necrosis factor in patients with congestive heart failure. Relation to nitric oxide-dependent vasodilation in the forearm circulation. *Circulation*, *90*, 12–16.

86. Kenchaiah, S., Gaziano, J. M., & Vasan, R. S. (2004). Impact of obesity on the risk of heart failure and survival after the onset of heart failure. *Med Clin North Am*, *88*, 1273–1294.

87. Komajda, M., et al. (2005). Adherence to guidelines is a predictor of outcome in chronic heart failure: the MAHLER survey. *Eur Heart J*, *26*, 1653–1659.

88. Kris-Etherton, P. M., Harris, W. S., & Appel, L. J. (2002). Fish consumption, fish oil, omega-3 fatty acids, and cardiovascular disease. *Circulation*, *106*, 2747–2757.

89. Krumholz, H. M., et al. (2002). Randomized trial of an education and support intervention to prevent readmission of patients with heart failure. *J Am Coll Cardiol*, *39*, 83–89.

90. Krumholz, H. M., et al. (2000). Evaluating quality of care for patients with heart failure. *Circulation*, *101*, E122–E140.

91. Krumholz, H. M., et al. (2000). Correlates and impact on outcomes of worsening renal function in patients ≥65 years of age with heart failure. *Am J Cardiol*, *85*, 1110–1113.

92. Lavie, C. J., et al. (2003). Body composition and prognosis in chronic systolic heart failure: the obesity paradox. *Am J Cardiol*, *91*, 891–894.

92a. Lennie, T. A., Moser, D. K., Heo, S., et al. (2006). Factors influencing food intake in patients with heart failure. *J Cardiovasc Nurs*, *21*, 123–129.

93. Levy, D., et al. (2002). Long-term trends in the incidence of and survival with heart failure. *N Engl J Med*, *347*, 1397–1402.

94. Linne, A. B., Liedholm, H., & Israelsson, B. (1999). Effects of systematic education on heart failure patients' knowledge after 6 months. A randomised, controlled trial. *Eur J Heart Fail*, *1*, 219–227.

95. Lloyd-Jones, D. M., et al. (2002). Lifetime risk for developing congestive heart failure: the Framingham heart study. *Circulation*, *106*, 3068–3072.

96. Lommi, J., et al. (1997). Haemodynamic, neuroendocrine and metabolic correlates of circulating cytokine concentrations in congestive heart failure. *Eur Heart J*, *18*, 1620–1625.

97. Maisel, A. S., et al. (2002). Rapid measurement of B-type natriuretic peptide in the emergency diagnosis of heart failure. *N Engl J Med, 347*, 161–167.

98. Mann, D. L. (2004). Activation of inflammatory mediators in heart failure. In D. L. Mann (Ed.), *Heart failure*. Philadelphia: Saunders.

99. McAlister, F. A., et al. (2001). A systematic review of randomized trials of disease management programs in heart failure. *Am J Med, 110*, 378–384.

100. McCarty, M. F. (1996). Fish oil and other nutritional adjuvants for treatment of congestive heart failure. *Med Hypotheses, 46*, 400–406.

101. McDonald, K., et al. (2001). Elimination of early rehospitalization in a randomized, controlled trial of multidisciplinary care in a high-risk, elderly heart failure population: the potential contributions of specialist care, clinical stability and optimal angiotensin-converting enzyme inhibitor dose at discharge. *Eur J Heart Fail, 3*, 209–215.

102. Michalsen, A., Konig, G., & Thimme, W. (1998). Preventable causative factors leading to hospital admission with decompensated heart failure. *Heart, 80*, 437–441.

103. Middlekauff, H. R. (1997). Mechanisms and implications of autonomic nervous system dysfunction in heart failure. *Curr Opin Cardiol, 12*, 265–275.

104. Milani, R. V., et al. (1996). The clinical relevance of circulating tumor necrosis factor-alpha in acute decompensated chronic heart failure without cachexia. *Chest, 110*, 992–995.

105. Mohamed-Ali, V., et al. (1999). Production of soluble tumor necrosis factor receptors by human subcutaneous adipose tissue in vivo. *Am J Physiol, 277*, E971–E975.

106. Moser, D. K. (1998). Pathophysiology of heart failure update: the role of neurohumoral activation in the progression of heart failure. *AACN Clin Issues, 9*, 157–171.

107. Moser, D. K. (2000). Heart failure management: optimal health care delivery programs. *Annu Rev Nurs Res, 18*, 91–126.

108. Moser, D. K., Doering, L. V., & Chung, M. L. (2005). Vulnerabilities of patients recovering from an exacerbation of chronic heart failure. *Am Heart J, 150*, 984.

109. Moser, D. K., et al. (2004). Aging with a broken heart: the effect of heart disease on psychological distress in the elderly. *Circulation, 110*, 416 (abstract).

110. Moser, D. K., et al. (2004). Symptom variability, not severity, predicts rehospitalization in patients with heart failure (abstract). *Circulation, 110*(suppl III), 738.

111. Moser, D. K., & Mann, D. L. (2002). Improving outcomes in heart failure: It's not unusual beyond usual care. *Circulation, 105*, 2810–2812.

112. Moser, D. K., & Riegel, B. (2004). Management of heart failure in the outpatient setting. In D. L. Mann (Ed.), *Heart failure. A companion to Braunwald's heart disease*. Philadelphia: Elsevier.

113. Moss, A. J., et al. (2002). Prophylactic implantation of a defibrillator in patients with myocardial infarction and reduced ejection fraction. *N Engl J Med, 346*, 877–883.

114. Mosterd, A., et al. (2001). The prognosis of heart failure in the general population: the Rotterdam study. *Eur Heart J, 22*, 1318–1327.

115. Naylor, M. D., et al. (1999). Comprehensive discharge planning and home follow-up of hospitalized elders: a randomized clinical trial. *JAMA, 281*, 613–620.

116. Neily, J. B., et al. (2002). Potential contributing factors to noncompliance with dietary sodium restriction in patients with heart failure. *Am Heart J, 143*, 29–33.

116a. Nelson, GS, et al. (2000). Left ventricular or biventricular pacing improves cardiac function at diminished energy cost in patients with dilated cardiomyopathy and left bundle-branch block. *Circulation, 102*, 3053–3059.

117. Ni, H., et al. (2000). Comparative responsiveness of Short-Form 12 and Minnesota Living With Heart Failure Questionnaire in patients with heart failure. *J Card Fail, 6*, 83–91.

118. Niebauer, J., et al. (1999). Endotoxin and immune activation in chronic heart failure: a prospective cohort study. *Lancet, 353*, 1838–1842.

119. Nieminen, M. S., et al. (2005). Executive summary of the guidelines on the diagnosis and treatment of acute heart failure: the task force on acute heart failure of the European Society of Cardiology. *Eur Heart J, 26*, 384–416.

120. Nohria, A., et al. (2003). Clinical assessment identifies hemodynamic profiles that predict outcomes in patients admitted with heart failure. *J Am College Cardiol, 41*, 1797–1804.

121. Olivetti, G., et al. (1997). Apoptosis in the failing human heart. *N Engl J Med, 336*, 1131–1141.

122. Opie, L. H. (2002). The neuroendocrinology of congestive heart failure. *Cardiovasc J S Afr, 13*, 171–178.

123. Opie, L. H., et al. (2006). Controversies in ventricular remodeling. *Lancet, 367*, 356–367.

124. Opie, L., & Gersh, B. (2004). *Drugs for the heart* (6th ed.). Philadelphia: Saunders.

125. Packer, M. (1996). New concepts in the pathophysiology of heart failure: beneficial and deleterious interaction of endogenous haemodynamic and neurohormonal mechanisms. *J Intern Med, 239*, 327–333.

126. Parameswaran, A. C., et al. (2005). Why do patients fail to receive beta-blockers for chronic heart failure over time? A "real-world" single-center, 2-year follow-up experience of beta-blocker therapy in patients with chronic heart failure. *Am Heart J, 149*, 921–926.

127. Pasini, E., et al. (2003). Malnutrition, muscle wasting and cachexia in chronic heart failure: the nutritional approach. *Ital Heart J, 4*, 232–235.

128. Paul, S. (2000). Impact of a nurse-managed heart failure clinic: a pilot study. *Am J Crit Care, 9*, 140–146.

129. Paul, S., & Paul, R. V. (2004). Anemia in heart failure: implications, management, and outcomes. *J Cardiovasc Nurs, 19*, S57–S66.

130. Pauly, D. F., & Pepine, C. J. (2003). The role of carnitine in myocardial dysfunction. *Am J Kidney Dis, 41*, S35–S43.

131. Piano, M. R. (2002). Alcohol and heart failure. *J Card Fail, 8*, 239–246.

132. Piepoli, M. F., et al. (2004). Exercise training meta-analysis of trials in patients with chronic heart failure (ExTraMATCH). *BMJ, 328*, 189.

133. Pouleur, H. G., et al. (1993). Changes in ventricular volume, wall thickness and wall stress during progression of left ventricular dysfunction: the SOLVD investigators. *J Am Coll Cardiol, 22*, 43A–48A.

134. Publication Committee for the VMAC Investigators (Vasodilation in the Management of Acute CHF). (2002). Intravenous nesiritide vs nitroglycerin for treatment of decompensated congestive heart failure: a randomized controlled trial. *JAMA, 287*, 1531–1540.

135. Rees, K., et al. (2004). Exercise based rehabilitation for heart failure. *Cochrane Database Syst Rev*, CD003331.

135a. Riegel, B., & Moser, D. K. (2007). Care of patients with chronic heart failure. In D. K. Moser & B. Riegel (Eds.), *Cardiac nursing: a companion to Braunwald's heart disease*. Philadelphia: Elsevier.

136. Rich, M. W. (1999). Multidisciplinary interventions for the management of heart failure: where do we stand? *Am Heart J, 138*, 599–601.

137. Rich, M. W. (1999). Heart failure disease management: a critical review. *J Card Fail, 5*, 64–75.

138. Rich, M. W. (2001). Heart failure disease management programs: efficacy and limitations. *Am J Med, 110,* 410–412.

139. Rich, M. W., et al. (1995). A multidisciplinary intervention to prevent the readmission of elderly patients with congestive heart failure. *N Engl J Med, 333,* 1190–1195.

140. Rich, M. W., et al. (1996). Effect of a multidisciplinary intervention on medication compliance in elderly patients with congestive heart failure. *Am J Med, 101,* 270–276.

141. Rich, M. W., et al. (1993). Prevention of readmission in elderly patients with congestive heart failure: results of a prospective, randomized pilot study. *J Gen Intern Med, 8,* 585–590.

142. Riegel, B., & Carlson, B. (2002). Facilitators and barriers to heart failure self-care. *Patient Educ Couns, 46,* 287–295.

143. Riegel, B., et al. (2000). Which patients with heart failure respond best to multidisciplinary disease management? *J Card Fail, 6,* 290–299.

144. Riegel, B., et al. (2002). Effect of a standardized nurse case-management telephone intervention on resource use in patients with chronic heart failure. *Arch Intern Med, 162,* 705–712.

145. Riegel, B., et al. (2004). Psychometric testing of the self-care of heart failure index. *J Card Fail, 10,* 350–360.

146. Riegel, B., et al. (2006). Nonpharmacologic care by heart failure experts. *J Card Fail, 12,* 149–153.

147. Roccaforte, R., et al. (2005). Effectiveness of comprehensive disease management programmes in improving clinical outcomes in heart failure patients. A meta-analysis. *Eur J Heart Fail, 7,* 1133–1144.

148. Roger, V. L., et al. (2004). Trends in heart failure incidence and survival in a community-based population. *JAMA, 292,* 344–350.

149. Roglieri, J. L., et al. (1997). Disease management interventions to improve outcomes in congestive heart failure. *Am J Manag Care, 3,* 1831–1839.

150. Rosamond, W., et al. (2007). Heart disease and stroke statistics—2007 update: a report from the American Heart Assocation statistics committee and stroke statistics subcommittee. *Circulation, 115,* e69.

151. Rosenfeldt, F., et al. (2003). Systematic review of effect of coenzyme Q10 in physical exercise, hypertension and heart failure. *Biofactors, 18,* 91–100.

152. Sackner-Bernstein, J., et al. (2005). Short-term risk of death after treatment with nesiritide for decompensated heart failure: a pooled analysis of randomized controlled trials. *JAMA, 293,* 1900–1905.

153. Schaffer, S. W., Lombardini, J. B., & Azuma, J. (2000). Interaction between the actions of taurine and angiotensin II. *Amino Acids, 18,* 305–318.

154. Serxner, S. M. M., & Jeffords, F. (1998). Congestive heart failure disease management study: a patient education intervention. *Congest Heart Fail, 4,* 23–28.

155. Seta, Y., et al. (1996). Basic mechanisms in heart failure: the cytokine hypothesis. *J Card Fail, 2,* 243–249.

156. Shah, M. R., et al. (2005). Impact of the pulmonary artery catheter in critically ill patients: meta-analysis of randomized clinical trials. *JAMA, 294,* 1664–1670.

157. Shah, N. B., et al. (1998). Prevention of hospitalizations for heart failure with an interactive home monitoring program. *Am Heart J, 135,* 373–378.

158. Shlipak, M. G., & Massie, B. M. (2004). The clinical challenge of cardiorenal syndrome. *Circulation, 110,* 1514–1517.

159. Silver, M. A. (2003). Dietary research in heart failure: beyond the salt shaker. *J Am Coll Cardiol, 42,* 1224–1225.

160. Simopoulos, A. P. (2002). The importance of the ratio of omega-6/omega-3 essential fatty acids. *Biomed Pharmacother, 56,* 365–379.

161. Sisk, J. E., et al. (2003). Cost-effectiveness of vaccination against invasive pneumococcal disease among people 50 through 64 years of age: role of comorbid conditions and race. *Ann Intern Med, 138,* 960–968.

162. Smith, L. E., et al. (1997). Symptomatic improvement and reduced hospitalization for patients attending a cardiomyopathy clinic. *Clin Cardiol, 20,* 949–954.

163. Sole, M. J., & Jeejeebhoy, K. N. (2000). Conditioned nutritional requirements and the pathogenesis and treatment of myocardial failure. *Curr Opin Clin Nutr Metab Care, 3,* 417–424.

164. Stevenson, L. (2004). Management of acute decompensation. In D. L. Mann (Ed.), *Heart failure: a companion to Braunwald's heart disease.* Philadelphia: Saunders.

165. Stevenson, L. W. (1991). Tailored therapy before transplantation for treatment of advanced heart failure: effective use of vasodilators and diuretics. *J Heart Lung Transplant, 10,* 468–476.

166. Stevenson, L., et al. (1990). Afterload reduction with vasodilators and diuretics decreases mitral regurgitation during upright exercise in advanced heart failure. *J Am Coll Cardiol, 15,* 174–180.

167. Stevenson, L. W., Massie, B. M., & Francis, G. S. (1998). Optimizing therapy for complex or refractory heart failure: a management algorithm. *Am Heart J, 135,* S293–309.

168. Stewart, S., et al. (2002). An economic analysis of specialist heart failure nurse management in the UK; can we afford not to implement it? *Eur Heart J, 23,* 1369–1378.

169. Stewart, S., & Horowitz, J. D. (2002). Detecting early clinical deterioration in chronic heart failure patients post-acute hospitalisation—a critical component of multidisciplinary, home-based intervention? *Eur J Heart Fail, 4,* 345–351.

170. Stewart, S., & Horowitz, J. D. (2002). Home-based intervention in congestive heart failure: long-term implications on readmission and survival. *Circulation, 105,* 2861–2866.

171. Stewart, S., & Horowitz, J. D. (2003). Specialist nurse management programmes: economic benefits in the management of heart failure. *Pharmacoeconomics, 21,* 225–240.

172. Stewart, S., et al. (2003). Heart failure and the aging population: an increasing burden in the 21st century? *Heart, 89,* 49–53.

173. Stewart, S., Marley, J. E., & Horowitz, J. D. (1999). Effects of a multidisciplinary, home-based intervention on unplanned readmissions and survival among patients with chronic congestive heart failure: a randomised controlled study. *Lancet, 354,* 1077–1083.

174. Stewart, S., Pearson, S., & Horowitz, J. D. (1998). Effects of a home-based intervention among patients with congestive heart failure discharged from acute hospital care. *Arch Intern Med, 158,* 1067–1072.

175. Stewart, S., et al. (1999). Prolonged beneficial effects of a home-based intervention on unplanned readmissions and mortality among patients with congestive heart failure. *Arch Intern Med, 159,* 257–261.

176. Sullivan, M., et al. (2002). Depression-related costs in heart failure care. *Arch Intern Med, 162,* 1860–1866.

177. Sutton, M. G., & Sharpe, N. (2000). Left ventricular remodeling after myocardial infarction: pathophysiology and therapy. *Circulation, 101,* 2981–2988.

178. Torre-Amione, G., et al. (1996). Proinflammatory cytokine levels in patients with depressed left ventricular ejection fraction: a report from the Studies of Left Ventricular Dysfunction (SOLVD). *J Am Coll Cardiol, 27,* 1201–1206.

179. Toussaint, J. F., et al. (2000). Biventricular pacing in severe heart failure patients reverses electromechanical dyssynchronization from apex to base. *Pacing Clin Electrophysiol, 23,* 1731–1734.

180. Tsuyuki, R. T., et al. (2001). Acute precipitants of congestive heart failure exacerbations. *Arch Intern Med, 161,* 2337–2342.

181. Vinson, J. M., et al. (1990). Early readmission of elderly patients with congestive heart failure. *J Am Geriatr Soc, 38,* 1290–1295.

182. WHO. (1997). Obesity: preventing and managing the global epidemic. *WHO Technical Report Series,* No. 894, Geneva, Switzerland: World Health Organization.

183. Weber, M., & Hamm, C. (2006). Role of B-type natriuretic peptide (BNP) and NT-proBNP in clinical routine. *Heart, 92,* 843–849.

184. Weinberger, M., Oddone, E. Z., & Henderson, W. G. (1996). Does increased access to primary care reduce hospital readmissions? Veterans affairs cooperative study group on primary care and hospital readmission. *N Engl J Med, 334,* 1441–1447.

185. West, J. A., et al. (1997). A comprehensive management system for heart failure improves clinical outcomes and reduces medical resource utilization. *Am J Cardiol, 79,* 58–63.

186. Witte, K. K., Clark, A. L., & Cleland, J. G. (2001). Chronic heart failure and micronutrients. *J Am Coll Cardiol, 37,* 1765–1774.

187. Yancy, C. W., & Fonarow, G. C. (2004). Quality of care and outcomes in acute decompensated heart failure: The ADHERE Registry. *Curr Heart Fail Rep, 1,* 121–128.

188. Young, J. B. (2004). The global epidemiology of heart failure. *Med Clin North Am, 88,* 1135–1143, ix.

189. Young, J. B., et al. (2003). Combined cardiac resynchronization and implantable cardioversion defibrillation in advanced chronic heart failure: the MIRACLE ICD Trial. *JAMA, 289,* 2685–2694.

190. Zambroski, C. H., et al. (2005). Impact of symptom prevalence and symptom burden on quality of life in patients with heart failure. *Eur J Cardiovasc Nurs, 4,* 198–206.

190a. Ziao, H. B., et al. (1996). Natural history of abnormal conduction and its relation to prognosis in patients with dilated cardiomyopathy. *Int J Cardiol, 53,* 163–170.

191. Zile, M. R., & Catalin, F. B. (2004). Alterations in ventricular function: diastolic heart failure. In D. L. Mann (Ed.), *Heart failure: a companion to Braunwald's heart disease.* Philadelphia: Saunders.

192. Zitter, M. (1994). Disease management: a new approach to health care. *Med Interface, 7,* 70–72, 75–76.

Peggy L. Kirkwood

Historically, cardiovascular disease (CVD) has been viewed as a man's disease. However, heart disease is now recognized as the number one cause of death of women in the United States.[85] One in four women has some form of CVD (coronary artery disease, stroke, heart failure, or hypertension). More women die of CVD than all forms of cancer combined, killing almost 500,000 women every year.[11] Coronary artery disease (CAD) typically becomes evident in men in their mid-50s, the prime of their life. However, in women it is generally not recognized until 10 to 20 years later. This delay has been attributed to the protection women receive from estrogen.[35,130] By the age of 75, the rates of cardiovascular (CV) morbidity and mortality in men and women are almost equal.[35]

The intent of this chapter is not to reiterate coronary artery disease in general (see Chapter 11). Instead, this chapter will focus on the evidence-based gender differences in etiology, prevention, assessment, and treatment of heart disease in women.

Women who develop heart disease experience more morbidity and disability than men. The clinical outcomes of women with heart disease are sobering. For example, in 2004 the American Heart Association (AHA) reported the following[11]:

- Within 1 year of a recognized myocardial infarction (MI), 38% of women (versus 25% of men) die. This is especially true in women younger than age 55.[130]
- 35% of women MI survivors will have another MI within 6 years, versus 18% of men.
- Within 6 years, 46% of women MI survivors become disabled with heart failure, versus 22% of men.
- 64% of women who died suddenly of an MI had no previous symptoms.

Until the last several decades, subjects in research studies on heart disease were primarily men. Our knowledge of the manifestations of heart disease in women has been extrapolated from these studies. Based on this research, improvements have been made in the treatment of heart disease, mostly in decreased mortality rates in men. However, similar gains have not been seen in decreasing mortality rates in women with heart disease. Further research is essential to truly understand the disparities in heart disease between women and men in an attempt to find better treatments for women.

PRIMARY PREVENTION

Because CAD is often fatal and because nearly two thirds of women who die suddenly have no previously recognized symptoms, risk identification and prevention are essential.[85] Most CV diseases are diagnosed in middle-aged women; therefore prevention must occur 20 to 30 years earlier to have an impact. Women are inclined to underestimate the importance of CAD and fail to implement practices that may prevent heart disease.[62,86] Society's gender roles and women's longer life span tend to make women caregivers to men,[123] and women take this caregiver role seriously. Consequently, they frequently discount their own health and well-being to fulfill these duties.[62,139] When women do attempt to make lifestyle changes, compliance has been shown to be very low[113] because of a variety of reasons, such as comorbid diseases (e.g., diabetes, obesity), older age at presentation, and depression.[89]

In 2004 the AHA and 11 other leading national health organizations published comprehensive guidelines for heart disease prevention in women.[85] These guidelines were updated in 2007.[85a] Information from many studies, including the Women's Health Initiative (WHI)[45,103] and the Heart and Estrogen/Progestin Replacement Study (HERS),[56] was used to make these evidence-based recommendations to lower heart disease risk in women. Strategies to implement the guidelines and prioritize risk-reducing therapies were summarized as saying "goodbye" (ALOHA) to heart disease in women (Box 13-1). This tool is a helpful way to assist women to better work with their healthcare providers not only to assess and decrease their risk of developing heart disease, but also to treat the CAD if it is present.

Box 13-1

ALOHA to Heart Disease

A—Assess risk and rank as high, intermediate, or low risk.

L—Lifestyle recommendations (e.g., smoking cessation, regular exercise, weight management, and heart-healthy diet) to prevent heart disease should be followed.

O—Other risk-reducing interventions are prioritized on the basis of strength of recommendation.

H—Highest priority for risk intervention is for women at highest risk.

A—Avoid medical therapies designated as class III (not useful and may be harmful).

From reference 86a.

Assess Risk

The first recommendation involves assessment of risk. Heart disease can be defined as an atherosclerotic plaque buildup in the blood vessels, which may significantly reduce the blood flow through an artery. Although a diagnosis of heart disease may be definite, heart disease *risk* is something people have to a greater or lesser degree and is commonly evaluated on a continuum. Although the Framingham Risk Assessment Calculator may be helpful in calculating a woman's 10-year risk of developing heart disease (Table 13-1), the more recent recommendations address a woman's lifetime risk, rather than focusing only on a 10-year risk.[72,85a] A Framingham global risk score of greater than 20% could be used to identify a woman at high risk, but a lower score is not sufficient to ensure low risk. The presence of a single risk factor at 50 years of age has been shown to substantially increase lifetime risk for CVD. Therefore medical and lifestyle history, Framingham risk score, family history of CVD, and genetic conditions should be considered when evaluating the "at risk" woman and recommending preventive therapies.[85a] Women with Framingham scores of less than 10% and a healthy lifestyle with no risk factors are considered to be at optimal risk. Once the percent of risk is calculated, lifestyle changes, diagnostic tests, and treatments are recommended based on the corresponding level of risk. Table 13-2 lists examples of clinical criteria and scenarios that healthcare providers might see with each risk group. This continuum helps to match the intensity of risk interventions to the baseline level of CVD risk. Table 13-3 lists priorities for prevention according to risk assessment. Diagnostic tests according to risk category will be discussed in a subsequent section of this text.

TABLE 13-1 The Framingham Risk Assessment Calculator: Estimate of 10-Year Risk for Women

Instructions: Find your point score in each of the five boxes on the left and then add the points to get your Point Total. Find that point value in the box on the right and you will also see an estimate of your 10-year risk as a percentage. A risk greater than 20% in 10 years is considered high risk. Intermediate risk ranges from 10% to 20%; low risk is less than 10%.

Age	Points
20-34	−7
35-39	−7
40-44	0
45-49	3
50-54	6
55-59	8
60-64	10
65-69	12
70-74	14
75-79	16

Total Cholesterol (mg/dl)	Age				
	20-39 years	40-49 years	50-59 years	60-69 years	70-79 years
	Points				
< 160	0	0	0	0	0
160-199	4	3	2	1	1
200-239	5	6	4	2	1
240-279	11	8	5	3	2
≥280	13	10	7	4	2

Smoking	Age				
	20-39 years	40-49 years	50-59 years	60-69 years	70-79 years
Nonsmoker	0	0	0	0	0
Smoker	9	7	4	2	1

HDL (mg/dl)	Points
≥60	−1
50-59	0
40-49	1
< 40	2

Systolic BP (mm Hg)	Untreated	Treated
< 120	0	0
120-129	1	3
130-139	2	4
140-159	3	5
≥160	4	6

Point total	10-year risk %
< 9	<1
9	1
10	1
11	1
12	1
13	2
14	2
15	3
16	4
17	5
18	6
19	8
20	11
21	14
22	17
23	22
24	27
≥25	≥30

From reference 86a.

TABLE 13-2 Classification of Cardiovascular Disease Risk in Women

RISK GROUP	CRITERIA
High risk	Established CHD Cerebrovascular disease[*] Peripheral arterial disease Abdominal aortic aneurysm Diabetes mellitus Chronic kidney disease[†] 10-year Framingham global risk greater than 20%
At risk	Evidence of subclinical CVD[‡] (e.g., coronary calcification) Metabolic syndrome One or more major risk factors for CVD[§] Markedly elevated levels of single risk factor[§] First-degree relative(s) with early-onset (age <55 yr in men and <65 yr in women) atherosclerotic CVD Poor exercise capacity on treadmill test and/or abnormal heart rate recovery after stopping exercise
Optimal risk	Framingham global risk less than 10% and a healthy lifestyle, with no risk factors

Modified from reference 85a.
CHD = Coronary heart disease, CVD = cardiovascular disease.
[*]Cerebrovascular disease may not confer high risk for CHD if the affected vasculature is above the carotids. Carotid artery disease (symptomatic or asymptomatic with >50% stenosis) confers high risk.
[†]As chronic kidney disease deteriorates and progresses to end-stage kidney disease, the risk of CVD increases substantially.
[‡]Some patients with subclinical CVD will have >20% 10-year CHD risk and should be elevated to the high-risk category.
[§]Patients with multiple risk factors can fall into any of the three categories by Framingham scoring.

TABLE 13-3 Priorities for Prevention According to Risk Group

	CLASS I RECOMMENDATIONS	CLASS IIA RECOMMENDATIONS	CLASS IIB RECOMMENDATIONS
High-risk women (>20% risk)	Smoking cessation Physical activity/cardiac rehabilitation Diet therapy Weight maintenance/reduction Blood pressure control Cholesterol control Aspirin therapy Beta-blocker therapy ACE inhibitor/ARB therapy Glycemic control in diabetic women	Treatment for depression	Omega-3 fatty-acid supplementation
At risk women (10%–20% risk)	Smoking cessation Physical activity Heart-healthy diet Weight maintenance/reduction Blood pressure control Cholesterol control	Aspirin therapy	
Optimal-risk women (<10% risk)	Smoking cessation Physical activity Heart-healthy diet Weight maintenance/reduction Treat individual heart risk factors as indicated		

Data from reference 85a.
ACE = Angiotensin-converting enzyme, ARB = angiotensin receptor blocker.

Lower Risk With Lifestyle Changes

The second recommendation involves strategies that may be initiated to lower heart disease risk with lifestyle changes. The five lifestyle changes that the AHA panel determined would have the greatest impact are listed.

1. **Stop smoking cigarettes and avoid secondhand tobacco smoke.**

Although 21% of all deaths from heart disease are attributable to smoking, that number is as high as 60% in women younger than 50 years.[15] Cigarettes adversely affect the lipid profile, causing women to lose the "natural" protection against CAD seemingly acquired from estrogen.[119] Women often smoke to relieve stress, anger, boredom, or depression, or as a strategy for weight loss.[115,126] It has also been shown that women who smoke and take oral contraceptives have a significantly higher risk of CAD.[44] The good news is that the risk of CAD decreases to equal that of nonsmokers by 3 years after smoking cessation.[100] Therefore stopping smoking can improve a woman's risk profile. In addition, there is a growing body of evidence demonstrating the impact of environmental (secondhand) smoke on a woman's CAD risk.[61,119] A review of nine cohort studies showed a 15% higher mortality rate among nonsmoking women who lived with a currently smoking spouse, as compared with nonsmoking women who lived with a nonsmoking spouse.[61]

2. **Get at least 30 minutes of physical activity each day.**

Given that inactivity and obesity are major contributors to CVD,[71] increased physical activity is clearly important to prevent heart disease from developing (primary prevention), as well as to prevent a second cardiac event when heart disease is known to be present (secondary prevention). Although the terms *exercise* and *physical activity* are sometimes used interchangeably, thus causing confusion, the definition of physical activity generally used in research studies is based on the definition by Caspersen et al. (p. 4)[27]: "any bodily movement produced by skeletal muscles that results in energy expenditure." This includes traditional exercise done to improve physical fitness, as well as occupational, household, and leisure time activities.[27] However, women tend to get insufficient amounts of physical activity as a result of many factors. Household chores and caretaking responsibilities contribute to the lack of leisure time needed to get the recommended amount of exercise.[117] Comorbid conditions, such as arthritis and obesity; lack of access to appropriate programs and facilities; and lack of an exercise companion also contribute to a more sedentary lifestyle.[117] The current recommendation is that women who are able

should get regular aerobic physical activity, such as brisk walking, at least 30 minutes per day most days of the week.[1] This will help not only to decrease CV disease risk but also to decrease or prevent hypertension.[1,140]

3. **Start a cardiac rehabilitation program after an MI or a coronary procedure.**

Exercise rehabilitation after an MI increases functional capacity and reduces mortality.[84] However, women are less likely than men to be referred for cardiac rehabilitation (CR) programs after an MI or coronary artery bypass surgery.[84] Even when referred, they are less likely to remain enrolled.[15,84] This is explained in part by the fact that cardiac events generally occur at an older age in women and comorbidities may interfere with their compliance. However, one study noted that older women were more inclined to stay in CR programs because there was less competition for their time (e.g., work and family obligations).[84] Another study reported that the presence of depression when starting a CR program was the main predictor of nonadherence, which also correlated with a poorer prognosis.[127]

4. **Eat a heart-healthy diet.**

Metabolic syndrome (defined as three or more of the following criteria: hypertension, hypertriglyceridemia, low high-density lipoprotein [HDL] cholesterol level, insulin resistance, and abdominal obesity) is highly prognostic of future CV risk and should be a targeted area for risk reduction.[2] The Women's Ischemia Syndrome Evaluation (WISE) study[48] identified metabolic syndrome, but not obesity, as a predictor of future CV events. Thus control of modifiable risk factors is recommended in both normal and overweight women to prevent the onset of metabolic syndrome and help prevent CVD.[48]

Dietary intake can affect lipid levels, systolic blood pressure, and the prevalence of metabolic syndrome.[2,7,91] Dietary recommendations are generally similar for men and women, as outlined in the Nutrition box on p. 280. Heart-healthy diets consist of total fat content that is less than 30% of total calories, saturated fats less than 10% of calories, and avoidance of trans fats altogether. Diets should consist of a variety of fruits, vegetables, legumes, nuts, soy products, low-fat dairy products, and whole-grain breads, cereals, and pastas. Keeping the sodium intake less than 2.4 grams per day is also recommended. A variety of fruits, vegetables, grains, low-fat or nonfat dairy products, fish, legumes, and sources of protein low in saturated fat should be encouraged. Omega-3 fatty acids have been associated with lower risk of nonfatal MI or fatal CAD in women.[55] Therefore omega-3 fatty acid (in the form of fresh fish, oils high in alpha-linolenic acid, or dietary supplement) is also recommended.[55,85,85a] One popular recommendation to meet these objectives is the Dietary Approaches to Stop Hypertension (DASH) diet, which has been shown to be effective in decreasing hypertension.[7,8] However, the DASH diet also has been shown to decrease levels of HDL (heart-protective lipid) and has no effect on triglycerides, both undesirable outcomes.[8] Recent research suggests that replacing carbohydrates with protein or monounsaturated fat in the DASH diet can further improve lipid risk factors.[8] Since dietary intervention for more than 2 years showed significant reductions in the rate of cardiovascular events,[54] these recommendations should be encouraged.

◆ NUTRITION

Recommended Nutrient Intake for Prevention and Treatment of Coronary Artery Disease in Women

WOMEN WITHOUT CAD

- Total fat: Less than 30% of total calories
- Saturated fat: Less than 10% of total calories
- Cholesterol: Less than 300 mg per day

WOMEN WITH CAD

- Total fat: 25%–30% of total calories
- Saturated fat and trans fatty acids: Less than 7% of total calories
- Polyunsaturated fat: up to 10% of total calories
- Monounsaturated fat: up to 20% of total calories
- Carbohydrate: 50%–60% of total calories
- Protein: approximately 15% of total calories
- Fiber: 20–30 g per day
- Cholesterol: Less than 200 mg per day
- Maximum sodium chloride: 2.4 g per day
- At least 5 servings of a variety of fruits and vegetables each day
- Whole grains, fibers, nuts, and seeds
- Low-fat or nonfat dairy products
- Fish with high omega-3 fatty acids, baked or broiled, 5 times per week
- Meats should be lean, broiled, or baked; red meat once per month
- Omega-3 fatty acids (flaxseed oil, flaxseeds, canola oil, soybean oil, English walnuts, olive oil)
- General suggestions:
  - Split restaurant entrees
  - Eat crunchy, healthy snacks
  - Keep high-calorie, high-fat, and refined-grain foods out of sight

Data from references 2 and 85.

---

5. Maintain a healthy weight.

Weight maintenance/reduction through an appropriate balance of calorie intake with physical activity is recommended. Body mass index (BMI) should be maintained between 17.5 and 24.9 kg/m^2 and waist circumference less than 35 inches.[85] Elevated BMI and obesity are associated with dyslipidemia, diabetes, and hypertension.[63] Overweight and obese adult women in the Framingham Heart Study had reduced survival when compared with women of normal weights, even after adjustments for hypertension, diabetes, physical activity, and education information at baseline.[96]

Other Risk-Reducing Interventions

The next recommendation is to prioritize other evidence-based interventions and recommend them as a standard of care. These include lowering blood pressure in all women with hypertension, encouraging healthy cholesterol levels in high- and intermediate-risk women, keeping diabetes under control, and receiving an influenza vaccination each year.

Hypertension. Blood pressure (BP) is optimal at less than 120/80 mm Hg.[28] BP values ranging from 120 to 139 mm Hg systolic or 80 to 89 mm Hg diastolic are said to be prehypertensive, identifying people at high risk of developing hypertension.[28] It has been shown in several studies[28,31,69] that both systolic hypertension and diastolic hypertension are major independent risk factors for CAD in both men and women. Cardiovascular deaths are significantly more common among women who have high BP.[28,69] Hypertension is less common among younger women than men; however, the incidence rises rapidly after age 50.[142] By the sixth decade, hypertension in women is equal to or exceeds that in men.[28] In addition, African Americans are more prone to hypertension, have it more severely, have more end-organ damage, and have a greater prevalence of other cardiovascular risk factors.[30] Hypertension treatment reduces the incidence of coronary artery disease by 15% to 33%.[28] Women who are prehypertensive should be counseled early to adopt lifestyle changes, primarily eating a heart-healthy diet and increasing physical activity.[140] Weight loss of as little as 10 pounds and adopting a low-sodium, low-cholesterol, and low saturated fat diet can reduce BP significantly.[49] If the blood pressure remains at or above 140/90 mm Hg, medications, such as diuretics, calcium channel blockers (CCBs), angiotensin-converting enzyme (ACE) inhibitors, or beta blockers, should be prescribed.[28] Women, however, are more likely than men to report adverse effects to medications, such as ACE inhibitor–induced cough, CCB-related peripheral edema, and diuretic-induced hypokalemia or hyponatremia.[70] Therefore follow-up must be provided to encourage adherence and provide support to reach BP goals.

Cholesterol Levels. Primary prevention of CAD starts with lifestyle changes to lower cholesterol levels, including reduced intake of saturated fats and cholesterol, increased physical activity, and weight control.[39] Adherence to these changes has been shown to have a positive impact on lipid levels, and thus on CVD risk.[39] The role of lipid-lowering medications in primary prevention is still controversial. Most major trials on primary prevention of CAD using cholesterol-lowering medications have not included women. One of the few that did is the 1998 Air Force/Texas Coronary Atherosclerosis Prevention Study.[36] The data presented on female patients do not show a strong benefit in preventing heart disease in healthy women (primary prevention). However, there is strong evidence to support lipid-lowering therapies for secondary prevention in women with known CAD.[95] The Heart Protection Study[29] also showed that high-risk women benefit from low-density lipoprotein (LDL) lowering with statins, for both primary and secondary prevention, as much as men. Lipid profiles can be improved upon by dietary modification and exercise, as well as drug therapy.[39]

Diabetes. Women with CVD have higher rates of diabetes compared to men.[37,116] Type 2 diabetes is the most important risk factor for heart disease, dramatically increasing the mortality of women after an MI.[52,68] CAD generally presents in women after menopause; however, diabetes eliminates the protective effect of estrogen.[88] In premenopausal women, type 2 diabetes contributes to endothelial dysfunction,[120] which has been implicated as a factor in CAD in women.[22] Glycemic control has been shown to reduce or delay diabetic complications, such as retinopathy, nephropathy, and neuropathy.[57] However, although there is a relationship between the level of hyperglycemia and the incidence of CAD, studies have not clearly shown that strict control of glucose levels in women with type 2 diabetes reduces the incidence of developing CAD.[19] Until more research is completed, it is recommended that women with diabetes keep their glycated hemoglobin levels (HbA_{1c}) near normal (less than 7%) with lifestyle changes and pharmacotherapy.[116]

Influenza Vaccination. The *2006 AHA/ACC Guidelines for Secondary Prevention for Patients With Coronary and Other Atherosclerotic Vascular Disease*[114] for the first time added a recommendation that anyone with chronic disorders of the CV system receive an annual influenza vaccine.

Highest Risk Priority Interventions

The fourth recommendation is that high-risk women should be treated aggressively with evidence-based therapies. Women at highest risk are those who already have CV disease, diabetes, chronic kidney disease, or a 10-year absolute CAD risk greater than 20%. Along with lifestyle changes, the medications listed in Table 13-4 have been shown to prevent MIs or increase survival. (See also the Medication table in Chapter 11 on pp. 218-221.) These medications include the following:

1. ACE inhibitor or angiotensin receptor blocker (ARB) therapy is recommended.
2. Aspirin (81 to 325 mg) is recommended unless contraindicated. Aspirin should not be used in women who have liver or kidney disease, stomach ulcers, other gastrointestinal problems, bleeding problems, or aspirin allergies.
3. Beta blockers are recommended for women who have had an MI or have ongoing angina or chest pain, unless contraindicated.
4. Statins [3-hydroxy-3-methylglutaryl coenzyme A (HMG CoA) reductase inhibitors] are effective in reducing total cholesterol and LDL levels. Recent studies have shown statins are helpful for prevention, even when the LDL level is below 100 mg/dL.[39]
5. Nicotinic acid (niacin) or fibric acids (gemfibrozil [Lopid], fenofibrate [Tricor]) are recommended for high-risk women with a low HDL.

Avoid Unhelpful Interventions

The fifth recommendation from AHA guidelines is to avoid interventions that have not shown benefit in research studies. They are the following:

1. Combined postmenopausal hormone replacement therapy (estrogen and progestin). The Women's Health Initiative showed no benefit from hormone replacement therapy (HRT) in preventing heart disease, and in some women, HRT is actually thought to cause heart attacks, stroke, or blood clots.[45,136]
2. Antioxidant supplements, such as vitamins C and E and beta carotene, have been shown to have no CVD prevention benefit;[34] some studies have shown unexpected increases in hemorrhagic stroke. They may also interfere with the beneficial effects of statin therapy.
3. Folic acid, with or without B_6 and B_{12} supplementation, should not be used for primary or secondary prevention of CVD.[85a]

TABLE 13-4	Strategies for the Secondary Prevention of Coronary Artery Disease in Women		
STRATEGY	**REDUCTION IN MORTALITY OR RECURRENT MI**	**UNDERUSE?**	**COMMENTS**

Lipid lowering
  Statins
  Nicotinic acid (niacin) or fibric acids (gemfibrozil [Lopid], fenofibrate [Tricor])
	30%–50%	Yes	Effective in reducing total cholesterol and LDL. Recommended for high-risk women with low HDL

Aspirin (81 or 325 mg)	20%–25%	Yes	Should not be used in women who have liver or kidney disease, stomach ulcers, other GI problems, bleeding problems. or aspirin allergies

Beta blockers
  After MI
  With LV dysfunction
	
	20%–30%
	10%–40%
		
		Yes
		Yes	

ACE inhibitors
  After MI
  With LV dysfunction
	
	5%–10%
	25%–30%
		
		Yes
		Yes	

Smoking cessation	65%	Yes	Risk of CAD decreases to equal that of nonsmokers by 3 years after smoking cessation
Hypertension	?	?	Both systolic and diastolic hypertension are major independent risk factors for CAD
Cardiac rehabilitation	?	Yes	Exercise rehabilitation after an MI increases functional capacity and reduces mortality
Hormone replacement therapy (HRT)	Increase	N/A	No benefit in preventing heart disease, and in some women is thought to cause heart attacks, stroke, or blood clot

Some data from reference 123.
ACE = Angiotensin-converting enzyme, CAD = coronary artery disease, GI = gastrointestinal, HDL = high-density lipoprotein, LDL = low-density lipoprotein, LV = left ventricular, MI = myocardial infarction.

4. Aspirin is not recommended for primary prevention of heart disease in healthy women younger than 65 years of age.[85a]

Evidence suggests that heart disease can be prevented. Using these guidelines can help women lower their risk of developing heart disease. A summary is given in the Multidisciplinary Plan of Care on pp. 283-284.

Depression

In addition to the AHA guidelines, there has been much research on the connection between depression and heart disease in women.[10,74,144] In women with no previous CVD, depression is closely linked to risk factors for CVD and CV morbidity, as well as an independent predictor of CVD and all-cause mortality.[45,138]

Postmenopausal women with established risk factors for CVD (such as smoking, obesity, low physical activity, hypertension, high cholesterol level, and diabetes) have a 20% to 50% higher occurrence of depression.[105,138] Depression is common in patients after an MI, and the prevalence of depression is found to be higher among women younger than age 60.[74] Depressed patients are at greater risk of cardiac death in the first few months after an MI and are less likely to adhere to recommended behavior and lifestyle changes to reduce their risk.[144]

Various biological mechanisms have been suggested that link depression to CVD mortality. One mechanism suggested is the altered sympathetic arousal in depressed patients.[138] This altered ratio between sympathetic and parasympathetic tone lowers the threshold for ventricular fibrillation and may make patients more susceptible to dysrhythmias and sudden death.[89]

MULTIDISCIPLINARY PLAN OF CARE FOR HEART DISEASE IN WOMEN

PROBLEM	INTERVENTION	RATIONALE	EXPECTED OUTCOME	SPECIAL CONSIDERATIONS
Risk of women developing heart disease	Assess risk.	Primary prevention is important to identify areas of concern to address.	CAD does not develop.	
	Adopt lifestyle changes.			
	Stop smoking and limit exposure to secondhand smoke.	Smoking is leading preventable cause of CVD in women. It causes a twofold to threefold increased risk of dying from CVD.[11]		18% of women smoke compared with 23% of men.[12]
	Strive for minimum of 30 min of physical activity each day.	Moderate-intensity physical activity substantially reduces risk of CVD.[140]		43% of women have a sedentary lifestyle.[118]
	Eat a heart-healthy diet (see Nutrition box on p. 280). Maintain a healthy weight	Abdominal obesity is a significant risk factor for women.	BMI between 18.5 and 24.9 kg/m^2 and a waist circumference smaller than 35 inches are maintained.	33% of adult women are classified as obese (BMI larger than 30 kg/m^2) and 62% are overweight (BMI larger than 25 kg/m^2).[11]
	Maintain optimal blood pressure.	Hypertension is a significant risk factor for CVD.[28]	Blood pressure is maintained at or below 120/80 mm Hg.[28]	60%–80% of women older than 55 have hypertension. Less than 30% of women with hypertension have it under control.[46] Hypertension is more common and more severe in African-American women.[30]
	Maintain optimal cholesterol levels.	Optimal cholesterol levels have been shown to decrease risk of heart disease.[39]	Strive for LDL lower than 100 mg/dL, HDL greater than 50 mg/dL, triglycerides lower than 150 mg/dL.	Low HDL appears to be a stronger predictor of heart disease in women than in men. High triglycerides may be an important risk factor in women.
	Maintain optimal glucose levels in diabetic patients.	Half of all deaths in persons with type 2 diabetes are caused by heart disease.[88]	Maintain HbA$_{1c}$ lower than 7%.	Diabetes is a stronger risk factor in women than in men.[88]

Table continues on page 284

PROBLEM	INTERVENTION	RATIONALE	EXPECTED OUTCOME	SPECIAL CONSIDERATIONS
Atypical presentation of heart disease in women	Maintain a high index of suspicion when women present with complaints of chest discomfort; peculiar feelings; neck, jaw, or back pain; dyspnea; nausea; and fatigue. Consider using McSweeney Symptom Survey[76] to assess symptoms.	43% of women do not experience chest discomfort with MI.[77] Typical angina is less predictive of CAD in women than in men.[35]	Women will be appropriately evaluated and treated for CAD.	Women present with CAD symptoms 10 years later than do men.[11]
Use of hormone replacement therapy	If HRT needed for menopausal symptoms, use lowest dose for shortest time around menopause, and then stop.	HRT is not indicated for primary or secondary prevention of heart disease in women.[85]		
Assessing heart disease in women	Exercise ECG recommended for women with low probability of CAD because of its high negative predictive value.[83] Stress echocardiography and nuclear scanning are effective noninvasive techniques in symptomatic women with intermediate to high risk of CAD.	Initial choice of testing is guided by risk assessment. Diagnostic testing is influenced by gender.	Women will be appropriately assessed.	Exercise ECG has a lower sensitivity and specificity, higher false-positive rates but high negative predictive value in women.[83]
Acute MI	Consider primary angioplasty and stenting; also consider coronary artery bypass surgery.	Blood flow needed for muscle viability.	Coronary artery blood flow restored. Termination of acute MI.	Women are more likely to die from first MI than are men. Women are less likely to undergo coronary intervention or bypass surgery.
Risk of reinfarction	Consider following treatment regimens: aspirin therapy, statin therapy, beta-blocker therapy, ACE inhibitor/ARB therapy, cardiac rehabilitation or regular physical activity, lifestyle changes as listed previously.	Use secondary prevention measures.	There is no reinfarction.	Women experience more long-term disability than men. Fewer women receive aspirin, beta blockers, or ACE inhibitors. Fewer women receive cardiac rehabilitation.[18]

BMI = Body mass index, CAD = coronary artery disease, CVD = cardiovascular disease, ECG = electrocardiogram, HDL = high-density lipoprotein, HRT = hormone replacement therapy, LDL = low-density lipoprotein, MI = myocardial infarction.

An increase in depressive symptoms may be an early warning sign of impending CV events. It is unknown, however, whether increasing depression is the cause of the CV event or if an impending CV event may be responsible for subclinical depressive symptoms.[138] It is also not known whether treating depressive symptoms will lower CV risk. It should be noted, however, that depression may influence patients' desire to adhere to their treatment plan and, thus, influence their overall prevention practices. In the WHI Observational Study,[138] there was a strong inverse correlation between depression and physical activity level, as well as other CV risk factor reduction practices, such as smoking cessation, weight management, and hypertension, hypercholesterolemia, and diabetes control. In addition, depression was a strong predictor of compliance with cardiac rehabilitation programs.[127]

APPLIED PATHOPHYSIOLOGY

CAD is characterized by an impairment of myocardial perfusion. Because most of the research on CAD has been done on males, the pathophysiology of CAD in women is just beginning to be understood. What is known so far is that several areas of pathogenesis may differ in women: vessel size, plaque characteristics, endothelial integrity, lipid profile, and effects of hormones. Each of these will be discussed. Further research is needed to clarify how differences are manifested, and thus how they should be treated.

Vessel Size

The dimensions of the coronary arteries providing oxygenated blood to the heart are directly proportional to the mass of the heart. Heart weight is determined by body size. Women generally have smaller body mass than men; therefore women's hearts weigh 50 to 100 g less than men's hearts. Both intravascular ultrasound and cardiac catheterization have demonstrated that the left main coronary artery and the left anterior descending artery are smaller in women.[112] This smaller artery dimension may contribute to the difficulty in diagnosing and treating CAD in women. Small coronary arteries have a higher prevalence of atherogenesis than larger arteries, possibly because volume flow rate, flow velocity, and shear stress increase as vessel radius decreases.[4]

Plaque

Fibrous plaques form the lesions of atherosclerosis. These plaques consist of a combination of lipid, cells, and connective tissue matrix. Several factors affect the formation of plaque, including endothelial injury, macrophage accumulation, platelet aggregation, smooth muscle proliferation, inflammatory cells, LDL accumulation, and local modification of LDL.[23] Chapter 11 provides further information on atherosclerotic buildup and the formation of plaque. Highlighted here is what is known about the differences in plaque formation in women. These differences seem to affect the presentation and identification of CAD in women.

Although coronary thrombosis is overwhelmingly the most likely cause of MI in both genders, the nature of the thrombus differs. Men more often have plaque *rupture* as the underlying cause of the infarction, whereas women are twice as likely to have plaque *erosion* as the underlying cause.[9,123] Plaque rupture is a disruption of the thin fibrous cap that lies over a large, necrotic core. In plaque erosion, a thrombus lies over a base of smooth muscle cells without a necrotic core. Lesions of plaque erosion are more often nonocclusive, eccentric, and not as calcified as ruptured plaque.[9]

Plaque morphology varies with menopausal status as well as with the presence of risk factors. For instance, plaque erosion is more often seen in women younger than 50 years, especially those who smoke.[24] However, plaque rupture is more often seen in women older than 50 and is correlated with elevated serum total cholesterol levels.[133] It appears that women younger than 50 years (premenopausal) may be protected from the development of lesions of plaque rupture by the plaque-stabilizing effects of hormones, but are not protected from developing plaque erosion.[133] More research is needed in this area to address these recent findings.

Endothelial Integrity

Vascular endothelium regulates vascular tone by producing a variety of vasoactive mechanisms, most of which promote vasodilation. Endothelial function is a key variable in the pathogenesis of atherosclerosis and its complications. Because of the suggested connection between endothelium dysfunction and CAD in women, studies are being directed toward identifying and evaluating coronary artery endothelial dysfunction as a primary mechanism for CAD.

Endothelial dysfunction produces inappropriate vasoconstriction because of a loss of response to acetylcholine.[22] Endothelial dysfunction has been correlated with impaired fibrinolysis, increased inflammation, and dyslipidemia.[19] This dysfunction leads to disturbances in coronary blood flow, which may increase myocardial ischemia and accelerate atherosclerosis and thrombosis.[22] Endothelial dysfunction seems to be a precursor of atherosclerosis and may cause major adverse cardiac events in patients with "normal" coronary arteries.[22,47,50] Currently, research is focusing on the best way to identify and diagnose endothelial dysfunction before a cardiac event.[22]

Inflammation may also play a role in endothelial dysfunction. Circulating inflammatory markers are strongly associated with cardiovascular event risk in women who have not had previous cardiovascular disease.[33,93] Tumor necrosis factor (TNF) receptors (receptors that mediate the effects of TNF, an inflammatory cytokine that induces the secretion of C-reactive protein in the liver[93]) are under investigation as a marker to evaluate inflammation. C-reactive protein (CRP) is another marker of an acute, low-grade inflammatory process that has been studied extensively.[14,109,111] An elevated level of CRP contributes to development of atherosclerotic lesions.[134] It has been reported that the level of CRP was a stronger predictor of heart disease than the LDL cholesterol level and that it should be incorporated into the Framingham risk score.[101] CRP levels have been shown to be reduced with statins, weight loss, and high-dose aspirin.[14,101] What is not known at this point is whether lowering the level of CRP decreases a woman's risk profile.

Lipids, Apolipoproteins, and Lipoproteins

Cholesterol and triglycerides are insoluble lipids unable to circulate in the blood unless combined with phospholipids called *lipoproteins*. The protein components of the lipoproteins are known as *apoproteins*, which play a role in the metabolism of lipid particles. Lipid metabolism includes the synthesis, transport, and functional activities of plasma lipoproteins, which include LDL, HDL, and very-low-density lipoproteins (VLDLs).

Studies have shown that increases in levels of total cholesterol and its subfractions (except for HDL) increase the risk of CAD. HDL levels seem to have a stronger link to CAD risk in postmenopausal women than in men.[110] Lipid profiles in women are affected by hormonal status and change at different ages. For instance, after age 55 years, LDL cholesterol and total cholesterol levels increase and HDL levels decrease—both of which increase the development of CAD. LDL levels peak between 55 and 65 years of age in women, about a decade later than in men.[15,17] HDL seems to have a protective effect even in patients with high total cholesterol levels. In fact, an HDL level greater than 60 mg/dl is considered a "negative risk factor," in that it offsets one of the other coronary risk factors.[15,17,123] In older women, triglycerides are also an independent predictor of CAD.[123]

Lp(a), an abnormal composite of LDL, is a known independent risk factor for the development of atherosclerosis, especially in women.[64,111] The synthesis of Lp(a) is primarily under genetic control. It has been proposed that estrogen and progestin may protect females to a large extent from the potentially deleterious effects of inherited high Lp(a) levels until menopause.[33] Unlike other lipid-rich particles, its levels are not significantly altered by conventional lipid-lowering therapies, diet, or exercise.[32] Although it has been reported that nicotinic acid and fibrates may decrease Lp(a) concentration,[26] lowering elevated Lp(a) concentration has not as yet been tied to decreasing heart disease.[15,111]

Hormones

Women spend on average 35 years of their lives in a postmenopausal, low-estrogen state. The majority of CAD is seen in women during this time,[125] which is about 10 years later than seen in men.[11] Estrogen has a variety of seemingly protective actions against ischemic or nonischemic injury of the heart and vessels.[90] The best-established mechanism involves its effects on lipid metabolism in the liver. Estrogen reduces total cholesterol and LDL cholesterol by 5% to 15%, increases HDL cholesterol by 10%, and reduces lipoprotein Lp(a) concentrations.[43] Estrogen also increases nitric oxide synthesis in the endothelial cells.[106] Nitric oxide causes the relaxation of the vascular smooth muscle cells and inhibits platelet activation,[125] both of which can be beneficial in decreasing cardiovascular events. These beneficial effects are absent after menopause. HRT has not been shown to produce similar effects.[103] In the large Women's Health Initiative (WHI) trial, it was reported that "overall health risks exceeded benefits from use of combined estrogen plus progestin for an average 5.2-year follow-up among healthy postmenopausal women" (p. 321).[103] Therefore HRT is not recommended to prevent CVD.

PRESENTATION

Women with heart disease present with different and more diverse symptoms than men. Women's initial manifestation of heart disease may be chest discomfort, rather than an MI.[35,94] However, that chest discomfort often does not predict prognosis in women.[25,35,77] Although women may describe classic chest pain, they may just as readily describe it as a "peculiar feeling" or a sensation in their chest or neck or left arm that "worries them."[35] Almost half (43%) do not experience any type of chest discomfort with an acute MI,[35,77] or they may describe the pain as more transient,[73] more sharp, or stabbing.[94] The most frequent acute symptoms reported are shortness of breath, weakness, and fatigue.[77] Women are also more likely to have neck pain, back pain, jaw pain, paroxysmal nocturnal dyspnea, nausea, vomiting, indigestion, and loss of appetite than are men.[35,73,94] In addition, women are less likely to report diaphoresis, but equally likely to report dizziness, fainting, or syncope.[94]

Women with heart disease tend to experience more noncardiac chest pain than men, and they seem to have it over a time.[77,81] It is thought that this may condition the heart muscle tissue to oxygen deprivation, which, in turn, may muddle the picture and make diagnosis more difficult.[81]

One study found that 95% of women experience symptoms more than 1 month before having an MI.[77] The most frequent prodromal symptoms include unusual fatigue, sleep disturbances, shortness of breath, indigestion, and anxiety. Only 30% reported chest discomfort in the prodromal period.[77] When women do experience prodromal symptoms, they often delay seeking care longer than men.[143] This may be because women perceive themselves to be less vulnerable to an MI; therefore they do not put as much emphasis on the symptoms or do not recognize the symptoms as indications of CAD.[143] Confounding the issue is that women tend to deny their symptoms might be heart-related by thinking their symptoms are not serious, waiting for symptoms to go away, and worrying about troubling others.[75,78,122] Also, women tend to place a different meaning on chest pain than do men. Some older women perceive angina as natural, and they may interpret the onset of exertional angina as a normal symptom of fatigue.[94] As a result, they may limit their physical activity without complaint or request for evaluation.[94] Women sometimes perceive cardiovascular disease as a natural way to end life.[94] Failure to recognize prodromal warning signs along with the less dramatic and nonspecific symptoms may be reasons that women, compared with men, experience a greater proportion of sudden cardiac deaths, have more unrecognized MIs, or are mistakenly diagnosed and discharged from emergency departments.[77]

Angina With "Normal" Coronary Arteries

Interestingly, women are less likely to have obstructive CAD than men.[25] There is a growing body of evidence to suggest that this phenomenon is not necessarily benign.[21,22] Women with "normal" coronary arteries (without angiographic evidence of CAD) or nonobstructive coronary disease frequently have persistent symptoms, rehospitalizations, and more adverse cardiac events.[25] Some women have noncardiac pain, others have chest pain of cardiac but nonischemic origin, and others have chest pain caused by myocardial ischemia related to coronary vascular abnormalities.[21] The WISE study documented that women who have angina and do not have obstructive CAD have a relatively poor prognosis compared with women who have obstructive coronary disease and no myocardial ischemia.[60] Therefore it would seem that this condition should be recognized early and addressed aggressively.

The chest pain from nonobstructive coronary disease is often similar in quality to classic angina, but usually more intense. It is usually described as "constricting" rather than "oppressive" and the pain may last 30 minutes or more.[22] Several consistencies in the patient's history that may indicate the presence of nonobstructive angina are the following: an extremely variable threshold of physical activity that produces the discomfort; radiation of the discomfort to the submammary areas; and the presence of features associated with pain, such as mental arousal or palpitation.[21]

The pathophysiology of women with angina and "normal" angiograms is unclear and diverse. One mechanism is thought to involve myocardial oxygen demand. Coronary flow reserve is the increase in blood flow in response to metabolic or pharmacologic stimulations. When this is impaired, increased myocardial oxygen demand may produce ischemia.[21,22] Coronary flow is regulated by several factors influencing vascular tone, including levels of nitric oxide.[21,22] After menopause, women experience decreased nitric oxide production, which decreases the vasodilation response, and thus decreases coronary flow reserve. This nonobstructive arteriolar narrowing may be a marker of endothelial dysfunction, from aging, hypertension, inflammation, or other processes.[22] Coronary artery spasm does not appear to play a major role.[21]

Unfortunately, there is no evidence to date from randomized trials suggesting appropriate treatment for women with angina and "normal" coronary arteries. Therefore lifestyle changes and risk factor management are essential components to prevent adverse coronary events. Exercise training has also been demonstrated to be beneficial.[38]

ASSESSMENT

Clinical evaluation of CAD has traditionally been more challenging in women compared with men. The initial assessment should consist of a careful history and physical examination. Atypical and prodromal symptoms are challenging to evaluate and link to an assessment of heart disease, as discussed in the Research Utilization box on p. 288. One instrument that has been developed to assist clinicians is the McSweeney Acute and Prodromal Myocardial Infarction

Symptom Survey (MAPMISS).[76,79] This survey is a comprehensive assessment tool developed to assist in the evaluation and earlier diagnosis of CAD in women.[76,79] The survey lists 33 prodromal and 37

◆ RESEARCH UTILIZATION

Prodromal Heart Disease Symptoms in Women

CLINICAL ISSUE

Women present with atypical symptoms of myocardial infarction days or weeks before the event. Little is known about early warning or prodromal heart disease symptoms in women. There is no clear connection between women's prodromal symptoms and how they relate to acute myocardial infarction (AMI) symptoms. Failure to recognize prodromal symptoms may be one reason women experience a greater proportion of sudden cardiac deaths than do men.

SUMMARY

This study identified the most frequent prodromal symptoms of an MI, how prodromal and acute symptoms relate to comorbidities and heart disease risk factors, and whether prodromal symptoms were predictive of AMI symptomatology. The study evaluated 515 white women diagnosed with AMI using the McSweeney Acute and Prodromal Myocardial Infarction Symptom Survey (MAPMISS) 4 to 6 months after discharge. Researchers found that 95% of the women experienced prodromal symptoms and those with more prodromal symptoms experienced more acute symptoms. The most frequent symptoms experienced *more than 1 month* before an AMI were unusual fatigue, sleep disturbance, and shortness of breath. Chest discomfort was reported in only 30% of the women. The most frequent *acute* symptoms were shortness of breath, weakness, and fatigue. Acute chest pain was reported in 67% of the subjects.

APPLICATION

Accurately describing women's prodromal and acute symptoms of CAD is important to provide a complete picture of women's typical symptoms. Thoroughly evaluating a woman's complaints of unusual fatigue, shortness of breath, and sleep disturbances may help with early recognition and treatment of heart disease. Also, when a woman experiences chest discomfort, she usually describes it as aching, tightness, or pressure. Women should have an in-depth assessment when these descriptors are used.

McSweeney, J. C., et al. (2003). Women's early warning symptoms of acute myocardial infarction. *Circulation, 108*(21), 2619–2623.

acute symptoms that have been identified in previous research studies.[76] Increased recognition of atypical symptoms in women by using this or some similar tool could help to improve the outcomes of women with heart disease. In addition, beginning evaluation should include assessment of coronary risk factors (see Table 13-2) and a resting ECG. If the 10-year risk of CAD exceeds 10%, further evaluation should be performed.[85] Initial test choice is guided by using the risk assessment to place women in low-, intermediate-, or high-risk categories.[83] For women with intermediate to high likelihood of CAD, noninvasive diagnostic studies, such as exercise ECG or cardiac imaging studies, are recommended[41] (Figure 13-1).

The accuracy and limitations of stress testing in women are confusing. This may be attributable to the higher prevalence of nonobstructive CAD and single-vessel disease in women, as well as the limitation of various forms of stress testing.[83] Standard exercise ECG is the most commonly used and least costly of the noninvasive testing. However, exercise ECG is not as predictive in women as men because of lower sensitivity and specificity and higher false-positive rates than in men.[53] Several factors account for this, including the effect of estrogen on the coronary arteries, an inadequate exercise response resulting from deconditioning or comorbidities, underlying ECG abnormalities, and altered hemodynamics.[132] Exercise ECG is, however, recommended in women with a low probability of CAD because it does have a high negative predictive value.[83]

When women have symptoms suggestive of CAD, stress echocardiography, either physiologically on a treadmill or pharmacologically with dobutamine (Dobutrex), can be effective to detect CAD and assess prognosis.[16] Echocardiography can detect regional wall motion abnormalities at rest. Dobutamine stress echocardiography is recommended for women with a normal or abnormal ECG who are incapable of exercise.[83]

Stress myocardial perfusion imaging using nuclear scanning provides direct imaging of the myocardium and is not dependent on the ECG to diagnose ischemia. Gated myocardial perfusion single-photon emission computed tomography (SPECT) is the most common nuclear imaging procedure used and can be performed with exercise or pharmacologically with adenosine. Technical limitations in women have been reported, including false-positive results because of breast attenuation and small left ventricular chamber size; however, current innovations have improved the accuracy of SPECT in high-risk women.[83]

Cardiac catheterization remains a valuable invasive tool for assessing the presence and severity of heart

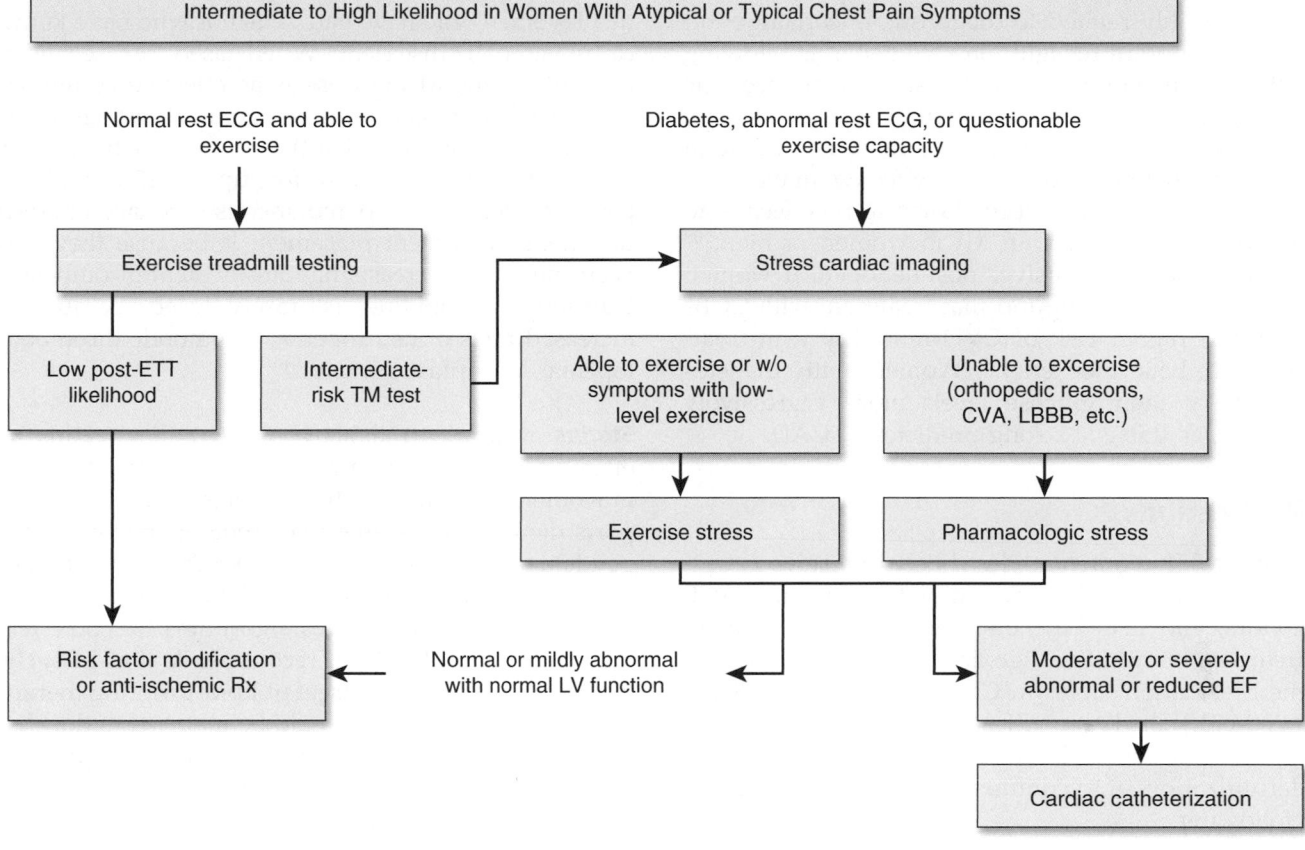

♦FIGURE 13-1 Algorithm for the evaluation of symptomatic women using exercise ECG or cardiac imaging. CVA = Cerebral vascular accident, ECG = electrocardiogram, EF = ejection fraction, ETT = exercise treadmill test, LBBB = left bundle branch block, LV = left ventricular, TM = treadmill.

disease. The same technique is used for men and women; however, because of the smaller vessel size, the technical difficulty is somewhat increased in women. This may lead to longer procedure times and more difficulties, such as bleeding, entry-site vascular problems,[59] neurologic complications, and hemodynamic instability.[6] Because of these complications, the benefit of invasive strategies in women with acute coronary syndrome (ACS) may be limited to high-risk women.[59]

Several emerging technologies warrant mentioning. Research has not clearly shown the benefit of computed tomography (CT) to detect coronary artery calcium as a marker of heart disease. At this time, testing for coronary artery calcium should be limited to clinically selected women at intermediate risk.[83] Limited data suggest a future role for cardiovascular magnetic resonance (CMR) imaging in patients with an intermediate likelihood of CAD.[83]

The emerging field of endothelial dysfunction may be best evaluated by perfusion-imaging studies with magnetic resonance imaging, positron emission tomography, or gated SPECT.[21] These techniques can detect abnormal flow-reserve patterns, suggesting that vascular dysfunction is present.[21] However, before recommendations can be made, more research is needed in this area.

When assessing for a myocardial infarction in women, the serum marker troponin seems to predict a worse outcome and is useful to guide early invasive management.[42] Guidelines recommend that any elevation in cardiac troponin T or troponin I above the 99th percentile of normal is sufficient to diagnose an MI. However, it has been found that, as with most guidelines, this diagnostic test is also less likely to be used in women.[141]

INTERVENTIONS

In 2002 the American College of Cardiology (ACC) and the AHA published guidelines for the management of patients with unstable angina and non–ST segment elevation (NSTEMI).[20] Even though these guidelines are "gender neutral," it was found that evidence-based treatments were less likely to be provided to women than to men with ACS.[18] This undertreatment is possibly related to diagnostic uncertainty and delays in symptom recognition.[18] In general, following an MI, women should receive the same pharmacologic and lifestyle interventions as men. These are aspirin, beta blockers, statins, and ACE inhibitors. Although calcium channel blockade may be effective in reducing hypertension, it has not been shown to be effective to improve outcomes after an MI in women or men.[108] In a study of hypertensive, postmenopausal women (ages 50 to 79), it was found that treatment with CCBs conferred a higher risk of CVD mortality than treatment with beta blockers.[137] Women with diabetes should have their glucose levels more aggressively controlled, as this is a strong predictor of CAD.

Medications

After an MI, women are less likely to receive thrombolytics, antidysrhythmics, antiplatelet agents, ACE inhibitors, and beta blockers, and are more likely to be treated with nitrates, digoxin, and diuretics.[18] (Refer to the Medication tables in Chapter 11 on pp. 218-219 and 220-221.) The known lifesaving treatments are consistently underused in women[85] Reasons for this underutilization of recommended guidelines include the following:

- Women are more often treated by a non-cardiologist.
- The older age of women at presentation seems to make practitioners more cautious about causing complications, such as increased bleeding and renal dysfunction.
- Women often choose to stop therapies on their own.[18]

Women seem to metabolize drugs differently than men, which may produce clinically relevant adverse drug reactions.[5] Women have a 50% higher risk of adverse drug reactions, which could be related to the response differences attributable to dosing not corrected for a lower body weight, the higher percent of body fat in women than in men, and a 10% lower glomerular filtration rate in women[5]—all of which should be accounted for when dosing medications for women.

Antiplatelet Agents. The platelet-inhibition properties of aspirin are widely known to decrease comorbidities (recurrent ischemic events) and mortality after an MI (secondary prevention).[13] However, in a large-cohort, 10-year study, aspirin did not reduce the risk of developing heart disease (primary prevention) in women.[102] Therefore the use of aspirin for primary prevention in women younger than 65 years old is not recommended

until further research is conducted, but should be used in all women who have had an MI or who have known cardiovascular disease.[85] When used for secondary prevention, the 81-mg dose is as effective as the 325-mg dose. The thienopyridine agents clopidogrel (Plavix) and ticlopidine (Ticlid) should also be used in combination with aspirin for up to 12 months in patients after ACS or percutaneous coronary intervention (PCI) with stent placement[114] because they have been shown to decrease the rates of stent thrombosis.[65] Currently, ticlopidine is rarely used because of increased rates of neutropenia, thrombotic thrombocytopenia, and aplastic anemia.[65]

Statins. Multiple trials have shown that statins are effective in secondary prevention of coronary events in women regardless of cholesterol levels.[36,39] This supports the theory that there are benefits of statins independent of LDL-lowering effects.[87] The National Cholesterol Education Program Adult Treatment Panel III (NCEP ATP III) provides algorithms for cholesterol management.[39] The Panel recommends that LDL cholesterol be the primary target of lipid-lowering therapy; the intensity of therapy should be matched to the absolute risk of the patient. Optimum levels of lipids and lipoproteins in women are the following:

- LDL less than 100 mg/dL
- HDL greater than 50 mg/dL
- Triglycerides less than 150 mg/dL
- Non-HDL (total cholesterol minus HDL cholesterol) less than 130 mg/dL[85]

In high-risk women or when LDL is elevated, saturated fat intake should be reduced to less than 7% of calories and cholesterol to less than 200 mg/dL, and trans fatty acid intake should be reduced (see Box 13-1). LDL-lowering therapy should be started along with lifestyle changes in high-risk women with LDL levels greater than 100 mg/dL, and statin therapy should be started in high-risk women with LDL levels less than 100 mg/dL, unless contraindicated.[39] Fibric acids and niacin can be used to treat high triglyceride levels,[15] as well as low HDL levels in high-risk women.[85] It should be noted that the dietary supplement niacin must not be used as a substitute for prescription niacin.[85] Because of the variability of the free nicotinic acid content in preparations that are not FDA regulated, over-the-counter niacin should be used only if approved and monitored by a physician; this is because OTC niacin has been found to be ineffective in raising HDL and can be hepatotoxic.[82]

ACE Inhibitors. ACE inhibitors after MI did not provide as much benefit in women as in men.[129] However, ACE inhibitors, as well as statins, may help improve endothelial dysfunction,[98] which is more prevalent in women and contributes to angina with "normal" coronary arteries, and therefore should be prescribed after an MI. ACE inhibitors should also be used to treat left ventricular dysfunction in anyone with left ventricular ejection fraction less than or equal to 40%.[114]

Beta Blockers. Studies show beta-blocking agents clearly provide substantial improvement in reducing chest pain episodes as well as promoting increased survival after MI; in fact, results in women were equal to, if not greater than, those seen in men.[123,135] These agents seem to accomplish this result by counteracting the effects of increased adrenergic tone, reducing myocardial oxygen demand, and promoting blood flow to vulnerable areas.

Hormone Replacement Therapy

HRT is used to treat menopausal symptoms (e.g., hot flashes and vaginal dryness). Although epidemiologic evidence was originally thought to be strong for postmenopausal use of estrogen in the prevention of heart disease, clinical trial evidence does not support these findings.[56,99,136]

HRT has a profound metabolic impact on the cardiovascular system, affecting arterial function.[121] These effects include an increased hypercoagulable state and increased levels of CRP, which is a marker for acute inflammation. Both of these effects may aggravate plaque instability and increase thrombotic risk and the potential for reinfarction.[3,81] Studies suggest that postmenopausal women who initiate HRT after a recent MI have an increased risk of cardiac events.[3,56]

It is important to remember that the primary indication approved by the FDA for the use of HRT is for the treatment of menopausal symptoms. Current recommendations are that HRT should not be used for primary or secondary prevention of CVD. If HRT is needed for treatment of menopausal symptoms, women should take the lowest dose for the shortest period of time.[97,136]

Percutaneous Coronary Interventions

Evidence demonstrating outcomes of women receiving PCI is conflicting. Women represent 15% to 38% of the population in studies of PCI, and relatively few sex-specific data exist.[65] While some studies report higher rates of mortality, nonfatal MI, and nonfatal disabling stroke in women than in men,[6,52,131] the GUSTO II-B PTCA study[124] and others[42,51] found no significant difference. More recently, studies have shown a 35% reduction in mortality in women treated with primary PCI after MI,[65,80] and a higher degree of myocardial salvage

after PCI than in men.[81] Outcomes after an intervention are somewhat explained by a higher risk profile for women,[65] including such variables as the following:

- Older age of women at presentation
- Hypertension
- Hypercholesterolemia
- Higher prevalence of risk factors, such as diabetes mellitus

In fact, women with diabetes are at particularly high risk of developing coronary restenosis after PCI, possibly because of an accelerated fibrotic response or enhanced hyperplasia.[88] In one study, diabetic women had more complex lesions and needed more stents than did nondiabetic women.[88]

Women have 1.5 to 4 times higher procedure-related vascular complications after PCI.[66] Procedural complications include retroperitoneal bleeds requiring transfusions,[59] vessel dissections, and perforations.[67] These have been attributed to the smaller body surface area (BSA), smaller coronary arteries, sheaths that are too large for the vessel, and non–weight-adjusted anticoagulant dosing.[67] Less aggressive anticoagulation regimens and increased use of weight-adjusted heparin dosing have helped to decrease the incidence of these complications.[65]

It has also been found that platelets in women seem to show an affinity to aggregation.[40] Even though it has been documented that women were less often treated acutely with glycoprotein (GP) IIb/IIIa inhibitors,[18] it seems they may benefit from effective antiplatelet inhibition.[42,65] As an adjunct to unfractionated heparin, IIb/IIIa inhibitors are not associated with an increased risk of bleeding complications.[67] It seems, therefore, that these drugs should be used more frequently in women.[42,65]

In observational registries, women are reported to have similar or lower target-lesion revascularization (TLR) rates after balloon angioplasty and stenting.[66] It has been shown that drug-eluting stents are effective in reducing restenosis and enhancing event-free survival in women as well as men.[67] Restenosis rates may be slightly higher in women because of the presence of other risk factors as previously described.[67]

Given the evidence at this point, it seems that early invasive management of ACS with a PCI in women is beneficial, especially in those with elevated troponin values, which puts them in a higher risk category.[65] In addition, the benefit of primary PCI over fibrinolytic therapy in women presenting with ST elevation MI has been clearly demonstrated.[65,124] Careful attention must be paid to appropriate dosing of adjunctive therapies, such as antiplatelet and anticoagulant medications, to minimize the incidence of side effects.

Coronary Artery Bypass Surgery

Coronary artery bypass graft (CABG) surgery is an effective method of treating CAD.[128] Approximately 30% of the total number of CABG surgeries in the United States are performed on women.[11] Data taken from the National Cardiovascular Network, adjusted for comorbidities, show that women have a higher in-hospital mortality rate and a higher 30-day mortality rate after CABG surgery.[129] In women under the age of 50, there is a three times greater risk of dying in the hospital after the procedure compared with men of similar age. This may be explained by the fact that only the most severe cases of CAD in younger women are recognized and treated with CABG surgery. Women are also less likely to receive internal mammary grafts as a bypass conduit, or to undergo complete revascularization.[129] Furthermore, they are more likely to experience the postoperative complications of heart failure, perioperative infarction, hemorrhage, and neurologic complications, and twice as likely to be rehospitalized in the first 60 days after surgery as are men.[129] The reason for these disparities is unknown. In one study, the women had less extensive vessel disease and better heart function than men and still had higher mortality.[74] Again, it is suggested that the smaller artery size could be a factor, but also advanced age and comorbidities, such as diabetes and hypertension, play a role. In addition, it is known that women are less likely to be closely followed up after CABG, less likely to receive the evidence-based medications, and less likely to be referred to a cardiac rehabilitation program.[129] After CABG, women have a lower likelihood of being free of angina and are more disabled.[58,92] They have more depression, slower recovery, more physical symptoms, and higher functional impairment.[107,123] Women tend to have more fatigue, shortness of breath, and chest discomfort than men,[107] causing readmission rates that can be 4.7 times higher than those of men.[104] Some of this may be explained by women being more likely than men to be single and living alone,[107] and therefore having limited sources of assistance after surgery.

Even though clinical and functional outcomes in women are not as positive as with men, it is still recommended that women have CABG surgery when it is indicated. However, recommendations are that women should be followed more closely after surgery than men, revascularization should be complete, internal mammary artery grafts should be used when appropriate, and a referral to cardiac rehabilitation should be made.[123] In addition, education specific to women's post-CABG recovery and assessment of social support systems are important to assist with a better quality of life after surgery.[104]

CONCLUSIONS

Effective management of heart disease in women requires early recognition of symptoms, knowledge of diagnostic testing, implementation of appropriate therapies, and recommendation of effective prevention strategies. Educating patients and clinicians about the known differences is critical to improving patient outcomes. For links to web sites concerning women and heart disease, see the end of the list of references in this chapter. There is compelling evidence that heart disease is largely preventable. Therefore, prevention of risk factors is imperative for women.

Much attention has been directed toward a better appreciation of the influence of gender on CV risk and management, but important gaps in knowledge are still evident. Recent research will have significant impact on prevention and care of women with heart disease. Continued research on the differences in pathophysiology, presentation, treatment, and prevention is essential to further our understanding and continue to improve outcomes.

REFERENCES

1. USDHHS. (2000). *Healthy people 2010*. Washington, DC: U.S. Government Printing Office.
2. Albert, N. M. (2005). We are what we eat: women and diet for cardiovascular health. *J Cardiovasc Nurs, 20*(6), 451–460.
3. Alexander, K. P., et al. (2001). Initiation of hormone replacement therapy after acute myocardial infarction is associated with more cardiac events during follow-up. *J Am College Cardiol, 38*(1), 1–7.
4. Alfaro-Franco, C. M., et al. (2002). Invasive diagnostic testing. In S. Wilansky & J. T. Willerson (Eds.), *Heart disease in women* (1st ed., pp. 175–177). Philadelphia: Saunders.
5. Anderson, G. D. (2005). Sex and racial differences in pharmacological response: where is the evidence? Pharmacogenetics, pharmacokinetics, and pharmacodynamics. *J Womens Health (Larchmt), 14*(1), 19–29.
6. Antoniucci, D., et al. (2001). Sex-based differences in clinical and angiographic outcomes after primary angioplasty or stenting for acute myocardial infarction. *Am J Cardiol, 87*(3), 289–293.
7. Appel, L. J., et al. (1997). A clinical trial of the effects of dietary patterns on blood pressure. DASH collaborative research group. *N Engl J Med, 336*(16), 1117–1124.
8. Appel, L. J., et al. (2005). Effects of protein, monounsaturated fat, and carbohydrate intake on blood pressure and serum lipids: results of the OMNIHEART randomized trial. *JAMA, 294*(19), 2455–2464.
9. Arbustini, E., et al. (1999). Plaque erosion is a major substrate for coronary thrombosis in acute myocardial infarction. *Heart, 82*(3), 269–272.
10. Ariyo, A. A., et al. (2000). Depressive symptoms and risks of coronary heart disease and mortality in elderly Americans. Cardiovascular health study collaborative research group. *Circulation, 102*(15), 1773–1779.
11. American Heart Association. (2004). *Heart disease and stroke statistics—2004 update*. Dallas, Tex: American Heart Association.
12. American Lung Association. (2006). *Trends in tobacco use—2006*, www.lungusa.org.

13. Baigent, C., et al. (1998). ISIS-2: 10 year survival among patients with suspected acute myocardial infarction in randomized comparison of intravenous streptokinase, oral aspirin, both, or neither. The ISIS-2 (second international study of infarct survival) collaborative group. *BMJ, 316*(7141), 1337–1343.

14. Ballantyne, C. M., et al. (2005). Lipoprotein-associated phospholipase A2, high-sensitivity C-reactive protein, and risk for incident ischemic stroke in middle-aged men and women in the atherosclerosis risk in communities (ARIC) study. *Arch Intern Med, 165* (21), 2479–2484.

15. Bedinghaus, J., et al. (2001). Coronary artery disease prevention: what's different for women? *Am Fam Physician, 63*(7), 1393–1400, 1405–1396.

16. Biagini, E., et al. (2005). Seven-year follow-up after dobutamine stress echocardiography: impact of gender on prognosis. *J Am Coll Cardiol, 45*(1), 93–97.

17. Bittner, V. (2002). Lipoprotein abnormalities related to women's health. *Am J Cardiol, 90*(8A), 77i–84i.

18. Blomkalns, A. L., et al. (2005). Gender disparities in the diagnosis and treatment of non-ST-segment elevation acute coronary syndromes: large-scale observations from the CRUSADE (can rapid risk stratification of unstable angina patients suppress adverse outcomes with early implementation of the American College of Cardiology/American Heart Association guidelines) national quality improvement initiative. *J Am Coll Cardiol, 45*(6), 832–837.

19. Brandenburg, S. L., et al. (2003). Cardiovascular risk in women with type 2 diabetes. *Med Clin North Am, 87*(5), 955–969.

20. Braunwald, E., et al. (2002). ACC/AHA 2002 guideline update for the management of patients with unstable angina and non-ST-segment elevation myocardial infarction—summary article: a report of the American College of Cardiology/American Heart Association task force on practice guidelines (committee on the management of patients with unstable angina). *J Am Coll Cardiol, 40*(7), 1366–1374.

21. Bugiardini, R., & Bairey Merz, C. N. (2005). Angina with "normal" coronary arteries: a changing philosophy. *JAMA, 293*(4), 477–484.

22. Bugiardini, R., et al. (2004). Endothelial function predicts future development of coronary artery disease: a study of women with chest pain and normal coronary angiograms. *Circulation, 109* (21), 2518–2523.

23. Buja, L. M., & Othman, M. O. (2002). Anatomy and pathophysiology. In S. Wilansky & J. T. Willerson (Eds.), *Heart disease in women* (1st ed., pp. 57–67). Philadelphia, Pa: Elsevier Science.

24. Burke, A. P., et al. (1998). Effect of risk factors on the mechanism of acute thrombosis and sudden coronary death in women. *Circulation, 97*(21), 2110–2116.

25. Cannon, R. O., III, & Balaban, R. S. (2000). Chest pain in women with normal coronary angiograms. *N Engl J Med, 342*(12), 885–887.

26. Carlson, L. A., et al. (1989). Pronounced lowering of serum levels of lipoprotein Lp(a) in hyperlipidemic subjects treated with nicotinic acid. *J Intern Med, 226*(4), 271–276.

27. Caspersen, C. J., et al. (1985). Physical activity, exercise, and physical fitness: definitions and distinctions for health-related research. *Public Health Rep, 100*(2), 126–131.

28. Chobanian, A., et al. (2003). The seventh report of the joint national committee on prevention, detection, evaluation, and treatment of high blood pressure: the JNC 7 report. *JAMA, 289*, 2560–2572.

29. Collins, R. (2002). MRC/BHF heart protection study of cholesterol lowering with simvastatin in 20,536 high-risk individuals: a randomized placebo-controlled trial. *Lancet, 360*(9326), 7–22.

30. Cooper, R., & Rotimi, C. (1997). Hypertension in blacks. *Am J Hypertens, 10*(7 Pt 1), 804–812.

31. Cushman, W. C., et al. (2002). Success and predictors of blood pressure control in diverse North American settings: the antihypertensive and lipid-lowering treatment to prevent heart attack trial (ALLHAT). *J Clin Hypertens (Greenwich), 4*(6), 393–404.

32. Davis, S. R., et al. (2002). Differing effects of low-dose estrogen-progestin therapy and pravastatin in postmenopausal hypercholesterolemic women. *Climacteric, 5*(4), 341–350.

33. Davison, S., & Davis, S. R. (2003). New markers for cardiovascular disease risk in women: impact of endogenous estrogen status and exogenous postmenopausal hormone therapy. *J Clin Endocrinol Metab, 88*(6), 2470–2478.

34. de Gaetano, G. (2001). Low-dose aspirin and vitamin E in people at cardiovascular risk: a randomised trial in general practice. Collaborative group of the primary prevention project. *Lancet, 357* (9250), 89–95.

35. DeVon, H. A., & Zerwic, J. J. (2003). The symptoms of unstable angina: do women and men differ? *Nurs Res, 52*(2), 108–118.

36. Downs, J. R., et al. (1998). Primary prevention of acute coronary events with lovastatin in men and women with average cholesterol levels: results of AFCAPS/TEXCAPS. Air Force/Texas coronary atherosclerosis prevention study. *JAMA, 279*(20), 1615–1622.

37. Elsaesser, A., & Hamm, C. W. (2004). Acute coronary syndrome. The risk of being female. *Circulation, 109*, 565–567.

38. Eriksson, B. E., et al. (2000). Physical training in syndrome X: physical training counteracts deconditioning and pain in syndrome X. *J Am Coll Cardiol, 36*(5), 1619–1625.

39. Executive summary of the third report of the national cholesterol education program (NCEP) expert panel on detection, evaluation, and treatment of high blood cholesterol in adults (adult treatment panel III). *JAMA, 285*(19), 2486–2497.

40. Faraday, N., et al. (1997). Gender differences in platelet Gp IIb-IIIa activation. *Thromb Haemostasis, 77*(4), 748–754.

41. Gibbons, R., et al. (2002). ACC/AHA 2002 guideline update for exercise testing: summary article: a report of the American College of Cardiology/American Heart Association task force on practice guidelines. *Circulation, 106*, 1883–1892.

42. Glaser, R., et al. (2002). Benefit of an early invasive management strategy in women with acute coronary syndromes. *JAMA, 288* (24), 3124–3129.

43. Godsland, I. F. (2001). Effects of postmenopausal hormone replacement therapy on lipid, lipoprotein, and apolipoprotein (a) concentrations: analysis of studies published from 1974–2000. *Fertil Steril, 75*(5), 898–915.

44. Goldbaum, G. M., et al. (1987). The relative impact of smoking and oral contraceptive use on women in the United States. *JAMA, 258*(10), 1339–1342.

45. Women's Health Initiative Study Group. (1998). Design of the women's health initiative clinical trial and observational study. The women's health initiative study group. *Control Clin Trials, 19*(1), 61–109.

46. Hajjar, I., & Kotchen, T. A. (2003). Trends in prevalence, awareness, treatment, and control of hypertension in the United States, 1988–2000. *JAMA, 290*(2), 199–206.

47. Halcox, J. P., et al. (2002). Prognostic value of coronary vascular endothelial dysfunction. *Circulation, 106*(6), 653–658.

48. Handberg, E., et al. (2006). Impaired coronary vascular reactivity and functional capacity in women: results from the NHLBI women's ischemia syndrome evaluation (WISE) study. *J Am Coll Cardiol, 47*(3 suppl), S44–S49.

49. He, J., et al. (2000). Long-term effects of weight loss and dietary sodium reduction on incidence of hypertension. *Hypertension, 35* (2), 544–549.

50. Heitzer, T., et al. (2001). Endothelial dysfunction, oxidative stress, and risk of cardiovascular events in patients with coronary artery disease. *Circulation, 104*(22), 2673–2678.

51. Hochman, J. S., et al. (1997). Outcome and profile of women and men presenting with acute coronary syndromes: a report from TIMI IIIb. TIMI investigators. Thrombolysis in myocardial infarction. *J Am Coll Cardiol*, *30*(1), 141–148.

52. Hochman, J. S., et al. (1999). Sex, clinical presentation, and outcome in patients with acute coronary syndromes. Global use of strategies to open occluded coronary arteries in acute coronary syndromes IIb investigators. *N Engl J Med*, *341*(4), 226–232.

53. Hoilund-Carlsen, P. F., et al. (2005). Usefulness of the exercise electrocardiogram in diagnosing ischemic or coronary heart disease in patients with chest pain. *Am J Cardiol*, *95*(1), 96–99.

54. Hooper, L., et al. (2001). Reduced or modified dietary fat for preventing cardiovascular disease. *Cochrane Database Syst Rev* (3), CD002137.

55. Hu, F. B., et al. (2002). Fish and omega-3 fatty acid intake and risk of coronary heart disease in women. *JAMA*, *287*, 1815–1821.

56. Hulley, S., et al. (1998). Randomized trial of estrogen plus progestin for secondary prevention of coronary heart disease in postmenopausal women. Heart and estrogen/progestin replacement study (HERS) research group. *JAMA*, *280*(7), 605–613.

57. Implications of the diabetes control and complications trial. *Diabetes Care*, *26*(suppl 1), S25–S27.

58. Jacobs, A. K. (2003). Coronary revascularization in women in 2003: sex revisited. *Circulation*, *107*(3), 375–377.

59. Jacobs, A. K., et al. (2002). Improved outcomes for women undergoing contemporary percutaneous coronary intervention: a report from the national heart, lung, and blood institute dynamic registry. *J Am Coll Cardiol*, *39*(10), 1608–1614.

60. Johnson, B. D., et al. (2004). Prognosis in women with myocardial ischemia in the absence of obstructive coronary disease: results from the National Institutes of Health-National Heart, Lung, and Blood Institute-sponsored women's ischemia syndrome evaluation (WISE). *Circulation*, *109*(24), 2993–2999.

61. Kaur, S., et al. (2004). The impact of environmental tobacco smoke on women's risk of dying from heart disease: a meta-analysis. *J Womens Health (Larchmt)*, *13*(8), 888–897.

62. King, K. B., & Arthur, H. M. (2003). Coronary heart disease prevention. *J Cardiovasc Nurs*, *18*(4), 274–281.

63. Kip, K. E., et al. (2004). Clinical importance of obesity versus the metabolic syndrome in cardiovascular risk in women. *Circulation*, *109*, 706–713.

64. Knopp, R. H. (2002). Risk factors for coronary artery disease in women. *Am J Cardiol*, *89*(12A), 28E–34E; discussion 34E-35E.

65. Lansky, A. J., et al. (2005). Percutaneous coronary intervention and adjunctive pharmacotherapy in women: a statement for healthcare professionals from the American Heart Association. *Circulation*, *111*(7), 940–953.

66. Lansky, A. J., et al. (2004). Comparison of differences in outcome after percutaneous coronary intervention in men versus women <40 years of age. *Am J Cardiol*, *93*(7), 916–919.

67. Lansky, A. J., et al. (2005). Gender differences in outcomes after primary angioplasty versus primary stenting with and without abciximab for acute myocardial infarction: results of the controlled abciximab and device investigation to lower late angioplasty complications (CADILLAC) trial. *Circulation*, *111*(13), 1611–1618.

68. Legato, M. J. (1998). Women's health: not for women only. *Int J Fertil Womens Med*, *43*(2), 65–72.

69. Lewington, S., et al. (2002). Age-specific relevance of usual blood pressure to vascular mortality: a meta-analysis of individual data for one million adults in 61 prospective studies. *Lancet*, *360*(9349), 1903–1913.

70. Lewis, C. E., et al. (1996). Efficacy and tolerance of antihypertensive treatment in men and women with stage 1 diastolic hypertension. Results of the treatment of mild hypertension study. *Arch Intern Med*, *156*(4), 377–385.

71. Li, T. Y., et al. (2006). Obesity as compared with physical activity in predicting risk of coronary heart disease in women. *Circulation*, *113*(4), 499–506.

72. Lloyd-Jones, D. M., et al. (1999). Lifetime risk of developing coronary heart disease. *Lancet*, *353*(9147), 89–92.

73. Lovlien, M., et al. (2006). Are there gender differences related to symptoms of acute myocardial infarction? A Norwegian perspective. *Prog Cardiovasc Nurs*, *21*(1), 14–19.

74. Mallik, S., et al. (2006). Depressive symptoms after acute myocardial infarction: evidence for highest rates in younger women. *Arch Intern Med*, *166*(8), 876–883.

75. McKinley, S., et al. (2000). Treatment-seeking behavior for acute myocardial infarction symptoms in North America and Australia. *Heart Lung*, *29*(4), 237–247.

76. McSweeney, J. (2001). *McSweeney acute and prodromal myocardial infarction symptom survey.*

77. McSweeney, J. C., et al. (2003). Women's early warning symptoms of acute myocardial infarction. *Circulation*, *108*(21), 2619–2623.

78. McSweeney, J. C., et al. (2005). What's wrong with me? Women's coronary heart disease diagnostic experiences. *Prog Cardiovasc Nurs, Spring*, *20*(2), 48–57.

79. McSweeney, J. C., et al. (2004). Development of the McSweeney acute and prodromal myocardial infarction symptom survey. *J Cardiovasc Nurs*, *19*(1), 58–67.

80. Mehilli, J., et al. (2002). Sex-based analysis of outcome in patients with acute myocardial infarction treated predominantly with percutaneous coronary intervention. *JAMA*, *287*(2), 210–215.

81. Mehilli, J., et al. (2005). Gender and myocardial salvage after reperfusion treatment in acute myocardial infarction. *J Am College Cardiol*, *45*(6), 828–831.

82. Meyers, C. D., et al. (2003). Varying cost and free nicotinic acid content in over-the-counter niacin preparations for dyslipidemia. *Ann Intern Med*, *139*(12), 996–1002.

83. Mieres, J. H., et al. (2005). Role of noninvasive testing in the clinical evaluation of women with suspected coronary artery disease: consensus statement from the cardiac imaging committee, council on clinical cardiology, and the cardiovascular imaging and intervention committee, council on cardiovascular radiology and intervention, American Heart Association. *Circulation*, *111* (5), 682–696.

84. Moore, S. M., et al. (1998). Women's patterns of exercise following cardiac rehabilitation. *Nurs Res*, *47*(6), 318–324.

85. Mosca, L., et al. (2004). Evidence-based guidelines for cardiovascular disease prevention in women. American Heart Association scientific statement. *Circulation*, *109*, 672–693.

85a.Mosca, L., et al. (2007). Evidence-based guidelines for cardiovascular disease prevention in women: 2007 Update, *J Am Coll Cardiol*, *49*(11), 230–250.

86. Mosca, L., et al. (2000). Awareness, perception, and knowledge of heart disease risk and prevention among women in the United States. American Heart Association women's heart disease and stroke campaign task force. *Arch Fam Med*, *9*(6), 506–515.

86a.Mosca, L., Appel, L. J., Benjamin, E. J., et al. (2004). Evidence-based guidelines for cardiovascular disease prevention in women. *J Am Coll Cardiol*, *43*, 900–941.

87. MRC/BHF heart protection study of cholesterol lowering with simvastatin in 20,536 high-risk individuals: a randomised placebo-controlled trial. *Lancet*, *360*(9326), 7–22.

88. Ndrepepa, G., et al. (2004). Sex-associated differences in clinical outcomes after coronary stenting in patients with diabetes mellitus. *Am J Med*, *117*, 830–836.

89. O'Connor, C. M., et al. (2000). Depression and ischemic heart disease. *Am Heart J, 140*(4 suppl), 63–69.

90. Ogita, H., et al. (2003). The role of estrogen and estrogen-related drugs in cardiovascular diseases. *Curr Drug Metab, 4*(6), 497–504.

91. Oh, K., et al. (2005). Dietary fat intake and risk of coronary heart disease in women: 20 years of follow-up of the nurses' health study. *Am J Epidemiol, 161*(7), 672–679.

92. Ott, R. A., et al. (2001). Conventional coronary artery bypass grafting: why women take longer to recover. *J Cardiovasc Surg (Torino), 42*(3), 311–315.

93. Pai, J. K., et al. (2004). Inflammatory markers and the risk of coronary heart disease in men and women. *N Engl J Med, 351*(25), 2599–2610.

94. Patel, H., et al. (2004). Symptoms in acute coronary syndromes: does sex make a difference? *Am Heart J, 148*(1), 27–33.

95. Pedersen, T. R. (1998). Coronary artery disease: the Scandinavian simvastatin survival study experience. *Am J Cardiol, 82* (10B), 53T–56T.

96. Peeters, A, et al. (2003). Improvements in treatment of coronary heart disease and cessation of stroke mortality rate decline. *Stroke, 34*(7), 1615–1616.

97. Penckofer, S. M., et al. (2003). Estrogen plus progestin therapy: the cardiovascular risks exceed the benefits. *J Cardiovasc Nurs, 18*(5), 347–355.

98. Pizzi, C., et al. (2004). Angiotensin-converting enzyme inhibitors and 3-hydroxy-3-methylglutaryl coenzyme A reductase in cardiac syndrome X: role of superoxide dismutase activity. *Circulation, 109*(1), 53–58.

99. Raza, J. A., et al. (2004). Ischemic heart disease in women and the role of hormone therapy. *Int J Cardiol, 96*(1), 7–19.

100. Rea, T. D., et al. (2002). Smoking status and risk for recurrent coronary events after myocardial infarction. *Ann Intern Med, 137*(6), 494–500.

101. Ridker, P. M., & Cook, N. (2004). Clinical usefulness of very high and very low levels of C-reactive protein across the full range of Framingham risk scores. *Circulation, 109*(16), 1955–1959.

102. Ridker, P. M., et al. (2005). A randomized trial of low-dose aspirin in the primary prevention of cardiovascular disease in women. *N Engl J Med, 352*(13), 1293–1304.

103. Rossouw, J. E., et al. (2002). Risks and benefits of estrogen plus progestin in healthy postmenopausal women: principal results from the women's health initiative randomized controlled trial. *JAMA, 288*(3), 321–333.

104. Sabourin, C. B., & Funk, M. (1999). Readmission of patients after coronary artery bypass graft surgery. *Heart Lung, 28*(4), 243–250.

105. Sauer, W. H., et al. (2001). Selective serotonin reuptake inhibitors and myocardial infarction. *Circulation, 104*(16), 1894–1898.

106. Schuit, S. C., et al. (2004). Estrogen receptor alpha gene polymorphisms and risk of myocardial infarction. *JAMA, 291*(24), 2969–2977.

107. Schulz, P., et al. (2005). Gender differences in recovery after coronary artery bypass graft surgery. *Prog Cardiovasc Nurs, Spring, 20* (2), 58–64.

108. Schwartz, L. M., et al. (1997). Treatment and health outcomes of women and men in a cohort with coronary artery disease. *Arch Intern Med, 157*(14), 1545–1551.

109. Shahar, E., et al. (2003). Plasma lipid profile and incident ischemic stroke: the atherosclerosis risk in communities (ARIC) study. *Stroke, 34*(3), 623–631.

110. Shai, I., et al. (2004). Multivariate assessment of lipid parameters as predictors of coronary heart disease among postmenopausal women: potential implications for clinical guidelines. *Circulation, 110*(18), 2824–2830.

111. Sharrett, A. R., et al. (2001). Coronary heart disease prediction from lipoprotein cholesterol levels, triglycerides, lipoprotein(a), apolipoproteins A-I and B, and HDL density subfractions: the atherosclerosis risk in communities (ARIC) study. *Circulation, 104*(10), 1108–1113.

112. Sheifer, S. E., et al. (2000). Sex differences in coronary artery size assessed by intravascular ultrasound. *Am Heart J, 139*(4), 649–653.

113. Silaste, M. L., et al. (2000). Dietary and other non-pharmacological treatments in patients with drug-treated hypertension and control subjects. *J Intern Med, 247*(3), 318–324.

114. Smith, S. C., Jr., et al. (2006). AHA/ACC guidelines for secondary prevention for patients with coronary and other atherosclerotic vascular disease: 2006 update endorsed by the National Heart, Lung, and Blood Institute. *J Am Coll Cardiol, 47*(10), 2130–2139.

115. Sorensen, G., & Pechacek, T. F. (1987). Attitudes toward smoking cessation among men and women. *J Behav Med, 10*(2), 129–137.

116. Sowers, J. R. (1998). Diabetes mellitus and cardiovascular disease in women. *Arch Intern Med, 158*(6), 617–621.

117. Speck, B. J., & Harrell, J. S. (2003). Maintaining regular physical activity in women. *J Cardiovasc Nurs, 18*(4), 282–291.

118. National Center for Health Statistics. (2000). Prevalence of sedentary leisure-time activity among overweight adults in the United States—1998. *MMWR, April 21, 49*(15), 326–330.

119. Steenland, K., et al. (1996). Environmental tobacco smoke and coronary heart disease in the American Cancer Society CPS-II cohort. *Circulation, 94*(4), 622–628.

120. Steinberg, H. O., et al. (2000). Type 2 diabetes abrogates sex differences in endothelial function in premenopausal women. *Circulation, 101*(17), 2040–2046.

121. Stevenson, J. C. (2004). The metabolic basis for the effects of HRT on coronary heart disease. *Endocrine, 24*(3), 239–244.

122. Svedlund, M., et al. (2001). Women's narratives during the acute phase of their myocardial infarction. *J Adv Nurs, 35*(2), 197–205.

123. Sweitzer, N. K., & Douglas, P. S. (2005). Cardiovascular disease in women. In D. P. Zipes (Ed.), *Braunwald's heart disease: a textbook of cardiovascular medicine* (7th ed., pp. 1951–1964). Philadelphia: Saunders.

124. Tamis-Holland, J. E., et al. (2004). Benefits of direct angioplasty for women and men with acute myocardial infarction: results of the global use of strategies to open occluded arteries in acute coronary syndromes angioplasty (GUSTO II-B) angioplasty substudy. *Am Heart J, 147*(1), 133–139.

125. Teede, H. J. (2002). Hormone replacement therapy and the prevention of cardiovascular disease. *Hum Reprod Update, 8*(3), 201–215.

126. Thanavaro, J. L. (2005). Barriers to coronary heart disease risk modification in women without prior history of coronary artery disease. *J Am Acad Nurse Practitioners, 17*(11), 487–493.

127. Turner, S. C., et al. (2002). Patient characteristics and outcomes of cardiac rehabilitation. *J Cardiopulm Rehabil, 22*(4), 253–260.

128. Vaccarino, V., et al. (2002). Sex differences in hospital mortality after coronary artery bypass surgery: evidence for a higher mortality in younger women. *Circulation, 105*(10), 1176–1181.

129. Vaccarino, V., et al. (2003). Gender differences in recovery after coronary artery bypass surgery. *J Am Coll Cardiol, 41*(2), 307–314.

130. Vaccarino, V., et al. (1999). Sex-based differences in early mortality after myocardial infarction. National registry of

myocardial infarction 2 participants. *N Engl J Med, 341*(4), 217–225.

131. Vakili, B. A., et al. (2001). Sex-based differences in early mortality of patients undergoing primary angioplasty for first acute myocardial infarction. *Circulation, 104*(25), 3034–3038.

132. Villareal, R. P., & Willerson, J. T. (2002). Noninvasive diagnostic testing. In S. Wilansky & J. T. Willerson (Eds.), *Heart disease in women* (1st ed.). pp. 148–174). Philadelphia: Saunders.

133. Virmani, R., et al. (2002). Pathophysiology, clinical recognition and diagnosis of coronary artery disease. In S. Wilansky & J. T. Willerson (Eds.), *Heart disease in women* (1st ed., pp. 67–85). Philadelphia: Saunders.

134. Visser, M., et al. (1999). Elevated C-reactive protein levels in overweight and obese adults. *JAMA, 282*(22), 2131–2135.

135. Vittinghoff, E., et al. (2003). Risk factors and secondary prevention in women with heart disease: the heart and estrogen/progestin replacement study. *Ann Intern Med, 138*(2), 81–89.

136. Wassertheil-Smoller, S., et al. (2003). Effect of estrogen plus progestin on stroke in postmenopausal women: the women's health initiative: a randomized trial. *JAMA, 289*(20), 2673–2684.

137. Wassertheil-Smoller, S., et al. (2004). Association between cardiovascular outcomes and antihypertensive drug treatment in older women. *JAMA, 292*(23), 2849–2959.

138. Wassertheil-Smoller, S., et al. (2004). Depression and cardiovascular sequelae in postmenopausal women. The women's health initiative (WHI). *Arch Intern Med, 164*(3), 289–298.

139. Wenger, N. K. (1998). Social support and coronary heart disease in women: the challenge to learn more. *Eur Heart J, 19*(11), 1603–1605.

140. Whelton, S. P., et al. (2002). Effect of aerobic exercise on blood pressure: a meta-analysis of randomized, controlled trials. *Ann Intern Med, 136*(7), 493–503.

141. Willingham, S. A., & Kilpatrick, E. S. (2005). Evidence of gender bias when applying the new diagnostic criteria for myocardial infarction. *Heart, 91*(2), 237–238.

142. Wolz, M., et al. (2000). Statement from the national high blood pressure education program: prevalence of hypertension. *Am J Hypertens, 13*(1 Pt 1), 103–104.

143. Zerwic, J. J., et al. (2003). Treatment seeking for acute myocardial infarction symptoms: differences in delay across sex and race. *Nurs Res, 52*(3), 159–167.

144. Ziegelstein, R. C., et al. (2000). Patients with depression are less likely to follow recommendations to reduce cardiac risk during recovery from a myocardial infarction. *Arch Intern Med, 160* (12), 1818–1823.

ELECTRONIC LINKS

For further information on women and heart disease, the following websites may be useful:

www.womenheart.org
www.americanheart.org
www.4woman.gov
www.nhlbi.gov/health/hearttruth/index.htm
www.cdc.gov
www.webmd.com

CHAPTER 14

Cardiac Surgery

Joni L. Dirks

More than 700,000 cardiac surgeries are performed in the United States each year.[6] As cardiac surgery has evolved over the last 5 decades, there have been improvements in traditional techniques, including myocardial protection, graft selection, and fast-track recovery as well as increasing opportunities for less invasive surgical procedures (e.g., port-access and off-pump or "beating heart" surgery). These advances, along with improvements in medical management and increased options for percutaneous intervention, have changed the characteristics of patients undergoing cardiac surgery. Today's patients are older, with more comorbid conditions and higher risk profiles than previous surgical candidates. As a result, the care of patients following cardiac surgery presents special challenges for the critical care team. This chapter will review surgical revascularization procedures as well as procedures performed for structural problems following myocardial infarction. Valvular surgery is addressed in Chapter 15.

CORONARY ARTERY BYPASS GRAFTING

Coronary artery bypass grafting (CABG) provides a new conduit for blood flow to a coronary artery distal to the site of an occlusion or stenosis. This procedure results in improved myocardial oxygen supply and is performed to improve both quality of life (by ameliorating symptoms) and length of life (by reducing mortality associated with coronary events). CABG may be performed alone or in conjunction with other surgical procedures (e.g., valve repair).

Indications

CABG is indicated for patients with refractory angina when a percutaneous coronary intervention (i.e., stenting or angioplasty) either is not feasible—because of lesion morphology or location—or is not successful. In addition, certain subsets of patients with coronary artery disease (CAD) have been found to have improved outcomes following surgical revascularization.[25] CABG is the treatment of choice for patients with significant stenosis of the left main coronary artery or the equivalent of left main stenosis, created by greater than 70% stenosis of both the proximal left anterior descending (LAD) and the circumflex arteries. CABG is also recommended for patients with diffuse coronary artery disease (three or more vessels), especially if there is evidence of ventricular dysfunction or inducible ischemia, or if the patient has diabetes. Surgery is also recommended for patients with two-vessel disease when there is involvement of the proximal LAD. Evidence-based indications for CABG have been well delineated and are described in joint guidelines published by the American College of Cardiology and the American Heart Association (Table 14-1).[25]

The decision to perform CABG is generally based on data obtained during cardiac catheterization. Atherosclerotic lesions narrowing the lumen of an artery by at least 50% are considered significant. Lesions of greater than 70% prevent increases in blood flow distal to the stenosis despite maximal coronary vasodilation, and thus are a priority for bypass. Target vessels for revascularization are also assessed during the cardiac catheterization to ensure that they are of adequate size (1 to 1.5 mm) to support flow through the graft. Other preoperative assessments may include stress testing to verify areas of ischemia, nuclear studies to determine myocardial viability and ventricular function, and echocardiography to evaluate for valvular problems and ventricular wall motion abnormalities.

Selection of Conduits

Conduits for bypass include either native arteries or veins. Sections of a vessel (free grafts) can be attached between an arterial blood source (e.g., the aorta) and the target vessel on the surface of the myocardium. Certain arteries can be left attached at their site of origin (in situ or pedicle grafts), dissected from the surrounding tissue, and reattached at the distal end to the coronary vessel. The selection of a particular conduit for

TABLE 14-1   ACC/AHA Guidelines: Class I Recommendations for Coronary Artery Bypass Graft Surgery

CLINICAL INDICATION	CORONARY ANATOMY OR SYMPTOMS
Asymptomatic or mild angina	Left main stenosis ≥50% Left main equivalent* 3-vessel disease, especially if EF <0.5
Stable angina	Left main stenosis ≥50% Left main equivalent* 3-vessel disease, especially if EF >0.5 2-vessel disease with >70% stenosis of proximal LAD and EF <50% or inducible ischemia 1–2-vessel disease without proximal LAD, but large area of ischemic myocardium Disabling angina on maximal medical therapy
Unstable angina or non–ST elevation MI	Left main stenosis ≥50% Left main equivalent* Refractory ischemia on maximal medical therapy
Emergent or urgent CABG following STEMI	Refractory ischemia and hemodynamic instability after failed PCI or in patients who are not candidates for PCI or fibrinolysis Performed in conjunction with repair of postinfarction mechanical defects Cardiogenic shock within 36 hr of STEMI, as long as surgery can be performed within 18 hr of developing shock and patient is <75 years
Poor left ventricular function	Left main stenosis ≥50% Left main equivalent* 2–3-vessel disease with >70% stenosis of proximal LAD
Ventricular dysrhythmias	Life-threatening ventricular dysrhythmias in presence of left main stenosis ≥50% or 3-vessel disease
Failed PCI	Ongoing ischemia, hemodynamic instability, threatened occlusion
Reoperation after prior CABG	Disabling angina despite optimal nonsurgical therapy No patent grafts with class I indications in native vessels (left main stenosis, left main equivalent, or 3-vessel disease) (class I: evidence shows CABG to be useful and effective)

Data from reference 25.
*Left main equivalent describes greater than 70% stenosis of both the left anterior descending and circumflex arteries.
CABG = Coronary artery bypass grafting, EF = ejection fraction, LAD = left anterior descending, MI = myocardial infarction, PCI = percutaneous coronary intervention, STEMI = ST elevation myocardial infarction.

CABG is influenced by several factors, including patient age, location of the vessel requiring bypass, conduit availability, and surgeon preference. Because improved patency rates and event-free survival have been shown with the use of arterial conduits, they are preferred over venous grafts whenever feasible.[25] Frequently, a combination of grafts is required to achieve the goal of total revascularization (Figure 14-1).

The saphenous vein is the most commonly used venous conduit. It may be harvested directly, through an open leg incision, or endoscopically, through small (3 to 4 cm) incisions (Figure 14-2). Although more time consuming, endoscopic vein harvesting (EVH) has been shown to decrease the incidence of postoperative leg wound complications (e.g., cellulitis and hematoma).[13] Patients also report less pain and improved appearance with EVH.[56] Other, lesser-used veins include the cephalic vein and the lesser saphenous vein. A major limitation of all venous grafts is progressive atherosclerosis. Patency rates have improved slightly with the aggressive use of statins and antiplatelet agents, but still remain at approximately 60% 10 years after surgery.[25]

The left internal mammary artery (LIMA) is the conduit of choice and is used in the majority of elective cases. It has long been shown to provide not only superior patency (greater than 90% at 10 years) but also

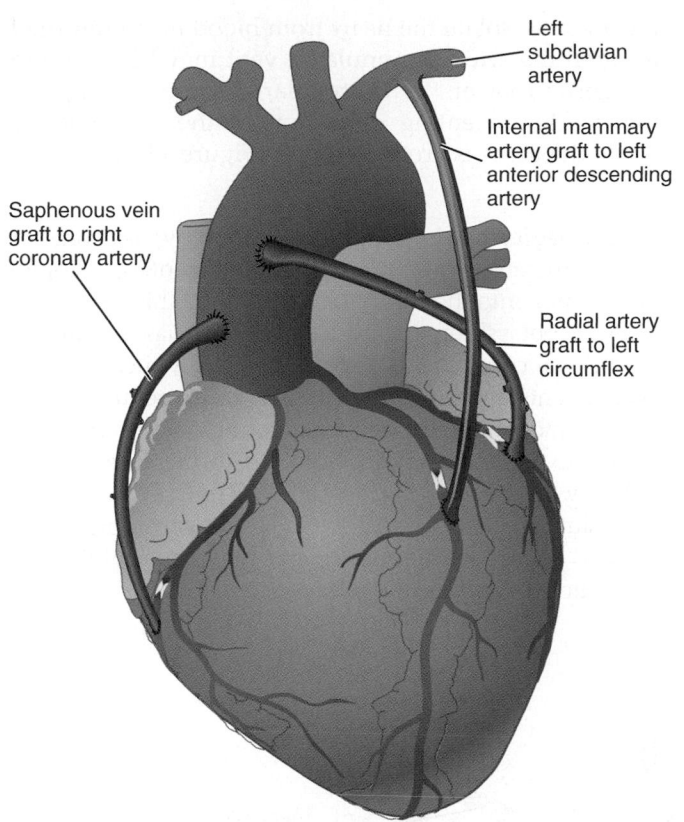

Saphenous vein graft to right coronary artery

Left subclavian artery

Internal mammary artery graft to left anterior descending artery

Radial artery graft to left circumflex

♦FIGURE 14-1 Coronary artery bypass grafting. Conduits for coronary artery bypass grafts may include segments of saphenous vein or radial artery that are anastomosed to the aorta and then to the coronary artery at a point distal to the lesion. The internal mammary artery may also be dissected from the chest tissue and attached directly to the coronary artery.

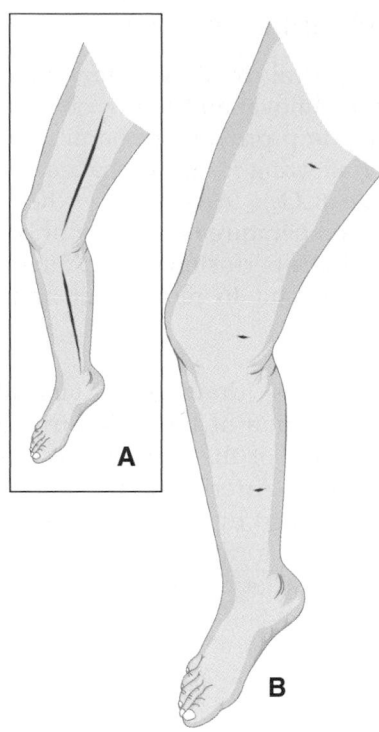

♦FIGURE 14-2 Techniques for harvesting the saphenous vein. Techniques for procuring saphenous veins include an open incision **(A)** and endovascular harvesting **(B)**. There may be one, two, or three incisions. There is usually one on the thigh and one near the knee.

improved survival with less risk of reoperation or myocardial infarction (MI).[44] Recent data suggest that LIMA grafting may have a protective effect on perioperative mortality as well.[41] The LIMA is anatomically well positioned to bypass lesions in the left anterior descending artery. The right internal mammary can be used as an in situ graft to bypass the right coronary artery or as a free graft to bypass other vessels. Because of superior patency rates, some surgeons advocate for bilateral use of the internal mammary artery, although this increases the length of the operation and has been associated with an increase in wound infections in diabetic patients.[25]

The use of the radial artery as a conduit for CABG has increased in the last decade, partially as a result of improved harvesting techniques and medications to prevent vasospasm. This artery is usually harvested from the nondominant hand, either through an open incision or endoscopically, and used as a free graft from the aorta or the LIMA.[17] Patency rates of greater

than 90% at 10 years have now been reported for radial artery grafts.[58]

Other options for arterial conduits include the gastroepiploic artery and the inferior epigastric artery. These may be used in younger patients when the goal of bypass is total arterial revascularization or in patients in whom other conduits are not available (e.g., patients undergoing reoperation).[68]

Surgical Procedure

Conventional CABG surgery is performed through a median sternotomy on an arrested heart. Cardiopulmonary bypass (CPB) is used to preserve end-organ function during the temporary absence of cardiac and pulmonary function. CPB involves diverting venous blood from the right atrium or vena cava to an extracorporeal oxygenator, and returning the oxygenated blood to the arterial system of the patient—bypassing the heart and lungs in the oxygenation process. The advantage of this approach is that it allows the surgeon to operate on a relatively bloodless, motionless heart. Currently the majority of CABG procedures are performed "on pump," using CPB.[25]

Cardiopulmonary Bypass

The extracorporeal circuit used for CPB consists of a cannula for the removal and return of blood, a centrifugal or roller pump providing nonpulsatile flow, and an oxygenator allowing for the exchange of oxygen and carbon dioxide (CO_2). In addition, a heat exchanger controls body temperature by heating or cooling blood passing through the perfusion circuit; filters are located throughout the circuit to remove air and particulate matter.

Cannulation. Venous drainage is usually accomplished by cannulation of the right atrial appendage, with the distal end of the cannula positioned in the inferior vena cava. Arterial return from the bypass pump is accomplished by inserting a cannula through purse-string sutures in the ascending aorta, proximal to the innominate artery. A cross-clamp is applied to the aorta to isolate the heart from blood being returned through the arterial cannula. A vent may be placed in the aortic root or the ventricular apex to decompress the heart, preventing distention of the left ventricle while the aorta is cross-clamped (Figure 14-3).

Cardioplegia. During cannulation for bypass, one or more catheters are also placed for infusion of a cardioplegic solution into the coronary circulation. This solution is high in potassium, to induce a rapid diastolic arrest. Additional components vary, but typically include buffering agents and substrates that optimize cellular metabolism and minimize cell damage. Frequently blood is added to the cardioplegia solution to increase oxygen delivery to the myocardial cells.[46] The temperature of the solution can be either 4° C ("cold" cardioplegia) or 37° C ("warm" cardioplegia), and may be administered continuously or intermittently.

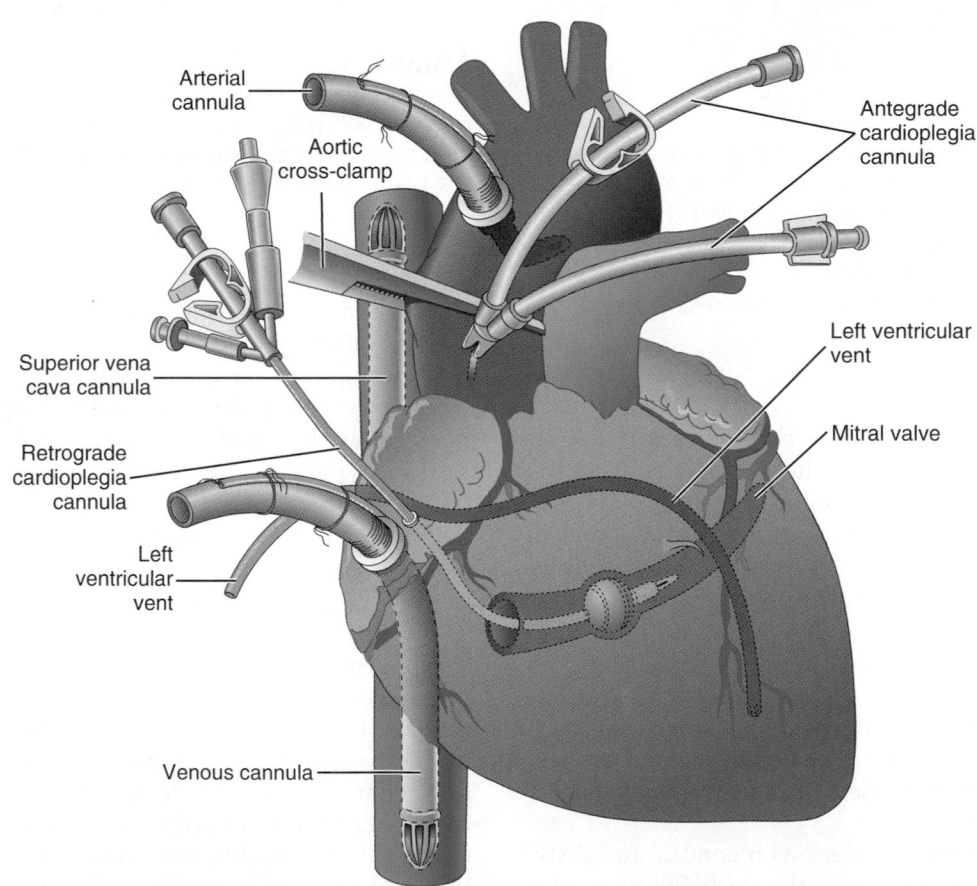

⬆FIGURE 14-3 Cannulation for cardiac surgery with cardiopulmonary bypass includes arterial and venous cannulas as well as cardioplegia cannulas (antegrade and possibly retrograde). A vent may be placed in either the left ventricle or the aortic root. The cross-clamp is applied to the aorta proximal to the arterial cannula but distal to the cannula that is used to deliver cardioplegia solution.

Antegrade cardioplegia is delivered under pressure through a catheter in the ascending aorta, positioned proximal to the aortic cross-clamp. The distribution of antegrade cardioplegia may be limited by severe coronary artery stenosis, leaving portions of the myocardium at risk for ischemic injury. As an alternative, retrograde cardioplegia allows for perfusion through the heart's venous system, and is accomplished through a catheter placed in the coronary sinus.

Cardiopulmonary Bypass Adjuncts. A number of adjuncts are used to enhance tissue perfusion while on bypass. Patients are anticoagulated with heparin to minimize clotting as the blood encounters the foreign components of the bypass machine. Adequate heparinization is verified by monitoring the activated clotting time (ACT). Generally the ACT is kept between 400 and 480 seconds during bypass. After weaning from CPB, protamine is administered to reverse the heparin effect. Systemic hypothermia is also used during bypass to protect the body's tissues by decreasing metabolic demands. The decreased metabolic rate allows the tissues to tolerate lower perfusion flow rates. Temperatures are usually decreased to between 28° and 32° C. Hemodilution, used during bypass, helps to counteract the increased blood viscosity normally produced by hypothermia. The extracorporeal circuit is primed with 1 to 1.5 liters of crystalloid solution, resulting in a hematocrit (Hct) of 20% to 25% while on bypass. Mannitol (Osmitrol) or furosemide (Lasix) may be administered to promote postoperative diuresis, which helps reverse the hemodilution.

Complications of Cardiopulmonary Bypass. Although bypass supports the body's tissues during the surgical procedure, it is associated with a number of undesired physiologic responses. During CPB the blood is exposed to a number of foreign surfaces, which damages blood elements (i.e., white cells, red cells, and platelets). In addition, extracorporeal circulation produces a generalized inflammatory response. This initiates a cascade of physiologic changes, including increased capillary permeability, increased circulating catecholamines, and impaired coagulation. The body's response to CPB contributes to the clinical problems encountered in the early postoperative period following surgery. Potential complications associated with CPB are summarized in Box 14-1.

"Off-Pump" Surgery

In an effort to avoid the adverse effects of CPB, there has been significant interest in developing technology to allow for surgical revascularization on a beating heart.

Box 14-1

Complications Related to Cardiopulmonary Bypass

- Bleeding
- Dysrhythmias
- Emboli (air, plaque, or denatured proteins)
- Electrolyte imbalances
- Fluid shifts
- Hypothermia
- Hemodynamic instability
- Myocardial depression
- Neurocognitive dysfunction
- Pulmonary dysfunction
- Systemic inflammatory response

Off-pump coronary artery bypass (OPCAB) is now performed in approximately 20% to 25% of cases.[16,47] In heart centers experienced in this approach, OPCAB can achieve revascularization results comparable to those obtained with conventional bypass.[63]

Unlike cardiac surgery performed with CPB, off-pump procedures require that the patient's own heart provide adequate perfusion to the body's tissue. The heart's hemodynamic performance may be compromised during the procedure secondary to positioning of the heart, dysrhythmias, or ischemia. Patients require vigilant monitoring during the operation, generally facilitated by transesophageal echocardiography (TEE). Pulmonary artery catheters that provide continuous cardiac output (CO) and mixed venous oxygen saturation (SvO_2) data are also frequently employed. Fluids, vasopressors, or inotropic agents may be needed during the operation to maintain an adequate CO and blood pressure (BP). At times, an intra-aortic balloon pump (IABP) may also be used for hemodynamic support.

A variety of incisional approaches can be used with "off-pump" surgery. In the minimally invasive direct coronary artery bypass graft (MIDCABG) procedure, a small left anterior thoracotomy incision is used to directly harvest the LIMA, which is then anastomosed to the LAD.[25] A standard median sternotomy approach with cardiac retraction and stabilizing systems is generally required for multivessel disease to allow for complete revascularization. Distal coronary vessels can be bypassed and proximal anastomoses performed with partial ascending aortic cross-clamping. Because a partial aortic clamp is required for this approach, the thromboembolic risks associated with manipulation of the aorta are still present.

Performing bypass surgery on a beating heart poses several technical difficulties. First, movement of the coronary artery hampers suturing. Second, blood flow to the segment of the artery chosen for anastomosis is temporarily halted, using specialized loops that occlude the vessel. This may result in ischemia, especially in patients with limited collateral flow and depressed ventricular function. Finally, to reach posterior and lateral targets, the heart has to be lifted; this may cause hemodynamic deterioration.

Several techniques are used to facilitate the surgical procedure during a beating heart operation. The pericardium is opened and a stabilizing device is used to minimize wall motion at the site of the anastomosis. These devices attach to a stabilizing arm and work by either compression or suction to create an immobile area (Figure 14-4). Drugs that temporarily decrease the heart rate (e.g., esmolol [Brevibloc]) or cause transient cardiac asystole (e.g., adenosine [Adenocard]) can further limit cardiac motion. Additional retracting sutures may be placed deeper in the pericardium to allow for elevation and rotation of the heart so that

posterior vessels may be bypassed. Other types of positioning apparatus use suction to pull the heart up and allow for better target vessel exposure. Occasionally intraluminal shunts may be placed within the vessel being bypassed, to allow for distal perfusion during the period of bypass grafting.[71]

Anesthetic requirements for off-pump surgery are similar to those for conventional bypass, but typically short-acting agents are used to facilitate early extubation—which may even be performed before transfer from the operating room. Anticoagulation is still needed during off-pump surgery to prevent clotting activated by the extrinsic pathway, but the amount of heparin is much less than that used for surgery with CPB. The patient's temperature will decrease as the chest is opened, so body temperature may need to be maintained with forced-air blankets and fluid warmers.

Some research has demonstrated improved mortality and morbidity with OPCAB, including decreased transfusion requirements, length of stay, and ventilator time, as well as reductions in the incidence of stroke and renal failure.[7,60] Other researchers were unable to demonstrate an advantage of OPCAB over conventional CABG in terms of morbidity.[32,42] This approach may have its greatest advantage in high-risk patients with significant comorbid conditions or those with contraindications to CPB (e.g., atherosclerotic disease in the ascending aorta).[48,71]

TRANSMYOCARDIAL REVASCULARIZATION

Transmyocardial revascularization (TMR) is a procedure in which transmural channels are created in the myocardium with a laser. Studies have confirmed that TMR is effective at decreasing angina, although the mechanism behind this effect is not clearly understood.[2,3] Initially the benefit of this procedure was believed to be that the channels allowed oxygenated blood from the left ventricle to provide additional perfusion to the myocardium. This idea has since been rejected because research has shown that the channels actually close over the first several months.[38] Two new theories have now been proposed as possible mechanisms for the effects obtained with TMR. The first is that the laser induces angiogenesis (growth of new vessels), improving regional blood flow to the myocardium. The other is that the laser induces denervation of the myocardium, resulting in a decrease in anginal symptoms even without improvement in myocardial oxygen delivery.[15]

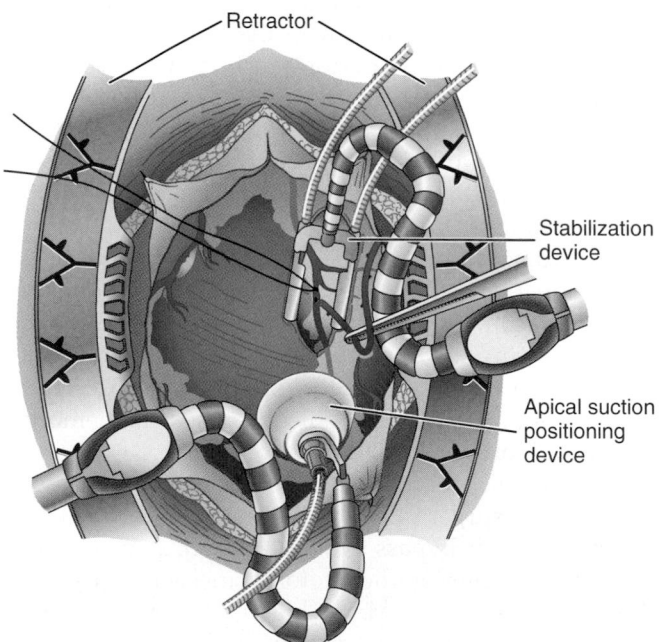

▲FIGURE 14-4 Off-pump positioning and stabilizing devices. Off-pump bypass grafting requires specialized equipment to position the heart and stabilize motion at the site of the anastomosis. Positioning aids include deep pericardial sutures and the use of apical suction devices. A mechanical foot can provide pressure to stabilize the anastomosis site.

Labels in figure: Retractor; Stabilization device; Apical suction positioning device

Indications

TMR is usually reserved for patients with severe angina who cannot be completely revascularized using CABG or percutaneous catheter interventions.[66] In this challenging patient population, TMR may be employed either as sole treatment or as an adjunct to CABG.[72] The Society for Thoracic Surgery has published guidelines with recommendations for patient selection for TMR.[15]

Procedure

TMR is performed with a laser device using infrared light to ablate myocardial tissue and create channels in the myocardium. The ischemic area may be accessed through a median sternotomy if the procedure is performed in conjunction with CABG, or via a thoracotomy if done in isolation. TMR is performed on a beating heart, with delivery of the energy pulses synchronized to the cardiac cycle. The presence of air bubbles in the left ventricle on the TEE is used to confirm transmural penetration. Bleeding from the newly created channels is controlled with mild pressure applied by the surgeon. There is also a potential for ventricular dysrhythmias resulting from myocardial irritation, but these are usually controlled with antidysrhythmic medications.[43]

VENTRICULAR ANEURYSM REPAIR

Ventricular aneurysms develop as a result of a large transmural MI, most commonly in the anterolateral wall of the left ventricle.[52] The damaged tissue becomes thin and less contractile, moving paradoxically during contraction. This results in a decrease in stroke volume; over time this may lead to dilation of the ventricle and symptoms of heart failure. In addition, thrombi may accumulate in this area. Finally, scar tissue at the border of the aneurysm may serve as a focus for dysrhythmias. When an aneurysm is associated with one or more of these problems, an aneurysmectomy may be performed.

Procedure

Aneurysmectomy is performed through a median sternotomy, with CPB. The standard approach to aneurysm repair is to open and excise the thin aneurysmal tissue, removing any visible thrombus at that time.

The healthy ventricular tissue is sutured together, using felt strips to reinforce the suture line. This linear approach may have suboptimal results for large aneurysms, because the normal shape of the ventricle is not maintained.[33] To create a more physiologic ventricular shape, a patch (composed of either Dacron or bovine pericardium) can be attached to the viable tissue at the edge of the aneurysm, with the ventricle closed over the patch. The Dor and Jantene procedures are a slightly modified version of this approach, in which a purse-string suture is placed around the entire circumference of the base of the aneurysm and then tightened to restore a normal ventricular cavity shape.

VENTRICULAR SEPTAL DEFECT

Necrosis and subsequent rupture of the ventricular septum is a rare and frequently fatal complication of an acute myocardial infarction. The frequency of postinfarction rupture of the septum has declined in the era of reperfusion and is now estimated to occur in less than 1% of patients with ST elevation MIs.[19] Ventricular septal defects (VSDs) allow shunting of blood from left to right, producing acute pulmonary edema and cardiogenic shock. Clinical signs of acute VSD include the presence of a holosystolic murmur and an increase in oxygen saturation in the right ventricle.[12] A cardiac echo can be done to confirm the diagnosis of VSD.

Surgical repair of an acute VSD is challenging, especially in patients who are hemodynamically unstable. However, because mortality for patients managed medically is greater than 90%, surgery is currently recommended for virtually all patients with postinfarction VSD.[8] Preoperatively, patients require inotropic support as well as afterload reduction to improve forward flow from the left ventricle. Generally an IABP is used to support the patient, both before and after the operation.

Procedure

Repair of a VSD is performed through a median sternotomy on an arrested heart. The ventricle is opened and a prosthetic patch is applied to the intraventricular septum. The ventriculotomy is then closed, using felt strips for reinforcement. Surgical repair is usually performed in conjunction with coronary artery grafting to improve myocardial perfusion. Surgical mortality with this procedure remains high and has been reported to be as high as 47%.[19]

MULTIDISCIPLINARY PLAN OF CARE

Initial postoperative management of patients following cardiac surgery is similar, regardless of the specific procedure performed. The primary goals of treatment during this time are to prevent complications associated with the surgery (e.g., hypothermia, bleeding, and dysrhythmias) and to optimize the patient's cardiac and pulmonary function. The patient requires frequent assessment, with interventions based on trends rather than absolute numbers. The Multidisciplinary Plan of Care on pp. 305-307 describes the general plan of care for patients following cardiac surgery.

♦ Case Study 14-1, Part A

Coronary Artery Bypass Grafting

J.P. is a 64-year-old man who was referred by his family physician to a cardiologist for evaluation of new-onset chest pain. He had a history of hypercholesterolemia and hypertension. He underwent a nuclear stress test that was stopped after 4 minutes secondary to ischemia. He was scheduled for a cardiac catheterization, which revealed 85% stenosis of the left main artery, 80% stenosis of the right coronary artery, and 70% stenosis of the circumflex artery. Based on these findings, J.P. was scheduled for urgent coronary artery bypass grafting the following morning.

J.P. underwent conventional CABG with a LIMA graft to his LAD, an SVG to his RCA, and a radial artery graft to his circumflex artery. Following bypass he was bradycardic, so AAI pacing was performed via epicardial wires at a rate of 90 ppm ok. He arrived in critical care intubated, with propofol (Diprivan) infusing at 30 mcg/kg/min. Vital signs on admission were as follows: HR 90 beats/min (paced), BP 120/62 mm Hg (MAP 76 mm Hg), PAWP 9 mm Hg, RAP 6 mm Hg, CI 2.6 L/min/m^2, SVR 980 dynes/sec/cm^{-5}, Svo$_2$ 0.62. He had two mediastinal chest tubes placed to −20 cm H$_2$O suction, with 90 ml of sanguineous drainage present from the OR. His Foley was draining clear yellow urine. J.P.'s chest tube output was 300 ml in the first hour after his return to critical care. His temperature had decreased to 35.9° C. The aPTT obtained with his initial postoperative labs rebounded at 45 seconds. He remained paced at a rate of 90 beats/min, with a BP of 140/76 mm Hg (98 mm Hg). Propofol continued to be infused and he appeared sedated.

Decision point: What interventions should be implemented at this time?

Case continues on page 308

In the immediate postoperative period the patient is at risk for hemodynamic instability as well as problems with oxygenation and ventilation. A team effort is needed to ensure that patient monitoring is continuous and treatments are not interrupted during transfer from the operating room (OR) to critical care. While initial report on the patient is called from the OR, an anesthesiologist generally accompanies the patient to the unit and is responsible for monitoring the patient and adjusting medications as necessary. The critical care nurse focuses on establishing cardiac and hemodynamic monitoring while a respiratory therapist ensures respiratory stabilization and attaches the patient to a ventilator at the prescribed settings, if the patient is still ventilated. The chest tubes are attached to suction, and proper functioning of the infusion pumps and the pacemaker (if present) is confirmed. Once monitoring is established, the critical care nurse receives any additional report regarding the patient's intraoperative course. The nurse obtains an initial assessment of the patient, including hemodynamic data, physical assessment, and diagnostic tests. Routine assessment criteria for patients immediately following cardiac surgery are described in Table 14-2.

Hypothermia

Although patients are generally rewarmed to 37° C before coming off of bypass, they frequently have mild hypothermia on arrival to critical care. This results from continued heat loss while the chest is open, cooler ambient temperatures in the OR, and peripheral vasoconstriction limiting heat distribution. Negative physiologic effects of hypothermia include impaired coagulation, an increased propensity for dysrhythmias, and increased systemic vascular resistance (SVR). In addition, hypothermia may precipitate shivering, resulting in increased oxygen demand and CO$_2$ production. Hypothermia has also been associated with prolonging time to extubation.

Measures to correct hypothermia include rewarming either with conventional or forced-air blankets. To avoid overwarming, blankets should be removed when the patient reaches 36.5° C. Fluid warmers may also be helpful, especially if large quantities of blood products are being administered. Shivering, if it occurs, may be effectively treated with meperidine (Demerol) administered intravenously in doses of 12.5 to 25 mg.[22]

MULTIDISCIPLINARY PLAN OF CARE FOR PATIENTS FOLLOWING CARDIAC SURGERY

PROBLEM	INTERVENTION	RATIONALE	EXPECTED OUTCOME	SPECIAL CONSIDERATIONS
Potential for hypothermia	Continuously monitor temperature. Apply warm-air blankets as needed for T <36° C. Administer meperidine (Demerol) as needed to treat shivering. Warm fluids as indicated.	Temperature "afterdrop" may occur after arrival in unit. Hypothermia has several negative consequences, including bleeding, vasoconstriction, and dysrhythmias. Shivering increases oxygen demand and CO_2 production.	Patient is normothermic.	Fluid warmers may be useful, especially if blood products are being administered.
Potential for bleeding	Maintain patency of chest tubes. Monitor postoperative lab results: Hct/Hgb,† aPTT, platelets. Obtain additional coagulation studies for continued bleeding. Administer blood products and medications for bleeding (see the Medication table on pp. 309-310) as warranted. Monitor for signs and symptoms of tamponade. Maintain MAP 65–75 mm Hg.	Facilitates drainage of mediastinal and pleural space. Laboratory tests help to guide treatment. For example, RBCs may be needed for low Hct/Hgb, whereas protamine may be required if aPTT is elevated. Blood that accumulates in mediastinum can compress heart and impair function. Increased pressure puts stress on suture lines and cannulation sites.	Chest tube output tapers to <90 ml in 8 hr. PT/aPTT within normal limits. Hct ≥24% or as ordered.	Decision to administer blood products should be based on clinical signs of impaired tissue oxygenation, rather than on a specific Hct value.[26,70]
Potential for dysrhythmias	Continuously monitor ECG, including ST segment monitoring. Attach pacing wires (if present) to pulse generator. Administer prophylactic beta blockers or other antidysrhythmics as ordered. Monitor serum K^+ and Mg^{++}; replace as needed.	Allows for early detection of ischemia or dysrhythmias. Pacemaker will be available in event patient has bradycardia or heart block. Prophylactic use of beta blockers has been shown to decrease incidence of atrial fibrillation.[25] Hypokalemia and hypomagnesemia may occur post-CPB and during periods of diuresis.	Sinus rhythm or paced rhythm adequate to maintain CO.	Nitroglycerin or diltiazem (Cardizem) infusions may be used to treat vasospasm in radial artery grafts. Pacing may be used to maintain AV synchrony for CO. If hemodynamically compromising dysrhythmias occur, they should be promptly treated based on ACLS protocols[5] or routine emergency orders.

Table continues on page 306

PROBLEM	INTERVENTION	RATIONALE	EXPECTED OUTCOME	SPECIAL CONSIDERATIONS
Depressed myocardial function	Monitor filling pressures and maintain preload with fluids as needed. Monitor BP or SVR if available. Alter afterload with vasodilators (Chapter 41 Medication table on pp. 1116-1121) or vasopressors as needed. Administer inotropic agents as needed (Chapter 41 Medication table on pp. 1116-1121). If above measures are inadequate, consider use of IABP.	Intravascular fluid deficits may occur post-CPB and decrease CO. Hypo- or hypertension may occur following surgery. Increased SVR may impair CO. Vasodilation may occur in some patients as part of inflammatory response.[1] Contractility is often decreased for 6–8 hr after CPB.	Adequate filling pressures for patient's LV function. MAP 65–85 mm Hg. SVR 800–1200 dynes/sec/cm.^{5} CI ≥ 2.2 L/min/m^2. Svo$_2$ greater than 65%.	Targeted filling pressures should be individualized to patient's preoperative ventricular function and hemodynamic response (Table 14-3). Patients without a pulmonary artery catheter should be assessed for evidence of adequate end-organ perfusion (e.g, LOC, urine output).
Pulmonary dysfunction	Maintain mechanical ventilation as needed until criteria for extubation are met. Monitor Sao$_2$ and provide supplemental O$_2$ as needed. Reposition frequently and get patient OOB to chair 1–2 × shift. Encourage use of IS every 1–2 hr. Instruct patient in use of cough pillow. Provide adequate analgesia to promote increased activity without inducing respiratory depression (Medication table on p. 316). Apply TEDS/SCDs as ordered.	Early extubation decreases pulmonary complications and facilitates mobility. Some degree of intrapulmonary shunting occurs postoperatively.[73] Mobilization and deep breathing help reverse atelectasis that occurs during surgery. Oversedation may lead to reintubation. Helps prevent DVT and pulmonary emboli.	Extubate within 12 hr of surgery if possible. Sao$_2$ maintained $\geq 92\%$.	Continuous infusions or PCAs may be helpful in providing adequate pain relief without oversedation.
Potential for pain and anxiety	Wean sedative agents and assess patient's LOC when ready to begin ventilator weaning. Assess level of pain every 1–2 hr, using an intensity scale (1–9) for comparison. Assess level of pain during activities, such as deep breathing and getting OOB.[53] Administer analgesics as needed per order.	Short-acting sedative agents may be used after surgery until patient is ready for extubation. Patients report varying levels of pain following cardiac surgery.[53] Pain has negative psychologic and physical effects.	Alert and able to participate in activities such as coughing, deep breathing, and getting OOB. Patient reports pain at a tolerable level.	When early extubation is anticipated, short-acting sedatives such as propofol may be used with small doses of narcotics. For prolonged intubation, longer acting agents like midazolam (Versed) may be used.

PROBLEM	INTERVENTION	RATIONALE	EXPECTED OUTCOME	SPECIAL CONSIDERATIONS
Risk of infection	Administer antibiotics as ordered. Treat hyperglycemia (if present) with an insulin infusion. Remove all lines and tubes as soon as possible. Assess patient for signs of infection (increased temperature and WBCs, redness, pain, or drainage from incisions).	Antibiotics are typically given for 24 hr, with first dose in OR. Hyperglycemia is associated with an increased risk for infection.[40]	Incisions clean, dry, and intact, without redness or discharge. Blood glucose level <110 mg/dl.[4] ETT removed within 12 hr postoperatively. CT removed when drainage is <90 ml in 8 hr. Arterial line and central lines removed when patient is stable and off vasoactive medications.	Tight hyperglycemic control has been shown to decrease incidence of mediastinitis.[30]

ACLS = Advanced cardiac life support, aPTT = activated partial thromboplastin time, AV = atrioventricular, BP = blood pressure, CI = cardiac index, CO = cardiac output, CPB = cardiopulmonary bypass, CT = chest tube, DVT = deep vein thrombosis, ECG = electrocardiogram, ETT = endotracheal tube, Hct = hematocrit, Hgb = hemoglobin, IABP, intra-aortic balloon pump, IS = incentive spirometer, K$^+$ = potassium, LOC = level of consciousness, LV = left ventricular, MAP = mean arterial pressure, Mg^{++} = magnesium, O$_2$ = oxygen, OOB = out of bed, OR = operating room, PCA = patient-controlled analgesia, RBCs = red blood cells, Sao$_2$ = arterial oxygen saturation, SCDs = sequential compression devices, Svo$_2$ = mixed venous oxygen saturation, SVR = systemic vascular resistance, T = temperature, TEDS = thromboembolic stockings, WBCs = white blood cells.

TABLE 14-2 Routine Postoperative Assessment Criteria

PARAMETER	CRITERIA ASSESSED
ECG	Select appropriate leads for dysrhythmia detection and ST analysis.
Hemodynamic measurements	Level and zero transducers. Obtain baseline measurements for BP, CVP, PAP, and CO. Calculate SVR and PVR.
Intravenous lines	Have medications infusing and properly labeled; dressings should be dry and occlusive.
Lab work	Obtain stat CBC, ABG, electrolytes, and blood glucose measurements. Obtain stat coagulation studies if bleeding (PT/aPTT, platelets).
Pacemaker	Verify correct lead attachment or ensure lead wires are electrically dressed and covered. If attached, confirm proper functioning of generator and settings as ordered.
Physical assessment	Auscultate heart sounds, noting murmurs or abnormal heart sounds. Auscultate breath sounds, noting absent or adventitious sounds. Assess capillary refill and peripheral pulses. Assess LOC, pupil reactivity, and ability to move extremities.
Portable chest x-ray	Review position of ETT, central lines, or pulmonary artery catheter. Note width of mediastinum, presence of pneumothorax or pleural effusion.
Pulse oximeter	Validate adequate signal. Correlate with current ABG.
Tubes	Ensure ETT tube secured. Confirm patency of chest tubes and placement to suction, noting character and quantity of output. Verify correct position of NG tube and placement to suction. Place Foley to gravity drainage, noting quantity of output.

ABG = Arterial blood gas, aPTT = activated partial thromboplastin time, BP = blood pressure, CBC = complete blood cell count, CVP = central venous pressure, CO = cardiac output, ECG = electrocardiogram, ETT = endotracheal tube, LOC = level of consciousness, NG = nasogastric, PAP = pulmonary artery pressure, PT = prothrombin time, PVR = pulmonary vascular resistance, SVR = systemic vascular resistance.

♦ Case Study 14-1, Part B

Coronary Artery Bypass Grafting

J.P.'s chest tube output decreased to 90 ml the next hour. As he rewarmed, his blood pressure decreased to 92/58 mm Hg (MAP 67 mm Hg). Warming blankets were removed and his nicardipine drip was discontinued. He remained AAI paced at a rate of 90 ppm, and measurements from his PA catheter were as follows: PAP 20/9 mm Hg, PAWP 8 mm Hg, RAP 4 mm Hg, CI 2.1 L/min/m², SVR 990 dynes/sec/cm⁻⁵, Svo₂ 0.54.

Decision point: What interventions might be prudent at this point?

Case continues on page 310

Bleeding

A number of factors place patients at risk for bleeding after cardiac surgery. Sequelae from bypass (i.e., dilution of clotting factors, damage to platelets,

hypothermia) may impair coagulation. Inadequate reversal of heparin may also contribute to a coagulopathy, or heparin rebound may occur with rewarming as heparin sequestered in the tissues is released into circulation. Postoperative hypertension can increase the risk of bleeding by placing additional stress on surgical suture lines and cannulation sites.

Chest tubes placed at the end of the operation allow for monitoring of mediastinal bleeding. These may be either conventional chest tubes (32 to 36 French [Fr]) or smaller Silastic (Blake) drains. The smaller drains provide comparable drainage efficiency and less discomfort for the patient.[29,39] Chest tubes are usually placed to suction (-20 cm H_2O), and patency is maintained by gently milking the tubes when clots are present. Vigorous stripping is avoided because the high pressures produced by stripping may exacerbate bleeding problems. Patients will typically have 50 to 150 ml of chest tube output for the first several hours following surgery, which gradually tapers over time.

Persistent, excessive bleeding (greater than 500 ml in 1 hour or greater than 300 ml/hr for 2 to 3 hours) requires surgical reexploration in the operating room, but this occurs in less than 3% of cases.

General measures used to promote hemostasis include rewarming and aggressive treatment of postoperative hypertension with vasodilators. Coagulation studies are obtained in patients who are actively bleeding, so that appropriate therapy can be instituted. This may include administration of blood products (packed red blood cells [PRBCs] or platelets), replacement of coagulation factors (fresh frozen plasma [FFP] or cryoprecipitate), or medications as needed.

Treatment of postoperative bleeding may be initiated before laboratory results are available, based on the most likely hemostatic disorder. For example, platelets may be administered empirically in patients who have received aspirin, clopidogrel (Plavix), or glycoprotein IIb/IIIa inhibitors preoperatively. FFP may be used to replenish clotting factors in patients with known hepatic dysfunction or those who have received multiple transfusions of PRBCs intraoperatively. Once coagulation studies become available, more definitive treatment of the bleeding disorder can be selected.

A number of pharmacologic agents are used in the management of postoperative bleeding. These agents are listed in the Medication table below. Protamine sulfate is administered at the end of the operation to neutralize circulating heparin. Additional protamine may be prescribed in critical care if the activated partial thromboplastin time (aPTT) remains elevated or if the patient receives additional cell-saver blood.[26] Antifibrinolytic agents, including aprotinin (Trasylol), aminocaproic acid (Amicar), and tranexamic acid (Cyklokapron), are administered intraoperatively to decrease blood loss by preventing normal clot breakdown. These agents may also be administered postoperatively when fibrinolysis is suggested by continued bleeding and abnormal coagulation studies—typically a prolonged prothrombin time (PT) or international normalized ratio (INR), increased aPTT, and decreased fibrinogen level. Desmopressin acetate (DDAVP) promotes platelet adhesion and may be beneficial in patients with disorders that affect platelet function (e.g., uremia or von Willebrand's disease).

MEDICATIONS USED TO PROMOTE HEMOSTASIS AFTER CARDIAC SURGERY

DRUG	ACTIONS	DOSE	SPECIAL CONSIDERATIONS
Aprotinin (Trasylol)	Serine protease inhibitor that helps block coagulation cascade that occurs from contact with bypass circuit Also preserves platelet adhesion and inhibits plasmin	2 million units IV over 20 min, followed by 0.5 million units/hr or 3.5 mg/kg IV bolus, then 3.5 mg/kg/hr × 1 hr, followed by 1 mg/kg/hr	Is given intraoperatively to attenuate response to bypass and decrease bleeding. This drug is expensive, so it is primarily used in high-risk patients. May also be used to treat postoperative bleeding. May cause transient renal dysfunction. May require dose adjustment for renal impairment. Elevates ACT.* Derived from bovine source, which is associated with higher risk of anaphylaxis.
Desmopressin acetate (DDAVP)	Synthetic form of vasopressin that promotes platelet adhesion by increasing release of factor VIII from tissue stores	0.3–0.4 mcg/kg IV over 20 min	Is beneficial in patients with disorders that affect platelet function (uremia, von Willebrand's disease) and in reoperations.
Aminocaproic acid (Amicar)	Antifibrinolytic agent that stabilizes clots by inhibiting conversion of plasminogen to plasmin	Bolus of 5–9 g IV while on CPB, followed by infusion of 1 g/hr for 5 hr	May be used if fibrinolysis is present (detected by low fibrinogen levels and high fibrin degradation products, or decreased clot lysis time). May require dose adjustment for renal impairment.

Table continues on page 310

DRUG	ACTIONS	DOSE	SPECIAL CONSIDERATIONS
Tranexamic acid (Cyklokapron)	Antifibrinolytic agent with actions similar to aminocaproic acid	100 mg/kg IV preop; if needed, can give 50 mg/kg postop 9–15 mg/kg IV or 0.5–1 g IV every 4–6 hr	Less expensive than aprotinin, so may be used in lower-risk patients. Adjust dose for renal impairment.
Protamine	Neutralizes heparin in a dose-related fashion (1 mg of protamine for every 90 units of heparin)	25–50 mg IV slowly,* at a rate of 5 mg/min Remainder of calculated dose can be administered by IV infusion over 8–16 hr	May be given postoperatively with reinfusion of cell-saver blood or if aPTT remains elevated. Half-life of protamine is only 5 min, so "heparin rebound" may occur if sequestered heparin is released from body tissues. Risk for anaphylaxis is greatest in patients with IDDM or fish allergies.

ACT = Activated clotting time, aPTT = activated partial thromboplastin time, CPB = cardiopulmonary bypass, IDDM = insulin-dependent diabetes mellitus.
*May cause hypotension if administered too rapidly.

Although the threshold for administering blood transfusions varies among practitioners, typically red blood cells are not replaced until the patient's Hct is less than 24% to 26%. The postoperative Hct is often decreased secondary to hemodilution in patients receiving nonblood infusions (e.g., colloids, crystalloids, FFP). The decision to transfuse should be based on the patient's clinical condition and signs of impaired tissue oxygenation, rather than on a specific Hct level.[26,70] In patients who are actively bleeding, red blood cell transfusion may be warranted to maintain a hemoglobin level that is adequate to maintain tissue oxygenation.

Autotransfusion of shed mediastinal blood can be used to provide the patient with volume and return of red cells. Autotransfusion can produce a coagulopathy, because the shed blood has lower levels of clotting factors and platelets, as well as elevated levels of fibrin split products. When performed, it is usually limited to the first 6 hours postoperatively to minimize the risk of infection.[21]

Patients are monitored for signs of cardiac tamponade that may occur if blood is not evacuated effectively from the mediastinal space. Signs of tamponade include decreased CO refractory to inotropes and hypotension along with elevated and equalized filling pressures. As blood accumulates in the pericardial space, pressure increases around the heart so that the right atrial, pulmonary artery wedge pressure (PAWP), and left atrial pressures equilibrate. Physical assessment may reveal jugular venous distention, diminished pulses, pulsus paradoxus, and muffled heart sounds. Tamponade usually occurs in a patient with significant mediastinal bleeding and is often preceded by a sudden cessation of chest tube drainage. If time permits, a widened cardiac silhouette on chest x-ray or evidence of pericardial fluid on an echocardiogram can provide additional confirmation of cardiac tamponade. Interventions for tamponade include returning to the OR for surgical evacuation of the clot or, if the patient exhibits extreme hemodynamic instability, emergency sternotomy in critical care.

▲ Case Study 14-1, Part C

Coronary Artery Bypass Grafting

Three hours after surgery, J.P. was normothermic, was hemodynamically stable on 3 mcg/kg/min of dobutamine, and had minimal chest tube drainage. His pacemaker was turned off and he had an underlying sinus rhythm with a rate approximately 80–90 beats/min. Other vital signs were as follows: MAP 76 mm Hg, PAP 28/15 mm Hg, PAWP 13 mm Hg, RAP 9 mm Hg, CI 2.6 L/min/m², SVR 984 dynes/sec/cm⁻⁵, SvO₂ 0.67.

His SaO₂ was 97% on an FiO₂ of 0.5. His propofol was discontinued and he awakened within 20 minutes and began overbreathing the ventilator. He was alert and able to move all four extremities on command. His IMV rate was decreased, and he had satisfactory ABGs after a 30-minute trial on CPAP. J.P. was extubated by the respiratory therapist, and his NG tube was removed. He was placed on 5 L of oxygen via nasal cannula.

Decision point: What are important nursing interventions for J.P. after extubation?

Dysrhythmias

Dysrhythmias occur frequently following cardiac surgery and include both supraventricular and ventricular rhythms. Rhythm disturbances may occur as a result of the patient's underlying cardiac disease or from surgical sequelae (i.e., edema of the conduction system, electrolyte imbalances, hypoxemia, or hypothermia). In addition, patients who have been taking beta blockers preoperatively may have an inadequate heart rate postoperatively.

Strategies for managing postoperative dysrhythmias include interventions targeting prevention as well as treatment. Serum potassium and magnesium levels should be monitored frequently, especially during periods of diuresis, and replaced to adequate levels. Continuous ST analysis should be performed so episodes of ischemia can be detected and treated. Arterial blood gases (ABGs) are monitored and ventilator settings adjusted as needed to correct hypoxemia and acidosis. Hemodynamically compromising dysrhythmias are treated immediately with temporary pacing, antidysrhythmic agents, cardioversion, or defibrillation, as described in advanced cardiac life support protocols.[5]

Atrial fibrillation is the most common dysrhythmia following cardiac surgery, occurring in 25% to 40% of patients.[20,35,37] Although initially it was theorized that atrial fibrillation would occur less frequently with off-pump procedures, studies have not shown a significant difference between the two approaches.[34] Because of its prevalence, a number of protocols have been developed for prophylaxis against atrial fibrillation. Preoperative or early postoperative (12 to 24 hours) administration of beta blockers has proven effective at decreasing the incidence of atrial fibrillation and is currently recommended as standard therapy in the American College of Cardiology/American Heart Association (ACC/AHA) guidelines.[25] Other strategies for managing postoperative atrial fibrillation are described in Box 14-2.

Pacing. Temporary epicardial pacing wires are frequently placed on the right atrium and ventricle at the conclusion of the surgical procedure and can be used for both therapeutic and diagnostic purposes in the postoperative period. Pacing can be used to optimize CO by providing a heart rate of 90 to 100 beats/min. If possible, patients are paced in synchronous modes that allow for maintenance of atrioventricular synchrony (e.g., AAI or DDD). If the patient has atrial fibrillation or flutter, ventricular pacing (VVI) is used.

A temporary pacemaker may also be used to terminate rapid reentrant supraventricular tachycardias (SVTs) that occur postoperatively (e.g., atrial flutter). This is accomplished with special pacemakers that can deliver impulses at rates of up to 800 pulses per

---

Box 14-2

Strategies for Managing Postoperative Atrial Fibrillation

PROPHYLAXIS

- Amiodarone
- Atrial pacing (AAI or biatrial)
- Beta blockers (metoprolol, propranolol)
- Magnesium sulfate
- Sotalol

TREATMENT

- Synchronized cardioversion
- Rapid atrial pacing
- Beta blockers
- Calcium channel blockers
- Procainamide

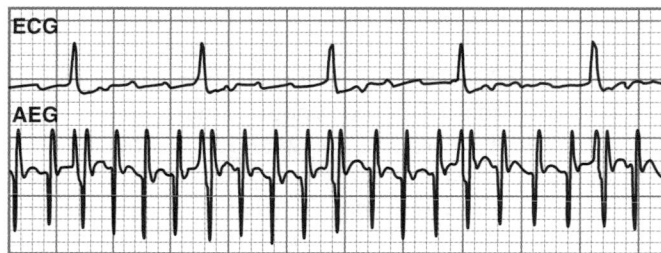

⬦FIGURE 14-5 Atrial electrogram. Atrial flutter with 4:1 AV block. The unipolar AEG demonstrates an atrial rate of about 300 with a ventricular response of about 75/min. AEG = Atrial electrogram.

---

minute. Atrial pacing is performed at a rate faster than the patient's intrinsic SVT to capture the atrial tissue, and then abruptly discontinued to allow the sinus node to resume control.

Atrial epicardial wires can be used for diagnostic purposes as well, by providing an amplified view of atrial electrical activity. Either one or both of the atrial wires can be attached to an ECG monitor to obtain an atrial electrogram (AEG), which can be helpful in differentiating among some of the more common postoperative dysrhythmias.[23] An example of an AEG is shown in Figure 14-5.

Myocardial Depression

Myocardial depression is common in the first 6 to 8 hours following surgery, as the heart recovers from a period of ischemia. Cardiac cellular function may be impaired by hypothermia, cellular edema, or inadequate myocardial protection during the operative procedure. Initial interventions are aimed at optimizing preload and afterload to enhance cardiac contractility, with the goal of maintaining a cardiac index (CI) greater than or equal to $2.2 \, L/min/m^2$ and an SvO_2 greater than 65%. Additional measures for CABG patients are directed at maintaining graft patency to ensure adequate myocardial perfusion. If optimizing these parameters fails to produce an adequate CI, inotropes may be used to enhance contractility. Finally, if pharmacologic interventions prove inadequate, patients may be supported with mechanical circulatory assist devices (e.g., IABP).

Preload. Although patients are usually total body fluid overloaded following CPB, they frequently require fluids to maintain adequate intravascular volume. This occurs in part because of the capillary leak induced by the systemic inflammatory response to bypass. In addition, a relative hypovolemia may occur as the patient vasodilates during rewarming or as a result of various medications. Patients with normal preoperative ventricular function can have their preload assessed with only a central venous catheter. For patients with more complex problems, a pulmonary artery catheter is helpful in evaluating postoperative problems. Because the ultimate goal of hemodynamic interventions is to provide adequate tissue oxygenation, catheters that continuously measure SvO_2 are particularly helpful. Rarely a left atrial line may be placed during surgery to monitor left-sided filling pressure in patients with severe pulmonary hypertension (HTN) or patients with a ventricular assist device (VAD). These lines require meticulous handling to minimize the risk of air emboli, including frequent assessment and aspiration of any bubbles, and use of an in-line air filter.

Fluids used to treat hypovolemia may vary based on institutional protocol and physician preference. Generally, crystalloids (e.g., normal saline or lactated Ringer's) are used first, and followed by colloids if the crystalloids are insufficient at raising the filling pressures to the required level. Either 5% albumin or hetastarch may be used, although hetastarch should be limited to 20 ml/kg in a 24-hour period to minimize the potential for bleeding.[10] The end point for fluid resuscitation should be based on achieving an adequate CO, rather than just reaching a target value for central venous pressure (CVP) or PAWP. Excessive fluid administration may increase lung water and delay extubation, as well as dilute clotting factors and Hct.

Preload requirements are usually influenced by the patient's preoperative ventricular function. The cardiac catheterization report can provide important information regarding the patient's preoperative function, including ejection fraction and right and left ventricular filling pressures. Patients with normal ventricular function will typically require lower filling pressures than those with dilated or hypertrophied ventricles. A comparison of postoperative care for patients with differing ventricular function is provided in Table 14-3.

Afterload. Afterload is frequently increased after cardiac surgery secondary to vasoconstriction induced by hypothermia and the catecholamines released as part of the sympathetic nervous system response to surgery. Patients with well-preserved ventricular function and preoperative hypertension are likely to manifest an elevated BP postoperatively. Other patients

---

TABLE 14-3 Implications of Ventricular Function on Filling Pressures

VENTRICULAR FUNCTION	ASSOCIATED CONDITIONS	POSTOPERATIVE IMPLICATIONS
Normal LV function		Usually require PAWP or LA pressures of 12–15 mm Hg. May need vasodilators short-term to decrease SVR.
Hyperdynamic LV	Aortic stenosis Hypertension Hypertrophic cardiomyopathy	Often require higher filling pressures (PAWP or LAP of 18–25 mm Hg). Pacing may be helpful to maintain AV synchrony, which optimizes stroke volume. Beta blockers may be used if patients are "hyperdynamic" (HTN and tachycardic) postoperatively.
Dilated LV	Congestive heart failure Aortic regurgitation Chronic mitral regurgitation	Usually require higher filling pressures (PAWP or LAP of 18–25 mm Hg). Afterload reduction is important to maintain CO.
RV failure	Pulmonary hypertension Acute RV infarct	Require high CVP (15–20 mm Hg) to increase RV output. Vasodilators may be needed to decrease PVR.

AV = Atrioventricular, CO = cardiac output, CVP = central venous pressure, HTN = hypertension, LAP = left atrial pressure, LV = left ventricle, PAWP = pulmonary artery wedge pressure, PVR = pulmonary vascular resistance, RV = right ventricle, SVR = systemic vascular resistance.

may have increased SVR accompanied by low or normal BP, secondary to impaired myocardial function. Treatment is usually required to prevent adverse effects of increased afterload, including increased myocardial work and risk of bleeding at surgical sites. Usually the goal is to keep the patient's systolic BP between 100 and 130 mm Hg and the mean arterial pressure (MAP) between 65 and 90 mm Hg. The target MAP must be individualized for patients with a history of HTN or cerebral or renal vascular disease. Lower MAPs are preferred if the patient is bleeding, to minimize pressure on the cannulation sites.

A number of interventions are used to manage postoperative vasoconstriction and hypertension. Hypothermic patients are rewarmed in an effort to decrease peripheral vasoconstriction. Analgesics and sedatives are administered as needed to minimize catecholamine outpouring associated with discomfort and emotional stress. A variety of vasodilators may be prescribed to maintain the desired BP and SVR. These agents may be used alone or in conjunction with inotropic agents in patients with marginal CO. Frequently used vasodilators are described in the Medication table on pp. 1116-1121 in Chapter 41. Agents that have an effect primarily on the arterial system may be more advantageous than mixed arterial and venous dilators, especially in the setting of hypovolemia.

Approximately 10% of patients may present with a profound vasodilation following cardiac surgery, presumed to be the result of the systemic inflammatory response to CPB.[1] These patients present with hypotension and low SVR, accompanied by signs of decreased perfusion (e.g., lactic acidosis and low urine output). Treatment usually includes volume resuscitation in conjunction with alpha-adrenergic agents (e.g., phenylephrine or norepinephrine). Vasopressin, which induces vasoconstriction through stimulation of V_1 receptors in vascular smooth muscle, has also been shown to be effective when administered as a continuous infusion at 0.01 to 1 unit/min.[1]

Inotropes. Because ventricular function is depressed following cardiac surgery, optimizing preload and afterload may not be sufficient to ensure adequate oxygen delivery to the tissues. Ventricular contractility often needs augmentation with inotropic agents. Inotropes can be initiated in the operating room to wean the patient off bypass or in the critical care unit to maintain a CI of greater than 2.2 L/min and an Svo_2 greater than 65%. First-line inotropic agents include catecholamines (e.g., epinephrine, dopamine, and dobutamine). If these fail to improve CO, phosphodiesterase inhibitors (e.g., milrinone [Primacor]) may be employed. Inotropic agents used in cardiac surgery patients are described in the Medication table on pp. 1116-1121 in Chapter 41.

Graft Patency. Ischemia may be a cause of impaired myocardial function in the immediate postoperative period. Patients are monitored for ST segment elevation, which may indicate acute vasospasm or graft closure. Intravenous nitroglycerin has been shown to dilate coronary arteries, increase coronary collateral blood flow, and relax areas of coronary artery spasm. Unfortunately, it may also worsen hypotension and decrease CO, especially in the setting of hypovolemia. For this reason, it should be administered cautiously in patients who are experiencing active ischemia. Prophylactic use of nitroglycerin has not been shown in studies to be effective at preventing myocardial ischemia in postoperative patients.[24] If a radial artery graft is used or spasm in other arterial conduits is suspected, calcium channel blockers (e.g., nicardipine [Cardene] or diltiazem [Cardizem]) may also be prescribed.

Aspirin inhibits platelet aggregation and has been shown to improve graft patency. The latest guidelines on antithrombotic therapy recommend that 75 to 162 mg of aspirin should be administered 6 hours after surgery, or as soon as mediastinal bleeding has decreased, and continued indefinitely.[67] A recent multicenter study showed that early use of aspirin (within 48 hours) following surgery not only decreased mortality but also reduced the incidence of ischemic complications in other organ systems (e.g., brain, kidneys, gastrointestinal tract).[50]

Cardiac Assist Devices. If the above measures fail to improve CO, an IABP or VAD may be inserted. These devices provide mechanical support to improve tissue perfusion, without placing additional demands on the injured myocardium. The selection of a cardiac assist device is influenced by patient condition, capabilities of a particular device, and availability of the equipment within the healthcare institution.

The IABP is the most commonly used assist device in cardiac surgery.[11] This device consists of a 40- to 50-ml polyurethane balloon positioned in the descending aorta and a console that controls inflation and deflation of the balloon in synchrony, but out of phase, with the cardiac cycle. Inflation of the balloon during diastole provides increased coronary perfusion while deflation just before systolic ejection decreases afterload. Indications for IABP insertion in cardiac surgery patients are described in Box 14-3.

The intra-aortic balloon is usually inserted percutaneously in the femoral artery, but for patients with severe vascular disease surgical insertion may be required. Nursing care involves assessment of proper IABP functioning to achieve the desired hemodynamic effects as well as monitoring the patient for potential complications. Details of nursing care are provided in the *AACN Protocol for Practice: Care of the Patient With an Intra-aortic Balloon Pump.*[61]

Box 14-3

Indications for Intra-Aortic Balloon Pump in Cardiac Surgery Patients

PREOPERATIVE

- Mechanical complications post–myocardial infarction (ventricular septal defect, papillary muscle rupture)
- Ongoing ischemia (despite medical management)
- Hemodynamic instability (cardiogenic shock)
- Prophylactic placement for high-risk patients
- Left main disease
- Severe left ventricular failure (ejection fraction less than 25%)

INTRAOPERATIVE

- High-risk patients undergoing off-pump coronary artery bypass
- Failure to wean from cardiopulmonary bypass

POSTOPERATIVE

- Low cardiac output unresponsive to moderate doses of inotropes
- Myocardial ischemia

increases CO by 10% to 20%, these devices can provide full perfusion to the tissues to allow the heart a period of rest.[11] Some devices are designed for short-term use, to allow a window of time for possible recovery of myocardial function. Others are more suitable for long-term use, if the chance for recovery is unlikely. Typically, long-term devices are used only in institutions that have transplant capabilities.

A VAD can be placed in either the left ventricle (LVAD) or the right ventricle (RVAD), or both (BiVAD), depending on where the ventricular failure is occurring. Figure 14-6 illustrates cannulation techniques for VADs. These patients typically require intensive nursing care, including maintaining adequate preload to allow for VAD filling and heparinization to prevent clotting in the device. Complications associated with VADs include bleeding, infection, and device failure.

Pulmonary Support

All patients will have some degree of pulmonary dysfunction postoperatively as a result of the effects of anesthesia, cardiopulmonary bypass, and surgical methods (dissection of the internal mammary, median sternotomy).[73] Postoperatively, patients experience varying degrees of ventilation/perfusion ($\dot{V}/\dot{Q}$) mismatch and intrapulmonary shunting. Despite these changes, early extubation (either in the operating room or within the first 4 to 6 hours) is feasible in the majority of patients. Studies have shown that early

VADs are used in patients who cannot be successfully weaned from CPB despite maximal support with medications and the IABP. Whereas an IABP only

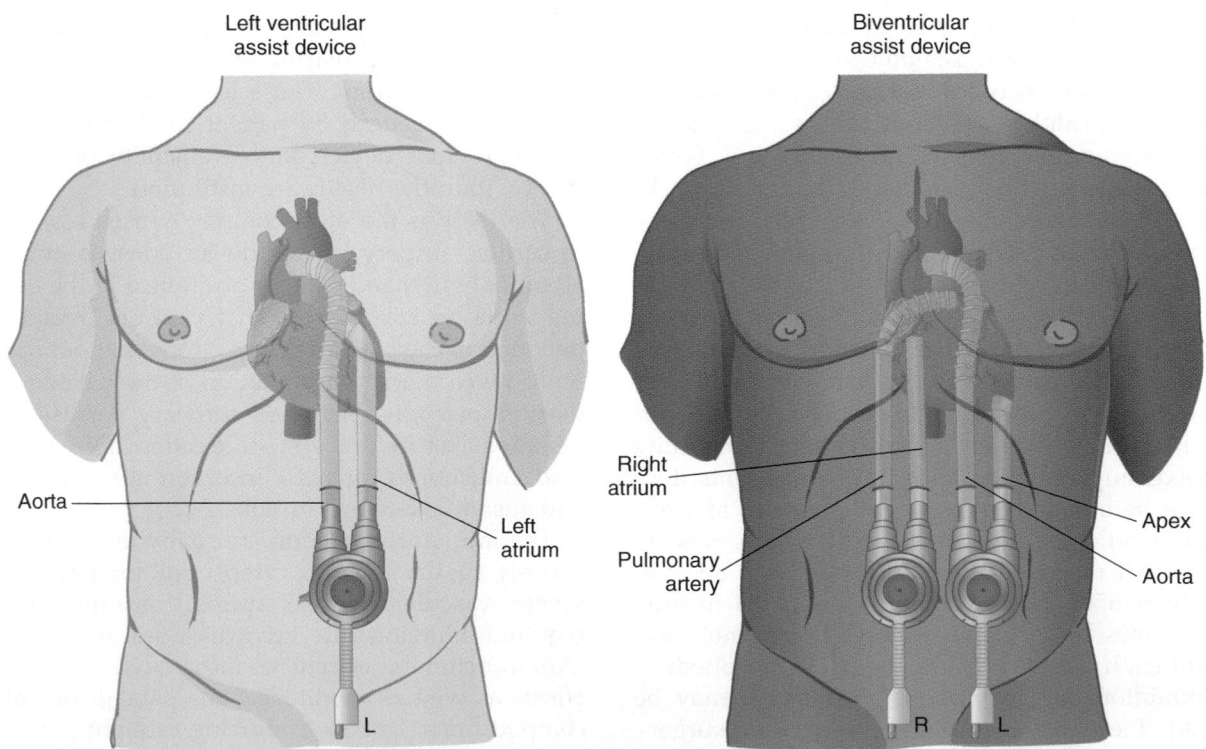

♦FIGURE 14-6 Cannulation for ventricular assist devices.

extubation shortens length of stay and can be achieved without an increase in pulmonary complications.[36,51] Protocols for anesthesia and immediate postoperative sedation have been developed to facilitate fast-tracking patients to extubation.

Initial ventilator settings in critical care usually include a tidal volume of 8 to 10 ml/kg, a respiratory rate of 8 to 10 breaths/min, a fraction of inspired oxygen (Fio_2) of 1, and low levels (5 cm H_2O) of positive end-expiratory pressure (PEEP) and pressure support (PS). The first ABG is obtained about 20 minutes after arrival in the critical care unit, to allow for equilibration after placement on the ventilator. The Fio_2 is usually weaned to maintain an Sao_2 of greater than 92%, the respiratory rate is adjusted based on the partial pressure of carbon dioxide ($Paco_2$) and pH results. When adjusting the ventilator settings, the patient's degree of hypothermia should be considered because the $Paco_2$ will generally rise as the patient rewarms, which can lead to acidosis. Ongoing assessment of the patient's ventilatory status can be accomplished with noninvasive measures of Sao_2 and end-tidal CO_2, with ABGs obtained only if the noninvasive data suggest a problem.

Criteria for weaning from the ventilator (see Chapter 20 for details) include awakening with minimal stimulation, reversal of neuromuscular blockade, satisfactory ABGs, hemodynamic stability, control of severe bleeding, and rewarming to normothermia. Patients need to be carefully assessed during the weaning process for signs of failure, which are described in Box 14-4. If the patient exhibits signs of failure, weaning should be stopped and ventilator settings resumed for a period of time. Prolonged ventilation may be required in patients with hemodynamic instability, advanced pulmonary disease, or severe neurologic damage.

After extubation, patients continue to require vigilant respiratory assessment. Oxygenation may be compromised by fluid overload or atelectasis. Most patients are provided supplemental oxygen via nasal cannula for the first 24 to 48 hours. Patients with a median sternotomy may tend to splint or take shallow breaths, thus retaining CO_2. Patients should be encouraged to cough, use the incentive spirometer every 1 to 2 hours, and get out of bed to a chair as soon as possible. Adequate pain medication and a "cough pillow" are important to facilitate these goals.[53]

A nasogastric (NG) tube may be used for gastric decompression, inserted either after the patient's transfer to critical care or on arrival in the OR. Insertion after admission may cause hypertension and dysrhythmias if the patient is not well sedated, or bleeding if the patient has a coagulopathy. The NG tube is removed

---

Box 14-4

Signs of Failure to Tolerate Ventilator Weaning

- Changes in neurologic status (agitation, somnolence)
- Diaphoresis
- Significant changes in heart rate or blood pressure
- Increase in respiratory rate >35 breaths/min
- Decrease in Pao_2 <60 mm Hg or Sao_2 <90% (on an Fio_2 of 0.5)
- Increased $Paco_2$ (>50 mm Hg) in conjunction with respiratory acidosis

Fio_2 = Fraction of inspired oxygen, $Paco_2$ = partial pressure of carbon dioxide in arterial blood, Pao_2 = partial pressure of oxygen in arterial blood, Sao_2 = oxygen saturation of arterial blood.

---

with extubation, and patients may gradually begin oral intake, usually with ice chips or clear liquids. Patients should be observed during initial oral intake to evaluate for the potential risk of aspiration. Although swallowing difficulties are rare in patients with short-term intubation, aspiration can have devastating consequences.

Antiembolic stockings are used routinely in cardiac surgery patients to decrease the risk of deep vein thrombosis and pulmonary embolism. Early mobilization is important to further reduce this risk. If the patient's condition requires prolonged periods of immobility (i.e., hemodynamic instability or prolonged intubation), sequential compression devices or low molecular weight heparin may also be used.

Sedation/Analgesia

Adequate analgesia and sedation are important to minimize the physiologic and psychologic problems associated with pain and anxiety. Myocardial function is impacted by the sympathetic nervous system response to pain, which includes an increase in myocardial oxygen demand and automaticity. Pulmonary function may also be adversely affected as a result of decreased lung expansion and retention of secretions.

Patients generally arrive in critical care sedated from agents they have received in the OR. Some institutions maintain patients on a propofol (Diprivan) infusion for a period of time postoperatively. When patients meet criteria for weaning, the propofol (or other sedative infusion) is discontinued and the patient is allowed to awaken. A bispectral index (BIS) monitor has been used in some institutions to evaluate the patient's level of sedation both during and immediately following the surgical procedure. The BIS provides a value derived from the patient's electroencephalograph (EEG), measured via a probe attached to the patient's forehead, that correlates with the patient's level of sedation.

The Medication table below describes some of the sedative and analgesic agents commonly prescribed for cardiac surgical patients. Most of these medications may be given in small bolus doses or by continuous infusion. Continuous infusions have the advantage of producing less respiratory depression and providing more consistent pain control. As patients progress, other pain options (e.g., patient-controlled analgesia, oral agents) can be used.

MEDICATIONS (SEDATIVES AND ANALGESICS) USED IN CARDIAC SURGERY PATIENTS

DRUG	ACTIONS	DOSE	SPECIAL CONSIDERATIONS
Fentanyl (Sublimaze)	Stimulates opiate receptors in central nervous system to produce analgesia and sedation	25–90 mcg IV bolus or 50–200 mcg/hr infusion	More rapid acting than morphine with a shorter duration of action. May cause chest wall rigidity.
Dexmedetomidine	Produces anxiolysis, analgesia, and sedation through its effects on alpha$_2$ receptors	1 mcg/kg IV loading dose over 9 min, followed by infusion at 0.2–0.7 mcg/kg/hr	Reduces anxiety and provides pain relief without sedation. Works synergistically with opioids to decrease dosage required.
Ketorolac (Toradol)	Nonsteroidal antiinflammatory with analgesic effects	30–60 mg IV every 6 hr (not to exceed 72 hr)	Avoid in patients with renal dysfunction. Inhibits platelet function. Does not produce respiratory depression or alter hemodynamics.
Midazolam (Versed)	Benzodiazepine that produces sedation, anxiolysis, and amnesia Does not produce analgesia, but may reduce analgesic requirements	2.5–5 mg IV every 1–2 hr or 0.5–4 mg/hr	Rapid onset and short duration of action, but may accumulate with prolonged infusion (48 hr) or in older adults. May cause respiratory depression in some patients.
Morphine sulfate	Stimulates opiate receptors in central nervous system to produce analgesia and sedation	2–9 mg IV every 2–4 hr or 1–5 mg/hr infusion	Active metabolite of morphine; can accumulate in renal failure. Promotes histamine release, which causes vasodilation (may cause hypotension).
Propofol (Diprivan)	Sedative-hypnotic that can be used for induction of anesthesia or sedation	5–50 mcg/kg/min	This agent has no analgesic effects. Short duration of action (5–9 min) allows for rapid reversal of effects. May cause hypotension, especially in hypovolemic patients. Lipid medium may increase triglyceride levels and presents a risk for bacterial growth. Prolonged sedation may occur in obese patients.

Adequate analgesia is essential to facilitate increasing activity levels and pulmonary exercises (e.g., coughing and deep breathing). An assessment of pain should be performed during activity as well as at rest, since researchers have found that pain levels are highest with coughing, turning, and getting out of bed.[53] In addition to promoting recovery activities, analgesics are also warranted during procedures (e.g., chest tube removal). Both opioids and nonsteroidal antiinflammatory agents have been found effective in reducing the pain associated with this procedure.[59]

Prevention of Infection

A number of strategies are used to decrease the risk of infection in cardiac surgery patients. Preoperative interventions include antiseptic skin prep and clipping (rather than shaving) hair at the surgical site. Prophylactic antibiotics are administered for the first 24 hours, beginning just before the surgical incision.[25] Prolonged use of antibiotics is not recommended, because it has been shown to increase the incidence of resistant organisms. Other interventions to decrease the risk of infection include prompt removal of intravenous lines and urinary catheters, and early extubation. Incisional dressings placed in the OR are usually removed on the first postoperative day. Subsequent coverage is usually not necessary unless drainage is present. All incisional sites are assessed daily for signs of infection (e.g., erythema, tenderness, drainage). In addition, patients with a median sternotomy should also be assessed for stability of the sternum.

Hyperglycemia and undiagnosed diabetes have been shown to pose a significant risk for the development of surgical site infections.[40] Within the past decade there has been increasing research to support the use of continuous insulin infusions to maintain blood glucose levels, particularly in diabetic cardiac surgery patients.[30] In addition to decreasing the incidence of infection, studies in the cardiac surgery population have shown reductions in both mortality and length of stay related to effective postoperative glucose control.[30] This research is further described in the Research Utilization box below.

Glucose control is ideally begun preoperatively and continued for a minimum of 48 hours postoperatively, with the goal of maintaining euglycemia (blood glucose levels of less than or equal to 110 mg/dl).[4]

◆ RESEARCH UTILIZATION

Diabetes Mellitus Risk Factors and Death After Coronary Artery Bypass Grafting

CLINICAL ISSUE

Diabetes mellitus (DM) is a well-established risk factor for death after coronary artery bypass grafting. It was long believed that the increased mortality was related to comorbid conditions associated with DM, such as more extensive atherosclerosis, peripheral vascular disease, renal insufficiency, obesity, and increased risk of infection.

SUMMARY

A total of 3554 diabetic patients undergoing CABG at one institution were treated aggressively with either subcutaneous (subQ) insulin every 4 hours (from 1987 to 1991) or a continuous intravenous (IV) insulin infusion (from 1992 to 2001). Continuous IV insulin yielded significantly better glucose control (177 ± 30 mg/dl) than subQ (213 ± 41 mg/dl) as well as significantly lower mortality (2.5% vs. 5.3%, $P < 0.0001$). Monitoring of glucose levels from blood obtained via fingerstick or the arterial line was performed every 30 minutes for 2 hours. The authors noted that target levels for glucose were decreased over the course of the study, from 150–200 mg/dl to 90–150 mg/dl, as caregivers became more comfortable using the protocol.

APPLICATION

Tight hyperglycemic control can be achieved with continuous insulin infusion, and should be the standard of care for diabetic patients undergoing cardiac surgery. Significant benefits associated with this intervention include decreased infection rates as well as improved mortality. Other researchers[69] have shown that the mortality benefit of controlling glucose levels extends to other critically ill patients as well.

NEED FOR FURTHER STUDY

A number of protocols have been devised for controlling blood glucose levels with continuous insulin infusions. Many of these are time-intensive for nurses, and there is a risk of inadequate glucose control (either hyper- or hypoglycemia) if patients are not adequately monitored or insulin coverage is inappropriate. Studies are needed to determine the best methodologies and hospital systems for improving glycemic control and clinical outcomes.

Furnary, A.P., et al. (2003). Continuous insulin infusion reduces mortality with diabetics undergoing coronary artery bypass grafting. *J Thorac Cardiovasc Surg, 125*, 1007–1021.

♦ NUTRITION

Nutritional Considerations for Postoperative Cardiac Surgery Patients

CALORIES

25 kcal/kg/day

PROTEIN

1.2–1.5 g/kg/day

FLUID

Fluid restriction may be required, especially for patients with CHF or renal failure.

ELECTROLYTES

Potassium replacement for level less than 4.5 mEq/L
Magnesium replacement for level less than 2 mEq/L
Sodium restriction of 2000–3000 mg/day

VITAMINS AND MINERALS

Multivitamins may be prescribed for patients with decreased intake.

SPECIAL CONSIDERATIONS

Generally a diet low in cholesterol and fat is prescribed. The diet may need to be less restrictive in the immediate postoperative period to ensure adequate nutritional intake to support healing. Diabetic patients will usually resume their preoperative diabetic diet.

Box 14-5

Predictors of Cardiac Surgery Mortality and Morbidity

- Emergent procedure
- Older age (>75)
- Poor ventricular function (ejection fraction <30% or elevated beta-type natriuretic peptide levels)
- Reoperation
- Female gender
- Left main disease
- Presence of comorbidities:
  Renal dysfunction (especially if dialysis dependent)
  COPD
  Diabetes mellitus
  Cerebrovascular disease

A number of standardized protocols have been developed to improve glycemic control, using both continuous insulin infusions and sliding-scale coverage. These protocols allow for titration of insulin based on frequent assessments of blood glucose level, as well as specifying interventions for hypoglycemia should it occur. Nursing care also includes increased frequency of blood glucose monitoring when alterations in metabolism are anticipated (such as an interruption of feeding or titration of catecholamine infusions).[45,62] The Nutrition box above outlines nutritional considerations for postoperative cardiac surgery patients.

Complications

The overall mortality associated with coronary artery bypass surgery is reported to be less than 3%.[65] Operative mortality is influenced by patient demographics, the extent of the cardiac disease, the urgency of the operation, and the presence of comorbid conditions. Factors found to be predictive of operative mortality and morbidity are listed in Box 14-5. These criteria are considered by surgeons during their preoperative assessment, to determine the patient's surgical risk.

Perioperative Myocardial Infarction. Perioperative MI is reported to occur in 2% to 4% of patients following surgical revascularization.[25] Potential causes include inadequate myocardial protection, arterial spasm in grafts or native arteries, or prolonged hypotension in the perioperative period. Diagnosis may be difficult because cardiac surgery is usually associated with nonspecific T wave and ST changes postoperatively, as well as elevations in myocardial-specific enzymes such as creatine kinase MB (CK-MB) and troponin. The diagnosis is frequently made based on new and persistent ECG changes and new regional wall abnormalities on echocardiogram.[14] While cardiac enzymes are elevated after surgery, marked elevations (CK-MB greater than 10 times normal) have been shown to be associated with adverse outcomes.[18,31] Other researchers have found that elevated troponin I levels (greater than 13 ng/dl) are also associated with an increased risk of cardiac death after CABG.[27] Patients in this high-risk group should receive aggressive medical management postoperatively, including administration of antiplatelet agents, beta blockers, angiotensin-converting enzyme (ACE) inhibitors, and statins.[25]

Renal Dysfunction. Renal dysfunction, defined by one large multicenter study as a postoperative serum creatinine level greater than 2 mg/dl or an increase from preoperative level of greater than 0.7 mg/dl, occurs in approximately 8% of patients.[49] Renal failure requiring dialysis occurs less frequently (1% to 2%), but is associated with mortality approaching 60%.[25] Risk factors for renal complications include preexisting renal disease, prolonged periods of hypotension or low CO perioperatively, and exposure to nephrotoxic agents.

Pulmonary Complications. Long-term pulmonary complications following cardiac surgery are rare and occur primarily in patients with severe underlying pulmonary disease. Patients with chronic lung disease may also require prolonged ventilation (i.e., greater than 48 hours) in the postoperative period. Acute lung injury progressing to acute respiratory distress syndrome occurs in less than 1% of patients, but carries a high mortality. Diaphragmatic failure may occur in a small number of patients secondary to intraoperative injury to the phrenic nerve. Signs include failure to wean from the ventilator, vital capacity of less than 500 ml, and paradoxical movement of the diaphragm. Pleural effusions are common but are generally small and left-sided and resolve spontaneously over time without treatment. Leaving a small Silastic (Blake) drain for several days following surgery has been shown to decrease the incidence of pleural effusions.[57]

Neurologic Complications. Neurologic complications after cardiac surgery have a reported incidence of between 0.4% and 80% depending on how they are defined.[25] Older adult patients (older than 70) and those with hypertension, diabetes, or preoperative neurologic dysfunction have an increased risk for adverse outcomes. The risk for altered cerebral tissue perfusion, with resultant neurologic dysfunction, is also increased with prolonged bypass times, perioperative hypotension, calcification of the aorta, and atrial fibrillation. More serious type 1 complications, which include fatal and nonfatal stroke and transient ischemic attacks, occur in approximately 3% of patients. Type 2 complications, which describe a more subtle impairment of cognitive function (i.e., concentration, short-term memory, and speed of mental or motor responses), occur more frequently, with some studies reporting an incidence of up to 80%.[55]

Gastrointestinal Complications. Gastrointestinal complications occur infrequently following cardiac surgery (less than 2%) but are associated with a high mortality when they do occur.[54] The most common problem encountered is gastroduodenal bleeding. The prophylactic use of H_2 blockers, proton pump inhibitors, or sucralfate (Carafate) may be prescribed by some physicians. Intestinal ischemia or infarction may occur secondary to compromised blood flow to the mesenteric arteries. Patients typically exhibit persistent acidosis despite correction of CO. Other signs include a persistently elevated white blood cell count, abdominal tenderness, and signs of sepsis.

Wound Infection. Superficial leg incision infections occur in 10% to 20% of patients who undergo open harvesting of saphenous vein grafts, with the highest risk occurring in patients who are obese, who have diabetes, or who have compromised peripheral circulation.[9] The risk for infection with endovascular vein harvest is much lower. Patients typically present with cellulitis at the incisional site, possibly with wound breakdown and purulent drainage. Treatment usually consists of antibiotics, drainage of the wound, and potential debridement.

Sternal wound infections may be superficial or deep; most cases present within the first 2 to 4 weeks of surgery. Deep sternal wound infection (i.e., mediastinitis and sternal osteomyelitis) occurs in 1% to 4% of patients and is associated with high mortality.[25] Risk factors include obesity, diabetes mellitus, chronic obstructive lung disease, longer CPB times, and use of both internal mammary arteries. Antibiotic use within 2 weeks before surgery, reexploration, and longer duration of autotransfusion may also place patients at increased risk for developing mediastinitis.[21]

Superficial infections are associated with symptoms of tenderness, erythema, and serous drainage, while the sternum remains stable. In deep infections, purulent discharge is generally present, along with increased pain and sternal instability. Symptoms of systemic infection (e.g., fever, leukocytosis, and bacteremia) are also common. Positive blood cultures, especially if the organism is *Staphylococcus aureus,* further support the diagnosis of mediastinitis.[28]

Treatment of mediastinitis includes opening of the incision to allow for drainage and irrigation of the wound, and possible sternal debridement if warranted. The wound is usually kept open for a period of time to allow for irrigation and packing. Negative-pressure wound therapy with a vacuum-assisted closure (VAC) system has also been used to help expedite wound healing.[64] After the infection clears, the wound may be closed by either primary closure or a reconstructive flap composed of muscle or omentum.

CONCLUSIONS

Mortality associated with cardiac surgery has not increased over the past several years, despite the fact that patients undergoing surgical procedures are increasingly sicker. This is in part attributable to the comprehensive care provided in the immediate postoperative period by the critical care team. The ability of skilled practitioners to anticipate problems and initiate prompt intervention remains an essential component of ensuring successful patient outcomes following cardiac surgery.

REFERENCES

1. Albright, T. N., et al. (2002). Vasopressin in the cardiac surgery intensive care unit. *Am J Crit Care, 11*(4), 326–332.

2. Allen, K. B., et al. (2004). Transmyocardial revascularization: 5-year follow-up of a prospective randomized multicenter trial. *Ann Thoracic Surg, 77*, 1228–1234.

3. Allen, K. B., et al. (2004). Adjunctive transmyocardial revascularization: five-year follow up of a prospective randomized trial. *Ann Thoracic Surg, 78*, 458–465.

4. American College of Endocrinology. (2004). Position statement on inpatient diabetes and metabolic control. *Endocr Practice, 9*, 77–82.

5. American Heart Association. (2005). Guidelines for cardiopulmonary resuscitation and emergency cardiovascular care. *Circulation, 112*(suppl IV), IV51–88.

6. American Heart Association. (2005). *Heart disease and stroke statistics—2005 update.* Dallas, Tex: American Heart Association.

7. Angelini, G. D., et al. (2002). Early and mid-term outcome after off-pump surgery in Beating Heart Against Cardioplegic Arrest Studies (BHACAS 1 and 2): a pooled analysis of two randomized controlled trials. *Lancet, 359*, 1194–1199.

8. Antman, E. M., et al. (2004). ACC/AHA guidelines for the management of patients with STEMI: executive summary. *J Am Coll Cardiol, 44*, 671–719.

9. Athanasiou, T., et al. (2003). Leg wound infections after coronary artery bypass grafting: a meta-analysis comparing minimally invasive versus conventional vein harvesting. *Ann Thoracic Surg, 76*, 2141–2146.

10. Avorn, J., et al. (2003). Hetastarch and bleeding complications after coronary artery surgery. *Chest, 124*, 1437–1442.

11. Baskett, R. J., et al. (2002). The intra-aortic balloon pump in cardiac surgery. *Ann Thoracic Surg, 74*, 1276–1287.

12. Birnbaum, Y., et al. (2002). Ventricular septal rupture after acute myocardial infarction. *N Engl J Med, 347*, 1426–1432.

13. Bitondo, J. M., et al. (2002). Endoscopic versus open saphenous vein harvest: a comparison of postoperative wound infections. *Ann Thoracic Surg, 73*, 523–528.

13. Botha, P., Nagarajan, D. V., & Lewis, P. J. (2004). *Best evidence topics: can cardiac troponins be used to diagnose perioperative myocardial infarction post cardiac surgery?* www.BestBETS.org.

15. Bridges, C. R., et al. (2004). The Society of Thoracic Surgeons practice guidelines series: transmyocardial revascularization. *Ann Thoracic Surg, 77*, 1494–1502.

16. Chen-Scarabelli, C. (2002). Beating heart coronary artery bypass surgery. *Crit Care Nurse, 22*(5), 44.

17. Connelly, M. W., et al. (2002). Endoscopic radial harvesting: results of the first 300 patients. *Ann Thoracic Surg, 74*, 502–505.

18. Costa, M. A., et al. (2001). Incidence, predictors, and significance of abnormal cardiac enzyme rise in patients treated with bypass surgery in the Arterial Revascularization Therapies Study (ARTS). *Circulation, 94*, 2689–2693.

19. Crenshaw, B. S., et al. 2000 for the GUSTO (Global Utilization of Streptokinase and TPA for Occluded Coronary Arteries) trial investigators. Risk factors, angiographic patterns, and outcomes in patients with ventricular septal defect complicating acute myocardial infarction. *Circulation, 91*, 27–32.

20. Crystal, E., et al. (2002). Interventions on prevention of postoperative atrial fibrillation in patient undergoing heart surgery: a meta analysis. *Circulation, 96*, 75–80.

21. Dial, S., Nguyen, D., & Menzies, D. (2003). Autotransfusion of shed mediastinal blood. A risk factor for mediastinitis after cardiac surgery? Results of a cluster investigation. *Chest, 124*, 1847–1851.

22. DeWitte, J., & Sessler, D. I. (2002). Perioperative shivering: physiology and pharmacology. *Anesthesiology, 96*, 467–484.

23. Drew, B. J., et al. (2004). Practice standards for electrocardiographic monitoring in hospital settings: an American Heart Association Scientific Statement from the Councils on Cardiovascular Nursing, Clinical Cardiology, and Cardiovascular Disease in the Young. *Circulation, 19*, 2721–2746.

24. Eagle, K. A., et al. (2002). ACC/AHA guideline update on perioperative cardiovascular evaluation for non-cardiac surgery. A report of the American College of Cardiology/American Heart Association task force on practice guidelines (committee to update the 1996 guidelines on perioperative cardiovascular evaluation for non-cardiac surgery). *Circulation, 95*, 1257–1267.

25. Eagle, K. A., et al. (2004). ACC/AHA 2004 guideline update for coronary artery bypass graft surgery: summary article. A report of the American College of Cardiology/American Heart Association task force on practice guidelines (committee to update the 1999 guidelines for coronary artery bypass graft surgery). *J Am Coll Cardiol, 44*, 1146–1154.

26. Erhman, B. L., & Moore, H. A. (2004). Blood conservation strategies in cardiovascular surgery. *Dimensions Crit Care Nurs, 23*(6), 244–252.

27. Fellahi, J. L., et al. (2003). Short- and long-term prognostic value of postoperative cardiac troponin I concentration in patients undergoing coronary artery bypass grafting. *Anesthesiology, 99*, 270–274.

28. Fowler, V. G., et al. (2003). *Staphylococcus aureus* bacteremia after median sternotomy: clinical utility of blood culture results in the identification of postoperative mediastinitis. *Circulation, 98*, 73–78.

29. Frankel, T. L., et al. (2003). Silastic drains vs. conventional chest tubes after coronary artery bypass. *Chest, 124*, 98–113.

30. Furnary, A. P., et al. (2003). Continuous insulin infusion reduces mortality in patient with diabetes undergoing coronary artery bypass grafting. *J Thoracic Cardiovasc Surg, 125*, 907–921.

31. Gavard, J. A., et al. (2003). Prognostic significance of elevated creatine kinase MB after coronary bypass surgery and after an acute coronary syndrome: results from the GUARDIAN trial. *J Thoracic Cardiovasc Surg, 126*, 807–813.

32. Gerola, L. R., et al. (2004). Off-pump versus on-pump myocardial revascularization in low risk patients with one or two vessel disease: perioperative results in a multicenter randomized controlled trial. *Ann Thoracic Surg, 77*, 569–573.

33. Gregoric, I. D., & Cooley, D. A. (2004). Ventricular aneurysms. In S. C. Yang (Ed.), *Current therapy in thoracic and cardiovascular surgery* (pp 675–677). Philadelphia: Mosby.

34. Guller, U., et al. (2004). Outcomes of early extubation after bypass surgery in the elderly. *Ann Thoracic Surg, 77*, 781–788.

35. Hogue, C. W., et al. (2005). American College of Chest Physicians guidelines for the prevention and management of postoperative atrial fibrillation after cardiac surgery. *Chest, 128*, 9S–16S.

36. Hravnak, M., et al. (2004). Short-term complications and resource utilization in matched subjects after on-pump or off-pump primary isolated coronary artery bypass. *Am J Crit Care, 13*, 499–508.

37. Kern, L. S. (2004). Postoperative atrial fibrillation: new directions in prevention and treatment. *J Cardiovasc Nurs, 19*(2), 93.

38. Krabatsch, T., et al. (2002). Factors influencing results and outcome after transmyocardial laser revascularization. *Ann Thoracic Surg, 73*, 1888–1892.

39. Lancey, R. A., Gaca, C., & Vander-Salm, T. J. (2001). The use of smaller, more flexible chest drains following open-heart surgery: an initial evaluation. *Chest, 119*, 19–24.

40. Latham, R., et al. (2001). The association of diabetes and glucose control with surgical-site infections among cardiothoracic surgery patients. *Infect Control Hosp Epidemiol, 22*, 607–612.

41. Leavitt, B. J., et al. (2001). Use of internal mammary artery graft and in-hospital mortality and other adverse outcomes associated with coronary artery bypass surgery. *Circulation, 93,* 507–512.

42. Legare, J. F., et al. (2004). Coronary bypass surgery performed off pump does not result in lower in-hospital morbidity than coronary artery bypass grafting on pump. *Circulation, 99,* 887–892.

43. Lindsay, M. R. (2003). Transmyocardial laser revascularization revisited. *Crit Care Nurs Q, 26*(1), 69.

44. Loop, F. D., et al. (1986). Influence of the internal-mammary-artery graft on 9-year survival and other cardiac events. *N Engl J Med, 314,* 1–6.

45. Lorenz, R. A., Lorenz, R. M., & Codd, J. E. (2005). Perioperative control of blood glucose during adult coronary artery bypass surgery. *AORN J, 81,* 125–150.

46. Louagie, Y. A., et al. (2004). Continuous cold blood cardioplegia improves myocardial protection: a prospective randomized study. *Ann Thoracic Surg, 77*(2), 664.

47. Mack, M. J. (2003). Advances in the treatment of coronary artery disease. *Ann Thoracic Surg, 76,* S2240.

48. Mack, M. J., et al. (2004). Comparison of coronary bypass surgery with and without cardiopulmonary bypass in patients with multivessel disease. *J Thoracic Cardiovasc Surg, 127*(1), 167.

49. Mangano, C. M., et al. for the Multicenter Study of Perioperative Ischemia Research Group. (1998). Renal dysfunction after myocardial revascularization: risk factors, adverse outcomes, and hospital resource utilization. *Ann Intern Med, 128,* 194–203.

50. Mangano, D. T., et al. for the Multicenter Study of Perioperative Ischemia Research Group. (2002). Aspirin and mortality from coronary bypass surgery. *N Engl J Med, 347,* 1309–1317.

51. Meade, M. O., et al. (2001). Trials comparing early vs. late extubation following cardiovascular surgery. *Chest, 120,* 445S–453S.

52. Mickleborough, L. L., et al. (2003). Ventricular reconstruction for ischemic cardiomyopathy. *Ann Thoracic Surg, 75,* S6–12.

53. Milgrom, L. B., et al. (2004). Pain levels experienced with activities after cardiac surgery. *Am J Crit Care, 13*(2), 116–125.

54. Musleh, G. S., et al. (2003). Off-pump coronary artery bypass surgery does not reduce gastrointestinal complications. *Eur J Cardiothoracic Surg, 23*(1), 170–174.

55. Newman, M. F., et al. (2001). Longitudinal assessment of neurocognitive function after coronary artery bypass surgery. *N Engl J Med, 344*(6), 395–402.

56. O'Hanlon, J. V. (2000). Minimally invasive saphenous vein harvesting. *Crit Care Nurs Q, 23*(1), 42.

57. Payne, M., et al. (2000). Left pleural effusions after coronary artery bypass decrease with a supplemental pleural drain. *Ann Thoracic Surg, 73,* 149–152.

58. Possati, G., et al. (2003). Long-term results of the radial artery used for myocardial revascularization. *Circulation, 98,* 1350–1354.

59. Puntillo, K., & Ley, J. (2004). Appropriately timed analgesics control pain due to chest tube removal. *Am J Crit Care, 13,* 292–302.

60. Puskas, J. D., et al. (2003). Off-pump coronary artery bypass grafting provides complete revascularization with reduced myocardial injury, transfusion requirements, and length of stay: a prospective randomized comparison of two hundred unselected patients undergoing off-pump versus conventional coronary artery bypass grafting. *J Thoracic Cardiovasc Surg, 125,* 797–808.

61. Quall, S. (2003). *AACN Protocol for Practice: Care of the Patient with an IABP.* Aliso Viejo, CA: American Association of Critical-Care Nurses.

62. Robinson, L. E., & van Soren, M. H. (2004). Insulin resistance and hyperglycemia in critical illness: role of insulin in glycemic control. *AACN Clin Issues, 15,* 45–62.

63. Sellke, F. W., et al. (2005). Comparing on-pump and off-pump coronary artery bypass grafting: numerous studies but few conclusions. A Scientific Statement from the American Heart Association Council on Cardiovascular Surgery and Anesthesia in collaboration with the Interdisciplinary Working Group on Quality of Care and Outcomes Research. *Circulation, 111,* 2858–2864.

64. Sjogren, J., et al. (2005). The impact of vacuum-assisted closure on long-term survival after post-sternotomy mediastinitis. *Ann Thoracic Surg, 80,* 1270–1275.

65. Society of Thoracic Surgeons. (2005). *Executive summary: adult cardiac surgery database.* www.STS.org.

66. Stanik-Hutt, J. A. (2005). Management options for angina refractory to maximal medical and surgical interventions. *AACN Clin Issues, 16,* 320–332.

67. Stein, P. D., et al. (2004). Antithrombotic therapy in patients with saphenous vein and internal mammary artery grafts. The seventh ACCP conference on antithrombotic and thrombolytic therapy. *Chest, 126,* 600S–608S.

68. Tavilla, G., et al. (2004). Long-term follow-up of coronary artery bypass grafting in three-vessel disease using exclusively pedicled bilateral internal thoracic and right gastroepiploic arteries. *Ann Thoracic Surg, 77*(3), 794.

69. Van den Berghe, G., et al. (2003). Outcome benefit of intensive insulin therapy in the critically ill: insulin dose versus glycemic control. *Crit Care Med, 31*(2), 359.

70. Van der Linden, P., et al. (2001). A standardized multidisciplinary approach reduces the use of allogenic blood products in patients undergoing cardiac surgery. *Can J Anesth, 48,* 894–901.

71. Verma, S., et al. (2004). Off-pump coronary artery bypass surgery: fundamentals for the clinical cardiologist. *Circulation, 99,* 1206–1211.

72. Wehberg, K. E., et al. (2003). Improved patient outcomes when transmyocardial revascularization is used as adjunctive revascularization. *Heart Surg Forum, 6*(5), 328–330.

73. Wynne, R., & Botti, M. (2004). Postoperative pulmonary dysfunction in adults after cardiopulmonary bypass: clinical significance and indications for practice. *Am J Crit Care, 13*(5), 384–393.

CHAPTER 15 Valvular Disease and Surgery

Barbara Leeper

The picture of valvular heart disease has changed significantly in the last 50 years. The impact of rheumatic heart disease as the most common cause of valve dysfunction was lessened by the widespread use of prophylactic penicillin.[33] In addition, breakthroughs in the medical management and surgical interventions for this potentially life-threatening situation have significantly changed patients' long-term outcomes. However, in spite of the improvements in medical management, the incidence of heart valve surgery and procedures has continued to increase.

The purpose of this chapter is to review the etiology and emerging trends in the management of valvular heart disease. The pathophysiology, assessment, medical management, and surgical interventions for each of the valve conditions will also be discussed.

PREVALENCE

The exact incidence of valvular heart disease is unknown. Some have suggested that more than 5 million people have some form (moderate to severe) of valvular regurgitation.[6] There has been as much as a fourfold increase in hospital discharge diagnoses of aortic and mitral regurgitation in the last 20 years.[6] In 2003 an estimated 95,000 heart valve surgical procedures were performed—the most frequent being aortic valve surgery, followed by surgery on the mitral valve, pulmonic valve, and tricuspid valve.[1]

ETIOLOGY

Disease processes of heart valves will cause either a "stenosis" or an "insufficiency" of the valve. Valvular insufficiency may also be called "regurgitation." A valve is said to be stenotic when it is narrowed and does not open properly. Pure stenosis will block the flow of blood from one heart chamber (atrium to ventricle) or may prevent adequate ejection of the blood from the ventricle into the circulation (pulmonary or peripheral). Insufficiency indicates the valve is leaking, allowing blood to leak back (or regurgitate) into the previous heart chamber. Frequently patients with valvular heart disease will have a combination of stenosis and regurgitation involving one or more valves. The most common diseases that cause valve problems are rheumatic fever and bacterial endocarditis.[5]

Rheumatic Fever

Rheumatic heart disease is one of the most common causes of valvular heart disease, especially mitral stenosis and aortic regurgitation.[5] The disease was thought to have been eradicated in the 1970s; however, there was a resurgence in the 1980s.[29] In 2003, 43,000 individuals diagnosed with rheumatic fever/rheumatic heart disease were discharged from U.S. hospitals, and the mortality rate was reported to be 1.2%.[1] In third-world countries, the incidence of chronic rheumatic disease is estimated to be 4.9 to 30 million in children and young adults.[36] African Americans, Puerto Ricans, Mexican Americans, and Native Americans have a higher incidence than other populations.[1]

Endocarditis

Endocarditis is a microbial infection of the lining of the heart, most commonly affecting the cardiac valves but also affecting the endocardium adjacent to an infected valve.[22] Congenital defects (such as patent ductus arteriosus, ventricular septal defect, and bicuspid aortic valves) or acquired defects from rheumatic heart disease are predisposing factors.[15,22] The lesion, or vegetation, is a mass of platelets and fibrin containing abundant microorganisms. The most common causative microorganisms are streptococci, staphylococci, enterococci, and gram-negative coccobacilli.[22] Patients with mitral valve prolapse and those with a history of intravenous drug abuse seem to be at the greatest risk.[22] Figure 15-1 shows an example of endocarditis affecting the aortic valve. Note the thickened valve leaflets from the vegetations.

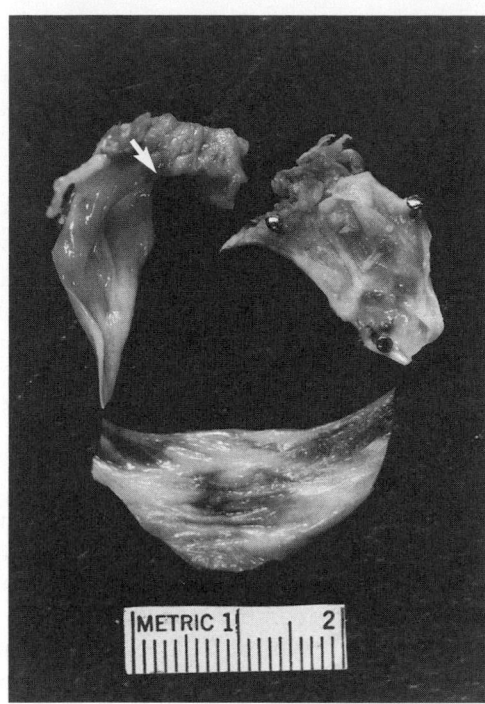

⇕FIGURE 15-1 Aortic valve with endocarditis. Note the vegetations on the thickened valve leaflets. The valve leaflet has been partially destroyed by the infectious process *(arrow)*.

Other Etiologies

Table 15-1 lists a variety of other etiologies for valvular heart disease. Of note are congenital defects, such as mitral valve clefts and unicuspid or bicuspid aortic valve, that may produce stenosis or insufficiency. In adults, aortic stenosis and regurgitation are often caused by the build-up of calcium on the valve leaflets, referred to as "senile degenerative" disease. In the setting of acute myocardial infarction, abrupt rupture of the chordae tendineae or papillary muscle will cause acute mitral regurgitation. A similar, but less frequent, event can occur with a right ventricular infarction causing acute tricuspid regurgitation.[5]

Appetite suppressants, including fenfluramine, dexfenfluramine, and phentermine, have also been linked to the development of valvular heart disease.[24,39] Some researchers have demonstrated a 31% incidence of valvular disease associated with one or more of these drugs.[39] The most common valvulopathies reported include (in order of frequency) aortic regurgitation, tricuspid regurgitation, and mitral regurgitation.[39] However, a systematic review of the literature demonstrated a wider variation, leading the investigators to conclude that the actual risk is undetermined and may be lower than once thought.[24]

EMERGING TRENDS IN SURGICAL MANAGEMENT OF VALVULAR HEART DISEASE

Valve Repair Versus Valve Replacement

With recent improvements in surgical techniques and devices, valve repair has become an important option for many patients. Valve repair offers patients the advantage of retaining the native valve, having a normal valve orifice, and avoiding the challenges that might be associated with long-term anticoagulation therapy normally required with mechanical valves.

TABLE 15-1 Etiologies of Valvular Heart Disease

MITRAL VALVE		TRICUSPID VALVE	
Stenosis:	**Insufficiency:**	**Stenosis:**	**Insufficiency:**
Rheumatic fever	Infective endocarditis	Rheumatic fever	Right ventricular dilation
Congenital	Myocardial infarction	Atrial myxoma	Pulmonary hypertension
	Systemic lupus erythematosus		Right ventricular infarction
	Rheumatoid arthritis		Bacterial endocarditis

PULMONIC VALVE		AORTIC VALVE	
Stenosis:	**Insufficiency:**	**Stenosis:**	**Insufficiency:**
Congenital	Pulmonary hypertension	Congenital bicuspid valve	Rheumatic fever
	Bacterial endocarditis	Rheumatic fever	Endocarditis
		Senile degenerative stenosis	Enlargement of aortic root, stretching valve cusps
		Atherosclerosis	

Data from reference 5.

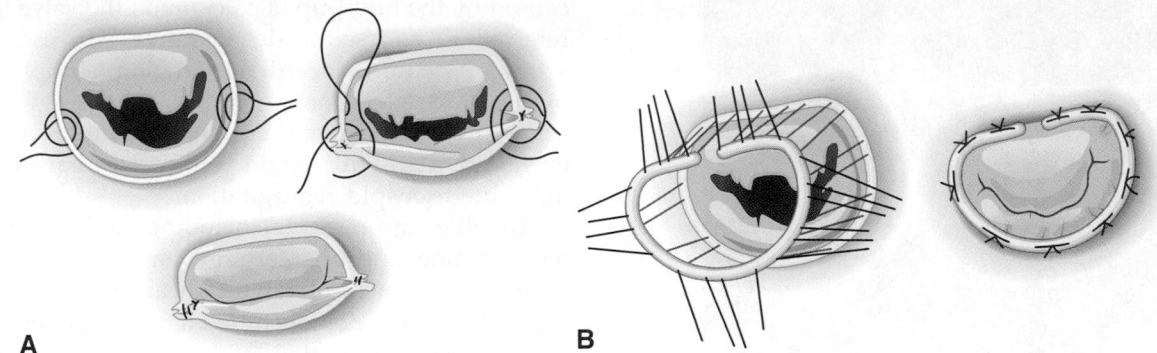

A   **B**

⬍FIGURE 15-2 Valve repair replacing the valve ring. **A,** Using valve annulus sutures, the mitral valve is repaired. **B,** This dilated mitral valve annulus is shown being reshaped by use of an annuloplasty ring.

Valve repair may include the insertion of a valve ring to repair the annulus, removal of abnormal tissue from the valve leaflets, restoration of the commissures, shortening of the chordae tendineae, or repair of the papillary muscle.[44] Figure 15-2 illustrates valve repair using a valve ring. Valve repair has been found to be an especially effective treatment for the mitral and aortic valves.[28,43–46]

Types of Prosthetic Valves. There are two types of prosthetic valves: mechanical valves and tissue valves (Box 15-1). Mechanical valves can be either caged-ball valves or bileaflet valves. There are three mechanical valves available: St. Jude, CarboMedics, and Medtronic-Hall valves. The most common mechanical valves used today are the low-profile bileaflet disk valves, which offer less impedance to blood flow through the orifice. Figure 15-3 shows the St. Jude bileaflet mechanical valve, one of the most commonly implanted valves in the United States.[3] Low-profile disk valves have leaflets that open anywhere from 55 to 80 degrees, depending on the type and maker of the valve.[3] The wider the opening, the less the obstruction of blood flow, which

is an important consideration when selecting the type of valve to be implanted. The advantage of a mechanical valve is longer durability—usually 20 years or more. In an effort to avoid reoperation for replacement of the valve, mechanical valves are usually implanted in younger individuals with a longer life expectation. The disadvantage of a mechanical valve is the need for long-term anticoagulation. Mechanical valves are associated with a higher risk of thrombosis and peripheral embolization, including stroke. As a result, these patients require close monitoring of prothrombin time (PT)/international normalized ratio (INR) to regulate their warfarin (Coumadin) dose.

There are also several types of tissue valves. These include the heterograft (porcine and bovine), homograft, and autograft valves. The porcine and the bovine heterograft valves are sterilized by glutaraldehyde, which stabilizes the collagen for durability. The glutaraldehyde also changes the tissue to be bioacceptable. The valve leaflets are mounted on a stent, which has a sewing ring.[19] The porcine valve is approved by the Food and Drug Administration (FDA) for use in both mitral and aortic positions. The durability of the

---

Box 15-1

Types of Prosthetic Heart Valves

MECHANICAL VALVES

- Caged-ball
- Bileaflet disk

TISSUE VALVES

- Heterograft valves
  - Porcine
  - Bovine pericardial
- Homograft valves
- Autograft valves

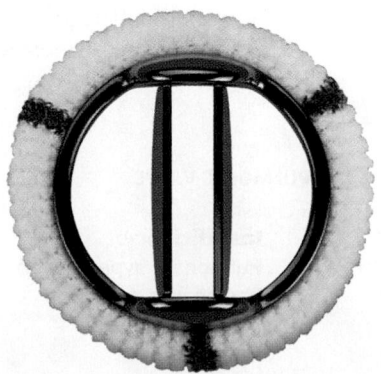

⬍FIGURE 15-3 The St. Jude bileaflet mechanical valve.

porcine valve is less than that of the mechanical valve. There are reports of porcine valves deteriorating 10 years after implant, requiring reoperation in 20% to 40% of patients who had a mitral bioprosthesis and in 15% to 20% who had an aortic bioprosthesis.[16]

Bovine valves are made from bovine pericardium and are approved for placement in the aortic position. Durability is somewhat longer than porcine valves, approximately 12 to 15 years, with reoperation occurring in 4% to 9% of patients at the 10-year mark.[16]

A homograft valve is a tissue valve that has been harvested from a donor, cleaned, mounted on a support device (with or without stent), and made available for implantation. The stentless valve that is implanted in the aortic position has a larger orifice, allowing for less impedance of blood flow. All prosthetic valves produce some stenosis, ranging from mild to moderate.[19] Therefore the stentless valve offers a little more opening for blood flow. Figure 15-4 shows the St. Jude homograft stentless valve. Structural valve deterioration is lower in this type of valve when compared with other tissue valves.[19] Pulmonary homografts have not been found to do well in the aortic position.[10] Studies show that this type of valve may not be as durable as the porcine valve.[14,19]

An autograft valve is one that is taken from the patient's pulmonic position and reimplanted in the aortic position as part of the Ross procedure. This procedure will be discussed in more detail later in this chapter. The pulmonic valve has been found to function extremely well in the aortic position, with 85% of patients being free from reoperation 20 years following placement.[19]

Older adult patients usually receive tissue valves because of the durability of the valve and the lack of anticoagulation needed. However, a recent study examining valve-related complications 15 years after mitral valve replacement found no difference in valve-related reoperation and mortality and thus favored mechanical prostheses in patients up to age 70.[21] There are some recent studies suggesting that some types of tissue valves may be better for younger age-groups, such as using a pulmonary autograft valve in younger and pediatric patients with the Ross procedure. More data with longer-term studies are needed to fully support this type of surgery.[12,14,32]

Complications of Prosthetic Valves. Complications associated with prosthetic heart valves include structural valve deterioration and peripheral embolization related to thrombus generation on the valve structure. Additional complications include prosthetic endocarditis, prosthetic dehiscence, bleeding, perivalvular regurgitation, and primary valve failure. Hemolysis also occurs with all mechanical prosthetic valves, but not with tissue valves. An increase in the concentration of lactic acid dehydrogenase (LDH) has been found to be reliable as an indicator of hemolysis. Prosthesis dysfunction, perivalvular leak, or cloth tear will produce a sudden increase in the LDH concentration;[19] therefore these patients should be closely monitored for these problems.

Surgical Approach. With the development of new instruments and technologies, the surgical approach to repairing or implanting a heart valve has changed. The traditional median sternotomy, considered to be the gold standard, is still routinely performed in many centers. However, this approach is being challenged because of the longer bone-healing time, requiring more time away from work and increased risk for deep sternal wound infections. Younger patients often prefer a less invasive surgical approach to avoid the more visible sternotomy scar. The advantage of the traditional approach is better visualization for the surgeon. Nevertheless, there is a trend to move toward less invasive approaches.

There are a variety of minimally invasive approaches that are being used. Some include a partial sternotomy with a lower transverse division (transsternal) for aortic and mitral valve procedures (Figure 15-5). Another approach is a parasternal incision for a mitral procedure. Mini-thoracotomies, either from the left or from the right side, are also being used. Many of these approaches require video assistance.[8] Proposed advantages of the minimally invasive approaches are reduction in patient morbidity and mortality. Generally, the literature suggests that the biggest benefit from the minimally invasive approach is the shorter length of hospital stay.[8]

One of the most recent developments is the use of robotics to perform minimally invasive valve surgery.

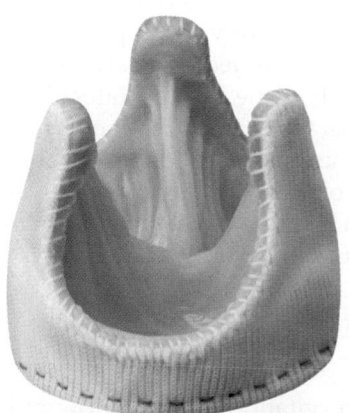

♦FIGURE 15-4 The St. Jude Toronto SPV homograft stentless valve.

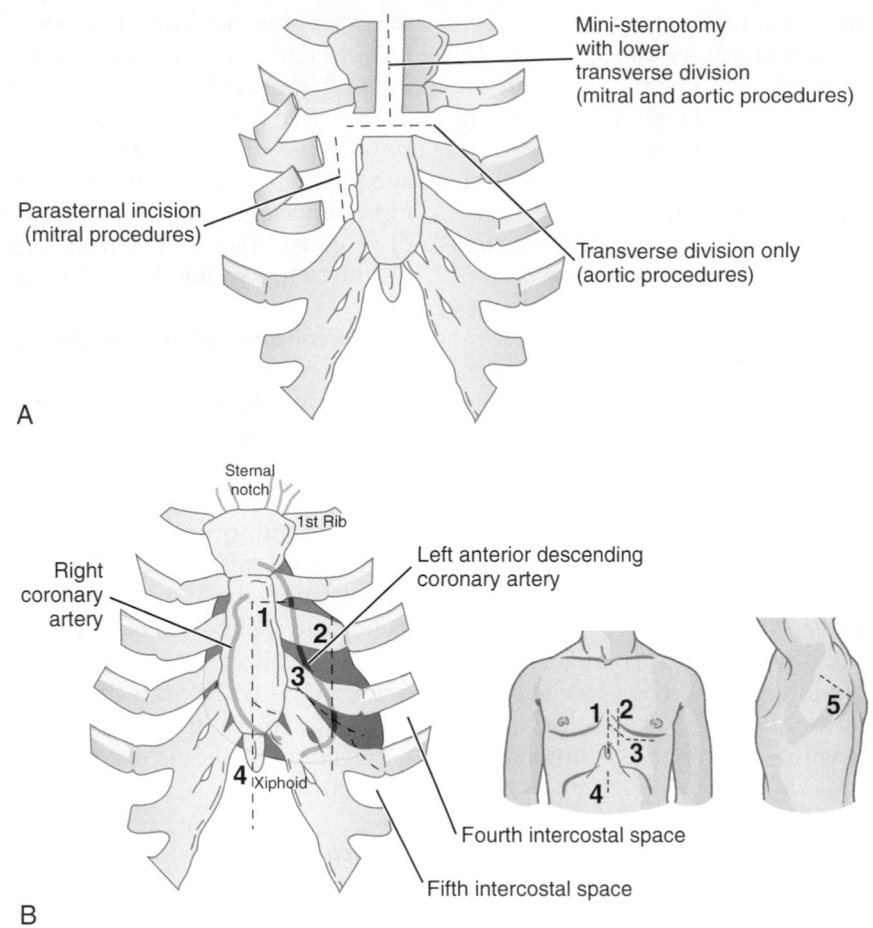

✦FIGURE 15-5 Minimally invasive surgical approaches. **A,** Incision lines. **B,** *1,* Mini-sternotomy approach; *2,* parasternal approach; *3,* anterior mini-thoracotomy approach; *4,* subxiphoid approach; *5,* posterolateral approach.

The da Vinci system (Intuitive Surgical, Inc.) is one example of this evolving technology (Figure 15-6). In addition, new instruments and clips have been developed to replace some suture material. The technology continues to undergo evaluation to determine its usefulness and impact on patient outcomes.[23]

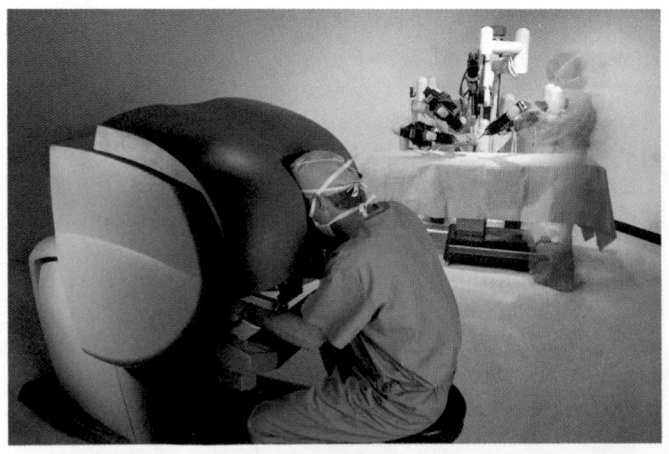

✦FIGURE 15-6 The Intuitive da Vinci robotic system.

Over the last 20 years, percutaneous approaches have been used to perform commissurotomies of the mitral valve and valvuloplasties of the aortic valve.[41] In the mid 1990s investigational work began on percutaneous catheter-based valve replacements of the aortic valve, in which a tissue valve is sutured into a stent and implanted in the aortic position just below the coronary orifices, and the native valve is pushed to the side. This procedure has continued to be studied in trials in Europe and recently in the United States.[41] While still investigational, this approach offers hope for some patients who are not surgical candidates but may benefit from replacement of their aortic valve.[7,41,42] Research is just beginning on percutaneous approaches for mitral valve repair and pulmonic valve replacement.

AORTIC REGURGITATION

Aortic regurgitation is a backflow of blood into the left ventricle after the ventricular contraction is complete because of an incompetent aortic valve. The incidence of aortic regurgitation is approximately 5% of the general population, increases with age, and is more common in men than in women.[13] Patients with aortic regurgitation tend to have higher mortality and morbidity rates than the general population. Heart failure usually occurs within 10 years after the onset.[5] The valvular disease process may be associated with primary disease of the valve or the aortic wall above the valve. Dilation of the aortic root (usually from age-related degeneration, Marfan syndrome, or aortic dissection[5]) occurs more commonly than a primary disease process of the valve leaflets.

Pathophysiology

Aortic root dilation causes the aortic annulus to enlarge, subsequently separating the valve leaflets and causing aortic regurgitation. The dilation causes tension and bowing of the individual valve cusps, further intensifying the regurgitation.[5]

The insufficient aortic valve allows a backflow of blood into the left ventricle during ventricular diastole, contributing to a larger left ventricular end-diastolic volume and end-diastolic pressure. This results in a larger stroke volume with the next ventricular ejection, causing an increased systolic pressure and wider pulse pressure. The large stroke volume can produce dilation of the ascending aorta. Left atrial pressure and pulmonary vascular pressures increase later in the disease process, resulting in a delay of the onset of symptoms of dyspnea and angina.[13]

Regardless of the cause, over time the left ventricle hypertrophies, increasing the patient's risk for sudden death. Patients with an ejection fraction (EF) less than 55% are also at greater risk for sudden cardiac death.[13]

Testing

Aortic regurgitation is identified by the presence of a diastolic murmur. Doppler echocardiography has proven to be indispensable, providing quantification of the regurgitant volume and determining the cause of the regurgitation and the degree of pulmonary hypertension.[4]

The ECG may reflect left ventricular hypertrophy, left axis deviation, and patterns consistent with diastolic overload, i.e., downsloping, depressed ST segments. The chest x-ray may show left ventricular enlargement; however, the actual changes are related to the severity of the regurgitation. Dilation of the aortic root may or may not be apparent. The presence of an aneurysm in the ascending aorta is suggestive of Marfan syndrome.[5]

Signs and Symptoms

A patient may have aortic regurgitation for many years before symptoms appear. Common symptoms the patient may experience include shortness of breath or chest tightness.[29] The patient will clinically present with bounding arterial pulses, sometimes described as a "water hammer" pulse, indicating an abrupt distention of the pulse followed by a quick collapse. Another classic sign is de Musset's sign, described as head bobbing with each heartbeat.[5,29]

A widened pulse pressure is also characteristic of aortic regurgitation. The large stroke volume increases the systolic pressure, and the insufficient valve allows backflow of blood into the left ventricle, causing the diastolic pressure to be very low. The Korotkoff sounds may be heard down to zero; however, one should note the point at which muffling of the Korotkoff sounds occurs. This point has been found to correlate with the diastolic pressure.[5]

A third heart sound may be present, along with the diastolic murmur. The murmur is best heard with the patient leaning forward in an upright position. Generally the murmur tends to be harsh sounding. The Austin Flint murmur occurs late in diastole, often described as a rumble, and is heard best at the apex.[5]

Management

Medical management consists of prophylactic antibiotic therapy for prevention of bacterial endocarditis. If the patient has signs and symptoms of volume overload, vasodilators, such as hydralazine (Apresoline), nifedipine (Procardia), felodipine (Plendil), and angiotensin-converting enzyme (ACE) inhibitors, seem to have beneficial effects.[5] If the regurgitation is severe, the patient should be managed similar to severe heart failure. However, beta blockers should be avoided to prevent bradycardia. The patient should be followed with echocardiograms at least annually and more frequently if symptomatic.[4,5] Serial radionuclide ventriculograms to assess left ventricular volume and function at rest have been found to be an accurate, cost-effective alternative to the echocardiogram.[4]

Surgery will relieve symptoms and correct the mechanical problem. Although there are no studies comparing nonsurgical therapy with surgical intervention, most experts agree that surgery is indicated for patients who have no contraindications.[11] The American Heart Association/American College of Cardiology (AHA/ACC) recommendations indicate that severe symptoms or a left ventricular end-diastolic volume (LVEDV) or dimension greater than or equal to 75 mm, an end-systolic diameter greater than or equal to 50 mm, and an EF less than 50% are indications for surgery (Class I recommendation).[4]

AORTIC STENOSIS

Aortic stenosis is an acquired or congenital narrowing of the aorta or its orifice attributable to lesions of the wall with scar formation. Congenital aortic stenosis is a condition in which there are two valve cusps versus the normal three. Acquired aortic stenosis can be caused by rheumatic heart disease or by calcification and degeneration of the valve cusps associated with the aging process. Degenerative aortic stenosis often coexists with calcification of the mitral valve. Statin medications have been shown to lower the rate of progression of senile aortic calcification, confirming that the process may have elements in common with the development of atherosclerosis.[5] Risk factors for the development of degenerative aortic stenosis include atherosclerosis, diabetes, and hypertension.[5]

Pathophysiology

In the setting of aortic stenosis, the left ventricle hypertrophies over time, maintaining an adequate cardiac output. Eventually, the valve becomes critically stenotic and cardiac output will fall. Severe aortic stenosis is defined as a peak systolic pressure gradient greater than 40 mm Hg and a valve area less than 1 cm^2, or less than one fourth of the normal aortic valve area (3 to 4 cm^2).[4,5] Figure 15-7 illustrates the pressure gradient that occurs with aortic stenosis. The left ventricle may develop a concentric hypertrophy as an adaptive response to the higher intracavitary pressures. Coronary blood blow may be reduced in relationship to the increased muscle mass. Additionally, as the heart rate increases with exercise, maldistribution of blood flow may occur, resulting in ischemia and the onset of chest pain.[4]

The left atrial waveform will have large "a" waves reflecting the higher end-diastolic pressure in the left ventricle. Atrial contraction is very important in the setting of aortic stenosis, as it serves to increase the LVEDP and support the pressure needed to eject the stroke volume. The cardiac output is generally normal at rest and will usually be diminished during exercise.[5]

Testing

The ECG may show signs of left ventricular and left atrial hypertrophy. The chest x-ray may reveal a heart that is slightly enlarged, with rounding of the left ventricular border and apex.[5] Left heart angiography is associated with some risk in these patients, in that it may be difficult to introduce a catheter across the valve if significant stenosis is present. Also, the injection of a large bolus of dye into a high-pressure left ventricle

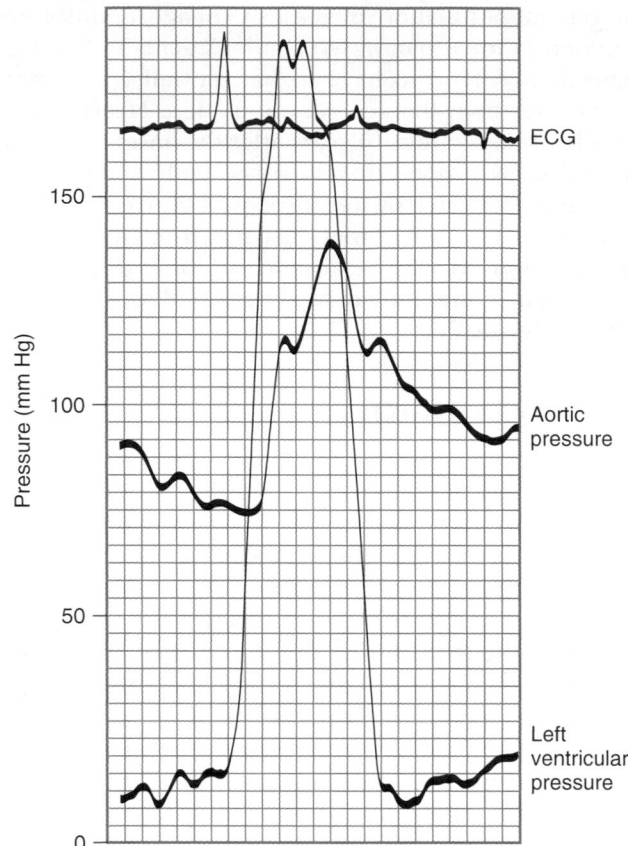

FIGURE 15-7 Left ventricular (LV) aortic pressure gradient associated with aortic stenosis. The LV systolic pressure is approximately 45 mm Hg higher than the aortic systolic pressure, which is a significant gradient.

can be hazardous because of the negative inotropic effect of the dye. Therefore left ventriculography is recommended only when noninvasive tests are inconclusive.[4] Right heart catheterization may be performed to assess the presence of pulmonary and right-sided hypertension.[5]

Echocardiography is considered to be the best assessment tool for aortic stenosis.[5] It provides reliable information about dimensions of the left ventricle and atrium, the size of the valve orifice, pressure gradients across the valve, and the dilation of the aortic root.

Signs and Symptoms

A murmur is often the first and only sign of aortic stenosis.[29] As the valve becomes more stenotic, the patient will begin to complain of dyspnea, angina, and dizziness or near-syncopal episodes. When the valve becomes critically narrowed, these patients are at risk for sudden death. The onset of atrial fibrillation with the loss of the atrial contribution to ventricular filling can cause syncope or sudden death.[29]

With senile aortic stenosis, the onset of symptoms usually occurs in the fifth or sixth decade. Patients will begin to experience shortness of breath with exertion, angina, syncope, and heart failure.[5] The arterial pulse waveform is characterized by *pulsus parvus et tardus*, in which the pressure rises slowly and is sustained (Figure 15-8). Aortic stenosis produces a systolic murmur heard best at the base of the heart, and may also be transmitted to the carotids.[5]

◆ Case Study 15-1, Part A

Acute Respiratory Distress and Pulmonary Edema

Mrs. J. is a 76-year-old female who was brought to the emergency department with acute respiratory distress and pulmonary edema. Significant history includes known aortic stenosis. She was last seen by her cardiologist 6 months before presentation. She reports that she has experienced some episodes of shortness of breath during the last 3 to 4 months while walking. She denies any episodes of chest pain or feeling faint. Her physical examination revealed a loud systolic murmur, grade V/VI, at the second intercostal space, right sternal border. Her blood pressure was 156/86 mm Hg, heart rate 110 beats/min and regular sinus rhythm, and respiratory rate 32 breaths/min. Her pulse oximetry was 88%. Oxygen was started at 5 L per nasal cannula and furosemide (Lasix) 40 mg was given intravenously. She was admitted to the cardiac telemetry unit.

Review of her prior medical records shows that she received an echocardiogram 6 months previously, which reported her aortic valve orifice was 1 cm². She was asymptomatic at that time, and her cardiologist recommended continued observation. The etiology of her aortic stenosis was thought to be senile degeneration with calcification of the valve.

On admission, orders were written for an echocardiogram and a left heart catheterization. The echocardiogram indicated her aortic valve orifice to be 0.5 cm² with significant thickening and hypertrophy of the left ventricular wall. The cardiac catheterization revealed normal circumflex and left anterior descending coronary arteries, and 60% proximal stenosis of her right coronary artery. The cardiologist was unable to advance a catheter across her aortic valve into the left ventricle because of the stenotic valve. She was referred for an aortic valve replacement the following day.

Decision point: When is the narrowed aortic valve considered to be critical?

Decision point: What are key symptoms patients with aortic stenosis should be taught to report to their healthcare provider?

Decision point: How frequently should patients with aortic stenosis be seen by their healthcare providers once the aortic valve orifice is 1 cm²?

Case continues on page 330

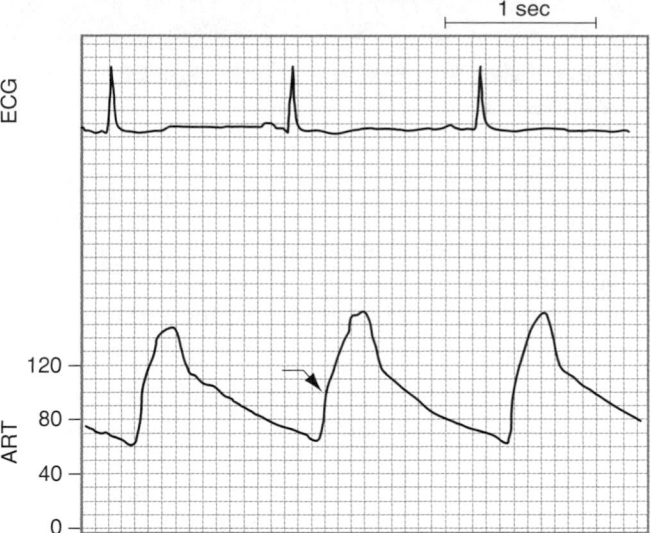

◆FIGURE 15-8 Arterial pressure waveform demonstrating aortic stenosis. The slurred upstroke of the systolic pressure and the delayed peak are characteristic of aortic stenosis. ART = arterial, ECG = electrocardiogram.

Management

Patients with aortic stenosis should be instructed to immediately report any onset of symptoms (angina, exertional dyspnea, dizziness, syncope), as well as to avoid vigorous physical activity.[5] Patients need to receive instruction about bacterial endocarditis prophylaxis. They should be followed closely with echocardiographic evaluations every 6 to 12 months, depending on the severity.[5] Generally, medical therapy offers very little for these patients. Therefore surgery becomes the treatment of choice for symptomatic patients (Class I recommendation).[4]

Surgical intervention usually involves replacement of the valve, although in some instances the valve may be repaired. The average perioperative mortality rate associated with isolated aortic valve replacement is 3% to 4%.[4] Since many of these patients are older, research has been done to determine outcomes and quality of life of these patients following surgery.[29] The Research Utilization box on p. 330 explores heart valve surgery in patients age 80 or older. Investigators have demonstrated that outcomes on individuals beyond 80 years of age undergoing aortic valve replacement were associated with a 30-day mortality rate of 11%. Survival at 1 and 5 years was 80% and 55%, respectively, and quality of life assessments were comparable to those predicted for the general population older than 75 years.[29] It was concluded that surgery should not be withheld from older adults if age is the only determining factor.[38]

♦ RESEARCH UTILIZATION

Heart Valve Surgery in Patients Age 80 Years or Older

CLINICAL ISSUE

Heart valve surgery in patients age 80 years or older is often considered to be futile. Some assume that this group of patients will have poorer outcomes than those who are younger and that there will be minimal improvement in functional outcome and survival rates.

SUMMARY

This study presented a series of 405 consecutive patients ≥80 years of age who underwent isolated or combined valve surgery over 5 years. The mean age of the group was 83 plus or minus 3 years, with 53% being female. Aortic valve replacement was performed in 59%, mitral valve repair in 16%, mitral valve replacement in 10%, and double valve replacement in 14% of the patients. The overall mortality was 6.4%, with isolated mitral valve replacement having the highest mortality at 10%. Atrial fibrillation was the most common postoperative complication, occurring in 38% of patients. Stroke occurred in 3.5% of patients. Aortic valve replacement was associated with higher survival rates when compared with mitral valve replacement at 1 and 5 years. Congestive heart failure and pneumonia were the most common causes of late deaths. At 2 years, 92% of patients exhibited New York Heart Association functional Class I or II heart failure symptoms, which is significantly better than predicted.

APPLICATION

Heart valve surgery should not be excluded as a potential intervention for a patient ≥80 years of age. This study demonstrates that this population of patients does experience an increase in functional class.

NEED FOR FURTHER STUDY

Future studies are needed to examine patients' perceptions of improvement in quality of life from preoperative to postoperative status as well as their perceptions of the surgical experience overall.

Unic, D., et al. (2005). Early and late results of isolated and combined heart valve surgery in patients ≥ 80 years of age. *Am J Cardiol*, 95, 1500–1503.

The Ross procedure is a surgical option for some adult patients who have isolated aortic valve stenosis. This procedure was first described by Donald Ross in 1967 and is done primarily in children. Recently, there has been growing acceptance of performing this procedure in adults up to 60 years and older. Additionally, it has proven to be beneficial for women of child-bearing age.[30] The procedure involves the removal of the native aortic root, aortic valve, pulmonic valve, and pulmonary artery root. The native pulmonary valve is implanted in the aortic position (autograft), and the coronary arteries are reimplanted into the trunk of the newly-implanted root. A prosthetic tissue (homograft) is implanted in the pulmonic position (Figure 15-9).[35] Preoperative evaluation includes right and left cardiac catheterization, as well as transesophageal echocardiography for the purpose of assessing the structure and size of the aortic and pulmonic valves. During the surgery, care must be taken to avoid injury to the coronary arteries, specifically the left main and left anterior descending coronary arteries. The left main coronary artery is near the posterior surface of the pulmonary artery, and the first septal branch of the left anterior descending coronary artery is adjacent to the pulmonary artery outflow tract.[35] Postoperatively, patient management is similar to that of any patient undergoing cardiac surgery.

MITRAL REGURGITATION

Mitral regurgitation is a backflow of blood from the left ventricle into the left atrium, resulting from imperfect closure of the mitral or bicuspid valve.

♦ Case Study 15-1, Part B

Acute Respiratory Distress and Pulmonary Edema

Mrs. J. went to surgery early the following morning. Her stenotic aortic valve was removed and replaced with a bovine pericardial tissue valve, and a single coronary bypass was completed to her proximal right coronary artery. On arrival to the cardiothoracic critical care unit, she was already intubated and sedated, with an arterial line in her right radial artery and a PAC in place. Her BP was 125/74 mm Hg, HR 106 beats/min, and respiratory rate 12 breaths/min. Her PAP was 34/16 mm Hg and RAP 6 mm Hg. Pulmonary artery wedge pressures (PAWPs) were not obtained. Her CO was 4.8 L/min and CI 2.6 $L/min/m^2$. Her BP was somewhat labile during the first few hours after surgery, and albumin was given to increase her intravascular volume and RAP. She was fully awake and extubated within 6 hours after arrival to critical care. Refer to the table on p. 331 for her initial postoperative hemodynamic profile.

Decision point: Why would the pulmonary artery pressures be elevated in this patient?

Decision point: Is sinus tachycardia common following cardiac surgery? Why?

Case continues on page 341

INITIAL POSTOPERATIVE HEMODYNAMIC PROFILE OF A PATIENT AFTER AORTIC VALVE REPLACEMENT SURGERY[*]

TIME	BP (mm Hg)	MAP (mm Hg)	P (beats/min)	RHYTHM	RR (breaths/min)	T (°C)	RAP (mm Hg)	PAP (mm Hg), S/D/M	CO/CI (L/min)/ (L/m/m²)	SVI (mL/m²)	SVR dynes•sec/ cm⁵/m²	SpO₂ (%)
1130	125/74	91	106	Sinus tachycardia	12/12	35.7	6	36/16/22	4.8/2.6	25	1350	96
1200	135/76	96	106	Sinus tachycardia	12/12	36.0	6	32/18/23				96
1300	126/72	93	102	Sinus tachycardia	14/10	36.2	7	31/15/21	4.1/2.4	24	1490	97
1400	120/72	88	100	Sinus tachycardia	14/10	36.5	11	31/15/21				96
1500	124/76	92	102	Sinus tachycardia	12/10	36.9	9	34/16/22	4.2/2.1	21	1177	96
1600	130/78	95	104	Sinus tachycardia	14/10	37.2	8	30/15/22				95
1700	128/70	89	108	Sinus tachycardia	16	37.6	11	29/15/22	4.5/2.3	22	1055	98
1800	122/68	86	98	Sinus	14	37.4	10	28/18/22				98
1900	120/68	85	96	Sinus	14	37.0	10	30/18/23	4.8/2.4	25	1105	96
2000	122/66	85	96	Sinus	12	37.0	12	29/15/20				97
2100	124/64	84	90	Sinus	12	37.2	10	32/18/23				96
2200	120/68	85	90	Sinus	12	37.4	10	30/14/22	4.6/2.4	27	1085	95
2300	126/72	90	86	Sinus	12	37.6	11	32/16/22				96

BP = Blood pressure, C = centigrade, CO/CI = cardiac output/cardiac index, MAP = mean arterial pressure, mm Hg = millimeters of mercury, P = pulse, PAP = pulmonary artery pressure, RAP = right atrial pressure, RR = respiratory rate, SpO₂ = oxygen saturation by pulse oximeter, SVI = stroke volume index, SVR = systemic vascular resistance, S/D/M = systolic/diastolic/mean, T = temperature.
[*]See Case Study 15-1, Part B.

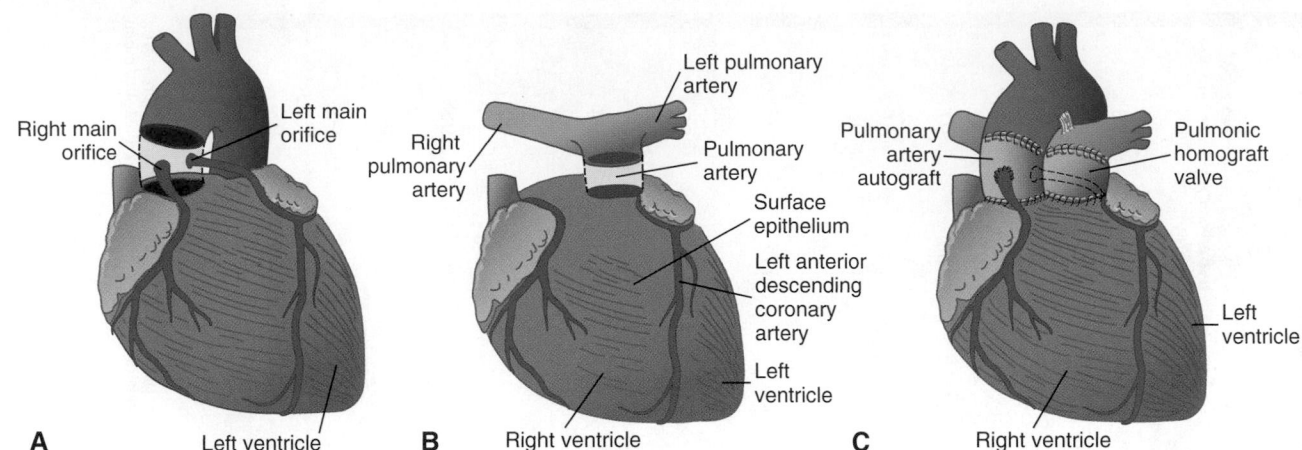

♦FIGURE 15-9   Ross procedure. **A,** The aortic valve and aortic root are removed. **B,** The pulmonic valve and pulmonary artery root are removed. **C,** The pulmonic autograft valve is implanted into the aortic position and the coronary arteries are reimplanted. A homograft valve is implanted in the pulmonic position.

Common causes of mitral regurgitation include rheumatic heart disease, bacterial endocarditis, mitral valve prolapse, dilated cardiomyopathy, and acute myocardial infarction.[5]

Pathophysiology

In dilated cardiomyopathy, the mitral valve annulus may dilate, or degenerate and become calcified. Calcification commonly occurs in patients with hypertension, diabetes, or atherosclerosis.[5]

In the presence of left ventricular dilation, the chordae tendineae may stretch, causing mitral regurgitation. In the setting of acute myocardial infarction, the chordae and the papillary muscle may rupture. The posterior papillary muscle is perfused by the posterior descending coronary artery and the anterior lateral papillary muscle is supplied by the left anterior descending and left circumflex coronary arteries. Rupture of the posterior papillary muscle occurs more frequently than rupture of the anterior lateral papillary muscle.[5]

The regurgitant flow of blood back into the left atrium during systole enhances left ventricular emptying. As the ventricle dilates and hypertrophies over time, the left ventricular end-diastolic volume will increase. This process can cause the mitral regurgitation to worsen by increasing the size of the valve annulus. Eventually, as compliance is reduced, the ventricle begins to decompensate, left ventricular filling pressures start to increase, and cardiac output falls.[5]

Testing

The ECG may indicate left atrial hypertrophy and, in some patients, signs of right ventricular hypertrophy are present. Lateral views of a chest x-ray will reveal left atrial hypertrophy.[5]

Echocardiography, including Doppler, two-dimensional, and transesophageal, is useful for assessing the presence and severity of mitral regurgitation (Class I recommendation).[4] The size of both the left atrium and the left ventricle can be determined, and the regurgitant volume and regurgitant orifice area can be measured. Echocardiography has proven to be more reliable than performing left heart angiography.[5] Magnetic resonance imaging (MRI) is useful in providing accurate measurements of the regurgitant flow as well.[5] Left ventriculography and hemodynamic assessments are recommended when noninvasive tests are inconclusive (Class I recommendation).[4]

Signs and Symptoms

Mitral regurgitation produces a holosystolic murmur and may resemble that of ventricular septal defect (VSD). The distinguishing factor is that the murmur of mitral regurgitation is heard loudest at the base of the heart, whereas the murmur of a VSD will be loudest at the sternal border. Mitral regurgitation produces a large "v" wave in the pulmonary artery wedge pressure (PAWP) waveform (Figure 15-10); therefore one must be careful to take the PAW reading at the "a" wave to avoid overestimation of the pressure.

Management

Acute versus chronic onset of mitral insufficiency will determine the best medical management of mitral regurgitation. With acute onset following myocardial infarction, afterload reduction is important. This can be

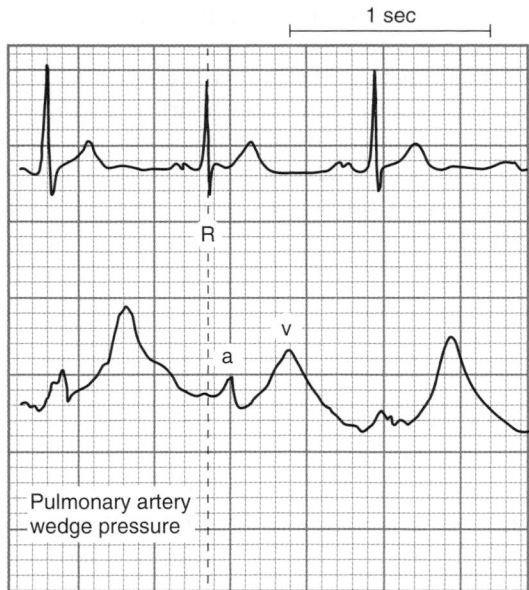

♦FIGURE 15-10 Pulmonary artery wedge pressure tracing with increased amplitude of "v" wave associated with mitral regurgitation.

TABLE 15-2 Recommendations for Anticoagulation Therapy in Mitral Valve Disease

	ANTITHROMBOTIC THERAPY	TARGET INR
Rheumatic heart disease plus atrial fibrillation or history of embolism	Long-term oral anticoagulation (warfarin [Coumadin])	INR 2.5 (range 2–3)
If systemic embolization develops	Add aspirin (ASA) 75–100 mg daily, or if unable to take ASA Dipyridamole (Persantine) 400 mg/day or Clopidogrel (Plavix) 75 mg/day	
Mitral valve prolapse	No therapy is recommended	
Mitral valve prolapse with unexplained TIAs	Long-term therapy is recommended: ASA 50–162 mg/day	

Data from reference 27.
INR = International normalized ratio, ASA = aspirin, TIA = transient ischemic attack.

accomplished pharmacologically with the use of sodium nitroprusside (Nipride), nitroglycerin, or ACE inhibitors.[4,5] Use of intra-aortic balloon pumping will provide mechanical unloading of the left ventricle.

Medical management of chronic mitral regurgitation is not as clear. Small studies indicate some benefit from the use of ACE inhibitors, but there has not been a large randomized trial supporting this as definitive therapy.[5] Some suggest that the use of beta blockers may be more beneficial than the use of ACE inhibitors.[5] Anticoagulation therapy should be considered if the patient has a history of rheumatic heart disease and atrial fibrillation or a history of embolism.[34] If the patient has mitral valve prolapse, anticoagulation therapy is not recommended unless there is a history of unexplained transient ischemic attacks. Table 15-2 outlines specific anticoagulation recommendations.

Surgical interventions should be considered for patients who have impaired activities of daily living (ADLs) from severe symptoms and for those who have progressive deterioration of the left ventricle.[4,5] Left ventricular EF is one of the best predictors for timing of surgery. Recommendations are to consider surgery if the EF falls below 55%.[6] The surgeon must consider whether to repair or replace the valve, weighing the costs and benefits of each procedure. Valve repair may consist of repairing the valve ring (annuloplasty) or using a prosthetic ring (see Figure 15-2). The chordae may be repaired and the surgeon can excise abnormal tissue material off of the valve leaflets, restoring

them to near-normal functioning. Recent data suggest mitral valve repair is applicable for all forms of mitral regurgitation and preferable over mitral valve replacement in patients with chronic severe mitral regurgitation (Class I recommendation).[4]

Replacement of the valve with a mechanical or tissue valve has been performed for many decades. The actual operative time for replacement may be shorter than when the valve is repaired, but the major disadvantage is the need for anticoagulation therapy.[4] Recent studies indicate, however, that repair of the valve is associated with better valve performance because of the intact chordae and papillary muscles.[5]

MITRAL STENOSIS

Mitral stenosis is a narrowing of the mitral orifice, obstructing free flow from the atrium to the ventricle. Rheumatic heart disease is the predominant cause of 99% of stenotic mitral valves excised at time of replacement.[5]

Pathophysiology

Following the initial rheumatic fever disease process, the mitral valve may become deformed by thickening and calcification of the valve leaflets. The pressure in the left atrium increases as higher pressures are needed to drive flow through the stenotic valve. Eventually the left atrium hypertrophies and becomes calcified, and the left main stem bronchus rises. Over time, the higher left atrial pressure causes increased pressure in the pulmonary vascular bed, resulting in moderate, and often severe, pulmonary hypertension. Clinically the patient will complain of exertional dyspnea.[5]

The normal mitral valve orifice is 4 to 6 cm^2. When the orifice is narrowed to 2.5 cm^2, a small pressure gradient will occur, in which the left atrial pressure will be higher than the left ventricular filling pressure.[5] A valve orifice of 1 cm^2 is considered critical mitral stenosis. In this situation, the left atrial to left ventricular pressure gradient is often as high as 20 mm Hg. The clinical implication is that a mean left atrial pressure of 25 mm Hg may be required to maintain a normal cardiac output at rest.[5]

It is interesting to note that the left ventricle (LV) may remain "protected" in the setting of isolated mitral stenosis. In 25% of patients with mitral stenosis, the LV EF and end-diastolic volumes are below normal.[5] This has been attributed to the chronic reduction in preload.

Hemodynamic changes associated with elevation of the left atrial pressure cause an increased amplitude of the "a" wave in the left atrial and PAWP tracings (Figure 15-11). Therefore the use of PAWP as an indicator of left ventricular filling pressure is misleading in this situation.

The left atrial hypertrophy will contribute to disorganized conduction velocities during depolarization and repolarization, contributing to the development of atrial fibrillation. The atrial fibrillation aggravates the atrial hypertrophy. The outcome is irreversible atrial fibrillation.[5]

Testing

Left atrial enlargement will be present in the lateral views of the chest x-ray. There may also be interstitial edema if PAWP is greater than 20 mm Hg.[5]

Right and left heart catheterization is often performed for the purpose of assessing the appearance of the mitral valve structures, the left ventricular performance, and the presence of coronary artery disease. Right heart catheterization will assess for high pulmonary vascular bed pressures.

The gold standard for assessment of mitral stenosis is 2D and Doppler echocardiography, which provides information about the thickened valve leaflets and hypertrophied left atrial chamber (Class I recommendation).[4] This exam also provides information about the presence of a left atrial thrombus and left ventricular contractile performance.[5]

Signs and Symptoms

The main symptom of mitral stenosis is dyspnea, which may be accompanied by a cough and wheezing. Orthopnea may develop as the disease progresses, and the patient is at risk for developing episodes of frank pulmonary edema with any increase in exertion. All of these can be attributed to the reduction in pulmonary compliance associated with the higher pressures. A few patients (15%) will complain of chest discomfort, which has been attributed to a marked increase in right ventricular pressure.[5]

Additional symptoms include the onset of hoarseness caused by the greatly enlarged left atrium and lymph nodes as well as a dilated pulmonary artery compressing the left recurrent laryngeal nerve. This is called *Ortner syndrome*.[5]

Physical examination will reveal a prominent "a" wave in the jugular venous pulse. With auscultation, an accentuated first heart sound (S$_1$) and a low-pitched, rumbling diastolic murmur, heard best at the apex using the bell of the stethoscope, may be heard.[5]

Management

Medical management focuses on prophylaxis for endocarditis, especially if the patient has a history of

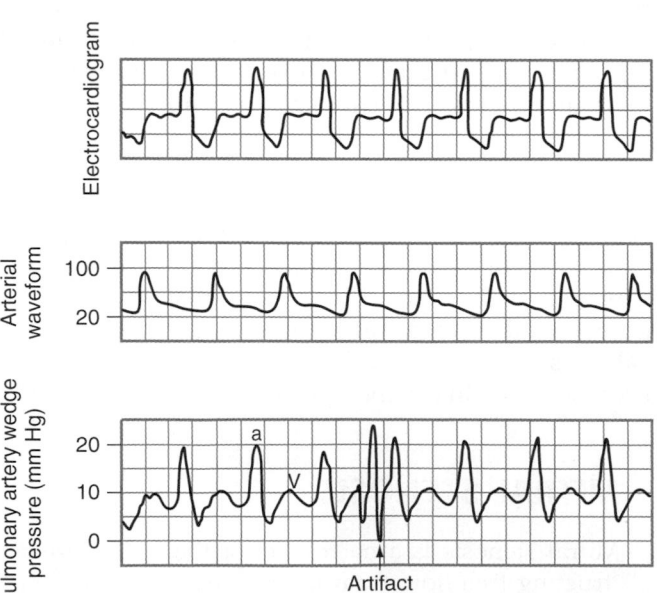

♦FIGURE 15-11 Pulmonary artery wedge waveform with large "a" wave associated with mitral stenosis.

rheumatic fever. Sodium restriction and use of diuretics have been shown to improve the symptoms.[5] Monitoring for the onset of atrial fibrillation is important, and, if present, beta blockers and calcium channel blockers may be used to slow the sinus rate or control the ventricular rate.[5] Also, anticoagulant therapy is indicated to prevent systemic embolization.[5]

Surgical interventions include a valvotomy, valve repair, and valve replacement. A balloon mitral valvotomy can be performed using a percutaneous approach. This has been found to be effective in younger patients who do not have marked thickening or calcification of the valve leaflets.[5] A surgical valvotomy can be performed with or without the use of cardiopulmonary bypass. This low-risk procedure is a palliative procedure, but will provide the patient with 10 to 15 years of clinical improvement.[5]

Mitral valve replacement is indicated for patients who have a mitral valve area less than 1.5 cm^2 and New York Heart Association (NYHA) Class III or IV symptoms of heart failure; it is also recommended for patients who have critical mitral stenosis (valve area less than 1 cm^2), NYHA Class II symptoms, and pulmonary artery pressure (PAP) greater than 70 mm Hg.[4]

TRICUSPID VALVE

Isolated tricuspid stenosis is rare. These patients usually have coexisting mitral or aortic valvular disease. Rheumatic heart disease is the most common cause (approximately 90%) of tricuspid stenosis. Other causes are right atrial myxomas and vegetations on the valve leaflets. Tricuspid regurgitation is most commonly caused by right ventricular dilation associated with right ventricular failure. When the right ventricular pressure exceeds 55 mm Hg, tricuspid regurgitation occurs. Other common causes include bacterial endocarditis, right ventricular infarction, and pulmonary hypertension.[5]

Pathophysiology

Tricuspid stenosis causes an elevated right atrial pressure (RAP), which causes a pressure gradient across the valve. If the disease becomes severe, there will also be a marked increase of peripheral venous pressures.

Tricuspid regurgitation worsens right ventricular failure. The insufficient valve contributes to an increased blood volume in the right atrium. Subsequently, the atrium delivers a higher volume of blood into the right ventricle and can contribute to further distention of the chamber.[5]

Testing

ECG changes seen in tricuspid stenosis are tall, peaked P waves when the patient is in a sinus rhythm. Tricuspid regurgitation produces an incomplete right bundle branch block. A chest x-ray will show marked cardiomegaly. Echocardiography is used to identify the presence and severity of tricuspid stenosis or regurgitation.[5]

Signs and Symptoms

The signs and symptoms of tricuspid stenosis may be masked because it is often associated with mitral valve disease. Auscultation will disclose a diastolic murmur at the lower left sternal border, which becomes louder on inspiration. Hemodynamically, the right atrial pressure is elevated, causing increased neck vein distention and an increased "a" wave on the right atrial waveform. Additional signs of peripheral venous congestion may be present, including hepatomegaly, ascites, and peripheral edema.

Generally, tricuspid regurgitation is well tolerated. However, when pulmonary hypertension is present, cardiac output falls and there are signs and symptoms of right heart failure. Hemodynamically, the right atrial waveform will have increased amplitude of the "v" wave (Figure 15-12). The patient will have a systolic

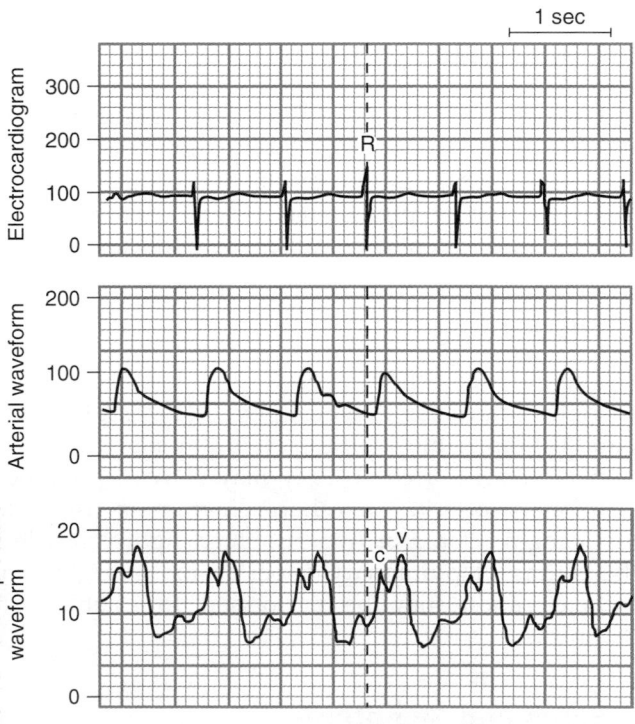

⬍**FIGURE 15-12** Central venous pressure (CVP) waveform and tricuspid regurgitation. Note the increased "v" wave amplitude in the CVP tracing.

murmur that is loudest in the fourth intercostal space, along the left sternal border, and may also be heard in the neck veins.[5] It is common for the patient to have a right ventricular S_3.

Management

Medical management of tricuspid stenosis includes restriction of sodium and administration of diuretics to relieve the venous congestion. The primary treatment, however, should be surgical intervention.

If pulmonary hypertension is present with tricuspid regurgitation, the intensity of symptoms of right heart failure is increased, and therefore more aggressive treatments should be considered. Surgical interventions may include an annuloplasty or valve replacement. Generally, an annuloplasty is performed using a prosthetic valve ring. However, it can also be done without a valve ring and is then called the *De Vega procedure*.[5] A recent study contradicts this practice of performing tricuspid valve annuloplasty, finding that the procedure does not consistently eliminate the regurgitation and, over time, the regurgitation increases.[26] The investigators suggest that they eventually require a high-risk reoperation and that they should be referred for surgery only when their symptoms are disabling.[26]

PULMONIC VALVE

Pulmonic stenosis is usually a congenital defect, and not the result of rheumatic fever. Pulmonic regurgitation is commonly caused by dilation of the valve ring in the setting of pulmonary hypertension. Pulmonic regurgitation can also be caused by endocarditis.[5]

Testing

The ECG may show signs of diastole overload, such as right ventricular hypertrophy or incomplete right bundle branch block (rSR').[5] If pulmonary hypertension is present, a chest x-ray may show a prominent pulmonary artery. An echocardiogram is useful for assessing a dilated or hypertrophied right ventricle in the setting of pulmonary hypertension. A right heart catheterization may be performed to establish the diagnosis.[5]

Signs and Symptoms

Pulmonic regurgitation causes volume overload of the right ventricle and, as a result, can worsen right ventricular failure. If pulmonary hypertension is not present, most patients will tolerate pulmonic regurgitation for many years.[5]

Auscultation will disclose a diastolic murmur heard best at the third or fourth intercostal spaces along the left sternal border. As PAP increases, a characteristic Graham Steell murmur may be heard. This is a high-pitched murmur that is loudest along the left sternal border between the second and fourth intercostal spaces.[5]

Management

Pure pulmonic regurgitation seldom requires medical intervention. Treatment should be directed toward the primary cause, e.g., antibiotic therapy if endocarditis is present. Inotropic agents have been shown to be beneficial if right ventricular failure is present.[5] Surgical replacement of the valve may be considered when right ventricular failure becomes severe.

MULTIVALVULAR DISEASE

Rheumatic fever and endocarditis are the most common causes of multivalvular disease. The patient's clinical presentation as well as the specific valves that are involved will determine the medical or surgical approach to be undertaken.

POSTOPERATIVE MANAGEMENT

Postoperative management of the patient following valvular surgery is similar to the postoperative management of any patient after cardiac surgery. The Multidisciplinary Plan of Care on pp. 337-339 outlines care of the patient undergoing cardiac valve surgery. Immediate postoperative issues specific to valve surgery patients may include the management of pulmonary hypertension and increased frequency of atrial dysrhythmias, such as atrial flutter and fibrillation.

Pulmonary hypertension may be present as a complication of aortic or mitral valve disease and may contribute to right ventricular failure. If pulmonary hypertension is severe, postoperative pulmonary artery systolic pressures may range from 70 to 100 mm Hg. The use of pulmonary artery vasodilator agents may be required to lower the pressures and reduce right ventricular afterload. The short-term use of nitric oxide in the immediate postoperative period has been shown to effectively lower PAPs and improve the hemodynamic performance of the heart.

The postoperative incidence of atrial flutter and fibrillation tends to be higher in this group of patients (60%) when compared with coronary artery bypass

MULTIDISCIPLINARY PLAN OF CARE FOR CARDIAC VALVE SURGERY

Plan of Care and Expected Outcomes

PROBLEM	CATEGORIES OF CARE	PREOPERATIVE	DAY OF SURGERY	FIRST POSTOP DAY	POSTOP DAYS 2 THROUGH 6	DISCHARGE OUTCOMES
Potential for decreased cardiac output	Assessment and monitoring	Obtain vital signs Weigh patient	Admit to ICU • Cardiac monitor • Vital signs (BP, P, R, Spo_2, Svo_2, CO) hourly with pressure readings • Obtain cardiac and pulmonary calculations hourly • Intake/output hourly Able to be weaned off inotropic and vasoactive agents with stable hemodynamic parameters	Cardiac monitor • Vital signs (BP, P, R, Spo_2, Svo_2, CO) hourly with pressure readings • Obtain cardiac and pulmonary calculations hourly • Intake/output hourly Maintains stable hemodynamics without pharmacologic support • Discontinue central lines, arterial line before transfer Maintains stable cardiac rhythm without pharmacologic or pacing support	Telemetry unit • Cardiac monitor • Vital signs 4 times per day	• Cardiac monitor • Vital signs 4 times per day	Heart rate and rhythm normal for patient
	Procedures and tests	CBC, CMP Type and cross-match for 2 units	• Arterial blood gases as needed • Stat chest x-ray • Stat BMP • Hct and K^+ 4 hr after admission	• Arterial blood gas • BMP • INR/PT • Chest x-ray	• INR/PT daily	INR levels therapeutic for patient
Potential for hypothermia Potential for impaired gas exchange High risk for fluid volume deficit Pain control	Treatments	• RT: patient will demonstrate deep breathing, coughing, and use of incentive spirometry	• Warming blanket as needed; temp <97.5° F • Volume ventilator: Initiate ventilator weaning protocol to be extubated within ___ hr	• Weight <u>• Chest tubes to −20-cm suction</u> • Urine catheter • Apply elastic stockings • Change chest dressings	O_2 per cannula Incentive spirometry tid	• Remove dressings from incisions and redress prn • Change pacing wire dressings until removed.	No evidence of respiratory distress at rest or with baseline ADLs Chest incisions clean and dry Pain-free or controlled with oral medications

Table continues on page 338

Plan of Care and Expected Outcomes

PROBLEM	CATEGORIES OF CARE	PREOPERATIVE	DAY OF SURGERY	FIRST POSTOP DAY	POSTOP DAYS 2 THROUGH 6	DISCHARGE OUTCOMES
		• Antimicrobial shower night before and morning preceding surgery	• After extubation: O_2 ___ L/min per face mask or ___ nasal canula • Incentive spirometry every 4 hr • Cough and deep breathe every 4 hr • Foley catheter • Chest tubes to −20-cm suction • IABP ___ Pulmonary status permits extubation	• Incentive spirometry every 4 hr • Cough and deep breathe every 4 hr Patient will demonstrate effective splinting of chest with coughing	• Following removal of pacing wires, monitor for signs and symptoms of cardiac tamponade • Change chest tube dressing prn • Remove and reapply elastic hose bid	
High risk for fatigue	Activity		Bed rest Dangle evening of surgery if hemodynamically stable	• If stable, out of bed to chair for breakfast	• Out of bed to chair for all meals • Orient to cardiac surgery ambulation protocol • Advance patient ambulation per protocol	Able to ambulate independently and perform ADLs at baseline
Potential for altered nutrition: less than body requirements Potential for drug-food interactions	Nutrition		NPO Clear liquids as tolerated after extubation	Advance diet as tolerated	Low-cholesterol, low-sodium diet	Low-cholesterol, low-sodium diet Verbalizes understanding of drug (warfarin)-food interactions

Plan of Care and Expected Outcomes

PROBLEM	CATEGORIES OF CARE	PREOPERATIVE	DAY OF SURGERY	FIRST POSTOP DAY	POSTOP DAYS 2 THROUGH 6	DISCHARGE OUTCOMES
Anxiety Potential for body image disturbance	Patient and family education	Patient and family to see preoperative cardiac surgery video Patient and family to verbalize understanding of procedure and follow-up care	Give family ICU fact sheet and nurse's business card Family will verbalize communication methods with patient while on ventilator	Patient/family will verbalize importance of cardiac surgery ambulation program, nutrition, and care of incision	Educate patient and family regarding warfarin, laboratory monitoring, and drug-food interactions Give patient cardiac valve surgery patient information book Day before discharge, patient and family to view cardiac surgery discharge video	Verbalizes understanding of discharge medications, including warfarin, and continued laboratory monitoring Verbalizes understanding of discharge instructions
	Discharge planning	Assess needs post-discharge (social work/care coordination)			Reevaluate for needs/resources post-discharge	Verbalizes necessary information for follow-up care with healthcare provider
Potential for spiritual distress	Psychosocial/spiritual/emotional needs	Chaplain to visit with patient/family Heart volunteer to visit with patient		Prepare for transfer to telemetry unit		Able to express feelings related to surgery Aware of support systems and resources

ADLs = Activities of daily living, BMP = basic metabolic panel, BP = blood pressure, CBC = complete blood cell count, CO = cardiac output, Hct = hematocrit, IABP = intra-aortic balloon pump, INR/PT = international normalized ratio/prothrombin time, K⁺ = potassium, P = pulse; R = respirations, RT = respiratory therapy, Spo₂ = oxygen saturation, Svo₂ = mixed venous oxygen saturation.

surgery patients (25% to 40%).[11] Atrial fibrillation has been found to increase hospital costs by as much as $10,000 and length of stay by 4.9 days.[11] Valvular heart disease is associated with atrial hypertrophy, affecting the pulmonary veins coming off the left atrium. This causes electrophysiologic changes to the area and increases the incidence of atrial fibrillation. There have been many studies investigating pharmacologic pro-phylaxis of atrial fibrillation.[11] The use of beta blockers before, during, and after surgery has been shown to have some effect. In recent years, the use of amiodar-one has increased. Atrial pacing in one or both atria has been used as a nonpharmacologic prevention. The rationale is that atrial fibrillation may be prevented by overdrive suppression of atrial ectopy. Investigators have shown that atrial pacing regardless of the site is safe and effective for preventing postoperative atrial fibrillation.[11]

Another difference is the initiation of anticoagulant therapy within 1 to 2 days following surgery, particu-larly if a mechanical valve has been implanted. The warfarin dosing will be regulated to achieve a target INR (Box 15-2). Caution must be used when initiating warfarin therapy in the older adult patient because of the increased risks for bleeding. There are published recommendations for warfarin dosing in this group of patients.[18,20,34]

Before discharge, patients should be encouraged to consider attending cardiac rehabilitation at a facility near where they reside. Cardiac rehabilitation in patients following heart valve surgery has been proven to have beneficial effects.[37] Researchers have demon-strated that women with mitral valve replacement improve their peak metabolic equivalent capacity by 19% and physical working capacity by 25%.[37] The increase in aerobic capacity in the exercise group was

---

Box 15-2

Warfarin Sodium (Coumadin) and Valvular Heart Disease

INDICATIONS

Prevention of thromboembolic complications associated with:
1. Cardiac valve replacement
2. Atrial fibrillation

PHARMACOKINETICS

1. Onset of action: 1 to 3 days
2. Duration of action: 4 to 5 days
3. Peak effect: 3 to 6 days
4. Half-life: 20 to 60 hours

METABOLISM

Metabolized by cytochrome P-450 enzymes in the liver. NOTE: This implies that the risk for drug-drug interaction is high. Patients should be educated regarding inform-ing their healthcare provider when taking new medica-tions, including those that are prescribed, over-the-counter, and herbal supplements. Impaired renal function will not significantly affect the excretion of warfarin.

DOSING

Recommended initial dosing is 2 to 10 mg daily to achieve a therapeutic INR, usually within 2 to 4 days. Adjust the dose thereafter to maintain the therapeutic INR.

LABORATORY MONITORING

Complete blood counts, international normalized ratio (INR), and prothrombin time (PT) should be monitored.

Daily INR levels are obtained until the desired level of anticoagulation is achieved, usually while an inpatient following surgery. Following stabilization of the INR, the duration between tests is gradually lengthened from weekly to every 3 to 4 weeks.

ADVERSE EFFECTS

Bleeding, microembolization, purple toe syndrome, gastro-intestinal disturbances, and elevated liver function tests can occur. Abnormal skin reactions, including dermatitis, alopecia, skin necrosis, vasculitis, and local thrombosis may occur.

SPECIAL GROUPS

1. Asians appear to be more sensitive than Cauca-sians to the effects.
2. Older adults are more sensitive to warfarin and may require smaller doses.
3. Hepatic insufficiency may intensify the effects of warfarin by inhibiting the metabolism of the drug. Warfarin should be used with caution in this group of patients and INR levels monitored closely.

OVERDOSE

1. Vitamin K may be used to reverse the effects of warfarin.
2. Blood transfusions, clotting factors, and fresh fro-zen plasma may be administered if significant bleeding is present.

Data from references 18 and 28.

38% higher when compared with a control group at 6 months and 37% higher after 12 months.[37] For most patients, participation in an outpatient cardiac rehabilitation program will improve their functional capacity and their ability to perform activities of daily living. The Centers for Medicare and Medicaid Services will reimburse cardiac rehabilitation costs for Medicare patients who have had only valve replacement.

Following discharge from the hospital, the first outpatient visit is usually within 3 to 4 weeks after the date of surgery. During this visit a chest x-ray, ECG, Doppler echocardiogram, and various laboratory tests are performed. The main focus is to evaluate the function of the repaired or prosthetic valve and assess for infection or valvular disorder. The Doppler echocardiogram will serve to provide baseline measurements for comparison of subsequent measurements.[4] Further follow-up outpatient visits are determined by the patient's needs. It is important to remember that replacement or repair of the valve is not curative. The patient must be followed carefully as with a patient before surgery. Annual visits are appropriate for those patients who are asymptomatic and uncomplicated.[4]

◆ Case Study 15-1, Part C

Acute Respiratory Distress and Pulmonary Edema

Mrs. J. continued to do well during the night following her surgery. The next morning, her arterial line and PAC were removed. She was prepared to transfer to the cardiac surgery telemetry unit. The nursing staff encouraged her to cough and deep breathe, providing her with a pillow for support. On the telemetry unit, she began to ambulate but complained of shortness of breath and the inability to cough. Her breath sounds were diminished in the lower bases, more so on the left than on the right. She remained in a sinus rhythm with a rate of 90 beats/min.

During her second postoperative night, she became increasingly short of breath and anxious. Her BP increased to 164/85 mm Hg while her respiratory rate was 32 breaths/min. Pulse oximetry was 91%. The physician was notified and a portable chest x-ray was obtained. It was noted that she had a significant left pleural effusion, and a thoracentesis was performed, with 750 ml of dark red fluid removed. The patient immediately stated she could breathe much better.

Following this event, she continued to increase her ambulation and improve clinically. Respiratory therapy worked with her to improve her coughing and deep breathing exercises. She was started on aspirin 325 mg daily. Additional medications included irbesartan (Avapro) 150 mg daily and furosemide 40 mg PRN. The decision was made not to start warfarin (Coumadin) because of her age.

She was discharged on her sixth postoperative day on the same medications as listed previously. Outpatient cardiac rehabilitation was encouraged with the suggestion that she begin after her follow-up visit to her surgeon 2 weeks postdischarge. She continued to improve clinically and functionally with no adverse events.

Decision point: What discharge instructions should be provided for this patient?

PATIENT EDUCATION ISSUES

Subacute Bacterial Endocarditis Prophylaxis

The risk for development of prosthetic valve endocarditis is greatest during the first 6 weeks to 6 months after surgery. *Staphylococcus epidermidis* is a common cause. Should valvular endocarditis occur, the infection often spreads beyond the valve into the surrounding tissue. Abscesses are formed and eventually the valve itself can dehisce.[22] General treatment guidelines for native valve endocarditis can be found in the Medication table on p. 342. There are additional recommendations for therapy based on the type of organism and resistance issues.

Prosthetic valve endocarditis is associated with higher mortality regardless of whether it is managed medically or surgically. Some recommend surgical management if the infection occurs within 3 months after valve replacement.[15] If the infection occurs later, medical management is appropriate. If the infection does not respond to antibiotic therapy, surgery may be required.

Box 15-3 provides a list of conditions associated with an increased risk of bacterial endocarditis. General recommendations for conditions that are associated with a higher risk for development of bacterial endocarditis are presented in Table 15-3. Patients should be instructed to contact their primary care provider or cardiologist for specific antibiotic prophylaxis that may be required. It is helpful to give patients written information about endocarditis and what their responsibility should be. Figure 15-13 is an example of such a tool. The American Heart Association has printed materials that are available as well.

Anticoagulation Issues

Patients receiving a mechanical valve will require chronic anticoagulation with warfarin for prevention of embolic events, such as ischemic stroke. General recommendations for a bileaflet aortic valve are an INR of 2 to 3, and for a bileaflet mitral valve, a slightly

MEDICATIONS FOR TREATMENT OF NATIVE VALVE BACTERIAL ENDOCARDITIS (ADULTS)

DRUG	DOSAGE/ROUTE	DURATION	COMMENTS
Penicillin Susceptible			
Aqueous crystalline penicillin G sodium OR	12–18 million units/24 hr IV continuously or in equally divided doses	4 weeks	Preferred in patients older than 65 years
Ceftriaxone sodium	2 g/24 hr IV/IM in 1 dose	4 weeks	
Patients without cardiac disease or extracardiac abscesses OR	Aqueous crystalline penicillin G sodium 12–18 million units/24 hr IV continuous infusion or in 6 equally divided doses	2 weeks	Not for those with creatinine clearance <20 ml/min, impaired eighth cranial nerve function
Ceftriaxone sulfate PLUS	2 mg/kg per 24 hr IV/IM in 1 dose	2 weeks	
Gentamicin sulfate	3 mg/kg per 24 hr IV/IM in 1 dose	2 weeks	
Vancomycin hydrochloride	30 mg/kg per 24 hr IV in 2 equally divided doses not to exceed 2 g/24 hr (unless vancomycin serum concentrations are not at target)	4 weeks	Recommended for patients unable to tolerate penicillin or ceftriaxone Recommended peak concentration 1 hour after administration = 30–45 mcg/ml Recommended trough concentration 10–15 mcg/ml
Penicillin Resistant*			
Aqueous crystalline penicillin G sodium OR	24 million units/24 hr IV continuously or in 4–6 equally divided doses	4 weeks	
Ceftriaxone sodium PLUS	2 g/24 hr IV/IM in 1 dose	4 weeks	
Gentamicin sulfate	3 mg/kg per 24 hr IV/IM in 1 dose	2 weeks	
Vancomycin hydrochloride	30 mg/kg per 24 hr IV in 2 equally divided doses not to exceed 2 g/24 hr (unless serum vancomycin concentrations are not at target)	4 weeks	Recommended for patients unable to tolerate penicillin or ceftriaxone Recommended peak concentration 1 hour after administration = 30–45 mcg/ml Recommended trough concentration 10–15 mcg/ml

Data from references 2 and 4.
*Therapy for penicillin-resistant streptococci including S. bovis and viridans group.

higher INR of 2.5 to 3.5.[31] Higher INR levels may be desirable if the patient has more than one prosthetic valve or if atrial fibrillation is present. Few randomized clinical trials examine the relationship between the risk/benefit and INR levels associated with anticoagulant therapy. One such study that reviewed the medical records of more than 1600 patients with a follow-up of more than 6000 patient-years demonstrated the optimal INR range to be 2.5 to 4.9.[9] Adverse events associated with this target range were 2 per 100 patient-years. If the INR level was higher than 4.9 or less than 2.5, the adverse event incidents rose sharply.[9] Figure 15-14 demonstrates the incidence of ischemic and hemorrhagic stroke according to the INR level.

TABLE 15-3 Recommendations for Anticoagulation Therapy for Patients With Prosthetic Heart Valves

	ANTITHROMBOTIC THERAPY	TARGET INR (RANGE)
All patients with mechanical heart valves St. Jude bileaflet valve in aortic position Tilting-disk valves and bileaflet mechanical valves in mitral position	Warfarin (Coumadin)	INR 2.5 (2–3) INR 3 (2.5–3.5) INR 3 (2.5–3.5)
Caged-ball or tilting-disk valves	Add ASA 75–100 mg/day	
Bioprosthetic valves	Warfarin for first 3 months after insertion in aortic and mitral position	INR 2.5 (2–3)
For patients in sinus rhythm and no atrial fibrillation	Long-term ASA 75–100 mg/day	

Data from reference 35.
INR = International normalized ratio, ASA = aspirin.

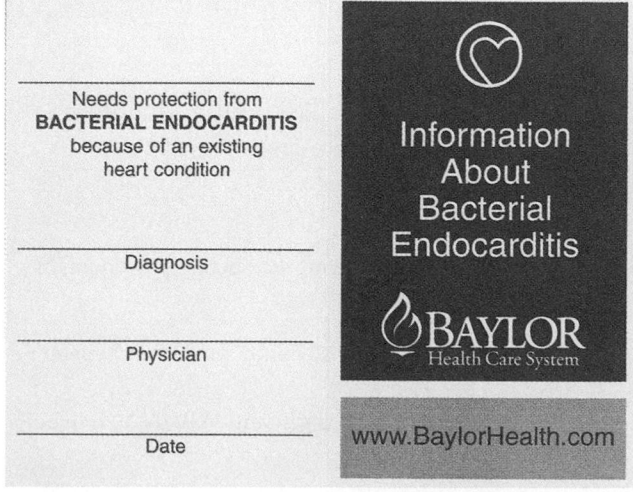

What Is Bacterial Endocarditis?

Bacterial Endocarditis is an infection of the heart's inner lining or heart valves. This can damage or even destroy heart valves.

How Does It Occur?

Bacterial Endocarditis occurs when bacteria in the bloodstream (bacteremia) lodge on abnormal heart valves or other heart tissue. Certain bacteria normally live on parts of the body, such as the mouth and upper respiratory system, the intestinal and urinary tracts, and the skin. Some surgical and dental procedures cause a brief episode of bacteremia. Although bacteremia is common after some invasive procedures, only certain bacteria commonly cause endocarditis.

Needs protection from
BACTERIAL ENDOCARDITIS
because of an existing
heart condition

_____
Diagnosis

_____
Physician

_____
Date

Information About Bacterial Endocarditis

BAYLOR
Health Care System

www.BaylorHealth.com

⬍**FIGURE 15-13** Bacterial endocarditis prophylaxis teaching tool.

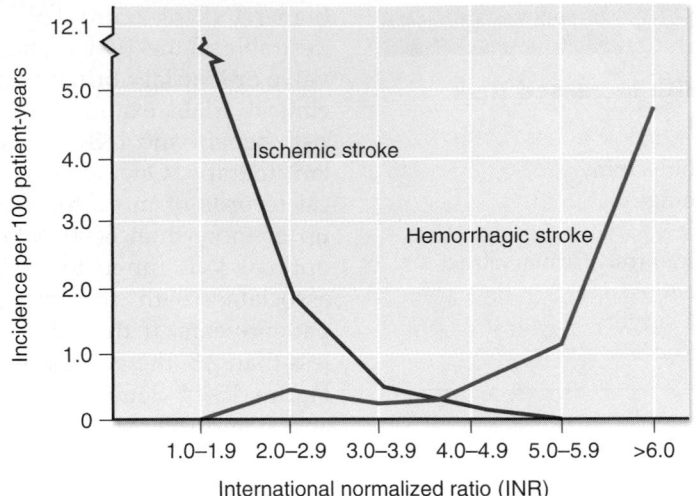

♦FIGURE 15-14 Incidence of ischemic and hemorrhagic stroke related to international normalized ratio (INR) levels.

Some suggest that close monitoring by an anticoagulation clinic will help ensure that the target INR range is maintained. Others report the use of home testing of the INR and patient self-monitoring using standardized protocols may be successful.[13] Regardless of the method, a systematic approach to patient management is essential to prevent bleeding complications. Table 15-4 provides a summary of anticoagulation recommendations for patients with prosthetic heart valves.

Patient and family education about the anticoagulation regimen is crucial. They should verbalize understanding of the purpose, dosing, side effects, and the need for close follow-up of lab testing for INR values. They should be taught which over-the-counter medications to avoid, and they should be encouraged to be aware of their dietary intake of foods high in vitamin K, such as green, leafy vegetables, as explained in the Nutrition box at right.

♦ NUTRITION

Nutritional Considerations for the Patient Taking Warfarin

Patients taking warfarin need to be cautious regarding their intake of the foods listed below. All of these contain vitamin K and may decrease the effect of the drug.

FOOD	MAXIMUM PORTION SIZE
Broccoli	$^1/_2$ cup
Brussels sprouts	5 sprouts
Cabbage	$1^1/_2$ cups
Collard greens	$^1/_2$ cup
Kale	$^3/_4$ cup
Lettuce	$1^3/_4$ cups
Liver (beef and pork)	4 oz
Mustard greens	$1^1/_2$ cups
Spinach	$1^1/_2$ cups
Turnip greens	$1^1/_2$ cups

Source: www.uspharmacist.com.

TABLE 15-4 General Recommendations for Conditions Associated With a Higher Risk for Development of Bacterial Endocarditis

PROCEDURE	RECOMMENDATION
Dental, oral, and upper respiratory tract procedures	Amoxicillin 2 g 1 hr before procedure, clindamycin 600 mg 1 hr before procedure, or azithromycin 500 mg 1 hr before procedure
Genitourinary and gastrointestinal procedures	Ampicillin 2 g IV/IM plus gentamicin 1.5 mg/kg within 30 min of procedure; repeat ampicillin 1 g IV/IM or give amoxicillin 1 g 6 hr later
	If allergic to penicillin: vancomycin 1 g IV over 1–2 hr plus gentamicin IM/IV 30 min before procedure; second dose not recommended

Data from references 4 and 23.
g = Grams, hr = hours, IM = intramuscular, IV = intravenous, mg = milligrams, min = minutes.

Echocardiography Following Valve Surgery

An echocardiogram is obtained 3 to 4 weeks after the surgical procedure to provide baseline information about the valve, heart chamber dimensions, and systolic function. It is suggested that repeat echocardiograms be obtained every 1 to 3 years initially. Patients with tissue valves that have been implanted for 10 years or longer should have repeat studies performed more frequently because of the limited durability of the valves.[31] Other routine follow-up visits should be dependent on the patient's needs.[4]

CONCLUSIONS

Valvular heart disease remains a significant cardiovascular problem with serious implications if the patient is not managed appropriately. Bacterial endocarditis prophylaxis is very important for both medically and surgically managed patients. Advances in surgical techniques and the development of newer types of heart valves offer promising treatment options for patients.

REFERENCES

1. American Heart Association. (2006). *Heart disease and stroke statistics—2006 update*. Dallas, Tex: American Heart Association.
2. Baddour, L. M., et al. (2005). Infective endocarditis: diagnosis, antimicrobial therapy, and management of complications. A statement for healthcare professionals from the committee on rheumatic fever, endocarditis, and Kawasaki disease, Council on Cardiovascular Disease in the Young, and the Councils on Clinical Cardiology, Stroke, and Cardiovascular Surgery and Anesthesia, American Heart Association—Executive summary. *Circulation, 111*, 3167–3184.
3. Bloomfield, P. (2002). Choice of heart valve prosthesis. *Heart, 87*, 583–589.
4. Bonow, R. O., et al. (2006). ACC/AHA guidelines for the management of patients with valvular heart disease. *J Am Coll Cardiol, 48*(3), e1–148.
5. Bonow, R. A., & Braunwald, E. (2005). Valvular heart disease. In D. P. Zipes, et al. (Eds.), *Braunwald's heart disease* (7th ed., pp. 1553–1632). Philadelphia: Elsevier Saunders.
6. Borer, J. S., & Bonow, R. O. (2003). Contemporary approach to aortic and mitral regurgitation. *Circulation, 108*, 2432–2438.
7. Boudjemline, Y., & Bonhoeffer, P. (2001). Percutaneous aortic valve replacement: will we get there? *Br Heart J, 86*(6), 705–706.
8. Caffarelli, A. D., & Robbins, R. C. (2004). Will minimally invasive valve replacement ever really be important? *Curr Opin Cardiol, 19*, 123–127.
9. Cannegieter, S. C., et al. (1995). Optimal oral anticoagulant therapy in patients with mechanical heart valves. *N Engl J Med, 333*(1), 11–17.
10. Dacey, L. J. (2000). Pulmonary homografts: current status. *Curr Opin Cardiol, 15, 8*, 6–90.
11. Daoud, E. G. (2004). Management of atrial fibrillation in the postcardiac surgery setting. *Cardiol Clin, 22*, 159–166.
12. Degenais, F., et al. (2004). Which biologic valve should we select for the 45- to 65-year-old age group requiring aortic valve replacement? *J Thorac Cardiovasc Surg, 129*(5), 1041–1049.
13. Ebell, M. H. (2005). A systematic approach to managing warfarin doses. *Family Pract Management.* www.aafp.org/fpm.
14. Enriquez-Sarano, M., & Tajik, A. J. (2004). Aortic regurgitation. *N Engl J Med, 351*(15), 1539–1546.
15. Fann, J. I., & Burdon, T. A. (2001). Are the indications for tissue valves different in 2001 and how do we communicate these changes to our cardiology colleagues? *Curr Opin Cardiol, 16*, 126–135.
16. Ferguson, E., Reardon, M. J., & Letsou, G. V. (2000). The surgical management of bacterial valvular endocarditis. *Curr Opin Cardiol, 15*, 82–85.
17. Finkelmeier, B. A. (2000). *Cardiothoracic surgical nursing* (2nd ed., pp. 169–188). Philadelphia: Lippincott Williams & Wilkins.
18. Frishman, W. H., Cheng-Lai, A., & Nawarskas, J. (2005). *Current cardiovascular drugs* (4th ed., pp. 114–116). Philadelphia: Current Medicine LLC.
19. Gage, B. F., Fihn, S. D., & White, R. (2001). Warfarin therapy for an octogenarian who has atrial fibrillation. *Ann Intern Med, 134*(6), 465–474.
20. Grunkemeier, G. L., Starr, A., & Rahimtoola, S. H. (2004). Clinical performance of bioprosthetic heart valves. In V. Fuster, R. W. Alexander & R. A. O'Rourke (Eds.), *Hurst's the heart* (11th ed., pp. 1723–1736). New York: McGraw-Hill.
21. Hamilton, R. J., & Sanchez, M. (2006). Oral anticoagulation management. *US Pharmacist, 27.* www.uspharmacist.com.
22. Jamieson, W. R. E., et al. (2005). Performance of bioprostheses and mechanical prostheses assessed by composites of valve-related complications to 15 years after mitral valve replacement. *J Thorac Cardiovasc Surg, 129*(6), 1301–1308.
23. Karchmer, A. W. (2005). Infective endocarditis. In D. P. Zipes, et al. (Eds.), *Braunwald's heart disease* (7th ed.). Philadelphia: Elsevier Saunders.
24. Kypson, A. P., et al. (2004). Robotics in valvular surgery: 2003 and beyond. *Curr Opin Cardiol, 19*, 128–133.
25. Deleted in proofs.
26. Mark, J. B. (1998). *Atlas of cardiovascular monitoring.* (p. 310). New York: Churchill Livingstone.
27. McCarthy, P. M., et al. (2004). Tricuspid valve repair: durability and risk factors for failure. *J Thorac Cardiovasc Surg, 127*, 674–685.
28. Messerli, F. H. (1996). *Cardiovascular drug therapy.* (pp. 1517–1521). Philadelphia: Saunders.
29. Minakata, K., et al. (2004). Is repair of the aortic valve regurgitation a safe alternative to valve replacement? *J Thorac Cardiovasc Surg, 127*(3), 645–653.
30. Nishimura, R. A. (2002). Aortic valve disease. *Circulation, 106*, 770–772.
31. Oswalt, J. D. (1999). Acceptance and versatility of the Ross procedure. *Curr Opin Cardiol, 14*(2), 90.
32. Otto, C. M. (2004). *Valvular heart disease* (2nd ed.). Philadelphia: Saunders.
33. Potter, D. D., et al. (2005). Operative risk of reoperative aortic valve replacement. *J Thorac Cardiovasc Surg, 129*, 94–103.
34. Rahimtoola, S. H., & Frye, R. L. (2000). Valvular heart disease. *Circulation, 102*, IV-24–IV-33.
35. Salem, D. N., et al. (2004). Antithrombotic therapy in valvular heart disease—native and prosthetic. The Seventh ACCP Conference on Antithrombotic and Thrombolytic Therapy. *Chest, 126*, 457S–482S.
36. Scott, C., Schactman, M., & Graver, L. M. (1997). Aortic valve replacement with a pulmonary autograft: case studies of the Ross procedure. *Am J Crit Care, 6*(6), 418–422.

37. Soler-Soler, J., & Gaive, E. (2000). Worldwide perspective of valve disease. *Heart*, *83*, 721–725.

38. Stewart, K. J., et al. (2003). Cardiac rehabilitation following percutaneous revascularization, heart transplant, heart valve surgery, and for chronic heart failure. *Chest*, *123*(2), 2104–2111.

39. Sundt, T. M., et al. (2000). Quality of life after aortic valve replacement at the age of > 80 years. *Circulation*, *102*(suppl III), III-70–III-74.

40. Deleted in proofs.

41. Unic, D., et al. (2005). Early and late results of isolated and combined heart valve surgery in patients ≥ 80 years of age. *Am J Cardiol*, *95*, 1500–1503.

42. Vahanian, A., & Palacios, I. F. (2004). Percutaneous approaches to valvular disease. *Circulation*, *109*, 1572–1579.

43. Vassiliades, T. A., et al. (2005). The clinical development of percutaneous heart valve technology. A position statement of the Society of Thoracic Surgeons (STS), the American Association for Thoracic Surgery (AATS), and the Society for Cardiovascular Angiography and Interventions (SCAI). *J Thorac Cardiovasc Surg*, *129*, 970–976.

44. Walkes, J. M., & Reardon, M. J. (2004). Status of mitral valve surgery. *Curr Opin Cardiol*, *19*, 117–122.

45. Wiegand, D. L. (2003). Advances in cardiac surgery: valve repair. *Crit Care Nurse*, *23*(2), 72–90.

46. Yacoub, M. H., & Cohn, L. H. (2004). Novel approaches to cardiac valve repair, from structure to function: Part I. *Circulation*, *109*, 942–950.

CHAPTER 16

Vascular Emergencies

Joni L. Dirks and June Howland-Gradman

Vascular emergencies occur as a result of an acute occlusion or disruption of blood flow to organs or tissues and can have catastrophic results. Disruption of flow in the aorta may be caused by dissection or rupture of an aneurysm, whereas occlusion of peripheral veins or arteries typically occurs secondary to acute thrombosis. The majority of patients who present with a vascular crisis have peripheral arterial disease (PAD), a broad term that encompasses the pathophysiologic processes that alter the structure and function of the aorta and its branch arteries. The prevalence of this disease increases with age and exposure to atherosclerotic risk factors such as smoking, diabetes, hyperlipidemia, and hypertension.[32] Regardless of the cause of the vascular emergency, prompt intervention is required to restore blood flow to the affected area and preserve end-organ function. This chapter will review the pathophysiology, diagnosis, and treatment of vascular emergencies that involve the aorta and the peripheral vessels.

EMERGENCIES INVOLVING THE AORTA

Vascular emergencies of the aorta can occur as a result of aortic dissection or rupture of an aneurysm. Although these two conditions are often described as a single entity—a dissecting aneurysm—they actually represent two different pathologies. Blunt trauma to the chest can also create a tear in the aorta. Although uncommon, all of these conditions are highly lethal. Aortic dissection and aneurysms result in approximately 15,000 deaths each year.[59] A significant number of patients with an acute aortic condition die before reaching the hospital.[45] For those who do present for treatment, accurate diagnosis may be hindered by the fact that the symptoms mimic other, more common conditions such as acute coronary syndrome or stroke.[29] Treatment strategies for these other conditions differ significantly, because anticoagulants and thrombolytics are contraindicated in the setting of acute dissection. Patient survival thus depends on accurate diagnosis and rapid intervention.

Aortic Dissection

Aortic dissection is the most common vascular emergency involving the aorta, with an incidence of approximately 2000 cases each year in the United States.[29] In most cases the aortic dissection results from a tear in the intimal layer of the aorta that allows blood to flow into the medial layer, creating a false channel. The rate of pressure change in the aorta (dP/dT) created by ejection of blood from the left ventricle plays a significant role in the propagation of the dissection.[15] With the force of pressure generated by ventricular contraction and systemic blood pressure (BP), the dissection can extend either proximally or distally.[45] As blood flows into the false lumen, perfusion to major arteries arising from that section of the aorta may be reduced or eliminated. Specific complications depend on the location and extent of the dissection, but many can be lethal, especially when the dissection impairs perfusion of the coronary arteries or the extracranial cerebral vessels (Figure 16-1). The dissection is described as "acute" for the first 2 weeks—the period associated with the greatest morbidity and mortality. For patients who survive this initial period, the dissection is referred to as chronic.[29]

Etiology. Aortic dissection occurs secondary to iatrogenic injuries, trauma, or disease processes that weaken the vessel wall. The vascular wall of the aorta consists of three layers—the intima, the media, and the adventitia. Weakening of the middle layer, or medial degeneration, is believed to contribute to the formation of aortic dissections and aneurysms.[85] Hereditary connective tissue disorders, such as Marfan syndrome and Ehlers-Danlos syndrome, affect the medial layer and are a primary cause of aortic dissection in younger people.[94] Atherosclerosis and long-standing hypertension are felt to be responsible for weakening of the medial layer in older adult patients. In a review of 464 patients from the International Registry of Acute Aortic Dissection (IRAD), hypertension was found to be the most common predisposing risk factor for aortic dissection.[29] A small percentage of aortic dissections are iatrogenic, caused by procedures such as retrograde catheter insertions,

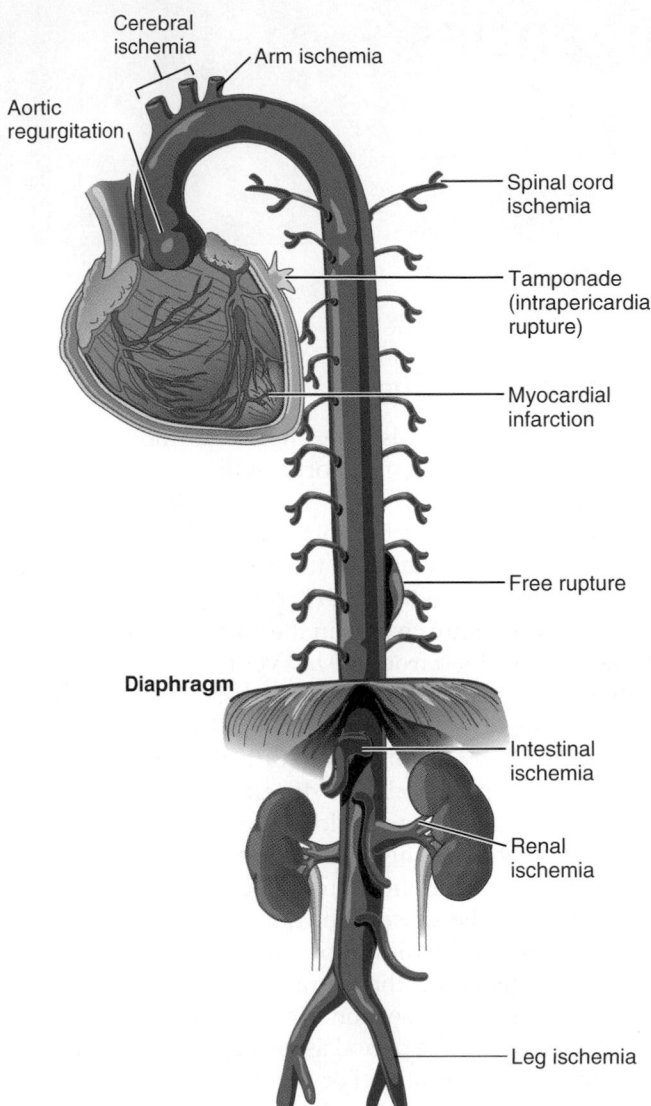

Cerebral
ischemia
Arm ischemia
Aortic
regurgitation
Spinal cord
ischemia
Tamponade
(intrapericardial
rupture)
Myocardial
infarction
Free rupture
Diaphragm
Intestinal
ischemia
Renal
ischemia
Leg ischemia

♦**FIGURE 16-1** Potential complications of aortic dissection.

cannulation for cardiopulmonary bypass, or aortic cross-clamping. Cocaine use has also been implicated as a cause in otherwise healthy people, presumably because of the acute rise in BP.[47] Other risk factors for aortic dissection are listed in Box 16-1.

Classification. Two types of classification systems are used to describe aortic dissections, based on anatomic location (Figure 16-2).[60] In the DeBakey system, aneurysms are classified as Type I if they involve the entire aorta; Type II, the ascending aorta only; and Type III, the descending aorta distal to the left subclavian artery. The Stanford system simplifies this somewhat, with Type A involving the ascending or proximal aorta (DeBakey Types I and II) and Type B including the descending or distal aorta (DeBakey Type III). The Stanford classification is widely used in determining both prognosis and a strategy for treatment.[95]

Box 16-1

Conditions Associated With Aortic Dissection

Atherosclerosis
Chronic hypertension
Congenital heart defects
- Bicuspid aortic valve
- Coarctation of the aorta
Connective tissue disorders
- Marfan syndrome
- Ehlers-Danlos syndrome
- Familial
Vascular inflammation
- Syphilis
- Takayasu's arteritis
Trauma
- Motor vehicle crashes
- Falls
Iatrogenic events
- Cardiac catheterization
- Cannulation for CPB
- Aortic cross-clamping
Pregnancy (rare)
Crack-cocaine use

CPB = Cardiopulmonary bypass.

The most common site of dissection is the ascending aorta (Stanford Type A), with the majority occurring just centimeters from the aortic valve.[31] Because the ascending aorta contains important structures such as the aortic valve and the coronary arteries, patients with Type A dissections are at significant risk for death from complications such as acute aortic regurgitation and pericardial tamponade. As a result, urgent surgical intervention is recommended to reduce mortality, which is estimated to be as high as 1% to 2% per hour from the time of symptom onset.[60] Generally, Type B dissections (distal aorta) are considered less lethal, and may be managed medically unless they are associated with ischemic complications.[24]

Clinical Presentation. The clinical presentation of an aortic dissection and its associated complications vary with the location of the dissection and stem from the resultant loss of perfusion to involved arteries or compression of adjacent tissues. The most common symptom of an aortic dissection is the sudden onset of severe pain, which occurs in up to 90% of patients.[24,47,48] The pain is usually described as tearing or ripping and is typically substernal in an ascending dissection and intrascapular if the descending aorta is affected. As the dissection progresses, the pain can propagate into the neck, lower back, abdomen, or flanks. Hypertension is present in up to 70% of patients with descending

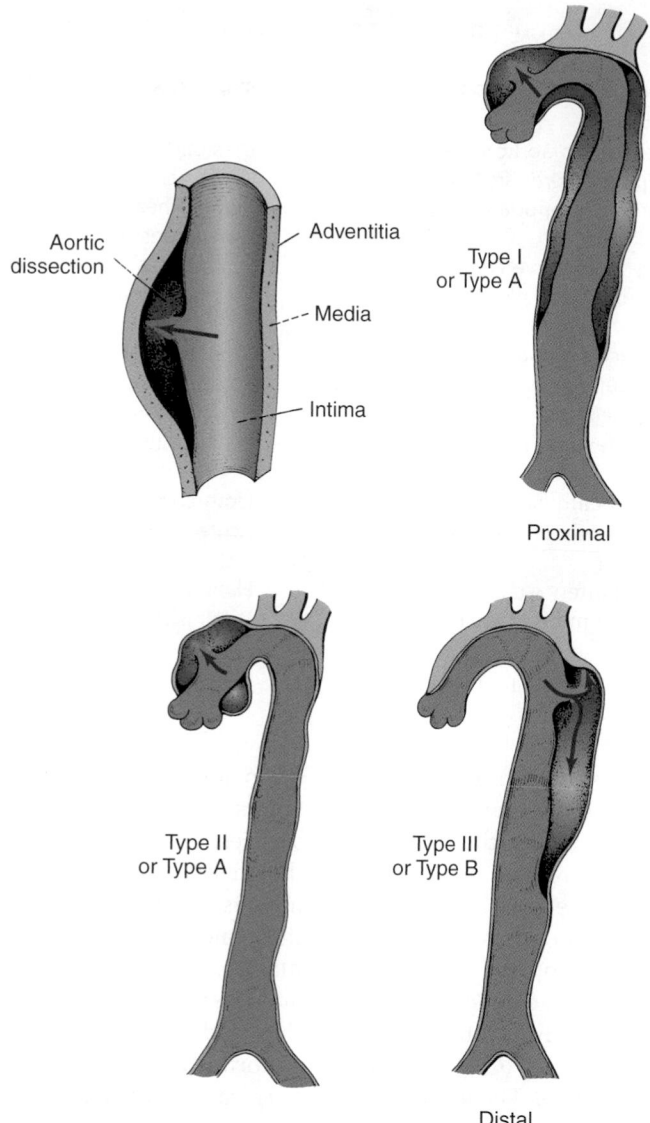

‡FIGURE 16-2 DeBakey classification of aortic dissection.

aneurysms, and hypotension may occur in up to 25% of ascending aneurysms.[29] A diastolic murmur secondary to aortic regurgitation may be present in up to 50% of patients with dissection of the ascending aorta.[60] If the dissection involves the brachiocephalic vessels, significant BP variation between the arms may be present. Table 16-1 outlines other possible symptoms based on the location of the dissection.

Diagnostic Tests. In a patient with suspected aortic dissection, one of the first priorities is to confirm or exclude the diagnosis so that appropriate therapy can be initiated. Because the presenting symptoms of aortic dissection are variable and often shared by other pathologies, an accurate diagnosis depends on clinicians maintaining a high level of suspicion for this disorder.[48,60] The physical examination may provide helpful clues—

such as pulse deficits or focal neurologic deficits—but is generally not sufficient to prove the diagnosis.[48] A number of diagnostic studies can be used to facilitate accurate diagnosis of aortic dissection, and frequently, more than one study is required.[29] The particular tests selected are generally influenced by the urgency of the patient's condition, physician preference, and institutional availability.

Common diagnostic tests, such as chest x-ray, 12-lead electrocardiogram (ECG), and laboratory studies, are generally a part of the initial diagnostic workup. A chest x-ray may show signs of acute dissection, such as changes in the aortic silhouette or a widened mediastinum, but in 10% to 40% of cases the radiograph may also be normal.[60] The 12-lead ECG may provide clues to the diagnosis, but often the findings are nonspecific. For example, a lack of ischemic changes on the 12-lead can

TABLE 16-1 Potential Signs and Symptoms of Aortic Dissection

LOCATION OF DISSECTION	IMPAIRMENT/PROBLEM	SYMPTOMS
Ascending aorta	Damage to aortic valve Impaired coronary blood flow Cardiac tamponade Laryngeal nerve compression Bleeding into pleural space	Diastolic murmur Chest pain indicative of MI Muffled heart sounds, pulsus paradoxus, JVD, hypotension Hoarseness Dyspnea, hemothorax
Aortic arch	Reduced blood flow to brain Interruption of cervical sympathetic ganglia Impaired brachiocephalic flow	Syncope, altered mental status Ptosis, miosis, anhidrosis (Horner syndrome) Blood pressure differential, asymmetric pulses in upper extremities
Descending aorta	Spinal cord ischemia Mesenteric artery ischemia	Limb paresthesia or paralysis Acute abdominal pain, melena, hyperactive bowel sounds
Thoracoabdominal aorta	Renal artery ischemia Lower limb ischemia	Flank pain, oliguria Diminished or absent pulses in lower extremities

JVD = Jugular venous distention, MI = myocardial infarction.

be helpful in differentiating between acute coronary syndrome and aortic dissection in some patients, but if the dissection compromises flow through the coronary arteries, ischemic changes will be present.[47] Similarly, troponin and creatine phosphokinase (CPK) levels can be elevated if the dissection has extended into the coronary arteries and caused myocardial injury.[47]

Because of the need for a definitive diagnosis, the presence of aortic dissection is usually established by either enhanced computed tomography (CT) or transesophageal electrocardiography (TEE). These imaging studies can confirm the diagnosis of dissection by visualization of an intimal flap that separates the two lumens. Other tests, such as magnetic resonance imaging (MRI), may be used in some settings. Advantages and disadvantages of imaging tests commonly used to diagnose aortic dissection are summarized in Table 16-2.

Research is ongoing for a test that will allow for more rapid diagnosis of acute aortic dissection. One small study suggested that serum D-dimer should be a part of the initial evaluation for suspected aortic dissection, in that a negative result made the presence of dissection unlikely.[91] Elevated levels of smooth muscle myosin heavy-chain proteins have been found to have a high sensitivity and specificity for identifying patients with acute dissection in some studies.[80,81] Unfortunately, this test is not readily available in most settings.

Aortic Aneurysm

An aortic aneurysm is a chronic dilatation of the vessel wall, typically 50% greater than the normal aortic diameter.[39] The progressive dilatation involves all three layers of the vasculature, and may occur in one or more segments of the aorta. As the aneurysm increases in size, the vessel wall weakens and the chance of rupture increases. The size of the aneurysm has proved to be the major risk factor for dissection, rupture, and, ultimately, survival.[39] As a result, patients with known aneurysms are followed with serial exams to determine the need for elective repair. Ruptured aneurysms carry a mortality estimated to be as high as 90%, and emergent surgical repair is the only chance for survival.[32]

Aneurysms are generally described based on their position in the aorta. Thoracic aneurysms occur in sections of the aorta above the diaphragm. Those that begin in the thorax but extend distally below the level of the diaphragm are referred to as *thoracoabdominal*.[94] Abdominal aneurysms occur below the diaphragm and may be located either above (suprarenal) or below (infrarenal) the renal arteries. Aneurysms may be further described based on their morphology, which includes either fusiform or saccular. Fusiform aneurysms are symmetrical and involve the entire circumference of the aorta, whereas saccular aneurysms involve a local ballooning of a portion of the vessel wall.

Thoracic aneurysms may occur in one or more segments of the thoracic aorta—the ascending aorta, the aortic arch, and the descending thoracic aorta—and are classified by location. When the aneurysm involves the aortic root, the term *annuloaortic ectasia* is used. Crawford and his colleagues developed a system for classifying thoracoabdominal aneurysms based on the extent of the aneurysm (Figure 16-3).[16] This

TABLE 16-2 Diagnostic Tests for Aortic Dissection

TEST	ADVANTAGES	DISADVANTAGES
Aortography	Allows for visualization of intimal tear as well as assessment of other involved arteries and aortic valve	False negatives can occur in patients with thrombosis of false lumen[31] Risk of further dissection secondary to placement of guidewire
Chest x-ray	May provide diagnostic evidence of AD, such as mediastinal widening or pleural effusions Performed at bedside	May be normal in 10%–40% of patients with AD[60]
Computed tomography (CT)	High sensitivity and specificity (>90%) for detection of AD[78] Widely available Not influenced by patient's body habitus[31]	Does not provide information regarding aortic valve and coronary artery involvement Requires use of IV contrast for improved accuracy
Magnetic resonance imaging (MRI)	No contrast dye required Multiple views facilitate diagnosis of determination of extent of aortic dissection Allows for evaluation of complications of AD, such as AR[31]	Not available on an emergent basis in some institutions May interfere with monitoring and medication infusions in unstable patients Contraindicated in patients with metallic implants, such as pacemakers
Transesophageal echocardiogram (TEE)	Complete visualization of ascending and descending aorta Allows for assessment of complications of AD, such as AR Performed at bedside No radiation or contrast exposure	Does not allow for visualization of abdominal aorta Requires use of procedural sedation that may induce hypotension Operator dependent Contraindicated in patients with esophageal varices or strictures
Transthoracic echocardiogram (TTE)	Noninvasive Performed at bedside	Limited visualization of descending thoracic aorta Suboptimal studies in obese patients and those with pulmonary emphysema[31]

AD = Aortic dissection, AR = aortic regurgitation, IV = intravenous.

classification has proved useful in defining treatment modalities, potential complications, and mortality associated with operative repair for various types of thoracoabdominal aneurysms.

Abdominal aortic aneurysms (AAA) are much more common than thoracic aneurysms, with the infrarenal location being the most common site.[1] Age is considered an important risk factor, with one study revealing an incidence of 5% in men over the age of 65 screened by ultrasound.[58] While AAAs are less common in women, one study showed the risk of rupture was four times greater in women than in men.[86] For this reason, recent guidelines suggest that elective repair of aneurysms in women should be performed earlier than in men, when the aneurysm diameter is less than 5.5 cm.[8]

Etiology. The causes of aortic aneurysm are similar to those for aortic dissection, and etiology tends to vary by location of the aneurysm. For example, atherosclerosis is the predominant cause of aneurysm formation in the descending aorta, whereas cystic medial degeneration is associated with ascending aneurysms.[39,94] Although atherosclerosis and its related risk factors (smoking, hypertension, hyperlipidemia) have long been considered the cause of abdominal aneurysms, new evidence suggests that genetic and immunologic factors probably contribute as well.[1,32,39] Smoking has been implicated as a significant risk factor for aortic aneurysm formation and has also been linked to accelerated rates of aneurysm expansion.[9,50] The incidence of chronic obstructive pulmonary disease (COPD) is also more prevalent in patients with aortic aneurysms and may be related to a common pathogenic mechanism for both diseases—elastin degradation caused by tobacco smoking.[70] Aneurysm formation secondary to chronic dissection can occur at any location along the aorta.

Clinical Presentation. Many patients with aortic aneurysms are asymptomatic; the aneurysm is detected during a routine chest x-ray or imaging study performed for

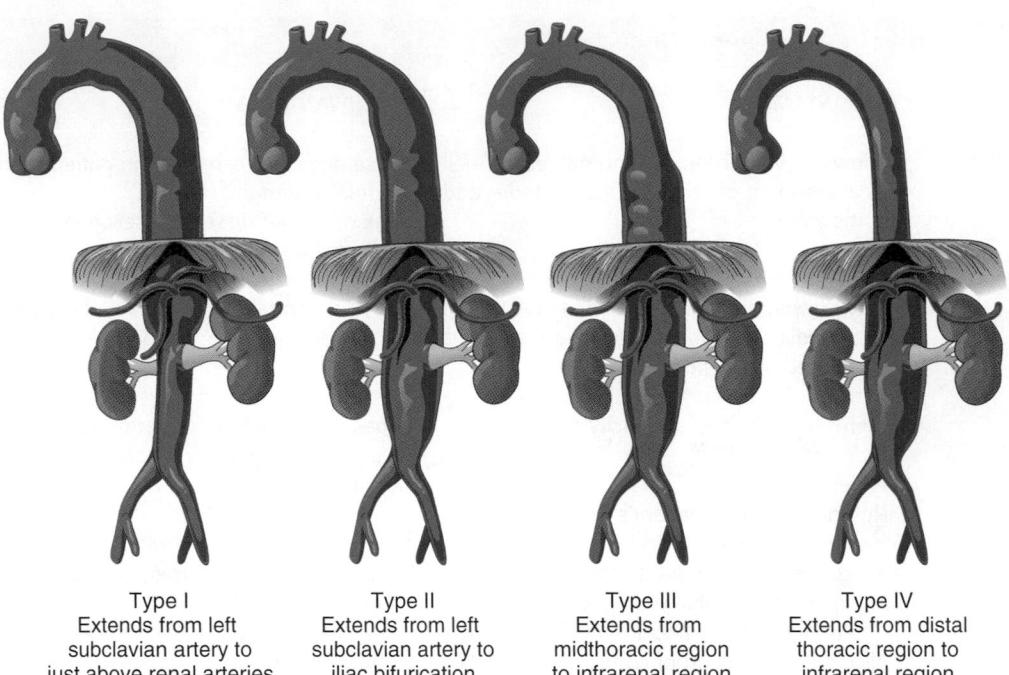

Type I	Type II	Type III	Type IV
Extends from left subclavian artery to just above renal arteries	Extends from left subclavian artery to iliac bifurication	Extends from midthoracic region to infrarenal region	Extends from distal thoracic region to infrarenal region

⬧FIGURE 16-3 Crawford classification of thoracoabdominal aneurysms.

some other reason. Patients may present with pain in the chest, back, or flank, depending on the location of the aneurysm. Other symptoms may result from compression of adjacent structures because of the size of the aneurysm or ischemia secondary to altered perfusion. Rupture of the aneurysm is generally associated with an abrupt onset of pain, unrelieved by changes in position. A ruptured thoracic aneurysm produces symptoms similar to those of an aortic dissection. The classic symptoms of a ruptured abdominal aneurysm include sudden onset of severe abdominal pain, hypertension, and the presence of a palpable pulsatile mass. It is recommended that patients who present with these symptoms undergo immediate exploratory surgery.[1] Unfortunately, this diagnostic triad of symptoms is only present in about one third of patients.[32]

Diagnostic Tests. A number of imaging tests can be performed to define the size and extent of an aortic aneurysm. Ultrasound of the aorta is preferred for initial diagnosis because it is noninvasive and readily available in most settings. If time permits, more detailed studies can be obtained with contrast-enhanced CT or MRI.

Traumatic Injury to the Aorta

Tears in the aorta may result from blunt trauma to the chest, such as a motor vehicle accident or a fall from a significant height.[73] The tear usually occurs at the aortic isthmus—the junction between the aortic arch and the descending aorta—or the aortic root. This type of

injury carries a high mortality as 80% to 85% of patients usually die at the scene of the accident or in transport, usually secondary to pericardial tamponade or massive exsanguination.[62] Of those who reach the hospital, 40% to 60% will die as a result of intrapleural surgical rupture before surgical repair can be accomplished.[72] If the rupture is contained by the adventitial layer of the aorta, the chance for survival is much improved.[72]

Clinical Symptoms. Patients who survive to the emergency department may have signs of hypovolemic shock, as well as evidence of injury to the ascending aorta (aortic valve insufficiency, coronary artery ischemia, tamponade) and impaired perfusion through the main branches of the thoracic aorta (upper extremity or cerebral ischemia). In addition, there may be signs of trauma to the chest wall such as bruising and fractures of the ribs or sternum. A chest x-ray may indicate a widened mediastinum and hemothorax. If the patient's condition allows, the diagnosis can be confirmed by CT scan. Urgent surgery is performed to repair the injury as soon as possible, but may not be feasible in light of other traumatic injuries, such as major intracranial damage.[84]

TREATMENT STRATEGIES

Surgical Treatment

Surgery on the aorta may be performed for dissection, aneurysm or traumatic tears. For aortic dissections, surgery involves resecting the area of the intimal tear, to "exclude" the false lumen from high-pressure blood flow, and positioning a graft to reinforce the damaged aorta.[41] Often, tissue adhesives or glue is used to repair the dissected layers or the aortic vasculature. The use of tissue glue has been associated with decreased bleeding and postoperative complications.[45,63] For aneurysm repair, surgery involves interposition of a Dacron graft and attaching it both proximally and distally to nondiseased segments of the aorta. If the aortic valve is damaged by either dissection or an aneurysm, it is repaired or replaced at the time of surgery. If the aneurysm is extensive and includes both the ascending and the descending segments of the aorta, the repair may take place in two stages.[69] Surgery for an aortic tear involves isolating the tear and anastomosing the aorta with or without a prosthetic graft. The procedure is usually performed through a left posterolateral incision with a "clamp and sew" technique to allow for rapid repair. A description of some of the surgical procedures performed on the aorta is provided in Table 16-3.

Indications. Surgery is performed urgently for Type A dissections, aortic tears, or any type of ruptured aneurysm. Generally Type B dissections are more stable and can either be managed medically or treated with elective surgery.[61] The exception to this is Type B dissections that present with a rapidly expanding aortic diameter or evidence of decreased perfusion to a major branch vessel.[82] Surgical repair of an aortic aneurysm is performed electively when an aneurysm reaches a critical size, to prevent the high mortality and morbidity associated with rupture. The decision to perform surgery is based on a number of factors, including the size and shape of the aneurysm, the rate of expansion, the type of aortic disease present (i.e., Marfan

TABLE 16-3 Surgical Procedures Performed on the Aorta

SURGICAL PROCEDURE	DESCRIPTION	INDICATIONS
Simple tube graft	Dacron tube graft is used to replace damaged portion of aorta.	May be used for aneurysms in ascending aorta in patients with a normal aortic root.
Composite graft (Bentall procedure)	Damaged section of ascending aorta is replaced with a Dacron graft, which has a valve incorporated into one end. Coronary arteries are removed from diseased aorta and reimplanted in graft.	Generally required in severe connective tissue disorders such as Marfan syndrome. It is also indicated whenever there is a combined dilation of aortic root, valve annulus, and ascending aorta or dissection of these structures.
Valve-sparing: reimplantation (David procedure[56])	Native aortic valve leaflets are reimplanted inside a Dacron tube graft, followed by reattachment of coronary arteries to graft.	Primarily suitable for patients with trileaflet aortic valves with minimal aortic insufficiency.
Valve-sparing: remodeling (Yacoub procedure[56])	Involves resecting aneurysmal sinus tissue while maintaining tissue along valve leaflets and scalloping Dacron graft to form new sinuses to reconstruct root. This procedure also requires reimplantation of coronary arteries.	Indicated for use in same group of patients as valve-sparing reimplantation procedure.
Pulmonary autograft (Ross procedure)	Native pulmonary valve is placed in aortic valve position, and a homograft (human donor) valve replaces pulmonary valve.	Ideal operation for a young or middle-aged patient who requires aortic valve replacement. Extensiveness of surgery may be beyond tolerance of unstable patients.
Staged repair of ascending and descending aorta ("elephant trunk" procedure[26])	First operation involves placement of a Dacron graft in ascending aorta, with an additional segment of graft left extending into distal lumen, like an elephant trunk. In second operation, distal end of graft is used to repair defect in descending thoracic aorta.	Used for extensive aneurysms involving ascending aorta, aortic arch, and descending thoracic or thoracoabdominal aorta. First procedure is done via median sternotomy and second via thoracotomy.

syndrome, bicuspid aortic valve, familial disease), and the general health and age of the patient.[1,39] Indications for aortic surgery are given in Box 16-2.

The risks of surgery increase with the urgency of the procedure. For example, operative risk for mortality with a ruptured AAA is approximately 50%, compared with 4% to 6% in elective repairs.[1,88] Mortality for elective repair of a thoracic aneurysm is somewhat higher, ranging from 8% to 15%.[20,39] For urgent repair of a dissection, the mortality can be as high as 26%. This is still considered an acceptable risk, however, as the mortality for patients managed medically is more than twice that of patients managed surgically.[29]

Surgical Procedures. Surgery on the aorta presents special challenges because of the risks associated with compromising circulation to major organs and tissues. Unlike traditional cardiac surgery, the use of cardiopulmonary bypass (CPB) may be limited in some cases because clamping of the aorta is hindered by the location of the injury. A number of techniques have been developed to minimize risks and improve outcomes associated with these high-risk procedures, including hypothermic circulatory arrest (HCA), left heart bypass, and separate cerebral perfusion catheters. The incisional approach, the use of CPB, and specialized techniques used to provide neurologic protection vary depending on the type of aortic surgery being performed.

When surgery is performed on the ascending aorta for repair of either a Type A dissection or an aneurysm, the goals are similar. These include maintaining myocardial blood flow via the coronary ostia, restoring function of the aortic valve, and preventing rupture into the pericardium, which could lead to tamponade and death.[61] The ascending aorta is accessed via a median sternotomy. The patient is placed on CPB, usually via cannulation of the right atrium and either the aorta distal to the surgical site or one femoral artery. The degree of damage to the aorta and the aortic valve is then assessed. If the dissection or aneurysm involves the aortic valve or the aortic tissue has deteriorated (common in Marfan syndrome), a composite graft is used for repair (Bentall procedure). This consists of a Dacron tube with an aortic valve sewn into one end. The graft is attached to the aortic annulus and the coronary arteries are then reimplanted in the graft. If the aortic tissue is structurally viable and the valve leaflets are intact, a valve-sparing procedure may be performed.[17,39] Although technically more demanding, this approach is preferred by some because it avoids the long-term anticoagulation therapy required with prosthetic valves.[41,61]

Surgical repair of dissections or aneurysms involving the aortic arch is more complicated, because the vessels branching from this area—the innominate, carotid, and subclavian arteries—supply blood flow to the upper body, including the brain. During repairs to the arch, the brachiocephalic vessels must first be removed from the diseased section of the aorta, and then reimplanted in the graft. This is typically performed with a period of circulatory arrest to allow for operation on a bloodless field.

Circulatory arrest is performed under deep hypothermia, with the patient cooled systemically to 15° to 18° C—the point at which electroencephalographic (EEG) silence occurs.[83] Systemic cooling is performed through the bypass circuit until the desired temperature is reached and EEG silence is confirmed. In emergent situations where EEG monitoring is not available, this cooling is performed over a period of 45 minutes, as research has shown this allows for EEG silence in most patients.[4] CPB is then halted and the surgical repair completed as quickly as possible. The goal is to perform the procedure in 40 minutes or less, because periods of HCA beyond this time are associated with increased neurologic dysfunction.[21]

During HCA, a variety of cerebral protection techniques are employed to minimize neurologic damage that can occur secondary to emboli or from global ischemia. These include packing the head in ice, providing antegrade or retrograde cerebral circulation with strategically positioned catheters, and administering cerebral protective medications.[18,21] These techniques are listed in Box 16-3. Of these methods, the use of antegrade

---

Box 16-2

Indications for Aortic Surgery

Ascending aorta/aortic arch
- Symptomatic or rapidly expanding aneurysm
- Aneurysm >5.5 cm (or >5 cm in Marfan syndrome patient)[20]
- Aneurysm >4–5 cm if surgery needed for AI or AS[20]
- All acute Type A dissections

Descending thoracic
- Symptomatic or rapidly expanding aneurysm
- Aneurysm >6.5 cm in diameter (or >6 cm in Marfan syndrome patient)[20]
- Complicated acute Type B dissections

Thoracoabdominal
- Symptomatic or rapidly expanding aneurysm
- Aneurysm >5.5–6 cm[32]

Abdominal
- Symptomatic or rapidly expanding aneurysm[32]
- Aneurysm >5.5 cm in low-risk patients[32]
- Aneurysm >4.5–5 cm in women[32]

AI = Aortic insufficiency, AS = aortic stenosis.

Box 16-3

Techniques for Cerebral Protection

Hypothermia
- Systemic cooling
- Packing the head in ice

Cerebral perfusion
- Antegrade via the innominate or carotid artery
- Retrograde via the superior vena cava

Pharmacologic
- Barbiturates
- Steroids
- Lidocaine
- Magnesium
- Mannitol

cerebral perfusion is currently believed to convey the most neurologic benefit, with some suggesting that this provides the ability to safely extend the period of HCA to 90 minutes for complicated repairs.[18]

Repairs to the descending aorta are typically done via a left thoracotomy and may be performed with full, partial, or no CPB in an attempt to minimize ischemia to the spinal cord and the kidneys. When full bypass is used, femoral cannulation is generally performed. Distal perfusion may be augmented with left heart bypass, in which a centrifugal pump is used to circulate oxygenated blood between the left atrium and a point in the aorta distal to the surgical repair. HCA is an alternative operative approach, with a recent study indicating improved mortality and fewer complications (renal failure and paraplegia) when this technique was used for repair of the distal aorta.[76] For traumatic injuries or aneurysm rupture, a "clamp and go" technique may be used in which clamps are applied on both sides of the damaged area and the graft is quickly interpositioned. This method may also be used for uncomplicated aneurysm repairs in which the anticipated period for clamping the aorta is 30 minutes or less.[14,18]

The most devastating complication of surgery on the distal aorta is paraplegia, which occurs secondary to interruption of blood flow to the spinal cord. Patients with extensive thoracoabdominal aneurysms (Crawford I and II) and those with active dissection are at greatest risk, with a reported incidence as high as 20% in some studies.[12,14] The process for injury to the spinal cord is complex, and involves several factors—perfusion, metabolic demand, and reperfusion injury.[12] Several interventions have been used in an attempt to mitigate the risk of spinal cord injury, including regional hypothermic cooling of the spinal cord, perioperative drainage

of cerebral spinal fluid, maintenance of distal aortic perfusion with left heart bypass, and reimplantation of critical intercostal arteries into the graft. These techniques are briefly described in Table 16-4.

Pulmonary complications are also common after surgery on the descending or thoracoabdominal aorta. This is partially attributable to the high prevalence of smoking and COPD in this patient population. In addition, the surgery typically requires a period of one-lung ventilation as well as a thoracotomy incision and the need to cut through the diaphragm to access the aorta. Newer surgical approaches that protect the phrenic nerve and preserve as much diaphragm as possible have helped to improve outcomes somewhat, but the number of patients requiring mechanical ventilation longer than 48 hours is still as high as 11% to 34% in some series.[37,49] The incidence of tracheostomy in patients with pulmonary complications has been reported to be between 7% and 11%.[11,49]

Risk of compromised flow to the kidneys occurs as a consequence of the dissection/aneurysm itself, from the absence of perfusion during cross-clamping, and because of hypotension during the perioperative period. In addition, preoperative renal insufficiency and ruptured aneurysms are known predictors of acute postoperative renal failure.[11] Outcomes can be improved with adequate hydration, judicious use of contrast dye, distal perfusion techniques, and renal artery reconstruction when needed.[37]

During repair of an AAA, access is obtained via a midline incision or through a retroperitoneal approach. The latter approach is associated with a decrease in pulmonary complications.[1] In elective cases, heparinization is used to minimize the risk of embolic complications, but this is not feasible for repair of a ruptured aneurysm. Open repair consists of clamping the aorta first distally and then proximally, to isolate the aneurysm. The aneurysm is then incised and a Dacron tube graft is anastomosed to the proximal and distal aorta. If the iliac arteries are involved, a bifurcated graft may be used. Cross-clamping the proximal aorta is associated with an increase in cardiac workload, while cross-clamping the distal aorta results in temporary ischemia to the lower body, including the kidneys. Complications for this procedure include myocardial infarction, colon ischemia, renal failure, and lower extremity emboli/thrombosis.[1]

Interventional Therapies

Within the past decade, a number of interventional options have become available for the treatment of aortic conditions. Options to restore flow through the aorta now include endovascular placement of stents and catheter-guided fenestration.[61] Recent studies have

TABLE 16-4 Perioperative Strategies to Reduce Paraplegia

INTERVENTION	DESCRIPTION	RATIONALE
Hypothermia	Local cooling of spinal cord is accomplished by a continuous infusion of cold (20° C) isotonic saline into an epidural catheter inserted at T11–12 level.	Hypothermia decreases metabolic demands of tissues and increases tolerance to decreased perfusion.
Steroids	Intravenous boluses of steroids may be administered intraoperatively as well as postoperatively if patient exhibits signs of neurologic deficit.	Stabilizes cell membranes and inhibits inflammatory cell mediators.
Naloxone (Narcan)	Naloxone infusions are administered intravenously throughout surgery.	Antagonizes effects of endogenous opiates, which are believed to play a role in development of spinal cord ischemia.
Reattachment of spinal arteries	Anterior radicular artery is believed to be primary artery supplying spinal cord, but there is significant variability in perfusion among patients.	All patent lower intercostal arteries from T8 to T12 are reattached at time of surgery to supplement perfusion to spinal cord.[22]
Left heart bypass	Centrifugal pump is used to circulate blood from a cannula placed in left atrium to one positioned in femoral artery or descending aorta.	Oxygenated blood from left heart can improve perfusion to spinal vessels from distal aorta during surgery.
Cerebrospinal fluid drainage	Lumbar catheter is inserted into subarachnoid space to allow drainage of CSF to maintain a prescribed pressure (usually <10 mm Hg).[14]	CSF pressure rises with aortic cross-clamping and may impair perfusion to spinal cord. Drainage of CSF during and after surgery may improve blood flow into spinal cord, by relieving opposing pressure created by pressure in subarachnoid space.

CSF = Cerebrospinal fluid, mm Hg = millimeters of mercury.

shown that these techniques may offer improved outcomes, even in high-risk patients.[51,61]

Percutaneous balloon fenestration is used to create a tear in the dissection flap between the true and the false lumen, to restore flow into the aorta. A needle attached to a guidewire is positioned within the false lumen at the desired location, and a balloon catheter is used to create a tear.[61] Although this may restore flow to compromised arterial branches, it carries the risk of embolism from thrombosis within the false lumen as well as an increased risk for future arterial rupture.[61] An alternative is to use a fenestrated stent graft designed with openings that can be positioned to allow flow into branch arteries while maintaining patency of the aortic lumen.

Endovascular stent grafts were first used in the abdominal aorta in 1990. Initially used only in the elective repair of abdominal aneurysms, stent use has now evolved to include treatment of thoracic aneurysm and Type B dissections as well.[39,51] Aortic stent grafts are available in a variety of configurations—straight tube, bifurcated, branch graft—depending on the area of the aorta that requires repair. All of the grafts are deployed via the femoral artery, and positioned with the use of fluoroscopy.[61] Figure 16-4 shows an endovascular graft positioned in the thoracic aorta.

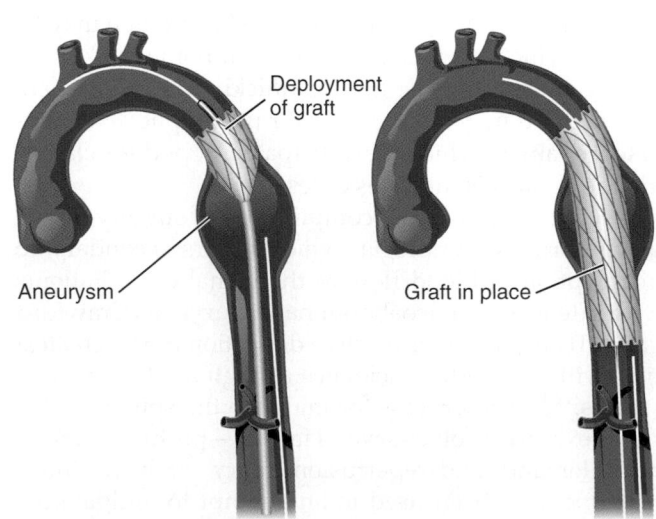

♦**FIGURE 16-4** Endovascular graft of the thoracic aorta.

Generally this procedure can be performed under epidural anesthesia, with minimal blood loss. As a result, these procedures may be performed in patients who would otherwise be deemed inoperable because of comorbid conditions. While the operative mortality and morbidity may be less with endovascular stents, randomized studies have shown no significant difference in long-term survival between open and endovascular interventions in patients with AAA.[6,27] Data on thoracic stents are more limited because of the newness of this technology, but a recent report indicated acceptable operative mortality and morbidity with stents placed for both elective and emergent repair of the thoracic aorta.[51,62]

Medical Management

Patients with uncomplicated Type B dissections, along with those patients with Type A dissections or aortic tears who are deemed too high a risk to undergo surgery, are usually managed medically. The goals of therapy include stabilizing the dissection or tear to prevent rupture and allow for healing, as well as reducing the risk of complications.[45] Treatment consists of BP control and reduction in the force of cardiac contraction, accomplished initially with intravenous agents such as beta blockers and vasodilators and later with oral medications. These pharmacologic options are listed in the Medication table below. Long-term therapy with beta blockers is considered important in patients with aortic aneurysms, to reduce the rate of aneurysm expansion. The beneficial effect of beta blockade on slowing aneurysmal growth has only been validated in patients with Marfan syndrome.[39] However, beta blockers are believed to be beneficial for the majority of patients with aortic disease, especially since they generally have concomitant hypertension and coronary artery disease—both well-established indications for beta-blocker therapy. BP control is essential and may include beta blockers, angiotensin-converting enzyme (ACE) inhibitors, or calcium channel blockers, to maintain the systolic pressure within a range of 100 to 110 mm Hg. Aggressive treatment of hypercholesterolemia and smoking cessation are also important management strategies for patients with either a dissection or an aneurysm.

Routine follow-up is performed both for medically managed patients and for those who have undergone either surgical or endovascular repair. This is to monitor for disease progression, as well as complications such as late dissection, development of additional aneurysms, and leaks from the endovascular stent.[61]

MEDICATIONS USED IN THE TREATMENT OF AORTIC EMERGENCIES

DRUG	DOSE	ACTIONS	SPECIAL CONSIDERATIONS
Enalapril (Vasotec)	0.625 mg IV over 5 min, then every 6 hr	Decreases blood pressure by inhibiting conversion of angiotensin I to angiotensin II (potent vasoconstrictor).	Especially useful in treatment of refractory HTN caused when AD impairs flow to kidneys, resulting in activation of RAAS.[31]
Esmolol (Brevibloc) Metoprolol (Lopressor)	0.25–0.5 mcg/kg bolus, followed by infusion of 50–200 mcg/kg/min OR 2.5–5 mg IV over 2 min; repeat up to total dose of 15 mg	Cardioselective agents block beta$_1$ receptors to decrease contractility and heart rate, thus decreasing BP.	Used alone or in combination with arterial vasodilators to decrease blood pressure and force of contraction.
Labetalol (Trandate)	Intermittent boluses of 20–40 mg administered over 2 min, or as infusion at 1–4 mg/min	Is a combined alpha and beta blocker. Blocks alpha receptors to decrease SVR and BP; blocks beta$_1$ receptors to prevent reflex tachycardia.	Helpful in setting of aortic dissection to decrease BP without reflexive increases in CO and HR. May be used intravenously in acute setting or as oral agent for long-term management. Maximum recommended cumulative dose per 24 hr is 300 mg.

Table continues on page 358

DRUG	DOSE	ACTIONS	SPECIAL CONSIDERATIONS
Diltiazem (Cardizem)	Bolus dose of 0.25 mg/kg IV over 2 min, followed by infusion of 5–15 mg/hr OR	Block calcium channels in myocardial tissue, decreasing both heart rate and contractility.	May be used to decrease heart rate and myocardial contractility in patients with contraindications to beta blockers.
Verapamil (Calan)	5–10 mg IV; may repeat in 15–30 min		
Nicardipine (Cardene)	2.5 mg over 5 min (may repeat × 4), followed by infusion at 2–4 mg/hr	Blocks transport of calcium into smooth muscle cells lining vasculature, causing vasodilation and decrease in SVR.	A titratable intravenous calcium channel blocker with onset of action between 5 and 15 min and duration of 4–6 hr.[87] May induce reflex tachycardia. Use cautiously in patients with renal/ hepatic impairment.
Fentanyl (Sublimaze)	25–100 mcg IV bolus OR 50–200 mcg/hr infusion	Stimulate opiate receptors in central nervous system to produce analgesia and sedation.	Pain control helps prevent exacerbations of tachycardia and hypertension.
Morphine sulfate	2–10 mg IV every 2–4 hr OR 1–5 mg/hr infusion		
Sodium nitroprusside (Nipride)	0.1–8 mcg/kg/min infusion	Relaxes arterial and venous smooth muscle to decrease both preload and afterload.	Commonly used because of rapid onset and short duration of action. May induce reflex tachycardia. May cause cyanide toxicity.
Phenylephrine (Neo-Synephrine)	10–100 mcg/min	Stimulates alpha receptors in vasculature to cause vasoconstriction.	May be used in setting of hypotension if fluid resuscitation fails to restore adequate blood pressure. Maximum rate is 300 mcg/min.

AD = Aortic dissection, CO = cardiac output, HTN = hypertension, SVR = systemic vascular resistance, RAAS = renin-angiotensin-aldosterone system.

MULTIDISCIPLINARY PLAN OF CARE

Patients with suspected aortic dissection or acute rupture of an aortic aneurysm are admitted to critical care for aggressive control of BP and vigilant monitoring. Frequent assessment, titration of vasoactive medications to targeted parameters, and pain management are essential nursing functions while the patient undergoes diagnostic tests and preparation for surgery as warranted. Support of the patient and family are important in light of the life-threatening nature of acute aortic syndromes.

Aortic aneurysms and dissection frequently occur in older adult patients with multiple comorbid conditions. At a minimum, most of these patients will have hypertension and diffuse atherosclerosis. Others may have diabetes mellitus, renal insufficiency, and chronic lung disease.[11] A plan of care must also address prevention of problems related to these conditions in order to optimize patient outcomes, as indicated in the Multidisciplinary Plan of Care on pp. 360-362.

Assessment

In the initial evaluation, the patient's hemodynamic status is assessed with the establishment of ECG monitoring and evaluation of BP in both arms. This allows for the detection of "pseudo" hypotension, which may occur in one arm if the dissection involves the brachiocephalic vessels.[78] An arterial line is then placed to allow for continuous monitoring of BP. Generally pressures are followed in the arm with the higher pressure, to allow for more accurate control of systemic BP.[64] Careful physical assessment is performed to assess for clues to the possible location of the dissection and to

Case Study 16-1, Part A

Thoracic Aortic Dissection

R.B. is a 62-year-old man who was transported to the emergency department after the sudden onset of tearing pain in his chest and upper back. The pain was unrelieved by changes in position and was not associated with shortness of breath, nausea, or vomiting. He had a history of hyperlipidemia and long-standing hypertension. Current medications included lovastatin (Mevacor) and captopril (Capoten). On admission, R.B.'s blood pressure was 168/92 mm Hg, his respiratory rate (RR) was 28 breaths/min, and he was afebrile. The ECG monitor showed sinus tachycardia without ectopy at a rate of 122 beats/min, and the pulse oximeter reading was 98% on room air. Lungs were clear to auscultation bilaterally, and there were no abnormal heart sounds or murmurs. Neurologically the patient was alert and oriented, but he presented with numbness and significant weakness in his left lower leg.

R.B. had two large-bore peripheral intravenous catheters inserted and was placed on oxygen via nasal cannula at 2 L/min. A 12-lead ECG was obtained, which showed nonspecific ST/T wave changes. Lab work was initiated immediately, and the troponin test was negative, whereas electrolytes, hematocrit, and hemoglobin were all within normal limits. A chest x-ray was also normal except for an abnormal aortic contour. A transesophageal echo performed at the bedside revealed a thoracic aortic dissection with true and false lumens extending from the left subclavian artery into the distal aorta. A CT scan of the aorta confirmed the presence of an aortic dissection that extended from the subclavian artery into the distal abdominal aorta. Vital signs at this time were as follows: heart rate (HR) 124 beats/min (sinus tachycardia), BP 176/92 mm Hg in the left arm and 184/88 mm Hg in the right arm, RR 30 breaths/min, Spo2 97%.

Decision point: What interventions should be implemented at this time?

Case continues on page 365

establish a baseline for comparison of ongoing assessment. Bilateral pulses are assessed and a rapid neurologic assessment is performed to detect gross motor or sensory deficits as well as signs of impaired cerebral circulation, such as confusion or decreased level of consciousness.[48] Cardiac assessment focuses on the presence of a diastolic murmur (indicative of an incompetent aortic valve) and the symptoms of cardiac tamponade, such as increased jugular venous pressure, muffled heart sounds, or pulsus paradoxus. Stable patients who are able to maintain adequate gas exchange are provided supplemental oxygen to optimize delivery to the tissues. Patients with respiratory compromise may require urgent intubation. A urinary catheter is inserted to measure hourly changes in urine output, which can provide clues to decreased renal perfusion.

Lab work typically includes hemoglobin and hematocrit to evaluate blood loss secondary to potential rupture and hemorrhage. Blood urea nitrogen (BUN) and creatinine levels are used to evaluate renal function. Cardiac enzymes can be used to detect myocardial damage secondary to involvement of the coronary arteries.

Blood Pressure Control

The initial therapeutic goal for a patient who presents with hypertension is reduction of systolic BP to the lowest level commensurate with adequate vital organ (e.g., cardiac, cerebral, renal) perfusion. Intravenous pharmacologic agents are used to reduce the systolic BP to around 100 to 110 mm Hg and the heart rate to 60 to 80 beats per minute.[31,78] Typically beta blockers such as esmolol (Brevibloc) or metoprolol (Lopressor) are used first, with the addition of vasodilators as needed to achieve the desired BP.[46] The sequence is important, because the initiation of a vasodilator before beta blockade can result in a reflexive increase in heart rate and contractility. This response, mediated by the sympathetic nervous system, could increase the dP/dT in the aorta and lead to extension of the dissection or aortic rupture. If beta blockers are contraindicated, calcium channel blockers that decrease heart rate and contractility, such as diltiazem (Cardizem) or verapamil (Calan), may also be used.[85]

Hypotensive patients require assessment for "pseudo" hypotension, which may occur if the dissection involves the brachiocephalic vessels. In this case there may be a significant difference in BP between the two arms; therefore bilateral BP should be evaluated in a patient with suspected aortic dissection. If hypotension is confirmed, then the patient is assessed for myocardial causes (acute ischemia, aortic regurgitation, or tamponade) as well as acute rupture (hypovolemia and decreased hematocrit). These patients typically require fluid resuscitation and may need vasopressor support until they can be taken to the operating room.

Pain Control

Pain control is often difficult in the setting of acute aortic emergencies because it occurs secondary to ischemia or pressure on adjacent organs. Morphine or fentanyl (Sublimaze) may be prescribed to help blunt

MULTIDISCIPLINARY PLAN OF CARE FOR AORTIC EMERGENCIES

PROBLEM	INTERVENTION	RATIONALE	EXPECTED OUTCOME	COMMENTS
Potential extension of aortic dissection or rupture of aorta	Establish baseline assessment of patient, followed by serial assessments to detect changes. Assessment should include: LOC, motor and sensory function Ischemic changes on ECG, presence of murmurs, signs of tamponade Bilateral pulses and BP Urine output, BUN, creatinine Breath sounds, Sao$_2$ In setting of HTN, administer intravenous agents to decrease blood pressure and HR. In setting of hypotension, administer volume and vasopressors as needed to support organ perfusion. Administer analgesics and sedation as needed.	Assessment provides clues to location of dissection and involvement of other structures, such as aortic valve, brachiocephalic vessels, vessels perfusing spinal cord, and renal arteries. Continued stress from blood pressure and force of contraction can propagate dissection. Patients with rupture or dissection involving critical structures (aortic valve, coronary arteries) may present with significant hypotension. Dissection creates pain, which can exacerbate blood pressure and tachycardia.	Significant changes noted and reported promptly. Systolic BP 100–110 mm Hg. HR 60–80 beats/min. Patient reports pain at tolerable level.	BP should be evaluated bilaterally before initiating treatment, to rule out "pseudo" hypotension created by dissection into brachiocephalic vessels.

Postoperative

PROBLEM	INTERVENTION	RATIONALE	EXPECTED OUTCOME	COMMENTS
Potential for complications related to use of hypothermic circulatory arrest, including hypothermia, bleeding, and neurologic injuries	*Hypothermia* Continuously monitor temperature. Apply warm-air blankets as needed for T <36° C. Administer meperidine as needed to treat shivering.	Temperature "afterdrop" may occur after arrival in unit. Hypothermia has several negative consequences, including bleeding, vasoconstriction, and dysrhythmias. Shivering increases oxygen demand and CO$_2$ production.	Patient is normothermic.	Fluid warmers may be useful, especially if blood products are being administered.
	Bleeding Maintain patency of chest tubes. Monitor postoperative lab results for Hct/Hgb, aPTT, and platelets; obtain additional coagulation studies for continued bleeding. Administer blood products and medications for bleeding as warranted (described in the	Facilitates drainage of mediastinal or pleural space. Laboratory tests help to guide treatment. For example, RBCs may be needed for low Hct/Hgb, while protamine may be required if aPTT is elevated. Increased pressure puts stress on suture lines and cannulation sites.	Chest tube output tapers to <100 ml in 8 hr. PT/aPTT within normal limits. Hct less than 28% or as ordered.	An acute increase in bleeding could signal leakage at graft anastomosis. Higher hematocrit and hemoglobin values may be needed in patients with vascular disease, to decrease risk of MI and spinal cord ischemia.[3] Risk of bleeding must be balanced

PROBLEM	INTERVENTION	RATIONALE	EXPECTED OUTCOME	COMMENTS
	Medication table on pp. 309-310). Maintain MAP 70–80 mm Hg in patients who are actively bleeding.			with need to optimize perfusion to vital organs.
	Neurologic Dysfunction Allow patient to awaken as soon as possible, to evaluate neurologic status. Complete assessment of cognitive function, as well as gross motor movement and sensation.	Impaired perfusion to brain and spinal cord may occur during period of circulatory arrest, or as result of emboli or debris from surgical procedure.	Alert and oriented ×3. Able to move all extremities to command. No sensory deficits.	
Potential for ischemic complications related to location of aortic injury, surgical approach, and preexisting disease	*Myocardial Ischemia* Continuously monitor ECG, including ST segment monitoring. Administer perioperative beta blockers as ordered.	Allows for early detection of ischemia or dysrhythmias. Perioperative use of beta blockers has been shown to decrease incidence of MI in patients with vascular disease.[7,44]	Sinus rhythm adequate to maintain cardiac output and blood pressure.	There is a high risk for cardiac ischemia in this population, secondary to preexisting CAD. Patients with defects in ascending aorta may also have involvement of coronary arteries.
	Spinal Cord Ischemia/Paraplegia Optimize perfusion to spinal cord by maintaining adequate blood pressure. If a lumbar drain is placed, maintain system at prescribed level and drain CSF as needed to maintain CSF pressure <10 mm Hg. Perform hourly assessments for neurologic impairment, including numbness, tingling, or weakness in lower extremities.	Patients undergoing repair of descending aorta are at increased risk for ischemia to spinal cord. CSF drainage can improve perfusion into spinal cord, by decreasing opposing pressure within spinal column. If neurologic deficits are detected, they may be reversed with interventions such as draining CSF, increasing SBP, and administering steroids as ordered.	MAP >80 mm Hg. SBP >100 mm Hg. CSF pressure <10 mm Hg.	Adequate hemoglobin and Sao_2 are also needed to optimize tissue perfusion. Patients should also be evaluated for complications related to CSF drain, such as infection (fever, headache, nuchal rigidity, or cloudy CSF).
	Renal Dysfunction Monitor urine output hourly. Monitor filling pressures and maintain preload with fluids as needed. Maintain adequate blood pressure for renal perfusion.	Renal failure may occur secondary to perioperative hypotension, hypovolemia, use of contrast dye, impaired perfusion during cross-clamping, or preexisting renal disease.	Urine output >50 ml/hr. CVP 8–10 mm Hg. MAP >80 mm Hg.	If acute renal failure occurs, CRRT may be used to remove fluid and wastes while avoiding hemodynamic instability.

Table continues on page 362

PROBLEM	INTERVENTION	RATIONALE	EXPECTED OUTCOME	COMMENTS
	GI Dysfunction Maintain NG tube to low continuous suction until bowel sounds are present. Monitor patient for signs of ischemic bowel, including abdominal pain and distention, persistent acidosis, elevated WBCs, and diarrhea.	Patients are at risk for an ileus postoperatively, especially with repairs of abdominal aorta. There is also a risk for ischemic colitis secondary to impaired perfusion to colon.	Bowel sounds present in all quadrants.	
	Distal Embolization Perform neurovascular checks to distal extremities: motor function, sensation, capillary refill, and pulses.	Cross-clamping or emboli may compromise flow to lower extremities.	Distal pulses present bilaterally by Doppler or palpation.	
Pulmonary dysfunction	Monitor Sao$_2$ and provide supplemental O$_2$ as needed. Maintain mechanical ventilation as needed until criteria for extubation are met. Reposition frequently and get patient out of bed to chair 1–2 × shift. Encourage use of IS every 1–2 hr. Instruct patient in use of cough pillow. Provide adequate analgesia to promote increased activity without inducing respiratory depression.	Early extubation decreases pulmonary complications and facilitates mobility. Mobilization and deep breathing help reverse atelectasis that occurs during surgery. Oversedation may lead to reintubation.	Sao$_2$ maintained greater than 92%. Extubate within 12 hr of surgery if possible.	Patients with poor preoperative pulmonary function may require prolonged mechanical ventilation and tracheostomy placement to facilitate weaning. Continuous infusions or PCAs may be helpful in providing adequate pain relief without oversedation.

aPTT = Activated partial thromboplastin time, BP = blood pressure, BUN = blood urea nitrogen, CAD = coronary artery disease, CO$_2$ = carbon dioxide, CRRT = continuous renal replacement therapy, CSF = cerebrospinal fluid, CT = chest tube, CVP = central venous pressure, ECG = electrocardiogram, GI = gastrointestinal, Hct = hematocrit, Hgb = hemoglobin, HTN = hypertension, HR = heart rate, IS = incentive spirometer, LOC = level of consciousness, MAP = mean arterial pressure, MI = myocardial infarction, NG = nasogastric, O$_2$ = oxygen, PCA = patient-controlled analgesia, PT = prothrombin time, RBCs = red blood cells, Sao$_2$ = arterial oxygen saturation, SBP = systolic blood pressure, T = temperature, mg/dl = milligrams per deciliter, mm Hg = millimeters of mercury.

the pain response, administered either intermittently or by continuous infusion. These may be combined with sedative agents such as midazolam (Versed) or propofol (Diprivan), especially if deeper sedation is required to achieve hemodynamic stability.

Postoperative Management

If the patient undergoes surgery for repair of the aorta, postoperative care will include monitoring for complications related to the procedure. This care is similar to that required for patients following cardiac surgery (Chapter 14), although the mortality and morbidity associated with surgery on the thoracic aorta, especially if performed urgently, is much greater.[74,75] This chapter will address primarily those postoperative issues that are unique to surgery performed on the aorta, including sequelae of HCA and ischemic risks related to interrupting blood supply to the distal aorta.

HCA Complications. Although patients are rewarmed at the end of the case, they may experience a significant drop in temperature after initial rewarming and present to critical care with hypothermia. To counteract the problems associated with hypothermia (hypertension, dysrhythmias, coagulopathy), aggressive interventions to rewarm the patient are used. The patient's core temperature is monitored continuously through the pulmonary artery catheter, and warming blankets and fluid warmers are used as needed. If the patient exhibits shivering, meperidine (Demerol) may be administered intravenously in doses of 12.5 to 25 mg every 20 minutes until shivering is controlled.

The extensive operative time required for cooling and warming the patient increases the risk for significant coagulopathy. Bleeding is monitored via chest tube drainage, and interventions include rewarming the patient, administering antifibrinolytic medications, and transfusing blood products as necessary. Hematocrit, platelet count, and coagulation studies are obtained in bleeding patients to guide appropriate therapy. The threshold for blood transfusion in this patient population is controversial, but many surgeons prefer to keep the hematocrit at 28% or the hemoglobin level between 9 and 10 g/dl to optimize tissue perfusion.[3]

Because HCA also increases the risk for neurologic deficits, patients are allowed to awaken as soon as feasible postoperatively to evaluate their neurologic status. After a gross assessment of central and peripheral neurologic function is performed, patients may be resedated to promote hemodynamic stability and facilitate hemostasis.

Neurologic Complications. Following surgical repair of the descending and thoracoabdominal aorta, patients

are assessed for potential injury to the spinal cord. A number of interventions are used to mitigate the risk of paraplegia. For example, the patient's mean arterial pressure (MAP) may be maintained somewhat higher than preoperative levels (80 to 90 mm Hg) to optimize organ perfusion, especially to the spinal cord.[12] Blood products are administered as needed to maintain a hemoglobin level that is adequate to supply oxygen to vital tissues. Supplemental oxygen is provided to prevent hypoxemia.[28]

If a lumbar drain is placed to improve spinal cord perfusion, nursing care includes maintaining the drain at the proper level (generally the level of the insertion site) and draining the cerebrospinal fluid (CSF) via gravity, either continuously or intermittently, to maintain the pressure within the subarachnoid space at the prescribed level.[71] One recent study, cited in the Research Utilization box below, showed improved neurologic outcomes when the pressure within the spinal column was maintained at 10 mm Hg.[14] Patients are also assessed for complications related to the lumbar drain (such as infection, elevated temperature, nuchal rigidity, headache, or cloudy CSF). Typically, the drain is maintained for 48 to 72 hours, but may be used longer if the patient presents with neurologic impairment. Delayed neurologic deficits may also occur, typically preceded by hypotension, hypoxemia, or a low hemoglobin level.[54] If recognized immediately, these deficits may sometimes be reversed by increasing MAP, draining CSF, and administering protective agents such as steroids.[28]

♦ RESEARCH UTILIZATION

Impact of Cerebrospinal Fluid Drainage on the Incidence of Spinal Cord Deficits

CLINICAL ISSUE

Despite the use of a number of strategies to prevent spinal cord ischemia, paraplegia remains one of the most devastating consequences of thoracoabdominal aortic aneurysm repair. Although drainage of cerebrospinal fluid (CSF) is often used as an adjunct to prevent spinal cord ischemia, its benefit is not proven. This study was performed to evaluate the impact of CSF drainage on the incidence of spinal cord deficits.

SUMMARY

A total of 145 patients undergoing surgery for Crawford Type I or Type II thoracoabdominal aneurysms were randomized to have the procedure performed with CSF drainage ($n = 76$) or without CSF drainage ($n = 69$). A consistent intraoperative strategy was used

Box continues on p. 364

that included moderate heparinization, mild hypothermia, left heart bypass, and reattachment of patent critical intercostal arteries. Patients who received CSF drainage had the therapy initiated intraoperatively and continued for 48 hours after surgery, with a target CSF pressure of 10 mm Hg. Nine patients (13%) in the control group had paraplegia or paraparesis develop, whereas only two patients (2.6%) in the CSF drainage group had deficits develop.

APPLICATION

There is some evidence that perioperative cerebrospinal fluid drainage can reduce the rate of paraplegia after surgical repair of Type I and Type II thoracoabdominal aneurysms. Based on this study, a reasonable target for CSF pressure would be 10 mm Hg, with either continuous or intermittent drainage to achieve this goal. Because the mechanism of spinal cord injury is not fully understood and is considered to be multifactorial, CSF drainage can be recommended as only one strategy for prevention of neurologic deficits. For example, other researchers have found that perioperative hypotension (MAP less than 70 mm Hg) is a significant predictor of spinal cord injury,[12] so maintaining an adequate blood pressure may be equally important in preventing paraplegia.

NEED FOR FURTHER STUDY

Additional randomized studies are needed on the efficacy of CSF drainage as well as on the mechanisms that lead to spinal cord injury. The optimum duration of catheter placement also warrants further study, as some investigators have reported delayed neurologic deficits in this patient population.[28,54]

Coselli, J. S., et al. (2002). Cerebrospinal fluid drainage reduces paraplegia after thoracoabdominal aortic aneurysm repair: results of a randomized clinical trial. *J Vasc Surg, 35,* 631–639.

Myocardial Infarction. Because atherosclerosis is a risk factor for aneurysm and dissection, patients with aortic disease generally have coronary artery disease as well. Patients are monitored for myocardial infarction (MI) during the perioperative period, with continuous ECG monitoring that includes ST segment analysis (Chapter 10). Perioperative beta blockers may also be prescribed, because they have been shown to decrease the risk of MI in the high-risk vascular patient population.[7,44] Postoperative patients are also at risk for atrial dysrhythmias and may receive additional benefits from the antidysrhythmic effects of beta blockers.

Pulmonary Dysfunction. Patients generally arrive in the critical care unit intubated, with the goal of weaning to extubation as soon as feasible. Unstable patients may

be sedated for a period of time until hemodynamic stability and hemostasis are achieved. As patients are allowed to awaken, adequate pain management is important to facilitate respiratory efforts, especially in patients who have undergone a thoracotomy.

Patients with poor preoperative pulmonary function may require prolonged mechanical ventilation and tracheostomy placement to facilitate weaning. In addition, patients who have received large quantities of blood products as a result of hemorrhage from the aortic injury or a perioperative coagulopathy are at increased risk for acute lung injury. These patients may develop signs of acute respiratory distress syndrome (ARDS) in the postoperative period and require complex ventilatory management.

Gastrointestinal Dysfunction. A nasogastric tube is usually placed intraoperatively, especially if the abdominal cavity is entered during surgery. Once patients are

---

▲▼ NUTRITION

Diet for Patients With Vascular Disease

CALORIES
- 25 kcal/kg/day

PROTEIN
- 1.2–1.5 g/kg/day

FLUID
- Fluid restriction may be required, especially for patients with renal failure.

ELECTROLYTES
- Potassium replacement for levels less than 4.5 mEq/L
- Sodium restriction of 2000–3000 mg/day

VITAMINS AND MINERALS
- Multivitamins may be prescribed for patients with decreased intake.
- Folate and vitamins B_{12} and B_6 have been found to correct high homocysteine levels and could be useful in hypertensive patients.[66]

SPECIAL CONSIDERATIONS
Generally a diet rich in fruits, vegetables, and grains with reduced saturated fats is recommended for patients with vascular disease. For patients with hypertension, the diet should also include foods that are rich in potassium, calcium, and magnesium as well as the incorporation of omega-3 fatty acids, such as those found in fish oil.[53] Salt restriction to less than 2400 mg (about 1 teaspoon) a day is also recommended for people with hypertension. Diabetic patients will usually resume their preoperative diabetic diet.

extubated, they can generally resume oral intake as long as bowel sounds are present (see the Nutrition box on p. 364). If the patient requires mechanical ventilation for a prolonged period, a feeding tube is placed to allow for enteral feeding when bowel activity returns.

Although rare, patients may develop a paralytic ileus postoperatively, especially when an abdominal aneurysm is repaired. Approximately half of the patients who survive a ruptured abdominal aneurysm will develop some degree of ischemic colitis, which may be limited to the mucosa or involve the full thickness of the colon.[3] Symptoms include abdominal distention, bloody diarrhea, leukocytosis, fever, and persistent acidosis. If the colitis is superficial, it usually resolves on its own. If necrosis occurs, rapid surgical repair is required to limit contamination of the peritoneal cavity.[1]

Renal Dysfunction. Urine output is monitored hourly, along with cardiac filling pressures such as central venous pressure (CVP) or pulmonary artery pressure (PAP), as available. Adequate hydration and maintenance of an adequate MAP are essential to preserving renal function. Some surgeons also advocate the use of mannitol (Osmitrol) or furosemide (Lasix) intraoperatively to promote adequate urine output.[1,3] Daily BUN and creatinine values are helpful in identifying renal dysfunction. If acute renal failure occurs, continuous renal replacement therapy is often employed to assist with fluid and waste removal while minimizing hemodynamic instability.

Lower-Extremity Thrombosis. Following surgery on the aorta, patients are also monitored for signs of embolization to the lower extremities. Thrombosis may occur in arterial vessels—leading to diminished or absent pulses—or in the microcirculation, where it causes cutaneous necrosis. Toes and feet are often affected, and the condition may be referred to as "trash foot."[1,3] Patients present with painful, mottled areas on the plantar surface of the feet or cyanotic toes. Treatment generally includes supportive wound care and pain control.

◆ Case Study 16-1, Part B

Thoracic Aortic Dissection

R.B. underwent surgical repair of the descending thoracic aorta via a left thoracotomy. The procedure was performed with left heart bypass. He arrived in critical care intubated and on a propofol (Diprivan) infusion. He had a pulmonary artery catheter in the right internal jugular vein and a left radial arterial line. His vital signs were as follows: HR 80 beats/min (sinus rhythm), BP 130/68 mm Hg (MAP 90 mm Hg), pulmonary artery wedge pressure (PAWP) 10 mm Hg, right atrial

(RA) pressure 6 mm Hg, cardiac index (CI) 2.3 L/min/m², systemic vascular resistance (SVR) 960 dynes/sec/cm⁻⁵. An esmolol (Brevibloc) drip was infusing at 100 mcg/kg/min. He had a cerebrospinal fluid (CSF) catheter in place with orders to drain as needed to maintain a CSF pressure of <10 mm Hg. His urine catheter was draining clear yellow urine. Pedal pulses were present by Doppler bilaterally.

During the first hour in critical care, R.B.'s chest tubes drained 200 ml of sanguineous drainage. His postoperative hematocrit was 24%, hemoglobin 8 g/dl, and PTT 37. He received fresh frozen plasma (FFP) and 1 unit of packed red blood cells (PRBC) per order. He was started on a nicardipine (Cardene) drip with orders to titrate to keep his MAP at 70 to 80 mm Hg. Ninety minutes after arrival in critical care, his propofol drip was weaned off and he was allowed to awaken. He moved all extremities to command. He was started on a fentanyl (Sublimaze) drip at 0.01 mcg/kg/min.

R.B. remained hemodynamically stable throughout the night. Urine output remained 50 to 100 ml/hr. The next morning he was extubated without difficulty and placed on oxygen 2 L per nasal cannula, with an SpO₂ value of 95%. Bowel sounds were present, so his NG tube was discontinued and he resumed a clear liquid diet. The nicardipine and esmolol drips were weaned off, and he was started on oral labetalol (Trandate). Two hours later R.B.'s BP decreased to 100/58 mm Hg (MAP 70 mm Hg). He complained of numbness in both legs, and he was unable to lift his left leg off the bed. Pedal pulses were palpable bilaterally.

Decision point:. What interventions should be performed at this time?

EMERGENCIES INVOLVING ARTERIES AND VEINS

Vascular emergencies may also occur when thrombi, emboli, or acute trauma compromise peripheral perfusion, resulting in a patient presenting with acute arterial or venous occlusion. The term *peripheral vascular disease* (PVD) is used to describe a group of diseases and syndromes that involve the arterial, venous, or lymphatic system. PVD of the lower extremities causes chronic disability and significantly decreases quality of life. The prevalence of arterial PVD is 10% for persons older than 65 years.[19] PVD can present as acute arterial or venous occlusion. Other disorders of the peripheral vascular system can result from traumatic injuries.

Acute Peripheral Arterial Occlusions

Etiology. Arterial disease restricts blood flow through the aorta and its branches and affects an estimated

8 to 10 million persons in the United States.[68] Atherosclerosis is the predominant underlying factor contributing to PVD. This disease affects the medium-size and large arteries, decreasing blood flow so that it becomes insufficient to meet metabolic demands. Atherosclerosis is an insidious and irreversible process. As the disease progresses, fatty streaks, fibroid plaque, calcification, and thrombus formation result in arterial wall thickening, hardening, and loss of elasticity. This process may lead to stenosis and eventual occlusion. Peripheral arterial occlusion may result in acute or chronic ischemia.

Acute ischemia is caused by a ruptured proximal atherosclerotic plaque; acute thrombosis on preexisting atherosclerotic disease; an embolism from the heart, aorta, or other large vessel; or a dissected aneurysm. Lower extremity arterial disease (LEAD) is associated with acute limb ischemia and may be a result of acute arterial occlusion or chronic arterial insufficiency. Multiple factors predispose patients for thrombosis. These include sepsis, hypotension, low cardiac output, aneurysms, aortic dissection, bypass grafts, atrial fibrillation, and underlying atherosclerotic narrowing of the arterial lumen.[32]

Atherothrombosis has been used to describe the unpredictable, sudden disruption of a plaque that leads to thrombus formation. The atherosclerotic plaque may be focal or diffuse, may grow slowly, or may rapidly occlude the lumen. Thromboses are often of an atheromatous nature and occur in the lower extremities more frequently than in the upper extremities. In the case of acute occlusion, there is insufficient time for collateral circulation to develop, resulting in sudden ischemic changes. The extent of arterial insufficiency is relative to the location and severity of the lesion and the presence of collateral vessels. Arterial insufficiency and ischemia occur acutely in patients with arterial embolism and spasm. Arterial occlusive disease can lead to chronic pain, nonhealing ulcers, gangrene, and amputation.

Emboli, the most common cause of sudden ischemia, usually originate in the heart (80%); on the other hand, they may also originate from proximal atheroma, tumor, or foreign objects.[77] Emboli tend to lodge at artery bifurcations or in areas where vessels abruptly narrow—the femoral artery bifurcation is the most common site (43%), followed by the iliac arteries (18%), the aorta (15%), and the popliteal artery (15%).[77] The severity of the acute manifestation is determined by the site of occlusion, the presence of collateral circulation, and the nature of the occlusion (thrombus or embolus). Emboli tend to carry higher morbidity because the extremity has not had time to develop collateral circulation.

The usual risk factors involved in development of atherosclerosis are seen in PVD patients. Patients with vascular disease often are older adults and may have one or more associated medical problems such as diabetes mellitus, chronic obstructive lung disease, coronary artery disease, or renal disease.[25,32] Smoking, hyperlipidemia, hyperhomocysteinemia, elevated C-reactive protein, and diabetes are also major risk factors associated with PVD.[32] Common sites of stenosis or occlusion include the aortoiliac, femoropopliteal, and tibial arteries. The most commonly affected site is the superficial femoral artery segment. The disease process is often bilateral because of its systemic nature and tends to manifest in the later years of life.

Patients with symptoms of PAD can be classified into one of five stages (Table 16-5). Patients in stages III and IV are those with "critical ischemia" whose

TABLE 16-5 Classification of Peripheral Arterial Disease: Fontaine's Stages and Rutherford's Categories

	Fontaine		Rutherford		
STAGE	CLINICAL	GRADE	CATEGORY		CLINICAL
I	Asymptomatic	0	0		Asymptomatic
IIa	Mild claudication	I	1		Mild claudication
IIb	Moderate-severe claudication	I	2		Moderate claudication
		I	3		Severe claudication
III	Ischemic rest pain	II	4		Ischemic rest pain
IV	Ulceration or gangrene	III	5		Minor tissue loss
		IV	6		Ulceration or gangrene

From reference 19.

limbs may be threatened. Invasive diagnostic procedures are justified for patients in these stages.[32]

Clinical Findings. Acute limb ischemia is a situation requiring prompt diagnosis and treatment to preserve the limb and prevent systemic illness or death that might result from the metabolic abnormalities associated with tissue necrosis.[32] Patients presenting with acute arterial occlusion leading to limb ischemia have the hallmark signs known as the "5 Ps": sudden onset of *pain, pulselessness, paresthesias, pallor,* and *paralysis.* A sixth P, *"polar,"* indicating a cold extremity, may also be included. A late finding may be poikilothermia, a skin condition characterized by pigmentation, telangiectasis, purpura, pruritus, and atrophy of the area.

Acute occlusion can cause severe ischemia with sensory and motor loss. Patients may present with a severely ischemic foot that is painful, cold, and often numb. Sudden onset or worsening of symptoms, a known embolic source, and the absence of previous claudication or other manifestations of obstructive arterial disease are suggestive of arterial embolism. A review of assessment priorities in a patient presenting with limb pain is included in Box 16-4. The presence of normal arterial pulses and Doppler systolic BP in the contralateral limb is another finding of acute occlusion.

An ischemic limb is often a marble white color, becoming more prominent in the lower leg and foot. Excessive deoxygenation of the blood in the skin capillaries gives the foot a purple-blue cyanosed appearance in the dependent position, but the blue fades to white when the leg is horizontal. The degree of elevation pallor can be assessed. The legs are elevated to about 60 degrees when the patient lies on the bed, and the color of the soles of the feet is observed. If the feet become pale, this confirms that the patient has peripheral arterial occlusive disease. The grading is based on how long it takes for the extremity to turn pale (Table 16-6). Unrelenting pain aggravated by leg elevation (preventing the patient from sleeping) along with pain relief from hanging the foot over the bedside can be other clues to disease progression. As ischemia worsens, ulcerations may form.

Another finding that can be found in an ischemic leg is called "dependency rubor." After elevating the leg, the patient is asked to sit up and hang his feet over the side of the bed. A normal leg will remain a healthy pink color. An ischemic leg will slowly turn from white to pink and then become a flushed purple-red color. This is caused by blood filling the dilated skin capillaries, and the color is attributable to deoxygenated blood. This indicates that the patient has critical limb ischemia.

Narrowing of the distal aorta indicating chronic peripheral arterial insufficiency can present as Leriche syndrome. Intermittent claudication, impotence, and

---

Box 16-4

Peripheral Vascular Assessment

History
- Myocardial infarction, angina, or cerebrovascular disease

Pain
- Intermittent claudication: cramping, burning, aching, pain caused by ambulation and relieved by rest
- Rest pain: cramping, burning, stinging, aching, or sharp pain in the toes, forefoot, or heel, often at night
- Location: buttock or thigh pain resulting from lesions in the abdominal aorta or iliac artery; calf pain caused by lesions in the superficial femoral artery

Circulation
- Decreased capillary refill >2 seconds, diminished pulses, cold/cool skin temperature in affected extremity, and decreased toe temperature because of arterial obstruction in the extremity
- Auscultation: bruits over the affected vessels as a result of turbulent blood flow caused by stenosis
- Color: persistent cyanosis, elevation pallor, increased pigmentation, or dependent rubor can indicate severe ischemia

Neurologic
- Paresthesia of extremity; syncope or alterations in level of consciousness resulting from cerebrovascular lesions

Genitourinary
- Impotence due to aortic iliac occlusion

Other
- Hair loss, thickened toenails, stasis dermatitis, gangrenous lesions, chronic ulcers caused by inadequate perfusion

---

significantly decreased or absent femoral pulses are seen with this syndrome. Advanced PVD may manifest as mottling in a "fishnet pattern" (livedo reticularis), pulselessness, numbness, or cyanosis of the involved extremity. Paralysis may follow, and the limb may become cold and gangrenous. Poorly healing injuries or ulcers in the extremities help provide evidence of preexisting PVD.[77]

Diagnosis. Diagnostic evaluation of critical limb ischemia (CLI) is used to confirm the diagnosis, localize the responsible lesion, gauge the relative severity, and assess the hemodynamic requirements for successful revascularization and endovascular or operative risk.

TABLE 16-6 Grading of Elevation Pallor

GRADING	DURATION OF ELEVATION
0	No pallor
1+	Pallor >60 sec
2+	Pallor 30–60 sec
3+	Pallor <30 sec
4+	Pallor at level

From www.umanitoba.ca/faculties/medicine/surgery/vascular/lectures/index.html

Patients should receive a resting ECG, as well as baseline hematologic and biochemical tests, including complete blood count (CBC), platelet count, fasting blood glucose, hemoglobin A_{1c}, creatinine, fasting lipid profile, and urinalysis to assess for glycosuria and proteinuria.

Continuous-wave Doppler ultrasound can be used to detect sound waves as blood moves through a vessel. This test is useful to determine lower extremity anatomy as well as the severity and progression of the disease. Diminished sound waves are caused by arterial obstruction. Pulse volume recordings can be used to monitor limb perfusion and predict the outcome in CLI and risk of amputation.[32] Duplex ultrasound can be used to define the severity of lower extremity arterial stenoses and is a useful tool for monitoring patients after surgical bypass. Arterial and venous Doppler signals can be useful in identifying the clinical category of acute limb ischemia (Table 16-7).[42]

Ankle/brachial index (ABI) is used to establish a PAD diagnosis in the lower extremities (Figure 16-5). After the patient is positioned supine, the brachial and ankle systolic pressure measurements are obtained. Measure the systolic brachial pressure in both the left and the right arms. There should be a difference of less than 10 mm Hg between each brachial pressure measurement. Select the higher of these two values as the brachial artery pressure measurement. Apply the BP cuff around the ankle above the malleolus and measure the pressure of both the anterior and posterior tibial arteries. Inflate to 20 mm Hg above the current brachial systolic BP. Note the reappearance of the Doppler signal as the cuff deflates. Normally, the ankle pressure is the same or higher than the brachial pressure. Divide the higher systolic pressure of the tibial measurement by the highest of the brachial pressures to determine the ratio. ABIs as high as 1.3 can be normal; abnormal values are those less than 0.9 (Table 16-8). Diabetes and heavily calcified vessels can produce an artifactually elevated ankle pressure, which can underestimate disease severity. In these patients, toe pressure determinations more accurately reflect perfusion.[68]

Segmental plethysmography can provide data to predict limb survival, wound healing, and patient survival. This test measures arterial blood volume changes that occur in the lower extremities during the cardiac cycle. BP cuffs are placed on the thigh, calf, and ankle and pulsed waveform recordings are obtained. Pulse

TABLE 16-7 Clinical Categories of Acute Limb Ischemia

CATEGORY	DESCRIPTION/PROGNOSIS	SENSORY LOSS	MUSCLE WEAKNESS	ARTERIAL DOPPLER SIGNAL	VENOUS DOPPLER SIGNAL
Viable	Not immediately threatened	None	None	Audible	Audible
Threatened marginally	Salvageable if promptly treated	Minimal (toes) or none	None	Often inaudible	Audible
Threatened immediately	Salvageable with immediate revascularization	More than toes Pain associated with rest	Mild, moderate	Usually inaudible	Audible
Irreversible	Major tissue loss or permanent nerve damage	Profound anesthetic	Profound paralysis (rigor)	Inaudible	Inaudible

Reprinted from reference 42.

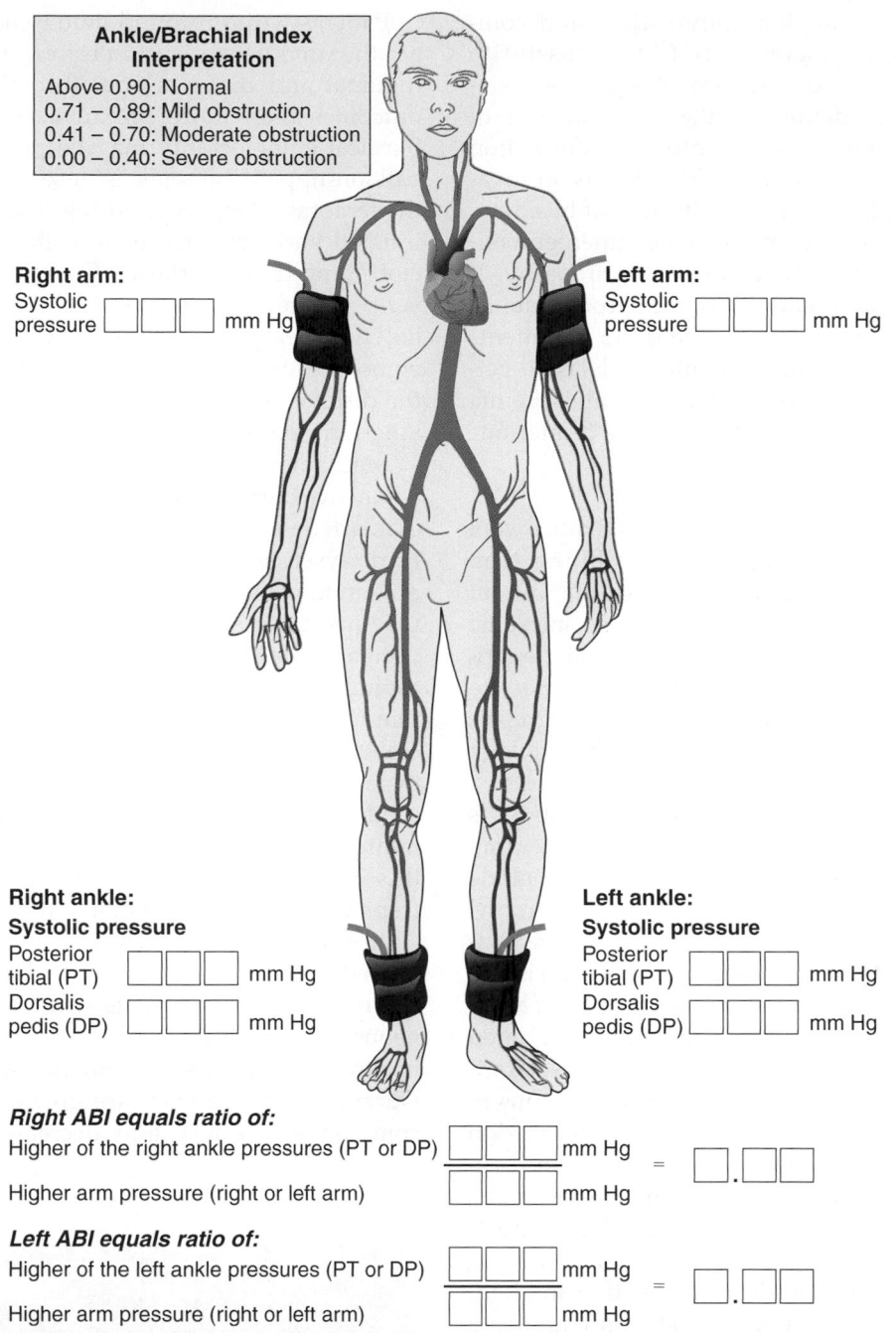

Ankle/Brachial Index Interpretation
Above 0.90: Normal
0.71 – 0.89: Mild obstruction
0.41 – 0.70: Moderate obstruction
0.00 – 0.40: Severe obstruction

Right arm:
Systolic pressure ☐☐☐ mm Hg

Left arm:
Systolic pressure ☐☐☐ mm Hg

Right ankle:
Systolic pressure
Posterior tibial (PT) ☐☐☐ mm Hg
Dorsalis pedis (DP) ☐☐☐ mm Hg

Left ankle:
Systolic pressure
Posterior tibial (PT) ☐☐☐ mm Hg
Dorsalis pedis (DP) ☐☐☐ mm Hg

Right ABI equals ratio of:
Higher of the right ankle pressures (PT or DP) ☐☐☐ mm Hg
Higher arm pressure (right or left arm) ☐☐☐ mm Hg = ☐.☐☐

Left ABI equals ratio of:
Higher of the left ankle pressures (PT or DP) ☐☐☐ mm Hg
Higher arm pressure (right or left arm) ☐☐☐ mm Hg = ☐.☐☐

⬍**FIGURE 16-5** Measuring ankle/brachial index.

TABLE 16-8 Values of Ankle/Brachial Index for Diagnosing Peripheral Arterial Disease

>1.3	Abnormal
1.30–0.91	Borderline and normal
0.9–0.3	Majority of patients with claudication
<0.2	Ischemic or gangrenous extremities

contour and amplitude correlate with the amount of obstruction.

Exercise testing is used to evaluate functional disability and lower extremity PAD when resting ABI values are normal.[32] The patient is placed on a treadmill for 5 minutes, or until maximum limit of exertion is reached or symptoms develop. Ankle waveforms and ABIs are obtained before and after the test. This test is used to assess patients with PAD but would not be used for acute occlusion.

Magnetic resonance angiography (MRA) and computed tomographic angiography (CTA) are useful to assess PAD anatomy and presence of significant stenoses. Arteriography delineates the proximal site of arterial occlusion and provides precise information about arterial inflow and outflow. This test is an invasive evaluation and is associated with risk of bleeding, infection, vascular access complications, atheroembolization, contrast allergy, and contrast nephropathy. It can be useful to differentiate thrombotic from embolic disease. ABI or ultrasound should be done in patients who present with acute limb ischemia. A delay in getting arteriography in the setting of acute limb ischemia can delay definitive treatment and have a deleterious effect.[19]

Treatment Options. Patients who present with a cool distal extremity, absent distal pulses, an ABI less than 0.4, flat pulse volume recording waveform, and absent pedal flow require an emergent vascular specialist referral to prevent limb loss. Immediate full heparinization with unfractionated heparin is required to prevent thrombotic propagation.[13] Lab and diagnostic tests should be considered to assess for the etiology behind the occlusion.

Revascularization can be achieved with thrombolysis and endovascular or surgical treatment. For acute limb ischemia, percutaneous interventions may include mechanical regional thrombolysis and thrombectomy, along with angioplasty and stents. Factors that are considered in choosing an intervention for acute limb ischemia are location and anatomy of lesion, duration of acute limb ischemia, type of clot, patient- and surgery-related risks, and any contraindications to thrombolysis. Gradual, low-pressure reperfusion may be advantageous in preference to the sudden, high-pressure reperfusion associated with surgical revascularization.[19] Intravenous administration of high-dose systemic thrombolysis in arterial occlusion is no longer recommended for treatment of arterial occlusion of the leg.[19]

Catheter-based thrombolysis is an effective and beneficial therapy and is indicated for patients with acute limb ischemia (Fontaine's Stages I and IIa: Table 16-5) of less than 14 days' duration.[32] Thrombolytic therapy offers a low-risk alternative to open surgery in complex patients with severe comorbidities. Immediate angiography with administration of regional thrombolytics helps delineate the arterial anatomy with visualization of both inflow and runoff vessels. Regional thrombolysis with tissue plasminogen activator (t-PA), streptokinase (Streptase), urokinase (Abbokinase), or reteplase (Retavase) can be used to treat the acute occlusion. Regional administration helps minimize systemic fibrinolysis. Patients are assessed for hemorrhagic complications with this therapy.

Patients with profound limb ischemia may not tolerate the time necessary to perform thrombolysis. Infrainguinal and distal arterial thrombolysis have worse outcomes than more proximal or iliofemoral lysis.[90] Surgical embolectomy may be performed, in which a balloon-tipped catheter is inserted, usually through the femoral artery, beyond the clot. The balloon is then inflated and the catheter is withdrawn, removing the clot. Long-term warfarin (Coumadin) is used to prevent recurrent embolism after the procedure. Thrombolytic therapy has the advantage over surgical embolectomy of clearing intra-arterial thrombus from the distal runoff vessels, thereby potentially enhancing long-term patency.

Mechanical thrombectomy devices can be used as adjunctive therapy for acute limb ischemia due to peripheral arterial occlusion (Figure 16-6). AngioJet, Oasis, Hydrolyser, and Amplatz devices have been studied in nonrandomized trials and small series.[32] These devices may avert the need for thrombolysis or permit use of decreased doses of thrombolytic drugs.[32] Percutaneous aspiration thrombectomy (PAT) is a technique that uses thin-wall, large-lumen catheters and suction to remove embolus or thrombus from femoropopliteal arteries, bypass grafts, and runoff vessels. Percutaneous mechanical thrombectomy (PMT) devices operate on the basis of hydrodynamic recirculation in which the device traps, dissolves, and evacuates the thrombus. Fresh thrombus responds better than old material.[19]

Nonsurgical approaches, known as endovascular procedures, to treat arterial disease are currently recommended for patients with claudication. Percutaneous transluminal angioplasty (PTA) and stents can improve results in symptomatic patients (Figure 16-7). Durability and patency are greatest for lesions in the common iliac artery and decrease distally and with

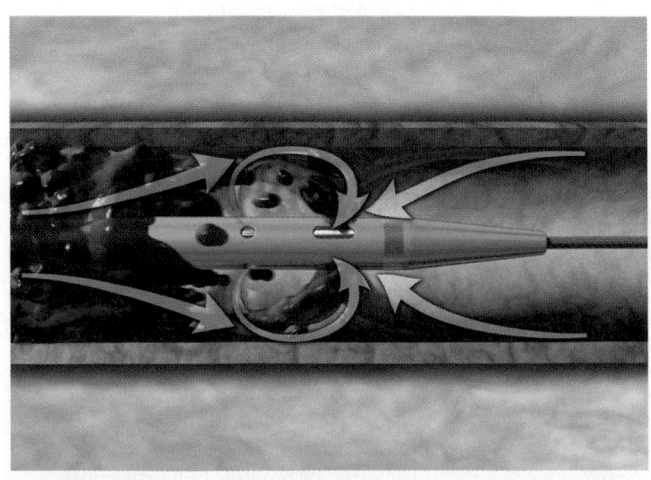

✦FIGURE 16-6 AngioJet thrombectomy device.

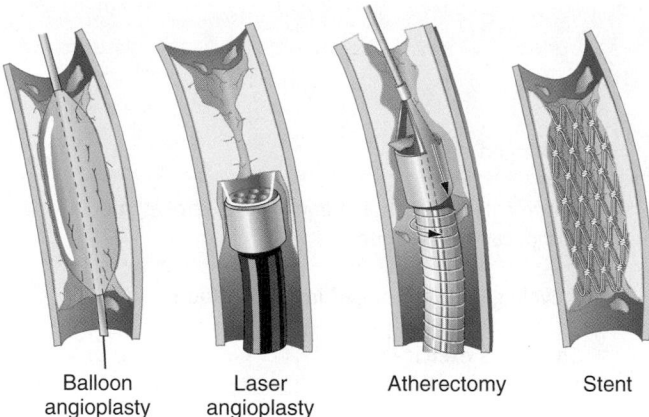

Balloon angioplasty   Laser angioplasty   Atherectomy   Stent

⬍FIGURE 16-7 Endovascular procedures.

increasing length of the stenosis occlusion, multiple and diffuse lesions, poor-quality runoff, diabetes, renal failure, smoking, and CLI.[32] Stenting is effective for common and external iliac artery stenosis and occlusion, and for salvage therapy in patients with suboptimal or failed results from balloon dilation.[32]

The nonsurgical procedures described require close vascular assessment. Patients are routinely placed on heparin infusions to maintain the partial thromboplastin time (PTT) 1.5 to 2.5 times the control. Monitoring BUN and creatinine levels is necessary to assess the renal effects of the contrast material used during diagnosis and intervention. Hydration is critical after treatment and accurate intake and output are recorded. Hemoglobin and hematocrit levels are important to monitor blood loss, especially less obvious bleeding that may occur into the peritoneal cavity.

Ischemic resting foot pain, gangrenous necrosis, or other limb-threatening symptoms signal the need for surgical intervention. Extensive disease involving a long segment of occlusion may also indicate the need for surgery. Individuals with claudication symptoms who have a significant functional disability and are unresponsive to other therapies may benefit from surgery. Patients who present with symptoms of claudication before age 50 have a poorer response to vascular surgical interventions, frequently requiring graft revisions or replacements.[32] Surgical intervention entails bypassing the occluded or ulcerated arterial segment by using autogenous vein or synthetic graft material such as Dacron or polytetrafluoroethylene (Teflon). The procedure involves the anastomosis of the graft from an area proximal to an area distal to the disease. Cardiac, pulmonary, and renal function are evaluated before surgery. A history of coronary or carotid artery disease may indicate the need for a more in-depth evaluation because of the added risk of acute MI and associated mortality.

Antiplatelet agents such as aspirin (ASA), clopidogrel (Plavix), ticlopidine (Ticlid), and aspirin/dipyridamole (Aggrenox) are used to prevent thrombus formation. Peripheral vasodilators, such as cilostazol (Pletal), are indicated if risk factor modification and an exercise program have not improved symptoms. Cilostazol should not be used in patients with heart failure. Agents that reduce blood viscosity, such as pentoxifylline (Trental), may be considered as a second-line therapy to improve walking distances.

Acute Peripheral Venous Occlusions

Etiology. *Venous thromboembolism (VTE)* refers to venous thrombosis and pulmonary embolism (PE).[32] Venous thrombosis can affect either the superficial veins (superficial thrombophlebitis) or the deep veins (deep vein thrombosis [DVT]). Prolonged venous thrombosis may lead to chronic venous insufficiency, with edema, pain, stasis pigmentation, stasis dermatitis, and stasis ulceration. Most venous thrombi begin in the valve cusps of deep calf veins. Most PEs originate from proximal DVT of the leg involving the popliteal, femoral, or iliac veins.[57]

Venous thrombus formation depends upon the interaction of three factors described as Virchow's triad: vessel wall trauma with endothelial injury, hypercoagulability, and stasis.[33,34] The presence of at least two of these three components leads to venous thrombus formation. Clinical risk factors include advanced age, prolonged immobility (bed rest or paralysis), previous VTE, cancer, extensive surgery, orthopedic surgery (hip or knee replacement), hip fractures, major trauma, stroke, obesity, varicose veins, heparin-induced thrombocytopenia (HIT), and heart failure (Table 16-9).[25]

Septic phlebitis is possible whenever a septic process is present in the extremity distal to or at the level of the venous obstruction. Septic thrombi may form separately from the infectious focus or along with the inflammatory area as part of a cellulitis.

The major risk associated with DVT is that it can lead to PE. PE has been estimated to cause death in more than 100,000 patients each year in North America and to contribute to death in another 100,000 patients per year.[33]

Clinical Findings. Superficial thrombophlebitis diagnosed by the symptoms: swollen, tender, superficial venous cord on examination.[25] Recent unilateral swelling and pain above or below the knee without explanatory bone or joint trauma is suspicious for DVT.[33] Clinical findings and patient history are important in diagnosis. Risk factors associated with DVT include previous history of VTE, family history of VTE, pregnant or postpartum, current estrogen use, recent trauma, surgery, immobilization, presence of cancer, presence of

TABLE 16-9 Causes of Venous Thromboembolism

ENDOTHELIAL INJURY	HYPERCOAGULABILITY	STASIS
Indwelling catheters	Malignant tumors	Prolonged bed rest
Injection of irritating substances	Blood dyscrasias	Chronic illness such as heart failure, stroke, and complications of trauma
Thromboangiitis obliterans	Oral contraceptives	Traveling with prolonged immobilization
Septic phlebitis	Idiopathic thrombosis	Strenuous exercise

varicosities, or immobilization on airline flight longer than 8 hours.[25]

DVT can be differentiated from acute arterial occlusion by physical examination. However, in greater than 50% of cases, acute DVT cannot be diagnosed by clinical findings alone. Erythema, warmth, unilateral edema, color change, and positive Homans' sign may be found. Specific limb findings (e.g., edema, dilated superficial veins) and evidence of pulmonary embolism will support the diagnosis.

Pulmonary emboli should be suspected if the patient presents with sudden onset of dyspnea, tachypnea, tachycardia, cough, pleuritic chest pain, hemoptysis, crackles, or hypoxemia. Massive PE can present with hemodynamic instability or cardiac arrest.

A well-validated clinical prediction rule known as the Wells model provides a reliable estimate of the pretest probability of DVT and PE. This tool can be used to help guide treatment (Boxes 16-5 and 16-6).

Box 16-5

Wells Model for Predicting Probability of DVT

Active cancer (treatment ongoing or within previous 6 months or palliative)	1
Paralysis, paresis, or recent plaster immobilization of lower extremity	1
Recently bedridden for more than 3 days or major surgery within 4 weeks	1
Localized tenderness along the distribution of the deep venous system	1
Entire leg swollen	1
Calf swollen by more than 3 cm when compared to asymptomatic leg (measured 10 cm below tibial tuberosity)	1
Pitting edema (greater in symptomatic leg)	1
Collateral superficial veins (nonvaricose)	1
Alternative diagnosis as likely or greater than that of deep vein thrombosis	1

Scoring:
If both legs are symptomatic, score the more severe side
High risk = 3 or more
Moderate risk = 1 or 2
Low risk = 0 or less

From reference 92.

Box 16-6

Wells Model for Predicting Probability of Pulmonary Embolism

Clinical signs and symptoms of deep vein thrombosis (DVT) (minimum of leg swelling and pain with palpation of deep veins)	3
An alternative diagnosis is less likely than pulmonary embolism (PE)	3
Heart rate >100 beats/min	1.5
Immobilization or surgery in previous 4 weeks	1.5
Previous DVT/PE	1.5
Hemoptysis	1
Malignancy (on treatment, treated in last 6 months, or palliative)	1

Score <2 = low clinical pretest probability
Score 2–6 = moderate clinical pretest probability
Score >6 = high clinical pretest probability

From reference 93.

Diagnostic Tests. D-dimer assays can be used in ambulatory care settings for patients with recent onset of symptoms who are not prescribed anticoagulation therapy.[25] This test may help reduce the need for subsequent tests. A negative D-dimer has been proven to have a strong negative predictive value for patients with a low probability of DVT or PE.[33] In patients with a low clinical pretest probability of DVT (Wells score of 0), a negative D-dimer can be considered as "ruled out for DVT and no further testing is needed."[25] Other lab tests may include a coagulation profile: aPTT, PT/INR, circulating fibrin, and fibrin degradation products (FDPs).

Duplex ultrasound with compression should be ordered as the first test for patients with moderate or high clinical probability.[10] Ultrasound is diagnostic in most cases in which thrombus involves the iliac, femoral, or popliteal veins. It may locate thrombi in the calf, although a negative test does not rule out the diagnosis of DVT and further testing may be needed.[25] A negative result can be followed by D-dimer, if it has not been done, to determine further radiologic testing needs.[25] Ultrasound assessment has several limitations: accuracy depends on the operator; it cannot distinguish between an old clot and a new clot; it is not accurate in detecting DVT in the pelvis or the small vessels of the calf; and it is not accurate in detecting DVT in the presence of obesity or significant edema.[65] In addition, false positives can be caused by superficial phlebitis, popliteal cysts, and abscess.[65]

If the diagnosis is in doubt, a venogram may be obtained. Venography with contrast is limited by the risk of pain, phlebitis, and hypersensitivity or toxic reactions to contrast agents; DVTs may also develop in a small number of patients who undergo this procedure.[65] When calf thrombosis is suspected but the initial ultrasound is negative, serial ultrasound can be repeated in 3 to 7 days as an acceptable alternative to venography.[10]

Diagnostic tests for PE include CT pulmonary angiography, ventilation/perfusion ($\dot{V}/\dot{Q}$) lung scan, and angiogram. Chest x-ray, arterial blood gases, ECG, and an echocardiogram can be performed to consider alternative diagnoses, such as angina, MI, pneumonia, or pericarditis.

An algorithm developed by the Institute for Clinical Systems Improvement (ICSI), an independent nonprofit collaboration of healthcare providers and insurance companies, incorporates evidence-based recommendations for the use of pretest clinical probability with prediction rules, D-dimer testing, and imaging in the diagnosis of DVT and PE (Figures 16-8 and 16-9).

Treatment Options. Treatment is aimed at preventing DVT. Identifying those patients at risk and starting anticoagulants can prevent thrombi from forming or extending. Despite intensive study, antiplatelet drugs have not proved to be effective for prevention. VTE can be prevented by counteracting increased blood coagulation with unfractionated heparin (UFH), low molecular weight heparin (LMWH), the pentasaccharide fondaparinux (Arixtra), warfarin, or other new anticoagulants, or by reducing venous stasis with external pneumatic compression, a venous foot pump, or graduated compression stockings.[32,33] In patients at moderate or high risk, anticoagulant prophylaxis (described in the Medication table on p. 376) is preferred to help prevent DVT and PE.

Heparin should be started in high-risk patients without delay. The main goal is to prevent PE and chronic venous insufficiency. Prophylactic dosing is 30 mg twice daily or 40 mg once daily; with renal dysfunction 30 mg once daily is recommended. For patients with DVT, LMWH is started at a dose of enoxaparin (Lovenox) 1 mg/kg twice daily or 1.5 mg once daily. For uncomplicated patients, once daily dosing is safe and effective. Obesity (greater than 100 kg), cancer, and chronic kidney disease are risk factors for failing once daily dosing. Therefore twice daily dosing is recommended for obese patients and patients with cancer.[33] If the patient has renal dysfunction the dose should be reduced to 1 mg/kg once daily. LMWH is the preferred heparin for initial anticoagulation for the patient with DVT. Other FDA-approved alternatives include tinzaparin (Innohep) 175 anti-Xa units/kg subcutaneous every day.

Heparin should be continued for at least 5 days after the initiation of warfarin therapy with the dosage adjusted to achieve an international normalized ratio (INR) greater than 2 for 2 consecutive days.[42] A therapeutic range of anticoagulation to keep the INR between 2 and 3 is recommended. Warfarin should be started at a dose of 5 mg daily. An initial dose of 10 mg has been associated with over-anticoagulation and is no more effective in achieving a therapeutic INR.[42]

When acute DVT is diagnosed, the patient may be hospitalized initially. However, because of advances in heparin therapy, selected patients with DVT can be treated at home, thereby reducing or eliminating hospitalization. Patients with uncomplicated VTE, good cardiorespiratory reserve, no excessive bleeding risks, and creatinine clearance greater than 30 ml/min can safely receive outpatient therapy.[10]

Both UFH and LMWH are associated with a risk for HIT, which is an immune-mediated reaction to heparin that occurs in 2% to 3% of patients receiving UFH and in 1% of patients treated with LMWH.[10] Patients who develop HIT are at increased risk for venous and arterial thrombosis. Patients who develop a skin lesion reaction at the injection site, have a reaction to a bolus administration of heparin, or develop a greater than 50% drop in platelet count should be tested for HIT. Direct thrombin inhibitors are the alternative

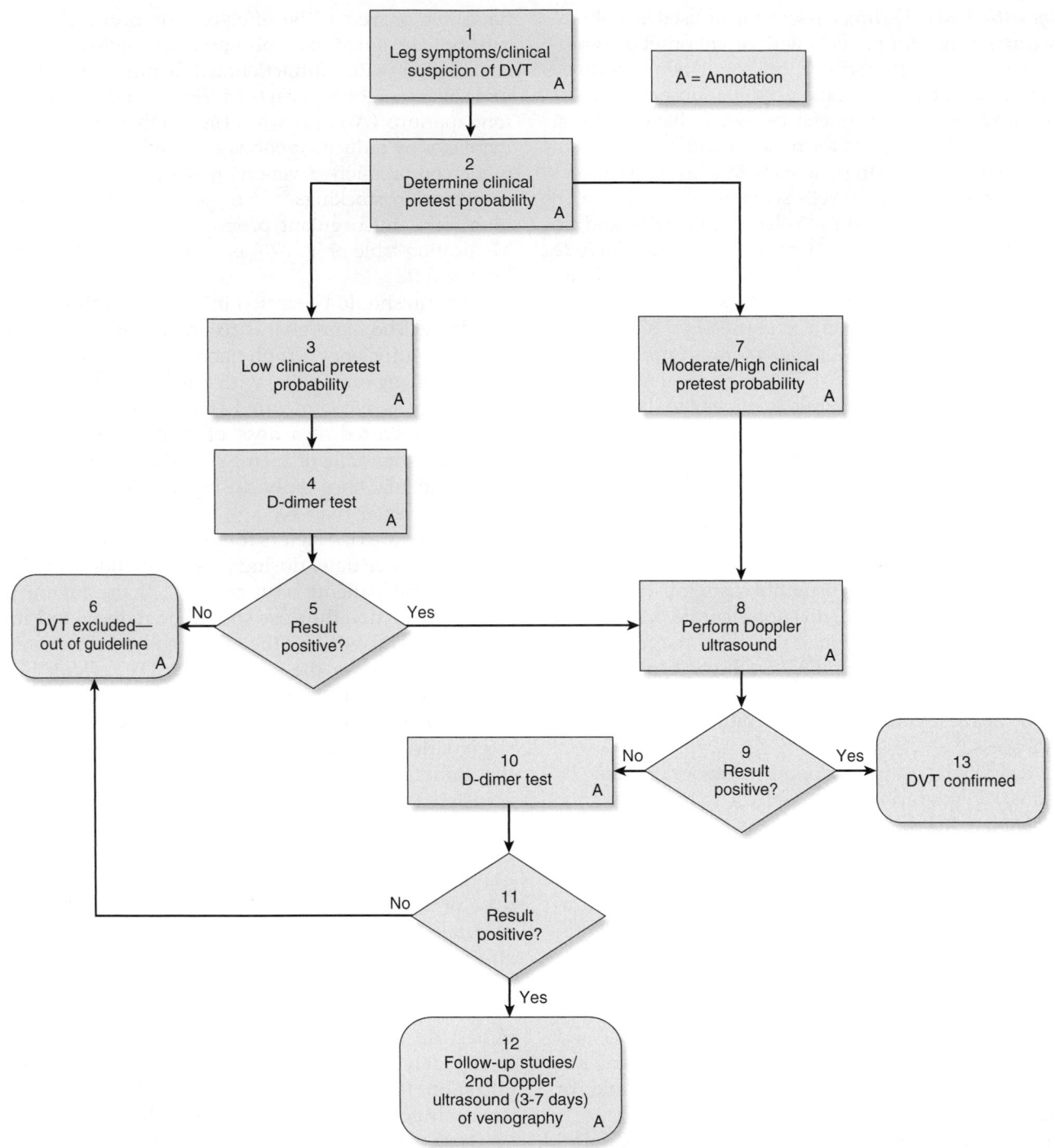

◆FIGURE 16-8 Diagnostic algorithm for deep vein thrombosis (DVT).

anticoagulant for patients with HIT. Lepirudin (Refludan), argatroban (Acova), or bivalirudin (Angiomax) can be used.[89]

Warfarin is contraindicated in pregnancy because it crosses the placenta and is associated with fetal abnormalities. Subcutaneous UFH, twice daily, or LMWH

has shown no increased fetal complications.[10] The postpartum period is a high-risk time for thrombosis, and anticoagulation is needed for 4 to 6 weeks after delivery.

Duration of anticoagulant therapy depends on the etiology of the condition. A single episode of thrombophlebitis subsiding clinically in 3 to 6 days in a young,

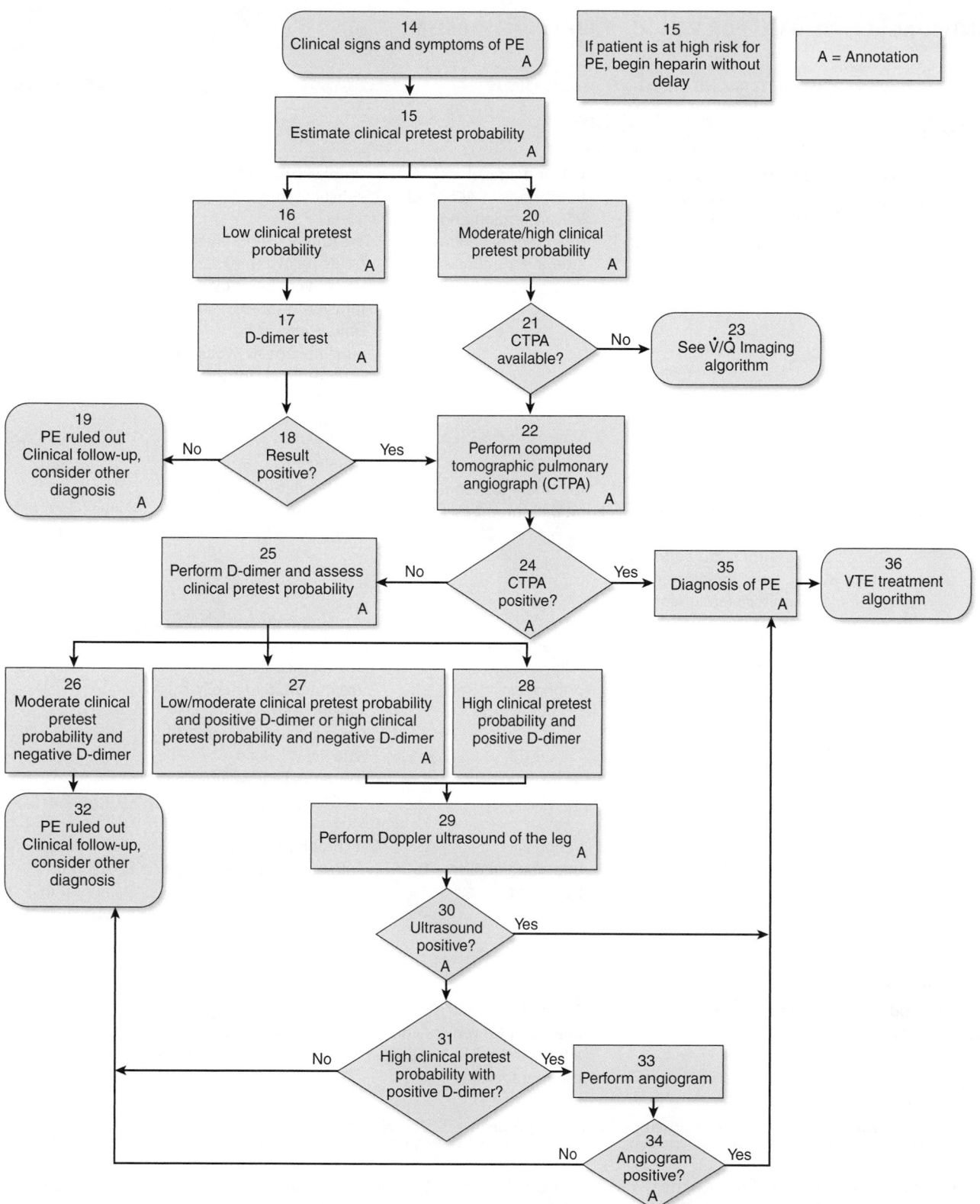

✦FIGURE 16-9 Diagnostic algorithm for pulmonary embolism (PE).

ANTICOAGULANTS USED FOR VENOUS THROMBOEMBOLISM

DRUG	TARGET/MONITORING	INDICATIONS	DOSAGES	SIDE EFFECTS
HEPARINS				
Unfractionated heparin (UFH)	Factors IIa and Xa. Adjust to maintain aPTT in therapeutic range. Monitor platelet count.	VTE and arterial thrombosis in ACS, and PCI prevention and treatment of venous and arterial thrombosis	Prophylaxis: 5000 units subcutaneously every 8 or 12 hr Treatment: 5000 units IV bolus followed by 32,000 units every 24 hr by IV infusion or 35,000–40,000 units every 24 hr subcutaneously (volume of drug required for this may be too high for a subcutaneous injection)	Bleeding; HIT with or without thrombosis; osteoporosis
Low molecular weight heparin (LMWH) (Lovenox)	Factors IIa and Xa Monitor factor Xa in renal failure and over- or underweight patients. Dose must be adjusted for renal impairment. Monitor platelet count.	Prevention of and treatment for venous and arterial thrombosis	Prophylaxis: 1 mg/kg subcutaneously bid Treatment: 1.5 mg/kg once daily for DVT treatment	Bleeding; lower incidence of HIT and osteoporosis
Fondaparinux sodium (Arixtra)	Factor Xa Monitor like LMWH. May need to adjust dose for renal impairment. Contraindicated if CrCl <30 ml/min.	Prevention of VTE following major orthopedic surgery	Prophylaxis: 2.5 mg subcutaneously daily Treatment: 5 mg daily if weight <50 kg; 7.5 mg daily if weight 50–100 kg; 10 mg daily if weight >100 kg	Bleeding
Tinzaparin (Innohep)	Factor Xa Monitor like LMWH.	Venous thromboembolism treatment	175 anti-Xa units/kg subcutaneously every day	Bleeding; use with caution in renal impairment
Vitamin K Antagonist				
Warfarin sodium (Coumadin)	Factors II, VII, IX, and X	Prevention of and treatment for venous and arterial thrombosis and cardioembolism	Start at low loading dose of 2.5–5 mg; monitor INR to adjust to between 2 and 3	Bleeding

ACS = Acute coronary syndrome, aPTT = activated partial thromboplastin time, CrCl = creatinine clearance, DVT = deep vein thrombosis, HIT = heparin-induced thrombocytopenia, INR = international normalized ratio, PCI = percutaneous cardiac intervention, VTE = venous thromboembolism.

active patient free of risk factors may require only 3 months of therapy; however, a patient with a demonstrable PE and persistent risk factors may require 6 to 12 months of therapy.[10] After more than two episodes of DVT, oral anticoagulant prophylaxis should be continued indefinitely. Follow-up of patients after discharge is required to minimize the risks of hemorrhagic and thrombotic complications. An INR target of 2.5 is recommended.[42]

Thrombolytic therapy using tissue plasminogen activator or urokinase in tandem with anticoagulants is effective for acute DVT of the popliteal and more proximal veins. The best results occur when the DVT has been present for greater than 48 to 72 hours. Complete or partial dissolution of thrombi usually occurs within 24 to 48 hours. Successful treatment restores venous anatomy and thus may prevent valvular damage and resulting chronic venous insufficiency. Before thrombolytic therapy is used, the diagnosis must be confirmed by venography. The contraindications and adverse effects, especially bleeding, and the details of treatment and monitoring must be understood. Thrombolytic therapy results in a more rapid clot resolution, but does not significantly reduce mortality or risk of recurrent PE.[19]

The patient should be measured for firm, below-knee elastic stockings (providing 30 to 40 mm Hg pressure) to control the edema that may occur with ambulation. Graduated compression stockings on the affected leg will reduce the risk of postphlebitic syndrome. Knee-high, 30 to 40 mm Hg, custom-fitted, graded compression stockings (not TEDS) help alleviate symptoms of edema and pain.[33] Improperly-fitted graduated compression stockings produce a reverse pressure gradient and are associated with a higher incidence of DVT.[36] The stocking should be worn while the patient is ambulatory to prevent the postphlebitic sequelae of chronic venous insufficiency: edema, pain, stasis pigmentation, and subsequent stasis dermatitis and stasis ulceration. Stockings and early ambulation do not cause any increase in PE and provide more rapid resolution of pain and swelling.[10]

Inferior vena cava (IVC) filters should not be used routinely for most patients with DVT. Placement of an IVC filter can be used as treatment for patients who cannot take anticoagulants or who have had recurrent thromboembolism despite adequate anticoagulation. Patients with underlying pulmonary hypertension in whom a PE would likely be fatal would also be candidates for IVC filters. Multiple filter types are available and all are effective in preventing PE. Surgical thrombectomy has been used for patients with extensive venous thrombosis who have contraindications for anticoagulation and lytic therapy.

VASCULAR INJURIES OF THE EXTREMITIES

Vascular injures are caused by penetrating or blunt trauma and are often associated with other neurologic, osseous, tendinous (involving the tendons), and visceral damage. If not treated rapidly these injuries can be life threatening. These injuries are seen more frequently in 20- to 40-year-old male patients. Often these patients can present with extensive musculoskeletal, nerve, and skin injury that can lead to a poor prognosis.[5]

Blunt trauma can result from motor vehicle accidents, falls, assaults, and crush injuries. Fractures of the long bones or dislocated joints can increase the chance for

vascular injuries. Penetrating trauma can be caused by gunshot and stab wounds, as well as industrial accidents and IV drug use. Vascular injuries can also be a result of iatrogenic complications of vascular access medical procedures, such as cardiac catheterization, arteriography, and balloon angioplasty.[2]

Clinical Presentation

Signs of hemorrhagic shock are clues to vascular trauma. Vessel injury may be nonsevered, partially severed, or completely severed. Patients may present with large lacerations or open wounds and hemorrhage. Signs include differences in BP between extremities, diminished or absent distal pulses, pallor, and paresthesias of the extremity. "Hard" and "soft" signs are used to identify treatment (Table 16-10). Hard signs identify patients requiring surgical intervention. A finding of a cool, cold, or pulseless extremity and variations in pulse quality can indicate underlying proximal vascular injury.[5] Neurologic deficits, delayed capillary refill, and bony abnormalities increase the suspicion of extremity vascular injury and the need for surgery. Hard signs indicate the need for further diagnostic evaluation. Soft signs require close observation and monitoring because serious vascular injury may not be overtly obvious.

Patients with hard and soft signs can present as an emergency with an open fracture. A careful clinical assessment of the vascular and neurologic status of the limb is required. The first decision is to determine whether limb salvage should be attempted. Poor prognostic signs for limb salvage are a major soft tissue injury, an ischemic time in excess of 6 hours, the presence of significant neurologic deficit, especially of the tibial nerve, and other major organ injuries.[43] There are a number of scoring systems that can be used in helping with decision making.

TABLE 16-10 Assessment of Vascular Injury

HARD SIGNS	SOFT SIGNS
Pulsatile hemorrhage	Pulse deficit without ischemia
Rapidly expanding hematoma	Neurologic deficit
Obvious arterial occlusion	Nonexpanding hematoma
Palpable thrill or audible bruit	History of hemorrhage, hypotension, fracture, or delayed capillary refill

Scoring Systems

Scoring systems have been developed to assist with the prediction of which limbs might be salvaged. They are utilized to evaluate the degree of injury and predict amputation and functional outcome.

The Mangled Extremity Severity Score (MESS) examines degrees of skeletal/soft tissue injury, limb ischemia, symptoms of shock, and patient age.[40] A score of less than 7 indicates a likelihood of successful limb salvage. A score of 7 or more is predictive of the need for amputation (Table 16-11).[30]

Other scoring systems in use include the Limb Salvage Index (LSI);[67] the Predictive Salvage Index (PSI);[35] the Nerve injury, Ischemia, Soft tissue injury, Skeletal injury, Shock, and Age index (NISSSA);[52] and the Hannover Fracture Scale-97 (HFS-97).[79] All of the scoring systems apply a numerical value to the severity of injury and can be used to predict the need for amputation.

The LSI exams limb trauma associated with vascular injury.[67] Seven components related to injury include arterial, nerve, bone, skin, muscle, deep venous injury, and warm ischemic time. Indication for amputation includes a score of 6 or more. The PSI looks at combined orthopedic and vascular injuries.[35] Level of vascular injury and degree of osseous and muscle injury along with warm ischemia time are weighted into a score that is used to look at limb salvage. NISSSA score has a nerve injury component (loss of plantar sensation) along with tissue injury that looks at soft and skeletal tissue variables.[52] This scoring system has also been found to be highly accurate in predicting the need for amputation. The HFS[79-97] is another tool orthopedic surgeons use in their decision making.

In general, low scores in any of the scales can be used to predict successful limb-salvage potential, but high scores do not have adequate sensitivity to predict amputation. Although scoring systems may be helpful, the treating surgeon must rely on clinical judgment in deciding how best to treat a mangled limb.[2]

TABLE 16-11 Mangled Extremity Severity Score

Skeletal/Soft Tissue Injury	
Low energy (e.g., stab, simple fracture, gunshot wound)	1
Medium energy (e.g., open or multiple fractures, dislocation)	2
High energy (e.g., shotgun, crush injury)	3
Very high energy (as above plus gross contamination, soft tissue avulsion)	4
Limb Ischemia	
Pulse reduced or absent but normal perfusion	1
Pulseless, paresthesias, reduced capillary filling	2
Cool, paralyzed, insensate limb (score doubled if longer than 6 hours)	3
Shock	
Systolic blood pressure maintained >90 mm Hg	0
Transient hypotension	1
Persistent hypotension	2
Age	
<30	0
30–50	1
>50	2

From reference 30.
See text for scoring instructions.

Diagnostic Workup

Lab studies include baseline blood work consisting of CBC, platelet count, electrolytes, BUN, and creatinine. Typing and cross-matching of 4 to 8 units of packed red blood cells (PRBCs) should be considered in a patient with obvious vascular trauma. In acute hemorrhage, the hematocrit and hemoglobin level may appear within the normal range even though there may be signs of cellular volume loss.

Diagnostic tests are used to evaluate the presence of vascular injury and the extent of injury. They are done to prevent unnecessary operations, document the presence of a surgical lesion, and localize the surgical lesion to plan an operative approach.[23] The ABI is used to evaluate vascular insufficiency resulting from the vascular injury. If the ABI is measured higher than 0.9 the patient can be observed, but an ABI lower than 0.9 warrants further evaluation. Transcutaneous oxygen monitoring of the extremity can also provide clues to decreased perfusion. Duplex ultrasonography is a rapid, noninvasive method of assessing vascular injury. Plain x-ray of the injured extremity can determine the presence of fractured bones and foreign bodies. Arteriogram can be performed in stable patients who do not have renal compromise. Unstable patients require surgical exploration. Arteriography can be performed by the surgeon in the emergency department or operating room.

MULTIDISCIPLINARY PLAN OF CARE FOR PERIPHERAL VASCULAR EMERGENCIES

PROBLEM	INTERVENTION	RATIONALE	EXPECTED OUTCOME	COMMENTS
Alterations in circulation to involved extremity related to acute arterial occlusion or VTE	Monitor vital signs. Palpate peripheral pulses, noting strength and equality. Assess capillary refill. Inspect for skin color and temperature changes, as well as edema. Note symmetry of calves; measure and record calf circumference; check for Homans' sign. Monitor closely for symptoms of pulmonary emboli: sudden or sharp chest pain, dyspnea, tachycardia, and apprehension.	Indicators of circulatory status and adequacy of perfusion. Peripheral arterial occlusion can cause pallor and coolness of extremities. Peripheral venous occlusion can present with redness, heat, tenderness, and localized edema and positive Homans' sign. Pulmonary embolism is a complication of DVT.	Maintain or enhance tissue perfusion in affected limb. Prevent or promptly detect pulmonary embolism.	Pulmonary embolism can also result from thrombosis associated with HIT.
Pain related to decreased peripheral perfusion resulting from PAD, acute arterial occlusion, or VTE	Assess level of discomfort or pain and medicate with prescribed analgesic. Evaluate effectiveness of pain medication after each dose. Assess distal perfusion of extremities. Note pulses, sensory and motor function.	Peripheral arterial disease presents with cramping or aching pain that increases with activity and is relieved by rest. Excruciating pain with sudden loss of distal pulses or decreased motor-sensory function requires immediate attention due to acute occlusion.	Patient is pain free or has pain controlled sufficiently to allow ADLs, rest, and sleep. Significant changes in perfusion noted and reported promptly.	
Risk for bleeding related to anticoagulant therapy	Administer anticoagulants as ordered. Assess for any evidence of bleeding. Monitor PTT for patients on heparin. Monitor anti-factor Xa (LMW factor) for patients on LWMH who have renal insufficiency, are overweight (>100 kg), or are underweight (<50 kg). Monitor INR for patients on warfarin.	Heparin is preferred initially to prevent further clot formation.	Absence of any serious signs of bleeding. Blood tests within prescribed therapeutic ranges: PTT 1.5–2 × normal INR 2–3	When converting from IV heparin to warfarin, warfarin should be started while patient is still on heparin. Once INR is therapeutic, heparin can be discontinued.
Knowledge deficit related to disease process and treatment recommendations	Provide information regarding disease process, risk factor reduction, drug therapy, activities, exercise program, infection control, and follow-up care. Recommend cessation of smoking. Offer referral resources for smoking cessation. Provide education regarding signs and symptoms that require medical evaluation: edema; redness; increased odorous drainage at incision or puncture site; changes in sensation, movement, skin color; pain or acute shortness of breath. Discuss purpose and dosage of prescribed anticoagulant, emphasizing importance of taking	Provides knowledge base so patient can understand disease process and complications. Smoking potentiates peripheral vasoconstriction and impairs circulation and tissue oxygenation. Prompt recognition allows for early intervention and may prevent serious complications. Warfarin interacts with a number of drugs and food products that can either increase or decrease INR levels.	Patient verbalizes knowledge of disease process, prescribed medications, and follow-up treatment. Absence of tobacco usage.	There is a high recurrence rate in patients with DVT. Acetaminophen and herbal products (ginkgo biloba, garlic, vitamin E) can prolong clotting times. ASA can decrease prothrombin activity.

Table continues on page 380

PROBLEM	INTERVENTION	RATIONALE	EXPECTED OUTCOME	COMMENTS
	drug as prescribed. Review possible drug interactions and stress need to check with pharmacist or doctor about OTC drugs. Identify safety precautions (e.g., use of soft toothbrush, electric razor for shaving, gloves for gardening, and avoidance of sharp objects, walking barefoot, or forceful blowing of nose).	Patients taking anticoagulants are at increased risk for bleeding.		
Self-care deficit related to lack of knowledge about proper foot care	Instruct patient regarding proper foot care, including keeping feet protected with shoes or slippers. Apply warm, moist compresses if indicated for VTE. Avoid heating pads or hot water bottles directly on skin in patients with arterial insufficiency. Use a bed cradle, sheepskin under the foot, and heel protectors/lambs wool in between toes. Avoid tape, if possible. Caution patient to avoid crossing legs or hyperflexion at knees. Instruct patient to avoid rubbing/massaging affected extremity.	Increased risk of leg ulcers with poor circulation. Warm, moist compresses may be prescribed for VTE to promote vasodilation and venous return and resolution of local edema. Heat should be avoided in arterial disease because it increases oxygen consumption. Protects skin integrity of lower extremities. Physical restriction of circulation impairs blood flow, increases venous stasis in vessels, and can increase swelling and discomfort. This activity potentiates risk of dislodging thrombus.	Patient verbalizes knowledge of proper foot care.	
Impaired mobility related to pain and recent intervention	Apply graduated compression stockings or intermittent pneumatic compression if indicated. Assist with frequent changes of position and get patient out of bed to ambulate as tolerated. Implement activity program for patient at home.	Properly fitted support hose can minimize or delay development of postphlebitic syndrome in patients with VTE. Turning and ambulation help prevent complications of bed rest. Increasing ambulation helps prevent thrombus formation.	Increased mobility.	Sequential compression devices improve blood flow velocity and empty vessels by providing artificial muscle-pumping action.
Impaired skin integrity related to decreased circulation or surgical incision	Assess for leg ulcers, gangrene, poor wound healing, and skin breakdown. Provide foot cradle.	Poor perfusion makes it difficult to heal and that may, as a result, develop infection or gangrene. Cradle keeps pressure off affected limb, reducing pressure and pain.	Skin and incisions intact, with healing of any peripheral ulceration.	

ADLs = Activities of daily living, ASA = acetylsalicylic acid (aspirin), DVT = deep vein thrombosis, HIT = heparin-induced thrombocytopenia, INR = international normalized ratio, IV = intravenous, LMW = low molecular weight, LMWH = low molecular weight heparin, OTC = over-the-counter, PAD = peripheral arterial disease, PTT = partial thromboplastin time, VTE = venous thromboembolism.

Management

The first priority of nursing care is to control the bleeding. Infusion of IV fluids and monitoring of BP are critical if the patient is actively bleeding. Monitoring vital signs and intake and output is required as preparations are made to evaluate the patient and prepare for surgery. Antibiotics, tetanus toxoid, and analgesics are provided to help with infection and pain. Patients need to be monitored for signs of compartment syndrome in the postoperative period.

Frequent monitoring—including the presence and quality of pulse, capillary refill, color and temperature of the extremity, and sensation and motor ability—should be continued for the first 24 to 48 hours. Vascular injury may be minimal (abnormal pedal pulse and no evidence of ischemia); moderate (abnormal pedal pulse examination and evidence of tissue ischemia); or severe (a cadaveric limb and no pedal pulse, cold foot, pale color, no capillary refill, and loss of motor and sensory function).[55] A high index of suspicion and a comprehensive, aggressive approach are required to achieve the best possible outcome.

CONCLUSIONS

Peripheral vascular emergencies can be attributable to a number of causes. Care involves prompt assessment and intervention to restore blood flow to the affected area and preserve limb function. The Multidisciplinary Plan of Care on pp. 379-380 summarizes the key components.

REFERENCES

1. Anderson, L. A. (2001). Abdominal aortic aneurysm. *J Cardiovasc Nurs, 15*(4), 1–14.
2. Austin, O. M. (1995). Vascular trauma—a review. *J Am Coll Surg, 181*, 91–108.
3. Barkhordarian, S., & Dardick, A. (2004). Preoperative assessment and management to prevent complications during high-risk vascular surgery. *Crit Care Med, 32*(suppl), S174–S185.
4. Bavaria, J. E., et al. (2002). Advances in the treatment of acute type A dissection: an integrated approach. *Ann Thorac Surg, 74*, S1848–S1852.
5. Bjerke H. *Extremity vascular trauma.* www.emedicine.com/med/topic2812.htm.
6. Blankensteijn, J., et al. (2005). Two-year outcomes after conventional or endovascular repair of abdominal aortic aneurysms. *N Engl J Med, 352*, 2398–2405.
7. Boersma, E., et al. (2001). Predictors of cardiac events after major vascular surgery: role of clinical characteristics, dobutamine echocardiography, and beta-blocker therapy. *JAMA, 285*, 1865–1873.
8. Brewster, D. C., et al. (2003). Guidelines for the treatment of abdominal aortic aneurysms: report of a subcommittee of the Joint Council of the American Association for Vascular Surgery and the Society for Vascular Surgery. *J Vasc Surg, 37*(5), 1106–1117.
9. Brown, L. C., & Powell, J. T. (1999). Risk factors for aneurysm rupture in patients kept under ultrasound surveillance. UK Small Aneurysm Trial Participants. *Ann Surg, 230*, 289–296; discussion 296–297.
10. Burnett, B., et al. (2006). *Health care guideline: venous thromboembolism* (7th ed.). Bloomington, MN: Institute for Clinical Systems Improvement.www.icsi.org.
11. Cambria, R. P., et al. (2002). Thoracoabdominal aneurysm repair: results with 337 operations performed over a 15-year interval. *Ann Surg, 236*, 471–479.
12. Chiesa, R., et al. (2005). Spinal cord ischemia after elective stent-graft repair of the thoracic aorta. *J Vasc Surg, 42*, 11–17.
13. Clagett, G. P., et al. (2004). Antithrombotic therapy in peripheral arterial occlusive disease: the Seventh ACCP Conference on Antithrombotic and Thrombolytic Therapy. *Chest, 126*(3 suppl), 609S–626S.
14. Coselli, J. S., et al. (2002). Cerebrospinal fluid drainage reduces paraplegia after thoracoabdominal aortic aneurysm repair: results of a randomized clinical trial. *J Vasc Surg, 35*, 631–639.
15. Coselli, J. S., & LeMaire, S. A. (2005). Thoracic aortic aneurysms and aortic dissection. In F. C. Brunicardi, et al. (Eds.), *Schwartz's principles of surgery* (8th ed.). New York: McGraw-Hill.
16. Crawford, E. S., et al. (1986). Thoracoabdominal aortic aneurysms: preoperative and intraoperative factors determining immediate and long-term results of operations in 605 patients. *J Vasc Surg, 3*, 389–404.
17. David, T. E., et al. (2002). Aortic valve sparing operations in patients with aneurysms of the aortic root or ascending aorta. *Ann Thorac Surg, 74*, S1758–S1761.
18. DiEusanio, M., et al. (2003). Brain protection using antegrade cerebral selective cerebral perfusion: a multicenter study. *Ann Thorac Surg, 76*, 1181–1189.
19. Dormandy, J. A., & Rutherford, R. B, for the TASC Working Group. (2001). TransAtlantic Inter-Society Consensus (TASC). Management of peripheral arterial disease (PAD). *J Vasc Surg, 31*, S1–S296.
20. Elefteriades, J. A. (2002). Natural history of thoracic aortic aneurysms: indications for surgery and surgical versus nonsurgical risks. *Ann Thoracic Surg, 74*, S1877–S1880.
21. Ehrlich, M. P., et al. (2003). Predicators of adverse outcome and transient neurological dysfunction following surgical treatment of acute Type A dissections. *Circulation, 108*(suppl), II318–II323.
22. Estrera, A. L., et al. (2001). Descending thoracic aortic aneurysm: surgical approach and treatment using the adjuncts cerebrospinal fluid drainage and distal aortic perfusion. *Ann Thorac Surg, 72*, 481–486.
23. Feliciano, D. (2002). *Management of peripheral vascular trauma.* American College of Surgeons Committee on Trauma, Subcommittee on Publication.
24. Finklemeier, B. A., & Marolda, D. (2001). Aortic dissection. *J Cardiovasc Nurs, 15*(4), 15–24.
25. Geerts, W. H., et al. (2004). Prevention of venous thromboembolism: the Seventh ACCP Conference on Antithrombotic and Thrombolytic Therapy. *Chest, 126*(3 suppl), 338S–400S.
26. Greenberg, R. K., et al. (2005). Hybrid approaches to thoracic aortic aneurysms: the role of endovascular elephant trunk completion. *Circulation, 112*, 2619–2626.
27. Greenhalgh, R. M., et al. (2005). Endovascular aneurysm repair versus open repair in patients with abdominal aortic aneurysm (EVAR trial 1): randomized controlled trial. *Lancet, 365*, 2179–2186.
28. Guerit, J. M., & Dion, R. A. (2002). State-of-the-art neuromonitoring for prevention of immediate and delayed paraplegia in thoracic and thoracoabdominal aorta surgery. *Ann Thorac Surg, 74*, S1867–S1869.

29. Hagan, P. G., et al. (2000). International registry of acute aortic dissection (IRAD): new insights into an old disease. *JAMA, 283,* 897–903.

30. Helfet, D. L., Howey, T., & Sanders, R. (1990). Limb salvage versus amputation. Preliminary results of the mangled extremity severity score. *Clin Orthop, July, 9256,* 80–86.

31. Henning, R. J., Eikman, E., & Patel, M. S. (2002). Acute and chronic aortic dissection. *Heart Disease, 4,* 231–241.

32. Hirsch, A. T., et al. (2005). *ACC/AHA guidelines for the management of patients with peripheral arterial disease (lower extremity, renal, mesenteric, and abdominal aortic): a collaborative report from the American Association for Vascular Surgery/Society for Vascular Surgery, Society for Cardiovascular Angiography and Interventions, Society of Interventional Radiology, Society for Vascular Medicine and Biology, and the American College of Cardiology/American Heart Association Task Force on Practice Guidelines.* Available at American College of Cardiology website:www.acc.org/clinical/guidelines/pad/index.pdf.

33. Hirsh, J. (Ed.) (Nov 2005). *A clinician's guide to thrombosis.* Dallas: American Heart Association and American Stroke Association through an educational grant by Astra Zeneca.

34. Hirsh, J., et al. (2004). The Seventh ACCP Conference on Antithrombotic and Thrombolytic Therapy: evidence-based guidelines, *Chest, 126*(3 suppl), 172S–696S.

35. Howe, H. R., et al. (1987). Salvage of lower extremities following combined orthopedic and vascular trauma. A predictive salvage index. *Am Surg, 52,* 205–208.

36. Hull, R. D., et al. (1990). Effectiveness of intermittent pneumatic leg compression for preventing deep vein thrombosis after total hip replacement. *JAMA, 263,* 2313–2317.

37. Huynh, T. T., et al. (2002). Determinants of hospital length of stay after thoracoabdominal aortic aneurysm repair. *J Vasc Surg, 35,* 648–653.

38. Deleted in proofs.

39. Isselbacher, E. M. (2005). Thoracic and abdominal aortic aneurysms. *Circulation, 111,* 816–828.

40. Johansen, K., et al. (1990). Objective criteria accurately predict amputation following lower extremity trauma. *J Trauma, 30,* 568–573.

41. Kallenbach, K., et al. (2004). Evolving strategies for treatment of acute aortic dissection type A. *Circulation, 110*(suppl II), 243–249.

42. Katzen, B. T. (2002). Clinical diagnosis and prognosis of acute limb ischemia. *Rev Cardiovasc Med, 3*(suppl 2), S2–S6.

43. Keating, J. F., Simpson, A. H., & Robinson, C. M. (2005). *Managing of fractures and bone loss,* http://findarticles.com/p/articles/mi_qa3767/is_200502/ai_n11827181.

44. Kertai, M. D., et al. (2004). A combination of statins and beta-blockers is independently associated with a reduction in the incidence of perioperative mortality and nonfatal myocardial infarction in patients undergoing abdominal aortic aneurysm surgery. *Eur J Vasc Endovasc Surg, 28,* 343–352.

45. Khan, I. A., & Nair, C. K. (2002). Clinical, diagnostic, and management perspectives of aortic dissection. *Chest, 122*(1), 311–328.

46. Khoynezhad, A., & Plestis, K. A. (2006). Managing emergency hypertension in aortic dissection and aortic aneurysm surgery. *J Card Surg, 21,* S3–S7.

47. Klein, D. G. (2005). Thoracic aortic aneurysms. *J Cardiovasc Nurs, 20*(4), 245–250.

48. Klompas, M. (2002). Does this patient have an acute thoracic dissection? *JAMA, 287*(17), 2262–2272.

49. Kouchoukos, N. T., et al. (2002). Hypothermic cardiopulmonary bypass and circulatory arrest for operations on the descending thoracic and thoracoabdominal aorta. *Ann Thorac Surg, 74,* S1885–S1898.

50. Lederle, F. A., et al. (2000). The aneurysm detection and management study screening program: validation cohort and final results. Aneurysm Detection and Management Veterans Affairs Cooperative Study Investigators. *Arch Intern Med, 160,* 1425–1430.

51. Leurs, L. J., et al. (2004). Endovascular treatment of thoracic aortic diseases: combined experience from the EUROSTAR and United Kingdom Thoracic Endograft registries. *J Vasc Surg, 40,* 670–679.

52. McNamara, M. G., Heckman, J. D., & Corley, E. G. (1994). Severe open fracture of the lower extremity: a retrospective evaluation of the Mangled Extremity Severity Score. *J Orthop Trauma, 8,* 81–87.

53. Maizes, V. (2002). Integrative approaches to hypertension. *Clin Fam Practice, 4,* 895–905.

54. Maniar, S. H., et al. (2003). Delayed paraplegia after thoracic and thoracoabdominal aneurysm repair: a continuing risk. *Ann Thorac Surg, 75,* 113–120.

55. McNutt, R., et al. (1989). Blunt tibial artery trauma: predicting the irretrievable extremity. *J Trauma, 29,* 1624–1627.

56. Milewicz, D. M., et al. (2005). Treatment of aortic disease in patients with Marfan syndrome. *Circulation, 111,* e150–e157.

57. Moser, K. M., & LeMoine, J. R. (1981). Is embolic risk conditioned by location of deep venous thrombosis? *Ann Intern Med, 158,* 585–593.

58. Multicentre Aneurysm Screening Study Group. (2002). Multicentre aneurysm screening study (MASS): cost-effectiveness analysis of screening for abdominal aortic aneurysms based on four year results from a randomized controlled trial. *BMJ, 325,* 1135–1138.

59. National Center for Health Statistics. (2005). Deaths: final data for 2002. *Natl Vital Stat Rep, 53*(5), 40.

60. Nienaber, C. A., & Eagle, K. A. (2003). Aortic dissection: new frontiers in diagnosis and management. Part I: From etiology to diagnostic strategies. *Circulation, 108,* 628–635.

61. Nienaber, C. A., & Eagle, K. A. (2003). Aortic dissection: new frontiers in diagnosis and management. Part II: Therapeutic management and follow-up. *Circulation, 108,* 772–778.

62. Ott, M. C., et al. (2004). Management of blunt thoracic aortic injuries: endovascular stents versus open repair. *J Trauma, 56,* 565–570.

63. Passage, J., et al. (2002). BioGlue surgical adhesive: an appraisal of its indications in cardiac surgery. *Ann Thorac Surg, 74,* 432–437.

64. Pickering, T. G., et al. (2005). Recommendations for blood pressure measurement in humans and experimental animals part 1: Blood pressure measurement in humans—a statement for professionals from the subcommittee of professional and public education of the American Heart Association council on high blood pressure research. *Hypertension, 45,* 142–161.

65. Ramzi, D., & Leeper, K. (2004). DVT and pulmonary embolism: part I. Diagnosis. *Am Fam Physician, 69*(12), 2829–2836.

66. Rodrigo, R., et al. (2003). Homocysteine and essential hypertension. *J Clin Pharmacol, 4,* 1299–1306.

67. Russell, V. L., et al. (1991). Limb salvage versus traumatic amputation. A decision based on a seven-part predictive index. *Ann Surg, 213,* 473–481.

68. Sacks, D., et al. (2003). Position statement on the use of the ankle brachial index in the evaluation of patients with peripheral vascular disease. A consensus statement developed by the Standards Division of the Society of Interventional Radiology. *J Vasc Interv Radiol, 14*(9 Pt 2), S389.

69. Safi, H. J., et al. (2004). Staged repair of extensive aortic aneurysms: long-term experience with the elephant trunk technique. *Ann Surg, 240,* 677–685.

70. Sakamaki, F., et al. (2002). Higher prevalence of obstructive airway disease in patients with thoracic or abdominal aortic aneurysm. *J Vasc Surg, 36,* 35–40.

71. Severance-Lossin, L., Blissitt, P. A., & Sullivan, J. (2005). Lumbar subarachnoid catheter insertion (assist) for cerebral spinal fluid pressure monitoring and drainage. In D. J. Lynn-McHale Wiegand

& K. K. Carlson (Eds.), *AACN procedure manual for critical care*. St. Louis: Elsevier Saunders.

72. Simon, B. J., & Leslie, C. (2001). Factors predicting early in-hospital death in blunt thoracic aortic injury. *J Trauma, 51*, 906–911.

73. Smith, J. G., & Butler, V. L. (2001). Perioperative care of the patient with aortic rupture. *Top Emerg Med, 23*, 47–52.

74. Society of Thoracic Surgeons. (2006). *STS adult CV surgery dational database—Fall 2005 executive summary*, www.sts.org.

75. Society of Thoracic Surgeons. (2006). *STS general thoracic surgery data summary January 2002 – June 2005 procedures*, www.sts.org.

76. Soukiasian, H. J., et al. (2005). Total circulatory arrest for the replacement of the descending and thoracoabdominal aorta. *Arch Surg, 140*, 394–398.

77. Stephens, E. *Peripheral vascular disease*. www.emedicine.com/emerg/topic862.htm.

78. Stulz, D. B., & Gupta, S. C. (2004). Rapid assessment and treatment of aortic dissection. *Emerg Med, 36*, 18–43.

79. Suedkamp, N. P., et al. (1993). The incidence of osteitis in open fractures: an analysis of 948 open fractures (a review of the Hannover experience). *J Orthop Trauma, 7*, 473–482.

80. Suzuki, T., et al. (1996). Novel biochemical method for aortic dissection. Results of a prospective study using an immunoassay of smooth muscle myosin heavy chain. *Circulation, 93*, 1244–1249.

81. Suzuki, T., et al. (2000). Diagnostic implications of elevated levels of smooth-muscle myosin heavy-chain protein in acute aortic dissection. *Ann Intern Med, 133*, 537–541.

82. Suzuki, T., et al. (2003). Clinical profiles and outcomes of acute type B aortic dissection in the current era: lessons learned from the International Registry of Aortic Dissection (IRAD). *Circulation, 108(suppl II)*, II312–II317.

83. Svensson, L. G. (2002). Progress in ascending and aortic arch surgery: minimally invasive surgery, blood conservation, and neurological deficit prevention. *Ann Thorac Surg, 74*, S1786–S1788.

84. Symbas, P. N., et al. (2002). Traumatic rupture of the aorta: immediate or delayed repair? *Ann Surg, 235*, 796–802.

85. Tsai, T. T., Nienaber, C. A., & Eagle, K. A. (2005). Acute aortic syndromes. *Circulation, 112*, 3802–3813.

86. United Kingdom Small Aneurysm Trial Participants. (2002). Long-term outcomes of immediate repair compared with surveillance of small abdominal aortic aneurysms. *N Engl J Med, 346*, 1445–1452.

87. Varon, J., & Marik, P. E. (2003). Clinical review: the management of hypertensive crises. *Crit Care, 7*, 374–384.

88. Veith, F. J., et al. (2003). Treatment of ruptured abdominal aneurysms with stent grafts: a new gold standard? *Semin Vasc Surg, 16*, 171–175.

89. Warken, T. E., & Greinacher, A. (2004). Heparin-induced thrombocytopenia: recognition, treatment, and prevention: the Seventh ACCP Conference on Antithrombotic and Thrombolytic Therapy. *Chest, 126*(3 suppl), 311S–317S.

90. Weaver, F. A., et al. (1996). For the STILE Investigators: surgery versus thrombolysis for ischemia of the lower extremity, surgical revascularization versus thrombolysis for non embolic lower extremity native artery occlusions: results for a prospective randomized trial. *J Vasc Surg, 24*, 413–521.

91. Weber, T., et al. (2003). D-dimer in acute aortic dissection. *Chest, 123*, 1375–1378.

92. Wells, P. S., et al. (1997). Value of assessment of pretest probability of deep vein thrombosis in clinical management, *Lancet, 350*, 1795–1798.

93. Wells, P. S., et al. (2000). Derivation of a simple clinical model to categorize patients' probability of pulmonary embolism: increasing the model's utility with the SimpliRED D-dimer. *Thromb Haemostasis, 83*, 416–420.

94. Wung, S. F., & Aouizerat, B. E. (2004). Newly mapped gene for thoracic aortic aneurysm and dissection. *J Cardiovasc Nurs, 19*(6), 409–416.

95. Yee, C. A. (2004). Aortic dissection: the tear that kills. *Nurs Manag, 35*(2), 25–32.

Nancy Albert

Cardiomyopathies are defined as diseases of the myocardium associated with cardiac dysfunction. It may seem the terms *cardiomyopathy* and *heart failure* (HF) are synonymous, but rather, HF is a clinical outcome of cardiomyopathy. Other outcomes of cardiomyopathy are cardiac dysrhythmias and sudden cardiac death occurring in the absence of clinical HF.[12] Thus HF is a clinical syndrome occurring subsequent to diseases of the heart muscle (see Chapter 12), whereas the classifications of cardiomyopathies refer to the underlying disease process and clinical phenotype itself. Cardiomyopathy may occur in the absence of symptoms or any clinical evidence of cardiac dysfunction. With aggressive treatment, advanced cardiomyopathy can be prevented or reduced, delaying the onset of clinical HF.

The overall incidence, prevalence, hospitalization, and mortality rates of cardiomyopathy in adults are not clearly identified. In the American Heart Association (AHA) *Heart Disease and Stroke Statistics—2005 Update,* incidence is not included.[1] The annual hospital cardiomyopathy discharge rate is 36,000 cases; the annual mortality rate is 28,863.[1] Knowing the burden of HF in the United States, these statistics seem low, but the data are misleading. When patients are discharged from the hospital after treatment for decompensated HF resulting from cardiomyopathy, the diagnosis-related group (DRG) code used is generally "HF" (i.e., DRG 127) rather than cardiomyopathy or another related medical circulatory system disease (e.g., myocarditis). In other reports of cardiomyopathy prevalence in the United States, it was estimated that 36.5 per 100,000 persons had dilated cardiomyopathy, 17.9 per 100,000 persons had hypertrophic cardiomyopathy, and 5000 persons had dysrhythmogenic right ventricular cardiomyopathy.[28,33,38] Data on restrictive cardiomyopathy were not listed because of its rare occurrence.[33] In the AHA statistical report, increased mortality from cardiomyopathy was associated with aging and being African American, similar to the data available on HF mortality.[1] One difference was that mortality was associated with male gender in cardiomyopathy and female gender in HF.[1]

In 1980 a task force was set up by the World Health Organization (WHO) and the International Society and Federation of Cardiology (ISFC) to establish consensus on cardiomyopathy definitions and nomenclature. By 1995 new advancements in research and higher level of awareness of heart disease led to a reconvening of the task force in Geneva.[32] At that time, new entities were defined and the group introduced changes in definitions and terminology.

A review of current definitions and nomenclature based on the 1995 WHO/ISFC report is presented.[32] Research findings that refute the current WHO/ISFC classifications report will be discussed as well as recommendations for change in practice. Finally, specific treatment strategies that differ from systolic HF consensus recommendations will be stated so that critical care nurses can better understand, communicate, and facilitate an optimized plan of care that provides the best opportunity to improve patient survival, morbidity, and quality of life. Chapter 12 provides more comprehensive details about HF pathophysiology, diagnosis, assessment, and management.

CARDIOMYOPATHY DEFINITIONS AND CLASSIFICATIONS

As stated previously, cardiomyopathy is simply defined as a disease of the myocardium associated with cardiac ventricular dysfunction. However, the simplicity ends with the basic definition. In the WHO/ISFC report,[32] cardiomyopathies were classified into four groups on the basis of their prevalent pathophysiology and, when possible, according to etiologic, genetic, and clinical features. Classification labels included dilated cardiomyopathy, hypertrophic cardiomyopathy, restrictive cardiomyopathy, and dysrhythmogenic right ventricular cardiomyopathy.[32] Table 17-1 presents characterizations of each of the four classifications of cardiomyopathies. About 30% to 50% of patients with hypertrophic cardiomyopathy have a left ventricular outflow tract obstruction. A normal heart is compared with hearts affected by dilated cardiomyopathy, hypertrophic cardiomyopathy, and restrictive cardiomyopathy in both systole and diastole in Figure 17-1.

TABLE 17-1 Characterizations of Each of the Four Classifications of Cardiomyopathy (As Defined by the World Health Organization and International Society and Federation of Cardiology)—cont'd

CARDIOMYOPATHY CLASSIFICATION	CARDIOMYOPATHY CHARACTERIZATIONS	PRESENTATION
Dilated cardiomyopathy[16,32]	Left or right cardiomyocyte dilation Increased size of ventricular cavity Left ventricular end-diastolic dimension ≥5 cm Left ventricular ejection fraction 50% or less Fractional shortening of 25% or less Impaired left or right ventricular contraction Nonspecific histology Myocardial fibrosis can be mild to severe	Any age (can affect young and old) Presentation: progressive congestive left- or right-sided HF May have dysrhythmias, thromboembolism, and sudden cardiac death
Hypertrophic cardiomyopathy[16,18,20,26,29,32]	Left or right cardiomyocyte hypertrophy, disarray, and interstitial fibrosis (increased collagen content) Usually asymmetric and involves interventricular septum and posterior wall Can be symmetric Maximum left ventricular wall thickness ≥15 mm Ventricle not dilated (small ventricular cavity) Exists when there is absence of an increased external load from other cardiac (e.g., aortic stenosis) or systemic disorders (e.g., hypertension) Usually left ventricle volume is reduced or normal Common to have systolic gradients (obstruction to left ventricular outflow) at rest and when provoked Obstruction is associated with hypertrophy of *basal portion* of ventricular septum and small outflow tract and an enlarged and elongated mitral valve Obstruction is either *subaortic,* caused by systolic anterior motion of mitral valve (known as SAM) and mid-systolic contact with ventricular septum, or *mid-cavity* Labeled "obstructive" when gradient is ≥30 mm Hg at rest or when provoked Normal or supernormal ejection fraction	Any age (can affect young and old) Presentation: dysrhythmias and sudden cardiac death (asymptomatic or with syncope, light-headedness/dizziness) common May present with fatigue and mild dyspnea and have progressive left-sided HF symptoms, including anginal chest pain May have embolic stroke as a complication of atrial fibrillation May have a stable and benign course (up to 25% achieve normal longevity) ECG: atrial fibrillation prevalence was 22% over a 9-year period of study Atrial fibrillation was associated with mortality, stroke, and severe functional disability; however, was benign in 35% of patients May see abnormal Q waves in leads I, aV$_L$, V$_5$, and V$_6$; right axis deviation and prolonged QRS duration in V$_5$ and V Left atrial overload common (terminal force of P wave is 0.04 mV) Signal-averaged ECG: ventricular late potentials and ventricular dysrhythmias, especially with abnormal functional properties of myocardium (increased collagen content) Outflow gradients cause a loud apical systolic ejection murmur
Restrictive cardiomyopathy[2,14,32,41]	Restrictive filling and reduced diastolic volume of right or left ventricle but normal ventricular wall motion or normal wall thickness and ventricular chamber dimensions (neither hypertrophy nor dilation) Can have endocardial thickening and ventricular cavity obliteration that hinders diastolic ventricular filling Dilated atria because of increased left ventricular end-diastolic pressures from derangement of ventricular filling Ischemic heart disease and specific heart	More common in elderly but can affect any age group Presentation: right-sided HF manifested by tachycardia, dyspnea, peripheral edema, ascites, and liver enlargement Sudden death is relatively common Mitral or tricuspid regurgitation often present; when advanced, S$_3$ gallop is common Atrial enlargement is usually pronounced ECG: P waves reflect right or left atrial hypertrophy or overload Peak right ventricular systolic pressure may

Table continues on page 386

Table 17-1 Characterizations of Each of the Four Classifications of Cardiomyopathy (As Defined by the World Health Organization and International Society and Federation of Cardiology)—cont'd

CARDIOMYOPATHY CLASSIFICATION	CARDIOMYOPATHY CHARACTERIZATIONS	PRESENTATION
	muscle disease (e.g., amyloidosis) can cause secondary restrictive cardiomyopathy	be around 40 mm Hg and can go up to 60 mm Hg
Dysrhythmogenic right ventricular cardiomyopathy[6,7,15,30,32,41]	Progressive replacement of myocytes by adipose and fibrous tissue (fibrofatty scarring and myocardial atrophy) of right ventricular free wall Causes global right ventricular dilation, thinning, and dysfunction in 54% Late: left ventricular involvement (10%), with relative sparing of septum Hypokinetic right ventricle; may have localized aneurysm (in up to 50% of cases) and dyskinesis	Age at onset of symptoms is generally 32 years; usually diagnosed by age 40 Presentation: ventricular tachydysrhythmias with left bundle branch block morphology (78.5%) and sudden cardiac death; may have palpitations (67%), syncope (32%), and atypical chest pain (27%) May present with progressive right-sided heart failure (less frequent) ECG: depolarization abnormalities—low voltage in QRS related to loss of right ventricular myocardium; prolongation of QRS in V_1–V_3 compared with V_6 Presence of epsilon wave (small-amplitude postexcitation electrical potentials that occur in 28% of cases at end of QRS complex and beginning of ST segment, reflecting delayed right ventricular activation) Repolarization abnormalities: precordial T wave changes

ECG = Electrocardiogram.

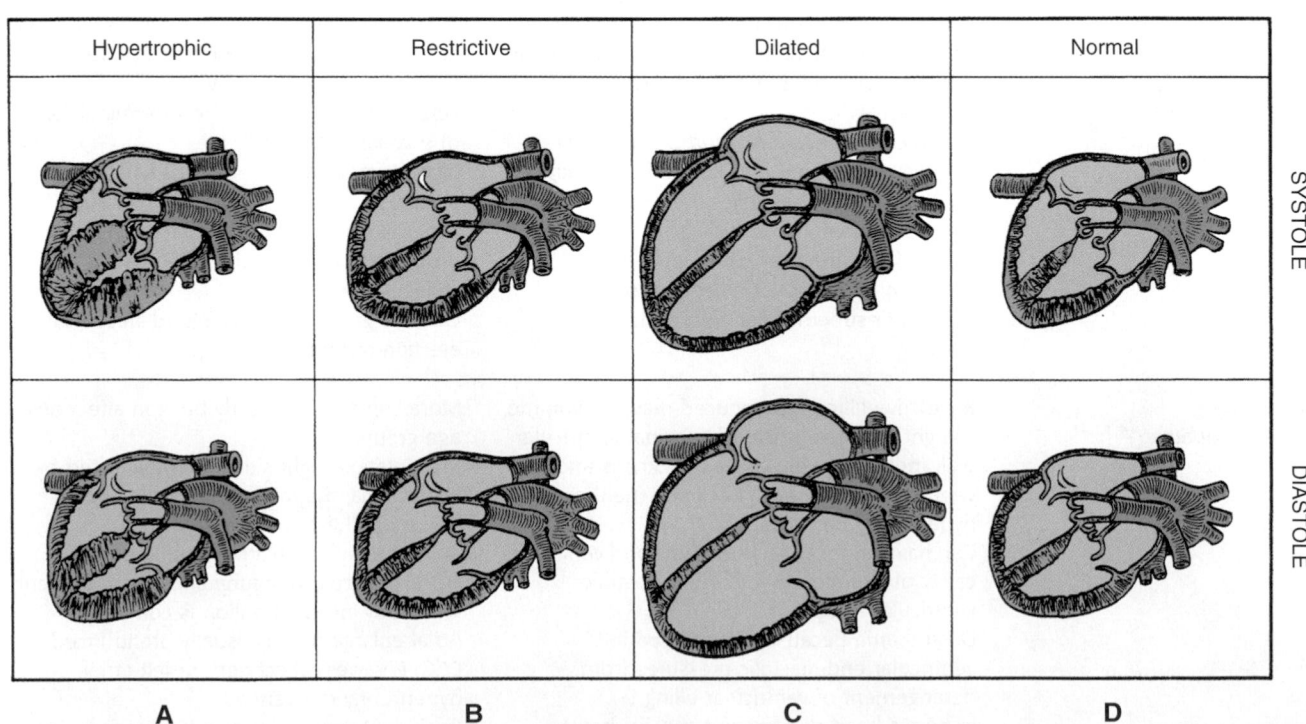

♦FIGURE 17-1 Types of cardiomyopathies and the differences in ventricular diameter during systole and diastole, compared with a normal heart. **A,** Hypertrophic. **B,** Restrictive. **C,** Dilated. **D,** Normal.

In addition, Figure 17-2 shows postmortem photographic images of a normal heart, a hypertrophic heart, and a heart diseased with dilated cardiomyopathy.

A fifth group, unclassified cardiomyopathies, was created to include cases that did not readily fit into one of the other four groups or cases that presented with features of more than one type of cardiomyopathy. Some examples include fibroelastosis and amyloidosis (generally considered restrictive cardiomyopathies), noncompacted myocardium (arrest of normal embryogenesis of the endocardium and myocardium, producing hypertrabeculation of the ventricles) that may occur with other congenital anomalies causing both systolic and diastolic dysfunction and ventricular dysrhythmias, systolic dysfunction with minimal dilation, and mitochondrial involvement.[32,43]

Cardiomyopathies can also be categorized as primary and secondary. *Primary* cardiomyopathies are those that are not the result of other diseases or consequent to disorders of other parts of the cardiovascular system. Primary cardiomyopathies may have many causes, but generally result from genetic defects that are isolated, are associated with skeletal muscle diseases, or are associated with neurologic diseases (Box 17-1). Table 17-2 provides a partial list of etiologies of primary cardiomyopathies and their classifications. Molecular genetic analyses of cardiomyopathies that are inherited as single-gene disorders have developed into a mature field as a result of completion of the Human Genome Project. The list of reported mutations associated with familial forms of cardiomyopathies is extensive. Gibbons et al.[11] reported selected genes associated with cardiovascular disease, classified by phenotype.

Cardiomyopathies that are the result of other diseases or are consequential to disorders of other parts of the cardiovascular system are labeled *secondary*

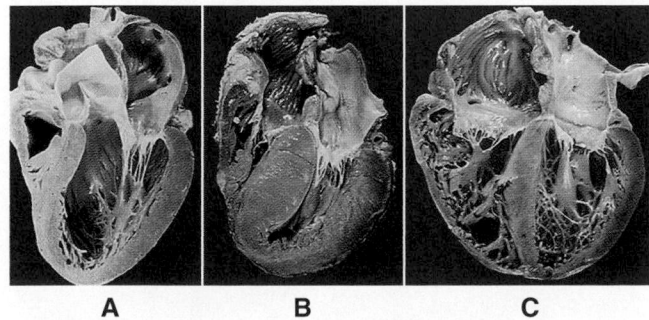

FIGURE 17-2 **A,** Normal heart, with normal left ventricular dimensions and thickness. **B,** Hypertrophic cardiomyopathy, showing a marked increase in myocardial mass and preferential hypertrophy of the interventricular septum. **C,** Dilated cardiomyopathy, showing marked increase in chamber size.

cardiomyopathies. Based on the 1995 WHO/ISFC report, secondary cardiomyopathies are termed *specific* cardiomyopathies.[32] These cardiomyopathies have many causes and may result from genetic and environmental interactions. The label given to each specific cardiomyopathy describes the specific cardiac and systemic diseases that caused the cardiomyopathy (e.g., ischemic, valvular, hypertensive, inflammatory, and metabolic cardiomyopathies). Also included in specific cardiomyopathies (even though some have a genetic basis and fit in the primary category) are general system diseases, muscular dystrophies, neuromuscular

TABLE 17-2 Etiologies of *Primary* Cardiomyopathies (Not Inclusive) and Their Pathophysiologic/Clinical Features Classification

ETIOLOGY	CLASSIFICATION
Isolated	
Viral	Dysrhythmogenic right ventricle (RV)
Autoimmune	Restrictive; hypertrophic; dilated
Postinfectious, autoimmune	Dilated
Cardiac myosin, troponin T or I, α-tropomyosin abnormalities	Hypertrophic; may progress to dilated
Cardiac troponin I abnormalities	Restrictive
Defects in cytoskeleton that impair force transmission; dystrophin, vinculin, or phospholamban abnormalities	Dilated
Long and short QT syndrome (sodium or potassium ion channel diseases of cell membrane); polymorphic ventricular tachycardia (abnormal ryanodine receptor 2 regulating calcium release from sarcoplasmic reticulum for electromechanical coupling); Brugada syndrome (sodium ion channel disease); Venetian cardiomyopathy (familial; Venice region of Italy); and Naxos disease (recessive form of abnormal cytoskeleton proteins regulating cell junctions, observed on the Greek island Naxos)	Dysrhythmogenic RV
Defective sarcomere proteins impairing force production	Hypertrophic; restrictive
Skeletal Diseases	
Viral	Dysrhythmogenic RV
Autoimmune	Restrictive; hypertrophic
Dystrophin, sarcoglycan abnormalities	Dysrhythmogenic RV; dilated
Bart's syndrome	Dilated
Emery-Dreifuss muscular dystrophy (emerin or lamin defect)	Dysrhythmogenic RV; dilated
Steinert's myodystrophy and other myodystrophies	Dysrhythmogenic RV; dilated
Neurologic Diseases	
Viral	Dysrhythmogenic RV; dilated
Ataxia (Friedreich's disease)	Hypertrophic; may progress to dilated
Kearns-Sayre syndrome	Dysrhythmogenic RV; dilated
Mitochondrial encephalomyopathy	Hypertrophic

Data from references 9, 27, and 41.

disorders, sensitivity and toxic reactions, and peripartum cardiomyopathy.[32] Characterizations of specific cardiomyopathies as defined by WHO/ISFC are described in the first column of Table 17-3.

Today, many scientists question the usefulness of the WHO/ISFC 1995 classifications of cardiomyopathies. The current classifications recognize only the advanced stages of the cardiomyopathic process when

TABLE 17-3   Characterization of Specific Cardiomyopathies*

SPECIFIC CARDIOMYOPATHY LABEL	DEFINITION OR LABEL OF SPECIFIC DISORDERS—WHO AND ISFC[32]	DEFINITION OR ETIOLOGIC CLASSIFICATION OR LABEL OF SPECIFIC DISORDERS—HFSC; *PROPOSED REVISIONS*[13]
Ischemic cardiomyopathy	Definition: dilated cardiomyopathy with impaired contractile performance *not explained by* extent of coronary artery disease or ischemic damage	Same label (*ischemic* cardiomyopathy) Definition: dilated cardiomyopathy with coronary atherosclerosis or vasculitis or resulting from anomalous coronary artery origin
Valvular cardiomyopathy	Ventricular dysfunction that is out of proportion to abnormal loading conditions	Classification label: *hyperergopathic* (referring to overwork) cardiomyopathies with two categories: (a) valvular heart disease; (b) hypertension
Inflammatory cardiomyopathy	Infectious, idiopathic, and autoimmune forms of myocarditis when associated with cardiac dysfunction, causing dilated and other cardiomyopathies	Inflammatory cardiomyopathy not listed Classification label: *infectious* cardiomyopathy includes viral, bacterial, rickettsial, and protozoal infections
Metabolic cardiomyopathy	Categories: (a) endocrine (thyrotoxicosis, hypothyroidism, adrenocortical insufficiency, pheochromocytoma, acromegaly, and diabetes mellitus); (b) familial storage disease and infiltrations (hemochromatosis, glycogen storage disease, and other deficiencies); (c) deficiency (potassium metabolism disturbances, magnesium deficiency, and nutritional disorders); (d) amyloid	Same label (*metabolic* cardiomyopathy) Categories a and c from WHO/ISFC metabolic cardiomyopathy classification are same in this classification Amyloid is listed in new classification: *neoplastic* cardiomyopathies (immunocytic dyscrasias) NOTE: familial disease (part of category b) is listed under muscular dystrophies
General system disease	Categories: (a) connective tissue disorders (systemic lupus erythematosus, polyarteritis nodosa, rheumatoid arthritis, scleroderma, and dermatomyositis); (b) infiltrations (sarcoidosis) and granulomas (leukemia)	*Collagen vascular disease* cardiomyopathy includes systemic lupus erythematosus, progressive systemic sclerosis, other connective tissue diseases
Muscular dystrophies	Includes Duchenne, Becker type, and myotonic dystrophies	*Genetic* cardiomyopathies with two categories: (a) familial (autosomal dominant, autosomal recessive, x-linked, and mitochondrial); (b) sporadic
Neuromuscular disorders		Neuromuscular disorder cardiomyopathies not listed; these would fall into genetic classification and *cardiomyopathy not otherwise specified (NOS)*
Sensitivity and toxic reactions	Includes alcohol, catecholamines, anthracyclines, irradiation, and miscellaneous	*Toxic* cardiomyopathies with four categories: (a) alcohol; (b) cocaine; (c) antineoplastic medications; (d) heavy metals *Physical agent* cardiomyopathies with three categories: (a) ionizing radiation; (b) electric shock; (c) trauma *Immunologically* mediated cardiomyopathies with two categories: (a) transplant rejection; (b) postvaccinal
Peripartal cardiomyopathy	Cardiomyopathy that may manifest in peripartum period	Cardiomyopathy *associated with pregnancy*

*As defined by the World Health Organization (WHO), the International Society and Federation of Cardiology (ISFC), and the Heart Failure Specialist Cardiologists (HFSC).

clinical dysfunction is present. Advanced cardiomyopathy may have a poor prognosis, especially if classified as dilated, restricted, or dysrhythmogenic right ventricular. The goal of management is not palliation; rather, the goal is to prevent or halt the progress of HF through interventions that interrupt (early on if possible) pathophysiologic processes.[12,13] Other limitations of the current classification system are that it does not include idiopathic (unknown etiology), hyperergopathic (overwork of cardiomyocytes with pathologic hypertrophy and cardiac remodeling), postgenomic (heredity and familial), and autoimmune classifications; it defines and describes ischemic cardiomyopathy in a manner paradoxical to common usage and does not allow for multiple etiologies (e.g., hypertension and diabetes).[4,10,12,40,41] In 2004 Giles et al.[13] recommended revisions to the WHO/ISFC classifications; the comparisons are shown in Table 17-3.

STAGES OF CARDIOMYOPATHY

In 2004 two groups[13,27] proposed pathways describing the evolution and progression of cardiomyopathy from the preclinical or latent period to the late or advanced period, using stages. Figure 17-3 represents the seven-stage process described by Nigro et al.[27] In this scheme, patients progress through five distinct stages. Stage one is a preclinical stage in which patients are asymptomatic but myocyte damage is detectable. Stages two through four represent the presence of

hypertrophic, dysrhythmogenic, or restrictive cardiomyopathy and are characterized by clinical, biochemical, electrocardiographic, echocardiographic, and nuclear investigation findings specific to each. Stage five represents the spotty fibrosis stage characterized by weakness, mild dyspnea, possible atypical angina, possible release of cardiac enzymes, ST and T wave changes on electrocardiogram, localized dyskinesis, increased acoustic densitometry, reduced ejection fraction below 50% on echocardiogram, and nonhomogeneous perfusion on nuclear investigations. Spotty fibrosis may develop into widespread fibrosis characterized by symptoms of congestive HF (i.e., dyspnea, liver enlargement, tachycardia, ventricular stiffness with reduction in ejection fraction, and electrocardiographic changes in T waves). Stage six, the dilated cardiomyopathy stage, is often the final stage of evolution of different cardiomyopathies. Patients have systolic ventricular dysfunction with a reduced ejection fraction below 45%, cardiac enlargement, and diffuse myocardial damage with spotty fibrosis. In stage six, HF is intractable. The final stage (stage seven) is labeled refractory HF, representing severe dilated cardiomyopathy no longer responsive to medical therapies, even when optimized. In stage seven, HF is irreversible. Myocardial fibrosis is extensive; patients have a very poor prognosis.[27] Nigro et al. believe that regular patient monitoring at least every 6 months is necessary to distinguish stages and assess progression through stages.[27]

The second pathway of cardiomyopathy evolution and progression is based on the presence of muscle

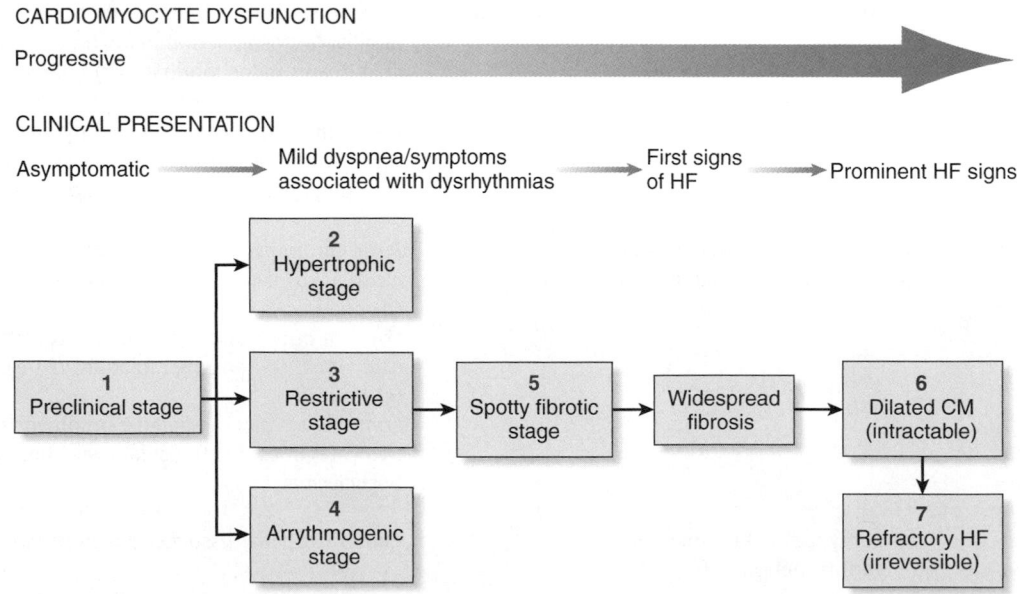

♦FIGURE 17-3 Representation of the seven stages of evolution from cardiomyopathy to heart failure. CM = Cardiomyopathy, HF = heart failure. (Data from reference 27.)

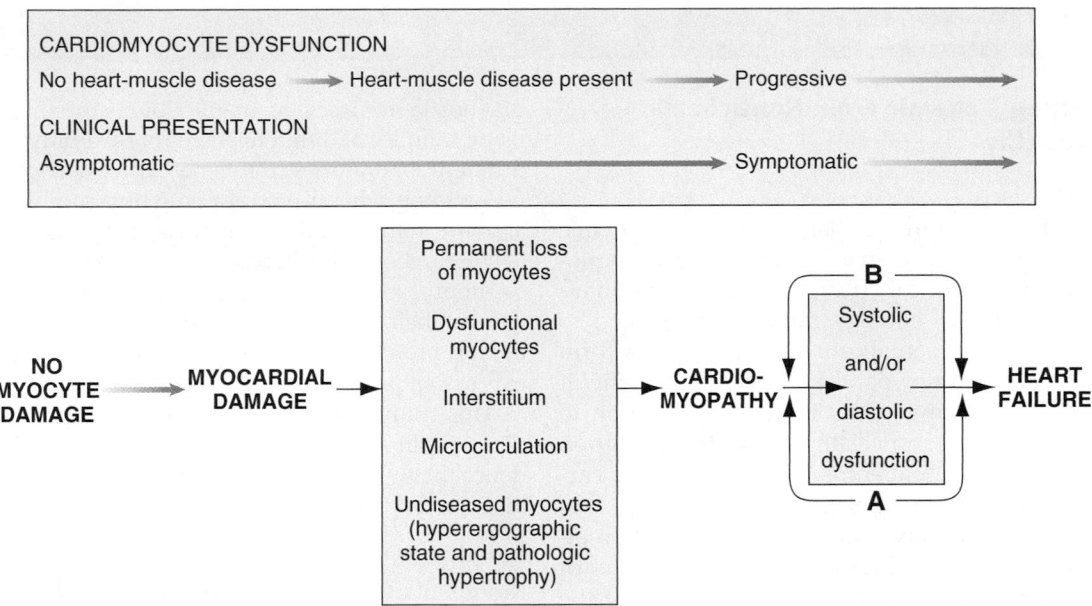

♦FIGURE 17-4 Representation of the *three* stages of evolution from cardiomyopathy to heart failure. Involves a vicious cycle that is set in motion by **(A)** neuroendocrine activation and **(B)** ventricular remodeling that perpetuate one another and prompt worsening of systolic and diastolic dysfunction, leading to symptoms (i.e., dyspnea, fatigue, edema, and cardiac dysrhythmias and dyssynchrony).

damage and symptoms and is represented graphically in three stages (Figure 17-4).[13] In this scheme, stage one is labeled *latent* or *potential* cardiomyopathy and represents precardiomyopathy; no evidence of heart disease is detected. In stage two, labeled *early* or *subclinical* cardiomyopathy, evidence of muscle disease is present; however, patients are still asymptomatic. In stage three, labeled *late* or *advanced* cardiomyopathy, heart muscle damage and symptoms are both present. The differing phenotypes of cardiomyopathy (i.e., dilated, restrictive, hypertrophic, and dysrhythmogenic) are used to classify patients. The following findings, typical of systolic HF, help describe the patient's clinical state: (1) an abnormal relationship between ventricular filling pressures and cardiac output, (2) abnormal cardiovascular autonomic function, (3) activation of neurohormonal systems, and (4) signs and symptoms of worsening HF (e.g., dyspnea, fatigue, edema) and disturbances in cardiac rhythm (e.g., dysrhythmias and cardiac dyssynchrony). Giles et al.[13] believe that the etiology and pathophysiology of the cardiomyopathy should be elucidated before clinical evaluation is completed.

Both of the proposed staging pathways are useful clinically. They move in only one direction, reflect the progressive nature of cardiomyopathy, and can be linked with treatment strategies. Communicating the current stage with patients might help them to recognize the progressive nature of cardiomyopathy, even when asymptomatic, especially if the communication is coupled with management strategies, including self-care. Of the two staging pathways, Nigro et al. have greater linearity in terms of expectations at various points in cardiomyopathy progression; these may be inconsistent with actual patient presentations.[27] The Giles et al. pathway uses a greater number of parallel tracks to reflect myocardial damage that precipitates cardiomyopathy before the development of HF.[13] Both are hypothesis-generating and require clinical utilization to determine their clinical applicability.

DIFFERENTIATING CARDIOMYOPATHY ETIOLOGY

Differentiation of ischemic and nonischemic cardiomyopathy is important since prognosis in coronary artery disease–induced cardiomyopathy is improved when the treatment plan includes revascularization in addition to medical management (see Chapter 12 for details of revascularization as part of HF management).[18,23,45] Segmental (and global) wall motion abnormalities visible by echocardiography are present in both dilated and ischemic cardiomyopathy; thus a definitive etiology cannot be determined by echocardiogram alone. The Research Utilization box on p. 392 highlights research in this area.

Distinguishing Ischemic From Nonischemic Cardiomyopathy

CLINICAL ISSUE

Accurately distinguishing ischemic and nonischemic cardiomyopathy aids in treatment planning and prognosis. In patients with clinical HF and a history of coronary artery disease, the HF etiology might be presumed to be ischemic, when the actual cause of HF may be a form of nonischemic cardiomyopathy. It is often difficult to determine if cardiomyopathy is out of proportion to coronary artery disease, especially when either condition is worsening while the patient is asymptomatic. As cardiomyopathy progresses, etiology is thought to be less important since pathophysiologic pathways and treatment modalities merge. However, at every stage of HF, management decisions can vary on the basis of the etiology of myocardial disease, and survival for ischemic cardiomyopathy is decreased in comparison with nonischemic cardiomyopathy.

SUMMARY

In this study, researchers attempted to identify a gene expression profile for 48 myocardial cell samples of patients with mild to advanced cardiomyopathy.[17] Endomyocardial biopsies were used for sample collection. The Prediction Analysis of Microassays statistical computing software was used to develop the etiology prediction profile in 16 samples from patients with end-stage cardiomyopathy (training set). The remaining samples were used to validate the profile. Patient characteristics differed at end-stage disease in those with nonischemic and ischemic cardiomyopathy. Patients with ischemic etiology were older, more likely to be male, more likely to be prescribed an angiotensin-converting enzyme inhibitor, and less likely to require intravenous inotropic agent support. In the training set of 16 samples of end-stage disease myocardial cells, researchers demonstrated 100% sensitivity and 100% specificity when developing their etiology prediction profile. When researchers tested the diagnostic accuracy of their etiology prediction profile using samples of different stages of cardiomyopathy from different laboratories, the gene expression profile classified all nonischemic cardiomyopathy samples correctly, and one in three of the ischemic samples correctly.[17]

Researchers concluded that patients with ischemic cardiomyopathy exhibited greater changes in gene expression as their disease progressed; thus stage-specific prediction profiles are necessary to ensure accuracy in gene expression profiling.[17]

This study represented the first report of gene expression profiling in cardiovascular disease and the first evidence that microassay experiments from endomyocardial biopsies are feasible.

APPLICATION

Results of studies on gene expression profiling of etiology to distinguish ischemic from nonischemic cardiomyopathy in newly diagnosed patients are under way. If the technology is validated, it can be applied to assist healthcare clinicians in patient management, in assessment of response to therapies, and in prognosis. Ultimately, it may refine diagnostic and prognostic accuracy. Individual patient profile information can be used by nurses in a variety of ways, including nursing research on the influence of etiology on self-care measures and clinical outcomes, recommendations for surgical options for HF, and education and care planning at the end of life.

NEED FOR FURTHER STUDY

Future studies are needed on molecular profiling to learn if the technology can distinguish cardiomyopathy patients by other clinical parameters of relevance. Accuracy in the diagnosis of etiology of cardiomyopathy may yield many strategies that can optimize the treatment plan, ease patient suffering, and improve healthcare provider efficiency.

Kittleson, M. M., et al. (2004). Identification of a gene expression profile that differentiates between ischemic and nonischemic cardiomyopathy. *Circulation, 110,* 3444–3451.

Researchers studied the results of noninvasive testing to differentiate ischemic versus nonischemic cardiomyopathy in patients with systolic left ventricular dysfunction and clinical HF. Electron beam tomography accurately detected the presence of atherosclerotic calcification in patients with obstructive coronary artery disease.[18] When compared with determining the etiology of cardiomyopathy by echocardiography findings, electron beam tomography had greater overall diagnostic accuracy (90% versus 70%, $P < 0.001$).[18] Another powerful diagnostic tool, gadolinium-enhanced cardiovascular magnetic resonance, distinguished dilated from ischemic cardiomyopathy in 90 patients with systolic HF. In addition, this technique showed that coronary angiogram results could lead to an incorrect assignment of dilated cardiomyopathy.[23] In another series of patients, dobutamine stress and pulsed-wave tissue Doppler echocardiogram had better accuracy than wall motion score index (calculated from resting echocardiogram data) in identifying coronary artery disease, especially in patients with left bundle branch block.[8] When single-photon emission computed tomography (SPECT) was used to differentiate ischemic and nonischemic cardiomyopathy, mixed results were found. In one study, the presence of a severe and extensive stress perfusion defect reliably identified ischemic cardiomyopathy; however, in another study, SPECT yielded only modest value in distinguishing the two cardiomyopathies.[44,45] Generally, researchers compared two diagnostic modalities to determine superiority rather than comparing all available types in the same study; thus tests used in the diagnosis of ischemic versus nonischemic cardiomyopathy are chosen based on equipment availability, radiologist expertise, and healthcare provider trust in test results.

Hibernating myocardium (defined as myocardium that fails to contract normally but is metabolically active when stimulated and may recover after revascularization) occurs in patients with ischemic cardiomyopathy from multivessel disease and low coronary artery blood flow. Imaging techniques for detection of myocardial viability are fluorodeoxyglucose positron emission tomography, transient ischemia modified thallium-201 (reinjection or rest-redistribution) studies, dobutamine echocardiography, or Tc-99m 2-methoxyisobutylisonitrile.[34] Once known, revascularization is a primary intervention. Patients with type 2 diabetes frequently have obesity and hypertension in their history. Diabetes is associated with concentric left ventricular remodeling, increased heart mass, perivascular fibrosis, and increased quantities of matrix collagen that are independent of myocardial ischemia.[39] These morphologic changes are believed to confer clinically significant impairment in diastolic compliance. It is unclear whether the myocardial energy metabolism alterations consistent with insulin resistance (type 2 diabetes) cause HF or if the HF causes insulin resistance. Sympathetic overactivity, sedentary lifestyle, endothelial dysfunction, and loss of skeletal muscle mass are all possible mechanisms by which HF causes insulin resistance.[39] These interactions are complex; it is hypothesized that the two conditions worsen each other.[39]

◆ Case Study 17-1, Part A

Etiology of Heart Failure

D.P., a 71-year-old female, complained of fatigue and dyspnea for 1 year. Initially, she was advised to lose weight (her body mass index was 30 kg/m²). Serum testing revealed dyslipidemia (high values of low- and very-low-density lipoproteins and low level of high-density lipoprotein). As a result, she was prescribed atorvastatin (Lipitor) 10 mg daily. After a second complaint of fatigue and dyspnea, she was

treated by her primary physician for an upper respiratory tract infection. When symptoms worsened, she was admitted to the emergency department of her local hospital and diagnosed with congestive heart failure. Her echocardiogram showed an ejection fraction of 15% to 20%, and she presented with 4+ mitral regurgitation. The electrocardiogram revealed normal sinus rhythm; D.P.'s heart rate was 92 beats/min with a PR interval of 150 ms and QRS duration of 84 ms. Blood pressure was 142/94 mm Hg and respirations were 22 per minute. Her history was positive for obesity, hypertension, type 2 diabetes (treated with diet), and coronary artery disease although she never had a myocardial infarction. In the emergency department she was treated with intravenous furosemide (Lasix) 40 mg. She watched a 12-minute video on managing HF and received written handouts that provided an overview of the same information. She was discharged on enalapril (Vasotec) 2.5 mg twice daily and the loop diuretic furosemide 40 mg daily. At discharge D.P. was instructed to visit her primary physician within 2 weeks.

Decision point: Based on the above findings, what is the most likely etiology of D.P.'s heart failure?

◆ Case Study 17-1, Part B

Etiology of Heart Failure

Two months later, D.P. is admitted to your unit with dyspnea on exertion after climbing one flight of stairs. Blood pressure was 110/72 mm Hg and pulse was 80 beats/min. Physical examination findings were negative for jugular venous distention and S₃ gallop, point of maximal impulse was normal, and an S₄ heart sound is auscultated.

Decision point: What diagnostic tests are key to determining etiology and developing an appropriate treatment plan?

Case continues on page 396

PREVENTION AND TREATMENT OF CARDIOMYOPATHY

As noted in both staging schemes, cardiomyopathy can occur without symptoms. It is often detected in the late (advanced) stage when symptoms appear and a call to action is raised. At this point, the patient typically has a known cardiovascular condition associated with symptoms, such as diabetes, hypertension, valve dysfunction, palpitations or syncope from atrial or ventricular dysrhythmias, or clinical HF. Treatments for each condition are discussed in other chapters. The Multidisciplinary Plan of Care on pp. 394-395 contains specific problems and treatments of the four cardio-myopathy classifications that are unique from HF management strategies found in Chapter 12. These recommendations include preventive therapies because their implementation may decrease the risk of adverse outcomes, most notably sudden cardiac death and worsening HF. It is important to note that there is lit-tle reference literature on certain recommendations. Recommendations are often made on the basis of expert practitioner experience and insights.

MULTIDISCIPLINARY PLAN OF CARE FOR PATIENTS WITH CARDIOMYOPATHY*

PROBLEM	INTERVENTION	RATIONALE	EXPECTED OUTCOME
Increased risk of sudden cardiac death with exercise in patients less than or equal to 40 years of age (HCM, ARVCM)	Prescribe and educate patients on activity and exercise restrictions (not inclusive): (1) *Not advised, especially if high intensity:* basketball, body building, weightlifting, ice hockey, rock climbing, racquetball, soccer, tennis, touch football, windsurfing, scuba diving, skiing (downhill and cross-country) (2) *Assess on an individual basis, especially if moderate intensity:* baseball/softball, skiing, surfing, hiking, sailing, jogging, motorcycling, horseback riding (3) *Probably permitted when low intensity:* bowling, golf, skating, weights, brisk walking, jogging, snorkeling, treadmill/stationary bicycle, doubles tennis, swimming (4) *Avoid:* burst exertion or sprinting, adverse environmental conditions, exercise programs that escalate in exertion, amusement park rides if intensely stressful or frightening[22]	Nonsustained ventricular tachycardia is associated with substantial increase in sudden cardiac death in young patients with HCM[25] Balance between vigorous activity that may trigger sudden cardiac death and allowing moderate exercise and fitness that have well-known health benefits Recommendations assume absence of important limiting cardiac symptoms and no implantable cardioverter-defibrillator Recommendations are aimed at preventing exercise-induced catecholamine release, inducing Valsalva maneuver, increasing left ventricular wall stress, or causing sudden acceleration in heart rate[22]	Avoidance of ventricular tachydysrhythmia–induced sudden cardiac death
	Implantation of an automatic defibrillator	Prevent sudden cardiac death; in ARVCM, ventricular tachycardia identified high-risk subjects for cardiovascular mortality[15]	Life-saving protection by terminating life-threatening ventricular tachydysrhythmias[6]
Concomitant use of substances that act as cardiac stimulants (HCM, ARVCM)	Educate patients *not* to use: (1) Dietary or nutritional supplement with ma huang (2) Compounds that enhance performance: cocaine and anabolic steroids[22]	(1) An herbal source of ephedrine that is potentially dysrhythmogenic	Decreased risk of adverse effects that cause dysrhythmogenesis
Left ventricular obstruction to outflow with symptoms refractory to	(1) Surgical treatment: Morrow operation, also know as myotomy-myectomy—proximal ventricular septum is incised and a small portion is resected	Outflow tract obstruction at rest is a strong predictor of progression to severe symptoms of HF and of death[21] In moderate-severe obstruction to	(1) Improved symptoms, improved forward blood flow during systole, thus decreasing ventricular wall stress

PROBLEM	INTERVENTION	RATIONALE	EXPECTED OUTCOME
pharmacology (HCM)	(2) Dual-chamber pacing: DDD pacing causes preexcitation of right ventricle that might prompt remodeling of ventricular wall; use before surgery, especially in older adults and those at high risk for surgery[5] NOTE: chronic DDD pacing impairs diastolic function in hypertrophic obstructive cardiomyopathy patients with normal diastolic function[3] (3) Alcohol septal ablation: after locating vessel that targets obstructing portion of proximal ventricular septum, absolute alcohol is injected to cause a myocardial infarction localized to ventricular septum[36] NOTE: often associated with procedure-related heart block, often requiring permanent pacing[5]	left ventricular outflow, when intraventricular pressure gradient greater than 50 mm Hg without stress, relief of obstruction leads to improved functional class in 90% of patients and decreases mitral regurgitation	(2) Reduces symptoms and left ventricular outflow pressure gradients (3) Reduces symptoms in patients at high risk for surgical morbidity and mortality (advanced age and pulmonary or renal disease) Procedural success occurs when ventricular outflow gradient is significantly reduced
Atrial fibrillation (all cardiomyopathies; however, greater risk of complications from atrial fibrillation in HCM)	(1) Implement prompt cardioversion to convert to normal sinus rhythm (2) Begin anticoagulation with warfarin (Coumadin) (3) Administer carvedilol (Coreg), metoprolol (Lopressor), or amiodarone to slow heart rate[28]	Atrial fibrillation can cause acute, severe hemodynamic compromise from tachycardia and loss of atrial contraction; paroxysmal or chronic atrial fibrillation exacerbates symptoms, especially in HCM	(1) Decreased risk of persistent or permanent atrial fibrillation (2) Decreased risk of embolization (3) Decreased in symptom severity
Acute changes in loading conditions causing volume depletion (HCM)	(1) If hypotensive, use intravenous phenylephrine infusion (direct-acting adrenergic agent); adult dose: 10 mg in 500 ml of D_5W, given at 100–170 mcg/min until hemodynamically stable, then 40–60 mcg/min as maintenance dose (2) Infuse fluids (generally D_5W or normal saline)[28]	(1) Slows heart rate and constricts blood vessels; other inotropic agents (dopamine, norepinephrine [Levophed], epinephrine, dobutamine [Dobutrex]) cause tachycardia (2) Need optimal diastolic filling to enhance cardiac output	Stabilize left ventricular loading conditions and optimize hemodynamics
Preclinical cardiomyopathy stage risk reduction (all cardiomyopathies)	Initiate familial counseling: educate families of patients to consider gene-based diagnosis for all relatives at risk when molecular cause of cardiomyopathy is defined for one family member[5]	Informative and efficient: gene-based testing identifies gene carriers before onset of clinical disease	Once detected, routine assessment can begin that may ultimately improve survival and decrease clinical outcomes (HF, tachydysrhythmias, or sudden cardiac death)

*This plan of care is specific to cardiomyopathy problems not associated with systolic HF (dilated cardiomyopathy). The type of cardiomyopathy in which the problem is seen is listed in parentheses after the problem, e.g., hypertrophic cardiomyopathy (HCM), dysrhythmogenic right ventricular cardiomyopathy (ARVCM), or all cardiomyopathies.

Exercise Restrictions

In young patients with genetic cardiovascular diseases, especially hypertrophic and dysrhythmogenic right ventricular cardiomyopathies, unexpected sudden cardiac death was found in those who engaged in leisure activities and competitive sports.[22] Triggers of life-threatening ventricular tachydysrhythmias and sudden cardiac death during sports were emotional stress, environmental factors, myocardial ischemia, sympathetic-vagal imbalance, and hemodynamic changes. Additionally, intense exercise and athletic training could promote disease progression or worsening of the dysrhythmia substrate.[22]

Pharmacologic Therapy in Hypertrophic Obstructive Cardiomyopathy

Pharmacologic therapy is the first line of treatment. Beta blockers (first choice) and the calcium channel blocker verapamil (Calan) (second choice) are used to block the effects of catecholamines that exacerbate the outflow tract obstruction. These medications also enhance diastolic filling by slowing the heart rate.[28] If symptoms are not controlled with a beta blocker, disopyramide (Norpace) should be considered to decrease inotropy and further decrease the outflow gradient, thereby improving or relieving symptoms.[28]

Interventional Therapy in Hypertrophic Obstructive Cardiomyopathy

Invasive treatments are considered when the resting outflow gradient is greater than 30 mm Hg and symptoms limit daily activities. Surgical septal myectomy is the gold standard invasive treatment because, if successful, the gradient and mitral regurgitation will be immediately and completely abolished, leading to near-normal exercise capacity and freedom of symptoms of dyspnea, angina, and exertional syncope.[28] The effects are long-lasting, without recurrence of outflow tract obstruction. Dual chamber pacemaker insertion is less invasive than myectomy, but the mechanism of therapeutic effect is unclear. In addition, in experimental studies the placebo effect was large and exercise capacity was not significantly improved in patients whose pacemakers were activated. This therapy is reserved for patients who have coexisting illnesses that are contraindications to other therapies or who require pacing for preexisting bradycardia.[28] Alcohol-induced septal ablation is performed in the cardiac catheterization laboratory. The rate of complete abolition of obstruction and relief of symptoms is less than with myectomy and has inherent risks, including complete heart block requiring permanent pacemaker therapy, large myocardial infarction, ventricular septal defect, intractable ventricular fibrillation, and myocardial perforation.[28]

◆ Case Study 17-1, Part C

Etiology of Heart Failure

On this current admission, D.P. had a new echocardiogram that showed an ejection fraction of 25%, with left ventricular systolic and diastolic internal diameters of 5.3 and 6.3 cm, respectively, mild right ventricular dysfunction, and a pseudonormal diastolic pattern. She was assigned New York Heart Association functional Class II-III. (Refer to Chapter 12 for assessment, signs and symptoms, diagnostic findings, and management strategies for patients with heart failure.) A cardiac catheterization was also performed, showing coronary artery disease with nine lesions in four vessels (diffuse disease in the right coronary artery: four lesions), each occluded between 60% and 70%.

Decision point: Should the diffuse obstructive coronary artery disease found on coronary angiography be the primary focus of treatment to halt progression of D.P.'s cardiomyopathy?

CONCLUSIONS

Cardiomyopathy can be the precursor to HF and other clinical outcomes (e.g., dysrhythmias and symptoms associated with fast heart rate) and sudden cardiac death. Cardiomyopathies are classified by their dominant pathophysiology and etiologic or pathogenetic factors. There are four broad classifications (i.e., primary cardiomyopathies) as well as categories for specific (i.e., secondary cardiomyopathies) and unclassified cardiomyopathies. Many cardiomyopathies are progressive and will shorten life. Diagnosis may be missed or delayed because of poor awareness of genetic predisposition and lack of clinically visible symptoms in the early stages. Once clinical signs and symptoms associated with cardiomyopathy are known or when the results of genetic testing are positive, risk assessment, preventive measures, and interventions that decrease morbidity and improve quality of life and survival must be implemented. Generally, interventions are those of HF management (see Chapter 12) except as noted in the Multidisciplinary Plan of Care on pp. 394-395.

Nurses work in tandem with other healthcare team members to educate patients and facilitate care so that outcomes are optimized. In addition to patient education, the critical care nurse should understand the rationale for interventions for specific cardiomyopathies and use this knowledge to ensure that optimal diagnostic testing and treatment strategies are implemented. Prevention, when possible, is an important aspect of prolonging survival. Even when asymptomatic, patients must be educated to understand the need for specific interventions that may prevent progressive left ventricular dysfunction. Critical care nurses must clearly communicate to their patients the normal progression of cardiomyopathy. Critical care nurses must also assess patient understanding of their cardiac condition(s) and clearly communicate self-care responsibilities to help avoid or, at least, slow progression, morbidities, and mortality.

REFERENCES

1. American Heart Association. (2005). *Heart disease and stroke statistics—2005 update*. Dallas, Tex: American Heart Association.
2. Ammash, N. M, et al. (2000). Clinical profile and outcome of idiopathic restrictive cardiomyopathy. *Circulation, 101*, 2490–2496.
3. Betocchi, S., et al. (2002). Dual chamber pacing in hypertrophic cardiomyopathy: long-term effects on diastolic function. *PACE, 25*, 1433–1440.
4. Boffa, G. M., et al. (2001). Ischemic cardiomyopathy: lack of clinical applicability of the WHO/ISFC classification of cardiomyopathies. *Ital Heart J, 2*, 778–781.
5. Braunwald, E., Seidman, C. E., & Sigwart, U. (2002). Contemporary evaluation and management of hypertrophic cardiomyopathy. *Circulation, 106*, 1312–1316.
6. Corrado, D., et al. (2000). Arrhythmogenic right ventricular dysplasia/cardiomyopathy. *Circulation, 101*(11), e101.
7. Davutoglu, V., et al. (2004). Arrhythmogenic biventricular dysplasia/cardiomyopathy masquerading as dilated cardiomyopathy with typical electrocardiographic features. *Int J Cardiol, 97*, 147–149.
8. Duncan, A. M., et al. (2003). Differentiation of ischemic from nonischemic cardiomyopathy during dobutamine stress by left ventricular long-axis function. *Circulation, 108*, 1214–1220.
9. Fontaine, G., Fontaliran, F., & Frank, R. (1998). Arrhythmogenic right ventricular cardiomyopathies. Clinical forms and main differential diagnoses. *Circulation, 97*, 1532–1535.
10. Fu, M., & Matsui, S. (2002). Is cardiomyopathy an autoimmune disease? *Keio J Med, 51*, 208–212.
11. Gibbons, G. H., et al. (2004). Genetic markers. Progress and potential for cardiovascular disease. *Circulation, 109*(suppl IV), IV-47–IV-58.
12. Giles, T. D. (1997). New WHO/ISFC classification of cardiomyopathies: a task not completed. *Circulation, 96*, 2081–2082.
13. Giles, T. D., et al. (2004). Definition, classification, and staging of the adult cardiomyopathies: a proposal for revision. *J Cardiac Failure, 10*, 6–8.
14. Hancock, E. W. (2001). Differential diagnosis of restrictive cardiomyopathy and constrictive pericarditis. *Heart, 86*, 343–349.
15. Hulot, J. S., et al. (2004). Natural history and risk stratification of arrhythmogenic right ventricular dysplasia/cardiomyopathy. *Circulation, 110*, 1779–1784.
16. Kamiyama, N., et al. (1997). Electrocardiographic features differentiating dilated cardiomyopathy from hypertrophic cardiomyopathy. *J Electrocardiol, 30*, 301–306.
17. Kittleson, M. M., et al. (2004). Identification of a gene expression profile that differentiates between ischemic and nonischemic cardiomyopathy. *Circulation, 110*, 3444–3451.
18. Le, T., et al. (2000). Comparison of echocardiography and electron beam tomography in differentiating the etiology of heart failure. *Clinical Cardiol, 23*, 417–420.
19. Deleted in proofs.
20. Maron, B. J., et al. (2003a). American College of Cardiology/European Society of Cardiology clinical expert consensus document on hypertrophic cardiomyopathy. *J Am Coll Cardiol, 42*, 1687–1713.
21. Maron, M. S., et al. (2003b). Effect of left ventricular outflow tract obstruction on clinical outcome in hypertrophic cardiomyopathy. *N Engl J Med, 348*, 295–303.
22. Maron, B. J., et al. (2004). Recommendations for physical activity and recreational sports participation for young patients with genetic cardiovascular diseases. *Circulation, 109*, 2807–2816.
23. McCrohon, J. A., et al. (2003). Differentiation of heart failure related to dilated cardiomyopathy and coronary artery disease using gadolinium-enhanced cardiovascular magnetic resonance. *Circulation, 108*, 54–59.
24. Milewicz, D. M., & Seidman, C. E. (2000). Genetics of cardiovascular disease. *Circulation, 102*(suppl IV), IV-013–IV-111.
25. Monserrat, L., et al. (2003). Non-sustained ventricular tachycardia in hypertrophic cardiomyopathy: an independent marker of sudden death risk in young patents. *J Am Coll Cardiol, 42*, 873–879.
26. Nanni, L., et al. (2003). Hypertrophic cardiomyopathy: two homozygous cases with "typical" hypertrophic cardiomyopathy and three new mutations in cases with progression to dilated cardiomyopathy. *Biochem Biophys Res Commun, 309*, 391–398.
27. Nigro, G., et al. (2004). Cardiomyopathies: diagnosis of types and stages. *Acta Myologica, 23*, 97–102.
28. Nishimura, R. A., & Holmes, D. R. (2004). Hypertrophic obstructive cardiomyopathy. *N Engl J Med, 350*, 1320–1327.
29. Olivotto, I., et al. (2001). Impact of atrial fibrillation on the clinical course of hypertrophic cardiomyopathy. *Circulation, 104*, 2517–2524.
30. Pinamonti, B., Sinagra, G., & Camerini, F. (2000). Clinical relevance of right ventricular dysplasia/cardiomyopathy. *Heart, 83*, 9–11.
31. Richard, P., et al. (2003). Hypertrophic cardiomyopathy. Distribution of disease genes, spectrum of mutations, and implications for a molecular diagnosis strategy. *Circulation, 107*, 2227–2232.
32. Richardson, P., et al. (1996). Report of the 1995 World Health Organization/International Society and Federation of Cardiology Task Force on the definition and classification of cardiomyopathies. *Circulation, 93*, 841–842.
33. Schwartz, K., et al. (1995). Molecular basis of familial cardiomyopathies. *Circulation, 91*, 532–540.
34. Schwartz, M. L., et al. (1996). Clinical approach to genetic cardiomyopathy in children. *Circulation, 94*, 2021–2038.
35. Deleted in proofs.
36. Shamim, W., et al. (2002). Nonsurgical reduction of the interventricular septum in patients with hypertrophic cardiomyopathy. *N Engl J Med, 347*, 1326–1333.
37. Spooner, P. M., et al. (2001). Sudden cardiac death, genes, and arrhythmogenesis. Consideration of new population and mechanistic approaches from a National Heart, Lung, and Blood Institute Workshop, Part II. *Circulation, 103*, 2447–2452.
38. Tabib, A., et al. (2003). Circumstances of death and gross and microscopic observations in a series of 200 cases of sudden death associated with arrhythmogenic right ventricular cardiomyopathy and/or dysplasia. *Circulation, 108*, 3000–3005.
39. Taegtmeyer, H., McNulty, P., & Young, M. E. (2002). Adaptation and maladaptation of the heart in diabetes: Part I General concepts. *Circulation, 105*, 1727–1733.
40. Tenenbaum, A., Fisman, E. Z., & Motro, M. (2002). Toward a redefinition of ischemic cardiomyopathy: is it an indivisible entity? *J Am Coll Cardiol, 40*, 205–206.

41. Thiene, G., Corrado, D., & Basso, C. (2004). Cardiomyopathies: is it time for a molecular classification? *Euro Heart J, 25,* 1772–1775.

42. Watkins, H. (2003). Genetic clues to disease pathways in hypertrophic and dilated cardiomyopathies. *Circulation, 107,* 1344–1346.

43. Weiford, B. C., Subbarao, V. D., & Mulhern, K. M. (2004). Noncompaction of the ventricular myocardium. *Circulation, 109,* 2965–2971.

44. Wu, Y., et al. (2003). TI-201 myocardial SPECT in differentiation of ischemic from nonischemic dilated cardiomyopathy in patients with left ventricular dysfunction. *J Nuclear Cardiol, 10,* 369–374.

45. Yao, S., et al. (2004). Prospective validation of a quantitative method for differentiating ischemic versus nonischemic cardiomyopathy by technectium-99m sestamibi myocardial perfusion single-photon emission computed tomography. *Clin Cardiol, 27,* 615–620.

CHAPTER 18

Heart and Lung Transplantation

Julie A. Stanik-Hutt, Debra J. Carter, and Diane Vail Skojec

For the last 20 years, transplantation has been the last therapeutic option for patients suffering end-stage heart or lung disease despite maximal medical therapy.[34] For these individuals, thoracic organ (i.e., heart, lung, or combined heart-lung) transplantation can prolong life, as well as enhance its quality. Over the years, improvements in donor and recipient selection, organ preservation, operative techniques, postoperative care, and immunosuppression have increased both patient and graft survival. Today, outcomes after heart transplant are generally good. Unfortunately, neither short-term nor long-term outcomes are as good after lung transplant.[68]

Optimal outcomes with thoracic transplantation require the collaborative efforts of a multidisciplinary team of healthcare professionals, including, but not limited to, critical care and transplant nurses; physicians; clinical pharmacists; respiratory, physical, occupational, and speech therapists; dietitians; social workers; psychologists; home care specialists; and financial coordinators. Medical specialties involved include cardiology, pulmonology, thoracic surgery, anesthesiology, pathology, immunology, and infectious disease specialists. The patient and the patient's family are also vital members of the team. They have a significant impact on the patient's preparation for and recovery from this major surgery. The multidisciplinary team approach is used to evaluate and select candidates for transplant, prepare them for the procedure, and provide care to the recipient after the transplant procedure.

This chapter will provide the critical care nurse with an understanding of the physiology and pathophysiology related to heart and lung transplantation, as well as implications for patient care during recovery from these procedures. Care of patients with end-stage heart or lung disease before transplantation, complex rules for posting candidates to national transplant lists, care of solid organ donors, and care of donor organs between harvest and implantation are not included. Information regarding long-term posttransplant monitoring, care, complications, and prognosis is also beyond the scope of this chapter.

More than 12,000 lung and 36,000 heart transplants have been performed since 1988. At any given time, more than 6000 Americans wait for a thoracic organ transplant: about 2900 for a heart and about 3100 for a lung.[73] Unfortunately, because of a shortage of usable donor organs, up to 20% of lung and 30% of heart transplant candidates die before a donor organ is found.[46] Out of 100 patients evaluated as a potential organ donor, only 15 can ultimately be used as a lung donor.[66] Ultimately, a little more than 2000 heart and 1000 lung transplants are performed in the United States annually.[73] While perioperative mortality after heart transplant is only 9%, early mortality after lung transplant can be as high as 24%.[27,47] One-year survival after lung transplant is only 73%, and by year 3, only 50% of lung transplant recipients are still alive.[71] Conversely, 1- and 5-year survival rates after heart transplant are 86% and 72%, respectively.[75a,b]

EVALUATION AND CANDIDACY FOR THORACIC TRANSPLANTATION

Because of the lack of an adequate number of thoracic organ donors, it is imperative that pretransplant conditions are optimized so that every transplanted thoracic organ, and recipient, has the highest chance for success and long-term survival. This process begins with careful evaluation of all potential thoracic transplant candidates before listing (Box 18-1).

The first goal of the evaluation is to confirm that the patient's disease is irreversible and would be likely to cause the individual's death within 2 years (Table 18-1 and Box 18-2).[72] It is also essential to determine that no conditions exist that would significantly increase the morbidity or mortality of the transplant procedure or the subsequent required immunosuppression (Box 18-3).[35]

The perfect thoracic transplant candidate is an individual who has life-threatening, irreversible heart or lung disease and no comorbidities. Debilitated patients with multiple comorbid conditions, those who are significantly overweight or underweight, and those colonized with pan-resistant microorganisms would be unlikely to survive the transplant procedure. They

Box 18-1

Heart and Lung Transplant Candidate Evaluation Procedures

DIAGNOSTIC TESTS

Electrocardiogram
Echocardiogram
MUGA scan[†]
Cardiac catheterization[‡]
Cardiopulmonary stress testing[*]
PA and lateral chest x-ray
Chest CT[†]
Complete pulmonary function tests (spirometry, volumes, and diffusion testing)
Differential quantitative ventilation/perfusion scan
Arterial blood gases
6-minute walk test[†]
Peripheral Doppler[*]
Carotid ultrasound[*]
TB skin testing with anergy testing if prescribed chronic steroids

CONSULTATIONS

Transplant cardiology/pulmonology
Transplant surgeon
Physical and occupational therapy
Dietitian
Social worker
Transplant psychologist
Transplant nurse coordinator
Financial/insurance adviser
Dental examination and clearance

LABORATORY TESTING

CBC, PT/PTT
Mammogram
Basic metabolic panel with liver function tests
Lipid profile
24-hour urine for creatinine clearance
Blood typing and antibody testing
Human leukocyte antigen tissue typing
Panel of reactive antibody testing
Antibody serologies: CMV, EBV, HSV, VZV, MMR
Screening for hepatitis B, hepatitis C, HIV, toxoplasmosis
Sputum for culture and sensitivity[†]

DISEASE PREVENTION SCREENING

Pelvic exam with Pap smear
Prostate-specific antigen[§]
Digital rectal exam[§]
Bone density scan
Colonoscopy/sigmoidoscopy[§]

[*]Heart candidates only.
[†]Lung candidates only.
[‡]All heart candidates; lung candidates older than 40 years of age or multiple risk factors.
[§]If older than 50 years of age.
CBC = Complete blood cell count, CMV = cytomegalovirus, CT = computerized tomography, EBV = Epstein-Barr virus, HIV = human immunodeficiency virus, HSV = herpes simplex virus, MMR = measles, mumps, rubella, MUGA = multiple gated acquisition, PA = posteroanterior, Pap = Papanicolaou, PT = prothrombin time, PTT = partial thromboplastin time, TB = tuberculosis, VZV = varicella zoster virus.

would probably be among the 14% of heart or 21% of lung recipients who do not survive the first year after transplantation.[74] Individuals with psychosocial characteristics (history of noncompliance, major uncontrolled psychiatric problems, active substance abuse, poor social support, and inadequate financial/insurance coverage) that would interfere with adherence to complex posttransplant regimens are also not good candidates. Age criteria may also be used to determine eligibility for thoracic transplantation. Although physiologic age may be taken into account, heart transplantation is generally not offered to individuals more than 65 years of age.[45] The age limits for combined heart and lung,

bilateral lung, and single lung transplants are 55, 60, and 65, respectively.[37]

Once accepted and listed, candidates are seen at the transplant center every few months to monitor their status and to be sure no new condition has developed that would preclude transplantation. At these visits, progression of the patient's disease may prompt a change in their listing status and move them higher on the priority list. However, candidates typically wait 2 years or more between listing and transplantation. During this time, it is not uncommon for a candidate to be requested to come to the hospital for transplant, only to be sent home when some problem with the donor organ is discovered.

TABLE 18-1   Indications of End-Stage Heart and Lung Disease

HEART

Maximum V_{O_2} <10 ml/kg/min with achievement of anaerobic metabolism

Severe ischemia consistently limiting routine activity and not amenable to revascularization

Recurrent symptomatic ventricular dysrhythmias refractory to all accepted therapeutic modalities

LUNG

Life expectancy of less than 2 years

Patients with COPD	
Patients with cystic fibrosis	FEV_1 <25% predicted $Paco_2$ >55 mm Hg Development of pulmonary hypertension in association with clinical deterioration
Patients with restrictive disease	Rapidly declining or FEV_1 <30% predicted Increased hospitalizations Massive hemoptysis Pao_2 <50 mm Hg or $Paco_2$ >55 mm Hg
Patients with pulmonary vascular disease	FVC <60% predicted DLCO <50% Severe hypoxemia Poor performance status Mean PAP >55 mm Hg Mean RA pressure >10 mm Hg Cardiac index <2 L/min/m^2 With congenital heart disease: progressive symptoms

From references 28a and 41a.
COPD = Chronic obstructive lung disease, FEV = forced expiratory volume, FVC = forced vital capacity, DLCO = carbon monoxide diffusion capacity, PAP = pulmonary artery pressure, mm Hg = millimeters of mercury, RA = right atrial.

Box 18-2

Diagnoses Amenable to Thoracic Transplantation

HEART DISEASES

- Ischemic cardiomyopathy
- Nonischemic cardiomyopathy (peripartum, inflammatory, familial, toxic, idiopathic)
- Miscellaneous (congenital, refractory ventricular dysrhythmias, valvular disease, retransplantation)

LUNG DISEASES

- Obstructive (COPD, emphysema, α_1-antitrypsin deficiency)
- Restrictive (sarcoidosis, scleroderma, idiopathic pulmonary fibrosis)
- Suppurative (cystic fibrosis, bronchiectasis)
- Pulmonary vascular (primary pulmonary hypertension, Eisenmenger's syndrome)

From references 28a and 41a.

Contraindications to Thoracic Transplantation

ABSOLUTE

- Age greater than 65 years
- Active malignancy in last 5 years
- Other significant irreversible organ system dysfunction

Renal: creatinine clearance <50 mg/ml/min

Hepatic

Bone marrow

Diffuse advanced cerebrovascular disease

Severe pulmonary hypertension (unless heart-lung transplant planned)

- Chronic colonization with pan-resistant microorganisms
- Active hepatitis or tuberculosis
- Human immunodeficiency virus
- Massive pulmonary mycetoma
- Active substance abuse including smoking
- Major psychiatric problems
- Weight greater than 130% or less than 70% of ideal body weight
- Severe debilitation
- Social/behavioral problems (e.g., noncompliance)
- Inadequate social support

RELATIVE

- Previous thoracic surgery or pleurodesis
- Chronic ventilator dependence
- Chronic high-dose steroids
- Symptomatic osteoporosis
- Financial problems

♦ Case Study 18-1, Part A

Post–Heart Transplant Care

M.J. is a 52-year-old male with diabetes mellitus (DM), hypertension, and a family history of coronary artery disease (CAD) who was diagnosed in 2001 with ischemic cardiomyopathy. He initially presented with complaints of decreased exercise tolerance and was treated medically. Despite optimal medical therapy, including percutaneous revascularization, M.J. continued to experience angina and his heart function continued to deteriorate. He was experiencing increasing episodes of heart failure and ventricular tachycardia.

He was referred for a transplant evaluation in 2004, which revealed an ejection fraction of 15% with severe global hypokinesis. A right heart catheterization showed right atrial (RA)

pressure 11 mm Hg, PAP 16/6 mm Hg, pulmonary artery wedge pressure (PAWP) 7 mm Hg, and CO 4.5 L/min. On exercise testing, his maximum oxygen consumption (V_{O_2}) was 11 ml/kg/min with achievement of anaerobic metabolism. Medical history was notable for DM for 8 years and hypertension for 6 years; no prior surgeries, no blood transfusions. Social history was notable for remote 10 pack-year smoking history, daily glass of red wine, and no other substance use or abuse. M.J. was disabled from his job in a manufacturing company sales office and is married to a woman who suffers from rheumatoid arthritis. Following completion of the evaluation, he was placed on the heart transplant waiting list as a status 2. After 6 months on the list, an appropriate donor was available and he underwent an orthotopic heart transplant.

Decision point: Is M.J. an appropriate heart transplant candidate?

Case continues on page 440

SURGICAL APPROACHES TO THORACIC TRANSPLANTATION

When an appropriate organ is identified, the patient is taken to the operating room (OR) to begin preparation for transplantation. Family members generally accompany the patient as far as possible and are reminded about the length of the surgery. At intervals, usually after specific landmarks in the procedure (for example, after the surgical incision is made, after organs arrive in the room, after implantation is complete, and after weaning from cardiopulmonary bypass [CPB]), someone from the surgical team will inform the family of the patient's condition and progress of surgery. After the completion of the surgery, the surgeon will meet the family to provide specific information about the procedure.

Heart Transplantation

The two surgical procedures used during heart transplantation are *orthotopic* and *heterotopic* implantation. The most common, orthotopic, requires explantation of all but parts of the atria of the recipient's native heart (Figure 18-1). This is followed by biatrial or bicaval implantation of the donor heart along with end-to-end anastomosis between the recipient and donor aorta and pulmonary artery (Figures 18-2 and 18-3). Heterotopic implantation occurs when the recipient's heart is not explanted. Rather, the donor heart is implanted alongside the recipient's native heart (Figure 18-4).

Once the donor organs have been inspected and accepted for transplantation, explantation of the native heart proceeds. The recipient's chest is opened via

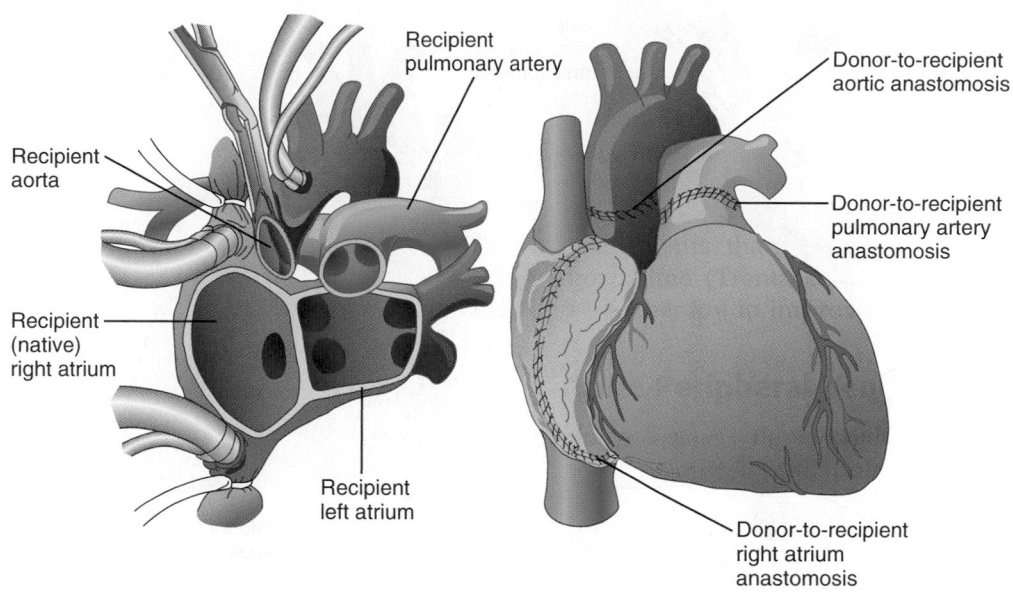

♦FIGURE 18-1 Before and after view of biatrial technique for donor heart implantation.

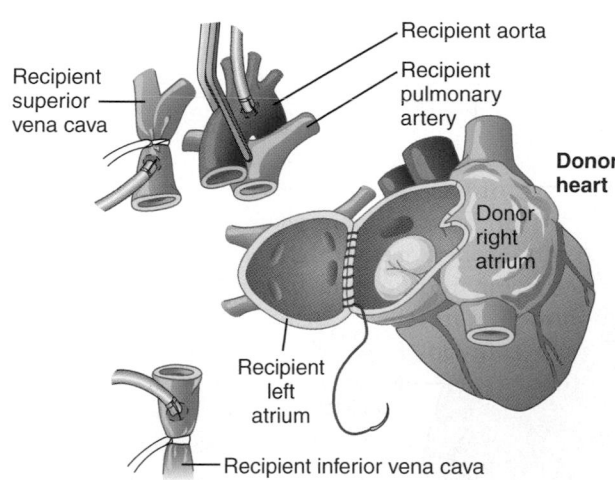

♦FIGURE 18-2 Bicaval anastomotic technique. Bicaval implantation proceeds with left atrial anastomosis followed by superior and inferior vena cava anastomoses. After the pulmonary arteries are joined, caval snares are released, air is vented from the heart, and blood is allowed to circulate through the heart and lungs. Finally, aortic anastomoses are performed.

sternotomy, which may be extended into the abdomen. The pericardium is opened, and preparations are made for CPB. At this point, adhesions formed after previous cardiac surgeries may present considerable challenges to dissection and cause significant hemorrhage. Dissection and preparation are necessary so that rapid explantation can proceed once the donor organs are in the room and ready for implantation. Precise timing

is important in order to limit the ischemic time to less than 6 hours for the donor organs. When both donor and native hearts are ready, the native heart is removed and the donor heart is placed into the thoracic cavity. CPB is used to support the patient while implantation of the donor heart is completed. Cooled lap pads and continuous cold pericardial irrigation are also used to insulate and preserve the unperfused organ.

The biatrial and bicaval approaches are the two most commonly used techniques for orthotopic heart transplant. The biatrial technique has been the standard method of implantation for more than 35 years.[33] This method requires the recipient's heart to be dissected, leaving cuffs of the right and left atria at the base of the heart. The donor and native atrial cuffs are joined and end-to-end anastomoses are performed on the aorta and pulmonary artery.[5] Postoperative atrial dysfunction and dysrhythmias are common after this procedure.

The second method of implantation, the bicaval technique, requires explantation of the entire native right atrium with subsequent bicaval anastomosis on the right. With this technique, the donor right atria are preserved intact. The left atrial anastomosis is performed in the traditional manner. This method reduces the incidence of postoperative dysrhythmias and atrioventricular valvular regurgitation,[5] as well as increases postoperative survival and decreases hospital length of stay.[44]

A third orthotopic technique, the total heart transplant procedure, is a new procedure being used at about 8% of the centers at this time.[44] This procedure requires total explantation of the recipient's native heart,

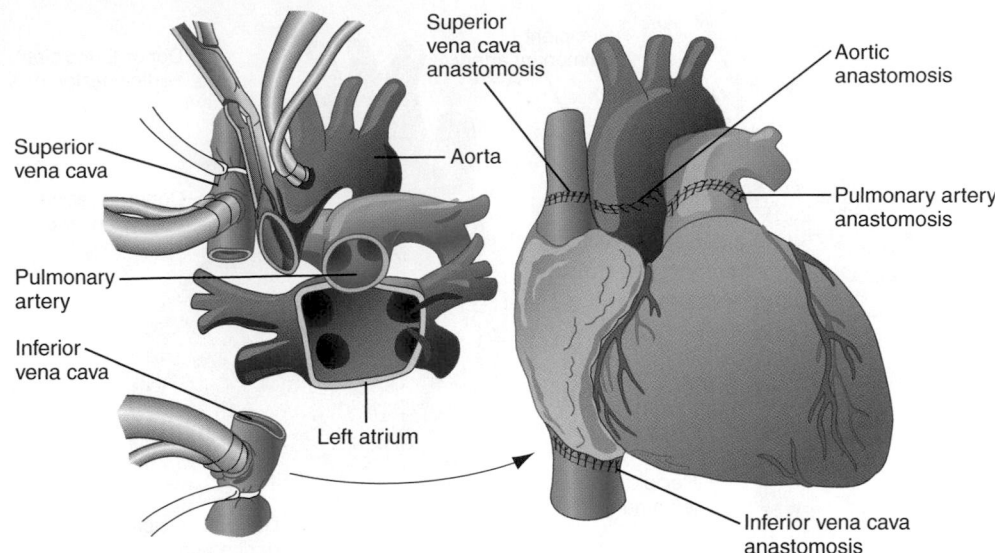

♦FIGURE 18-3 Before and after view of bicaval technique for donor heart implantation. Bicaval technique proceeds with left atrial anastomoses followed by superior and inferior vena caval anastomoses.

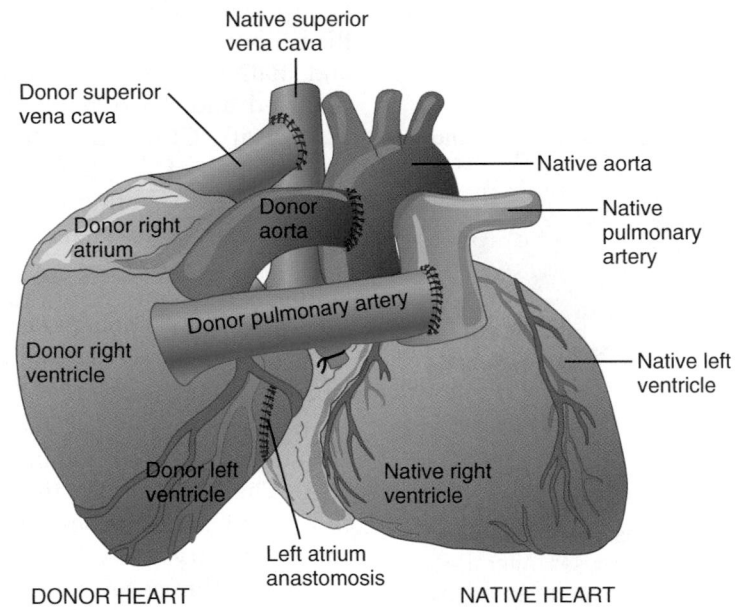

♦FIGURE 18-4 Heterotopic heart transplantation. The donor heart is placed in the recipient chest and positioned next to the native heart. The superior vena cava, aorti, pulmonary arteries, and left atrial anastomoses join the donor heart to that of the recipient.

preserving only a small amount of common atrial tissue surrounding the two left and right pulmonary veins (Figure 18-5). The bicaval technique is used to anastomose the right atrium, and the donor heart left atrium is anastomosed to the preserved patch of the recipient's left atrial tissue adjacent to the pulmonary veins. Because there are six anastomoses, operative time is significantly increased. The posterior pulmonary vein anastomosis sites are difficult to reach and may result in pulmonary vein stenoses.[44] Heterotopic implantation may be used for recipients who have fixed pulmonary hypertension, or if the donor heart is too small to fully support the recipient. The donor heart is implanted without explanting the native heart. Anastomoses are performed with the superior vena cava, pulmonary artery, and aorta. This technique requires lifelong

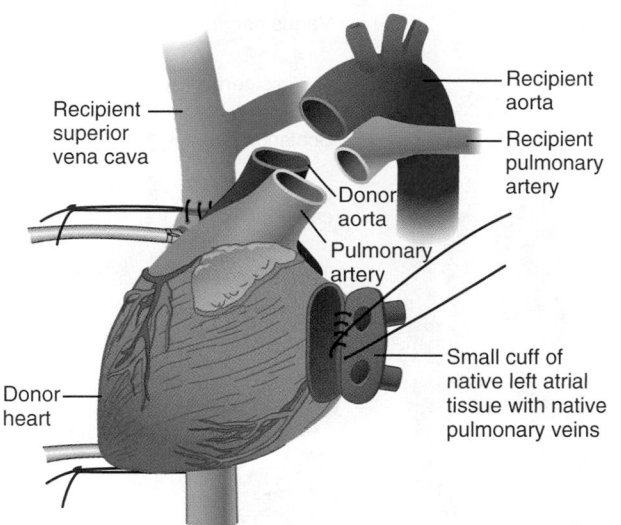

FIGURE 18-5 Total orthotopic heart transplantation proceeds after total excision of the recipient heart, leaving only a very small amount of native atrial tissue surrounding the pulmonary vein insertion sites of left atrial "cuffs" on the native pulmonary veins. Consequently, the native pulmonary veins must be anastomosed directly to the donor heart, requiring four pulmonary vein anastomoses.

anticoagulation and, because the native heart is not removed, the patient may still experience debilitating anginal pain. This technique is rarely used, and accounts for less than 1% of heart transplants.[8]

After implantation is complete, the patient is weaned from CPB. Once the patient is stabilized, transported, and settled in critical care, the family is invited to visit.

Lung Transplantation

Lung implantation procedures differ based on the number of lungs being transplanted. Single lung transplant is accomplished via a standard posterolateral thoracotomy incision. Double lung transplant requires a much larger anterior thoracosternotomy, also called a clamshell incision (Figure 18-6). Patients may or may not require support from CPB during lung implantation.

During the surgery, the recipient's native pulmonary artery, left atrium, and bronchi are dissected away from supporting structures. Great care is taken to avoid injury to the heart, aorta, thoracic duct, and thoracic nerves (phrenic, vagus, and recurrent laryngeal nerves) (Figures 18-7 and 18-8). This dissection is necessary in order to mobilize the native structures and facilitate their rapid explantation once the donor organs are in the room so that ischemic time can be limited to less than 6 hours.[70] As the tissues are dissected, adhesions from previous thoracic or cardiac surgery may cause significant hemorrhage. Once the donor organs are prepared for implantation, the native lung is removed and the donor organ placed into the thoracic cavity. Ice slush or cold surgical lap pads are used to cool the organs in the chest while the donor bronchus and pulmonary artery are anastomosed to corresponding recipient structures (Figures 18-9 and 18-10).[12] Finally, the donor pulmonary veins and the area adjacent to the recipient's left atrial-pulmonary vein junction are incised to create one large donor pulmonary vein and one large atrial-pulmonary cuff. These two reshaped structures are then joined, completing the transplantation (Figure 18-11).

After implantation is complete, the surgeon inspects the bronchial anastomosis and clears any blood or debris from the airway via bronchoscopy. Unless independent

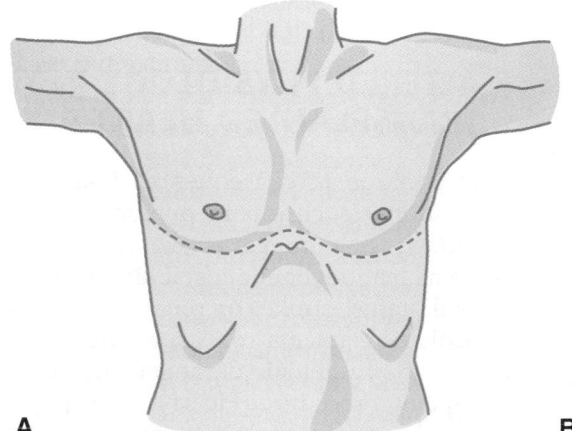

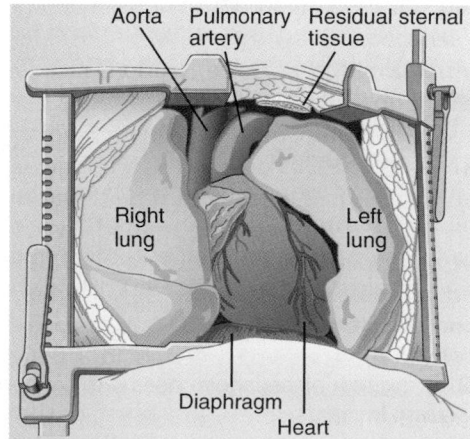

FIGURE 18-6 Clamshell incision for lung transplantation. **A,** Bilateral thoracosternotomy or "clamshell" incision used for bilateral lung transplantation, **B,** Exposed right and left lungs, heart, and great vessels with retraction of ribs and soft tissue via clamshell incision. Sternum has been transected and temporarily removed during the procedure.

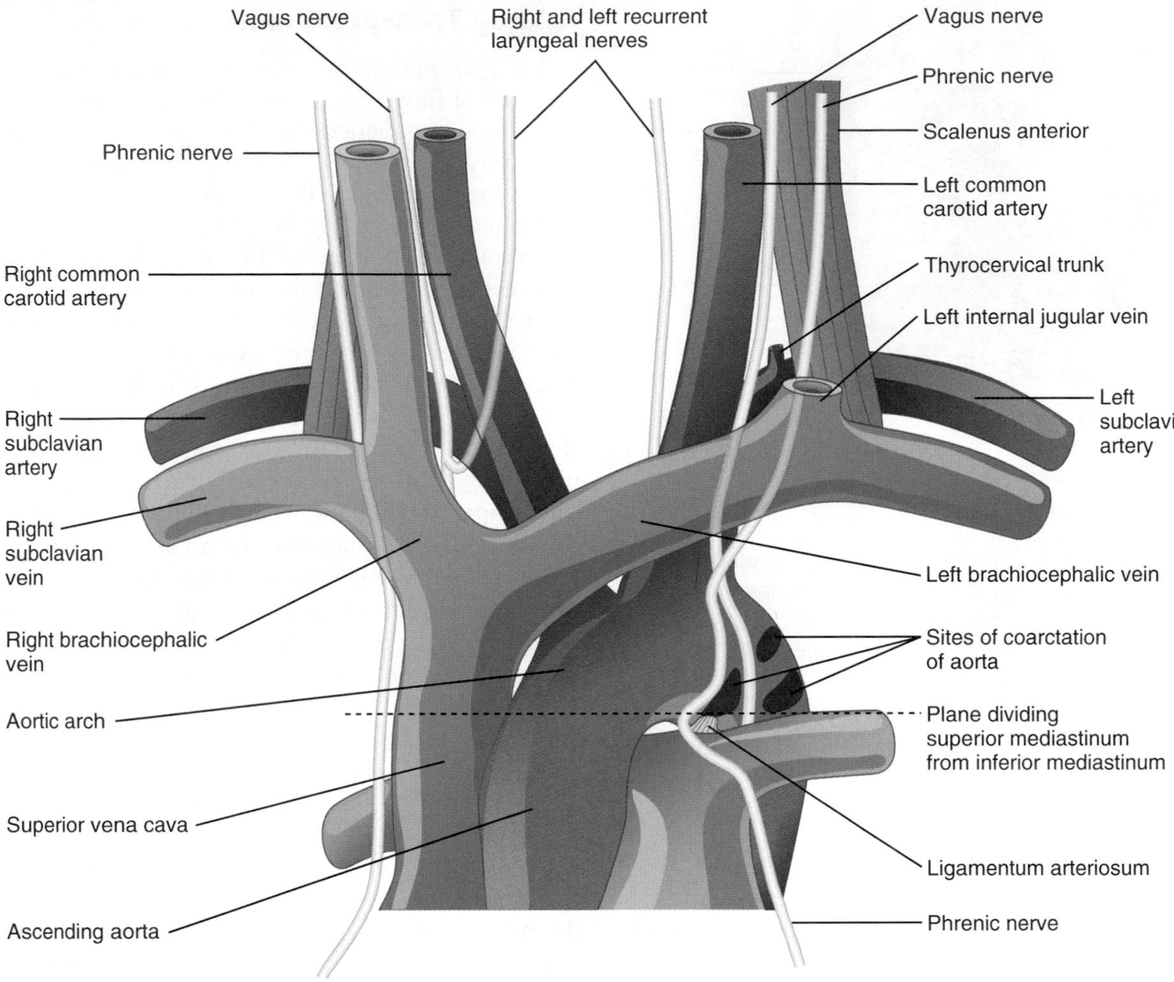

Vagus nerve

Right and left recurrent laryngeal nerves

Vagus nerve

Phrenic nerve

Scalenus anterior

Phrenic nerve

Left common carotid artery

Right common carotid artery

Thyrocervical trunk

Left internal jugular vein

Right subclavian artery

Left subclavian artery

Right subclavian vein

Left brachiocephalic vein

Right brachiocephalic vein

Sites of coarctation of aorta

Aortic arch

Plane dividing superior mediastinum from inferior mediastinum

Superior vena cava

Ligamentum arteriosum

Ascending aorta

Phrenic nerve

⬥**FIGURE 18-7**   Neurovascular structures in the superior mediastinum. Note close proximity of vagus and phrenic nerves to the heart, great vessels, and lungs. These nerves can easily be injured during heart or lung transplantation.

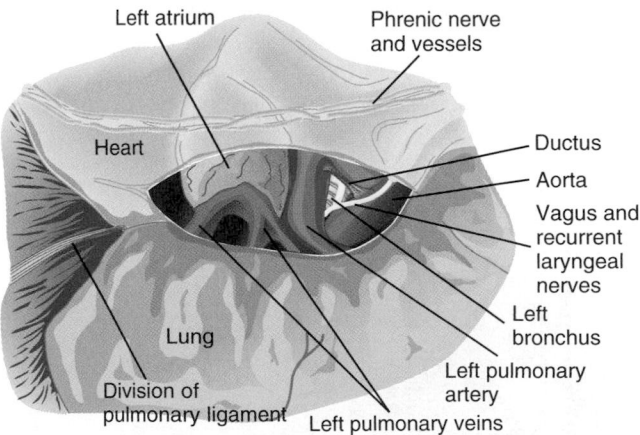

Left atrium

Phrenic nerve and vessels

Heart

Ductus

Aorta

Vagus and recurrent laryngeal nerves

Left bronchus

Lung

Left pulmonary artery

Division of pulmonary ligament

Left pulmonary veins

⬥**FIGURE 18-8**   Proximity of peripheral nerves to cardiopulmonary and vascular structures.

lung ventilation is planned, the double-lumen endotracheal tube used during the surgery is exchanged for a single-lumen tube. The patient is then transported intubated, with mechanical ventilator support, to critical

care. The family is informed of the outcome of surgery. Once the patient has been stabilized, the patient's family is encouraged to visit.

ALTERED PHYSIOLOGY IN THE TRANSPLANTED HEART AND LUNG

In addition to consequences that may accompany thoracotomy (such as pain, pneumothorax, hemothorax, atelectasis, pneumonia, or wound infection) and CPB (such as hemodynamic instability, bleeding, change in mental status, stroke, or renal insufficiency), thoracic transplant recipients can experience untoward effects related to physiologic derangements as a result of the transplant procedure. Heart transplant recipients are vulnerable to postoperative problems related to denervation of the heart. Postoperative problems specifically related to lung transplantation include pulmonary denervation, disruption of lymphatic drainage, and ciliary paralysis.[48]

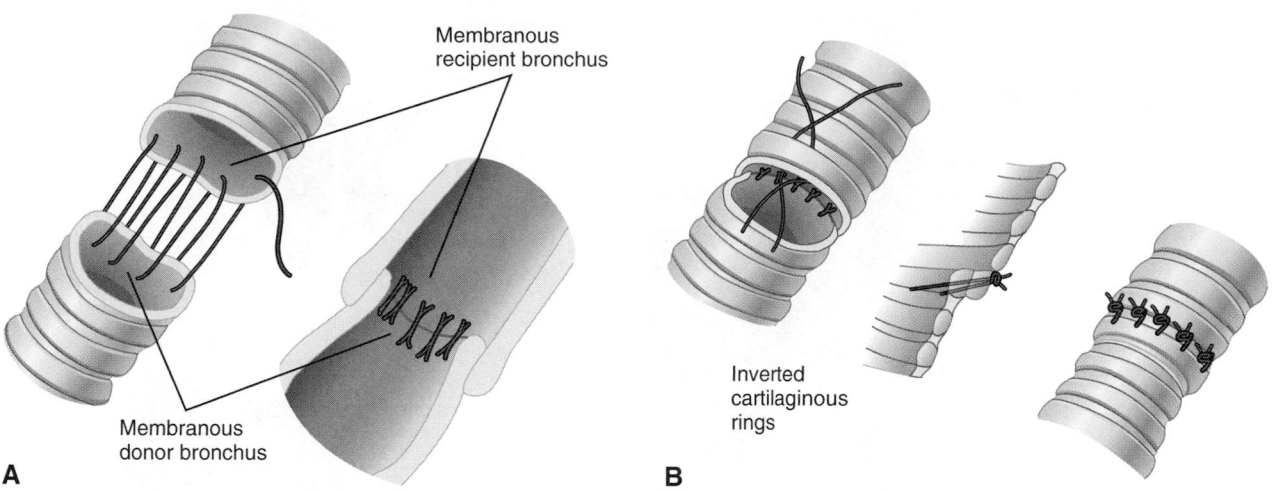

FIGURE 18-9   Techniques for membranous and cartilaginous bronchial anastomoses. **A,** Bronchial anastomosis is shown here using an inverted technique that uses continuous sutures on the membranous bronchus and interrupted sutures on the cartilaginous bronchus. **B,** The interrupted sutures used on the cartilaginous bronchus are sewn in a figure eight pattern. The donor and recipient bronchi are drawn together when the sutures are tightened. Sutures are tied on the external surface.

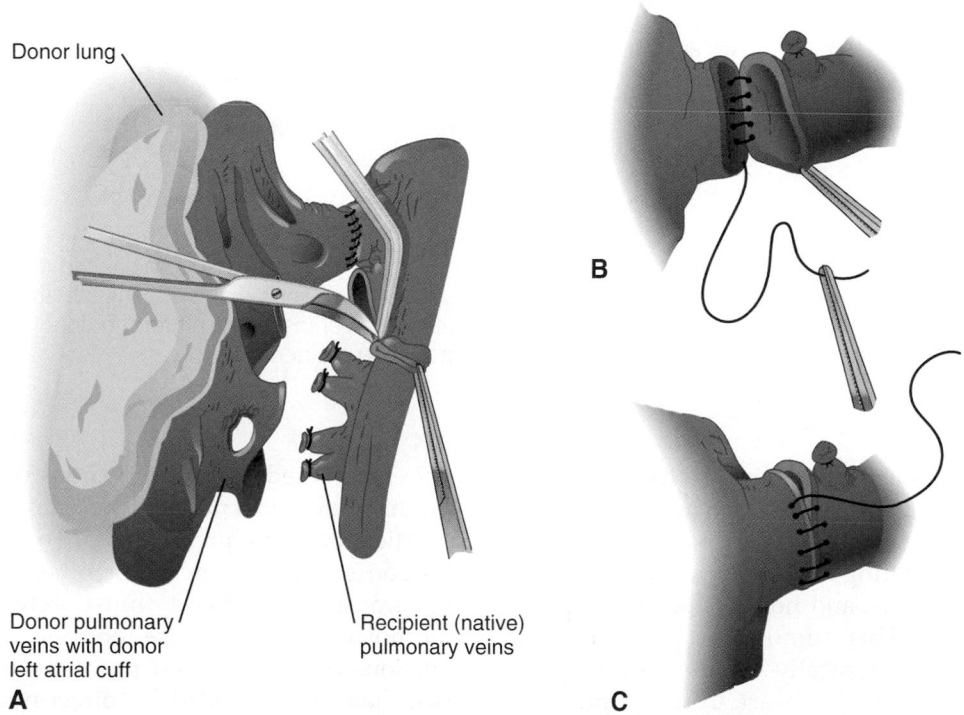

FIGURE 18-10   Techniques for pulmonary artery anastomosis in lung transplantation. **A,** Donor and recipient arteries are trimmed to appropriate lengths. **B** and **C,** End-to-end anastomoses of donor to recipient pulmonary arteries.

The Denervated Transplanted Heart

During harvesting, connections between the donor heart and nerves are severed. As a result, the donor heart is denervated and abnormalities of heart rhythm and contractility occur. Normally, heart rate (HR) is regulated via neural and hormonal systems. The parasympathetic and sympathetic nervous systems maintain HR within certain limits and produce an increase in the rate when metabolic demand is increased. These systems control the rate of firing of the sinoatrial (SA) node as well as depolarization and repolarization of the myocardium. They also modulate the contractility of the heart to meet metabolic demands.

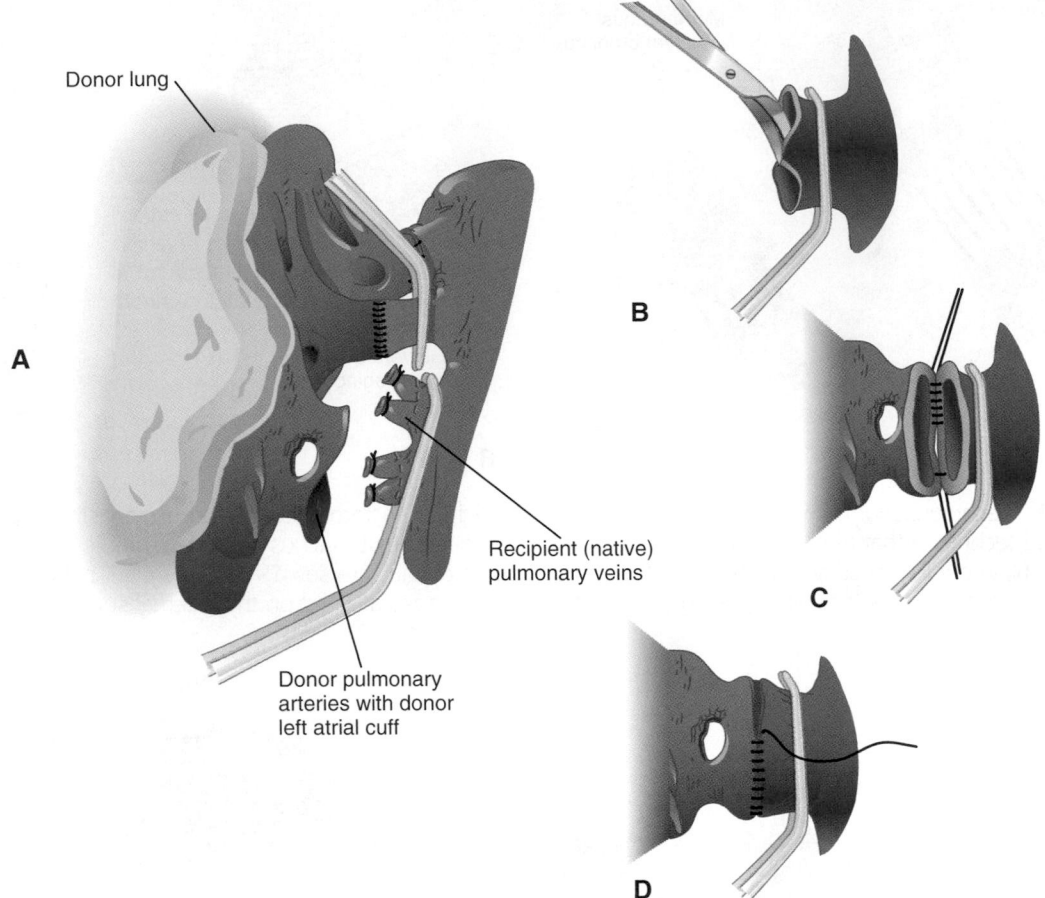

Donor lung

A

B

Recipient (native)
pulmonary veins

Donor pulmonary
arteries with donor
left atrial cuff

C

D

⬍FIGURE 18-11 Technique for anastomosis of donor pulmonary vein cuff and recipient left atrial cuff in lung transplantation. **A,** Large recipient left atrial cuff is created by trimming remaining pulmonary vein tissue and incising left atrial tissue between the superior and inferior pulmonary vein insertions into left atria, creating a larger insertion cuff for the donor pulmonary vein cuff. **B, C,** and **D,** The donor and newly created recipient pulmonary vein cuffs are joined.

The denervated heart is not subject to direct efferent neural stimulation. Vagal tone is lost, causing a resting HR of between 90 and 110 beats per minute (beats/min). However, circulating hormones, such as the catecholamines, epinephrine, and norepinephrine, can still stimulate the heart. This stimulation proceeds at a much slower pace than typically seen with direct autonomic stimulation of a native heart. Consequently, the chronotropic response that typically increases the HR during stress and exercise is blunted.[79] Because these chronotropic responses are slow, reliance on tachycardia as an indication of hypovolemia, hemorrhage, hypoxia, and fever can delay recognition of these problems and, subsequently, delay life-saving interventions.

Cardiac output (CO) is the product of heart rate and stroke volume. Stroke volume (SV) is determined by preload, afterload, and contractility. If one of the contributors to CO is reduced, another must increase or CO will fall and the patient will experience symptoms.

Preload is reduced when venous return to the heart is reduced. When a patient rises from the recumbent to a vertical position, preload falls. To maintain CO with position changes, exercise, or other physical stresses, the transplanted heart must rely on circulating catecholamines to increase inotropic and chronotropic function. This stimulation proceeds at a much slower pace than that provided by direct neural stimulation. Consequently, a heart transplant recipient must allow the transplanted heart time to "warm up" before activities, such as position changes or exercise. Conversely, after stress or activity, the HR will return to resting levels more slowly because of the time required for circulating catecholamines to decline. As a result, "cool down" periods must be extended.

Afferent and efferent sensory fibers are also severed. This prevents the transmission of nociceptive impulses associated with cardiac ischemia. Without these afferent impulses, the experience of ischemic angina is absent. Patients may not be aware of episodic myocardial ischemia and therefore may fail to seek medical attention when needed. The loss of these afferent impulses also explains the lack of reflex autonomic responses to position changes (i.e., peripheral vasoconstriction), which normally maintain blood pressure (BP).[41]

Standard medications used to manipulate cardiac function may not have the desired effect on a denervated transplanted heart. The treatment of atrial tachydysrhythmias and bradycardias requires careful drug choices. For example, the use of digoxin (Lanoxin) to control atrial fibrillation or paroxysmal atrial tachycardia has little or no effect on the SA or atrioventricular (AV) nodes after heart transplant. Adenosine (Adenocard) may still be used to treat a paroxysmal supraventricular tachycardia, but an exaggerated response and profound bradycardia may occur. If atrial fibrillation occurs, intravenous diltiazem (Cardizem) is the drug of choice to slow the HR because of its direct effect on the AV node.[63,67]

More importantly, after heart transplant, atropine's vagolytic effects are lost and may actually cause asystole or AV block if used to treat bradycardia.[6] In the past, isoproterenol (Isuprel) was the preferred treatment for symptomatic bradycardia. It may still be used in addition to oral or intravenous aminophylline (for persistent bradycardia). However, these beta stimulant medications have been associated with increased myocardial oxygen demand and can precipitate myocardial ischemia. Therefore the current treatment of choice for posttransplant bradydysrhythmias is temporary atrial or AV sequential pacing.[32]

Compensatory reflex tachycardia, which maintains CO when anti-hypertensive medications such as hydralazine (Apresoline) are used, may not occur. As a result, the use of these medications after heart transplant may produce more profound decreases in CO and BP than are typically expected. If hypotension should occur with the use of these medications, epinephrine would be the drug of choice.[32]

Interrupted Pulmonary Lymphatics After Lung Transplant

Under normal conditions, the lymphatic system drains 10% of pulmonary interstitial fluid, including an average of 100 ml/hr through the thoracic duct.[24] These lymphatic drainage systems can be interrupted during the lung transplant surgical procedure.[25,43] Consequently, excess interstitial fluid can only leave the lung parenchyma via the capillary networks.

According to Starling's law of fluid dynamics, movement of fluids between intravascular to extravascular spaces is dependent on the relationships between intravascular and extravascular oncotic and hydrostatic pressures.[24] In order for interstitial (extravascular) fluid to enter the capillary (intravascular space), either interstitial hydrostatic pressure must exceed capillary hydrostatic pressure or capillary oncotic pressure must exceed interstitial oncotic pressure. These circumstances rarely occur. The loss of lymphatic drainage, therefore, leaves the transplanted lung vulnerable to interstitial fluid retention.

Interstitial fluid retention causes altered gas diffusion, loss of compliance, and increased work of breathing. The loss of lymphatic drainage also interferes with elimination of infectious organisms from the interstitial space, predisposing the lung to infection.

Pulmonary Ciliary Dysfunction After Lung Transplant

Pulmonary cilia in transplanted lungs do not function properly.[25,75a,b] The cause of this dysfunction is not clearly understood; however, epithelial abnormalities, specifically ciliary depletion and cellular death, have been described.[60] As a result, mucus does not move up out of the small terminal airways and can accumulate, causing mucous plugs. Small airways become obstructed, resulting in postobstructive atelectasis and ultimately loss of gas-exchanging units. The result may be hypoxemia and hypercarbia. Accumulated mucus also creates media for bacterial growth and predisposes to infection.[21]

The Denervated Transplanted Lung

Nerve supply to the native lung is severed during explantation.[25] When the donor lung is implanted, these thoracic nerves cannot be anastomosed. As a result, the transplanted lung does not transmit or respond to nervous impulses from the central nervous system. Bronchial reflex responses to mechanical stimulation below the level of the bronchial anastomosis are absent.[4,26] Consequently, the patient does not spontaneously cough to expel materials that are aspirated below the bronchial anastomosis. This places the patient at increased risk for silent aspiration. This risk is greatest in patients with preexisting gastroesophageal reflux disease or esophageal disorders related to scleroderma. Patients also have problems sensing, and therefore clearing, accumulated secretions and mucous plugs. Aggressive pulmonary hygiene is used to overcome these problems.

Peripheral Nerve Injuries. During transplant surgery, peripheral nerve injuries may also occur. The phrenic, vagus, and recurrent laryngeal nerves are all vulnerable to injury during dissection and reimplantation (see Figures 18-7 and 18-8). Injury to the phrenic nerve can produce diaphragmatic paralysis. This complication may present as poor inspiratory volumes or weaning parameters on the ventilator, or after extubation as a very weak cough. Phrenic nerve injuries can be detected with a fluoroscopic sniff test or peripheral nerve conduction studies. They may be permanent or may resolve after weeks or months. Patients with a phrenic nerve injury may require prolonged mechanical ventilation or intermittent noninvasive respiratory assistance via intermittent positive pressure breathing (IPPB) or bilevel continuous positive airway pressure (BiPAP). Upright positioning, for example, chair rest (rather than bed rest), helps to decrease the impact of this injury by reducing intra-abdominal pressure on the thorax, thus allowing the diaphragm to move more freely.

Laryngeal or vagal nerve injuries may also occur, producing problems with gastroesophageal reflux, gastroparesis, vocal cord function, and dysphagia.[68,80] Injuries to these nerves are more difficult to detect, and although they usually resolve after a few days to weeks, they can produce significant problems.

Injury to the recurrent laryngeal nerve can produce vocal cord paralysis, leaving the patient's airway unprotected. Vocal cord paralysis causes hypophonia or a hoarse voice. It can also interfere with airway protection reflexes, especially during swallowing. After extubation, and before oral hydration or nutrition is started, patients undergo bedside swallow evaluation by a speech therapist. If evidence of vocal cord dysfunction, aspiration, or inability to clear laryngeal penetrations is found, the patient continues without oral intake. A video swallow can be performed to further evaluate functional swallowing. Postpyloric or parenteral nutrition and appropriate speech therapy (swallowing instructions and maneuvers, and recommendations regarding dietary consistency) are provided until the patient can safely swallow. Ear, nose, and throat consult for direct laryngoscopy and vocal cord injection may also be required.

Injuries to the vagus nerve can be more difficult to identify. The patient may complain of heartburn, nausea, early satiety, bloating, or abdominal pain. Patients may present with hoarseness, vomiting, or ileus. Direct laryngoscopy sometimes reveals inflamed vocal cords as a result of acid reflux. Barium swallow or endoscopy may be required to rule out esophageal emptying problem or reflux. Gastric emptying studies can determine if emptying times are prolonged. If new to the patient, any of these findings could be evidence of vagal nerve injury. However, the symptoms, signs, and test findings could also have a variety of other causes. Levels of serum electrolytes, especially potassium, magnesium, and calcium, are monitored and maintained within normal limits. Patient mobility should be encouraged. Time in bed is minimized to periods of sleeping, and the patient is assisted out of bed to a chair for all meals. Gastric acid can be controlled with proton pump inhibitors or histamine-2 blockers, and promotility agents can be used to provide symptomatic relief. Small, frequent feedings may be needed to ensure adequate nutrition.

THE IMMUNE SYSTEM AND TRANSPLANTATION

A basic understanding of the immune system is essential when caring for patients who have undergone heart or lung transplantation. Increased survival in this population may be attributed in part to the improved understanding of transplant immunology and the development of more specific immunosuppressive agents to prevent and treat rejection.

The immune system functions to allow the recognition of "self" vs. "non-self." In this context a transplanted organ is viewed as a foreign pathogen or antigen, which initiates the immune response directed at the allograft.[24] The location of the major histocompatibility complex (MHC) that codes for the antigens on all cell surfaces is chromosome 6. In humans these antigens are called human leukocyte antigens (HLAs).[69] HLAs are divided into class I and class II antigens. Class I antigens (HLA A, B, and C) are located on all nucleated cells. Class II antigens (HLA DP, DQ, and DR) are found only on antigen-presenting cells (i.e., B lymphocytes, macrophages), activated T lymphocytes, and endothelial cells.[24]

Before being listed for transplantation, patients are HLA typed to identify their preexisting class I and II antigens. A panel-reactive antibody (PRA) assessment is also obtained to identify preformed antibodies that may have developed after a previous blood transfusion, pregnancy, use of left ventricular assist devices, or a previous transplant.

The immune response to foreign antigens consists of a cellular response and a humoral response. The cellular response is mediated by the T lymphocytes, and the humoral response is mediated by the B lymphocytes. In order for the immune response to be initiated, the foreign antigen must be recognized as non-self by presenting it in the context of the MHC by antigen-presenting cells (APCs). A transplanted organ is different from a foreign pathogen in that it has two sets of APCs capable of stimulating the activation of a recipient's T lymphocytes.[54,69] One mechanism, called the indirect pathway, involves the recipient's APCs activating T lymphocytes due to the recognition of the donor cell as non-self MHC.

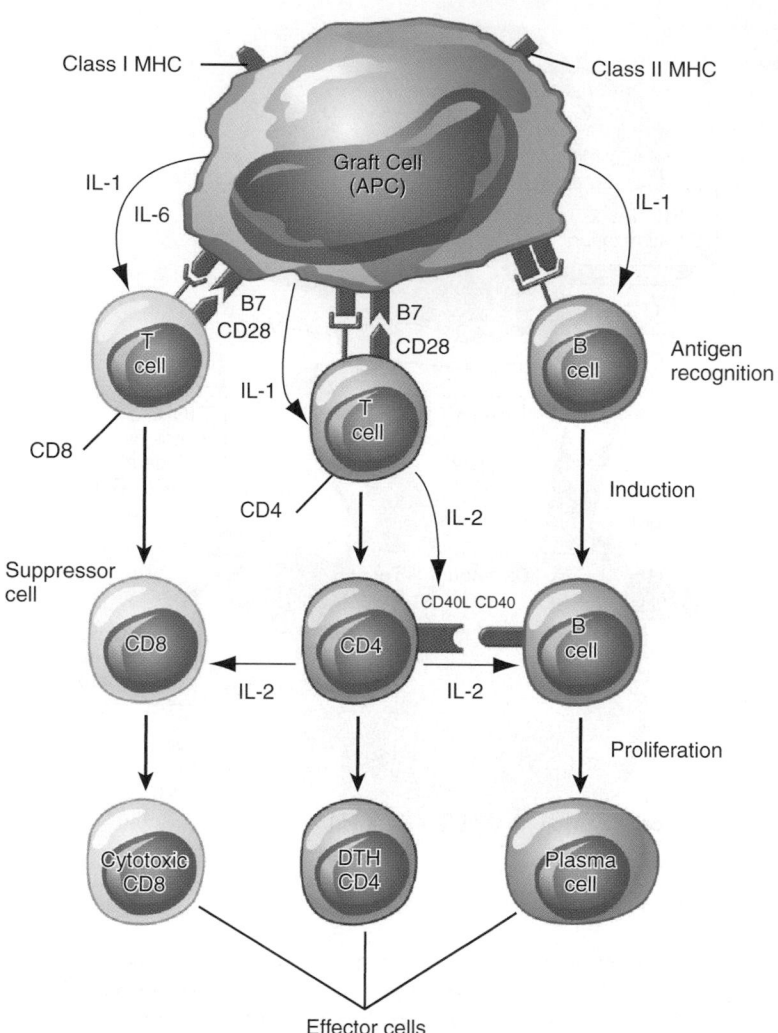

◆FIGURE 18-12 Generation of primary allograft rejection responses. APC = Antigen-presenting cell, MHC = major histocompatibility, DTH = delayed-type hypersensitivity, IL = interleukin, T cell = T lymphocyte; B cell = B lymphocyte.

The direct pathway is unique to transplantation and is a result of the donor's APCs directly stimulating the recipient's T cells. The intensity of the rejection response is believed to be related to this direct pathway. Figure 18-12 illustrates the rejection response that occurs when an allograft cell is identified by the immune system.[54]

IMMUNOSUPPRESSION

Management of immunosuppression is critical to long-term outcomes after transplantation. Intense immunosuppression prevents rejection, but increases the risk of infection and malignancy, and may contribute to dysfunction of other organ systems.[20] Weak immunosuppression decreases the risk of infection

and malignancy, but increases the risk of rejection and subsequent transplanted organ dysfunction. Consequently, appropriate immunosuppression requires careful attention and close monitoring and is always individualized.

It was not until the introduction of cyclosporine in the 1980s that thoracic transplantation became a viable option for individuals with end-stage heart and lung disease. During the ensuing 25 years, the development of stronger and more specific immunosuppressive agents has allowed clinicians to individualize medication regimens.[52] This has resulted in decreased side effects from the various agents. Immunosuppression regimens are divided into three forms: induction, maintenance, and rescue therapy (Figure 18-13). Agents in each category are listed in the Medication table on pp. 412-413.

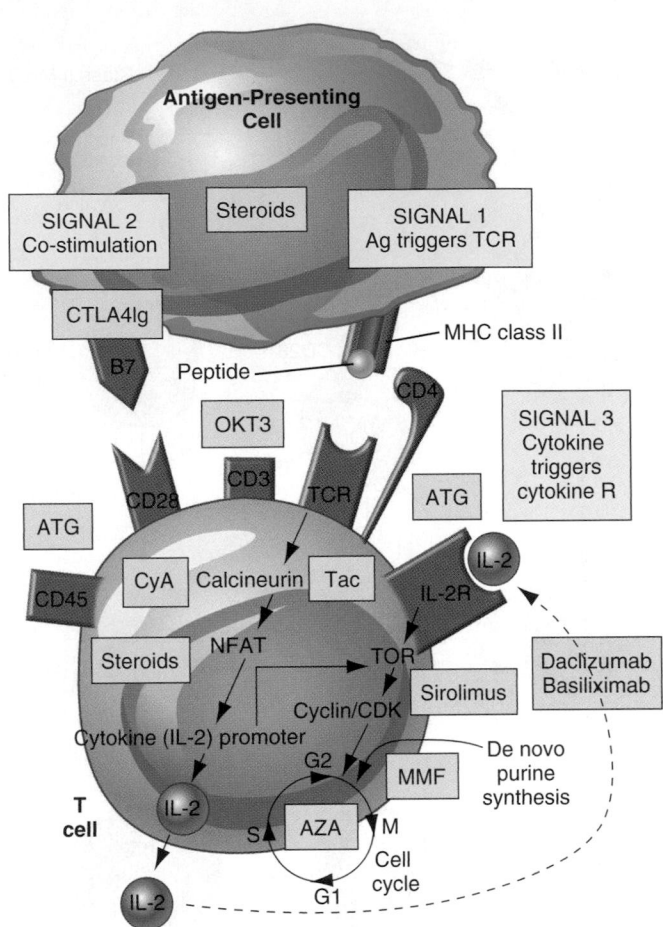

FIGURE 18-13 U.S. Food and Drug Administration–approved immunosuppressive agents and sites of action. APC = Antigen-presenting cell, MHC = major histocompatibility, IL = interleukin, TOR = target of rapamycin, TCR = T-cell receptor, ATG = polyclonal antithymocyte globulin, AZA = azathioprine, CyA = cyclosporine, MMF = mycophenolate mofetil, Tac = tacrolimus.

MEDICATIONS USED AFTER HEART OR LUNG TRANSPLANT

MEDICATION	ACTIONS	DOSAGE	SPECIAL CONSIDERATIONS
Cyclosporine (Neoral, Gengraf, Sandimmune)	Inhibition of T lymphocytes through suppression of interleukin-2 production and release	On call to the OR: PO dose based on baseline creatinine (creatinine <1.4 = 10 mg/kg to max of 800 mg; creatinine 1.4–2 = 5 mg/kg; creatinine >2 = none) *Many centers choose to delay initiating calcineurin inhibitors until after transplantation. Postop: IV infusion 0.25–1 mg/kg/min or 1 mg/hr and then adjust dose daily to reach goal blood level before transition to PO. Rising creatinine may preclude aggressive titration to goal. PO dosing adjusted to reach goal level based on morning 12-hr trough levels	Monitor serum concentrations Monitor for nephrotoxicity (25%-37% incidence); hepatotoxicity (4%-7% incidence); usually responsive to dose reduction. May cause hypertension, tremors, confusion, seizures, hyperkalemia, hypomagnesemia hemolytic-uremic syndrome, hyperlipidemia. Multiple drug, food, and herbal interactions. Brands are not bioequivalent and should not be used interchangeably. Oral dose will depend on formulation.

MEDICATION	ACTIONS	DOSAGE	SPECIAL CONSIDERATIONS
Tacrolimus (Prograf)	Inhibition of T lymphocytes through suppression of interleukin-2 production	*Many centers choose to delay initiating calcineurin inhibitors until after transplantation. Postop: IV tacrolimus: 0.01 mg/kg/day as continuous infusion: dose based on trough levels *Many centers start postop immunosuppression with IV infusion of cyclosporine (see above) to goal blood level before transition to tacrolimus PO. PO: 0.015–0.03 mg/kg/day given bid: based on 12-hour trough levels	Monitor serum concentrations. Monitor for nephrotoxicity, glucose intolerance. May cause hypertension, tremors, confusion, seizures, hyperkalemia hemolytic-uremic syndrome, hyperlipidemia.
Sirolimus (Rapamycin)	Inhibition of T lymphocytes activation and proliferation by IL-2, IL-4 and IL-5	PO: 6-mg loading dose. Maintenance: 2–5 mg/day. Doses adjusted based on 24-hour trough levels Not typically recommended for lung transplant due to risk of bronchial anastomotic dehiscence.	Monitor serum concentrations. Monitor CBC, renal function tests, and lipids. May cause hypertension and hyperlipidemia, bone marrow suppression, hemolytic-uremic syndrome, brochiolitis obliterans organizing pneumonia
Mycophenolate mofetil (CellCept)	Inhibits inosine monophosphate dehydrogenase in purine synthesis pathway, thereby inhibiting T and B lymphocytes	Cardiac: 1–1.5 g bid IV/PO Lung: 1 g bid IV/PO	Compatible only with D_5W infusions. May cause bone marrow suppression, diarrhea and vomiting. Monitor CBC, LFTs. Blood levels may be monitored.
Azathioprine (Imuran)	Interferes with DNA and RNA synthesis, inhibition differentiation and proliferation of both T and B lymphocytes	Lung: 2 mg/kg/day to max of 200 mg daily IV/PO	May cause bone marrow suppression, hepatotoxicity, nausea and vomiting. Monitor CBC and LFTs.
Methyl-prednisolone (Solu-Medrol)	Suppression of migration of leukocytes; inhibits lymphokine-mediated amplification of macrophages and lymphocytes	Induction protocols are frequently a set dose, e.g., 250–1000 mg IV intraoperatively, followed by POD1–125 mg IV q 8 hr, POD2–125 mg IV q 12 hr, POD3–switch to prednisone PO dosing 0.1–0.5 mg/kg daily or in divided doses, etc.	Monitor for hyperglycemia, hypokalemia, fluid retention, hypertension, impaired wound healing, myopathy, osteoporosis, gastric ulcers, sleep disturbances and psychosis.
Prednisone	Suppression of migration of leukocytes; inhibits lymphokine-mediated amplification of macrophages and lymphocytes	PO: 0.1 to 0.5 mg/kg daily or in divided doses Dose will depend on time since transplant, rejection history, infection history	Monitor for same adverse effects as for methylprednisolone.

CBC = Complete blood cell count, LFTs = liver function tests, POD = postoperative day.

During an induction regimen, potent intravenous medications are used to initiate immunosuppression.[42] Induction immunosuppression is provided at the time of surgery, and its goal is to delay the onset of the first episode of acute rejection. Induction protocols are controversial, and they are used in only 52% of lung transplant centers.[35] When used, induction protocols begin either in the OR or on the day after surgery.

Intravenous steroids such as methylprednisolone sodium (Solu-Medrol) are used to begin induction and are commonly administered intraoperatively just before removal of arterial cross-clamps. Other agents commonly used for induction include cytolytic agents, such as the polyclonal antibodies antithymocyte immune globulin (equine, Atgam; rabbit, Thymoglobulin) and the newer interleukin-2 (IL-2) receptor blockers, such as basiliximab (Simulect) or daclizumab (Zenapax). Induction agents are also used early after transplant as "renal sparing" therapies to allow for the delay in initiating the use of a calcineurin inhibitor. Calcineurin inhibitors frequently contribute to renal dysfunction. By delaying the use of calcineurin inhibitors until the kidneys have recovered from intraoperative insults, renal function may be preserved or "spared." They are also used for high-risk individuals when donor or recipient characteristics place the recipient at greater than usual risk for rejection.

Antithymocyte cytolytic agents can be associated with several adverse effects, including pancytopenia and bronchospasm. During therapy, patients are monitored closely with daily complete blood counts (CBCs) and CD3 counts to guide dosing. These agents may produce a serum sickness–like syndrome, which presents as fever, chills, and hypotension. It is difficult to differentiate this syndrome from the onset of infection. Premedication with a steroid, acetaminophen (Tylenol), and diphenhydramine (Benadryl) can minimize the severity of this syndrome. In addition, the use of cytolytic agents increases the risk of infection and malignancy.[55,69] Another cytolytic agent, orthoclone OKT3 (Muromonab-CD3), is rarely used with thoracic transplantation because of the risk of flash pulmonary edema, which would be devastating in this population. It is also associated with poor long-term outcomes.[42]

The IL-2 receptor blockers primarily affect the activated T lymphocytes and are generally well tolerated. They have been found to reduce cellular rejection without increasing infections or malignancy.[19,55]

The second regimen, maintenance immunosuppression, is a daily medication cocktail designed to allow long-term graft survival and prevent acute rejection episodes. Maintenance immunosuppression is usually lifelong and begins immediately after surgery or after initial induction therapy. Most institutions use what is called "triple therapy" for maintenance immunosuppression.[35] Triple therapy consists of simultaneous use of medications from three drug categories: a corticosteroid, a calcineurin inhibitor, and an antimetabolite. Abnormal renal and hepatic function during the immediate postoperative period, as well as low blood cell counts from the use of cytolytic induction agents, requires careful attention when using maintenance immunosuppressants. Dosages are reduced over time, and consideration of rejection history, time since transplant, and other rejection risk factors are used to determine the tapering of each agent.

The most common steroid used for long-term maintenance therapy is prednisone. Cyclosporine (Sandimmune, Neoral, Gengraf) and tacrolimus (Prograf, FK-506) are calcineurin inhibitors. Azathioprine (Imuran) and mycophenolate mofetil (CellCept) are antimetabolites. Many institutions begin maintenance immunosuppression by administering an oral loading dose of a calcineurin inhibitor and an antimetabolite preoperatively. The addition of sirolimus (Rapamune), another immunosuppressant, is avoided early after lung transplant because of evidence of increased incidence of tracheobronchial anastomosis dehiscence.[23,31]

The use of immunosuppressive agents to reverse an established rejection is called rescue therapy. Rescue immunosuppression often employs the addition of potent immunosuppression medication to enhance existing immunosuppression levels. It typically employs the use of short-course intravenous or increased dose of oral steroids.[35] Depending on the patient's history, severity of the rejection, and clinical findings, cytolytic agents may be employed. Rescue immunosuppression is not used during the initial post-transplant period unless acute rejection is suspected or diagnosed.

REJECTION

Rejection occurs when the recipient's immune system recognizes the transplanted tissue as foreign and activates complex processes to attack the grafted organ. Rejection can damage and ultimately destroy the transplanted organ. Despite the advances in management of individuals undergoing transplant and the improved survival statistics, rejection continues to be a major cause of morbidity and mortality. Rejection occurring early after transplant can be divided into three categories: hyperacute, acute cellular, and acute humoral rejection.[5,76] Signs and symptoms of rejection may be subtle, such as fatigue or fever, or may be more specific signs of organ dysfunction (Box 18-4). Chronic rejection, manifested as accelerated vasculopathy in heart transplants and as bronchiolitis obliterans in lung transplants, develops over several months to years and is not a

Box 18-4

Signs and Symptoms of Acute Rejection in Thoracic Transplant Recipients

Heart Transplant	Lung Transplant
Fatigue	Fatigue
Shortness of breath	Increased shortness of breath
Low-grade fever	More than 10% decrease in FEV_1
Atrial dysrhythmias	Low-grade fever
Decreased ejection fraction	Increased cough or sputum production
Peripheral edema	Decreased exercise tolerance
Third heart sound	Hypoxemia
Increased jugular venous pressure	Pulmonary infiltrates on CXR
	New pleural effusion

From reference 28.
CXR = Chest x-ray, FEV_1 = forced expiratory volume at 1 second.

problem in the acute and critical care recovery period after thoracic transplant surgery.

Hyperacute rejection is an antibody-mediated or humoral response that may occur within minutes to hours following graft revascularization.[69] This type of rejection is a result of preformed antibodies to donor HLA. These antibodies react to the endothelia of the graft, resulting in the development of microemboli that leads to graft thrombosis and necrosis. Because hyperacute rejection leads to rapid graft dysfunction and loss, it is often fatal.[13,78] Retransplantation is the only treatment option, and death from heart or pulmonary failure typically occurs before another organ can be found. Fortunately, because of the intense screening pretransplant for preformed antibodies, this type of rejection is rare.

Acute cellular rejection is a cell-mediated response to an allograft. It is uncommon during the acute and critical care recovery periods after thoracic transplant surgery and accounts for only 1.3% and 4.9% of early deaths after heart and lung transplant, respectively.[36,68] It is the most prevalent within the first few months post-transplant, and the incidence decreases dramatically after the first year[69] (see the Medication table on pp. 412-413). Despite a decrease in the incidence of acute cellular rejection after the first year, recipients will always be susceptible to the development of this form of rejection and, therefore, will require lifelong immunosuppression.

The most reliable method of detecting acute rejection in heart transplant recipients is endomyocardial biopsy, and in lung transplant recipients is transbronchial biopsy. Because many patients do not experience symptoms until rejection is advanced, many transplant centers perform surveillance biopsies on a specific schedule.[35] Heart transplant recipients undergo biopsy as early as 1 week after transplant. However, pulmonary biopsy is rarely performed this early after transplant, as tissue will invariably show diffuse alveolar damage related to ischemia and reperfusion, and therefore is of little help in guiding further treatment.

Initial treatment of acute rejection (rescue immunosuppression) includes corticosteroids, either intravenous (IV) methylprednisolone or an increased dose of oral prednisone. If treatment with IV methylprednisolone is used, it is followed by increased doses of oral prednisone that are then rapidly tapered back to the baseline dose over several days (e.g., methylprednisolone 500–1000 mg IV daily for 3 doses, then prednisone 40 mg orally daily for 7 days, followed by a 5 mg/day taper back to the previous daily prednisone dose). If the rejection is steroid resistant or there is severe cardiopulmonary or hemodynamic compromise, cytolytic agents (antithymocyte immune globulin, Thymoglobulin, OKT3) may be used (see Figure 18-13). In addition, the maintenance immunosuppression is maximized.

For many years the clinical significance of acute humoral rejection was disputed. Recently, however, the International Society for Heart Lung Transplantation has recognized antibody-mediated or humoral rejection as a distinct clinical entity.[55] It is usually seen in the early post-transplant phase. This type of rejection may be correlated with the development of HLA antibodies to the donor but has also been seen without identified HLA antibody formation. It is manifested by vascular inflammation and damage.[40] Biopsy immunofluorescence stains disclose immunoglobulin G (IgG) or IgM depositions with C3 or C1q.[13] This type of rejection may occur in the presence or absence of acute cellular rejection. It is often manifested in heart recipients by hemodynamic compromise and in lung recipients by pulmonary dysfunction. Treatment may include the use of corticosteroids, the employment of plasmapheresis, and the administration of intravenous immunoglobulin.

SURGICAL COMPLICATIONS AFTER THORACIC TRANSPLANT

Common complications and causes of perioperative mortality after thoracic transplant include hemorrhage, infection, early graft failure, cardiac rhythm disturbances, right ventricular failure, acute renal failure, and gastrointestinal disturbances. In addition, lung transplant recipients may also suffer complications related to bronchial, arterial, or venous anastomoses[68,72] (Table 18-2; Figure 18-14).

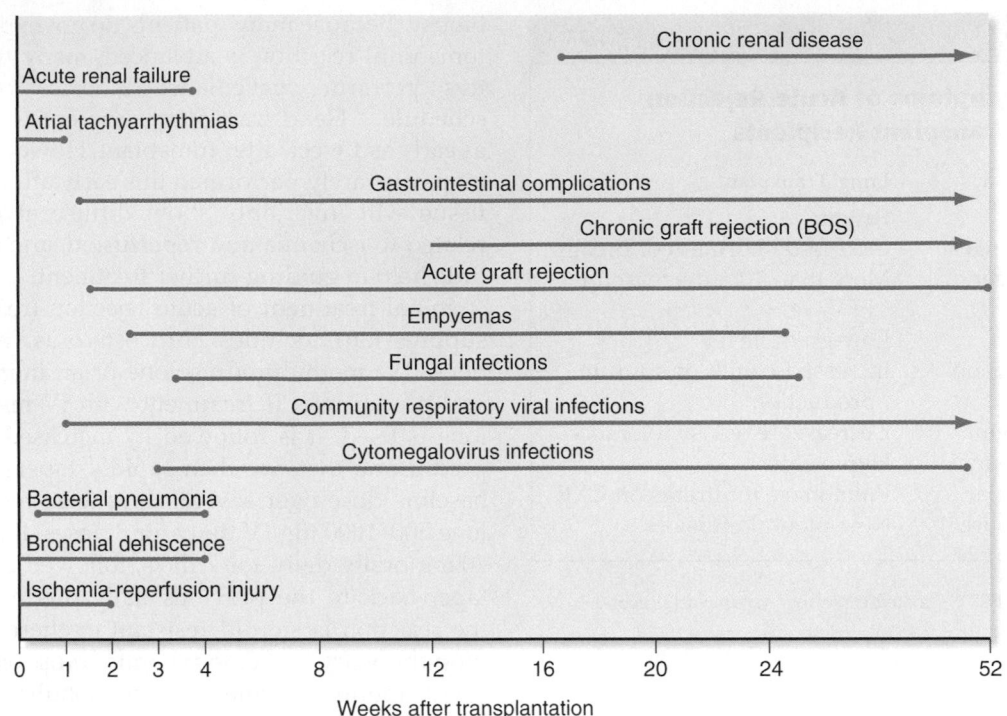

✛FIGURE 18-14 Complications timeline after lung transplantation. BOS = Bronchiolitis obliterans syndrome.

Hemorrhage and infection can occur after any surgical procedure. Patients who have had previous thoracic surgeries (e.g., open heart surgery, lobectomy) are at higher risk for bleeding because of the presence of vascular-rich scar tissue from previous surgeries. This may increase bleeding during the dissection required to remove the diseased native lung. CPB, with associated anticoagulation use, also contributes to hemorrhage.

Infections

Infection is a leading cause of early death (within 1 year of transplant) for both heart and lung transplant recipients.[73] Infection control procedures are incorporated into processes for patient evaluation before patients are listed for transplantation. These include surveillance activities that occur while the patient is waiting for transplant as well as protocols followed during the perioperative period to minimize infectious exposures and risks. At the time of surgery, infectious risks include incisions, the transplanted organ, systems breached with invasive devices (bloodstream, bladder), and unrelated preoperative infections.

Before being listed for transplantation, transplant candidates are carefully evaluated for the presence of infections or conditions that would increase their risk of infection. Some preexisting infections, such as tuberculosis and hepatitis C, contraindicate transplantation

and subsequent immunosuppression. Patients with these potentially life-threatening organisms are deferred from listing. Candidates are also tested for antibodies to common viral infections (such as herpes simplex virus [HSV]; varicella-zoster virus [VZV]; mumps, rubella, rubeola [MMR]; cytomegalovirus [CMV]; Epstein-Barr virus [EBV]; and hepatitis B virus [HBV]). Patients who lack immunity to viruses that can be prevented with immunization (VZV, MMR, and HBV) are immunized during the waiting period. Identification of CMV status is used to select appropriate post-transplant prophylaxis. Some centers avoid transplanting EBV-positive organs into an EBV-negative recipient because of the increased risk for post-transplant lymphoproliferative disorder.

Patients found to be chronically colonized with pan-resistant organisms are also deferred from listing. Patients with preexisting septic lung processes, such as cystic fibrosis and bronchiectasis, provide sputum specimens for culture at intervals during routine preoperative clinic visits. This culture and sensitivity information is available at the time of transplant and is incorporated into decision making regarding antibiotic therapies.

The use of a ventricular assist device (VAD) to bridge a failing heart to transplantation can also present infectious risks. Implanted devices increase the incidence of subacute, device-related (VAD hardware, pocket, and percutaneous driveline) infections, and the risk of

TABLE 18-2 Causes of and Complications After Thoracic Transplantation

COMPLICATION	HEART TRANSPLANT CAUSES	LUNG TRANSPLANT CAUSES
Hemorrhage	Adhesions from previous cardiac surgery Anticoagulation from CPB	Adhesions from previous thoracic surgery Adhesions from previous pneumothoraces Adhesions from previous pleurodeses High pulmonary artery or venous pressures ECMO
Infections	Sternal wound Invasive lines or drains	Thoracic wound Pneumonia from donor organisms Pneumonia from preoperative recipient colonization with organisms or septic lung disease Bronchial anastomosis site infections or dehiscence Silent aspiration Inability to clear secretions because of poor cough reflex and ciliary paralysis Invasive lines or drains
Early graft failure	Pericardial tamponade Poor myocardial preservation Myocardial stunning, ischemia, or infarction Donor-recipient size mismatch Hypertension-related increased afterload	Ischemia reperfusion injury Poor preservation Volume overload Flooding grafted lung with entire cardiac output because of high pulmonary artery pressures in native lung Compression of grafted lung from overexpanded native lung Pulmonary arterial or venous anastomosis stenosis or kinking Dehiscence of bronchial anastomosis Phrenic nerve injury related diaphragmatic paralysis
Disturbances of cardiac rhythm	Poor preservation Surgical trauma during implantation Interruption of sinoatrial node blood supply Loss of direct neural control Electrolyte imbalance Preoperative use of amiodarone	Post-thoracotomy atrial irritability Irritability of pulmonary veins Volume overload and dilation of atria Hypoxemia, hypercarbia, or acidosis Circulating catecholamines Electrolyte imbalance
Right ventricular failure	Preexisting pulmonary hypertension Poor preservation Hypoxemia Acute hypercapnia Left ventricular dysfunction Pericardial tamponade Pulmonary embolism	Ischemia reperfusion injury Persistent pulmonary hypertension Pulmonary arterial or venous anastomosis stenosis or kinking Pulmonary embolism
Renal failure	Preexisting renal insufficiency Ischemia during CPB Nephrotoxic medications	Ischemia during CPB Hypoxia because of early graft failure Nephrotoxic medications
Gastrointestinal problems	Pancreatitis "Shock liver," bowel ischemia/infarction because of CPB	Paralytic ileus, gastroparesis, and gastroesophageal reflux disease related to vagal nerve injury Cystic fibrosis patients: malabsorption resulting from failure to provide pancreatic enzymes, distal intestinal obstruction syndrome

CPB = Cardiopulmonary bypass, ECMO = extracorporeal membrane oxygenation.

colonization with nosocomial microorganisms that may be resistant to standard antibiotics.[77] Multidrug resistance can also be a problem if the patient has required hospitalization or has been exposed to long-term antibiotic therapy before transplantation.

At the time of transplant, the presence of any active infection can significantly increase surgical morbidity and mortality. Most transplant centers will defer the offer of transplantation until an infection is cleared. During the postoperative period, nosocomial infections, caused by the same organisms that plague all critically ill patients, are frequent in solid organ recipients.[73] To minimize the risk of these infections, scrupulous attention is paid to infection control procedures during this period of profound immunosuppression. To minimize exposure to pathogens in critical care after the procedure, the patient is admitted to a private room; careful hand washing is essential; protective equipment, such as gowns, gloves, and masks, is worn during patient contact; and staff and visitors who are ill are asked to avoid patient contact. Strict sterile technique must be observed during line or drain placement and during dressing changes.

Institutional protocols specify initial empiric surgical antibiotic prescriptions. Cephalosporins or vancomycin (Vancocin) is typically used for surgical prophylaxis with heart transplantation to prevent *Staphylococcus aureus* wound infections. Sternal wound infections are very serious and carry a 25% mortality rate in this population.[2]

Lung transplant recipients can develop nosocomial pulmonary infections related to donor microorganisms. During the period of ventilatory support before the determination of donor brain death and organ harvest, donor lungs frequently become colonized with gram-negative bacteria. During donor evaluation, sputum is collected for culture to determine if colonization has occurred. At the time of implant, donor and recipient bronchi are swabbed for culture specimens.[12]

In the absence of preexisting recipient septic lung disease, broad-spectrum antibiotics are administered during the perioperative period to minimize the risk of infection caused by donor organisms. If gram-negative organisms, such as *Pseudomonas,* are found in the sputum cultures, inhaled tobramycin (Tobi) or colistin (Polymyxin E) is often added to intravenous antibiotics. Once available, the results of both donor and recipient cultures are used to guide specific antibiotic therapy. If all cultures remain negative, and the recipient remains free of signs or symptoms of infection, these empiric antibiotics may be discontinued after 1 week.

Use of multiple invasive devices also increases the risk of infection (such as central vascular catheters or urine catheters) and should be removed as soon as possible. Patients are monitored for any sign or symptom

of infection (i.e., temperature elevation, leukocytosis, purulent sputum, inflammation of any wounds). Any evidence of possible infection should prompt an immediate search for a cause with blood, urine, sputum, and drainage specimens for culture, and chest x-ray for infiltrates. Potentially contaminated devices should be removed or replaced using sterile technique. Early consultation with the transplant infectious disease team should also occur to further evaluate the patient and obtain recommendations regarding appropriate antimicrobial therapies.

Opportunistic infection is a well-known complication of immunosuppression in heart and lung transplant recipients. Risk of opportunistic infection is greatest during the period starting around 4 weeks after transplant and continuing until approximately 6 months after transplant. Therefore antibiotic prophylaxis for opportunistic infections is instituted during critical care hospitalization (Box 18-5).[42] Prophylactic antimicrobial protocols include medications to prevent *Pneumocystis jiroveci* pneumonia and oral *Candida albicans.* Lung recipients are also vulnerable to aspergillus, particularly at the bronchial anastomosis site;[50] nebulized amphotericin B (Fungizone) is used as prophylaxis.[35,43]

CMV infection can be particularly devastating to heart and lung recipients and contributes to long-term graft loss. Most transplant centers have specific prophylaxis protocols based on the donor and recipient antibody status for this disease (Table 18-3). CMV immune globulin (CytoGam) is used in the highest-risk patients, in addition to intravenous ganciclovir (Cytovene) or oral valacyclovir (Valtrex) used for lower-risk patients.

EARLY GRAFT FAILURE

Early graft failure or graft dysfunction is a problem for both heart and lung transplant recipients and accounts for up to 30% of deaths within the first 30 days of heart transplantation.[2] It may occur during weaning from CPB in the operating room and can produce right or left ventricular failure. Pharmacologic support may be necessary to successfully wean from bypass. In cases of severe graft dysfunction, atrial pacing, intra-aortic balloon counterpulsation, or single or bilateral VAD may be required. Cardiac graft dysfunction can also present in the initial postoperative phase,[7] and may be caused by poor myocardial protection at the time of procurement, hyperacute cardiac rejection, or pericardial tamponade.

In lung transplant recipients, early graft failure presents as ischemia reperfusion injury (IRI). It is a common syndrome that occurs within hours after lung transplant, is similar to adult respiratory distress syndrome (ARDS), and is associated with high mortality (Figure 18-15).[10,30]

Box 18-5

Alternatives for Opportunistic Infection Prophylaxis After Thoracic Transplant

- *Candida albicans* esophagitis (until daily prednisone dose less than 5 mg)

  Nystatin (Mycostatin) solution 5000 units swish and swallow 4 times a day

  Clotrimazole (Mycelex) troches 10 mg after meals and before bed

- *Pneumocystis jiroveci* pneumonia (lifelong)

  SS (trimethoprim/sulfamethoxazole [Bactrim]) daily or DS (trimethoprim/sulfamethoxazole) every other day

  Dapsone 100 mg PO daily

  Atovaquone (Mepron) 750 mg PO bid

  Pentamidine (NebuPent) nebulization monthly

- CMV infection or reactivation (varies by risk stratification)

- CytoGam cytomegalovirus immune globulin 150-100 mg/kg for 7 doses

- Ganciclovir IV 5 mg/kg bid for 14 days induction followed by 5 mg/kg daily for maintenance period (dose adjusted based on creatinine clearance)

- Valganciclovir 900 mg PO bid for 14 days induction followed by 900 mg PO daily for maintenance period (dose adjusted based on creatinine clearance)

- Acyclovir 800 mg tid or valacyclovir 500–1000 mg daily (after GCV/valganciclovir completed)

From reference 57a.

The causes of IRI are not fully understood; however, it is associated with procedural risks, such as prolonged (more than 6 hours) ischemic time, inadequate lung preservation, hyperinflation between harvest and implant, and use of CPB,[1] and with donor-related risks, such as increased age, aspiration pneumonia, and lung contusions before harvest.[34,43,56,70] Loss of lymphatic pulmonary drainage in the transplanted lung and volume overload may also contribute.

IRI presents as a progressive, sometimes rapid decline in lung function. On biopsy, pathologic changes indicative of increased pulmonary capillary permeability, increased interstitial lung water, and occasionally diffuse alveolar damage can be seen.[68] Clinical signs and symptoms include decreased lung compliance, hypercapnia, hypoxemia, increased pulmonary artery pressures, right ventricular failure, and even systemic shock.[43] The chest radiograph usually resembles the diffuse pulmonary infiltrates seen in pulmonary edema or ARDS.

The appearance of IRI demands immediate attention, including ensuring a negative fluid balance, maximal ventilator support, and occasionally use of inhaled nitric oxide (iNO) and extracorporeal membrane oxygenation (ECMO).[17,34,39,53,59]

Airway Problems

After lung transplantation, the area of bronchial anastomosis is particularly vulnerable to injury and infection because it has a poor blood supply and is dependent on retrograde flow from the pulmonary circulation.[62,72] Consequently, the bronchial anastomosis is a relatively ischemic wound, with necrotic tissue subject to infection and dehiscence. Use of sirolimus has also been associated with bronchial wound healing problems.[23] IRI and early episodes of acute rejection have also been found to be associated with problems at the bronchial anastomosis.[62]

To decrease the interstitial edema related to the interruption to pulmonary lymphatics, patients are

TABLE 18-3 Cytomegalovirus Prophylaxis Protocol Based on Recipient and Donor CMV Status

	RECIPIENT CMV NEGATIVE	RECIPIENT CMV POSITIVE
Donor CMV negative	Low risk: IV ganciclovir or oral valganciclovir × 6 weeks	Moderate risk: reactivation recipient strain CMV IV ganciclovir or oral valganciclovir × 12 weeks
Donor CMV positive	Highest risk: active new CMV infection during immunosuppression IV ganciclovir or PO valganciclovir × 12 weeks plus full course CMV immune globulin: CytoGam 150 mg/kg IV on days 0, 14, 28, 42, 56 CytoGam 100 mg/kg IV on days 84 and 112	Moderate risk: reactivation of recipient strain or new infection with donor strain IV ganciclovir or oral valganciclovir × 12 weeks plus full course CMV immune globulin

From reference 57a.

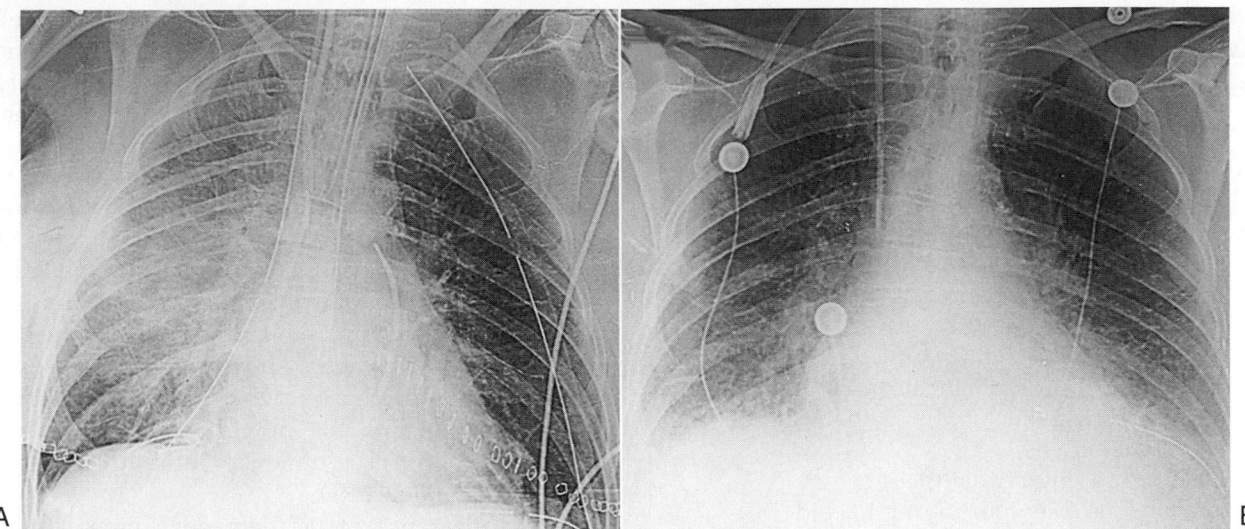

♦FIGURE 18-15 Unilateral ischemia-reperfusion lung injury. **A,** Significant unilateral lung edema and diffuse interstitial infiltrates characteristics of ischemia reperfusion injury. **B,** Same patient several days later with complete resolution of ischemia reperfusion injury after supportive care.

actively diuresed, fluid intake is restricted, and pulmonary hypertension is avoided, which will reduce the capillary hydrostatic pressure and allow interstitial fluid to return to the intravascular compartment. Nursing and respiratory therapy interventions focus on facilitating coughing to assist with mucus clearance, necessary because of the ciliary dysfunction. Specific therapies include chest physiotherapy with postural drainage; cupping and clapping; endotracheal suctioning; and therapeutic bronchoscopy. Patients are encouraged to cough and use the incentive spirometer 10 times hourly while awake. They are also taught other mucus mobilization techniques, such as use of a flutter valve and huffing. A flutter valve is a handheld, pipe-shaped device through which the patient exhales. As the patient exhales, a ball inside the device moves up and down, creating airway resistance and a slight vibration. This vibration helps to break up respiratory secretions.[58] Huffing is a coughing technique used to move airway secretions to large airways where they can be cleared by coughing. To huff, the patient inspires deeply and then breathes out forcefully through an open mouth and without closing the glottis, causing a blowing "huh" sound.[38] Once mobilized to the upper airway, secretions can be cleared by expectoration.

Dehiscence presents as abrupt respiratory distress, new air leak, subcutaneous emphysema or expanding pneumothorax, and hemoptysis. Sepsis frequently follows these symptoms. Dehiscence is diagnosed with direct bronchoscopy and, if very small, may be repaired with topical fibrin glue. However, if the area of dehiscence is large, surgical repair may be required.[57]

Dysrhythmias

After heart and lung transplantation, supraventricular dysrhythmias are the most frequent dysrhythmia. After heart transplant, inadequate atrial protection during procurement or surgical trauma during implantation can produce sinus node dysfunction (SND), resulting in a bradydysrhythmia. Additional causes of SND include intraoperative disturbance in blood supply to the SA node or the preoperative use of amiodarone (Cordarone).[22] Because of its long half-life, the antidysrhythmogenic and negative chronotropic effects of amiodarone can persist for some time after the last dose. AV sequential pacing, and less often intravenous isoproterenol or aminophylline, may be required to support the HR until the bradycardia resolves. If the bradycardia does not resolve on its own, the insertion of a permanent pacemaker may be required.

AV disturbances can also occur, but the AV node's response to exogenous agents is altered from denervation. In addition, any new onset of dysrhythmia, especially atrial flutter, may signify an acute rejection episode in heart recipients.[15] A right bundle branch block caused by surgical trauma is associated with right ventricular dysfunction.[65] Wenckebach rhythm has been seen with acute graft failure or rejection.[29] Second-degree AV block and complete heart block are also consequences of surgical injury.[14]

For lung transplant patients, uncontrolled tachycardia can degenerate into atrial fibrillation. Vasopressors, such as dopamine (Intropin), and continued endogenous catecholamine discharge resulting from unrelieved pain can increase the risk of supraventricular tachycardias.[49] Electrolyte imbalances can also increase the risk for dysrhythmias. If present, supraventricular tachycardia in lung recipients should be rate controlled with beta blockers or calcium channel blockers, and treated with amiodarone.

Right Ventricular Failure

Right ventricular (RV) failure in the newly transplanted heart can have devastating effects on the postoperative recovery. Because preexisting pulmonary hypertension contributes to this complication, routine right heart catheterizations are done to assess the pulmonary pressures during pretransplant evaluation. Ideally, the pulmonary vascular resistance (PVR) should be well below 5 Wood's units and the transpulmonary gradient less than 12–15 mm Hg. Progression of congestive heart failure can lead to an increased PVR as the pressures on the left side of the heart rise. The patient may require continuous intravenous milrinone (Primacor) or dobutamine (Dobutrex) therapy, or implantation of a left or bilateral (right and left) VAD to optimize pulmonary pressures before transplantation.

RV failure can also be the result of hypoxemia, acute hypercapnia, pericardial tamponade, pulmonary embolus, or inadequate preservation of the RV during procurement. Treatment involves optimizing RV output and decreasing pulmonary resistance to RV outflow, with a goal of maintaining a transpulmonary gradient of 5–10 mm Hg.[11] A systolic murmur in the tricuspid area and prominent V waves when assessing the jugular venous pressure are indicative of tricuspid regurgitation, which is a complication of RV failure. Lower extremity edema with or without hepatomegaly and abdominal bloating may also be present.

Correcting hypoxemia, acidosis, and electrolyte imbalances can improve RV function. Pharmacologic agents of choice include IV preparations of milrinone, nitroprusside (Nipride), nitroglycerin (Tridil), isoproterenol, and dobutamine. Inhaled NO decreases pulmonary resistance and exerts a positive chronotropic influence on the denervated heart.[11] It is preferred over using of epoprostenol (Flolan) because of its selective pulmonary vasodilator effects and should be made available both perioperatively and postoperatively. Sildenafil (Revatio) used orally twice daily has also been shown in clinical trials to reduce pulmonary hypertension and has now been FDA approved for this purpose.[81] If the failure is severe, an RV assist device may be required to support the ailing ventricle until the cause can be corrected or minimized.

Renal Failure. Acute renal insufficiency or renal failure can occur during the initial postoperative phase after heart transplant due to effects of preexisting renal insufficiency, CPB, or a compromised postoperative CO.[51] In lung transplant recipients, aggressive diuresis to decrease interstitial lung water also is a contributing factor. Careful attention detects decreases in urine output, indicating inadequate renal perfusion, or decreased effectiveness of diuretics, signifying worsening renal function.

If renal dysfunction is present, diuretics may be used to keep the urine output greater than 50 ml/hour. Calcineurin inhibitors (cyclosporine, tacrolimus) may be temporarily avoided because of their nephrotoxic effects. The Research Utilization box below discusses the role of calcineurin inhibitors in chronic renal failure. In this case, induction therapy with cytolytic antibodies is essential in order to prevent early cellular rejection. When calcineurin inhibitors are used, serum creatinine and 12-hour trough drug levels are monitored daily. Based on these data, the dose is adjusted to achieve therapeutic levels and avoid toxic levels.

⬧ RESEARCH UTILIZATION

Chronic Renal Failure After Transplantation

CLINICAL ISSUE

New-onset chronic renal failure (CRF) is a common cause of morbidity and mortality after nonrenal solid organ transplantation. Calcineurin inhibitor immunosuppression is frequently implicated as a major contributor to this complication. Data are limited regarding the overall incidence of, risk factors for, and long-term survival in nonrenal solid organ recipients who develop CRF. Most studies of this problem have restricted their sample to recipients of only one type of solid organ transplant or to only brief follow-up periods, or the studies used conflicting definitions of chronic renal failure.

SUMMARY

This retrospective analysis of data from the Centers for Medicare and Medicaid Services included information from nearly 70,000 nonrenal transplant recipients over a 10-year period ending in 2000. A standard definition of CRF as glomerular filtration rate (GFR) less than 29 ml/min/1.73 m^2 of body surface area or initiation of dialysis or preemptive renal transplant was used. The authors found that the incidence of chronic renal failure was 16.5%, with nearly one third of those patients (28.9%) requiring chronic dialysis or transplantation.

(Continued)

▲ **RESEARCH UTILIZATION—CONT'D**

Five-year risk of CRF varied by type of organs transplanted, with the highest risk among intestinal transplant recipients (21.3%) and the lowest among heart-lung recipients (6.9%) (liver, 18.1%; lung, 15.8%; heart, 10.9%). The high incidence of CRF associated with intestinal transplant may have been biased by the small number of patients receiving these types of organ transplants. Female gender and increased age as well as pretransplant diabetes, hypertension, and hepatitis C were associated with increased risk of post-transplant CRF. Postoperative acute renal failure occurred in 7.6% of recipients and also conferred increased risk. The risk of CRF for all patients increased with time. Although between 86% and 93% of patients received a calcineurin inhibitor early after transplantation, no association was found between the use of these medications and CRF. However, data on use of these drugs were missing for 11.6% of the patients, and data regarding plasma levels of calcineurin inhibitors were not available. In addition, up to 23.8% of the patients, including 1.5% with preexisting end-stage renal disease (ESRD), had some degree of decreased renal function before transplantation. For every 10-ml decrease in preoperative GFR, patients had a 9% increased risk of developing CRF. The impact of potential improvements in surgical techniques or patient management over the 10-year period was not controlled.

APPLICATION

The results of this study can be used to identify patients at increased risk for CRF after transplantation. They also support efforts to reduce risks of CRF, such as careful selection of patients for transplantation and use of strategies that might reduce postoperative acute renal failure (e.g., prevention of hypoxemia and hypoperfusion during and immediately after transplantation, avoidance of nephrotoxic drugs). These data can also be used to better inform patients of the long-term complications associated with transplantation. Since survival after transplant has been increased by improved immunosuppression and technologies, it is important that efforts to minimize risk factors for CRF be enhanced.

NEED FOR FURTHER STUDY

Prospective randomized trials are needed to examine interventions to decrease the risk of CRF after nonrenal transplant. Data on outcomes of control of calcineurin inhibitor levels, improved renal perfusion during and after surgery, avoidance of nephrotoxic agents, and control of diabetes and hypertension are specifically needed.

Ojo, A., et al. (2003). Chronic renal failure after transplantation of a nonrenal organ. *N Engl J Med, 349*(10), 931–940.

Other nephrotoxic agents must also be avoided if at all possible. All nonsteroidal antiinflammatory drugs, with the possible exception of aspirin, are contraindicated. Aminoglycoside antibiotics, intravenous contrast, and systemic amphotericin are avoided unless absolutely necessary. Doses of renally eliminated drugs, such as trimethoprim/sulfamethoxazole (Bactrim) and ganciclovir (Cytovene), are adjusted daily based on fluctuations in creatinine clearance.

Consultation with a transplant nephrologist is warranted for more than minor changes in renal function. Ultrafiltration, continuous veno-veno hemodialysis, or hemodialysis (Chapter 33) may be required in order to control fluid balance and provide adequate nutrition and necessary IV medications until renal function improves.

Gastrointestinal Complications. Gastrointestinal complications occur frequently after thoracic transplantation. Symptoms include nausea, vomiting, diarrhea, and abdominal pain or discomfort. The cause may be difficult to determine and may stem from residual effects of anesthesia, the surgery itself, infection, immunosuppressant, or other medication side effects. Mycophenolate mofetil and azathioprine can cause anorexia, nausea, vomiting, dyspepsia, abdominal pain, diarrhea, and elevated levels of liver transaminases. Cyclosporine can also contribute to nausea and vomiting. Hypoperfusion to the gut and bowel ischemia or infarction during bypass can also lead to diarrhea. Pancreatitis can be caused by preexisting pancreatic disease, perioperative hypoperfusion, direct trauma, or drugs such as trimethoprim/sulfamethoxazole or azathioprine. Corticosteroids can mask an acute abdominal process, making diagnosis difficult. Prompt evaluation with blood work and radiographic studies is necessary to rule out an acute process. If one is found, immediate gastrointestinal surgical consultation should be obtained and surgical intervention considered.

ADDITIONAL POSTOPERATIVE PROBLEMS AFTER THORACIC TRANSPLANTATION

Diabetes Mellitus

Both heart and lung transplant recipients are vulnerable to short- or long-term diabetes from the immunosuppressant drugs. Post-transplant hyperglycemia and insulin resistance are significant risk factors for cardiovascular disease and postoperative infections. New postoperative hyperglycemia may be steroid-induced and sometimes disappears once steroids are weaned to minimal doses. The incidence of new diabetes during immunosuppression with tacrolimus is five times greater than that with cyclosporine.[18]

Blood glucose levels are monitored several times a day throughout the postoperative period. If results are significantly elevated, treatment with a continuous insulin drip is indicated. Once glycemic control is attained, the insulin drip can be replaced with long-acting insulin. Short-acting insulin is added as needed before meals on the basis of monitoring results. If only mild hyperglycemia is present, patients are taking oral nutrition, and no renal insufficiency exists, oral agents (sulfonylureas, insulin sensitizers) may be used. Chapter 34 provides comprehensive information about glycemic control.

Nutrition

End-stage lung disease and transplant surgery significantly increase metabolic needs. Nutrition should be provided via the enteral or parenteral route within 48 hours of transplant, as indicated in the Nutrition box below. If the enteral route is used, a postpyloric tube is preferred to minimize the risk of aspiration of gastric contents. Patients should be cleared for oral intake with a swallow evaluation. Because of the risks of delayed esophageal and gastric emptying, patients should be out of bed for all meals and should not resume recumbent position for at least 1 hour after eating.[9] If a patient encounters nausea or vomiting, promotility agents and nonsedating anti-emetics should be used.

♦ NUTRITION

Diabetic Guidelines for the Heart or Lung Transplant Patient

GENERAL CONSIDERATIONS

- All diabetic patients need to follow an American Dietetic Association (ADA) diet to control carbohydrate content. A "no concentrated sweets" or a "cardiac" diet is not sufficient and will make glucose control very difficult and increase the risk of postoperative complications.
- Correction regimens should be written for aspart (NovoLog) insulin AC only. A low-dose regimen is 1 unit/50 mg/dl greater than 150; a medium-dose regimen is 2 units/50 mg/dl greater than 150.
- Glucose control parameters for the inpatient setting are the following:
  - Fasting: less than 110 mg/dl
  - Preprandial: 80–120 mg/dl
  - Postprandial: less than 180 mg/dl

- Measurements higher than these levels will increase the risk of infection and other complications in a hospitalized diabetic patient.

POSTOPERATIVE GUIDELINES

1. Transplant patients will be managed with a basal/nutritional/correction insulin regimen until their creatinine levels, liver function tests, and steroid regimens are stable. Only at the point where these parameters are stable will they be transitioned to an oral regimen.
2. Transplant patients should be taught glucometer skills, insulin administration, and basic insulin instruction while they are recovering from their surgery. They may need to be discharged on insulin as their steroid taper is continued on an outpatient basis.
3. Unless a patient is already followed by an endocrinologist preoperatively, follow-up either with an endocrinologist locally or with an endocrine fellow should be arranged.
4. Transplant patients who are NPO for biopsy or bronchoscopy:
   a. Standing aspart (NovoLog) should be held and one half the dose of basal insulin (which is usually NPH) given, even if the patient has no preoperative history of diabetes. Prednisone stimulates the liver to release glycogen regardless of food intake and also increases insulin resistance at the cellular level.
   b. If you are notified that the patient is to be scheduled for a study, in addition to ordering the patient to be NPO, please have a physician or nurse practitioner write for the above insulin regimen.
5. Transplant patients who are ordered pulse or stress dose steroids for rejection:
   a. Each component of the insulin regimen needs to be increased to prevent hyperglycemia while receiving an increased steroid regimen. The transplant endocrine team should be notified when increased corticosteroids are initiated.

To provide adequate nutritional substrate without increasing carbon dioxide production, dietary protein and fat may need to be increased and carbohydrate consumption decreased. Dietary consultation and guidance are necessary for exact diet prescriptions. Calorie counts and levels of albumin, prealbumin, and transferrin are monitored to determine adequate nutritional intake. Cystic fibrosis (CF) patients must be given their pancreatic enzymes before meals. Special attention is required to avoid severe constipation in patients with CF, who are prone to distal intestinal obstruction syndrome.

CHAPTER 19

Acute Respiratory Failure and Acute Lung Injury

Laurie Baumgartner

Acute respiratory failure (ARF) is the most common type of organ failure and a major cause of morbidity and mortality in the adult critical care unit.[28,30] The incidence of adult primary respiratory failure in the United States accounts for 137 hospitalizations per 100,000 residents annually.[6] ARF alone has a good prognostic outcome; however, when a patient has dysfunction in multiple organs, the chance of mortality rises exponentially per dysfunctional organ.

DEFINITION

ARF is the inability of the respiratory system to maintain gas exchange. One of two phenomena may occur. In type 1 failure, the body fails to deliver an adequate supply of oxygen to the arterial blood. Type 1 is also known as *hypoxemic failure* or *oxygenation failure*. In type 2 respiratory failure, the body ineffectively eliminates carbon dioxide (CO_2) from the arterial blood. Type 2 is also known as *hypercapnic respiratory failure* or *ventilatory failure*.[28,30]

Defining objective measurements for ARF is a challenge for healthcare professionals. The most common clinical definition of ARF uses set partial pressure of arterial oxygen tension (Pao_2) and partial pressure of arterial carbon dioxide ($Paco_2$) values. Many patients display clinical manifestations of ARF before reaching these targeted values. Therefore it is crucial that each patient undergo a comprehensive assessment versus the practitioner's relying solely on laboratory values. The definition of hypoxemic ARF is a Pao_2 value less than 60 mm Hg. Hypercapnic ARF is defined as a $Paco_2$ level greater than 50 mm Hg with a pH less than or equal to 7.30. Others have defined ARF based on the Pao_2/fraction of inspired oxygen (Fio_2) [P/F] ratio. The Acute Lung Injury (ALI)/Acute Respiratory Distress Syndrome (ARDS) section later in the chapter provides a comprehensive review of P/F ratio.

MECHANISM OF HYPOXEMIC ACUTE RESPIRATORY FAILURE

The respiratory system consists of the lungs (the gas-exchanging unit), the chest wall including the respiratory muscles, the respiratory controllers in the central nervous system (CNS), and the spinal and peripheral nerves that connect the central nervous system to the respiratory muscles. During hypoxemic ARF, the gas-exchange unit becomes dysfunctional, resulting in the inability to diffuse oxygen across the alveoli to the arterial blood supply. Conditions that often result in hypoxemic ARF include chronic obstructive pulmonary disease (COPD), asthma, bronchiolitis, cystic fibrosis, pneumonia, pulmonary emboli, inhalation of toxic gases, and near drowning.[72]

There are five primary mechanisms of hypoxemic ARF. A brief discussion of each will follow.

Ventilation/Perfusion Mismatching

Under normal physiologic conditions, pulmonary blood flows to ventilated areas, resulting in a matching of ventilation ($\dot{V}$) and perfusion ($\dot{Q}$). Hypoxemia causes a compensatory localized capillary vasoconstriction, preventing pulmonary blood from flowing past hypoxic alveoli.[39] $\dot{V}/\dot{Q}$ mismatch occurs when some perfused alveoli are flooded or collapsed, as occurs with pneumonia and congestive heart failure (pulmonary edema) ($\dot{V} < \dot{Q}$); some alveoli are ventilated but not perfused because of capillary thrombosis, as occurs in pulmonary embolism ($\dot{V} > \dot{Q}$). Some are relatively unaffected ($\dot{V} = \dot{Q}$) (Figure 19-1).

Intrapulmonary Shunt

Depending on the amount of blood that does not take part in gas exchange in the lungs, oxygenation may be greatly affected. Shunt refers to the state in which pulmonary capillary perfusion is normal, but

PROBLEM	INTERVENTION	RATIONALE	EXPECTED OUTCOME	COMMENTS
	Administer NMB, analgesics, and sedation as required by patient response to the mode of respiratory support provided.	Intubation and mechanical ventilation is an uncomfortable procedure. Analgesia and sedation minimize anxiety and pain. NMB may be required when patient is fighting the ventilator.	Patient will exhibit decreased pain, decreased agitation, and decreased potential for self-extubation; also will show decreased posttraumatic stress disorder.	
	Monitor for effectiveness of ventilator treatment and medication.	Treatments may be adjusted based on results.	Indexes of infection will show improvement over time.	
Potential for nosocomial infections and adverse events	Assess for readiness to wean daily.	Early weaning and extubation decrease length of stay and ventilator-associated events.	Pao_2 >60 mm hemoglobin, Fio_2 <0.5, PEEP ≤5 cm H_2O, intact ventilatory drive, cardiovascular stability, afebrile, adequate nutritional status, and absence of organ failure. Assess predictors of weaning outcome: VC >10 ml/kg, MIP <−30, M_E <10 L/min, RR <30 breaths/min	
	Ensure patient has DVT prophylaxis and PUD prophylaxis.	Decrease DVT and PUD adverse events.	No gastrointestinal bleeds, gastritis, or deep vein thrombotic and pulmonary embolic events.	See www.ihi.org for information on a ventilator bundle to decrease adverse events.
	Maintain head of bed >30 degrees and <45 degrees.	Decrease ventilator-associated nosocomial infections.	Patient has 0/1000 ventilator days nosocomial infection rate.	See www.ihi.org for information on a ventilator bundle to decrease ventilator-associated pneumonias.
	Provide oral care every 8–12 hours with toothbrush and toothpaste, provide oral care every 2 hours with moisture swab, and provide continuous supraglottic suctioning while intubated.	Decreased oral bacterial burden.	Decreased passage of contaminated supraglottic secretions to bronchioles, with resultant pneumonia.	See AACN practice alerts for ventilator-associated pneumonia prevention and oral care at www.aacn.org.

AACN = American Association of Critical-Care Nurses, ABG = arterial blood gas, CXR = chest x-ray, DVT = deep vein thrombosis, Fio_2 = fraction of inspired oxygen, MIP = maximal inspiratory pressures, M_E = minute ventilation, NMB = neuromuscular blockade, Pao_2 = partial pressure of arterial oxygen tension, $Paco_2$ = partial pressure of arterial carbon dioxide, PEEP= positive end-expiratory pressure, PFTs = pulmonary function tests, PUD = peptic ulcer disease, RR = respiratory rate, Sao_2 = arterial oxygen saturation, Spo_2 = arterial oxygen saturation by pulse oximetry, VC = vital capacity, V_t = tidal volume.

While the cerebral cortex controls voluntary ventilation, control of the muscles of respiration occurs in the spinal cord. The phrenic nerve controls the diaphragm. There are central and peripheral chemoreceptors that sense the chemical composition of the blood and extracorporeal fluids and provide information to the CNS about oxygenation, pH, and CO_2 concentrations. Conditions that inhibit these sensors and pneumotaxic and chemotaxic centers include narcotic or sedative overdose, CNS abnormalities such as tumor or congenital abnormalities, infections of the brain, infections or disruption of the spinal cord, botulism, Guillain-Barré syndrome, myxedema, and obesity (pickwickian syndrome).

Lungs: Airways/Alveoli. Alterations in the airways or alveolar-blood interface (such as from pneumonia, chronic bronchitis and emphysema [COPD], severe asthma, cystic fibrosis, pulmonary edema, pulmonary fibrosis, ALI, and adult respiratory distress syndrome) cause significant alterations of carbon dioxide diffusion. The Multidisciplinary Plan of Care on pp. 450-452 outlines the potential for inadequate airway patency. Both high and low $\dot{V}/\dot{Q}$ ratios limit gas exchange. When additional stressors materialize in patients with chronic respiratory conditions (hypoxic or hypercapnic), the patient may succumb to ARF. A Cochrane database meta-analysis of randomized control trials in COPD patients found that noninvasive positive pressure ventilation (NIPPV) reduces the incidence of and morbidities associated with endotracheal intubation and mechanical ventilation.[62]

ACUTE LUNG INJURY/ACUTE RESPIRATORY DISTRESS SYNDROME

ALI and ARDS are life-threatening inflammatory diseases of the lung that manifest in a continuum (Figure 19-2). Characteristics of ALI and ARDS include bilateral pulmonary infiltrates, hypoxemia unresponsive to increasing oxygen supplementation, and decreased

TABLE 19-1 Definition of ALI and ARDS

ONSET	ACUTE AND PERSISTENT
Oxygenation criteria	Pao_2/Fio_2 greater than 200; less than or equal to 300 for ALI
	Pao_2/Fio_2 less than or equal to 200 for ARDS
Exclusion criteria	PAWP greater than or equal to 18 mm Hg
	Clinical evidence of left atrial hypertension
Radiographic criteria	Bilateral opacification representative of pulmonary edema

Data from reference 8.

pulmonary compliance. In ALI the P/F ratio falls between 200 and 300 mm Hg, and in ARDS the P/F ratio is less than 200 mm Hg.[8]

Vietnam War physicians first described ARDS in the 1960s using names such as *shock lung, wet lung, post-traumatic respiratory distress syndrome,* and *Da Nang lung.*[4] These physicians described a clinical presentation consisting of acute onset of hypoxia resistant to supplemental oxygen, tachypnea, diffuse pulmonary infiltrates, and decreased alveolar compliance.[5] Before 1994 a lack of consensus on the defining characteristics of ALI and ARDS impeded epidemiology and outcome research. This problem was partially ameliorated when the North American-European Consensus Conference (NAECC) on ALI and ARDS established the criteria for diagnosis (Table 19-1).[8] The issue is not completely resolved because the definitions provide sensitivity, but still lack specificity, making it difficult to ensure a homogeneous population. The exclusion criterion helps to ensure the absence of heart failure as the cause of pulmonary edema.

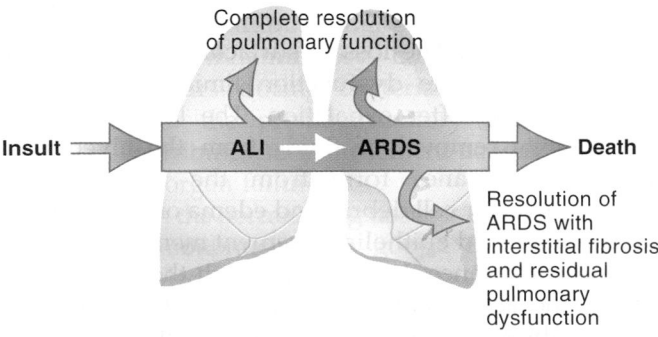

◆FIGURE 19-2 Continuum of lung injury.

EPIDEMIOLOGY AND RISK OF ACUTE LUNG INJURY/ACUTE RESPIRATORY DISTRESS SYNDROME

The incidence and prevalence of ALI and ARDS have historically proven to be elusive numbers, due in part to the lack of definitive definition. A recent study estimates the annual U.S. ALI incidence to be 64.2 cases per 100,000 persons.[34] The authors of a single hospital study done in Spain using American-European census criteria reported the incidence of ARDS (in cases per 100,000

CPAP: CPAP level and oxygen are the main settings. BiPAP: Inspiratory pressure level (IPL, I-PAP), expiratory pressure level (PEEP, E-PAP), FiO_2 (may be a dial on the ventilator but most require that oxygen is bled into the system [e.g., 6 L] at the mask interface or between the ventilator and circuit).

- Mode names also vary with manufacturer and include spontaneous (PSV), spontaneous/timed (S/T or AC), and timed (control) modes. With the timed modes, fx and T_i are also set.

RESPIRATORY WAVEFORM MONITORING

A relatively new assessment skill for nurses and respiratory therapists working with mechanically ventilated patients is the interpretation of respiratory waveforms. Years ago, respiratory waveform monitoring was rare; today it is widely available on ventilators. Unfortunately, the waveforms are poorly understood, and as a result, the technology is not used to full advantage. This section describes the most common waveforms available on ventilators today. The reader is reminded that waveform configurations may vary, dependent on the manufacturer; however, the concepts are broadly applicable.

Respiratory waveform monitoring is most helpful in monitoring volume or pressure modes of mechanical ventilation. Respiratory waveform monitoring is non-invasive, is undetectable by the patient, and does not interfere with normal ventilator function; no special patient considerations are required for its use. Once the visual display is set up, selected waveforms are available and may be graphed (depending on the equipment). Commonly available waveform graphics include pressure-time, flow-time, volume-time, and "loop" configurations (pressure-volume and flow-volume loops). Respiratory waveform monitoring may be helpful to identify appropriate modes of ventilation (and patient/ventilator dyssynchrony), detect auto-PEEP and air leaks, evaluate changes in compliance and resistance, identify end-expiration during hemodynamic monitoring, and monitor spontaneous respiratory effort when muscle relaxants are being used. A description of the waveforms and selected applications follows.

Pressure-Time and Flow-Time Waveforms

Volume modes are associated with *accelerating pressure* waveforms (see Figure 20-1), because pressure gradually builds as the volume of gas is delivered. Examples of pressure waveforms from volume modes of ventilation include AC (Figure 20-7) and IMV (Figure 20-8). Flow waveforms with volume ventilation are generally a *square* configuration (see Figure 20-2) because flow is stable throughout the breath.

With *pressure modes,* a high flow of gas is delivered until a predetermined pressure is reached. The pressure is maintained throughout inspiration, and the associated waveform is called a *square pressure waveform* (see Figure 20-4). Examples of pressure waveforms from pressure modes include PSV (Figure 20-9), PC/IRV (Figure 20-10), and volume-guaranteed pressure options (Figures 20-11 and 20-12). Pressure waveforms of mixed volume and pressure modes, such as IMV plus PSV, demonstrate a combination of the two (Figures 20-13 and 20-14). In all pressure modes, flow is initially high but tapers as the chest fills; thus the

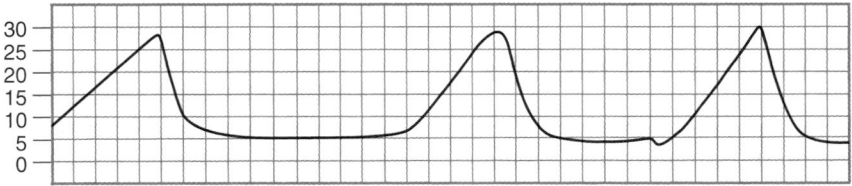

✦FIGURE 20-7 Pressure waveform of the assist-control mode. Note that the third waveform starts with a negative deflection indicative of patient effort.

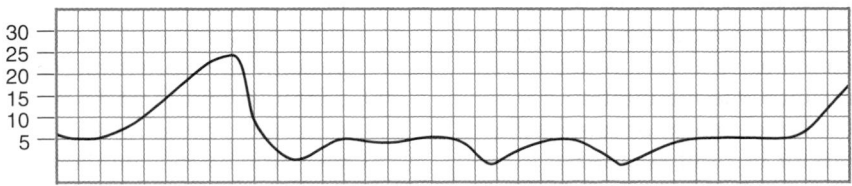

✦FIGURE 20-8 Pressure-time waveform of intermittent mandatory ventilation.

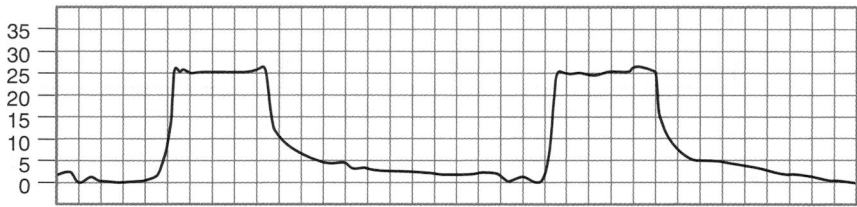

◆FIGURE 20-9 Pressure-time waveform of pressure support ventilation. All breaths have square pressure configuration.

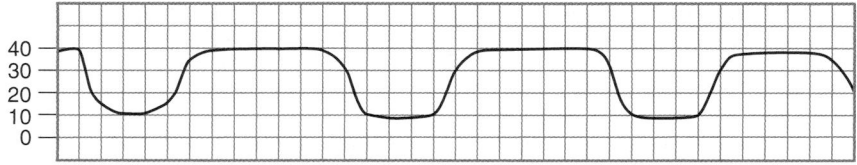

◆FIGURE 20-10 Pressure-time waveform of pressure-controlled inverse-ratio ventilation (2:1 ratio).

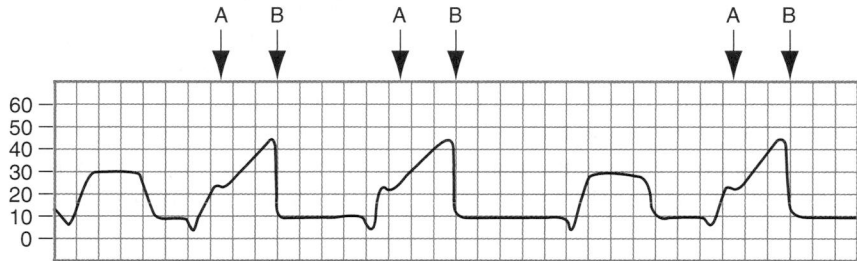

◆FIGURE 20-11 Pressure-time waveform of pressure-controlled inverse-ratio ventilation (2:1 ratio). The breath starts as a pressure breath (*A* = square pressure waveform) but ends as a volume breath (*B* = accelerating pressure waveform).

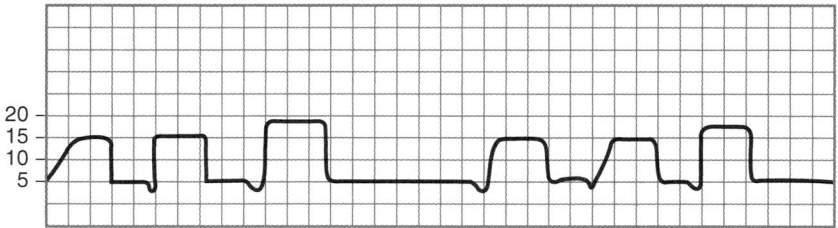

◆FIGURE 20-12 Pressure-time waveform of a volume-guaranteed pressure option: "volume support." The mode adjusts the pressure level to ensure the desired volume.

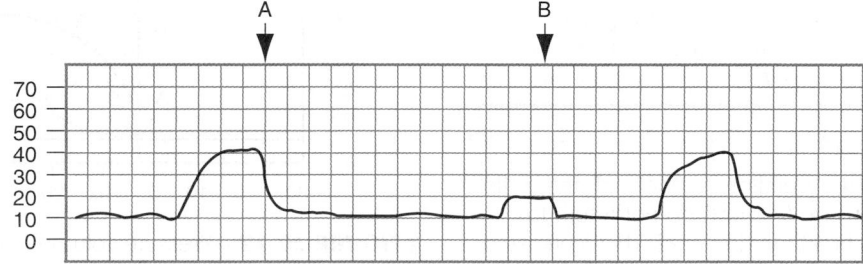

◆FIGURE 20-13 Pressure-time waveform of mixed modes: IMV plus PSV. *A* = IMV and *B* = PSV. IMV = Intermittent mandatory ventilation; PSV = pressure support ventilation.

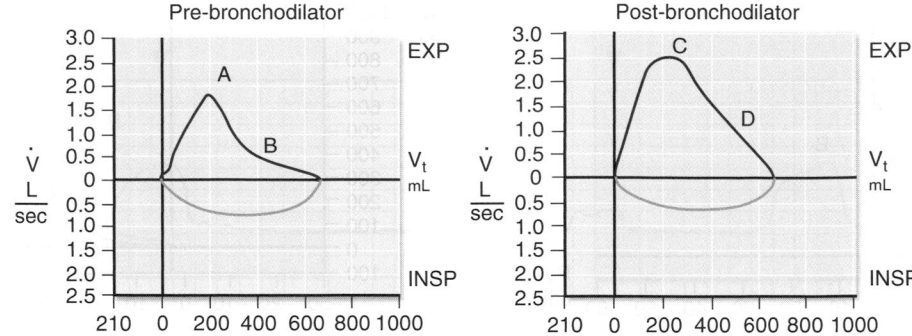

FIGURE 20-22 Flow-volume loops demonstrate the difference in peak expiratory flow rate before and after bronchodilator therapy (*A* and *C*). In addition, the scalloped shape near the end of exhalation (*B*) is characteristic of poor airway conductivity before bronchodilator use, which is markedly improved after using the bronchodilator (*D*).

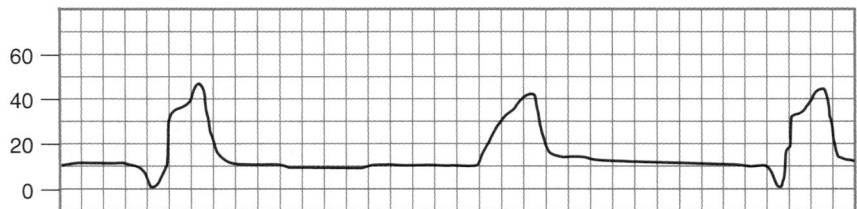

FIGURE 20-23 Pressure-time waveform of the AC mode. Note the first and third waveforms, which are initiated by the patient. The deep negative pressure drop preceding the patient-initiated breaths indicates significant work of breathing. The scooped portion of the accelerating waveform suggests that flow is not adequate. The patient is dyssynchronous.

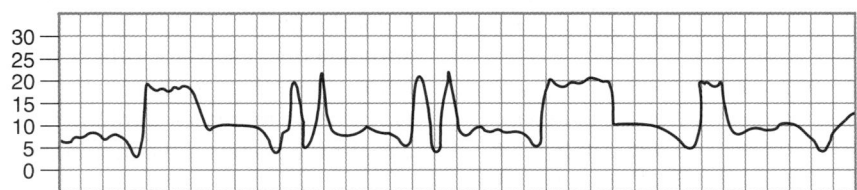

FIGURE 20-24 Pressure-time waveform of PSV. The short, choppy waveforms indicate poor inspiration (the patient was hiccoughing). The patient is dyssynchronous.

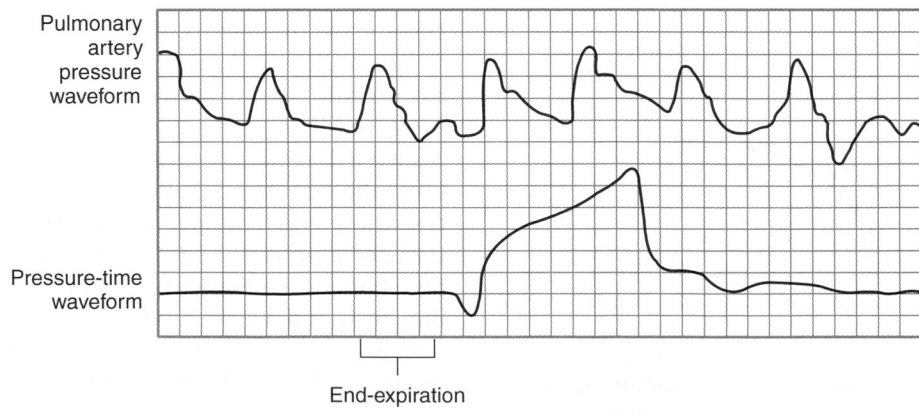

FIGURE 20-25 Simultaneous pulmonary artery tracing and pressure-time waveform. Measurement of end-expiration is easy to perform.

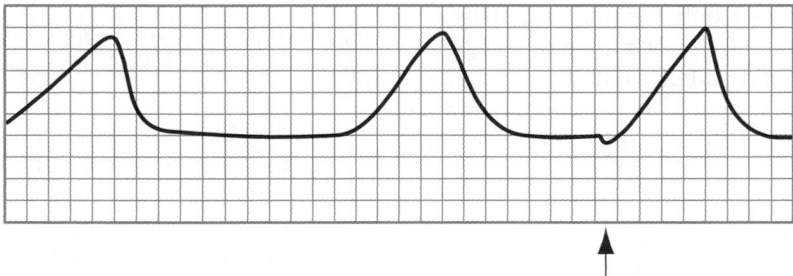

♦FIGURE 20-26 Pressure-time waveform indicating breakthrough breathing *(arrow)* on a patient receiving neuromuscular blockade.

Assessment

Assessment of the weaning patient begins with an evaluation of stability and determination that the condition necessitating mechanical ventilation has resolved.

In the past, "traditional" or "standard" weaning indexes were relied on to identify weaning readiness (Box 20-6).[87,88] While the indexes are helpful to assess respiratory muscle strength and endurance, they are not good

---

Box 20-6

Traditional Weaning Indexes

NEGATIVE INSPIRATORY PRESSURE (NIP)

Before beginning, the endotracheal or tracheal tube cuff is inflated. Attach a one-way valve and a pressure manometer to the patient's artificial airway, making sure the cuff is inflated. Instruct the patient to try to exhale maximally before attaching the measurement device (this is an attempt to begin at residual volume). Once the measurement device is attached, instruct the patient to inhale forcefully against the closed system. The best effort (most negative number) is recorded in 20 seconds. Abort the test if the patient becomes unduly agitated or experiences dysrhythmias or desaturation.

$$NIP\ threshold = \leq20\ cm\ H_2O$$

POSITIVE EXPIRATORY PRESSURE (PEP)

Inflate the endotracheal or tracheal tube cuff. Measurement is as in NIP, but the measurement device is adapted to allow the patient to inhale but not exhale. The patient is instructed to exhale forcefully against the closed system. The best effort, in this case the most positive number, is recorded in 20 seconds.

$$PEP\ threshold = \geq30\ cm\ H_2O$$

SPONTANEOUS TIDAL VOLUME (V_tsp)

Attach a respirometer or other volume-measuring device to the expiratory side of a two-way valve and instruct the patient to breathe normally for 1 minute. Average V_t is calculated by dividing the patient's spontaneous RR into the minute ventilation. This measurement may also be done with the patient on the ventilator at a CPAP level of zero. Observe the digital tidal volume readout to determine the average V_t.

$$V_tsp\ threshold = 5\ ml/kg$$

VITAL CAPACITY (VC)

Obtained by using the same equipment as with V_tsp (or on the ventilator as described), but the technique is markedly different and difficult to perform on the intubated patient. The patient must be able to understand and follow the instructions. First, ask the patient to inhale maximally before the measurement device is attached. Once the device is attached, the patient is asked to exhale maximally and forcefully. The maneuver is usually attempted more than once and the patient is allowed to rest between attempts. Record the best effort.

$$VC\ threshold = \geq15\ ml/kg$$

MINUTE VENTILATION ($\dot{V}_E$)

Minute ventilation is obtained by multiplying RR times V_t. It may be measured manually (after 1 minute of spontaneous breathing) using a respirometer (as described for V_tsp). More commonly, the exhaled minute ventilation (also known as minute volume) may be observed on the ventilator displays.

$$\dot{V}_E threshold = 5 - 10\ L/min$$

From reference 18a.

positive predictors.[68,69] In fact, only the negative inspiratory pressure (NIP) measurement is non–effort-dependent; studies have demonstrated that it is highly variable, dependent on technique.[106] However, the traditional indexes may be useful as negative predictors; a poor value, especially of the NIP, is associated with inability to wean successfully.

Because of the poor positive predictive value of the traditional weaning indexes, investigators have developed other indexes integrating additional variables.* An example is the index of rapid, shallow breathing (Box 20-7).[107] Unfortunately, the index has not proven to be predictive in many cases and is sporadically used.[62] Regardless, the ratio does represent a pattern of breathing that may indicate respiratory muscle fatigue (i.e., rapid, shallow breathing) and subsequently unsuccessful weaning trials.[99,100] The information may be effectively used as part of a more comprehensive assessment.

Perhaps the best approach to ensure that the patient is physiologically and psychologically ready to begin weaning trials is to assess both pulmonary and nonpulmonary factors regularly. An example of an assessment tool that has been designed to accomplish this goal is the Burns Weaning Assessment Program (BWAP) (Box 20-8). The BWAP, which consists of a bedside checklist and a PDA application, is designed to prompt the clinician to systematically assess factors important to weaning[60] and to encourage interventions to improve them. In addition, the BWAP score may be used to track progress, or lack thereof, and to determine the level of weaning readiness.[15,17]

Box 20-7

Rapid Shallow Breathing Ratio*

To calculate the rapid shallow breathing ratio, divide spontaneous respiratory fx in 1 minute by tidal volume (V_t) in liters:

$$\text{Threshold} < 105 = \text{weaning success}$$
$$> 105 = \text{weaning failure}$$

*Also known as frequency to tidal volume (fx/V_t) ratio.

◆ Case Study 20-2

Weaning

T.G. is a 55-year-old woman admitted to the thoracic ICU for a coronary artery bypass graft. Her medical history is significant for smoking and type 2 diabetes mellitus (DM). Although her postoperative course is uneventful, attempts

---

*References 15, 75, 78, 89, 90, 107.

at weaning are unsuccessful, and she is transferred to the medical intensive care unit (MICU) for weaning on hospital day 5.

T.G.'s ventilator settings on transfer are as follows: mode = A/C, Fio_2 = 0.4, V_t = 600 ml (she weighs 40 kg), fx = 20 breaths/min (total rate is 30), T_i = 1 sec, sensitivity = −2 cm H_2O, and PEEP = 5 cm H_2O. ABG results are the following: pH = 7.33, $Paco_2$ = 50 mm Hg, and Pao_2 = 90 mm Hg.

The multidisciplinary team evaluates T.G. using the BWAP and recognizes that a number of factors are present that may impede T.G.'s weaning progress. They include hematocrit of 22%, overhydration (weight is up 5 kg), tachypnea, wheezing, and anxiety. A chest x-ray demonstrates the presence of bilateral pleural effusions and pulmonary edema. Auto-PEEP is measured at 10 cm H_2O and is being exacerbated by the large V_t and the high RR on the A/C mode.

Decision point: How should these issues be addressed?

Decision point: Is she ready for extubation or is additional information needed?

The effects of sedation (sedation infusions) on weaning outcomes have recently been clarified and point to the importance of assessing sedation requirements routinely.[13,60] In two randomized controlled trials by Brook et al.[13] and Kress et al.,[60] a nurse-managed algorithm for sedation management and a protocol for daily interruption of sedative infusions, respectively, resulted in shorter ventilator duration and LOS. Both trials suggested that the use of intermittent bolus sedation may obviate the need for sedation by infusion. A follow-up study to the Kress project was done to determine if the abrupt discontinuance of the sedation infusion resulted in negative psychological outcomes for the patients.[61] Interestingly, patients assigned to the sedative interruption group were less likely to have symptoms of posttraumatic stress disorder than the control group. The studies suggest that the rapid removal of the sedatives is both psychologically and clinically beneficial and should be incorporated into the weaning assessment and plan. The use of intermittent bolus sedative administration is suggested to decrease the potential use of infusions of the agents.

RESPIRATORY MUSCLE FATIGUE, REST, WORK, AND CONDITIONING

Respiratory muscles, like all muscles, fatigue, and once fatigued 12 to 24 hours are required to recuperate.[6] When the muscles are required to work to excess, mitochondrial stores deplete, the muscles do not contract optimally, and

Box 20-8

Burns Weaning Assessment Program (BWAP)*

Patient_____

Yes	No	N/A	

GENERAL ASSESSMENT

1. Hemodynamically stable (pulse rate, cardiac output)?
2. Free from factors that increase or decrease metabolic rate (seizures, fever, sepsis, bacteremia, hypo/hyperthyroid)?
3. Hematocrit >25% (or baseline)?
4. Systemically hydrated (weight at or near baseline, balanced intake and output)?
5. Nourished (albumin >2.5 g/dl, parenteral/enteral feedings maximized)? (If albumin is low and anasarca or third spacing is present, score for hydration should be No.)
6. Electrolytes within normal limits (including Ca^{++}, Mg^+, PO_4)? (Correct Ca^{++} concentration for albumin level.)
7. Pain controlled (subjective determination)?
8. Adequate sleep/rest (subjective determination)?
9. Appropriate level of anxiety and nervousness (subjective determination)?
10. Absence of bowel problems (diarrhea, constipation, ileus)?
11. Improved general body strength/endurance (i.e., out of bed in chair, progressive activity program)?
12. Chest roentgenograph improving?

RESPIRATORY ASSESSMENT

Gas Flow and Work of Breathing

13. Eupneic respiratory rate and pattern (spontaneous respiratory rate <25 breaths/min, without dyspnea, absence of accessory muscle use)? (*This is assessed off the ventilator while measuring #20–23.)
14. Absence of adventitious breath sounds (rhonchi, rales, wheezing)?
15. Secretions thin and minimal?
16. Absence of neuromuscular disease/deformity?
17. Absence of abdominal distention/obesity/ascites?
18. Oral endotracheal tube ≥7.5 mm ID or trach ≥6.5 mm/ID?

Airway Clearance

19. Cough and swallow reflexes adequate?

Strength

20. Negative inspiratory pressure less than or equal to 20 cm H_2O?
21. Positive expiratory pressure greater than +30 cm H_2O?

Endurance

22. Spontaneous tidal volume >5 ml/kg?
23. Vital capacity >10–15 ml/kg?

Arterial Blood Gases

24. pH between 7.30 and 7.45?
25. $Paco_2$ approximately 40 mm Hg (or baseline) with minute ventilation <10 L/min (evaluated while on ventilator)?
26. Pao_2 >60 mm Hg on Fio_2 <40%?

From Burns, S. M., Fahey, S. A., Barton, D. M., Slack, D. (1991). Weaning form mechanical ventilation: a method for assessment and planning. *AACN Clin Issues, 2,* 372-387.
*To score the BWAP: divide the number of "yes" responses by 26.
N/A = Not assessed.

hypercarbic respiratory failure ensues.[6,20] Dyspnea, rapid shallow breathing, and chest abdominal asynchrony appear to be compensatory signs heralding fatigue and should be heeded.[6,20] To that end, decreasing the workload is essential; mechanical ventilation in these cases is life-saving. However, the method of applying mechanical ventilation to ensure respiratory muscle rest is dependent on the mode and application of ventilation.

Studies by Marini et al. have demonstrated that for muscle work to cease while ventilated, patient effort must cease.[72] For example, consider the case of a patient on a volume mode of ventilation. If the patient on the AC mode of ventilation initiates breaths between the set (i.e., control) breaths, the patient's respiratory muscles will continue to work throughout the machine-delivered patient-initiated breaths. To ensure respiratory muscle rest with volume ventilation, patient effort must be eliminated. Often, increasing the set rate to eliminate spontaneous effort or the judicious use of sedatives accomplishes this goal.

With a spontaneous mode of pressure ventilation such as PSV, off-loading of muscles may occur with an increase in the PSV level.[10] With this mode, absence of accessory muscle use, eupneic breathing pattern, and a spontaneous respiratory rate less than 20 breaths/min are signs of decreased workload.

Closely related to the concepts of respiratory muscle work and rest are those of conditioning and deconditioning. It is known that respiratory muscles can become deconditioned and in some cases may atrophy. This is especially true if paralytic agents, steroids, or high levels of sedation are used. Though possible under these conditions, it is indeed rare that a patient does not work at all while on the ventilator. Studies suggest that the type of muscle work (endurance or strengthening) may dictate the application of conditioning regimens.[65,67]

In weight lifting, *strength conditioning* works muscles to extreme, indeed to fatigue. The muscle fibers sustain small muscle tears, and lactic acid production is expected. The fatigued muscles are then rested for more than 24 hours to optimize the training effect. In the ventilated patient, modes and methods that require high-pressure, low-volume work most closely simulate such conditioning. CPAP, t-piece, or "blow-by" are examples of modes and methods that provide this type of work.[65,67]

Endurance conditioning requires that the workload be gradually increased over time. The muscle work is increased slowly and steadily as endurance increases. A form of ventilatory endurance conditioning is PSV, which can be gradually decreased as the patient assumes more and more of the workload. The mode, used in this manner, provides high-volume, low-pressure work.[65,67]

These concepts, borrowed from the discipline of exercise physiology, are useful. However, the specifics related to how long training intervals should be, how fast to progress them, and what type of conditioning is best are yet to be determined. Studies exploring the superiority of weaning modes and methods (described below) suggest that short-duration CPAP or t-piece trials (1 hour, once per day) followed by rest

may be a superior method. These methods are discussed in the next section on modes and methods of weaning.

MODES AND METHODS

Recent studies suggest that protocols for weaning are essential to attain positive outcomes.[22,37,68] In addition, the use of a "wean screen" is an integral component because it ensures early testing of readiness. While most of the studies used spontaneous breathing modes such as CPAP or t-piece for the trials, others used PSV, and still others used volume modes such as IMV.[12,37,40,59,104] It is as yet unclear that any one mode is better than the other for weaning; however, how they are used does make a difference. The point is to construct the protocol so that a wean trial is attempted as soon as the patient is "ready" as identified by wean screen criteria. Protocol components include the wean screen, the trial mode or method, criteria defining wean trial intolerance, and how to rest the patient between trials (Box 20-9).[12,37,40,59] The components of weaning protocols follow.

COMPONENTS OF WEANING PROTOCOLS

Criteria for Entry ("Wean Screen")

The "wean screen" consists of physiologic criteria that suggest patient stability and readiness to begin a weaning trial. A minimum of criteria are selected (e.g., FiO_2, PEEP levels, $\dot{V}_E$, hemodynamic status, secretions). Patients who have been ventilated for a long time are generally more debilitated than those ventilated short-term. In these patients, the use of a more comprehensive assessment tool (e.g., the BWAP) may be helpful.

Weaning Trial Protocol. Weaning trials vary by method, and duration is dependent on many factors. For example, patients with tracheostomies may use a tracheostomy collar and have longer trials of spontaneous breathing than those with endotracheal tubes (ETTs). The end point of a trial with an ETT is extubation, whereas the goal with a tracheostomy trial may be extension of the spontaneous breathing interval.

Evidence suggests that long-duration spontaneous breathing trials are not necessary in the majority of patients (except as noted previously with the tracheostomy patient who requires very prolonged ventilator duration). In a follow-up study, Esteban et al., using spontaneous breathing trials of 2-hour duration, demonstrated that a 30-minute to 1-hour spontaneous

Box 20-9

Example of a Weaning Protocol

Weaning Trial Screen: Assessed Daily

1. Hemodynamic stability (no dysrhythmias, heart rate [HR] $\leq$120 beats/min, absence of vaso-pressors—low-dose dopamine and dobutamine are exceptions).
2. FiO_2 $\leq$50%.
3. Positive end-expiratory pressure $\leq$8 cm H_2O.
4. BWAP >45% (in patients ventilated less than 3 days, a BWAP assessment is not necessary).
5. *If the patient meets all these criteria, a **weaning trial protocol** is initiated following discussion with the multidisciplinary team.*

Weaning Trial Protocol: Continuous Positive Airway Pressure (CPAP) (1 Trial, 1-hr Duration)

1. One trial of CPAP is attempted daily. The trial may last *no more than* 1 hour total unless previously negotiated with healthcare team.
2. With any signs of intolerance (see definition below), the trial is discontinued and the patient is returned to a resting mode until the next trial.
3. When the complete trial is sustained without signs of intolerance, the team is approached and extubation is discussed.
4. Full respiratory muscle rest is provided between trials and at night.

Or

Weaning Trial Protocol: Pressure Support Ventilation (PSV) (2 Trials, 4-hr Duration)

1. Start at PSV_{max} level (level to attain RR $\leq$20 breaths/min with V_t of 8–10 ml/kg).
2. Decrease PSV by 5 cm H_2O.

3. If no signs of intolerance are evident during the first 4-hour trial, the PSV is decreased by another 5 cm H_2O for the second trial.
4. With any signs of intolerance during trials, the patient is returned to previous level for the next 4-hour trial.
5. If unable to tolerate, the patient is fully rested until the next day, when the process begins again.
6. Once the patient is able to sustain 5–6 cm PSV without signs of intolerance (for 4 hr), the team is approached and extubation is discussed.

Intolerance for Either Protocol Is Defined as Any of the Following (3–5 min Sustained)

1. RR $\geq$35 breaths/min for 5 min.
2. O_2 saturation $\leq$90% or a decrease of 4%.
3. HR $\geq$140 beats/min or a 20% sustained change of HR in either direction.
4. Systolic BP $\geq$180 and $\leq$90 mm Hg.
5. Excessive anxiety or agitation.
6. Diaphoresis.

Rest for Either Protocol

1. PSV_{max}: PSV_{max} is that pressure level required to attain an RR of 20 breaths/min or less and a V_t of 8–10 ml/kg. Respiratory pattern should be synchronous, and there should be no accessory muscle use.
2. Other modes: With volume modes such as assist control (A/C) or intermittent mandatory ventilation (IMV), respiratory muscle rest is not ensured unless there is cessation of respiratory muscle activity. Therefore rest is considered that level of support required to prevent patient-initiated breaths. When IMV is used, PSV may be added for protection (i.e., as "safety"). Regardless, the goal is cessation of spontaneous effort.

Adapted from University of Virginia Health System MICU weaning protocol. (© 2002 by the Rector and Board of Visitors of the University of Virginia).

breathing trial was as effective in determining weaning trial outcome as the longer trials.[41] The authors noted that signs of fatigue (e.g., intolerance) generally appear within the first 0.5 hour, and additional time at that workload may be counterproductive. CPAP and t-piece both employ high-pressure, low-volume work. As described earlier, short-duration trials with full rest between attempts may optimize the training effect.

When PSV is used, the PSV level is gradually decreased and the trials are gradually lengthened. Extubation is attempted once the lowest desired PSV level is reached. PSV is an especially good mode option for endurance conditioning. Examples of patients who may be good candidates for this mode include those who are profoundly weak and those with poor cardiac

reserves. In patients with cardiac problems (e.g., CHF), the rapid removal of positive pressure results in an increase in venous return that may overwhelm the heart's ability to compensate.[64,92] Attention to preload and afterload reduction in these patients is the key to good outcomes. Gradual reductions of PSV may be better tolerated than the more dramatic spontaneous trials with CPAP or t-piece.

Combined modes (e.g., IMV with PSV) for weaning trials, at least in one study, were found to prolong the duration of weaning.[39] To date, no studies have been done to test the validity of this finding; it may be that the use of combined modes may simply add unintended variability to the weaning process. Decisions about how to decrease either the PSV or the IMV tend to be somewhat arbitrary and based on clinician preference. Further, the plan tends to be less aggressive than when a protocol using CPAP is used, and clear intolerance thresholds for the combination modes are difficult to identify. If the combined modes are used, it is important to carefully construct the protocol so that the patient is advanced as aggressively as possible.

Signs of Intolerance and How to Rest. For protocols to be easily interpreted and implemented effectively, intolerance must be defined so that a weaning trial is not continued inappropriately. As discussed in the section on respiratory muscle fatigue, signs of impending failure include tachypnea, dyspnea, and chest-abdomen asynchrony. However, other signs of stress also emerge (e.g., diaphoresis, tachycardia, and blood pressure changes). The protocol not only defines the criteria for stopping a trial but also describes how to rest the patient. Refer to the content on rest described earlier and Box 20-9 for an example of a weaning protocol that includes all these components.

Timing of Tracheostomy and Weaning Trials

In a study by Rumbak et al., 120 patients projected to require mechanical ventilation for greater than 14 days were randomly assigned to percutaneous tracheostomy within 48 hours.[86] Mortality, incidence of pneumonia, and accidental extubations were all statistically significantly improved in the early tracheostomy group compared to the controls. They also had shorter critical care LOS, shorter ventilator duration, and less damage to the mouth and larynx.[86] It is unclear from the results of the study, however, whether the more expedient weaning may have resulted from less reliance on sedation in those with tracheostomies versus those without. Before the Rumbak study, tracheostomy was often only considered after 10 to 12 days (or longer) had elapsed. Exceptions included those conditions in which the need for a tracheostomy was obvious (e.g., spinal cord injury, trauma). While this early

timing (e.g., 48 hours) is unlikely to enjoy widespread application, at a minimum, tracheostomy should be considered earlier in the course of mechanical ventilation than has traditionally been the case.

Weaning with a tracheostomy tube in place affords an element of safety not possible with an ETT. Because the goal is not extubation but rather spontaneous breathing for at least 24 hours, the trials can be more aggressive (e.g., longer). However, in very difficult cases, trials are best progressed gradually while other rehabilitation plans are also activated (e.g., physical mobility). Often a plan incorporating daytime trials, with nighttime rest on the ventilator, works well. Progression to spontaneous breathing during the night is accomplished once daytime goals are attained. Concepts of respiratory muscle rest, work, and fatigue apply as does the need for systematic assessment (and correction) of impediments.

Multidisciplinary Plan of Care

System initiatives are programs incorporating many evidence-based elements of care into a formalized approach. These models vary in scope and design, but the common focus is a systematic, progressive approach to weaning, decreasing variation in the process. In many models, evidence-based clinical pathways are used to clarify when to initiate selected care elements (see the Nutrition box below), mobility, prophylaxis (e.g., gastrointestinal bleeding, deep vein thrombosis, sinusitis), weaning trials, and other aspects of care that affect weaning (e.g., glucose control and sedation management).[13,18,60,94,103] Importantly, clinicians (often advanced practice nurses) are identified to manage the process, coordinate the multidisciplinary approach, and monitor the outcomes.[16,18] To date these multidisciplinary approaches have resulted in positive clinical and financial outcomes and are to be encouraged. However, it is clear that few processes of care are successful unless sustained attention to monitoring and managing the processes of care are ensured.[16,18,38]

Managing the ventilated patient is complex and requires an in-depth understanding of the modes and

---

♠ NUTRITION

Nutritional Concerns in the Mechanically Ventilated Patient

CALORIC REQUIREMENTS

- Each patient's calorie needs should be individualized based on previous nutritional status and current medical condition.

- Estimated patient calorie needs:
  - Patients with severe malnutrition/refeeding risk require approximately 15–25 kcal/kg.
  - Most patients require between 25 and 35 kcal/kg.
  - Patients with mild stress or surgery require 25–30 kcal/kg.

- Patients with moderate to severe stress require 30–35 kcal/kg.
- Patients in the rehabilitation phase of illness with increased physical activity require 35–45 kcal/kg (or more).

PROTEIN REQUIREMENTS

- Each patient's protein needs should be individualized based on previous nutritional status and current medical condition.
- Patients with mild to moderate stress require 1.2–1.3 g/kg (of body weight).
- Patients with moderate to severe stress need 1.4–1.5 g/kg.
- Patients with severe stress and wound healing require 1.6–2 g/kg.
- Hemodialysis patients require 1.4–1.8 g/kg.
- Peritoneal dialysis patients require 1.4–1.8 g/kg.
- Continuous renal replacement therapy patients require 1.5–2.5 g/kg.
- Patients with hepatic coma/severe encephalopathy need 1–1.2 g/kg.
- Patients in the rehabilitative phase require 1.2–1.5 g/kg.

CARBOHYDRATE REQUIREMENTS

- Amount of carbohydrates should not exceed the physiologic capacity for carbohydrate oxidation (7 g/kg [5 mg/kg/min] of body weight).
- Carbohydrates should compose 40% to 60% of total calories.
- Consider hidden sources of carbohydrates (e.g., 5% dextrose in IVs, dextrose in dialysate).

FAT REQUIREMENTS

- Limit fat intake to 1.5 g/kg of body weight.
- Fats should compose 20% to 40% of total calories.

- Fat should provide 4% of total fat calories to prevent essential fatty acid deficiency.
- Consider fat sources in medications (e.g., Diprivan is delivered in 10% lipid emulsion).
- Monitor serum triglycerides in patients on IV lipids or Diprivan if patient has a history of dyslipidemia.

ELECTROLYTES

- Maintain normal serum phosphorus levels.
- Maintain glucose level at or below 110 mg/dl.
- Monitor patient's arterial Pa_{CO_2}. Increase in levels *may* be caused by increased CO_2 production secondary to overfeeding—expect other causes first, however.

SPECIAL CONSIDERATIONS

- Gastric feeding is the preferred route for nutrition.
- Institute feedings within 72 hours of mechanical ventilation.
- Percutaneous endoscopic gastrostomy (PEG) is recommended for patients requiring enteral feeding for longer than 4–6 weeks.
- Attempt to prevent aspiration during gastric feeding with the mechanical ventilated patient:
  - Elevate head of bed 30–40 degrees.
  - Provide oral care.
  - Decrease use of narcotics.
  - Verify feeding tube placement.
  - Assess GI tolerance (e.g., abdominal distention, fullness, discomfort, vomiting).
  - Assess for excessive residual volumes.
- Parenteral nutrition should be reserved for patients with nonfunctional or inaccessible gastrointestinal tract resulting from intestinal hemorrhage, acute abdominal condition, ileus, bowel obstruction, or pancreatitis who are not tolerating jejunal feeding and are experiencing moderate to severe malnutrition.

From reference 79a.

methods in addition to the evidence that guides application. Further, collaboration among the many disciplines caring for aspects of the patients' well-being is necessary if outcomes are to be positive.

CONCLUSIONS

Caring for the mechanically ventilated patient requires that the clinician understand the pathophysiology of pulmonary conditions that necessitate the therapy as well as how to monitor and intervene when appropriate. Knowledge of ventilator parameters and modes, in conjunction with the use of respiratory

waveform monitoring, is essential if application is to produce favorable outcomes from the acute to the weaning stages of ventilation.

REFERENCES

1. Afessa, B., Hogans, L., & Murphy, R. (1999). Predicting 3-day and 7-day outcomes of weaning from mechanical ventilation. *Chest, 116,* 456–461.
2. Amato, M. B. P., et al. (1995). Beneficial effects of the "open lung approach" with low distending pressures in acute respiratory distress syndrome. *Am J Respir Crit Care Med, 152,* 1835–1846.
3. Amato, M. B. P., et al. (1998). Effect of protective ventilation strategies on mortality in the acute respiratory distress syndrome. *N Engl J Med, 338,* 347–354.

4. Banner, M. J., Blanch, P. B., & Kirby, R. R. (1993). Imposed work of breathing and methods of triggering a demand-flow continuous positive airway system. *Crit Care Med, 21,* 183–190.

5. Bear Medical Systems (Palm Springs, Calif). www.bearmedical. com/Bear/Default.htm.

6. Bellemare, F., & Grassiino, A. (1982). Evaluation of human diaphragm fatigue. *J Appl Physiol, 53,* 1196–1206.

7. Bellomo, R., et al. (1994). Asthma requiring mechanical ventilation: a low morbidity approach. *Chest, 105,* 891–896.

8. Beydon, L., et al. (1988). Inspiratory work of breathing during spontaneous ventilation using demand values and continuous flow systems. *Am Rev Respir Dis, 138,* 300–304.

9. Bidani, A., et al. (1994). Permissive hypercapnia in acute respiratory failure. *JAMA, 272,* 957–962.

10. Brochard, L., Pluskwa, F., & Lemaire, F. (1987). Improved efficacy of spontaneous breathing with inspiratory pressure support. *Am Rev Respir Dis, 136,* 411–415.

11. Brochard, L., et al. (1989). Inspiratory pressure support prevents diaphragmatic fatigue during weaning from mechanical ventilation. *Am Rev Respir Dis, 139,* 513–521.

12. Brochard, L., et al. (1994). Comparison of three methods of gradual ventilatory support during weaning from mechanical ventilation. *Am J Respir Crit Care Med, 150,* 896–903.

13. Brook, A. D., et al. (1999). Effect of a nursing-implemented sedation protocol on the duration of mechanical ventilation. *Crit Care Med, 27,* 2609–2615.

14. Burns, S. M., et al. (1995). Weaning from long-term mechanical ventilation. *Am J Crit Care, 4,* 4–22.

15. Burns, S. M., Burns, J. E., & Truwit, J. D. (1994). Comparison of five clinical weaning indices. *Am J Crit Care, 3,* 342–352.

16. Burns, S. M., et al. (1998). Design, testing, and results of an outcomes-managed approach to patients requiring prolonged mechanical ventilation. *Am J Crit Care, 7,* 45–57.

17. Burns, S. M., Ryan, B., & Burns, J. E. (2000). The weaning continuum: use of APACHE III, BWAP, TISS, and WI scores to establish stages of weaning. *Crit Care Med, 28,* 2259–2267.

18. Burns, S. M., et al. (2003). Implementation of an institutional program to improve clinical and financial outcomes of patients requiring mechanical ventilation: one year outcomes and lessons learned. *Crit Care Med, 31,* 2752–2763.

18a. Burns, S. M. (2007). AACN protocols for practice: Care of mechanically ventilated patients, (2nd ed). Boston: Jones and Bartlett.

19. Cohen, I. L., et al. (1991). Reduction of duration and cost of mechanical ventilation in an intensive care unit by use of a ventilatory management team. *Crit Care Med, 19,* 1278–1284.

20. Cohen, C. A., et al. (1982). Clinical manifestations of inspiratory muscle fatigue. *Am J Med, 73,* 308–316.

21. Combes, A., et al. (2003). Morbidity, mortality, and quality-of-life outcomes of patients requring ≥14 days of mechanical ventilation. *Crit Care Med, 31,* 1373–1381.

22. Cook, D. (Nov 1999). *Evidence report on criteria for weaning from mechanical ventilation.* Contract No. 290-97-0017. Rockville, Md: Agency for Health Care Policy and Research.

23. Craven, D., et al. (1986). Risk factors for pneumonia and fatality in patients receiving mechanical ventilation. *Am Rev Respir Dis, 133,* 792–796.

24. Darioli, R., & Perret, C. (1984). Mechanical controlled hypoventilation in status asthmaticus. *Am Rev Respir Dis, 129,* 385–387.

25. Davis, K., et al. (1996). Comparison of volume control and pressure control ventilation: is flow waveform the difference? *J Trauma, 41,* 808–814.

26. De Jonghe, B., et al. (1998). Acquired neuromuscular disorders in critically ill patients: a systematic review. *Intensive Care Med, 24,* 1242–1250.

27. Derdak, S., et al. (2002). High-frequency oscillatory ventilation for acute respiratory distress syndrome in adults. *Am J Respir Crit Care Med, 166,* 801–808.

28. Douglas, S. L., et al. (1997). Outcomes of long-term ventilator patients: a descriptive study. *Am J Crit Care, 6,* 99–105.

29. Douglas, S. L., et al. (2002). Survival and quality of life: short-term versus long-term ventilator patients. *Crit Care Med, 30,* 2655–2662.

30. Douglas, P. S., et al. (1987). DRG payment for long term ventilator dependent patients: implications and recommendations. *Chest, 91,* 413–417.

31. Dreyfuss, D., et al. (1985). Intermittent positive-end expiratory pressure hyperventilation with high inflation pressures produces pulmonary microvascular injury in rats. *Am Rev Respir Dis, 132,* 880–884.

32. Dreyfus, D., et al. (1988). High inflation pressure pulmonary edema: respective effects of high airway pressure, high tidal volume, and positive end-expiratory pressure. *Am Rev Respir Dis, 137,* 1159–1164.

33. Dreyfuss, D., & Saumon, G. (1993). The role of tidal volume, FRC and end-inspiratory volume in the development of pulmonary edema following mechanical ventilation. *Am Rev Respir Dis, 148,* 1194–1203.

34. Dreyfus, D., & Saumon, G. (1998). Ventilator induced lung injury. *Am J Respir Crit Care Med, 157,* 294–323.

35. Durante, G., et al. (2002). ARDS Net lower tidal volume ventilatory strategy may generate intrinsic positive end-expiratory pressure in patients with acute respiratory distress syndrome. *Am J Respir Crit Care Med, 165,* 1271–1274.

36. Elpern, E. H., et al. (1991). The non-invasive respiratory care unit: patterns of use and financial implications. *Chest, 99,* 205–208.

37. Ely, E. W. (1996). Effect on the duration of mechanical ventilation of identifying patients capable of breathing spontaneously. *N Engl J Med, 335,* 1864–1869.

38. Ely, E. W., et al. (1999). Large scale implementation of a respiratory therapist-driven protocol for ventilator weaning. *Am J Respir Crit Care Med, 159,* 439–446.

39. Esteban, A., et al. (1994). Modes of mechanical ventilation and weaning: a national survey of Spanish hospitals. *Chest, 106,* 1188–1193.

40. Esteban, A. (1995). A comparison of four methods of weaning patients from mechanical ventilation. *N Engl J Med, 332,* 345–350.

41. Esteban, A., et al. (1999). Effect of spontaneous breathing trial duration on outcome of attempts to discontinue mechanical ventilation. *Am J Respir Crit Care Med, 159,* 512–518.

42. Fagon, J., et al. (1989). Nosocomial pneumonia in patients receiving continuous mechanical ventilation. *Am Rev Respir Dis, 139,* 877–884.

43. Fiastro, J. F., Habib, M. P., & Quan, S. F. (1988). Pressure support compensation for inspiratory work due to endotracheal tubes and demand continuous positive airway pressure. *Chest, 93,* 499–505.

44. Foti, G., et al. (2000). Effects of periodic lung recruitment maneuvers on gas exchange and respiratory mechanics in mechanically ventilated acute respiratory distress syndrome (ARDS) patients. *Intensive Care Med, 26*(5), 501–507.

45. Fu, Z., et al. (1992). High lung volume increases stress failure in pulmonary capillaries. *J Appl Physiol, 73,* 123–133.

46. Fujino, Y., et al. (2001). Repetitive high-pressure recruitment maneuvers required to maximally recruit lung in a sheep model of acute respiratory distress syndrome. *Crit Care Med, 29*(8), 1579–1586.

47. Gattinoni, L., et al. (1986). Adult respiratory distress syndrome profiles by computed tomography. *J Thorac Imaging, 1,* 25–30.

48. Gattinoni, L., et al. (1987). Pressure volume curve of total respiratory system in acute respiratory failure: computed tomographic scan study. *Am Rev Respir Dis, 136*, 730–736.

49. Gattinoni, L., et al. (1991). Body position changes redistribute lung computertomographic density in patients with acute respiratory failure. *Anesthesiology, 74*, 15–25.

50. Gattinoni, L., et al. (2001). Effect of prone positioning on the survival of patients with acute respiratory failure. *N Engl J Med, 345*, 568–573.

51. Gibney, N. R. T., Wilson, R. S., & Pontoppidan, H. (1982). Comparison of work of breathing on high gas flow and demand valve continuous positive airway pressure systems. *Chest, 82*, 692–695.

52. Goodnough-Hanneman, S. K., et al. (1994). Weaning from short-term mechanical ventilation: a review. *Am J Crit Care, 3*, 421–443.

53. Grap, M. J., et al. (2003). Collaborative practice: development, implementation and evaluation of a weaning protocol for patients receiving mechanical ventilation. *Am J Crit Care, 12*, 454–460.

54. Henneman, E., et al. (2001). Effect of a collaborative weaning plan on patient outcome in the critical care setting. *Crit Care Med, 29*, 297–303.

55. Henneman, E., et al. (2002). Using a collaborative weaning plan to decrease duration of mechanical ventilation and length of stay in the intensive care unit for patients receiving long-term mechanical ventilation. *Am J Crit Care, 11*, 132–140.

56. Hickling, K. G., Henderson, S. J., & Jackson, R. (1990). Low mortality associated with low volume pressure-limited ventilation with permissive hypercapnia in severe adult respiratory distress syndrome. *Intensive Care Med, 16*, 372–377.

57. Hickling, K. (1992). Low volume ventilation with permissive hypercapnia in the adult respiratory distress syndrome. *Clin Intensive Care, 3*, 67–78.

58. Hoo, G. W. S., & Park, L. (2002). Variations in the measurement of weaning parameters: a survey of respiratory therapists. *Chest 121*, 1947–1955.

59. Kollef, M. H., et al. (1997). A randomized, controlled trial of protocol-directed versus physician-directed weaning from mechanical ventilation. *Crit Care Med, 25*, 567–574.

60. Kress, J. P., et al. (2000). Daily interruption of sedative infusions in critically ill patients undergoing mechanical ventilation. *N Engl J Med, 342*, 1471–1477.

61. Kress, J. P., et al. (2003). The long-term psychological effects of daily sedative interruption on critically ill patients. *Am J Respir Crit Care Med, 168*, 1457–1461.

62. Krieger, B. P., et al. (1997). Serial measurements of the rapid-shallow-breathing index as a predictor of weaning outcome in elderly medical patients. *Chest, 112*(4), 1029–1034.

63. Lachmann, B. (1992). Open up the lung and keep the lung open. *Intensive Care Med, 18*, 319–321.

64. Lemaire, F., et al. (1988). Acute left ventricular dysfunction during unsuccessful weaning from mechanical ventilation. *Anesthesiology, 69*, 171–179.

65. MacIntyre, N. R. (1986). Respiratory function during pressure support ventilation. *Chest, 89*, 677–683.

66. MacIntyre, N. R., Cheng, K.-C. G., & McConnell, R. (1997). Applied PEEP during pressure support reduces the inspiratory threshold load of intrinsic PEEP. *Chest, 111*, 188–193.

67. MacIntyre, N. R. (1988). Weaning from mechanical ventilatory support: volume-assisting intermittent breaths versus pressure-assisting every breath. *Respir Care, 83*, 1121–1225.

68. MacIntyre, N. R., et al. (2001). Evidence-based guidelines for weaning and discontinuing ventilatory support: a collective task force facilitated by the American College of Chest Physicians; the American Association for Respiratory Care; and the American College of Critical Care Medicine. *Chest, 120*(6 suppl), 375S–395S.

69. Mador, M. J. (1992). Weaning parameters: are they clinically useful? *Chest, 102*, 1642.

70. Maquet Critical Care. www.maquet.com/criticalcare.

71. Marelich, G. P., et al. (2000). Protocol weaning of mechanical ventilation in medical and surgical patients by respiratory care practitioners and nurses: effect on weaning time and incidence of ventilator associated pneumonia. *Chest, 118*, 459–467.

72. Marini, J. J., Rodriguez, M., & Lamb, V. (1986). The inspiratory workload of patient-initiated mechanical ventilation. *Am Rev Respir Dis, 134*, 902–909.

73. Marini, J. J. (2001). Recruitment maneuvers to achieve an "open lung"—whether and how? *Crit Care Med, 29*, 1647–1648.

74. Mehta, S., & Hill, N. S. (2001). Noninvasive ventilation. *Am J Respir Crit Care Med, 163*, 540–577.

75. Mensies, R., Gibbons, W., & Goldberg, P. (1989). Determinants of weaning and survival among patients with COPD who require mechanical ventilation for acute respiratory failure. *Chest, 95*, 398–405.

76. Menitove, S. M., & Golring, R. A. (1983). Combined ventilator and bicarbonate strategy in the management of status asthmaticus. *Am J Med, 74*, 889–901.

77. Messerole, E., et al. (2002). The pragmatics of prone positioning. *Am J Respir Crit Care Med, 165*, 1359–1363.

78. Morganroth, M. L., et al. (1984). Criteria for weaning from prolonged mechanical ventilation. *Arch Intern Med, 144*, 1012–1016.

79. Pappert, D., et al. (1994). Influence of positioning on ventilation-perfusion relationships in severe adult respiratory distress syndrome. *Chest, 106*, 1511–1516.

79a. Parrish, C., & Krenitsky, J. (2007). In S. M. Burns (Ed.), *AACN protocols for practice: Care of mechanically ventilated patients* (2nd ed.). Boston: Jones and Bartlett.

80. Pepe, P. E., & Marini, J. J. (1982). Occult positive end-expiratory pressure in mechanically ventilated patients with airflow obstruction. *Am Rev Respir Dis, 126*, 166–170.

81. Petrof, B. J., et al. (1990). Continuous positive airway pressure reduces work of breathing and dyspnea during weaning from mechanical ventilation in severe chronic obstructive pulmonary disease. *Am Rev Respir Dis, 141*, 281–289.

82. Puritan Bennett. www.puritanbennett.com.

83. Ranieri, V. M., et al. (1993). Physiologic effects of positive end-expiratory pressure in patients with chronic obstructive pulmonary disease during acute ventilatory failure and controlled mechanical ventilation. *Am Rev Respir Dis, 147*, 5–13.

84. Rappaport, S. H., et al. (1994). Randomized, prospective trial of pressure-limited versus volume-controlled ventilation in severe respiratory failure. *Crit Care Med, 22*, 22–32.

85. Respironics. Available at www.respironics.com.

86. Rumbak, M. J., et al. (2004). A prospective, randomized study comparing early percutaneous dilational tracheotomy to prolonged translaryngeal intubation (delayed tracheotomy) in critically ill medical patients. *Crit Care Med, 32*, 1689–1694.

87. Sahn, S. A., & Lakshminarayan, S. (1973). Bedside criteria for discontinuation of mechanical ventilation. *Chest, 63*, 1002–1005.

88. Sahn, S. A., Lakshminarayan, S., & Petty, T. L. (1976). Weaning from mechanical ventilation. *JAMA, 235*, 2208–2212.

89. Sassoon, C. S. H., et al. (1987). Airway occlusion pressure: an important indicator for successful weaning in patients with chronic obstructive pulmonary disease. *Am Rev Respir Dis, 135*, 107–113.

90. Sassoon, C. S. H., & Mahutte, C. K. (1993). Airway occlusion and breathing pattern as predictors of weaning outcome. *Am Rev Respir Dis, 143*, 860–866.

91. Scheinhorn, D. J., et al. (1997). Post-ICU mechanical ventilation: treatment of 1,123 patients at a regional weaning center. *Chest, 111*, 1654–1659.

92. Sereika, S. M., & Clochesy, J. M. (1996). Left ventricular dysfunction and duration of mechanical ventilatory support in the chronically critically ill: a survival analysis. *Heart Lung, 25*, 45–51.

93. Slutsky, A. S. (1994). Consensus conference on mechanical ventilation—January 28–30, 1993, at Northbrook, Ill. Parts 1 and 2. *Intensive Care Med, 20,* 64–79150–162. See the published erratum: *Intensive Care Med, 20,* 378.

94. Smyrnios, N. A. (2002). Effects of a multifaceted, multidisciplinary, hospital-wide quality improvement program on weaning from mechanical ventilation. *Crit Care Med, 30,* 1224–1230.

95. Stewart, T. E., et al. (1998). Evaluation of a ventilation strategy to prevent barotrauma in patients at high risk for acute respiratory distress syndrome: pressure- and volume-limited ventilation strategy group. *N Engl J Med, 338,* 355–361.

96. Tablan, O. C., et al. (2004). Guidelines for preventing health-care–associated pneumonia, Recommendations of CDC and the Healthcare Infection Control Practices Advisory Committee. *MMWR, 53*(RRO3), 1–36.

97. The Acute Respiratory Distress Syndrome Network. (2000). Ventilation with lower tidal volumes as compared with traditional tidal volumes for acute lung injury and the acute respiratory distress syndrome. *N Engl J Med, 342,* 1301–1307.

98. The ARDS Clinical Trials Network; National Heart, Lung, and and Blood Institute: National Institutes of Health. (2003). Effects of recruitment maneuvers in patients with acute lung injury and acute respiratory distress syndrome ventilated with high positive end-expiratory pressure. *Crit Care Med, 31,* 2592–2597.

99. Tobin, M. J., et al. (1986). The pattern of breathing during successful and unsuccessful trials of weaning from mechanical ventilation. *Am Rev Respir Dis, 134,* 1111–1118.

100. Tobin, M. J., et al. (1987). Konno-Mead analysis of ribcage-abdominal motion during successful and unsuccessful trials of weaning from mechanical ventilation. *Am Rev Respir Dis, 135,* 1320–1328.

101. Tremblay, L. (1997). Injurious ventilatory strategies increases cytokines and c-fos m-RNA expression in an isolated rat lung model. *J Clin Invest, 99,* 944–952.

102. Tuxen, D. (1994). Permissive hypercapina. In M. J. Tobin (Ed.), *Principles and practice of mechanical ventilation.* New York: McGraw-Hill..

103. Van den Berghe, G., et al. (2003). Outcome benefits of intensive insulin therapy in the critically ill: insulin dose versus glycemic control. *Crit Care Med, 31,* 359–366.

104. Vitacca, M., et al. (2001). Comparison of two methods for weaning COPD patients requiring mechanical ventilation for more than 15 days. *Am J Respir Crit Care Med, 164,* 225–230.

105. West, J. B. (1990). *Ventilation/blood flow and gas exchange* (5th ed.). Philadelphia: Lippincott.

106. Yang, K. L. (1992). Reproducibility of weaning parameters. A need for standardization. *Chest, 102,* 1829–1832.

107. Yang, K. L., & Tobin, M. J. (1991). A prospective study of indexes predicting the outcomes of trials of weaning from mechanical ventilation. *N Engl J Med, 324,* 1445–1450.

Jo Ann Brooks

General thoracic surgery, a subspecialty within cardiothoracic surgery, is a major growth area in cardiothoracic surgery. On a national level, adult cardiac surgery procedures are decreasing; however, the demands for general thoracic surgical procedures are increasing as a specialty as a result of lung cancer, aerodigestive cancers, and other pulmonary, esophageal, and mediastinal diseases.[50]

General thoracic surgery has a fortuitous and long history. Pulmonary resection techniques developed slowly in the late 1800s in hospitals and surgical clinics throughout the world. In 1912 the first lobectomy was performed using a new dissection technique; however, it received little attention for many years.[52] Between 1900 and 1930 surgeons began to specialize and perform resections using a variety of techniques, often with poor outcomes. By 1930 thoracic surgery had become an established specialty; surgeons throughout the world were involved in a collaborative effort that culminated in safe, one-stage thoracic resections. Before this time, multiple-stage resections were often performed unsuccessfully.[52] In 1933 the first successful one-stage pneumonectomy was performed and by mid-century it became a standard operation for lung cancer.[29]

General thoracic surgery involves the lung, pleural space, airways, mediastinum, diaphragm, and esophagus. Surgeries involving the great vessels are usually classified under cardiac or vascular procedures; however, extensive thoracic procedures may also involve the great vessels and heart. Surgeries can be classified as pulmonary, tracheobronchial, pleural, diaphragm, and chest wall. Esophageal procedures may be divided into procedures for malignancy or benign conditions. Cardiac/pericardium/great vessel procedures may include procedures such as pericardial window, pericardiectomy, or repair/reconstruction of the thoracic aorta, abdominal aorta, superior or inferior vena cava, pulmonary artery/veins, or subclavian artery.

This chapter will be divided into sections discussing general thoracic surgery topics; specific surgeries related to the lung, pleura, mediastinum, diaphragm, and chest wall; and then surgeries of the esophagus. Because general thoracic surgery is a large field, only those surgeries that are commonly performed will be discussed in detail, with other procedures receiving a brief description.

THORACIC SURGERIES
PULMONARY RESECTION
Indications

Lung cancer is the most common reason for performing lung resection; however, resective surgery may be performed for benign masses/tumors, acute or chronic infection, or congenital abnormalities.[43] In 2005 there were an estimated 172,500 new cases of cancer of the lung and bronchus (93,000 men and 79,500 women). In the same year, it was estimated that 163,500 would die from this disease.[42] For men, the incidence of lung cancer has remained relatively constant. In women, the incidence of lung cancer has begun to plateau after a continuous rise over the past 30 years.[42] Two thirds of the U.S. population with lung cancer are 65 years and older.[40] In approximately 70% of lung cancer patients, the disease has spread to regional lymphatics and other sites by the time of diagnosis; these patients are not candidates for surgical resection. Because of the large number of patients presenting with advanced disease, the long-term survival rate for lung cancer patients is low.

There are two general classifications of lung cancer: non–small cell lung cancer (NSCLC) and small cell lung cancer. NSCLC accounts for 85% of cases and small cell 15%. For the 25% to 30% of patients diagnosed with early-stage NSCLC, surgical resection is the mainstay of treatment.[64] One type of NSCLC is squamous cell carcinoma, which is usually more centrally located, arising more commonly in the segmental and subsegmental bronchi. Adenocarcinoma is the most prevalent carcinoma of the lung for both men and women; it presents more peripherally as peripheral masses or nodules and often metastasizes. Large cell carcinoma (also called undifferentiated carcinoma) is a fast-growing tumor that tends to arise peripherally. Bronchioalveolar cell cancer is found in the terminal bronchus and alveoli and is usually slower growing as compared to other bronchogenic carcinomas. Small cell lung carcinomas occur primarily as a proximal lesion or lesions, but may arise in any part of the tracheobronchial tree. Most small cell carcinomas develop in the major bronchi and spread by infiltration along the bronchial wall. Small cell carcinoma is usually a nonsurgical diagnosis and is treated with other modalities.

In addition to cell type, lung cancers are also clinically staged. The stage of an NSCLC refers to the size of the tumor, its location, whether lymph nodes are involved, and whether the cancer has spread.[2] NSCLC is staged as I to IV. Stage I is the earliest stage, with the highest cure rates, while stage IV designates metastatic spread. Estimated 5-year survival rates for the stages of NSCLC are as follows: stages IA and IB, 50%-80%; stages IIA and IIB, 30%-50%; stage IIIA, 10%-40%; stage IIIB, 5%-20%; and stage IV, less than 5%.[5] Small cell lung cancers are classified as limited or extensive.

Stages of NSCLC that may be amenable to surgical intervention include stages I through IIIA.[57] Recent data support that stage IA NSCLC should be treated with surgery alone, while higher stages may have improved survival if treated with surgical resection followed by adjuvant (following surgery) chemotherapy or radiation therapy.[36] For higher staged cancers and depending upon the stage, location, and nodal involvement, patients may benefit from neoadjuvant (before surgery) chemotherapy or radiation therapy.[57]

Diagnostic Evaluation

As part of the diagnostic workup before determination of surgical candidacy, a variety of tests may be ordered as part of the clinical staging process. Most often, the staging begins with computed tomography (CT) of the chest to further delineate nodules and masses not easily visualized on a chest radiograph and to examine the mediastinum for lymphadenopathy. Preferably, the CT is done with contrast in order to examine both the lung and soft tissue areas (e.g., lymph nodes). Flexible fiberoptic bronchoscopy is sometimes used and provides a detailed study of the tracheobronchial tree and allows for brushings, washings, and biopsies of suspicious areas. For peripheral lesions not amenable to bronchoscopic biopsy, a transthoracic fine-needle aspiration may be performed under CT guidance to aspirate cells from a nodule or mass. An endoscopy with esophageal ultrasound (EUS) may be used to obtain a transesophageal biopsy of enlarged subcarinal lymph nodes that are not easily accessible by other means.

A variety of other scans may be used to assess for metastasis of the cancer. These may include bone, abdominal, positron emission tomography (PET), and fusion CT/PET scans. PET scans are now widely used as part of the staging process. CT scanning is an anatomic imaging tool while PET is based on the biological activity of the tumor cells in response to an injection of 18-fluorodeoxyglucose.[38] Cancer cells usually demonstrate a higher glucose uptake and utilization compared with normal lung or lymphatic tissue. However, false-positive results may occur in granulomatous inflammatory diseases and in infection. CT of the head and magnetic resonance imaging procedures are used to detect central nervous system metastases.

Mediastinoscopy or mediastinotomy may be used to obtain biopsy samples from certain lymph node areas in the mediastinum. Using a general anesthetic, a cervical mediastinoscopy is done via a small 1.5- to 2-cm incision made just above the manubrium. A scope is passed into the upper mediastinal area and precarinal nodes can be biopsied. An anterior mediastinotomy (Chamberlain procedure—usually on left side) allows for assessment of nodes in the aortopulmonary window and left para-aortic area. It can be used to obtain tissue from an anterior mediastinal mass or a centrally located mass within the hilum.[43] A small incision is made usually through the bed of the second costal cartilage or at the level of the second intercostal space. Two other staging procedures are video-assisted thoracoscopic surgery (VATS) and thoracotomy. The VATS procedure will be described in more detail later, but may be used to diagnose and stage NSCLC as well as to resect specific areas. In the past, an open thoracotomy was sometimes used to stage lung cancer; however, with newer staging modalities, this more invasive procedure is not necessary for staging.

Surgical resection is the preferred method of treating patients with localized NSCLC, no evidence of metastatic spread, and adequate cardiopulmonary function. The cure rate of surgical resection depends on the type and NSCLC stage. Surgery is primarily used for NSCLC because small cell cancer of the lung grows rapidly and metastasizes early and extensively. Unfortunately, in many patients with bronchogenic cancer, the lesion is inoperable at the time of diagnosis.

Other malignant tumors of the pulmonary system that may require pulmonary resection include carcinoid and sarcoma.[43] Examples of benign lung tumors include papilloma, fibroma, leiomyoma, hamartoma, teratoma, and inflammatory pseudotumors. Diseases or problems that might require pulmonary resection are empyema, necrotizing pneumonia, other infectious processes, granulomatous disease, and bronchiectasis.

◆ Case Study 21-1, Part A

Pulmonary Resection

M.R. is a 46-year-old Caucasian male referred to the thoracic oncology clinic. He is a truck driver presenting with complaints of increasing shortness of breath and intermittent hemoptysis. He has smoked three packs of cigarettes per day for the past 31 years, has tried to cut back, and is now smoking 2 packs per day. He reports daily alcohol intake. Over the past 3 months, he has lost approximately 20 pounds. He had gone to his primary care physician: a chest x-ray was obtained demonstrating an abnormality in the right apex of the lung. A bronchoscopy was done, and biopsies and washings demonstrated NSCLC: squamous cell-moderately differentiated.

Decision point: With a mass in the right apex of the lung, what additional signs and symptoms should be evaluated?

Case continues on page 496

Preoperative Evaluation

Before making a decision regarding surgical intervention, it must be determined whether the patient is physiologically capable of tolerating resectional surgery and whether or not the lesion/mass can be completely resected. An algorithm for preoperative pulmonary evaluation is shown in Figure 21-1. Preoperative evaluation and preparation of patients for surgery involve a multidisciplinary approach. The type and complexity of the preoperative evaluation are dependent upon the patient's history, physical assessment findings, social history (e.g., smoking), and the extent of the planned surgery (amount of lung tissue to be resected or amount of expected lung compromise). Specific diagnostic tests are key in the preoperative evaluation of the patient to evaluate if the patient can tolerate the pulmonary physiologic impairment resulting from the surgery. Box 21-1 lists common diagnostic tests used to evaluate

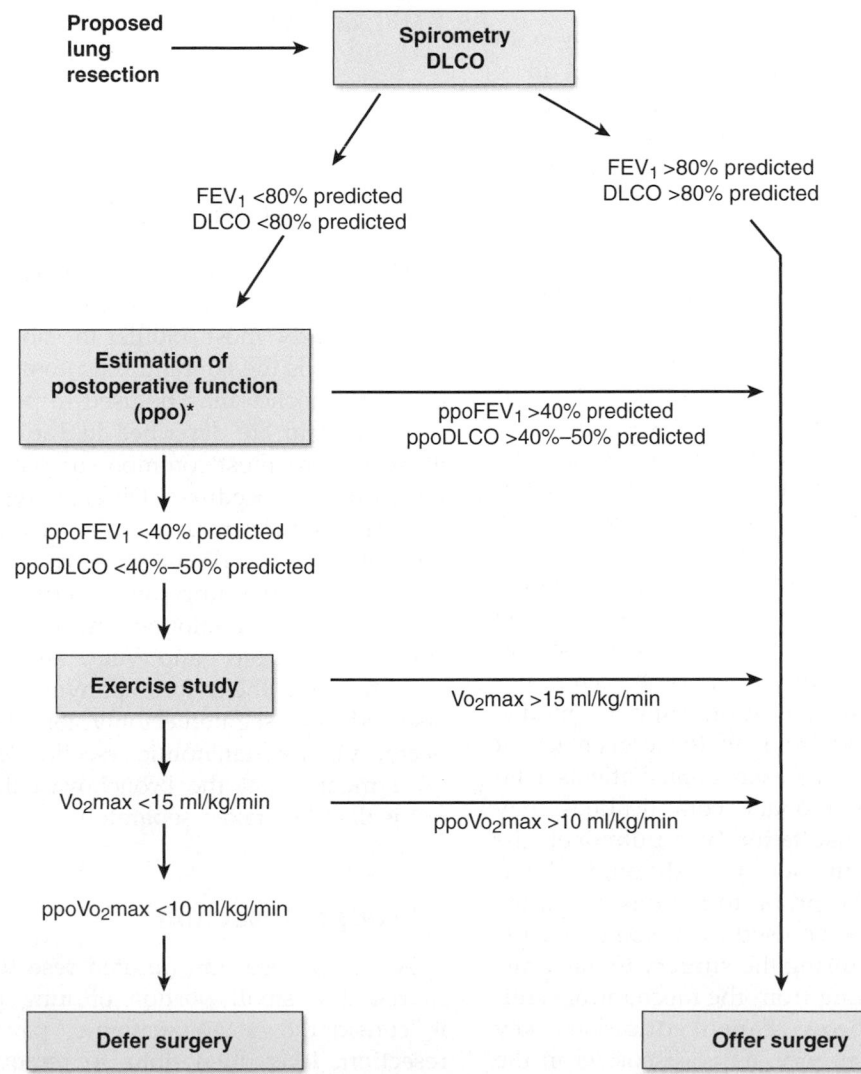

◆FIGURE 21-1 Algorithm for preoperative pulmonary evaluation. DLCO = Diffusing capacity of the lung for carbon monoxide, FEV_1 = forced expiratory volume in 1 second, ppo = predicted postoperative, Vo_2 = oxygen consumption.

Box 21-1

Common Diagnostic Tests to Evaluate Pulmonary Function and Predictors of Poor Outcome

DIAGNOSTIC TEST	PREDICTOR OF POOR OUTCOME
Basic spirometry	
FEV_1	<0.8 ml
DLCO	<40%
Arterial blood gas analysis	
Pa_{CO_2}	>46 mm Hg
Pa_{O_2}	<70 mm Hg
Cardiopulmonary exercise testing (V_{O_2max})	<15 ml/min/kg

DLCO = Diffusing capacity, FEV_1 = forced expiratory volume in 1 sec, Pa_{CO_2} = partial pressure of arterial carbon dioxide, Pa_{O_2} = partial pressure of arterial oxygen tension.

preoperative cardiopulmonary function, along with values cited as predictors of poor outcome. Not all of the diagnostic tests may be evaluated for each patient, and the decision of which tests should be ordered is dependent upon the patient's history and planned surgery. Spirometry is often evaluated, and critical values examined include the forced vital capacity (FVC) and forced expiratory volume in 1 second (FEV_1). In addition, a diffusing capacity (DLCO) may be evaluated to examine the lung's ability to diffuse a test gas across the alveolar-capillary membrane. As part of the evaluation of spirometry, predicted postoperative values for FEV_1 and DLCO may be determined. These values are calculated by determining the amount of lung to be resected and then evaluating the predicted postoperative values. Specific calculations are available to determine predicted postoperative values.[30]

Other tests of pulmonary function are arterial blood gas (ABG) analysis, quantitative ventilation/perfusion ($\dot{V}/\dot{Q}$) scan, and formal cardiopulmonary exercise testing. The quantitative ventilation/perfusion scan evaluates differing regions of the lung (upper, middle, lower) and allows comparisons of the percentage of ventilation and perfusion in each area. Patients who are at high risk for pulmonary complications may undergo preoperative consultation by a pulmonologist to optimize pulmonary function. In addition, for high-risk patients who may be prone to sputum retention, a mini tracheostomy may be used or in some patients a tracheostomy is done during the surgery to make airway clearance and weaning from the mechanical ventilator a more efficient process.[7] Patient education is key in the preparation for surgery, as is discussed in the section titled Multidisciplinary Care.

◆ Case Study 21-1, Part B

Pulmonary Resection

For M.R., the diagnostic test results were as follows:

- Chest CT demonstrates a 3.5-cm right upper lobe NSCLC centrally located that appears to encroach upon the mainstem bronchus. No lymphadenopathy is noted. PET scan demonstrates hypermetabolic activity in the right upper lobe area and a questionable area in the right upper abdominal quadrant. No lymph node activity is noted. Split ventilation/perfusion quantitative function demonstrates nearly equal distribution between both lungs.
- Physical exam—weight, 146 pounds; height, 70 inches; blood pressure, 136/90 mm Hg; respirations, 16 breaths/min.
- Breath sounds—apical areas left > right but severely decreased at bases with expiratory prolongation and moderate wheezing bilaterally.

Decision point: What other disciplines should be involved in M.R.'s care? Provide your rationale.

Case continues on page 519

APPROACHES AND PROCEDURES

The most common thoracic surgical procedures in the adult are for resection of lung cancer (often a lobectomy), and the most popular incision for open thoracic procedures is the lateral thoracotomy. A variety of surgical approaches may be used in pulmonary resective surgeries and are described in Table 21-1. Figure 21-2 illustrates the most common surgical approaches used for thoracic procedures. Different types of lung resections/procedures may be performed and may be done for malignant or nonmalignant conditions (Table 21-2). Resections of the lung can be termed *anatomic* or *nonanatomic*. In an anatomic resection, the lung parenchyma, the artery and vein, and also any related bronchi with their accompanying lymph nodes are resected (e.g., segmentectomy, lobectomy, or pneumonectomy). A nonanatomic resection (e.g., wedge resection) means that the bronchovascular structures are not isolated or taken separately.

Wedge Resection

A wedge resection (limited resection) is performed to resect a small portion of lung parenchyma and is considered a nonanatomic, parenchymal-sparing resection. It is often done to remove a small, well-circumscribed peripheral pulmonary nodule or

TABLE 21-1 Definitions of Common Thoracic Approaches

APPROACH	DEFINITION
Thoracoscopy (VATS)	Also known as VATS: Minimally invasive approach that uses two or more "ports" or small incisions in chest. Openings used to place instruments into chest, including video camera and other instruments for grasping, cutting, or stapling. Used for diagnostic purposes, pleurodesis, staging procedures, or partial/total lung resection.
Thoracotomy	Incision made between two ribs to gain access to the thoracic cage for exploration or definitive surgical therapy. Location and extent of incision are dependent on specific operation to be performed. Types: lateral posterolateral, anterior, and muscle-sparing.
Thoracoabdominal	Large incision that provides exposure to both upper abdominal cavity and thorax. Starts in upper abdomen and sweeps up in a crescent shape into thorax and between ribs.
Median sternotomy	Widely used in cardiac surgery, but may be used in thoracic procedures. Sternum is cut in half lengthwise from suprasternal notch to xiphoid process. Sternum reconnected with wires.
Partial sternotomy	Like a sternotomy but only a portion of sternum is cut in a vertical fashion. Example: upper portion of sternum is cut to access thymus for thymectomy.
Hemiclamshell ("trapdoor")	Provides wide access to one side of chest. Incision begins mid-axillary in fourth or fifth intercostal space and continues across chest to sternum. Incision then moves vertically upward as a partial sternotomy.
Transverse sternotomy (clamshell)	Provides access to mediastinum and both lungs. Incision begins mid-axillary in fourth or fifth intercostal space and continues across chest (transversely) following line of fourth or fifth rib, through sternum to opposing mid-axillary line.
Cervical	Oblique incision of neck that begins at sternal notch and continues along anterior border of sternocleidomastoid muscle.
Subxiphoid	Vertical incision over lower sternum and xiphoid process with or without removal of xiphoid to gain access to pericardium or lower mediastinum.

VATS = Video-assisted thoracoscopic surgery.

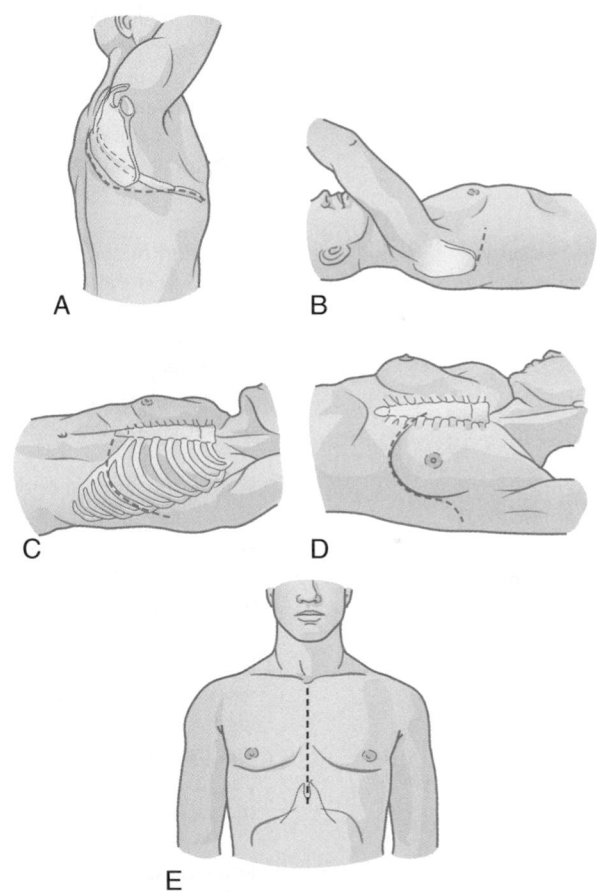

▲**FIGURE 21-2** Common surgical approaches for thoracic surgery. **A,** Posterolateral approach; **B,** lateral approach; **C,** thoracoabdominal approach; **D,** anterior approach; **E,** median sternotomy approach.

nodules (benign or metastatic). Although lobectomy is still considered the conventional surgery for localized cancer, a wedge resection may be used in patients with diminished pulmonary reserve. Studies, however, have demonstrated that local recurrence rates are higher following wedge resection for cancer as compared to a lobectomy.[43] Usually a VATS

TABLE 21-2 Definitions of Common Thoracic Procedures

PROCEDURE	DEFINITION
Pulmonary	
Wedge resection, single	Removal or resection of a small, wedged-shape area of lung parenchyma. Indicated for well-circumscribed benign tumors, pulmonary metastasis in select patients with small peripheral nodule(s), or a biopsy. Performed by either VATS or thoracotomy.
Segmentectomy	Resection of an anatomic subdivision of a pulmonary lobe (bronchopulmonary segment). Procedure is indicated for a nodule/mass with segmental distribution. Other indications: bronchiectasis, hamartoma, lung abscess. Usually performed using thoracotomy approach.
Lobectomy	Resection of a lobe of lung. Frequently performed for treatment of NSCLC, but may also be used for nonmalignant conditions. Performed by either thoracotomy or VATS.
Sleeve lobectomy	Procedure used to save lung parenchyma because of location of a mass that directly involves or protrudes into a major airway. A section of the airway and lobe is removed. Reanastomosis of airway proximal and distal to resected area is performed. Procedure is primarily used for malignancy, but may also be used for more benign conditions such as carcinoid tumors or trauma. Usual approach is thoracotomy.
Bilobectomy	Resection of two lobes of the lung. Is most frequently performed for treatment of NSCLC. Usual approach is thoracotomy.
Pneumonectomy, standard	Removal of entire lung. Primary indication is NSCLC. Other indications: multiple lung abscesses, bronchiectasis, or extensive infection. Occasionally performed for extensive involvement of lung in diseases such as sarcoma, mesothelioma, or metastatic disease to lung. Standard incision is posterolateral thoracotomy. Other approaches are median sternotomy and, rarely, VATS.
Pneumonectomy, intrapericardial	Similar to standard pneumonectomy, but one or more of the principal lung vessels within pericardial sac must be ligated. May occur when a tumor encroaches on hilum to extent that a standard pneumonectomy is not otherwise possible, the dissection is extremely difficult because of inflammatory tissue, or a vessel is torn close to pericardium. Standard incision is thoracotomy.
Pneumonectomy, sleeve (carinal)	Used when a tumor involves mainstem airway (right, rarely left). Carina and entire lung are resected in one piece. Remaining mainstem bronchus then gets sewn end-to-end to trachea. Right-sided carinal pneumonectomy is usually done either through a right thoracotomy or by a median sternotomy. Left-sided carinal pneumonectomy requires bilateral thoracotomies because left mainstem bronchus cannot be sewn into trachea from left chest (aortic arch is in the way).
Pneumonectomy, extrapleural	Removal of lung within envelope of the parietal pleura. Parietal pleura is separated from chest wall and diaphragm. Indications include malignant disease such as NSCLC, mesothelioma, or extensive infectious processes. Standard incision is thoracotomy and often a rib is resected as well to gain adequate exposure.
Pneumonectomy, completion	Removal of all remaining lung following previous removal of a portion of a lung. Standard incision is thoracotomy and often a rib is resected as well to gain adequate exposure.
Lung volume reduction	Removal of lung tissue damaged by emphysema. Provides room for expansion of better functioning lung tissue. Usually upper lobes are targeted. Bilateral approach is generally preferred to provide maximum benefit in one operation. Approaches used are sternotomy, VATS, or thoracotomy.
Bullectomy	Removal of bullae from the lung. Bullae are opened and fibrous septa excised. Walls of bulla used to reinforce staple line at base of resected bulla. Usually thoracotomy is used.

PROCEDURE	DEFINITION
Pleura	
Pleurodesis	Procedure to create adhesions between visceral and parietal pleurae. Usually done to prevent recurrent pneumothoraces or reaccumulation of pleural effusion. A sclerosing agent such as talc is instilled to cause inflammation and adhesion between pleurae. VATS or muscle-sparing thoracotomy is used.
Pleurectomy	Removal/excision of lining along inside of chest wall (parietal) and the lung (visceral). Thoracotomy is used.
Decortication	Removal of exudate/scar tissue in pleural space that traps lung. Done when lung is constricted and cannot be totally expanded. Approach used is VATS or thoracotomy.
Clagett procedure	Resection of rib(s) for drainage of an empyema; skin flap created to maintain an open window for access.
Chest Wall	
Chest wall resection	Performed to remove masses/tumors that invade into/through chest wall. Both ribs and muscular areas adjacent to affected ribs may be removed. Indications include neoplasm, infection, trauma, and radiation burns. Approach is highly dependent upon location and depth of resection required. Following chest wall resection, some type of reconstructive surgery may be necessary.
Chest wall reconstruction	Done to reestablish structural integrity of chest (stabilization) and protect underlying chest organs. Indications for reconstruction are trauma, reconstruction following chest wall resection for infection, radiation burns, and congenital anomalies. Plates or struts, synthetic materials (Prolene or Vicryl mesh), solid prostheses, or composites may be sutured over defect area to bridge defects in rib cage. Skin or muscle coverage of the mesh may also be used.
Thoracoplasty	Removal of two or more ribs to promote inward collapse of an area of chest wall. Although widely used in past to treat diseases such as tuberculosis, thoracoplasty is used today only to treat patients with chronic pleural space infection where lung cannot be reexpanded.
Sternectomy, complete	Complete removal of sternum. Performed because of a mass or malignancy involving sternum, infection, or severe trauma. Both rigid and soft materials may be used to cover area.
Sternectomy, partial	Partial removal of sternum. Done because of a mass or malignancy involving sternum, chronic infection, or severe trauma.
Diaphragm	
Diaphragmatic plication	Plicating the diaphragm is tucking the muscle or making folds in the membrane to make it smaller and more functional with respiration.
Diaphragmatic hernia repair	Repair of diaphragm following injury, trauma, or congenital defect. Hole or opening in diaphragm allows abdominal contents to protrude into chest; abdominal contents are repositioned into abdomen and opening in diaphragm is closed by suturing or using a patch.
Mediastinum	
Mediastinoscopy	Use of a rigid scope to examine mediastinum and biopsy tissue anterior to trachea; an incision is made at the base of the neck, above sternal notch, and mediastinoscope is passed along trachea.
Anterior mediastinotomy (Chamberlain)	Small horizontal incision between ribs usually to the left, but sometimes to the right of sternum. This approach is often used to examine lymph nodes in aortopulmonary window or anterior mediastinal masses.

Table continues on page 500

Table 21-2 Definitions of Common Thoracic Procedures—cont'd

PROCEDURE	DEFINITION
Mediastinal lymph node dissection	Removal of lymph nodes in mediastinum; this procedure indicates removal of most lymph nodes on one side of mediastinum, at all nodal stations. Done for pathologic staging of NSCLC.
Mediastinal lymph node sampling	Same as above, but sampling of lymph nodes on one side of mediastinum. Done for pathologic staging of NSCLC.
Resection, mediastinal mass	Removal of a mass in mediastinum. Type of approach is dependent upon location of mass.
Thymectomy	Excision/removal of thymus gland. Thymus is in anterior mediastinum. Usual approaches are transcervical, VATS, transthoracic (median sternotomy).
Thoracic duct ligation	Tying off of main lymph channel in chest; usually performed at level of diaphragm on right side and commonly done for a chyle leakage (chylothorax); duct is usually visualized near L2 vertebra and is approached using thoracotomy or VATS.

NSCLC = Non–small-cell lung cancer, VATS = video-assisted thoracoscopic surgery.

(Figure 21-3) or a limited thoracotomy approach procedure is used.

Minimal physiologic effects subsequent to a wedge resection are experienced. Morbidity following a wedge resection is also minimal and similar to that of segmentectomy.[48] Most often complications are a result of retention of secretions or pleural problems. A persistent pleural air space may occur in up to 10% of cases. Often, the space produces no symptoms and does not require treatment.[48] Mortality rate following a wedge resection is less than 1%.[48]

Segmentectomy

A segmentectomy is an anatomic resection to excise a bronchopulmonary segment or segments of the lung. There are 8 segments in the left lung and 10 segments in the right lung. A segmentectomy is used to remove small lesions or disease that has a segmental distribution. The standard incision for a segmentectomy is a thoracotomy. Physiologic effects are similar to those from a lobectomy.

Complications following a segmentectomy are prolonged air leak (peripheral alveolar pleural fistula or bronchopleural fistula), empyema, and persistent pleural air space.[48] Persistent pleural air space may be as high as 33% in specialized populations, such as those with pulmonary tuberculosis. As compared with a lobectomy, persistent pleural air spaces following segmentectomy are small. They may be conservatively treated with prolonged chest tube drainage and, if necessary, talc pleurodesis may be used. However, when problems in the pleural space arise, they are often septic in nature. Mortality rate following segmentectomy is around 1%, but may be higher (4% to 6%) in

patients with poor pulmonary function or previous pulmonary resection.[48]

Lobectomy

Lobectomy is the most common pulmonary resection procedure and is an anatomic resection. There are three lobes in the right lung and two lobes in the left lung.

Occasionally, two lobes are removed on the right side; this is termed a *bilobectomy*. Approaches used for a lobectomy include thoracotomy and VATS.[32] For lung cancer resective surgeries, mediastinal lymph node sampling or dissection will be done on the operative side. This allows additional pathologic staging information.

A sleeve lobectomy may also be performed. A sleeve lobectomy involves the removal of a portion of the main bronchus in conjunction with the involved lobar bronchus and associated lung tissue (Figure 21-4). A sleeve lobectomy is an alternative to a pneumonectomy, preserves lung tissue, and has a lower morbidity and mortality rate as compared to pneumonectomy. Approximately 6% to 8% of resections for primary lung cancer are sleeve resections.[27]

Physiologic changes following lobectomy include overinflation of both the contralateral tissue and the remaining lung tissue on the operated side. Functional loss of lung function is dependent upon the individual patient, preoperative lung function, and presence/absence of postoperative complications. Mortality following lobectomy is cited between 2% and 3% and may be increased in older adult patients and those with comorbid conditions.[55] Mortality rates for sleeve lobectomy vary depending upon the series cited, from

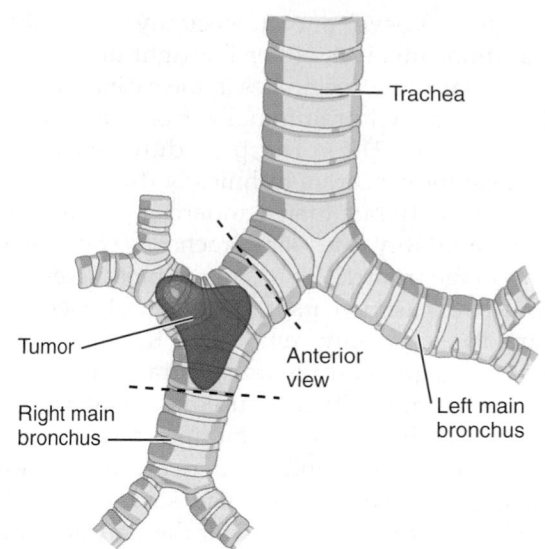

✦FIGURE 21-4 Sleeve lobectomy removing a right main bronchus tumor.

Pneumonectomy

Pneumonectomy is most commonly done for malignant disease. Tumors that extend deep into hilar structures, tumors that invade the main pulmonary artery or veins, and tumors extending across a major fissure may all be indications for a pneumonectomy. A lobectomy may be contemplated; however, once the chest is open, it becomes clear that a pneumonectomy is required. Also, should damage to a pulmonary artery occur when a lobectomy is being performed, this may also necessitate a more involved procedure.

Benign inflammatory diseases that may be an indication for a pneumonectomy include tuberculosis, mycobacteria other than tuberculosis, extensive fungal infections, necrotizing pneumonia, lung abscess, or bronchiectasis. Other potential indications for pneumonectomy may be penetrating trauma to the lung or congenital malformations. An anterior or lateral thoracotomy approach is frequently used for a pneumonectomy; however, a sternotomy may also be used.

There are different types of pneumonectomy. A standard pneumonectomy involves removal of the lung, and the remaining mainstem bronchus is sutured closed. Mortality rates for a standard pneumonectomy are cited at 3% to 8%.[55] A complete pneumonectomy entails reoperation to remove the remaining partially resected lung. Indications for complete pneumonectomy in the acute setting include bronchial dehiscence, venous infarction, pulmonary artery thrombosis, and positive tumor margin. More delayed indications include recurrent tumor, secondary primary cancer, benign disease progression, or bronchial stenosis.

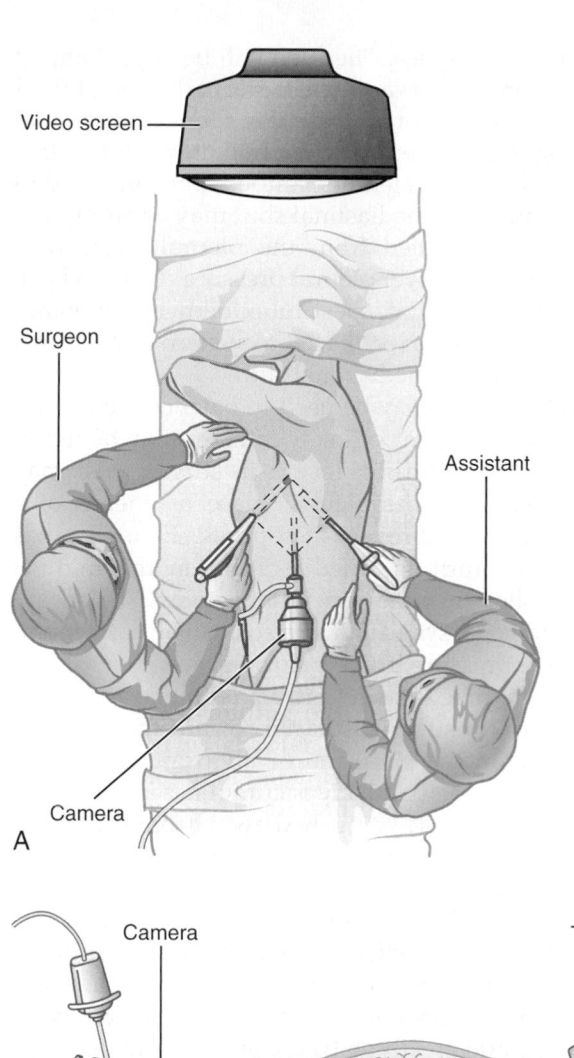

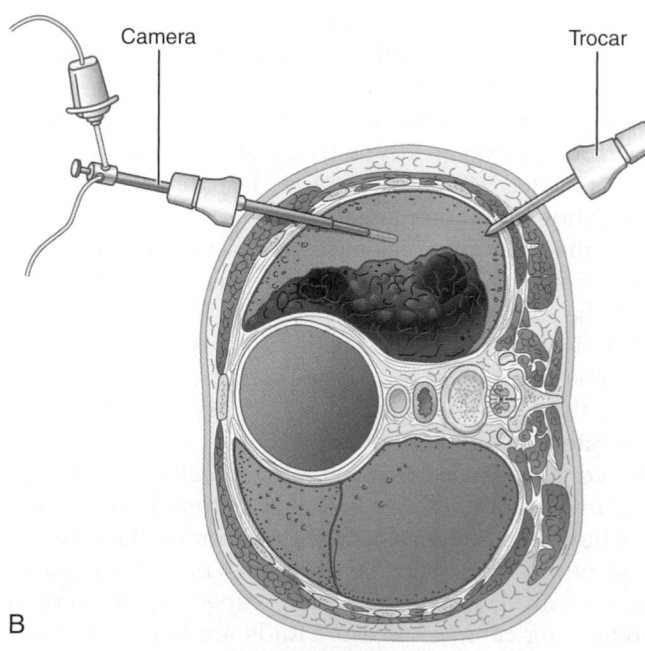

✦FIGURE 21-3 **A** and **B,** Different views of video-assisted thoracic surgery (VATS).

1% to 12%. Usually a mortality of around 5% is noted but may be higher depending upon the patient's preoperative cardiopulmonary condition and comorbid factors.[27]

A tracheal sleeve pneumonectomy is considered when a tumor involves either the right or the left tracheobronchial angle, originates in the carina, or invades the distal trachea intraluminally from the mainstem bronchus (Figure 21-5). The procedure is most commonly done for cancer, is technically difficult, and has a higher mortality rate than standard pneumonectomy. Operative mortality rates for a tracheal sleeve pneumonectomy range from 4% to 8% in the most recent series cited over the past 5 years.[73] Extrapleural pneumonectomy involves not only removal of the lung but also removal of the parietal pleura (pleura lining the chest wall). Most commonly it is used to treat malignant pleural mesothelioma. Lastly, intrapericardial pneumonectomy involves entry into the pericardium and examination and dissection of cardiac structures that are involved in the disease process. If the pericardium has been incised or opened, careful closure is required to prevent constriction of the heart and prevent herniation of the heart into the pneumonectomy space.[43]

Functional changes following pneumonectomy are extensive and can be classified as acute or chronic. In contrast to other types of lung resections, the pneumonectomy space following surgery is not routinely drained of air and fluid. Dry closure with perhaps a small amount of antibiotic solution left in the space is the simplest method. However, a chest tube may be left in for up to 24 hours to monitor for bleeding into the

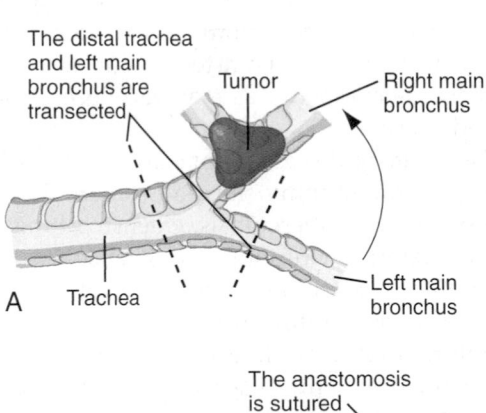

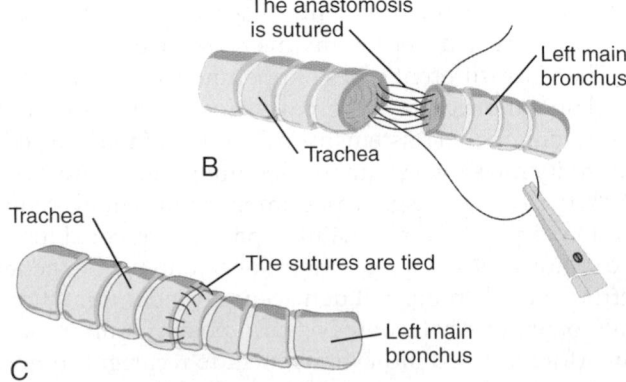

⬥**FIGURE 21-5** Sleeve pneumonectomy.

pneumonectomy space. The tube will be kept clamped except to monitor or evacuate pleural collection of fluid or readjust pleural pressures. If an underwater seal drainage system is used in the immediate postoperative period and the tube is left unclamped and connected to an underwater seal, mediastinal shift may occur rapidly as air will be expelled from the pleural space with coughing, causing lower pleural pressure. This can have drastic consequences. A chest tube following pneumonectomy should never be placed to suction because this may cause an acute mediastinal shift.

Several methods may be used to balance the pleural space following surgery. A soft catheter may be left in the pleural space during closure in surgery. Air may be evacuated from the pleural space by means of a large syringe and three-way stopcock. Enough air is removed to return the mediastinum to the midline position following the pneumonectomy. Balancing pleural drainage systems are also available to monitor/manage pressure in the pleural space.

During the first 24 hours after pneumonectomy, the mediastinum is usually displaced toward the operated side because of the extrusion of air from the pleural space. If fluid (blood) quickly accumulates in the space, the mediastinum may be pushed away from the operative side. If either of these two opposing forces becomes unbalanced or if pressure changes occur too quickly following surgery, this may severely impair the patient's cardiopulmonary function. When the mediastinum is shifted toward the remaining lung, this may compromise pulmonary function and impair venous return. If the mediastinum greatly shifts toward the operated side, this may lead to dysrhythmias, hypotension, cardiac herniation, or pulmonary edema.

In the early postpneumonectomy period, there is a reduction in all lung volumes in the remaining lung and the diaphragm is elevated on the operative side. There is a shift of the mediastinum and a narrowing of the intercostal spaces on the operated side. Serosanguineous fluid accumulates in the empty pleural space. The rate of accumulation is variable, but the space is usually completely opacified by 3 to 6 weeks. Following a pneumonectomy, all the cardiac output is traversing one lung. The right heart dilates to accommodate the cardiac output. Thus the patient is at high risk for postpneumonectomy pulmonary edema, especially if there is preexisting cardiac disease. Fluids are kept to a minimum to keep the patient relatively "dry." Whether fluid administration is causally related to postpneumonectomy pulmonary edema, it is apparent that in the presence of increased pulmonary capillary permeability, unnecessary crystalloid administration exacerbates the degree of pulmonary edema. Restricting fluids to less than 20 ml/kg for the first 24 hours postoperatively is generally possible without hemodynamic instability.[37]

Potential signs of developing postpneumonectomy pulmonary edema include increasing airway peak pressures (if mechanically ventilated), increased respiratory distress (if spontaneously breathing without mechanical ventilation or "fighting the ventilator"), increasing oxygenation needs, tachycardia, and restlessness or confusion.

Chronic changes following pneumonectomy include hyperinflation or an increase in the lung volumes of the remaining lung. The fluid within the pleural space of the operated lung is gradually absorbed; a potential space exists. The trachea, heart, and mediastinum shift toward the operated side, and the remaining lung expands anteriorly and partially into the pneumonectomy space.

Pneumonectomy is associated with a higher risk of operative morbidity and mortality than other lung resections; reported operative morality ranges from 4% to 8%.[37,43,58,73] Most operative deaths from pneumonectomy are associated with pulmonary complications, with the other major causes including cardiovascular or surgical technical problems. Right-sided pneumonectomy has a much higher risk of morbidity and mortality because of a variety of factors.[37] Bronchopulmonary fistula and potential stump dehiscence are more common with a right-sided pneumonectomy as compared to the left. This is due to several factors, including the fact that the right bronchial stump closure is completed in the "open" as opposed to the left-sided stump, which gets buried in the mediastinal tissues immediately after surgical closure. A small dehiscence of the left stump is usually inconsequential. Also, an important factor related to increased bronchopulmonary fistula on the right is that the right mainstem is shorter than the left and suture closure is under increased tension. When closing the right mainstem near the origin, there is much more radial tension distracting the suture line as compared to the left side. A pedicle of pleura or intercostal muscles may be used to buttress the pneumonectomy stump closure.[43]

Lung Volume Reduction Surgery. Not all resective surgeries are done for lung cancer. Treatment options for patients with end-stage chronic obstructive pulmonary disease (stage IV) with a primary emphysematous component are limited, although lung volume reduction surgery (LVRS) is an option for a select subset of patients. This subset includes patients with homogeneous disease or disease that is focused in one area and not widespread throughout the lungs. LVRS involves the removal of a portion of the diseased lung parenchyma. This reduces hyperinflation and allows the functional tissue to expand, resulting in improved elastic recoil of the lung and improved chest wall and diaphragmatic mechanics. This type of surgery does not cure the disease or

improve life expectancy, but it may decrease dyspnea, improve lung function, and improve the patient's overall quality of life.[35] Careful selection of patients for this procedure is essential to decrease morbidity and mortality.

The National Emphysema Treatment Trial (NETT) found that the addition of LVRS to optimal medical management and rehabilitation led to overall improvement in exercise tolerance and survival in a subgroup of patients with predominantly upper lobe disease.[54] LVRS is paid for by Medicare in centers that meet specific criteria.[10] All patients must be able to complete a preoperative rehabilitation program in preparation for surgery. The ideal candidate for LVRS is one with heterogeneous disease with defined targets in the diseased lung. Specific criteria for LVRS are shown in Table 21-3. In addition, debate surrounds the type of procedure (unilateral vs. bilateral) and the incisional technique used (median sternotomy vs. VATS). Regardless of technique, the diseased lung is identified and a staple line is used to excise one half to two thirds of the upper lobes. Depending upon the amount of lung excised, there is the potential for a residual postoperative air space that may result in prolonged air leak. A pleural tent may be used, which means dissecting the parietal pleura from the chest wall and reducing the size of the pleural space by promoting apposition of the pleural surfaces. Operative mortality following LVRS varies from 5% to 10%, with most deaths related to pulmonary insufficiency, lung infection, or cardiac problems.[23]

Of the information available regarding LVRS, the following can be concluded at this time: (1) in a select group of patients, this procedure offers an improved quality of life; (2) bilateral resection may provide better results than unilateral resection; (3) VATS results in lower postoperative morbidity; (4) stapling of the tissue may provide more consistent results than laser ablation; (5) pulmonary rehabilitation before and after surgery is key; and (6) LVRS is a palliative procedure.[23]

PLEURAL SURGERY

A variety of surgical procedures may be done for disease or problems relating to the pleural space (see Table 21-2). Some of these conditions may be the result of thoracic surgery and are described under Complications of Thoracic Surgery. Pleural conditions are disorders that involve the membranes covering the lungs (parietal and visceral pleura) or disorders affecting the pleural space. The lungs are covered by a thin serous membrane. The visceral pleura covers the surfaces of the lungs and extends into the fissures between the lobes. The parietal pleura lines the inner surface of the chest wall, covers the diaphragm, and reflects over

TABLE 21-3 Centers for Medicare and Medicaid Services (CMS) Criteria for Lung Volume Reduction Surgery

ASSESSMENT	CRITERIA
History and physical examination	Consistent with emphysema BMI $\leq$31.1 kg/m^2 (men) or $\leq$32.3 kg/m^2 (women) Stable with $\leq$20 mg of prednisone (or equivalent) daily
Radiographic	High-resolution CT scan evidence of bilateral emphysema
Pulmonary function (pre-rehabilitation)	FEV$_1$ $\leq$45% predicted ($\geq$15% predicted if age $\geq$70 years) TLC $\geq$100% predicted post-bronchodilator RV $\geq$150% predicted post-bronchodilator
Arterial blood gas level (pre-rehabilitation)	Paco$_2$ $\leq$60 mm Hg (Paco$_2$ $\leq$55 mm Hg if 1 mile above sea level) Pao$_2$ $\geq$45 mm Hg on room air (Pao$_2$ $\geq$30 mm Hg if 1 mile above sea level)
Cardiac assessment	Approval for surgery by cardiologist if any of following are present: unstable angina; LVEF cannot be estimated from echocardiogram; LVEF <45%; dobutamine-radionuclide cardiac scan indicates coronary artery disease or ventricular dysfunction; dysrhythmia (>5 premature ventricular contractions per minute; cardiac rhythm other than sinus; premature ventricular contractions on ECG at rest)
Surgical assessment	Approval for surgery by pulmonary physician, thoracic surgeon, and anesthesiologist post-rehabilitation
Exercise	Post-rehabilitation 6-min walk of $\geq$140 m; able to complete 3 min of unloaded pedaling in exercise tolerance test (pre- and post-rehabilitation)
Consent	Signed consents for screening and rehabilitation
Smoking	Plasma nicotine level $\leq$13.7 ng/ml (or arterial carboxyhemoglobin $\leq$2.5% if using nicotine products) Nonsmoking for 4 months before initial interview and throughout evaluation for surgery
Preoperative diagnosis and therapeutic program adherence	Must complete assessment for and program of preoperative services in preparation for surgery

From reference 10.
BMI = Body mass index, FEV$_1$ = forced expiratory volume in 1 sec, LVEF = left ventricular ejection fraction, Paco$_2$ = partial pressure of arterial carbon dioxide, Pao$_2$ = partial pressure of arterial oxygen tension, TLC = total lung capacity, RV = residual volume.

the structures occupying the middle of the thorax (the mediastinum). The potential space between the pleurae is known as the pleural space/cavity. A small amount of fluid lies between the two pleurae. Pleural fluid is continuously produced and reabsorbed, and at any given time there is less than 10 ml in the pleural space. Also, the parietal pleura has nerve endings; the visceral pleura does not.

Problems of the Pleural Space

Pneumothorax. A simple pneumothorax causing respiratory impairment is usually treated via conventional means with chest tube insertion and evacuation of air from the pleural space. However, surgery may be indicated for patients who require definitive management of a pneumothorax with a persistent air leak or a pneumothorax that will not resolve. Indications include massive air leak that prevents lung reexpansion, persistent air leak, and recurrent pneumothorax. VATS may be used for examination of the pleural space and the achievement of pleural symphysis.

Pleural Effusion. Pleural effusion is a collection of fluid in the pleural space and is rarely a primary disease process, but is usually secondary to other diseases. It may be a complication of heart failure, tuberculosis, pneumonia, pulmonary infections (particularly viral infections), nephrotic syndrome, connective tissue disease, pulmonary embolism, and neoplastic tumors. Lung cancer is the most common malignancy associated with a pleural effusion. Once the pleural space is adequately drained, a chemical pleurodesis may be performed to obliterate the pleural space and prevent reaccumulation of fluid. Other treatments for malignant pleural effusions include surgical pleurectomy, insertion of a small catheter attached to a drainage bottle for outpatient management (Pleur-X catheter), or implantation of a pleuroperitoneal shunt.

Empyema. An empyema is an accumulation of thick, purulent fluid within the pleural space (an infection in the pleural space), often with fibrin development and a loculated (walled-off) area where infection is located. Most empyemas occur as complications of bacterial pneumonia or lung abscess. Other causes include penetrating chest trauma, hematogenous infection of the pleural space, nonbacterial infections, or iatrogenic causes (following thoracic surgery or thoracentesis). Treatment of an empyema includes fluid evacuation, pleural space obliteration, nutrition, and antimicrobial support.[43] An acute empyema may be drained by thoracentesis or placement of a chest tube if/when fluid reaccumulates. Chronic empyemas may require either rib resection and drainage or decortication. Open chest drainage is usually performed via thoracotomy and includes potential rib resection to remove the thickened pleura, pus, and debris and to remove the underlying diseased pulmonary tissue.

With long-standing inflammation, an exudate can form over the lung, trapping the lung and interfering with its normal expansion. This exudate, or pleural peel, must be removed surgically in a process called *decortication* (Figure 21-6). A chest tube is left in place until the pus-filled space is completely obliterated. The complete obliteration of the pleural space is monitored by serial chest x-rays, and the patient should be informed that treatment may be long term. Patients are frequently discharged from the hospital with a chest tube in place, with instructions to monitor fluid drainage at home.

Pleural Tumors. Approximately 95% of pleural tumors are due to metastatic disease.[43] The most common primary pleural tumor is mesothelioma. Two surgical options exist for the management of malignant mesothelioma: (1) pleurectomy (removal of parietal pleura) with or without decortication of the visceral pleura and (2) extrapleural pneumonectomy.

However, only 20% of patients with mesothelioma are candidates for surgery.[43] Usually, the mainstay of treatment for this disease is chemotherapy, radiation, immunotherapy, or gene therapy.[43]

Pleural Space Procedures

Pleurodesis. Pleurodesis is a procedure used to cause inflammation of the pleurae and the formation of adhesions. This inflammation causes apposition of the parietal and visceral pleurae and assists in the reexpansion of the lung or to minimize the possibility of recurring pleural effusions. Pleurodesis is performed either through mechanical means (direct abrasion) or by chemical abrasion with talc, tetracycline, or doxycycline instilled into the pleural space.

Pleurodesis may be performed using a VATS or via a chest tube. Initially, fluid must be removed from the pleural space. A chemically irritating agent (e.g., talc) is instilled or aerosolized into the pleural space. The technique of chemical pleurodesis is critical for a

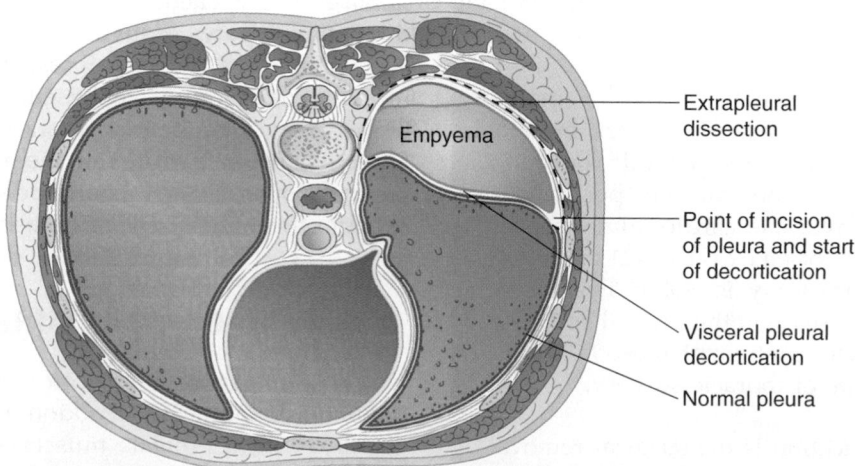

Empyema

Extrapleural dissection

Point of incision of pleura and start of decortication

Visceral pleural decortication

Normal pleura

⬥FIGURE 21-6 Cross section of thorax with empyema and operative techniques.

successful outcome. The pleural surfaces must be juxtaposed at the time of inflammation and remain in close contact for the next 48 to 72 hours.[65] With the chest tube approach, after the agent is instilled, the chest tube is clamped for 60 to 90 minutes, and the patient is assisted to assume various positions to promote uniform distribution of the agent and to maximize its contact with the pleural surfaces. However, one study has suggested that patients need not be rotated to enhance distribution, and there are no studies evaluating the optimal time for the tube to be clamped.[65] The tube is unclamped as ordered, and chest drainage may be continued several days longer to prevent reaccumulation of fluid and to promote the formation of adhesions between the visceral and parietal pleurae. With the VATS procedure, the pleural space is examined and drained, and the sclerosing agent is instilled or aerosolized. A chest tube is left in place following this procedure as well.

Pain with this procedure has not been well studied. As the parietal pleura has pain fibers, patients may complain of discomfort with the instillation of a chemical agent. One recommendation is the use of small doses of intravenous narcotic and midazolam (Versed) with the chest tube instillation procedure.[65]

Pleurectomy. In a pleurectomy, the parietal pleura is removed by careful dissection via a thoracotomy approach. Care must be taken to avoid damage to the phrenic, recurrent laryngeal, and sympathetic nerves, and to stellate ganglion as well as the vascular structures. Depending upon the patient, some visceral dissection may be indicated. A pleurectomy can control fluid accumulation (recurrent nonmetastatic pleural effusion) and decrease pain. In early stages of malignant mesothelioma, when a pleurectomy is combined with other treatments such as radiation and chemotherapy, it may improve the length of survival. However, once the disease has penetrated the parietal pleura, pleurectomy may not be beneficial because of the spread of disease.

An advantage of pleurectomy is its low mortality rate compared to more invasive, complex mesothelioma surgery such as an extrapleural pneumonectomy.[43] Also, the operation can be performed in patients with a less favorable cardiopulmonary function than that required for an extrapleural pneumonectomy. However, pleurectomy is not indicated if the patient has extensive disease in the pleural space. Only 20% of all patients with malignant mesothelioma are candidates for any type of thoracic surgery.[43]

Decortication. Decortication is the surgical removal of a loculated exudate between the pleurae or a pleural peel of adhesions. The approach may be VATS or thoracotomy, depending upon the extent of surgery planned. Decortication may be used to treat an organizing or chronic empyema. Early decortication usually results in better control of the infection and potential reexpansion of lung tissue.

MEDIASTINAL DISEASE

The mediastinum can be divided into three anatomic subdivisions: anterior, middle, and posterior. A variety of diseases may invade the mediastinum. Approximately 25% to 42% of mediastinal masses are malignant, and in the adult the most common masses in order of decreasing frequency are neurogenic tumors, primary cysts, thymomas, lymphomas, and germ cell tumors.[33] Anterosuperior mediastinal masses are most likely malignant, followed by tumors of the middle mediastinum and posterior mediastinum. Superior vena cava syndrome is caused by compression or obstruction of the venous outflow tract in the mediastinum from the head, neck, and upper extremities. This results in swelling of the face, neck, arms, and upper chest.[33] Treatment focuses on shrinking, debulking, or removing masses or the cause of the compression or obstruction.

Diagnostic tests for evaluating mediastinal disease include CT scans of the chest, magnetic resonance imaging, EUS, radionuclide agents (e.g., iodine-131 or iodine-123), and biochemical markers (e.g., alpha-fetoprotein, human chorionic gonadotropin beta-subunit, carcinoembryonic antigen). A mediastinoscopy may be used to biopsy nodes or masses anterior to the trachea in the mediastinum, and a mediastinotomy may be used to biopsy masses in the aortopulmonary window area. CT-guided fine-needle aspiration or core biopsies may also be done, if the mass is accessible via this technique.

Surgical approaches to the mediastinum are dependent upon the area of involvement of the mediastinum and the amount of disease present. The anterosuperior mediastinum is accessed by either a median sternotomy or an anterolateral thoracotomy; the superior aspect of the anterosuperior mediastinum via a transcervical approach; and the middle or posterior mediastinum through a posterolateral thoracotomy.

DIAPHRAGMATIC SURGERY

The diaphragm serves both anatomically as a separation of the thoracic and abdominal cavities and functionally as the major muscle of respiration. The diaphragm has two distinct parts—the costal muscle and the crural aspect. The costal muscle is thin and provides some of the downward displacement of the diaphragm on inspiration. The crural aspect is thicker and supports the heart. In reality the diaphragm is made of two hemidiaphragms divided by a central tendon and innervated by the phrenic nerve.

Diaphragmatic Abnormalities

There are different types of diaphragmatic hernias. These are briefly described in Table 21-4. Any herniation in the diaphragm may allow abdominal contents to extrude into the thoracic cavity. Diaphragmatic hernias may be repaired through either an abdominal or a thoracic approach often using laparoscopy or VATS.

Diaphragm eventration (upward displacement of the diaphragm) may be congenital or acquired. Diaphragmatic plication may be performed when there is paralysis of either the left or the right diaphragm. The goal of plication is to lower the diaphragm into a flat position to reduce the paradoxical motion and associated shift in the mediastinum during respiration.[43] Usually a thoracotomy or thoracoabdominal approach is used for plication, but a VATS may also be performed.

Primary tumors of the diaphragm are rare. More often, tumors spread from the lung, upper abdominal viscera, or pleura and invade the diaphragm. Benign diaphragmatic tumors include lipoma, cystic masses, and bronchogenic, mesothelial, and teratoid tumors. Examples of malignant tumors include sarcoma, schwannoma, chondroma, pheochromocytoma, and endometriosis. Mesothelioma may be benign or malignant, and the primary site of origin may be the diaphragm. Surgical resection is not indicated for all tumors.[43] The diaphragm and its pleural and peritoneal layers are excised en bloc. The defect is closed via sutures, a prosthetic soft tissue patch of Gore-Tex, or polypropylene mesh.

CHEST WALL DISORDERS

Tumors are the most common disorder of the chest wall observed in adults. Approximately 5% of thoracic neoplasms are primary chest wall tumors, and approximately 85% of these occur in the ribs.[43] Chest wall tumors can be classified as benign or malignant tumors of the bone or soft tissue. Examples of benign tumors are lipomas, osteochondroma, chondroma, and fibrous dysplasia. Malignant tumors of the chest wall include chondrosarcoma, fibrosarcoma, multiple myeloma, and Ewing's sarcoma. Solid tumors may metastasize to the chest wall and include lung, breast, pancreatic, gastric, and colon cancers. Treatment of a chest wall tumor is dependent on the specific tumor and the extent of involvement. Some chest wall tumors are treated in a palliative fashion with radiation therapy. If surgery is indicated, a variety of procedures may be performed, depending on the location and the involvement with surrounding tissues and ribs. Rib resection may be indicated as well. Chest wall reconstruction is performed using a mesh such as polypropylene or Gore-Tex. In addition, muscle flaps may be used to cover the defect and provide added protection and structure.

COMPLICATIONS OF THORACIC SURGERY

Intraoperative

In addition to problems related to anesthesia, the four primary intraoperative problems related to any type of thoracic surgery include injury to a major vessel resulting in hemorrhage, cardiac dysrhythmias, myocardial ischemia, and development of a contralateral pneumothorax.[58] Intraoperative cardiac complications most often occur in patients with preexisting cardiac disease. A contralateral pneumothorax is a rare complication, with an incidence of less than 1%. It may occur during the positive pressure ventilation of the nonoperative lung because of a spontaneous rupture of a bleb. Air accumulates in the pleural space on the nonoperative side and impairs expansion.

TABLE 21-4 Types of Diaphragmatic Hernias

TYPE	DESCRIPTION
Morgagni	Retrosternal anterior diaphragmatic defect. Usually on right side (90%). Hernia sac may contain omentum, colon, stomach, liver. Surgically repaired when symptomatic.
Paraesophageal	Upward dislocation of gastric fundus alongside a normally (type II) positioned gastroesophageal junction. Less common than sliding hernias. Potential for serious complications such as gastric volvulus/obstruction, gastric necrosis. Surgery indicated because of seriousness of potential complications.
Sliding (type I)	Dome-shaped upward migration of gastroesophageal junction into posterior mediastinum. Treated when symptomatic.

Postoperative

The majority of complications related to thoracic surgical procedures are pulmonary in origin. Table 21-5 describes functional changes and complications related to various types of thoracic procedures.

Pulmonary Complications

Prolonged Air Leak or Drainage. An air leak may occur from a residual raw or stapled parenchymal surface and is relatively common. As the lung reexpands completely and the pleural space is obliterated, the leak often stops in 2 to 3 days. Persistence of an air leak beyond 7 days is considered a prolonged air leak. Air leaks are common after lobectomy, especially when incomplete fissures have been divided during the operation and in LVRS.[68] Most resolve upon reexpansion of the lung and stop within 2 weeks.

There is a lack of evidence-based practice for management of chest tubes following pulmonary resection. Recent studies have shown that although the majority of physicians favor placing chest tubes to suction when a patient has an air leak following resection, water seal is superior.[11,13,15,16,49]

The use of tissue glue has been suggested to reduce the incidence and duration of air leak. Fabian et al. conducted a prospective, blinded study and randomized patients to aerosolized spraying of 5 ml of fibrin glue onto raw lung surface. Patients receiving the aerosolized fibrin glue had a reduction in the incidence of air leak, duration of air leak, and duration of chest tube use.[28] Additional studies are needed to support these results.

For patients with prolonged air leak who are otherwise ready for discharge from the hospital, options are available. Patients can be discharged with small one-way valves (Heimlich Chest Drain Valve, BD Bard-Parker, Franklin Lakes, NJ; Pneumostat Chest Drain Valve, Atrium Medical Corp., Hudson, NH). In addition, a small 500-ml chest tube drainage device that also monitors air leak is available (Express Mini 500, Atrium Medical Corp.). If the air leak continues for 2 to 3 weeks, other options should be discussed and may include returning to surgery with a VATS procedure either to apply fibrin glue or some type of sealant or possibly to perform a pleurodesis.

Bronchopleural Fistula. Tracheal or bronchopleural fistula complications are difficult to prevent and manage in the postoperative patient. Prevention focuses on vigilant management of the tracheobronchial anastomosis. Frequent bronchoscopic evaluation to assess the area for ischemia or necrosis may be used. Some surgeons advocate minimization of deep endobronchial suctioning so that the integrity of the suture line will not be compromised. However, secretion management is key in the care of this population.

Failure of the bronchial stump to heal following an anatomic lung resection may occur and either result in a minor complication or progress to a major, life-threatening event. It is more common after pneumonectomy (right greater than left) and is a more severe problem following pneumonectomy than lobectomy or segmentectomy. Risk factors for this complication include the following: type of resection, reason for resection (such as resection performed for infection or inflammation), timing of resection (such as following full-dose radiation

TABLE 21-5 Functional Effects and Complications Related to Specific Thoracic Procedures

PROCEDURE	PHYSIOLOGIC EFFECTS	COMPLICATIONS
Wedge resection	Minimal	Retention of secretions Persistent pleural air space
Segmentectomy	Overinflation of contralateral lung and remaining tissue on operated side	Retention of secretions Prolonged air leak Empyema Persistent pleural space
Lobectomy	Similar to segmentectomy	Similar to segmentectomy
Pneumonectomy	Residual pneumonectomy space Mediastinal/tracheal shift toward remaining lung Functional loss of lung tissue Diaphragm elevation on resected side Cardiac output transversions: one pulmonary and one lung	Retention of secretions Bronchopulmonary fistula Empyema Noncardiac pulmonary edema

therapy or prolonged mechanical ventilation), post resection infected space, or technical factors.[58]

Management of this complication depends upon the time of development following surgery. Very early in the postoperative period, reoperation and repair may be indicated. If the fistula occurs later in the postoperative recovery, the patient will expectorate serosanguineous, frothy fluid from the pleural space. Prompt attention to this complication is needed so that the remaining lung is not flooded with the pleural drainage. The patient should be positioned with the operative side down to protect the remaining lung, and a chest tube should be placed or a portion of the previous incision site should be opened and a tube placed.

If the bronchopleural fistula persists or occurs in the presence of infection (empyema), more aggressive measures may be indicated. Drainage may be performed by establishing an Eloesser flap or reopening a portion of the original thoracotomy. A flap of skin is sutured to the pleura, creating an epithelium-lined opening into the empyema area to assist in drainage. The bronchial stump is resutured and reinforced. A Clagett maneuver is used to sterilize the pleural space. This involves open drainage and irrigation of the pleural cavity with antibiotics for several months. The chest wall is then closed once the infection has been thoroughly treated and has resolved.

Severe Atelectasis. Atelectasis occurs in all patients in the postoperative period; however, severe atelectasis leading to respiratory insufficiency occurs in 7% to 10% of patients following resection. Table 21-6 describes the pathogenesis of atelectasis, and Table 21-7 lists risk factors frequently identified in thoracic surgery patients. Treatment includes adequate volume while the patient is on mechanical ventilation and intensive volume expansion measures, including secretion management, turning/mobilization, and bronchoscopy once the patient is extubated.

Pneumonia. Pulmonary infection may occur in association with unresolved atelectasis, with aspiration, and in the setting of mechanical ventilation. The incidence with thoracic surgery is cited between 2% and 22%, with larger series ranging from 5% to 8%.[58] Thoracic surgery is listed as a risk factor for nosocomial pneumonia.[70] In the thoracic surgery patient, risk factors for postoperative pneumonia include increased age, preexisting pulmonary disease (chronic lung disease, smoking), poor nutritional status, aspiration, prolonged anesthesia duration, use of transfusions, presence of a nasogastric tube, prolonged mechanical ventilation, poor volume expansion, poor secretion management, poor pain management, and lack of mobilization.

Pneumonia is often misdiagnosed in the postoperative setting. Treatment includes early identification of patients at risk, early extubation, early identification of pneumonia, appropriate antibiotic treatment, lung volume expansion maneuvers, and aggressive secretion management. For ventilator-associated pneumonia,

TABLE 21-6 Pathogenesis of Atelectasis

"PURE" HYPOVENTILATION*	INCREASED/MODIFIED SECRETIONS	Decreased Clearance	
		INEFFICIENT COUGH	MECHANICAL IMPEDIMENTS
Pain	COPD/chronic infection	Pain	Bronchial stenosis
General anesthesia	Active smoking	Lack of cooperation	Deficient glottic occlusion
Diaphragmatic dysfunction	Bronchial denervation	Unstable chest wall	
Chest wall alterations	"Open bronchus" surgery	Diaphragmatic palsy	
Partial pneumothorax	Previous head and neck surgery		
Pleural effusion			
Bronchial stenosis			
Abdominal distention			

From reference 49a.
*Hypoventilation per se, not related to bronchial obstruction.

TABLE 21-7 Risk Factors for Postoperative Atelectasis

1. Medical History	2. Operative Details
Swallow disorders*	Chest wall resection
Neurologic disease	Diaphragmatic palsy
Previous head and neck surgery	Sleeve lobectomy
Low performance status	
Active smoking	
Increased secretions	**3. Postoperative Management**
Chronic obstructive pulmonary disease	Failure of pain control
Infectious lung disease	Lack of cooperation

From reference 49a.
*Swallow disorders are a major risk factor; preventive tracheostomy should be considered as a planned approach.

key measures to prevent this complication include initiation of the ventilator bundle of care. Chapter 9 provides more comprehensive information on ventilator-associated pneumonia prevention.

Early identification of this complication is important. Mortality in the postoperative patient can be as high as 30%, and unfortunately, pneumonia may lead to acute respiratory failure or acute respiratory distress syndrome.[3,17]

Acute Respiratory Failure and Acute Respiratory Distress Syndrome. Respiratory failure and acute respiratory distress syndrome are discussed in detail in Chapters 19 and 20.

Postpneumonectomy Pulmonary Edema. Postpneumonectomy pulmonary edema is difficult to predict, prevent, or treat successfully. It is a rapidly occurring, lethal complication that happens in 2% to 5% of cases and, when unrecognized, carries a mortality of 60% to 90%.[58] Although the complication is similar to noncardiogenic pulmonary edema, it is refractory to standard therapy and may have devastating consequences for the pneumonectomy patient. The pathophysiologic mechanisms are similar to those for acute respiratory distress syndrome and include the factors of contralateral pulmonary hyperinflation, alveolar rupture and interstitial emphysema, damage to the alveocapillary

membrane, and decreased lymphatic resorption of fluid.[58]

Prevention of postpneumonectomy pulmonary edema involves minimization of fluid infusion in the operative and early postoperative periods, early use of diuretics, and use of vasopressors if fluid volume appears adequate.[58] Prolonged high-pressure ventilation should be minimized if at all possible.

Pleural Effusion. In the acute postoperative period, a small effusion at the base of the lung is common after lobectomy or a lesser resection. Small to moderate effusions are drained via the chest tube or reabsorbed over time. A chronic or recurring effusion that causes symptoms of pulmonary impairment in the postoperative setting may require ultrasound-guided thoracentesis or a return to surgery for drainage and pleurodesis.

Chylothorax. A chylothorax is an accumulation of lymphatic fluid within the pleural space. Chylothorax may occur after pneumonectomy, lobectomy, or extensive hilar and mediastinal dissection. Injury to the thoracic duct may occur anywhere along its course. Because of its anatomic location, injuries to the thoracic duct in the lower chest often result in right-sided chylothorax, and injuries to the upper portion of the duct result in left-sided chylothorax. When observed in the chest tube drainage system or tubing, the effusion is usually a whitish, milky fluid. Conservative management includes continued drainage and avoidance of oral alimentation in conjunction with total parenteral nutrition. In approximately 50% of cases, the lymphatic fistula will close on its own.[37,43] Surgical repair should be considered in patients with continuous drainage lasting more than 2 weeks or with large-volume drainage. With surgical repair, the chest is opened and the leaking thoracic duct identified and ligated. To assist in identifying the duct, a patient may be given a fatty substance (e.g., cream, half and half) by mouth or through a nasogastric tube 2 to 3 hours before surgery. This provides increased visualization of the leak.

Lobar Torsion. A rotation of a lobe on its bronchovascular components may occur postoperatively. If unrecognized and not corrected, this results in infarction of the lobe and potential gangrene. This complication can be observed on chest radiograph as the lobe fails to reexpand and is opacified. Also, depending upon the patient's preoperative pulmonary function, differing degrees of hypoxemia may be present. Bronchoscopy is usually performed to evaluate the airways. When possible, torsion of a lobe is identified and immediate reoperation is indicated to release the torsion and hopefully save the viability of the lobe.

Cardiac Complications

Cardiac Dysrhythmias. Atrial fibrillation (AF) is the most common dysrhythmia following noncardiac thoracic surgery, with a reported incidence of 10% to 20% occurring after lobectomy and up to 40% after pneumonectomy.[9,18] Risk factors for development of AF following noncardiac thoracic surgery include age greater than 65 years, extrapleural or intrapericardial pneumonectomy, right-sided procedures, extent of pulmonary resection, and chronic obstructive pulmonary disease, as defined by results of preoperative pulmonary function tests. The peak incidence of AF following pulmonary procedures is most frequently reported as occurring 48 to 72 hours after surgery.

Although the dysrhythmia is often self-limiting and transient, there can be serious consequences associated with developing this dysrhythmia. Postoperative AF can lead to disabling symptoms and may have consequences such as stroke and hemodynamic instability, prolonged hospital and critical care stay, increased monitoring time, and added patient discomfort. Atrial fibrillation occurring after thoracic surgery has been associated with increased mortality.[66,72]

Despite speculation, the direct cause of atrial fibrillation after thoracic operation remains unclear. However, most believe that it is multifactorial and results from the synergistic action of increased vagal tone, atrial inflammation, pulmonary hypertension, dilation of the right side of the heart, and hypoxemia. Several drugs have been used for the prevention of atrial fibrillation after thoracic surgery, including digoxin, flecainide, diltiazem, verapamil, propranolol, atenolol, and amiodarone. Unfortunately, because of the pulmonary issues in many of the patients undergoing thoracic surgery, beta blockers are relatively contraindicated or are poorly tolerated in this patient population.

Myocardial Ischemia and Infarction. Ischemia and infarction are not common following thoracic procedures. Patients with preexisting cardiac problems are at a higher risk of these complications. Appropriate cardiac evaluation before surgery is important in preventing or minimizing cardiac problems. It is suggested that following recent myocardial infarction under medical management, thoracic surgery should be delayed.[69]

Cardiac Herniation. If a thoracic resection requires opening the pericardium, cardiac herniation can occur regardless of the location of pulmonary resection (left vs. right). Cardiac herniation usually occurs in the early postoperative period and may be associated with a change in the patient's position. Signs and symptoms include increased venous pressure, sudden hypotension, tachycardia, displaced cardiac impulse, and cardiovascular collapse.[58]

Herniation can be identified on chest radiograph, and prompt surgical repair is required. Mortality from this complication is high at approximately 50%.[58]

Cardiac Tamponade. When the pericardium has been opened and closed during surgery, tamponade is a possibility. Undetected bleeding may occur in the pericardium. Signs and symptoms include hypotension, increased central venous pressure, a paradoxical pulse, and slowly developing cardiac failure. Treatment includes drainage of the fluid via a transthoracic, subxiphoid incision, or by a percutaneous catheter.

Neurologic Complications

Phrenic Nerve Injury. Although rare, injury to the phrenic nerve may occur during thoracic surgery. Most patients can tolerate a unilateral loss of diaphragmatic function and the resultant loss in ventilation, but in some with limited pulmonary reserve the consequences may be significant.[58]

Recurrent Laryngeal Nerve Injury. This injury occurs more frequently on the left side and results from injury during the surgery or invasion of tumor into the area of the aortopulmonary window. Right-sided injury is rare and is seen only in very extensive lymph node dissection. Unilateral damage to the nerve results in hoarseness and in some patients may cause problems with cough, aspiration, and secretion clearance. Treatment includes a "watch and wait" philosophy to see if the injury is transient because of traction on the nerve during surgery, or a minor procedure for medialization of the vocal cords may be performed.

Other Complications

Pulmonary Embolism. Pulmonary embolism occurs in between 1% and 5% of patients following thoracic surgery.[58] It is more frequent following pneumonectomy (right greater than left) than other types of thoracic surgeries. The usual site of origin is the lower extremities. The Institute for Clinical Systems Improvement published a patient algorithm for risk and prophylaxis of venous thromboembolism (Chapter 16).[41] Few studies are available to support specific prophylaxis regimens following thoracic surgery.[24] The American College of Chest Physicians 7th Consensus Conference recommended early initiation of prophylaxis; if elastic stockings or sequential compression devices (SCDs) are used, they should be applied before surgery and continued until the patient is ambulatory, with the same plan for the use of intermittent compression devices. There are several types of SCDs including foot, calf, and thigh-high compression as well as graduated, asymmetric, and circumferential compression.[8,51] Studies comparing foot, calf, and thigh-high compression found little difference in effectiveness. However, to achieve adequate compression, foot compression devices required pressures of 130 mm Hg, compared with 40 mm Hg necessary for calf compression. There is little evidence favoring the type of compression used.[1,61] Pharmacologic prophylaxis should be used in addition to mechanical means in patients undergoing thoracic surgery.

MULTIDISCIPLINARY CARE

Principles of Care

The goal of postoperative management is to prevent or minimize the effects of the most common problems that may lead to poor outcome.[48] Prevention begins in the preoperative setting. The Multidisciplinary Plan of Care on pp. 515-516 describes the aspects of multidisciplinary care of the thoracic surgery patient throughout the entire episode of care, beginning with preoperative preparation and ending with discharge from the hospital. Wright et al. identified the most common problems that delayed discharge from the hospital. These included inadequate pain control, prolonged air leak, severe nausea, fever, debility, and atrial dysrhythmia.[77] The most common reasons

patients are readmitted after thoracotomy include pulmonary complications, wound problems, cardiac complications, and deep venous thrombosis.[48]

Preoperative Preparation

Preoperative patient education is critical for the thoracic surgery population but is sometimes compromised because of lack of time or lack of personnel to prepare the patient and family. Written materials or some way to communicate information (web-based or CD, for example) is important, but nothing surpasses face-to-face discussion with a healthcare provider. Preparation includes preoperative teaching, "prehabilitation" with lung volume expansion maneuvers and exercises, smoking cessation, nutritional evaluation and repletion if possible, evaluation of preoperative medications, and psychological preparation of the patient. Psychological preparation of the patient includes realistic expectations of the immediate postoperative period, including the need for mechanical ventilation, functional compromise, and pain management, as well as expectations in the postoperative period. Long-term outcomes to address may include functional status, the potential need for supplemental oxygen, and expectations regarding the recovery from the surgery and specific needs following discharge.[75] A summary of key patient education topics is given in Box 21-2.

DRUGS AND DOSAGES FOR INTRAVENOUS PATIENT-CONTROLLED ANALGESIA (PCA)

	EQUIPOTENT DOSES	HALF-LIFE	IV PCA RANGES*	RECEPTOR	COMMENTS
Morphine	1 mg	2.5–3.5 hr	1–3 mg q 10 min	Alpha agonist	Histamine release
Hydromorphone (Dilaudid)	0.125 mg	2–3 hr	0.1–0.3 mg q 10 min	Alpha agonist	
Meperidine (Demerol)	8 mg	1.5–2.5 hr	10–25 mg q 10 min	Alpha and beta agonist	Rarely used because of risk of seizures in patients with renal insufficiency
Fentanyl (Sublimaze)	20 mcg	3 hr in steady state, but extreme lipophilicity makes first doses have shorter effect	15–35 mcg q 10 min	Alpha agonist	Preferred in patients with renal insufficiency

From reference 56.
*Doses are approximate and need to be adjusted for many factors, including but not limited to patient weight, age, central nervous system disease, concomitant medications, opioid tolerance, renal function, and hepatic function.

Key Preoperative Patient Education Topics in Thoracic Surgery

- General preoperative education
  - Verbal instruction
  - Written materials
  - Web-based material
  - Audio-visual material
- Specific procedure information
- Respiratory volume expansion maneuvers
  - Volume expansion maneuvers—incentive spirometry
  - Mobilization
- Secretion management techniques
  - Effective coughing techniques
- Smoking cessation
- Nutrition
- Pain management strategies
- Potential clinical research protocols

"Prehabilitation" has been advocated in patients deemed high-risk candidates for thoracic surgery. Goals are to optimize quality of life, functional capacity, and overall surgical outcomes.[71] Historically, presurgery rehabilitation and postoperative rehabilitation have been used with positive results in lung volume reduction surgery and lung transplantation. Lung resection surgery has been added to the list that may benefit from such a program. However, little information is available regarding descriptions of these programs, and minimal data exist to support the use of "prehabilitation" in patients undergoing lung resection surgery.[6,71,76] One reason that few data exist is due to the time constraint between diagnosis with NSCLC and the urgency of surgical resection. A modified or compressed rehabilitation needs to take place within a short period of time (2 to 3 weeks maximum) for this population and often is done in the outpatient or home setting.

Intraoperative Management

The type of surgical approach may affect the patient's pain and potentially length of stay. A muscle-sparing thoracotomy is less invasive than a standard posterolateral thoracotomy because it preserves the latissimus dorsi and serratus anterior muscles.[47] Even more so, compared with a thoracotomy, a VATS decreases the amount of chest wall involvement and decreases postoperative pain. In addition, following VATS, pulmonary function is less impaired compared to that after a thoracotomy.

VATS has been associated with improved postoperative immune response by reducing the body's inflammatory response, decreasing length of hospital stay, and producing an earlier return to normal functions as compared with a thoracotomy.[44,46,53]

Chest Drainage Management

Chest tubes and drainage systems are used to reexpand the lung and keep the lung expanded as well as to prevent the development of a space infection. In the past, all chest tubes were placed to suction at -20 cm H_2O; however, in more recent years this practice has been questioned.[4,13] An important role of the nurse is to assess the drainage tubes regularly for patency, function, air leak, and drainage. A functioning tube is one that shows fluctuation in the fluid within the tubing as the patient breathes quietly.[48] This demonstrates pressure changes within the pleural space.

Air leaks are best assessed by observing the water seal chamber drainage during quiet respiration off suction. The patient is requested to cough and the chamber is assessed. The suction can be applied and then the patient is requested to cough again. Air leaks are assessed by the amount of cough required to expel air. A small leak is one that is intermittent and may only be assessed while on suction. A large leak is a continuous air leak. Differing systems are made by different manufacturers. Some include a water seal and some are considered dry systems. In addition, the chest tube is evaluated for the extent of air leak and changes that may occur.

Cerfolio and colleagues have developed a qualitative and quantitative method to measure postoperative air leaks.[14,15] This classification system evaluates an air leak based on when it occurs in the respiratory cycle (qualitative) and how large the air leak appears (quantitative). The air leak is classified as continuous, inspiratory, expiratory, or forced expiratory, and the air leak is scored by evaluating in which chamber on the water seal drainage the bubbles from the air leak appear. Leaks are assigned a numerical value from 1 to 28.[14,15]

The amount, consistency, and character of drainage should be closely monitored. A change from sanguineous to serous is a good sign, while a change from sanguineous to purulent could indicate the development of an empyema or infection. Also, milky colored fluid may indicate a chylothorax.

Once air leak and drainage have decreased to acceptable levels, the chest tube can be removed. There is little evidence to guide this practice. Different criteria for removal of the tube are used by surgeons, ranging anywhere from 100 to 400 ml of drainage per 24 hours. Lack of an air leak and a volume of 100 to 150 ml of fluid output per 24 hours are often used as criteria that the chest tube may be removed while the patient performs a

Valsalva maneuver or during the expiratory phase of mechanical ventilation.[37,39] Routine chest radiographs are not necessary after uncomplicated chest tube removal, and the decision to reinsert a chest tube can be based on the patient's clinical examination.[37,39] Newer small chest drainage systems are available (500-ml capacity) that facilitate patient ambulation, and patients may be discharged home with such a device if drainage or an air leak persists.

Pain Management

Thoracic surgery can produce some of the most intense postoperative pain in the acute setting; it sometimes continues into a chronic problem as well. Pain is an area of great concern for patients in the postoperative setting.[56] Current treatment options for acute postoperative pain include epidural analgesia, intravenous patient-controlled analgesia, intercostal and paravertebral nerve blocks, and oral medications. A multimodality approach with a smooth transition between pain medications should be chosen with the focus of minimizing and preventing pain. The Department of Defense, Veterans Health Administration (DOD), has identified evidence-based pain management strategies in thoracic (noncardiac) surgery[22] (Box 21-3).

Several considerations must be taken into account when choosing a pain management regimen, route, frequency, and dosage of medications, such as the patient's medical history, age, and type of surgery. Systemic opioids administered intravenously via patient-controlled mechanisms are a mainstay for acute pain management. Typical medications used in patient-controlled analgesia are shown in the Medication table on p. 512. Epidural analgesia is frequently used in the postoperative setting. Studies have demonstrated that patients receiving epidural analgesia following thoracic surgery have less pain, are extubated sooner, have fewer pulmonary complications, and have decreased length of stay.[20,56] Questions remain regarding the optimal use of epidural analgesia and include optimal location for placement of the catheter, medications used, timing of the initiation of medications, use of patient control, and use of adjuvant analgesics.

A newer method of providing continuous infusion of local anesthetic is called the ON-Q catheter (ON-Q Pain Buster, I-Flow Corp., Lake Forest, Calif). This device delivers anesthetic to the surgical wound site to reduce postoperative pain. The device consists of a small balloon pump that holds a local anesthetic and delivers it through a small catheter directed into the surgical site at the end of surgery. This catheter can

---

Box 21-3

Evidence-Based Practice for Pain Management After Thoracic Surgery*

- Effective postoperative pain control may be achieved by delivering an opioid or a combination of opioid and local anesthetic into the thoracic epidural space.
- The addition of local anesthetic to epidural opioid allows a significant reduction in the total dose of opioid required to produce equivalent analgesia.
- Preoperative initiation of continuous local anesthetic epidural block has been associated with reduced long-term pain (at 6 months).
- There is no significant difference between epidural and intravenous administration of highly lipid-soluble opioids.
- Intrapleural local anesthetics can be delivered via catheter between the parietal and visceral pleurae and a local anesthetic can be injected every 4 to 6 hours or infused continuously to produce analgesia.

From reference 22.
*All of these interventions are categorized as I and A interventions.
I = evidence exists from studies of strong design for answering the question addressed; A = randomized, controlled trial.

---

be used alone or in conjunction with other pain management strategies.[74] At discharge, patients should be given explicit instructions regarding how and when to use these medications. Pain will exist during the recovery process, but adequate pain management should facilitate the patient's recovery by assisting in increasing ambulation and walking and improving the patient's mental outlook regarding progress.

Nutrition

Fluid management in the thoracic surgery patient is focused on limiting free water that may produce interstitial edema and limit oxygenation. During the first 24 to 48 hours, urine output will be lower than following other types of surgical procedures (concern if less than 20 ml/hr), and it is important to evaluate the patient's preoperative renal status. Fluid intake is monitored closely in the pneumonectomy patient to prevent fluid overload in the early postoperative period. Physiologically, the body has to adapt to the loss of 50% of the pulmonary capillary bed.

MULTIDISCIPLINARY PLAN OF CARE OF THE THORACIC SURGERY PATIENT

PROBLEM	INTERVENTION	RATIONALE	EXPECTED OUTCOME	COMMENT
Postoperative pulmonary dysfunction	Maintain mechanical ventilation as needed until criteria for extubation are met. Reintubate if patient experiences pulmonary compromise not responsive to immediate interventions. If high risk for complications, prophylactic tracheostomy during surgery. While on mechanical ventilation, head of bed elevated minimum of 30 degrees, higher if possible. Reposition frequently; turn a minimum of every 2 hr. Mobilization to chair as soon as possible, ambulate when possible. Once extubated, encourage volume expansion measures: incentive spirometry every 1–2 hr; if inspiratory volumes not adequate, consider other interventions (e.g., CPAP, PEP). Provide adequate analgesia to promote awareness, ability to follow commands without inducing respiratory depression. Aggressive secretion management interventions (i.e., suctioning, bronchoscopy if needed).	Early extubation decreases pulmonary complications (e.g., VAP). Thoracic surgery patient is at risk of rapidly occurring pulmonary compromise that may be life-threatening. Facilitate airway management and weaning from mechanical ventilation. Minimize risk factors for VAP. Repositioning, volume expansion maneuvers, and mobilization assist in secretion management, change V̇/Q̇ ratios in lung, and enhance ventilation to reverse/minimize atelectasis, pneumonia. Oversedation may lead to slow weaning from mechanical ventilation and potential need to reintubate. Thoracic surgery patients are at high risk for retention of secretions, blockage of airways.	Low incidence of acute respiratory failure, VAP. Decrease in pulmonary complications. Decrease in critical care and total length of stay in hospital. Maintain Sao_2 greater than 92%.	
Pain	Closely evaluate Sao_2 and hemodynamics with any changes in positioning or interventions. Evaluate patient's preoperative pain management (if applicable). Assess level of pain every 1–2 hr using a reliable/valid scale; once extubated,	At risk of pulmonary and hemodynamic compromise with changes in positioning. Pain from thoracic surgery is often profound and protracted. In addition to resected lung tissue, pain further decreases pulmonary function,	Adequate pain management as gauged by pain scale. Alert and able to follow commands and participate in activities. Adequate pain	

Table continues on page 516

PROBLEM	INTERVENTION	RATIONALE	EXPECTED OUTCOME	COMMENT
Pain, *continued*	assess pain at rest and with activities (i.e., volume expansion maneuvers, mobilization). Use multimodal analgesia regimens.	leading to atelectasis, pneumonia, and potentially acute respiratory failure. Pain may also affect stress response of other systems. Multimodal strategies may target different pain pathways and provide optimal pain management.	management as patient transitions through episode of care to oral pain medications.	
Deep venous thrombosis leading to pulmonary embolism	Assess for patient risk factors for DVT. Initiate thromboprophylaxis as soon as risk of DVT begins (preoperatively or intraoperatively). Application of mechanical means of thromboprophylaxis: graduated compression stockings, intermittent pneumatic compression devices. Continue mechanical means until patient is fully ambulatory. Use of pharmacologic thromboprophylaxis: unfractionated heparin, low molecular weight heparin. (Chapter 9 provides detailed information about prevention of DVT.)	Early initiation of thromboprophylaxis will prevent or minimize risk of DVT and development of pulmonary embolism.	Low incidence of DVT and pulmonary embolism.	

CPAP = Continuous positive airway pressure, DVT = deep venous thrombosis, PEP = positive expiratory pressure, Sao$_2$ = arterial oxygen saturation, VAP = ventilator-associated pneumonia, V/Q = ventilation/perfusion.

Depending upon the surgical procedure and the progress of the patient following extubation, the patient may begin oral fluids with a quick transition to a regular diet. Patients should be monitored closely for sedation, overzealous pain management, and the potential for aspiration. Roberts et al. studied patients undergoing thoracic operations and found that pre-emptive gastrointestinal tract management (nothing by mouth [NPO] the day of surgery, clear liquids on day 1, and regular diet on day 2) reduced the incidence of aspiration and respiratory failure versus patients who had nutritional orders to "advance as tolerated."[63]

Pneumonectomy patients are generally kept NPO for 24 to 48 hours because of risk of aspiration resulting from mediastinal shift, diaphragmatic elevation, alteration of the esophageal hiatus, and possible damage to the vagus and recurrent laryngeal nerves.[39] For complex patients with hemodynamic instability, ventilatory dependency, preoperative cachexia, and those expected to be NPO for greater than 48 hours, early nutrition should be established via enteral or parenteral routes.[39]

Mechanical Ventilation

Following thoracic surgery, the goal is to extubate the patient in the operating room if at all possible.[37,39] However, high-risk patients may require continued intubation and ventilatory support. Potential indications for mechanical ventilation following thoracic surgery include the following: poor preoperative pulmonary function (predicted postoperative FEV_1 less than 30%), prolonged intraoperative course, massive fluid administration or blood infusions under anesthesia, cardiac failure, need for postoperative chest wall immobilization/stabilization, inadequate respiratory drive or incomplete recovery of neuromuscular function, FiO_2 requirement greater than 0.50 or 50%, and visible respiratory distress.[39] In addition, specific types of surgery may require mechanical ventilation in the postoperative period in order to facilitate healing and recovery (e.g., tracheal resection, sleeve resection, pneumonectomy).

The specific ventilatory needs of the patient will dictate the mode of ventilation; however, the most common mode of ventilation used in the thoracic surgical patient postoperatively is spontaneous intermittent mandatory ventilation (SIMV) with pressure support ventilation (PSV). Additional information on mechanical ventilation and weaning can be found in Chapter 20.

Respiratory Care

Early extubation is a priority in the thoracic surgery patient to minimize the risk of ventilator-associated pneumonia and to speed the recovery process. Following extubation, it is critical to promote frequent volume expansion maneuvers (e.g., incentive spirometry, continuous positive airway pressure). Atelectasis is a common complication following thoracic surgery and if left untreated can potentially lead to pneumonia.

Secretion management is also key in this population. Vigilant observation and management of the secretions regarding amount, color, and consistency are important. If standard secretion management techniques do not help to clear the airways, then more aggressive measures such as bronchoscopy are indicated. Positioning may cause an increase in secretions, and the patient must be closely monitored when changing positions.

Continuous lateral rotation therapy may be of assistance in this population as well. If the patient requires prolonged ventilation, this intervention may be considered.

Mobilization

Early mobilization and ambulation are important in the thoracic surgery patient, as they are in any postoperative patient. Mobilization helps to increase ventilation, improve ventilation/perfusion, enhance secretion clearance, prevent lower extremity blood stasis, and build stamina in the recovering patient.

Along with mobilization in the postoperative period, it is important for patients to begin physical therapy exercises, both passive and active. Before discharge, the patient should be instructed regarding basic upper extremity and shoulder exercises to assist in mobilization on the operated side. In addition, the patient should be provided with a progressive walking program with daily goals. The triad for optimal postoperative management to prevent pulmonary complications includes optimal pain management, volume expansion/secretion management, and early mobilization.

Critical Pathway

Critical pathways have been designed to guide postoperative care and facilitate early discharge. Table 21-8 shows one example of a clinical pathway for pulmonary resection. Cerfolio et al. demonstrated that in 500 consecutive pulmonary resections they were able to improve quality and cost-effectiveness by streamlining care with use of a critical pathway.[12] By scrutinizing all aspects of the episode of care, inevitably areas can be identified for improvement in this population.

TABLE 21-8 Sample Clinical Pathway for Elective Pulmonary Resection

	PREOPERATIVE	DAY OF OPERATION	POSTOPERATIVE DAY 1	POSTOPERATIVE DAY 2	POSTOPERATIVE DAYS 3–4
Education	Expected course, possible complications	Review pathway*	Review pathway, discharge plans	Review pathway, discharge plans	Discharge instructions
Interventions	Smoking cessation	Muscle-sparing thoracotomy or VATS, extubate in OR, transfer to floor if stable	Discontinue central line, wean O_2, place chest tube to water seal	Discontinue epidural, Foley 8 hr later, first chest tube if no air leak	Discontinue second chest tube if no air leak and output <400 ml/day; if air leak use Heimlich valve
Assessment	History and physical examination	Monitor chest tube output, cardiac rhythm	O_2 saturation	O_2 saturation	Adequate oxygenation, pain control
Tests	Preoperative laboratory tests, pulmonary function tests	Laboratory tests PRN, chest x-ray	Laboratory tests PRN, chest x-ray	Laboratory tests PRN, chest x-ray	Laboratory tests PRN, chest x-ray
Activity	Exercise program if appropriate	Ambulate with assistance	Ambulate, physical therapy consult PRN	Ambulate	Ambulate
Medications	Nicotine patch PRN	Preoperative antibiotics, epidural, incentive spirometer	Inhalers, chest PT, anti-emetics PRN, discontinue antibiotics	Oral pain medication PRN	Oral pain medication PRN
Nutrition	NPO after midnight	Evening after operation: full liquids	Resume preoperative diet		
Discharge planning	Identify patients for case manager	Confirm home support	Identify need for rehabilitation or home oxygen		Set up close follow-up visit

From reference 47.
*Clinical pathways are general guidelines, and variances in individual patient needs and responses are to be expected.
NPO = Nothing by mouth, OR = operating room, PRN = as needed, PT = physical therapy, VATS = video-assisted thoracic surgery.

Case Study 21-1, Part C

Pulmonary Resection

M.R. wanted to think about the options of surgery. After a long discussion with the patient and his wife regarding the risk of right pneumonectomy with a bronchoplasty procedure, surgical resection was selected. M.R. was admitted the morning of surgery for a rigid bronchoscopy, right upper lobe sleeve lobectomy (possible pneumonectomy), prophylactic tracheostomy, and gastrostomy tube. The following procedures were performed: right thoracotomy, resection of the right sixth rib, right upper lobectomy with an extended sleeve bronchoplasty with complete peribronchial and mediastinal lymph node dissection, temporary prophylactic tracheostomy, and gastrostomy.

Decision point: Why would a temporary tracheostomy be placed in M.R?

Decision point: What are the potential postoperative complications (pulmonary and nonpulmonary) M.R. may experience?

Once M.R. was in critical care, he received 2 units of blood for a low hematocrit (Hct). On several occasions (4), he had a flexible bronchoscopy for retained secretions. He remained on mechanical ventilation for 8 days and was slowly weaned. His chest tube was removed on postoperative day 9. After a slow recovery, he was discharged from the hospital on supplemental oxygen. He was to return to the hospital in 1 week for an outpatient bronchoscopy. His final pathology demonstrated the presence of NSCLC involving the right upper lobe, with an unusual area of endobronchial metastasis.

One might expect that M.R. would have some difficulty in weaning from mechanical ventilation (poor pulmonary function, smoking history, type of surgery, nutritional status). The tracheostomy assisted with the secretion management and weaning; however, several bronchoscopy procedures were still required. Also, since MR had a history of alcohol intake on a daily basis, he was under precautions for withdrawal. He had a gastrostomy tube placed during surgery, so he received nutritional support in the postoperative period. Several months later, M.R. was re-admitted for a completion pneumonectomy because of a continuing bronchial anastomotic stricture. He had undergone more than 15 bronchoscopy procedures since his original surgery for continuing anastomotic stricture. The procedure performed was a redo right thoracotomy, completion extrapleural pneumonectomy with cardiopulmonary bypass standby, placement on an ON-Q pump for pain management, and flexible bronchoscopy. He left the operating room intubated and was returned to critical care on mechanical ventilation. A red rubber tube was inserted for 24 hours in the residual pleural space for drainage; it was then removed. He remained on the ventilator for 6 days and was slowly, but successfully, extubated on postoperative day 7. He was discharged from the hospital on oxygen, ambulating with the help of a walker.

Decision point: What issues may M.R. face in the immediate postoperative period?

Decision point: Given M.R.'s long and complicated hospitalizations, what issues may need to be addressed before discharge?

ESOPHAGEAL SURGERIES

ESOPHAGEAL DISEASE

The esophagus is approximately 23 to 25 cm long and is a long muscular channel. It extends from the pharynx inferiorly to the stomach. Anatomically it originates in the neck at the inferior border of C6, descends anteriorly to the vertebral column, passes through the superior and posterior mediastinum and then through the diaphragm, and enters the abdomen opposite T11. The narrowest part of the esophagus is where it passes into the diaphragm.

Other structures located near the esophagus and sometimes involved in surgery include the recurrent laryngeal nerves, ascending between the esophagus and the trachea (tracheoesophageal groove), and the thoracic duct, located on the left side of the esophagus. The thoracic duct carries the majority of the lymph and chyle into the blood and is the end point for most of the lymphatic vessels of the body except for some of the vessels on the right side. Both of these structures may be involved or injured during the surgical process.

Important in esophageal cancer are the layers of the esophagus. The esophagus has four layers: mucosa, submucosa, muscularis propria, and adventitia. Part of the staging process for esophageal cancer includes determining the extent of mucosal invasion of the tumor with an endoscopic ultrasound. Where the esophagus enters the stomach is the gastroesophageal junction. This area is often involved in adenocarcinoma of the esophagus. There are multiple regional lymph nodes surrounding the esophagus as well as nonregional nodes that are assessed in the staging process (e.g., celiac, cervical).

Esophageal disorders may be malignant (esophageal cancer) or benign. Esophageal cancer will be discussed in more detail in the next section, with a brief review of benign esophageal disease at the end of the chapter.

ESOPHAGEAL CANCER

Esophageal cancer is the second most common solid intrathoracic malignancy behind lung cancer. In 2005 there were an estimated 14,500 new cases of cancer of the esophagus (11,200 men and 3300 women). In the same year, it was estimated that 13,500 would die from this disease.[42] The two main histologic types of esophageal cancer are squamous cell and adenocarcinoma, which account for more than 90% of these cancers.[26] Squamous cell is usually located in the upper two thirds of the esophagus; adenocarcinoma is found in the distal third and in the gastroesophageal junction. While the incidence of squamous cell carcinoma has remained relatively stable over the past 30 years, the incidence of adenocarcinoma of the esophagus has increased rapidly at an alarming rate.[21] It now accounts for more than half of all esophageal cancers.[21] Barrett's esophagus is thought to be a precursor to esophageal adenocarcinoma. Associations have been demonstrated between Caucasian race, increasing age, increased frequency and duration of gastroesophageal reflux disease, and an increased incidence of Barrett's esophagus.[21]

Esophageal cancer occurs in mid to late adulthood, and the rates rise with age. This cancer is 2.7 times more common in males than in females. Squamous cell cancer is more prevalent in African-American males, while Caucasian males have a higher prevalence of adenocarcinoma. Risk factors of squamous cell carcinoma include smoking, alcohol intake, diet, and nutritional deficiencies. In the United States, the two common predisposing factors are tobacco consumption and heavy alcohol intake, and these two risk factors exhibit a multiplicative effect. Barrett's esophagus is a risk factor for adenocarcinoma, and the risk is further increased with smoking.

Diagnosis

The diagnosis of esophageal cancer is usually done via an esophagogastroduodenoscopy (EGD). The patient is instrumented with a flexible endoscope, and the lining of the esophagus can be directly visualized for abnormalities and biopsies taken. A CT scan of the chest and abdomen is done to grossly evaluate tumor size and invasion of adjacent structures, potential nodal involvement, and metastatic disease to the chest and abdomen. An endoscopic esophageal ultrasound (EUS) is a staging technique and has provided a significant advancement in the evaluation of esophageal cancer. The EUS provides specific information regarding the depth of tumor invasion through the wall of the esophagus and the lymph nodes involved in proximity to the gastrointestinal wall. With this technique, lymph nodes proximal to the esophagus can be biopsied. A variety of other scans may be used to assess for metastasis of the cancer. These may include bone scans, abdominal scans, PET scans, fusion CT/PET scans, and liver ultrasound. PET scans are now widely used as part of the staging process.

As with lung cancer, esophageal cancer is staged by the TNM system. The T evaluates the tumor invasion

through the wall of the esophagus, the N evaluates lymph node involvement, and the M is metastasis. Once esophageal cancer develops, it may spread rapidly. At the time of diagnosis, more than 50% of patients have either unresectable disease or metastases.[26] The overall survival at 5 years for esophageal cancer is approximately 14%. Five-year survival rates for the differing stages are as follows: stage I, 50%–80%; stage IIA, 30%–40%; stage IIB, 10%–30%; stage III, 10%–15%. Stage IV disease has a median survival of less than 1 year.[26]

Esophageal Resection Procedures

Patients who present with localized esophageal cancer are treated with surgery alone or with neoadjuvant chemoradiation therapy followed by surgery. Differing surgical procedures can be used to perform an esophagectomy (removal of all or part of the esophagus) or esophagogastrectomy (removal of all or part of the esophagus and removal of a portion of the gastric cardia). Esophagectomy may also be performed following damage to the esophagus from caustic injuries or achalasia that does not respond to more conservative medical or surgical management.

The surgery is most commonly performed through an open approach; however, thoracoscopic and robotic procedures are also done. No single esophagectomy approach is ideally suited for all patients. There is controversy regarding the optimal surgical approach and the extent and need of regional lymph node dissection. The four common surgical approaches for an esophagectomy are the Ivor-Lewis, 3-field, thoracoabdominal approach, and transhiatal approach (blunt dissection of the thoracic esophagus). Usually, the stomach or remaining portion of the stomach is pulled up to take the place of the esophagus (gastric pull-up) (Figure 21-7). However, colon and jejunum may also be used. Table 21-9 describes the approaches and explains why a specific approach may be chosen. The video-assisted thoracoscopic esophagectomy is performed with the patient in the left lateral position and usually four trocars are inserted.[19] The Research Utilization box on p. 522 discusses postoperative morbidity and mortality associated with esophageal resection.

Preoperative Evaluation

An esophageal resection is a major thoracic procedure and a patient must be thoroughly evaluated to determine surgical candidacy. Factors to consider regarding surgical risk include age, pulmonary function, cardiac function, nutritional status, presence of preoperative chemotherapy or radiation therapy, and the patient's understanding of the complexity and long-term recovery from the surgery.

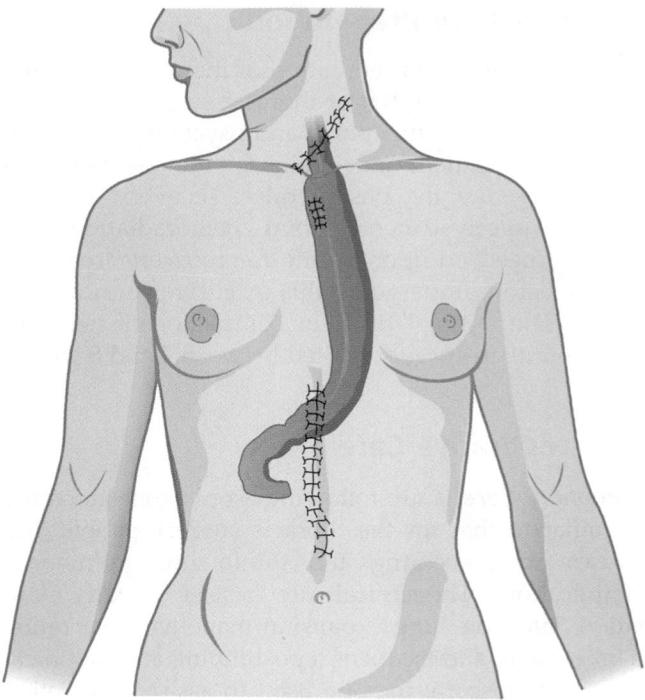

◆FIGURE 21-7 Gastric conduit placement after transhiatal esophagectomy.

Although age is difficult to set as a criterion, the age of greater than or equal to 70 years has been identified as an indicator of increased risk by some patients.[25,31] Pulmonary complications are the most common complication following esophagectomy and result in increased length of stay, increased morbidity, and increased mortality. Potential reasons the patient is at increased risk include the opening into two body cavities, disruption of the lymphatic system, disruption of pulmonary muscles, placement of a conduit in the chest, and potential recurrent laryngeal nerve injury.[25] Preexisting impaired pulmonary function, smoking history, alcohol abuse, and poor functional status all contribute to potential complications. As with pulmonary resection surgery, careful evaluation of pulmonary and cardiac function is important.

Weight loss and dysphagia are common presenting symptoms in esophageal cancer. Poor nutrition, decreased immune function as a result of poor nutrition or preoperative chemotherapy or radiation therapy, and decreased functional status may all contribute to poor outcomes. An extensive nutritional evaluation should be performed and preoperative nutritional supplementation considered orally or via a jejunal feeding tube or percutaneous gastrostomy tube. Optimizing nutritional status before surgery is important.

TABLE 21-9 Description of Approaches for Esophageal Resection

APPROACH	DESCRIPTION	ADVANTAGES	DISADVANTAGES
Ivor-Lewis	Laparotomy and right thoracotomy; Broadly applicable to differing tumor sites	Precise esophageal and lymph node dissection under direct vision; Anastomosis in chest (low incidence of leaks); Infrequent recurrent laryngeal nerve injury	Anastomosis in chest (leaks may be highly morbid); Pain from thoracotomy
3-Field	Ivor-Lewis approach plus left cervical incision	Precise esophageal and lymph node dissection under direct vision; Anastomosis in neck	Pain from thoracotomy
Thoracoabdominal	Combined laparotomy and left thoracotomy; Best suited for tumors of gastric cardia	Excellent exposure to stomach and distal esophagus	Painful incision; Anastomosis in chest
Transhiatal	Laparotomy and left cervical incision; Best suited for tumor of distal esophagus, but may be used for mid-thoracic tumors	Near-total esophagectomy; Anastomosis in neck (less severe leaks)	Imprecision in esophageal and lymph node dissection; Reduced pain (no thoracotomy); Risk of recurrent laryngeal nerve injury

◆ RESEARCH UTILIZATION

Reducing Morbidity and Mortality From Respiratory Complications After Esophagectomy

CLINICAL ISSUE

An esophagectomy is a complex procedure with significant morbidity and mortality. Respiratory complications—including respiratory insufficiency, pneumonia, and potential aspiration because of swallowing disorders—are widely recognized problems following esophagectomy.

SUMMARY

This study identified prognostic variables that might be used to optimize care and outcomes following esophagectomy. These investigators reviewed the medical records of approximately 400 patients who underwent an esophagectomy. Operative mortality was 5.8%, and 64% experienced complications (pulmonary, 28.5%; anastomotic stricture, 25%; and anastomotic leak, 14%). Increasing age, anastomotic leak, a higher comorbidity index, poor swallowing scores, and pneumonia were all associated with increased risk of mortality. However, in the multivariate analysis only age ($P = 0.002$) and pneumonia ($P = 0.0008$) were independently associated with mortality. Pneumonia in this sample was associated with a 20% incidence of death.

APPLICATION

A multidisciplinary approach is needed among nursing, medicine, respiratory care, speech therapy, and physical therapy to prevent these pulmonary complications. Interventions include early extubation and avoidance of prolonged mechanical ventilation to prevent ventilator-associated pneumonia; use of the ventilator bundle to prevent ventilator-associated pneumonia; intensive respiratory care following extubation, including voluntary expansion maneuvers (use of incentive spirometry); secretion management; adequate pain management to facilitate secretion management and mobilization; early mobilization of patients to improve ventilation and perfusion of the lungs and to mobilize secretions; and assessment of swallowing abnormalities that might lead to aspiration.

NEED FOR FURTHER STUDY

Understanding those physiologic variables placing patients at risk for complications following different types of surgery would be helpful in establishing best practices for postoperative care.

Atkins, Z., Shah, A., Hutcheson, K., et al. (2004). Reducing hospital morbidity and mortality following esophagectomy. *Ann Thorac Surg, 78,* 1170–1176.

Preoperative Preparation

The preoperative preparation of the esophagectomy patient is similar to that of thoracic surgery, with key elements being the functional and psychological preparation of the patient and family for the complexity of the surgery and the postoperative recovery. Patients who have received neoadjuvant chemoradiation therapy may need additional time for recovery from this therapy before undergoing this extensive surgical procedure. The optimal time for completion of neoadjuvant therapy to surgery is cited between 4 and 8 weeks.

Postoperative Care

Pulmonary Care. Care following esophagogastrectomy is similar to that for the thoracic surgery patient and focuses on preventing and minimizing pulmonary complications. The clinical care focuses on early extubation, intensive lung expansion maneuvers, secretion management, and frequent repositioning and mobilization. Bronchoscopy may be used to assist in secretion management.

Gastrointestinal Care. The patient is maintained on an NPO status for usually 5 to 7 days after surgery and a nasogastric tube is in place. The nasogastric tube should be well secured and placed on intermittent suction. The tube should be checked regularly to make sure it is not obstructed. On postoperative day 5 to 7, the patient is tested by using a Gastrografin swallow or EGD to assess the anastomotic integrity, and the nasogastric tube may then be pulled. Oral intake is subsequently started on an incremental basis, beginning with liquids and then slowly progressing to solids. Surgeon preference determines when solid foods are started. Some surgeons will also have a jejunostomy tube in place, and feeding will commence once the nasogastric tube is removed.

Depending upon the surgical technique used, the patient may have one or two chest tubes in place. These patients are managed similarly to thoracic surgery patients with chest tubes. If a cervical incision has been made, the patient may also have a drain placed and the amount and type of drainage should be noted every 8 hours. Lastly, early mobilization of the patient is important, just as it is with thoracic surgery patients.

Pain Management. Pain management techniques are similar to those used in thoracic surgery. With the differing esophageal approaches, pain may be an important issue in the recovery of the patient. Pain management is also key in assisting the patient in the progression of mobilization and frequent ambulation.

Discharge Instructions. The major areas to cover in patient and family education and nutritional support before discharge are listed in Box 21-4 and in the Nutrition box below. These areas are key in facilitating the recovery of the patient with realistic expectations.

Box 21-4

Key Postoperative Patient Education Topics in Esophageal Resection

- Nutrition
  - Caloric intake
  - Choice of foods
  - Delayed gastric emptying and reflux
  - Dumping syndrome and diarrhea
- Pain management
- Mobilization—progressive ambulation
- Dysphagia
- Psychological support

♦ NUTRITION

Nutritional Considerations for Esophageal Resection

- Patient should eat in a relaxed state while sitting up and avoid eating 3 hours before bedtime to avoid reflux.
- Patient may expect weight loss following discharge as the body adapts to the new gastrointestinal conduit.
- Weight should be monitored at home and reported to the healthcare provider at visits or phone follow-ups.
- Foods may not taste or smell appealing as a result of anesthesia and chemotherapy. With time, normal taste and smell will return.
- Appetite may be poor and food intake may be a difficult topic at times, and patient will require strong support from caregivers.
- Increasing activities will help to stimulate appetite and gastrointestinal motility.
- Predischarge nutritional education by the dietitian is key:
  - Need to eat multiple (6) small meals per day
  - Information regarding dumping syndrome and avoidance of concentrated sweets, which may cause postprandial diarrhea
  - Intake of high-calorie foods and liquid supplementation if necessary
  - Consultation via phone with dietitian once patient is discharged

Complications Related to Esophageal Surgery

The morbidity and mortality following esophagectomy are high because of the complexity of the surgery. Mortality rates at major centers range from 3% to 7%.[25] The major complications following esophagectomy are primarily pulmonary in origin, with pulmonary complications accounting for 25% to 35% of complications in some series.[25,67] In addition, respiratory failure is a significant cause of death.

Complications following esophagectomy are listed in Box 21-5. Pulmonary complications related to esophagectomy are similar to those seen following thoracic surgery, and the reader should review the previous information presented in the chapter. Patient risk factors and the complexity of the procedure performed (minimally invasive vs. 3-port) may also predict the degree of pulmonary complications.[45]

Anastomotic Leaks. Anastomotic leakage is a problem after esophagectomy. Cervical anastomotic leaks may occur and gastric drainage may be noted at the cervical incision or through the drain. Usually, the cervical incision is opened and wound care administered. Cervical anastomotic leak usually heals with conservative approaches and rarely requires surgical closure. Conservative management of an anastomotic leak would include radiologic confirmation of leak, restriction of oral intake, decompression with nasogastric tube, provision of enteral or parenteral nutrition, and administration of antibiotics as indicated. Intrathoracic leaks present a more complex problem. They are less likely to heal spontaneously, and definitive surgical repair may be necessary.

Box 21-5

Complications Associated With Esophageal Resection

- Anastomotic leak
- Anastomotic stricture
- Cardiovascular complications
  - Atrial dysrhythmias
  - Myocardial infarction
- Pulmonary complications
  - Acute respiratory failure
  - Pneumonia
  - Acute respiratory distress syndrome
  - Empyema
  - Aspiration
- Recurrent laryngeal nerve injury

Anastomotic Stricture. Although often not considered a complication, anastomotic strictures occur following esophagectomy. Strictures are cited as frequently as in 30% to 50% of patients in the first 3 months following surgery.[59] This is due to scar tissue formation at the site of the anastomosis. Patients complain of increasing dysphagia or food "sticking." Treatment includes an endoscopy with dilation of the stricture site. Some patients may require many dilations during the initial postoperative period following discharge.

Necrosis of Conduit. Rarely, there is ischemia with necrosis of the conduit (stomach, colon, or jejunum) because of poor blood flow. Signs include septic toxemia, fever, and foul-smelling secretions. Endoscopy is used to confirm the diagnosis. Once identified, the patient is returned to surgery and the conduit removed. A cervical esophagostomy is performed in which the stomach and the esophageal stump are closed and the remainder of the esophagus is exteriorized at the neck. An appliance is placed over the opening for drainage of saliva and secretions. A feeding tube is placed (often jejunal), and placement is dependent upon which area will be used for the subsequent reconstruction of the esophagus. Reconstruction is not attempted for at least 3 to 6 months following this event.

Other Esophageal Surgery

Disorders of esophageal motility are benign in origin. Achalasia is a motor disorder of the esophagus characterized by functional obstruction of the distal esophagus because of incomplete relaxation of the lower esophageal sphincter. This causes a lack of progressive peristalsis in the body of the esophagus. Secondary achalasia (pseudoachalasia) may be caused by a distal obstruction (carcinoma, lymphoma) or be neuropathic in origin. Assessment for achalasia includes a thorough history and physical, barium swallow (demonstrates a bird's beak appearance of esophagus), and esophageal manometry. Symptoms include dysphagia, regurgitation of undigested food, and retrosternal pain. Surgical treatment is usually attempted following failed medical management. Surgical treatment includes an esophagomyotomy, which has a success rate between 75% and 90%.[62] A short 5- to 7-cm myotomy or cutting of the muscle is performed on the distal esophagus. A variety of approaches may be used to accomplish a myotomy: VATS, laparoscopic incision, left thoracotomy, or laparotomy.

Esophageal diverticula are pouches arising from the esophageal lumen. Zenker's diverticulum is the most commonly recognized of the esophageal diverticula. Symptoms include dysphagia, halitosis, retrosternal pain, alterations in voice tone or character, and coughing or wheezing following episodes of aspiration.[60] Treatment of Zenker's diverticulum is a cricopharyngeal myotomy.

CONCLUSIONS

The thoracic surgery patient provides both challenges and opportunities for the experienced critical care nurse to combine both advanced knowledge of pathophysiology and specific interventions to prevent or minimize complications following surgery. In addition, the preoperative education of the patient and the preoperative evaluation of risk are crucial to guiding the care of this population.

REFERENCES

1. Agu, O., Hamilton, G., & Baker, D. (1999). Graduated compression stocking in the prevention of venous thromboembolism. *Brit J Surg, 86*, 992–1004.
2. American Joint Committee on Cancer (AJCC). (2002). *Cancer staging manual* (6th ed.). New York: Springer-Verlag.
3. American Thoracic Society. (2005). Guidelines for the management of adults with hospital-acquired, ventilator-associated, and healthcare-associated pneumonia. *Am J Respir Crit Care Med, 171*, 388–416.
4. Antanavicius, G., Lamb, J., Papasavas, P., et al. (2005). Initial chest tube management after pulmonary resection. *Am Surgeon, 71*, 416–419.
5. Baldwin, P. D. (2003). Lung cancer. *Clin J Oncol Nurs, 7*, 699–702.
6. Bisson, A., Stern, M., & Caubarrere, I. (1998). Preparation of high-risk patients for major thoracic surgery. *Chest Surg Clin North Am, 8*, 541–555.
7. Bonde, P., Papachristos, I., McCraith, A., et al. (2002). Sputum retention after lung operation: prospective, randomized trial shows superiority of prophylactic minitracheostomy in high-risk patients. *Ann Thorac Surg, 74*, 196–203.
8. Byrne, B. (2001). Deep vein thrombosis: the effectiveness and implications of using below knee or thigh-length graduated compression stockings. *Heart Lung, 30*, 277–284.
9. Cardinale, D., Martinoni, A., Cipolla, C. M., et al. (1999). Atrial fibrillation after operation for lung cancer: clinical and prognostic significance. *Ann Thorac Surg, 68*, 1827–1831.
10. Centers for Medicare and Medicaid Services. (2004). *National coverage determination for lung volume reduction surgery.* Jan 1, 2004.
11. Cerfolio, R. J., Tummala, R. P., Holman, W. L., et al. (1998). A prospective algorithm for the management of air leaks after pulmonary resection. *Ann Thorac Surg, 66*, 1726–1731.
12. Cerfolio, R. J., Pickens, A., Bass, C., et al. (2001). Fast-tracking pulmonary resections. *J Thorac Cardiovasc Surg, 122*, 318–323.
13. Cerfolio, R. J., Bass, C., Katholi, C. R., et al. (2001). A prospective randomized trial compares suction versus water seal for air leaks. *Ann Thorac Surg, 71*, 1613–1617.
14. Cerfolio, R. J. (2002). Chest tube management after pulmonary resection. *Chest Surg Clin North Am, 12*, 507–527.
15. Cerfolio, R. J. (2002). Advances in thoracostomy tube management. *Surg Clin North Am, 82*, 833–848.
16. Cerfolio, R. J., Bryant, A. S., Singh, S., et al. (2005). The management of chest tubes in patients with a pneumothorax and an air leak after pulmonary resection. *Chest, 128*, 816–820.

17. Chastre, J., & Fagon, J. Y. (2003). Ventilator-associated pneumonia. *Am J Respir Crit Care Med, 165*, 867–903.

18. Curtis, J. J., Parker, B. M., McKenney, C. A., et al. (1998). Incidence and predictors of supraventricular dysrhythmias after pulmonary resection. *Ann Thorac Surg, 66*, 1766–1771.

19. deHoyos, A., Litle, V. R., & Luketich, R. (2005). Minimally invasive esophagectomy. *Surg Clin North Am, 85*, 531–647.

20. deLima, N. F., & Carvalho, A. L. (2003). Early discharge following major thoracic surgery: identification of related factors. *Rev Port Pneumol, 9*, 205–213.

21. Dellon, E. S., & Shaheen, J. J. (2005). Does screening for Barrett's esophagus and adenocarcinoma of the esophagus prolong survival? *J Clin Oncol, 23*, 4478–4482.

22. Department of Defense, Veterans Administration Hospital. (2002). *Clinical practice guideline for the management of postoperative pain. Version 1.2.* Washington, DC: Department of Defense, Veterans Health Administration.

23. Deslauriers, J., & LeBlanc, P. (2005). Emphysema of the lung and lung volume reduction operations. In T. Shields, J. Locicero III, R. Ponn, et al. (Eds.), *General thoracic surgery* (6th ed.). Philadelphia: Lippincott Williams & Wilkins.

24. Donahue, D. M. (2005). Pulmonary embolism prophylaxis: evidence for utility in thoracic surgery. *Thorac Surg Clin, 15*, 237–242.

25. Donnington, J. S. (2005). Preoperative preparation for esophageal surgery. *Thorac Surg Clin, 15*, 277–285.

26. Enzinger, P. C., & Mayer, R. J. (2003). Esophageal cancer. *N Engl J Med, 349*, 2241–2252.

27. Faber, L. P. (2005). Sleeve lobectomy. In T. Shields, J. Locicero III, R. Ponn, et al. (Eds.), *General thoracic surgery* (6th ed.). Philadelphia: Lippincott Williams & Wilkins.

28. Fabian, T., Federico, J. A., & Ponn, R. B. (2003). Fibrin glue in pulmonary resection: a prospective, randomized blinded study. *Ann Thorac Surg, 75*, 1587–1592.

29. Fell, S. C. (1999). A history of pneumonectomy. *Chest Surg Clin North Am, 9*, 267–290.

30. Ferguson, M. (2005). Pulmonary physiologic assessment of operative risk. In T. Shields, J. Locicero III, R. Ponn, et al. (Eds.), *General thoracic surgery* (6th ed.). Philadelphia: Lippincott Williams & Wilkins.

31. Ferguson, M. K., & Durkin, A. E. (2002). Preoperative prediction of the risk of pulmonary complications after esophagectomy for cancer. *J Thorac Cardiovasc Surg, 123*, 661–669.

32. Flores, R. M. (2003). *VATS lobectomy for early stage lung cancer.* CTSNet,www.ctsnet.org.

33. Flummerfelt, P. M. (2001). Tumors of the mediastinum. In H. L. Karamanoukian, P. R. Soltoski & T. A. Salerno (Eds.), *Thoracic surgery secrets.* Philadelphia: Hanley & Belfus.

34. Geerts, W. H., Pineo, G. F., Heit, J. A., et al. (2004). Prevention of venous thromboembolism: the 7th ACCP conference on antithrombotic and thrombolytic therapy. *Chest, 126*(3 suppl), 338S–400S.

35. Global Initiative for Chronic Obstructive Lung Disease (GOLD), World Health Organization (WHO), National Heart, Lung and Blood Institute (NHLBI). (2004). *Global strategy for the diagnosis, management, and prevention of chronic obstructive pulmonary disease* (100 pages). Bethesda, Md: GOLD, WHO, and NHLBI.

36. Green, M. R., Andrews, M., Leff, R., et al. (2005). Adjuvant therapy choices in patients with resected non-small-cell lung cancer: correlation of doctor's treatment plans and relevant phase III trial data. *J Oncol Pract, 1*, 37–42.

37. Hartigan, P. M., Body, S. C., & Sugarbaker, D. J. (2005). Pulmonary resection. In J. A. Kaplan & P. D. Slinger (Eds.), *Thoracic anesthesia* (3rd ed.). Philadelphia: Churchill Livingstone.

38. Hetzel, J., Hetzel, M., & Babiak, A. (2005). Staging and early diagnosis of patients with non-small cell lung cancer. *New Directions Treatment Lung Cancer, 1*, 1–10.

39. Higgins, T. L. (2005). Postthoracotomy complications. In J. A. Kaplan & P. D. Slinger (Eds.), *Thoracic anesthesia* (3rd ed.). Philadelphia: Churchill Livingstone.

40. Hurria, A., & Kris, M. G. (2003). Management of lung cancer in older adults. *CA: Cancer J Clinicians, 53*, 325–341.

41. Institute for Clinical Systems Improvement (ICSI). (2003). *Venous thromboembolism prophylaxis for surgical/trauma patients.* Bloomington, Minn: ICSI.

42. Jenal, A., Murray, T., Ward, E., et al. (2005). Cancer statistics, 2005. *CA: Cancer J Clinicians, 55*, 10–29.

43. Kaiser, L. R., & Singhal, S. (2004). *Surgical foundation: essentials of thoracic surgery.* Philadelphia: Mosby.

44. Kaseda, S., Aoki, T., Hangai, N., et al. (2000). Better pulmonary function and prognosis with video-assisted thoracic surgery than with thoracotomy. *Ann Thorac Surg, 70*, 1644–1646.

45. Law, S., Wong, K. H., Kwok, K.F, et al. (2004). Predictive factors for postoperative pulmonary complications and mortality after esophagectomy for cancer. *Ann Surg, 240*, 791–800.

46. Leaver, H. A., Craig, S. R., Yap, P. L., et al. (2000). Lymphocyte responses following open and minimally invasive thoracic surgery. *Eur J Clin Invest, 30*, 230–238.

47. Lin, J., & Iannettoni, M. D. (2005). Fast-tracking: eliminating roadblocks to successful early discharge. *Thorac Surg Clin, 15*, 221–228.

48. LoCicero, J. (2005). Segmentectomy and lesser pulmonary resections. In T. Shields, J. Locicero III, R. Ponn, et al. (Eds.), *General thoracic surgery* (6th ed.). Philadelphia: Lippincott Williams & Wilkins.

49. Marshall, M. B., Deeb, M. E., Bleier, J. I. S., et al. (2002). Suction vs. water seal after pulmonary resection: a randomized prospective study. *Chest, 121*, 831–835.

49a.Massard, G., & Wihlm, J-M. (1999). Postoperative atelectasis. *Chest Surg Clin North Am, 8*(3), 507.

50. Mathiesen, D. J. (2001). What's new in general thoracic surgery. *J Am Coll Surg, 192*, 737–749.

51. Morris, R. J., & Woodcock, J. P. (2004). Evidence-based compression: prevention of stasis and deep vein thrombosis. *Ann Surg, 239*, 162–171.

52. Mountain, C. F. (2000). The evolution of the surgical treatment of lung cancer. *Chest Surg Clin North Am, 10*, 83–104.

53. Nakajima, J., Takamoto, S., Kohno, T., et al. (2000). Cost of videothoracoscopic surgery vs. open resection for patients with lung cancer. *Cancer, 89*(11 suppl), 2497–2501.

54. National Emphysema Treatment Trial Research Group. (2003). A randomized trial comparing lung-volume reduction surgery with medical therapy for severe emphysema. *N Engl J Med, 348*, 2059–2073.

55. Nwogu, C. E. (2001). Primary malignant neoplasms of the lung. In H. L. Karamanoukian, P. R. Soltoski & T. A. Salerno (Eds.), *Thoracic surgery secrets.* Philadelphia: Hanley & Belfus.

56. Ochroch, E. A., & Gottschalk, A. (2005). Impact of acute pain and its management for thoracic surgical patients. *Thorac Surg Clin, 15*, 105–121.

57. Patel, V., & Shrager, J. B. (2005). Which patients with stage III non-small lung cancer should undergo surgical resection? *The Oncologist, 10*, 335–344.

58. Ponn, R. B. (2005). Complications of pulmonary resection. In T. Shields, J. Locicero III, R. Ponn, et al. (Eds.), *General thoracic surgery* (6th ed.). Philadelphia: Lippincott Williams & Wilkins.

59. Port, J. L., Korst, R., & Altorki, N. K. (2005). Transthoracic resection of the esophagus. In T. Shields, J. Locicero III, & R. Ponn, et al. (Eds.), *General thoracic surgery* (6th ed.). Philadelphia: Lippincott Williams & Wilkins.

60. Powers, C. J., & Karamanoukian, H. L. (2001). Esophageal diverticula. In H. L. Karamanoukian, P. R. Soltoski & T. A. Salerno (Eds.), *Thoracic surgery secrets*. Philadelphia: Hanley & Belfus.

61. Proctor, M. C., Greenfield, L. J., Wakefield, T. W., et al. (2001). A clinical comparison of pneumatic compression devices: the basis for selection. *J Vasc Surg, 34*, 459–464.

62. Ricci, M., & Karamanoukian, R. L. (2001). Achalasia. In H. L. Karamanoukian, P. R. Soltoski & T. A. Salerno (Eds.), *Thoracic surgery secrets*. Philadelphia: Hanley & Belfus.

63. Roberts, J. R., Shyr, Y., Christian, K. R., et al. (2000). Preemptive gastrointestinal tract management reduces aspiration and respiratory failure after thoracic operations. *J Thorac Cardiovasc Surg, 119*, 449–452.

64. Sack, S. Z., & Glatstein, E. (2005). Non-small cell lung cancer: importance of locoregional tumor control in the era of emerging adjuvant chemotherapy. *Principles Practice Updates Oncol, 19*, 1–15.

65. Sahn, S. A. (2005). Malignant pleural effusions. In T. Shields, J. Locicero III, R. Ponn, et al. (Eds.), *General thoracic surgery* (6th ed.). Philadelphia: Lippincott Williams & Wilkins.

66. Sekine, Y., Kesler, K. A., Behnia, M., et al. (2001). COPD may increase the incidence of refractory supraventricular arrhythmias following pulmonary resection for non-small cell lung cancer. *Chest, 120*, 1783–1790.

67. Sherry, K. M. (2001). How can we improve the outcome of oesophagectomy? *Brit J Anaesthesia, 86*, 611–613.

68. Shields, T. W. (2005). General features of pulmonary resections. In T. Shields, J. Locicero III, R. Ponn, et al. (Eds.), *General thoracic surgery* (6th ed.). Philadelphia: Lippincott Williams & Wilkins.

69. Slinger, P. D., & Johnston, M. R. (2005). Preoperative assessment and management. In J. A. Kaplan & P. D. Slinger (Eds.), *Thoracic anesthesia* (3rd ed.). Philadelphia: Churchill Livingstone.

70. Tablan, O. C., Anderson, L. J., Besser, R., et al. (2004). Healthcare infection control practices advisory committee, Centers for Disease Control and Prevention. Guidelines for preventing healthcare-associated pneumonia, 2003: recommendations of the CDC and Healthcare Infection Control Practices Advisory Committee. *MMWR Recomm Rep, 53*(RR-3), 1–36.

71. Takaoka, S. T., & Weinacker, A. B. (2005). The value of preoperative pulmonary rehabilitation. *Thorac Surg Clin, 15*, 203–211.

72. Vaporciyan, A., Correa, A., Rice, D., et al. (2004). Risk factors associated with atrial fibrillation after noncardiac thoracic surgery: analysis of 2588 patients. *J Thorac Cardiovasc Surg, 127*, 779–786.

73. Watanabe, Y. (2005). Tracheal sleeve pneumonectomy. In T. Shields, J. Locicero III, R. Ponn, et al. (Eds.), *General thoracic surgery* (6th ed.). Philadelphia: Lippincott Williams & Wilkins.

74. Wheatley, G. H., Rosenbaum, D. H., Paul, M. C., et al. (2005). Improved pain management outcomes with continuous infusion of a local anesthetic after thoracotomy. *J Thorac Cardiovasc Surg, 130*, 464–468.

75. Whyte, R. I., & Grant, P. D. (2005). Preoperative patient education in thoracic surgery. *Thorac Surg Clin, 15*, 195–201.

76. Wilson, D. J. (1997). Pulmonary rehabilitation exercise program for high-risk thoracic surgical patients. *Chest Surg Clin North Am, 7*, 697–706.

77. Wright, C. D., Wain, J. C., Grillo, H. C., et al. (1997). Pulmonary lobectomy patient care pathway: a model to control cost and maintain quality. *Ann Thorac Surg, 64*, 299–302.

NERVOUS SYSTEM

CHAPTER 22

Head Injury and Dysfunction

Jan Powers and Christine Smith Schulman

Traumatic brain injury (TBI) results from any mechanical disruption of brain tissue from an impact or injury to the head.[119] Severe head injury can be one of the most complex and challenging conditions with which clinicians must contend, requiring a coordinated, comprehensive, and multidisciplinary approach.[124]

In the United States at least 1.4 million people sustain TBIs each year. Of these, about 50,000 die, 235,000 are hospitalized, and 1.1 million are treated and released from emergency departments. Children, older adolescents, and adults age 75 years and older are more likely than others to sustain a TBI.[36] Adults age 65 years and older sustain 155,000 TBIs each year. Adults age 75 or older have the highest rates of TBI-related hospitalization and deaths. In every age-group, males have a higher incidence of TBI than females. The most common cause of traumatic brain injuries is motor vehicle crashes (MVCs), accounting for the greatest number of TBI hospitalizations; MVCs account for 30% of TBIs. Falls are the leading cause in the age-groups from birth to 4 years and 75 years and older, accounting for 28% of TBIs.[37]

Unfortunately, many traumatic brain injuries result in serious long-term problems. Even if mortality can be decreased, the morbidity and long-term disabilities associated with TBI can be devastating, leaving the patient in a persistent vegetative state or with other significant impairments requiring constant care. The consequences of TBI are much farther reaching than the initial physical and mental impact to the affected person. The long-term disability related to brain injuries is associated with significant financial and societal burdens. Approximately 80,000 to 90,000 people with TBIs sustain permanent disabilities from their injury.[37] However, because the Centers for Disease Control and Prevention (CDC) report is based only on hospital and emergency department data, the actual number of injuries is probably underestimated; it does not account for those treated in a primary care setting, physician's office, or other outpatient clinic. An estimated 25% of patients with mild to moderate TBI do not receive medical attention.[3]

Severity of TBI is generally classified according to the Glasgow Coma Scale (GCS) score (Table 22-1). A GCS score of 3 to 8 represents severe TBI, 9 to 12 signifies moderate TBI, and a score of 13 to 15 is considered mild TBI. Approximately 10% of hospitalized TBI patients are classified on admission as severe, another 10% as moderate, and the remaining 80% of injuries are mild.[207]

The GCS is a commonly used tool providing a standardized approach for assessment of level of consciousness (LOC) and is used for determination of TBI severity. The GCS has become the most widely used and accepted tool for outcome prediction; however, there are many limitations to the use of this tool and the GCS does not necessarily reflect the extent of injury associated with the TBI. It does not assess pupil response or account for subtle changes with strength or movement of extremities. Skewed assessments and inaccurate scoring can result when patients are intubated or have received medications that alter level of consciousness. Trauma patients often have concomitant spinal or other orthopedic injuries that can affect the accuracy of the GCS. The GCS, although useful in determining LOC, needs to be used in conjunction with other neurologic assessment methods.[65]

Our understanding of the underlying mechanisms of injury and the associated intracranial pathophysiology of TBI has been rapidly advancing. Outcomes following TBI can be significantly improved when the activities of all disciplines are integrated into a coordinated systematic approach to the patient.

APPLIED PHYSIOLOGY

Ongoing, continual neurologic assessment is of utmost importance for any patient with neurologic injuries and is especially true for patients who have sustained a TBI. Because patients with brain injuries can exhibit neurologic changes from moment to moment, it is extremely important for the critical care nurse to be aware of how these changes may be consistent with brain dysfunction and increased intracranial pressure (ICP).

TABLE 22-1 Glasgow Coma Scale

Eyes	Open	Spontaneously	4
		To verbal command	3
		To pain	2
		No response	1
Best motor response	To verbal command	Obeys	6
	To painful stimulus	Localizes pain	5
		Flexion—withdrawal	4
		Flexion—abnormal (decorticate rigidity)	3
		Extension (decerebrate rigidity)	2
		No response	1
Best verbal response		Oriented and converses	5
		Disoriented and converses	4
		Inappropriate words	3
		Incomprehensible sounds	2
		No response	1
Total			3–15

From reference 211.

The purpose of this chapter is not to review the basics of neurologic assessment or anatomy; however, Tables 22-2, 22-3, and 22-4 and Figures 22-1 and 22-2 review basic findings associated with traumatic brain dysfunction.

The brain comprises only 2% of body weight, yet accounts for 18% of resting energy consumption.[133] It receives 15% of cardiac output and uses 20% of total body oxygen and 25% of total body glucose supplies. With normal cerebral blood flow (CBF), the brain extracts about 50% of the oxygen and 10% of the glucose from arterial blood. Because neuronal cytoplasm does not contain any glycogen reserves, the brain is totally dependent on a continuous and reliable supply of both oxygen and glucose from the blood. If circulation to an area is interrupted, even for just a few seconds, neurons in that region will be injured. The longer the interruption of circulation, the more severe the neuronal injury.[133] High-energy phosphates, predominantly adenosine triphosphate (ATP), are the most important energy source for the brain. Neurons derive ATP from intracellular mitochondrial processes solely dependent upon aerobic mechanisms and almost entirely produced through the oxidative metabolism of glucose. The brain is highly dependent on this energy source.[235] ATP is expended to maintain normal ion concentrations; when cellular energy demands are increased, available ATP can be quickly depleted.[133]

Cerebral Hemodynamics

Cerebral blood flow (CBF) is influenced and regulated by a number of factors. These factors include systemic arterial blood pressure (BP), ICP, venous outflow, blood viscosity, the partial pressure of arterial carbon dioxide ($PaCO_2$), the partial pressure of arterial oxygen tension (PaO_2), collateral flow, vasoreactivity, and the ability of the brain to autoregulate. The primary sites for regulating vascular resistance are the arterioles and precapillary segments.[6] The major determinant of regional blood flow is cerebral metabolism.[219] Measurements of cerebral ischemia within 12 hours of injury have shown that more than 30% of patients exhibit global CBF reductions below accepted ischemic thresholds (less than 18 ml/100 g/min).[26]

CBF averages 50 ml/100 g of brain tissue per minute. CBF may be markedly reduced within the first few hours after severe brain injury. Irreversible neuronal damage occurs if CBF drops below 18 ml/100 g of brain tissue per minute. The net driving force for the cerebral circulation is cerebral perfusion pressure

TABLE 22-2 Primary Functions of Brain Lobes

LOBE	FUNCTION
Frontal	Prefrontal
	Short-term memory
	Emotional responsiveness
	Abstract thinking
	Foresight/judgment
	Behavior/tactfulness
	Primary motor cortex
	Broca's speech area (dominant hemisphere)*
	Expressive speech/vocalization
	Intellect
	Personality
Temporal	Primary auditory cortex
	Visual task learning
	Dominant hemisphere*
	Wernicke's speech area
	Receptive speech/comprehension
	Interpretive area
	Intellect
	Emotion
	Long-term memory
	Dominant hemisphere: verbal
	Nondominant hemisphere: sensory
Parietal	Primary sensory cortex
	Sensory interpretation
	Tactile and kinesthetic sense
	Body awareness
	Body image
	Spatial orientation/relations
	Dominant hemisphere
	Language
	Object perception recognition
	Nondominant hemisphere
	Neglect syndrome
Occipital	Primary visual cortex
	Visual association

From reference 141.
*Dominance: The majority (80%) of both right- and left-handed people have left hemispheric dominance for speech. A small percentage of left-handed people have both right and left hemispheric speech control. The preponderance of left cerebral dominance is felt to be due to anatomic asymmetry of the human brain. Sixty-five percent of people have a larger speech area (Wernicke's area) surface on the left hemisphere, in 11% the right is larger, and in 24% the right and left sides are equal in size. Hemispheric lateralization or dominance is also found in functions related to mood and affect, as well as verbal, auditory, and visuospatial tasks.

(CPP), which is defined as the difference between mean arterial pressure (MAP) and ICP.[85]

Cerebral autoregulation is the brain's ability to keep cerebral blood flow relatively constant despite changes in CPP. Autoregulation allows the brain to maintain a constant blood flow even in the face of wide variations in systemic mean arterial pressures. When ICP increases, blood flow is maintained by narrowing the diameter of the cerebral blood vessels, thus increasing MAP to maintain an adequate CPP and CBF.[190] When compensatory mechanisms fail, the autoregulatory capacity of the brain is lost.[190] There is a close relationship between dysautoregulation, abnormal cerebral metabolism, and increased mortality.[188]

As a result of autoregulation, depicted in Figure 22-3, CBF remains relatively constant when CPP is between 40 and 140 mm Hg, due to changes in cerebrovascular resistance.[101] Low-flow states leading to hypoxia or hypercapnia result in acidosis and cause cerebral vasodilation and increased blood flow.[124] The opposite of a decrease in CBF is cerebral hyperemia, defined as CBF in excess of metabolic demand. It is frequently seen in severely head-injured patients, particularly children. Hyperemia can be caused by metabolic derangements, vasodilation resulting from loss of vasomotor tone, or severe tissue acidosis.[27]

MECHANISM OF INJURY

All types of severe cranial injury involve the transmission of kinetic energy through the brain. Pressure waves of varying magnitude and duration, or direct-impact damage to small and large vascular structures and neurons close to the cortical surface, determine the extent of brain injury sustained.[141]

Common mechanisms of injury related to TBI can be divided broadly into two categories: blunt or penetrating injuries. Mechanisms of blunt TBI within these categories include acceleration-deceleration injury, deformation, and rotation (Figure 22-4).[141] Most blunt injuries are a result of motor vehicle crashes, motorcycle crashes, pedestrian injuries, falls, or assaults. The most common causes of blunt injuries are motor vehicle collisions. In the elderly, falls are a frequent etiology of blunt injuries. In the pediatric population, shaken baby syndrome and other causes of nonaccidental trauma are a major concern. Tissue damage from blunt injuries is caused by several mechanisms, most commonly acceleration-deceleration or rotational forces (see Figure 22-4).[141]

Acceleration injury occurs when the skull and brain are rapidly set into motion. Deceleration injury occurs when the head hits a stationary object, causing the skull to decelerate rapidly.[141] The brain moves within the skull and collides with the inner

TABLE 22-3 Pupil Abnormalities Related to Brain Dysfunction*

PUPIL FINDINGS	RELATED DYSFUNCTION	OTHER POTENTIAL CAUSES
Unilateral fixed and dilated pupil	Ipsilateral oculomotor (CN III) compression or injury	Instillation of mydriatics (e.g., scopolamine, atropine) Orbital injuries
Bilateral fixed and dilated pupils	Severe brain anoxia and ischemia; bilateral CN III compression	Medications (e.g., dopamine, amphetamines, atropine)
Pinpoint, nonreactive pupils	Pons damage	Miotic agents, opiates Overdose
Small, equal, reactive pupils	Bilateral diencephalic damage affecting sympathetic innervation originating from hypothalamus	Metabolic dysfunction
Nonreactive, midpositioned pupils	Midbrain damage	

*Data from references 85, 142.

TABLE 22-4 Respiratory Patterns Associated With Brain Dysfunction

NAME	DESCRIPTION	NEUROANATOMIC BRAIN LESIONS
Cheyne-Stokes respirations	Regular cycles of respirations that gradually increase in depth to hyperpnea and then decrease in depth to periods of apnea	Usually bilateral lesions deep within cerebral hemispheres, diencephalon, and basal ganglia
Central neurogenic hyperventilation	Deep, rapid respiration	Midbrain, upper pons
Apneustic respirations	Prolonged inspirations followed by a 2- to 3-second pause; occasionally may alternate with an expiratory pause	Pons
Cluster respirations	Clusters of irregular breaths followed by an apneic period lasting a variable amount of time	Lower pons and upper medulla
Ataxic or Biot's respirations	Irregular, unpredictable pattern of shallow and deep respirations and pauses	Medulla

From reference 141.

cranial surface and its rough bony prominences. The brain may also bounce backward from the point of impact, causing a collision with the contralateral skull surface (Figure 22-5).[141] Rotation may also occur with acceleration-deceleration injuries, resulting in a twisting of the brain within the skull. Rotational forces produce shearing that injures brain tissue or vascular structures.[32,62] Injury severity is dependent upon the speed, direction, and force of rotation and impact.[108]

Penetrating injuries are most commonly related to gunshot or stab wounds. Penetrating injuries are most

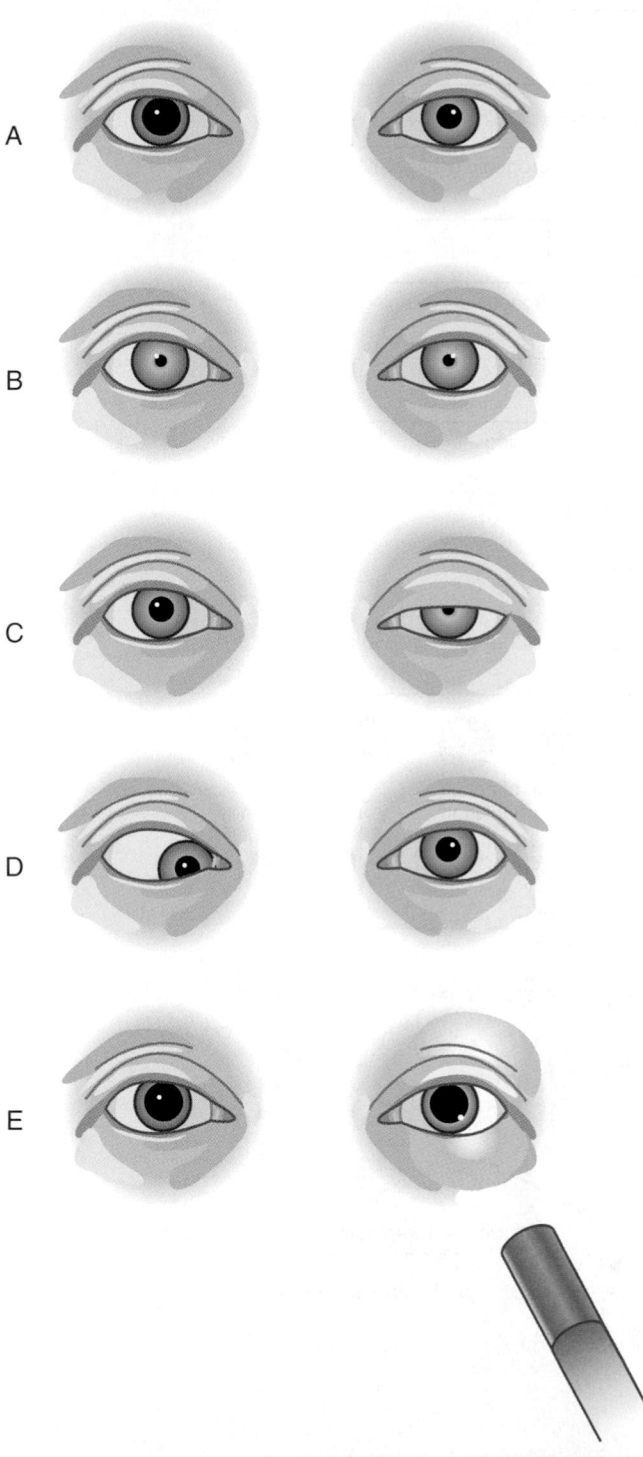

⬍FIGURE 22-1 Pupil response. **A,** Unilateral fixed dilated pupil: pressure on cranial nerve (CN) III. **B** Pinpoint pupils: brain stem hemorrhage. **C,** Unilateral small pupil and ptosis: Horner syndrome with sympathetic/parasympathetic dysfunction. **D,** Failure of eyes to look downward and inward (left eye is normal eye): CN IV palsy. **E,** Bilateral fixed dilated pupils: brain herniation.

commonly caused by missile injuries from bullets. However, any object that penetrates the skull into the brain tissue can result in penetrating trauma; other objects such as shrapnel, arrows, and metal pipes have also been reported to cause penetrating trauma. Some objects or missiles responsible for penetrating injuries may have low mass, but they strike the cranium at high or very high velocity. In a penetrating injury the area of damage is localized to the path of the object.[32,62,108] Stab wounds are low-velocity injuries that can cause damage to vascular structures, cranial nerves, and white matter fiber tracts.

TYPES OF TRAUMATIC BRAIN INJURY

Regardless of the underlying mechanism, damage to the brain typically results in focal or diffuse lesions. Diffuse brain injury and focal brain injury can coexist, especially in the severely injured patient.[154]

Focal Injuries

Focal injuries are generally associated with a direct impact to the head. These localized brain injuries are easy to identify and can occasionally be surgically removed. They generally produce hematomas or contusions, including focal cortical contusions with or without associated intracerebral hematoma formation. Hematomas are categorized by their location in relation to the brain tissue and meningeal layers. Symptomatology, morbidity, and mortality from focal injuries are affected by the size, location, and progression of the lesion.[32,33,108]

Skull Fractures

Although not technically brain injuries, many skull fractures can cause or accompany underlying brain injury. Skull fractures occur in about half of all persons with severe traumatic brain injuries (Figure 22-6).[108] The more severe the brain injury, the greater likelihood an associated skull fracture may be present.[108]

A simple linear fracture is the most benign type of fracture and typically does not require any specific treatment.[108] However, it is helpful to perform a computed tomography (CT) scan to assess for any associated brain injuries, especially if the fracture is in the temporal region where underlying arteries are present and easily torn.[108]

Depressed skull fractures are more complex, resulting in the cranial bone being forced below the normal plane of the skull, impinging on the brain tissue. Depressed skull fractures result in lacerations and hematomas from bone fragments. Surgical treatment of this injury is required for debridement and

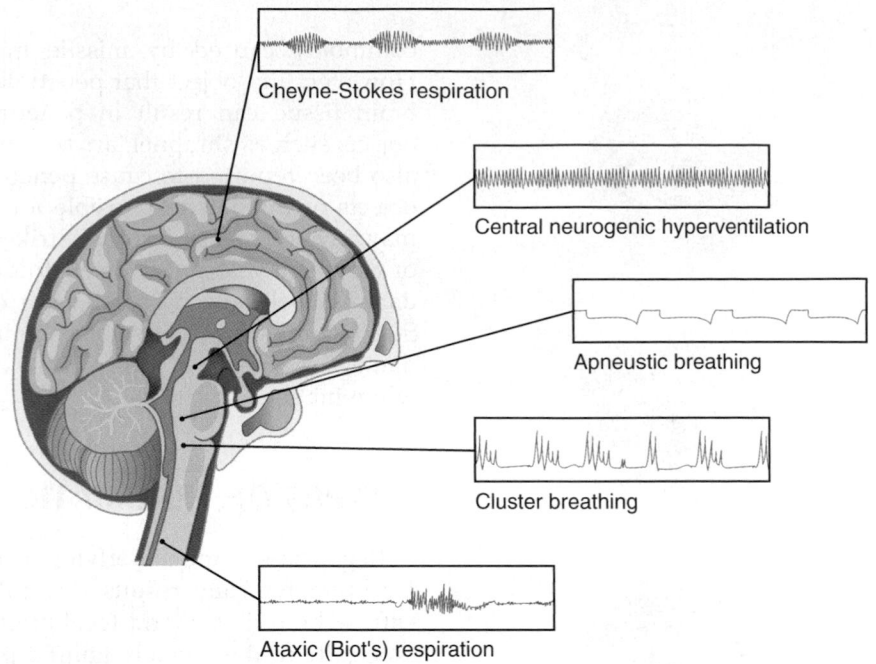

♦FIGURE 22-2 Increased intracranial pressure-associated changes in respiratory patterns.

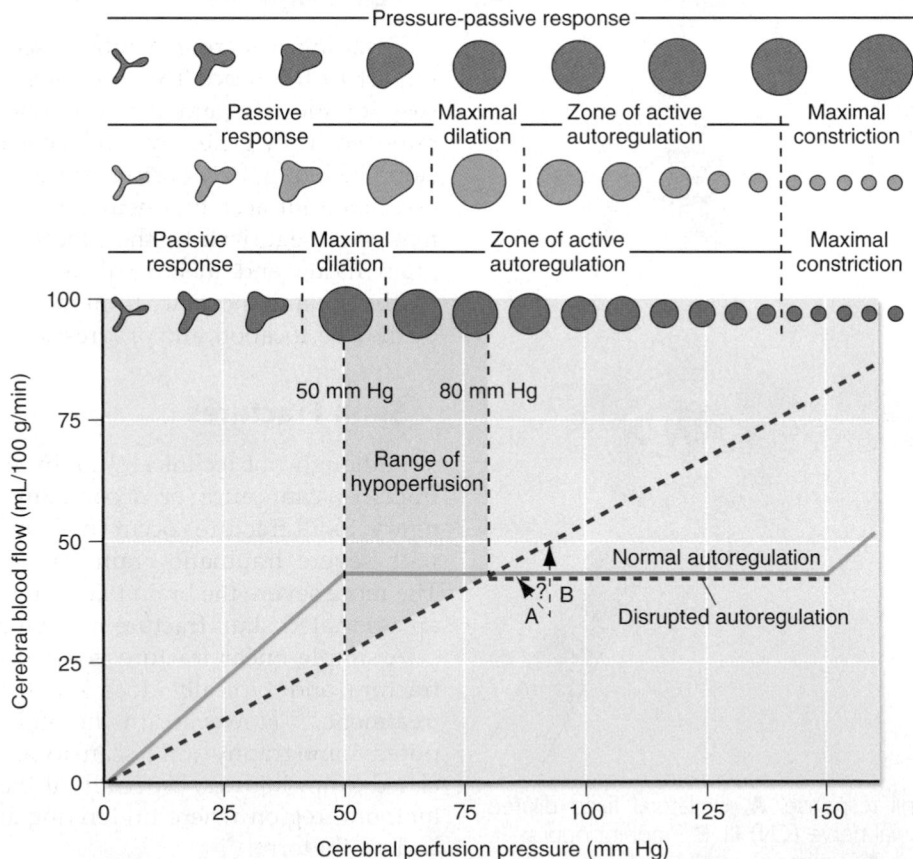

♦FIGURE 22-3 Mechanisms of normal and disrupted autoregulation. The top three rows represent the vascular system. *Bottom row:* Intact autoregulation (AR). *Middle row:* Partially disrupted AR. *Top row:* Complete disruption of AR. On the graph, the *solid line* represents normal pressure AR in the range of 50 to 150 mm Hg *(bottom row above)*. The *broken line* represents disrupted pressure AR and illustrates its pressure-passive nature (line *B*) where cerebral blood flow is directly proportional to cerebral perfusion pressure (CPP). In partial disruption (line *A*), the system is pressure-passive up to 80 mm Hg, followed by pressure AR occurring until pressure exceeds 150 mm Hg. NOTE: The range of hypoperfusion between 50 and 80 mm Hg may represent ischemia even when CPP appears to be normal.

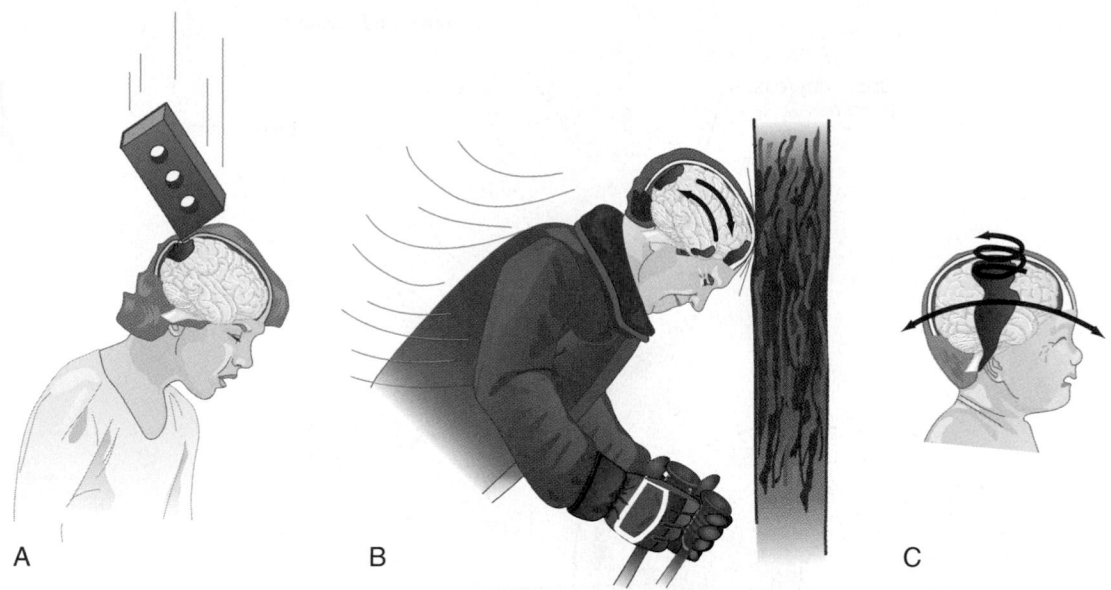

♦FIGURE 22-4   Mechanisms of injury. **A,** Deformation. **B,** Acceleration-deceleration. **C,** Rotation.

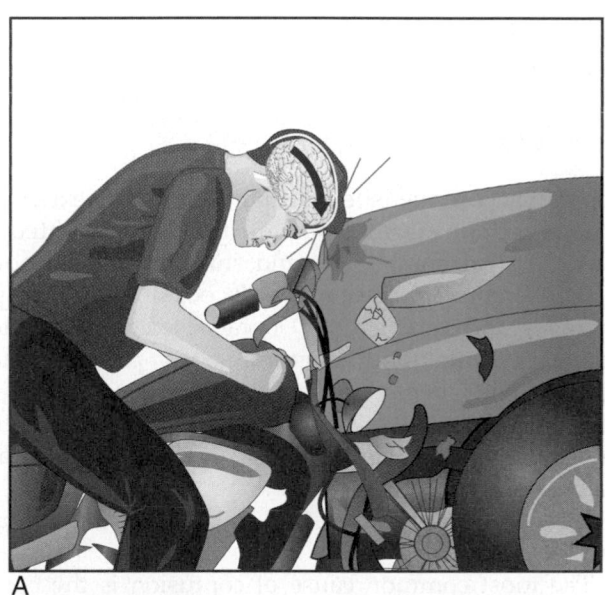

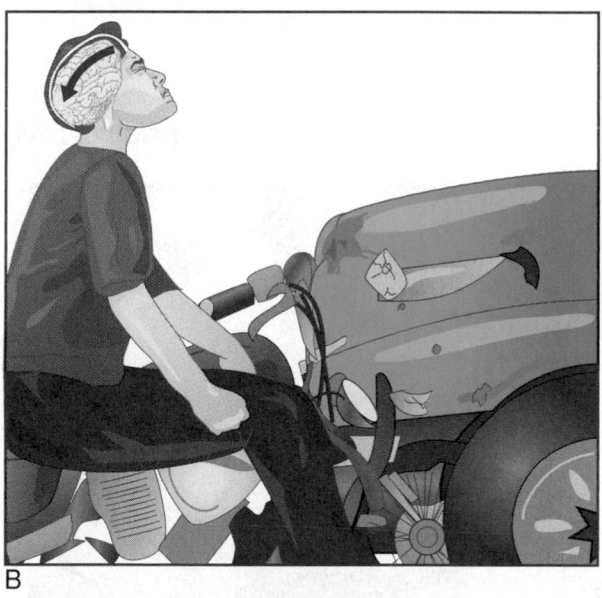

♦FIGURE 22-5   Acceleration-deceleration injuries. **A,** The brain strikes the skull. **B,** The brain rebounds.

evacuation of associated clots or bone fragments, repair of dural lacerations, and elevation of the depressed bone fragment.[108]

Basilar skull fractures are located at the base of the cranium, generally in the anterior or middle fossa. These fractures are difficult to detect with routine radiographs, and diagnosis is often based on clinical findings. Signs include periorbital ecchymosis (raccoon eyes), extensive subconjunctival hemorrhage, cerebrospinal fluid (CSF) otorrhea, CSF rhinorrhea, and ecchymosis over the mastoid process (Battle's sign).[108] Otorrhea and rhinorrhea are concerning because they indicate the presence

of a dural tear, which places patients at risk for meningitis.[32,108]

Contusions

Cerebral contusions are focal injuries that occur when localized forces damage the small blood vessels and other tissue components of the neural parenchyma (Figure 22-7). Injury occurs when brain tissue moves across the irregular bony surfaces of the anterior and middle cranial fossa during rapid deceleration. Bleeding from damaged blood vessels is usually the most obvious

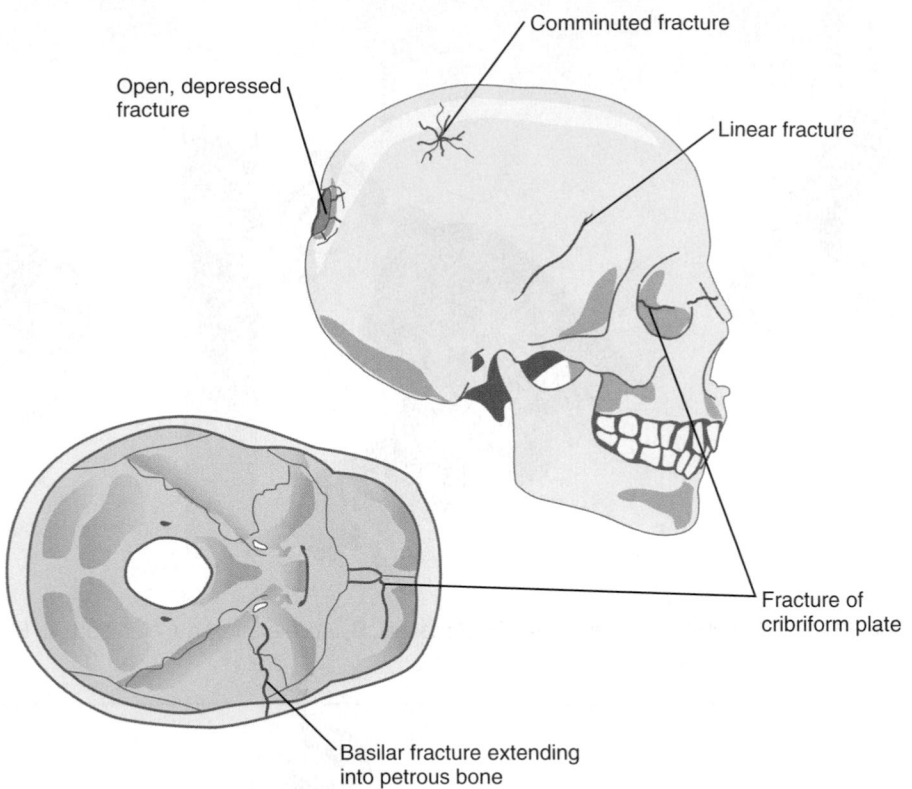

⬍FIGURE 22-6 Types of skull fractures.

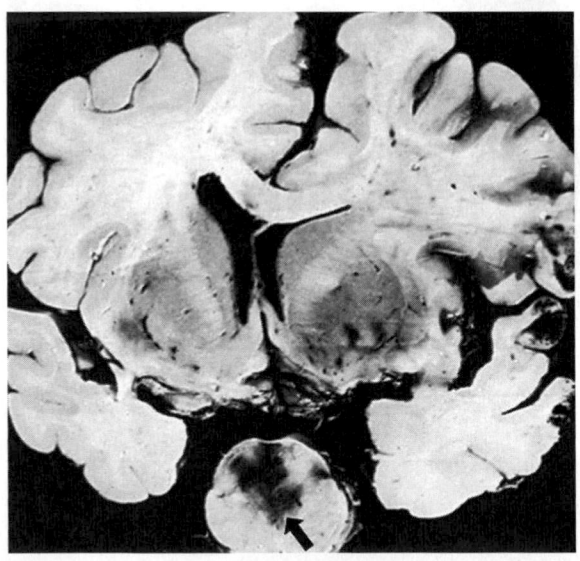

⬍FIGURE 22-7 Recent contusions of frontal and temporal lobes, with displacement of cingulate gyrus and lateral ventricles. Secondary hemorrhages are evident.

dependent on the site of injury and the extent of contused brain. Contusions are frequently located in the inferior frontal lobes and inferolateral temporal lobes. Cerebral contusions rarely occur in the occipital lobes and cerebellum.[23] Because contusions often occur in frontal and temporal lobes, patients often present with behavior and personality changes as well as speech and motor deficits. Contusions can resolve with little consequence or lead to significant brain edema. However, expanding lesions may lead to increased mass effect and increased intracranial pressure.[24]

The most common cause of contusion is the coup-contrecoup injury. Injury results from direct impact (coup) and from impact on the opposite site of the cranium (contrecoup).[11] As a result of acceleration-deceleration injury, the brain moves inside the cranial cavity in response to the impact (see Figure 22-5). The brain collides with the inner cranial surface and moves over its rough bony prominences.[11] It may also bounce backward from the point of impact, colliding with the contralateral skull surface as well.

Hematomas

Epidural, subdural, and intracerebral hematomas are illustrated in Figure 22-8 and discussed in the sections that follow.

feature on examination, resulting in a spectrum of abnormalities ranging from microhemorrhages to multiple confluent hemorrhages that disrupt brain tissue.[24] Essentially bruises of the brain, contusions are problematic for the area of brain affected. Severity of injury is

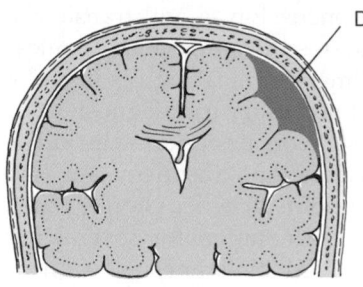

Dura

Subdural hematoma

Epidural hematoma

Intracerebral hematoma

⬍FIGURE 22-8 Hematomas.

Epidural Hematoma. An epidural hematoma (EDH) is located outside the dura mater but inside the skull, giving the EDH its classic smooth, convex shape (Figure 22-9). An EDH is an uncommon injury, occurring in less than 1% to 2% of TBI patients;[117,124] however, up to 15% of fatal head injuries are a result of EDH.[70] The most common location for an EDH is the temporal-parietal region, most commonly associated with laceration of the middle meningeal artery as a result of a temporal skull fracture. The classic presentation of the patient with an EDH is an initial loss of consciousness, followed by a period of lucidity, and then by progressive loss of consciousness. Even though this has been described as the classic presentation, it only occurs in about 40% of all EDH patients.[124] If the clot is evacuated immediately, recovery is generally favorable. However, if surgery is delayed, this injury can be fatal because of rapid arterial bleeding that leads to cerebral herniation.[70]

Subdural Hematoma. A subdural hematoma (SDH) involves bleeding or clot formation under the dura mater, yet outside the surface of the brain itself (see Figure 22-8). This produces a classic crescent-shaped collection of blood, with irregular edges visible (Figure 22-10). SDHs are more common than EDHs, occurring in about 30% of severe head injuries.[124] SDHs most commonly result from tearing of the tiny bridging veins located between the cerebral cortex and the venous sinus, and are often the result of acceleration-deceleration injuries. Mortality ranges from 30% to 90%, with the lowest mortality occurring in patients who undergo surgery within 4 hours of injury.[193] Eighty percent of patients presenting with an SDH have an adjacent parenchymal contusion. This underlying brain injury most strongly influences the patient's course and outcome.[124]

SDHs can be classified based on time from injury to presentation of symptoms. Acute SDH contains clotted blood and occurs either immediately upon impact or up to several days later. Subacute hematoma contains a mixture of clotted blood and fluid and occurs within several days of the injury up to 3 weeks afterward.[63] Chronic SDH occurs 3 weeks or more after injury and

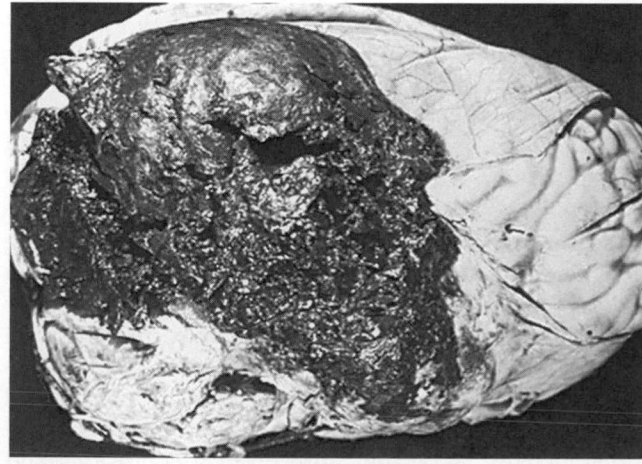

⬍FIGURE 22-9 Acute epidural hematoma. Skull fracture with tear of middle meningeal artery and vein.

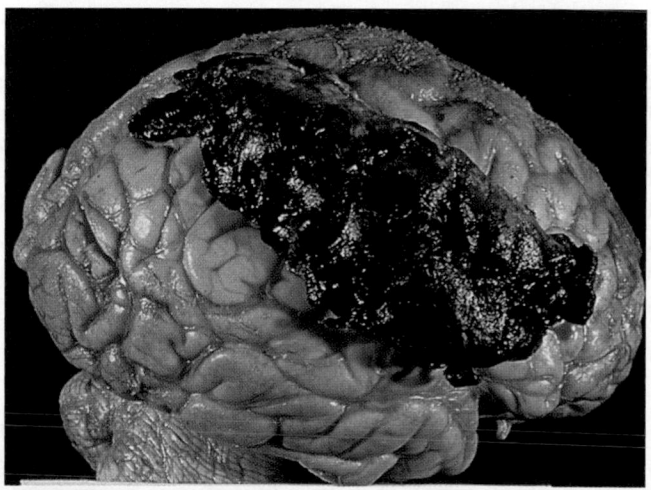

⬍FIGURE 22-10 Acute subdural hematoma (dura removed).

consists of mostly fluid. Older adults, chronic alcohol abusers, or those taking anticoagulants will have a greater incidence of this type of SDH.[63]

Intracerebral Hematoma. Intracerebral hematomas (ICHs) are areas of bleeding within the brain parenchyma that are approximately 2 cm or greater in size and do not contact the surface of the brain (see Figure 22-8).[199] ICHs are produced by bleeding within the parenchyma of the brain, causing a mass lesion. When caused by trauma, most of these lesions occur in the frontal and temporal lobes.[124] Bleeding is caused by rupture of parenchymal blood vessels at the time of injury, and ICHs are noted on CT scan as hyperdense areas representing intraparenchymal hemorrhage. These hematomas are found in 15% of autopsy cases of severe head injury patients and they are often multiple. Twenty-eight percent of ICHs are associated with SDHs and 10% are associated with EDH.[199] One third to one half of the patients with an ICH are unconscious on admission, and up to 20% demonstrate a lucid interval between the time of injury and the onset of coma.[199] Development of ICHs may be delayed, not appearing on CT scan for more than 24 hours after the initial insult.[124] For this reason, any neurologic deterioration or increasing intracranial pressure necessitates prompt repeat CT scanning.[124]

Traumatic Basal Ganglia Hemorrhage. One other type of hemorrhage that may be seen in patients with TBI is a traumatic basal ganglia hemorrhage (TBGH). It is generally associated with a poor prognosis. In one study, 88% of patients with TBGH and an elevated ICP had a poor outcome (severe disability, vegetative state, or death); 50% of those with normal ICP had poor outcomes.[171] Lee and Wang[114] reported 53.8% of the patients in their study with TBGH had a functional survival; those with poor outcomes had concomitant intraventricular or brain stem hemorrhage. This hemorrhage results from two mechanisms: the first is from stretching or shearing of the anterior choroidal vessels against the edge of the tentorium; the second is from stretching or perforation of branches of the middle cerebral arteries.[117,156] Deep blood vessels shear as a result of acceleration-deceleration forces. Intracerebral hemorrhages in the thalamus or basal ganglia have been noted in about 10% of patients with fatal head injuries, and they are associated with an increased incidence of diffuse axonal injury.[108]

Diffuse Injuries

Diffuse injuries are not limited to a localized area and can therefore be difficult to detect and treat. The most common types of diffuse injuries are concussions and diffuse axonal injuries.

Concussion. A concussion is any transient neurologic dysfunction that results after a mechanical force or impact. The hallmark clinical sign is loss of consciousness, but it is not necessary for diagnosis of concussion. Other symptoms of concussion may include confusion, headache, disorientation, dizziness, and disturbances with vision. Symptoms of concussion are typically mild confusion and disorientation for several minutes and may be accompanied by amnesia.[11] Concussions are typically diagnosed clinically and do not present with any identifiable lesions on CT scan. Concussions do not result in cell death like other brain injuries, but rather cause temporary neuronal dysfunction from alterations in metabolism, neurotransmitter function, and ionic shifts. They often completely resolve over time.[74]

Diffuse Axonal Injuries. Diffuse axonal injury (DAI) is defined as the presence of diffuse damage to axons of the cerebral hemispheres, corpus callosum, brain stem, or cerebellum.[24] DAI often results in immediate and prolonged unconsciousness.[24] The pathophysiology of DAI is not completely understood. It is thought that since DAI results from stretching or shearing of the neuronal axons, this leads to an influx of extracellular ions such as calcium.[24] This influx of calcium ultimately disrupts the cytoskeleton and causes focal swelling, detaching axons at the point of focal swelling. Tissue damage may continue to occur for several hours to days after the injury.[24]

DAI is not readily visible on CT scans and often requires magnetic resonance imaging (MRI) for detection. CT scans may reveal small punctate hemorrhages, but often CT scans appear negative and diagnosis is based on clinical exam in which there is a lack of radiographic findings to explain the patient's loss of consciousness. MRI is required to identify and qualify the injury as mild, moderate, or severe. The extent and location of axonal damage will determine the outcome associated with this type of injury. High morbidity and mortality have been associated with DAI, and these patients are often left in a persistent vegetative state.[173]

Subarachnoid Hemorrhage. Subarachnoid hemorrhage (SAH) is another type of diffuse injury. SAH is commonly associated with rupture of aneurysms or arteriovenous malformations (AVMs), but also occurs as a result of traumatic injury to the brain.[24] This injury involves bleeding into the subarachnoid space; SAH is the most common abnormality in TBI, although in most cases it is minor and of little clinical significance. SAH may interfere with the normal circulation and reabsorption of CSF, precipitating hydrocephalus and subsequent intracranial hypertension. Significant SAH can occur following injury and is usually associated with cortical contusions and lacerations; the accumulation of blood may become so massive that it acts as a local space-occupying lesion.[24]

PATHOPHYSIOLOGY

Regardless of the type of injury, damage from TBI can occur via two mechanisms. The initial traumatic injury to the brain results in an area of hemorrhage or compression, referred to as the primary brain injury. The primary injury may be associated with a simple hematoma or with more complex diffuse lesions. This initial injury produces immediate neuronal dysfunction and death as a result of damage to blood vessels, axons, and neurons. Neuronal destruction caused by the initial impact is irreversible.[78]

Surrounding the area of primary brain injury is a zone of impaired and ischemic cells called the penumbra. Brain tissue in this region is viable and may be salvaged, or it could die at some point after the initial impact.[145] Specific neuroprotective strategies are designed to target the cells in the penumbra, preserve cellular function, and limit the area of neuronal death. Some of these strategies will be discussed later in this chapter.

When cell damage occurs within or even beyond the borders of the penumbra, secondary brain injury has occurred. Multiple mechanisms lead to secondary brain damage after TBI, including hypotension, hypoxemia, hyperthermia, increased intracranial pressure, and electrolyte imbalances.[145] At the cellular level, the process leading to secondary brain injury involves a cascade of complex molecular events that, if not recognized and reversed, produce cellular damage and cerebral edema.[78] This can result in increased ICP, inadequate tissue perfusion, neuronal cell death, permanent neurologic impairment,[43,155] and the initiation of a self-perpetuating cycle of neuronal damage. However, this secondary damage is potentially preventable and reversible with early recognition and adequate treatment.[145]

The downward trajectory often associated with the cellular ischemic cascade and subsequent secondary brain injury begins immediately after the primary impact.[24] Ischemia, excitotoxicity, impaired metabolism, blood-brain barrier (BBB) disruption, and inflammatory factors have all been implicated in secondary brain injury.[24,64,79,145] These varied mechanisms are closely interrelated in the causation of secondary brain injury.

Calcium plays a major role in both primary and secondary brain injury. TBI triggers various cellular processes that lead to an excess of intracellular calcium.[138] Calcium concentration increases tenfold within seconds of onset of severe ischemia, causing a rapid and massive increase of intracellular free calcium ions within minutes of the initial injury.[64] This overabundance of intracellular calcium activates and sustains additional mechanisms that lead to secondary brain injury via multiple metabolic pathways.[78] The net result is a dangerous increase in intracellular ion concentrations, furthering and perpetuating inflammation, ischemia, and neural damage.[138] Figure 22-11 outlines the mechanisms activated by an increase in intracellular calcium concentration. The common final end points of the processes described earlier are neurotoxicity, the release of cellular contents, and neuronal death (Figures 22-12 and 22-13).[24,32,79]

Ischemia

Cerebral ischemia is the predominant cause of secondary brain injury. In one study, 90% of patients with a fatal TBI showed evidence of regional and global cerebral ischemia on autopsy.[77] Hypotension associated with primary ischemia tends to affect focal areas supported by arterial blood flow. Patients with multisystem trauma are particularly susceptible because of decreased cerebral perfusion from systemic hemorrhage related to other injuries or shock. CBF is further reduced at the tissue level by such processes as astrocytic swelling, hypotension, and elevated ICP, all of which cause cellular dysfunction and potentiation of secondary brain injury.[32] Hypoxemia tends to have a more global effect.

Cerebral ischemic and metabolic changes result in widespread cell membrane depolarization and release of neurotransmitters into the extracellular space.[6] The associated failure of cellular membrane pumps, excess intracellular calcium, and reduction in available ATP (adenosine triphosphate) provide additional pathways that lead to neuronal swelling (cytotoxic edema) or death. The cumulative effects of these pathologic mechanisms affect patients with severe head injury to varying degrees.[32]

Excitotoxicity. Ischemic damage causes the release of excitatory amino acids (EAAs) and can lead to excitotoxicity. This phenomenon is characterized by excessive EAA release, generally glutamate and aspartate.[32,64,144] These amino acids act as excitatory neurotransmitters to influence receptor-operated calcium channels in damaged brain tissue,[184] thereby altering intracellular concentrations of sodium and calcium and leading to neuronal cell death (see Figure 22-13).[5]

Glutamate initiates cell membrane depolarization, allowing movement of calcium and sodium into the cell and an efflux of potassium out of the cell through ion channels such as NMDA (N-methyl-D-aspartate) receptors.[59] Activation of glutamate receptors also causes the generation of highly reactive free radical molecules[133] like nitric oxide. Neurotoxicity from activation of glutamate receptors is due to excessive intracellular calcium levels and the subsequent production of toxic levels of nitric oxide.[160,184]

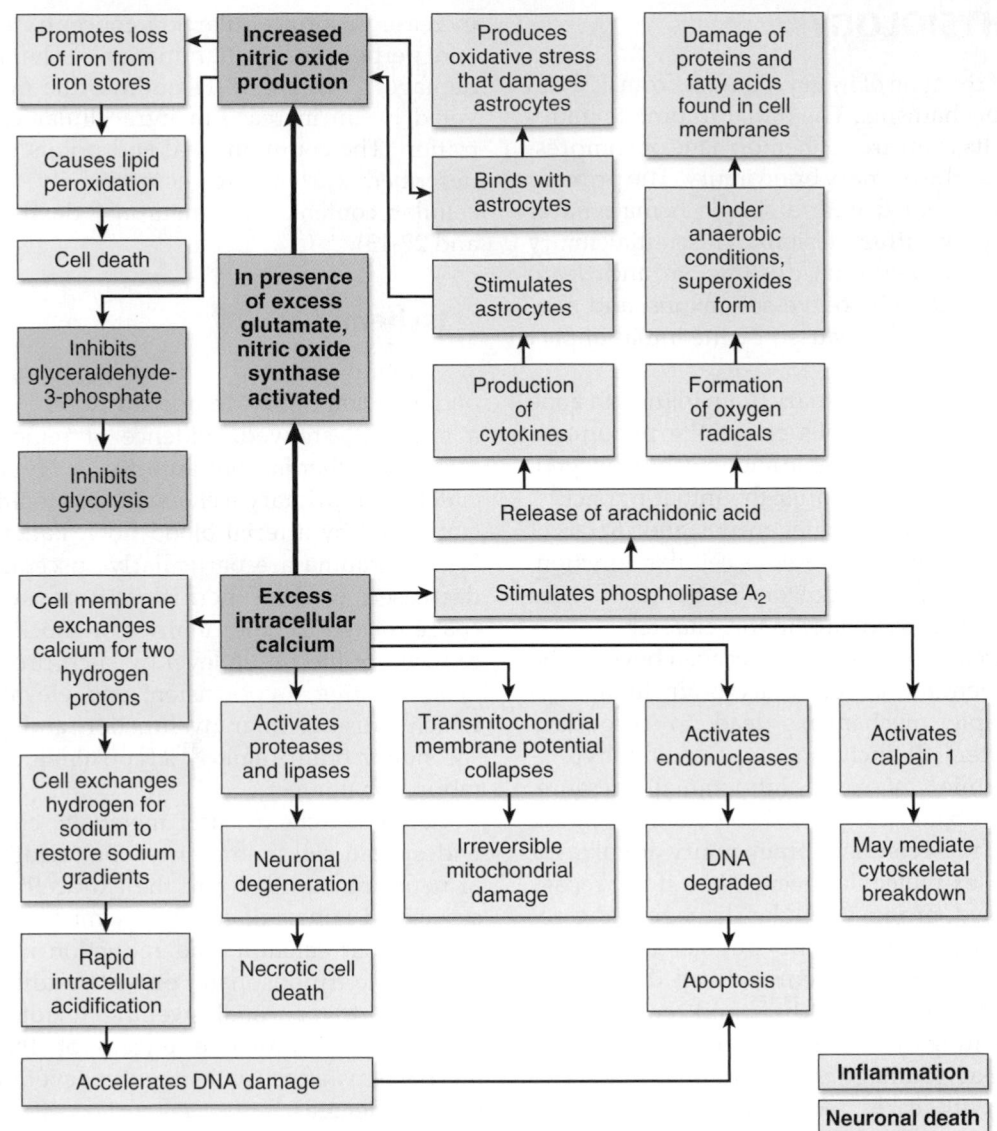

♦FIGURE 22-11 Effects of calcium on brain injury.

Free radicals are active in many chemical reactions and are necessary for life, but can also result in cell damage via unwanted side effects. In TBI, they are associated with the inhibition of cell membrane-mediated ion exchange activity, the release of arachidonic acid, and neuron apoptosis.[226] Associated ATP depletion leads to increased calcium levels, triggering further ion permeability at the mitochondrial membrane level.[226] The mitochondria swell and trigger oxidative phosphorylation, resulting in more free radicals and cell death.[226]

Impaired Metabolism

The brain depends on the delivery of oxygen and glucose for aerobic metabolism and the production of ATP.

Impairment of perfusion and oxygenation frequently follows severe head injury, most likely related to hypermetabolism. This metabolic derangement is a common and important consequence of TBI.[5] Accelerated metabolism further depletes already inadequate oxygen and glucose supplies, potentiating hypoxia, anaerobic metabolism, and secondary brain injury.[32] The Nutrition box on p. 541 highlights enteral and parenteral nutrition for TBI patients.

Neuronal cell death can also be related to an increase in regional glucose utilization usually noted in the first few days after injury.[59] This early posttraumatic hyperglycolysis may result from cellular efforts to reestablish normal ionic gradients.[89] Hyperemic zones, or areas of increased CBF, may represent an appropriate response to metabolic needs.[87] An increase

◆ NUTRITION

Enteral and Parenteral Nutrition for Patients With Severe Traumatic Brain Injury

Patients with severe TBI experience a significant hypermetabolic and hypercatabolic state and require nutrition via enteral or parenteral routes. The goal of nutritional support is to provide nutrients without adversely influencing morbidity. The parenteral route has been associated with hyperglycemia and an increased risk of infections. Early enteral feeding has been associated with preservation of gastrointestinal mucosal integrity and reduced hypermetabolic response. Institution of early enteral feeding is important for supporting immunocompetence and has been associated with decreased complications.[56] Nutritional support should support metabolic alterations, minimize catabolism, and optimize caloric delivery to meet metabolic demands. Daily assessment of caloric goals, protein requirements, patient response, and nutritional lab values is essential. Caloric assessments need to be determined using indirect calorimetry or a predictive equation such as the Harris-Benedict equation, which is used to estimate basal energy expenditure (BEE). The most accurate method to measure energy expenditure in mechanically ventilated critically ill patients is indirect calorimetry.[58] Using this strategy, neurotrauma patients will have the greatest opportunity for a positive outcome.

	DAILY DOSE RANGE	SPECIAL CONSIDERATIONS
Calories	25–35 kcal/kg/day	
Protein	2–2.5 g/kg/day	
Fluid	30–40 ml/kg/day	
Electrolytes		May need to alter intake with gastrointestinal losses or when renal failure is present.
Na	100–120 mEq	
K	80–120 mEq	
Ca	4–10 mEq	
Mg	12–15 mEq	
PO$_4$	10–15 mEq	
Vitamin supplements	Especially in the presence of a history of alcohol abuse	
Glucose	600–900 g	Hyperglycemia adversely affects outcomes by causing further damage to ischemic cells.[67]

Data from reference 58.

in local lactate production has also been noted after TBI. Lactate levels tend to normalize within a few days in those that survive, but are 5 to 10 times greater than normal in those who eventually die.[89] When lactate levels increase, extracellular fluid (ECF) glucose declines to extremely low levels.[87,89]

Lactate generation and anaerobic cerebral metabolism occur even when blood flow is adequate, suggesting that trauma incapacitates mitochondrial activity and causes a shift toward anaerobic metabolism.[87,89] Evidence suggests a link between increased ECF glutamate and increased anaerobic glycolysis.[89] Depending on the extent and severity of tissue damage, brain cells may be unable to restore ionic homeostasis despite a maximal increase in glycolytic activity.[30] If tissue blood flow is reduced during an episode of maximal metabolic need, tissue glucose and oxygen levels fall to subthreshold levels.[89] When glucose and oxygen levels fall, tissue swelling is exacerbated and ischemic necrosis will occur.[59]

Blood-Brain Barrier Disruption. The BBB functions to restrict or facilitate the passage of substances from blood to brain.[134] Endothelial cells of the cerebral capillaries in the BBB are sealed together by tight junctions and contain a large number of mitochondria that facilitate the transport of substances into the brain.[234] Only lipid-soluble compounds (e.g., CO_2, O_2, ammonia, steroids, prostaglandins, and small alcohols) can diffuse across the membranes of endothelial cells into the interstitial fluid of the brain and spinal cord.[234] Larger, water-soluble compounds can cross the capillary walls only by active or passive transport. These processes are dependent upon astrocytes that secrete chemicals to control the permeability of the endothelium.[138] If the astrocytes are damaged or stop stimulating the endothelial cells, the BBB becomes compromised.

Brain injury disrupts astrocytic activity and the BBB, resulting in edema formation driven primarily by capillary hydrostatic pressure.[32] Hyperthermia has also been linked to an increased permeability of the BBB.[138]

Inflammatory Factors

The inflammatory response and the role of cytokines are critical factors in the pathophysiology of TBI. Cytokines are proteins that function as inflammatory

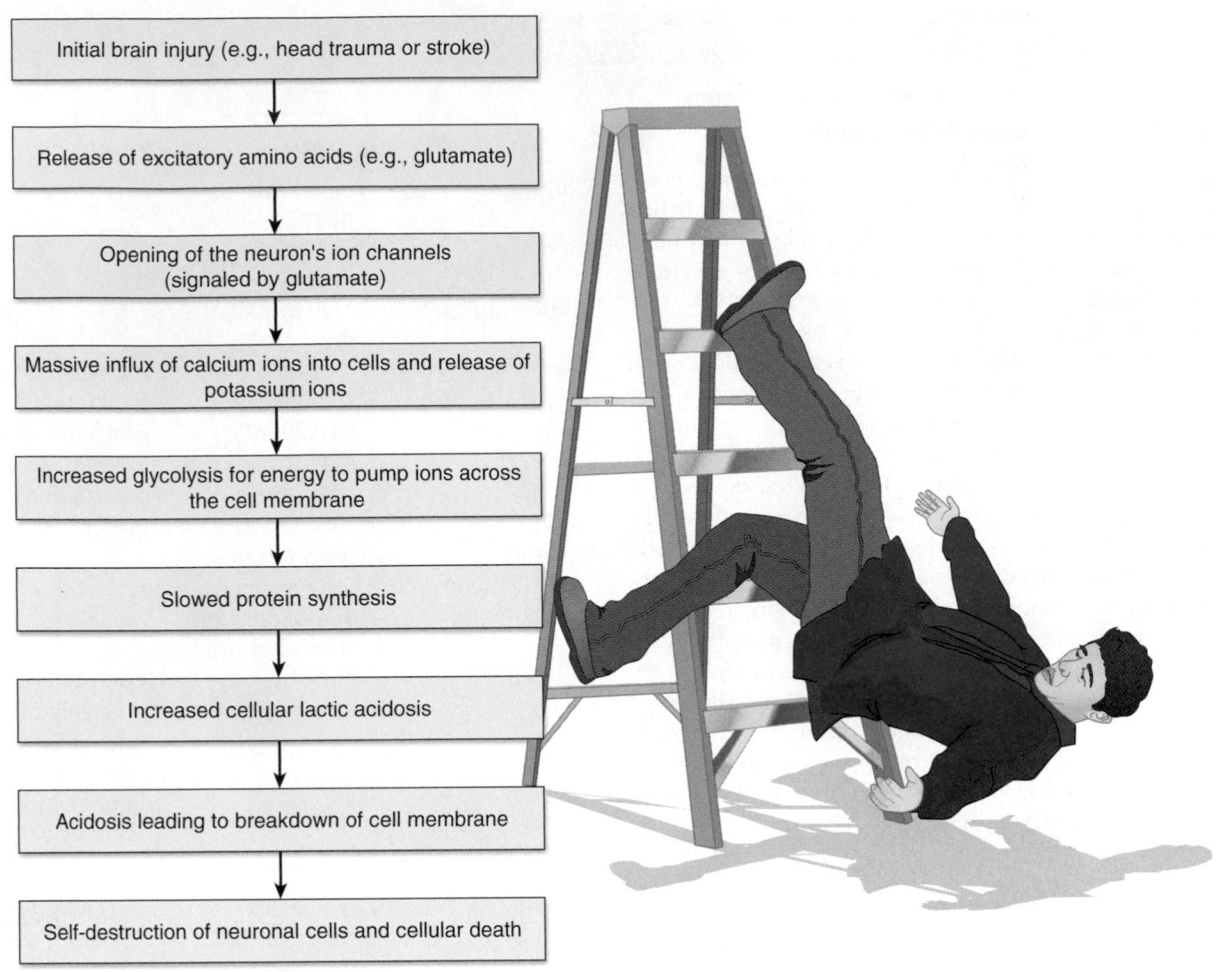

FIGURE 22-12 Metabolic cascade of brain injury.

mediators and act as intracellular communicators, playing a role in regulating cell function while attempting to maintain homeostasis.[154] They are stored intracellularly as precursor proteins and are eventually modified into active molecules.[210] Cytokines are released as a defense response to infection, inflammation, trauma, and ischemia within minutes of TBI.[154] Cytokine production following TBI occurs via intrinsic and extrinsic mechanisms. Intrinsic mechanisms produce cytokines from neurons, astrocytes, and microglia, whereas extrinsic mechanisms generate cytokines by infiltrating leukocytes.[210]

Overexpression of cytokines can be harmful to injured tissue and may even cause cell death.[224] Conversely, in the recovery phase, low levels of cytokines can enhance the repair process.[224] While information regarding cytokines involved in brain injury continues to evolve, the most commonly known cytokines are interleukin-1 (IL-1) and tumor necrosis factor (TNF). Both of these molecules act as mediators in neuronal apoptosis, causing neuronal loss in brain-injured patients.[154,224]

In addition, IL-1 and TNF can disrupt many endothelial cell activities, resulting in vascular endothelial damage and increased permeability.[224] Normally, the vascular endothelium regulates coagulation and inflammatory responses, allowing lymphocytes and monocytes to efficiently adhere and penetrate vessel walls.[224] When the vascular endothelium is damaged, however, the resulting prothrombotic condition causes intravascular coagulation. Furthermore, an overwhelming response by lymphocytes and monocytes causes injury to the vascular endothelium, leading to interstitialization of fluids and additional cytokine release.[119]

Types of Cerebral Edema

Progressive edema may result from leukotrienes released from white blood cells and platelets.[79] Leukotrienes are chemoattractant agents primarily involved in the activation of inflammatory and immune responses.[79] Brain swelling after head injury results

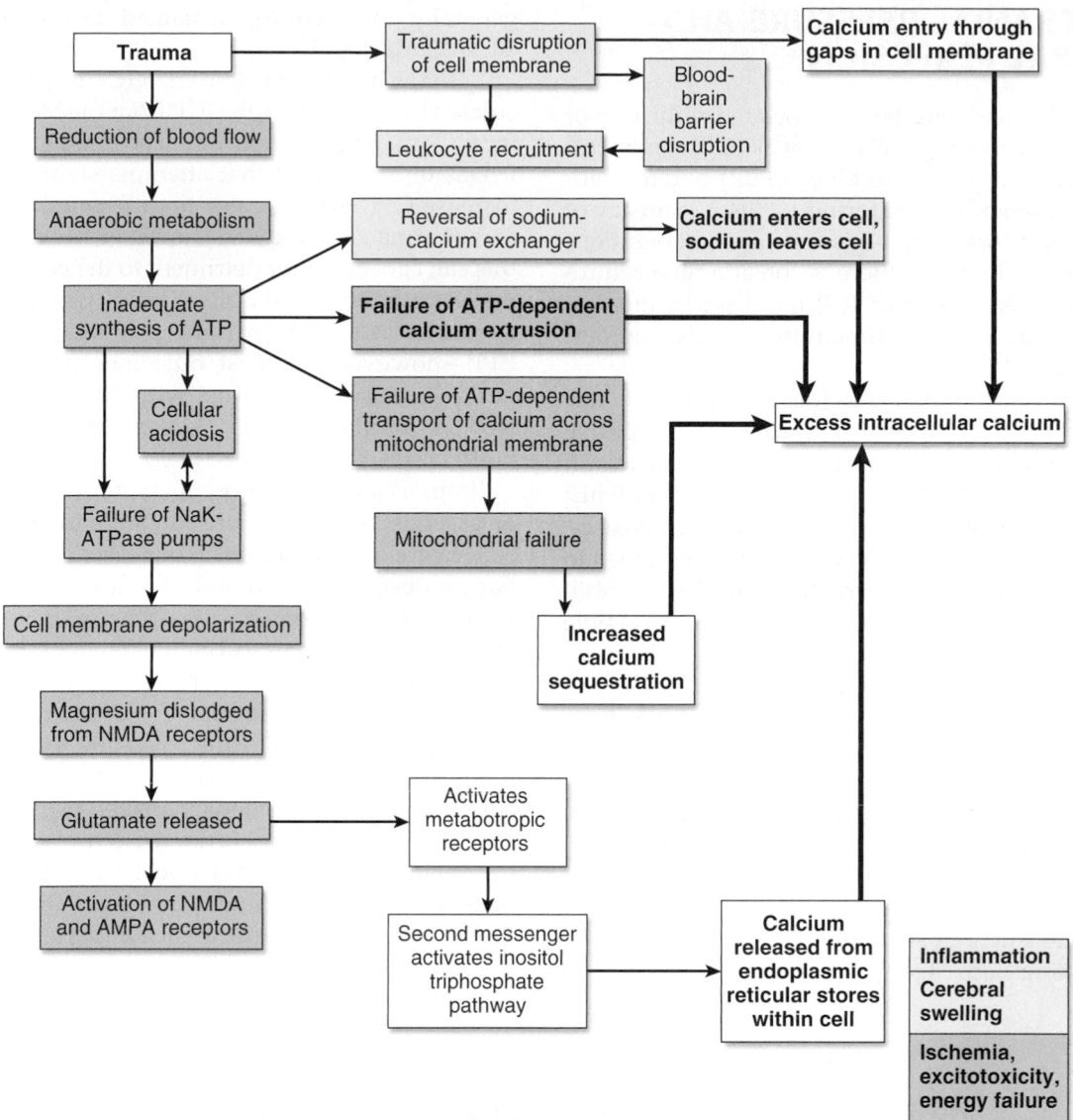

✦FIGURE 22-13 Pathophysiology of secondary brain injury.

from cerebral cellular edema, an increase in intravascular blood volume, or a combination of the two.[24]

Cerebral edema can be classified into five types:[148]

1. Vasogenic edema involves impairment of the BBB leading to accumulation of protein-rich fluid in the extracellular space. Vasogenic edema produces localized swelling around contusions or hematomas.[148]

2. Cytotoxic edema occurs with hypoxic-ischemic damage when there is an ionic gradient disturbance leading to accumulation of intracellular fluid.[148]

3. Hydrostatic edema results from a sudden increase in intravascular pressure in an intact vascular bed, causing extracellular accumulation of protein-poor fluid. Hydrostatic edema may follow the sudden decompression of a mass lesion or may occur when autoregulation is defective following head injury.[148]

4. Osmotic brain edema is caused by critical reductions in serum osmolality, resulting in increased intracellular water. The etiology may be due to iatrogenic hemodilution from excessive use of intravenous dextrose/water solutions, or the syndrome of inappropriate secretion of antidiuretic hormone secretion (SIADH).[148]

5. Interstitial brain edema is produced by periventricular extravasation of water. This uncommon event occurs as a result of high-pressure obstructive hydrocephalus.[148]

INTRACRANIAL PRESSURE AND CEREBRAL PERFUSION

Elevated ICP has long been associated with a poor outcome. ICP levels (especially the peak ICP) can be correlated with poorer prognosis for mortality and morbidity.[131,149,171] Currently, monitoring ICP is a mainstay of TBI therapy and forms the basis for most interventions and treatments. However, there is considerable controversy over the usefulness of ICP monitoring, monitor types, site of placement, treatment thresholds, and outcome measures.[131,171]

According to the Monro-Kellie doctrine, the key determinations of ICP are pressure and volume (Figure 22-14). This doctrine states that the cranial vault is a nondistensible structure with three basic contents: blood, brain, and CSF. If one of these contents increases, another must decrease to allow room for the other to expand. If this does not happen, the brain tissue within the cranial vault will compress, resulting in irreversible damage of the brain until herniation occurs.[124]

Normal ICP is 0 to 15 mm Hg. Elevated ICP can occur even without brain injury. For example, brief increases in intrathoracic pressure as seen with coughing or sneezing can cause ICP to increase greater than 30 to 50 mm Hg. In these situations the brain is normal and homeostasis returns within seconds. However, with TBI, ICP increases as a result of swelling of the brain tissue. Transient elevations in ICP also occur with activities such as suctioning, turning, and other routine nursing care. Treatment for increased ICP is generally initiated for sustained levels greater than 20 to 25 mm Hg.[33]

Perhaps more important than ICP is CPP. CPP is calculated by subtracting the ICP from the MAP.[11] The goal for CPP management in TBI is 60 mm Hg or greater.[228] It was once thought that attempts should be made to increase CPP even greater than 70 mm Hg with fluids and pharmacologic agents; however, we now know that this can cause further detriment to the patient by resulting in pulmonary complications.[33] Controversy exists as to what is the best parameter to treat in TBI—ICP or CPP—however, the best outcomes probably involve multimodality monitoring with these parameters as well as jugular venous oxygen saturation (SjvO₂) or brain tissue oxygen levels (BtO₂).[160]

Brain tissue damage results from increasing pressure on essential brain structures. In brain injuries with associated cerebral edema, small increases in volume are not harmful because blood and CSF flow out of the cranial vault to accommodate increased brain tissue volume.[124] However, if there is further edema or swelling, the increased pressure compresses vascular structures, reducing cerebral perfusion.[163] When cerebral perfusion falls below a critical value, cerebral ischemia occurs (Figure 22-15). Ischemia leads to neuronal injury and aggravates cerebral edema, further increasing ICP.[124] As the ICP continues to increase, pressure gradients eventually displace brain tissue from areas of higher pressure to areas of lower pressure. Displacement of the brain from one intracranial compartment to another is known as herniation.[11]

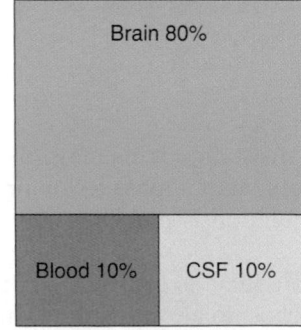 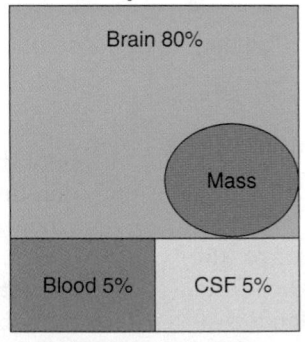 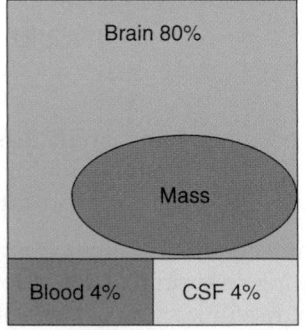

FIGURE 22-14 Monro-Kellie doctrine.

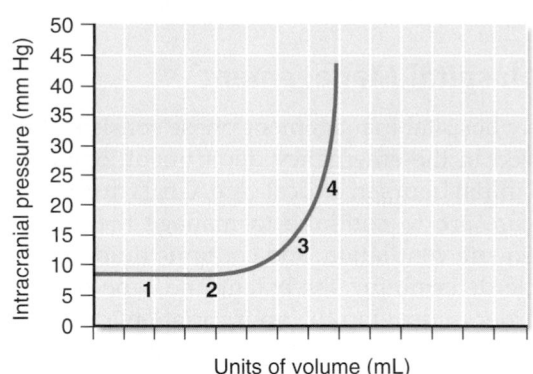

STAGES ON THE PRESSURE-VOLUME CURVE

Stage 1: There is high compliance and low elastance. The brain is in total compensation, with accommodation and autoregulation intact. An increase in volume does not increase ICP.

Stage 2: The compliance is lower and elastance is increasing. An increase in volume places the patient at risk of increased ICP.

Stage 3: There is high elastance and low compliance. Any small addition of volume causes a great increase in pressure. There is a loss of autoregulation, and there may be symptoms indicating increased ICP, such as systolic hypertension with an increasing pulse pressure, bradycardia, and slowing of respiratory rate (Cushing's triad). With the loss of autoregulation and the rise in the systolic blood pressure as a result of the Cushing response, decompensation occurs. The ICP passively mimics the blood pressure.

Stage 4: Finally, when the patient reaches stage 4, the ICP rises to terminal levels with little increase in volume. Herniation occurs as the brain tissue shifts from the compartment of greater pressure to the compartment of lesser pressure.

✦**FIGURE 22-15** Pressure-volume curve.

HERNIATION

Four main types of herniation can occur: cingulate, uncal, transtentorial, and central (Figure 22-16). They may occur in isolation from one another or in combination as intracranial pressure gradients can displace brain tissue laterally and downward at the same time. Herniation syndromes are life-threatening occurrences and can progress rapidly.[85]

To understand the different types of herniation, it is important to briefly review the basic anatomy within the intracranial cavity. The cavity is divided into smaller compartments by fibrous dura mater; folds in the dura are the falx cerebri and the tentorium cerebelli. The falx cerebri divides the supratentorial space into a left and right side along a longitudinal fissure.[85] The tentorium cerebelli separates the occipital lobes from the cerebellum and most of the brain stem.[85]

Cingulate herniation occurs as increasing pressure from an expanding lesion in one cerebral hemisphere pushes brain tissue beneath the falx cerebri.[85,141] Intracranial volume is displaced across the midline and compresses brain tissue on the opposite side of the brain as well as vascular structures, potentiating cerebral edema and ischemia.[85] This results in an increase in ICP, but little else is known about the signs and symptoms associated with cingulate herniation.[85] Uncal herniation occurs when brain tissue is shifted toward the midline and then over the edge of the tentorium cerebelli.[141] Classic signs of uncal herniation include rapid deterioration of consciousness, an ipsilateral fixed and dilated pupil, contralateral hemiparesis, and progressive dysfunction of cranial nerves III through

XII.[85,141] This type of herniation is associated with unilateral lesions and can cause life-threatening brain stem compression.[141]

Transtentorial herniation, the most common form of herniation,[85] involves compression of the brain stem, anteroposterior elongation of the midbrain, buckling of the tectum, downward stretching of the basilar artery and its branches, and displacement of the medulla into the foramen magnum.[85] This is a life-threatening event when brain stem structures are involved. Signs are coma, abnormal respiratory patterns, pupillary changes, and abnormal posturing progressing to flaccidity.[85] Central herniation is transtentorial herniation associated

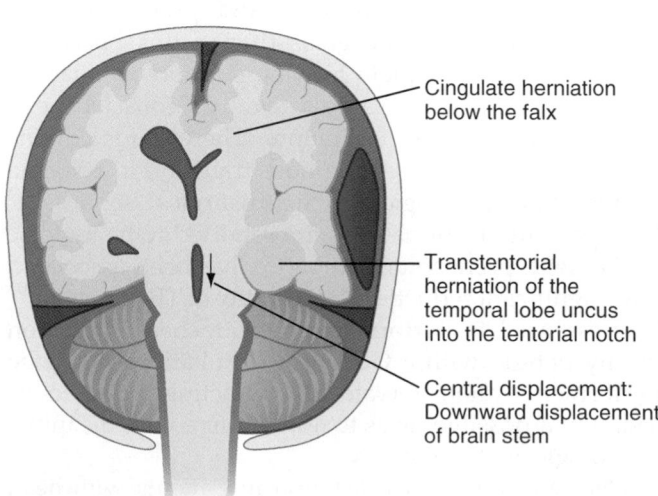

Cingulate herniation below the falx

Transtentorial herniation of the temporal lobe uncus into the tentorial notch

Central displacement: Downward displacement of brain stem

✦**FIGURE 22-16** Brain displacement from supratentorial herniation.

with medullary compression and ultimately brain stem death.[85]

A compensatory hemodynamic response to herniation is the Cushing's phenomenon. Life-threatening increased ICP, as seen with herniation, reduces CBF, which initiates autoregulatory mechanisms to restore adequate perfusion to the brain. Cushing's phenomenon, seen in patients with intact cerebral autoregulation, refers to the triad of cardiovascular symptoms indicative of herniation: hypertension, bradycardia, and respiratory irregularity.[52–54,91,94]

MULTIDISCIPLINARY PLAN OF CARE FOR THE TRAUMATIC BRAIN INJURY PATIENT

In TBI, the goal of treatment is to limit the extent of secondary damage using hemodynamic and pharmacologic neuroprotective strategies. Determining optimal methods for achieving this goal has been the focus of most research in the last decade related to managing brain injuries. Current treatment of TBI involves supportive therapy, neuroprotection, control of ICP, and hemodynamic stabilization; ongoing research continues to identify new treatment options.[119] Management of the patient with TBI can be divided into various phases of care. These management phases, summarized below, are prehospital, early hospital, critical care, and rehabilitation.

Prehospital Phase

The prehospital phase starts immediately after injury and continues until emergency department (ED) arrival. This is probably the most important time interval for determining eventual outcome and preventing irreversible damage.[124] The goals during this phase are to maintain an adequate airway, support ventilation, immobilize the spine, assess level of consciousness, and initiate fluid resuscitation. These interventions should be followed by expeditious transport to a trauma center with neurologic and neurosurgical services.[124] Fifty percent of TBI patients are reported to be hypoxic in the field; prehospital intubation has been associated with significant reduction in mortality of TBI patients.[204] It is essential to perform early orotracheal intubation in any patient with a GCS ≤8.[33] Intubation should be performed without the aid of long-acting paralytics or sedation if possible, so as to not interfere with the initial neurologic evaluation.[126]

Delayed volume resuscitation in patients with head injuries has been shown to affect the extent of secondary brain injuries.[124] Early volume resuscitation with Ringer's lactate is important if systolic BP is less than 110 mm Hg.

Alternatively, small volume resuscitation with a hypertonic saline solution (HTS) may be appropriate.[197,220] Research regarding the use of HTS continues. The use of HTS will be discussed fully later in this section.

Early Hospital Management

The early hospital management phase consists of the care received in the emergency department, operating room, and initial hours in critical care. Goals during this phase of care are to continue to manage the airway, ensure adequate ventilation, and continue fluid resuscitation while determining the extent and type of brain injury in order to develop the appropriate plan of care. Patients with GCS ≤8, and those who are otherwise unable to protect their airway, require immediate intubation if this was not previously performed. The incidence of concomitant spinal cord injury (SCI) with TBI is 6% to 8%;[86,146] therefore cervical spine precautions need to be maintained at all times, especially during intubation. Cervical spine precautions include using a rigid cervical collar and back boards and log-rolling the patient until any damage to the spine is ruled out radiographically.[86,146]

Unless essential, drugs that have a hypnotic effect and those that reduce vascular tone should be avoided to ensure accurate neurologic exams and adequate cerebral blood flow. Initially, all TBI patients should be placed on 100% oxygen; the fraction of inspired oxygen (FiO_2) can then be titrated down to maintain an adequate PaO_2.[33,159] The $PaCO_2$ should be maintained between 35 and 40 mm Hg. The use of prophylactic hyperventilation ($PaCO_2$ ≤35 mm Hg) should be avoided in the first 24 hours following TBI.[31] Although this practice can rapidly reduce ICP, it does so by decreasing CBF through severe vasoconstriction. The decreased CBF quickly leads to ischemic damage. Clinical studies have demonstrated that patients hyperventilated after head injury experienced worse neurologic outcomes compared to patients kept normocarbic.[33,159]

After securing an airway and oxygenation, maintaining a BP and restoring normal circulating volume are essential. The current Brain Trauma Foundation (BTF) guidelines[33] for management of severe head injury state that maintaining a MAP of ≥90 mm Hg should be the goal for the TBI patient in order to ensure a cerebral perfusion pressure of 60 mm Hg.[228] A single episode of hypotension is associated with a doubling of mortality and an increase in morbidity following TBI.[33] Therefore it is extremely important to aggressively restore normal circulating volume to avoid hypotensive episodes. The optimal method for restoring circulating volume is through the use of isotonic fluids. Other fluid options may include the use of packed red blood cells (PRBCs) if the patient has experienced blood loss, HTS, and

◆ Case Study 22-1, Part A

Head Injury and Dysfunction

M.P., a 34-year-old male, was working on the roof of his house when he fell approximately 20 feet from a ladder and hit his head on the ground. His wife saw him fall and immediately called 9-1-1. Emergency medical technicians (EMTs) arrived within 5 minutes. Upon their arrival, M.P. was walking around his yard disoriented and combative and had a GCS of 14. M.P. had an unremarkable medical history. As the EMTs tried to calm the patient, he suddenly lost consciousness and had difficulty maintaining his airway. His left pupil was 5 mm in size and reacted sluggishly. The right pupil was 3 mm and briskly reactive. M.P.'s GCS was now 7; he was orally intubated and quickly rushed to the ED.

Soon after arrival to the ED, the patient experienced a grand mal seizure. He was treated for the seizure activity with 4 mg of intravenous lorazepam and then given a loading dose of 1000 mg of phenytoin. His pupils were still unequal, with the left now 6 mm and the right 4 mm, and both were reacting sluggishly. M.P. was somnolent and had decreased movement of his right arm and leg. His BP was 130/78 mm Hg, telemetry indicated sinus rhythm at a rate of 64 beats/min, and respirations were being controlled by the ventilator at a rate of 14 per minute.

Following initial stabilization in the ED, M.P. was immediately taken to the radiology department for a CT scan of the head that revealed a left SDH and a small left temporal SAH. Additional CT findings included a left temporal nondepressed skull fracture and a left linear basilar skull fracture.

He was taken to the OR for evacuation of the SDH, and a fiberoptic intraparenchymal ICP monitor was placed in his right cerebral hemisphere. M.P. was then admitted to neuroscience critical care.

The plan of care for M.P. included continued mechanical ventilation. His initial settings were 100% Fio_2, PRVC mode, rate 16, tidal volume 650 ml, PEEP 5 cm H_2O, pressure support 10 cm H_2O. His arterial blood gas (ABG) on these settings yielded the following results: pH 7.42, $Paco_2$ 41 mm Hg, Pao_2 185 mm Hg. Fio_2 was quickly weaned down to 40%, maintaining oxygen saturation (Sao_2) >95%. Vital signs were stable in critical care: heart rate 98 beats/min in normal sinus rhythm, respiratory rate 18 breaths/min, BP 118/74 mm Hg, temperature 97.2° F, ICP 8–12 mm Hg with a CPP of 76–80 mm Hg.

Clinical findings included bilateral periorbital ecchymosis (raccoon eyes). His initial neurologic exam was limited because of anesthesia, but after 2 hours the patient became agitated, he localized to pain, and he had no eye opening and no verbal response because of intubation. The patient's pupils were 4 mm and briskly reactive to light bilaterally.

Decision Point: What is the patient's current GCS?

Decision Point: What caused the changes noted in M.P.'s pupils?

Decision Point: What clinical assessment criteria will the critical care nursing staff need to monitor on an ongoing basis?

Case continues on page 555

---

albumin. Should the patient with TBI be unresponsive to fluid resuscitation, norepinephrine may be used to increase MAP without resulting in hyperemia if pressure autoregulation is preserved.[135] Aggressive attempts to maintain CPP greater than 70 mm Hg with fluids or vasopressors should be avoided because of the increased risk of pulmonary complications.[33]

Isotonic fluids, such as normal saline (NS) or lactated Ringer's solution, are appropriate for volume resuscitation of hypotensive, hypovolemic patients. Hypotonic solutions (e.g., 0.45% NS or 2.5% D_5W) are dangerous to use because sudden fluid shifts from the intravascular space into brain cells increases cerebral edema and elevates ICP. They should not be administered to head-injured patients.[208]

HTS has been identified as beneficial in head-injured patients. The effects of HTS include expansion of intravascular volume, extraction of water from the intracellular space into the intravascular space, ICP reduction, and increased cardiac contractility.[13,98,137] Some studies have found its use associated with significantly improved survival.[13,99,137,220] Administration of HTS will cause an increase in serum sodium concentrations, but levels as high as 170 mEq/L are well tolerated in

the head-injured patient.[82,104,168,223] Although HTS use appears promising, optimal timing, appropriate concentration, and ideal volume have yet to be determined. During this phase of care, the prophylactic use of mannitol is not recommended unless the patient is exhibiting signs of transtentorial herniation[175] because of its volume-depleting diuretic effect.[30]

Continued Critical Care Management

Once the patient is stabilized and transferred to critical care, it is important to implement further physiologic monitoring in order to facilitate and direct the ongoing management of these patients.[124] Continued hemodynamic and respiratory resuscitation may be required to manage associated injuries as well as protect cerebral perfusion. Because early priorities for managing the patient's neurologic injuries are to control intracranial pressure and limit secondary brain injury, ICP monitoring should be instituted as soon as possible in ED, operating room (OR), or critical care. Treatment of TBI patients in critical care is guided by ICP monitoring and focused on reducing elevated pressures according to accepted guidelines.[30] Extended critical care management of these patients will require ongoing fluid resuscitation, ventilator management, and nutritional support (see the Nutrition box on p. 541). Attention must also be focused on preventing and treating complications such as electrolyte derangements, pulmonary problems, deep vein thrombosis, and stress ulcers. Some of these will be discussed later in this chapter, beginning on p. 562.

Rehabilitation

The last phase of care with the TBI patient is rehabilitation. This is necessary for the majority of severely injured patients and often for those with moderate brain injuries as well. The goal of rehabilitation is to improve the patient's functional and cognitive status as much as possible with the goal of returning to preinjury status. Because this phase of care is outside the scope of this publication, the reader is referred to a rehabilitation text for further information on this topic area.

MONITORING

There are several techniques for monitoring brain tissue for signs of damage related to TBI. Monitoring devices measure ICP, oxygenation of the brain tissue, electroencephalogram (EEG) activity, CBF, and even electrolytes and other substrates in the brain tissue. It is the prevalent thought that there is not one method that should be solely relied upon for all treatment decisions, but rather a multimodality approach will best serve the patients with TBI.[160]

Intracranial Pressure Monitoring

The most common monitoring technique is ICP monitoring. ICP can be monitored in the intraparenchymal tissue, epidural space, subdural space, and intraventricular sites (Table 22-5 and Figure 22-17).[11] Intraventricular monitoring has been considered the gold standard for ICP measurement and allows for drainage of CSF.[11] However, the catheter used for this method is also the most difficult to place, especially if the ventricles are small or displaced. Intraventricular monitoring also has the highest risk of infection and other complications such as occlusion or tissue or vascular injury.[11] Therefore other monitoring methods may be preferred. The most commonly used technique is intraparenchymal monitoring. Placement of an intraparenchymal ICP probe is quick and easy, with very few associated complications. However, if CSF drainage is required, a separate intraventricular catheter will be required (Figure 22-18).[85]

TABLE 22-5 Comparison of Intracranial Pressure Monitors			
TYPE	**SITE**	**ADVANTAGES**	**DISADVANTAGES**
Intraventricular catheter	Ventricles	Most accurate, CSF cultures can be collected, CSF can be withdrawn to control ICP, contrast materials can be injected for radiologic studies	Risk of hemorrhage, increased risk of infection, risk of CSF leak at site, artifacts may cause dampening of recordings, more difficult to insert
Subarachnoid bolt	Subarachnoid space	Can be used with small or collapsed ventricles, does not penetrate brain parenchyma, low infection rates, low cost, ease and safety of insertion	Does not allow CSF drainage or withdrawal, becomes occluded, may dampen and give unreliable readings after a few days, brain tissue may herniate into bolt
Epidural sensor	Epidural space	Ease of insertion, least invasive, recommended in cases of meningitis and CNS infections, less risk of infection, does not require recalibration	Slower response time, fragile, can become wedged against skull, affected by heat or febrile patient, diaphragm can rupture, less accurate, unable to drain CSF
Intraparenchymal catheter	Intraparenchymal tissue	Very accurate, yields good waveform patterns, second only to intraventricular based on accuracy and stability, easy and quick to insert even with small ventricles	Fiberoptic catheters can break if kinked or stretched, does not allow CSF drainage or withdrawal, potential complications of infection or hemorrhage

Data from references 11, 85.

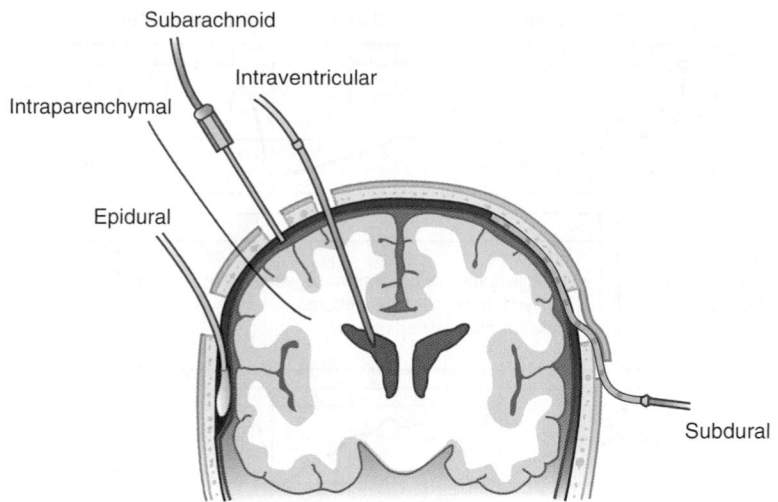

FIGURE 22-17 Potential sites for intracranial pressure monitoring devices.

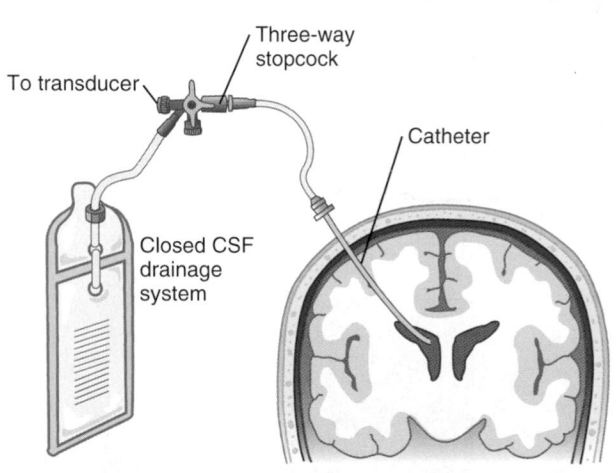

FIGURE 22-18 Intraventricular catheter system.

ICP waveform interpretation is an important aspect of monitoring patients. The relationship between CPP and exhaustion of autoregulation can be identified through analysis of ICP waveforms. Compliance related to brain compression is also identified by waveform interpretation. Physiologic compliance of the intracranial system is related to cerebrovascular alterations, particularly venous outflow resistance.[41] Waveforms represent intracranial and arterial pulsations reflecting the cardiac and respiratory cycles. Waveforms have three peaks: P_1, P_2, and P_3 (Figure 22-19). P_1 is the percussion wave and is thought to originate from pulsations of the intracranial arteries and the choroid plexus.[41] P_2 is the tidal wave and has a lower and more variable amplitude than P_1.[41] P_3, the dicrotic wave, has the lowest amplitude and usually tapers back to baseline.[41] Wave amplitude changes as the brain's volume and compliance change. If P_1 and P_2 are equal,

compliance is poor, indicating an inability to compensate for additional increases in volume.[41] It is important to be able to identify these waveforms and their variations in order to most appropriately treat the TBI patient. For example, if P_1 and P_2 are of equal amplitude, meaning the compliance is poor, it would be best to limit care activities or space interventions. Nursing activities such as turning may need to be modified based on waveform interpretation. Suctioning may also need to be kept brief or require premedication with lidocaine to limit ICP response during this activity. Performing these and other nursing interventions guided by waveform interpretation and assessment of compliance changes may prevent dangerous elevation in ICP that might precipitate herniation syndromes.[41]

ICP waveforms generally fall into one of three different types: A, B, or C. A waves are plateau waves of large amplitude (50 to 100 mm Hg) and variable duration (5 to 20 min). These waves are clinically significant and indicate dangerously reduced intracranial compliance. 'A' waves indicate increased ICP and demand immediate attention because, if unalleviated, cerebral ischemia and neurologic deterioration will result.[41] B waves are smaller (up to 50 mm Hg), sharper waves with a dominant frequency (0.5 to 2/min).[41] C waves are small (up to 20 mm Hg), rhythmic oscillations with a frequency of 4 to 8/min.[41] These are of little clinical significance (Figure 22-20).

Neuroimaging

Early identification of intracranial pathology is essential to determine whether surgery is needed and to guide additional interventions. The most commonly used method for neuroimaging is CT scan. The CT is

INTRACRANIAL PRESSURE WAVEFORM ANALYSIS

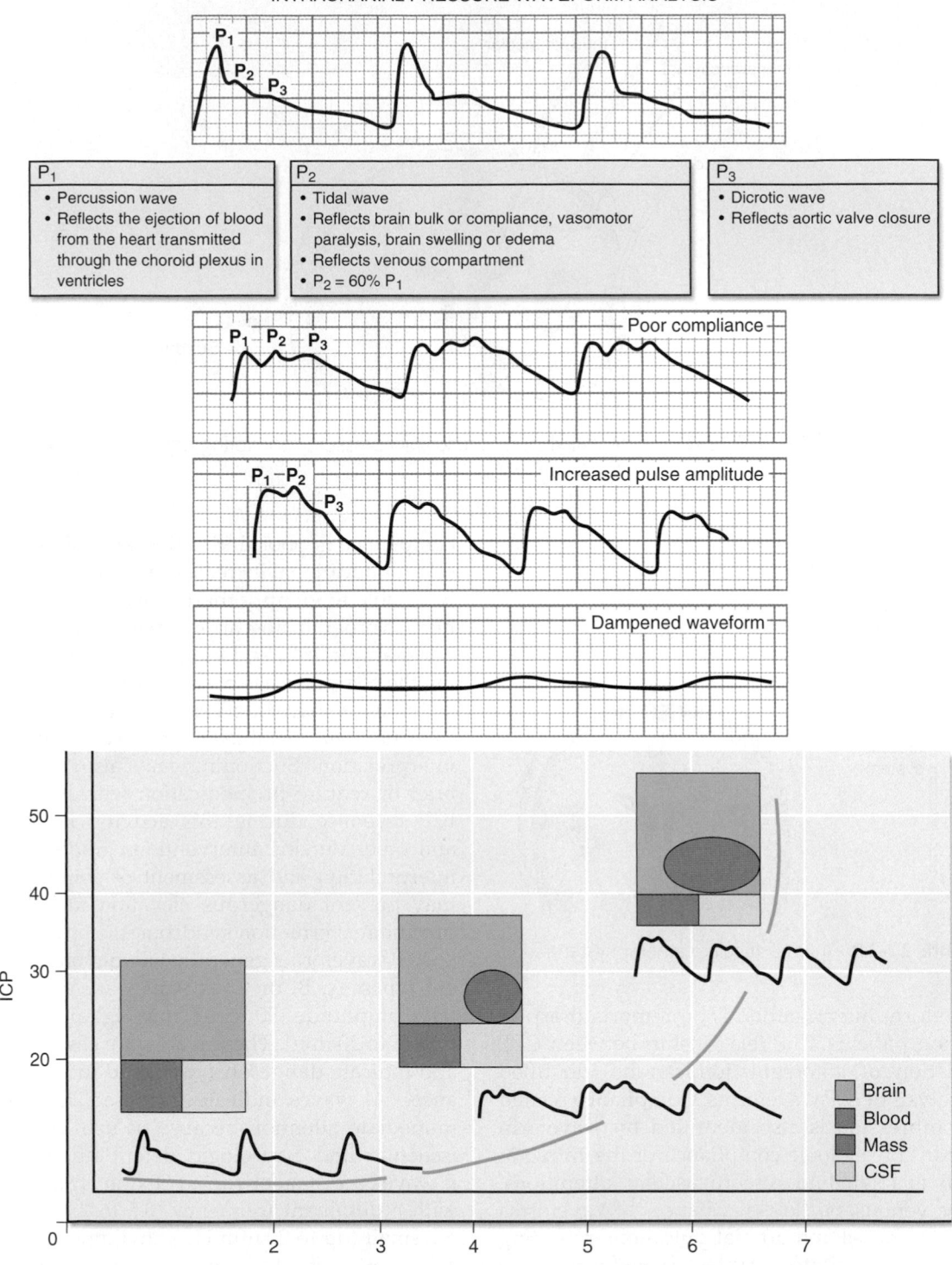

P₁	P₂	P₃
• Percussion wave • Reflects the ejection of blood from the heart transmitted through the choroid plexus in ventricles	• Tidal wave • Reflects brain bulk or compliance, vasomotor paralysis, brain swelling or edema • Reflects venous compartment • $P_2 = 60\%\ P_1$	• Dicrotic wave • Reflects aortic valve closure

✦FIGURE 22-19 Normal intracranial pressure waveform.

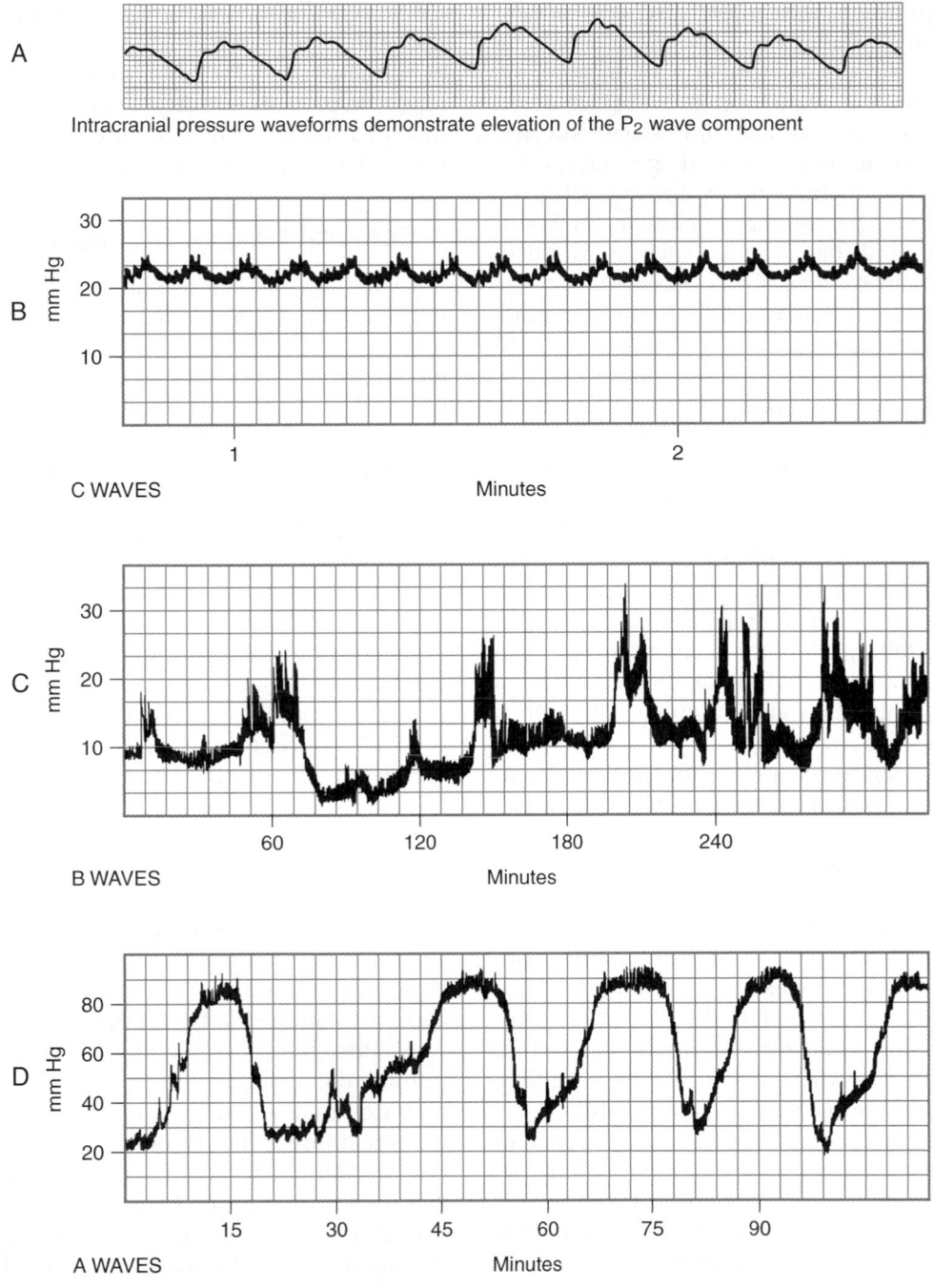

Intracranial pressure waveforms demonstrate elevation of the P₂ wave component

$\blacklozenge$**FIGURE 22-20** Types of intracranial pressure waveforms.

helpful for identifying gross abnormalities, bleeding, fractures, hydrocephalus, and edema.[124] MRIs may be used later in the patient's course to identify more subtle lesions such as shearing and ischemic changes.[124] The patient is unavailable for interventions during the MRI; therefore these exams may be deferred until later in the hospital course when the patient is determined to be more stable.

A CT scan is the diagnostic procedure of choice for the evaluation of acute head trauma. CT scanners are quick and readily available in most institutions. A head CT should be performed on anyone who has a GCS less than 15 with focal neurologic deficits, clinical signs of a basilar or depressed skull fracture, or any loss of consciousness (LOC).[33] It is important to remember that a normal initial CT scan does not exclude the presence of significant intracranial hypertension.[124] Therefore it is important to review the CT scan in context with the clinical examination of the patient. Emergent neurosurgical evaluation is critical for determining whether to proceed with immediate surgical evacuation of hematomas. General guidelines for surgical intervention include the following: all acute traumatic extra-axial hematomas ≥1 cm in thickness; subdural or epidural hematomas >5 mm in thickness with equivalent midline shifts; comatose patients (GCS ≤8); intracerebral hematomas >20 ml with mass effect; and depressed, compound skull fractures.[124,194]

One technique that is available for measuring CBF quantitatively is xenon-enhanced CT. This scan uses xenon to quantify the brain's uptake and clearance of this diffusible gas.[166] Because xenon is a lipid-soluble gas, it diffuses freely across the BBB, allowing it to be used as a tracer to measure CBF. Xenon is administered most commonly by inhalation, but can also be used intravenously. This is a relatively easy method that can be used to determine global and regional CBF. This technique can be affected by patient movement, resulting in artifact and inaccurate results. The xenon concentration can also cause vasodilation and augment CBF, which can also affect the study results.[165]

Other types of imaging techniques for functional neuroimaging include positron emission tomography (PET) and single-photon emission computed tomography (SPECT). PET and SPECT scanning techniques use radionuclide tracers injected into the patient and then employ different scanning techniques to assess cerebral blood flow and metabolism.[36,112] These techniques are helpful in determining changes in CBF and metabolism during recovery. These scans may detect areas of cerebral dysfunction and brain ischemia that may not be detected on CT scan or MRI.[36,112] For this reason, they are helpful in determining prognosis after TBI.[36,112,178] Because these techniques only provide a snapshot of CBF, they are not routinely used in the acute setting.

Monitoring techniques used for other neurologic dysfunctions are currently being investigated for use in TBIs as well. Transcranial Doppler ultrasonography (TCD) penetrates thin areas of the cranium using a low-frequency ultrasonic signal to measure velocity and direction of blood flow in the intracranial arteries.[57,121] This is most commonly used to detect vasospasm following aneurysms and other vascular disorders, but it may also be helpful in detecting posttraumatic cerebral hemodynamic changes and complications such as hyperemia, vasospasm, decreased CBF, and intracranial hypertension.[57,121] Magnetic resonance angiography (MRA) is another technique that may be beneficial with TBI. MRA, typically used for identification of location of vascular lesions such as aneurysms and AVMs, utilizes flow measurement by oxyhemoglobin spectral

shifts and contrast indication transit times to detect flow through the vasculature to identify any vascular abnormalities.[232] This is currently being investigated for use in patients with acute severe head injuries. These methods and their value in the critical care management phase require further evaluation.

Cerebral Oxygen Monitoring

Extremely valuable methods for monitoring patients with TBI include the use of devices that measure cerebral oxygenation. Methods for monitoring oxygenation include continuous monitoring of jugular venous oxygen and brain tissue oxygen sensors. Monitoring the partial pressure of brain tissue oxygen ($Pbto_2$) has recently emerged as a promising therapeutic guide for patients with severe TBI.[7] Still in its infancy, monitoring $Pbto_2$ is emerging as a preferred method for predicting unfavorable patient outcomes that result from decreased levels of brain oxygenation.[160,217] Many experts now believe that oxygen monitoring may be even more important than pressure monitoring for guiding therapeutic support in the TBI patient.[7,33,160,217] This issue is explored in the Research Utilization box on p. 553. $Pbto_2$ represents local brain tissue oxygenation; a $Pbto_2$ of 15 mm Hg is accepted as the critical lower limit in patients with severe TBI.[7] Low $Pbto_2$ levels have been described in up to 50% of patients within 24 hours after TBI.[34] Some controversy still exists as to whether the most appropriate placement site for the probe is within injured tissue, penumbral, or uninjured tissue.[161,218] Future clinical studies will continue to clarify these issues. Two devices used to monitor $Pbto_2$ are currently commercially available.

Another means of monitoring brain oxygenation is through the use of a jugular venous bulb catheter. $Sjvo_2$ provides an assessment of global cerebral oxygenation and an indirect indication of CBF.[76] This catheter is inserted into the jugular vein in a retrograde fashion so that the tip rests in the jugular bulb. Placement is confirmed by plain radiograph film. Much like mixed venous oxygen saturation (Svo_2) monitoring, $Sjvo_2$ is thought to represent global brain oxygenation and cellular oxygen utilization.[160] Normal $Sjvo_2$ in an adult is approximately 65% (ranging from 55% to 71%).[76] In comatose patients, values greater than 50% are considered normal.[51,195] Whenever $Sjvo_2$ drops below 50% for more than 15 minutes, the etiology must be sought. A decline in $Sjvo_2$ may be caused by low Pao_2, prolonged hyperventilation, decreased CPP (less than 70 mm Hg), vasospasm, or low hemoglobin concentration.[76] An increase in $Sjvo_2$ reflects an increased supply of oxygen to the brain (i.e., hyperemia) or decreased oxygen utilization from sedation, barbiturates, hypothermia, or large areas of cerebral infarction.[7,76,160]

◆ **RESEARCH UTILIZATION**

Monitoring of Brain Tissue Oxygenation via $Sjvo_2$ or Bto_2

CLINICAL ISSUE

Research continues to evolve regarding the use of Bto_2 monitoring. As research in this area continues to develop, it will be important for nurses to appropriately use this technology. It is important to monitor brain tissue oxygenation via $Sjvo_2$ or Bto_2. Measurement of brain tissue oxygenation via a Bto_2 probe is important with hyperventilation to ensure that any further reduction in $Paco_2$ (values <30 mm Hg) does not compromise blood flow and cause brain tissue death. A fundamental principle in caring for TBI patients is to ensure adequate cerebral oxygenation and perfusion. This monitoring and appropriate interventions based on these data may be shown to improve outcomes of patients with TBI.

SUMMARY

van den Brink and colleagues (2000) studied 101 comatose, head-injured patients with a GCS ≤8. Patients were treated according to nationally accepted guidelines with a brain tissue oxygen probe inserted. Depth and duration of brain tissue hypoxia were related to outcome, and brain tissue hypoxia was an independent predictor of unfavorable outcome and death at 6 months after injury. This study demonstrates the need to increase CPP and decrease ICP in TBI patients, and the importance of instituting interventions that increase brain tissue oxygen levels.

APPLICATION

- Develop procedures for managing patients using Bto_2 as a parameter to guide resuscitation.
- Develop protocols with treatment algorithms for management of Bto_2.
- Goal of therapy should be to maintain the following: Sao_2 100%, optimal MAP, $Pbto_2$ >20 mm Hg or $Sjvo_2$ >55% and <75%, ICP <20 mm Hg.
- If $Pbto_2$ drops <15 mm Hg, place on Fio_2 at 100% until $Pbto_2$ >20.
- Continue with other interventions for ICP management including fluids, vasopressors (if needed), sedation, and maintenance of normothermia.

NEED FOR FURTHER STUDY

Future studies are needed to monitor outcomes of TBI patients based on clinical management of $Pbto_2$ levels.

van den Brink W. A., et al. (2000). Brain oxygen tension in severe head injury. *Neurosurgery*, 46(4): 868–878.

Arterio-jugular venous difference of oxygen ($Avjdo_2$) is calculated by subtracting the content of jugular venous oxygen from the arterial oxygen content.[141] This provides an overall picture of cerebral blood flow and oxygen consumption. Normal $Avjdo_2$ levels range from 4.5 to 8.5 ml/dl. Elevations occur as a result of inadequate cerebral blood flow or decreased oxygen consumption. Decreased values reflect an excessive oxygen delivery over the demand for oxygen.[141]

$Sjvo_2$ reflects global cerebral blood flow and is therefore unable to detect focal ischemic episodes. Because jugular bulb and local oxygen pressure monitoring complement each other by providing distinctly different information, many facilities use these modalities in conjunction with each other.[7] Still, many unanswered questions remain regarding the use of brain oxygen monitoring (Table 22-6); additional studies regarding placement, critical values, and use of values as resuscitation guides are needed.

Microdialysis

Microdialysis has been used as a research tool to identify neurochemical and metabolic changes following TBI.[93] Microdialysis involves the insertion of a tubular dialysis membrane into the brain tissue to measure lactate, glucose, pyruvate, and glutamate.[18] Correlations have been noted between reduced cerebral oxygenation and elevations in lactate concentration. Microdialysis has currently been used only in experimental settings and is not yet widely accepted for routine clinical practice.[18,93]

Continuous Electroencephalography

Continuous EEG monitoring has limited applications in TBI, but indications for monitoring are expanding as more possibilities are being explored. The most routine and well-accepted application of continuous EEG monitoring is in the patient with induced barbiturate coma for refractory increased ICP.[63,178] EEG monitoring facilitates assessment of the extent of burst suppression. Other applications for EEG monitoring may include diagnosis of seizure activity and verification of the absence of brain activity in the diagnosis of brain death.[63]

Another type of EEG monitoring that may have future applications in TBI is the use of bispectral index

TABLE 22-6 Monitoring Parameters

PARAMETER	SOURCE	NORMAL VALUE	CRITICAL LEVELS
Parameters Used in TBI			
ICP	Directly measured	0–15 mm Hg	>20 mm Hg
CPP	Calculated: MAP − ICP	60–100 mm Hg	<60 mm Hg
CBF	Directly measured Calculated	50–55 ml/100 g/min	<28–20 ml/100 g/min
CMR_{O_2}		3.2 ml/100 g/min	
Pbt_{O_2}	Directly measured	25–40 mm Hg	Low: <20 mm Hg *Ischemic values:* <15 mm Hg for 30 min <10 mm Hg for 10 min
Sjv_{O_2}	Directly measured	55%–75%	<50% for 10 min
Cerebral Extraction			
Of oxygen (CE_{O_2})	Calculated: $Sa_{O_2} - Sjv_{O_2}$	24%–40%	<24% oxygen, supply greater than demand >40% oxygen, supply less than demand
Avj_{DO_2}	Calculated: $Ca_{O_2} - Cjv_{O_2}$ $Ca_{O_2} = (Sa_{O_2} \times 1.34 \times Hb) + (Pa_{O_2} \times 0.0031)$ $Cjv_{O_2} = (Sjv_{O_2} \times 1.34 \times Hb) + (Pjv_{O_2} \times 0.0031)$	4.5–8.5 ml/dl	<4.5 ml/dl, oxygen supply greater than demand >8.5 ml/dl, oxygen supply insufficient for demand

Data from references 7, 11, 142.
ICP = Intracranial pressure, CPP = cerebral perfusion pressure, MAP = mean arterial pressure, CBF = cerebral blood flow, CMR_{O_2} = cerebral metabolic rate of oxygen, Pbt_{O_2} = partial pressure of brain tissue oxygen, Sa_{O_2} = arterial oxygen saturation, Sjv_{O_2} = jugular venous oxygen saturation, CE_{O_2} = cerebral extraction of oxygen, Avj_{O_2} = arterio-jugular venous oxygen difference, Ca_{O_2} = arterial oxygen content, Cjv_{O_2} = jugular venous oxygen content, Hb = hemoglobin, Pjv_{O_2} = partial pressure of jugular venous oxygen.

(BIS) monitoring. BIS monitoring is a newer technology integrating electromyography (EMG) and EEG waveforms to assess sedation levels.[179] This has been used in operative situations to assess sedation levels and absence of recall.[69] Another potential use for BIS is monitoring of sedated patients and those in pentobarbital-induced coma.[8,179] The BIS value provides a numerical representation from 0 to 100, with 100 being wide awake. Typically, a BIS value of 40 to 60 represents the absence of recall, and this is the goal in operative situations and in critical care sedation. An additional index on the BIS monitor is the suppression ratio (SR)—a measurement of the percentage of EEG in the last 60 seconds that is completely suppressed or isoelectric.[69] This number is a measure from 0 to 100, with 0 being no burst suppression of the EEG and a measure of 100 indicating the complete absence of electrical activity.[69] When used for therapeutic barbiturate coma, the goal of therapy is to keep BIS less than 20 and SR greater than 70.[179] Recent data suggest that BIS may be a potentially viable assessment tool that is easily applied and interpreted at the bedside and may be particularly valuable to guide titration of barbiturates.[8,179] Other tools for monitoring patients with TBI are currently under investigation.

Decision Point: What interventions would be appropriately instituted for decreased Sjvo$_2$ values?

Decision Point: What additional interventions could be used to help control the patient's ICP?

Case continues on page 569

Case Study 22-1, Part B

Head Injury and Dysfunction

The next day, M.P. experienced ICP spikes to 30 mm Hg on two separate occasions. He had orders to receive bolus doses of 150 ml of 20% mannitol whenever his ICP remained elevated above 20 mm Hg for greater than 10 minutes (usual dose is 0.25–0.5 g/kg; repeat every 3–5 hours for treatment of elevated ICP). He received mannitol and aggressive nursing interventions to decrease his ICP. Nursing interventions for prevention and control of ICP included elevating head of bed at 30 degrees, maintaining body alignment, and ensuring that the ETT tape and cervical collar were not constricting. The patient's vital signs remained stable. M.P. was now on a continuous propofol infusion with fentanyl as needed. He was also started on enteral feedings per his orogastric (OG) tube.

On day 3, M.P. continued to have intermittent elevations in his ICP from 28 to 32 mm Hg with a CPP of 54 mm Hg, and required more frequent dosing of mannitol. His serum osmolality was now 302 mOsm/L. When propofol was turned off for a neurologic exam, he would move his extremities to noxious stimuli; there was no attempted verbal response and no eye opening. His pupils remained 4 mm and reactive to light. M.P.'s temperature had increased to 102.3° F. M.P. was given acetaminophen (Tylenol) 325 mg both per OG tube and per rectum. External cooling measures were also instituted.

M.P. continued to have an elevated ICP in the range of 30–39 mm Hg despite sedation and multiple doses of mannitol. On day 4, an external ventricular drain was placed to facilitate CSF drainage in an attempt to lower ICP. Despite appropriate drainage of CSF, the patient's ICP increased to 34 mm Hg with a CPP of 57 mm Hg. His neurologic exam, although limited by sedation and intubation, demonstrated no verbal response, no eye opening, and minimal movement of all four extremities to noxious stimuli. M.P.'s pupils remained equal and reactive to light. Vital signs remained stable with the exception of increased temperature and sinus tachycardia of 128 beats/min.

In an effort to control the elevated ICP, M.P. was next placed in a pentobarbital-induced coma. Eight hours after initiation, serum pentobarbital levels were 54 mcg/ml. A BIS monitor was applied with a BIS reading of 12–20 and an SR maintained greater than 70%. The patient's ICP continued to spike, so the Paco$_2$ was further decreased with hyperventilation while simultaneously monitoring Sjvo$_2$ and Pbto$_2$ to ensure that brain tissue was receiving adequate oxygenation despite hyperventilation.

Decision Point: Why is it important that M.P. have only oral endotracheal and nasogastric tubes rather than nasal intubation?

Decision Point: What laboratory values are most important in M.P.'s care?

TREATMENT OF TRAUMATIC BRAIN INJURY

MANAGEMENT OF HYPOXIA AND HYPOTENSION

The first goal in treating the TBI patient is to reduce initial hypoxic ischemic damage by following standard trauma resuscitation principles. The most important component of early care is prevention of hypoxia and hypotension. Any hypotension and hypoxia must be treated aggressively.[30] Hypoxemia with a Pao$_2$ less than 60 mm Hg at the scene of injury has a reported incidence of as high as 55%.[204] Supplemental oxygen and mechanical ventilation may be needed to maintain Pao$_2$ greater than 60 mm Hg and Paco$_2$ between 35 and 40 mm Hg.[141] Even brief episodes of hypotension are associated with an increased risk of death in trauma patients and may result in a longer critical care recovery phase for those patients who survive.[235] A single episode of hypotension has been shown to double mortality and increase morbidity in patients with severe TBI.[39] The goal of BP management should be to keep SBP greater than 90 mm Hg with fluids and vasopressors.[141]

Fluids and vasopressor agents are given to augment CPP and increase blood flow to the brain, preventing ischemic etiologies of increased ICP. The goal for CPP management in TBI is 60 mm Hg or greater. Although it was once thought that attempts should be made to increase CPP greater than 70 mm Hg with fluids followed by pharmacologic agents, it is now known that excessive fluid resuscitation can result in pulmonary complications. Therefore if TBI patients remain hypotensive despite seemingly adequate fluid resuscitation and filling pressures (i.e., central venous pressure [CVP] greater than 12 mm Hg, pulmonary artery wedge pressure [PAWP] greater than 14 mm Hg), vasopressors may be needed to keep BP greater than 90 mm Hg.[30]

MANAGEMENT OF INTRACRANIAL PRESSURE

Management of traumatic brain injuries is primarily aimed at prevention and reduction of elevated ICP to preserve brain function. Figure 22-21 shows a hierarchy

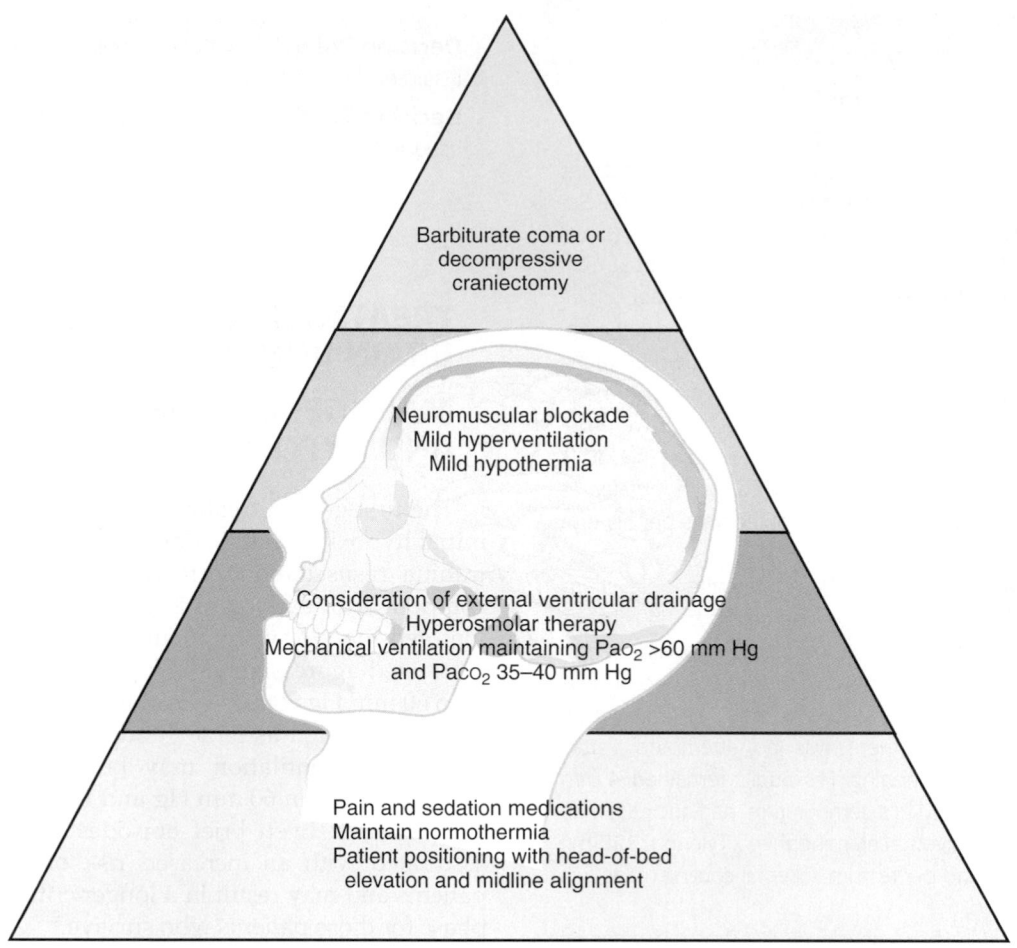

Barbiturate coma or
decompressive
craniectomy

Neuromuscular blockade
Mild hyperventilation
Mild hypothermia

Consideration of external ventricular drainage
Hyperosmolar therapy
Mechanical ventilation maintaining Pao_2 >60 mm Hg
and $Paco_2$ 35–40 mm Hg

Pain and sedation medications
Maintain normothermia
Patient positioning with head-of-bed
elevation and midline alignment

◆FIGURE 22-21 Treatment pyramid for increased intracranial pressure.

for treating patients with ICP. Treatment of elevated ICP should be initiated when levels are sustained ≥20 mm Hg for greater than 5 to 10 minutes.[30] ICP management involves a tiered approach using the TBI guidelines.

First-Level Approaches for Intracranial Pressure Management

The most basic approach to decreasing ICP is to facilitate venous drainage and prevent constriction of venous outflow;[33] this is easily accomplished with appropriate patient positioning. Patients should be positioned with the head of the bed elevated 30 to 45 degrees, avoiding hyperextension, flexion, or rotation of the head and neck; the legs should be straight, and sharp hip flexion must be avoided. Use of reverse Trendelenburg's (RT) position may be helpful to facilitate venous drainage by preventing femoral constriction. The nurse should also ensure there is no constriction of the jugular veins from endotracheal tube tape, tracheostomy ties, or cervical collars that are too tight.[30]

It is also important to consider other causes of increased ICP unrelated to TBI. Abdominal compartment syndrome (ACS), for example, will cause problems not only from compression of the abdominal contents but also from restricted jugular venous outflow due to increased abdominal pressure, increasing ICP.[35] ACS is characterized clinically by the evolution of a tense, distended abdomen, progressive oliguria, and progressive respiratory compromise.[35] Increased levels of positive end-expiratory pressure (PEEP) to treat pulmonary conditions such as acute respiratory distress syndrome (ARDS) can also cause an increase in the ICP.[48] This increased PEEP and the resultant increased intrathoracic pressure also obstruct venous return and increase ICP.[48] Therefore it is important to cautiously monitor the ICP while carefully titrating increased PEEP to improve oxygenation.

Other basic measures for preventing increased ICP are to focus on factors that decrease stimuli and decrease cerebral metabolic demand in order to optimize oxygen delivery/consumption ratio. Interventions include decreasing environmental stimuli and the use of sedation and pain medication.

Sedation and Analgesia. Pain control and use of sedation are important interventions in TBI patients. The goals of sedation are to maintain CPP and control ICP by decreasing cerebral metabolic demands, facilitating effective ventilation, and reducing ICP.[141] Pain and agitation result in BP elevations that can cause increased ICP,[162] and severe agitation increases intrathoracic pressure and reduces venous outflow.[42] Furthermore, agitation increases cerebral metabolism and subsequently increases CBF, ultimately resulting in an elevated ICP.[42] Any noxious stimuli, commonly seen with nursing activities such as turning and suctioning, can increase cerebral metabolic demands and elevate ICP. Pain control and sedation decrease the cerebral metabolic rate of oxygen consumption and reduce CBF by decreasing cerebral vascular resistance, thereby decreasing ICP.[162] Because these agents can also limit the neurologic exam, they need to be administered judiciously, especially in patients without intracranial monitoring devices. If possible, a complete neurologic exam should be performed before administration of sedatives or analgesic agents.[141] Short-acting agents or the use of daily sedation wake-ups allows for adequate opportunities to obtain a thorough neurologic exam in patients requiring sedation and analgesia. Common medications, dosages, and contraindications for the administration of sedation and analgesic agents are presented in the Medication table on p. 78 in Chapter 4.

Propofol. Propofol (Diprivan) is an intravenous sedative-hypnotic that is lipid soluble and rapidly crosses the BBB. Because of its short effective half-life of less than 1 hour, rapid onset, and short recovery time, propofol can be quickly discontinued in order to assess a patient's neurologic status.[42] It can then be restarted, with a rapid onset of action. It is also theorized that there may be a dose-dependent decrease in CBF and cerebral metabolic rate (CMR), thus decreasing ICP.[162] Patients with head injury may be at higher risk of cardiac failure at doses higher than 5 mg/kg/hr; starting the infusion at 0.3 mg/kg/hr, increasing every 5–10 minutes to a maximum of 3 mg/kg/hr as needed, may avoid cardiac complications. Because of the lipid component of propofol, it is important to monitor triglyceride levels and monitor liver and pancreatic functions when prolonged high doses are used.[11] Prolonged use of propofol has been associated with adverse effects of metabolic acidosis, rhabdomyolysis, hypotension, and bradycardic events.[109]

Benzodiazepines. Benzodiazepines have sedative and anticonvulsant properties, making them very useful for the management of TBI patients during anesthesia and intensive care treatment.[85] Benzodiazepines commonly used are midazolam (Versed) and lorazepam (Ativan).

Narcotics. Pain has a direct effect on cerebral metabolic rate and subsequent problems of elevated ICP. The healthcare team needs to balance the management of pain versus interference with neurologic assessment and adverse hemodynamic effects.[85] Morphine or fentanyl (Duragesic, Sublimaze) may be given to patients for their analgesic effects. Morphine, however, may cause vasodilation, which threatens adequate cerebral perfusion. Fentanyl and other synthetic opioids may cause carbon dioxide–independent ICP increases.[30]

Osmotherapy. Osmotic diuretics are frequently used to decrease ICP. The ideal osmotic agent produces a favorable osmotic gradient by remaining largely in the intravascular compartment, is inert and nontoxic, and has minimal systemic side effects.[22] The most common osmotic diuretic used is mannitol.

Mannitol (Osmitrol) is usually given as a 20% solution in bolus doses of 0.25 to 1 g/kg and not as a continuous infusion. ICP will typically decrease within 5 to 10 minutes, with maximum effect occurring in about 60 minutes and lasting up to 4 hours.[206] A powerful osmotic diuretic, mannitol draws fluid from the intracellular and interstitial spaces into the vascular compartment. The resulting hemodilution reduces blood viscosity, which improves CBF and cerebral oxygen delivery.[33] Another beneficial effect of mannitol is a reduction in red blood cell (RBC) rigidity, which also facilitates RBC movement into small vessels.[208]

An intact BBB is relatively impermeable to the effects of mannitol.[15,177] However, in high concentrations or after prolonged use, the normal BBB may open, allowing mannitol and other large molecules to enter the extracellular space.[177,208] Thus it can cause a reverse osmosis and actually draw fluid into brain cells, causing a rebound rise in ICP (Figure 22-22).[97] A high serum osmolality from too much mannitol can damage the BBB and reverse the direction of the osmotic gradient.[15] A serum osmolality of 300 to 320 mOsm/L has been recommended for patients with poor intracranial compliance.[181] However, in an attempt to obtain maximal benefit from osmotherapy in patients with brain injuries, a serum osmolality greater than 320 mOsm/L can be permitted if used with caution.[22,187]

When diuretics are being used frequently, close monitoring of serum osmolality is essential to prevent inadvertent volume depletion. As osmolality rises, increased blood viscosity causes a decrease in CPP, which subsequently leads to cerebral vasodilation and a rise in ICP.[208] With repeated doses, mannitol may become less effective in reducing ICP. Consequences of prolonged or repeated doses of mannitol include dehydration, hypotension, hypokalemia, and renal failure.[15,208] It is important to maintain euvolemia with adequate fluid replacement when administering mannitol.[30]

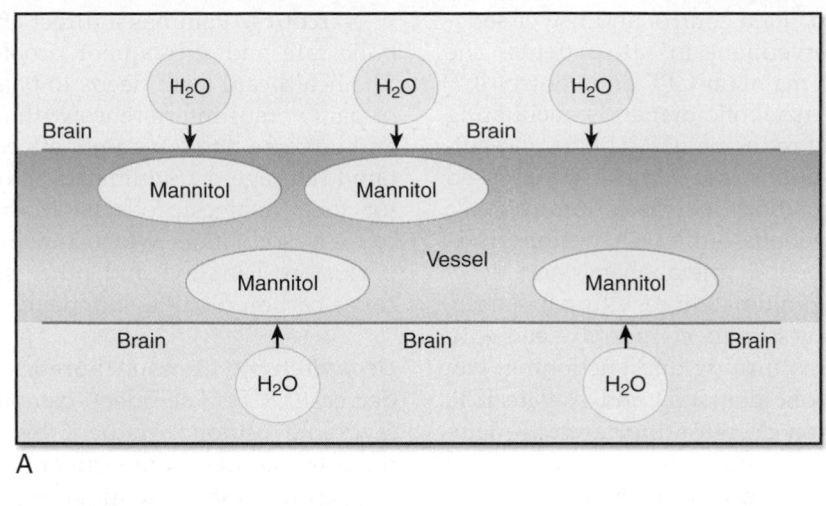

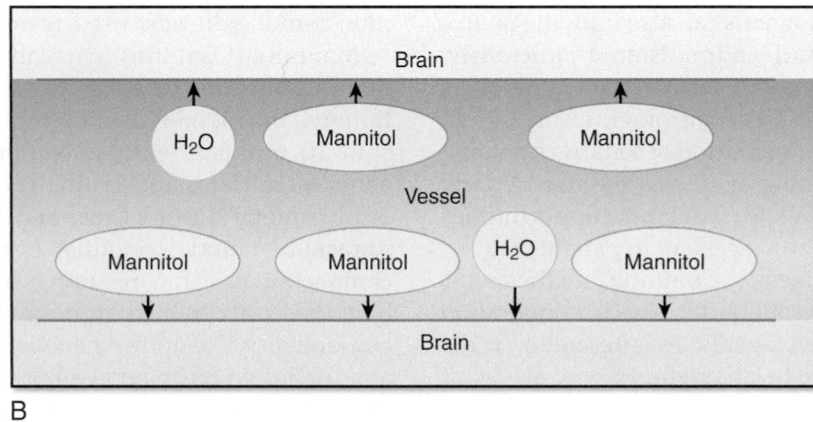

FIGURE 22-22 Effect of mannitol on fluid movement in the brain. **A,** Normal effect of mannitol. **B,** Reverse effect of mannitol.

Another agent that has been recently explored as an alternative to the use of mannitol is HTS, and these two options are compared in Table 22-7. The mechanism of action of HTS is based on the high tonicity of the fluid, which draws water from the cells and interstitial tissues into the vascular spaces.[23,60] The dose and concentration of HTS most effective for the treatment of increased ICP remain to be determined through ongoing clinical research. In the patient with refractory increased ICP despite maximal osmotic therapy, other therapies to reduce ICP must be initiated.[30]

Cerebrospinal Fluid Drainage. Use of external ventricular drains (EVDs) is helpful for several reasons; they can be used to monitor ICP, to monitor the color and amount of CSF, and to serve as an adjunct to treatment by facilitating drainage of CSF. By draining CSF, one of the contents of the cranial vault, more space is created within the cranium and ICP will decrease. Removing CSF too quickly can result in ventricular collapse and deterioration in the patient's neurologic status, and even lead to brain stem herniation.[85] Complications of

EVDs and CSF drains that must be considered are dislodgment of the catheter, clotting of the catheter, and infectious complications.[123] The EVD should be leveled and zeroed at the foramen of Monro.[123] The external auditory canal, or the tragus of the ear, can be used as a visible landmark for this structure. Placement of the drainage chamber is determined by the physician, and may be level with the external auditory meatus (EAM), or 5 to 20 cm above the EAM. The nurse must vigilantly monitor the EVD for appropriate positioning and drainage; CSF drainage decreases if the collection unit is raised and drainage increases if the collection unit is lowered.[85] The physician's orders should clarify whether the EVD is to remain open to continuous drainage at all times or to intermittent drainage at scheduled intervals or when an ICP measurement is higher than a certain value. To avoid infectious complications such as ventriculitis and meningitis, it is imperative that the system remains closed and strict aseptic technique is utilized when any interruption of the system is necessary[85] (e.g., whenever samples are removed or when tubing is changed).

TABLE 22-7 Comparison of Mannitol and Hypertonic Saline Solution

MEDICATION	MANNITOL	HYPERTONIC SALINE SOLUTION
Bolus dosing	0.25–1 g/kg rapid bolus	None
Infusion dose		0.1–1 ml/kg/hr
Maximum serum osmolality	320 mOsm/L	360 mOsm/L
Diuretic effect	Osmotic diuretic; may necessitate volume replacement to avoid hypovolemia	Diuresis through action of atrial natriuretic peptide (ANP)
Proposed beneficial effect	Antioxidant effects	Restoration of resting membrane potential and cell volume, inhibition of inflammation
Adverse effects	Renal failure, hypotension, rebound elevation in ICP	Rebound elevation in ICP, central pontine myelinolysis, bleeding, electrolyte abnormalities

Data from reference 106.

Neuromuscular Blocking Agents. The use of neuromuscular blocking agents (NMBAs) is appropriate to facilitate mechanical ventilation and to control intracranial hypertension related to muscle movement such as posturing and coughing.[141] The use of NMBAs is only a temporary bridge to more definitive treatments that control problems with agitation and should always be used in conjunction with analgesics and sedation.[85,141]

NMDAs can only be used in mechanically ventilated patients. They may be especially helpful in the first 24 to 48 hours following injury to prevent coughing and other activities that increase intracranial pressure or increase cerebral oxygen demand.[161] Depolarizing and nondepolarizing agents are available as short- and long-acting agents.[161] For routine intubations, depolarizing, short-acting agents, such as succinylcholine (Anectine), are typically the drugs of choice. However, succinylcholine can cause increased ICP and should be avoided in patients with TBI. Depolarizing agents should also be avoided for patients who have been immobile or in critical care for a long period of time because these agents cause release of intracellular potassium, and may lead to profound cardiac complications such as ventricular tachycardia and asystole.[134] The best choice for prolonged ICP management is provided by longer-acting, nondepolarizing agents such as cisatracurium or vecuronium. Chapter 4 reviews commonly used NMBAs along with dosing recommendations and duration of action. Previously believed not to penetrate into the brain, it is now known that these agents do cross the BBB and may activate brain acetylcholine receptors.[161] This could lead to central autonomic dysfunction, weakness, and seizures.[161] If used, patients should be carefully monitored using a peripheral nerve stimulator to minimize resistance caused by receptor upregulation.[85] Caution must be taken when used in conjunction with corticosteroids because the combination of NMBA and concomitant use of steroids has been associated with critical care polyneuropathy.[66]

Second-Level Approaches for Intracranial Pressure Management

For patients with ICP refractory to conventional, conservative approaches, there are various second-tier therapeutic options. These include induced barbiturate coma, controlled hyperventilation, mild hypothermia, and surgical decompression (Figure 22-23).[170]

Barbiturates. Barbiturates, such as thiopental or pentobarbital, are used as second-tier therapies to treat patients with refractory ICP. Intravenous administration of barbiturates produces an anesthetic response along with a dose-dependent fall in CBF and CMR,[147] thus decreasing ICP. The administration of barbiturates to induce coma has been used to decrease the cerebral metabolism in order to limit swelling and cellular damage.[130] Cerebral vasoconstriction induced by barbiturates is effective in controlling elevated ICP refractory to other treatments.[130] Barbiturates may improve blood flow to underperfused areas of the injured brain that have lost or reduced vasoreactivity.[116,130] There may also be an effect on decreasing secondary brain injury by stabilizing plasma and lysosomal membranes and reducing the release of excitotoxic amino acids and intracellular calcium concentrations.[75]

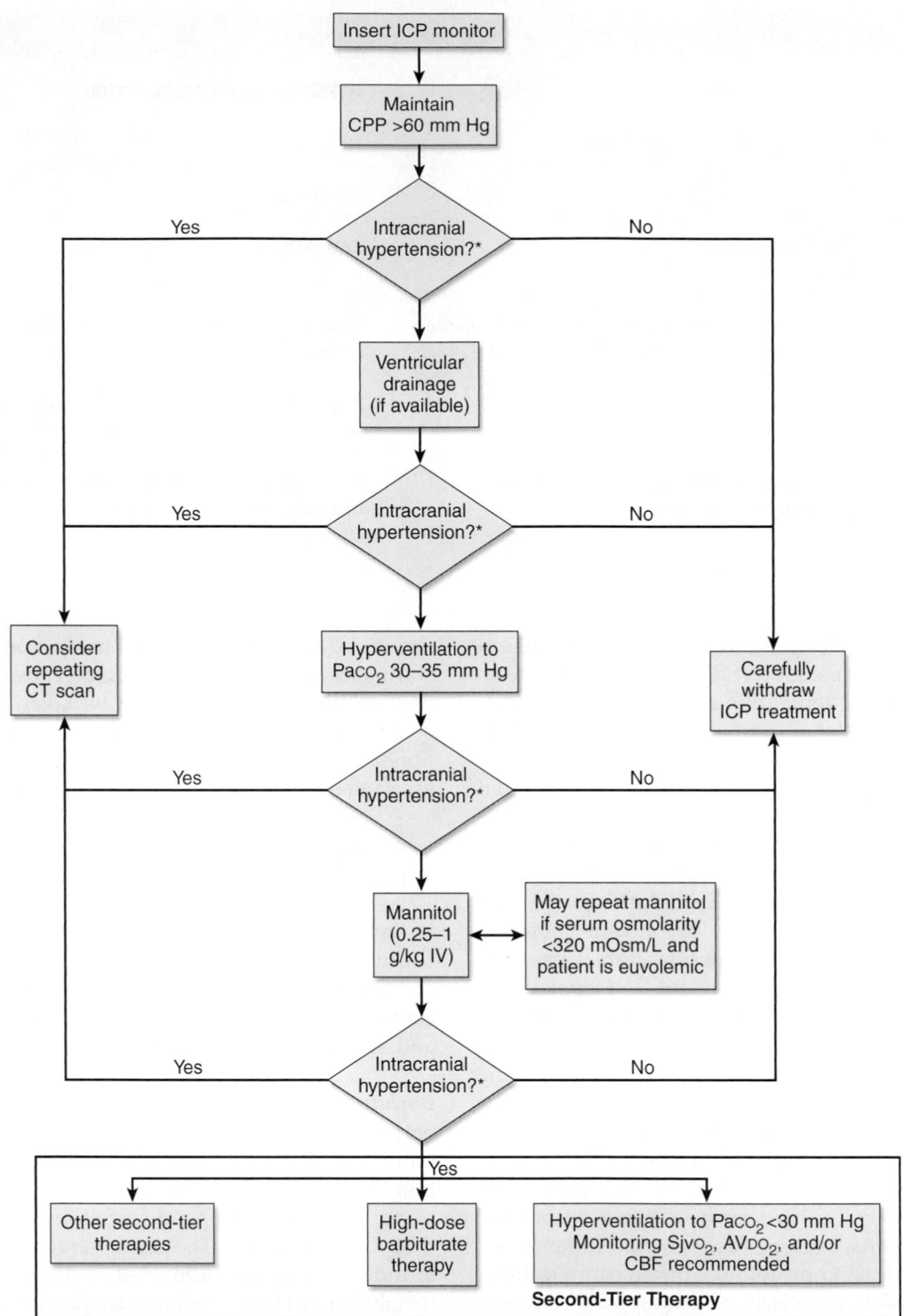

FIGURE 22-23 Algorithm for treatment of increased intracranial pressure. AV_{DO_2} = Arteriovenous oxygen content difference, CBF = cerebral blood flow, CPP = cerebral perfusion pressure, CT = computed tomography, ICP = intracranial pressure, mOsm/L = milliosmoles per liter, $Paco_2$ = partial pressure of arterial carbon dioxide, $Sjvo_2$ = jugular venous oxygen saturation.

Despite evidence of cerebral protection in experimental models, there is little evidence that barbiturates improve outcome after severe head injuries.[225] There are many negative consequences to the use of barbiturates, including decreased gastrointestinal motility, decreased protective mechanisms (i.e., suppression of cough and gag reflexes), and immunosuppression, that lead to increased susceptibility to pulmonary complications such as pneumonia.[205] High doses of pentobarbital can cause myocardial depression, necessitating the use of vasopressors to maintain BP and CPP.[40,205] Serum pentobarbital levels must be monitored in order to ensure that levels are adequate and to avoid toxicity with increased serum pentobarbital levels. Induction of barbiturate coma should be supported by continuous EEG or BIS monitoring.[7]

Hypothermia. Temperature regulation is another important intervention to consider in managing increased ICP in TBI patients. Hyperthermia is detrimental to the brain because it impairs energy metabolism, disrupts the BBB, and increases the release of excitatory neurotransmitters and free radicals, all of which contribute to increased ICP.[214] Increased body temperature has also been associated with increased cytokine release and worse outcomes in TBI.[214] Animal models and small clinical studies of therapeutic hypothermia have produced mixed results. Although preliminary data suggested that this may be an effective therapy, larger randomized clinical trials have failed to demonstrate improved outcomes using induced hypothermia.[44,125,172] Side effects of hypothermia include shivering, dysrhythmia, and increased blood viscosity.[111] Hypothermia can cause or exacerbate coagulopathy and acidosis in the trauma patient because of platelet alterations, enzyme inhibition, and fibrinolysis.[111] This is the reason that hypothermia should be used only in patients with primary central nervous system injury.

In a study of hibernating animals, it is interesting to note that profound degrees of ischemia and oligemia can be tolerated. One study demonstrated that hemoglobin level remains normal during hibernation but severe leukopenia and thrombocytopenia occur.[145] Thus it is possible that depletion of platelets and leukocytes may be a "natural" form of neuroprotection during hypothermia. Leukopenia and thrombocytopenia may therefore offer some form of protection by limiting the progressive edema that follows ischemia.[145]

Although the impact of induced hypothermia in TBI is not fully known, there is ample evidence to demonstrate that preventing hyperthermia and maintaining normothermia can help prevent increased ICP.[33,34] Early treatment and diagnosis of the underlying cause of fever are critical in TBI patients to minimize its effect on secondary brain injury.[33,145] Several techniques are available for both external and internal cooling (see Chapter 7). Currently, there is not enough data to support the selection of one therapy over another.

Controlled Hyperventilation. Hyperventilation, once thought to be an effective treatment of increased ICP, has been shown to be detrimental to the patient and brain tissue.[3] Because decreased $PaCO_2$ is a potent vasoconstrictor, the premise behind hyperventilation is that hyperventilation causes vasoconstriction, which subsequently leads to a decrease in intracranial blood volume and ICP. Negative consequences of hyperventilation result from overconstriction of cerebral blood vessels, severely compromising blood flow to the point of causing ischemia. Current research based recommendations from the National Brain Trauma Foundation suggest maintaining normocarbia in the low-normal level of $PaCO_2$ 35 to 40 mm Hg.[30] The use of prophylactic hyperventilation ($PaCO_2$ less than or equal to 35 mm Hg) during the first 24 hours after TBI should be avoided because of the potential for compromised cerebral perfusion.[33,176] Further hyperventilation can severely reduce blood flow and is not recommended without some additional monitoring of brain tissue oxygenation via $SjvO_2$ or BtO_2[33] to ensure that any further reduction in $PaCO_2$ (values less than 30 mm Hg) does not compromise blood flow and cause brain tissue ischemia. $PaCO_2$ of 20 to 25 mm Hg may reduce the CBF by 40% to 50%, and, conversely, an increase to greater than 50 mm Hg increases CBF by more than 50%.[176] These changes occur almost immediately in a healthy human, but responses may be altered after head injury.[27]

Decompressive Craniectomy. Decompressive craniectomy is an additional treatment for severe, refractory intracranial hypertension that does not respond to conventional therapeutic measures.[170] Removal of a large area of the skull allows an increase in the volume of intracranial contents without increasing pressure. When it is indicated, decompressive craniectomy should be performed in a protocol-driven fashion, only after conventional treatment approaches have failed to relieve refractory elevations of ICP.[170] There remain several unanswered questions regarding which patients are appropriate for this surgery and which surgical technique should be used. Currently, there are no prospective randomized controlled trials that examine the risks and benefits or suggest that decompressive craniotomy improves outcomes.[164] There is an ongoing study, and it is hoped that the results of this multicenter RESCUEicp study (Randomized Evaluation of Surgery with Craniectomy for Uncontrollable Elevation of Intra-Cranial Pressure; website http://rescueicp.com)[164] will shed new light on this area.

STRATEGIES FOR NEUROPROTECTION

All the interventions described previously are aimed at reducing cerebral edema and preventing secondary injury. More definitive treatment strategies for neuro-protection are still in the experimental stages. As this research evolves, treatment may include the use of free radical scavengers to prevent lipid peroxidation, N-methyl-D-aspartate (NMDA) and alpha amino-3-hydroxy-5-methylisoxazole-4-propionic acid (AMPA) receptor antagonists to limit damage from excitatory amino acids such as glutamate, and calcium antago-nists to prevent influx of calcium into cells.[5,14,17,22]

Preventing calcium influx into the cells is the goal of many neuroprotective agents, such as nimodipine, that are designed to block voltage-operated calcium chan-nels[152] or receptor-operated channels.[83] Unfortunately, patients with nontraumatic SAH have shown a better response to nimodipine in clinical trials than those with traumatic brain injuries.[152]

COMPLICATIONS AFTER TRAUMATIC BRAIN INJURY

Unfortunately, many complications can occur follow-ing a TBI that further complicate the patient's course. It is important for the nurse to be aware of these complica-tions in order to prevent their occurrence or be able to identify them early so that proper treatment can be insti-tuted. Complications result from the injury itself, immune dysfunction resulting from TBI, and problems related to the patient's immobility.

Immunosuppression

New information is continually emerging that sug-gests the immune dysfunction associated with TBI adversely affects patient outcomes.[26] After any traumatic injury, a stress response occurs involving a cascade of metabolic and neurohormonal changes. Induced immu-nosuppression following TBI originates from a variety of abnormalities including a reduced number of circ-ulating lymphocytes, depressed T-cell activation, and proliferation and production of immunosuppressive fac-tors.[142] These changes initially occur to ensure survival of the body, but when prolonged, they can become life-threatening.[142] The prolonged immunosuppression is accompanied by a hypermetabolic, hypoperfused state, thus setting the stage for subsequent infections, sepsis, and multiple organ failure.[189] Figure 22-24 offers a more thorough explanation of the immune consequences fol-lowing traumatic injury.

Coagulopathy

TBI and severe traumatic injuries are associated with activation of the coagulation system. This activa-tion results from the inflammatory response and damage to the endothelium. Activation of the coagu-lation system results in increased clotting and con-sumption of clotting factors that ultimately lead to excessive bleeding. Coagulation abnormalities can lead to delayed intracranial hemorrhage. The severity of coagulopathy has been correlated with the severity of morbidity from TBI.[136] It is important to monitor coagulation parameters and replace blood products such as RBCs, plasma, and platelets as indicated by laboratory tests.[136] A new emerging therapy, factor VIIa, may be beneficial in patients with hemorrhagic strokes, and may also be beneficial in TBI.[96] However, definitive studies are yet to be completed on this therapy.

Electrolyte Disturbances

An understanding of fluid and electrolyte imbal-ances associated with head injury is important for opti-mal patient management. The reader is referred to Chapter 31 for detailed discussions of electrolyte man-agement. This chapter will address these issues as they relate to TBI.

Hyponatremia. A serum sodium (Na) concentration less than 135 mEq/L is seen in approximately 5% to 12% of patients with severe head injury.[202] In this population, hyponatremia is often due to excess antidiuretic hormone (ADH) secretion secondary to hypovolemia, fluid restriction, or hemorrhage. While excess ADH secretion is an appropriate response to hypovolemia, it is inappropriate in the presence of hyponatremia.[10] Uncorrected hyponatremia may lead to reduced levels of consciousness and even seizures.[202]

Pathogenesis of hyponatremia has many etiologies, including a shift of water out of the cell, as seen with hyperglycemia or mannitol infusion. It is also present with an intracellular shift of sodium that accompa-nies potassium loss. Sodium loss also occurs through the kidneys, gastrointestinal (GI) tract, and skin.[10,202,213] Hyponatremia following head injury is often due to the SIADH.

Syndrome of Inappropriate Antidiuretic Hor-mone. SIADH is defined as hyponatremia resulting either from increased ADH secretion initiated by stim-ulation of baroreceptors or from a reduction in non-ADH renal water excretion mechanisms. It is a form

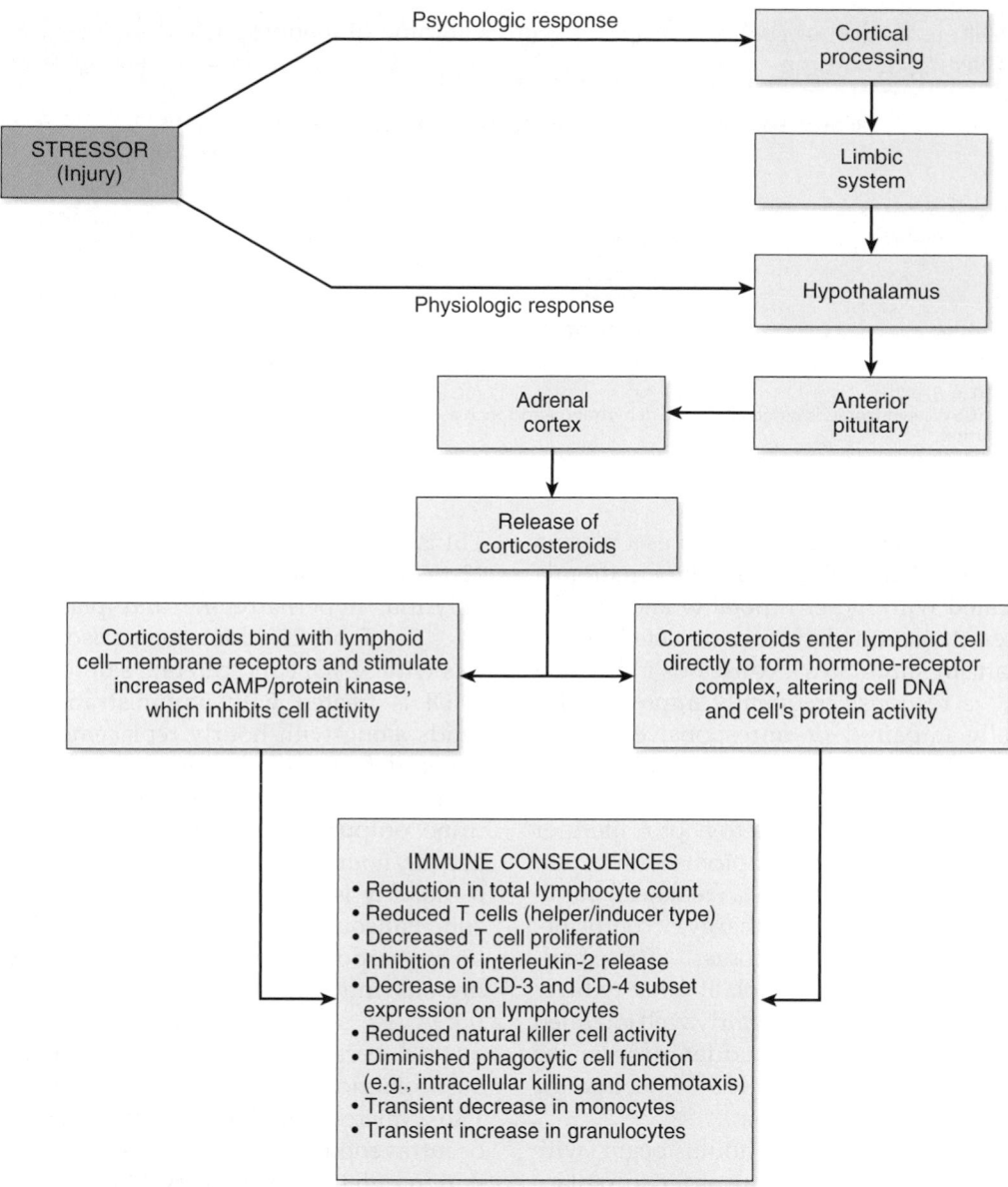

FIGURE 22-24 Immune consequences of traumatic brain injury.

of dilutional hyponatremia, with increases in ECF of 3 to 4 liters without peripheral edema. The glomerular filtration rate is increased, causing a decrease in the renal absorption of sodium.[10] Criteria for diagnosis of SIADH include hypotonic hyponatremia, urine osmolality greater than plasma osmolality, urine sodium excretion greater than 20 mEq/L in the absence of hypotension, hypovolemia, edema, or drug events.[10,202] Conservative treatment involves fluid restriction; more aggressive therapy may include judicious administration of HTS and possibly furosemide for diuresis.[141] Table 22-8 compares SIADH with cerebral salt wasting and diabetes insipidus.

Cerebral Salt Wasting. Another form of hyponatremia associated with TBI is cerebral salt wasting. It is hypothesized that this condition occurs when brain injury triggers the stress response and a surge of sympathetic nervous system hormones and catecholamines acts on the kidneys to excrete sodium. There is an inability to conserve sodium and this, in turn, leads to hypovolemia. The resultant hyponatremia and hypovolemia are treated with a conservative plan of intravenous NS if the patient is asymptomatic. In more severe cases, HTS and fludrocortisone (Florinef) may be used. See Table 22-8 for a comparison of cerebral salt wasting with SIADH and diabetes insipidus.

TABLE 22-8 Differentiation of Diabetes Insipidus from Syndrome of Inappropriate Antidiuretic Hormone and Cerebral Salt Wasting Syndrome

	SERUM SODIUM	SERUM OSMOLALITY	URINE SODIUM	URINE OSMOLALITY	URINE SPECIFIC GRAVITY
Diabetes insipidus*	↑	↑	↓	↓	↓
SIADH	↓	↓	↑	↑	↑
Salt wasting syndrome	↓	↑ or normal	↑	↑	↑

Data from references 10 and 142.

*Cerebral salt wasting (CSW) syndrome is associated with dehydration and increased BUN levels, whereas dehydration is absent in SIADH and BUN levels are normal.

Hypernatremia. Hypernatremia is defined as a plasma sodium level greater than 145 mEq/L. Hypernatremia is always associated with hyperosmolality and may be caused by water depletion. In water-depleted states, the thirst mechanism stimulates a conscious individual to drink water,[10] a response frequently impossible for the neurologically impaired or unresponsive patient. Hypernatremia is generally not symptomatic unless plasma sodium concentration is 155 to 160 mEq/L or greater (this equates to water depletion of 6 liters or more in a 70-kg man).[181] Clinical symptoms with hypernatremia include pyrexia, restlessness, weakness, paralysis, irritability, drowsiness, lethargy, confusion, tremor, hyperreflexia, seizures, and coma.[181] These findings are the result of increased osmolality that reduces brain cell volume. Hypernatremia is fairly well tolerated if it develops slowly. However, a sudden drop in the osmolality of the ECF can cause a shift of water into the brain cells, producing cerebral edema.[213]

Treatment for hypernatremia should begin with isotonic fluids (i.e., normal saline) in order to replace intravascular volume and improve tissue perfusion, especially when hypotension is present. Hypotonic solutions, such as D_5W or hypotonic saline solutions (0.45% saline), must be used cautiously with severely hypernatremic and volume-depleted patients. Hypernatremia caused by excess sodium intake is treated with water and diuretic administration.[168,181]

Diabetes Insipidus. Diabetes insipidus (DI) is characterized by polyuria and polydipsia resulting either from a complete or partial failure of ADH secretion (central or neurogenic DI) or from a decrease in the renal response to ADH (nephrogenic DI).[182] Head injury is a common cause of central DI. Early-onset DI is typical following major hypothalamic damage and is associated with a high mortality.[182,213] Head-injured patients with fractures involving the base of the skull and sella turcica are at an increased risk for DI.[50] Time of onset of DI in

TBI is commonly 5 to 10 days,[102] but can be as early as 12 to 24 hours following injury. DI is characterized by polyuria, hypernatremia, and plasma hyperosmolality.[10] See Table 22-8 for a comparison of diabetes insipidus with SIADH and cerebral salt wasting.

DI is treated with administration of maintenance fluids along with hourly replacement of both the free water deficit and the urine output with a dextrose solution.[102] Aqueous vasopressin (AVP) is given if urine output remains excessive (greater than 200 to 250 ml/hour) in the absence of diuretics or if hyperosmolality is present. The usual dose is 5 to 10 units subcutaneously or intramuscularly (IM). Patients who do not respond after the initial dose may require a continuous intravenous vasopressin drip. Desmopressin (DDAVP), a synthetic analog of AVP, may be used instead because it has a longer half-life and fewer vasoconstrictive effects. The usual dose of DDAVP is 1 to 2 micrograms (mcg) administered subcutaneously or intravenously every 12 to 24 hours or by nasal insufflation of 5 to 20 mcg every 12 hours. It is important to monitor urine output and to watch for water excess, evidenced by hyponatremia and elevated urinary osmolality.[10]

Volume Depletion

Dehydration increases sympathetic stimulation, metabolism, and oxygen demand.[16] The aim of therapy is to maintain euvolemia and normal physiologic indexes, especially CPP. Because there is no evidence to support fluid restriction as a means of limiting cerebral edema following brain injury, it is no longer considered appropriate to keep TBI patients "dry."[33,155]

Tonicity defines effective osmolality, i.e., the osmotic force caused by the particles, which cannot permeate between compartments. All body fluids must be in osmotic equilibrium. Changes in tonicity, regardless of their cause, will result in fluid shifts between the ECF and the intracellular fluid (ICF) in order to reestablish osmotic equilibrium. Patients with osmotic hypertonicity will have a contracted intracellular compartment.[16] Because brain expansion is limited by the confines of the cranial vault, severe hyponatremia will result in increased ICP. Urea increases osmolality but will not affect tonicity, and because it passes freely through biological membranes, it will not alter the intracellular volume.[155]

Fluid used for initial resuscitation efforts should include isotonic fluids such as NS or lactated Ringer's solution. Both solutions are freely permeable across the vascular membrane and distribute evenly.[186] Hypotonic solutions will increase cerebral edema and should not be administered to head-injured patients.[208] They decrease serum osmolality, causing water to move from the vascular compartment into the interstitial compartment. As the interstitial fluid is diluted, its osmolality decreases, which, in turn, encourages water movement into the adjacent brain cells.[186] While helpful in dehydrated states after the establishment of adequate intravascular volume, hypotonic fluids can be dangerous because the sudden fluid shift from the intravascular space into cells increases ICP.[11] D_5W should not be used; in the vascular space it acts as a hypotonic solution, encouraging fluid movement into the cells and increasing cerebral edema.

Because hypertonic solutions have higher osmolality than serum, they pull fluid and electrolytes from the intracellular and interstitial compartments into the intravascular compartment. This helps stabilize BP, increase urine output, and reduce edema. HTS has shown beneficial effects in head-injured patients, including expansion of intravascular volume, extraction of water from the intracellular space, decreased ICP, and increased cardiac contractility, and is associated with significantly improved survival.[13,99,137,220] Use of HTS will cause an increase in serum sodium concentration, but this may be well tolerated with a sodium level as high as 170 mEq/L in head-injured patients.[82,104,168,223] Although HTS appears to be promising in the resuscitation of head-injured patients, the optimal timing, appropriate concentration, and correct volume have yet to be determined.

Colloid solutions (e.g., albumin) do not cross capillary membranes readily and are confined mainly to the intravascular spaces. Colloid molecules are too large to pass out of the capillary membranes and remain in the vascular compartment. The large protein molecules give colloid solutions a very high osmolality, drawing fluid from the interstitial and intracellular compartments into the vascular compartments.[186] If the solution has a higher oncotic pressure than plasma, interstitial fluid will move into the intravascular space and expand the plasma volume.[186] Colloids can produce dramatic

fluid shifts, and therefore need to be administered in controlled settings.

The use of packed RBCs, which are colloids, can be an important consideration in TBI, especially in patients with acute blood loss from associated injuries. Global tissue perfusion exacerbates cerebral hypoxia, cerebral ischemia, and increased ICP. RBCs expand circulating volume and may improve oxygen-carrying capacity to the injured brain.[85,207]

Metabolic Response

As described earlier, the brain is highly dependent on oxygen and is unable to store glucose as energy. There are adverse consequences when the supply of oxygen and glucose is inadequate to support the increased metabolic requirements of the injured brain.[110] Therefore a continuous replenishment of oxygen is required via the cerebral circulation.

Glucose is the main substrate for energy metabolism and is used aerobically to provide the brain with significant energy. The energy is supplied from ATP synthesized through glycolysis, the Krebs cycle, and the respiratory chain. During aerobic metabolism each molecule of glucose produces 36 molecules of ATP.[133] However, during anaerobic metabolism only 2 molecules of ATP are produced.[133] When ATP molecules are inadequate to fuel the sodium-potassium pump, lactic acid accumulates within the cell, causing the mitochondria to lose their ability to contain calcium ions. This results in a subsequent rise in intracellular calcium levels, ultimately killing the cell and causing neuronal death.[2]

Interestingly, hyperglycemia also adversely affects patient outcomes with TBI, and is associated with more pronounced cerebral edema and a deterioration of brain energy metabolism.[56] Worse neurologic outcomes have been associated with glucose levels of 150 to 200 mg/dl than those with glucose levels less than 150 mg/dl.[110] Therefore it is important to maintain serum glucose levels less than 150 mg/dl with insulin administered subcutaneously or by continuous intravenous infusion.[110]

Infectious Complications

TBI patients are prone to infectious complications such as urinary tract infections (UTIs), bloodstream infections, pneumonia, and other systemic infections.[141] Yet another infectious complication that may afflict TBI patients is development of a brain abscess or meningitis resulting from a breach of the dura mater. Urinary tract infections can occur from urinary stasis associated with immobility and from use of indwelling urinary catheters necessary for monitoring fluid status and management of incontinence. Indwelling urinary catheters are significantly associated with an increased rate of UTI.[9]

MULTIDISCIPLINARY PLAN OF CARE FOR PATIENTS WITH RESPIRATORY COMPLICATIONS AND INCREASED INTRACRANIAL PRESSURE

PROBLEM	GOAL	INTERVENTIONS	RATIONALE
Potential or actual increased ICP	Maintain physiologic parameters: Pao_2 >60 mm Hg $Paco_2$ 35–40 mm Hg Sao_2 92%–100% MAP 90–100 mm Hg CPP >60 mm Hg ICP <20 mm Hg Serum osmolality <320 mOsm Glucose <150 mg/dl Normothermia Adequate urinary output Hct >10 g/Hct <32%	Elevate HOB 30 degrees Maintain neutral body alignment Ensure ETT or cervical collars are not constricting Maintain patent airway, suction as needed, oxygenate before and after suctioning, do not hyperventilate when suctioning Control noxious stimuli Treat elevated temperature aggressively; maintain normothermia Prevent shivering Administer mannitol (0.25–1 g/kg) bolus Administer sedation, analgesics, NMBA Treat seizures, high-risk prophylaxis × 7 days ICP monitoring: possible ventriculostomy for drainage if ICP >20 mm Hg	Interventions should prevent any increase in cerebral metabolic rate and facilitate optimal venous drainage.
	Second-tier interventions: Barbiturate coma Mild hypothermia Controlled hyperventilation Decompressive craniectomy	For ICP refractory to other measures, these therapies may provide additional benefit in decreasing cerebral metabolic response and decreasing ICP	
Potential risk of development of pneumonia or other respiratory complications from immobility	Pao_2 at least >60 mm Hg with goal of 80–100 mm Hg $Paco_2$ 35–40 mm Hg Sao_2 92%–100% Maintain mechanical ventilator plateau pressures <30 mm Hg	HOB elevated at least 30 degrees Turn patient minimally q 2 hr Frequent oral care: brush teeth q 12 hr with swabbing/moisturizing q 2–4 hr	Pneumonia can be prevented by aggressive maintenance of HOB elevation, oral care, and mobility.
Potential for DVT		Apply mechanical devices for DVT prophylaxis	
Prevent complications of immobility		Turn patient q 2 hr, log-roll if concomitant SCI present Use pressure-relieving surfaces to prevent skin breakdown: PROM PT/OT OOB activity as soon as possible	

Data from references 11, 35, 85, and 141.
ICP = Intracranial pressure, Pao_2 = partial pressure of arterial oxygen tension, $Paco_2$ = partial pressure of arterial carbon dioxide, Sao_2 = arterial oxygen saturation, MAP = mean arterial pressure, CPP = cerebral perfusion pressure, HOB = head of bed, ETT = endotracheal tube, Hct = hematocrit, NMBA = neuromuscular blocking agents, q = every, DVT = deep vein thrombosis, SCI = spinal cord injury, PROM = passive range of motion, PT = physical therapy, OT = occupational therapy, OOB = out of bed.

Bloodstream infections occur from the use of multiple intravascular access devices; in particular, catheters used for parenteral nutrition have been associated with a greater incidence of bloodstream infections. The nurse must be diligent in providing care for patients with invasive access and lines and ensure that appropriate aseptic techniques are used during insertion and with each subsequent access of the lines.

Pulmonary Complications

Any process that impairs oxygenation will in turn affect the oxygen available for adequate brain cell functioning. Pulmonary complications associated with head injury include prolonged or permanent inadequate airway protection, ventilator-acquired pneumonia (VAP), ARDS and acute lung injury (ALI), and neurogenic pulmonary edema (NPE). The last two problems are discussed here as they relate to TBI.

Very few studies have attempted to identify the incidence of ALI in patients with TBI. A 1969 autopsy series of Vietnam combat casualties noted that 85% of those who died from isolated head injuries had pulmonary edema.[198] In a more recent study that examined the incidence of ALI in comatose patients following isolated TBI, the researchers found that 20 of every 100 patients developed ALI. These patients also demonstrated a higher incidence of poor neurologic outcome or death.[28]

Because severe TBI generally requires endotracheal intubation and mechanical ventilation, respiratory complications following TBI are common and extremely problematic. The most common complication is pneumonia, either caused by aspiration at the time of the initial injury or acquired in the hospital. VAP has the highest incidence in neurotrauma patients, probably related to immobility, loss of protective reflexes, and the immune suppression associated with trauma.[25]

Patients with TBI can also develop ALI or ARDS that negatively impacts positive outcomes. In one study evaluating the use of CPP to direct goal-oriented management of TBI, the risk of ARDS was reported to be five times greater in the CPP-targeted group than in the ICP-targeted group.[33] Therefore attempts to maintain CPP greater than 70 mm Hg with aggressive administration of fluids or vasopressors should be avoided because of the increased risk of ARDS. Furthermore, TBI patients are more prone to ARDS because of the central neurogenic mechanism for increased sympathetic activity. TBI patients who develop ARDS are more likely to develop refractory elevations of ICP and are three times more likely to be in a vegetative state or dead at 6 months post-injury.[218] The multidisciplinary plan of care on p. 566 outlines care of head injury patients with ICP.

The treatment of ARDS includes the use of protective lung ventilation with the use of low tidal volume (6 ml/kg) and PEEP. Low tidal volume ventilation commonly results in an increase in $Paco_2$, which is problematic for the TBI patient and can result in an elevated ICP. Use of PEEP with ARDS patients is a mainstay of treatment but has been controversial in those with head injuries.[48] Although PEEP improves oxygenation in the head-injured patient,[48,162] it also alters systemic hemodynamics by increasing intrathoracic pressure, which, in turn, increases CVP and decreases cardiac filling. This results in decreased MAP, reduced CPP, and, subsequently, increased ICP.[150,158] In patients with intact cerebral autoregulation, the responses to MAP reduction can be tolerated without development of cerebral ischemia. However, when autoregulation is impaired, there is a greater risk of ischemia.[150]

NPE is an infrequent complication following head trauma and occurs in the absence of cardiogenic etiologies.[227] NPE also occurs with other neurologic processes such as subarachnoid hemorrhage (SAH), stroke, tumors, meningitis, and Guillain-Barré syndrome in addition to TBI. The exact mechanisms of NPE are unclear, although it is hypothesized that it results from sympathetic stimulation as a result of the massive alpha-adrenergic discharge immediately after injury.[227] This sympathetic outpouring leads to a redistribution of blood flow from the systemic to pulmonary vasculature, increasing systemic and pulmonary vascular resistances. The subsequent increases in left atrial pressure and PAWP disrupt pulmonary capillary membranes.[227] Endothelial injury may also contribute to NPE[151] because damage to the pulmonary endothelium causes a persistent permeability defect,[212] leading to the accumulation of pulmonary edema fluid with a high protein content. Treatment of NPE is mostly supportive, aimed at improving oxygenation. Experimental therapies are currently being explored (Figure 22-25).[212]

Complications Related to Immobility

Other complications related to immobility include venous stasis resulting in deep vein thrombosis (DVT) and pulmonary embolus (PE). TBI patients are also prone to GI complications such as stress ulcers, ileus, and constipation that can result from immobility and use of narcotic medications.[25] These complications are discussed in multiple chapters throughout this text.

Seizures

Seizures are a known complication in TBI, occurring in 22% of patients with TBI, with an incidence of up to 50% in penetrating injuries.[222] Seizure activity increases cerebral metabolism and CBF, exacerbating cerebral

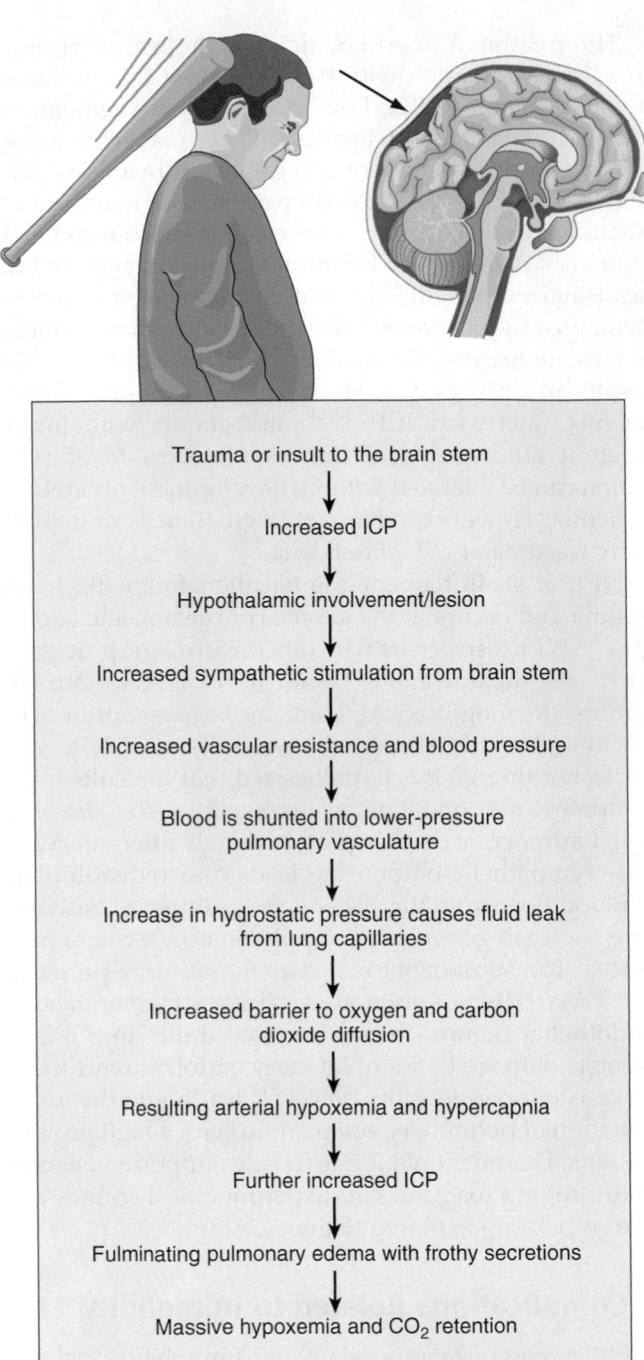

Trauma or insult to the brain stem

↓

Increased ICP

↓

Hypothalamic involvement/lesion

↓

Increased sympathetic stimulation from brain stem

↓

Increased vascular resistance and blood pressure

↓

Blood is shunted into lower-pressure
pulmonary vasculature

↓

Increase in hydrostatic pressure causes fluid leak
from lung capillaries

↓

Increased barrier to oxygen and carbon
dioxide diffusion

↓

Resulting arterial hypoxemia and hypercapnia

↓

Further increased ICP

↓

Fulminating pulmonary edema with frothy secretions

↓

Massive hypoxemia and CO_2 retention

⬍FIGURE 22-25 Development of neurogenic pulmonary edema in traumatic brain injury. CO_2 = Carbon dioxide, ICP = intracranial pressure.

ischemia and secondary brain injury in TBI patients. Benzodiazepines reduce cerebral metabolism and increase the seizure threshold, making them useful agents for treating and preventing seizures. Anticonvulsant agents such as phenytoin (Dilantin) or fosphenytoin (Cerebyx) are indicated for seizure prophylaxis for the first 7 days post-injury.[33] Phenytoin is given as a loading dose of 15 mg/kg followed by a maintenance dose of 100 mg every 6 to 8 hours based on serum phenytoin levels.[38] There is no support for continued treatment after 7 days unless a seizure has occurred in the patient.[38] For adult patients with severe TBI, prophylactic treatment with phenytoin, beginning with an IV loading dose, should be initiated as soon as possible after injury to decrease the risk of posttraumatic seizures occurring within the first 7 days. Prophylactic treatment with phenytoin, carbamazepine (Tegretol), or valproate (Depakote) should not be routinely used beyond the first 7 days after injury.[38] Adverse effects associated with the use of phenytoin are rash, Stevens-Johnson syndrome, leukopenia, and elevated levels of liver enzymes.[38]

OTHER MEDICATIONS USED FOR TRAUMATIC BRAIN INJURY

Lidocaine

Lidocaine, a local anesthetic, may be given to prevent ICP spikes during intubation.[215] The dose is 1 to 1.5 mg/kg IV given within 60 to 90 seconds of intubation or as a 4% intratracheal aerosol. Bolus doses of 1 mg/kg lidocaine can be given intravenously or via endotracheal tube before suctioning to blunt the increased ICP response to suctioning.[61,141]

Furosemide

Furosemide (Lasix) is a nonosmotic diuretic that can be used alone or in combination with osmotic agents to potentiate the effect. Furosemide acts rapidly and reduces ICP to a lesser extent than mannitol or other osmotic agents but is not associated with increased cerebral blood flow.[61]

Steroids

Because of the effectiveness of steroids in the treatment of edema associated with brain tumors and abscesses, it was once believed that there would be the same response in patients with edema after TBI. However, several clinical trials failed to demonstrate a benefit from the use of steroids within this population.[49,55,185] Steroids have been shown to increase death rate when given after severe brain injury.[3,46] The recent findings of the CRASH trial (effect of intravenous corticosteroids on death within 14 days in 10,008 adults with clinically significant head injury) suggest that steroids should no longer be routinely used in people with traumatic head injury.[3,46]

▲ Case Study 22-1, Part C

Head Injury and Dysfunction

On day 5, M.P. was no longer tolerating gastric feedings and had a transpyloric feeding tube placed at the bedside in order to continue enteral nutrition. The patient had temperature spikes as high as 105.2° F. He developed bilateral pulmonary infiltrates on chest x-ray and had purulent sputum. Cultures were obtained from sputum, blood, and urine, and he was subsequently diagnosed with pneumonia. External cooling mechanisms were initiated with ice packs and cooled circulating ambient air. An endovascular cooling device was also inserted for more aggressive cooling. The patient's pulmonary status continued to decline. The diagnosis of ARDS was made with the following ABG results: pH 7.52, $Paco_2$ 28 mm Hg, Pao_2 92 mm Hg on 80% Fio_2. The patient was placed on a rotating/turning bed surface in order to aid in mobilizing secretions and improve ventilation/perfusion matching.

M.P.'s pulmonary status slowly but progressively improved over the next 7 days, and his temperature was controlled. His ICP remained stable without further spikes over the following week.

Hyperventilation was discontinued, $Paco_2$ was normalized, and the jugular venous catheter was removed. ICP remained stable during this process. Pentobarbital was then weaned and discontinued, with no further spikes in ICP. The EVD was progressively raised and clamped, again with no increases in ICP. M.P.'s neurologic status progressively improved after pentobarbital was discontinued, and his ICP remained less than 20 mm Hg with a CPP of 68 mm Hg. His neurologic status now consisted of eye opening to noxious stimuli and combative behavior. Even though he required intermittent bolus doses of sedatives for his combativeness, he was beginning to follow simple commands. He was unable to respond verbally because of the ETT but he was starting to mouth some words. Ventilator weaning was started and M.P. was extubated. His allowed activity was gradually increased with physical therapy involvement for strengthening. The patient was eventually discharged to a rehabilitation facility for aggressive traumatic brain injury rehabilitation.

Throughout his hospital stay, the patient's wife was informed of treatment being instituted; she asked appropriate questions and remained very supportive. She attended a weekly traumatic brain injury support group that was offered at the institution.

Decision Point: Why is it important to avoid hyperthermia in the care of M.P.?

Decision Point: What are the potential complications of barbiturate-induced coma?

Decision Point: What interventions should be in place to minimize long-term complications of TBI?

OUTCOMES

Outcomes following TBI are often predicted based on initial GCS and functional level. However, an accurate prognosis cannot be determined for up to 12 months after injury and improvement may continue for 3 to 5 years after injury.[36] Because of the heterogeneity of brain injuries, differing age responses, and varying extent of secondary injuries, it is difficult to accurately predict patient outcomes.[39] Two factors shown to negatively impact outcomes following TBI are the presence of hypotension and hypoxia at any point following TBI.[39] Hypotension and hypoxia occurring in the early posttraumatic period are primary determinants of outcome.[124] Even one episode of hypotension increases the morbidity and mortality associated with TBI.[124] The Traumatic Coma Data Bank confirmed this finding when data analysis demonstrated that prehospital hypotension was an independent predictor of poor outcome.[39]

Family decision-making related to prognosis of TBI is extremely difficult because of the differing responses and outcomes. It is extremely difficult for families facing the potential reality of a loved one being left in a persistent vegetative state and making the decision to withdraw life-saving supportive measures. In the cases of TBI resulting in brain death, families are also faced with the decision of organ donation; even if brain death is not determined and the decision to withdraw support is made, the possibility of donation after cardiac death exists. Brain death and organ donation will be discussed more fully in Chapter 54. It is important for families to understand fully the implications of all care alternatives in order to make the most informed decisions. Family support regarding all potential options related to outcomes is essential. This is also true when patients are left with long-term disabilities. Family access to community resources is indispensable in assisting with physical, psychological, emotional, and social needs.

CONCLUSIONS

Patients who recover from severe head injury often have significant mental and physical handicaps producing social disability. The distinction between primary brain damage and that which develops from secondary events is helpful in explaining the apparent paradox of one patient whose initial injury was relatively mild yet ends up with severe brain damage, whereas another patient whose early condition was life-threatening recovers completely. Patients with the same type of lesion may have markedly different outcomes, depending on the causative lesion and treatment received.

The most reliable predictor of outcome is based on post-resuscitation GCS score, pupil reaction, age, and type of head injury.[141] TBI is not limited to an isolated event or impact. It is instead an aggregate of many mechanisms involving both primary and secondary damage. It is essential that the critical care nurse be knowledgeable of events contributing to ongoing damage in order to aggressively prevent and treat potential causes of further deterioration. Early hemorrhage control, volume resuscitation, tissue oxygenation, optimization of cerebral perfusion, adequate treatment of increased intracranial pressure, and prevention of complications are essential components of TBI patient care.[207]

REFERENCES

1. Aaslid, et al. (2003). Dynamic pressure-flow velocity relationships in the human cerebral circulation. *Stroke, 34,* 1645–1649.
2. Albano, C., Comandante, L., & Nolan, S. (2005). Innovations in the management of cerebral injury. *Crit Care Nurs Q, 28*(2), 135–149.
3. Alderson, P., & Roberts, I. (2005). Corticosteroids for acute traumatic brain injury. *Cochrane Database Syst Rev, 4,* CD000196; PMID:10796701.
4. Anderson, J. T., et al. (1997). Initial small-volume hypertonic resuscitation of shock and brain injury: short- and long-term effects. *J Trauma, 42*(4), 592–601.
5. Arundine, M., & Tymianski, M. (2004). Molecular mechanisms of glutamate-dependent neurodegeneration in ischemia and traumatic brain injury. *Cell Mol Life Sci, 61,* 657–668.
6. Auer, L. M., & Loew, F. (1983). *The cerebral veins. An experimental and critical update.* Vienna: Springer-Verlag.
7. Bader, M. K., March, K. S., & Littlejohns, L. (2002). *Cerebral oxygenation: how do we manage it and how will the patient benefit from targeted therapy?* Preconference Workshop, National Teaching Institute and Critical Care Exposition, Atlanta, May 2002.
8. Bader, M. K., & Arbour, R. (2005). Refractory increased intracranial pressure in severe traumatic brain injury: barbiturate coma and bispectral index monitoring. *AACN Clin Issues, 16*(4), 526–541.
9. Bagshaw, S. M., & Laupland, K. B. (2006). Epidemiology of intensive care unit-acquired urinary tract infections. *Curr Opin Infect Dis, 19,* 67–71.
10. Barker, E. (2002). Metabolic disorders. In E. Barker (Ed.), *Neuroscience nursing, a spectrum of care* (2nd ed.). St Louis: Mosby.
11. Barker, E. (2002). Intracranial pressure and monitoring. In E. Barker (Ed.), *Neuroscience nursing, a spectrum of care* (2nd ed.). St Louis: Mosby.
12. Blank-Reid, C., & Barker, E. (2002). Neurotrauma: traumatic brain injury. In E. Barker (Ed.), *Neuroscience nursing, a spectrum of care* (2nd ed.). St Louis: Mosby.
13. Battistella, F. D., & Wisner, D. H. (1991). Combined hemorrhagic shock and head injury: effects of hypertonic saline (7.5%) resuscitation. *J Trauma, 31,* 182–188.
14. Bayir, H., Clark, R. S. B., & Kochanek, P. M. (2003). Promising strategies to minimize secondary brain injury after head trauma. *Crit Care Med, 31*(1 suppl), S112–S117.
15. Becker, D. P., & Vries, J. K. (1972). The alleviation of increased intracranial pressure by the chronic administration of osmotic agents. In M. Brock & H. Kietz (Eds.), *Intracranial pressure* (pp 309–315). Berlin: Springer.
16. Beckstead, J. E., et al. (1978). Cerebral blood flow and metabolism in man following cardiac arrest. *Stroke, 9*(6), 569.
17. Belayev, L., et al. (1995). HU-211, a novel non-competitive NMDA antagonist, improves neurological deficit and reduces infarct volume after reversible focal cerebral ischemia in the rat. *Stroke, 26,* 2313–2320.
18. Bellander, B. M., et al. (2004). Consensus meeting on microdialysis in neurointensive care. *Intensive Care Med, 30,* 2166–2169.
19. Benmalek, F., et al. (1999). Renal effects of low-dose dopamine during vasopressor therapy for posttraumatic intracranial hypertension. *Intensive Care Med, 25,* 399–405.
20. Bergen, J. M., & Smith, D. C. (1997). A review of etomidate for rapid sequence intubation in the emergency department. *J Emergency Med, 15,* 221–230.
21. Bernert, H., & Turski, L. (1996). Traumatic brain damage prevented by the non-*N*-methyl-D-aspartate antagonist 2,3-dihydroxy-6-nitro-7-sulfamoylbenzol[*f*]quinoxaline. *Proc Natl Acad Sci USA, 93,* 5235–5240.
22. Bhardwaj, A., & Ulatowski, J. A. (2004). Hypertonic saline solutions in brain injury. *Curr Opin Crit Care, 10,* 126–131.
23. Biegon, A., et al. (1993). MRI study of rat brain edema after head trauma: effects of HU-211, a nonpsychotropic cannabinoid. *Am Soc Neurosci, 19*(abstract), 1485.
24. Blumbergs, P. C. (1997). Pathology. In P. Reilly & A. B. Ross (Eds.), *Head injury; pathophysiology and management of severe closed injury.* London: Chapman & Hall.
25. Boddie, D., et al. (2003). Immune suppression and isolated severe head injury: a significant clinical problem. *Brit J Neurosurg, 17,* 405–417.
26. Bouma, G. J., et al. (1991). Cerebral circulation and metabolism after severe traumatic brain injury: the elusive role of ischemia. *J Neurosurg, 75,* 685–693.
27. Bouma, G. J., et al. (1992). Ultra-early evaluation of regional cerebral blood flow in severely head-injured patients using xenon-enhanced computed tomography. *J Neurosurg, 77,* 360–368.
28. Bratton, S. L., & Davis, R. L. (1997). Acute lung injury in isolated traumatic brain injury. *Neurosurgery, 40*(4), 707–712.
29. Bullock, M. (2000). Initial management. *J Neurotrauma, 17,* 463–469.
30. Bullock, M. (2000). Intracranial pressure treatment threshold. *J Neurotrauma, 17,* 493–495.
31. Bullock, R., Butcher, S., & McCullough, J. (1990). Changes in extracellular glutamate concentration after acute subdural haematoma in the rat—evidence for an "excitotoxic" mechanism. *Acta Neurochirurgica (Suppl), 57,* 274–276.
32. Bullock, R. (1997). Pathology. In P. Reilly & A. B. Ross (Eds.), *Head injury; pathophysiology and management of severe closed injury.* London: Chapman & Hall.
33. Bullock, R., et al. (2000). Guidelines for the management of severe traumatic brain injury. In *Brain Trauma Foundation and American Association of Neurological Surgeons: management and prognosis of severe traumatic brain injury.* New York: Brain Trauma Foundation.
34. Bullock, R. M., Chestnut, R., & Clifton, G. (2001). Management and prognosis of severe traumatic brain injury. *J Neurotrauma, 17*(6–7), 451–627.
35. Burch, J. M., et al. (1996). The abdominal compartment syndrome. *Surg Clin North Am, 76,* 833–842.
36. Caron, M. J. (1996). PET/SPECT imaging in head injury. In R. K. Narayan, J. E. Wilberger, Jr., & J. T. Povlishock (Eds.), *Neurotrauma* (pp. 163–168). New York: McGraw-Hill.
37. Centers for Disease Control and Prevention, Department of Health and Human Services. (2004). *Traumatic brain injury in the United States, emergency department visits, hospitalizations, and deaths.* Atlanta: Division of Injury and Disability Outcomes and Programs, National Center for Injury Prevention and Control, Centers for Disease Control and Prevention, Department of Health and Human Services.

38. Chang, B. S., & Lowenstein, D. H. (2003). Practice parameter: antiepileptic drug prophylaxis in severe traumatic brain injury. *Neurology, 60,* 10–16.

39. Chestnut, R., Marshall, L. F., & Klauber, M. R. (1993). The role of secondary brain injury in determining outcome from severe head injury. *J Trauma, 34,* 216–222.

40. Chestnut, R. M. (1996). Treating raised intracranial pressure in head injury. In R. K. Narayan, J. E. Wilberger, Jr., & J. T. Povlishock (Eds.), *Neurotrauma* (pp 445–469). New York: McGraw-Hill.

41. Chopp, M., & Portnoy, H. D. (1983). Hydraulic model of cerebrovascular bed: an aid to understanding the volume-pressure test. *Neurosurgery, 13,* 5–11.

42. Citerio, G., & Cormio, M. (2003). Sedation in neurointensive care: advances in understanding and practice. *Curr Opin Crit Care, 9,* 120–126.

43. Clark, R. S. B., & Kochanek, P. (Eds.) (2001). *Brain injury.* Boston: Kluwer Academic Publishers.

44. Clifton, G. L., et al. (2001). Lack of effect of induction of hypothermia after acute brain injury. *N Engl J Med, 344,* 556–563.

45. Coles, J. P. (2004). Regional ischemia after head injury. *Curr Opin Crit Care, 10,* 120–125.

46. CRASH Trial Collaborators. (2004). Effect of intravenous corticosteroids on death within 14 days, 10008 adults with clinically significant head injury (MRC CRASH trial): randomised placebo-controlled trial. *Lancet, 364,* 1321–1328.

47. Cooper, D., et al. (2004). Prehospital hypertonic saline resuscitation of patients with hypotension and severe traumatic brain injury: a randomized controlled trial. *JAMA, 291,* 1350–1357.

48. Cooper, K. R., Boswell, P. A., & Choi, S. C. (1985). Safe use of PEEP in patients with severe head injury. *J Neurosurg, 63,* 552–555.

49. Cooper, P. R., et al. (1979). Dexamethasone and severe head injury. A prospective double-blind study. *J Neurosurg, 51,* 307–316.

50. Crompton, M. R. (1971). Hypothalamic lesions following closed head injury. *Brain, 94,* 165–172.

51. Cruz, J. (1993). Cerebral oxygenation—monitoring and management. *Acta Neurochirurgica (Suppl), 59,* 415–430.

52. Cushing, H. (1901). Concerning a definite regulatory mechanism of the vasomotor center which controls blood pressure during cerebral compression. *Bull Johns Hopkins Hospital, 12,* 290–292.

53. Cushing, H. (1902). Some experimental and clinical observations concerning states of increased intracranial tension. *Am J Med Sci, 124,* 375–400.

54. Cushing, H. (1903). The blood pressure reaction of acute cerebral compression, illustrated by cases of intracranial haemorrhage. *Am J Med Sci, 125,* 1017–1044.

55. Dearden, N. M., et al. (1986). Effect of high-dose dexamethasone on outcome from severe head injury. *J Neurosurg, 64,* 81–88.

56. Diaz-Parejo, P., et al. (2003). Cerebral energy metabolism during transient hyperglycemia in patients with severe brain trauma. *Intensive Care Med, 29,* 544–550.

57. Doberstein, C., & Martin, N. A. (1996). Transcranial Doppler ultrasonography in head injury. In R. K. Narayan, J. E. Wilberger, Jr., & J. T. Povlishock (Eds.), *Neurotrauma* (pp 539–552). New York: McGraw-Hill.

58. Donaldson, J., Borzatta, M. A., & Matossian, D. (2000). Nutrition strategies in neurotrauma. *Crit Care Nurs Clin North Am, 12*(4), 465–473.

59. Doppenberg, E. M. R., Choi, S. C., & Bullock, R. (2004). Clinical trials in traumatic brain injury: lessons for the future. *J Neurosurg Anesthesiol, 16*(1), 87–94.

60. Doyle, J. A., Davis, D. P., & Hoyt, D. B. (2001). The use of hypertonic saline in the treatment of traumatic brain injury. *J Trauma, 50,* 367–383.

61. Duhaime, A. C. (1996). Conventional drug therapies for head injury. In R. K. Narayan, J. E. Wilberger, Jr., & J. T. Povlishock (Eds.), *Neurotrauma.* New York: McGraw-Hill.

62. Dutton, R. P., & McCunn, M. (2003). Traumatic brain injury. *Curr Opin Crit Care, 9,* 503–509.

63. Farrar, J. A. (1998). Trauma. In M. R. Kinney et al. (Ed.), *AACN clinical reference for critical care nursing* (4th ed.). St Louis: Mosby.

64. Fineman, I., Hovda, D. A., & Smith, K. (1993). Concussive brain injury is associated with a prolonged accumulation of calcium: a 45 calcium autoradiographic study. *Brain Res, 624,* 94–102.

65. Fischer, J., & Mathieson, C. (2001). The history of the Glasgow coma scale: implications for practice. *Crit Care Nurs Q, 23*(4), 52–58.

66. Fisher, J. R., & Baer, R. K. (1996). Acute myopathy associated with combined use of corticosteroids and neuromuscular blocking agents. *Ann Pharmacother, 30*(12), 1437–1445.

67. Flakoll, P., Wentzel, L., & Hyman, S. (1995). Protein and glucose metabolism during isolated closed-head injury. *Am J Physiol, 269,* 636.

68. Foulkes, M., Eisenberg, H. M., & Jane, J. A. (1991). The Traumatic Coma Data Bank: design, methods and baseline characteristics. *J Neurosurg, 75,* S8–S13.

69. Fraser, G. L., & Riker, R. R. (2005). Bispectral index monitoring in the intensive care unit provides more signal than noise. *Pharmacotherapy, 25*(5), 19S–27S.

70. Freytag, E. (1963). Autopsy findings in head injuries from blunt force. Statistical evaluation of 1,367 cases. *Arch Pathol, 75,* 402–413.

71. Fritz, H. G., & Bauer, R. (2004). Secondary injuries in brain trauma: effects of hypothermia. *J Neurosurg Anesthesiol, 16*(1), 43–52.

72. Gabriel, E. J., et al. (2002). Guidelines for prehospital management of traumatic brain injury. *J Neurotrauma, 19,* 111–174.

73. Gennarelli, T. A., et al. (1982). Influence of the type of intracranial lesion on outcome from severe head injury. *J Neurosurg, 56,* 26–32.

74. Giza, C. C., & Hovda, D. A. (2001). The neurometabolic cascade of concussion. *J Athletic Training, 36*(3), 228–235.

75. Goodman, J. C., et al. (1996). Lactate and excitatory amino acids measured by microdialysis are decreased by pentobarbital coma in head-injured patients. *J Neurotrauma, 13,* 549–556.

76. Gopinath, S. P., et al. (1994). Jugular venous desaturation and outcome after head injury. *J Neurol, Neurosurg Psychiatry, 57,* 717–723.

77. Grahama, D. I., et al. (1989). Ischaemic brain damage is still common in fatal non-missile head injury. *J Trauma, 52,* 346–350.

78. Guha, A. (2004). Management of traumatic brain injury: some current evidence and applications. *Postgrad Med J, 80,* 650–653.

79. Hallenbeack, J., et al. (1986). Polymorphonuclear leucocyte accumulation in brain regions with low blood flow during the early postischaemic period. *Stroke, 17,* 246.

80. Hanley, D. F., & Varelas, P. (1999). Glutamate in parenteral nutrition. *Crit Care Med, 27*(10), 2319–2320.

81. Harder, D. R., et al. (1998). Functional hyperemia in the brain: hypothesis for astrocyte-derived vasodilator metabolites. *Stroke, 29*(1), 229–234.

82. Hartl, R., et al. (1997). Hypertonic/hyperoncotic saline reliably reduces ICP in severely head injured patients with intracranial hypertension. *Acta Neurochirurgica, 70*(suppl), 126–129.

83. Hatfield, R., & Gill, R. (1992). Dose response relationship and therapeutic window from Dizocilpine (MK801) in a rat focal ischaemia model. *Eur J Pharmacol, 216*:1–7.

84. Henderson, W., et al. (2003). Hypothermia in the management of traumatic brain injury: a systematic review and meta-analysis. *Intensive Care Med, 29,* 1637–1644.

85. Hickey, J. V. (2002). Intracranial pressure: theory and management of increased intracranial pressure. In J. V. Hickey (Ed.),

The clinical practice of neurological and neurosurgical nursing (5th ed). Philadelphia: Lippincott, Williams & Wilkins.

86. Hills, M. W., & Deane, S. A. (1993). Head injury and facial injury: is there an increased risk of cervical spine injury? *J Trauma, 34,* 549–553.

87. Hovda, D. A., et al. (1995). The neurochemical and metabolic cascade following brain injury: moving from animal models to man. *J Neurotrauma, 12,* 903–906.

88. Hutchinson, P., & Kirkpatrick, P. J. (2004). Decompressive craniectomy in head injury. *Curr Opin Crit Care, 10,* 101–104.

89. Inao, S., et al. (1988). Production and clearance of lactate from brain tissue, cerebrospinal fluid, and serum following experimental brain injury. *J Neurosurg, 69,* 736–744.

90. Jamieson, K. G., & Yelland, J. D. N. (1968). Extradural haematoma: report of 167 cases. *J Neurosurg, 29,* 13–23.

91. Jennet, W. B. (1961). Experimental brain compression. *Arch Neurol, 4,* 599–607.

92. Johnston, A. J., et al. (2004). Effect of cerebral perfusion pressure augmentation with dopamine and norepinephrine on global and focal brain oxygenation after traumatic brain injury. *Intensive Care Med, 30,* 791–797.

93. Johnston, A. J., & Gupta, A. J. (2002). Advanced monitoring in the neurology intensive care unit: microdialysis. *Curr Opin Crit Care, 2,* 121–127.

94. Johnston, I. H., & Rowan, J. O. (1974). Raised intracranial pressure and cerebral blood: 3. Venous outflow tract pressures and vascular resistances in experimental intracranial hypertension. *J Neurol Neurosurg Psychiatry, 37,* 392–402.

95. Jones, P. A., et al. (1994). Measuring the burden of secondary insults in head-injured patients during intensive care. *J Neurosurg Anaesthesiol, 6,* 4–14.

96. Kase, C. S. (2005). Hemostatic treatment in the early stage of intracerebral hemorrhage: the recombinant factor VIIa experience. *Stroke, 36*(10), 2321–2322.

97. Kaufmann, A. M., & Cardoso, E. R. (1992). Aggravation of vasogenic cerebral edema by multiple-dose mannitol. *J Neurosurg, 77,* 584–589.

98. Kawamata, T., et al. (1995). Lactate accumulation following concussive brain injury: the role of ionic fluxes induced by excitatory amino acid. *Brain Res, 674,* 196–204.

99. Kein, N. D., Reitan, J. A., & White, D. A. (1991). Cardiac contractility and blood flow distribution following resuscitation with 7.5% hypertonic saline in anesthetized dogs. *Circ Shock, 35,* 109–116.

100. Kellie, G. (1824). An account of the appearances observed in the dissection of two of three individuals presumed to have perished in the storm of the third and whose bodies were discovered in the vicinity of Leith on the morning of the 4th, November, 1821, with some reflections on the pathology of the brain. *Transact Medico-Chirugical SocEdinburgh, 1,* 84–169.

101. Kelly, B., & Luce, J. M. (1993). Current concepts in cerebral protection. *Chest, 103,* 1246–1254.

102. Kern, K., & Meislin, H. (1984). Diabetes insipidus: occurrence after minor head trauma. *J Trauma, 24,* 69–72.

103. Khaldi, A., et al. (2002). The significance of nitric oxide production in the brain after injury. *Ann NY Acad Sci, 962,* 53–59.

104. Khanna, S., et al. (2000). Use of hypertonic saline in the treatment of severe refractory posttraumatic intracranial hypertension in pediatric traumatic brain injury. *Crit Care Med, 28,* 1144–1151.

105. Kirkness, C. J. (2005). Cerebral blood flow monitoring in clinical practice. *AACN Clin Issues, 16*(4), 476–487.

106. Knapp, J. M. (2005). Hyperosmolar therapy in the treatment of severe head injury in children. *AACN Clin Issues, 16*(2), 199–211.

107. Knoller, N., et al. (2002). Dexanabinol (HU-211) in the treatment of severe closed head injury: a randomized, placebo-controlled, phase II clinical trial. *Crit Care Med, 30,* 548–554.

108. Kraus, J. F., et al. (1996). Epidemiology of brain injury. In R. K. Narayan, J. E. Wilberger, Jr., & J. T. Povlishock (Eds.), *Neurotrauma* (pp 13–30). New York: McGraw-Hill.

109. Kumar, M. A., et al. (2005). The syndrome of irreversible acidosis after prolonged propofol infusion. *Neurocrit Care, 3*(3), 257–259.

110. Lam, A. M., et al. (1991). Hyperglycemia and neurological outcome in patients with head injury. *J Neurosurg, 75,* 545–551.

111. Lapointe, L. A., & Von Rueden, K. T. (2002). Coagulopathies in trauma patients. *AACN Clin Issues, 13*(2), 192–203.

112. Lautsch, L., et al. (1999). Incorporation of SPECT imaging in a longitudinal cognitive rehabilitation therapy programme. *Brain Injury, 13,* 555–570.

113. Le Roux, P., et al. (1997). Cerebral arteriovenous difference of oxygen: a predictor of cerebral infarction and outcome in severe head injury. *J Neurosurg, 87,* 1–8.

114. Lee, J. P., & Wang, A. D. (1991). Post-traumatic basal ganglia hemorrhage: analysis of 52 patients with emphasis on the final outcome. *J Trauma, 31*(3), 376–380.

115. Leker, R. R., & Shohami, E. (2002). Cerebral ischemia and trauma—different etiologies yet similar mechanisms: neuroprotective opportunities. *Brain Res Rev, 39,* 55–73.

116. Levin, A. B., et al. (1979). Treatment of increased intracranial pressure. *Neurosurgery, 5*(5), 570–575.

117. Lindenberg, R. (1971). Trauma of meninges and brain. In J. Minkler (Ed.), *Pathology of the nervous system* (Vol 2, pp 1705–1765). New York: McGraw Hill.

118. Littlejohns, L., & Badar, M. K. (2005). Prevention of secondary brain injury: targeting technology. *AACN Clin Issues, 16*(4), 501–514.

119. Lovasik, D., Kerr, M. E., & Alexander, S. (2001). Traumatic brain injury research: a review of clinical studies. *Crit Care Nurs Q, 23*(4), 24–41.

120. Macmillan, C. S. A., et al. (2002). Traumatic brain injury and subarachnoid hemorrhage: in vivo occult pathology demonstrated by magnetic resonance spectroscopy may not be ischaemic. A primary study and review of the literature. *Acta Neurochirugica, 144,* 853–862.

121. Manno, E. M. (1997). Transcranial Doppler ultrasonography in the neurocritical care unit. *Crit Care Clin, 13,* 79–104.

122. March, K. (2000). Application of technology in the treatment of traumatic brain injury. *Crit Care Nurs Q, 23*(3), 26–37.

123. March, K. (2005). Intracranial pressure monitoring: why monitor? *AACN Clin Issues, 16*(4), 456–475.

124. Marik, P. E., Varon, J., & Trask, T. (2002). Management of head trauma. *Chest, 122*(2), 699–711.

125. Marion, D., et al. (1997). Treatment of traumatic brain injury with moderate hypothermia. *N Engl J Med, 336,* 540–546.

126. Marion, D. W., & Carlier, P. M. (1994). Problems with initial Glasgow Coma Scale assessment caused by prehospital treatment of patients with head injuries: results of a national survey. *J Trauma, 36,* 89–95.

127. Marion, D. W., et al. (2002). Effect of hyperventilation on extracellular concentrations of glutamate, lactate, pyruvate, and local cerebral blood flow in patients with severe traumatic brain injury. *Crit Care Med, 30*(12), 2619–2625.

128. Marmarou, D. W., et al. (1993). The contribution of brain edema to brain swelling ICP and craniospinal dynamic. In C. J. J. Avezaat, J. H. M. van Eindhoven, A. I. R. Maas et al. (Eds.), *Intracranial pressure VIII* (pp 525–528). Berlin: Springer-Verlag.

129. Marmarou, A. (1994). Traumatic brain edema: an overview. *Acta Neurochirugica, 60*(Suppl), 421–424.

130. Marshall, L. F. (1978). Pentobarbital therapy for intracranial hypertension and metabolic coma. *Crit Care Med, 6*(1), 1–5.

131. Marshall, L. F., Smith, R. W., & Shapiro, H. M. (1979). The outcome with aggressive treatment in severe head injuries. Part 1: The significance of intracranial pressure monitoring. *J Neurosurg, 50*, 832–840.

132. Marshall, R. S. (2004). The functional relevance of cerebral hemodynamics: why blood flow matters to the injured and recovering brain. *Curr Opin Neurol, 17*, 705–709.

133. Martini, F. H. (2004). *Fundamentals of anatomy & physiology*. San Francisco: Pearson Education.

134. Martyn, J. A., & Richtsfeld, M. (2006). Succinylcholine-induced hyperkalemia in acquired pathologic states: etiologic factors and molecular mechanisms. *Anesthesiology, 104*(1), 158–169.

135. Mascia, L., et al. (2000). Cerebral blood flow and metabolism in severe brain injury: the role of pressure autoregulation during cerebral perfusion pressure management. *Intensive Care Med, 26*, 202–205.

136. May, A. K., et al. (1997). Coagulopathy in severe closed head injury: is empiric therapy warranted? *Am Surg, 63*, 233–236.

137. Mazzoni, M. C., et al. (1988). Dynamic fluid redistribution in hyperosmotic resuscitation of hypovolemic hemorrhage. *Am J Physiol, 255*(3 pt 2), H629–H637.

138. Mcilvoy, L. H. (2005). The effect of hypothermia and hyperthermia on acute brain injury. *AACN Clin Issues, 16*(4), 488–500.

139. McIntyre, L., et al. (2003). Prolonged therapeutic hypothermia after traumatic brain injury in adults: a systematic review. *JAMA, 289*, 2992–2999.

140. McKee, J. A., et al. (2005). Analysis of the brain bioavailability of peripherally administered magnesium sulfate: a study in humans with acute brain injury undergoing prolonged induced hypermagnesemia. *Crit Care Med, 33*(3), 651–666.

141. McQuillan, K. A., & Mitchell, P. H. (2002). Traumatic brain injuries. In K. A. McQuillan, K. T. Von Rueden & M. B. Hartsock, R. L. et al. (Eds.), *Trauma nursing* (3rd ed.). Philadelphia: Saunders.

142. Meert, K. L., et al. (1995). Alterations in immune function following head injury in children. *Crit Care Med, 23*(5), 822–828.

143. Meixensberger, J., et al. (2003). Brain tissue oxygen guided treatment supplementing ICP/CPP therapy after traumatic brain injury. *J Neurol Neurosurg Psychiatry, 74*, 760–764.

144. Meldrum, B. (1990). Protection against ischaemic neuronal damage by drugs acting on excitatory neurotransmission. *Cerebrovasc Brain Metab Rev, 2*(1), 27–57.

145. Mendelow, A. D., & Crawford, P. J. (1997). Primary and secondary brain injury. In P. Reilly & A. B. Ross (Eds.), *Head injury: pathophysiology and management of severe closed injury*. London: Chapman & Hall.

146. Michael, D. B., Guyot, D. R., & Damody, W. R. (1989). Coincidence of head and cervical spine injury. *J Neurotrauma, 6*, 177–189.

147. Michenfelder, J. D. (1974). The interdependency of cerebral function and metabolic effects following massive doses of thiopental in the dog. *Anesthesiology, 41*, 231.

148. Miller, J. D. (1993). Traumatic brain swelling and edema. In P. R. Cooper (Ed.), *Head injury*. Baltimore: Williams & Wilkins.

149. Miller, J. D., et al. (1981). Further experience in the management of severe head injury. *J Neurosurg, 79*, 60–64.

150. Miller, J. I., et al. (1998). Continuous intracranial multimodality monitoring comparing local cerebral blood flow, cerebral perfusion pressure, and microvascular resistance. *Acta Neurochir Suppl, 71*, 82–84.

151. Minnear, F. L., et al. (1987). Endothelial injury and pulmonary congestion characterize neurogenic pulmonary oedema in rabbits. *J Appl Physiol, 63*(1), 335–341.

152. Mohamed, A., et al. (1985). Effect of pretreatment with the calcium antagonist, nimodipine on local cerebral blood flow and histopathology after middle cerebral artery occlusion. *Ann Neurol, 18*, 705.

153. Monro, A. (1783). *Observations on the structure and function of the nervous system*. Edinburgh: Creech & Johnston.

154. Morganti-Kossmann, M. C., et al. (2002). Inflammatory response in acute traumatic brain injury: a double-edged sword. *Curr Opin Crit Care, 8*, 101–105.

155. Morse, M. L., et al. (1985). Effect of hydration on experimentally induced cerebral edema. *Crit Care Med, 13*(7), 563.

156. Mosberg, W. H., & Lindenberg, R. (1959). Traumatic haemorrhage from the anterior choroidal artery. *J Neurosurg, 16*, 209–221.

157. Moulton, R. J. (2001). Abdominal compartment syndrome in the head-injured patient. *Crit Care Med, 29*(7), 1487–1488.

158. Muench, E., et al. (2005). Effects of positive end-expiratory pressure on regional cerebral blood flow, intracranial pressure, and brain tissue oxygenation. *Crit Care Med, 33*(10), 2367–2372.

159. Muizelaar, J. P., Marmarou, A., & Ward, J. D. (1991). Adverse effects of prolonged hyperventilation in patients with severe head injury: a randomized clinical trial. *J Neurosurg, 75*, 731–739.

160. Mulvey, J. M., et al. (2004). Influence of cerebral oxygenation following severe head injury on neuropsychological testing. *Neurol Res, 26*(4), 414–417.

161. Murray, M. J., et al. (2002). Clinical practice guidelines for sustained neuromuscular blockade in the critically ill adult patient. *Crit Care Med, 30*, 142–156.

162. Myburgh, J. A. (1997). Respiratory and cardiovascular support. In P. Reilly & R. Bullock (Eds.), *Head injury: pathophysiology and management of severe closed injury*. London: Chapman & Hall.

163. Narayan, R. K., & Wilberger, J. E., Jr (1996). Computed tomography of closed head injury. In R. K. Narayan, J. E. Wilberger & J. T. Povlishock (Eds.), *Neurotrauma*. New York: McGraw-Hill.

164. Nortje, J., & Menon, D. K. (2004). Traumatic brain injury: physiology, mechanisms, and outcome. *Curr Opin Neurol, 17*, 711–718.

165. Obrist, W. D., & Marion, D. W. (1997). Xenon techniques for CBF measurements in clinical head injury. In R. K. Narayan, J. E. Wilberger & J. T. Povlishock (Eds.), *Neurotrauma*. New York: McGraw-Hill.

166. Olesen, J., Paulson, O. B., & Lassen, N. A. (1971). Regional cerebral blood flow in man determined by the initial slope of the clearance of intra-arterially injected ^{133}Xe. *Stroke, 2*, 51, 9–540.

167. Pellerin, L., & Magistretti, P. J. (1994). Glutamate uptake into astrocytes stimulates aerobic glycolysis: a mechanism coupling neuronal activity to glucoutilization. *Proc Natl Acad Sci USA, 91*, 10625–10629.

168. Peterson, B., et al. (2000). Prolonged hypernatremia controls elevated intracranial pressure in head-injured pediatric patients. *Crit Care Med, 28*, 1136–1143.

169. Phillis, J. W., & Goshgarian, H. G. (2001). Adenosine and neurotrauma: therapeutic perspectives. *Neurol Res, 23*, 183–189.

170. Piek, J. (2002). Decompressive surgery in the treatment of traumatic brain injury. *Curr Opin Crit Care, 8*, 13, 4–138.

171. Pitts, L. H., et al. (1980). ICP and outcome in patients with severe head injury. In K. Shulman, A. Marmarour, J. D. Miller, et al. (Eds.), *Intracranial pressure IV*. Berlin: Springer-Verlag.

172. Polderman, K. H., et al. (2002). Effects of therapeutic hypothermia on intracranial pressure and outcome in patients with severe head injury. *Intensive Care Med, 28*, 1563–1573.

173. Povlishock, J. T., & Katz, D. I. (2005). Update of neuropathology and neurological recovery after traumatic brain injury. *J Head Trauma Rehabil, 20*(1), 76–94.

174. Prough, D. S., & Bedell, E. A. (2001). Cerebral ischemia in humans after traumatic brain injury. *Crit Care Med, 29*(2), 456–457.

175. Qureshi, A. I., et al. (2000). Long-term outcome after medical reversal of transtentorial herniation in patients with supratentorial mass lesions. *Crit Care Med, 28,* 1556–1564.

176. Raichle, M. E., & Plum, F. (1972). Hyperventilation and cerebral blood flow. *Stroke, 3,* 566–575.

177. Reilly, P., & Bullock, R. (1997). *Head injury: pathophysiology and management of severe closed injury.* London: Chapman & Hall.

178. Riker, J. H., & Zafonte, R. D. (2000). Functional neuroimaging and quantitative electroencephalography in adult traumatic head injury: clinical applications and interpretive cautions. *J Head Trauma Rehabil, 15,* 859–868.

179. Riker, R. R., Fraser, G. L., & Wilkins, M. L. (2003). Comparing the bispectral index and suppression ratio with burst suppression of the electroencephalogram during pentobarbital infusions in adult intensive care patients. *Pharmacotherapy, 23,* 1087–1093.

180. Ropper, A. H., & Rockoff, M. A. (1993). Physiological and clinical aspects of raised intracranial pressure. In A. H. Ropper (Ed.), *Neurological and neurosurgical intensive care* (3rd ed.). New York: Raven Press.

181. Ross, E. J., & Christie, S. B. M. (1969). Hypernatremia. *Medicine, 48,* 441–472.

182. Roth, P., & Farls, K. (2000). Pathophysiology of traumatic brain injury. *Crit Care Nurs Q, 23*(3), 14–25.

183. Rothoeri, R. D., Woertgen, C., & Brawanski, A. (2004). Hyperemia following aneurysmal subarachnoid hemorrhage: incidence, diagnosis, clinical features, and outcome. *Intensive Care Med, 30,* 1298–1302.

184. Sanchez, P. C. (1996). How neurotrophic factors protect brain against excitotoxicity. *Surg Neurol, 46,* 152–153.

185. Saul, T. G., et al. (1981). Steroids in severe head injury: a prospective randomized clinical trial. *J Neurosurg, 54,* 596–600.

186. Scalea, T. M., & Boswell, S. A. (2002). Initial management of traumatic shock. In K. A. McQuillan, K. T. Von Rueden, M. B. Hartsock, et al. (Eds.), *Trauma nursing* (3rd ed.). Philadelphia: Saunders.

187. Schell, R. M., Applegate, R. L., II, & Cole, D. J. (1996). Salt, starch, and water on the brain. *J Neurosurg Anaesthetics, 8,* 178–182.

188. Schmidt, E., et al. (2003). Asymmetry of pressure autoregulation after traumatic brain injury. *J Neurosurg, 99,* 991–998.

189. Schrader, K. A. (1996). Stress and immunity after traumatic injury: the mind-body link. *AACN Clin Issues, 7*(3), 351–358.

190. Schroder, M., & Muizelaar, J. (1993). Regional ischemia and regional cerebral blood volume (CBV) after severe head injury in man. *J Neurotrauma, 10*(suppl 1), 557.

191. Schubert, A. (2002). Cerebral hyperemia, systemic hypertension, and perioperative intracranial morbidity: is there a smoking gun? *Anesth Analg, 94*(3), 485–487.

192. Seckl, J. R., Dunger, D. B., & Lightman, S. L. (1897). Neurohypophyseal function during early post-operative diabetes insipidus. *Brain, 110,* 737–746.

193. Seelig, J. M., et al. (1981). Traumatic acute subdural haematoma. Major mortality reduction in comatose patients treated within four hours. *N Engl J Med, 304,* 1511–1518.

194. Sharp, S. J., Thompson, S. G., & Altman, D. G. (1996). The relation between treatment benefit and underlying risk in meta-analysis. *BMJ, 313,* 735–738.

195. Sheinberg, M., et al. (1992). Continuous monitoring of jugular venous oxygen saturation in head-injured patients. *J Neurosurg, 76,* 212–217.

196. Shohami, E., et al. (1997). Cytokine production in the brain following closed head injury: dexabinol (HU-211) is a novel TNF-alpha inhibitor and an effective neuroprotectant. *J Neuroimmunol, 72,* 169–177.

197. Simma, B., et al. (1998). A prospective, randomized, and controlled study of fluid management in children with severe head injury: lactated Ringer's solution versus hypertonic saline. *Crit Care Med, 26,* 1265–1270.

198. Simmons, R. L., et al. (1969). Respiratory insufficiency in combat casualties: II—pulmonary edema following head injury. *Ann Surg, 170,* 39–44.

199. Soloniuk, D., et al. (1986). Traumatic intracerebral haematomas: timing of appearance and indications for operative removal. *J Trauma, 26,* 787–794.

200. Soukup, J., et al. (2002). Relationship between brain temperature, brain chemistry and oxygen delivery after severe human head injury: the effect of mild hypothermia. *Neurol Res, 24,* 161–168.

201. Stahl, N., Ungerstedt, U., & Nordstrom, C. H. (2001). Brain energy metabolism during controlled reduction of cerebral perfusion pressure in severe head injuries. *Intensive Care Med, 27,* 1215–1223.

202. Steinbok, P., & Thompson, G. B. (1987). Metabolic disturbances after head injury: abnormalities of sodium and water balance with special reference to the effects of alcohol intoxication. *Neurosurgery, 3*(1), 9–15.

203. Steiner, L. A., et al. (2004). Direct comparison of cerebrovascular effects of norepinephrine and dopamine in head-injured patients. *Crit Care Med, 32*(4), 1049–1054.

204. Stochetti, N., Furlan, A., & Volta, F. (1996). Hypoxemia and arterial hypotension at the accident scene in head injury. *J Trauma, 40,* 764–767.

205. Stover, J. F., & Stocker, R. (1998). Barbiturate coma may promote reversible bone marrow suppression in patients with severe isolated traumatic brain injury. *Eur J Clin Pharmacol, 54,* 529–534.

206. Stuart, F. P., et al. (1970). Effects of single, repeated and massive mannitol infusion in the dog: structural and functional changes in kidney and brain. *Ann Surg, 172,* 190–204.

207. Sumann, G., et al. (2002). Early intensive care unit intervention for trauma care: what alters the outcome? *Curr Opin Crit Care, 8,* 587–592.

208. Tanno, H., et al. (1992). Breakdown of the blood-brain barrier after fluid percussive brain injury in the rat; part 1: distribution and time course of protein extravasation. *J Neurotrauma, 9,* 21–32.

209. Tasker, R. C. (1999). Pharmacological advance in the treatment of acute brain injury. *Arch Dis Child, 81*(1), 90–95.

210. Taski, A., et al. (2003). Prognostic value of interleukin-1 beta levels after acute brain injury. *Neurol Res, 25,* 871–874.

211. Teasdale, G. M., & Graham, D. I. (1998). Craniocerebral trauma: protection and retrieval of the neuronal population after injury. *Neurosurgery, 43*(4), 723–737.

212. Theodore, J. R. (Ed.) (1976). Speculations on neurogenic pulmonary edema (NPE). *Am Rev Respir Dis, 113,* 405–411.

213. Thomas, P. D. (1997). Fluid, electrolyte and metabolic management. In P. Reilly & R. Bullock (Eds.), *Head injury: pathophysiology and management of severe closed injury.* London: Chapman & Hall.

214. Thompson, H. J., et al. (2003). Hyperthermia following traumatic brain injury: a critical evaluation. *Neurobiol Disease, 12,* 163–173.

215. Thurman, D., & Guerrero, J. (1999). Trends in hospitalization associated with traumatic brain injury. *JAMA, 282,* 954–957.

216. Traystman, R. J. (2004). Anesthetic mediated neuroprotection. *J Neurosurg Anesthesiol, 16*(4), 308–312.

217. van den Brink, W. A., et al. (2000). Brain oxygen tension in severe head injury. *Neurosurgery, 46,* 868–878.

218. Valadka, A. B., et al. (1998). Relationship of brain tissue P_{O_2} to outcome after severe head injury. *Crit Care Med, 26,* 1576–1581.

219. Vassar, M. J., et al. (1993). A multicenter trial for resuscitation of injured patients with 7.5% sodium chloride: the effect of added dextran 70; The Multicenter Group for the Study of Hypertonic Saline in Trauma Patients. *Arch Surg, 128,* 1003–1011.

220. Vassar, M. J., et al. (1991). 7.5% sodium chloride/dextran for resuscitation of trauma patients undergoing helicopter transport. *Arch Surg, 126,* 1065.

221. Vavilala, M. S., et al. (2001). The influence of inhaled nitric oxide on cerebral blood flow and metabolism in a child with traumatic brain injury. *Anesth Analg, 93*(2), 351–353.

222. Vespa, P. M., et al. (1999). Increased incidence and impact of nonconvulsive and convulsive seizures after traumatic brain injury as detected by continuous electroencephalographic monitoring. *J Neurosurg, 91,* 750–760.

223. Wade, C. E., et al. (1997). Individual patient cohort analysis of the efficacy of hypertonic saline/dextran in patients with traumatic brain injury and hypotension. *J Trauma, 42*(5 suppl), S61–S65.

224. Wang, C. X., & Shuaib, A. (2002). Involvement of inflammatory cytokines in central nervous system injury. *Prog Neurobiol, 67,* 161–172.

225. Ward, J., et al. (1985). Failure of prophylactic barbiturate coma in the treatment of severe head injury. *J Neurosurg, 62,* 383–388.

226. Wilson, J. X., & Gelb, A. W. (2002). Free radicals, antioxidants, and neurologic injury: possible relationship to cerebral protection by anesthetics. *J Neurosurg Anesthesiol, 14*(1), 66–79.

227. Wray, N. P., & Nicotra, M. B. (1978). Pathogenesis of neurogenic pulmonary oedema. *Am Rev Respir Dis, 118,* 783–786.

228. www.braintrauma.org

229. www.Globalrph.com

230. Yano, M., et al. (1986). Effect of lidocaine on the ICP response to endotracheal suctioning. *Anesthesiology, 64,* 651–653.

231. Yoshino, A., et al. (1991). Dynamic changes in local cerebral glucose utilization following cerebral concussion in rats: evidence of a hyper- and subsequent hypo-metabolic state. *Brain Res, 561,* 106–119.

232. Yucel, E. K., et al. (1999). Magnetic resonance angiography, update on applications for extracranial arteries. *Circulation, 100,* 2284–2301.

233. Zafonte, R. D., & Mann, N. R. (1997). Cerebral salt wasting syndrome in brain injury patients: a potential cause of hyponatremia. *Arch Phys Med Rehabil, 78,* 540–542.

234. Zauner, A., & Muizelaar, J. P. (1997). Brain metabolism and cerebral blood flow. In P. Reilly & R. Bullock (Eds.), *Head injury: pathophysiology and management of severe closed injury.* London: Chapman & Hall.

235. Zenati, M. S., et al. (2002). A brief episode of hypotension increases mortality in critically ill trauma patients. *J Trauma, 53,* 232–237.

CHAPTER 23 Cerebrovascular Disorders

Patricia Ann Blissitt

Stroke is a neurologic emergency requiring prompt recognition and timely implementation of effective interventions for the best possible outcome.[178,325] While stroke has long been recognized as the third leading cause of death and the first leading cause of disability in the United States (with similar statistics worldwide), failure to respond to the concept that "time is brain" in an efficient and effective manner is all too common, even in an acute care setting.[8,144] Stroke is defined by both the National Institute of Neurologic Disorders and Stroke (NINDS) and the World Health Organization (WHO) as loss of brain function related to inadequate cerebrovascular blood flow for a duration of at least 24 hours.[85,322] A stroke occurs every 45 seconds in the United States, and up to 15% of all strokes may occur in the inpatient setting.[8,28] Critical care patients are particularly vulnerable to stroke, frequently having predisposing conditions such as hemodynamic instability, cardiac disease, and coagulopathy. The critically ill also undergo interventions that result in vascular injury, embolism, hypotension or hypertension, and prothrombotic or anticoagulated states.[28] Stroke may be the presenting and primary diagnosis, secondary to another illness or injury, or related to a much needed intervention for another disease or condition.[28]

In the past 15 years, interest in stroke care and research has flourished. New technologies, pharmacologic agents, and procedures have been developed or adapted for stroke intervention. The American Heart Association became the American Heart Association/American Stroke Association (AHA/ASA). In recognition of the need for excellence in stroke care, The Joint Commission (TJC), formerly known as the Joint Commission on the Accreditation of Healthcare Organizations, developed a certification program for primary stroke centers in collaboration with the Brain Attack Coalition and the ASA.[4,218] While some strokes may be inevitable, the critical care nurse working in a collaborative manner with the multidisciplinary team is key in minimizing secondary injury and maximizing resources available to lessen death and disability.

PATIENTS AT RISK

In 2006 the Stroke Council of the AHA/ASA updated previous evidence-based consensus statements regarding risk factors.[112,267] The task force categorized stroke risk factors into one of three categories: nonmodifiable; modifiable and well documented; and potentially modifiable or less well documented.[112,267] Risk factors identified as nonmodifiable are age, sex, birth weight, race/ethnicity, and genetics.[8,112,127,267] In regard to age, stroke risk doubles every 10 years after 55 years.[112,267] Overall, stroke is more common in men, although certain subtypes, such as aneurysmal subarachnoid hemorrhage, are more common among women.[8,112,127,266] Birth weight, a new risk factor, refers to stroke in adults, not perinatal stroke. Low birth weight as a nonmodifiable risk factor is based on both European and North American studies. The risk of stroke doubles for individuals who weighed less than 2500 g (5.5 lb) at birth compared to those who weighed more than 4000 g (8.8 lb) at birth.[112] The relationship of birth weight to stroke is not clear.[112] African Americans, Hispanic Americans, and Asians have a higher incidence of stroke than Caucasians, in part related to the prevalence of hypertension, diabetes, and obesity in these ethnicities.[112] Genetics not only contributes to stroke incidence in regard to one's familial predisposition to hypertension, diabetes, and hyperlipidemia, but also is related to inherited coagulopathies and vascular disease.[210,216] Two apolipoprotein E alleles, E2 and E4, have been associated with stroke, in regard not only to incidence but also to sequelae and outcome.*

The modifiable and well-documented risk factors include hypertension, smoking, diabetes, atrial fibrillation and other cardiac conditions, dyslipidemia, high-grade carotid artery stenosis (defined as greater than 70% and less than 100%), sickle cell disease, postmenopausal hormone therapy with estrogen, a diet high in fat and lacking in fruits and vegetables, physical inactivity, and obesity with abdominal fat. Hypertension and diabetes increase the risk of stroke related to

---

*References 6, 37, 173, 216, 221, 323.

angiopathy.[189,203] Atrial fibrillation increases the risk of an acute ischemic stroke (AIS) fivefold.[95,112,189] Dyslipidemia refers to increased levels of total cholesterol, total triglycerides, and low-density lipoprotein (LDL) cholesterol, and decreased levels of high-density lipoprotein (HDL) cholesterol. In men, low HDL is a risk factor for ischemic stroke.[112] However, the associated risk for women and older adults needs additional clarification.[112]

Individuals who have transient ischemic attacks (TIAs), previous stroke, and symptomatic carotid or intracranial disease are also at increased risk for stroke.[40,111,112,139,267] TIAs are defined as focal neurologic deficits related to inadequate cerebral blood flow that lasts less than 24 hours and generally less than 10 minutes.[31,266,267] A revised definition of TIA under consideration at this time includes a focal neurologic deficit with a time limit of less than 1 hour, rather than 24 hours, without evidence of infarction.[267] The risk of stroke after a TIA may be as high as 10.5%, with the greatest incidence of stroke occurring during the first week after the TIA.[267]

The less well-documented or potentially modifiable risk factors designated by the AHA/ASA include metabolic syndrome, alcohol and drug abuse, use of oral contraceptives, sleep-disordered breathing, migraine headaches, hyperhomocysteinemia, elevated levels of lipoprotein and lipoprotein-associated phospholipase, hypercoagulability, inflammation, and infection.* A diagnosis of metabolic syndrome requires three or more of the following: obesity based on abdominal circumference of greater than 102 cm (40 inches) for men and 88 cm (35 inches) for women; hyperlipidemia defined as levels of triglycerides greater than 150 mg/dl and of HDL cholesterol less than 40 mg/dl; blood pressure (BP) equal to or greater than 130/85 mm Hg; and a fasting glucose level greater than 110 mg/dl.[112] Vascular headaches classified as migraines are associated with stroke only before age 60. The mechanism is not clear.[112]

Many individuals with sleep-disordered breathing, formerly known as sleep apnea, have established risk factors for stroke, including age, male gender, smoking, and alcohol consumption. However, sleep-disordered breathing may also increase the probability of stroke independent of these risk factors. Sleep-disordered breathing has been found to reduce cerebral blood flow, alter vascular tone and cerebral autoregulation, and contribute to systemic hypertension.[333,339]

A number of other systemic diseases/conditions increase stroke risk. While cardiac disease is a well-documented risk factor for stroke,[28,47,112,196] other diseases also increase risk, including hepatic and renal

disease and cancer.[41,168,261,262] Patients with hepatic disease, particularly end-stage liver disease, are at great risk for hemorrhagic stroke. Associated coagulopathies include impaired synthesis of clotting factors, excessive fibrinolysis, disseminated intravascular coagulation (DIC), thrombocytopenia, and platelet dysfunction.[168]

Ischemic stroke in patients with chronic renal failure is primarily the result of atherosclerosis, thromboembolic disease, or hypotension during dialysis.[41] Hyperhomocysteinemia, an independent risk factor for atherosclerosis, is estimated to be present in 85% to 100% of the patients with chronic renal failure.[41] High doses of folic acid and vitamin B may reduce homocysteine levels, but endothelial function is not improved in this patient population.[41] Hemorrhagic stroke in patients with chronic renal failure is multifactorial, including the following: impaired platelet dysfunction and platelet-vessel wall interaction associated with uremia; systemic hypertension; the use of anticoagulation during hemodialysis;[219] and a 10% increased risk of cerebrovascular anomalies in polycystic kidney disease compared to the general population.[41]

Stroke in oncology patients may be the result of a coagulopathy induced by the cancer, cerebral metastasis, or therapy. Coagulopathic mechanisms resulting in ischemic stroke include nonbacterial thrombotic endocarditis, intravascular coagulation, and cerebral venous thrombosis (CVT).[261,262] Coagulopathic mechanisms resulting in hemorrhagic stroke include DIC, thrombocytopenia, and microangiopathic hemolytic anemia. Radiation may cause carotid atherosclerosis and cerebral vasculopathy, and chemotherapy may result in arterial or venous sinus thrombosis or hemorrhage.[261,262]

Stroke Across the Life Continuum

Although increasing age is a well-documented risk factor in stroke,[70,112,127] stroke also occurs during pregnancy and childhood.[48,282] A number of alterations in maternal physiology contribute to stroke in pregnancy. Pregnancy is, in many respects, a hypercoagulable state as a result of platelet hyperaggregability and decreased fibrinolysis; increased clotting factors V, VII, VIII, IX, X, and XII and fibrinogen; decreased levels of proteins C and S and antithrombin III during the last trimester; and increased resistance to protein C.[282] This hypercoagulability continues 2 to 3 weeks after childbirth. However, subarachnoid hemorrhage (SAH) and intracerebral hemorrhage (ICH) can occur as well as AIS. Hypertension associated with eclampsia is present in up to 47% of all AIS cases and 44% of all ICH cases during pregnancy.[282] Other pregnancy-related causes of ischemic stroke include choriocarcinoma, amniotic fluid embolism, and peripartum cardiomyopathy. Most aneurysmal SAH occurs during the third trimester.[282]

---

*References 70, 107, 112, 139, 179, 181, 294.

Fortunately, stroke in the pediatric population is rare. The first 30 days of life and even up to the first year have a disproportionate incidence of both ischemic and hemorrhagic stroke, compared to ages 1 to 14 years.[7,48] Unlike adults, risk factors for stroke, including diabetes, hyperlipidemia, and cardiovascular disease, are not common in the pediatric population. However, the increasing trend of childhood obesity in the United States may result in these risk factors beginning at a much younger age.[7] Congenital heart disease and sickle cell anemia are the most common etiologies of pediatric stroke.[7,48] Other etiologies of pediatric stroke include hematologic disorders such as leukemia and polycythemia; prothrombotic states related to decreased levels of protein C, protein S, or antithrombin III, or the presence of antiphospholipid antibodies; arteriovenous malformations (AVMs), aneurysms, CVT, patent foramen ovale (PFO), moyamoya disease, and other intracranial vascular anomalies; metabolic syndromes such as hyperhomocysteinemia; migraine and substance abuse–related vasospasm; and trauma.[48] Unlike adults, the ratio of ischemic stroke to hemorrhagic stroke is approximately equal, and long-term outcome in ischemic and hemorrhagic pediatric stroke survivors is the same.[48]

PREVENTION

Stroke is not entirely preventable. However, concerted efforts to lessen modifiable risk factors decrease one's stroke risk.[127] Hypertension has been associated with ischemic and hemorrhagic stroke.* Strong evidence exists that smoking may contribute to 50% of all strokes, and smoking cessation is strongly encouraged.[169] Glycemic control in diabetes, particularly in conjunction with a reduction in BP, has been well substantiated as an effective measure in reducing stroke risk.[189,203] Statins are also recommended for patients with abnormally high levels of LDL and total cholesterol, and for patients with diabetes, especially after ischemic stroke or TIA.[9,111] Though not well substantiated, a diet high in folate and vitamin B_{12}, or supplementation with these vitamins, may provide some protection against hyperhomocysteinemia-related stroke.[112,179] Patients with prothrombotic and cardioembolic conditions may require antiplatelet agents or anticoagulation for primary and secondary stroke prevention. However, these agents may also increase the risk of intracranial hemorrhage.[248,276,279]

Some neurologic and cardiovascular conditions such as valvular disease and high-grade carotid stenosis are amenable to surgery or endovascular surgery, and correction of these abnormalities may provide greater

---

*References 18, 79, 88, 140, 180, 190, 191, 260.

Box 23-1

American Heart Association/American Stroke Association Levels of Evidence and Recommendations

The AHA/ASA has established levels of evidence and recommendation grades for their clinical practice guidelines regarding management of patients with AIS, SAH, and ICH.

Five levels of evidence exist, with I being the highest and V being the lowest.

- Level I evidence constitutes data from randomized trials with low false-positive and low false-negative errors. Grade A recommendations are based on Level I evidence.
- Level II evidence is data from randomized trials with high false-positive or high false-negative errors. Grade B recommendations are supported by Level II evidence.
- Level III evidence is obtained from nonrandomized concurrent cohort studies.
- Level IV evidence is from nonrandomized cohort studies using historical controls.
- Level V is data from anecdotal case series.

Grade C recommendations are based on Levels III, IV, and V evidence.

From references 1, 2, 36, 198, 267.
AHA/ASA = American Heart Association/American Stroke Association, AIS = acute ischemic stroke, ICH = intracerebral hemorrhage, SAH = subarachnoid hemorrhage.

---

benefit than risk to the patient in regard to stroke prevention.[2,112,267] Indications for carotid endarterectomy have been well defined by a number of multicenter prospective randomized controlled trials. Carotid endarterectomy is recommended for high-grade, 70% to 99% asymptomatic carotid stenosis (Box 23-1).[112]

Carotid endarterectomy is also recommended for patients with recent TIAs or ischemic stroke and moderate to severe, 50% to 99%, carotid artery stenosis (Level I evidence).[267] However, the patient's comorbidities and life expectancy and the surgeon's mortality and morbidity rates must be taken into consideration.[112,267]

DEFINITION

Stroke is a heterogeneous disease. The two major subtypes are ischemic and hemorrhagic. Hemorrhagic stroke refers to SAH and ICH. Approximately 85% to 88% of all strokes are ischemic. Approximately 9% to 10% of strokes are the result of ICH, with SAH contributing another 3% to 7%.[7,117] Each subtype has a number of mechanisms (Figure 23-1).

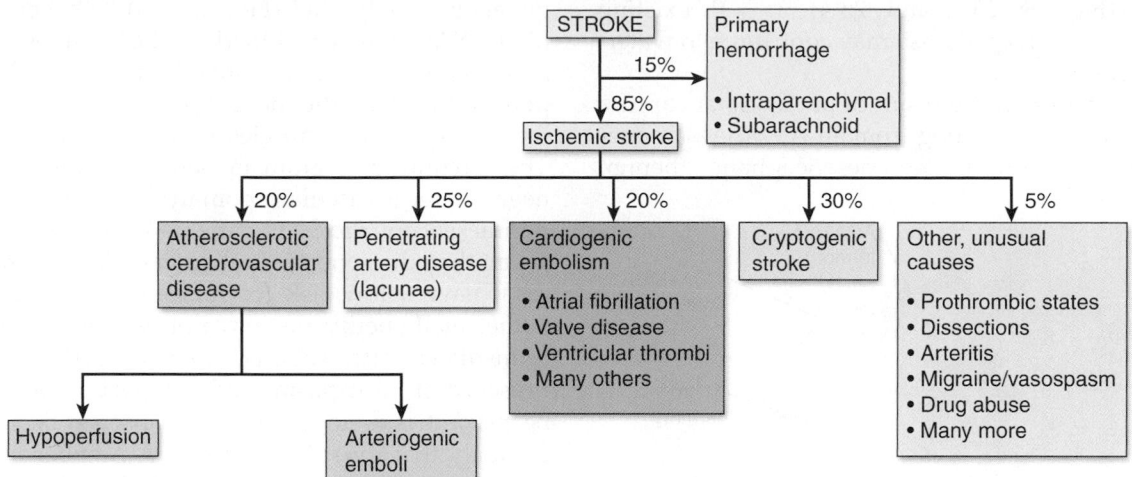

FIGURE 23-1 Classification of stroke by mechanism with frequency estimates.

Ischemic stroke may occur as a result of athero-thrombotic events, including large-vessel stenosis; artery-to-artery plaque embolization with occlusion of smaller vessels distal to the original site of plaque formation; and small-vessel disease in deep penetrating arteries supplying the basal ganglia, cerebral white matter, thalamus, and pons.*

Risk factors for small-vessel ischemic stroke, also referred to as lacunar infarct or stroke, are hypertension and diabetes.[47,304] Without known trauma, the carotid or vertebral arteries may dissect and shower emboli distal to the dissection.[326] In CVT, one or more of the cerebral veins or sinuses occlude, resulting in cerebral edema, impaired cerebrospinal fluid (CSF) absorption, and hemorrhagic or nonhemorrhagic infarcts.[291,292] Cardiac-related stroke refers to cardio-embolic atrial fibrillation, valvular disease or mechanical valve thrombogenesis, and paradoxical emboli associated with PFO (Figure 23-2).† Approximately 30% of all strokes are ischemic strokes of undetermined etiology, or cryptogenic. However, every attempt should be made to determine the etiology of a stroke before declaring it cryptogenic.[47,104,111]

Cardiac or respiratory arrest and generalized hypotensive states may result in a more global ischemia. Patients with systemic hypotension are at risk for watershed infarctions. Watershed infarction is the term used to describe a subtype of ischemic stroke in non-anastomosing/terminal arterial border zone areas between major vessels of the circle of Willis. Normally, blood flow to the most distal branches of the circle of Willis is under a lower amount of arterial pressure than that to the more proximal branches. During hypotensive states, the cerebral perfusion pressure and

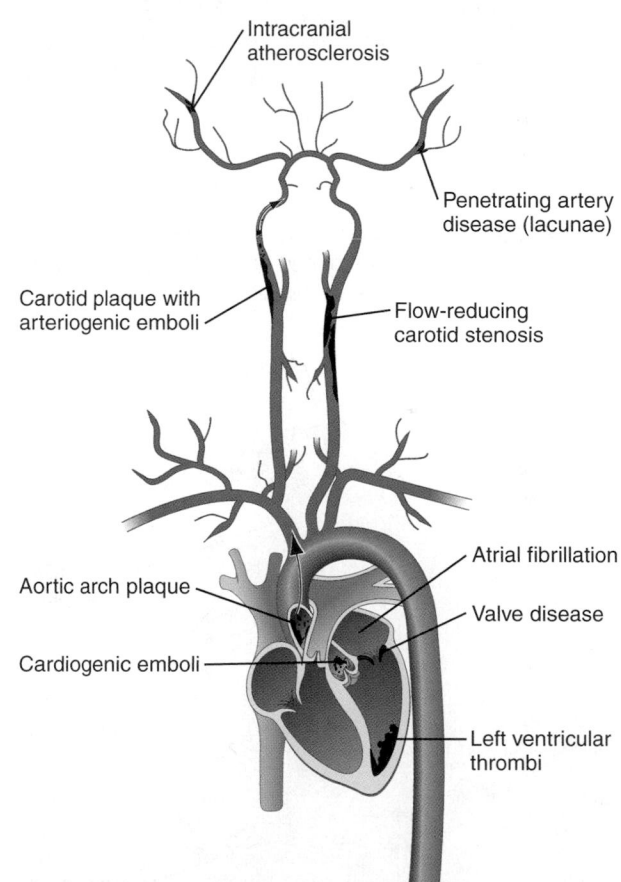

FIGURE 23-2 Common sites of arterial and cardiac lesions causing ischemic stroke.

collateral blood flow to these areas may be inadequate, resulting in infarction.[30,215] The junction of the distal branches of the middle cerebral artery (MCA) and the anterior cerebral artery (ACA) and the junction of the distal branches of the MCA and the posterior cerebral artery (PCA) are two areas prone to watershed

*References 47, 85, 204, 236, 242, 304, 322.
†References 47, 68, 112, 127, 156, 196, 234.

infarction (Figures 23-3 and 23-4).[30,215] Preexisting internal carotid artery disease may contribute to watershed infarction.[215]

SAH is most often the result of aneurysmal rupture or, less commonly, bleeding from an AVM. An innocuous form of SAH is perimesencephalic (benign nonaneurysmal) SAH (Figure 23-5).[97,313] Perimesencephalic SAH refers to blood in the perimesencephalic and prepontine cisterns, anterior to the midbrain and pons, rather than the more typical location of aneurysmal SAH in the ventricles or lateral sylvian fissures. The cerebral angiogram in perimesencephalic SAH is negative for a vascular anomaly.[97,313] Up to 95% of all perimesencephalic SAH patients have a second angiogram that does not reveal a vascular anomaly, and most have a low risk for rebleed or vasospasm.[97,313] Some small aneurysms may not be seen on angiogram immediately after subarachnoid hemorrhage or in the presence of vasospasm, and a repeat angiogram may be needed later to confirm the absence of a vascular anomaly that must be repaired. A number of connective tissue diseases are associated with aneurysms, including polycystic kidney disease, Marfan syndrome, and Ehlers-Danlos syndrome.[18,190]

ICH is most often associated with systemic hypertension or cerebral amyloid angiopathy. Cerebral amyloid angiopathy is associated with lobar, cortical, or subcortical ICH, whereas hypertensive ICH typically occurs in deep structures such as the basal ganglia and thalamus (Figure 23-6).[87,279]

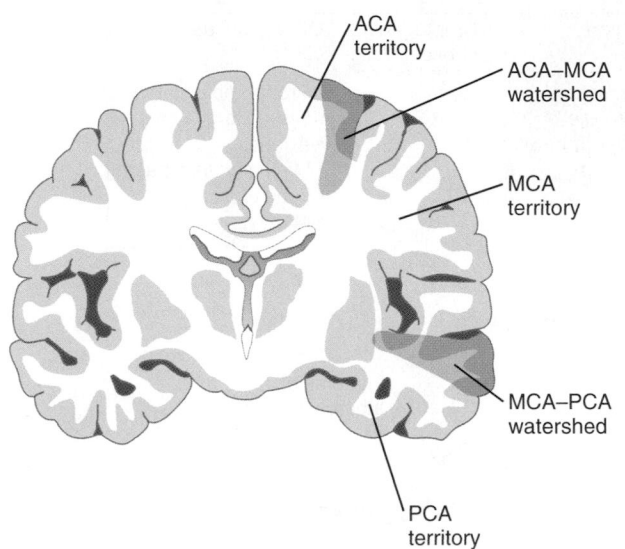

♦FIGURE 23-3 Watershed zone for the major arteries: coronal section. ACA = Anterior cerebral artery, MCA = middle cerebral artery, PCA = posterior cerebral artery.

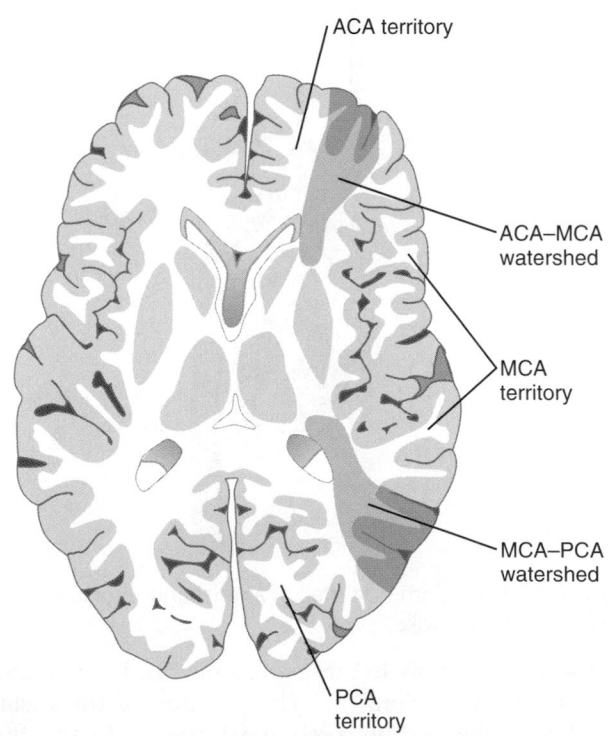

♦FIGURE 23-4 Watershed zone for the major arteries: axial section. ACA = Anterior cerebral artery, MCA = middle cerebral artery, PCA = posterior cerebral artery.

PATHOPHYSIOLOGY

All subtypes present according to anatomic and clinical correlation (Tables 23-1 and 23-2; Figure 23-7).[31,280] In addition, large artery or posterior fossa infarcts and infarcts with hemorrhagic transformation in AIS, SAH, and ICH may present with additional signs and symptoms related to increased intracranial pressure (ICP) from edema, mass effect, or hydrocephalus. The clinical presentation of stroke is also impacted by the biochemical events of the ischemic cascade, impaired autoregulation, or uncoupling of the cerebral blood flow (CBF) and cerebral metabolism. Autoregulation, the ability of the cerebral blood vessels to dilate and constrict as needed to maintain adequate cerebral perfusion, is only operational at a mean arterial BP of approximately 50 to 150 mm Hg and may be impaired in chronic hypertension.[240,263] Autoregulation is also impaired to varying degrees as a result of stroke. With impaired autoregulation, the CBF passively follows the systemic BP, resulting in ischemia or hyperemia. Both may cause increased ICP. In chronic hypertension, the BP necessary to adequately perfuse the brain is shifted to the right, requiring a higher-than-normal BP (Figure 23-8).[241,245,263,293]

Ischemic Stroke

Glucose is the brain's only energy substrate. As a result, the brain depends on a constant supply of glucose

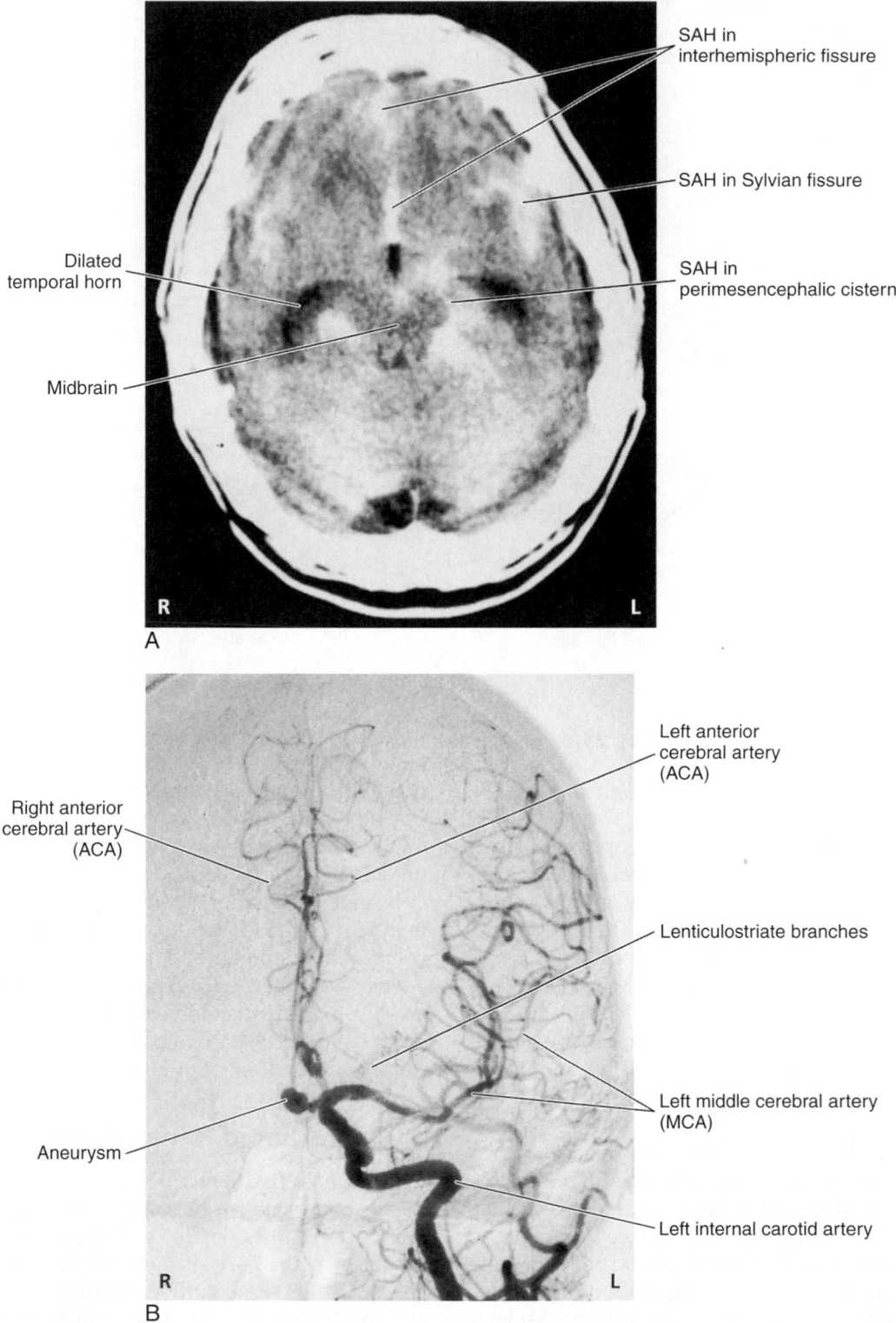

SAH in interhemispheric fissure

SAH in Sylvian fissure

Dilated temporal horn

SAH in perimesencephalic cistern

Midbrain

R   L

A

Right anterior cerebral artery (ACA)

Left anterior cerebral artery (ACA)

Lenticulostriate branches

Left middle cerebral artery (MCA)

Aneurysm

Left internal carotid artery

R   L

B

⬍**FIGURE 23-5**   Aneurysmal subarachnoid hemorrhage (SAH). **A,** CT axial image showing subarachnoid blood and hydrocephalus. **B,** Angiogram, anteroposterior view.

and oxygen for aerobic metabolism. When a blood vessel is occluded, oxygen and glucose delivery to the area of the brain perfused by that vessel is critically decreased or stopped altogether.[115,170]

The events that follow, referred to as the ischemic cascade, begin with the depletion of adenosine triphosphate (ATP), membrane depolarization, and the release of extracellular potassium. These processes are followed

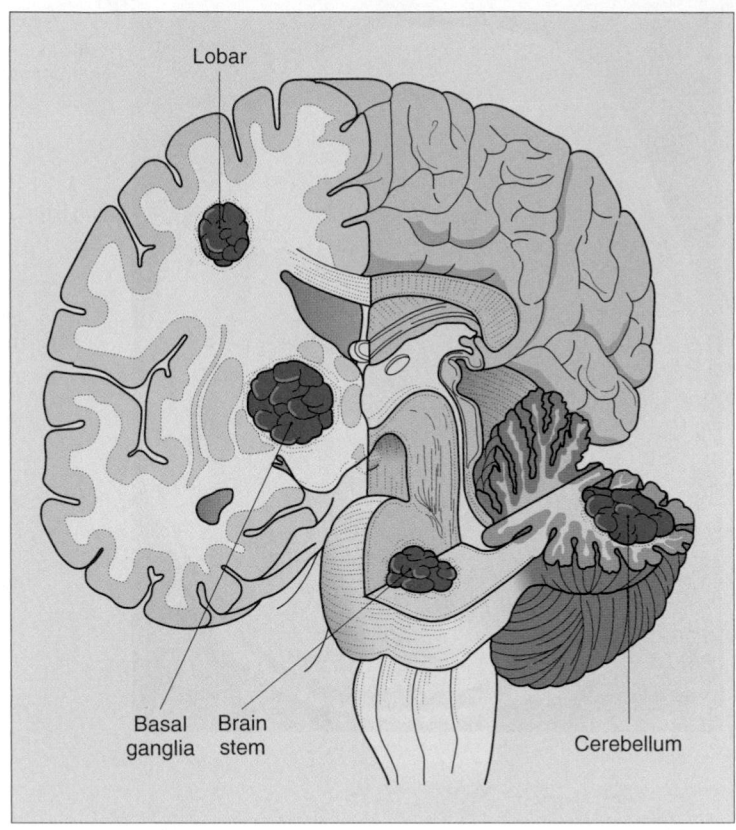

Lobar

Basal
ganglia

Brain
stem

Cerebellum

♦FIGURE 23-6 Locations of intracerebral hemorrhage.

by an increase in oxygen extraction and glucose metabolism with the formation of lactic acid. Depolarization of neuronal membranes results in the opening of calcium channels and an influx of intracellular calcium. In addition, the release of toxic excitatory neurotransmitters, such as glutamate, activates N-methyl-D-aspartate (NMDA) receptors to increase the neuron's sodium permeability and cellular swelling. NMDA receptors mediate additional movement of calcium into the cells. Glutamate-activated alpha-amino-3-hydroxy-5-methyl-4-isoxazolepropionic acid (AMPA) and metabotropic receptors also participate in the influx of calcium.[115,170]

Calcium activates enzymes such as lipases to produce arachidonic acid and free radicals, and stimulates neuronal nitric oxide synthase (nNOS) to increase nitric oxide production. Nitric oxide is a free radical. The production of free radicals and enzymatic perturbations result in lipid peroxidation with disruption of the neuronal and endothelial membrane, loss of cytoskeletal integrity, and mitochondrial damage resulting in cell death (Figure 23-9).[115,170]

The core tissue, the area immediately around the blood vessel, infarcts and is no longer salvageable. However, tissue just outside the core area, referred to as the ischemic penumbra, is injured but potentially viable. The ischemic penumbra can be restored to normal function if reperfused within an adequate time.[64,120,194] Over the next 4 to 5 days, cerebral edema will increase in the injured and especially the infarcted area (Figure 23-10).[170] In AIS, this may result in some ICP; however, unless the infarct involves the cerebellum or more than 50% of the MCA, the increased ICP will not likely result in herniation.[51,295] The mass effect and additional edema associated with hemorrhagic transformation of an AIS may further increase ICP and risk of herniation.[15,117] Infarcts, particularly in the cerebellum or brain stem, may result in respiratory impairment.[15,51,117]

Subarachnoid Hemorrhage

SAH most frequently occurs as a result of an intracranial aneurysm rupture. Intracranial aneurysms most often occur on the circle of Willis or its major arterial branches at the base of the brain in the subarachnoid space. The greatest number of intracranial aneurysms are located at the anterior communicating cerebral artery, followed by the posterior communicating and the middle cerebral arteries.[190,225,330] As a result of the aneurysm's rupture, blood is forced into the subarachnoid space and basal cisterns, mixing with CSF. The blood may form thick layers or clots intraventricularly but also may extend intraparenchymally and subdurally.[163,313,315,330]

TABLE 23-1 Arterial Supply to the Brain

ARTERY	TERRITORY SUPPLIED BY ARTERY
ANTERIOR CIRCULATION (AND BRANCHES)	
Internal Carotid Artery (ICA)	
Anterior choroidal	Optic tract, choroid plexus, internal capsule, basal ganglia, hippocampus, cerebral peduncle
Ophthalmic artery	Eye orbits and optic nerves
Middle Cerebral Artery (MCA)	
M1	Sylvian fissure
Lenticulostriate	Basal ganglia, internal capsule
M2	Cerebral cortex in lateral sulcus (insula)
M3	Cerebral cortex above and below the lateral sulcus (opercula)
M4	Lateral cortical surface of brain (except occipital pole), precentral (motor) gyrus supplying arm and face, postcentral (sensory) gyrus supplying arm and face
Anterior Cerebral Artery (ACA)	
A1	Junction of anterior communicating artery (AComA)
A2	
A1 and A2	Corpus callosum
Recurrent artery of Huebner	Medial surfaces of frontal and parietal lobes, cingulate gyrus and precentral (motor) gyrus supplying leg, postcentral (sensory) gyrus supplying leg
	Basal ganglia and internal capsule
Anterior communicating artery (AComA)	Connects two anterior cerebral arteries
Posterior communicating artery (PComA)	Connects carotid (anterior) circulation with vertebrobasilar (posterior) circulation
POSTERIOR CIRCULATION	
Vertebral Artery (VA)	
Posteroinferior cerebellar artery (PICA)	Undersurface of cerebellum, medulla, and choroid plexus of fourth ventricle
Anterior and posterior spinal arteries	Anterior two thirds and posterior one third of spinal cord
Basilar Artery (BA)	
Posterior cerebral artery (PCA)	Thalamus, hypothalamus, medial and inferior surface of temporal lobes, occipital lobes, midbrain, choroid plexuses of third and fourth ventricles
Choroidal artery	Tectum, choroid plexus of third ventricle, medial/superior thalamus
Superior cerebellar artery (SCA)	Undersurface of cerebellum and midbrain
Anterior inferior cerebellar artery (AICA)	Undersurface of cerebellum and lateral pons

From references 31, 281.

TABLE 23-2 Anatomic and Clinical Correlation: Circle of Willis

CEREBRAL VESSEL/AREA	CLINICAL PRESENTATION
I. Anterior Circulation (frontal lobe, temporal lobes, parietal lobes, occipital lobe)	
Internal carotid artery (ICA)	Contralateral arm and leg weakness/paralysis and sensory loss; contralateral homonymous hemianopsia; expressive and receptive aphasia/dysphasia
Anterior cerebral artery (ACA)	Contralateral leg weakness/paralysis and sensory loss (leg worse than arm); frontal lobe behavioral abnormalities; contralateral hemineglect if lesion on nondominant side
Middle cerebral artery (MCA)	Contralateral arm weakness/paralysis and sensory loss (arm worse than leg); frontal lobe behavioral abnormalities; contralateral homonymous hemianopsia; contralateral lower facial motor and sensory loss; expressive/receptive dysphasia if dominant side
II. Posterior Circulation (occipital lobe, cerebellum, and brain stem)	
Posterior cerebral artery (PCA)	Contralateral hemiplegia and sensory loss; homonymous hemianopsia
Vertebral basilar (VB) arteries	Hemiplegia, ipsilateral facial weakness/numbness; dysarthria, dysphagia, vertigo, nausea, dizziness, ataxic gait, locked-in syndrome
Posterior inferior cerebellar artery (PICA)	Wallenberg syndrome: ataxia, vertigo, nausea and vomiting; contralateral body pain and temperature loss; ipsilateral facial pain and temperature loss; nystagmus, dysarthria, dysphagia, dysphonia, Horner syndrome
Cerebellum	Ataxia, dysarthria, disconjugate gaze, nystagmus
Brain stem	Quadriplegia and sensory loss; ataxia, dysarthria, disconjugate gaze, nystagmus
III. Lacunar Syndromes	Pure motor or pure sensory deficits limited to one side of body only

From references 30, 47, 243, 281.

Severe headache, classically described as "the worst headache of my life," seizures, loss of consciousness, or herniation may occur at the time of the rupture. Patients with chronic headaches such as migraines may describe a change in the character of the headache. The pathogenesis of aneurysm is not completely known.[18,81,190,330] Although aneurysms are congenital, their growth and rupture are thought to be influenced by such conditions as hypertension and smoking. They are frequently found at the bifurcation of the vessel, and 20% to 30% of individuals with an aneurysm have more than one (Figure 23-11).[80,147] An area of infarcted tissue may occur at the site of the rupture.[18,81,190,315] The patient is at risk for rebleeding if the vessel is not repaired, with the greatest risk of rebleeding within the first 24 hours.[223] In addition, the extravascular blood and blood clots in the subarachnoid space and ventricles frequently result in hydrocephalus and increased ICP. Hydrocephalus occurs as a result of the blood in the CSF impairing

reabsorption of the CSF. The hydrocephalus may resolve over the first couple of weeks after the SAH, or the patient may require a shunt.[109] After 3 days, cerebral vasospasm may occur and continue for up to 3 or 4 weeks.[190,330]

Cerebral vasospasm is sustained constriction of the blood vessel related to the biochemical and histologic changes induced by extravascular blood and may occur at multiple sites simultaneously, at the site of the rupture, but also on the contralateral side. Vasospasm may be present radiographically, clinically, or both. Approximately 70% of all aneurysmal patients have cerebral vasospasm, but only 20% to 30% are symptomatic.[190,330] Clinical cerebral vasospasm is also referred to as delayed ischemic neurologic deficit (DIND).[3,81,140,184] Vasospasm, if allowed to progress, may result in secondary infarct, permanent deficits, and increased mortality and morbidity.[17] The pathogenesis of vasospasm is not entirely known but is thought to be related to the sustained extraluminal

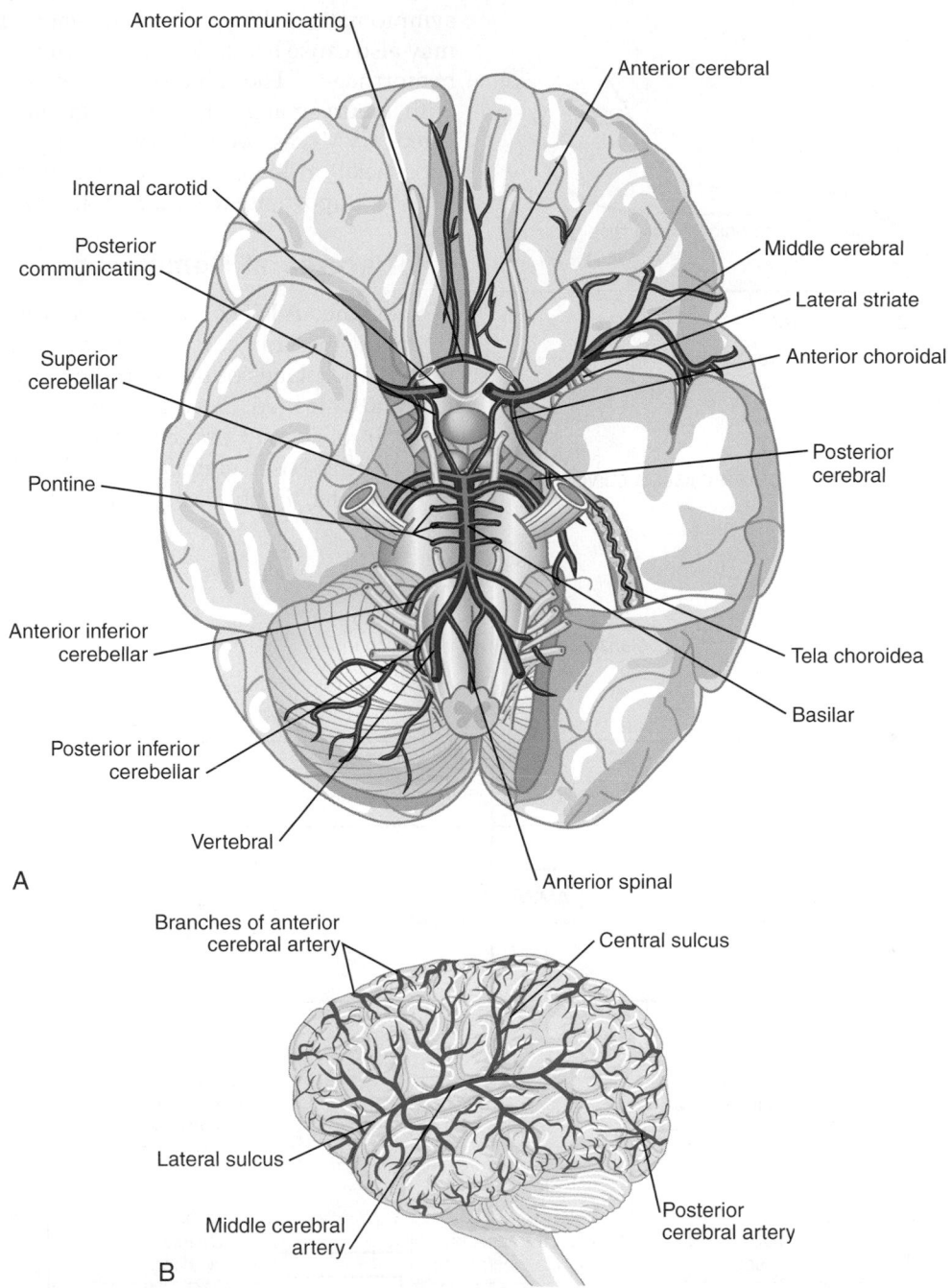

FIGURE 23-7 Cerebral circulation **A,** Cerebral arterial circulation at the base of the brain. **B,** Blood vessel distribution on the lateral surface of the cerebral hemisphere.

exposure of subarachnoid blood. The blood and its constituents provoke an inflammatory response and morphologic changes in the vessels.[3,18,140] Following aneurysmal SAH, cerebral autoregulation is impaired, related to ischemic damage at the time of the hemorrhage, decreased CBF, increased ICP, vasospasm, and preexisting chronic hypertension in some patients.*

An AVM is an abnormal cluster of blood vessels that lack the normal capillary connection between arteries and veins necessary for tissue perfusion. The blood is said to be shunted and the area around the shunt, the core of the AVM, is referred to as the nidus.[56] Progressive neurologic deficits may occur as a result of the shunting. In addition, the arterial blood flowing to the venous side under arterial pressure may result in hemorrhage, especially SAH. Most AVMs become

*References 21, 76, 162, 164, 184, 190.

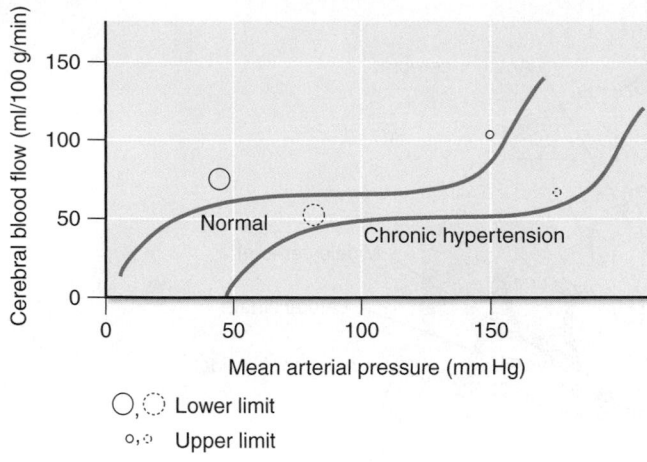

⬧FIGURE 23-8 Cerebral autoregulation curve.

symptomatic following hemorrhage. However, they may also cause headaches and seizures before and after hemorrhage.[56] Though thought to be less common than with aneurysmal SAH, vasospasm may occur with ruptured AVMs as well.[56] AVMs vary in size, may be superficial or deep, and may or may not involve functionally important structures of the brain.[56,140]

Intracerebral Hemorrhage

Spontaneous ICH occurs with bleeding into the parenchyma of the brain. As the bleeding occurs, additional vessels and planes of tissue in the surrounding area are torn and damaged. Bleeding may be lobar (cortical, subcortical), or it may occur in deeper cerebral structures such as the basal ganglia or thalamus, or it may be infratentorial, in the cerebellum or brain stem. Lobar

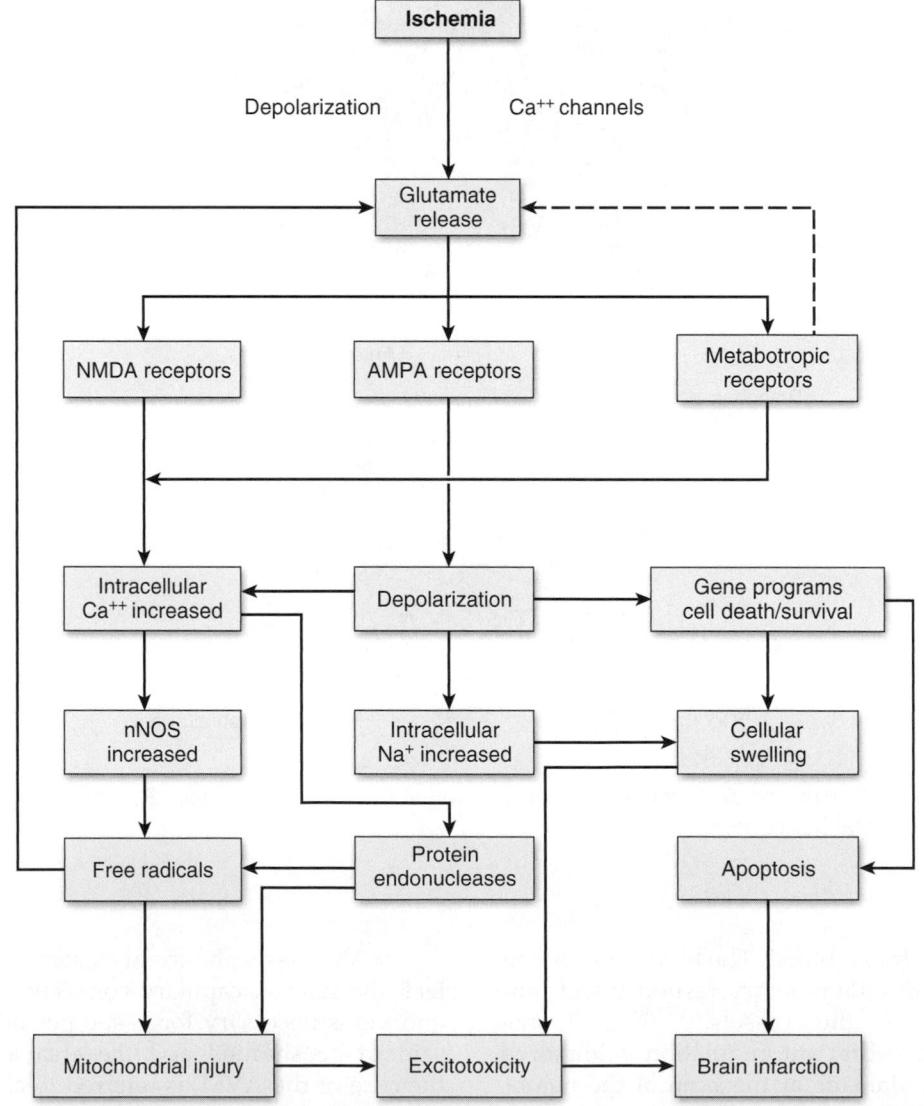

⬧FIGURE 23-9 Neurodegenerative cascade. AMPA = Alpha-amino-3-hydroxy-5-methyl-4-isoxazolepropionic acid, Ca^{++} = calcium, ICH = intracerebral hemorrhage, IPH = intraparenchymal hemorrhage, nNOS = neuronal nitric oxide synthase.

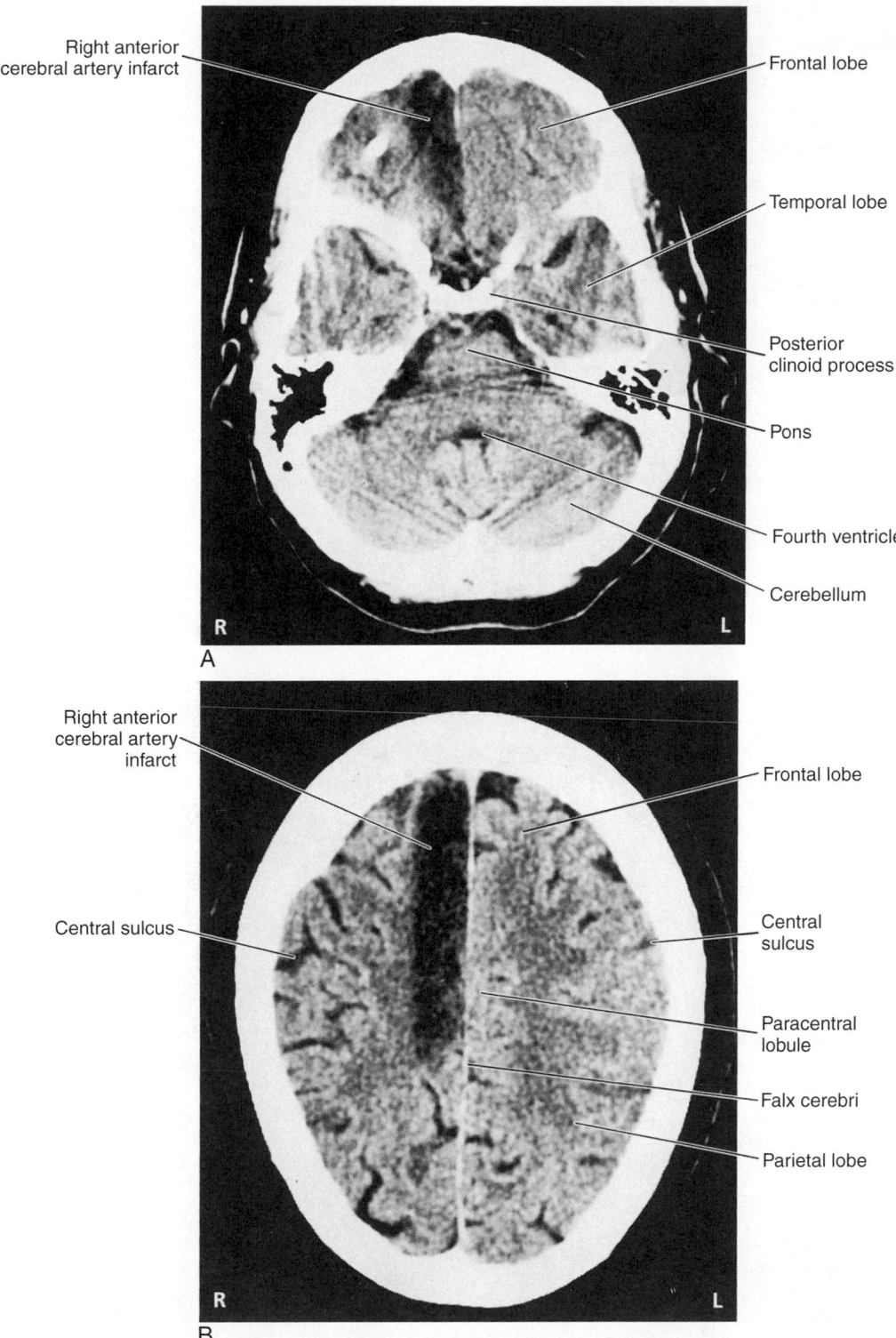

✦FIGURE 23-10 Right anterior cerebral artery infarction: axial CT images progressing from inferior **(A)** to superior **(B).**

bleeds are associated with cerebral amyloid angiopathy that increases with age.[87,117,140,186,279] The intracerebral blood may dissect through brain parenchyma and the walls of the ventricles, causing intraventricular extension (Figure 23-12). Intraventricular blood carries a poorer prognosis related to obstruction of CSF flow, distention of the ventricles, and compression of adjacent brain tissue, resulting in hydrocephalus and increased ICP.[92] Herniation sometimes occurs at the time of the bleed. Hydrocephalus and increased ICP are common.[92,140]

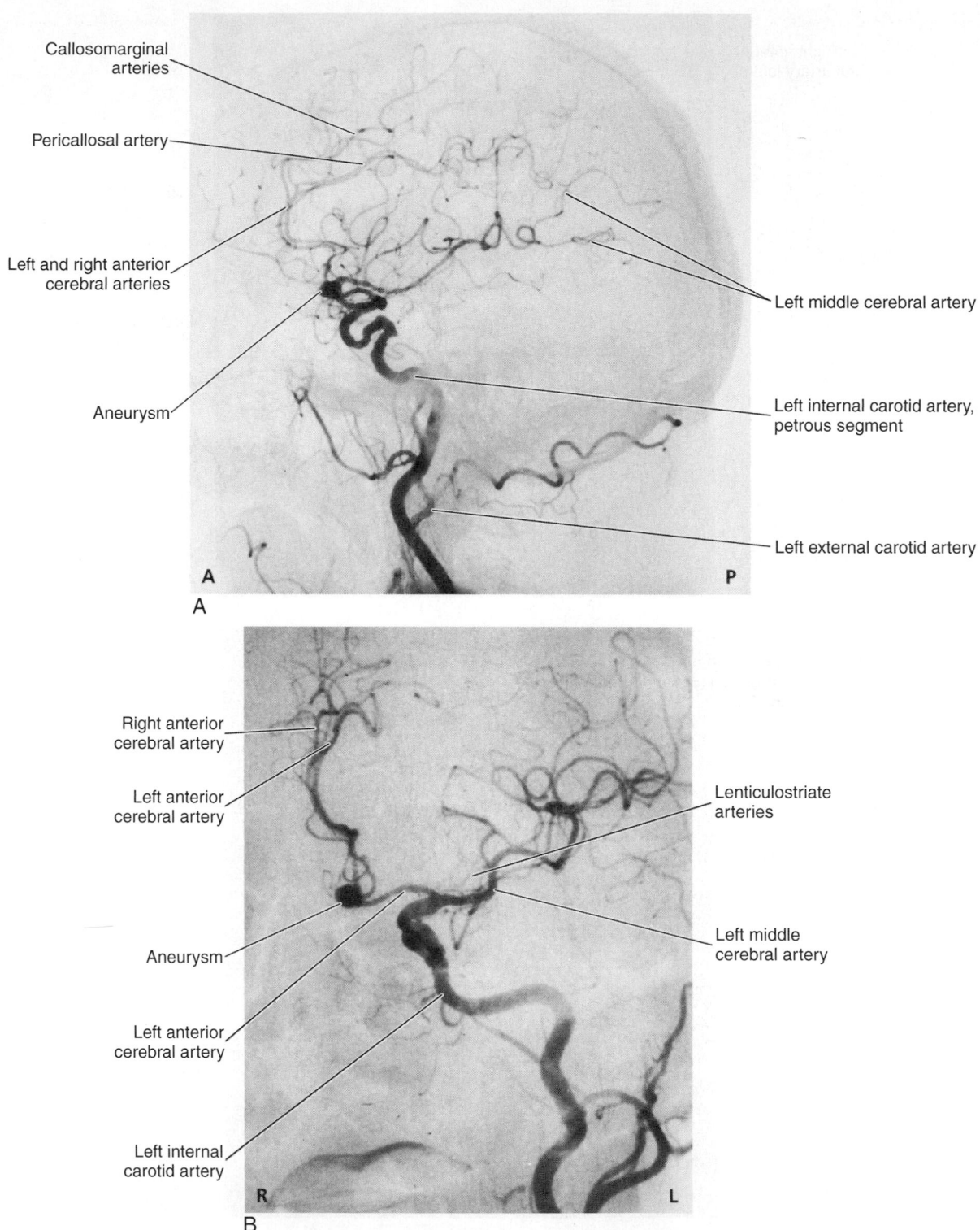

Callosomarginal
arteries

Pericallosal artery

Left and right anterior
cerebral arteries

Aneurysm

Left middle cerebral artery

Left internal carotid artery,
petrous segment

Left external carotid artery

A

A   P

Right anterior
cerebral artery

Left anterior
cerebral artery

Lenticulostriate
arteries

Left middle
cerebral artery

Aneurysm

Left anterior
cerebral artery

Left internal
carotid artery

B

R   L

♦FIGURE 23-11   Anterior cerebral artery aneurysm.

ICH is frequently the result of hypertension, and secondary enlargement of the hematoma may occur with continued uncontrolled hypertension.[39] The optimal systemic BP has yet to be established.[36,100,241,343] If the ICH is related to coagulopathy, the hematoma may continue to enlarge until the coagulopathy is reversed.* A potentially salvageable area of tissue may exist around the hemorrhage. However, whether the penumbra is ischemic or

_____

*References 11, 84, 117, 140, 230, 279.

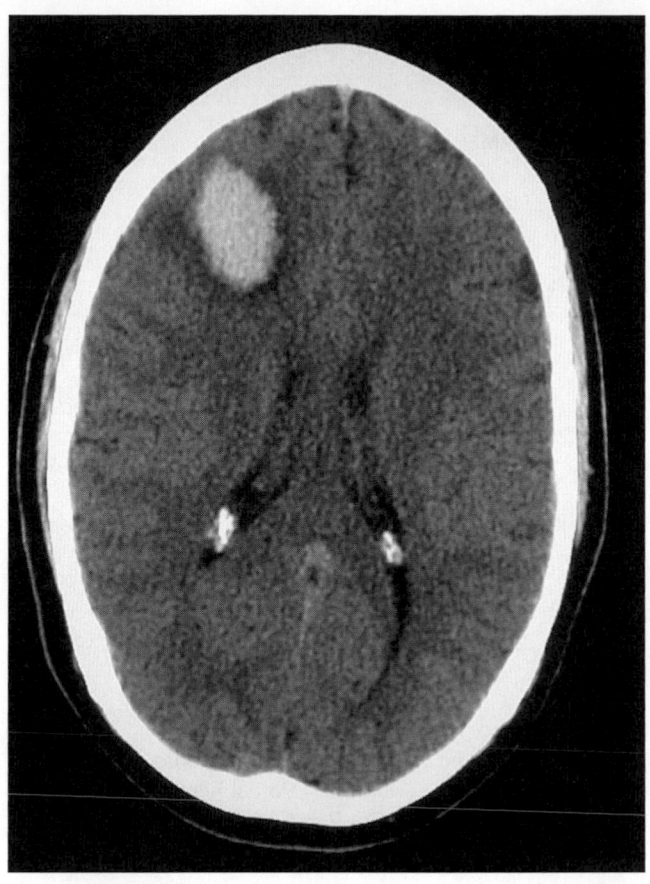

⬦FIGURE 23-12 Intracerebral hemorrhage.

altered as a result of biochemical changes—such as disruption of the blood-brain barrier, activation of the complement system, and the release of hemoglobin, oxyhemoglobin, or free radicals—is controversial.[241,319,338] Autoregulation is impaired, and attempts at normalization of the BP may result in secondary injury.[118,241,319,338]

ASSESSMENT

While the definitive diagnosis will be made by a neurodiagnostic study, a bedside assessment with attention to the cardiopulmonary status; airway, breathing, and circulation (ABCs); and neurologic deficits (D) is imperative for the stroke patient. The components of a thorough neurologic exam include level of consciousness, mental status, language and speech, cranial nerves, movement and strength of extremities, sensation, and vital signs. A number of validated scoring tools are also applicable to the acute stroke patient, including the Glasgow Coma Scale (GCS), the National Institutes of Health Stroke Scale (NIHSS), Hunt and Hess SAH classification, World Federation of Neurological Surgeons (WFNS) SAH scale, Fisher SAH scale, Spetzler and Martin AVM Classification, and the Hemphill ICH score, in combination with the Kothari method of determining intracerebral hemorrhage volume on CT.*

The GCS is a level of consciousness assessment scale, originally developed as a research tool for the assessment of severe traumatic brain injury but later applied to nontraumatic injury as well.[94] Patients are scored based on stimuli required for eye opening, and their best verbal and motor responses to stimuli. GCS values range from 3 to 15; a high GCS score is associated with a better outcome. A GCS score of equal to or less than 8 is associated with severe neuronal injury (Table 23-3).[140]

The NIHSS was originally developed to screen and follow patients who receive recombinant tissue

---

*References 49, 53, 89, 117, 131, 140, 164, 172.

TABLE 23-3 Glasgow Coma Scale

RESPONSE	SCORE
Eye Opening	
Spontaneous	4
To sound	3
To pain	2
None	1
Motor Response	
Obeys commands	6
Localizes pain	5
Normal flexion (withdrawal)	4
Abnormal flexion	3
Extension	2
None	1
Verbal Response	
Oriented	5
Confused conversation	4
Inappropriate words	3
Incomprehensible sounds	2
None	1

From reference 297a.

plasminogen activator (rt-PA) for AIS but is also used for SAH and ICH.[101] An NIHSS score of greater than 16 is predictive of severe disability, and a score less than 6 is associated with good recovery.[340] Videos and online training and certification to ensure correct use of the NIHSS are available through the AHA/ASA (Table 23-4).

The Hunt and Hess classification scale, WFNS scale, and Fisher scale are specific to aneurysmal SAH. The Hunt-Hess classification is based on the initial assessment. Despite the patient's outcome, the Hunt-Hess classification does not change. The patient's clinical status is rated from 0 to V, with 0 (unruptured) to II being good grades and IV to V being considered poor grades (Table 23-5). The WFNS scale combines the GCS, Hunt-Hess classification, and the presence of any neurologic deficits. Similar to the Hunt-Hess classification, lower grades (0–I) are associated with better outcomes and grades IV to V have a worse prognosis (Table 23-6). [140] The Fisher scale is based on the amount of blood visualized by computed tomography (CT) scan. The Fisher score was developed to predict vasospasm based on the amount of SAH blood. A Fisher score of 3 is associated with the greatest risk of vasospasm. However, a Fisher score of 4, denoting intraventricular or intracerebral clot, is also associated with a poor outcome.[49,164] Fisher scores range from 1 (no blood) to 4 (clot) (Table 23-7).[140]

A guide to predict surgical risk, the Spetzler and Martin score is a 1 to 5 ranking based on angiogram size of the AVM, the pattern of venous drainage (e.g., deep or superficial), and the functional importance of the AVM. The larger the nidus, the deeper the venous drainage; and the greater the functional importance of the area supplied by the AVM, the higher the score and the greater the surgical risk.[140]

The ICH score ranges from 0 to 6 and combines the GCS with the ICH volume, the location of blood, and the age of the patient.[131] The lower the score, the better the predicted outcome.[131] None of these instruments is comprehensive, but each provides a standardized and validated format for assessing and communicating the stroke patient's condition and has been found to be helpful in predicting the patient's outcome.[49,140,172,340]

Laboratory Findings

The most basic laboratory workup of the stroke patient consists of serum chemistry, complete blood count, coagulation, and toxicology studies. Other tests may be indicated, depending on the patient's systemic disease, general condition, and potential etiologies, including arterial blood gas, creatine kinase-myocardial bands (CK-MB), troponin, cholesterol and triglycerides, fibrinogen, glycosylated hemoglobin (HbA_{1c}),

TABLE 23-4 National Institutes of Health Stroke Scale

ITEM	NAME	RESPONSE
1a	Loss of consciousness	0 = Alert 1 = Not alert, arousable 2 = Not alert, obtunded 3 = Unresponsive
1b	Questions	0 = Answers both correctly 1 = Answers one correctly 2 = Answers neither correctly
1c	Commands	0 = Performs both tasks correctly 1 = Performs one task correctly 2 = Performs neither task correctly
2	Gaze	0 = Normal 1 = Partial gaze palsy 2 = Total gaze palsy
3	Visual fields	0 = No visual loss 1 = Partial hemianopsia 2 = Complete hemianopsia 3 = Bilateral hemianopsia
4	Facial palsy	0 = Normal 1 = Minor paralysis 2 = Partial paralysis 3 = Complete paralysis
5a	Left motor arm	0 = No drift 1 = Drifts before 10 seconds 2 = Falls before 10 seconds 3 = No effort against gravity 4 = No movement
5b	Right motor arm	0 = No drift 1 = Drifts before 10 seconds 2 = Falls before 10 seconds 3 = No effort against gravity 4 = No movement
6a	Left motor leg	0 = No drift 1 = Drifts before 10 seconds 2 = Falls before 10 seconds 3 = No effort against gravity 4 = No movement
6b	Right motor leg	0 = No drift 1 = Drifts before 10 seconds 2 = Falls before 10 seconds 3 = No effort against gravity 4 = No movement

ITEM	NAME	RESPONSE
7	Ataxia	0 = Absent 1 = One limb 2 = Two limbs
8	Sensory	0 = Normal 1 = Mild loss 2 = Severe loss
9	Language	0 = Normal 1 = Mild aphasia 2 = Severe aphasia 3 = Mute or global aphasia
10	Dysarthria	0 = Normal 1 = Mild 2 = Severe
11	Extinction/ inattention	0 = Normal 1 = Mild 2 = Severe

From reference 222a.

TABLE 23-5 Hunt and Hess Clinical Classification of Subarachnoid Hemorrhage

CATEGORY*	CRITERIA
Grade I	Asymptomatic or minimal headache and slight nuchal rigidity
Grade II	Moderate to severe headache, nuchal rigidity, no neurologic deficit other than cranial nerve palsy
Grade III	Drowsiness, confusion, or mild focal deficit
Grade IV	Stupor, moderate to severe hemiparesis, possibly early decerebrate rigidity and vegetative disturbances
Grade V	Deep coma, decerebrate rigidity, moribund appearance

From reference 137a.
*Serious systemic disease such as hypertension, diabetes, severe arteriosclerosis, chronic pulmonary disease, and severe vasospasm seen on arteriography results in placement of the patient in the next less favorable category.

TABLE 23-6 World Federation of Neurological Surgeons Subarachnoid Hemorrhage Scale

WFNS GRADE	GCS SCORE	MOTOR DEFICIT
I	15	Absent
II	14–13	Absent
III	14–13	Present
IV	12–7	Present or absent
V	6–3	Present or absent

From reference 75a.
GCS = Glasgow Coma Scale, WFNS = World Federation of Neurological Surgeons.

TABLE 23-7 Fisher Grading System of Severity of Subarachnoid Hemorrhage

FISHER GROUP	BLOOD ON COMPUTED TOMOGRAPHY
1	No subarachnoid blood detected
2	Diffuse or vertical layers ≤1 mm thick
3	Localized clot or vertical layer >1 mm thick
4	Intracerebral or intraventricular clot with diffuse or no subarachnoid hemorrhage

From reference 94a.

antiphospholipid antibodies (anticardiolipin), hemoglobin electrophoresis, lipid profile, lupus anticoagulant, homocysteine, disseminated intravascular coagulation panel, partial thromboplastin time, platelet assays, proteins C and S, prothrombin time, sickle cell test, and an antithrombin III study (Table 23-8).[15,28,47,52] A 12-lead electrocardiogram (ECG) is recommended for all critically ill stroke patients because cardiac disease or myocardial injury may be the cause or the result of a stroke.[1,2,204] Signs and symptoms of cardiac-related stroke, myocardial infarction, or hemodynamic instability warrant additional studies including serial CK-MB and troponin laboratory assessments, transthoracic echocardiogram (TTE), transesophageal echocardiogram (TEE), and cardiac catheterization.* TTEs reveal valvular disease, left ventricular dysfunction and a low ejection fraction, atrial or ventricular thrombi, or a PFO as possible sources of stroke.[52] A TEE is more sensitive in the detection of left atrial thrombi, a PFO, some

*References 18, 47, 52, 152, 155, 322, 326.

TABLE 23-8 Laboratory Testing in Stroke

LABORATORY TEST	NORMAL VALUES	ABNORMAL VALUES AND SIGNIFICANCE IN STROKE
Antiphospholipid antibodies	Negative	Present in hypercoagulability; increases risk of ischemic stroke
Anticardiolipin antibody	Negative	Most common antiphospholipid antibody; present in hypercoagulability; increases risk of ischemic stroke
Antithrombin III	Plasma: 21–30 mg/dl; 85%–115% of standard; greater than 50% of control value	Decreased in ischemic stroke; increased in hemorrhagic stroke
Disseminated intravascular coagulation panel		Underlying etiology may be malignancy, sepsis, surgical or obstetric complications, or trauma Stroke may be thromboembolic or hemorrhagic
• Fibrin degradation products	2–10 mcg/ml	Increased
• Fibrin split products	Negative	Positive
• Fibrinogen level	150–400 mg/dl	Decreased
• Partial thromboplastin time	20–36 sec	Prolonged
• Platelets	150,000–400,000	Decreased
• Prothrombin time	10–15 sec	Prolonged
Factor assays		Increased clotting factors associated with hypercoagulability and increased risk of ischemic stroke
• V, VII, VIII, IX, X, XII	50%–150% of normal (control sample)	
• XI	65%–135% of normal (control sample)	
• XIII	Clot is insoluble for 24 hours	Decreased or absent factor VIII or IX with hemophilia
Glucose (fasting)	Adult: 70–115 mg/dl Child: 60–100 mg/dl	Diabetes is associated with increased risk of ischemic stroke
Glycosylated hemoglobin (HgA$_{1c}$)	Normal: 5.5%–8.8% Well-controlled diabetes: 3.5%–6.0%	Poorly controlled diabetes associated with atherosclerosis and microangiopathy of cerebral arteries; increases risk of thromboembolic strokes
Hemoglobin electrophoresis	Hemoglobin S: negative	Sickle cell hemoglobin greater than 30%, 80%–100%
Homocysteine	3–4.7 μmol/L	Increased homocysteine levels are associated with increased ischemic stroke risk related to atherosclerosis

LABORATORY TEST	NORMAL VALUES	ABNORMAL VALUES AND SIGNIFICANCE IN STROKE
Lipid profile	Recommended coronary heart disease risk levels	Low HDL is associated with ischemic stroke in men
• Total cholesterol	<200 mg/dl	
• HDL cholesterol	>35 mg/dl	
• LDL cholesterol	<130 mg/dl	
• Total triglyceride	<190 mg/dl	
Lupus anticoagulant	Negative	Present with hypercoagulability; increases risk of ischemic stroke
Partial thromboplastin time	20–36 sec	Prolonged on heparin therapy and hypercoagulability; increases risk of hemorrhagic stroke
Platelet aggregation	60%–100% (depends on assay used and laboratory-specific normal values)	Increased values may indicate greater risk of thrombosis, ischemic stroke May be used to monitor effectiveness of antiplatelet agents for primary or secondary prevention of ischemic stroke
Protein C	58%–148%	Deficiency increases risk of thrombosis, ischemic stroke
Protein S	74–112 units/dl	Deficiency increases risk of thrombosis, ischemic stroke
Prothrombin time International Normalized Ratio	10–15 sec INR 1.0	Prolonged with warfarin therapy; increases risk of hemorrhagic stroke
Sickle cell test	Negative	Positive in sickle cell disease or trait; screening test for sickle cell; definitive test is hemoglobin electrophoresis Sickle cell disease increases risk of ischemic stroke
Toxicology screen	Negative	Positive for amphetamines and cocaine metabolites in intracerebral hemorrhage and subarachnoid hemorrhage

From references 34, 52, 105, 149, 324, 325.
HDL = High-density lipoprotein, INR = international normalized ratio, LDL = low-density lipoprotein.

valvular dysfunction, and aortic arch plaques that may be the cardioembolic source for a stroke.[52,304] TEE requires the insertion of an esophageal probe, which may not be well tolerated by the patient.[52]

Radiographic Findings

The radiographic workup of the stroke patient consists of a number of well-established and newer neuro-imaging modalities, utilizing CT, angiography, magnetic resonance imaging (MRI), single photon emission computed tomography (SPECT), and positron emission tomography (PET) (Table 23-9).* The noncontrast CT scan is universally considered a first-line neuro-diagnostic tool for stroke.† While the noncontrast CT will not demonstrate an AIS in its earliest stages, it will show the presence of blood as a hemorrhagic stroke subtype, providing quick information regarding a patient's ineligibility for rt-PA administration if blood is present. If a CT scan is negative for hemorrhage but SAH is suspected and no mass effect/signs of increased ICP are

*References 52, 175, 176, 306, 317, 319, 333.
†References 1, 2, 8, 15, 18, 28, 36, 47, 52, 71, 87, 92, 104, 113.

TABLE 23-9 Radiographic Tests for Stroke

RADIOGRAPHIC STUDY	INDICATION	ADVANTAGES	DISADVANTAGES
Cerebral angiography	Demonstrates structure of cerebral vasculature, vascular anomalies, and vasospasm	Detailed Direct arterial access allows endovascular therapy including stenting, embolization, and intra-arterial injection of rt-PA and papaverine Gold standard for outline of cerebral vasculature and vasospasm	Requires arterial puncture, risk of dissection of arteries, plaque rupture with embolization, retroperitoneal hemorrhage Contrast material that is potentially nephrotoxic is injected
CT without contrast	Differentiates ischemic vs hemorrhagic stroke Demonstrates infarction (less acutely), edema, herniation	Rapid Portable scanners are available Does not require injection of contrast material	Less informative regarding infratentorial structures
CT angiography (CTA)	Demonstrates structure of cerebral vessels	Does not require arterial puncture	Requires peripheral IV access Contrast material that is potentially nephrotoxic is injected
Perfusion CT	Demonstrates qualitative and quantitative maps of CBF, cerebral blood volume, and mean transit time	Allows rapid evaluation of stroke; distinguishes infarcted tissue from ischemic penumbra	Contrast material that is potentially nephrotoxic is injected
Xenon-enhanced CT	Provides quantitative measurement of cerebral blood flow	Does not require arterial or venous puncture (xenon is inhaled) Rapid	Utilizes xenon gas, which may cause transient euphoria, light-headedness, sensory changes, and respiratory depression Requires FDA authorization for use Uses x-ray
MRI	Identifies infarct and hemorrhage, especially in posterior fossa and deep cerebral structures		Longer duration than CT Ferromagnetic metals are not allowed in room (requires special precautions or equipment for monitoring and care during MRA/MRI) Patient has to be screened for MRI Compatible/incompatible metals or devices in body Patient may experience claustrophobia
MRA	Demonstrates structure of cerebral vessels	Does not use x-ray Greater detail in regard to infratentorial area	Longer duration than CT Ferromagnetic metals are not allowed in room (requires special precautions or equipment for monitoring and care during MRA/MRI)

RADIOGRAPHIC STUDY	INDICATION	ADVANTAGES	DISADVANTAGES
			Patient has to be screened for MRI Compatible/incompatible metals or devices in body
Magnetic resonance imaging			
• Perfusion-weighted imaging (PWI)	Identifies area of ischemic tissue (area that is still potentially salvageable)	If area of decreased perfusion (PWI) is significantly larger than area of decreased diffusion (DWI), a PWI-DWI mismatch, patient may be less likely to hemorrhage with rt-PA administration and possibly eligible for rt-PA beyond 3-hour limit	Same as MRI Best method to determine volume of salvageable tissue has not been determined
• Diffusion-weighted imaging (DWI)	Identifies area of infarcted tissue (core of stroke)		
Fluid-attenuated inversion recovery (FLAIR) MRI	May detect even more detail regarding infarction than T2 gradient spin-echo sequences		Same as MRI
T2 gradient spin-echo sequences MRI	Detects small lobar ICH related to cerebral amyloid angiography		Same as MRI
PET	Demonstrates areas of infarcted as well as hypoperfused brain tissue with intact oxygen consumption Demonstrates three-dimensional quantitative and qualitative CBF values	Performs high-resolution scans and serial scans Determines glucose and oxygen metabolism	PET is expensive; requires arterial blood sampling; requires transport; limited to few major medical centers
SPECT	Provides qualitative information regarding early ischemia (as in early vasospasm)	Noninvasive; radioisotope is injected through an intravenous catheter Nurse may stay in room during scan	Provides qualitative information; scan must be performed within a few hours of injection

From references 136, 175, 176, 270, 271, 337.
CBF = Cerebral blood flow, CT = computed tomography, FDA = Food and Drug Administration, ICH = intracerebral hemorrhage, IV = intravenous, MRA = magnetic resonance angiography, MRI = magnetic resonance imaging, PET = positron emission tomography, rt-PA = recombinant tissue plasminogen activator, SPECT = single photon emission computed tomography.

seen, a lumbar puncture is indicated.[104,166,213] Perfusion CT quickly quantifies ischemia and may provide information about the cerebral vasculature.[136]

Xenon CT uses inhaled xenon gas to detect early ischemia (Figure 23-13). Inhalation of xenon has been reported to cause transient euphoria, light-headedness, sensory changes, and respiratory depression.[146] However, adverse effects have been reported in less than 0.1% of AIS patients receiving a 32% concentration of xenon.[175,176] A combination of 28% xenon and 72% oxygen is the most commonly used mixture.[175,176] Previously, xenon for cerebral perfusion imaging was in limited supply. It is currently approved through the U.S. Food and Drug Administration for clinical research, requiring an Investigational New Drug (IND) authorization.[176]

While the noncontrast CT scan is more efficient at identifying intracranial blood and less costly than an

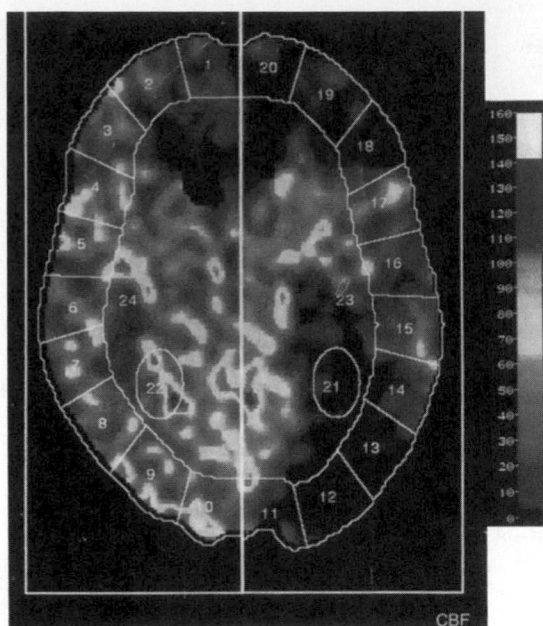

FIGURE 23-13 Xenon CT scan: a transverse slice from a xenon computed tomography scan with designated regions of interest *(numbers)* and color-coded information indicating the level of cerebral blood flow *(scale on the right)*.

MRI, T2-weighted MRI images are better than CT at detecting acute brain stem and lacunar ischemic stroke.[52,319] However, some patients cannot undergo MRI because of internal ferromagnetic devices/objects. Intraocular foreign bodies from welding or firearms, heart valves made before 1964, and older aneurysm clips, shunts, pacemakers, medication pumps, and middle ear prosthetics are contraindications for MRI.[52] The presence of ferromagnetic intraocular foreign bodies may be determined with a plain skull x-ray. Medication patches with foil or metal components may burn the patient and must be removed before the test. Monitoring and care of the critically ill patient in MRI is difficult because of the inability to use the usual ferromagnetic-containing equipment and signal interference on the ECG.[120,317,319,320]

Other MRI modalities such as diffusion-weighted imaging (DWI) and perfusion-weighted imaging (PWI) are gaining favor in regard to sensitivity and specificity relative to the character of an AIS. However, most institutions cannot efficiently complete most of these new modalities for the critically ill patient within the window of opportunity for rapid intervention such as the standard 3-hour time limit for intravenous rt-PA administration. Completion and interpretation of DWI and PWI MRIs require more time than noncontrast CT, and assessment and management of the patient are more difficult while they are being scanned.[120,187,317,319,320]

As two of the newer, more clinically valuable MRI modalities, DWI and PWI MRIs may allow intravenous

rt-PA to be safely administered beyond the 3-hour window from onset of symptoms in patients with a PWI-DWI mismatch. In AIS, PWI identifies the tissue that is hypoperfused (the penumbra) and DWI examines the area that has already infarcted and cannot be salvaged (the core).[64,66,158] The difference between the two, PWI minus DWI, is referred to as the PWI-DWI mismatch. If the area of decreased perfusion, PWI, is significantly larger than the diffusion abnormality, DWI, the patient may be at lower risk for hemorrhage from rt-PA administration; more likely to benefit from reperfusion therapy; and possibly eligible for rt-PA up to 6 hours after symptom onset without worsening outcome.[64,66,157,273,325] The intricacies of mapping the best PWI and calculating the volume of the hypoperfused but salvageable tissue have not been determined.[65] Research continues in this area.*

T2 gradient spin-echo MRI sequences have been found to be valuable in detecting small lobar hemorrhages related to cerebral amyloid angiography in ICH and may, in the future, determine treatment in regard to stroke that initially appears to be ischemic in origin.[176] Fluid-attenuated inversion recovery (FLAIR) MRI may provide information beyond T2 gradient spin-echo images in regard to infarction.[133]

Both CT angiography (CTA) and MR angiography (MRA) provide useful information regarding the cerebral vasculature. Carotid ultrasound and duplex also identify atherosclerotic lesions at the bifurcation of the carotid arteries. However, the four-vessel angiogram or digital subtraction angiography is still considered the gold standard for large-vessel and intracranial vascular anomalies, stenosis, and vasospasm.[175,176]

A nuclear medicine study that utilizes an intravenously injected radioisotope—the SPECT scan (Figure 23-14)—provides qualitative information regarding ischemia and is sometimes used to demonstrate early ischemia related to vasospasm.[175,176,319,331]

The value of transcranial Doppler (TCD) in cerebral ischemia related to sickle cell anemia and aneurysmal SAH vasospasm is substantial.[283] TCD is also used in emboli detection in carotid dissection and PFO.[14,283] Although angiography remains the gold standard for assessing vasospasm, TCD has the advantage of being performed at the bedside, being noninvasive, and not requiring injection of potentially nephrotoxic contrast materials (Figures 23-15 and 23-16).[283] TCD does not directly measure cerebral blood flow. Rather, it measures cerebral blood flow velocity (in centimeters per second). Mean flow velocities (MFVs) are used in the interpretation of TCD (Table 23-10). Upright waveforms indicate the flow of blood toward the probe (e.g., MCA), and inverted waveforms reveal flow away from

---

*References 65, 66, 156, 157, 195, 273.

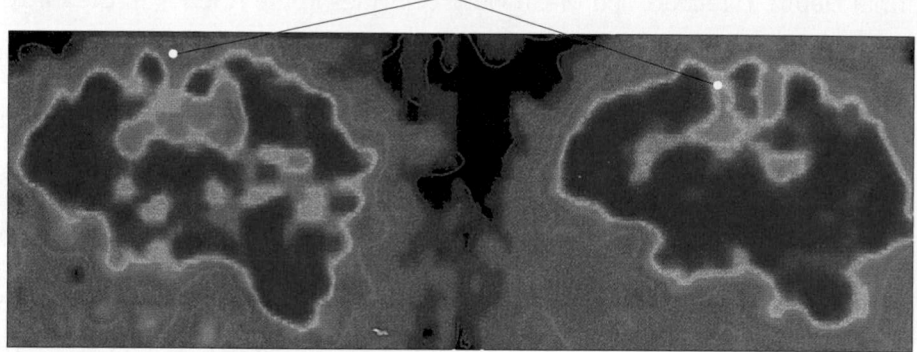

Areas of hypoperfusion in
the watershed zone

FIGURE 23-14 Single photon emission computed tomographic (SPECT) cerebral blood flow scan in a patient with carotid occlusion and frequent spells of hemiparesis but no evidence of infarction on CT or MRI scan.

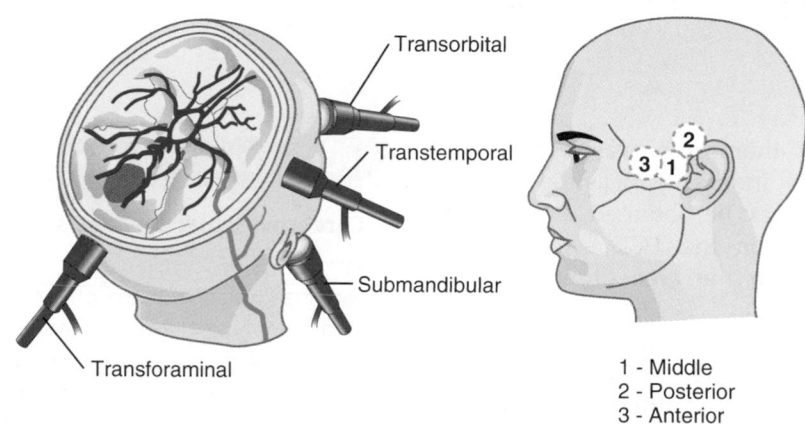

1 - Middle
2 - Posterior
3 - Anterior

FIGURE 23-15 Transcranial Doppler views. The temporal view has three aspects.

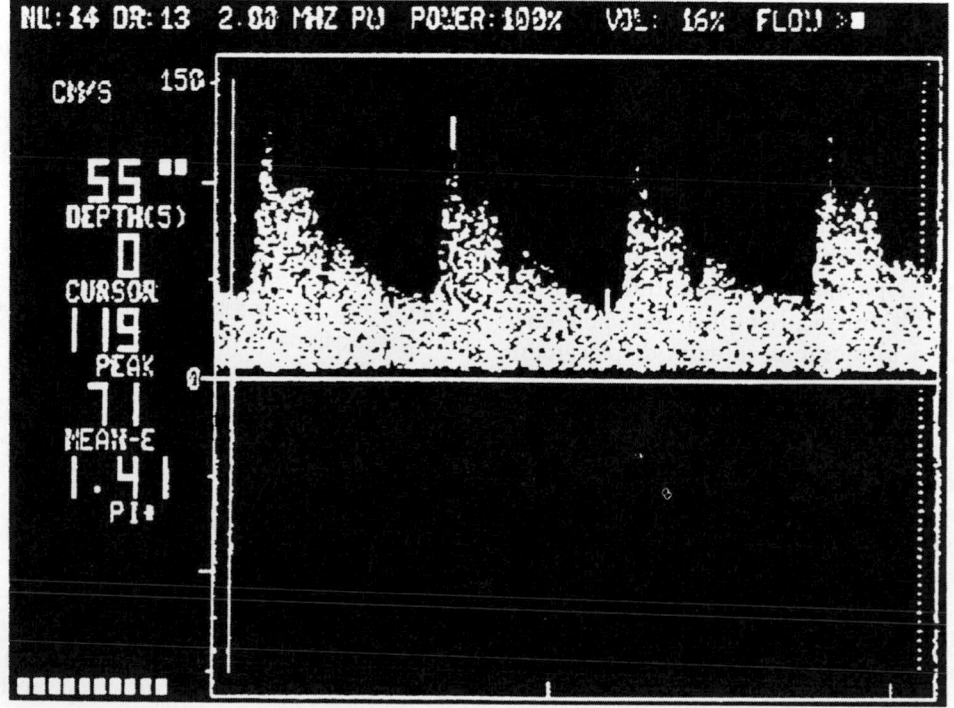

FIGURE 23-16 Normal transcranial Doppler waveform. Note the similarity to an arterial pressure waveform.

TABLE 23-10 Normal Depth, Direction, and Mean Flow Velocities in the Arteries of the Circle of Willis

ARTERY	DEPTH (mm)	DIRECTION	CHILDREN	ADULTS
M1 MCA	45–65	Toward	<170 cm/sec	32–82 cm/sec
A1 ACA	62–75	Away	<150 cm/sec	18–82 cm/sec
ICA siphon	60–64	Bidirectional	<130 cm/sec	20–77 cm/sec
OA	50–62	Toward	Variable	Variable
PCA	60–68	Bidirectional	<100 cm/sec	16–58 cm/sec
BA	80–100+	Away	<100 cm/sec	12–66 cm/sec
VA	45–80	Away	<80 cm/sec	12–66 cm/sec

From reference 334.

the probe (e.g., ACA). Other cerebrovascular parameters such as pulsatility index—a measure of cerebrovascular resistance—may be obtained. Emboli can be heard and visualized on the TCD screen. Some research has been done in the area of noninvasive ICP recording utilizing TCD.[334] TCD may be repeated daily, and serial recordings, especially by the same experienced sonographer, are advantageous.[283,332]

Limitations of TCD include limited expertise and inadequate bone windows to insonate vessels. TCD technology relies on areas of the cranium with sufficiently thin bone or naturally occurring foramina to allow transmission of the ultrasound beam. The following are naturally occurring cranial windows: transtemporal for insonation of the MCA, ACA, PCA, anterior communicating artery, and posterior communicating artery; transforaminal (suboccipital) for insonation of the vertebral artery and basilar artery; transorbital for insonation of the ophthalmic artery and internal carotid artery (ICA) siphon; and retromandibular (submandibular) to insonate the ICA before it enters the skull. Surgical burr holes or craniotomy flaps may serve as additional intracranial windows.[103,201] Surgical staples, burr hole covers, extracranial and intracranial edema, displacement of vessels from mass effect, patient movement, and naturally occurring hyperostosis of the cranium may complicate transmission of the ultrasound signal.[103]

In the pregnant patient, a brain CT may be safely performed with shielding of the abdomen. Brain MRI may be performed as well. Avoidance of CT and MRI contrast agents is preferable; however, if cerebral angiography is necessary, it may be performed with abdominal shielding. TCD may certainly be performed as it is an application of the same ultrasound technology used in monitoring the fetus.[282]

◆ Case Study 23-1, Part A

Cerebrovascular Disorders

Mrs. S.P. is a 55-year-old Caucasian female who presents with the "worst headache of her life" (10/10), nausea and vomiting, photophobia, and increasing drowsiness. She has a history of migraines but she states that this headache is much worse than her typical migraine. Other pertinent medical history includes smoking two packs per day for 30 years, and mild hypertension. Mrs. S.P. is neurologically intact except for a headache 10/10, nuchal rigidity, slight drowsiness, and a slight right lower facial weakness (asymmetric smile). Her vital signs are as follows: temperature, 37.5° C (99.5° F); heart rate, 78 beats/min (normal sinus rhythm); respirations, 16 breaths/min; BP, 160/88 mm Hg; Sao$_2$, 95%.

Mrs. S.P.'s GCS is 14 (opens eyes to name call, but not spontaneously), NIHSS 1 (not alert, requires minor stimuli), Hunt and Hess grade II (moderate to severe headache, unequal pupils), WFNS grade II (GCS 14 and no major focal deficit), and Fisher grade 3 (localized clot of subarachnoid blood on CT scan greater than 1 mm). She is sleepy but arouses to name call, oriented × 4, moves all extremities without difficulty 5/5. She has slightly unequal pupils, with the left being 4 mm and the right being 3 mm, but both are briskly reactive to light and accommodation. Both she and her family claim her pupils are usually equal. No other cranial nerve deficits are detected. Mrs. S.P. has nuchal rigidity and continues to complain of a severe headache with nausea and vomiting. A stat CT reveals diffuse subarachnoid blood, a localized clot of subarachnoid blood greater than 1 mm (Fisher 3), and slightly enlarged ventricles. An angiogram reveals a left middle cerebral artery aneurysm. Her vital signs now are as follows: temperature, 37.8° C (100° F); heart rate, 74 beats/min (normal sinus rhythm); respirations,

16 breaths/min; Sao$_2$, 92%; BP, 170/110 mm Hg. Her laboratory workup is negative for toxicology and coagulopathy.

Decision point: What pathophysiology is associated with this stroke?

Decision point: What are the initial priorities for her care?

Case continues on page 627

MANAGEMENT

Initial Management

Before admission to critical care, a number of interventions for patients with stroke may have occurred—before arrival at the hospital, in the emergency department, or elsewhere in the hospital if they are already inpatients. Airway, breathing, and circulation are always of higher priority than the neurologic insult because failure to promptly recognize and emergently and aggressively treat respiratory and cardiac instability may worsen the cerebral ischemia or infarct. Some stroke patients will require intubation and mechanical ventilation, particularly if they have a decreased level of consciousness, are unable to maintain their airway, or have aspirated. Others may only need supplemental oxygen with a nasal cannula or face mask. The goal oxygen saturation is greater than 95%.[325] Intravenous access is essential for administration of normal saline and medications as needed. ECG rate and rhythm are monitored, and hemodynamically compromising dysrhythmias are treated according to Advanced Cardiac Life Support (ACLS) protocols.[8] BP is monitored as well; however, it is only treated initially if the BP exceeds 220/120 mm Hg.[1,2]

As soon as the patient's cardiopulmonary status is stabilized and new neurologic deficit(s) is (are) recognized, a systematic approach, including a brief history and physical examination, laboratory tests, and radiographic workup, must be conducted. Each of the following must be determined: When did stroke signs and symptoms begin? Has the patient had a stroke in the past; is the patient having a stroke now? If so, is the stroke ischemic or hemorrhagic? If the stroke is ischemic, does the patient meet inclusion criteria to receive rt-PA? The sudden onset of numbness or weakness in an extremity or face; difficulty with speech or dysarthria; visual disturbance in one or both eyes; severe headache; and clumsiness or loss of balance are among the most common assessment findings suggestive of a stroke.* However, stroke mimics conditions such as hypoglycemia and alcohol/drug ingestion, which must be ruled out as well.† A stroke code is called in some facilities

---

*References 1, 2, 104, 113, 128, 129, 334.
†References 47, 104, 113, 128, 129, 165, 333.

when the possibility of a stroke is recognized; the stroke code team members are a multidisciplinary group of first responders dedicated to assessing and managing stroke during the first few hours after onset.[12] While certain signs and symptoms, such as complaints of "the worst headache of my life," seizures, nausea and vomiting, and a decreased level of consciousness, may strongly suggest hemorrhagic stroke, differentiation of an ischemic stroke from a hemorrhagic stroke can only be confirmed by noncontrast brain CT.[175,319] An AIS within the first few hours after onset will not be seen on CT scan, but blood will be evident.[1,2,333]

Since delays in care may worsen the prognosis and limit treatment options, time targets suggested by NINDS include a goal of 1 hour after arrival in the emergency department or recognition of an in-hospital stroke to assess, obtain initial labs and CT, and determine type of stroke and treatment. If the patient meets criteria for rt-PA administration, it should begin at the end of the first hour but only after the BP is within the acceptable range of less than 185/110 mm Hg[1,2] and after all invasive lines are inserted. Recommended devices include a minimum of two intravenous catheters and a Foley catheter.[243] Because of time constraints, rt-PA administration typically begins in the emergency department or in the patient's original room if an inpatient. Invasive devices must be inserted before administration of rt-PA. However, the infusion may be completed in critical care. A neurosurgical consult, as appropriate, is to be completed by the second hour. If the stroke is determined to be hemorrhagic, oral or intravenous anti-hypertensives, as a bolus or continuous infusions, may be administered before transfer to critical care to prevent additional hemorrhage. In general, the remainder of the neurodiagnostic evaluation and most additional interventions, such as insertion of invasive monitoring devices (for patients not receiving rt-PA), will occur after admission to critical care. Transfer to the appropriate level of care, such as critical care, progressive care, or, at minimum, a telemetry floor, is to be completed by the third hour.[8]

Critical Care Management

Many of the interventions for stroke are the same regardless of the stroke subtype. Before a discussion of interventions specific to each subtype—AIS, SAH, and ICH—interventions common to all stroke subtypes are presented in the Multidisciplinary Plan of Care on pp. 600-604.

Neurologic Interventions. Following stroke, the patient is at risk for secondary neuronal injury related to a number of mechanisms. Cerebral edema occurs with all strokes, and the patient may experience further

MULTIDISCIPLINARY PLAN OF CARE FOR PATIENTS WITH CEREBROVASCULAR DISORDERS

PROBLEM	INTERVENTION	RATIONALE	EXPECTED OUTCOME
At risk for secondary neuronal injury	• Monitor and maintain BP within prescribed parameters. • Use vasoactive agents as prescribed. • Initiate and monitor ICP/CPP. • Maintain ICP/CPP and other multimodality parameters ($Sjvo_2$, bto_2) as prescribed (CPP at least 60 mm Hg) using: (1) pharmacologic agents (osmotic diuretics [mannitol, furosemide]), HTS, sedation (propofol, opioids/benzodiazepines, barbiturate coma); and (2) nonpharmacologic measures such as ventriculostomy, position (monitor effect of head of bed position on intracranial dynamics), cooling measures to maintain normothermia, preoxygenation before suctioning, and adequate oxygenation. • Avoid hyperventilation. • Monitor pain and nausea and administer analgesics and anti-emetics (non-phenothiazines) as needed. • SAH: Maintain aneurysm precautions before endovascular coiling/clipping. • AIS: Administer rt-PA. • SAH: Administer nimodipine, HHH therapy, assist with angioplasty. • ICH: Correct coagulopathies; maintain BP parameters to minimize hematoma enlargement. • Maintain hemodynamic and cardiac stability. • Administer blood products as needed. • Seizure prophylaxis with SAH and lobar (cortical) ICH. • Craniotomy/craniectomy/hemispherectomy for malignant intracranial hypertension in AIS, SAH, and ICH.	Patient with stroke has impaired autoregulation, potential for increased intracranial pressure, inadequate cerebral perfusion pressure but an area of injured but potentially salvageable tissue. AIS patient is at risk for hemorrhagic transformation. SAH patient is at risk for rebleed and vasospasm. ICH patient is at risk for hematoma expansion, rebleed.	Patient at risk will experience minimal neurologic injury.

PROBLEM	INTERVENTION	RATIONALE	EXPECTED OUTCOME
At risk for pulmonary deterioration	• Monitor ABGs, Sao_2, end-tidal CO_2, CXR, respirations, breath sounds, CVP, PAP/PAWP, and sputum cultures. • Maintain ABGs within normal limits. • Perform pulmonary hygiene; antibiotics as needed. • Maintain head of bed at 30 degrees as intracranial dynamics allow. • Provide oral care. • Check tube-feeding residuals and hold as needed. • Administer DVT prophylaxis. • Consider tracheostomy for long-term mechanical ventilation. • Perform ventilation/pulmonary hygiene in a patient with impaired cough/gag or decreased level of consciousness.	Decreased respiratory effort and decreased ability to protect airway related to neurologic disease and bed rest. Risk of infection related to intubation, mechanical ventilation. Aspiration risk. Previous smoking history associated with increased likelihood of pulmonary complications. SAH: HHH therapy: HTS and neurologic disease may result in pulmonary edema. ICH: Neurologic disease and hypertonic saline may result in pulmonary edema.	Patient will maintain/attain normal ABGs and pulmonary status. Patient will wean from mechanical ventilation as soon as possible.
At risk for hemodynamic instability	• Monitor vital signs, ECG, heart sounds. • Monitor parameters obtained from pulmonary artery catheter or central venous catheter; obtain/maintain prescribed parameters. • Follow ACLS protocols as needed for rate and rhythm disturbances. • Obtain and monitor serial CK-MB and troponin levels, 12-lead ECGs, and other cardiac diagnostic studies. • Monitor and replace electrolytes as needed. • Administer, as prescribed, any cardiac medications given to patient before or after stroke. Monitor levels. Monitor for adverse effects.	Stroke and interventions for stroke may compromise hemodynamic stability.	Maintain/attain hemodynamic stability.
At risk for fluid and electrolyte imbalance	• Monitor fluid and electrolyte status, including intake and output, daily weight, and hemodynamic parameters. • Replace electrolytes as needed. Treat hyponatremia related to SIADH or CSW. • AIS: If SIADH, restrict fluids and administer sodium. • SAH: Do not restrict fluids (most likely CSW). • Administer sodium and fludrocortisone. • Replace other electrolytes as needed.	Stroke patient is at risk for fluid and electrolyte imbalances related to neurologic disease, pharmacologic agents, and decreased ability to drink and eat.	Maintain/attain normal electrolytes and fluid status appropriate to stroke subtype (AIS, ICH: euvolemia; SAH: euvolemia to hypervolemia during vasospasm).

Table continues on page 602

PROBLEM	INTERVENTION	RATIONALE	EXPECTED OUTCOME
At risk for undernutrition	• See Nutrition box on p. 613. • Start nutrition as soon as possible. • If patient is able to participate, obtain a swallow evaluation as soon as possible after admission to minimize risk of aspiration. • Otherwise, initiate enteral (preferred) or parenteral nutrition by day 3. • Attain and maintain normoglycemia. • Minimize use of dextrose-containing intravenous solutions. • Achieve and maintain goal rates of administration. • Administer GI prophylaxis (H-blockers or proton pump inhibitors). • Administer metoclopramide or erythromycin to enhance motility as needed. • Assess gastric contents and stool for occult bleeding. • Administer stool softeners/fiber as needed.	Stroke is a stress state with a hypermetabolic response. Stroke patients may be undernourished. As stroke increases with age, the patient's geriatric status and any preexisting special dietary needs must be taken into consideration. Hyperglycemia is associated with worse neurologic outcomes, impaired healing, and decreased immune status and may even impair recanalization after rt-PA administration.	Attain/maintain adequate nutrition.
At risk for bowel and renal/bladder dysfunction	• Monitor urine and stool elimination. • Administer stool softeners/fiber/mild laxatives as needed. • Monitor renal function and effect of potentially nephrotoxic pharmacologic agents such as radiologic contrast agents and vancomycin. • Remove Foley catheter and attempt timed voiding if patient is able to participate and fluid intake is not excessive related to HHH therapy or other needs. • Monitor urinalysis and urine culture and treat as needed.	The stroke patient is at risk for neurogenic bowel and bladder with incomplete emptying, incontinence, or retention; diarrhea or constipation.	Attain and maintain normal gastrointestinal and genitourinary elimination.
At risk for musculoskeletal impairment	• Initiate PT and OT consults (as soon as intracranial dynamics and vital signs have stabilized). • Monitor for footdrop and wristdrop, contractures. • Assist with protective positioning. • Assist with progressive activity as condition permits, including getting in and out of bed and pivoting into chair.	The stroke patient may have varying degrees of paresis to complete paralysis in one or more extremities. A delay in therapy increases the consequences of immobility and impedes recovery.	Experience minimal musculoskeletal deformity. Attain and maintain maximum mobility.

PROBLEM	INTERVENTION	RATIONALE	EXPECTED OUTCOME
At risk for skin breakdown	• Assess skin and mucous membranes for evidence of pressure and breakdown. • Keep skin clean and dry. • Reposition at least every 2 hours. • Collaborate with dietitian in regard to nutrition needs.	The stroke patient may be at increased risk for skin breakdown related to age, diabetes, peripheral vascular disease, and prestroke undernutrition.	Maintain skin and mucous membrane integrity.
At risk for infection and sepsis	• Monitor temperature, white blood cell count and differential, and culture and sensitivity results. • Observe for signs and symptoms of infection, particularly from invasive devices such as intravenous and arterial catheters, urinary catheter, intracranial monitoring devices, and incisions. • Maintain sterile technique during bedside insertion procedures (e.g., ventriculostomy, intravenous and arterial lines, and tracheostomy), dressing changes, obtaining specimens, and changing drainage bags. • Administer antimicrobial agents as prescribed. • Monitor antimicrobial levels as ordered.	The critically ill stroke patient is at increased risk of infection related to multiple invasive devices and other factors such as advanced age, nutritional status, diabetes, comorbidities, and related treatments that may influence immune status.	Experience minimal infection.
Impaired communication	• Assess patient for receptive, expressive, or global aphasia; anomia; and dysarthria. • Speak clearly, slowly, and at normal volume (unless hearing impaired); minimize distractions during communication. • Present one idea at a time when talking to patient. • Provide visual cueing as needed. • Speak to patient in visual field, from nonimpaired side or midline. • Minimize environmental distractions when talking to patient. • Collaborate with speech therapy in regard to communication techniques and use of assistive devices such as a communication board.		Patient will communicate as effectively as possible given language/speech deficits.

Table continues on page 604

PROBLEM	INTERVENTION	RATIONALE	EXPECTED OUTCOME

Impaired vision; perceptual deficits	• Assess visual acuity, visual fields with patient's corrective lenses as available.
	• Approach patient in visual field, from nonimpaired side or midline initially.
	  • Place objects, such as food, in visual field.
	  • As condition permits, teach patient to scan environment.
	  • Assess for diplopia.
	  • If diplopia is present, consider eye patch, alternating eyes.
		The stroke patient may have a variety of visual defects, including visual field cut and diplopia.	Attain maximum awareness of surrounding environment.

At risk for depression	• Monitor patient for depression and emotional distress. • Mobilize patient as soon as possible. • Educate patient and family regarding possibility of poststroke depression. • Promote sleep; provide comfort measures. • Praise progress and encourage family participation in stroke support group as available. • Consider pharmacologic agents (e.g., SSRIs) once neurologic status has stabilized.	Poststroke depression has a physiologic and psychosocial basis.	Experience highest quality of life possible. Experience minimal feelings of hopelessness and despair.
At risk for knowledge deficit	• Communicate with patient and family in regard to stroke diagnostic workup, diagnosis, plan of care, and progress. • Provide written materials to patient and family as appropriate to reinforce teaching. • Educate patient and family about basic pathophysiology, signs and symptoms, emergency action for a stroke, risk factors, and strategies for modification of those risk factors.	The stroke patient and family may be uninformed about stroke and current management. Knowledge increases cooperation and possibly deters feelings of hopelessness and despair.	Patient and family will have necessary knowledge to cope with stroke.

From references 1, 2, 13, 23, 24, 36, 67, 73, 100, 114, 122, 160, 178, 180, 190, 198, 204, 224, 230, 231, 242, 243, 267, 268, 273, 278, 279, 303, 304, 310, 321, 344.
ABG = Arterial blood gas, ACLS = advanced cardiac life support, AIS = acute ischemic stroke, BP = blood pressure, bto$_2$ = brain tissue oxygen, CK-MB = creatine kinase-myocardial bands, CO$_2$ = carbon dioxide, CSW = cerebral salt wasting, CPP = cerebral perfusion pressure, CVP = central venous pressure, CXR = chest x-ray, DVT = deep venous thrombosis, ECG = electrocardiogram, GI = gastrointestinal, HHH = hypervolemia, hypertension, and hemodilution therapy, HTS = hypertonic saline, ICH = intracerebral hemorrhage, ICP = intracranial pressure, OT = occupational therapy, PAP = pulmonary artery pressure, PAWP = pulmonary artery wedge pressure, PT = physical therapy, rt-PA = recombinant tissue plasminogen activator, SAH = subarachnoid hemorrhage, Sao$_2$ = arterial oxygen saturation, SIADH = syndrome of inappropriate antidiuretic hormone, Sjvo$_2$ = jugular venous oxygen saturation, SSRI = selective serotonin reuptake inhibitors.

neurologic deterioration from edema and increased ICP for 96 hours or more after the stroke. Increased ICP may result in further ischemia, infarction, and herniation.[117,206,325] Detailed serial neurologic assessment, including level of consciousness, orientation and mentation, language and speech, cranial nerves, movement, sensation, and vital signs every 1 to 2 hours, is paramount. Deterioration may be subtle or dramatic but must be detected as soon as possible and evaluated with consideration of additional interventions as appropriate.[117,206,325] Signs and symptoms of increased ICP include a decrease in level of consciousness; headache; nausea and vomiting; change in pupil size, shape, and reactivity; and impaired extraocular movements.[109,243]

Nursing interventions to decrease the ICP and maintain an adequate cerebral pressure include elevation of the head of the bed at 30 degrees or as needed to maintain an ICP less than 20 mm Hg and an acceptable cerebral perfusion pressure (CPP).[277] Specific recommendations for CPP in stroke have not been established. A goal of 60 to 70 mm Hg is used based on evidence from traumatic brain injury guidelines.[32] Depending on the type of stroke, interventions to prevent additional stroke, and the time since stroke onset, vasopressors or antihypertensive agents may be needed to achieve a target BP adequate to maintain the goal CPP without increasing the risk of additional ischemia, hemorrhagic transformation, rebleed, or hyperemia. More specific BP-related interventions are addressed later in this chapter with regard to each stroke subtype. In general, no attempt should be made to normalize the BP, particularly in a patient with a known history of hypertension.[148] Attempts to scientifically determine the optimal BP for a particular stroke patient or perhaps a subgroup of stroke patients utilizing autoregulatory testing and multimodality monitoring are being conducted.[138,263,286–288]

Other position-related measures to decrease ICP include maintaining the trunk and neck in alignment to minimize intrathoracic and intra-abdominal pressure and promote jugular venous return. Spacing of nursing activities such as turning, hygiene, and venipunctures may also reduce sustained increases in ICP. Small doses of analgesics such as morphine or fentanyl (Sublimaze) for headache or other discomfort may decrease ICP as well as assist with BP management if the patient is hypertensive. Nausea and vomiting, which may occur as a result of intracranial hemorrhage or increased ICP, also aggravate ICP. Non-phenothiazines such as ondansetron (Zofran) are recommended for nausea and vomiting; agents such as promethazine (Phenergan) and prochlorperazine (Compazine) lower the seizure threshold and may produce extrapyramidal symptoms with repeated dosing.[109,134] Routine administration of stool softeners will also assist with comfort and prevent increased ICP and bleeding or rebleeding associated with Valsalva and straining with bowel evacuation.*

Hyperthermia increases the cerebral metabolic rate (CMR), the brain's oxygen and energy requirements. Brain temperature is normally $1°$ C ($1.8°$ F) greater than core temperature and may be even higher when systemic hyperthermia is present.[238,295,299] Increased CMR is associated with increased CBF, which increases ICP.[202] At the cellular level, fever has been shown to contribute to the ischemic cascade by depleting ATP stores, promoting the release of glutamate, contributing to the synthesis of oxygen free radicals, and facilitating breakdown of the blood-brain barrier.[126,299] Every attempt should be made to attain and maintain normothermia in the care of the acute stroke patient.[123,229,318] Interventions to achieve normothermia include administering antipyretics, obtaining and monitoring cultures and sensitivities with administration of appropriate antimicrobials, monitoring serum antimicrobial levels, and implementing additional cooling measures. Reduction of ambient temperature, cool baths, and the use of such technologies as intravascular cooling catheters may also facilitate achieving normothermia.[16,193] Shivering associated with cooling measures will increase the ICP and the CMR, and negate the benefits of fever reduction.[5] A limited number of studies of various research designs have been conducted regarding the use of therapeutic hypothermia in acute stroke.[106,123,168,238] However, methodologies have differed, and Level I evidence for controlled hypothermia in stroke is lacking. Many questions remain regarding the optimal cooling process, target temperature, duration, and risks versus benefits.[167,329]

A number of pharmacologic agents, as detailed in the Medication table on pp. 608-611, may be administered to decrease ICP in acute stroke, including mannitol (Osmitrol), furosemide (Lasix), hypertonic saline (HTS), barbiturates, propofol (Diprivan), and opioids and benzodiazepines. Repeated dosing of mannitol may result in rebound edema and hypovolemia. Renal failure may occur if the serum osmolality exceeds 320 mOsm/L.[135,280] HTS acts rapidly and may be given after maximum serum osmolality has been reached with mannitol. HTS increases the serum sodium concentration, which results in a rapid movement of fluid out of the edematous tissues and into the intravascular compartment. However, pulmonary edema, congestive heart failure, and rebound edema may occur with its use. The target serum sodium level has not been established, although a goal of 145 to 155 mg/dl has been used by some clinicians.[26,227] Concentrations of 7% to 23.4% HTS have been used;[26,227] however, the optimal concentration has not been determined, and conclusive evidence regarding

---

*References 15, 87, 243, 322, 324, 325.

its efficacy is lacking.[26,227] Propofol and barbiturates decrease the CMR.[109,206]

The short half-life of propofol makes serial neurologic assessment possible. Barbiturates are generally reserved for refractory increased ICP because they depress the myocardium, induce hypotension, and impede neurologic assessment. Barbiturate coma is associated with an increased risk of pneumonia, sepsis, and hepatic failure.[109,206] Continuous electroencephalogram monitoring is also required to titrate the barbiturate to burst suppression.[109,206] Both propofol and barbiturates require intubation and mechanical ventilation and often a vasopressor to maintain adequate cerebral perfusion pressure. Barbiturates may also lower body temperature.[109,206]

In addition to ICP and CPP monitoring, cerebral oxygenation monitoring may guide therapy as well. A jugular venous oxygen saturation ($SjvO_2$) bulb catheter measures global oxygenation.[288] Acceptable values for $SjvO_2$ are 55 to 75 mg/dl. A brain tissue oxygenation catheter (btO_2) measures regional brain oxygenation.[141,208] Two btO_2 catheter monitoring systems were previously available: Licox (Integra Neurosciences, Plainsboro, NJ) and Neurotrends (Codman, Rayham, Mass). Acceptable values varied by manufacturer. Currently, only the Licox brain tissue oxygen catheter is available. Goal parameters specific to the Licox brain tissue oxygen catheter are 20 to 25 mm Hg.[141,208] The $SjvO_2$ catheter and the btO_2 catheter may be used together. The $SjvO_2$ catheter may allow judicious use of hyperventilation in increased ICP refractory to other measures and placement of the btO_2 catheter in the ischemic penumbra may facilitate prompt recognition and aggressive treatment of salvageable tissue adjacent to infarction or vasospasm.[208,288]

In supratentorial ischemic or hemorrhagic stroke with massive edema, surgical decompression with removal of cranial bone and infarcted tissue may be life-saving (Figure 23-17).[63,290,297] However, the procedure is controversial; the optimal time for surgery is unknown, and improvement of outcome in stroke patients has been unsubstantiated.[63,290,297,325] In contrast, emergent surgical decompression in cerebellar stroke may result in a good outcome.[143,171,205,279,293]

Pulmonary Interventions. Following stroke, the patient may have a number of pulmonary complications that can contribute to additional neurologic deterioration. These must be managed aggressively because systemic hypoxia worsens cerebral ischemia. Acute stroke patients are at high risk for aspiration, which may result in respiratory distress, pneumonia, or respiratory failure.[224]

A head of bed elevation of 30 degrees or more is preferable to minimize risk of aspiration.[93,202,249] Stroke patients who exhibit any signs or symptoms of dysphagia must not receive anything by mouth (NPO) until they are evaluated and deemed safe for oral intake with

or without restrictions (Box 23-2). Unilateral hemispheric AIS patients rarely require intubation unless they experience a decreased level of consciousness related to cerebral edema.[15] However, brain stem or bilateral hemispheric strokes with cranial nerve dysfunction may require intubation to protect the airway.[243] Intubation and mechanical ventilation is indicated with any of the following:

1. GCS less than or equal to 8
2. Inability to clear oral secretions
3. Absent cough and gag reflexes
4. Airway obstruction related to loss of tongue and pharyngeal muscle control
5. Respiratory distress or failure as evidenced by apnea, tachypnea, hypercapnia, oxygen desaturation, and use of accessory muscles
6. Partial pressure of arterial oxygen tension (PaO_2) less than 70 mm Hg despite oxygen therapy by nasal cannula or mask
7. Partial pressure of arterial carbon dioxide ($PaCO_2$) greater than 60 mm Hg, or severe respiratory acidosis[24,109,166,188]

In some cases, bronchoscopy may be needed to remove secretions.[206,242] Other measures to minimize an increase in ICP and cerebral ischemia include preoxygenation with 100% oxygen before suctioning and limiting suctioning to 10 to 15 seconds.[243]

For other patients, supplemental oxygen by nasal cannula or face mask may be the only oxygen therapy needed. Patients with sleep-disordered breathing may benefit from continuous positive airway pressure (CPAP) or bi-level positive airway pressure. The goal for arterial oxygen saturation (SaO_2) is 95% or greater.[1,2] Serial chest x-rays indicate worsening of the pulmonary status. Aggressive treatment of infection based on the culture and sensitivity is imperative. For patients who can participate, deep-breathing exercises and use of an incentive spirometer may be effective in minimizing atelectasis. If ICP, CPP, and other intracranial parameters permit, chest physiotherapy may facilitate pulmonary hygiene as well.[109,242]

Cardiac Interventions. Critically ill patients with acute stroke are at risk for cardiac complications for several reasons, including preexisting cardiac disease (a risk factor for stroke), acute myocardial infarction, and dysrhythmias related to autonomic nervous system dysfunction.

The most common dysrhythmia is atrial fibrillation.[206] A 12-lead ECG is recommended for all acute stroke patients.[1,2] Chest pain, unexplained hypotension, and hemodynamically unstable dysrhythmias indicate the need for serial cardiac enzymes, CK-MB, and troponin. An echocardiogram may be beneficial to determine ejection fraction and structural abnormalities,

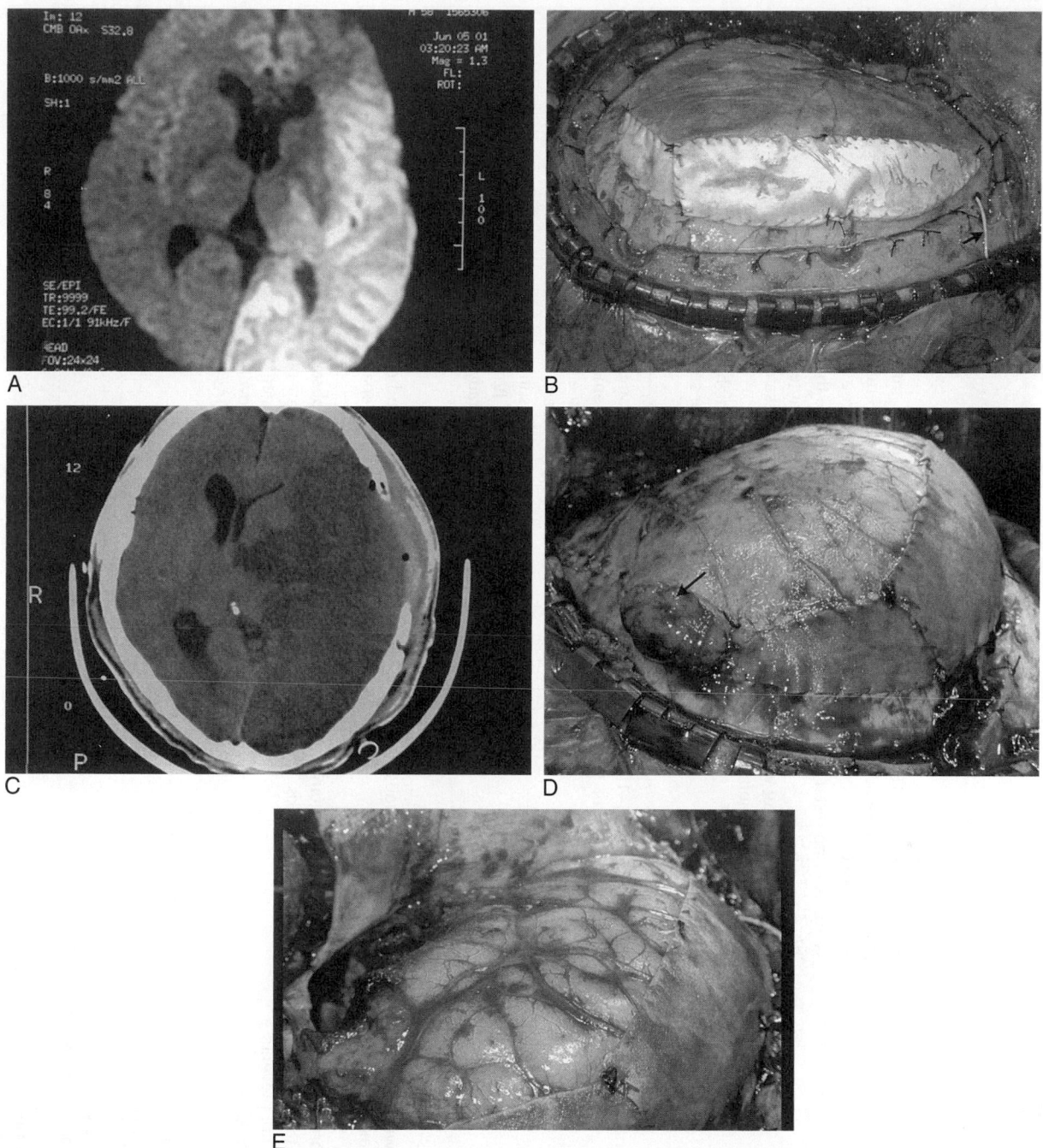

♦FIGURE 23-17 Radiographic changes in a patient with a sudden loss of consciousness and right hemiplegia. **A,** Magnetic resonance imaging (MRI) 4 hours after onset showing large hypersensitivity area at middle and posterior cerebral arteries. **B,** Decompressive craniotomy with duraplasty performed. **C,** Computed tomography (CT) scan shows larger and extended low density with midline shift of the brain at 36 hours. **D,** With return to surgery, brain herniated from the weak point of duraplasty. **E,** Brain edema subsided after the opening of the dura, an enlarged craniotomy, and an anterior temporal lobectomy were performed.

such as PFO, valvular defects, or vegetations. Serial doses of low-dose beta blockers such as metoprolol (Lopressor) may be administered in the absence of bradycardia, atrioventricular blocks, and relative hypotension to blunt the deleterious effects of catecholamines on the heart.[224]

The patient with acute stroke is also at risk for deep venous thrombosis (DVT). Ten percent of deaths in stroke patients occur as a result of pulmonary embolus.[1,2] Factors contributing to DVT include immobility, paralysis, atrial fibrillation, and advanced age.[1] Because administration of subcutaneous prophylactic heparin or

MEDICATIONS USED TO TREAT CEREBROVASCULAR DISORDERS

MEDICATION	ACTION	DOSAGE	SPECIAL CONSIDERATIONS
Anticonvulsants			
Phenytoin (Dilantin)	Stabilizes neuronal membranes in motor cortex	Loading dose: 15–18 mg/kg IV; maintenance dose: 300–400 mg IV/PO/NG daily Administer no faster than 50 mg/min IV Use an in-line filter when administering as infusion	Prophylactic use of anticonvulsants in stroke is controversial; recommended in hemorrhagic stroke Monitor total and free levels: total therapeutic range, 10–20 mcg/ml; free therapeutic range, 0.1–0.2 mcg/ml Avoid peripheral IV injection (irritating to vein and surrounding tissues with extravasation) or use fosphenytoin (a phenytoin prodrug) Since phenytoin is highly protein bound, it interacts with many other drugs. Monitor serum levels closely when initiating other medications.
Fosphenytoin (Cerebyx)	Stabilizes neuronal membranes in motor cortex	Loading dose: 15–18 mg/kg IV; maintenance dose: 300–400 mg IV	Prophylactic use of anticonvulsants in stroke is controversial; recommended in hemorrhagic stroke Monitor total and free levels: total therapeutic range, 10–20 mcg/ml; free therapeutic range, 0.1–0.2 mcg/ml Fosphenytoin is less irritating to tissues than phenytoin when given by peripheral IV injection; may also cause less hypotension and bradycardia than phenytoin
Anticoagulants			
Enoxaparin (Lovenox)	Low molecular weight heparin for DVT prophylaxis	40 mg subcutaneous daily	Monitor platelets and observe for signs and symptoms of bleeding. Monitor renal function.
Heparin	Blocks conversion of prothrombin to thrombin and fibrinogen to fibrin; prevents formation of new clots DVT prophylaxis Prevention of cardioembolic stroke related to prosthetic heart valves, atrial fibrillation Prevention of artery to artery emboli, e.g., carotid or vertebral dissections Management of DVT and pulmonary emboli	5000 units subcutaneously bid to tid for DVT prophylaxis	Monitor aPTT and observe for signs and symptoms of hemorrhage; monitor platelet count for HIT Antidote for prolonged aPTT: protamine sulfate Heparin is of no proven benefit in management of atherothrombotic TIAs

MEDICATION	ACTION	DOSAGE	SPECIAL CONSIDERATIONS
Warfarin (Coumadin)	Interferes with synthesis of vitamin K–dependent clotting factors Prevents formation of new clots Prevention of cardioembolic stroke associated with prosthetic heart valves and atrial fibrillation Prevention of artery-to-artery emboli; e.g., carotid or vertebral dissections Management of DVT/pulmonary emboli	5–15 mg PO daily initially; then 2–10 mg daily with adjustments according to PT/INR	Monitor PT/INR and observe for signs and symptoms of hemorrhage Repeated and intense patient/family education regarding compliance, PT/INR monitoring, precautions, and food-drug interactions Antidote is vitamin K
Antihypertensives			
Hydralazine (Apresoline)	Directly dilates arterioles	10–20 mg IV bolus every 4–6 hr as needed. Maximum dose is 300 mg/day	May produce lupus-like syndrome
Labetalol (Trandate)	Blocks alpha$_1$-, beta$_1$-, and beta$_2$-adrenergic receptor sites	20 mg IV bolus given over 2 min. Can repeat with boluses of 40–80 mg at 10-min intervals as needed up to 300 mg. Alternatively, can give IV infusion of 1 mg/ml labetalol at rate of 2 mg/min; max dose is 300 mg	Contraindicated in asthma, AV heart block and bradycardia Effects should be observed within 5 min of IV dose
Nicardipine (Cardene)	Calcium channel blocker, depresses cardiac and vascular smooth muscle	Continuous infusion: 25 mg/250 ml or 50 mg/250 ml (central venous catheter concentration); infuse at 5–15 mg/hr	Abrupt discontinuation may result in chest pain, particularly in patients with angina
Nifedipine (Procardia)	Calcium channel blocker; depresses cardiac and vascular smooth muscle	30–120 mg PO extended-release formulation daily	Monitor closely for hypotension Avoid sublingual dosing due to risk of profound hypotension
Antiplatelets			
Acetylsalicylic acid (aspirin)	Inhibits platelet aggregation and prostaglandin synthesis	80–325 mg PO daily	May cause gastric irritation

Table continues on page 610

MEDICATION	ACTION	DOSAGE	SPECIAL CONSIDERATIONS
	For primary and secondary ischemic stroke prevention		
Aspirin/ dipyridamole (Aggrenox)	Aspirin: see above Dipyridamole: inhibits platelet aggregation by inhibiting activity of adenosine deaminase and phosphodiesterase, enzymes that cause adenosine and cyclic AMP accumulation	Each capsule consists of 200 mg dipyridamole and 25 mg aspirin Dose is typically one capsule twice daily	GI distress: heartburn, nausea Alters platelet for life of platelet (approximately 10 days) Patients should avoid aspirin or other products containing aspirin while on Aggrenox therapy
Clopidogrel (Plavix)	Inhibits platelet aggregation by inhibiting binding of ADP to its platelet receptor and ADP-mediated activation of a glycoprotein complex	75 mg PO daily	GI distress: heartburn, nausea Increased risk of gastrointestinal hemorrhage when administered with aspirin
Dipyridamole (Persantine)	See above	75–400 mg PO daily	May prolong bleeding time; observe for bleeding Monitor platelet count for thrombocytopenia Not typically used as solo therapy
Ticlopidine (Ticlid)	Inhibits platelet aggregation by inhibiting ADP-induced platelet-fibrinogen binding	250 mg PO bid	GI distress: heartburn, nausea Monitor closely during the first 3 months of therapy due to risk of life-threatening neutropenia/agranulocytosis, thrombotic thrombocytopenic purpura and aplastic anemia
Colloids			
5% Albumin	Increases intravascular volume, reduces hemoconcentration, reduces blood viscosity	500 ml infusion; can give as rapidly as tolerated May repeat in 30 min if needed	Fluid overload, heart failure, pulmonary edema Increases intravascular volume, reduces hemoconcentration, reduces blood viscosity
Plasma protein fraction (Plasmanate)	Increases intravascular volume, reduces hemoconcentration, reduces blood viscosity	250–500 ml IV; not to exceed 10 ml/min	Fluid overload, congestive heart failure, pulmonary edema Increases intravascular volume, reduces hemoconcentration, reduces blood viscosity
Fludrocortisone (Florinef)	Mineralocorticoid that works at distal renal tubules to increase sodium reabsorption and water retention	0.2 mg NG daily	May aggravate HF Monitor sodium and potassium carefully

MEDICATION	ACTION	DOSAGE	SPECIAL CONSIDERATIONS
Mannitol (Osmitrol)	Osmotic diuretic; pulls cerebral edema into intravascular space Use for increased intracranial pressure	0.25–1 g/kg IV Use inline filter of less than 5 microns if given as infusion (rather than bolus)	Renal failure; monitor serum osmolality; risk increases with serum osmolality greater than 320 mmol/L Hypotension Hypokalemia Monitor electrolytes
Nimodipine (Nimotop)	Cerebroselective calcium channel blocker; protects neurons during vasospasm	60 mg NG/PO every 4 hr; use 18-gauge needle to withdraw solution from the capsule. After adding drug to NG tube, flush with 30 ml NS. Adjust dose to 30 mg NG/PO every 2 hr if hypotension occurs	Observe for hypotension; avoid sublingual dosing to minimize large decreases in BP
Recombinant tissue plasminogen activator (Alteplase)	Thrombolytic: enzyme binds to fibrin in clot, converting plasminogen to plasmin, initiating fibrinolysis	Bolus: 10% of 0.9 mg/kg dose over 1 min followed by 90% of 0.9 mg/kg dose over 60 min Recommended within 3 hr of onset of symptoms	Obtain head CT before administration Obtain baseline labs, CBC, coagulation studies, including fibrinogen, and type and screen before administration Monitor for signs and symptoms of hemorrhage; hemorrhagic transformation of AIS Do not administer heparin, warfarin, or aspirin for at least 24 hr Avoid venipunctures, arterial punctures, and insertion of invasive devices after administration
Saline: isotonic (0.9%) and hypertonic	Pulls cerebral fluid into intravascular space for renal elimination Used for refractory increased intracranial pressure IV bolus amounts vary from 10 to 30 ml 0.9% to 3% used for hyponatremia in CSW or SIADH	Use central venous catheter for 3% or greater concentration	Hypernatremia; transient intravascular fluid overload Calculate sodium deficit to guide dosing Goal serum sodium level is 145–155 mEq/L Caution if serum sodium level exceeds 160 mEq/L HTS is irritating to veins and tissues; administer through central venous catheter

From references 36, 135, 224, 226, 280, 294, 310, 321, 325, 327, 330, 332, 345.
ADP = Adenosine diphosphate, AIS = acute ischemic stroke, AMP = adenosine monophosphate, aPTT = activated partial thromboplastin time, AV = atrioventricular, CBC = complete blood count, CSW = cerebral salt wasting, CT = computed tomography, DVT = deep venous thrombosis, HF = heart failure, HIT = heparin-induced thrombocytopenia, HTS = hypertonic saline, ICH = intracerebral hemorrhage, INR = international normalized ratio, NS = normal saline, PT = prothrombin time, SIADH = syndrome of inappropriate antidiuretic hormone, TIA = transient ischemic attack.

Box 23-2

Signs and Symptoms of Dysphagia During and Between Meals

- Drooling, excessive secretions
- Excessive tongue movement, tongue thrusting, or spitting food out of the mouth
- Poor control of tongue
- Facial weakness
- Pocketing of food in cheek, under tongue, or on hard palate
- Slurred speech
- Coughing or choking while eating*
- Regurgitation through nose, mouth, or tracheostomy tube
- Wet "gurgly" voice after eating or drinking, or frequent throat clearing
- Hoarse or breathy voice
- Complaints of food getting stuck in the throat
- Delay or absence of laryngeal (Adam's apple or thyroid cartilage) elevation
- Recurrent pneumonia (because of aspiration)
- Prolonged chewing or eating time
- Reluctance to consume particular food consistencies or to eat at all

*Caution: Aspiration commonly occurs without coughing. The presence or absence of the gag reflex does not indicate whether the swallowing reflex is intact.

---

low-dose heparinoid may be delayed following hemorrhagic stroke or administration of rt-PA, mechanical devices such as sequential compression devices should be initiated on admission.[1,2] Anti-embolism stockings are of unproven value[1,2] although they are frequently used, sometimes in addition to sequential compression devices. DVT may occur in the upper extremities as well. Central venous catheters may promote upper extremity thrombosis and emboli formation.[65] Venous Doppler studies are indicated for stroke patients with any unilaterally swollen, inflamed, and painful extremity.[65]

A well-documented risk factor, many stroke patients have a known history of hypertension before their stroke. A number of intravenous and oral anti-hypertensive agents are used in the management of acute stroke, as indicated in the Medication table on pp. 608-611. Hypertension must be controlled but with consideration for cerebral perfusion. Hypotension and rapid fluctuations in the BP may result in additional ischemia and infarct.*

Gastrointestinal Complications. The impact of stroke on the gastrointestinal system may increase the risk of aspiration related to nausea and vomiting, gastric

*References 1, 2, 36, 62, 190, 206, 263.

hypomotility, impaired swallow, and enteral nutrition. Stroke patients with an abnormal gag, impaired or absent cough, inability to swallow saliva, dysphonia, and cranial nerve palsies are at increased risk of aspiration.[93,249] In addition to elevation of the head of the bed, preventive interventions include the following:

1. Maintaining NPO status until a dysphagia evaluation is completed
2. Adhering to dietary restrictions based on swallow evaluation
3. Allowing oral intake only when the patient is alert and head is elevated
4. Monitoring gastric residuals
5. Administering metoclopramide (Reglan) to facilitate gastric emptying[109,206]

While bedside swallowing assessments are helpful in dysphagia screening, video fluoroscopy and fiberoptic endoscopy during feeding may provide more definitive information.[1,2,153,249] Collaboration with speech therapy for dysphagia assessment and management is prudent. Techniques that facilitate swallow include tucking the chin and turning the head, and checking for pocketing of food. Maintaining head of bed elevation for 30 minutes to 1 hour after eating, particularly for individuals with gastroesophageal reflux, may minimize aspiration.[243]

Nasogastric tubes for gastric emptying and enteral feeding offer only limited protection against aspiration.[78] If tube feedings are required to attain adequate nutrition and minimize the risk of aspiration, small-bowel feedings may lessen the aspiration risk and enable attainment of caloric and protein requirements more quickly.[206] If long-term enteral feeding is required, percutaneous endoscopic placement of a feeding tube is indicated.[1,2]

Failure to provide the stroke patient with adequate nutrition may negatively impact outcome; however, the benefit of supplemental nutrition has not been substantiated.[1,2] While studies have shown traumatic brain injury patients to be hypermetabolic and hypercatabolic, the exact requirements specific to stroke have not been determined beyond basic energy expenditure requirements with possibly the addition of a stress factor.[1,2,153,166] However, monitoring intake and output, weight, caloric intake, serum proteins, fluids and electrolytes, and blood count is recommended at a minimum.[77,153] Collaboration with a registered dietitian is essential in regard to dietary requirements as well as modifications based on other risk factors such as heart disease, renal disease, or diabetes.[1,2,50,77] Nutritional considerations for patients with cerebral vascular disorders are discussed in the Nutrition box on p. 613.

Stroke patients are at risk for stress ulcers and gastrointestinal hemorrhage, particularly if they have

NUTRITION

Nutritional Considerations for Patients With Cerebral Vascular Disorders

- Special Considerations: Stroke patients are at tremendous risk for aspiration. Assess for dysphagia, including silent aspiration; consult speech pathologist for bedside swallowing evaluation as soon as patient is able to participate. Dysphagia modifications must be based on the individual's swallowing impairment and may include thick or thin liquids, pureed food, or mechanical soft food in the diet.
- Calories: Utilize indirect calorimetry (metabolic cart) if available. The Harrison-Benedict energy expenditure equation may be used in calorie determination. This equation is based on gender, age, weight, and height. A stress factor may be added, e.g., 1.2. Consider other comorbidities.
- Maintain normoglycemia.
- Protein: Monitor prealbumin level; 24-hour urine collections for urea nitrogen level and creatinine clearance. Consider diets (including tube feeding) formulated for renal and hepatic insufficiency as appropriate. Protein/albumin levels may be influenced by albumin administration in hypervolemia, hemodilution, and hypertension therapy.
- Fat: Include propofol administration in calculation of calories. Monitor triglycerides.
- Fluid: Attain and maintain euvolemia for acute ischemic stroke and intracerebral hemorrhage. Attain and maintain euvolemia to hypervolemia for subarachnoid hemorrhage. Consider insensible water loss from diarrhea, fever, and perspiration. Avoid IV solutions containing glucose.
- Monitor intake and output; daily weights.
- Electrolytes: Replace electrolytes as needed. Be alert for decreasing serum sodium level and replace. Attain and maintain normoglycemia. Use sliding-scale insulin and an insulin drip as needed to maintain blood glucose level at 70 to 150 mg/dl.
- Vitamins and Minerals: Supplement as needed, particularly with individuals at risk before admission.

From references 1, 2, 93, 109, 153, 166.

received anticoagulation, antiplatelet, or thrombolysis agents or experience repetitive vomiting.[3,325,345] While oral intake or enteral feeding may provide some protection against stress ulcers, prophylaxis with histamine blockers or proton pump inhibitors is recommended. Constipation is to be avoided. Straining during a stool may result in intracranial hemorrhage and increased ICP. Most patients benefit from stool softeners during the acute phase of stroke.[243]

Genitourinary Complications. Initially, many critically ill stroke patients will require an indwelling urinary catheter to minimize the risk of retention and incontinence and to maintain accurate intake and output records. Retention may increase the risk of infection, add to the patient's discomfort, and increase the ICP. Incontinence may increase the risk of skin breakdown. However, the catheter should be removed as soon as possible to decrease the risk of infection and to reestablish voiding.[1,2] Voiding may be facilitated by placing the patient on the bedpan or bedside toilet or offering the urinal at scheduled times.[243] Signs and symptoms of urinary tract infections warrant investigation and appropriate antimicrobial management based on the culture and sensitivity.[15,178,204]

Endocrine Support. Hyperglycemia has been associated with poor outcomes after ischemic and hemorrhagic stroke.[1,2,207,224] Hyperglycemia is thought to increase acidosis, edema, and glutamate release, which results in greater neuronal injury. Hyperglycemia may also contribute to hemorrhagic transformation.[325] However, the findings of research to date have been inconsistent. Furthermore, the acceptable range of blood glucose level varies from publication to publication, ranging from 80 to 300 mg/dl.[1,2,207,224] Since hypoglycemia is also detrimental to neurons, attaining and maintaining a normal blood glucose level, approximately 80 to 120 mg/dl, is desirable. Because intravenous solutions containing dextrose may aggravate hyperglycemia and cerebral edema, some clinicians advocate minimizing their use.* If the glucose level cannot be managed with a sliding-scale regimen or a sliding-scale regimen with a base dose, then an infusion of regular insulin with hourly glucose monitoring is appropriate (Level II evidence).[207,224,243]

Musculoskeletal Interventions. Following stroke, weak or paralyzed extremities are extremely vulnerable to injury.[77] At a minimum, care must be taken to maintain the arm or leg in proper alignment when turning and positioning to avoid musculoskeletal complications. Orthotic devices may assist in maintaining alignment of the extremities as well. Although evidence is lacking regarding the best time to start physical therapy and occupational therapy, the nurse has a role in assessing the patient's tolerance to passive range of motion and performing those exercises once the intracranial dynamics and vital signs have stabilized.[73,77] After an initial period of flaccidity, spasticity is likely, which may be uncomfortable and also increase the risk of permanent deformities. Antispasticity medications may be warranted and enhance benefits received from physical

*References 1, 2, 207, 231, 243, 255, 325.

and occupation therapy.[73,77] If shoulder subluxation, footdrop, external hip rotation, or contractures occur, they may severely compromise the patient's rehabilitation potential and affect the patient's quality of life.[73,77]

Skin Care Interventions. Paralysis, diabetes or peripheral vascular disease, bed rest, incontinence, and poor nutrition may all contribute to skin breakdown. Keeping the skin clean and dry and turning with attention to alleviating pressure points are essential. Use of pressure-alleviating beds may assist in maintaining skin integrity.[206,325]

Rest and Comfort Interventions. Initially following stroke, pain presents primarily as headache. If the patient has had an SAH, the headache is frequently accompanied by a painful and stiff neck and backache from the blood in the CSF irritating the meninges. Photophobia may also be present with subarachnoid blood. Hypertension and increased ICP may also contribute to headache.[104] Invasive monitoring and therapeutic devices add to the patient's discomfort. If surgical or endovascular therapy is performed, those procedures cause additional discomfort. Analgesics may make neurologic assessment more difficult; however, their judicious use is appropriate as needed for comfort. Failure to alleviate pain and discomfort may cause further deterioration in the patient's status.[243,322]

Once the patient is stable, uninterrupted sleep of at least 1- to 2-hour intervals is essential and may result in an improved neurologic assessment. Fatigue and impaired sleep are common manifestations after stroke, and a prolonged stay in intensive care with repeated neurologic assessments and interventions further deprives the stroke patient of much-needed sleep and rest.[67,274]

Communication Interventions. Following stroke, up to 40% of all stroke patients have impaired communication.[77,116] The communication disorder may be a language disorder, aphasia, or a problem with the mechanics of speech, such as dysarthria. The term *aphasia* is used interchangeably with the word *dysphasia*. Aphasia may be one of the following: receptive, also referred to as Wernicke's or fluent; expressive, also referred to as Broca's or nonfluent; or global, a combination of fluent and nonfluent. Anomia is difficulty with word finding. Broca's area, responsible for expressive speech (verbalization), is located in the motor strip of the frontal lobe; Wernicke's area, responsible for receptive speech (understanding the spoken word), is located at the junction of the temporal and parietal lobes (Figure 23-18).[30,289,322] A speech therapy consult may be beneficial before and after extubation to assist with communication in acute stroke patients. Hand-held

boards with the alphabet or pictures and visual cueing may facilitate communication and decrease anxiety in the patient with receptive ability.[116,322]

Perception and Sensory Interventions. Following stroke, patients may have both sensory and perceptual deficits, including visual field cuts and neglect. The field cut most associated with supratentorial strokes is homonymous hemianopsia, in which half of the visual field, contralateral to the side of the brain lesion, is missing. Neglect is also contralateral to the brain lesion. A visual field cut and neglect may exist separately or simultaneously. Immediately after a stroke, communication is most effective if the patient is approached from the side without the deficit or at least from the midline. Later, during recovery, the stroke patient can be taught to compensate for the visual deficit by turning the head from the intact visual field to the missing visual field. Occupation, physical, and speech therapy also work with the patient to teach compensation for visual and perceptual deficits.[77,116,243]

Psychosocial Support. The reasons for depression following stroke are psychosocial as well as physiologic. Most stroke patients have neurologic deficits from which they may never completely recover, and many have difficulty communicating because of cranial nerve deficits, dysphasia/aphasia, intubation, cognition, or sedation. Furthermore, they may not feel well and are sleep-deprived as a result of their stroke and the critical care environment. In addition, some researchers have shown that pathophysiologic changes as a result of left hemispheric infarcts may contribute to poststroke depression.[86] Antidepressants such as selective serotonin reuptake inhibitors (SSRIs) may be helpful

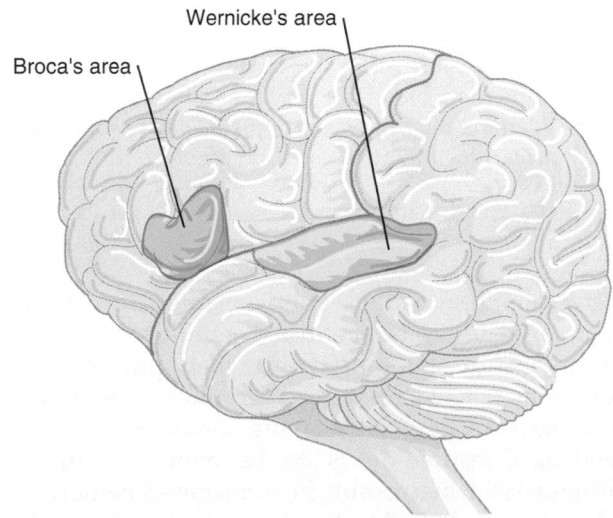

Wernicke's area

Broca's area

⬧**FIGURE 23-18** Territories of language areas.

by blocking the reuptake of serotonin.[322] Depression, in general, has been associated with low serotonin levels.[122] Initiating physical, occupational, and speech therapy as soon as possible may decrease depression as well, particularly if the patient is made aware of his or her progress.[77] Collaboration with the patient's family and a clinical psychologist may provide insight into the patient's thoughts and needs.[243]

Providing Education. Following stroke, the educational needs are great for both the family and the patient if the patient is cognitively aware of the diagnosis. Both family and patient need basic information about stroke pathophysiology, emergency action during stroke, stroke management and rehabilitation, risk factors, and strategies for modification of risk factors. Education of the patient and family may empower them to better cope with the illness and to look to the future.[243]

Ischemic Stroke

Most AIS patients may not need or benefit from intensive care. However, if they have oxygenation issues, require intubation or mechanical ventilation, experience cardiac instability, require continuous infusions of vasoactive agents, or have neurologic instability, admission to a critical care unit is warranted. A patient who has sustained a large MCA infarct with massive edema definitely needs intensive care.[295] Other more stable AIS patients may benefit from an acute care unit with an aggressive multidisciplinary approach to stroke care, including early involvement of occupational, physical, and speech therapy. Dedicated stroke units, which are frequently classified as progressive care units, have been shown to have better outcomes than nonneurologic acute care units.[72]

Following AIS, BP is a major consideration. BP that is too high may contribute to cerebral edema and hemorrhagic transformation. However, BP that is too low may inadequately perfuse the brain, resulting in an even larger infarct.[1,2] Optimal BP for this subgroup of stroke patients has not been scientifically substantiated. Based on AHA/ASA guidelines for AIS, BP is only to be treated if it exceeds a systolic of greater than 220 mm Hg or a diastolic of greater than 120 mm Hg unless the patient is a candidate for rt-PA (level V evidence).* If rt-PA is to be administered, the BP must then be lowered cautiously to 185/110 mm Hg or less and maintained below that level.[1,2]

Scientific support for the use of intravenous rt-PA for thrombolysis in AIS is based on a large multicenter randomized controlled trial conducted by NINDS. The use of intravenous rt-PA in eligible AIS patients is based on Level I evidence.[1,2] If a patient is given intravenous rt-PA, inclusion and exclusion criteria and guidelines for follow-up care must be strictly adhered to in order to minimize the risk of bleeding. Contraindications to rt-PA administration are intracranial and systemic hemorrhage (Box 23-3).[71,151,273,312,345] Anticoagulants and antiplatelet agents must not be given for at least 24 hours. Risk factors associated with hemorrhage following rt-PA administration include a high NIHSS score, longer time to treatment, hyperglycemia, decreased platelet count, and increased age. Hyperglycemia also decreases recanalization, reopening of the occluded artery.[43,102] BP is maintained within parameters for post rt-PA administration, and invasive monitoring, arterial and venous punctures, is minimized. BP is carefully lowered with antihypertensives such as intermittent IV doses of labetalol or continuous nicardipine (Cardene). The use of continuous intravenous infusions of nitroprusside (Nipride), a vasodilator, is controversial because some clinicians feel it may contribute to increased ICP.[135,263,280]

In addition to intravenous rt-PA, intra-arterial rt-PA (at the clot), a combination of intravenous rt-PA and intra-arterial rt-PA, or a clot retrieval device may be utilized to unblock the artery.*

However, at this time administration of intra-arterial rt-PA and the use of mechanical devices to open arteries in AIS are still considered investigational.

Recombinant t-PA is clot-specific yet may result in hemorrhagic tendencies, intracranial or systemic.* Following rt-PA administration, the patient must be closely watched for signs of hemorrhage, intracranial or systemic. Neurologic deterioration related to intracranial hemorrhage after rt-PA may be subtle or dramatic, such as a sudden loss of consciousness, seizure, onset of severe headache, or sudden increase in systemic BP. Tachycardia, a decrease in BP, and a downward trend in the hematocrit and hemoglobin levels as well as visible bleeding may indicate systemic hemorrhage.†

Recombinant t-PA has not been approved for use during pregnancy. However, low-dose aspirin, subcutaneous low-dose heparin, low molecular weight heparin, and warfarin have been safely used during pregnancy to prevent thrombosis in hypercoagulable states or to prevent cardiac-related embolization.[282]

Surgical carotid endarterectomy or interventional carotid angioplasty with stenting has been shown to be beneficial with asymptomatic carotid stenosis of greater than 70% but less than 100% or symptomatic (recent TIA or AIS) carotid stenosis of greater than

---

*References 1, 2, 79, 101, 151, 180, 235, 243, 272, 273.

*References 66, 74, 102, 151, 159, 177, 187, 272, 273, 314.
†References 71, 235, 273, 304, 312, 345.

Box 23-3

TPA Stroke Study Group: Protocol Guidelines[*,†] for the Administration of rt-PA to Patients With Acute Ischemic Stroke

These protocol guidelines represent only one possible approach to the treatment of eligible patients with acute ischemic stroke. Healthcare practitioners and institutions will need to exercise their own professional judgment in creating or adopting treatment protocols or guidelines, as well as in the treatment of each individual patient.

1. ELIGIBILITY FOR IV TREATMENT WITH rt-PA

- Age 18 years or older
- Clinical diagnosis of ischemic stroke causing a measurable neurologic deficit
- Time of symptom onset well established to be less than 180 minutes before treatment would begin

2. PATIENT SELECTION: CONTRAINDICATIONS[(C)] AND WARNINGS[(W)]

- Evidence of intracranial hemorrhage on pretreatment CT[c]
- Only minor or rapidly improving stroke symptoms[w]
- Clinical presentation suggestive of subarachnoid hemorrhage, even with normal CT findings[c]
- Active internal bleeding[c]
- Known bleeding diathesis, including but not limited to the following:
  - Platelet count $<100,000/mm^{3c}$

- Receipt of heparin within 48 hours and an elevated activated partial thromboplastin time (greater than upper limit of normal for laboratory)[c]
- Current use of oral anticoagulants (e.g., warfarin sodium) or recent use with an elevated prothrombin time >15 seconds[c‡]
- Major surgery or serious trauma excluding head trauma in the previous 14 days[w]
- Intracranial surgery, serious head trauma, or previous stroke within 3 months[c]
- History of gastrointestinal or urinary tract hemorrhage within 21 days[w]
- Recent arterial puncture at a noncompressible site[w]
- Recent lumbar puncture[w]
- On repeated measurements, systolic blood pressure >185 mm Hg or diastolic blood pressure >110 mm Hg at the time treatment is to begin, and aggressive treatment required to reduce blood pressure to within these limits[c]
- History of intracranial hemorrhage[c]
- Abnormal blood glucose level (<50 or >400 mg/dl)[w]
- Post–myocardial infarction pericarditis[w]
- Seizure observed at the same time the onset of stroke symptoms[w]
- Known arteriovenous malformation or aneurysm[c]

3. TREATMENT

- rt-PA 0.9 mg/kg (maximum of 90 mg) infused over 60 minutes with 10% of the total dose administered as an initial IV bolus over 1 minute

Courtesy Genentech, Inc., South San Francisco, Calif.
[*]This protocol is based on research supported by the National Institute of Neurological Disorders and Stroke.
[†]Reference should also be made to the manufacturer's prescribing information for alteplase.
[‡]In patients without recent use of oral anticoagulants or heparin, treatment with rt-PA can be initiated before the availability of coagulation study results but should be discontinued if either the prothrombin time is greater than 15 seconds or the partial thromboplastin time is elevated by local laboratory standards.
CT = Computed tomography, rt-PA = recombinant tissue plasminogen activator.

50% but less than 100%.[*] Carotid endarterectomy is based on Level I evidence, whereas interventional carotid angioplasty with stenting is based on Level II evidence.[111,267] Recanalizing an ICA that is already 100% stenosed may result in ICH because collateral circulation has compensated for the closure of the ICA and reestablishment of ICA flow may result in hyperemia with hemorrhage.[111,112,119]

Both approaches, surgical and endovascular, have advantages and disadvantages. Surgery is associated with a greater of risk of myocardial infarction, DVT, and pulmonary embolism as well as the complications associated with general anesthesia, including intubation, the systemic effects of muscle relaxants and anesthesia, and

pneumonia. Although carotid endarterectomy may be performed under local anesthesia, general anesthesia is more common (Figure 23-19).[15,40,42]

In endarterectomy, the artery distal to the stenosis is temporarily clamped to protect the brain from embolic material. Similarly protective filters and occlusive balloons are used during angioplasty and stenting to prevent embolism. The surgical incision in carotid endarterectomy may injure cutaneous and cranial nerves, result in hematoma formation with life-threatening tracheal compression, or become infected.[40,42]

In contrast, angioplasty with stenting is usually performed under local anesthesia and conscious sedation.[42] Angioplasty with stenting carries the usual risks of angiography. In addition, plaque debris may extrude through the struts of the stent during placement and is

---

[*]References 15, 40, 42, 111, 112, 159, 267.

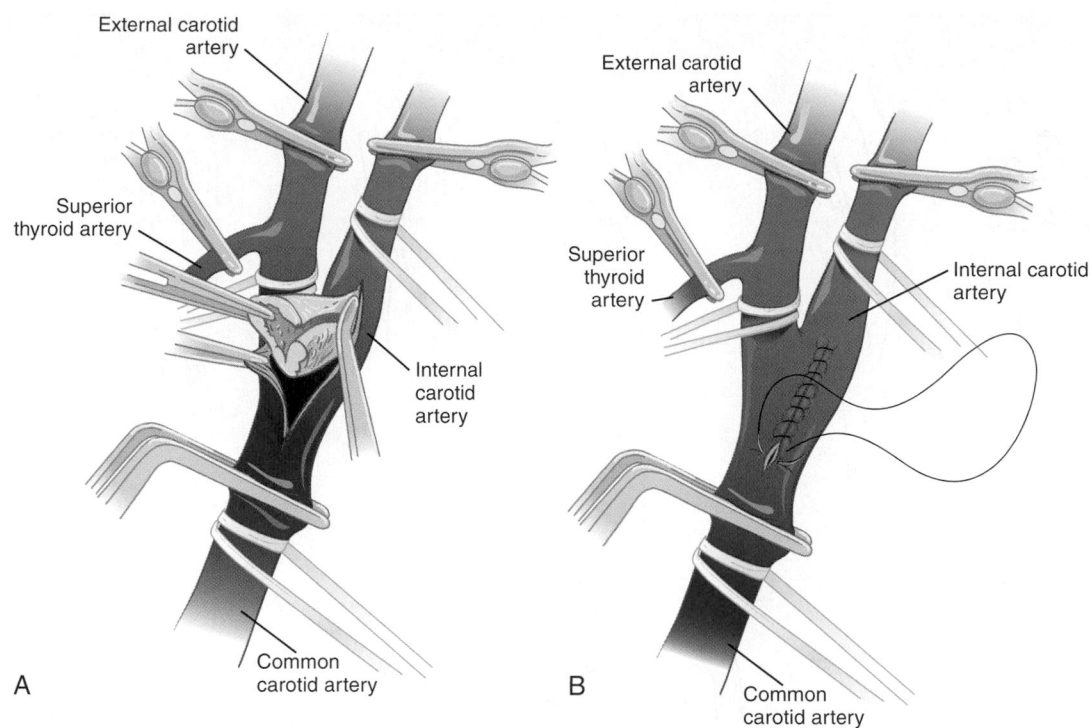

✦FIGURE 23-19 Cross-clamping with carotid endarterectomy **A,** Dissection of plaque within the common carotid artery with extension into the internal carotid artery. **B,** Carotid artery closure following plaque removal.

potentially thrombogenic until endothelium covers the stent. Restenosis is more common after angioplasty with stenting than with carotid endarterectomy, and the long-term efficacy of endovascular therapy is not known.[40,42] Drug-eluting carotid stents are now available and may deter restenosis. Similar to the drug-eluting stents used in interventional cardiology, carotid stents are covered with a polymer that releases antiplatelet, antithrombotic, or antiproliferative agents, such as paclitaxel (Taxol), to reduce stenosis.[265] Following angioplasty with stenting, the patient may be placed on a heparin or abciximab (ReoPro) infusion and then discharged home on aspirin or clopidogrel (Figure 23-20).[42]

An extracranial-intracranial (EC-IC) bypass of the anterior circulation may be successfully performed for selected patients with such conditions as moyamoya disease.[305,342] Most often a branch of the superficial temporal artery (STA) is anastomosed to a branch of the MCA to provide blood flow distal to the ICA occlusion (Figure 23-21). Complications include ischemic or hemorrhagic stroke.[119] Immediate postoperative care may include positioning the patient on the side opposite the bypass to avoid compromising flow and auscultation of blood flow over the temporal area with a Doppler to assess patency.[119]

Revascularization procedures may also be performed to restore blood flow to the posterior circulation when pharmacologic therapy, including antiplatelet agents,

has failed. Treatment options such as vertebrobasilar angioplasty and stenting, endarterectomy, arterial reimplantation, and EC-IC bypass may be performed. The STA, occipital artery, and external carotid artery can be used to increase blood flow to the superior cerebellar artery, PCA, posterior inferior cerebellar artery, and anterior inferior cerebellar artery.[60]

Malignant MCA infarction may result in refractory increased intracranial pressure and herniation.[295] If the increased ICP cannot be treated with the usual mannitol, furosemide, HTS, or barbiturate coma, a craniectomy or a decompressive craniotomy with removal of infarcted brain may be life-saving. However, if delayed, such heroic surgical efforts may not result in an improved quality of life.[51,99,246,259] Prophylactic anticonvulsants are not recommended with acute ischemic stroke. However, seizures must be treated emergently with a benzodiazepine and long term with an anticonvulsant.[46,90]

Anticoagulation with intravenous heparin followed by oral Coumadin has not been shown to be effective after an AIS (Level I evidence) with the exception of cardioembolic sources such as mechanical valves or atrial fibrillation or CVT.* In addition to diet and drug interactions, compliance, gender, and ethnicity/race may affect prothrombin time/International Normalized Ratio (PT/INR) levels.[82] The goal INR for prevention of

---

*References 1, 2, 22, 95, 192, 234, 248, 292.

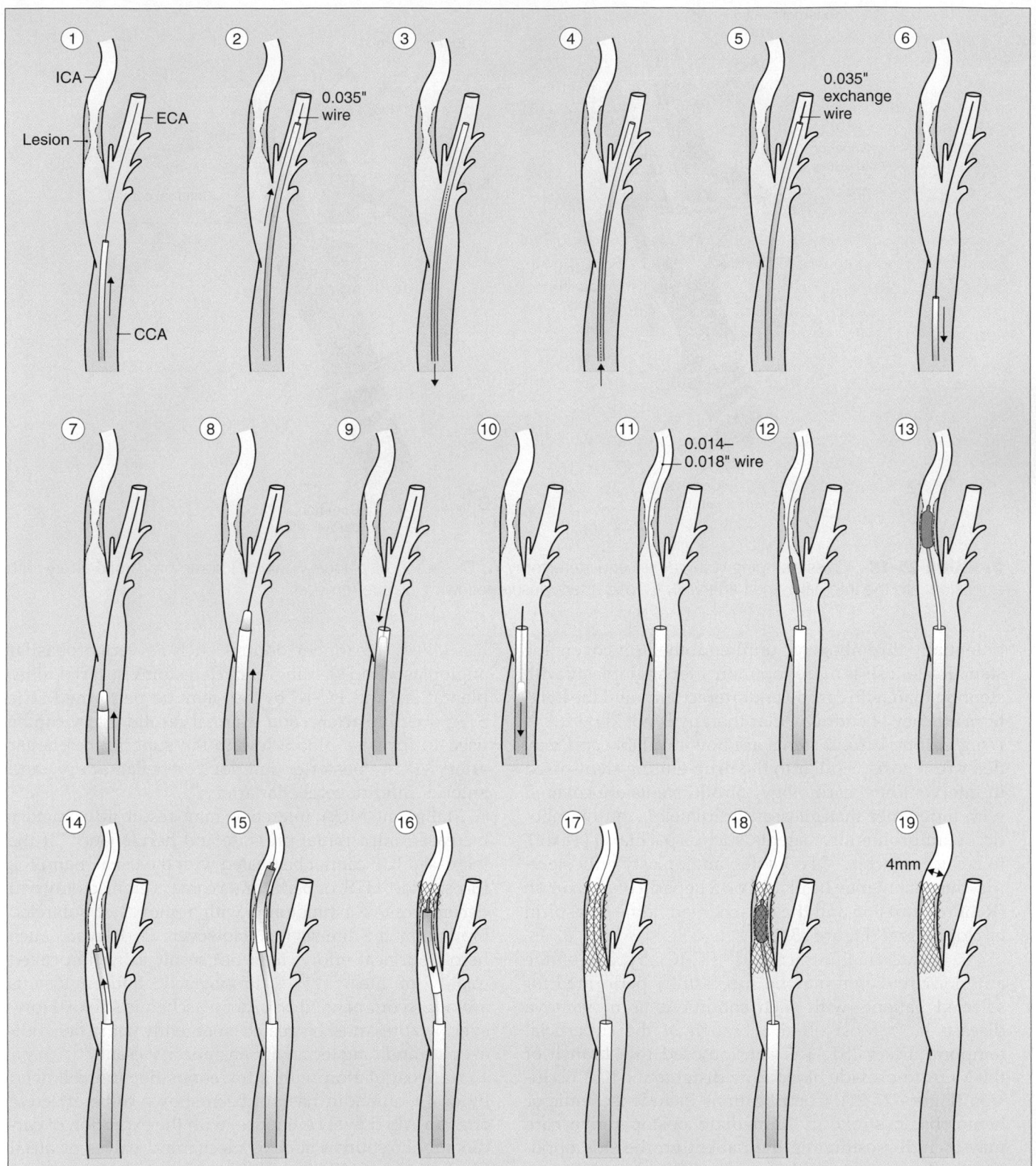

♦FIGURE 23-20 Placement of a carotid stent. *12* and *13*, An angioplasty balloon is advanced across the lesion and inflated. *14*, The balloon is removed. *15*, The stent is advanced over the wire, across the lesion. *16*, Following positioning, the stent is unsheathed. *17*, Completed stent deployment. *18*, Post-stent angioplasty is performed to remove any remaining areas of in-stent stenosis. *19*, Final view showing the carotid following stent-assisted angioplasty.

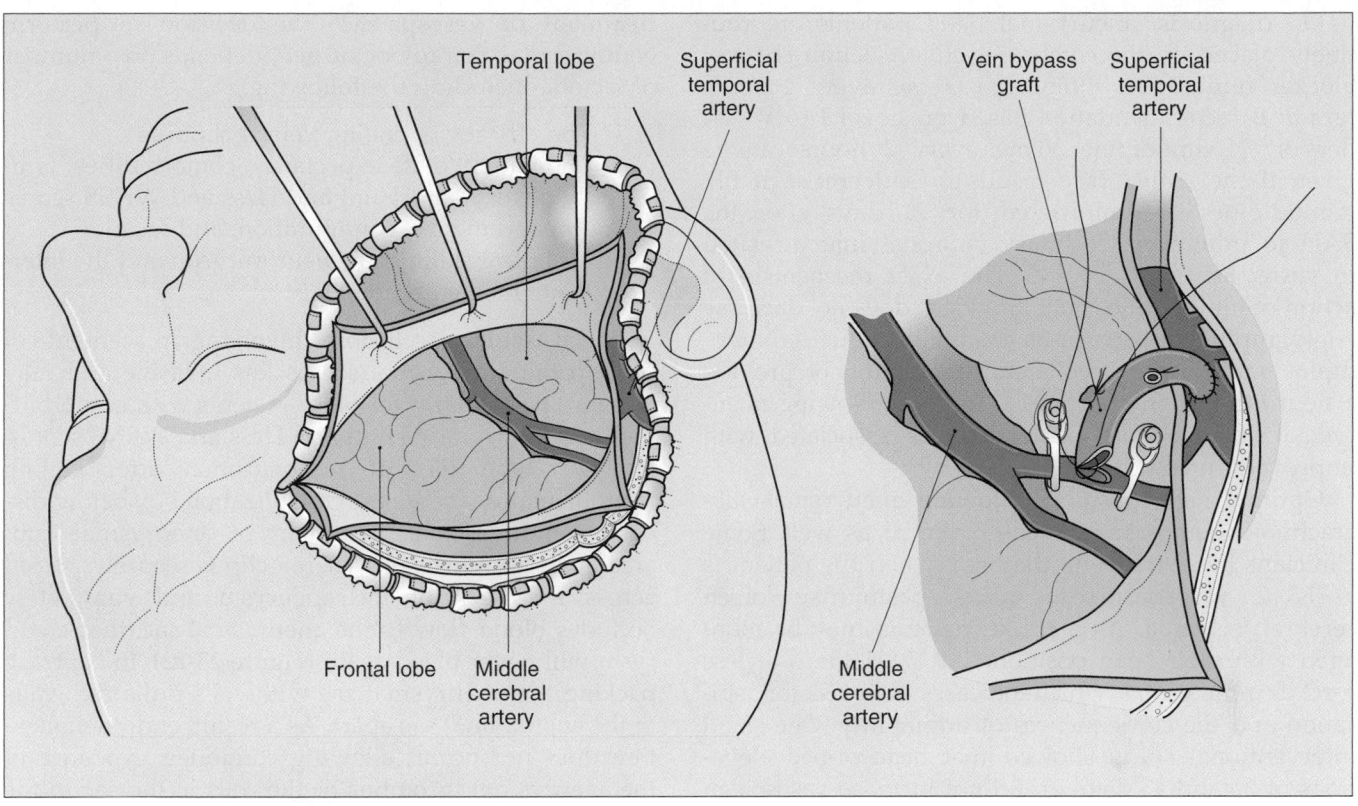

⇕FIGURE 23-21 Superficial temporal artery to middle cerebral artery bypass technique.

cardioembolic stroke related to atrial fibrillation and bio-prosthetic valves is 2.0 to 3.0, or 2.5.[1,2,210] The target INR for patients with mechanical heart valves is 2.5 to 3.5, or 3.0.[1,2,210] Attaining and maintaining a therapeutic PT/INR is not straightforward.[275] Patient and family education is critical. Following ischemic stroke, antiplatelet therapy with aspirin, an aspirin and dipyridamole combination (Aggrenox), clopidogrel (Plavix), or aspirin and clopidogrel is generally prescribed.[267,276] The combined use of clopidogrel and aspirin increases the risk of hemorrhage.[266,267]

Subarachnoid Hemorrhage

Following rupture, aneurysmal SAH patients are at risk for rebleed, hydrocephalus, seizures, and vasospasm.[256] Blood in the subarachnoid space and ventricles frequently impairs the reabsorption of CSF, resulting in hydrocephalus. Placement of an external ventricular device (EVD), a ventriculostomy, for hydrocephalus frequently results in an improvement in neurologic status. EVDs remain the gold standard for intracranial pressure monitoring and allow for CSF drainage.[3,18,140,198,250] Overdrainage, generally not more than 20 to 25 ml/hr, must be avoided. Particularly in the setting of an unrepaired aneurysm, overdrainage may result in rebleeding by dramatically lowering the ICP and altering the pressure across the arterial wall.[18,140] Studies are currently being conducted to investigate the utility of cisternal irrigation via a ventriculostomy and whether the use of a lumbar drain to remove additional blood will decrease vasospasm.[162,250,311]

Infection is a significant complication of external ventricular drainage. Sterile technique at the time of insertion, dressing and drainage bag change, and sampling of CSF is essential. Tunneling of the drain at the insertion site and prophylactic intravenous antibiotics are also thought to be beneficial.[109]

Before repair of the ruptured aneurysm, noxious stimuli must be minimized as much as possible to avoid elevations in BP that may contribute to rebleeding.[18,198] Before endovascular coiling or surgical resection with clipping, the BP must be modestly reduced and sudden increases and decreases in BP avoided.[58,62] Current AHA/ASA guidelines do not include specific parameters for BP management before surgical clipping or coil embolization.[198] Updated guidelines are currently being developed.[60] A maximum systolic BP of 140 to 160 mm Hg is recommended as the upper limit by some clinicians.[23,58,166,190]

On diagnosis, aneurysmal SAH patients are routinely placed on the cerebroselective calcium channel blocker nimodipine (Nimotop) 60 mg every 4 hours (grade B recommendation based on Level I to V evidence).[198] Nimodipine 30 mg every 2 hours can be given if the larger dose results in a decrease in BP. Nimodipine is administered for 21 days after the SAH to minimize secondary neuronal injury related to vasospasm.[18,140,191,313,330] The exact mechanism of action of nimodipine is not known; it does not decrease angiographic vasospasm as originally thought. Nimodipine may improve collateral circulation or provide a neuroprotective effect.[190,330] Its use following aneurysmal subarachnoid hemorrhage is associated with improved outcomes.[223,258]

Optimal head position following aneurysmal subarachnoid hemorrhage is controversial as well. Some clinicians believe raising the head when the patient is at risk for vasospasm, or is in vasospasm, may worsen cerebral ischemia. As a result, patients may be managed with their head positioned at 30 degrees or less for 2 or more weeks, which increases their risk for aspiration and the consequences of immobility. One small interventional study showed that head-of-bed elevations of 20 and 45 degrees did not increase vasospasm or cause neurologic deterioration. However, additional research is needed.[29]

The use of prophylactic anticonvulsants after SAH is controversial. The risk of SAH-related seizures has been reported to be as high as 25% with many, if not most, occurring at the time of the initial hemorrhage.[253] Anticonvulsants are given to minimize the risk of the deleterious intracranial and systemic effects of a seizure or status epilepticus, including rebleed and increased ICP.[200] However, no research has been published that refutes or substantiates the value of prophylactic anticonvulsants after SAH.[3,166,198] If anticonvulsants are prescribed, phenytoin (Dilantin) is commonly used. A loading dose of 1000 mg or higher is typical. Phenytoin is protein-bound, and both free and total levels may be monitored for therapeutic efficacy. Administration of intravenous phenytoin is associated with hypotension and bradycardia. Purple glove syndrome may occur when phenytoin is given peripherally. Extravasation of dilantin into a limb may result in tissue necrosis, ischemia, and possibly loss of the extremity. Fosphenytoin (Cerebyx), a phenytoin prodrug, may be preferable for peripheral intravenous administration because it is less likely to injure local tissues. A rare but potentially fatal side effect of phenytoin and fosphenytoin is Stevens-Johnson syndrome.[135,280]

Early surgical resection of the aneurysm with placement of a clip, or coil embolization with or without stenting, is standard practice to allow more aggressive treatment of vasospasm.* The decision to perform endovascular therapy or surgery depends on a number of factors, including the following:

1. The efficacy of coiling versus clipping
2. The patient's life expectancy, comorbidities, family history, and Hunt and Hess and WFNS scores
3. Aneurysm size, configuration, and location
4. Technical skills of the neurosurgeon and the interventional neuroradiologist[35,145]

Endovascular occlusion, involving placement of coils in the aneurysmal sac, is less invasive and may be safer, particularly for older patients with comorbidities and poor grade Hunt and Hess and WFNS scores. However, the risk of recanalization after coiling is problematic. The Research Utilization box below discusses endovascular treatment of aneurysmal subarachnoid hemorrhage. When a clip is securely placed across the neck of the aneurysm and completely occludes blood flow to the aneurysmal sac, that aneurysm will never bleed again (Figure 23-22). In contrast, packing the aneurysmal sac with coils pulls the walls of the aneurysmal sac apart. As a result, endothelialization does not occur, allowing continued exposure of the aneurysmal thrombus or the coils in the sac to the circulating blood. The coils may compress and compartmentalize, allowing blood to flow around their periphery into the aneurysmal sac. This recanalization of the aneurysm makes the patient vulnerable to the possibility of rebleed because blood flow to the aneurysmal sac is no longer blocked by the coils.[35]

*References 110, 137, 145, 183, 247, 284.

▲ RESEARCH UTILIZATION

Endovascular Treatment of Aneurysmal Subarachnoid Hemorrhage

CLINICAL ISSUE

Though far less common than ischemic stroke, the loss of potential life years from aneurysmal subarachnoid hemorrhage before the age of 65 years is comparable. Early repair of the ruptured aneurysm is necessary to prevent rebleed and to allow aggressive therapy of vasospasm. A craniotomy with placement of an aneurysm clip or endovascular coiling may be performed. However, endovascular coiling is a newer option that has not been thoroughly substantiated as superior, comparable, or inferior to surgical repair. An open craniotomy allows for removal of blood and clot around the vasculature; however, endovascular coiling is less traumatic. Endovascular coiling may not provide protection from further rebleeding.

SUMMARY

A prospective randomized trial including 42 neurosurgical centers and 2143 patients demonstrated a greater independent survival from endovascular coiling at 1 year than surgical clipping. This benefit continued for up to 7 years. The risk of rebleed was slightly more common after endovascular coiling than surgical clipping. The risk of seizures was significantly lower in the patients who were treated with coils.

APPLICATION

Aneurysmal subarachnoid hemorrhage patients may now be treated surgically or endovascularly. Endovascular treatment now provides an option for individuals who cannot undergo general anesthesia and craniotomy related to other morbidities. However, just like craniotomy with application of an aneurysm clip, endovascular treatment may not be possible for all aneurysms. Outcomes utilizing either procedure are highly dependent on the physician's skill and the patient's clinical condition before the aneurysm repair.

NEED FOR FURTHER STUDY

Long-term protection from additional bleeding using endovascular coiling is not known at this time. Patients with endovascular coiling need long-term follow-up.

Johnston, S.C., et al. (2002). Recommendations for the endovascular treatment of intracranial aneurysms. A statement of healthcare professionals from the Committee on Cerebrovascular Imaging of American Heart Association Council on Cardiovascular Radiology. *Stroke, 33*(10), 2536–2544.

Molyneux, A. J., et al. (2005). International Subarachnoid Aneurysm Trial (ISAT) of neurosurgical clipping versus endovascular coiling in 2143 patients with ruptured intracranial aneurysms: a randomized comparison of effects on survival, dependency, seizures, rebleeding, subgroups, and aneurysm occlusion. *Lancet, 366*(9488), 809–817.

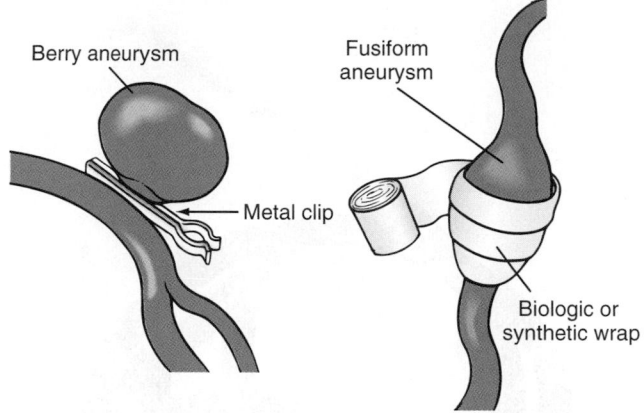

⬦FIGURE 23-22   Aneurysm clipping.

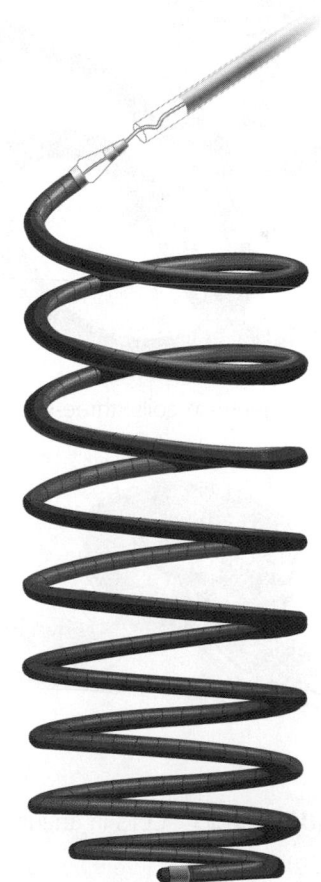

⬦FIGURE 23-23   Aneurysm coils: microcoil.

Placement of coils in the sac of the aneurysm may be performed with general anesthesia or conscious sedation.[33,35] Coils come in various configurations (Figures 23-23 and 23-24). Consideration must be given to the size of the aneurysm, the configuration, and the dome-to-neck ratio before coiling is performed. A small neck, a small dome size, and a large dome-to-neck ratio are optimal for coiling.[35] Several coils may be placed into the aneurysmal sac to prevent rebleed.[31] Placement of a stent at the neck of the aneurysm may prevent migration of coils and lessen the possibility of rebleed (Figure 23-25).[35]

If clipping or coiling of the aneurysm is not possible and collateral circulation is adequate, the parent vessel may be sacrificed by surgical ligation or embolization to prevent rebleed. Before permanently occluding the parent artery surgically or in interventional neuroradiology, blood flow through that vessel may be temporarily stopped utilizing an endovascular balloon during cerebral angiography to determine collateral flow. The patient remains awake and is assessed during the balloon occlusion test so that any neurologic deterioration will be detected.[315]

Patients with SAH may benefit from multimodality monitoring, including ICP, CPP measurement, btO_2, brain temperature, $SjvO_2$ as a measure of global oxygenation, and, ideally, daily TCD to quantify

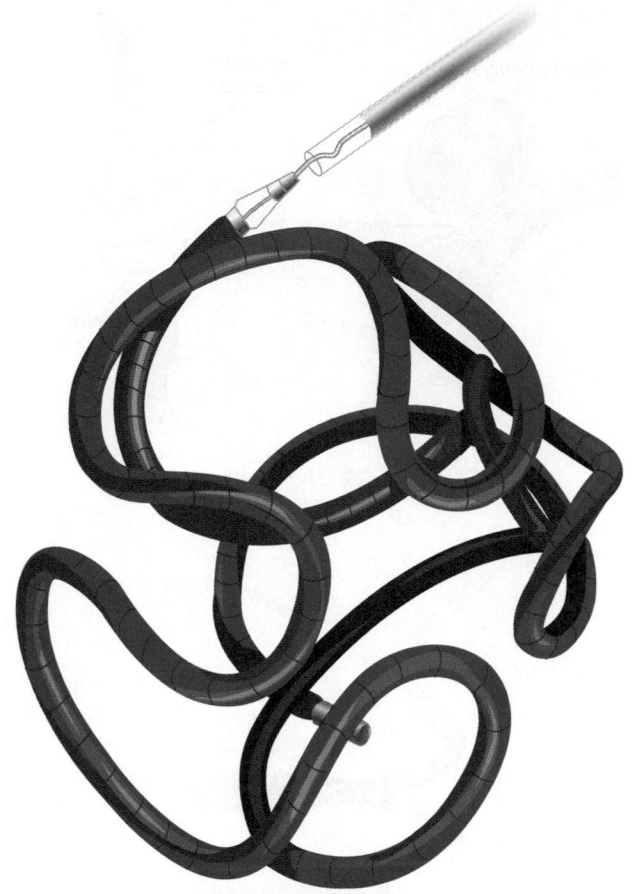

FIGURE 23-24 Aneurysm coils: three-dimensional spherical coils.

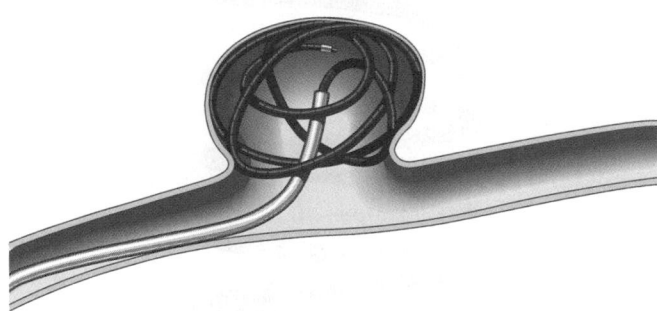

FIGURE 23-25 Coils in aneurysm.

vasospasm.[140,190,208,288] Sensitivity and specificity for middle cerebral artery vasospasm are high; however, they are less so for the other vessels.[121,197] Diagnosis of MCA vasospasm requires measurement of the MFV not only of the MCA but also of the ICA to determine the MCA/ICA ratio. Abnormally high values for grading the severity of the vasospasm in the circle of Willis vessels vary in the literature. Generally, MCA MFV values of 120 cm/sec or greater and MCA/ICA ratios of 3 or greater indicate vasospasm. MCA values of greater than 200 cm/sec and MCA/ICA ratios of

greater than 6 are considered severe vasospasm of the MCA (Figure 23-26).[121,190,197,283,334]

Clinical signs and symptoms of vasospasm correlate with the functional area supplied by the constricted vessel(s) and may be subtle or profound. Extremity weakness, for example, may range from pronator drift to complete paralysis. Vasospasm typically begins after day 3 but may continue for a total of 3 or 4 weeks.[184,190,247,258] The peak incidence of vasospasm is approximately days 5 through 14 after the hemorrhage.[184,190,247,330] Hypervolemic hemodilution with or without controlled hypertension therapy (HHH) (Table 23-11) is routinely used in the treatment of vasospasm despite the lack of evidence regarding its benefit.[257] The rationale for HHH therapy is based on the brain's impaired autoregulatory status after SAH. The CBF is passively dependent on the mean arterial pressure (MAP). By increasing the intravascular volume, diluting the blood, and increasing the systemic BP, an adequate MAP and CBF may be achieved to prevent secondary ischemia and infarct associated with vasospasm.[183,184] However, a prospective randomized controlled multicenter trial has yet to be published to substantiate the value of HHH therapy in improving

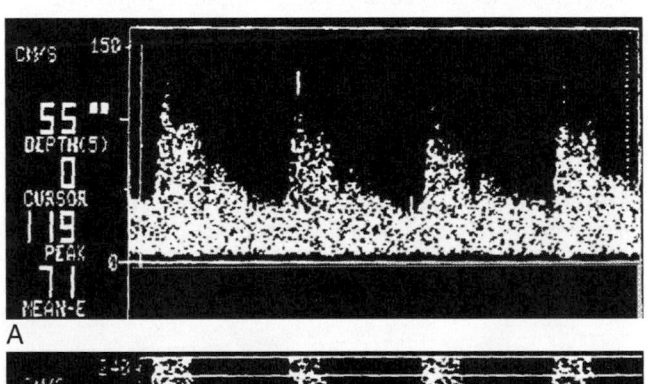

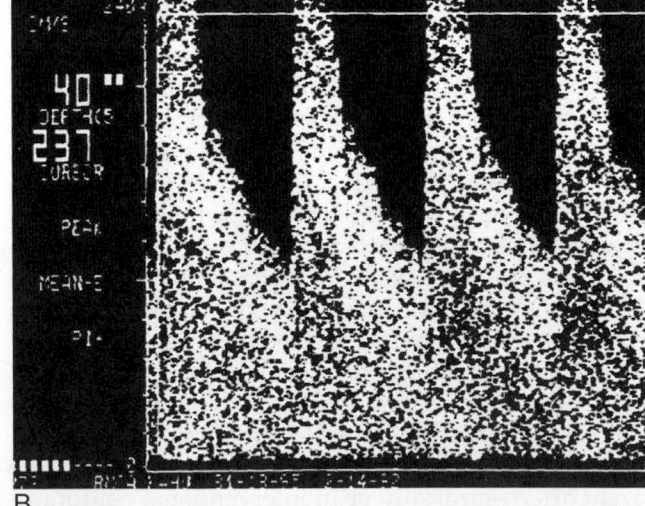

FIGURE 23-26 Transcranial Doppler showing severe vasospasm.

TABLE 23-11 Hypervolemic Hemodilution Therapy, With or Without Controlled Hypertension*

PROBLEM	INTERVENTION	RATIONALE	EXPECTED OUTCOME	COMMENTS
At risk for secondary neuronal injury related to cerebral vasospasm	Hemodilution with crystalloids will also result in a decrease in hematocrit and hemoglobin	Decreased RBCs in blood will enhance flow through constricted vessels	Maintain hematocrit and hemoglobin at approximately 30% and 10 gm/dl, respectively	Crystalloid of choice is normal saline Albumin or plasma fractionate is used as the colloid
	Controlled hypertension with vasopressors (such as Neo-Synephrine, dopamine, norepinephrine, or dobutamine)	Pharmacologic augmentation of BP facilitates flow through cerebral vessels with impaired autoregulation	Attain/maintain prescribed BP (systolic or mean arterial BP) such as systolic BP 140–160 mm Hg (mild vasospasm); 160–180 mm Hg (moderate vasospasm); and 180–200 mm Hg (severe vasospasm)	

From references 36, 163, 263, 278, 302, 332, 336.
*Use cautiously if unsecured aneurysms are present.
BP = Blood pressure, RBC = red blood cell.

outcomes, and the pharmacologic agents and the parameters used vary from publication to publication (Level III-V evidence).[190,264,278,302,332] At a minimum, the patient must maintain euvolemia if not hypervolemia.[190] If HHH therapy is used, in addition to intra-arterial BP monitoring, central venous pressure (CVP) or pulmonary artery pressure monitoring is recommended to assess the patient's hemodynamic status and guide management.[190,198] Goal parameters are generally related to the degree of vasospasm.[184,190,198] For example, following surgical clipping or endovascular coiling, the target parameters in mild vasospasm might be the following: systolic BP 140–160 mm Hg, CVP 8–10 mm Hg, or pulmonary artery wedge pressure (PAWP) 12–14 mm Hg; in moderate vasospasm, systolic BP 160–180 mm Hg, CVP 10–12 mm Hg, or PAWP 14–16 mm Hg; and in severe vasospasm, systolic BP 180–200 mm Hg, CVP 12–14 mm Hg, or PAWP 16–18 mm Hg.* Normal saline is the typical crystalloid used. The colloids are albumin and plasma fractionate (Plasmanate). Hetastarch (Hespan) is avoided because its use may result in coagulopathy.[135,280] Crystalloids and colloid solutions are used in variable amounts. The vasopressor of choice may be phenylephrine (Neo-Synephrine), dopamine (Intropin), norepinephrine (Levophed), and even dobutamine (Dobutrex) (see Chapter 41). Phenylephrine is usually the first choice because it is an alpha agonist and thought to work primarily on extracranial vasculature to increase flow to vasospastic cerebral vessels and minimize risk of secondary infarction.[135,190,278,280,336]

Dopamine may result in unacceptable tachycardia. To evaluate effectiveness, dobutamine is ideally used with a pulmonary artery catheter with continuous cardiac output measurement capability.[278,285,303,313,336] All are ideally administered through a central venous catheter to prevent injury to peripheral tissues.[135,280] Since approximately 20% to 30% of patients with intracranial aneurysms have more than one aneurysm,[80,147,244,313] clinicians must be cognizant of this in regard to the risk of increasing BP to treat vasospasm.

SAH patients are at high risk for hyponatremia, more often thought to be related to cerebral salt wasting (CSW) rather than syndrome of inappropriate antidiuretic hormone (SIADH). The mechanism by which SAH leads to CSW is not completely understood. Central nervous system (CNS)–mediated input to the kidneys is thought to be impaired as a result of the SAH, and atrial and brain natriuretic peptides are released, resulting in hypovolemia, hemoconcentration, and hyponatremia.[75,130,252]

As serum sodium level drops, patients are also at increased risk for seizures below 125 mEq/L, and hyponatremia may impair the patient's level of consciousness.[18,75,130] Supplemental enteral salt may be given as well as fludrocortisone (Florinef) to increase the serum sodium level and maintain a balanced to positive fluid status.[313] Free water is restricted and saline is used to flush feeding tubes.[75] HTS of varying percentages may be given to increase the serum sodium level as well as decrease intracranial pressure,[18,75,130,313] although large human studies demonstrating efficacy have not been published at this time. Rapid correction of

*References 18, 140, 184, 190, 198, 302, 330.

hyponatremia may result in central pontine myelinolysis. Therefore the serum sodium should not be corrected more rapidly than 10 mEq/L in a 24-hour time period.[18] Hypervolemia and HTS may already push a patient prone to neurogenic pulmonary edema or acute respiratory distress syndrome into additional pulmonary compromise.[227]

In contrast, SIADH is the CNS-mediated release of excess antidiuretic hormone (ADH) or increased renal sensitivity to ADH, resulting in hypervolemia and hyponatremia.[75,130] Treatment for SIADH is fluid restriction, which is generally thought to be harmful to patients at risk for cerebral vasospasm (Level III-IV evidence) (Box 23-4).[198]

If nimodipine and HHH therapy are insufficient to prevent DIND related to vasospasm, selective cerebral angioplasty may be performed (Figure 23-27). However, distal vasospasm often cannot be reached without vessel injury, and intra-arterial vasodilators such as papaverine are injected into the vasospastic artery to open the vessel.[44,109,145,190,336] Cerebral angioplasty may be repeated, but sometimes once is all that is required. Unfortunately, the results of intra-arterial vasodilators are short-lived, generally lasting less than 24 hours.[44,190,336] Attention to the ICP is necessary during the intra-arterial injection of vasodilators because it may result in a massive cerebral vasodilation and a sudden rise in ICP, increasing the risk of hemorrhage or herniation.*

Recent studies in regard to vasospasm include the use of nicardipine implants, cisternal irrigation, hypermagnesemia, microdialysis, and the role of nitric oxide.* Nicardipine implants,[150] cisternal irrigation and intraventricular thrombolysis,[83] hypermagnesemia,[307] and nitric oxide[232,237,251,298] are intended to directly decrease vasospasm or protect the neurons from vasospasm-induced ischemia and infarction. Cisternal irrigation, intraventricular thrombolysis, and CSF drainage using a lumbar drain may assist in the removal of blood from the ventricles and around the blood vessels, which in turn may lessen vasospasm.[83,161,174,298] A nitric oxide deficiency may contribute to vasospasm. In two small studies, intrathecal administration of sodium nitroprusside, a nitric oxide donor, resulted in the prevention or reversal of severe vasospasm and improved outcomes.[237,251] In contrast, microdialysis is a monitoring modality aimed at analyzing biomarkers of cerebral ischemia in vasospasm, including pH, lactate-to-pyruvate ratio, and levels of lactate, pyruvate, and glutamate.[18,233,288]

In addition to neurologic interventions, many aneurysmal SAH patients will require intubation and mechanical ventilation associated with decreased level of consciousness, impaired respiratory effort, or neurogenic pulmonary edema.[18] They may also present with neurogenic dysrhythmias and 12-lead ECG changes suggestive of a myocardial infarction. ECG changes associated with aneurysmal SAH have been reported

---

*References 3, 18, 44, 109, 163, 190, 332.

*References 76, 134, 150, 233, 237, 251, 298.

Box 23-4

Differentiating Cerebral Salt Wasting and Syndrome of Inappropriate Antidiuretic Hormone

Cerebral Salt Wasting

Serum sodium level less than 135 mEq/L
Decreased extracellular fluid volume
Increased hematocrit
Increased plasma albumin concentration
Normal or increased serum potassium level
Normal or decreased plasma uric acid level
Increased blood urea nitrogen/creatinine level
Signs of dehydration:
    Orthostatic changes
    Flat neck veins
    Dry mucous membranes
    Poor skin turgor
    Tachycardia
    Weight loss
    Negative fluid balance
    Central venous pressure less than 6 mm Hg or
        pulmonary artery wedge pressure less than 8 mm Hg

Syndrome of Inappropriate Antidiuretic Hormone

Serum sodium level less than 135 mEq/L
Increased extracellular fluid volume
Normal hematocrit
Normal plasma albumin concentration
Normal serum potassium level
Decreased plasma uric acid level
Urine sodium level greater than 25 mEq/L
Serum osmolality less than 280 mOsm/L
Urine osmolality greater than serum osmolality
Decreased urine output (400–500 ml/24 hr)
Signs of hypervolemia:
    Increased body weight
    Elevated central venous pressure and
        pulmonary artery wedge pressure readings

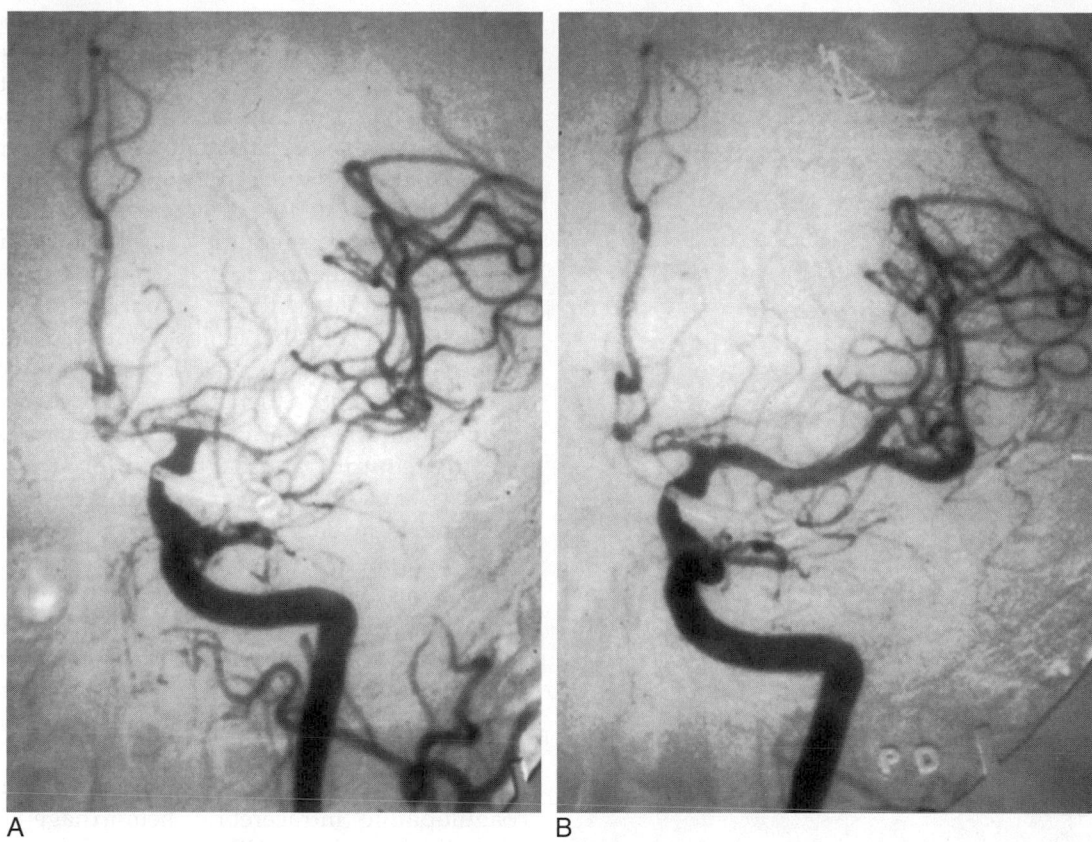

♦FIGURE 23-27 Angioplasty for vasospasm. **A,** Anteroposterior left internal carotid artery angiogram of a patient 5 days after subarachnoid hemorrhage, demonstrating severe spasm of the anterior cerebral and middle cerebral arteries. **B,** Same patient after balloon angioplasty, showing marked improvement in the middle cerebral artery size.

to occur from 50% to 100% of the time and include rhythm, P wave, repolarization, and conduction abnormalities and pathologic Q waves.[142,185,199,269] Disturbances in rhythm are usually benign and are treated only if the patient is hemodynamically compromised.[330,338] A cardiac workup may reveal actual coronary artery occlusion with infarction and abnormal CK-MB and troponin levels, but cardiac damage is more frequently the result of the catecholamine and sympathetic release at the time of the bleed.[212,308] Pathologic changes, though different from true myocardial ischemia, may occur with neurogenic cardiac injury and contribute to pulmonary edema, hypotension, and decreased cardiac output. The myocardium is referred to as "stunned,"[141] and the neurogenic-induced cardiac changes may reverse over time.*

Critical care management of AVMs, ruptured or unruptured, is similar to management of aneurysms. Patients with AVMs are also at risk for rebleed, seizures, vasospasm, and hydrocephalus. Definitive treatment of AVMs includes surgical resection, endovascular embolization, and radiosurgery.[56,239] Surgical resection alone

was the only definitive treatment for years, and complications were common, including hemorrhage during and after surgery, cerebral edema, and stroke. Endovascular therapy allows embolic agents (such as polyvinyl alcohol), detachable coils, or liquid polymer to be injected into the feeder arteries at the arteriovenous junction. This halts the flow of blood to the venous side of the AVM, where most AVM bleeding occurs. This procedure may also be conducted before surgical resection or radiosurgery to decrease circulation to the AVM and facilitate eradication of the AVM.[239] Stereotactic radiation, using gamma knife or linear accelerator with or without endovascular therapy, usually requires several treatments and a time span of up to 2 years before obliteration of the AVM (Figure 23-28).[56]

Aneurysmal or AVM SAH may be treated surgically or endovascularly during pregnancy using an abdominal shield during radiographic procedures. Treatment of the ruptured aneurysm or AVM hemorrhage to minimize the risk of rebleed should take precedence over obstetric concerns if the patient is not in labor and the fetus is not in distress.[282] However, the risk of using prophylactic anticonvulsants, nimodipine, and papaverine in pregnancy may outweigh the benefits.[282]

*References 20, 54, 55, 142, 152, 185, 208.

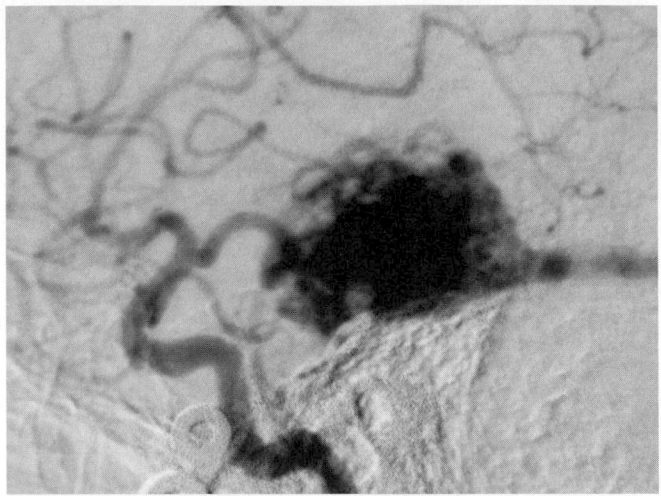

A

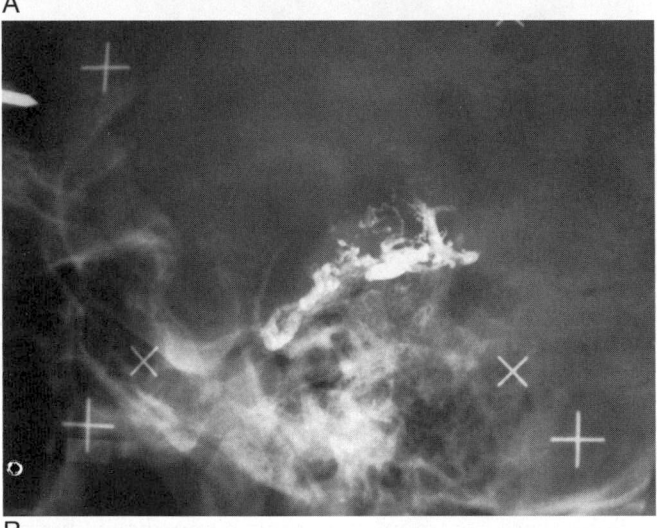

B

♦FIGURE 23-28 Arteriovenous malformation. **A,** Preoperative angiogram. **B,** After radiation and embolization.

Intracerebral Hemorrhage

As in aneurysmal SAH, the patient with ICH frequently presents with impaired level of consciousness and inability to protect the airway or inadequate respiratory effort. Also as in SAH, if the patient was found supine, aspiration is a concern.* ICH stroke patients may also present with neurogenic cardiac dysrhythmias and 12-lead ECG changes as well as neurally mediated pulmonary edema, and the initial cardiopulmonary workup/treatment is similar to that for SAH. ECG changes in patients with ICH have been less documented than those in SAH, but their incidence has been reported as high as 60% to 70%.[54,55,155,338] The most common ICH-related abnormalities are rhythm disturbances, QT prolongation, T wave inversion,

U waves, ST depression, and pathologic Q waves, and similar to the dysrhythmias and ECG changes associated with SAH, they are left untreated unless the patient is hemodynamically unstable.[54,55,155] ICH of the deep structures, such as the thalamus and basal ganglia or the posterior fossa, brain stem, or cerebellum, places the patient at increased risk of increased ICP and herniation, or respiratory arrest requiring emergency intubation and mechanical ventilation.*

ICH may occur with or without coagulopathy. If the patient with ICH is being given anticoagulants or antiplatelet agents, they must be discontinued immediately, even if the patient is at risk for cardioembolic events, until the neurologic condition has stabilized.[268] Patients requiring anticoagulation for atrial fibrillation are at less risk for cardioembolic events than those with mechanical cardiac valves.[84,96] If coagulopathy is present, it must be corrected as soon as possible. Fresh frozen plasma and vitamin K have been most commonly used to correct a coagulopathy. Prothrombin complex concentrate has also been used with some success, but availability is limited.[25,341] However, recombinant activated factor VII (rfVIIa [Novo-7]) may be more effective in correcting the coagulopathy than fresh frozen plasma and vitamin K and may even have a place in noncoagulopathic intracerebral hemorrhage.[90] Recombinant activated factor VII does not carry risk of blood transfusion reaction and does not require a large-volume administration; however, repeat administration may be necessary. Use of rfVIIa, particularly for use in noncoagulopathic ICH, is currently under study.†

Enlargement of the hematoma may be associated with hypertension; however, the optimal BP is not exactly known.[228,335,343] AHA/ASA guidelines for intracerebral hemorrhage were recently revised.[36] Previous guidelines recommended a MAP of less than 130 mm Hg or a systolic BP of less than 180 mm Hg.[36] Other clinicians recommended a 15% to 30% reduction in the patient's baseline MAP.[87,100,217] Evidence to support the recommendation of a specific BP threshold is contradictory. Current guidelines for intracerebral hemorrhage do not include a specific BP parameter.[36] Prescribed antihypertensives include hydralazine, labetalol, and nicardipine.[36,87,100,217]

Mannitol and furosemide are used to reduce intracranial pressure. Monitoring the ICP with a ventriculostomy allows drainage of CSF and blood (if ventricular extension of the hemorrhage has occurred). If the patient has a coagulopathy, it must be corrected before insertion of the ventriculostomy. Patients with supratentorial lesions may benefit from ICP/CPP monitoring and perhaps bto_2 monitoring in ICH.

---

*References 23, 36, 45, 87, 100, 140, 171, 230.

*References 36, 45, 87, 140, 143, 171, 230.

†References 27, 38, 91, 154, 191, 200, 338.

Anticonvulsant therapy is reasonable in lobar and especially cortical lesions.*

Medical versus surgical management is controversial.[154,300,301] Surgical management is generally considered appropriate in the young person with a moderate to large lobar hemorrhage and good GCS or early in a cerebellar hemorrhage before long-standing herniation (Level II-V evidence).[36,61,211] However, a craniotomy or blind aspiration to evacuate a deep hematoma may only worsen the patient's condition.[209] The International Surgical Treatment of ICH (ISTICH) study, a large multicenter prospective randomized controlled trial, was recently conducted comparing surgical with nonsurgical management of ICH. Surgery was not found to be more beneficial than medical management; however, the study had several design flaws.[209] New, less invasive surgical techniques have been developed and may improve outcomes. Current surgical procedures under investigation include endoscopic hematoma evacuation using ultrasound and laser coagulation; stereotactic endoscopic ultrasonic aspiration; and stereotactic aspiration with thrombolytics used at the clot.[†] When anticoagulation administration should be restarted is controversial. AHA/ASA guidelines recommend 2 to 4 weeks after the ICH before restarting anticoagulation.[268,276]

An aggressive approach to the management of the patient with ICH may result in better outcomes. Care of the critically ill ICH patient in a designated neuroscience critical care unit has been associated with improved outcomes.[72] In contrast, if the ICH patient is managed in an environment where some diagnoses are promptly associated with "do not resuscitate" (DNR) status, attempts to aggressively treat the sequelae of ICH may be viewed as futile and the resulting outcome poor. In one study, the single most important factor in regard to an ICH patient's outcome was the hospital's percentage of all patients with DNR orders. The higher the hospital's percentage of all patients with DNR orders, the higher the mortality rate for patients with ICH.[132]

EVIDENCE-BASED CARE

The AHA/ASA has published practice guidelines and advisory statements on the prevention, diagnosis, acute management, and rehabilitation of stroke for more than 20 years. Several of these guidelines have been referenced in this chapter. At this time, nearly 30 guidelines exist.[‡] These documents are evidence-based

consensus statements from task force experts who have reviewed the current evidence. Many of these guidelines include the grade of the recommendation and the level of the evidence.*

---

*References 1, 2, 4, 9, 36, 77, 112, 145, 183, 198, 267.

◆ Case Study 23-1, Part B

Cerebrovascular Disorders

Mrs. S.P. became increasingly sleepy after admission (GCS 13). A CT scan revealed hydrocephalus, and she underwent a bedside ventriculostomy. The patient's initial ICP with insertion of the ventriculostomy was 25 mm Hg. The ICP stabilized around 15 mm Hg, with the ventriculostomy set to drain at 15 mm Hg and an hourly output around 5–10 ml/hr. Within 24 hours she underwent a craniotomy for clipping of the left MCA aneurysm. Surgical resection with clipping of the aneurysm was chosen over embolization with Guglielmi detachable coils by the patient. The neurosurgeon explained both procedures to her and her family and together they decided to proceed with the craniotomy with clipping. The long-term possibility of recanalization of the aneurysm after coiling and the subsequent risk for another SAH in the future were worrisome to Mrs. S.P., and she had no other major organ dysfunction that would increase her surgical risk. Once the aneurysm was secured, the patient was encouraged to cough and deep breathe every 1–2 hours to improve her atelectasis. Her legs were wrapped with sequential compression devices on admission to neuroscience critical care. However, prophylactic subcutaneous heparin was not started until 24 hours after surgery to minimize bleeding.

By day 7 post SAH, daily TCDs were reflecting increasing vasospasm, not only in the left MCA but also in the right MCA as well. The left MCA mean flow velocity and MCA/ICA ratio were 178 cm/sec and 4.2, respectively; the right MCA mean flow velocity and MCA/ICA ratio were 152 cm/sec and 3.6, respectively. Mrs. S.P. required gentle shaking to arouse for orientation questions, and her answers were slower than they had been earlier; she was having difficulty with stating her age (NIHSS 2) and performing simple mathematical calculations. She would not use the incentive spirometer despite the nurse's coaching. The pupils remained unequal, with the right 3 mm and the left 4 mm. The left pupil was sluggish. Her GCS was 13. However, at that time she was moving all four extremities without focal weakness. Her vital signs were stable with a temperature of 37.2° C (98.8° F), heart rate 80 beats/min (sinus rhythm), respirations 20 breaths/min, and BP 156/80 mm Hg.

Decision point: What clinical signs and symptoms indicated the need for HHH therapy?

Case continues on page 628

Case Study 23-1, Part C

Cerebrovascular Disorders

A pulmonary artery catheter was inserted and HHH therapy started, utilizing normal saline and albumin fluid boluses and phenylephrine. The target parameters for the systolic BP were 180 mm Hg and 16 mm Hg for the PAWP. On day 10, her left MCA mean flow velocities on TCD increased to 220 cm/sec with MCA/ICA ratio 6.2, she remained sleepy and could not state her age, and she had developed right upper extremity pronator drift, right lower facial paralysis, and slight slurring of her speech (GCS 13, NIHSS 5) despite nimodipine and HHH therapy. Mrs. S.P.'s systolic BP parameter was increased to 200 mm Hg, and a goal PAWP of 18 mm Hg was ordered.

Angiography revealed severe MCA vasospasm, left greater than right, and she underwent angioplasty of the left MCA with interarterial papaverine injection of the right MCA and left ACA. The following day her left MCVs had decreased to 156 cm/sec with a ratio of 3.6, she no longer had a RUE pronator drift, and she had only mild right lower facial weakness and dysarthria. She was awake, alert and oriented, and following commands (GCS 15, NIHSS 2). Mrs. S.P. continued to improve over the next week, and HHH therapy was continued until day 13. Once her vasospasm had decreased to the mild range and her neurologic assessments and vital signs were stable, the phenylephrine and then fluid boluses were weaned off. Physical, occupational, and speech therapy were asked to evaluate and treat Mrs. S.P. as needed. Her ventriculostomy was raised to 20 mm Hg on day 14 and clamped on day 15. She remained neurologically stable, and the drain was removed on day 16. Mrs. S.P. was transferred to the progressive neurologic unit on day 16. She was discharged home on day 21.

Decision point: What signs and symptoms would indicate that Mrs. S.P. is not tolerating raising and clamping of the ventriculostomy?

ETHICAL CONSIDERATIONS

Many critically ill patients with stroke have a poor prognosis. Regardless of the clinicians' best efforts, the primary injury may be too devastating to restore a quality life. Some patients may present on admission or within the next few hours or days as brain dead. Often, however, when to consider withdrawal of life support or "do not attempt to resuscitate" status is not clear cut and is emotionally laden for both clinicians and family. Neurologic assessment tools have been shown to be of some help in predicting outcome. A GCS less than 8, Hunt-Hess grades IV–V, and an NIHSS greater than 16, for example, are associated with poor prognosis.[49,53,69,172,328] However,

some stroke patients improve unexpectedly if aggressive care with a proactive multidisciplinary approach to the prevention of secondary neuronal injury and the sequelae of stroke is undertaken.[328,340]

CONCLUSIONS

Stroke is a heterogeneous disease with many clinical presentations as well as variable outcomes. A number of pharmacologic agents and technologies are available today that were not available 20 years ago to enhance care. In addition, more is known today about stroke than was known previously. However, none of these advances are of value if they are not utilized by knowledgeable, skilled, and caring clinicians, especially and including the critical care or progressive care nurse. The acute/critical care nurse is key in the assessment, planning, intervention, and evaluation of care.

REFERENCES

1. Adams, H. P., et al. (2003). Guidelines for the early management with acute ischemic stroke. A scientific statement from the Stroke Council of the American Stroke Association. *Stroke, 34*(4), 1056–1083.
2. Adams, H., et al. (2005). Guidelines for the early management of patients with ischemic stroke: 2005 update. A scientific statement from the Stroke Council of the American Heart Association/ American Stroke Association. *Stroke, 36*(4), 916–923.
3. Adams, H. P., & Davis, P. H. (2004). Aneurysmal subarachnoid hemorrhage. In J. P. Mohr, et al. (Eds.), *Stroke: pathophysiology, diagnosis and management* (4th ed.). Philadelphia: Churchill Livingstone.
4. Adams, R., et al. (2002). Recommendations for improving the quality of care through stroke centers and systems: an examination of stroke identification options: multidisciplinary consensus recommendations from the Advisory Working Group on Stroke Center Identification Options of the American Stroke Association. *Stroke, 33*(1), e1–e7.
5. Albano, C., Comandante, L., & Nolan, S. (2005). Innovations in the management of cerebral injury. *Crit Care Nurs Q, 28*(2), 135–149.
6. Alexander, S., et al. (2005). Apolipoprotein E genotype in the subarachnoid hemorrhage. *Nurs Health Sci, 7*(2), 143–144.
7. American Heart Association and American Stroke Association. (2006). Stroke and stroke in children. *Heart disease and stroke statistics: 2006 update.* (pp. 14–17). Dallas, Tex: American Stroke Association/American Heart Association.
8. American Heart Association. (2004). Stroke. *ACLS provider manual.* Dallas, Tex: American Heart Association.
9. American Heart Association and American Stroke Association. (2004). Statins after ischemic stroke and transient ischemic attack. An advisory statement from the Stroke Council, American Heart Association and the American Stroke Association. *Stroke, 35*(4), 1023.
10. Andrews, C. O., & Engelhard, H. H. (2001). Fibrinolytic therapy in intraventricular hemorrhage. *Ann Pharmacother, 35*(11), 1435–1448.

11. Aronowski, J., & Hall, C. (2005). New horizons for primary intracerebral hemorrhage. *Neurol Res, 27*(3), 268–279.

12. Asimos, A. W., et al. (2004). Therapeutic yield and outcomes of a community teaching hospital code stroke protocol. *Acad Emerg Med, 11*(4), 361–370.

13. Ayata, C., & Ropper, A. H. (2003). Intensive care management of specific stroke treatment. *Adv Neurol, 92,* 361–377.

14. Babikian, V. L., & Wijman, C. A. (2003). Brain embolism monitoring with transcranial Doppler ultrasound. *Curr Treat Options Cardiovasc Med, 5*(3), 221–232.

15. Badjatia, N., Nguyen, T. N., & Koroshetz, W. J. (2004). Neurointensive care of the acute ischemic stroke patient. In J. I. Suarez (Ed.), *Critical care neurology and neurosurgery.* Totowa, NJ: Humana Press.

16. Badjatia, N., et al. (2004). Achieving normothermia in patients with febrile subarachnoid hemorrhage: feasibility and safety of a novel intravascular catheter. *Neurocrit Care, 1*(2), 145–156.

17. Baldwin, M. E., et al. (2004). Early vasospasm on admission angiography patients with aneurysmal subarachnoid hemorrhage is a predictor for in-hospital complications and poor outcome. *Stroke, 35*(11), 2506–2511.

18. Bambakidis, N. C., & Selman, W. R. (2004). Subarachnoid hemorrhage. In J. I. Suarez (Ed.), *Critical care neurology and neurosurgery.* Totowa, NJ: Humana Press.

19. Banerji, M. A. (2005). Statins and the prevention of stroke in diabetes. *Curr Diab Rep, 5*(1), 1–3.

20. Banki, N. M., & Zaroff, J. G. (2003). Neurogenic cardiac injury. *Curr Treat Options Cardiovasc Med, 5*(6), 451–458.

21. Beck, J., et al. (2004). Tissue at risk concept for endovascular treatment of severe vasospasm after aneurysmal subarachnoid hemorrhage. *J Neurol Neurosurg Psychiatry, 75*(12), 1779–1781.

22. Benatar, M. (2005). Heparin use in acute ischaemic stroke: Does evidence change practice? *QJM, 98*(2), 147–152.

23. Bernardini, G. L., & DeShaies, E. M. (2001). Critical care of intracerebral and subarachnoid hemorrhage. *Curr Neurol Neurosci Rep, 1*(6), 568–576.

24. Bernstein, R., & Hemphill, J. (2001). Critical care of acute ischemic stroke. *Curr Neurol Neurosci Rep, 1*(6), 587–592.

25. Bertram, M., et al. (2000). Managing the therapeutic dilemma: patients with spontaneous intracerebral hemorrhage and urgent need for anticoagulation. *J Neurol, 247*(3), 209–214.

26. Bhardwaj, A., & Ulatowski, J. A. (2004). Hypertonic saline solutions in brain injury. *Curr Opin Crit Care, 10*(2), 126–131.

27. Birchall, J., et al. (2006). Recombinant factor VIIa for the prevention and treatment of bleeding in patients without haemophilia. *Cochrane Database Syst Rev, 2,* CD 00075320.

28. Blacker, D. J. (2003). In-hospital stroke. *Lancet Neurol, 2*(12), 741–746.

29. Blissitt, P. A., et al. (2006). Cerebrovascular dynamics with head of bed elevation in patients with mild or moderate vasospasm after aneurysmal subarachnoid hemorrhage. *Am J Crit Care, 15* (2), 206–216.

30. Blumenfeld, H. (2002). Higher order cerebral function. In H. Blumenfeld (Ed.), *Neuroanatomy through clinical cases.* Sunderland, Mass: Sinauer.

31. Blumenfeld, H. (2002). Cerebral hemispheres and vascular supply. In H. Blumenfeld (Ed.), *Neuroanatomy through clinical cases.* Sunderland, Mass: Sinauer.

32. Brain Trauma Foundation, American Association of Neurological Surgeons. (2003). *Guidelines for the management of severe traumatic brain injury update: cerebral perfusion pressure.* New York: Brain Trauma Foundation.

33. Brettler, S. (2005). Endovascular coiling for cerebral aneurysms. *AACN Clin Issues, 16*(4), 515–525.

34. Brey, R. L., & Coull, B. M. (2005). Coagulation abnormalities in stroke. In J. P. Mohr, et al. (Eds.), *Stroke: pathophysiology, diagnosis and management* (4th ed.). Philadelphia: Churchill Livingstone.

35. Britz, G. W. (2005). Clipping or coiling of cerebral aneurysms. *Neurosurg Clin North Am, 16*(3), 475–485.

36. Broderick, J. P., et al. (2007). Guidelines for the management of spontaneous intracerebral hemorrhage. 2007 update. A guideline from the American Heart Association, American Stroke Association Stroke Council, High Blood Pressure Research Council, and the Quality of Care and Outcomes in Research Interdisciplinary Working Group. *(Dallas): American Stroke Association.*

37. Broderick, J., et al. (2001). Apolipoprotein E phenotype and the efficacy of intravenous tissue plasminogen activator in acute ischemic stroke. *Ann Neurol, 49*(6), 736–744.

38. Brody, D. L., et al. (2005). Use of recombinant factor VIIa in patients with warfarin-associated intracranial hemorrhage. *Neurocrit Care, 2*(3), 263–267.

39. Brott, T., et al. (1997). Early hemorrhage growth in patients with intracerebral hemorrhage. *Stroke, 28*(1), 1–5.

40. Brott, T. G., et al. (2004). Carotid revascularization for prevention of stroke: carotid endarterectomy and carotid artery stenting. *Mayo Clin Proc, 79*(9), 1197–1208.

41. Brouns, R., & De Deyn, P. P. (2004). Neurological complications in renal failure. *Clin Neurol Neurosurg, 107*(1), 1–16.

42. Brown, M. M. (2003). Angioplasty and stenting. *Adv Neurol, 92,* 335–345.

43. Bruno, A., Williams, L., & Kent, T. A. (2004). How important is hyperglycemia during acute brain infarction? *Neurologist, 10*(4), 195–200.

44. Burry, M. V., & Mericle, R. A. (2004). Basic endovascular neurosurgery and neuroradiology. In A. J. Layon, A. Gabrieli, & W. A. Friedman (Eds.), *Textbook of neurointensive care.* Philadelphia: Saunders.

45. Butcher, K., & Laidlaw, J. (2003). Current intracerebral haemorrhage management. *Clin Neurosci, 10*(2), 158–167.

46. Camilo, O., & Goldstein, L. B. (2004). Seizures and epilepsy after ischemic stroke. *Stroke, 35*(7), 1769–1775.

47. Caplan, L. R., & Hon, F. K. S. (2004). Clinical diagnosis of patients with cerebrovascular disease. *Prim Care, 31*(1), 95–109.

48. Carlin, T. M., & Chanmugam, A. (2002). Stroke in children. *Emerg Med Clin North Am, 20*(3), 671–685.

49. Cavanagh, S. J., & Gordon, V. L. (2002). Grading scales used in the management of aneurysmal subarachnoid hemorrhage: a critical review. *J Neurosci Nurs, 34*(6), 288–295.

50. Chalela, J. A. (2004). Acute stroke patients are being underfed: a nitrogen balance study. *Neurocrit Care, 1*(3), 331–334.

51. Chen, C., & Carter, B. S. (2004). Hemicraniectomy for massive cerebral infarction. *Top Stroke Rehabil, 11*(2), 7–11.

52. Chernecky, C. C., & Berger, B. J. (2004). *Laboratory test and diagnostic procedures* (4th ed.). St Louis: Saunders.

53. Cheung, R., & Zou, L. (2002). Use of the original, modified or new intracerebral hemorrhage score to predict mortality and morbidity after intracerebral hemorrhage. *Stroke, 34*(7), 1717–1722.

54. Cheung, R. T. F., & Hachinski, V. (2003). Cardiac rhythm disorders and muscle changes with cerebral lesions. *Adv Neurol, 92,* 213–220.

55. Cheung, R. T., & Hachinski, V. (2004). Cardiac effects of stroke. *Curr Treat Options Cardiovasc Med, 6*(3), 199–207.

56. Choi, J. H., & Mohr, J. P. (2005). Brain arteriovenous malformations in adults. *Lancet Neurol, 4*(5), 299–308.

57. Chong, J. Y., & Mohr, J. P. (2005). Anticoagulation and platelet antiaggregation therapy in stroke prevention. *Curr Opin Neurol, 18*(1), 53–57.

58. Claassen, J., et al. (2004). Effect of acute physiologic derangements on outcome after subarachnoid hemorrhage. *Crit Care Med, 32*(3), 832–838.

59. Clarke, J. L., et al. (2004). External validation of the ICH Score. *Neurocrit Care, 1*(1), 53–60.

60. Coert, B. A., et al. (2005). Revascularization of the posterior circulation. *Skull Base, 15*(1), 43–62.

61. Cohen, Z. R., et al. (2002). Management and outcome of non-traumatic cerebellar haemorrhage. *Cerebrovasc Dis, 14*(3–4), 207–213.

62. Coplin, W. M. (2005). Management of hypertension in acute subarachnoid hemorrhage. *Blood pressure management in critically ill neurologic patients: correcting cerebral autoregulation impairment.* (Monograph, pp. 12–13). Des Plaines, Ill: Society of Critical Care Medicine.

63. D'Ambrosio, A. L., et al. (2005). Decompressive hemicraniectomy for poor-grade aneurysmal subarachnoid hemorrhage patients with associated intracerebral hemorrhage: clinical outcome and quality of life assessment. *Neurosurg, 56*(1), 12–19.

64. Davalos, A., et al. (2004). The clinical-DWI mismatch: a new diagnostic approach to the brain tissue at risk of infarction. *Neurology, 62*(12), 2187–2192.

65. Davidson, B. L. (2000). Risk assessment and prophylaxis of venous thromboembolism in acutely and/or critically ill patients. *Haemostasis, 30*(suppl 2), 77–81.

66. Davis, S. M., et al. (2005). Selection of thrombolytic therapy beyond 3 h using magnetic resonance imaging. *Curr Opin Neurol, 18*(1), 47–52.

67. De Groot, M. H., Phillips, S. J., & Eskes, G. A. (2003). Fatigue associated with stroke and other neurologic conditions: implications for stroke rehabilitation. *Arch Med Rehabil, 84*(11), 1714–1720.

68. Demaerschalk, B. M. (2003). Diagnosis and management of stroke (brain attack). *Semin Neurol, 23*(3), 241–252.

69. Dennis, M. S. (2003). Outcome after brain haemorrhage. *Cerebrovasc Dis, 16*(suppl 1), 9–13.

70. Diaz, J., & Sempere, A. (2004). Cerebral ischemia: new risk factors. *Cerebrovasc Dis, 17*(suppl 1), 43–50.

71. Diez-Tejedor, E., & Fuentes, B. (2004). Acute care in stroke: the importance of early intervention to achieve better brain protection. *Cerebrovasc Dis, 17*(suppl 1), 130–137.

72. Diringer, M. N., & Edwards, D. F. (2001). Admission to a neurology/neurosurgical intensive care unit is associated with reduced mortality rate after intracerebral hemorrhage. *Crit Care Med, 29*(3), 635–640.

73. Dobkin, B. H. (2005). Rehabilitation after stroke. *N Engl J Med, 352*(16), 1677–1684.

74. Donnan, G., et al. (2003). Can the time window for administration for thrombolytics in stroke be increased? *CNS Drugs, 17*(14), 995–1011.

75. Dooling, E., & Winkelman, C. (2004). Hyponatremia in the patient with subarachnoid hemorrhage. *J Neurosci Nurs, 36*(3), 130–135.

75a. Drake, C. G. (1998). Report of the World Federation of Neurological Surgeons Committee on a Universal Subarachnoid Hemorrhage Grading Scale. *J Neurosurg, 68*, 985–986.

76. Dumont, A. S., et al. (2003). Cerebral vasospasm after subarachnoid hemorrhage: putative role of inflammation. *Neurosurgery, 53*(1), 123–133.

77. Duncan, P. W., et al. (2005). Management of adult stroke rehabilitation care: a clinical practice guideline. *Stroke, 36*(9), e100–e143.

78. Dziewas, R., et al. (2004). Pneumonia in acute stroke patients fed by nasogastric tube. *J Neurol Neurosurg Psychiatry, 75*(6), 852–856.

79. Eames, P., et al. (2005). Acute stroke hypertension: current and future management. *Expert Rev Cardiovasc Ther, 3*(3), 405–412.

80. Ellamushi, H. E., et al. (2001). Risk factors for the formation of multiple intracranial aneurysms. *J Neurosurg, 94*(5), 728–732.

81. Ellegala, D. B., & Day, A. L. (2005). Ruptured cerebral aneurysms. *N Engl J Med, 352*(2), 121–124.

82. El Rouby, S., et al. (2004). Racial and ethnic differences in warfarin response. *J Heart Valve Dis, 13*(1), 15–21.

83. Engelhard, H. H., et al. (2003). Current management of intraventricular hemorrhage. *Surg Neurol, 60*(1), 15–21.

84. Estol, C. J., & Kase, C. S. (2003). Need for continued use of anticoagulants after intracerebral hemorrhage. *Curr Treat Options Cardiovasc Med, 5*(3), 201–209.

85. Fahy, B. G., & Sivaraman, V. (2002). Current concepts in neurocritical care. *Anesthesiol Clin North Am, 20*(2), 441–462.

86. Farrell, C. (2004). Poststroke depression in elderly patients. *Dimens Crit Care Nurse, 23*(6), 264–269.

87. Feen, E. S., Lavery, A. W., & Suarez, J. I. (2004). Management of nontraumatic intracerebral hemorrhage. In J. I. Suarez (Ed.), *Critical care neurology and neurosurgery.* Totowa, NJ: Humana, Press.

88. Feldmann, E., et al. (2005). Major risk factors for intracerebral hemorrhage in the young are modifiable. *Stroke, 36*(9), 1881–1885.

89. Fernandes, H., et al. (2001). Testing the ICH score. *Stroke, 33*(6), 1455–1456.

90. Ferro, J., & Pinto, F. (2004). Post stroke epilepsy: epidemiology, pathophysiology, and management. *Drugs Aging, 21*(10), 639–653.

91. Fewel, M. E., & Park, P. (2004). The emerging role of recombinant-activated factor VII in neurocritical care. *Neurocrit Care, 1*(1), 19–29.

92. Findlay, J. M. (2005). Intraventricular hemorrhage. In J. P. Mohr, et al. (Eds.), *Stroke: pathophysiology, diagnosis and management* (4th ed.). Philadelphia: Churchill Livingstone.

93. Finestone, H. M., & Greene-Finestone, L. S. (2003). Rehabilitation medicine: 2. Diagnosis of dysphagia and its nutritional management for stroke patients. *CMAJ, 169*(10), 1041–1044.

94. Fischer, J., & Mathieson, C. (2001). The history of the Glasgow Coma Scale: implications for practice. *Crit Care Nurs Q, 23*(4), 52–58.

94a. Fisher, C. M., Kistler, J. P., & Davis, J. M. (1980). Relation of cerebral vasospasm to subarachnoid hemorrhage visualized by CT scanning. *Neurosurgery, 6*(1), 1–9.

95. Fitzgerald, B. T., Cohn, S. L., & Klein, A. L. (2005). Stroke prevention in atrial fibrillation. *Cleve Clin J Med, 72*(supp 1), S24–S30.

96. Flaherty, M. L. (2005). Anticoagulant-associated intracerebral hemorrhage. *Issues Hemost Manag, 1*(4), 1–9.

97. Flaherty, M. L., et al. (2005). Perimesencephalic subarachnoid hemorrhage: incidence, risk factors, and outcome. *J Stroke Cerebrovasc Dis, 14*(6), 267–271.

98. Flemming, K. D., Wijdicks, E. F. M., & Li, H. (2001). Can we predict poor outcome at presentation in patients with lobar hemorrhage? *Cerebrovasc Dis, 11*(3), 183–189.

99. Foerch, C., et al. (2004). Functional impairment, disability, and quality of life outcome after decompressive hemicraniectomy in malignant middle cerebral artery infarction. *J Neurosurg, 101*(2), 248–254.

100. Frank, J. I. (2005). Management of acute intracerebral hemorrhage. *Blood pressure management in critically ill neurologic patients: correcting cerebral autoregulation impairment.* (Monograph, pp. 8–11). Des Plaines, Ill: Society of Critical Care Medicine.

101. Frankel, M. R., et al. (2000). Predicting prognosis after stroke: a placebo group from the National Institute of Neurological Disorders and Stroke rtPA Stroke Trial after acute stroke. *Neurology, 55*(7), 952–959.

102. Frey, J. L. (2005). Recombinant tissue plasminogen activator (rtPA) for stroke. *Neurologist, 11*(2), 123–133.

103. Fujioka, K. A., & Douvillle, C. M. (1992). Anatomy and freehand examination techniques. In D. W. Newell & R. Aaslid (Eds.), *Transcranial Doppler*. New York: Raven Press.

104. Gaini, S. M., et al. (2004). The headache in the emergency department. *Neurol Sci, 25*(suppl 3), S196–S201.

105. Gandolfo, C., & Conti, M. (2003). Stroke in young adults: epidemiology. *Neurol Sci, 24*(suppl 1), S1–S3.

106. Gasser, S., et al. (2003). Longterm hypothermia in patients with severe brain edema after poor-grade subarachnoid hemorrhage. *J Neurosurg Anesthesiol, 15*(3), 240–248.

107. Gatenby, P. A. (2004). Controversies in the antiphospholipid syndrome. *Thromb Res, 114*(5–6), 483–488.

108. Gebel, J. M., et al. (2002). Natural history of perihematomal edema in patients with hyperacute spontaneous intracerebral hemorrhage. *Stroke, 33*(11), 2631–2635.

109. Georgiadis, D., Schwab, S., & Hacke, W. (2004). Critical care of the patient with acute stroke. In J. P. Mohr, et al. (Eds.), *Stroke: pathophysiology, diagnosis and management* (4th ed.). Philadelphia: Churchill Livingstone.

110. Goddard, A. J. P., Raju, P. P. J., & Gholkar, A. (2004). Does the method of treatment of acutely ruptured intracranial aneurysms influence the incidence and duration of cerebral vasospasm and clinical outcome? *J Neurol Neurosurg Psychiatry, 75*(6), 868–872.

111. Goldstein, L. B. (2003). Extracranial carotid artery stenosis. *Stroke, 34*(11), 2767–2773.

112. Goldstein, L. B., et al. (2006). Primary prevention of ischemic stroke: a statement for healthcare professionals from the American Heart Association/American Stroke Association Stroke Council of the American Heart Association. *Stroke, 37*(6), 1583–1633.

113. Goldstein, L. B., & Simel, D. L. (2005). Is this patient having a stroke? *JAMA, 293*(19), 2391–2402.

114. Good, D. C. (2003). Promising neurorehabilitation interventions and steps toward testing them. *Am J Phys Med Rehabil, 82*(10 suppl), S50–S57.

115. Green, A. R., Hainsworth, A. H., & Jackson, D. M. (2000). GABA potentiation: a logical pharmacological approach for the treatment of acute ischaemic stroke. *Neuropharmacology, 39*(9), 1483–1494.

116. Greener, J., Enderby, P., & Whurr, R. (2000). Speech and language therapy for aphasia following stroke. *Cochrane Database Syst Rev, 2*, CD000425.

117. Greer, D. M. (2004). Acute stroke and other neurologic emergencies. In A. J. Layon, A. Gabrielli, & W. A. Friedman (Eds.), *Textbook of neurointensive care*. Philadelphia: Saunders.

118. Grotta, J. C. (2004). Management of primary hypertensive hemorrhage of the brain. *Curr Treat Options Neurol, 6*(6), 435–442.

119. Grubb, R. L. (2004). Extracranial-intracranial arterial bypass for treatment of occlusion of the internal carotid artery. *Curr Neurol Neurosci Rep, 4*(1), 23–30.

120. Guadagno, J. V., et al. (2004). Imaging the ischaemic penumbra. *Curr Opin Neurol, 17*(1), 61–67.

121. Gupta, C., et al. (2004). Transcranial Doppler sonography evaluation in patients with vasospasm following subarachnoid hemorrhage. *J Indian Med Assoc, 102*(4), 191–192.

122. Hackett, M. L., Anderson, C. S., & House, A. O. (2005). Management of depression after stroke. *Stroke, 36*(5), 1092–1097.

123. Hajat, C., Hajat, S., & Sharma, P. (2000). Effects of poststroke pyrexia on stroke outcome: a meta-analysis of studies in patients. *Stroke, 31*(2), 410–414.

124. Hall, C. E., & Grotta, J. C. (2005). New era for management of primary hypertensive intracerebral hemorrhage. *Curr Neurol Neurosci Rep, 5*(1), 29–35.

125. Hallevy, C., et al. (2002). Spontaneous supratentorial intracerebral hemorrhage: criteria for short-term functional outcome prediction. *J Neurol, 249*(12), 1704–1709.

126. Hammer, M. D., & Kreiger, D. W. (2003). Hypothermia for acute ischemic stroke: not just another neuroprotectant. *Neurologist, 9*(6), 280–289.

127. Hankey, G. J. (2003). Risk management to prevent stroke. *Adv Neurol, 92*, 179–185.

128. Hanley, D. F. (2005). Review of critical care and emergency approaches to stroke. *Stroke, 36*(2), 362–364.

129. Hanley, D. F., & Hacke, W. (2004). Critical care and emergency medicine in neurology. *Stroke, 35*(2), 205–207.

130. Harrigan, M. R. (2001). Cerebral salt wasting syndrome. *Crit Care Clin, 17*(1), 125–138.

131. Hemphill, J. C., et al. (2001). The ICH score: a simple, reliable grading scale for intracerebral hemorrhage. *Stroke, 32*(4), 891–897.

132. Hemphill, J. C., et al. (2004). Hospital usage of early do-not-resuscitate orders and outcome after intracerebral hemorrhage. *Stroke, 35*(5), 1130–1134.

133. Hermier, M., et al. (2001). MRI of acute post-ischemic cerebral hemorrhage in stroke patients: diagnosis with T2-weighted gradient-echo sequences. *Neuroradiology, 43*(10), 809–815.

134. Hillered, L., Vespa, P. M., & Hovda, D. A. (2005). Translational neurochemical research in acute human brain injury: the current status and potential future for cerebral microdialysis. *J Neurotrauma, 22*(1), 3–41.

135. Hodgson, B. B., & Kizior, R. J. (2006). *Saunders nursing drug book*. St Louis: Saunders.

136. Hoeffner, E. G., et al. (2004). Cerebral perfusion CT: technique and clinical applications. *Radiology, 231*(3), 632–644.

137. Hoh, B. L., et al. (2004). Effect of clipping, craniotomy, or intravascular coiling on cerebral vasospasm and patient outcome after aneurysmal subarachnoid hemorrhage. *Neurosurgery, 55*(4), 779–786.

137a. Hunt, W. E., & Hess, R. M. (1968). Surgical risk as related to time of intervention in the repair of intracranial aneurysms. *J Neurosurg, 28*, 14–20.

138. Immink, R. V., et al. (2005). Dynamic cerebral autoregulation in acute lacunar and middle cerebral artery territory ischemic stroke. *Stroke, 36*(12), 2595–2600.

139. Ionita, C., et al. (2005). What proportion of stroke is not explained by classic risk factors? *Preven Cardiol, 8*(1), 41–46.

140. Jabbour, P. M., Awad, I. A., & Huddle, D. (2004). Hemorrhagic cerebrovascular disease. In A. J. Layon, A. Gabrielli, & W. A. Friedman (Eds.), *Textbook of neurointensive care*. Philadelphia: Saunders.

141. Jaeger, M., et al. (2005). Correlation of continuously monitored regional cerebral blood flow and brain tissue oxygen. *Acta Neurochir (Wien), 147*(1), 51–56.

142. Jain, R., Deveikis, J., & Thompson, B. G. (2003). Management of patients with stunned myocardium associated with subarachnoid hemorrhage. *AJNR Am J Neuroradiol, 25*(1), 126–129.

143. Jensen, M. B., & St. Louis, E. K. (2005). Management of acute cerebellar stroke. *Arch Neurol, 62*(4), 537–544.

144. John, M., et al. (2005). Factors causing patients to delay seeking treatment after suffering a stroke. *W V Med J, 101*(1), 12–15.

145. Johnston, S. C., et al. (2002). Recommendations for the endovascular treatment of intracranial aneurysms. A statement of healthcare professionals from the Committee on Cerebrovascular Imaging of American Heart Association Council on Cardiovascular Radiology. *Stroke, 33*(10), 2536–2544.

146. Jungreis, C. A., & Goldstein, S. (2004). Computed tomography-based evaluation of cerebrovascular disease. In J. P. Mohr, et al. (Eds.), *Stroke: pathophysiology, diagnosis and management* (4th ed.). Philadelphia: Churchill Livingstone.

147. Juvela, S. (2000). Risk factors for multiple intracranial aneurysms. *Stroke, 31*(2), 392–397.

148. Kanji, S., Corman, C., & Douen, A. G. (2002). Blood pressure management in acute stroke: comparison of current guidelines with prescribing patterns. *Canad J Neurol Sci, 29*(2), 125–131.

149. Kasner, S. E. (2000). Stroke treatment: specific considerations. *Neurol Clin, 18*(2), 399–417.

150. Kasuya, H., et al. (2005). Application of nicardipine prolonged-release implants: analysis of 97 consecutive patients with acute subarachnoid hemorrhage. *Neurosurgery, 56*(5), 895–902.

151. Katzan, I. L., et al. (2004). Utilization of intravenous tissue plasminogen activator for acute ischemic stroke. *Arch Neurol, 61*(3), 346–350.

152. Kawahra, E., et al. (2003). Role of autonomic nervous dysfunction in electrographic abnormalities and cardiac injury in patients with acute subarachnoid hemorrhage. *Circ J, 67*(9), 753–756.

153. Kedlaya, D., & Brandstater, M. E. (2002). Swallowing, nutrition, and hydration during acute stroke care. *Top Stroke Rehabil, 9*(2), 23–38.

154. Keep, R. F., et al. (2005). The deleterious or beneficial effects of different agents in intracerebral hemorrhage: think big, think small, or is hematoma size important. *Stroke, 36*(7), 1594–1596.

155. Khechinashvili, G., & Asplund, K. (2002). Electrocardiographic changes in patients with acute stroke: a systematic review. *Cerebrovasc Dis, 14*(2), 67–76.

156. Kidwell, C. S., & Warach, S. (2003). Acute ischemic cerebrovascular syndrome: diagnostic criteria. *Stroke, 34*(12), 2995–2998.

157. Kidwell, C. S., Alger, J. R., & Saver, J. L. (2003). Beyond mismatch: evolving paradigms in imaging the ischemic penumbra with multimodal magnetic resonance imaging. *Stroke, 34*(11), 2729–2735.

158. Kidwell, C. S. (2004). Evolving paradigms in neuroimaging of the ischemic penumbra. *Stroke, 35*(11 suppl 1), 2662–2665.

159. Kirmani, J. F., et al. (2005). Therapeutic advances in interventional neurology. *NeuroRx, 2*(2), 304–323.

160. Klijn, C. J. M., & Hankey, G. J. (2003). Management of acute ischaemic stroke: new guidelines from the American Stroke Association and European Stroke Initiative. *Lancet Neurol, 2*(11), 698–701.

161. Klimo, P., et al. (2004). Marked reduction of cerebral vasospasm with lumbar drainage of cerebrospinal fluid after subarachnoid hemorrhage. *J Neurosurg, 100*(2), 215–224.

162. Klopfenstein, J. D., et al. (2004). Comparison of rapid and gradual weaning from external ventricular drainage in patients with aneurysmal subarachnoid hemorrhage: a prospective randomized trial. *J Neurosurg, 100*(2), 225–229.

163. Kosty, T. (2005). Cerebral vasospasm after subarachnoid hemorrhage: an update. *Crit Care Nurs Q, 28*(2), 122–134.

164. Kothari, R. U., et al. (1996). The ABCs of measuring intracerebral hemorrhage volume. *Stroke, 27*(8), 1304–1305.

165. Kowalski, R. G., et al. (2004). Initial misdiagnosis and outcome after subarachnoid hemorrhage. *JAMA, 291*(7), 866–869.

166. Kraus, J. J., Metzler, M. D., & Coplin, W. M. (2002). Critical care issues in stroke and subarachnoid hemorrhage. *Neurol Res, 24*(suppl 1), S47–S57.

167. Krieger, D. W., et al. (2001). Cooling for acute ischemic brain damage (cool-aid): an open pilot study of induced hypothermia in acute ischemic stroke. *Stroke, 32*(8), 1847–1854.

168. Kujovich, J. L. (2005). Hemostatic defects in end stage liver disease. *Crit Care Clin, 21*(3), 563–587.

169. Kurth, T., et al. (2003). Smoking and risk of hemorrhagic stroke in women. *Stroke, 34*(12), 2792–2795.

170. Labiche, L. A., & Grotta, J. C. (2004). Pharmacologic modification of acute cerebral ischemia. In J. P. Mohr, et al. (Eds.), *Stroke: pathophysiology, diagnosis and management* (4th ed.). Philadelphia: Churchill Livingstone.

171. Labovitz, D. L., & Sacco, R. L. (2001). Intracerebral hemorrhage: update. *Curr Opin Neurol, 14*(1), 103–108.

172. Lagares, A., et al. (2005). A comparison of different grading scales for predicting outcome after subarachnoid hemorrhage. *Acta Neurochir (Wien), 147*(1), 5–16.

173. Lanterna, L., et al. (2005). APOE influences vasospasm and cognition of noncomatose patients with subarachnoid hemorrhage. *Neurology, 64*(7), 1238–1244.

174. Lapointe, M., & Haines, S. (2002). Fibrinolytic therapy for intraventricular hemorrhage in adults. *Cochrane Database Syst Rev, 3,* CD003692.

175. Latchaw, R. E. (2004). Cerebral perfusion imaging in acute stroke. *J Vasc Interv Radiol, 15*(1, pt 2), S29–S46.

176. Latchaw, R. E., et al. (2003). Guidelines and recommendations for perfusion imaging in cerebral ischemia. A scientific statement for healthcare professions by the writing group on perfusion imaging from the Council on Cardiovascular Radiology of the American Heart Association. *Stroke, 34*(4), 1084–1104.

177. Leary, M. C., et al. (2003). Beyond tissue plasminogen activator: mechanical intervention in acute stroke. *Ann Emerg Med, 41*(6), 838–846.

178. Lees, K. R. (2002). Management of acute stroke. *Lancet Neurol, 1*(1), 41–50.

179. Lentz, S. R., & Haynes, W. G. (2004). Homocysteine: is it a clinically important cardiovascular risk factor? *Cleve Clin J Med, 71*(9), 729–734.

180. Lindenauer, P. K., et al. (2004). Use of antihypertensive agents in the management of patients with acute ischemic stroke. *Neurology, 63*(2), 318–323.

181. Lindsberg, P. J., & Grau, A. J. (2003). Inflammation and infections as risk factors for ischemic stroke. *Stroke, 34*(10), 2518–2532.

182. Little, K. M., & Alexander, M. J. (2002). Medical versus surgical therapy for spontaneous intracerebral hemorrhage. *Neurosurg Clin N Am, 13*(3), 339–347.

183. Lorenzi, L., et al. (2003). Influence of delaying treatment after symptoms develop from subarachnoid hemorrhage: a preliminary analysis. *J Neurosci Nurs, 35*(4), 210–214.

184. Macdonald, R. L. (2005). Cerebral vasospasm. In J. P. Mohr, et al. (Eds.), *Stroke: pathophysiology, diagnosis and management* (4th ed.). Philadelphia: Churchill Livingstone.

185. Macrea, L. M., Tramer, M. R., & Walder, B. (2005). Spontaneous subarachnoid hemorrhage and serious cardiac dysfunction: a systematic review. *Resuscitation, 65*(2), 139–148.

186. MacWalter, R. S., Ersoy, Y., & Wolfson, D. R. (2001). Cerebral haemorrhage. *Gerontology, 47*(3), 119–130.

187. Madden, K. (2002). Optimal timing of thrombolytic therapy in acute ischemic stroke. *CNS Drugs, 16*(4), 213–218.

188. Mahanes, D., & Lewis, R. (2004). Weaning of the neurologically impaired patient. *Crit Care Nurs Clin North Am, 16*(3), 387–393.

189. Mankovsky, B. N., & Ziegler, D. (2004). Stroke in patients with diabetes mellitus. *Diabetes Metab Res Rev, 20*(4), 268–287.

190. Manno, E. M. (2004). Subarachnoid hemorrhage. *Neurol Clin, 22* (2), 347–366.

191. Manno, E. M., et al. (2005). Emerging medical and surgical management strategies in the evaluation and treatment of intracerebral hemorrhage. *Mayo Clin Proc, 80*(3), 420–433.

192. Marcos, Z., & Sundararajan, S. (2004). Cerebral venous sinus thrombosis. In J. I. Suarez (Ed.), *Critical care neurology and neurosurgery.* Totowa, NJ: Humana Press.

193. Marion, D. W. (2004). Controlled normothermia in neurologic intensive care. *Crit Care Med, 32*(2 suppl), S43–S45.

194. Markus, H. S. (2004). Cerebral perfusion and stroke. *J Neurol Neurosurg Psychiatry, 75*(3), 353–361.

195. Markus, H. S. (2005). Current treatments in neurology: stroke. *J Neurol, 252*(3), 260–267.

196. Mas, J. L. (2003). Specifics of patent foramen ovale. *Adv Neurol*, *92*, 197–202.

197. Mascia, L., et al. (2003). The accuracy of transcranial Doppler to detect vasospasm in patients with aneurysmal subarachnoid hemorrhage. *Intensive Care Med*, *29*(7), 1088–1094.

198. Mayberg, M. R., et al. (1994). Guidelines for the management of aneurysmal subarachnoid hemorrhage. A statement for health-care professionals from a special writing group of the Stroke Council, American Heart Association. *Stroke*, *25*(11), 2315–2328.

199. Mayer, S. A., et al. (1999). Myocardial injury and left ventricular performance after subarachnoid hemorrhage. *Stroke*, *30*(4), 780–786.

200. Mayer, S. A., et al. (2005). Recombinant activated factor VII for acute intracerebral hemorrhage. *N Engl J Med*, *352*(8), 777–785.

201. McCartney, J. P., Thomas-Lukes, K. M., & Gomez, C. R. (1997). Examination techniques. *Handbook of transcranial Doppler*. New York: Springer.

202. McDonald, D., & Carter, B. S. (2002). Medical management of increased intracranial pressure after spontaneous intracerebral hemorrhage. *Neurosurg Clin N Am*, *13*(3), 335–338.

203. McFarlane, S. I., Sica, D., & Sowers, J. R. (2005). Stroke in patients with diabetes and hypertension. *J Clin Hypertens (Greenwich)*, *7*(5), 286–292.

204. McGovern, R., & Rudd, A. (2003). Management of stroke. *Postgrad Med J*, *79*(928), 87–92.

205. McNaughton, H., et al. (2005). Management problems of spontaneous ICH. *Hosp Med*, *66*(4), 229–234.

206. Meena, A. K., Suvarna, A. K., & Kaul, S. (2002). Critical care management of acute stroke. *Neurol India*, *50*(suppl 1), S37–S49.

207. Mees, S. M. D., et al. (2003). Glucose levels and outcome after subarachnoid hemorrhage. *Neurology*, *61*(8), 1132–1133.

208. Meixensberger, J., et al. (2003). Monitoring of brain tissue oxygenation follow severe subarachnoid hemorrhage. *Neurol Res*, *25*(5), 445–450.

209. Mendelow, A. D., et al. (2005). Early surgery versus initial conservative treatment in patients with spontaneous supratentorial intracerebral haematomas in the International Surgical Trial in Intracerebral Haemorrhage (STICH): a randomized trial. *Lancet*, *365*(9457), 387–397.

210. Meschia, J. F., Brott, T. G., & Brown, R. D. (2005). Genetics of cerebrovascular disorders. *Mayo Clin Proc*, *80*(1), 122–132.

211. Minematsu, K. (2003). Evacuation of intracerebral hematoma is likely to be beneficial. *Stroke*, *34*(6), 1567–1568.

212. Miss, J. C., et al. (2004). Cardiac injury after subarachnoid hemorrhage is independent of the type of aneurysm therapy. *Neurosurgery*, *55*(6), 1244–1250.

213. Mohr, J. P., et al. (2004). Arteriovenous malformations and other vascular anomalies. In J. P. Mohr (Ed.), *Stroke: pathophysiology, diagnosis and management* (4th ed.). Philadelphia: Churchill Livingstone.

214. Molyneux, A. J., et al. (2005). International Subarachnoid Aneurysm Trial (ISAT) of neurosurgical clipping versus endovascular coiling in 2143 patients with ruptured intracranial aneurysms: a randomized comparison of effects on survival, dependency, seizures, rebleeding, subgroups, and aneurysm occlusion. *Lancet*, *366*(9488), 809–817.

215. Momjian-Mayor, I., & Baron, J.-C. (2005). The pathophysiology of watershed infarction internal carotid artery disease: review of cerebral perfusion studies. *Stroke*, *36*(3), 567–577.

216. Morgan, L., & Humphries, S. E. (2005). The genetics of stroke. *Curr Opin Lipidol*, *16*(2), 193–199.

217. Morgenstern, L. B., & Yonas, H. (2001). Lowering blood pressure in acute intracerebral hemorrhage: safe but will it help? *Neurology*, *57*(1), 5–6.

218. Morrison, K. (2005). The road to JCAHO disease-specific care certification: a step-by-step process log. *Dimens Crit Care Nurs*, *24*(5), 221–227.

219. Murakami, M., et al. (2004). Clinical features and management of intracranial hemorrhage in patients undergoing maintenance dialysis treatment. *Neuro Med Chir (Tokyo)*, *44*(5), 225–233.

220. Naff, N. J., et al. (2004). Intraventricular thrombolysis speeds blood clot resolution: results of a pilot, prospective, randomized, double-blind, controlled trial. *Neurosurgery*, *54*(3), 577–583.

221. Naidech, A. M., et al. (2005). Predictors and impact of aneurysm rebleeding after subarachnoid hemorrhage. *Arch Neurol*, *62*(3), 410–416.

222. Nakano, T., & Ohkuma, H. (2005). Surgery versus conservative treatment for intracerebral haemorrhage: is there an end to the long controversy? *Lancet*, *365*(9457), 361–362.

222a. National Institute of Neurological Disorders and Stroke. (2003). *National Institutes of Health Stroke Scale*. Glenview, Ill: U.S. Department of Health and Human Services.

223. Naval, N. S., et al. (2006). Controversies in the management of aneurysmal subarachnoid hemorrhage. *Crit Care Med*, *34*(2), 511–524.

224. Nguyen, T., & Koroshetz, W. (2003). Intensive care management of ischemic stroke. *Curr Neurol Neurosci Rep*, *3*(1), 32–39.

225. Niskanen, M., et al. (2005). Complications and postoperative care in patients undergoing treatment for unruptured intracranial aneurysms. *J Neurosurg Anesthesiol*, *17*(2), 100–105.

226. Norris, J. W., & Beletsky, V. (2003). Cervical artery dissection. *Adv Neurol*, *92*, 119–125.

227. Ogden, A. T., Mayer, S. A., & Connolly, E. S. (2005). Hyperosmolar agents in neurosurgical practice: the evolving role of hypertonic saline. *Neurosurgery*, *57*(2), 207–215.

228. Ohwaki, K., et al. (2004). Blood pressure management in acute intracerebral hemorrhage. Relationship between elevated blood pressure and hematoma enlargement. *Stroke*, *35*(6), 1364–1367.

229. Otawara, Y., et al. (2003). Brain and systemic temperature in patients with severe subarachnoid hemorrhage. *Surg Neurol*, *60*(2), 159–164.

230. Panangos, P. D., Jauch, E. C., & Broderick, J. P. (2002). Intracerebral hemorrhage. *Emerg Med Clin North Am*, *20*(3), 631–655.

231. Paolino, A. S., & Garner, K. M. (2005). Effects of hyperglycemia on neurologic outcome in stroke. *J Neurosci Nurs*, *37*(3), 130–135.

232. Pathak, A., et al. (2003). Intermittent low dose intrathecal sodium nitroprusside therapy for treatment of symptomatic aneurysmal SAH-induced vasospasm. *Br J Neurosurg*, *17*(4), 306–310.

233. Peerdeman, S. M., van Tulder, M. W., & Vandertop, W. P. (2003). Cerebral microdialysis as a monitoring method in subarachnoid hemorrhage patients and correlation with clinical events. *J Neurol*, *250*(7), 797–805.

234. Pengo, V. (2003). Oral anticoagulant therapy in patients with atrial fibrillation. *Semin Vasc Med*, *3*(3), 333–338.

235. Perler, B. (2005). Thrombolytic therapies: the current state of affairs. *J Endovasc Ther*, *12*(2), 224–232.

236. Pinto, A., et al. (2004). Cerebrovascular risk factors and clinical classification of stroke. *Semin Vasc Med*, *4*(3), 287–303.

237. Pluta, R. M. (2005). Delayed cerebral vasospasm and nitric oxide: review, new hypothesis, and proposed treatment. *Pharmacol Ther*, *105*(1), 23–56.

238. Polderman, K. H., et al. (2005). Induction of hypothermia in patients with various types of neurologic injury with use of large volumes of ice-cold intravenous fluid. *Crit Care Med*, *33*(12), 2744–2751.

239. Pollock, B. E., & Flickinger, J. C. (2002). A proposed radiosurgery-based grading system for arteriovenous malformations. *J Neurosurg*, *96*(1), 79–85.

240. Powers, W. J. (1993). Acute hypertension after stroke: the scientific basis for treatment decisions. *Neurology, 43*(3, pt 1), 461–467.

241. Powers, W. J., et al. (2001). Autoregulation of cerebral blood flow surrounding acute (6 to 22 hours) intracerebral hemorrhage. *Neurology, 57*(1), 18–24.

242. Provencio, J. J., Bleck, T. P., & Connors, A. F. (2001). Critical care neurology. *Am J Respir Crit Care Med, 164*(3), 341–345.

243. Pugh, S., et al. (2004). *Guide to the care of the patient with ischemic stroke.* (Monograph). Glenview, Ill: American Association of Neuroscience Nurses.

244. Qu, F., et al. (2004). Untreated subarachnoid hemorrhage: who, why, and when? *J Neurosurg, 100*(2), 244–249.

245. Qureshi, A., et al. (2002). Cerebral blood flow changes associated with intracerebral hemorrhage. *Neurosurg Clin N Am, 13*(3), 355–370.

246. Qureshi, A. I., et al. (2003). Timing of neurologic deterioration in massive middle cerebral artery infarction: a multi-center review. *Crit Care Med, 31*(1), 272–277.

247. Rabenstein, A. A., & Wijdicks, E. F. (2005). Cerebral vasospasm in subarachnoid hemorrhage. *Curr Treat Options Neurol, 7*(2), 99–107.

248. Rahimi, A. R., et al. (2004). Clinical correlation between effective anticoagulants and risk of stroke: are we using evidence-based strategies? *South Med J, 97*(10), 924–931.

249. Ramsey, D. J. C., Smithard, D. G., & Kalra, L. (2003). Early assessments of dysphagia and aspiration risk in acute stroke patients. *Stroke, 34*(5), 1252–1257.

250. Reilly, C. (2004). Clot volume and clearance rate as independent predictors of vasospasm and aneurysmal subarachnoid hemorrhage. *J Neurosurg, 101*(2), 255–261.

251. Reinert, M., et al. (2004). Transdermal nitroglycerin in patients with subarachnoid hemorrhage. *Neurol Res, 26*(4), 435–439.

252. Revilla-Pacheco, F., et al. (2005). Cerebral salt wasting syndrome in patients with aneurysmal subarachnoid hemorrhage. *Neurol Res, 27*(4), 418–422.

253. Rhoney, D. H., et al. (2000). Anticonvulsant prophylaxis and timing of seizures after aneurysmal subarachnoid hemorrhage. *Neurology, 55*(2), 258–265.

254. Rhoney, D. H. (2005). Pharmacokinetics and pharmacodynamics of vasoactive therapy in the patient with acute cerebrovascular disease. *Blood pressure management in critically Ill neurologic patients: correcting cerebral autoregulation impairment.* (Monograph, pp. 4–7). Des Plaines, Ill: Society of Critical Care Medicine.

255. Ribo, M., et al. (2005). Acute hyperglycemia state is associated with lower tPA-induced recanalization rates in stroke patients. *Stroke, 36*(8), 1705–1709.

256. Rinkel, G. J. E. (2003). Treatment of patients with aneurysmal subarachnoid hemorrhage. *Lancet Neurol, 2*(1), 12.

257. Rinkel, G. J. E., et al. (2004). Circulatory volume expansion therapy for aneurysmal subarachnoid hemorrhage. *Cochrane Database Syst Rev, 1*, CD000483.

258. Rinkel, G. J. E., et al. (2005). Calcium antagonists for aneurysmal subarachnoid hemorrhage. *Cochrane Database Syst Rev, 1*, CD000277.

259. Robertson, S. C., et al. (2004). Clinical course and surgical management of massive cerebral infarction. *Neurosurgery, 55*(1), 55–62.

260. Robinson, T. G., & Potter, J. F. (2004). Blood pressure in acute stroke. *Age Ageing, 33*(1), 6–12.

261. Rogers, L. R. (2003). Cerebrovascular complications in cancer patients. *Neurol Clin, 21*(1), 167–192.

262. Rogers, L. R. (2004). Cerebrovascular complications in patients with cancer. *Semin Neurol, 24*(4), 453–460.

263. Rose, J. C., & Mayer, S. A. (2004). Optimizing blood pressure in neurological emergencies. *Neurocrit Care, 1*(3), 287–299.

264. Rothoerl, R. D., Woertgen, C., & Brawanski, A. (2004). Hyperemia following aneurysmal subarachnoid hemorrhage: incidence, diagnosis, clinical features, and outcome. *Intens Care Med, 30*(7), 1298–1302.

265. Roubin, G. S., et al. (2004). Carotid stenting. In J. P. Mohr, et al. (Eds.), *Stroke: pathophysiology, diagnosis, and management* (4th ed.). Philadelphia: Churchill Livingstone.

266. Sacco, R. L. (2004). Risk factors for TIA and TIA as a risk factor for stroke. *Neurology, 62*(8, suppl 6), S7–S11.

267. Sacco, R. L., et al. (2006). Guidelines for prevention of stroke in patients with ischemic stroke or transient ischemic stroke: a statement for healthcare professionals from the American Heart Association/American Stroke Association Council on Stroke. *Stroke, 37*(2), 577–617.

268. Sacco, S., Marini, C., & Carolei, A. (2004). Medical treatment of intracerebral hemorrhage. *Neurol Sci, 25*(suppl 1), S6–S9.

269. Sakr, Y. L., et al. (2004). Relation of EKG changes to neurological outcome in patients with aneurysmal subarachnoid hemorrhage. *Int J Cardiol, 96*(3), 369–373.

270. Schellinger, P. D., et al. (2003). Stroke MRI in intracerebral hemorrhage. Is there a perihemorrhagic penumbra? *Stroke, 34*(7), 1674–1679.

271. Schellinger, P. D., & Fiebach, J. B. (2004). Intracranial hemorrhage: the role of magnetic resonance imaging. *Neurocrit Care, 1*(1), 31–45.

272. Schellinger, P. D., & Hacke, W. (2005). Stroke: advances in therapy. *Lancet Neurol, 4*(1), 2.

273. Schellinger, P. D., Kaste, M., & Hacke, W. (2004). An update on thrombolytic therapy for acute stroke. *Curr Opin Neurol, 17*(1), 69–77.

274. Schuiling, W. J., et al. (2005). Disorders of sleep and wake in patients after subarachnoid hemorrhage. *Stroke, 36*(3), 578–582.

275. Schulman, S. (2003). Clinical practice. Care of patients receiving long-term anticoagulant therapy. *N Engl J Med, 349*(7), 675–683.

276. Schulman, S. (2003). Unresolved issues in anticoagulant therapy. *J Thromb Haemostasis, 1*(7), 1464–1470.

277. Schwarz, S., et al. (2002). Effects of body position on intracranial pressure and cerebral perfusion in patients with large hemispheric stroke. *Stroke, 33*(2), 497–501.

278. Sen, J., et al. (2003). Triple-H therapy in the management of aneurysmal subarachnoid hemorrhage. *Lancet Neurol, 2*(10), 614–621.

279. Skidmore, C. T., & Andrefsky, J. (2002). Spontaneous intracerebral hemorrhage: epidemiology, pathophysiology, and medical management. *Neurosurg Clin N Am, 13*(3), 281–288.

280. Skidmore-Roth, L. (2006). *Mosby's nursing drug reference.* St Louis: Mosby.

281. Slazinski, T., & Littlejohns, L. R. (2004). Anatomy of the nervous system. In M. K. Bader & L. R. Littlejohns (Eds.), *AANN core curriculum for neuroscience nursing* (4th ed.). St Louis: Saunders.

282. Sloan, M. A., & Stern, B. J. (2003). Cerebrovascular disease in pregnancy. *Curr Treat Options Neurol, 5*(5), 391–407.

283. Sloan, M. A., et al. (2004). Assessment: transcranial Doppler ultrasonography. Report of the Therapeutic and Technology Assessment Subcommittee of the American Academy of Neurology. *Neurology, 62*(9), 1468–1481.

284. Sluzewski, M., et al. (2003). Endovascular treatment of ruptured intracranial aneurysms with detachable coils; long-term clinical and serial angiographic results. *Radiology, 227*(3), 720–724.

285. Smith, M. J., et al. (2005). Packed red blood cell transfusion increases local cerebral oxygenation. *Crit Care Med, 33*(5), 1104–1108.

286. Soehle, M., et al. (2004). Continuous assessment of cerebral auto-regulation in subarachnoid hemorrhage. *Anesth Analg, 98*(4), 1133–1139.

287. Soehle, M., Jaeger, M., & Meixensberger, J. (2003). Online assessment of brain tissue oxygen autoregulation in traumatic brain injury and subarachnoid hemorrhage. *Neurol Res, 25*(4), 411–417.

288. Springborg, J. B., et al. (2005). Trends in monitoring patients with aneurysmal subarachnoid hemorrhage. *Br J Anaesth, 94*(3), 259–270.

289. Steele, R. D., Aftonomos, L. B., & Munk, M. W. (2003). Evaluation and treatment of aphasia among the elderly with stroke. *Top Geriatric Rehabil, 19*(2), 98–108.

290. Stiefel, M. F., et al. (2004). Cerebral oxygenation following decompressive hemicraniectomy for the treatment of refractory intracranial hypertension. *J Neurosurg, 101*(2), 241–247.

291. Stam, J. (2003). Cerebral venous and sinus thrombosis: Incidence and causes. *Adv Neurol, 92*, 225–232.

292. Stam, J. (2003). The treatment of cerebral venous sinus thrombosis. *Adv Neurol, 92*, 233–240.

293. Sterzi, R., & Vidale, S. (2004). Treatment of intracerebral hemorrhage: the clinical evidences. *Neurol Sci, 25*(suppl 1), S12.

294. Stroke Council, American Heart Association/American Stroke Association. (2004). Statins after ischemic stroke and transient ischemic stroke. *Stroke, 35*(4), 1023.

295. Subramaniam, S., & Hill, M. D. (2005). Massive cerebral infarction. *Neurologist, 11*(3), 150–160.

296. Tan, S. H., et al. (2001). Hypertensive basal ganglia hemorrhage: a prospective study comparing surgical and nonsurgical management. *Surg Neurol, 56*(5), 287–293.

297. Tazbir, J., et al. (2005). Decompressive hemicraniectomy with duraplasty: a treatment for large-volume ischemic stroke. *J Neurosci Nurs, 37*(4), 194–199.

297a. Teasdale, G., & Jennett, B. (1974). Assessment of coma and impaired consciousness: a practical scale. *Lancet, 2*, 81–84.

298. Thomas, J. E., & Rosenwasser, R. H. (1999). Reversal of severe cerebral vasospasm in three patients after aneurysmal subarachnoid hemorrhage: initial observations regarding the use of intraventricular sodium nitroprusside in humans. *Neurosurgery, 44*(1), 48–57.

299. Thome, C., Schubert, G., & Schilling, L. (2005). Hypothermia as a neuroprotective strategy in subarachnoid hemorrhage: a pathophysiological review focusing on the acute phase. *Neurol Res, 27*(3), 229–237.

300. Thompson, R. C. (2005). Intracerebral hemorrhage: the least treatable form of stroke. *South Med J, 98*(8), 760.

301. Tomson, J., & Lip, G. (2005). Blood pressure changes in acute haemorrhagic stroke. *Blood Press Monit, 10*(4), 197–199.

302. Treggiari, M. M., et al. (2003). Systematic review of the prevention of delayed ischemic neurological deficits with hypertension, hypervolemia, and hemodilution therapy following subarachnoid hemorrhage. *J Neurosurg, 98*(5), 978–984.

303. Tuhrim, S. (2002). Management of hemorrhagic stroke. *Curr Cardiol Rep, 4*(2), 158–163.

304. Tuhrim, S. (2002). Management of stroke and transient ischemic attack. *Mt Sinai J Med, 69*(3), 121–130.

305. Tummala, R. P., Chu, R. M., & Nussbaum, E. S. (2003). Extracranial-intracranial bypass for symptomatic occlusive cerebrovascular disease not amenable to carotid endarterectomy. *Neurosurg Focus, 14*(3), e8.

306. U-King-Im, J. M., et al. (2005). Current diagnostic approaches to subarachnoid hemorrhage. *Eur Radiol, 15*(6), 1135–1147.

307. van den Bergh, W. M., Dijkhuizen, R. M., & Rinkel, G. J. E. (2004). Potentials of magnesium treatment in subarachnoid hemorrhage. *Magnes Res, 17*(4), 301–313.

308. van den Bergh, W. M., Algra, A., & Rinkel, G. J. E. (2004). Electrocardiographic abnormalities and serum magnesium in patients with subarachnoid hemorrhage. *Stroke, 35*(3), 644–648.

309. van Gijn, J., & Rinkel, G. J. E. (2001). Subarachnoid hemorrhage: diagnosis, causes, and management. *Brain, 124*(Part2), 249–278.

310. Varelas, P. N., & Mirski, M. A. (2004). Management of seizures in critically ill patients. *Curr Neurol Neurosci Rep, 4*(6), 489–496.

311. Varelas, P., et al. (2005). Intraventricular hemorrhage after aneurysmal subarachnoid hemorrhage: pilot study of treatment with intraventricular tissue plasminogen activator. *Neurosurgery, 56*(2), 205–213.

312. Vatankhah, B., et al. (2005). Thrombolysis for stroke in the elderly. *J Thromb Thrombolysis, 20*(1), 5–10.

313. Vates, G. E., et al. (2004). Intracranial aneurysm. In J. P. Mohr, et al. (Eds.), *Stroke: pathophysiology, diagnosis and management* (4th ed.). Philadelphia: Churchill Livingstone.

314. Versnick, E. J., et al. (2005). Mechanical thrombectomy for acute stroke. *AJNR Am J Neuroradiol, 26*(4), 875–879.

315. Vespa, P. M. (2004). The golden day after subarachnoid hemorrhage. *Crit Care Med, 32*(3), 902–904.

316. Vespa, P., et al. (2005). Frameless stereotactic aspiration and thrombolysis of deep intracerebral hemorrhage is associated with reduction of hemorrhage volume and neurologic improvement. *Neurocrit Care, 2*(3), 274–281.

317. Vo, K. D., Lin, W., & Lee, J.-M. (2003). Evidence-based neuroimaging in acute ischemic stroke. *Neuroimag Clin N Am, 13*(2), 167–183.

318. Wagner, K., & Zuccarello, M. (2005). Local brain hypothermia for neuroprotection in stroke treatment and aneurysm repair. *Neurol Res, 27*(3), 238–245.

319. Warach, S. (2003). Is there a perihematomal ischemic penumbra? More questions and an overlooked clue? *Stroke, 34*(7), 1680.

320. Warach, S. (2003). Stroke neuroimaging. *Stroke, 34*(2), 345–347.

321. Wardlaw, J. M., et al. (2003). Thrombolysis for acute ischaemic stroke. *Cochrane Database Syst Rev, 3*, CD000213.

322. Warlow, C., et al. (2003). Stroke. *Lancet, 362*(9391), 1211–1224.

323. Waters, R., & Nicoll, J. A. R. (2005). Genetic influences on outcome following acute neurological insults. *Curr Opin Crit Care, 11*(2), 105–110.

324. Wechsler, L. R. (2002). Innovative strategies in the management of acute stroke. *Curr Treat Options Cardiovasc Med, 4*(5), 421–428.

325. Wechsler, L. R., & Barch, C. A. (2005). Management of acute ischemic stroke. In M. P. Fink, et al. (Eds.), *Textbook of critical care* (5th ed.). St Louis: Elsevier.

326. Wein, T. H., & Bornstein, N. M. (2000). Stroke prevention: cardiac and carotid-related stroke. *Neurol Clin, 19*(2), 321–341.

327. Weinberger, J. (2005). Adverse effects and drug interactions of antithrombotic agents used in prevention of ischemic stroke. *Drugs, 65*(4), 461–471.

328. Wijdicks, E. F. M., & Rabinstein, A. A. (2002). Absolutely no hope? Some ambiguity of futility of care in devastating acute stroke. *Crit Care Med, 32*(11), 2332–2342.

329. Wijdicks, E. F. (2004). Induced hypothermia in neurocatastrophes: feeling the chill. *Rev Neurol Dis, 1*(1), 10–15.

330. Wijdicks, E. F. M., et al. (2005). Subarachnoid hemorrhage: neurointensive care and aneurysm repair. *Mayo Clin Proc, 80*(4), 550–559.

331. Wilby, M. J., et al. (2003). Cost-effective outcome for treating poor-grade subarachnoid hemorrhage. *Stroke, 34*(10), 2508–2511.

332. Wilson, S. R., Hirsh, N. P., & Appleby, I. (2005). Management of subarachnoid haemorrhage in a non-neurosurgical centre. *Anaesthesia, 60*(5), 470–485.

333. Wityk, R. J., & Beauchamp, N. J. (2000). Diagnostic evaluation of stroke. *Neurol Clin, 18*(2), 357–378.

334. Wojner-Alexandrov, A. W., & Alexandrov, A. V. (2005). Transcranial Doppler monitoring. In D. J. McHale-Wiegand & K. K. Carlson (Eds.), *AACN procedure manual for critical care* (5th ed.). St Louis: Mosby.

335. Woo, D., et al. (2004). Effect of untreated hypertension on hemorrhagic stroke. *Stroke, 35*(7), 1703–1708.

336. Wu, C., et al. (2004). Treatment of cerebral vasospasm after subarachnoid hemorrhage: a review. *Acta Anaesthesiol Taiwan, 42*(4), 215–222.

337. Xavier, A. R., et al. (2003). Neuroimaging of stroke: a review. *South Med J, 96*(4), 367–379.

338. Xi, G., et al. (2004). Intracerebral hemorrhage: pathophysiology and therapy. *Neurocrit Care, 1*(1), 5–18.

339. Yaggi, H., & Mohsenin, V. (2003). Sleep-disordered breathing and stroke. *Clin Chest Med, 24*(2), 223–237.

340. Yamamoto, L., & Magalong, E. (2003). Outcome measures in stroke. *Crit Care Nurs Q, 26*(4), 283–293.

341. Yasaka, M., et al. (2003). Correction of INR by prothrombin complex concentrate and vitamin K in patients with warfarin related hemorrhagic complication. *Thromb Res, 108*(1), 25–30.

342. Yonekawa, Y., & Kahn, N. (2003). Moyamoya disease. *Adv Neurol, 92*, 113–118.

343. Zarulia, A. R., et al. (2001). Hypoperfusion without ischemia surround acute intracerebral hemorrhage. *J Cereb Blood Flow Metab, 21*(7), 804–810.

344. Zuccarello, M., Andaluz, N., & Wagner, K. R. (2002). Minimally invasive therapy for intracerebral hematomas. *Neurosurg Clin N Am, 13*(3), 349–354.

345. Zweifler, R. M. (2003). Management of acute stroke. *South Med J, 96*(4), 380–385.

CHAPTER 24

Spinal Cord Injury

Patricia Ann Blissitt

More than 11,000 new spinal cord injuries occur in the United States annually.[61,83] While the international incidence of spinal cord injury (SCI) varies widely, from 15 to 40 cases per million population, the United States has one of the highest incidence rates at 40 cases per million.[1,61] In addition, an unknown number of spinal cord injured are found dead at the scene.[1,61,83] Many, if not most of those who survive the initial injury, have physiologic and psychosocial needs that require the focused, detailed, and comprehensive approach attainable in a critical care environment. Few injuries or illnesses present a bigger challenge to the critical care nurse and the multidisciplinary team than the patient with a traumatic SCI.

PATIENTS AT RISK

Traumatic SCI occurs most commonly among 16- to 30-year-olds.[61,83] However, in the last 30 years, an upward trend in the mean age at injury has been noted from 28.7 to 37.7 years.[83] This may be a reflection of individuals living longer; improved prehospital resuscitation efforts increasing survival of older persons with SCI at the scene; or an actual increased incidence of SCI among older persons.[61,83] Males have consistently been more likely to sustain traumatic SCI than females, at a ratio of 4:1, possibly related to greater risk-taking behavior among males.[61,83] In regard to ethnicity in the United States, Caucasians continue to be the highest percentage of spinal cord–injured individuals, at approximately 67.4%, with African Americans at 19.4%, Hispanics at 10.1%, and the remaining racial/ethnic groups at 3.2%.[61] The three leading causes of traumatic SCI are motor vehicle crashes, falls, and violence, especially gunshot wounds. Other significant causes of traumatic SCI include sports and work-related accidents.[61,83]

PREVENTION

An estimated two thirds to three fourths of all traumatic spinal cord injuries are preventable.[89,109] Obvious preventive strategies include avoiding alcohol intoxication when driving; wearing seat belts; and driving within speed limits congruent with legal restrictions, weather, and road conditions.[111] Several trauma prevention programs have been initiated in an attempt to modify risk-taking behavior of young people. Some, such as Mothers Against Drunk Driving and Students Against Drunk Driving, are nonspecific to SCI. Others, such as the Think First program, specifically target central nervous system (brain and spinal cord) injury. The Think First program, developed by the American Association of Neurological Surgeons in 1986, introduces students in elementary and high school to individuals with SCI as well as members of the multidisciplinary team who care for them.[93] The combined efforts of the spinal cord–injured individual and the healthcare provider give the young person a personal and professional perspective on living with SCI. A recent evaluation of the Think First program included efficacy studies that showed evidence of increased knowledge and changes in attitude and behavior as a result of attending a Think First program.[93] However, the success of prevention programs, defined as a decrease in the number of injuries, is unknown.

Efforts to prevent injuries in the home include having adequate lighting, particularly at steps, using grab bars and other safety measures in the bathroom, and minimizing slippery floor surfaces. Properly worn protective sport gear, player and coach education, and appropriate training, such as physical conditioning and safe defensive strategies, may prevent some sport injuries.[108] Additional efforts include limiting sporting activities for those individuals with a previous SCI, degenerative spine disease, and/or a congenital narrowing of the spinal canal.[108]

DEFINITION

From a broader perspective, SCI may include nontraumatic etiologies such as infection, tumors, and nontraumatic vascular events.[35] However, this discussion is limited to traumatic SCI. For a fortunate few, damage to the spine, the vertebrae, and their supporting structures—the intervertebral disks and ligaments—does not necessarily result in an injury to the cord. Conversely, an injury to the cord may occur in the absence of damage to the spine and its supporting structures. Spinal cord injury without radiographic abnormality (SCIWORA) is the term used to describe neurologic impairment in the absence of fracture or ligamentous injury on plain spine films and computed tomography (CT) scan.[6,55] SCIWORA has historically been primarily associated with pediatric SCI. However, up to 10% to 15% of adults in the past have been diagnosed with SCIWORA.[53,109] This percentage may continue to decrease as magnetic resonance imaging (MRI) is increasingly used to detect ligamentous/soft tissue injuries.[6,14,52,55,91,107,113]

Traumatic SCI may be defined based on the level of injury: cervical, thoracic, lumbar, cervicothoracic, thoracolumbar, lumbosacral, sacral, and multilevel (not necessarily contiguous). The cervical spine and the thoracolumbar areas are most vulnerable to injury because they are the most mobile. The thoracic spine is supported by the anterior and posterior rib cage.[89] Cervical spinal cord injuries comprise approximately 50% to 55% of all spinal cord injuries, with thoracic and thoracolumbar spinal cord injuries following at 10% to 15% and 15% to 20%, respectively.[35] Approximately 10% are lumbosacral or pure sacral insults.[35] Approximately 20% of all spinal cord–injured patients have injury at more than one level.[35] The neurologic level, which may be different or the same as the level of spine injury, is the lowest level of the spinal cord with normal bilateral motor strength and sensation, as shown in Figure 24-1. Quadriplegics, also referred to as tetraplegics, are those with injuries at or above C7, and paraplegics are those with injuries below C7.[63,105]

In addition to level, SCI is classified as complete or incomplete. A complete injury occurs when all sensory and motor function below the level of spinal cord lesion is absent (Figure 24-2). An incomplete injury is defined as residual neurologic function, motor or sensory, noncontiguous below the level of neurologic injury.

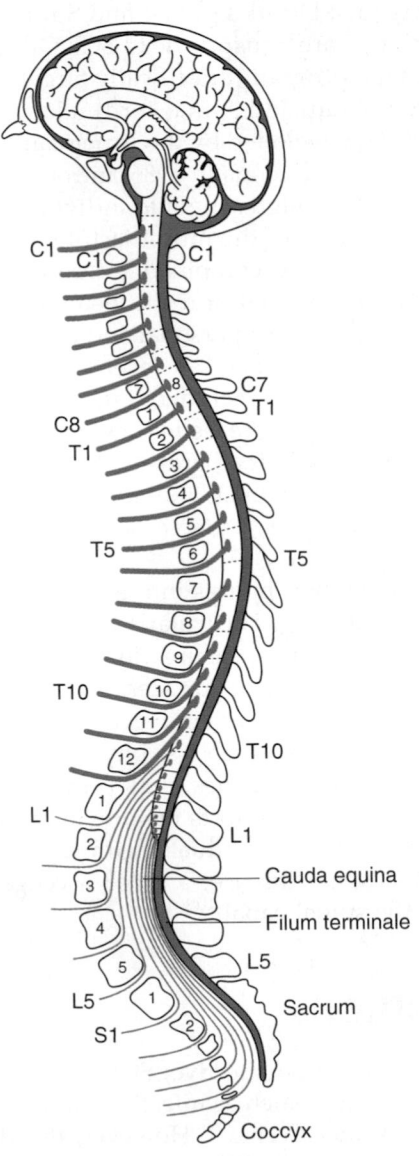

◆FIGURE 24-1 Spinal nerves emerging from the spinal cord through the intervertebral foramina.

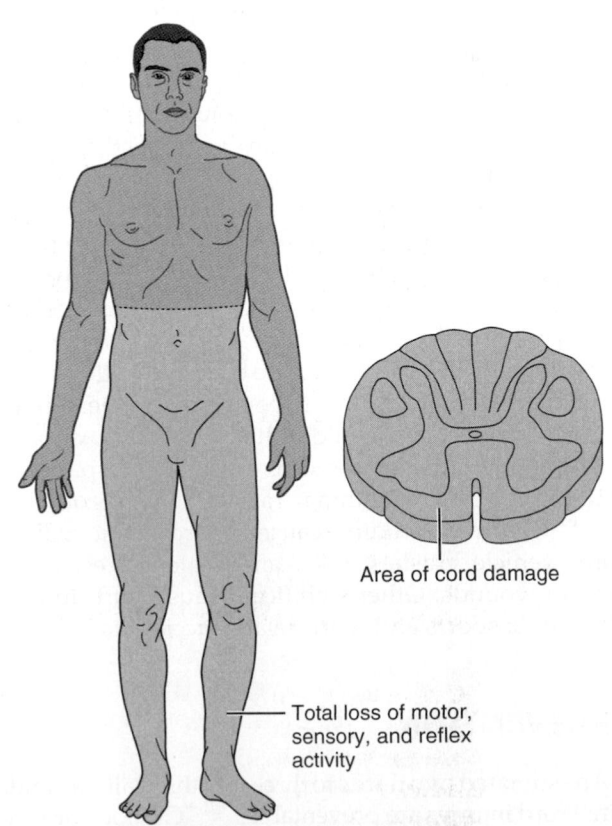

Area of cord damage

Total loss of motor, sensory, and reflex activity

◆FIGURE 24-2 Complete lesion.

A number of incomplete syndromes with characteristic clinical findings exist, including anterior cord, posterior cord, Brown-Séquard, central cord, conus medullaris, and cauda equina. These syndromes are summarized in Table 24-1.

Anterior cord syndrome results when the anterior motor and sensory pathways of the spinal cord are injured (Figure 24-3). Voluntary movement, pain and temperature sensation, and light touch are impaired, while proprioception, vibration, and tactile discrimination are retained.[74,89,107] In contrast, posterior cord injury (dorsal column syndrome) impairs proprioception, vibration, and tactile discrimination (Figure 24-4).[35,74,107] Brown-Séquard syndrome is a physiologic hemi-transection of the spinal cord with (1) ipsilateral voluntary motor loss; (2) ipsilateral impairment of proprioception, vibration, and discriminatory touch; and (3) contralateral impairment of pain and temperature sensation (Figure 24-5).[74,89,107] Central cord syndrome, an injury to the cervical region, is characterized by greater motor impairment and sensory deficits in the arms than the legs (Figure 24-6). Central cord syndrome is associated with sacral sparing.[74,89,107] Sacral sparing refers to noninvolvement of the sacral nerve roots, which control bowel, bladder, and sexual function. Recovery from an incomplete injury is variable. However, the potential for a better outcome is greater with incomplete injury than with complete injury.[88]

In contrast, both conus medullaris syndrome and cauda equina syndrome result in loss of bowel and bladder function and sexual dysfunction (Figure 24-7). Injury to the conus medullaris, the cauda equina, and lumbar nerve roots may also impact lower limb movement to variable degrees. The cauda equina syndrome involves not only the lumbosacral nerve roots but also the peripheral nerve roots that extend beyond the conus medullaris at the end of the spinal cord.[17,58,89,107] In the adult, the spinal cord ends at vertebral levels L1-L2.[17,107]

As with trauma in general, particular mechanisms of injury in spinal cord trauma are associated with and

TABLE 24-1 Spinal Cord Syndromes

SYNDROME	COMMON MECHANISMS OF INJURY	FEATURES
Complete	Multiple	Disruption of all voluntary movement and sensory function below level of lesion Quadriplegia/tetraplegia: cervical spinal cord injury Paraplegia: thoracic spinal cord injury
Incomplete		Some movement or sensation below level of lesion
Anterior	Anterior cord compression/flexion Interruption of blood supply to anterior two thirds of spinal cord	Paralysis with loss of pain and temperature and light touch below injury
Posterior	Posterior cord compression/extension	Loss of vibration, proprioception, and tactile discrimination below injury
Central cord	Hyperextension to cervical spine	Motor loss greater in upper extremities than lower extremities; variable sensory and bladder function loss
Brown-Séquard	Penetrating injury; hemi-transection of spinal cord	(1) Ipsilateral paralysis (lateral corticospinal tract disruption) (2) Ipsilateral loss of tactile discrimination, vibration, and proprioception (dorsal column disruption) (3) Contralateral loss of pain and temperature sensation (lateral spinothalamic tract)
Conus medullaris	Compression at distal end of spinal cord, approximately L1-L2	Bowel, bladder, sexual dysfunction; motor impairment variable but may include flaccid paralysis
Cauda equina	Compression of lumbosacral nerve roots below L1	Areflexic bowel and bladder, radicular pain, variable (lower) motor and sensory loss

Data from references 17, 35, 89, 96.

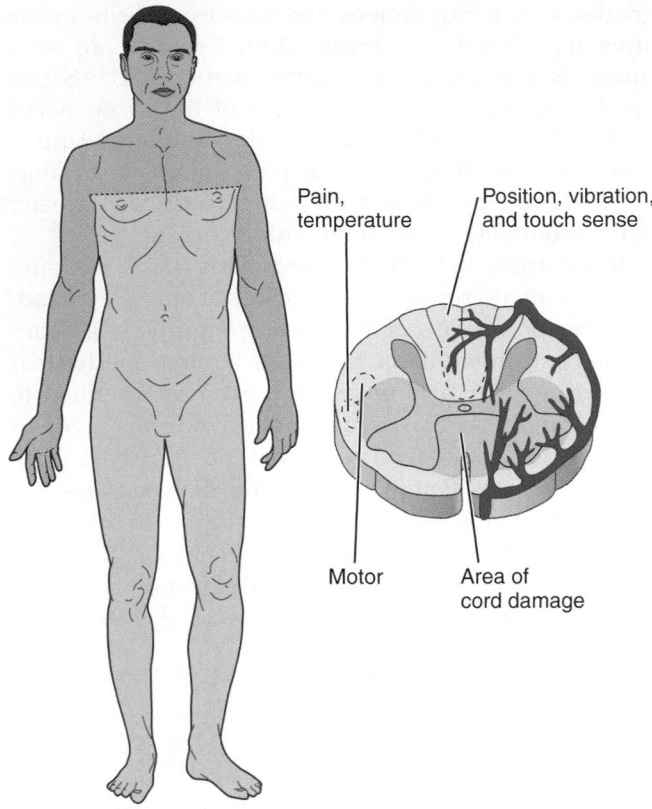

FIGURE 24-3 Anterior cord syndrome.

Pain, temperature

Position, vibration, and touch sense

Motor

Area of cord damage

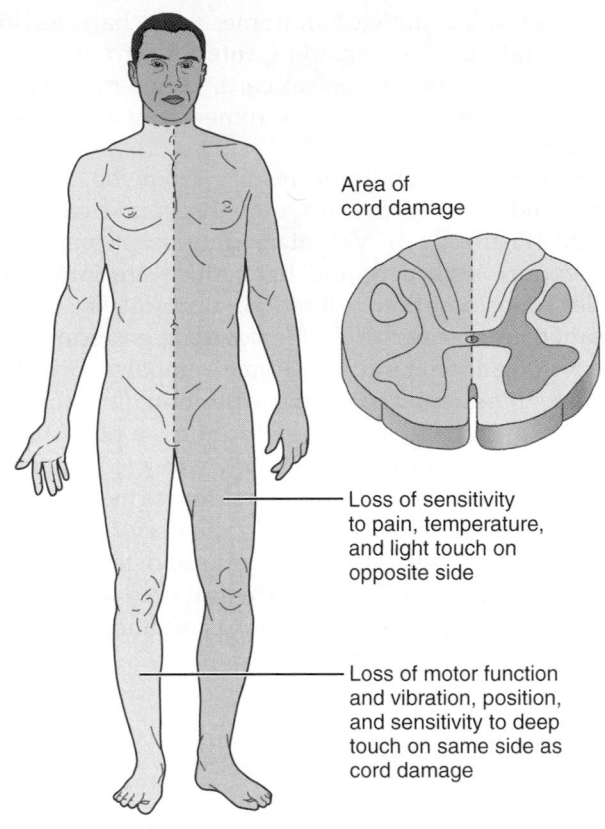

FIGURE 24-5 Brown-Séquard syndrome.

Area of cord damage

Loss of sensitivity to pain, temperature, and light touch on opposite side

Loss of motor function and vibration, position, and sensitivity to deep touch on same side as cord damage

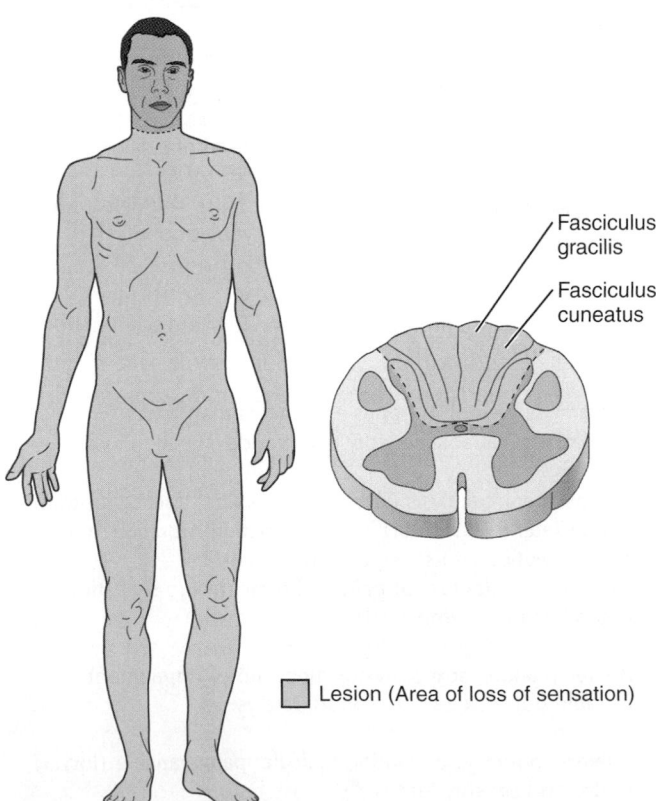

FIGURE 24-4 Posterior cord syndrome.

Fasciculus gracilis

Fasciculus cuneatus

Lesion (Area of loss of sensation)

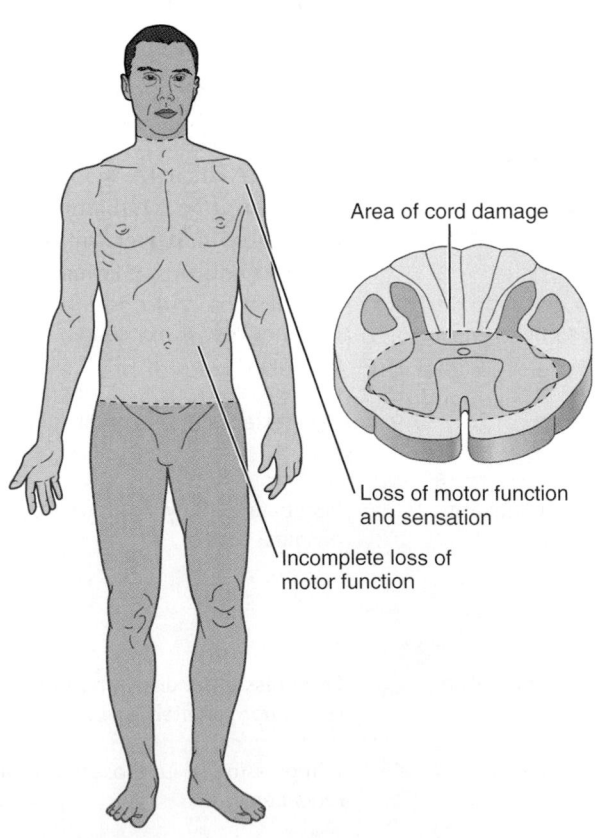

FIGURE 24-6 Central cord syndrome.

Area of cord damage

Loss of motor function and sensation

Incomplete loss of motor function

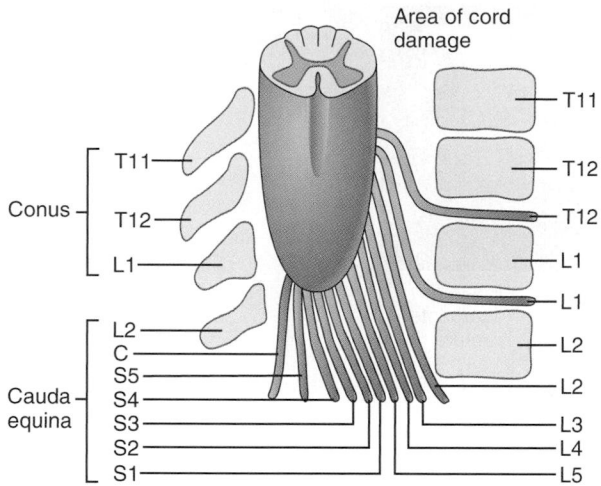

Area of cord damage

Conus — [T11, T12, L1]

Cauda equina — [L2, C, S5, S4, S3, S2, S1]

T11, T12, T12, L1, L1, L2, L2, L2, L3, L4, L5

◆**FIGURE 24-7** Conus medullaris and cauda equina syndromes: motor and sensory function is lost in a variety of patterns. There is potential for recovery of function.

are predictive of specific clinical presentations. Typical mechanisms of injury in spinal cord trauma include hyperflexion, hyperextension, flexion-extension with rotation, distraction, compression, axial loading, or penetrating (Figure 24-8).[17,35,96,105] The sudden stop of a moving vehicle may result in an acceleration-deceleration mechanism with resultant hyperflexion and hyperextension injuries.[89,96] Hyperflexion injuries fracture the vertebrae anteriorly, causing anterior cord injury and disrupting posterior ligaments. Hyperflexion injuries are seen in diving accidents and front impact motor vehicle crashes. Hyperextension disrupts the anterior ligaments and may fracture the spinous processes, facets, or lamina. Falls and rear impact motor vehicle crashes result in hyperextension injury. Axial loading or vertical compression is associated with burst fractures from falls on the head or jumping. Rotation injuries tear the posterior ligaments.[89,96] Penetrating injuries such as stab wounds cause vascular injury and actual cutting of the spinal cord. Missiles cause injury at the point of impact but also cause additional trauma through kinetic energy, involving more than the area of direct impact.[70,89]

Injury to the vertebrae and ligaments may be classified as well. Vertebral fractures are described as simple, wedged or compressed, burst or comminuted, or teardrop. A simple fracture occurs at the spinous or transverse process without cord involvement. A wedge fracture results in anterior compression of the vertebral body. Burst or comminuted fractures frequently result in a shattered vertebral body with fragments compressing the spinal cord. A piece of the vertebra separates and lodges in the spinal canal in teardrop fractures. In teardrop fractures the vertebral body is displaced

and the spinal cord is compressed. The vertebral injury may also be described as a dislocation, subluxation, or fracture-dislocation.[40,49,62,86] In a dislocation, one vertebra slides over another, one or both facets dislocate and lock, and the vertebrae are misaligned. Locked facets require traction or surgical reduction.[14,17,35,55,72] Subluxation is a partial dislocation of one vertebra. Subluxation or dislocation may result in an unstable injury. A fracture-dislocation is associated with cord and ligament injury. An unstable injury does not necessarily involve bony disruption but refers to the integrity of the ligaments.[62] Vertebral facets may move out of alignment and become locked into position, requiring traction or surgical reduction.[62]

The first two cervical vertebrae are associated with specific bony injuries. C1 and C2 are referred to as the atlas and axis, respectively. Atlanto-occipital dislocation (AOD) refers to the area where the cervical spine joins with the cranium. AOD is often fatal as a result of brain stem injury and respiratory arrest.[106] A Jefferson fracture of C1 is a burst injury involving both the anterior and the posterior arches and may include a ligament tear (Figure 24-9). This fracture sometimes results in death as well.[106] Injury to C2, also known as the axis, may present as an odontoid (dens) fracture of types I, II, or III (Figure 24-10). It may also present as a hangman's fracture involving bilateral pedicles. A type I odontoid fracture is an oblique fracture through the upper aspect of the odontoid. It is rare but usually stable. Type II occurs where the body of C2 meets the odontoid process. It is typically unstable and may not fuse. Type III involves the body of C2 but is typically more stable and fuses. A hangman's fracture occurs at C2 as a result of axial loading and extension (Figure 24-11). A hangman's fracture consists of bilateral fractures, ligamentous disruption, and subluxation. It is referred to as traumatic spondylolisthesis but may be asymptomatic.[62,86]

Anatomic differences associated with both ends of the life continuum, pediatric and geriatric, may contribute to SCI. Incomplete ossification of vertebrae, greater elasticity of the stabilizing ligaments, and the larger size of the head in relationship to the body contribute to SCI in children.[6,55,73] Osteoporosis and degenerative spine disease with narrowing of the spinal canal or deformation of the spine may increase the risk of SCI in older adults.[116]

APPLIED PATHOPHYSIOLOGY

The architecture of the spinal column affords the spinal cord and spinal nerves with some degree of protection. The spinal column consists of 7 cervical, 12 thoracic, 5 lumbar, 5 (fused) sacral, and 4 (fused) coccyx

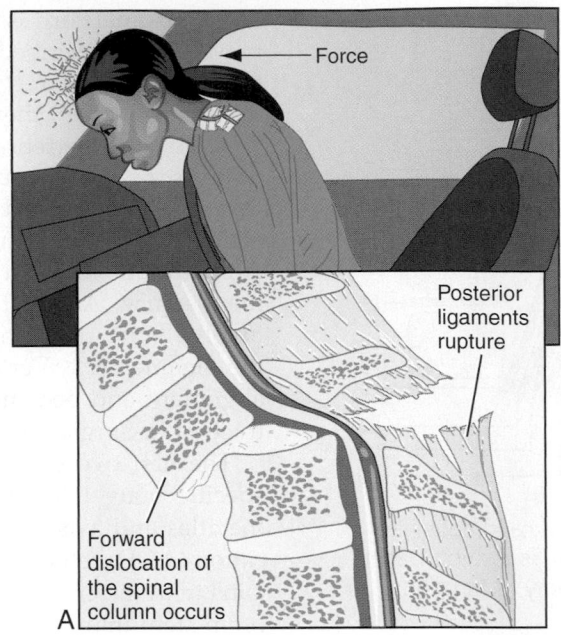

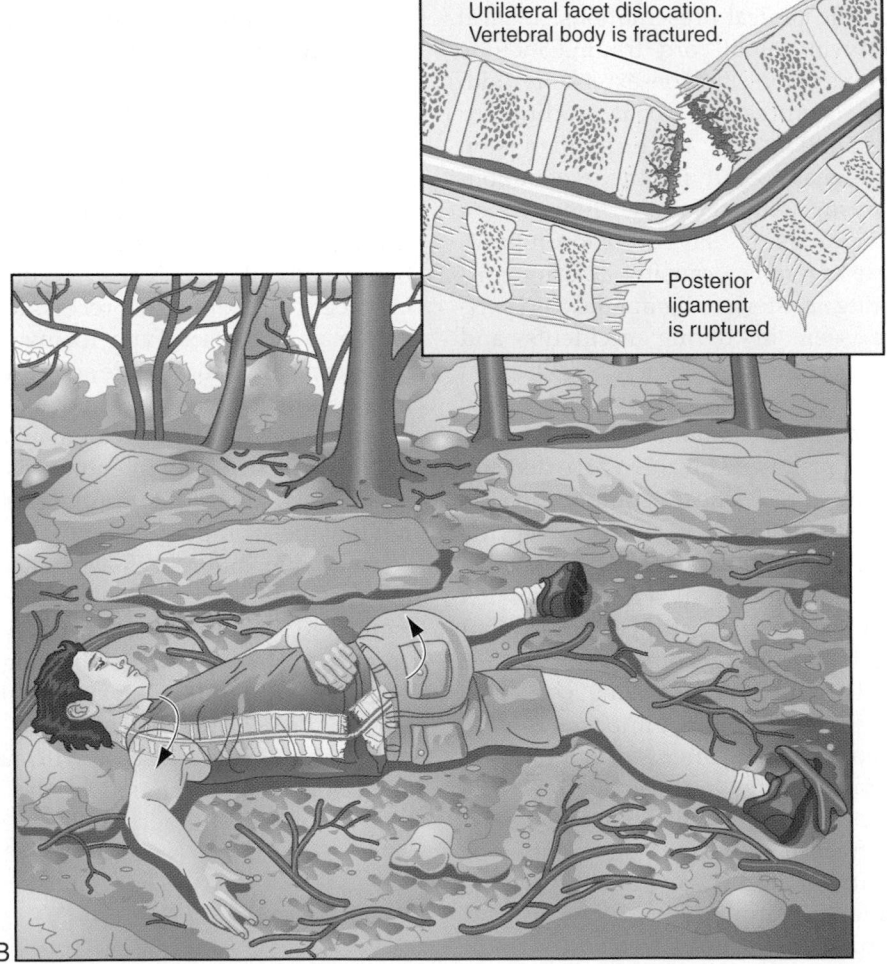

‡FIGURE 24-8 Mechanisms of vertebral column injury. **A,** Flexion in a forward-moving victim. **B,** Flexion in a rotating victim.

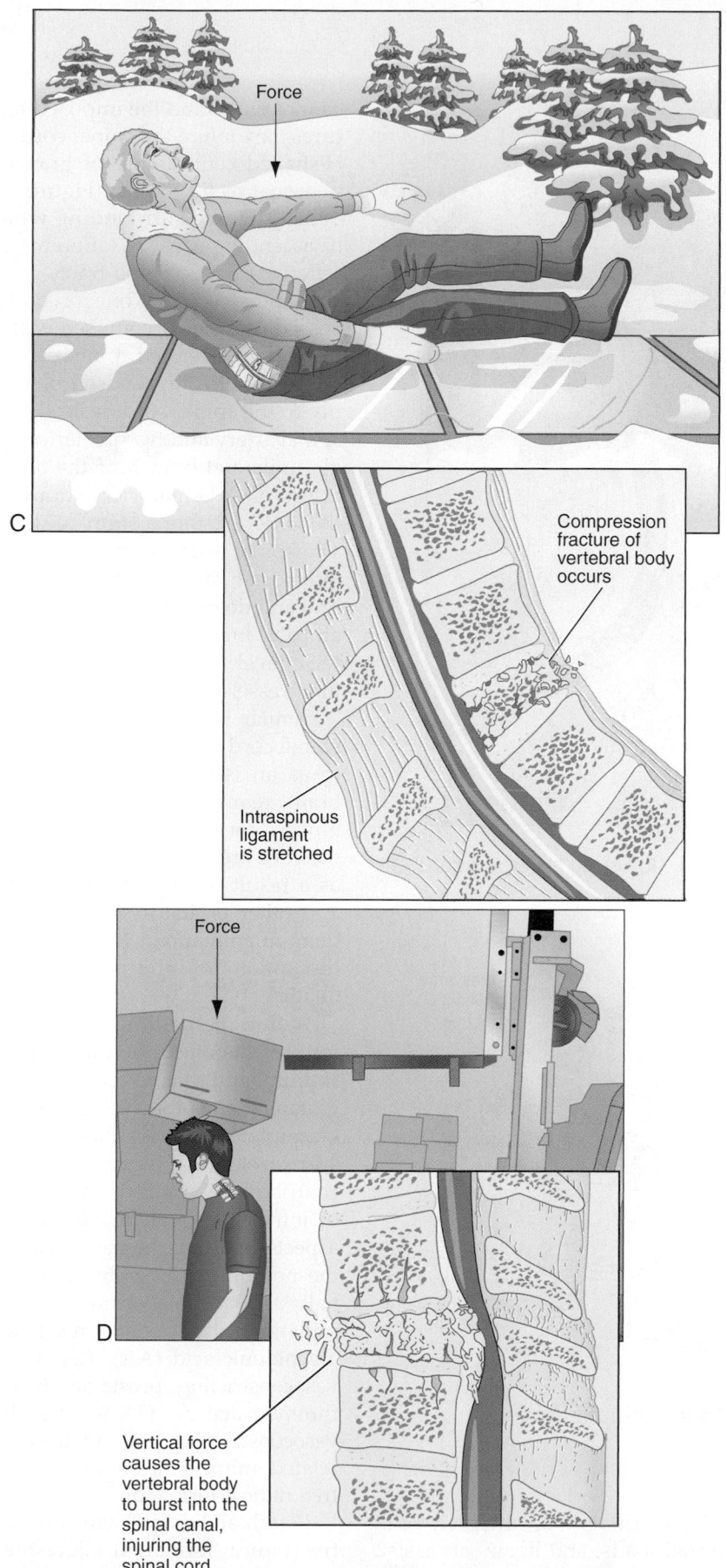

FIGURE 24-8, cont'd **C,** Flexion-axial compression. **D,** Flexion-axial compression with vertical compression.

Continued

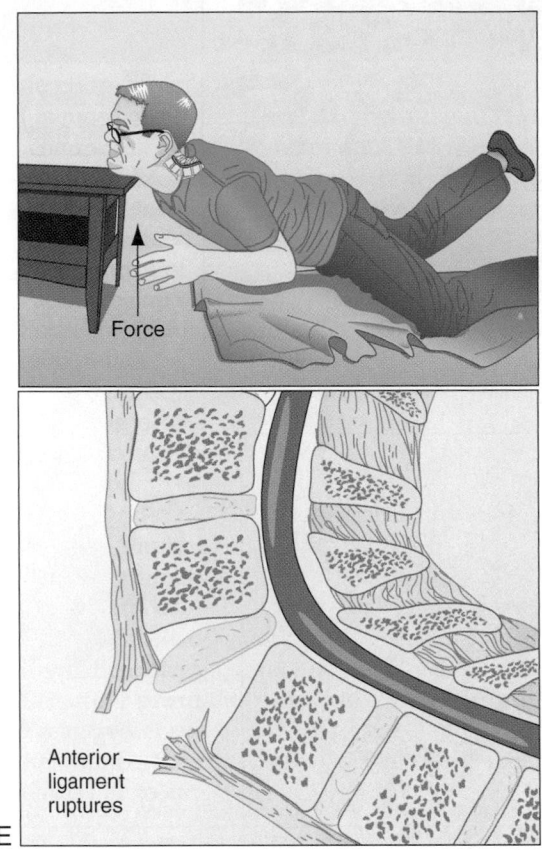

✦FIGURE 24-8, cont'd   E, Forced hyperextension.

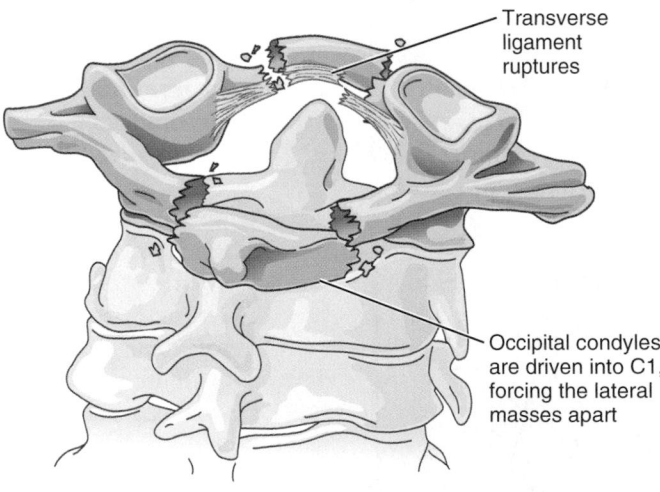

Transverse
ligament
ruptures

Occipital condyles
are driven into C1,
forcing the lateral
masses apart

✦FIGURE 24-9   Jefferson fracture.

vertebrae (Figure 24-12). Cartilaginous intervertebral disks absorb some external loads, and ligaments assist in maintaining alignment and stabilizing the spine.[89,96] However, if the spinal column or its adjacent structures

cannot withstand the imposed forces, these same structures may injure the spinal cord. The spinal cord has an H-shaped central core of gray matter that consists of neuronal cell bodies (Figure 24-13). As shown in Table 24-2, the surrounding white matter is composed of ascending sensory (afferent) and descending motor (efferent) tracts. Some tracts cross; others do not.[17,101] The spinal cord at one or more levels may be concussed (transient), contused with or without hematoma formation, lacerated, transected (rare), or compressed. All result in compromised blood flow. The blood supply to the spinal cord basically consists of one anterior spinal artery and two posterior spinal arteries.[105] A single unilateral branch of the anterior spinal artery, the artery of Adamkiewicz, supplies up to two thirds of the anterior thoracolumbar (T5-L4) blood supply.[101] The spinal arteries arise from vertebral, deep cervical, intercostal, and iliac arteries and the aorta. The vertebral and deep cervical arteries supply the cervical cord, and the intercostals and aorta send blood to the thoracic level. The lumbosacral region is perfused by the iliac vessels.[17,101]

Similar in many aspects to the brain, injury to the spinal cord results in a sequence of events also referred to as an ischemic cascade. The spinal cord, like the brain, requires a near-constant source of oxygen and glucose for metabolism. When the metabolic needs of the cord are not met, similarly, secondary injury occurs as a result of calcium influx, the release of glutamate and other excitatory amino acids, free radical formation, inflammation, edema, and lipid peroxidation with disruption of the neuronal membrane and cell death.[56,96,105]

Within the first few minutes, the mechanical injury induces depolarization and opening of the potassium, sodium, and calcium channels. Depolarization releases glutamate and other neurotransmitters to open N-methyl-D-aspartate (NMDA) and α-amino-3-hydroxy-5-methyl-4-isoxazolepropionic acid (AMPA) channels, which also contribute to increased intracellular calcium. The influx of intracellular calcium is one of the more damaging aspects of the ischemic cascade. Calcium overload in the neuron causes mitochondrial damage that in turn halts aerobic metabolism and results in lactic acid accumulation, nitric oxide production, and the release of arachidonic acid (AA). AA is converted to deleterious vasoconstricting prostaglandins, such as $PGF_{2\alpha}$, and thromboxane A_2 (TXA_2), which results in additional vasoconstriction and platelet aggregation. Calcium-related mitochondrial dysfunction also contributes to free radical formation.[56]

Petechial hemorrhage, anaerobic metabolism, and free radical formation injure the lipid cell membranes and contribute to microvascular, axonal, and myelin damage and ischemia. Axons and myelin are further

Type I

Located at superior tip of the odontoid process

Type II

Occurs at the junction of the odontoid process and the vertebral body

Type III

Extends into the body of the atlas

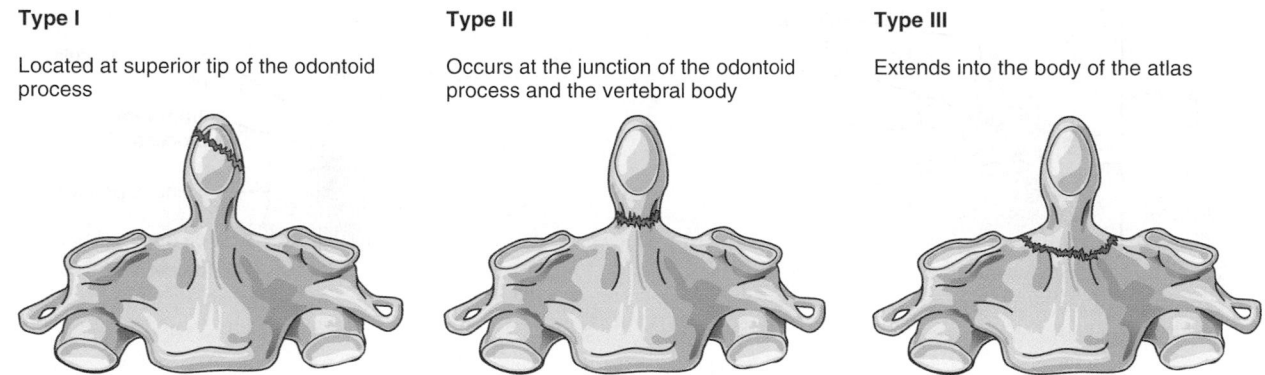

⬍**FIGURE 24-10**   Odontoid fractures. Type I odontoid fracture: rare but usually stable. Type II: typically unstable and may not fuse. Type III: more stable and fuses.

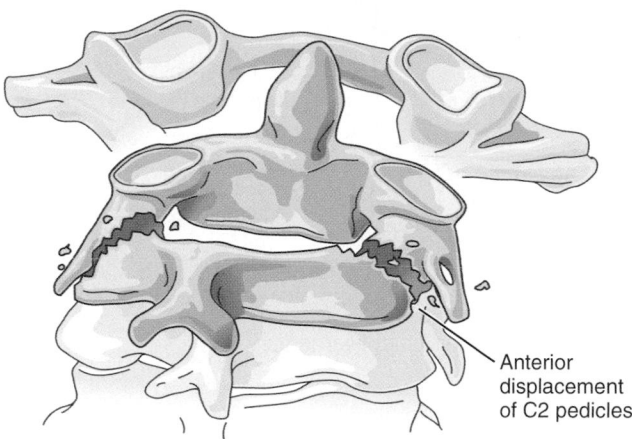

Anterior displacement of C2 pedicles

⬍**FIGURE 24-11**   Hangman's fracture.

damaged by the activation of calpain, which results from the influx of calcium. Leukotrienes (LTs) induce polymorphonuclear leukocyte and macrophage influx, which causes inflammation and additional microvascular damage. Another contributor to secondary injury is the release of endogenous opiates associated with traumatic injury. Endorphins activate opiate receptors. The opiate receptors also contribute to ischemia by compromising vascular and metabolic function (Figure 24-14).[56]

Also, like the brain, the spinal cord is thought to autoregulate to maintain adequate cord perfusion, with its vasculature constricting and dilating as needed. However the mean arterial pressure (MAP) range at which autoregulation is functional may be lower in the spinal cord than in the brain—50 to 120 mm Hg rather than 60 to 150 mm Hg.[92] Autoregulation is impaired in SCI. As a result, cord perfusion passively follows, to varying extents, increases and decreases in systemic blood pressure.[92,105]

Immediately following an injury, spinal shock occurs. Spinal shock is characterized as a flaccid paralysis with loss of sensation, autonomic dysfunction, areflexia, and bowel and bladder impairment below the level of the SCI. Spinal shock may resolve in 48 hours or persist as long as 6 weeks after the injury; shock is replaced with spasticity and hyperreflexia.[35,96] Spinal shock is *not* synonymous with neurogenic shock. Neurogenic shock is the bradycardia, hypotension, and impaired thermoregulation that occurs secondary to the autonomic dysfunction of spinal shock. Neurogenic shock is the result of interrupted sympathetic outflow and subsequent unopposed vagal activity, venous pooling, decreased venous return, and decreased cardiac output with spinal cord injuries at T6 and above.[8,63,96,105] Interruption of input from the hypothalamus results in disturbances in temperature regulation, including the ability to shiver and sweat as needed to maintain a normal body temperature. A state of poikilothermy occurs in which the systemic temperature changes with the ambient temperature.[35,96,105]

Disruption of supraspinal input from above the level of the injury also results in autonomic dysreflexia/hyperreflexia (AD), a neurologic emergency usually occurring after the resolution of spinal and neurogenic shock. The following series of events occurs in AD:

1. Intact sensory peripheral nerves carry noxious input to the spinal cord
2. Sympathetic reflexes are stimulated by the peripheral input
3. The peripheral arteries constrict as a result of the sympathetic input
4. The blood pressure increases in response to the vasoconstriction
5. Aortic arch and carotid baroreceptors send the brain stem input regarding the blood pressure increase

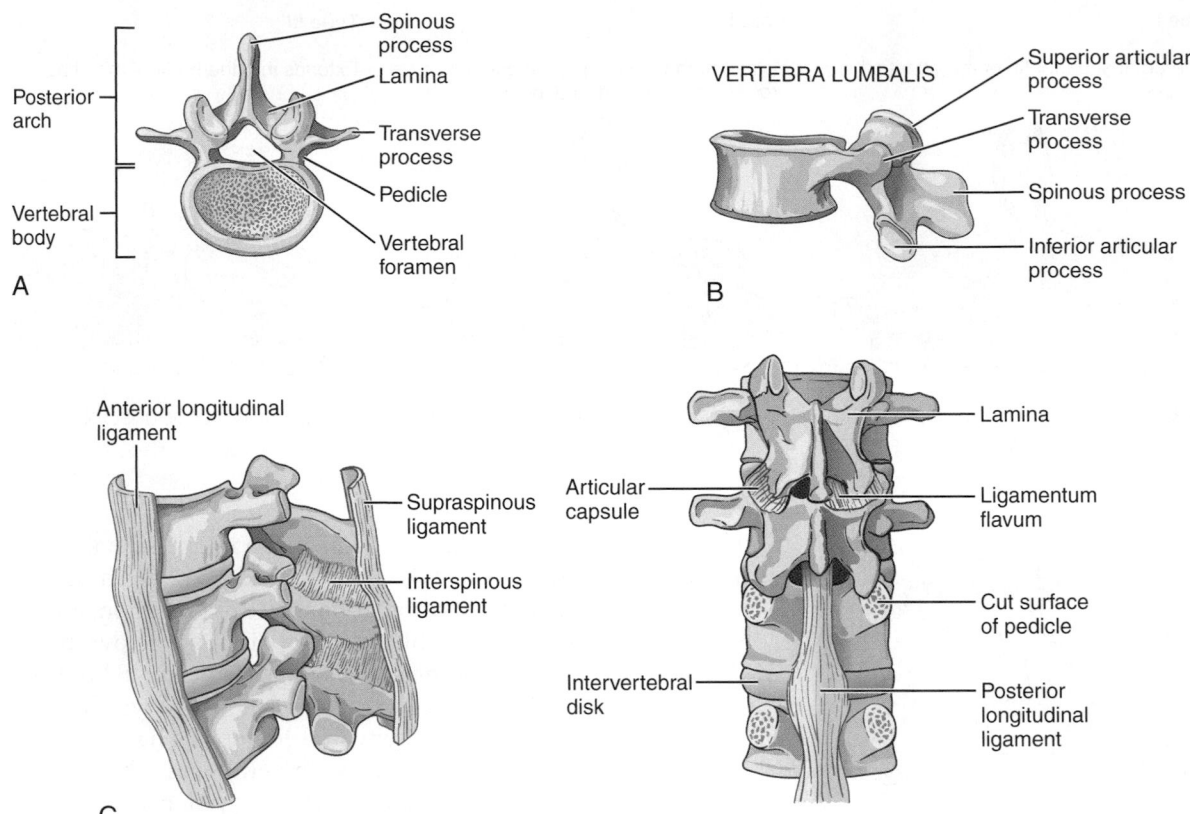

FIGURE 24-12 Different views of the vertebrae and their chief ligaments.

TABLE 24-2 Major Spinal Cord Tracts and Function

TRACT	AFFERENT/EFFERENT ORIGIN/DESTINATION CROSSED/UNCROSSED	FUNCTION
Motor		
Corticospinal tract	Efferent (descending) Origin: motor cortex Crosses where it terminates in spinal cord Destination: motor neurons in anterior horn	Voluntary movement
Lateral corticospinal tract	Efferent (descending) Origin: parietal lobe Crosses in medulla (decussation of pyramids) Destination: motor neurons in anterior horn	Voluntary movement
Rubrospinal tract	Efferent (descending) Origin: red nucleus in midbrain Crosses immediately Destination: motor neurons in anterior horn	Voluntary movement of upper extremities, especially distal musculature Inhibition of extensors and influence on muscle tone and posture

TRACT	AFFERENT/EFFERENT ORIGIN/DESTINATION CROSSED/UNCROSSED	FUNCTION
Vestibulospinal tract	Efferent (descending) Origin: vestibular nuclei Uncrossed Destination: motor neurons of cervical spine	Posture and balance in response to body position changes, especially head and neck
Lateral and medial reticulospinal tracts	Efferent (descending) Origin: reticular formation in brain stem Uncrossed Destination: motor neurons in posterior neuron	Posture, balance, and ambulation
Tectospinal tract	Efferent (descending) Origin: superior colliculus in midbrain Crosses soon after origin Destination: motor neurons in anterior horn of spinal cord	Coordination of head and eye movement in response to visual or auditory stimuli
Sensory		
Anterior spinothalamic tract	Afferent (ascending) Origin: posterior horn of spinal cord Crosses 1–2 segments above origin in spinal cord Destination: thalamus	Light touch
Lateral spinothalamic tract	Afferent (ascending) Origin: posterior horn of spinal cord Destination: thalamus	Pain and temperature
Posterior (dorsal) columns	Afferent (ascending)	Proprioception, vibration, tactile discrimination
Fasciculus gracilis	Origin: posterior lumbar and sacral spinal cord	Impulses from lower extremities
Fasciculus cuneatus	Origin: posterior cervical and thoracic spinal cord	Impulses from upper extremities
	Both cross in medulla Destination: sensory strip of parietal lobe	
Posterior (dorsal) spinocerebellar tract (Clarke's column)	Afferent (ascending) Origin: posterior horn of spinal cord Uncrossed from sacrum and lower lumbar area Destination: cerebellum	Reflex proprioception, detailed control of movement and coordination; posture
Anterior spinocerebellar tract	Afferent (ascending) Origin: posterior horn of spinal cord Crossed and uncrossed Destination: cerebellum	Reflex proprioception, detailed control of movement and coordination; posture
Spinotectal tract	Afferent (ascending) Origin: posterior horn of spinal cord Crossed Destination: tectum of midbrain	Eye and head movement in response to visual stimuli

Data from references 17, 101.

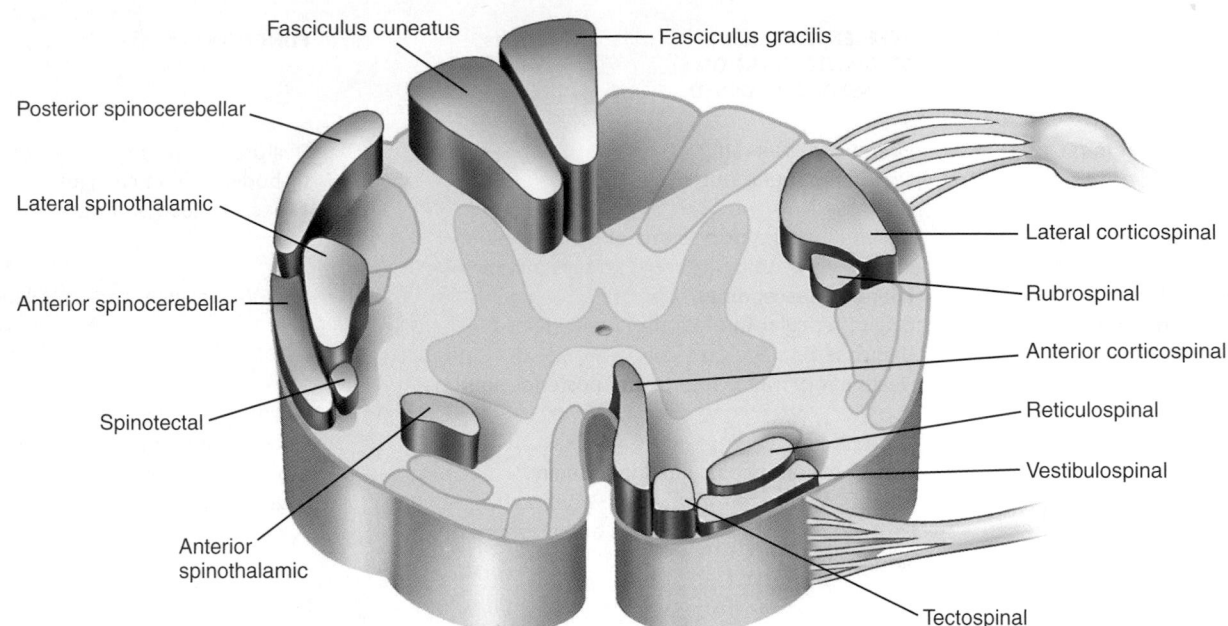

⬆FIGURE 24-13 Cross section of the spinal cord.

6. A compensatory decrease in heart rate occurs in an ineffective attempt to decrease the blood pressure

7. The blood pressure remains elevated because the sympathetic outflow above the SCI cannot provide feedback to the area below the level of the injury.

The clinical manifestations of hypertension, bradycardia, headache, facial flushing, piloerection, and sweating above (and possibly below)[29] the lesion persist as long as the noxious peripheral stimulation continues. The noxious stimuli of AD are most often an overdistended bladder, a fecal impaction, uterine contractions, or a pressure ulcer, and they may result in a hypertensive crisis that causes an intracerebral hemorrhage, seizures, or a myocardial infarction.[29,76]

As with cerebral insults, spinal cord edema persists for several days following injury. Spinal cord edema may result in a neurologic deterioration for up to 1 week.[8,105,112] Much later, the spinal cord may also develop a syrinx (a cystic cavity in the spinal cord), a tethered cord, or a surgical abscess, all contributing to neurologic deterioration. Syringomyelia may present subtly with a change in sensory level, increased spasticity, or pain.[35,114]

Often of greater priority than the motor, sensory, and cardiovascular effects of traumatic SCI are the effects on the respiratory system. The diaphragm is innervated by the phrenic nerve between C3 and C5. If input from the spinal cord to the diaphragmatic nerve is impaired, intubation and mechanical ventilation will be required.

Many persons with spinal cord injuries found dead at the scene die from respiratory arrest. However, injuries as low as T6-T12 may be associated with pulmonary complications. T1 through T6 innervate the intercostal muscles required for deep breathing and coughing. T7 through T12 innervate the abdominal muscles used in expiration and coughing. Respiratory impairment results in hypoventilation, hypoxemia, hypercarbia, atelectasis, and pneumonia. Pulmonary complications are the primary cause of mortality and morbidity in SCI.* Neurogenic pulmonary edema or pulmonary edema aggravated by volume resuscitation may compromise pulmonary status initially. Up to 44% of all patients with acute SCI exhibit neurogenic pulmonary edema.[72,99,102] The mechanism is thought to be sudden, increased sympathetic activity resulting in pulmonary capillary leakage.[99,102] Other pulmonary complications include pulmonary emboli, adult respiratory distress syndrome, and sleep apnea. Venous stasis as a result of impaired mobility of the extremities places the SCI patient at greatest risk for deep vein thrombosis and pulmonary emboli.[47,105,112] Sleep apnea associated with SCI is obstructive or central and may be related to obesity or neurologic changes.[30,71]

Immediately following SCI, the patient experiences gastric atony with hypoactive bowel sounds and delayed gastric emptying. This places the patient at risk for vomiting and aspiration. Later, the patient will require a bowel training program to make elimination

---

*References 7, 14, 30, 52, 65, 105, 112.

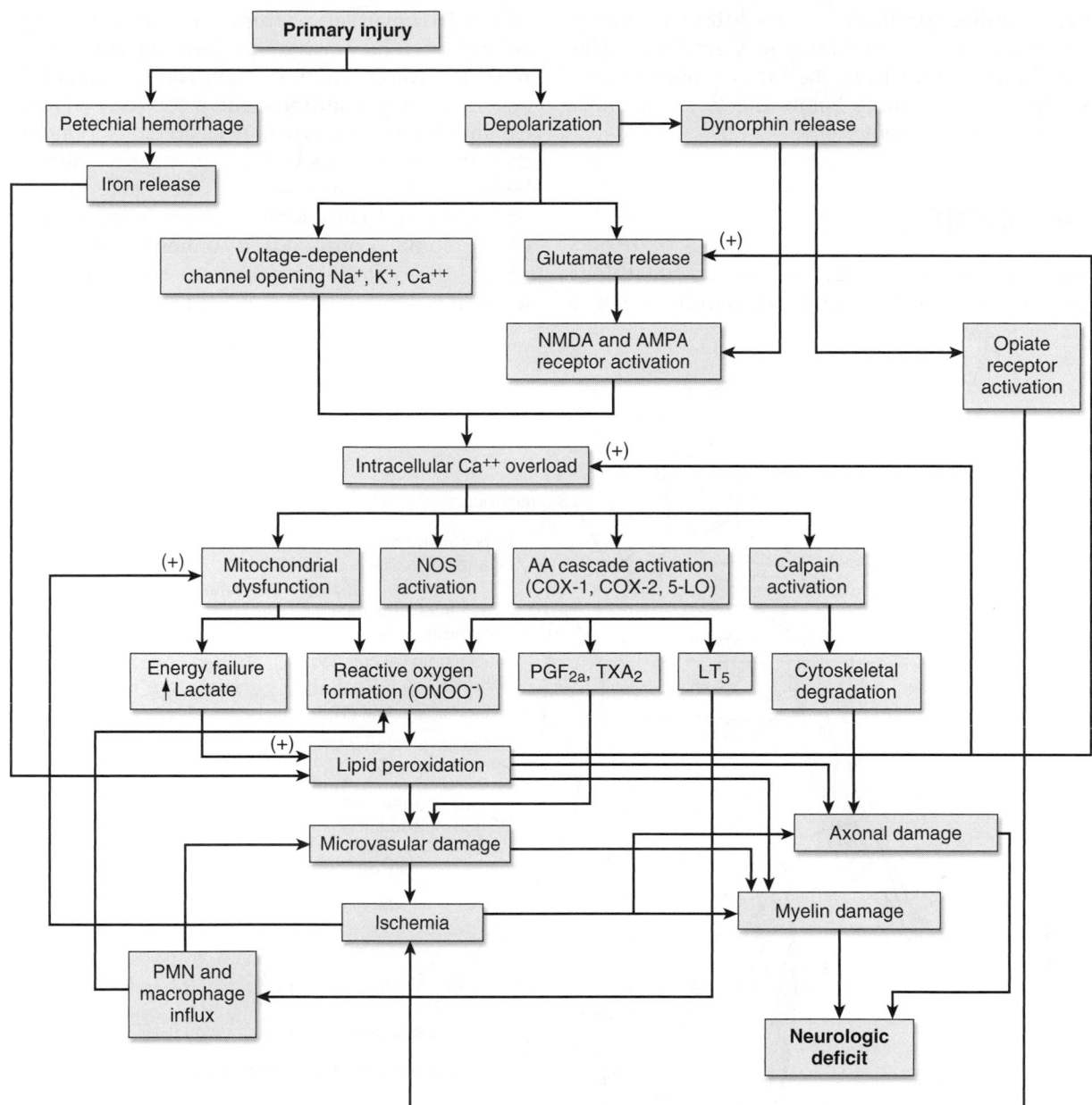

♦FIGURE 24-14 Neuroprotection algorithm for spinal cord injury. AMPA = α-amino-3-hydroxy-5-methyl-4-isoxazolepropionic acid, Ca^{++} = calcium, COX = cyclooxygenase, K^+ = potassium, 5-LO = 5-lipoxygenase, LT_5 = leukotrienes, Na^+ = sodium, NMDA = N-methyl-D-aspartate, NOS = nitric oxide synthase, $ONOO^-$ = peroxynitrite anion, PGF_{2a} = prostaglandin F_{2a}, PMN = polymorphonuclear leukocyte, TXA_2 = thromboxane A_2.

regular and predictable and minimize the risk of ileus or AD.[25] Spinal cord patients are also at increased risk for acute acalculous cholecystitis.[45,117] The increased incidence of cholecystitis is thought to be related to decreased gastrointestinal motility, parenteral nutrition, mechanical ventilation with positive end-expiratory pressure, and use of opiates.[3,45]

Urinary elimination is impaired as well. The flaccidity of the bladder requires the insertion of an indwelling catheter in the early stages of the injury. Once spinal shock has resolved, some SCI patients reflex void.[85,99,106] Loss of neural input, bone demineralization, and immobilization following SCI result in an increased risk of renal calculi.[35]

Following the resolution of spinal shock, spasticity of musculature below the level of the spinal cord lesion occurs. Reflexive movement, not under the patient's volition, may be mistaken as a sign of recovery by the patient and family. Spasticity is the result of an imbalance between excitatory and inhibitory impulses. The normal inhibitory input from the brain cannot modulate the excitatory impulses below the lesion to limit the spinal reflex movement.[116]

ASSESSMENT

As with other critically ill patients, airway, breathing, and circulation are of higher priority than the neurologic injury. However, all attempts must be made to prevent secondary injury while performing interventions to resolve cardiopulmonary compromise. Immobilization efforts, spine precautions, and a cervical collar are critical until the spine is officially cleared.[6,43,55] Once the cardiopulmonary status of the patient is stabilized, serial bedside clinical assessment must take place in an organized and consistent manner. Because up to 50% of all spinal cord–injured patients also experience TBI,[105] the neurologic exam must be comprehensive, including mental status and cranial nerves as well as

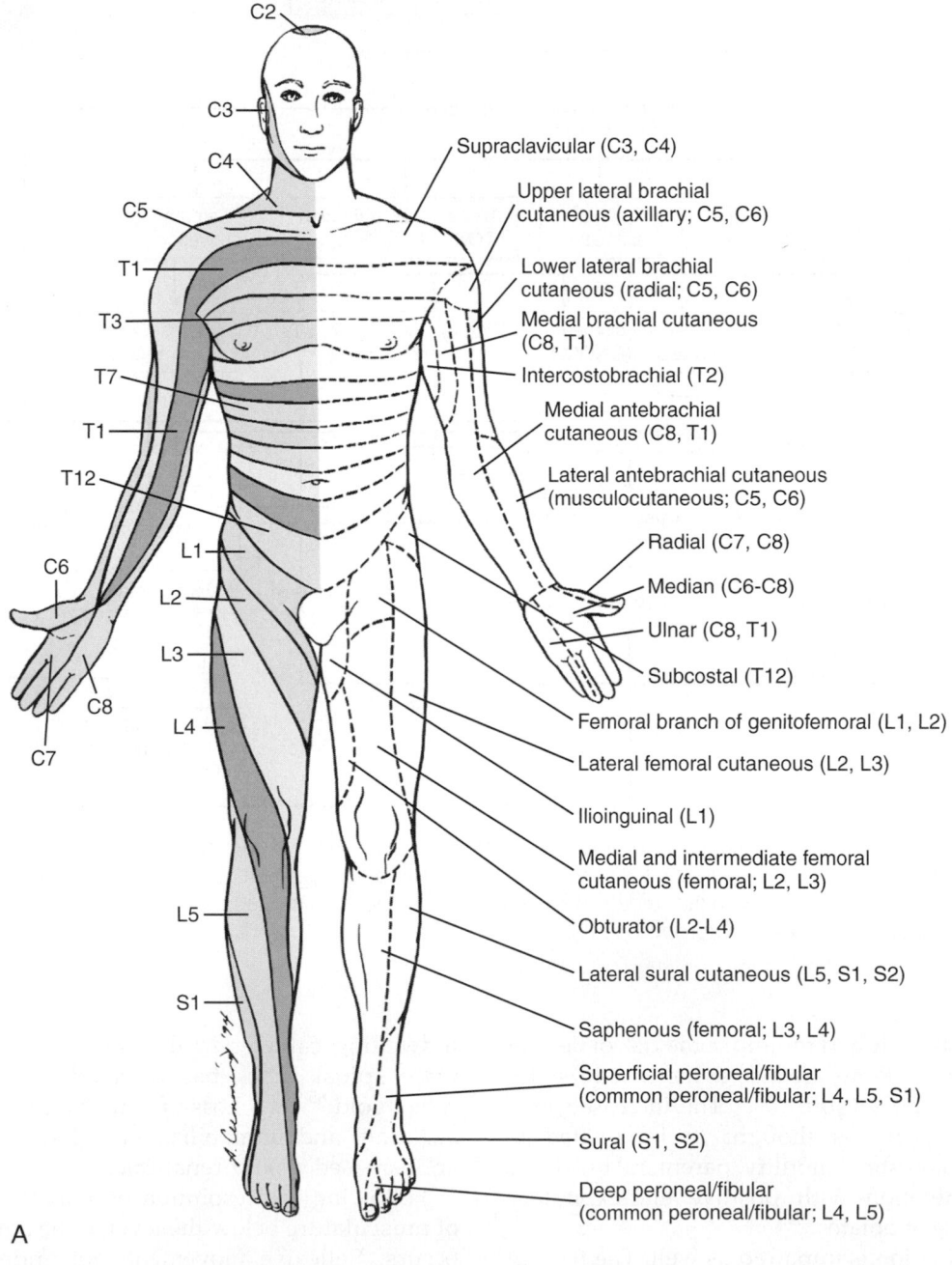

Supraclavicular (C3, C4)

Upper lateral brachial cutaneous (axillary; C5, C6)

Lower lateral brachial cutaneous (radial; C5, C6)

Medial brachial cutaneous (C8, T1)

Intercostobrachial (T2)

Medial antebrachial cutaneous (C8, T1)

Lateral antebrachial cutaneous (musculocutaneous; C5, C6)

Radial (C7, C8)

Median (C6-C8)

Ulnar (C8, T1)

Subcostal (T12)

Femoral branch of genitofemoral (L1, L2)

Lateral femoral cutaneous (L2, L3)

Ilioinguinal (L1)

Medial and intermediate femoral cutaneous (femoral; L2, L3)

Obturator (L2-L4)

Lateral sural cutaneous (L5, S1, S2)

Saphenous (femoral; L3, L4)

Superficial peroneal/fibular (common peroneal/fibular; L4, L5, S1)

Sural (S1, S2)

Deep peroneal/fibular (common peroneal/fibular; L4, L5)

A

⬍FIGURE 24-15 Dermatomes. **A,** Anterior view.

attention to the spinal cord assessment. Until proven otherwise, all traumatic patients are assumed to have an SCI.

The spinal cord assessment is performed in a standardized and consistent format, making bilateral comparisons, moving down the body from head to toe. Muscle groups, dermatome level testing of sharp and dull sensation, and proprioception are included (Figure 24-15). Superficial cutaneous reflexes and deep tendon reflexes, if included, will be hyporeflexic or areflexic. Priapism may be present initially but usually resolves spontaneously.[107] Tables 24-3 through 24-7 summarize assessment of the spinal cord.

A standardized internationally recognized scoring system for delineating SCI is the American Spinal Cord Injury Association (ASIA) classification, shown in Figure 24-16).[6,74,105,107] The ASIA score consists of a motor score composed of 10 muscle groups innervated from C5 through T1 and from L2 through S1 (the upper and lower extremities, respectively) as well as 28 dermatomes, as indicators of sensation. The ASIA Impairment Scale categorizes the injury as normal, as complete, or as variable degrees of incomplete.[74,105,107] The ASIA classification combines the severity (ASIA Score) and the completeness of the injury (ASIA Impairment Scale) and has been found to correlate with outcome.[74,105,107]

Factors that may influence the patient's response in addition to the SCI include TBI, alcohol or other drug use, pain, preexisting illness/injury, and other injuries

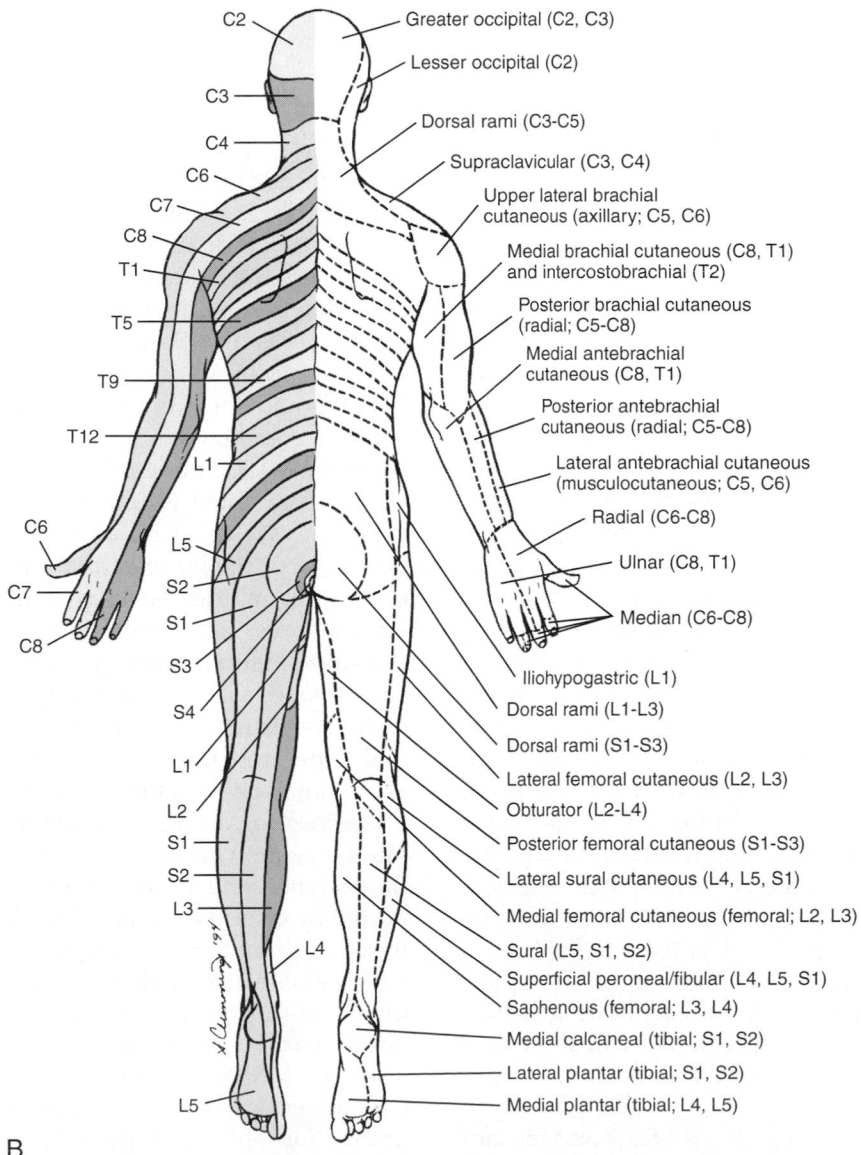

B

✦FIGURE 24-15, cont'd Dermatomes. **B,** Posterior view.

TABLE 24-3 Cutaneous Reflexes, Level of Spinal Cord Innervation, and Method of Stimulation and Response

REFLEX	SPINAL INNERVATION	STIMULUS	RESPONSE
Upper abdominal	T8-T9-T10	Stroke upper abdomen	Abdominal wall contraction causes umbilicus to move toward stimulus
Lower abdominal	T10-T11-T12	Stroke lower abdomen	Abdominal wall contraction causes umbilicus to move toward stimulus
Cremasteric	L1-L2	Stroke medial thigh	Testicular elevation
Bulbocavernosus	S3-S4	Pressure to glans penis	Contraction of anus
Anal wink	S2-S3-S4	Stroke perianal area	Contraction of external anal sphincter

From reference 6a.

such as chest and abdominal injuries and long bone fractures.[107] A routine laboratory workup includes arterial blood gases, serum chemistries, complete blood count, coagulation studies, and urine/blood ethanol and drug screens.

Of great priority is the radiologic evaluation. The first film to be obtained should be a cross-table lateral cervical spine film. Cross-table lateral cervical spine films are accurate approximately 70% to 83% of the time and will reveal an atlanto-occipital or atlanto-axial dissociation.[62] In addition to the lateral cross-table cervical spine view, the routine radiologic workup includes anteroposterior spine films and an open-mouth view of the cervical spine to visualize the odontoid process of C2. A complete cervical spine film series requires visualization of all seven cervical vertebrae, C1 through C7. To facilitate visualization of C7, a swimmer's view may be required. The swimmer's view requires the patient to be turned slightly more than laterally, with one arm extended toward the head and abducted 180 degrees while the other arm is extended posteriorly and toward the feet. This maneuver moves the shoulder away from the cervicothoracic junction.[62] If the patient is able to cooperate, flexion-extension films under the direction of a physician may aid in clearing the cervical spine.[62] Flexion-extension radiographic evaluation can also be performed under fluoroscopy.[62] CT is used to confirm or dispel questionable areas of fracture on the plain films.[62] If the patient is unable to cooperate in a bedside assessment to clear the spine, MRI will show ligamentous injury. However, false-positives may result.[6,55,91,113]

Because of the devastating effects of SCI and the lack of well-designed prospective randomized controlled trials (Class I evidence) (Box 24-1), clearance of the cervical spine continues to be an area of great anxiety and debate without universally applied standards.[86,91,121] As a result, some trauma patients are subjected to additional x-ray exposure; transport out of the critical care unit to radiology with the increased possibility of disruption of life-sustaining interventions; and the added discomfort and potential skin breakdown from wearing a cervical collar that may not be necessary. Based on current evidence in 2002, the American Association of Neurological Surgeons (AANS) and the Congress of Neurological Surgeons (CNS) recommended, as a standard (Class I evidence based on 40,000 patients), radiographic evaluation of the cervical spine is unnecessary in trauma patients who are awake, alert, and not intoxicated; without neck pain or tenderness; and without other significant distracting injuries such as long bone fractures, visceral injuries, large lacerations, or burns.[6,55] In regard to symptomatic trauma patients, the AANS and CNS recommend, as a standard, a three-view cervical spine series consisting of anteroposterior, lateral, and odontoid films and CT scan for any suspicious areas or areas not well visualized by plain x-rays. However, guidelines regarding discontinuation of cervical spine immobilization are only an option (supported by Class III evidence, the weakest) and not a standard (supported by Class I evidence, the highest). Cervical spine immobilization for symptomatic awake trauma patients with neck pain or tenderness may be discontinued with normal cervical spine films (and CT as needed) and either normal flexion-extension x-rays or a normal MRI within 48 hours of injury. Discontinuation of cervical spine immobilization is also only an option for obtunded patients with normal cervical spine films (and CT as needed) and at least one of the following: normal flexion-extension studies under

TABLE 24-4 Muscle Groups and Associated Level of Spinal Cord Innervation and Method of Testing

MUSCLE TESTED	INNERVATION	METHOD OF TESTING
Deltoids	C5	Raise arms
Biceps	C5	Flex elbow
Wrist extensors	C6	Extend wrist
Triceps	C7	Extend elbow
Hand intrinsics	C8-T1	Hand squeeze, flex finger, abduct finger
Iliopsoas	L2	Flex hips
Hip adductors	L2-L3-L4	Adduct hips (squeeze legs together)
Hip abductors	L4-L5-S1	Abduct hips (separate hips)
Quadriceps	L3-L4	Extend knee
Hamstrings	L4-L5-S1-S2	Flex knee
Tibialis anterior	L4	Dorsiflex foot
Extensor hallucis longus (EHL)	L5	Extend great toe
Gastrocnemius	S1	Plantar flex foot

From reference 6a.

TABLE 24-5 Muscle Strength Grading Scale

SCORE	MUSCLE FUNCTION
0	Absent; no muscular contraction detected
1	Flicker or palpable muscle contraction
2	Poor; active movement of muscle with gravity eliminated
3	Fair; active muscle movement against gravity
4	Good; muscle movement against some resistance (± may be used with this score to indicate degree of strength against resistance)
5	Normal strength; movement against resistance

From reference 6a.

TABLE 24-6 Deep Tendon Reflexes and the Associated Level of Spinal Cord Innervation

REFLEX	SPINAL INNERVATION
Brachioradialis (supinator)	C5-C6
Biceps	C5-C6
Triceps	C7-C8
Patellar (knee)	L2-L3-L4
Achilles (ankle)	S1-S2

From reference 6a.

TABLE 24-7 Scoring Strength of Deep Tendon Reflexes

SCORE	REFLEX RESPONSE
4+	Hyperreactive, clonus
3+	Very brisk
2+	Normal, average
1+	Diminished
0	No response, flaccid

From reference 6a.

fluoroscopy; normal MRI within 48 hours; or the physician's discretion.[6,55]

Thoracic and lumbar radiographic evaluation is not addressed by AANS/CNS standards. However, anteroposterior and lateral thoracic and lumbar films are generally considered warranted in patients with neurologic deficits, pain, or a likely mechanism of injury. CT scans of the spine are generally more demonstrative in regard to bony abnormalities, while MRI is more likely to reveal soft tissue pathology or ligamentous injuries.[40,113]

The spinal column stability of the thoracic and lumbar regions can be assessed using at least three different classification systems. One such method is the Denis three-column injury model (Figure 24-17). The damaged vertebra is divided vertically into anterior, middle, and posterior one thirds. The anterior column consists of the anterior longitudinal ligament, anterior half of the vertebral body, and the intervertebral disk. The middle column includes the posterior longitudinal ligament, posterior half of the vertebral body, and the

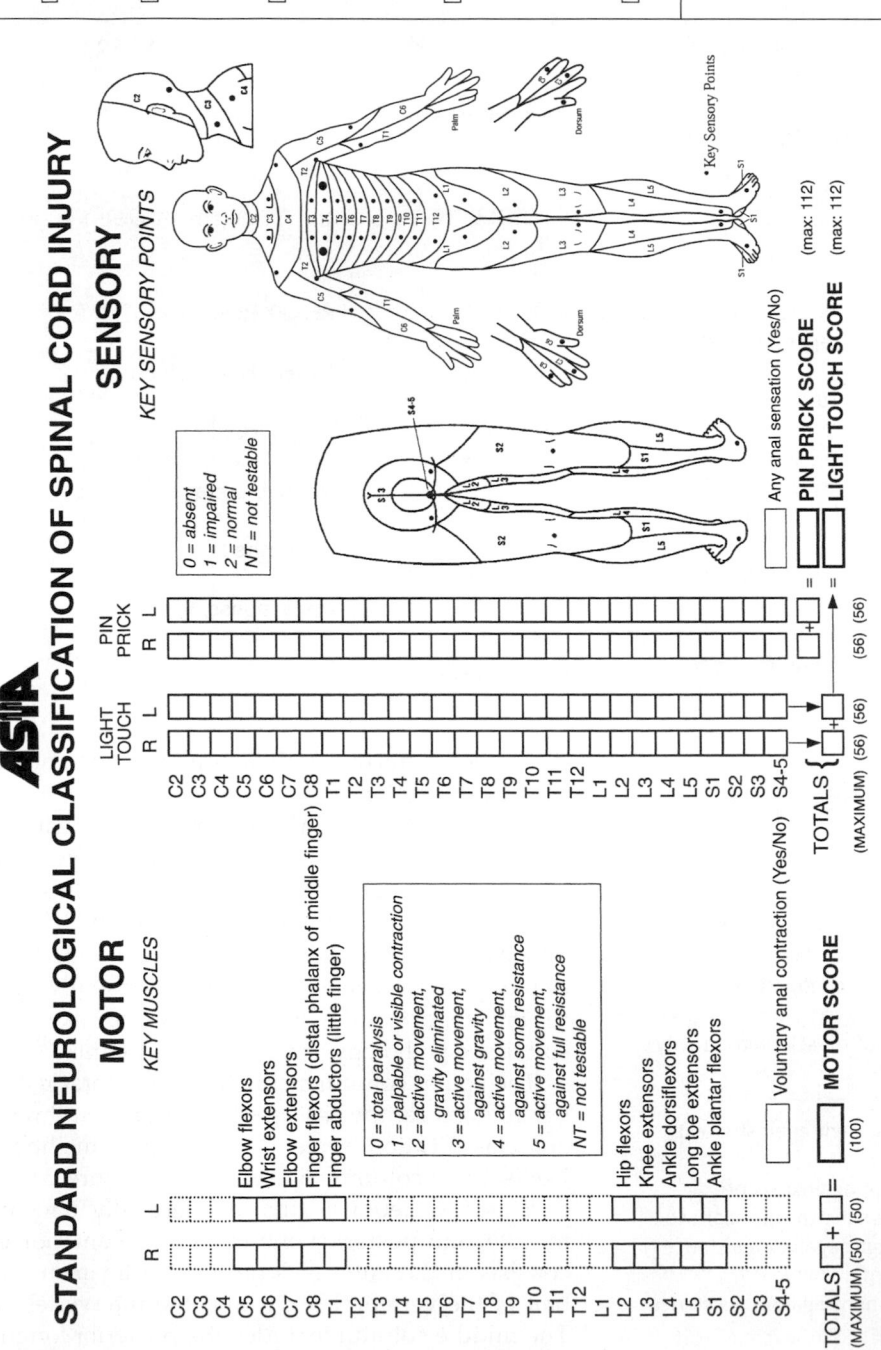

FIGURE 24-16 American Spinal Injury Association (ASIA) scale. Standard neurologic classification of spinal cord injury: sensory and motor worksheet.

Classification of Evidence*

CLASS I

- AANS/CNS: Evidence from at least one well-designed, randomized controlled clinical trial, including trial overviews. Class I evidence supports the strongest type of recommendations, practice *standards.*
- CSCM: Evidence from large randomized trials with obvious results and low risk of error. Class I evidence supports a *grade A* clinical practice guidelines, the strongest type.

CLASS II

- AANS/CNS: Evidence from at least one well-designed comparative clinical study, such as nonrandomized cohort studies, case-control studies, and less well-designed randomized controlled studies. Class II evidence supports practice *guidelines,* which indicate a moderate degree of certainty.
- CSCM: Evidence from small randomized trials with less certain results and moderate to high risk of error. Class II evidence supports *grade B* clinical practice guidelines, with an intermediate level of certainty.

CLASS III

- AANS/CNS: Evidence from case series; comparative studies using historical controls, case reports, and expert opinion; and significantly flawed randomized controlled trials. Class III evidence supports practice *options,* which reflect a lack of clinical certainty.
- CSCM: Evidence from nonrandomized trials with concurrent controls. Class III evidence supports *grade C* clinical practice guidelines, with the lowest degree of certainty.

CLASS IV AND CLASS V (CSCM ONLY)

- CSCM: Evidence from nonrandomized trials with historical controls (Class IV) or case series with no controls (Class V). Class III evidence supports *grade C* clinical practice guidelines, with the lowest degree of certainty.

*As defined by the American Association of Neurological Surgeons and Congress of Neurological Surgeons (AANS/CNS)[6] and the Consortium for Spinal Cord Medicine (CSCM).[24–31]

intervertebral disk. The posterior one third is comprised of facet joints, the ligamentum flavum, and intraspinous and supraspinous ligaments. If two or more columns are damaged, the injury is classified as unstable.[40,77]

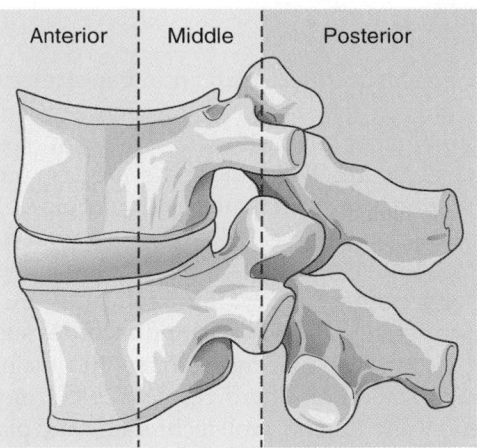

FIGURE 24-17 Three-column theory of spinal stability. This theory is based on the overlap between columns, with the integrity of the middle column most important. If there is injury to the anterior and middle columns or to the posterior and middle columns, the resulting fracture is unstable.

Case Study 24-1, Part A

Evidence-Based Management of a Patient With Traumatic Spinal Cord Injury

J.G., a 22-year-old Caucasian male, was an unrestrained driver involved in a rollover motor vehicle crash. The car broke the guardrail and rolled down a hill, and J.G. was found lying on the ground at the bottom of the embankment. His blood alcohol level was 0.15 mg%, consistent with intoxication and over the legal limit at 0.08 mg%. J.G. was complaining of neck pain and difficulty breathing, and his skin was dry and cool. He was confused but responsive. J.G. was able to follow commands with his face, shrug his shoulders, and move his arms weakly. He had no obvious signs of hemorrhage.

J.G.'s temperature was 35° C. He exhibited shallow respirations at 12 breaths/min with a blood pressure of 80/40 mm Hg and a heart rate of 45 beats/min. He could raise both arms, flex elbows, and extend wrists (functional deltoids, biceps, wrist extensors). He had bicep and brachioradialis deep tendon reflexes but no triceps reflexes. J.G. was unable to extend his elbows or grip and could not move his lower extremities. He had a flaccid paralysis of his lower extremities without patellar or ankle deep tendon reflexes. He had no abdominal or bulbocavernous reflexes. Priapism was present initially. His sensory level was approximately C5-C6. C5-C6 fractures were visualized on spine films. His ASIA motor score was 16 and his ASIA sensory score was 28, for a total of 44. His ASIA Impairment Scale category was A, complete.

Decision point: What mechanisms of injury are likely to be associated with this injury?

Decision point: What associated injuries are likely?

Decision point: What are the initial priorities for his care?

Case continues on page 675

MANAGEMENT

Before arrival in critical care, a number of interventions will have already taken place in the prehospital field and in the emergency department. Although basic and advanced measures to support the airway, breathing, and circulation take precedence over neurologic trauma, trauma resuscitation must be carried out with consideration for potential or actual SCI to minimize the risk of primary or secondary injury. Immobilization and stabilization of the spine is imperative and includes such maneuvers as modified jaw thrust to open and maintain the airway, application of a hard cervical collar, movement of the patient as a unit (log-roll technique), and placement on a backboard.

In the emergency department, the patient may be placed on a methylprednisolone protocol. Considerations for this protocol are discussed in the Research Utilization box below. While corticosteroids are definitely contraindicated in TBI,[19] they are an option in SCI.[6] In 2000 the Brain Trauma Foundation and AANS published guidelines for the management and prognosis of severe TBI, including a standard regarding the role of steroids. Their review of multiple prospective randomized controlled clinical trials, Class I evidence, led them to conclude that the use of steroids in severe head injury does not reduce intracranial pressure or improve outcome and is therefore not recommended.[19] In contrast, though acknowledged to be the most controversial recommendation, AANS classified methylprednisolone for 24 to 48 hours as an option (Class III evidence) that should be used only with the understanding that the detrimental effects may outweigh the benefits in acute cervical SCI. The methylprednisolone protocol is weight-based and must be initiated within 3 hours of injury for the 24-hour regimen or within 3 to 8 hours of injury for the 48-hour course of therapy. The methylprednisolone protocol is not indicated in penetrating SCI.[6,55]

◆ RESEARCH UTILIZATION

Considerations for Use of Methylprednisolone Protocol

CLINICAL ISSUE

Since the mid-1980s, steroids, specifically a methylprednisolone protocol, have been used to minimize secondary neuronal injury following acute spinal cord injury. However, despite three prospective randomized controlled trials—National Acute Spinal Cord Injury Studies (NASCIS) I, II, and III—the controversy of risk versus benefit continues. After a review of the evidence published from 1996 to 2001, the American Association of Neurological Surgeons guidelines recommended methylprednisolone only as an option with consideration for possible adverse effects. Methylprednisolone is thought to stabilize the neuronal cell membrane, inhibit lipid peroxidation, reduce free radicals, improve spinal cord blood flow, reduce cord edema and inflammation, and possibly salvage some ischemic but not permanently damaged neurons. However, high-dose weight-based steroids for 24 hours (if treatment initiated within 3 hours) or 48 hours (if treatment initiated between 3 and 8 hours) may further impair damaged neurons if hyperglycemia results; decrease immune status, resulting in increased risk of infection; and increase the risk of gastrointestinal hemorrhage.

SUMMARY

This meta-analysis included all published randomized controlled trials—NASCIS I, II, and III and Japanese and French trials. Design, methodological, and analytical flaws were cited, and NASCIS III could not be replicated. NASCIS I did not obtain data from placebo-treated groups. NASCIS I results were replicated in Japan using randomization but not placebo. NASCIS II did not report any motor function data. NASCIS III used unequal motor impaired/unimpaired treatment groups, and results were statistically significant only in 1 subgroup analysis, despite 36 subgroups. In addition, NASCIS trials could not be replicated in two smaller randomized trials in France and Japan.

APPLICATION

A standardized protocol of an initial intravenous bolus (30 mg/kg over 15 minutes) followed by a continuous infusion of methylprednisolone (5.4 mg/kg/hr) for 23 hours (if initiated within the first 3 hours) or 47 hours (if initiated from 3 to 8 hours post-injury) remains common practice. Clinicians who care for patients on this protocol must be aware of potential benefits as well as complications, and include prophylactic management strategies that minimize risk of gastric hemorrhage, hyperglycemia, and infection and provide aggressive treatment if they occur.

NEED FOR FURTHER STUDY

Methylprednisolone continues to be used despite the lack of conclusive scientific evidence. However, several other neuroprotective strategies continue to be investigated.

Bracken, M. B. (2002). Steroids for acute spinal cord injury. *Cochrane Database Syst Rev, 3,* CD001046.
Other data from references 5, 6, 41, 50, 55, 56, 78, 90.

Additional realignment of the spine and reduction of a fracture dislocation include the initiation of cervical traction or surgical decompression of the cervical, thoracic, or lumbar spine. These interventions may occur before or after admission to critical care. Tong traction for cervical spine injury consists of metal tongs with a weight and pulley system (Figure 24-18). Gardner-Wells tongs are spring-loaded for ease of insertion and maintenance and do not require drilling of pin sites before insertion. Crutchfield and Vinke tongs require drilling before pin insertion.[72,120] The ring of the halo brace may be used instead of tongs. Gardner-Wells and Vinke tongs as well as the halo ring are available in nonferrous MRI-compatible styles. The amount of weight to be used initially for traction is 5 pounds per vertebral level above and including the level of the fracture or dislocation. For example, a C5 fracture would have 25 pounds of traction initially.[72] Up to 10 pounds or more per level may be added gradually per vertebral segment, with serial neurologic assessment and radiographic evaluation to assess realignment of the spinal vertebrae.[119]

Tong traction is not without potential harm. Increasing neurologic deficits may occur, particularly in people with distraction injuries and ankylosing spondylitis, a degenerative disease characterized by calcification of soft and ligamentous tissues.[72] Other sequelae of tong traction include pin site infections, osteomyelitis, skull penetration, increased patient discomfort related to muscle spasms, and consequences of imposed bed rest, including aspiration. Analgesics and muscle relaxants may be of benefit. To be effective, the weights must be hanging freely and the knot on the rope used to connect the weights to the tongs cannot be resting on the wheel of the pulley system.[72,120] The use of tong traction is at best controversial if not absolutely contraindicated in AOD because of the risk of medullary injury. A 10% risk of neurologic deterioration with cervical tong traction has been reported.[6,57]

Cervical traction may be placed on a regular hospital bed. However, a bed that allows greater turning of the patient is preferable. Two types of turning beds are an automatic rotating table, such as the Roto Rest kinetic treatment table (Kinetic Concepts, San Antonio, Tex), and a manual wedge frame, such as the Stryker frame (Stryker Corp., Kalamazoo, Mich) (Figures 24-19 and 24-20).[120] Both beds have been studied extensively in regard to benefits and shortcomings. Patients on the manual turning frame may fall off the bed if the locking pin is not replaced securely after each turn, if the frames are not securely tight before turning prone or supine, or if the patient is restless or agitated. The automatic turning table will rotate the bed up to a 125-degree arc approximately every 5 minutes,[120] which may aggravate the bradycardia and hypotension associated with neurogenic shock; result in respiratory compromise/desaturation; hamper incontinence and back care; shear the skin if the torso moves during rotation; and dislodge invasive monitoring and therapeutic devices. Turning with either bed may potentially allow an unstable fracture or dislocation to move out of alignment.[120] Requirement of an order to use either bed to turn the patient is appropriate and legally prudent.[120]

For individuals not requiring the more stabilizing effect of cervical traction either because of early

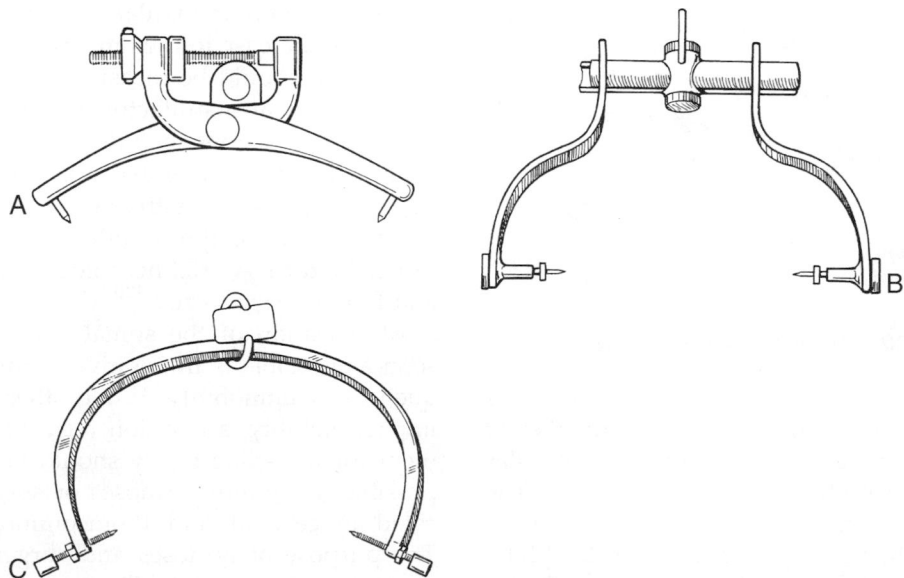

FIGURE 24-18 Three types of cervical tongs. All types have a stainless-steel body with sharp tips at each end. **A,** Crutchfield tongs. **B,** Vinke tongs. **C,** Gardner-Wells tongs.

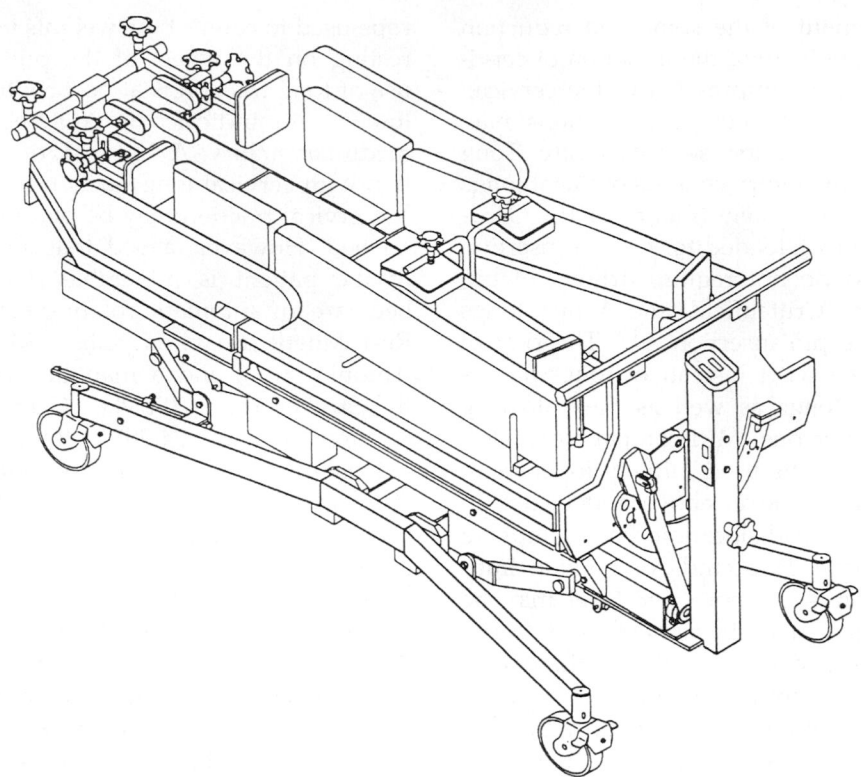

◆FIGURE 24-19 Rotating kinetic treatment table. The table allows the patient to be rotated side to side, displacing weight to assist in pressure relief. It also facilitates pulmonary care.

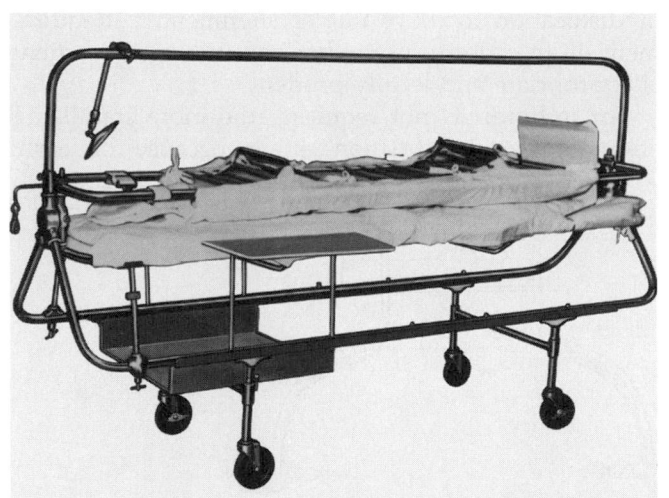

◆FIGURE 24-20 Stryker wedge turning frame.

surgery or because of lack of indication, a number of hard cervical collars are available. A soft cervical collar provides minimal protection against cord injury. The typical first-responder cervical collar is a rigid collar providing maximum immobilization, such as the Philadelphia collar (Philadelphia Cervical Collar Co., Thorofare, NJ). Some cervical collars such as the Aspen (Aspen Medical Products, Irvine, Calif) and Miami J

(Ossur, Aliso Viejo, Calif) have removable and cleanable padding for comfort and provide some protection against skin breakdown. However, skin breakdown is a significant problem, especially at the occiput and chin. A cervical collar is only as good as its fit, which must be secure but not constricting. A tight cervical collar may impair jugular venous outflow from the brain and increase intracranial pressure in TBI. Ideally, the patient should be measured for proper fit according to the collar manufacturer's guidelines.[120]

Spine precautions include not only the use of a cervical collar but also transfer of the patient as a unit (log-rolling), ideally with five people, two on each side and one at the head to stabilize the head and neck and direct the turn. A brief neurologic assessment precedes and follows each turn.[43,120,121]

Mobilization of the spinal cord–injured patient as soon as possible is imperative to minimize the consequences of immobility. While other injuries may also impact mobility, a decision regarding definitive treatment for the spine injury should be made as soon as possible. Long-term orthoses or surgery may be indicated in cervical and thoracolumbar spine injuries. The purpose of orthoses and surgery is realignment, decompression, and stabilization of the spine. A number of considerations and controversies exist in regard to surgery. The following questions should be asked:

Is surgery indicated or will an orthotic device suffice? When is the best time for surgery? What is the best surgical approach/procedure? Will the patient need orthoses in addition to surgery?*

Based on AANS/CNS guidelines, surgical fixation is recommended in: atlanto-occipital dislocations; type II and III odontoid fractures; some C1 hangman's fractures; C3-C7 facet dislocations; central cervical SCI; and pediatric ligamentous injury.[6,55] Either internal or external fixation are options in C3-C7 fractures without facet dislocations. External fixation alone is recommended as an option in occipital condyle fractures; isolated atlas fractures with intact transverse ligaments; and isolated fractures of the axis body.[6,55] In penetrating SCI, surgery is indicated for incomplete injuries, persistent cerebrospinal fluid (CSF) fistula, infection, and cauda equina injuries.[6,70] While evidence-based recommendations regarding thoracolumbar injuries have not been published, indications for surgery include spine instability, neural compression, and risk of complications such as neurologic deterioration, deformity, and pain.[49] A number of surgical procedures exist, including anterior and posterior approaches, corpectomy, decompressive laminectomy, and fusions using bone or instrumentation. Instrumentation consists of wiring, rods, rods and hooks, and plates and screws.[40,49,52,62,77] An anterior corpectomy in which a bone graft is placed is shown in Figure 24-21. A posterior approach using pedicle screws is illustrated in Figure 24-22.

Locked facets that cannot be realigned with increasing traction and serial radiographic evaluations in association with neurologic deterioration require urgent surgery. However, the optimal timing of other surgeries is less clear. One advantage of early surgery is prompt mobilization and initiation of aggressive occupational and physical therapy.[49,62] The urgency of surgery in the presence of a complete SCI is debated. Furthermore,

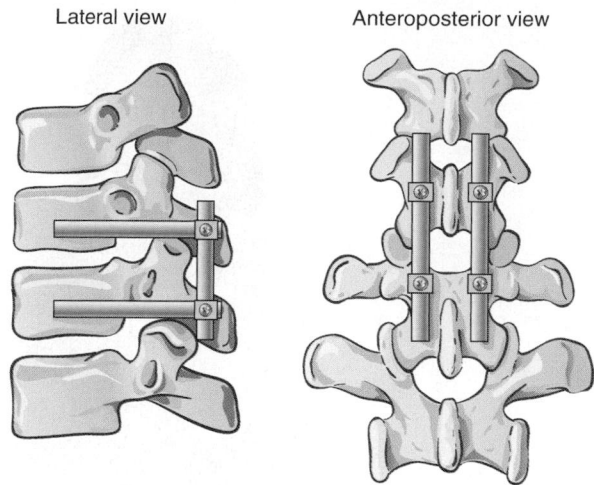

♦FIGURE 24-22 Lateral and anteroposterior views of pedicle screw placement.

because of an increased risk of secondary injury to the edematous spinal cord, surgery after the first 24 hours up to 8 days may be more harmful than postponement.[13] Possible complications of spine surgery include worsening of neurologic deficit related to additional surgical trauma and postoperative edema, cord compression with instrumentation, and interruption of vascular supply; worsening of pulmonary status related to anesthesia, an anterior thoracic approach, or postoperative immobilization and pain; CSF fistula; infection; hardware failure; and pseudoarthrodesis, an abnormal fibrous fusion between bone.[49,62,77] Intraoperative monitoring of somatosensory-evoked potentials (SSEPs) and motor evoked potentials (MEPs) is used to alert the surgeon to potentially injurious changes during the surgical procedure.[34] Somatosensory-evoked potentials measure electrical activity of the dorsal columns, and motor-evoked potentials measure anterior and lateral corticospinal tract electrical activity.[34] Decrements in evoked-potential amplitude are associated with spinal cord compromise.[110] Ultrasound is also used during surgery to detect bone fragments in the spinal canal.[49]

Cervical orthoses are available in a number of styles, including collars, poster-type, and the halo. The halo is the gold standard, providing the most protection against motion from the occiput through C3. Hard collars and poster collars are generally for nondisplaced C1-C2 fractures. The sterno-occipital mandibular immobilization (SOMI) brace provides three-point fixation and prohibits flexion-extension more effectively than a hard collar (Figure 24-23). However, it is less restrictive than a halo (Figure 24-24). A Minerva cervicothoracic orthotic is available for middle to lower cervical spine injuries (Figure 24-25).[62,120] Examples of thoracolumbosacral orthoses (TLSO) include the custom-made rigid plastic body jacket (clamshell) TLSO and the metal Jewett brace

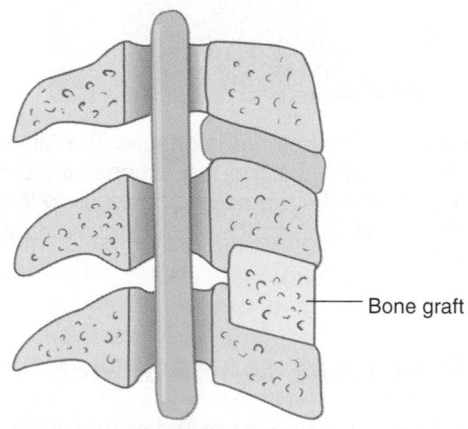

♦FIGURE 24-21 Anterior corpectomy.

Bone graft

*References 5, 40, 49, 52, 62, 66, 106.

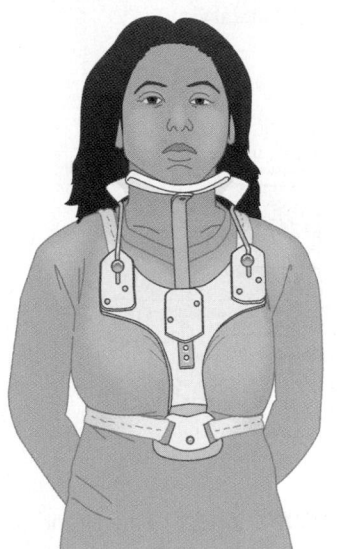

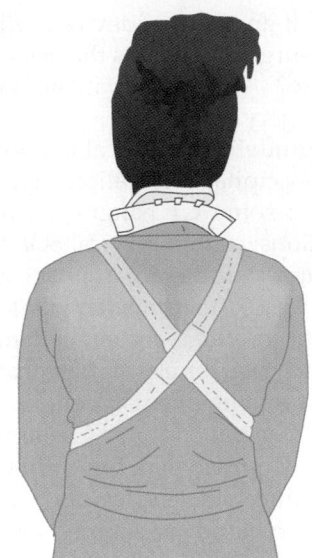

◆FIGURE 24-23 SOMI brace.

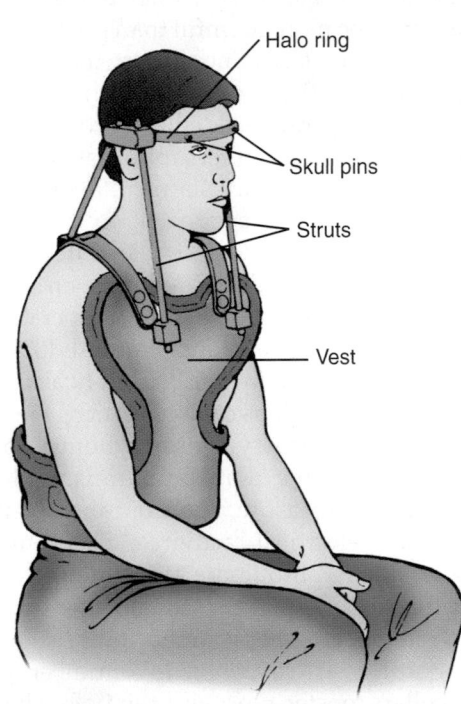

Halo ring

Skull pins

Struts

Vest

◆FIGURE 24-24 Halo external fixator.

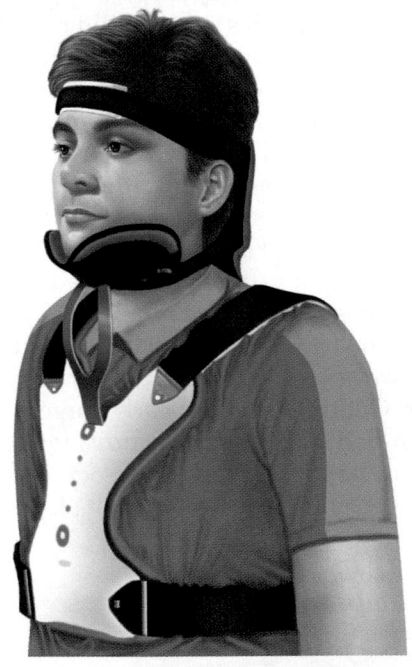

◆FIGURE 24-25 Cervicothoracic orthotic. The Minerva brace is a custom-molded jacket that supports the chin and posterior skull. It encloses the pelvis or extends to the costal margins, depending on the stability required by the patient.

(Florida Brace Corp., Winter Park, Fla), depicted in Figure 24-26. All of these have the potential to cause skin breakdown.[120] The risk of injury from cervical orthoses is even greater, with complications ranging from skin breakdown to aspiration.[57,81,104] Additional complications of the halo include pin site infection and osteomyelitis, penetration of the skull, subdural abscess, periorbital edema, scarring, cranial nerve palsies, fracture overdistractions, and persistent instability.[57]

CRITICAL CARE MANAGEMENT

Critical care management of the spinal–cord injured patient requires attention to each and every system. The pulmonary, cardiac, and neurologic sequelae are the most immediately life-threatening but each and

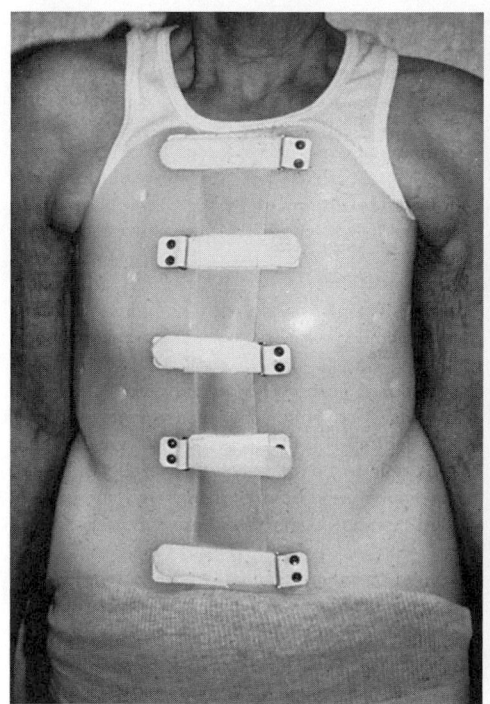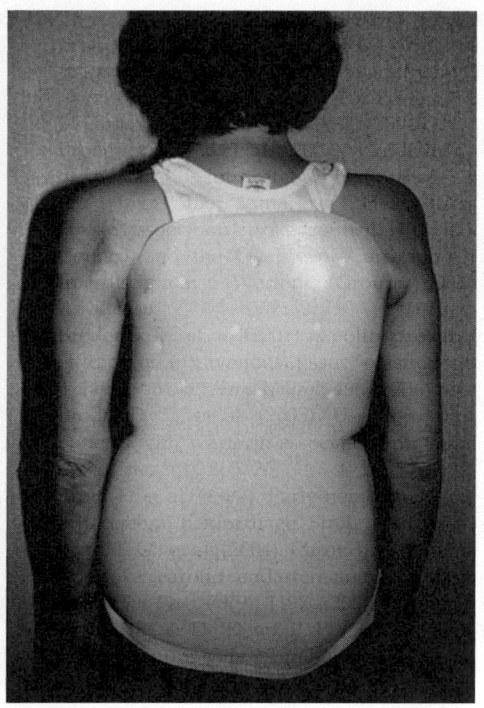

♦FIGURE 24-26 Jewett brace.

every system can pose risk to the patient both acutely and chronically. The multidisciplinary care plan must include consideration for each system as well as a rehabilitation perspective on a consistent, ongoing basis from admission to discharge. A multidisciplinary clinical pathway may provide an efficient and effective framework for organizing care and goal-setting for the patient.[79] A Multidisciplinary Plan of Care is shown on pp. 662–665.

Neurologic

The continuum of care for SCI begins prehospital and continues in the emergency department (ED) and possibly even in the operating room (OR) before the patient's admission to critical care. The care provided before the patient's arrival to the intensive care unit is the foundation from which the nurse and multidisciplinary team initiate their care. Continued serial monitoring of the patient's neurologic status by detailed clinical assessment is paramount.

Unlike the brain, technology to measure spinal cord perfusion at the bedside is lacking. In addition to their application in surgery, somatosensory and motor-evoked potentials are sometimes used intermittently at the bedside in determination of a prognosis. Evoked potentials measure electrical activity, not blood flow.[34] By stimulating an extremity below the spinal cord lesion and recording the response from scalp electrodes, neuronal conduction can be assessed. However, evoked-potential monitoring presents too many technical difficulties to be conducted continuously and utilized in the day-to-day management of the patient.[34]

Neurologic deterioration may occur for a number of reasons such as loss of alignment with or without surgery or traction; cord edema; and a change in the level of consciousness and mental status related to TBI, other injuries, a decline in oxygenation, medications, and sleep deprivation. Even subtle changes may warrant additional investigation. Use of a detailed SCI flow sheet and a neurologic assessment performed jointly by both the oncoming nurse and the offgoing nurse may facilitate prompt detection of neurologic deterioration. Spine precautions are to be maintained until prescribed otherwise.[43] These may include maintaining the patient on a backboard; using a cervical collar; positioning the patient in reverse Trendelenburg to elevate the head of the bed; turning as a unit; and waiting to turn manually on a wedge turning frame or an automatic turning table bed.[43] Though controversial, strict adherence to the methylprednisolone protocol is essential for maximum benefit.[56] Delays and incomplete administration related to lack of intravenous access are to be avoided.[56]

Other neurologic injuries in addition to the SCI may be present. TBI and peripheral injuries complicate

MULTIDISCIPLINARY PLAN OF CARE FOR PATIENTS WITH TRAUMATIC SPINAL CORD INJURY*

PROBLEM	INTERVENTION	RATIONALE	EXPECTED OUTCOME	COMMENTS
Risk for development of secondary neuronal injury	Strictly adhere to spine precautions. Maintain orthotics. Maintain activity and position restrictions, including restrictions regarding interruption and application of orthotics. Maintain traction as prescribed. Maintain alignment postoperatively after surgical reduction and fixation with bony fusion or instrumentation. Administer methylprednisolone per protocol. Monitor vital signs. Maintain MAP at 85–90 mm Hg for at least first 7 days. Monitor neurologic status; report any change in neurologic status, motor or sensory.	Loss of innervation	Maintain or improve immediate post-injury level of neurologic function	Methylprednisolone is treatment option, not a standard or guideline. Observe for adverse reactions such as hyperglycemia, gastrointestinal hemorrhage, infection, and poor wound healing. Failed stabilization procedures, spinal cord infections/abscesses, syrinx formation, or other abnormalities may initially present with subtle changes such as sensory level alterations or increased spasticity or discomfort.
Risk for inadequate oxygenation	Monitor respiratory status, including physical assessment, Sao₂, end-tidal CO_2, CXR, ABGs, sputum, pulmonary function parameters (vital capacity, negative inspiratory pressure, minute ventilation, and tidal volume). Maintain chest tubes and monitor drainage. Intubate and mechanically ventilate as needed; provide oxygen therapy. Perform and assist patient with pulmonary hygiene, including positioning and application of abdominal binder when sitting; quad-assist coughing; brochodilators; suctioning; tracheostomy care; and bronchoscopy as needed. Administer antibiotic therapy for positive sputum cultures. Wean mechanical ventilation as possible. Assist with tracheostomy if unable to wean from mechanical ventilation. Maintain aspiration precautions.	Impairment of respiratory musculature	Maintain adequate oxygenation on minimal support	If patient has or develops a pneumothorax or a thoracotomy is performed for an anterior approach to spinal cord, patient will have chest tubes. Quadriplegics may experience improved ventilatory effort with head of bed limited to 45 degrees (rather than higher) and use of an abdominal binder when sitting. Mini-dose heparin or low molecular weight heparinoid alone is not adequate. Mechanical compression is needed as well. Insertion of a vena cava filter is an option if patient develops a deep vein thrombosis or pulmonary embolus.

PROBLEM	INTERVENTION	RATIONALE	EXPECTED OUTCOME	COMMENTS
	Perform swallow evaluation, especially if patient is in cervical orthoses and has had recent cervical surgery or tracheostomy. Administer prophylactic subcutaneous heparin/low molecular weight heparinoid *and* application of mechanical device such as pneumatic compression leg wraps. Apply anti-embolism stockings. Administer blood products as needed.			
Risk for cardiovascular instability	Monitor heart rate, rhythm, and blood pressure and other hemodynamics as available. Minimize vagal stimulation; preoxygenate before suctioning. Administer atropine or assist with insertion of pacemaker if patient has symptomatic bradycardia. Administer fluids and vasoactive agents as needed to maintain normovolemia and goal blood pressure. Monitor and maintain acceptable hematocrit and hemoglobin. Apply abdominal binder, antiembolism stockings, and elastic wraps before raising head. Administer ephedrine or midodrine an hour before sitting. Monitor for orthostatic hypotension. Observe for autonomic dysreflexia/hyperreflexia. Patients with lesions at T6 or above are at risk. Treat aggressively. Raise head of bed and remove noxious stimuli.	Spinal shock is related to disruption of sympathetic outflow and unopposed vagal tone. The acute spinal cord–injured patient in neurogenic shock typically presents with bradycardia and hypotension. Other hemodynamic findings may include decreased CVP, PCWP, SVR, SV, and CO related to vasodilation.	Hemodynamic stability	Dopamine and norepinephrine (with alpha, beta, and chronotropic properties) are preferred over phenylephrine (pure alpha properties), which may worsen bradycardia. Dobutamine may be added as an adjuvant therapy to improve cardiac output but administered by itself may produce hypotension. Autonomic dysreflexia is a neurologic emergency. Common causes include a distended bladder, fecal impaction, uterine contractions, skin irritation, or poor wound care.

Table continues on page 664

PROBLEM	INTERVENTION	RATIONALE	EXPECTED OUTCOME	COMMENTS
At risk for gastrointestinal complications and under- or overnutrition	Assess GI system, nutritional status, including nutritional indicators: indirect calorimetry, labs (prealbumin, transferrin, 24-hour urine for urea nitrogen), daily weights. Maintain nasogastric decompression as needed to prevent vomiting. Administer histamine blocker or proton pump inhibitors. Administer enteral or parenteral nutrition (see Nutrition box on p. 670). Monitor stools, occult blood, and gastric pH. Perform daily bowel training regimen.	Gastric atony, ileus, neurogenic bowel	Maintain gastrointestinal integrity; adequate nutrition	Use enteral nutrition whenever possible to promote gut motility, decrease risk of infection and central venous catheter complications. A gastric pH of 4 or greater has been associated with decreased risk of gastrointestinal hemorrhage. Best bowel training results are obtained after enteral nutrition boluses/eating.
Impaired thermoregulation	Use warming and cooling methods to maintain normal body temperature.	Loss of hypothalamic input to area below injury; temperature varies with environment	Maintain normothermia	
At risk for genitourinary complications	Monitor intake and output, renal function, urinalysis/urine culture and sensitivity results. Use continuous bladder drainage initially. Once spinal shock has resolved, attempt intermittent catheterization. Avoid bladder overdistention; alter fluid intake or intermittent catheterization schedule as needed.	Neurogenic bladder	Urinary elimination with minimal support and infection; maintain normal renal function	
At risk for musculoskeletal discomfort, pain, deformity	Consult PT/OT for ROM and splinting/protective positioning strategies as soon as possible. Administer antispasticity agents and analgesics as needed.	Loss of innervation	Minimize deformity, discomfort/pain	
At risk for integumentary injury	Minimize initial backboard time to a maximum of 2 hours. Change position at least every 2 hours or use rotating bed when stable. Assess pressure points of orthotic devices and underlying skin.	Impaired mobility and ischemia to integumentary system with sustained pressure	Intact skin; absence of pressure ulcers	

PROBLEM	INTERVENTION	RATIONALE	EXPECTED OUTCOME	COMMENTS
	Provide pin site care. Apply soft cotton knit shirt under removable orthotics (e.g., TLSO); change halo vest lining when wet or soiled. Assist with pressure relief every 15 minutes while up in chair. Use protective seat cushions/bed mattresses. Ensure adequate nutrition. Keep skin clean and dry.			
At risk for pain	Assess for pain and treat patient's perceptions of pain seriously. Administer antispasticity medications, CNS agents for paresthesias, and analgesics as needed.	Multifactorial pain: SCI, surgery and diagnostic procedures, orthotics, spasticity, and neurogenic pain	Minimal pain; able to participate in physical and occupational therapy	
At risk for emotional distress and ineffective coping	Establish communication method with patient as soon as possible. Assess for stages of grief; depression and suicidal ideation. Provide emotional support to patient/family. Answer questions honestly. Provide positive reinforcement. Offer patient some choice in regimen. Mental health consultation as appropriate. Facilitate undisturbed sleep/rest periods as possible. Patient/family education.	Impaired mobility	Acceptance; effective coping; highest quality of life	

Data from references 4, 7, 8, 18, 23–26, 28–31, 35, 43, 44, 46, 48, 57, 63–65, 72, 76, 89, 90, 92, 97–100, 105, 112, 116, 117, 120.
ABGs = Arterial blood gases, CNS = central nervous system, CO = cardiac output, CO_2 = carbon dioxide, CVP = central venous pressure, CXR = chest x-ray, GI = gastrointestinal, MAP = mean arterial pressure, Sao_2 = arterial oxygen saturation, OT = occupational therapy, PAWP = pulmonary artery wedge pressure, PROM = passive range of motion, PT = physical therapy, SCI = spinal cord injury, SV = stroke volume, SVR = systemic vascular resistance, TLSO = thoracolumbosacral orthoses.

spinal cord assessment and management. For example, Horner syndrome, which is sometimes seen with acute SCI, is related to disruption of the cervical sympathetic chain and presents with ptosis and miosis. These findings may be mistakenly interpreted as an indicator of intracranial pathology.[72,105]

By virtue of their close anatomic proximity, trauma to the cervical spine may also result in damage to the carotid and vertebral arteries. Cerebral angiography and magnetic resonance angiography (MRA) are recommended as options in complete cervical SCI, cervical fractures, facet dislocation, or vertebral subluxation.[6,55] Vascular injury may result in transient ischemic stroke or a complete stroke if it is unrecognized and treatment with anticoagulation or repair of the vessel is delayed.[6]

Pulmonary

Hypoventilation as a direct result of the SCI is of major concern in cervical and thoracic cord injuries. Many if not most cervical cord–injured patients with or without other pulmonary injuries will be intubated before arrival in the critical care unit. With C3-C5 or higher injuries, the diaphragm is affected and apnea results. Lower cervical spinal cord injuries at C5-C7 and T1-T12 have impaired intercostal muscle function that may result in shallow but ineffective breathing.[71,80] The forced vital capacity and maximum inspiratory and expiratory forces are reduced up to 70%.[8] Respirations are shallow and the patient exhibits decreased ability to cough and clear secretions. Some cervical and thoracic SCI patients will not require intubation immediately but within the first 24 hours related to cord edema or neurogenic pulmonary edema following resuscitation. Others will require immediate intubation at the scene related to their SCI, other injuries, or aspiration of gastric contents. Aspiration of gastric contents continues to be a risk factor for the SCI patient related to the supine position; cervical traction or orthotics;[57,81,84,104] intubation, including tracheostomy; and impaired gastric motility related to spinal shock.[7,100] Continuous monitoring of oxygen saturation and serial arterial blood gases, especially a rising Paco$_2$, and physiologic parameters such as vital capacity will detect a gradual deterioration of pulmonary status. Non-emergent intubation is preferable as care must be taken to avoid secondary neurologic injury. Sedation, analgesia, and neuromuscular blockade may facilitate oral intubation.[7,8] However, the paralytic medication succinylcholine is to be avoided following SCI. The massive denervation in SCI in combination with the depolarizing action of succinylcholine will result in a massive and potentially deadly release of potassium into the circulation.[7] Nasal intubation is contraindicated in the presence of basilar skull fractures and some facial trauma.[7]

Once intubated, mechanical ventilation simplifies maintenance of the airway and clearance of secretions. However, the patient is at increased risk for pneumonia. The leading cause of death of SCI patients is respiratory complications primarily resulting from pneumonia. The risk of ventilator-associated pneumonia increases by 1% to 3% a day each day a patient is intubated.[33] Pulmonary status—including chest auscultation, respiratory rate and character, arterial blood gases, oxygen saturation, end-tidal carbon dioxide monitoring, chest x-rays, sputum, white blood cell count, and temperature—must be closely monitored. Antibiotics should be prescribed based on the culture and sensitivity of the sputum. Pulmonary hygiene is critical. Frequent turning and early mobilization, suctioning of secretions as needed, and assisted cough may decrease the need for prolonged mechanical ventilation, antibiotics, and repeated bronchoscopy to clear secretions.* Quadriplegics may have more effective breathing while lying supine or wearing an abdominal binder when the head is up. These interventions displace some of the weight of the abdomen away from the weakened diaphragm and chest muscles.[8] Assisted cough, also referred to as "quad coughing," can be performed with a fist below the xiphoid process in a Heimlich-type maneuver or with open hands at the anterolateral base of each lung, pushing upward as the patient repeatedly coughs[4] (Figure 24-27). Improper placement of the hand may result in a rib or xiphoid process fracture. Migration and deformation of vena cava filters and small bowel perforation have been reported as well with assisted coughing.[9,87]

For patients with injuries at C4 or below, weaning from mechanical ventilation is a priority. Resolution of spinal shock with an associated increase in forced vital capacity, negative sputum cultures, fraction of inspired oxygen (Fio$_2$) requirement of 50% or less, and a minute ventilation of less than 10 L may facilitate weaning 2 weeks or more after the injury.[7,8] A tracheostomy frequently improves pulmonary mechanics, eases suctioning, and is more comfortable than prolonged nasal or oral intubation. However, if an anterior surgical approach is taken to stabilize the cervical injury, the tracheostomy may be delayed to allow wound healing.[7] A number of weaning modalities are used, including pressure support, positive airway support, and increasingly longer T-piece or tracheostomy collar trials during the day while allowing the patient to rest on the ventilator at night. The higher the level of injury, the longer the length of time to successfully wean from the ventilator and the greater likelihood of

*References 4, 7, 8, 30, 32, 71, 97, 105.

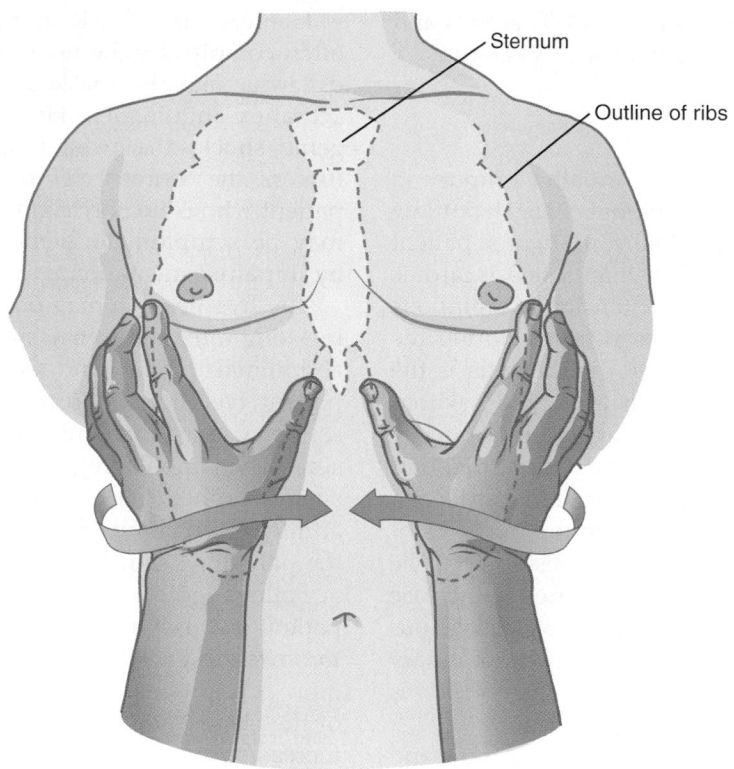

Sternum

Outline of ribs

◆FIGURE 24-27 Technique for quad coughing. Open hands at anterolateral base of each lung, pushing upward.

pulmonary complications.[32] Aggressive pulmonary hygiene remains a priority during and after successful ventilator weaning.

For patients with injuries at C4 and above, especially complete injuries, weaning from mechanical ventilation may not be possible and ventilator dependence will be a part of life. However, DiMarco and others have experienced some success with combined intercostal and diaphragm pacing in quadriplegics.[36–38] Electrical stimulation of the phrenic nerve allows the diaphragm to contract and produce sufficient inspiratory volumes to potentially wean some patients from the ventilator. However, if the motor neurons in the spinal cord or either phrenic nerve are injured, pacing is ineffective. Pacing of a unilaterally functional phrenic nerve and intercostals may provide another alternative to ventilator dependence. Traditionally, placement of these electrodes has required a thoracotomy, but they may now be placed laparoscopically.[36–38] Clinical trials are currently under way to restore expiratory muscles using high-frequency magnetic stimulation, surface stimulation of abdominal musculature, and electrical stimulation in the lower thoracic spinal cord.[36]

In addition to hypoventilation, pulmonary edema, and pneumonia, thromboembolic disease from impaired mobility of the extremities poses a constant threat to the lungs. Deep vein thrombosis (DVT) prophylaxis includes mechanical devices, such as sequential compression devices and elastic compression stockings, and anticoagulation, including low-dose heparin and low molecular weight heparinoids (enoxaparin). Low-dose heparin or low molecular weight heparinoid alone has been found to be insufficient for DVT prophylaxis in SCI.[6,55] Clinicians often delay anticoagulation because of concern for SCI or systemic hemorrhage or the need for surgery in the near future. Intravenous heparin sufficient to increase the activated partial thromboplastin time (APTT) 1.5 to 2 times the control is effective but substantially increases the risk of bleeding and is usually reserved for patients with a confirmed DVT or pulmonary embolus. Low-dose subcutaneous heparin or enoxaparin (Lovenox) is safe and effective. Placement of a vena cava filter is an option if anticoagulation is contraindicated.[7,8,26,47]

Diagnosis of DVT by physical assessment alone is difficult because of impaired sensation in SCI patients. However, the use of bedside ultrasound is safe and reliable. If pulmonary emboli are suspected, angiography remains the gold standard. However, limitations of pulmonary angiography include availability, expense, and complications. Ventilation/perfusion ($\dot{V}/\dot{Q}$) scans and spiral CT of the chest are more widely used.

The sensitivity and specificity of spiral CT, at 94% and 96%, respectively, are greater than those of $\dot{V}/\dot{Q}$ scans.[115]

Cardiac

At the time of injury, the loss of sympathetic input and subsequent unopposed parasympathetic (vagal) outflow place the cervical or thoracic spinal cord–injured patient at risk for hemodynamic instability manifested as cardiac dysrhythmias and systemic hypotension. Continuous cardiac and arterial monitoring is prudent during the first 1 to 2 weeks following injury. Bradycardia is the most common dysrhythmia and usually occurs within 2 weeks after injury. Hypoxia or vagal stimulation by manipulation of a suction catheter or nasogastric/orogastric tube may induce a symptomatic bradycardia evidenced by a decrease in blood pressure or level of consciousness.[7,8,52,65] Oxygenation and cessation of the vagal stimulation may be all that is required to increase the heart rate. However, administration of intravenous atropine in symptomatic bradycardia may be necessary and is effective. Occasionally a temporary pacemaker is needed until resolution of the neurogenic shock.[7,8,52,100]

The loss of tone in the peripheral vasculature and venous pooling as a result of cervical and thoracic SCI result in hypotension. Unlike hypovolemic shock, neurogenic shock is accompanied by bradycardia as described previously. However, first-line treatment for both is fluid resuscitation. One to two liters of a non–glucose-containing intravenous solution is administered initially in an attempt to bring the blood pressure into the desired parameter. Too much fluid may aggravate cord edema and neurogenic pulmonary edema. The desired parameter is not known with certainty. The current recommendation based on available evidence is a MAP of 85 to 90 mm Hg the first 7 days after injury.[6,55]

If the initial fluid is ineffective in raising the blood pressure, a vasopressor may be added. Ideally, vasopressors are added after the placement of a central venous catheter or preferably a pulmonary artery catheter. In neurogenic shock, the preload, heart rate, left ventricular end-diastolic pressure, stroke volume, systemic vascular resistance, and cardiac output are all decreased. Therefore ideal vasopressors for SCI have chronotropic and alpha and beta properties. Phenylephrine (Neo-Synephrine) is not recommended because of its pure alpha-adrenergic action and reflex bradycardic effect. Effective choices in cervical and thoracic SCI include dopamine (Intropin) or norepinephrine (Levophed). Both agents have alpha- and beta-adrenergic effects and increase heart rate. Dobutamine (Dobutrex) can be used with dopamine or Levophed to increase cardiac output but may cause hypotension. Therefore it is probably not the best agent to be used alone.[7,8,65,105]

Hemorrhagic shock in the presence of acute SCI often complicates the neurogenic picture, and the bradycardia may be masked by tachycardia related to actual exsanguination. However, in the case of neurogenic shock, the patient is usually dry and warm (unless the ambient temperature is low), while the patient who is hemorrhaging is clammy and cold. Both may be symptomatic hemodynamically as evidenced by impaired mentation and low urine output.[72]

The hypotension may persist with upright positioning long after the initial injury. The application of an abdominal binder and elastic leg wraps after the patient has stopped receiving intravenous vasopressors may assist in maintaining the systemic blood pressure when mobilizing the patient. Oral vasopressors such as ephedrine or midodrine (Amatine) are often administered about 45 minutes to 1 hour before raising the patient's head.[11,15]

Following resolution of neurogenic shock, the patient is at risk for AD. Prevention includes attention to bowel and bladder elimination and other less common precipitants. Prompt recognition and treatment of the classic paroxysmal hypertension or more subtle increase in blood pressure and other symptomatology associated with AD is critical to prevent severe disability or death from intracerebral hemorrhage, seizures, and myocardial infarction. Initial management includes raising the head of the bed unless contraindicated and removing the noxious stimulation, such as alleviating a distended bladder or evacuating a rectal vault containing stool. Short-acting antihypertensives such as nitroglycerin (Nitrol) and nifedipine (Procardia) may be given as well to assist in lowering the blood pressure[29,76](Box 24-2).

Pregnant patients with an injury at T6 or above who deliver after their spinal shock has resolved are at risk for AD related to uterine contractions. Regional anesthesia at the onset of labor may allow for a vaginal delivery without risk to the mother. However, a cesarean section is indicated if the AD is uncontrollable.[29] The hypertension and subjective symptoms of AD may be mistakenly diagnosed as preeclampsia.[63] As with all high-risk obstetrics, the general principle is to take care of the mother first.[63]

Gastrointestinal

Following SCI, the gastrointestinal system is atonic. Bowel sounds may not be auscultated. Abdominal distention results from lack of motility and possibly from air swallowing or from attempts to provide supplemental oxygen and rescue breaths with a bag-valve-mask apparatus. The patient is at risk for emesis and aspiration. If not already inserted in the emergency department, an orogastric or nasogastric tube (in the absence

Box 24-2

Autonomic Dysreflexia

PATHOPHYSIOLOGY

In autonomic dysreflexia (AD)/hyperreflexia, sensory nerves below a spinal cord injury from C1 to T6 transmit noxious ascending impulses to the spinal cord. Sympathetic neurons are stimulated. However, the usual inhibitory impulses above T6 are blocked by the SCI. As a result, sympathetic outflow from T6 to L2 is unopposed. Autonomic dysreflexia occurs after spinal shock resolves and reflexes become hyperreflexic.

PREVENTION

The best prevention for autonomic dysreflexia is compliance with bowel and bladder training and patient/family education.

SIGNS AND SYMPTOMS

Autonomic dysreflexia symptoms include the following:
1. Sudden large increase in systolic and diastolic blood pressures (e.g., systolic >200 mm Hg) or an increase in blood pressure 20 to 40 mm Hg above baseline
2. Pounding headache
3. Bradycardia or a relative bradycardia compared to the patient's baseline heart rate
4. Profuse perspiration, especially above the lesion but also possible below the lesion
5. Piloerection above or possibly below the level of the lesion
6. Flushing, especially above the lesion but also possible below the lesion
7. Nasal congestion
8. Visual changes
9. Anxiety and apprehension

SIGNIFICANCE

AD is a true neurologic emergency. Failure to recognize and treat the symptoms of AD promptly, especially the hypertension, may result in myocardial infarction, seizures, or hemorrhagic stroke.

CAUSES

Autonomic dysreflexia may be caused by any noxious stimulus. Bowel and bladder problems are the most frequent causes, including bladder distention, an occluded catheter, urinary tract infection, catheterization, renal calculi, urologic or gastrointestinal instrumentation, fecal impaction, gastric ulcers, gallstones, and appendicitis. Pressure ulcers, blisters and burns, constrictive clothing, labor and delivery, sexual intercourse, deep vein thrombosis, pulmonary emboli, surgical and diagnostic procedures, and stimulants are other causes.

TREATMENT

Definitive treatment for AD is removing the noxious stimulation. However, while determining the noxious stimulation and continuing to monitor the patient's signs and symptoms, other interventions that may improve the clinical presentation temporarily include elevating the head of the bed unless contraindicated; loosening any constrictive clothing or devices; using a topical anesthetic such as 2% lidocaine lubricant when catheterizing the patient or removing a fecal impaction; and administering a short-acting antihypertensive such as nitroglycerin or nifedipine to resolve hypertension.

Data from references 7, 29, 76.

of basilar skull fracture or other contraindication) is needed. After auscultation, aspiration, or radiographic exam to verify proper placement, the gastric tube is attached to low constant suction to minimize gastric content.[7,8] Measurement of gastric pH monitors the effectiveness of gastrointestinal prophylaxis to prevent stress ulceration. A gastric pH of 4 or greater may decrease the risk of gastrointestinal bleeding.[23] Discontinuation of a histamine blocker and initiation of a proton pump inhibitor may increase the gastric pH.[82,100] If the impaired motility continues for 3 or more days, total parenteral nutrition is required to prevent malnutrition. Gradual introduction of enteral feedings at low rates may be effective.[94] Withholding enteral feedings for high residuals is imperative to decrease the risk of aspiration.[40] The Nutrition box on p. 670 discusses the nutritional considerations for patients with spinal cord injuries.

The bowel is innervated by the sacral segments of the spinal cord. In incomplete spinal cord injuries with sacral sparing, normal bowel function is preserved. At the time of a complete SCI, the bowel is flaccid. With the resolution of spinal shock, the bowel with an SCI above the sacrum, an upper motor neuron lesion, will become reflexic. This reflex activity may facilitate regular consistent bowel evacuation.[29] Initially, a suppository and digital evacuation will be required for bowel training. However, with repeated consistent efforts at the same time each day, the bowel may eventually automatically expel stool at a predictable time or require only digital stimulation or a glycerin suppository. Bowel training is frequently begun with a bisacodyl (Dulcolax)

♦ NUTRITION

Nutrition for Patients With Traumatic Spinal Cord Injuries

CALORIES

Serial indirect calorimetry performed at the bedside in collaboration with the respiratory therapist and registered dietitian is preferred over Harris-Benedict equation estimate (HBEE) calculations for resting energy expenditure. HBEE is based on gender, age, weight, and height, and a stress factor may be added. Calculations using the HBEE may overestimate energy requirements. Isolated acute spinal cord injury patients have increased metabolic needs that may vary depending on the level, the extent, and the time since injury. Age, preexisting illness, other comorbidities, injuries, infection, wounds, or surgery will also affect requirements. (For example, traumatic brain injury patients in general require a resting energy expenditure 140% greater than basal energy expenditure.) Maintaining normoglycemia is essential for optimal neurologic outcome. Obesity is a problem in chronic spinal cord injury.

PROTEIN

Acute spinal cord injury is associated with obligatory large nitrogen losses for up to 2 months related to denervated musculature.

FLUID

Glucose-containing intravenous solutions are to be avoided. Enteral fluids are to be administered as soon as possible. Normovolemia is to be achieved and maintained.

ELECTROLYTES

Electrolytes within normal limits are to be achieved and maintained.

VITAMINS AND MINERALS

Provide supplementation as needed.

No research has been published that confirms the composite nutritional needs of the spinal cord patient. Recommended percentage of calories from carbohydrates is 50% to 60%, calories from protein 20% to 30%, and calories from fat 20% to 30%. Overfeeding may negatively impact mechanical ventilator weaning. Increased fat intake may result in hypoxia, cholestasis, and hyperlipidemia.

SPECIAL CONSIDERATIONS

The patient must be assessed for aspiration risk before oral feeding. A dysphagia evaluation by speech therapy is appropriate. Enteral nutrition is to be administered as soon as possible. However, nutrition should not be delayed if the patient is unable to use the enteral route. Initiate parenteral nutrition and convert to enteral nutrition as condition permits.

Data from references 2, 6, 7, 12, 39, 42, 81, 84, 93, 104, 105.

suppository[25,102] or digital stimulation. Digital stimulation may induce AD after spinal shock resolves. A local anesthetic agent such as lidocaine ointment may prevent the onset of AD during bowel training. Bowel training is most effective if performed when the gastrocolic reflex is most active, immediately after a meal. Bowel care after the evening meal may be least disruptive in regard to interference with other rehabilitation efforts including physical and occupational therapy in critical care. Supplemental fiber with adequate fluid intake and stool softeners may facilitate bowel training. Large-volume enemas are to be avoided.[7,25]

In a complete SCI at the sacral segments, a lower motor neuron lesion, the bowel remains areflexic after spinal shock is resolved. Bowel care with a lower motor neuron lesion may be more problematic than with an upper motor neuron lesion. Retention of formed stool with incontinence of liquid stool frequently occurs, with stool softeners and suppositories being less effective. Digital stimulation is ineffective and manual removal of stool may be necessary.[7,25]

With either a reflexic or an areflexic bowel, constipation in the spinal cord patient is a serious complication that is potentially life-threatening as it impairs gastrointestinal motility; increases the risk of aspiration with high gastric residuals; and is a frequent cause of autonomic dysreflexia with injuries above T6.[7,25]

Genitourinary

Like the gastrointestinal tract, the genitourinary system is flaccid immediately after the injury. Following the resolution of spinal shock, the upper motor neuron bladder, with injury above the sacral segments of the cord, will regain tone, which may facilitate reflex voiding. Over time some patients will reflex void sufficiently to empty the bladder; others will require intermittent catheterization completely or for high residuals. Some patients are able to facilitate reflex voiding with the use of Credé, Valsalva, abdominal massage, or pubic hair pulling maneuvers.[58,85] As soon as fluid intake and output is stable, an effort to remove the indwelling catheter is prudent to minimize the risk of urinary tract infection and sepsis. However, overdistention of the bladder is to be avoided. The normal adult bladder capacity is 400 to 500 ml.[58] To avoid overdistention, fluid intake may be limited or the frequency of intermittent catheterization increased. Urinalysis and culture and sensitivity are monitored on a routine basis and antibiotics are prescribed based on those results only. Prophylactic antibiotic therapy is not effective and may be detrimental.[46] In the case of women who void incontinently, an indwelling catheter or urinary diversion procedure may continue to be necessary in critical care to avoid skin breakdown.

Patients with a lower motor neuron lesion continue to have an areflexic bladder after the resolution of spinal shock and will not void. An indwelling catheter with conversion to an intermittent catheterization regimen will be necessary. With a lesion at the junction of the conus medullaris and the cauda equina, a mixed upper and lower neuron presentation also exists in which the patient may or may not void spontaneously. In incomplete injuries with sacral sparing, spontaneous voiding and urinary control are possible.[48,58,85]

While removal of the indwelling urinary catheter as soon as possible is ideal, large-volume urinary retention is to be avoided because of the risk of autonomic dysreflexia in patients with SCI above T6. Urinary retention also increases the risk of infection and renal disease.[48,58,85]

Endocrine

Following SCI and the release of catecholamines as well as the administration of methylprednisolone, the patient is prone to hyperglycemia.[6,14,60,102] Though less investigated than the negative effects of glucose in TBI, hyperglycemia in SCI is associated with poor neurologic outcomes.[14,105] A sliding scale insulin regimen or an intravenous infusion may be needed initially to maintain normoglycemia.

Musculoskeletal

As soon as the patient is stable, physical and occupational therapy are consulted. Early mobilization is the goal. However, actual range of motion may be immediately contraindicated related to other injuries such as extremity fractures or increased intracranial pressure. Nevertheless, a prompt consult with these therapies provides assistance with preventive positioning and the early minimization of contractures and deformities associated with SCI. During spinal shock the extremities are flaccid. With the resolution of spinal shock, spasticity occurs. Upper and lower extremity orthotics are frequently prescribed to promote normal alignment and minimize contractures.[31,44] Spasticity may actually assist in rehabilitation goals; however, spasticity and the pain associated with spasticity can also deter rehabilitation efforts. Spasticity also contributes to contractures and skin breakdown.[20] Enteral baclofen (Lioresal) , dantrolene (Dantrium), and diazepam (Valium) have been found to be beneficial.[60,100,116] However, some patients may eventually require an intrathecal baclofen medication pump.[20] The Medication table below outlines pharmacologic treatment of spasticity and related problems. Nonpharmacologic interventions for spasticity include range-of-motion exercise and functional electrical stimulation (FES).[31,116]

SELECTED MEDICATIONS FOR PATIENTS WITH TRAUMATIC SPINAL CORD INJURIES

MEDICATION	ACTIONS	DOSAGE	SPECIAL CONSIDERATIONS
Antispasticity			
Baclofen (Lioresal)	Skeletal muscle relaxant, antispasticity agent	5 mg PO/NG tid; can increase dose by 15 mg/day every 3 days as needed Maximum total daily dose is 80 mg	May cause drowsiness and hypotension; increase gradually; withdrawal seizures, hallucinations Use caution in renal impairment Do not discontinue abruptly; may result in rebound spasticity Also available as solution for intrathecal infusion
Dantrolene (Dantrium)	Skeletal muscle relaxant, antispasticity	25–400 mg PO/NG daily, given as divided doses tid May increase dose weekly if needed. Start with 25 mg daily for 7 days, followed by 25 mg tid for	May cause drowsiness, weakness, fatigue, and seizures; increase gradually Monitor liver function tests closely; high risk of liver toxicity if hepatic

Table continues on page 672

MEDICATION	ACTIONS	DOSAGE	SPECIAL CONSIDERATIONS
		7 days, 50 mg tid for 7 days, then 100 mg tid. Maximum dose is 400 mg/day, given as four divided doses.	impairment, age older than 35, and/or for female patients If no additional relief is obtained at higher doses, decrease dose to next lower dose
Corticosteroids			
Methylprednisolone (Solu-Medrol)	Stabilizes neuronal membranes	Infuse intravenous bolus of 30 mg/kg over 15 min; wait 45 min If injury is within 3 hr, follow bolus with 5.4 mg/kg/hr for 23 hr If time from injury is greater than 3 hr but less than 8 hr, 5.4 mg/kg/hr for 47 hr	May cause hyperglycemia, impair wound healing, impair immune function, and promote gastric (stress) ulceration Administer GI prophylaxis Not indicated in penetrating SCI
Blood Pressure Control			
Ephedrine	Vasoconstriction; prevention of orthostatic hypotension	2.5 mg PO/NG daily	May cause tachycardia, hypertension, tremors, and anxiety Administer 45 min to 1 hr before raising head
Midodrine (Amatine, ProAmatine)	Vasoconstriction; prevention of orthostatic hypotension	2.5–10 mg/NG tid	May cause hypertension, flushing, and restlessness; administer 45 min to 1 hr before raising head May need to adjust dose for renal dysfunction
Nifedipine (Procardia)	Vasodilation; treatment of hypertension associated with AD	10–20 mg sublingual	Capsule must be opened and liquid contents (bite and chew) in contact with oral mucosa for rapid onset (1–5 min) May cause hypotension and headache
Nitroglycerin (Nitrostat, sublingual tablets)	Treatment of hypertension associated with AD	0.4% tablet sublingual	Onset is 1–3 min (sublingual)
Nitrol, Nitrobid (ointment)		½–2 inches topical	Onset 15 min to 1 hr (topical)
Stool Softeners/ Stimulants	Soften stool and stimulate colon to facilitate bowel training		May cause diarrhea, abdominal cramping
Docusate (Colace)		100 mg PO/NG tid	
Senna-docusate (Senokot-S)		2 tablets PO/NG bid	
Bisacodyl (Dulcolax)		10 mg (1 suppository) per rectum daily after meal or bolus tube feeding	

Data from references 6–8, 18, 25, 26, 29, 60, 78, 102.

Exercise may also minimize long-term musculo-skeletal complications of SCI, including osteoporosis, pathologic fractures, and heterotopic ossification—the abnormal deposition of bone around the joints of paralyzed extremities. Fitting the patient with a wheelchair and mobilizing while in critical care provide benefits physiologically and psychosocially as well as opportunity for patient/family education.[44]

Integumentary

The potential for skin breakdown starts from the time the patient is placed in a collar and on a back-board during prehospital care.[28] While this does not preclude their use, every effort should be made to remove the patient from the backboard as soon as possible. Backboard time should not exceed 2 hours.[14] Once the spine has been stabilized, turning the patient in bed every 1 to 2 hours is a priority.[28,54] Pads that support and position the patient in a kinetic treatment table must be secure to preventing shearing with turning. In regard to sitting, an appropriate cushion and position changes are essential every 15 to 20 minutes.[98,103] Tilting the patient backward to alleviate pressure while up in a chair is facilitated with the use of a wheelchair rather than a cardiac chair or a regular chair. Turns and hygiene measures provide opportunities for skin assessment. Keeping the skin clean and dry and minimizing pressure are critical. Skin under orthotic devices and at pin insertion sites needs attention as well. Any evidence of skin breakdown must be treated aggressively.[7,28,120] Early collaboration with a skin and wound specialist is warranted.

Pain

Though SCI patients may not be able to perceive touch, discriminate between sharp and dull, or demonstrate vibratory or proprioceptive ability, their pain is real. Pain may be associated with spasticity, visceral injury, or acute illness, or be neuropathic. Neuropathic pain is distal to the injury and may be characterized as paresthesias or dysesthesias and described by the patient as burning, stinging, tingling, piercing, stabbing, or cutting.[122] Antispasmodic medications, anticonvulsants, and analgesics and sedatives may be effective. Central-acting nonnarcotic agents such as phenytoin (Dilantin), carbamazepine (Tegretol), gabapentin (Neurontin), clonazepam (Klonopin), and amitriptyline (Elavil) have decreased discomfort for many patients.[122] However, long-term use of sedation and medications that are psychologically and physiologically addicting interferes with rehabilitation efforts and eventually detracts from the patient's quality of life. These medications also complicate bowel and bladder elimination.[7,25]

Pain is an important indicator of disease. However, pathology usually identifiable by the location and character of the pain may be misdiagnosed in patients with SCI. For example, gastrointestinal pathology related to hemorrhage may present as referred pain rather than abdominal discomfort. Alternatively, a patient with preexisting coronary artery disease may experience a myocardial infarction without the usual chest discomfort. Any hypotension and bradycardia may be mistakenly attributed only to neurogenic shock.[7]

Psychosocial

The spinal cord–injured patient faces a myriad of physical and psychosocial obstacles. They may vacillate among different stages of the grief process—denial, anger, bargaining, depression, and acceptance—in addition to disturbances in body image and self-concept. Because many SCI patients are young male teenagers and adults, they may be especially vulnerable to these psychosocial ramifications. Feelings of powerlessness may pervade as well.[10,24,75] This is frequently manifested by the patient repeatedly calling the nurse into the room as an attempt to control the environment. Even their ability to communicate their concerns is hampered by intubation and their inability to write messages. Initiation of a communication system as soon as possible is important. Collaboration with the speech therapist and the respiratory therapist in the initiation of a tracheostomy speaking valve may be a significant step in the patient's psychosocial well-being and rehabilitation. One such valve, the Passy-Muir tracheostomy speaking valve, opens during inspiration, allowing air into the lungs, and closes during expiration, redirecting the exhaled air through the vocal cords, mouth, and nose to allow the patient to speak (Figure 24-28).[13,64] The tracheostomy cuff must be completely deflated and this may put the patient at increased risk for aspiration. Close monitoring of the patient's pulmonary status is necessary. The valve is not to remain in the airway when the patient is asleep. Vocal cord paralysis, excessive and thick pulmonary secretions, and tracheal or laryngeal obstructions are contraindications to its use.[13,64]

Over time research has demonstrated that acceptance and positive adaptation to the SCI may occur with some individuals.[75] However, life satisfaction studies are contradictory and inconclusive. The person's age, age at injury, and level and duration of the injury are factors that may influence their perception.[10]

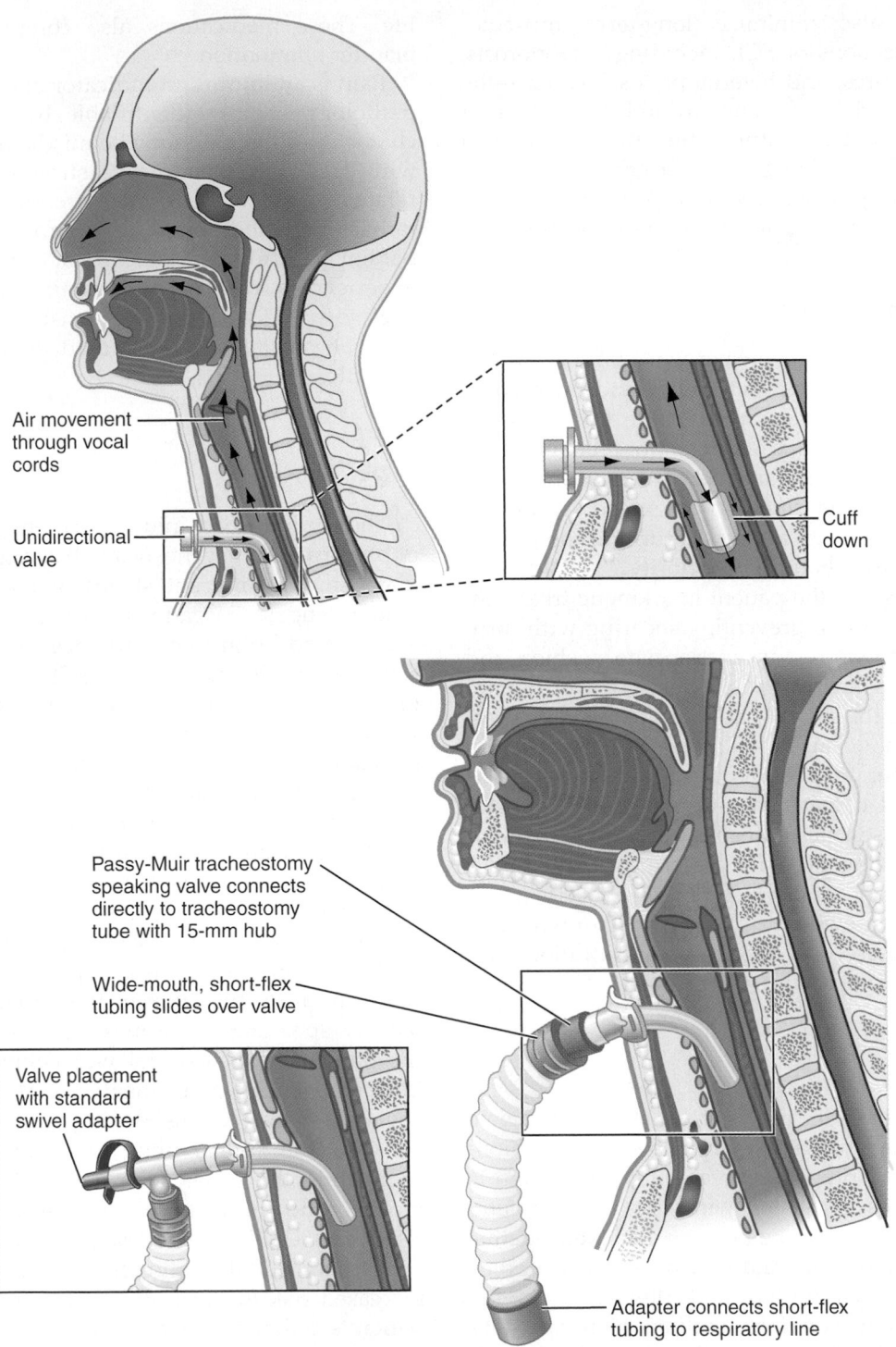

Air movement through vocal cords

Unidirectional valve

Cuff down

Passy-Muir tracheostomy speaking valve connects directly to tracheostomy tube with 15-mm hub

Wide-mouth, short-flex tubing slides over valve

Valve placement with standard swivel adapter

Adapter connects short-flex tubing to respiratory line

◆FIGURE 24-28 Passy-Muir tracheostomy speaking valve.

Case Study 24-1, Part B

Evidence-Based Management of a Patient With Traumatic Spinal Cord Injury

J.G. was placed on the standard 24-hour methylprednisolone protocol. Low-dose dopamine was infused to maintain a mean blood pressure of 85 to 90 mm Hg. He was placed in cervical tong traction, and his C5-C6 burst fracture with posterior ligament injury was later stabilized with open reduction internal fixation (ORIF) using instrumentation. A halo brace was placed for 3 months. He required intubation and mechanical ventilation 2 days postoperatively, aggressive pulmonary hygiene, bronchoscopy twice, antiembolism stockings, pneumatic compression devices, and low-dose enoxaparin (Lovenox). Elastic leg wraps and an abdominal binder were used to support his blood pressure and facilitate respiratory efforts when up in a chair. J.G. was maintained on enteral nutrition until he was weaned from the ventilator and cleared for a regular diet after a swallow evaluation (while in the halo). He was placed on a bowel training regimen at night after the evening meal. With the return of reflexes, the indwelling Foley catheter was discontinued. An external catheter was applied, and a post-voiding intermittent catheter residual check was performed every 4 to 6 hours until the residuals were consistently less than 100 ml. Physical and occupational therapists were consulted during the first week of his critical care stay, and they continued to follow and provide positioning, orthotic, and exercise management throughout his stay in acute care. He was transferred to the progressive care unit for continued pulmonary hygiene, family/patient education, and physical and occupational therapy, and then transferred to the rehabilitation unit for a more aggressive program.

Decision point: What are the priorities in caring for J.G. during his stay in critical care?

Case continues on page 677

EVIDENCE-BASED CARE

Major components of the care of the critically ill SCI patient have been addressed in evidence-based guidelines developed by the Consortium of Spinal Cord Medicine (CSCM), consisting of several multidisciplinary professional organizations who work with spinal cord patients and the AANS/CNS.[6,24,25,27–31] Many of the recommendations are stated as guidelines and options (levels II and III to V evidence) rather than standards (level I). Much is yet to be substantiated by well-designed scientific inquiry. CSCM originally developed recommendations beginning in the late 1990s on the sequelae and long-term management of SCI, including respiratory, thromboembolism, bowel,

autonomic dysreflexia, depression, upper extremity function, and outcome issues.[24–31] In 2002 the AANS/CNS published the first guidelines that focus on the immediate management of the cervical spine and cord injury itself in addition to some of the sequelae, including thromboembolism and nutritional concerns.[6]

RESEARCH

Research is ongoing in acute SCI. While the controversy regarding the benefits of methylprednisolone persists, as explained in the Research Utilization box on p. 656, a number of other pharmacologic trials have resulted in even less optimistic findings or inconclusive results. Over the past 30 years, clinical trials have been conducted with GM-1 gangliosides (Sygen), thyrotropin-releasing hormone (TRH), nimodipine, and autologous macrophages (ProCord), to name a few.[5,41,69] Gangliosides are chemicals abundant in the neuron's outer membrane. They accelerate neurite outgrowth and decrease edema while facilitating peripheral nerve regeneration. While the initial trials were promising, a larger multicenter trial in North America did not show any improvement over the control group. Both the treatment and control groups received methylprednisolone. The AANS/CNS considers GM-1 ganglioside an option without proven benefit. Sygen is used in Europe but is not approved by the FDA in the United States.[69]

TRH has neuroprotective qualities as an antiinflammatory agent, antioxidant, and membrane stabilizer and is thought to increase spinal cord blood flow. Patients receiving TRH experienced improved recovery, but many research participants were lost to follow-up and additional research is needed.[69] Intravenous nimodipine was investigated based on its neuroprotective calcium channel blocking properties, but no difference was seen in the treatment or placebo groups. Both groups received methylprednisolone.[5,69]

In the ProCord study, activated autologous macrophages are injected into the spinal cord of patients with complete lesions in the area of the injury to boost the body's own antiinflammatory actions. Enrollment for Phase II of this FDA-approved international clinical trial for patients with single lesions from C5 to T11 less than 14 days after the injury began in 2003 and was ongoing in 2006.[67]

OUTCOMES

Functional outcomes are predictable based on the level and completeness of injury (Table 24-8). A C5-C6 injury such as J.G.'s (see Case Study 24-1) would most

TABLE 24-8 Functional Goals for Spinal Cord–Injured Patients

SPINAL CORD LEVEL	MUSCLE FUNCTION	FUNCTIONAL GOALS
C3-C4	Neck control Scapular elevators	Manipulate electric wheelchair with mouth stick Feed self with limitations using ball-bearing feeders Dress upper trunk Turn self in bed with arm slings Depend on others for bowel and bladder care
C5	Fair to good shoulder control Good elbow function	Propel wheelchair with hand rim projections Feed self with hand splint Require assistance getting to and from bed Depend on others for bowel and bladder care
C6	Good shoulder control Wrist extension Supinators	Transfer from wheelchair to bed and car with or without minimal assistance Feed self with tenodesis hands Assist getting to and from commode chair Require assistance with bladder care Drive with adapted van
C7	Weak shoulder depression Weak elbow extension Some hand function	Independently transfer to bed, car, and toilet Dress independently Propel wheelchair without hand rim projections Feed self without assistive devices Perform bowel and bladder care independently Drive car or adapted van with hand controls
C8-T4	Good to normal upper extremity muscle function	Transfer from chair or bed to wheelchair and return Maneuver wheelchair up and down curb Maneuver wheelchair to tub and return self to wheelchair
T5-L2	Partial to good trunk stability	Maneuver wheelchair independently Ambulate with limitations using long leg braces and crutches

L3-L4	All trunk-pelvic stabilizers intact
	  Hip flexors
	  Adductors
	  Quadriceps
		Ambulate with short leg braces with or without crutches, depending on level

L5	Hip extensors, abductors, knee flexors, ankle control	Do not require any equipment if plantar flexion is sufficiently strong to initiate steps after standing

Modified from reference 80a.

likely allow him to perform some activities of daily living with assistance or orthotic devices. Aggressive rehabilitation beginning in critical care assists spinal cord patients to maximize their quality of life. Improvement in motor function may occur for up to 2 years post-injury.[27,119] However, the late complication of syringomyelia may result in deterioration.[26,118]

Currently approximately 200,000 Americans are living with SCI.[83] Life expectancy is variable depending on the level (including ventilator dependency), the completeness of the injury, and the age at the time of injury. High-level ventilator-dependent quadriplegics are likely to be dead in 10 to 15 years.[83] As a group, young paraplegics are expected to live up to 45 years after injury.[82] However, individuals 60 years and older who sustain SCI may only survive about 10 years post-injury.[83] The consequences of immobility secondary to the SCI dramatically impact the disease processes associated with aging, and spinal cord patients are at increased risk for ischemic cardiovascular disease, stroke, and cancer as well as pulmonary disease and infections.[10,22,83] Respiratory diseases and infection are the leading causes of death, with hypertension, ischemic heart disease, and cancer following.[22,83] Individuals living with SCI have an increased risk of bladder cancer, reportedly as much as 16 to 28 times higher, related to chronic indwelling catheters and infection.[51,59]

ETHICAL CONSIDERATIONS

Acute SCI, particularly high-level complete cervical and ventilator-dependent quadriplegia, presents a number of ethical dilemmas, including the right to die, the right to refuse treatment, and the use of advance directives. Most acute SCI patients, in part because of their young age, will not have an advance directive already in place. Furthermore, the multidisciplinary team will be successful in stabilizing and maintaining the acute spinal cord–injured patient. However, long-term quadriplegia, ventilator dependence, and multiple complications may prolong the initial hospitalization, require frequent readmissions, delay rehabilitation, and require around-the-clock care by the family at home or in an assisted living facility. Pulmonary complications, such as pneumonia and pulmonary emboli, urinary tract infections, pressure ulcers, and sepsis are common reasons for readmission to the hospital or critical care.[83] The quality of life is forever devastatingly compromised.

Acutely spinal cord–injured patients may experience profound depression and suicidal ideation, and may or may not express a desire to die. However, perceptions of their life may improve over time. As the patient's advocate, nurses have a responsibility to communicate the patient's stated wishes to the multidisciplinary team and to help the patient and family work through their feelings.[68] Butt and Scofield developed guidelines for dealing with ethical dilemmas in quadriplegia.[21] They recommend the following:

1. Involving healthcare providers with neutral opinions regarding right to die/right to live issues
2. Following the patient's thoughts and decisions for consistency regarding wishes
3. Introducing the patient to another spinal cord–injured patient to answer questions if possible
4. Moving the patient to less acute levels of care as soon as condition permits
5. Evaluating congruence in the thoughts of the patient and the patient's family
6. Establishing the patient's competency
7. Obtaining informed consent for those who persist in their desire to withdraw life support

8. Providing comfort measures and palliative care during the dying process while also attending to family.

An ethics committee consult is recommended.[21,28,95] In addition to the ethical issues, the multidisciplinary team must also act within the law.

If the patient is determined to be competent and withdrawal of support is decided, but the nurse or another member of the multidisciplinary team is uncomfortable participating in withdrawal of support, the environment must be conducive to the team member's expressing discomfort and being excused from the process. For SCI patients who choose life before leaving acute care, a discussion regarding advance directives is warranted. Blackmer and Ross determined that post-acute spinal cord–injured individuals are interested in establishing advance directives for themselves.[16]

◆ Case Study 24-1, Part C

Evidence-Based Management of a Patient With Traumatic Spinal Cord Injury

J.G. develops a headache (pain scale 10/10) about a month after his injury. His face is flushed and his blood pressure is 160/90 mm Hg. He states that he feels like he is dying. Piloerection (gooseflesh) is noted on his upper extremities. Reflex movement of his lower extremities is noted. His usual blood pressure is between 110–120/60–70 mm Hg. His heart rate, which is usually in the 60–70 beats/min range, is sinus bradycardia in the 50–60 beats/min range. He no longer has an indwelling catheter because he has been reflex voiding with residuals of 30 ml or less.

Decision point: What is most likely occurring and what are the appropriate interventions?

CONCLUSIONS

Care of the critically ill patient with SCI requires utmost attention to the neurologic injury to minimize secondary neuronal injury. However, once the neurologic injury is stabilized, the major causes of mortality and morbidity are rarely the SCI but commonly the impact of the SCI on other systems. The time after the initial stabilization is just as challenging and critical to the spinal cord–injured patient's outcome as the first few days in the critical care environment. Much of the care is directed toward minimizing complications and assisting the patient to cope with the neurologic deficits that remain. Care of the critically ill traumatic SCI patient is truly the work of the critical care nurse.

REFERENCES

1. Ackery, A., Tator, C., & Krassioukov, A. (2004). A global perspective on spinal cord injury epidemiology. *J Neurotrauma, 21*(10), 1355–1370.

2. Agarwal, N. (2002). Nutrition in spinal cord injured patients. In B. L. Lee & L. E. Ostrander (Eds.), *The spinal cord injured patient* (pp 317–325). New York: Demos.

3. Ahmed, H. U., et al. (2002). Cholecystectomy in patients with previous spinal cord injury. *Am J Surg, 184*(5), 452–459.

4. Alexander, T. T., Hiduke, R. J., & Stevens, K. A. (1999). Cough enhancement. In *Rehabilitation nursing procedures manual* (pp 276–281). New York: McGraw-Hill.

5. Amador, M., & Guest, J. D. (2005). An appraisal of experimental procedures in human spinal cord injury. *J Neurol Phys Ther, 29*(2), 70–86.

6. American Association of Neurological Surgeons and Congress of Neurological Surgeons. (2002). Guidelines for management of acute cervical spine injuries. *Neurosurgery, 50*(suppl 3), S1–S178.

6a. Bader, M. K., & Littlejohns, L. R. (2004). *AANN core curriculum for neuroscience nursing*. 4th ed. Philadelphia: Saunders.

7. Ball, P. A., Chicoine, R. E., & Gettinger, A. (2000). Anesthesia and critical care management of spinal cord injury. In C. H. Tator & E. C. Benzel (Eds.), *Contemporary management of spinal cord injury: from impact to rehabilitation* (pp 99–108). Park Ridge, Ill: American Association of Neurological Surgeons.

8. Ball, P. A. (2001). Critical care of spinal cord injury. *Spine, 26* (24 suppl), S27–S30.

9. Balshi, J. D., Cantelmo, N. L., & Menzoian, J. O. (1989). Complications of caval interruption by Greenfield filter in quadriplegics. *J Vasc Surg, 9*(4), 558–562.

10. Banko, L. (2005). Aging with spinal cord injury: a review of the literature. *SCI Nurs, 22*(3), 138–145.

11. Barber, D. B., et al. (2000). Midodrine hydrochloride and the treatment of orthostatic hypotension in tetraplegia: two cases and a review of the literature. *Spinal Cord, 38*(2), 109–111.

12. Barco, K. T., et al. (2002). Energy expenditure assessment and validation after acute spinal cord injury. *Nutr Clin Practice, 17*(5), 309–313.

13. Bell, S. D. (1996). Use of Passy-Muir tracheostomy speaking valve in mechanically ventilated neurological patients. *Crit Care Nurse, 16*(1), 63–68.

14. Bernhard, M., et al. (2005). Spinal cord injury (SCI)—prehospital management. *Resuscitation, 66*(2), 127–139.

15. Blackmer, J. (1997). Orthostatic hypotension in spinal cord injured patients. *J Spinal Cord Med, 20*(2), 212–217.

16. Blackmer, J., & Ross, L. (2002). Awareness and use of advance directives in the spinal cord injured population. *Spinal Cord, 40* (11), 581–594.

17. Blumenfeld, H. (2002). *Neuroanatomy through clinical cases* (pp 13–46, 213–301). Sunderland, Mass: Sinauer Associates.

18. Bracken, M. B. (2002). Steroids for acute spinal cord injury. *Cochrane Database Syst Rev, 3*, CD001046.

19. Brain Trauma Foundation and the American Association of Neurological Surgeons. (2000). Role of steroids. In *Management and prognosis of severe traumatic brain injury* (pp 131–138). New York: Brain Trauma Foundation.

20. Britton, D., et al. (2005). Baclofen pump intervention for spasticity affecting pulmonary function. *J Spinal Cord Med, 28*(4), 343–347.

21. Butt, L., & Scofield, G. (1997). The bright line reconsidered: the issue of treatment discontinuation in patients with ventilator-dependent tetraplegia. *Top Spinal Cord Inj Rehabil, 2*(3), 85–94.

22. Capoor, J., & Stein, A. B. (2005). Aging with spinal cord injury. *Phys Med Rehabil Clin N Am, 16*(1), 129–161.

23. Chan, K., et al. (1995). Prospective double-blind placebo-controlled randomized trial of the use of ranitidine in preventing postoperative gastroduodenal complications in high-risk neurosurgical patients. *J Neurosurg, 82*(3), 413–417.

24. Consortium for Spinal Cord Medicine. (1998). *Depression following spinal cord injury: a clinical practice guideline for primary care physicians*. Washington, DC: Paralyzed Veterans of America.

25. Consortium for Spinal Cord Medicine. (1998). *Neurogenic bowel management in adults with spinal cord injury*. Washington, DC: Paralyzed Veterans of America.

26. Consortium for Spinal Cord Medicine. (1999). *Prevention of thromboembolism in spinal cord injury* (2nd ed.). Washington, DC: Paralyzed Veterans of America.

27. Consortium for Spinal Cord Medicine. (1999). *Outcomes following traumatic spinal cord injury: clinical practice guideline for health-care professionals*. Washington, DC: Paralyzed Veterans of America.

28. Consortium for Spinal Cord Medicine. (2000). *Pressure ulcer prevention and treatment following spinal cord injury: a clinical practice guideline for health-care professionals*. Washington, DC: Paralyzed Veterans of America.

29. Consortium for Spinal Cord Medicine. (2001). *Acute management of autonomic dysreflexia: individuals with spinal cord injury presenting to health-care facilities* (2nd ed.). Washington, DC: Paralyzed Veterans of America.

30. Consortium for Spinal Cord Medicine. (2005). *Respiratory management following spinal cord injury: a clinical practice guideline for health-care professionals*. Washington, DC: Paralyzed Veterans of America.

31. Consortium for Spinal Cord Medicine. (2005). *Preservation of upper limb function following spinal cord injury: a clinical practice guideline for health-care professionals*. Washington, DC: Paralyzed Veterans of America.

32. Cotton, B. A., et al. (2005). Respiratory complications and mortality risk associated with thoracic spine injury. *J Trauma, 59*(6), 1400–1409.

33. Craven, D. E. (2000). Epidemiology of ventilator-assisted pneumonia. *Chest, 117*(4 suppl 2), 186S–187S.

34. Daube, J. R. (2002). Spinal cord monitoring. In J. R. Daube (Ed.), *Clinical neurophysiology* (2nd ed., pp 539–554). New York: Oxford.

35. Derwenskus, J., & Zaidat, O. O. (2004). Spinal cord injury and related diseases. In J. I. Suarez (Ed.), *Critical care neurology and neurosurgery* (pp 417–432). Totowa, NJ: Humana Press.

36. DiMarco, A. F. (2005). Restoration of respiratory muscle function following spinal cord injury: review of electrical and magnetic stimulation techniques. *Respir Phys Neurobiol, 147*(2–3), 273–287.

37. DiMarco, A. F., et al. (2005). Phrenic nerve pacing via intramuscular diaphragm electrodes in tetraplegic subjects. *Chest, 127*(2), 671–678.

38. DiMarco, A. F., Takaoka, Y., & Kowalski, K. E. (2005). Combined intercostal and diaphragm pacing to provide artificial ventilation in patients with tetraplegia. *Arch Phys Med Rehabil, 86*(6), 1200–1207.

39. Dvorak, M. F., et al. (2004). Early versus late enteral feeding in patients with acute cervical spinal cord injury. *Spine, 29*(9), E175–E180.

40. Fassett, D. R., & Dailey, A. T. (2005). Thoracolumbar spine fractures. In S. S. Rengachary & R. G. Ellenbogen (Eds.), *Principles of neurosurgery* (2nd ed., pp 381–385). Edinburgh: Elsevier Mosby.

41. Fehlings, M. G., & Baptiste, D. C. (2005). Current status of clinical trials for acute spinal cord injury. *Injury, 36*(suppl 2), S-B113–S-B122.

42. Fine, C. K., & Nelson, A. (2001). Nutrition. In A. Nelson & C. P. Zejdlik (Eds.), *Nursing practice related to spinal cord injury and disorders: a core curriculum* (pp 189–202). Jackson Heights, NY: Eastern Paralyzed Veterans' Association.

43. Freeborn, K. (2005). The importance of maintaining spinal precautions. *Crit Care Nurs Q, 28*(2), 195–199.

44. Fries, J. M. (2005). Critical rehabilitation of the patient with spinal cord injury. *Crit Care Nurs Q, 28*(2), 179–187.

45. Ganuza, F. J. R., et al. (1997). Acute acalculous cholecystitis in patients with acute traumatic spinal cord injury. *Spinal Cord, 35*(2), 124–128.

46. Garcia, L. M. E., & Esclarin, D. R. A. (2003). Management of urinary tract infection in patients with spinal cord injuries. *Clin Microbiol Infect, 9*(8), 780–785.

47. Geerts, W. H., et al. (2004). Prevention of venous thromboembolism: the Seventh ACCP Conference on Antithrombotic and Thrombolytic Therapy. *Chest, 126*(3 suppl), 338S–400S.

48. Giroux, J. A. (2001). Bladder elimination and continence. In A. Nelson & C. P. Zejdlik (Eds.), *Nursing practice related to spinal cord injury and disorders: a core curriculum* (pp 163–188). Jackson Heights, NY: Eastern Paralyzed Veterans Association.

49. Gokaslan, Z. L., & McCormick, P. (2000). Surgical techniques: thoracic and lumbar. In C. H. Tator & E. C. Benzel (Eds.), *Contemporary management of spinal cord injury: from impact to rehabilitation* (pp 173–187). Park Ridge Ill: American Association of Neurological Surgeons.

50. Gomes, J. A., et al. (2005). Glucocorticoid therapy in neurologic critical care. *Crit Care Med, 33*(6), 1214–1224.

51. Groah, S. L., et al. (2002). Excess risk of bladder cancer in spinal cord injury: evidence for an association between indwelling catheter use and bladder cancer. *Arch Phys Med Rehabil, 83*(3), 346–351.

52. Gunnarsson, T., & Fehlings, M. G. (2003). Acute neurosurgical management of traumatic brain injury and spinal cord injury. *Curr Opin Neurol, 16*(6), 717–723.

53. Gupta, S. K., et al. (1999). Spinal cord injury without radiographic abnormality in adults. *Spinal Cord, 37*(10), 726–729.

54. Gutierrez, P. A., Young, R. R., & Vulpe, M. (1993). Spinal cord injury—an overview. *Urol Clin N Am, 20*(3), 373–382.

55. Hadley, M. N., et al. (2002). Guidelines for the management of acute cervical spine and spinal cord injury. *Clin Neurosurg, 49,* 407–498.

56. Hall, E. D., & Springer, J. E. (2004). Neuroprotection and acute spinal cord injury: a reappraisal. *NeuroRx, 1*(1), 80–100.

57. Hayes, V. M., et al. (2005). Complications of halo fixation of the cervical spine. *Am J Orthop, 34*(6), 271–276.

58. Herschorn, S., & Ordorica, R. C. (2000). Urological management of the spinal cord injury patient. In C. H. Tator & E. C. Benzel (Eds.), *Contemporary management of spinal cord injury: from impact to rehabilitation* (pp 273–284). Park Ridge, Ill: American Association of Neurological Surgeons.

59. Hess, M. J., et al. (2003). Bladder cancer in patients with spinal cord injury. *J Spinal Cord Med, 26*(4), 335–338.

60. Hodgson, B. B., & Kizior, R. J. (2006). *Saunders nursing drug handbook 2006.* St Louis: Saunders.

61. Jackson, A. B., et al. (2004). A demographic profile of new traumatic spinal cord injuries: change and stability over 30 years. *Arch Phys Med Rehabil, 85*(11), 1740–1748.

62. Jenkins, A. L., Vollmer, D. G., & Eichler, M. C. (2005). Cervical spine trauma. In H. R. Winn (Ed.), *Youmans neurological surgery* (5th ed., pp 4885–4914). Philadelphia: Saunders.

63. Kang, A. H. (2005). Traumatic spinal cord injury. *Clin Obstet Gyn, 48*(1), 67–72.

64. Kaut, K., Turcott, J. C., & Lavery, M. (1996). Passy-Muir speaking valve. *Dimens Crit Care Nurs, 16*(6), 298–306.

65. King, B. S., Gupta, R., & Narayan, R. K. (2000). The early assessment and intensive care management of patients with severe traumatic brain and spinal cord injuries. *Surg Clin North Am, 80*(3), 855–870.

66. Kishan, S., Vives, M. J., & Reiter, M. F. (2005). Timing of surgery following spinal cord injury. *J Spinal Cord Med, 28*(1), 11–19.

67. Knoller, N., et al. (2005). Clinical experience using incubated autologous macrophages as a treatment for complete spinal cord injury. Phase study results. *J Neurosurg Spine, 3*(3), 173–181.

68. Kraft, M. R. (1999). Refusal of treatment: an ethical dilemma. *SCI Nurs, 16*(1), 9–13, 20.

69. Lammertse, D. P. (2004). Invited review: update on pharmaceutical trials in acute spinal cord injury. *J Spinal Cord Med, 27*(4), 319–325.

70. Landy, H. J., Arias, J., & Green, B. A. (2000). Penetrating injuries. In C. H. Tator & E. C. Benzel (Eds.), *Contemporary management of spinal cord injury: from impact to rehabilitation* (pp 199–207). Park Ridge Ill: American Association of Neurological Surgeons.

71. Ledsome, J. R., & Sharp, J. M. (1981). Pulmonary function in acute cervical cord injury. *Am Rev Respir Dis, 124*(1), 41–44.

72. Lee, T. L., & Green, B. A. (2002). Immediate management of the spinal cord injured patient. In B. Y. Lee & L. E. Ostrander (Eds.), *Spinal cord injured patient: comprehensive management* (2nd ed.). New York: Demos Medical Publishing.

73. Lennarson, P. J., & Menezes, A. H. (2000). Pediatric spinal cord injury. In C. H. Tator & E. C. Benzel (Eds.), *Contemporary management of spinal cord injury: from impact to rehabilitation* (pp 209–229). Park Ridge, Ill: American Association of Neurological Surgeons.

74. Levi, A. D. O. (2005). Approach to the patient and diagnostic evaluation. In H. R. Winn (Ed.), *Youmans neurological surgery* (5th ed., pp 4869–4884). Philadelphia: Saunders.

75. Livneh, H., & Martz, E. (2005). Psychosocial adaptation to spinal cord injury: a dimensional perspective. *Psychol Rep, 97*(2), 577–586.

76. Love, L. (2001). Cardiovascular and thermoregulatory control. In A. Nelson & C. P. Zejdlik (Eds.), *Nursing practice related to spinal cord injury and disorders: a core curriculum* (pp 145–161). Jackson Heights, NY: Eastern Paralyzed Veterans Association.

77. Madsen, P. W., Eismont, F. J., & Green, B. A. (2005). Diagnosis and management of thoracic spine fractures. In H. R. Winn (Ed.), *Youmans neurological surgery* (5th ed., pp 4951–4985). Philadelphia: Saunders.

78. McCutcheon, E. P., et al. (2004). Acute traumatic spinal cord injury, 1993–2000. A population-based assessment of methylprednisolone administration and hospitalization. *J Trauma, 56*(5), 1076–1083.

79. McIlvoy, L., Meyer, K., & Vitaz, T. (2000). Use of an acute spinal cord injury clinical pathway. *Crit Care Nurs Clin North Am, 12*(4), 521–530.

80. McMichan, J. C., Michel, L., & Westbrook, P. R. (1980). Pulmonary dysfunction following traumatic quadriplegia. *JAMA, 243*(6), 528–531.

80a. McQuillen, K. A., Von Rueden, K. T., Hartsock, R. L. (2002). Trauma nursing: From resuscitation through rehabilitation, 3rd ed. Philadelphia: Saunders.

81. Morishima, N., Ohota, K., & Miura, Y. (2005). The influences of halo-vest fixation and cervical hyperextension on swallowing in healthy volunteers. *Spine, 30*(7), 179–192.

82. Mossner, J., & Caca, K. (2005). Developments in the inhibition of gastric acid secretion. *Eur J Clin Invest, 35*(8), 469–475.

83. National Spinal Cord Injury Statistical Center. (2004). *The 2004 annual statistical report for the model spinal cord injury care systems.* Birmingham, Ala.

84. Odderson, I. R., & Lietzow, D. (1997). Dysphagia complications of the Minerva brace. *Arch Phys Med Rehabil, 78*(12), 1386–1388.

85. Owens, G. F. (2002). Urologic evaluation and management of spinal cord injured patients. In B. Y. Lee & L. E. Ostrander (Eds.), *The spinal cord injured patient* (pp 47–57). New York: Demos.

86. Pateder, D. B., & Carbone, J. J. (2005). Cervical spine trauma. *J Surg Ortho Adv, 14*(1), 8–16.

87. Pearl, J., et al. (2001). Small bowel perforation after a quad cough maneuver. *J Trauma, 51*(1), 162–163.

88. Pollard, M. E., & Apple, D. F. (2003). Factors associated with improved neurologic outcomes in patients with incomplete tetraplegia. *Spine, 28*(1), 33–39.

89. Prendergast, V., & Sullivan, C. (2000). Acute spinal cord injury: nursing considerations for the first 72 hours. *Crit Care Nurs Clin North Am, 12*(4), 499–508.

90. Provencio, J. J., Bleck, T. P., & Connors, A. F. (2001). Critical care neurology. *Am J Respir Crit Care Med, 164*(3), 341–345.

91. Richards, P. J. (2005). Cervical spine clearance: a review. *Injury, 36*(2), 248–269.

92. Rose, J. C., & Mayer, S. A. (2004). Optimizing blood pressure in neurological emergencies. *Neurocrit Care, 1*(3), 287–299.

93. Rosenberg, R. I., Zirkle, D. L., & Neuwelt, E. A. (2005). Program self-evaluation: the evaluation of an injury prevention foundation. *J Neurosurg, 102*(5), 847–849.

94. Rowan, C. J., et al. (2004). Is early enteral feeding safe in patients who have suffered spinal cord injury? *Injury, 35*(3), 238–242.

95. Rundquist, J. (2002). The right to die—ethical dilemmas in persons with spinal cord injury. *SCI Nurs, 19*(1), 7–10.

96. Sheerin, F. (2005). Spinal cord injury: causation and pathophysiology. *Emerg Nurse, 12*(9), 29–38.

97. Sheerin, F. (2005). Spinal cord injury: acute care management. *Emerg Nurse, 12*(10), 26–34.

98. Shenaq, S. M., & Dinh, T. A. (1990). Decubitus ulcers: how to prevent them and intervene should prevention fail. *Postgrad Med, 87*(4), 91–95.

99. Singh, R. V., Suys, S., & Villaneuva, P. A. (2000). Prevention and treatment of medical complications. In C. H. Tator & E. C. Benzel (Eds.), *Contemporary management of spinal cord injury: from impact to rehabilitation* (pp 253–272). Park Ridge Ill: American Association of Neurological Surgeons.

100. Singhal, A., Baker, A., & Fehlings, M. G. (2003). Spinal cord injury management. In B. T. Andrews (Ed.). *Intensive care in neurosurgery*. New York: Thieme.

101. Slazinski, T., & Littlejohns, L. R. (2004). Anatomy of the nervous system. In M. K. Bader & L. R. Littlejohns (Eds.), *AANN core curriculum for neuroscience nursing*. St Louis: Saunders.

102. Skidmore-Roth, L. (2006). *2006 Mosby's nursing drug reference*. St Louis: Mosby.

103. Staas, W. E., & LaMantia, J. G. (1982). Decubitus ulcers and rehabilitation medicine. *Intern J Derm, 21*(8), 437–444.

104. Stambolis, V., et al. (2003). The effects of cervical bracing upon swallowing in young, normal, healthy volunteers. *Dysphagia, 18*(1), 39–45.

105. Stevens, R. D., et al. (2003). Critical care and perioperative management of traumatic spinal cord injury. *J Neurosurg Anesthesiol, 15*(3), 215–229.

106. Taggard, D. A., & Traynelis, V. C. (2005). Treatment of occipital C1 injury. In H. R. Winn (Ed.), *Youmans neurological surgery* (5th ed., pp 4925–4937). Philadelphia: Saunders.

107. Tator, C. H. (2000). Clinical manifestations of acute spinal cord injury. In C. H. Tator & E. D. Benzel (Eds.), *Contemporary management of spinal cord injury: from impact to rehabilitation* (pp 21–32). Park Ridge, Ill: American Association of Neurological Surgeons.

108. Tator, C. H. (2000). Sports and recreation as causes of spinal cord injury: epidemiology, screening, injury, management, and return to play. In C. H. Tator & E. D. Benzel (Eds.), *Contemporary management of spinal cord injury: from impact to rehabilitation* (pp 231–235). Park Ridge, Ill: American Association of Neurological Surgeons.

109. Tewari, M. K., et al. (2005). Diagnosis and prognostication of adult spinal cord injury without radiographic abnormality using magnetic resonance imaging: analysis of 40 patients. *Surg Neurol, 63*(3), 204–209.

110. Tsirikos, A. I., et al. (2004). Spinal cord monitoring using intraoperative somatosensory evoked potentials for spinal trauma. *J Spinal Disord Tech, 17*(5), 385–394.

111. Tyroch, A. H., et al. (1997). Spinal cord injury. A preventable public burden. *Arch Surg, 132*(7), 778–781.

112. Urdaneta, F., & Layon, A. J. (2003). Respiratory complications in patients with traumatic cervical spine injuries: case report and review of the literature. *J Clin Anesthesia, 15*(5), 398–405.

113. Van Goethem, J. W. M., et al. (2005). Imaging in spinal trauma. *Eur Radiol, 15*(3), 582–590.

114. Vannemreddy, S. S., Rowed, D. W., & Bharatwal, N. (2002). Posttraumatic syringomyelia: predisposing factors. *Brit J Neurosurg, 16*(3), 276–283.

115. Van Rossum, A. B., et al. (1996). Pulmonary embolism: validation of spiral CT angiography in 149 patients. *Radiology, 201*(2), 467–470.

116. Veit, N., & Quigley, P. (2001). Spasticity. *Rehabilitation in nursing practice related to spinal cord injury and disorders: a core curriculum* (pp 279–284). Jackson Heights, NY: Eastern Paralyzed Veterans Association.

117. Villanueva, N. E. (2000). Spinal cord injury in the elderly. *Crit Care Nurs Clin North Am, 12*(4), 509–519.

118. Wang, D., et al. (1996). A clinical magnetic resonance imaging study of the traumatised spinal cord more than 20 years following injury. *Paraplegia, 34*(2), 65–81.

119. Waters, R. L., et al. (1994). Motor and sensory recovery following incomplete paraplegia. *Arch Phys Med Rehabil, 75*(1), 67–72.

120. Wilberger, J. E. (2000). Immobilization and traction. In C. H. Tator & E. C. Benzel (Eds.), *Contemporary management of spinal cord injury: from impact to rehabilitation* (pp 91–98). Park Ridge, Ill: American Association of Neurological Surgeons.

121. Wollard, S. (2003). Cervical spine clearance in adult trauma patients. *JAAPA, 16*(4), 19–20, 23.

122. Yarkony, G. M., & Gittler, M. (2002). Spinal cord injury rehabilitation. In B. Y. Lee & L. E. Ostrander (Eds.), *The spinal cord injured patient*. New York: Demos.

CHAPTER 25

Special Neurologic Patient Populations

Jeannette Richardson

Patients with neurologic concerns in critical care include not only those who have acute disorders of the central nervous system (CNS) but also those who have exacerbations or sequelae from chronic neurologic illnesses. Some of the more common neuroscience diagnoses encountered by critical care nurses are addressed in this chapter. A brief discussion of neurodiagnostic testing frequently performed in the critically ill neuroscience patient is provided in Table 25-1 and in the Medication table on pp. 684-686 to assist in the critical analysis and evaluation of patient diagnosis and management.

The disease processes addressed include seizure disorders, CNS infections and tumors, and specific neuromuscular diseases or syndromes such as Guillain-Barré, the myopathies and neuropathies of critical illness, and the exacerbation of chronic myasthenia gravis. Determination of death by neurologic criteria and the use of therapeutic hypothermia for improved neurologic outcome are also included.

In addition to these diagnoses, selected high-risk/low-volume neuroscience patient populations of current interest will be included. These patient groups, representing increasingly familiar diagnoses in some facilities, include those with neurocysticercosis and Creutzfeldt-Jakob disease.

Many critically ill neuroscience patients have complex diseases and limited treatment options. Supportive care secondary to the disease process is a mainstay in this patient population and often includes mechanical ventilation; monitoring and treatment of altered hemodynamic parameters; ongoing assessment of the patient's neurologic status; and often palliative and end-of-life measures. Nursing care of the critically ill neuroscience patient can present a challenge to even the most experienced practitioner.

NEURODIAGNOSTIC TESTING

Patients with known or suspected disorders within the CNS often undergo different types of diagnostic testing. With the continuously advancing technology available to healthcare providers today, newer and better tests are rapidly emerging. The critical care nurse must have a working knowledge of various neurodiagnostic tests in order to better prepare, assist, and recover patients. Additionally, the nurse will be better able to help patients understand and interpret test results and plan for treatment as needed. Selected types of neurodiagnostic testing are presented here and in Table 25-1.

Computed Tomography Scan

Computed tomography (CT) scans are accomplished with the use of a large scanning machine that takes a series of x-rays and creates a computerized composite picture based on the densities of the various tissues visualized.[106] Unenhanced or noncontrast CT scans are often done to detect acute hemorrhage. When performed on an emergent basis in a facility with protocols in place, the scan can often be completed and read within 10 minutes. Although the scanner is somewhat confining and can be difficult for patients with claustrophobia, most scans are completed quickly enough so sedation is unnecessary. Nonetheless, some neuroscience patients with disorientation, an altered level of consciousness (LOC), or involuntary motor movements will require some sedation for the procedure. It is critical that the patient is able to lie still so that the scans are clear and not marred by artifact. Artifact can also occur from intracranial or nearby extracranial metallic foreign objects such as aneurysm clips, intracranial pressure (ICP) monitors, or tongs.[106] For comparison, Figure 25-1 shows an example of a patient who has had a CT and other complementary scanning procedures completed on the same day.

Contrast dye is used to highlight different types of brain tissue and can be extremely helpful in specific situations such as CNS infection and tumor.[184] However, iodinated contrast is associated with both allergic reactions and acute renal failure.[157] Allergic reactions can be anaphylactic and must be aggressively treated using advanced life support principles.[157] Episodes of acute renal failure have been associated with contrast media. Iso-osmolar nonionic contrast media appear to have the least nephrotoxicity.[141] Patients at risk include

681

TABLE 25-1 Neurodiagnostic Tests

NAME OF TEST	MECHANISM	INDICATION/SPECIAL CONSIDERATIONS
Computed tomography (CT) scan	CT scans are generated by a series of noninvasive x-rays that are processed to create a computerized image based on densities of various tissues visualized.[106]	Details specific areas of brain and spine, vascular changes, edema, shift, and hydrocephalus.[51] Gives information about structure but not function.[106] Superior to MRI for diagnosing skull fracture and subarachnoid hemorrhage.[51] Potential for allergic reaction or renal failure when iodine-based contrast is given.[51]
Computed tomography angiography (CTA)	High-speed CT images are obtained during contrast injection to visualize vessels reconstructed in three-dimensional images.[51]	For visualization of vessels or vascular abnormalities. Quicker, less expensive, and less invasive than cerebral angiography but tends to overestimate degree of vessel stenosis.[51]
Magnetic resonance imaging (MRI)	Noninvasive magnetic fields and radio-frequency waves are used to align protons (hydrogen atoms) in tissue. The computer reconstructs signals from the resonance or vibration of protons into video images based on signal intensity.[106] Different types of images (T1, T2, Flair, DWI) are used to detect specific lesions or abnormalities.[51]	Used to diagnose structural and biochemical abnormalities of brain and neural tissue including tumors, inflammation, infection, degenerative disorders, and traumatic brain injury.[184] MRI has greater sensitivity than CT for contusions, hematomas, intraparenchymal injury, and edema.[51] Electronic devices and magnetizable materials (including some intracranial devices) preclude MRI scanning.[106] The optional contrast agent used with MRI, gadolinium, has a low incidence of allergies. No radiation is used. The length of time necessary for image construction makes MRI susceptible to motion artifact. Claustrophobia and noise level can make MRI scanning uncomfortable; sedation may be indicated.[106]
Magnetic resonance angiography (MRA)	As with MRI, this is a noninvasive test (IV gadolinium is optional) using magnetic fields sensitive to proton movement. For MRA, focus is on proton oscillations within bloodstream that are magnetically manipulated for signal alteration and creation of desired video image.[78]	Used in evaluation of intra- and extracranial vasculature. Newest generation contrast-enhanced MRA scans are comparable to cerebral angiography in sensitivity in detection of carotid stenosis but lower in specificity.[78] As with MRI, patients with electronic devices and metallic implants are not candidates and sedation may be indicated.
Cerebral angiography	Catheter is inserted to site of interest. After injection of a radiopaque contrast medium, vessels are visualized through a series of radiographs[51] and examined for patency, narrowing and occlusion.[106]	Gold standard for vascular evaluation to determine degree of narrowing or obstruction of a blood vessel in brain, head, or neck.[51,184] Used to diagnose and localize stroke, aneurysm, arteriovenous malformations, and brain tumors.[184]

NAME OF TEST	MECHANISM	INDICATION/SPECIAL CONSIDERATIONS
Positron emission tomography (PET)	Images result from use of IV or inhaled substances that are labeled with radioisotopes (e.g., glucose, oxygen).[279] Provides images of quantitative parameters of brain hemodynamics including regional cerebral blood flow, regional cerebral blood volume, regional oxygen extraction fraction, and regional metabolic rate of oxygen or glucose.[279]	Used to diagnose chronic cerebrovascular disorders, dementia and psychiatric diseases, epilepsy, and brain tumors and for functional mapping studies.[279]
Single photon emission CT (SPECT)	Tomographic images are generated of three-dimensional distribution of a radioisotope to reflect regional cerebral blood flow.[270]	Used to diagnose acute and chronic cerebrovascular diseases, trauma, dementia and psychiatric diseases, and epilepsy; especially for presurgical localization of epileptic foci. May be helpful in diagnosing viral encephalitis and to confirm brain death.[279]
Electroencephalography (EEG)	Scalp electrodes monitor electrical brain activity from standard sites on scalp according to an international placement system. Electrical brain activity is recorded as a measurement of voltage between two electrode sites.[128]	Used to help diagnose seizure disorders, brain damage, encephalitis, and other metabolic and degenerative disorders of brain. Also useful in evaluation of sleep disorders and coma, and in determination of brain death.[184]
Electromyography (EMG)	Patterns of electrical activity of skeletal muscle are assessed during voluntary muscle activity or at rest. Accomplished using a system of very fine wire electrodes inserted into muscle and connected to a recording device.[51,184]	Provides information to help differentially diagnose neural from muscular disorders and to determine lesion site.[51] Often done in conjunction with nerve conduction studies.[184]
Nerve conduction studies	Assessment of nerve's ability to generate a signal: measurement of conduction velocity and amplitude of neural action potentials.[51] Two sets of flat electrodes are connected to patient over area of interest. A small electrical current is transmitted through one electrode and assessed at second electrode for appropriateness of response.[184]	Evaluates presence and extent of peripheral nerve damage.[51]
Somatosensory evoked potentials (SSEP)	Small electrical shocks are delivered via a needle electrode to a nerve in arm or leg. Responses are recorded by another electrode attached to patient's scalp.[184]	For evaluation of neural pathways involving spinal cord, brain stem, thalamus, and cerebral cortex. Used as an adjunct in diagnosing multiple sclerosis, brain tumor, and spinal cord injury. Also helpful in evaluating patients in coma and in determining brain death.[184]

CTA = Computed tomography angiography, CT = computed tomography, EEG = electroencephalogram, EMG = electromyography, MRA = magnetic resonance angiography, MRI = magnetic resonance imaging, PET = positron emission tomography, SPECT= single photon emission computed tomography, SSEP = somatosensory evoked potentials.

MEDICATIONS FREQUENTLY USED IN THE CARE OF CRITICALLY ILL NEUROSCIENCE PATIENTS

DRUG	ACTION	INDICATION AND USUAL DOSAGE	SPECIAL CONSIDERATIONS
Phenytoin (Dilantin)	Limit repetitive firing of action potentials through slowing of sodium channels[171]	*Status epilepticus (SE) and maintenance therapy for seizure prophylaxis:* Loading dose 20 mg/kg IV at 50 mg/min Maintenance dose 1.5 mg/kg IV three times per day[149] Therapeutic range 10–20 mcg/ml Many patients in SE may require serum levels of 25-30 mcg/ml to achieve seizure control[221]	Risk of hypotension and cardiac dysrhythmias, especially with rapid infusion Risk of infusion site reactions and soft tissue injury including "purple glove syndrome"[161] Allergic reactions and side effects are not uncommon and can include confusion, diplopia, lymphadenopathy, rash, Stevens-Johnson syndrome, and toxic epidermal necrolysis[218]
Fosphenytoin (Cerebyx)		Fosphenytoin ordered as "phenytoin equivalent" units	Water-soluble prodrug of phenytoin; less likely to cause infusion site reactions but much more expensive[149] Anticonvulsant medications are not effective in preventing first seizures in patients with newly diagnosed brain tumors[86]
Benzodiazepines			
Lorazepam (Ativan)	Act at benzodiazepine binding sites near GABA receptors to decrease neuronal firing and transmission of impulses[161]	*Status epilepticus:* Loading dose 0.1–0.15 mg/kg IV Follow with maintenance anti-epileptic drug[76]	Slightly slower onset but longer acting than diazepam[76] Needs refrigeration Can be administered rectally or sublingually but these routes have not been extensively studied[161]
Diazepam (Valium)		*Status epilepticus:* Loading dose 0.15 mg/kg IV Maintenance 4–8 mg/hr IV Follow with maintenance anti-epileptic drug[76]	Available as a rectal preparation when IV access inadequate[76] Not typically used as maintenance therapy[149]
Midazolam (Versed)		*Status epilepticus:* Loading dose 0.2 mg/kg IV Maintenance 0.2–2.9 mg/kg/hr[29] IV	Unlike other benzodiazepines, is water soluble and therefore can be given intramuscularly; also available for intranasal, buccal, or rectal administration Rapid onset of action but short half-life requires frequent dosing[76]
Barbiturates			
Phenobarbital (Luminal)	Act on GABA receptor complex and limit synaptic transmission[28]	*Status epilepticus:* Loading dose 20 mg/kg[76,149] IV Maintenance 2–4 mg/kg/day[149] IV	High risk of respiratory depression; higher doses result in stupor and coma Cardiovascular collapse can occur at high levels

DRUG	ACTION	INDICATION AND USUAL DOSAGE	SPECIAL CONSIDERATIONS
			Long half-life of 90 hr prolongs effects of drug for days or weeks[149]
Pentobarbital (Nembutal)		*Status epilepticus:* Loading dose 3–15 mg/kg IV over 1 hr[76] Maintenance 1–10 mg/kg/hr IV to achieve desired effect on EEG Breakthrough seizures: Additional 3–5 mg/kg IV bolus[28]	High risk of hypotension; long half-life of 10–20 hr[149] Pentobarbital levels are not as helpful during treatment as EEG effect[76]
Propofol (Diprivan)	General anesthetic; GABA receptor site agonist[28]	*Status epilepticus:* Loading dose 1–5 mg/kg IV Maintenance 2–15 mg/kg/hr[149,236] IV	Rapid onset and offset of action[29] High cost Significant lipid component in IV admixture; rarely, pancreatitis[149] Rapid discontinuation of drug may precipitate seizures[28] Risk for propofol infusion syndrome: profound hypotension, lipidemia, and metabolic acidosis[76]
Corticosteroids			
Dexamethasone (Decadron)	Mode of action in reduction of peritumoral edema unclear: proposed mechanisms include inhibition of phospholipase A₂, stabilization of lysosomal membranes, and improvement of peritumoral microcirculation[122]	*Treatment for peritumoral edema:* Loading dose 10 mg PO Maintenance 4 mg PO every 6 hr[192] Dosage varies between 4 and 100 mg/day[122] *Treatment for bacterial meningitis (begin with first dose of antibiotics):* 10 mg IV every 6 hr for 4 days[262] *Myasthenia gravis:* Steroid therapy reserved for patients with moderate or severe disease[253] *Guillain-Barré:* Corticosteroids proved to be of no benefit[92]	Dexamethasone is preferred corticosteroid for treatment of brain tumors because of minimal mineralocorticoid effect and lower rates of infection and psychosis[19,130] Side effects include immunosuppression, altered glucose metabolism, gastrointestinal irritation, mood swings, myopathy, fat redistribution, and peripheral edema[228] Steroids for bacterial meningitis are contraindicated in septic shock, immunosuppression, and postneurosurgical meningitis[262]
Desmopressin acetate (DDAVP)	Form of vasopressin	*Diabetes insipidus:* 10–40 mcg (0.1–0.4 ml) intranasally once or twice daily *or* 2–4 mcg IV or subcutaneously once or twice daily *or* 0.1–0.8 mg/day divided into 2 or 3 doses in oral tablets[230]	Side effects are uncommon and dose related: headache, nausea, nasal congestion or rhinitis, flushing, and cramping In high doses, can cause hypertension[230]

Table continues on page 686

DRUG	ACTION	INDICATION AND USUAL DOSAGE	SPECIAL CONSIDERATIONS
Intravenous immunoglobulin (IVIG)	Acts to modulate immune system through multiple mechanisms involving immunoglobulin class G (IgG) and receptors on macrophages and B cells; enhances T cell function[216]	*Myasthenia gravis:* 400 mg/kg IV for 5 days[253] *Guillain-Barré syndrome:* 400 mg/kg IV daily for 5 days[186]	IVIG and plasmapheresis are equally effective in treatment of MG and GBS[108,253] When compared to plasmapheresis, IVIG has fewer complications and may be more comfortable for patient[186] Side effects of IVIG include expansion of plasma volume and self-limiting fever, myalgia, headache, nausea, and vomiting[142]
Acyclovir (Zovirax)	Inhibits viral replication[42]	*Herpes simplex and varicella-zoster encephalitis:* 10 mg/kg three times daily for 14 days[42]	Most effective when given early in course of encephalitis[42]
Anthelmintics (Antiparasitics)			
Albendazole (Albenza)	Cesticidal drugs	*Neurocysticercosis:* 15 mg/kg/day for 1 week[80]	Albendazole superior to praziquantel in destroying brain cysts[231] Adverse effects include headaches, increased seizure frequency, increased ICP, cerebral infarction, hyperthermia, hypotension, dysrhythmias, and death[247] Anthelmintics should be given in conjunction with steroid/immunosuppressive therapy to decrease inflammatory reaction to dying parasites[227,231] Patients with calcified cysts do not require anthelmintics[231]
Praziquantel (Biltricide)		*Neurocysticercosis:* 10–100 mg/kg administered every 8 hr for 3–21 days[27] *or* 25–30 mg/kg every 2 hr times 3 doses[49]	
Acetylcholinesterase Inhibitors			
Pyridostigmine (Mestinon)	Inhibits acetylcholinesterase and thus increases availability of acetylcholine to act on ACh receptors	*Myasthenia gravis:* Started at 30 mg three times per day Can be gradually increased to 60–90 mg four times per day based on response and tolerance[253] Onset of action in 15–30 min with duration of about 4 hr[253]	Side effects include abdominal pain, diarrhea, and excessive salivation[253] Cholinesterase crisis involving an excess of acetylcholine at neuromuscular junction is characterized by worsening of weakness and abdominal pain, and hypersalivation Treatment involves reduction of dose[253]

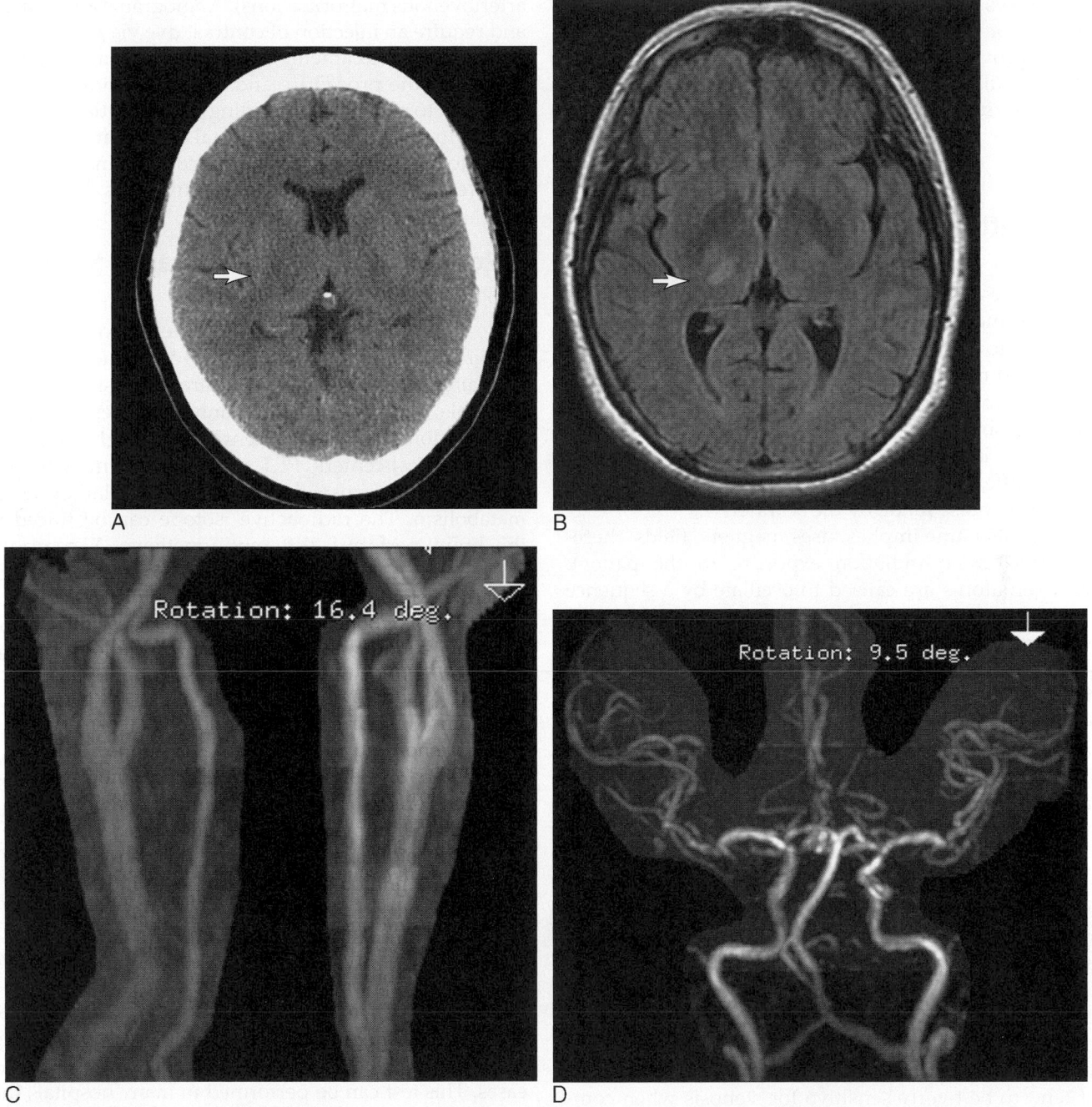

♦FIGURE 25-1 CT, MRI, and MRA on the same patient with acute ischemic stroke. **A,** Unenhanced CT scan showing subtle hypodensity in the right thalamus indicative of early cerebral infarct. **B,** MRI Flair image of acute right thalamic infarct. **C,** Normal MRA of neck vessels. **D,** Normal MRA of brain/intracranial vessels.

those with diabetes who have an elevated serum creatinine level of 2 mg/dl or higher before contrast administration.[141,208] There is also some evidence of a link with the medication metformin.[185] Adequate hydration with intravenous (IV) saline before the procedure is critical in preventing acute renal failure.[88] Hydration with sodium bicarbonate has been shown to have some effectiveness, but more study is indicated.[175] The benefit of pharmacologic agents appears limited, but *N*-acetylcysteine has

been used with some success to prevent contrast medium nephropathy.[88] Chapter 33 provides more details on the prevention of acute renal failure.

Computed Tomography Angiography

Computed tomography angiography (CTA) is a quick imaging technique that utilizes an injection of contrast medium to create angiographic images of the vascular system. Although this technology has been available for several decades, later generation scanners have improved the speed and quality of the images that are available in three dimensions.[78] The ease of use and improving reliability of this test have put it in the forefront to replace magnetic resonance angiography (MRA) and cerebral angiography in some cases.[243]

Magnetic Resonance Scan

Magnetic resonance imaging (MRI), MRA, and magnetic resonance venography (MRV) are all done with the same large piece of scanning equipment. When compared to the CT scanner, the MR scanner is bigger, louder, and more confining. An MR scan can take considerably longer than CT, often 1 hour or more. Many claustrophobic patients require some sort of anxiolytic medication in order to tolerate the scan time. Many facilities offer earphones with music to drown out the hammering noise made by the scanner.

MR, as its name implies, uses magnetic fields; therefore there is no radiation exposure to the patient. Hydrogen atoms are caused to oscillate by a sequence of radiofrequency pulsations. The computer measures these oscillations to create an image.[106] Because the equipment is based on magnets, patients who have implanted devices that are magnetic are usually not able to undergo MR imaging. Currently, many implants that used to be magnetic (e.g., orthopedic joint replacement hardware) are being recreated with materials that are not magnetic so that patients can still undergo MRI testing in the future.

MRI scans create a graphic image of bone, fluid, and soft tissue structures. They often are used to give a more defined image of anatomic details and may help diagnose small tumors or early infarction syndromes. Without contrast, an MRI is a valuable, noninvasive diagnostic tool. When contrast is required, nonnephrotoxic gadolinium, which is metabolized by the liver, is used.[18]

MRA and MRV are studies of cerebral blood flow in various vessels. The images are fast and noninvasive but tend to be overly sensitive for stenosis when compared with conventional angiograms.[18] Correlation with ultrasound evaluations or angiography is occasionally indicated. Figure 25-1 shows examples of MRI and MRA scans.

Cerebral Angiogram

Cerebral angiography is the gold standard of diagnostic tools for evaluation of the vasculature of the brain. It is used to determine vessel patency, narrowing, and occlusions as well as structural abnormalities (aneurysms or dissections), vessel displacement (tumors or edema), and alterations in blood flow (tumors and arteriovenous malformations). Angiograms are invasive and require an injection of contrast dye via a catheter. A common site for catheter insertion is the femoral artery. Following the procedure and catheter removal, nurses will need to monitor for bleeding and potential impaired circulation to the extremity distal to the catheter insertion site. Additionally, the use of contrast may compromise renal status in susceptible individuals.[106]

Positron Emission Tomography Scan

Positron emission tomography (PET) scans use radioactive isotopes that are injected into the bloodstream to provide a two- or three-dimensional picture of brain activity. The scanners are expensive and less available than CT or MRI scanners, so testing is frequently done on an outpatient basis at highly sophisticated medical centers. PET scans are extremely helpful and unique because they measure cellular or tissue metabolism. The radioactive isotope can be traced as the brain performs different functions. A computer processes the information and displays it as an image. PET scans are useful in detecting tumors and diseased tissue and in evaluating patients with seizure disorders, memory disorders, and brain changes secondary to injury or chemical abuse.[184]

Single Photon Emission Computed Tomography Scan

A single photon emission computed tomography (SPECT) scan is a nuclear imaging test that, like the PET scan, involves injection of a radioactive isotope (some facilities use inhaled isotopes[106]). The isotope will travel to areas of increased blood flow, and therefore the SPECT scan also tests physiologic functioning. A gamma camera circles the patient and records the areas where isotope has collected, and a computer converts this information into a three-dimensional image. SPECT scans are useful in diagnosing tumors, infections, and some degenerative diseases. This test can be performed in many hospitals that have nuclear imaging departments.[184] PET and SPECT scans, because of their ability to test for physiologic brain function, can be used to diagnose structural abnormalities but also may help in clarifying some behavioral disturbances, such as dementia and schizophrenia, that may have a physiologic basis.[106]

Electroencephalogram

An electroencephalogram (EEG) is performed to evaluate the electrical activity of the brain. EEGs are generally done with electrodes pasted to the scalp but can also be done intracranially using electrode grids, strips, or depth electrodes. Intracranial electrodes are useful in reducing signal interference from the skull.[184]

Analysis of EEG recordings can help detect specific areas of abnormal electrical activity such as seizures, tumors, and abscesses. Generalized processes such as metabolic disturbances, coma, and brain irritation secondary to infection can also be noted on EEG. A recording done to determine electrical activity in the brain can be useful in the clinical determination of brain death.[18]

Electromyography, Nerve Conduction Studies, and Neuromuscular Junction Studies

Testing done on nerves, muscles, and the junction between them is performed to evaluate nerve conduction and subsequent skeletal muscle function. The tests are often done together to evaluate, diagnose, or monitor nerve and muscle dysfunction and spinal cord disease.

Generally, electrodes are used to either electrically stimulate or record responses to the stimulation. The electrodes may be pasted on or inserted as needles into the muscle. Muscle and nerve activity can be recorded at rest or with voluntary activity.[184]

Evoked Potentials

Evoked potentials (EPs) are a specific electrodiagnostic test used to evaluate nerve conduction. They measure the electrical signals in the brain that are generated by hearing (auditory evoked potentials), sight (visual evoked potentials), and touch (somatosensory evoked potentials). The patient has a set of electrodes pasted to the scalp and is then stimulated with noise, visual testing, or tiny electrical shocks. Responses to the stimuli are recorded from the brain electrodes and used to assess sensory nerve problems or confirm neurologic conditions such as multiple sclerosis, brain tumor, acoustic neuroma, and spinal cord injury. In critical care, EPs are helpful in predicting prognosis, especially in situations of hypoxic brain damage or an altered LOC. EPs are also used to monitor brain activity in patients in coma and to confirm brain death.[184]

SEIZURE DISORDERS

Seizures are a common and frequent reason for patient visits to the emergency department (ED) and for hospital admissions. Occasionally, seizure activity requires monitoring and interventions available only within critical care. Status epilepticus, continuous video/EEG monitoring for seizure activity with or without intracranial electrodes, and postoperative care

for epilepsy patients are some of the seizure-related situations with which critical care nurses should be familiar.

Status Epilepticus

Definition and Epidemiology. Status epilepticus (SE) has been traditionally defined as continuous seizure activity lasting greater than 30 minutes or as two or more discrete seizures between which consciousness is not fully regained.[283] This definition is based on pathologic evidence that suggests that neuronal damage begins after 30 minutes of continuous seizure activity and on epidemiologic data noting increased morbidity and mortality with seizures that last longer than 30 minutes.[147,282] Current investigators have been interested in amending the definition based on clinical experience that seizures in adults rarely last longer than 2 minutes; virtually all practitioners agree that initiation of treatment should be as early as possible to avoid neuronal or systemic injury and complications.[63] A suggested contemporary definition for SE includes all adult patients whose seizures continue longer than 5 minutes or who have two or more seizures with incomplete recovery between them.[152] This new definition, not yet universally accepted, is primarily operational and is designed to encourage the initiation of early treatment strategies in the course of prolonged seizures.

Refractory status epilepticus (RSE) is a particularly resistant form of SE defined as seizures lasting longer than 60 minutes despite treatment with a benzodiazepine and an adequate loading dose of a standard IV anticonvulsant drug. RSE, which shares the same treatment algorithms as SE, occurs in approximately 30% of patients with SE and is associated with increased length of hospital stay and functional disability.[169] The most common etiology for RSE is CNS infection (encephalopathy or Creutzfeldt-Jakob disease [CJD]), but many other etiologies are possible.[29] Complications associated with RSE include fever, pneumonia, hypotension, bacteremia, and anemia treated with blood transfusion.[169]

There are approximately 100,000 to 160,000 episodes of SE in the United States annually, most of which are experienced by patients with epilepsy;[62] approximately 5% of adults with epilepsy will have at least one episode of SE.[226,248] Among adults, stroke accounts for almost 50% of cases of SE and is the most common cause of SE in older adults.[62,271] Survivors of SE are at significant risk for another episode, and 13% of all patients will have a recurrent bout.[75] Up to 10% of SE patients may be left with disabling neurologic deficits.[46]

Mortality from SE is often a direct result of the underlying cause, but the seizures themselves, as well as the treatment, may contribute.[76] The etiology is the most important determinant of outcome. The mortality rate for adults who present with a first episode of SE is roughly 20%. This estimate is a function not only of underlying etiology but also of age and duration of SE.[145] Mortality is higher in older adult patients or when SE is secondary to an acute event such as stroke, anoxia, trauma, intracranial infections, or metabolic derangements. These diagnoses can be life-threatening in and of themselves and contribute to the mortality rate.[256] Anoxia and hypoxia associated with SE lead to very high mortality rates, 71% and 53%, respectively.[62] SE resulting from low anti-epileptic drug levels has a mortality rate of approximately 4%. In general, SE secondary to alcohol or anticonvulsant withdrawal, tumors, or epilepsy has a more benign prognosis than SE secondary to the aforementioned acute events.[256]

Clinical Presentation. Just as there are many different seizure types, so are there many clinical presentations of SE. In general, SE can be classified broadly into generalized convulsive status epilepticus (GCSE) and nonconvulsive status epilepticus (NCSE) on the basis of clinical and electrographic criteria.[41] GCSE is the most easily recognizable form of SE, in which generalized convulsive activity presents as tonic or clonic movement of the extremities. This disorder is associated with complete loss of consciousness and is frequently accompanied by incontinence and tongue biting. Afterward, the patient is stuporous but returns to full alertness with time.[76] If seizure activity is prolonged, these clinical manifestations become muted and less apparent.[161] The subtle features of late-stage GCSE may consist of only small-amplitude twitching of the face, hands, or feet, ocular deviation, or fine nystagmus before progressing to only electrical activity without physical correlation.[151,258] Figure 25-2 shows an example of an EEG with characteristic polyspike and wave discharges in evolving seizure activity.[267]

NCSE refers to continuous or near-continuous generalized electrical seizure activity without the typical tonic-clonic physical motor manifestations.[75] Diagnosis can be extremely difficult because typical presentations range from an alteration of awareness with bizarre behaviors to mild confusion to coma. NCSE occurs commonly following treatment for GCSE. In GCSE, if the patient does not recover from postictal stupor within 20 to 60 minutes, the possibility of continuing epileptic brain activity should be considered. An EEG is helpful in confirming the diagnosis, but treatment may be started empirically if clinical suspicion is high.[76] There is some evidence that the use of continuous EEG monitoring in critical care allows detection of a higher incidence of nonconvulsive seizures and SE than suspected previously through clinical examination

Generalized seizure

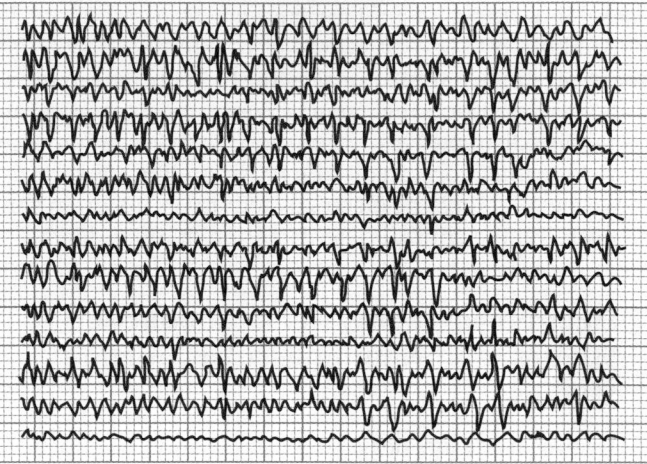

Evolving generalized seizure

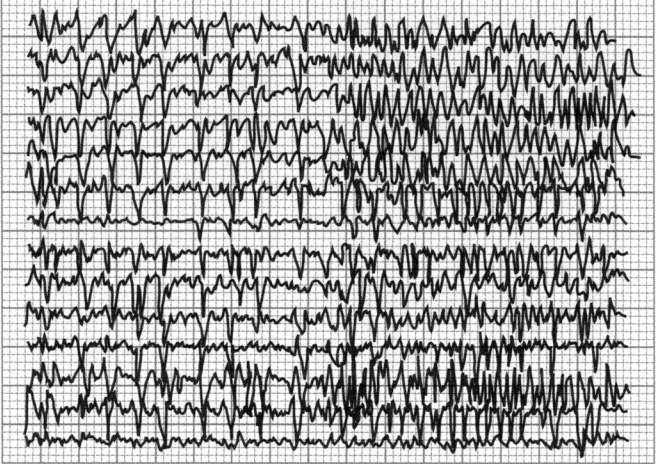

Seizure ends

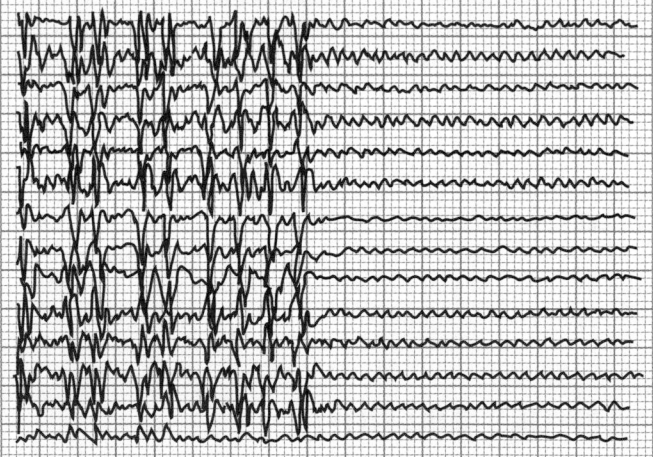

⬧FIGURE 25-2 EEG study of a generalized electroencephalographically detected seizure that evolves over time.

(noted in 20% to 25% of patients following traumatic brain injury).[177,267]

Pathophysiology. Seizures are the result of an imbalance of neurotransmitters in the CNS. *N*-Methyl-D-aspartate (NMDA) receptors are activated by the excitatory neurotransmitter glutamate and are believed to be required for the propagation of seizure activity. Gamma-aminobutyric acid (GABA) is the major inhibitory neurotransmitter and is hypothesized to be responsible for the normal termination of a seizure.[50] SE represents a failure of inherent cellular mechanisms that allows for persistent excitation or prevents sustained activity.[161]

The brain's internal mechanisms fail secondary to an imbalance between excitability and suppression, and subsequently a reverberating circuit is created.[164] Seizures can become self-sustaining after 15 to 30 minutes of stimulation.[161] As seizures persist, the GABA receptors change and become less susceptible to the GABA agonist effects of some medications.[123] These alterations in the function of neurotransmitters lay the basic groundwork for the choices in and use of pharmacologic agents for SE.

In humans and animals, sustained seizures cause selective neuronal loss in vulnerable regions such as the hippocampus, cortex, and thalamus. The degree of neuronal injury is closely related to the duration of seizures, emphasizing the need for rapid control of SE.[66]

SE is a major medical emergency associated with significant morbidity and mortality.[161] It has the potential to cause injury both because of the metabolic stress of repeated muscular convulsions noted in GCSE and because of the intense neuronal activity within the CNS. Neuronal death can occur after 30 to 60 minutes of continuous seizure activity,[235] and the longer an episode of SE continues, the greater the neurologic damage.[164]

Systemically, GCSE prompts changes in a multitude of body systems. Initially, the increased metabolic demands of the brain for glucose and oxygen are met by a compensatory increase in the production of catecholamines with subsequent elevations in blood pressure, heart rate, and cardiac output. This facilitates the desired effect of an increase in cerebral blood flow. Preservation of serum glucose is accomplished through an increase in the production of glucagon and stimulation of glycogenolysis in the liver.[41,76]

After approximately 30 minutes of seizure activity, these same compensatory mechanisms can become harmful and cause transient or permanent sequelae. Cerebral autoregulation becomes impaired as there is increased difficulty in meeting the metabolic demands of the brain. Rhabdomyolysis leads to lactic acidosis and a decrease in serum pH. As seizure activity progresses, blood pressure falls because of a loss of vessel responsiveness to circulating catecholamines, in turn leading to a reduction in cerebral perfusion and oxygen and glucose supplies to the brain. The elevated blood glucose levels eventually lead to increased insulin production and hypoglycemia.[76]

Hyperthermia is common during SE and is generally a result of seizure activity rather than an infectious process.[229] Lactic acid accumulates, and glucose and bicarbonate levels decrease. Metabolic acidosis and hyperkalemia may develop as a consequence of rhabdomyolysis[164] and could lead to cardiac dysrhythmias. Hypoxia results from increased metabolic and neuronal oxygen demands. A combination of hypoxia, hypoglycemia, and chemical synaptic alterations results in neuronal damage.[35] Additionally, the patient outcome may be further compromised by resultant aspiration pneumonitis, neurogenic pulmonary edema, and respiratory failure.[41]

Assessment and Diagnosis. Assessment of seizure activity should take all aspects into consideration. Any aura that may have occurred, the ictal phase, and the postictal period should be included. Mental status, motor features (body parts involved, tone, vocalizations), vital signs, and autonomic signs (pupils, gastrointestinal activity, and skin condition) should be included. After the episode, the patient should be questioned regarding somatosensory (psychic, sensory, or autonomic) symptoms. Postictal data should consider the time it takes the patient to return to baseline, the presence of headache, and any residual neurologic deficit.[5]

The diagnosis of SE may be straightforward but ultimately rests primarily upon the neurologic examination and the EEG. The neurologic exam includes an assessment of the LOC and observations for convulsive tonic-clonic activity, automatic movements or myoclonic activity, and any asymmetric features that might indicate a focal structural lesion. Many cases of SE can be diagnosed on the basis of the neurologic examination alone.[164]

An EEG is diagnostic of SE if it reveals continuous seizure activity. However, some limitations in the use of EEGs include the fact that some EEG patterns are difficult to recognize. An EEG obtained over a short time and between seizures can miss intermittent seizure activity.[165] The patient who continues to be obtunded or comatose after treatment of generalized convulsive SE poses a particular challenge. Epileptiform discharges on EEG, typically a 3-hertz spike and slow wave discharges,[76] are diagnostic of continued "subtle" SE.[165] However, patients with "subtle" SE often have EEG patterns of various types that may not conclusively show epileptic discharges. Clinicians have controversial opinions as to whether or not these patterns should require further aggressive therapeutic measures.[165]

Patients who are being treated with sedation or barbiturate coma for RSE are often monitored with continuous EEG recordings for a burst-suppression pattern. However, there is no consensus as to the duration of "burst" and "flat" periods for optimal medication dosing; most clinicians consider that establishing and maintaining any degree of suppression-burst pattern is adequate.[165] To further complicate treatment decisions, several investigators have noted that seizures can recur even in burst-suppression patterns.[29,133] Some clinicians feel that the goal of therapy should be seizure suppression independent of EEG background activity.[28]

Despite the controversial nature of EEG analysis, many clinicians believe that continuous EEG monitoring, or at least a follow-up standard EEG, is warranted in any patient requiring prolonged therapy for RSE or those remaining unconscious after the initial phase of anti-epileptic drug treatment. These practitioners report that electroencephalography is underused in these patients.[150]

The bispectral index (BIS) monitor is another EEG-derived tool used to assess sedation levels in patients who are chemically paralyzed or in a barbiturate-induced coma. The four-electrode sensor adheres to the patient's forehead and provides continuous EEG readings.[105] There has been some preliminary study in the use of this device to correlate the suppression ratio score with EEG burst-suppression, but further research is indicated.[85]

Diagnostic radiologic imaging is not a first-line test for SE but may reveal potential focal areas of interest. MRI can show areas of increased signal intensity and possible structural lesions.[45] SPECT may demonstrate areas of increased perfusion during SE that can persist for weeks after the termination of seizures.[250] Functional MRI (fMRI) can also assist in mapping areas of interest for future diagnostic and therapeutic purposes, but it is not generally used for the diagnosis of SE.[12]

Management and Treatment. The primary goal in the treatment of SE is the rapid termination of seizure activity.[161] It is believed that early administration of medication leads to the termination of seizures with much smaller doses and less risk to the patient than would be required if seizures were allowed to progress.[28] However, therapy for SE should proceed simultaneously along three fronts: termination of SE, prevention of recurrence, and treatment of complications.[28] The healthcare team must address airway protection, the prevention of aspiration, the management

of potential precipitating causes, and the treatment of any underlying conditions.[164] As noted earlier, the etiology of the episode of SE is usually the most important determinant for patient outcome.[76] Optimal management of SE requires prompt and accurate identification and correction, if possible, of any predisposing factors that may be present. These factors are listed in Box 25-1.[7,235,256]

There are four main categories of drugs used to treat SE: benzodiazepines, phenytoin (Dilantin) (or fosphenytoin [Cerebyx]), barbiturates, and propofol (Diprivan). Other drugs such as lidocaine, paraldehyde, ketamine (Ketalar), carbamazepine (Tegretol), and etomidate (Amidate) are less effective[283] or less well studied and so should not be considered as routine treatment strategies for SE.[235]

Benzodiazepines are considered the first-line treatment for SE because of their rapid onset of action and bioavailability. This class of drugs acts at the benzodiazepine binding site near the GABA receptors, resulting in an opening of chloride channels and influx of intracellular chloride, enhanced hyperpolarization of the cell

---

Box 25-1

Predisposing Factors for Status Epilepticus

- Anti-epileptic drug noncompliance or discontinuation
- Withdrawal syndromes associated with the discontinuation of alcohol, barbiturates, baclofen, or benzodiazepines
- Acute structural injury (e.g., encephalitis, tumor, stroke, head trauma, subarachnoid hemorrhage, cerebral anoxia, or hypoxia)
- Remote or long-standing structural injury (e.g., prior head injury, cerebral palsy, previous neurosurgery, perinatal cerebral ischemia, arteriovenous malformations)
- Metabolic abnormalities (e.g., hypo- or hyperglycemia, hepatic encephalopathy, uremia, pyridoxine deficiency, hyponatremia, hypocalcemia, hypomagnesemia)
- Use of, or overdose with, drugs that lower the seizure threshold (e.g., theophylline, imipenem, high-dose penicillin G, quinolone antibiotics, metronidazole, isoniazid, tricyclic antidepressants, lithium, clozapine, flumazenil, cyclosporine, lidocaine, bupivacaine, metrizamide, and phenothiazines)
- Chronic epilepsy; status epilepticus may present as an exacerbation of a patient's underlying epileptic syndrome

Data from references 7, 235, 256.

membrane, and reduction of neuronal firing and transmission of impulses.[161] The three most commonly used benzodiazepines are lorazepam (Ativan), diazepam (Valium), and midazolam (Versed). Although individual patient scenarios must always be taken into consideration, lorazepam has emerged as the treatment of choice for many episodes of SE[47,149] because of its ability to control seizures for an extended length of time with fewer recurring seizures.[47] Advantages and disadvantages of various benzodiazepines are listed in Table 25-2.[76,257]

Phenytoin is one of the most commonly used treatments for SE. Benzodiazepines offer faster cessation of seizures, but phenytoin is well suited to maintenance therapy and is often used after initial benzodiazepine administration. Phenytoin is a barbiturate-like drug that limits the repetitive firing of action potentials through the slowing of sodium channels.[171] Phenytoin is formulated with a propylene glycol carrier that is responsible for occasional infusion reactions, some of which can be extremely dangerous.[149] IV administration of phenytoin is associated with cardiac dysrhythmias, hypotension, and "purple glove" phlebitis. Fosphenytoin is the prodrug of phenytoin that is converted to its active state within the body. It lacks the propylene glycol carrier that causes many of the side effects of phenytoin. It seems prudent to use the drug

that causes fewer side effects, yet fosphenytoin is not universally used because of its higher cost.[76]

Barbiturates have been a mainstay in the traditional treatment of seizures. This drug group acts on the GABA receptor complex in a fashion similar to that of the benzodiazepines, and they are effective in limiting synaptic transmission. Phenobarbital (Luminal), pentobarbital (Nembutal), or thiopental (Pentothal) continue to be considered as options for therapy after lorazepam or phenytoin.[28] However, studies have indicated that any second-line agent will have a small chance of terminating SE[257] and because the barbiturates have a similar mode of action as the benzodiazepines, the usefulness of this drug group is brought into question. Barbiturates can often lead to sedation, and higher doses can result in stupor, coma, and respiratory and CNS depression. They have a long half-life but do help prevent seizure recurrence. Pentobarbital has emerged as one of the standard choices used in the treatment of RSE. Continuous EEG monitoring for burst-suppression patterns is used to adjust the dosage of the drug.[28]

Propofol, a rapidly acting general anesthetic, was first used for SE in the late 1980s. Its clinical effect has a rapid onset, and recovery is within 20 to 30 minutes after a single bolus dose. Propofol is a pharmacologically unique GABA agonist that may also have other mechanisms of anticonvulsant action.[28] It seemed

TABLE 25-2 Benzodiazepines Commonly Used in Status Epilepticus

DRUG	ADVANTAGES	DISADVANTAGES
Lorazepam (Ativan)	Initial drug of choice for most SE. Duration of action is as long as 4–6 hours; longer acting than diazepam. Does not have metabolites that contribute to drug toxicity. Less lipid soluble than diazepam. Less risk of respiratory depression than with diazepam.	Takes up to 2 min after IV injection for maximum effect.
Diazepam (Valium)	Rapidly crosses BBB; effect on seizure activity can be seen 10–20 seconds after IV administration. Stable and readily accessible in liquid form. Available as rectal gel formulation when no IV access.	Subsequent redistribution of drug into adipose tissue leads to <20-min duration of anticonvulsant effect; must be followed by maintenance anticonvulsant. Undesirable metabolites have prolonged half-lives and can result in toxicity.
Midazolam (Versed)	Terminates seizures quickly, frequently in less than 1 minute. Can be administered IM, through oral mucosa, or intranasally (it is affected by nasal secretions). Can be used as continuous IV drip with minimal cardiovascular side effects.	Short half-life in CNS. Continuous IV administration probably less effective than high-dose barbiturates or propofol.

Data from references 76, 149, 176, 257.

like the ideal drug for neurologic critical care use with its rapid onset and offset of action.[236] However, soon after its introduction, there were concerns over a proconvulsant effect. This apparently represented myoclonus rather than seizure activity.[28] Currently, the concern regarding the propofol infusion syndrome (profound hypotension, lipidemia, and metabolic acidosis) has somewhat reduced enthusiasm for prolonged use of this agent.[76,134] Intubation is frequently required, and the risk of relapse into SE is substantial when the drug is withdrawn.[76]

A growing body of basic science and clinical work supports the concept that SE becomes more difficult to control as its duration increases. In retrospective studies, out-of-hospital treatment has been shown to shorten the duration of SE.[3] A landmark study that compared four conventional treatment options (lorazepam, phenobarbital, diazepam plus phenytoin, and phenytoin alone) indicated that regardless of the group of the study into which a patient was randomized, the first conventional agent used was the only one that had a reasonable chance of terminating SE.[257] In this study, 45% of patients responded to first-line therapy.[164] Subsequent treatment of patients who did not respond to first-line therapy resulted in a response rate of 7% to second-line agents and 2.3% to third-line agents.[28]

Pharmacologic choices may be less important than the implementation of an established treatment protocol. Protocols can shorten the time needed to control seizures and typically include the sequential administration of benzodiazepines, phenytoin, phenobarbital, or pentobarbital for patients with refractory seizures.[84,226] Figure 25-3 is an example of an algorithm that addresses target goals in the care of the patient in SE.[164]

Understanding of the pathophysiologic mechanisms of SE remains quite limited; therefore healthcare providers are challenged to design and implement new treatment strategies.[149] There is evidence from animal studies that neurotransmitter receptors undergo changes in their sensitivities to benzodiazepines as seizures become more and more prolonged.[123] The following results were found in at least two animal models: Although SE was initially controlled by GABA agonists, over time these drugs lose their efficacy. In addition, NMDA antagonists, which are not useful initially, later become effective.[225] Combinations of drugs with different mechanisms may be required. For this reason, some practitioners have begun to use ketamine, the only clinically available NMDA antagonist, for SE that is refractory to both conventional agents and the more potent GABA agonist agents (benzodiazepines, propofol, or barbiturates).[225]

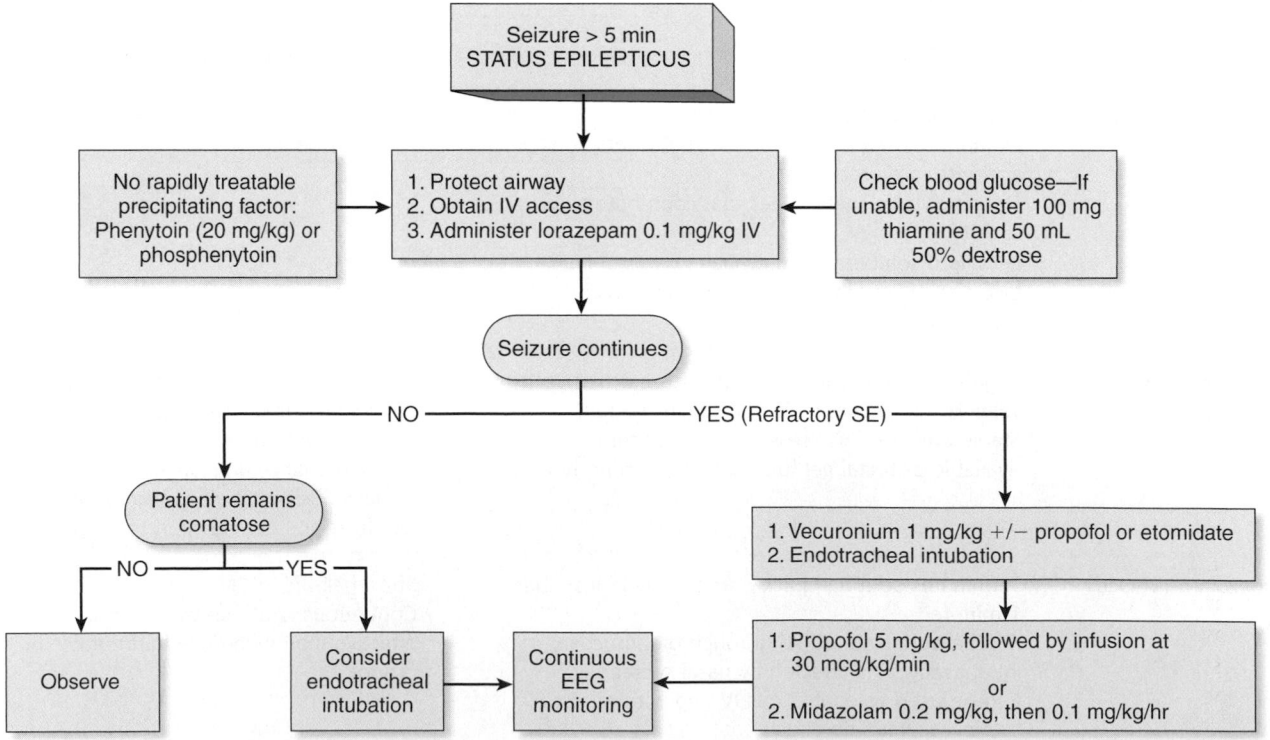

♦**FIGURE 25-3** Example of an algorithm for treatment of patient in SE.

Other clinically available agents with neuroprotective potential, such as topiramate (Topamax) and lamotrigine (Lamictal), may also be studied in the near future if IV formulations for their drug delivery that allow for rapid administration can be developed.[149]

Although treatment of SE and cessation of seizure activity tend to focus on anticonvulsant pharmacologic management, attention to the fundamentals of airway, breathing, and circulation must not be neglected. Nursing care of a patient during status epilepticus is focused not only on emergent cessation of seizure activity through the administration of medications but also on patient assessment and safety.

The patient at risk for SE should have precautionary measures taken. The bed should be equipped with padded side rails, and immediate access to an oxygen source and suction equipment must be available. The patient should be continuously monitored, if not by EEG then within the field of the nurse's vision, for recurrence of seizures until that threat has passed. Code carts should be nearby. Critical care nurses must be familiar with the potential side effects from anticonvulsant medications and be prepared to deal with the sequelae. Certain drugs, such as phenytoin, often have hospital policies written to guide medication administration.[35]

The patient should be placed in a side-lying position to facilitate drainage of secretions. Nurses should guide the patient's movements to prevent injury but should not try to restrain the patient. Adequate airway protection using the head-tilt/chin-lift maneuver may be necessary as well as the administration of oxygen as needed; suctioning may be warranted to prevent aspiration.[103] Prolonged or frequent seizures may require intubation for adequate oxygenation.[103]

IV fluid or vasoactive medication administration may be warranted to offset the effects of continued seizure activity or anticonvulsant medications. The patient's temperature must be monitored closely, and any hyperthermia should be treated with passive cooling or an antipyretic. Blood glucose levels should be normalized. Laboratory assessment of anti-epileptic drug levels as well as pH, lactic acid, creatine kinase, or myoglobin should be monitored.[150,161]

The patient may need to have any constrictive clothing loosened, and staff should remove any sharp objects from the patient and the immediate vicinity (e.g., eyeglasses). Patients are not in danger of swallowing their tongue. Forcing anything into the patient's mouth might cause damage to the teeth, the oral cavity, or the healthcare provider.[103] After seizure activity has ended, the patient should be allowed to sleep.[103] Nurses should assess the patient for any injury, including the oral cavity, and document the duration and characteristics of the seizure activity as well as the postictal status of the patient.

OTHER SEIZURE-RELATED ADMISSIONS TO CRITICAL CARE

Approximately 20% to 25% of all patients with epilepsy are medically intractable such that seizures persist, despite trials of multiple anti-epileptic drugs.[16] These patients may be admitted for continuous EEG/video monitoring of seizure activity. This monitoring is done to confirm the diagnosis of epileptic seizures, to locate the origin of the seizure activity in order to optimize drug treatment, or to evaluate the patient for epilepsy surgery. Patients may have individual or grids of electrodes temporarily placed in the epidural or subdural spaces, or they may have depth electrodes placed in deeper structures in an effort to locate the area in which the seizures originate.[48,224] If the seizure focus is localized in an area that is amenable to surgical resection with a low risk of postoperative neurologic deficit, then the patient could be a candidate for epilepsy surgery (e.g., temporal lobectomy or multiple subpial transection).[67,125] In some cases, seizures are frequent or severe and impose a devastating effect on the individual's quality of life and yet a definitive seizure focus cannot be identified. Some of these patients may still be candidates for surgical procedures that ablate or interrupt the electrical pathways of the seizures to decrease clinical frequency or severity (e.g., corpus callosotomy).[48] These patients usually receive care in epilepsy centers and may require critical care monitoring because of the potential risks involved in placement and complications of the electrodes. After the epilepsy surgery, these patients will be critical care residents during the immediate postoperative period.[16]

Another treatment used to control medically intractable seizures is vagal nerve stimulation (VNS). After surgical placement of the VNS system, the patient may be a resident in critical care for routine monitoring and observation. The mechanism for preventing a seizure is not completely understood, but it may be through the interruption of the seizure by sending an electrical stimulus through the vagal nerve to the brain. Patients who are VNS candidates have failed medical treatment and do not qualify for epilepsy surgery.[16]

The VNS system has two components: an implanted pulse generator with a battery and computer chip approximately the size of a cardiac pacemaker; and two electrodes that are tunneled under the skin during the surgical procedure and attached to the mid-cervical portion of the left vagal nerve,[125] as illustrated in Figure 25-4. Postoperatively, the patient is taught to interrupt seizure activity by manually passing a magnet over the pulse generator, but the system is not activated until several days or weeks after implantation.[16]

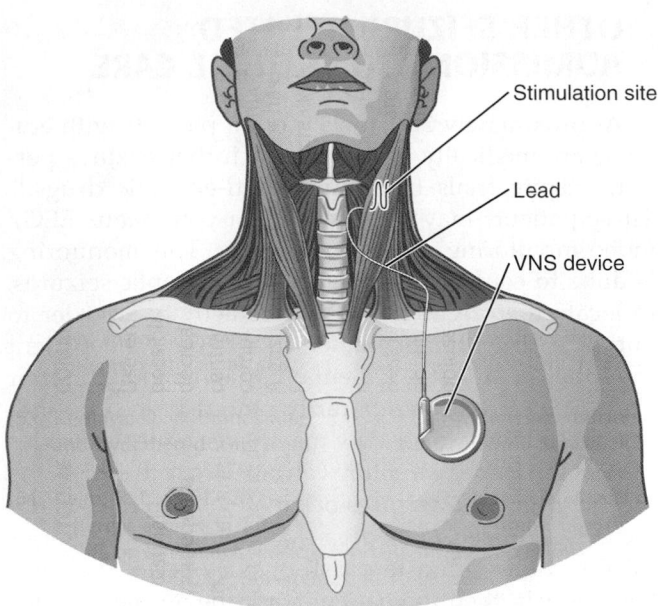

♦FIGURE 25-4 Vagal nerve stimulator.

Labels: Stimulation site, Lead, VNS device

♦ Case Study 25-1, Part A

Status Epilepticus

S.B., a 54-year-old woman, is transported to the emergency department in an unconscious state. Earlier in the day she had told her family that she was feeling "strange." The family reported that the patient had been complaining of increasing fatigue for the last 6 months, which she had attributed to menopause. She also complained of occasional tingling on the right side of her face. She has no remarkable medical history and sees her physician annually. She has smoked two packs of cigarettes per day for the last 35 years and she has a chronic dry cough.

Approximately 15 minutes before arrival in the ED, the family reports that the patient was working at the kitchen sink when they heard a high-pitched scream; the family saw S.B. slide to the ground and shake all over in what they assumed was seizure activity. They did not think that she had hit her head. Her husband immediately called 911 and an ambulance arrived after the episode had ended; the family guessed that it had lasted for 5 minutes. The emergency medical technicians (EMTs) quickly established that S.B.'s airway was patent and there were no foreign bodies present, although they did suction frothy saliva from her mouth. S.B. had not yet regained consciousness and was experiencing myoclonic-type jerking of all four extremities. Pupils were equal and reactive but deviated to the left. Blood pressure was noted to be 152/88 mm Hg with sinus tachycardia of 125 beats/min and labored respirations of 32 breaths/min. Her temperature was 37.3° C and the oxygen saturation

(O_2 sat) level was 95%. A fingerstick capillary blood glucose level was 88 mg/dl. The EMTs administered oxygen at 2 liters/min per nasal cannula and established an IV line. They loaded the patient into the ambulance and quickly made the trip to the ED.

Upon arrival to the ED, S.B. experienced a tonic-clonic convulsive seizure. Staff positioned the patient for safety and administered 7 mg of lorazepam intravenously (patient's weight = 155 pounds). The seizure activity decreased in amplitude, but the patient continued to have generalized tonic-clonic activity. At this point, S.B. was determined to be in status epilepticus. The patient was then loaded with 1 g of IV phenytoin without any further change in her neurologic status. It had now been approximately 45 minutes since the initial seizure activity in the patient's home. S.B. was given a loading dose of 75 mg of propofol IV and then started on a propofol drip at a rate of 150 mg/hr. Within 5 minutes her clinical seizure activity had stopped. She remained unconscious and was exhibiting sonorous respirations with an O_2 sat of 76%, so the ED team intubated the patient and placed her on a ventilator. A stat CT scan was unremarkable. Laboratory specimens were drawn and sent for arterial blood gases, basic chemistries, complete blood cell counts, creatine kinase, myoglobin, and a toxicology panel. A call was made to the neurology service for an emergent consult. Plans were made to admit S.B. to critical care. The critical care nursing staff prepared for her arrival using seizure safety precautions, including padded side rails and having suction equipment available.

Decision point: Does the patient have any risk factors for developing SE?

Decision point: Did the patient have any premorbid symptoms that might indicate neurologic pathology and a potential for seizure activity?

Case continues on page 705

BRAIN TUMORS

Patients who have brain tumors are seen in critical care when an acute neurologic event leads to diagnosis, when undergoing procedures for treatment, or when complications arise. This population of patients requires a sensitive and compassionate approach to what is often a devastating diagnosis with neurologic changes that compromise quality of life and mortality. Because of the various treatment modalities for brain tumors currently available, critical care nurses see these patients only sporadically, but general information may help nurses provide better care to this patient population. A brief overview of brain tumors, complications, and interventions is presented here.

Incidence and Classification

Cancer is the second leading cause of death in the United States, and 2003 statistics indicated that 556,902 people died of all types of cancer, accounting for 22.7% of all deaths.[6] In 2002 it was predicted that an estimated 39,550 new cases of both malignant and benign brain tumors would be diagnosed in the United States.[244] The exact incidence is unknown because patients often are undiagnosed or underreported.[130] Although brain tumors account for only 2% of all cancers and are about one fifth as common as breast or lung cancer, they account for a disproportionate share of cancer morbidity and mortality.[244] The 5-year relative survival rate (percentage of patients who live at least 5 years after their cancer is diagnosed) for all people with brain cancer varies with age and tumor type. For young adults from ages 15 to 44, it is 55%. For those between the ages of 45 and 64, it is 16%, and for adults older than 65, it is 5%.[6]

Many studies have noted an increasing trend over the last several decades in the incidence rates for brain tumors in industrialized countries. It is hypothesized that at least part of this increase is the result of improved diagnostic capabilities with the advent of CT scanners in the 1970s and MRI in the 1980s. Additionally, management of common illnesses may allow for longer life spans and the subsequent emergence of brain tumors that would not have been evident if the patient had died earlier.[54] However, these factors do not fully account for the increased rates and, hence, exposure to environmental factors must be considered.[198] Of particular note, the incidence rate for primary CNS lymphoma has tripled in the last several decades. This form of cancer occurs most often in immunocompromised patients, but the incidence is also increasing in immunocompetent patients.[217]

There are several different classification systems for brain tumors. Brain tumors can be classified based on tissue of origin, cell type (histology), location, whether they are primary or metastatic (secondary), or whether they are malignant or benign. Primary brain tumors originate in the brain and are derived from cells or structures found in or adjacent to the CNS. Metastatic brain tumors originate in other organs and disseminate systemically through hematogenous spread of circulating tumor cells or frank tumor emboli.[130] Metastatic brain lesions are approximately tenfold more common than primary brain tumors.[8] However, up to half of the patients with brain metastases die from systemic disease progression.[263]

It is extremely important to determine if a tumor is metastatic because treatment is based on the primary site. Biopsy is often indicated. The most common forms of cancer that spread to the brain originate as lung cancer (responsible for 48% of metastatic brain tumors) and breast cancer (15%). Because the brain does not have a lymphatic system, it is unlikely that tumors will migrate from the brain into other body areas.[30]

Brain tumors are also classified by their degree of differentiation. Many tumors are well differentiated and are referred to as "benign." Tumors that are completely resected during surgery may in fact be cured and require no further therapy. There are also many well-differentiated tumors that cannot be completely removed because of their anatomic location. Deep tumors, brain stem lesions, and tumors that blend with normal brain tissue may not be cured with surgery. Although these may be classified histologically as low grade or benign, they are considered by many neuro-oncologists to be malignant because of their ability to recur, cause neurologic deficits, and even cause death. Many "benign" brain tumors recur in spite of multiple treatment modalities. In addition, even low-grade tumors can become lethal because of their infiltrating properties and their tendency to undergo malignant transformation over time.[21]

Cell type or histology is another classification system for brain tumors, which are named for the cell or structure from which they have developed (e.g., an astrocytoma is a tumor derived from astrocytes, a type of supporting cell in the CNS). The World Health Organization (WHO) Classification of Tumors of the CNS is frequently used. There are more than 100 different WHO classifications and grades of tumors. The major WHO categories of brain tumors are listed in Box 25-2.[21,195] Of all primary brain tumors, the most frequently noted are gliomas (46%), meningiomas (27%), pituitary tumors, and schwannomas (together 15%). These four types account for approximately 90% of primary brain tumors.[30,148] Table 25-3 describes characteristics of these most common brain tumors.[30,100]

Clinical Presentation and Diagnosis

Patients with brain tumors experience signs and symptoms that can be either generalized and related to increased ICP or focal, based on the tumor location. Generalized signs might include headaches, decreased LOC, seizures, weakness, cognitive/behavioral changes, nausea, and vomiting.[180] Focal signs and symptoms, based on brain location, are listed in Table 25-4.[30,100] Figure 25-5 shows the brain anatomy associated with the clinical presentation.

Whatever the type of brain tumor, there are four general circumstances that lead to diagnosis. Patients who have intracranial neoplasms will present with partial or generalized seizures; increased ICP with accompanying headache, nausea, vomiting, dizziness, or visual disturbances; focal neurologic deficits reflecting the tumor site; or cognitive dysfunction of variable severity.[21]

Box 25-2

World Health Organization Classification of Brain Tumors

TUMORS OF NEUROEPITHELIAL TISSUE

- Astrocytic tumors (grades I-IV)
- Oligodendroglial tumors
- Mixed gliomas
- Ependymal tumors
- Choroid plexus tumors
- Neuronal and mixed neuronal-glial tumors
- Neuroblastic tumors
- Pineal parenchymal tumors
- Embryonal tumors

TUMORS OF PERIPHERAL NERVES

- Schwannoma (neuroma)
- Neurofibroma
- Perineuroma
- Malignant peripheral nerve sheath tumor

TUMORS OF THE MENINGES

- Tumors of meningothelial cells
  - Meningioma

- Atypical meningioma
- Anaplastic meningioma
- Mesenchymal, nonmeningothelial tumors
- Primary melanocytic lesions

LYMPHOMAS AND HEMATOPOIETIC NEOPLASMS

- Malignant lymphomas
- Plasmacytoma
- Granulocytic sarcoma

GERM CELL TUMORS

- Germinoma
- Embryonal carcinoma
- Yolk sac tumor
- Choriocarcinoma
- Teratoma
- Mixed germ cell tumors

TUMORS OF THE SELLAR REGION

- Craniopharyngioma
- Granular cell tumor

METASTATIC TUMORS

From reference 195.

TABLE 25-3 Commonly Occurring Primary Brain Tumors

TUMOR TYPE	SUBTYPES	CLINICAL PRESENTATION	COMMENTS/TREATMENT	PROGNOSIS
Glioma	Grade I: Pilocytic astrocytoma	Related to brain area involved or generalized signs Contrast enhancing	85% are cerebellar Slow growing; cystic Surgical removal can be curative	5–6 year survival on average
	Grade II: Diffuse astrocytoma	Symptoms subtle or acute Seizures common Typically does not enhance on CT/MRI	Slow growth; infiltration of brain tissue Biopsy or craniotomy for diagnosis Positive prognosis related to younger age and near-to-total surgical resection; may need radiation in follow-up	
	Grade III: Anaplastic astrocytoma	Focal or generalized signs Some tumors enhance; likely to have edema	Cellular proliferation Biopsy or craniotomy for diagnosis or resection Radiation with or without chemotherapy needed Younger patients have better prognosis	15–28 month survival

TUMOR TYPE	SUBTYPES	CLINICAL PRESENTATION	COMMENTS/TREATMENT	PROGNOSIS
	Grade IV: Glioblastoma multiforme	Neurologic symptoms including increased ICP Contrast enhancing with central area of necrosis	Poorly differentiated; highly mitotic Biopsy or craniotomy for diagnosis or resection Radiation with or without chemotherapy Gross total resection and younger patients have better prognosis	12-month survival
Meningioma	Less common, aggressive subtypes: Atypical meningioma Malignant meningioma	Related to compression of brain structures May cause headache, seizures Enhancing dural mass; may have calcification or edema	Slow growing; usually benign; attached to dura mater Falx cerebri most common location Amount of tumor resection related to favorable prognosis	"Cure" with total removal Many years with partial excision and radiation
Pituitary adenoma	Classified by hormonal content/ structure	Visual loss Headache Cranial nerve deficits Symptoms related to imbalances of pituitary hormones	Benign Pharmacologic management of hormone imbalances Transsphenoidal hypophysectomy is usual surgical approach Radiation occasionally for residual tumor	Cure with complete resection; very good outcome in others
Schwannoma	Vestibular schwannoma is "acoustic neuroma"	Often present with hearing loss or tinnitus Enhancing lesion	Slow growing; benign Surgically curable Cranial nerve deficits can result	Cure with total resection; tumor regrowth possible

Data from references 30, 100.
ICP = Intracranial pressure.

TABLE 25-4 Brain Tumor Location and Associated Signs and Symptoms

BRAIN TUMOR LOCATION	ASSOCIATED NEUROLOGIC SIGNS AND SYMPTOMS
Frontal lobe	Contralateral paresis/plegia; cognitive/behavioral/personality changes; emotional lability; memory deficits; loss of self-restraint
Temporal lobe	Seizures; aphasia; memory problems; visual field cut
Parietal lobe	Sensory deficits; visual field cut; language deficits; neglect syndromes; seizures
Occipital lobe	Visual loss or hallucinations
Cerebellum	Ipsilateral ataxia; nystagmus; vertigo; nausea
Brain stem	Dysphagia/gag reflex dysfunction; motor and sensory deficits; vertigo; hiccups; nystagmus; nausea and vomiting
Intraventricular	Symptoms related to obstruction of cerebrospinal fluid flow/hydrocephalus (gait disturbance, cognitive deficits, urinary incontinence); sudden death

Data from references 30, 100.

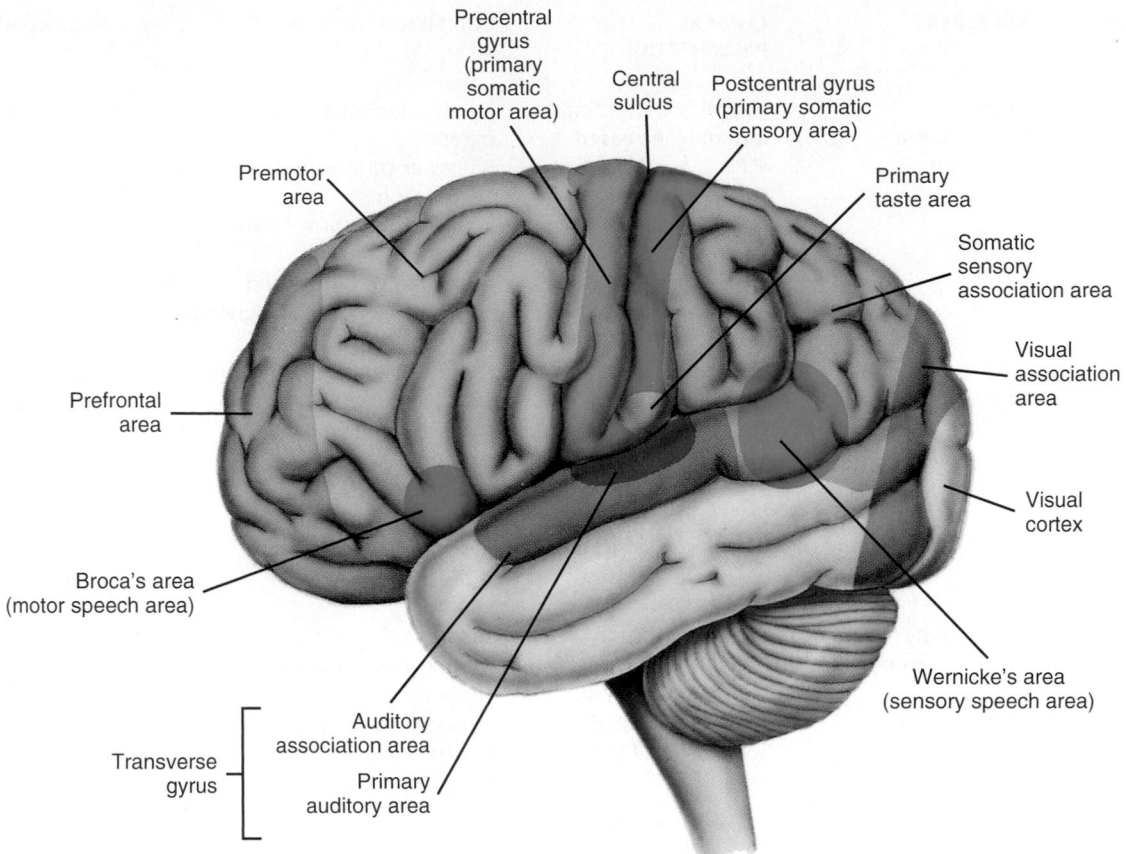

Precentral
gyrus
(primary
somatic
motor area)

Central
sulcus

Postcentral gyrus
(primary somatic
sensory area)

Premotor
area

Primary
taste area

Somatic
sensory
association area

Prefrontal
area

Visual
association
area

Visual
cortex

Broca's area
(motor speech area)

Wernicke's area
(sensory speech area)

Transverse
gyrus

Auditory
association area

Primary
auditory area

‡FIGURE 25-5 Lateral view of the brain.

Depending upon the nature of these symptoms, a patient may require admission to critical care. Most often, admission is required because the patient is having complications caused by increased ICP, hydrocephalus, or seizures.

Diagnostic imaging for brain tumors is relatively straightforward and involves MRI with gadolinium enhancement. CT scans are less reliable. Examples of various imaging techniques are seen in Figure 25-6. Unfortunately, these imaging patterns are not specific to tumor type, and diagnosis must be confirmed by histologic biopsy or surgically resected samples. Accurate pathologic grading is essential because it defines treatment and prognosis. Tumors are graded on the basis of the most malignant area identified.[21]

Occasionally, a PET scan is used to identify the most hypermetabolic area of a tumor in order to select that area for surgical resection or biopsy.[54] Additionally, patients with brain tumors occasionally present with an intracranial hemorrhage (ICH). Diagnostic workup of suspicious sites for ICH or unusual presentation may disclose a tumor underlying the hemorrhage.[209] It may be necessary to perform a biopsy to determine if a tumor is present.[245]

Management and Treatment

The goals of treatment for the patient with a brain tumor are to alleviate neurologic symptoms, to improve quality of life, and to achieve a cure when possible.[130] The plan of care depends largely upon the location, size, and number of tumors, the prognosis, any existing neurologic deficits, and the current and anticipated quality of life. A combination of surgery, radiation, chemotherapy, and other medical modalities can be utilized.[140]

Surgical options include total or near-total resection specific to the type and location of the tumor, or debulking and removal of tumor mass to alleviate ICP concerns. Radiation therapy can be whole-brain or focused-beam utilizing the gamma knife, linear accelerator photon knife (LINAC), or stereotactic systems.[263]

Chemotherapy must be tapered to the cancer cell type. This modality has exhibited limited efficacy. Controversy exists regarding the role of the blood-brain barrier (BBB) in allowing chemotherapeutic agents to cross into the tumor mass.[140,189] Alternative treatment options that are being investigated include the use of BBB disrupting agents before or concurrent with chemotherapeutic treatments[126] and implantation into brain tissue of wafers saturated with highly focused chemotherapy, in conjunction with surgery.[33]

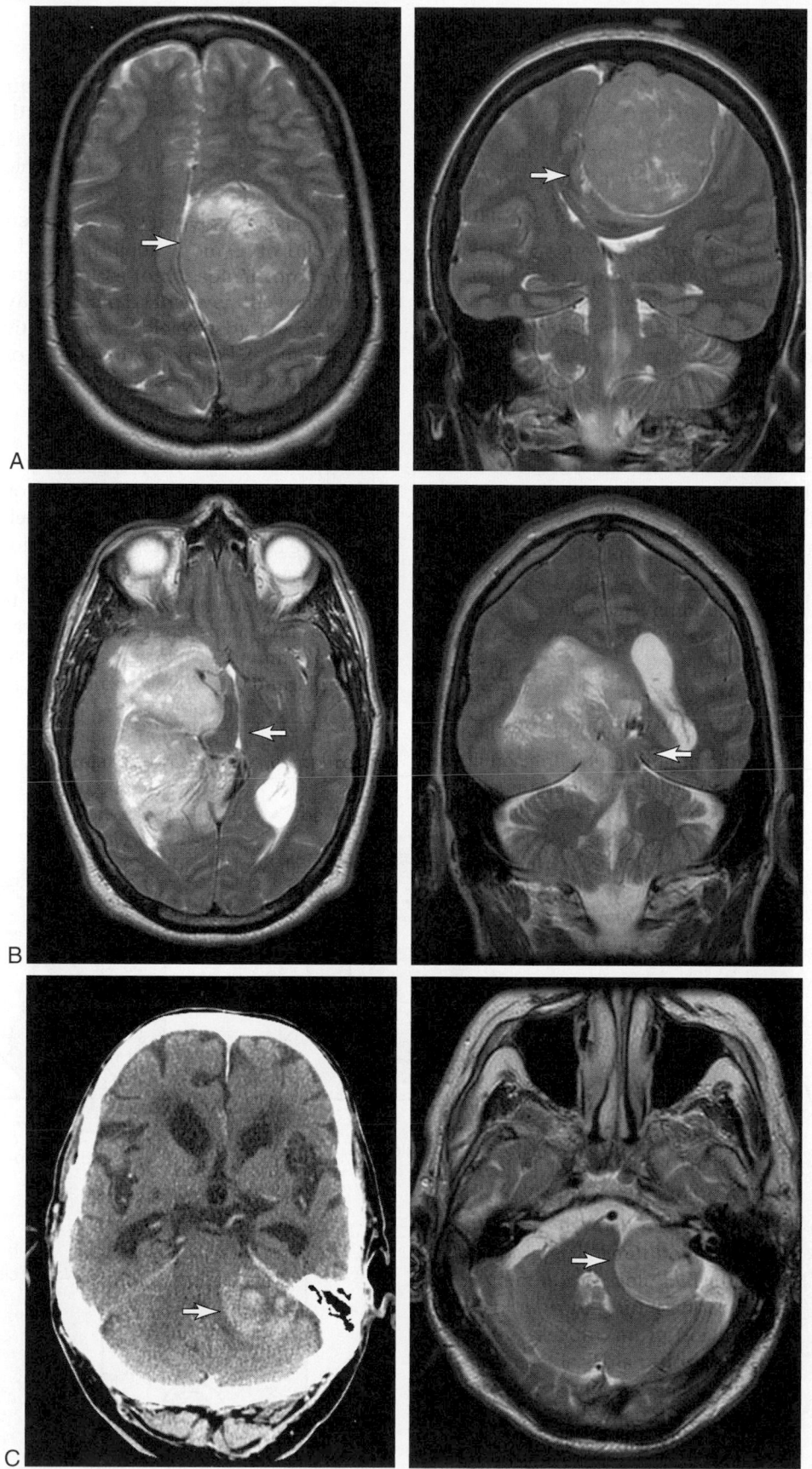

✦FIGURE 25-6 Diagnostic imaging of brain tumors. **A,** Axial and coronal views on T2 MRI of left posterior frontal meningioma with considerable compression of the ventricles. **B,** Axial T2 and coronal T2 MRI images of anaplastic oligoastrocytoma in the right temporal lobe with extensive uncal herniation of tumor. **C,** Unenhanced CT and MRI T2 of a large left vestibular schwannoma.

Craniotomy. Nurses in critical care come into contact with patients who have brain tumors after surgical procedures involving biopsy or surgical resection. Often, these abbreviated stays in critical care are for observation for postoperative complications including increased ICP, bleeding at the surgical site, seizures,[228] infarction, infection,[64] and cerebrospinal fluid (CSF) leak.[220] Similar to the diagnosis of tumors, postoperative signs and symptoms are often related to the particular brain area involved.

There are two common methods of craniotomy used in the majority of patients. The most common approach to supratentorial tumors consists of a curving incision behind the hairline in front of the ear and arching above the eye (Figure 25-7). This incision exposes the cerebrum, especially the lateral aspects of the frontal, temporal, and parietal lobes. The most common approach to infratentorial tumors is at the nape of the neck, near the occipital lobe and the cerebellum.[14] Generally, entry into the skull begins by drilling burr holes. A window of bone, known as a "bone flap," is then removed by sawing between the burr holes. The dura mater is separated from the undersurface of the bone flap and opened for access to the brain tissue. After the procedure, the dura is closed with sutures or dural substitute and the bone flap is secured back into position with plates, sutures, or wires. The bone flap is not physiologically necessary and may not be replaced if tumor has invaded the bone, if the bone is infected, or if the potential for increased ICP is high. If the bone is not replaced, the area will need to be protected in some way with an artificial plate or perhaps a helmet. The bone flap may be replaced at a later time after the critical period is over. Drains can be placed to reduce subdural, epidural, or subgaleal (scalp) fluid accumulation.[199]

Transsphenoidal Hypophysectomy. Pituitary adenomas are one of the most common tumors of the CNS.[30,148] Critical care nurses routinely care for patients who have undergone surgical resection of these tumors. The tumors themselves present a unique challenge to the healthcare team because of their medical presentation and location. The microsurgical transsphenoidal approach is the most common surgical treatment (Figure 25-8).[201] Postoperatively, patients must be

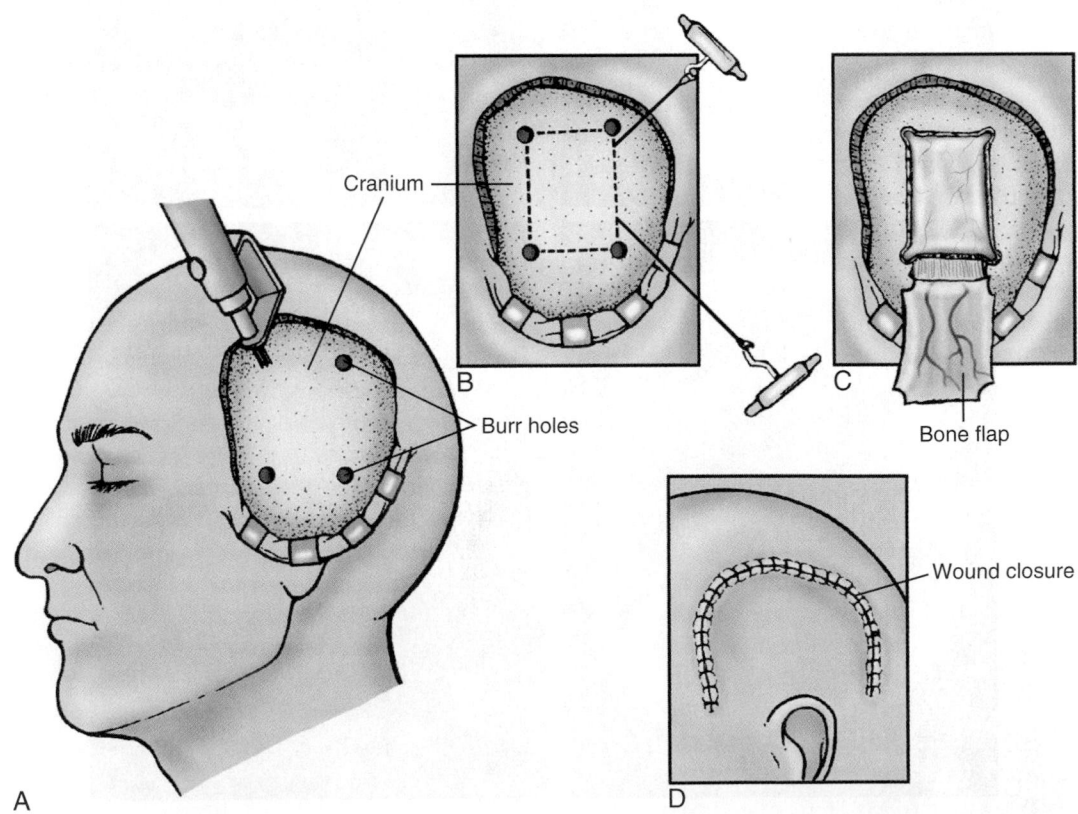

Cranium

Burr holes

Bone flap

Wound closure

A

B

C

D

⬥FIGURE 25-7   Craniotomy procedure. **A,** Burr holes are drilled into the skull. **B,** A surgical saw is used to cut an aperture between the burr holes. **C,** The cranial contents are exposed. **D,** The bone is replaced and the wound is closed.

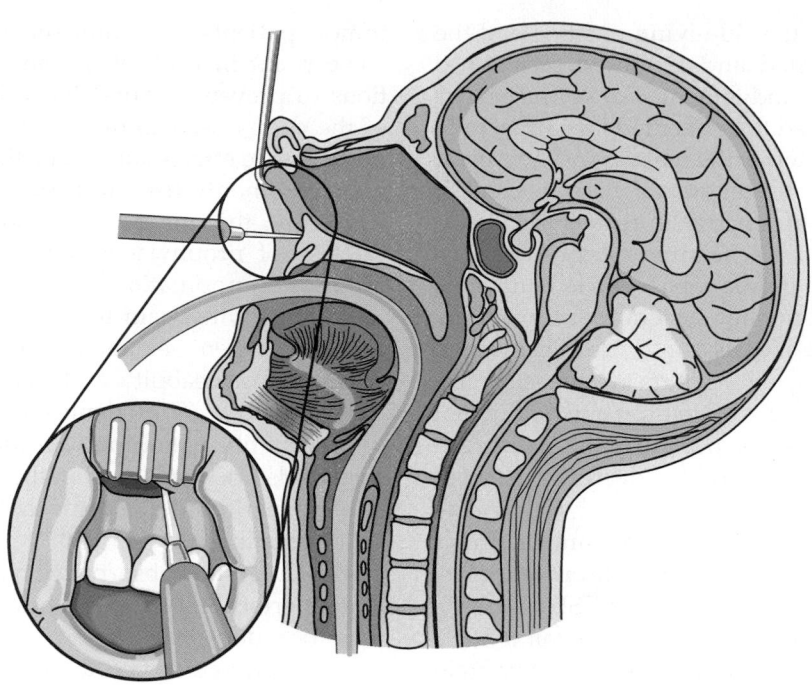

⬍FIGURE 25-8 Transsphenoidal approach to hypophysectomy: anterior pituitary surgery with incision in the gingival mucosa.

observed for CSF leaks, visual deficits, and hormonal imbalances.[201] CSF leaks may present as rhinorrhea (fluid from the nose) or the patient may report fluid running down the back of the throat and describe a "salty" taste. It can be difficult to differentiate CSF drainage from other body fluids. A large volume of nasal drainage when the patient is brought up into a sitting position is suspicious for a CSF leak.[201]

CSF on bed linens may exhibit the "halo" sign—clear or pale yellow fluid surrounded by a reddish bloody border or ring. However, this is not a reliable test for CSF. Glucose strip testing is occasionally done for CSF determination, but a positive result could indicate either CSF, blood, or any other fluid containing glucose and is not reliable.[201] If there is enough fluid, it can be captured in a test tube and sent to the laboratory for tau transferrin analysis, which can determine whether CSF is a component of the body fluid collected.[10]

Hormonal imbalances typically noted after transsphenoidal hypophysectomy include diabetes insipidus (DI)—polyuria of dilute urine related to a decrease in antidiuretic hormone. DI is diagnosed when urine specific gravity is less than 1.005, urine output is greater than 200 ml/hour, serum sodium level is elevated above 148 mEq/L, and serum osmolality is elevated. Patients are encouraged to drink fluids to keep up with the diuresis, are given IV fluids, and are treated with desmopressin acetate (DDAVP) as necessary. This is usually a transient problem for the patient, but fluids and electrolytes must be monitored closely during the immediate postoperative period.[17]

A more recently utilized tool for resection of pituitary adenomas is the endoscope. This mononostril or binasal approach may lend itself to better visibility of the surgical field and less postoperative discomfort for the patient, who will rarely need nasal packing. However, the endoscope does not have the zoom capabilities of the microscope and it may require the addition of an ear, nose, and throat surgeon in the operating suite.[116] Further comparison studies of these approaches are needed to guide practice.

Lumbar Cerebrospinal Fluid Drains. Occasionally after craniotomy for tumor resection and other reasons for which the dura mater needs to be opened, drainage or monitoring of CSF through a temporary external system is desired to decrease pressure from CSF and allow the surgical site to heal. This can be done via an intraventricular catheter (discussed in Chapter 22), generally placed in one of the lateral ventricles, or with a lumbar drain. Drainage systems are also used for patients after repair of cerebral aneurysms, and for patients with acute hydrocephalus, traumatic brain injury, CSF leaks or fistulas,[237] and CSF infections.[163] In addition, lumbar drains are used for CSF drainage in thoracoabdominal aortic aneurysm repairs.[26]

Lumbar drains can be inserted in the operating room or at the patient's bedside using aseptic technique.

The patient is placed in the side-lying position and the lumbar catheter is inserted and anchored securely to prevent possibility of dislodgement. The drainage system is attached and zeroed to a specified level, generally the insertion site or the "top of the mattress." The patient must be instructed not to get out of bed or even sit upright without calling for assistance because the drainage could abruptly increase, leading to complications such as hemorrhage or herniation. It may be possible to temporarily clamp a drainage system at times to allow for closely monitored activity.[237,255] Physicians will determine the type and specifics of the drainage parameters, as listed in Table 25-5.[255] Dressing and equipment changes should be done as per hospital policy but generally only when needed to decrease chances of infection.

Complications related to the use of lumbar drains include pneumocranium, hematoma, hemorrhage, infection, nerve root irritation, and persistent CSF leak.[163,255] Some facilities are now using endoscopic repair for CSF leaks related to elective craniotomies and traumatic brain injuries.[143] Since results for CSF leak closure are comparable and successful both with[162] and without lumbar drainage, use of lumbar drains may decrease in some patient populations in the future.[139,143]

Medical Management. The most frequently noted medical complications in patients with brain tumors include seizures, peritumoral edema, and venous thromboembolism (VTE).[272] Prophylactic and supportive care for these common complications can significantly impact the patient's quality of life.

Seizures are the presenting symptom in 10% to 40% of patients with brain tumors, and the need for anti-epileptic medications in this population is clear—they should be prescribed one of the first-line anticonvulsants.[86,272] However, another 20% to 45% of brain tumor patients will ultimately develop seizures at some point in their illness and the need for medications to prevent seizures has not been clarified. Many of the drugs used to treat seizures have clinically significant side effects and interactions with other medications commonly used to treat brain tumor patients.[272] Currently, there is no consensus statement regarding the use of prophylactic anti-epileptic medications in this patient population.[86]

Patients with brain tumors are prone to the formation of vasogenic edema as a result of increased brain capillary permeability and plasma leaking into brain parenchyma.[122] This edema contributes significantly to the morbidity noted in brain tumor patients.[272] Corticosteroids are a standard in the management of symptomatic peritumoral edema associated with primary or metastatic brain tumors.[130,131] They act by enhancing extracellular fluid absorption and decreasing tumor capillary permeability. Headaches usually improve more than focal deficits.[130]

The preferred corticosteroid is dexamethasone (Decadron) because of minimal mineralocorticoid effect and lower rates of infection and psychosis.[19,130] Although this class of drugs is associated with significant side effects including an immunocompromised state, altered glucose metabolism, gastrointestinal irritation, mood swings, myopathy, fat redistribution, and peripheral edema,[228] some of these complications can be decreased by using the lowest possible doses.[266]

Patients with cancer are six times more likely to experience VTE than those without cancer.[98] The pathophysiology is not clearly understood, but a hypercoagulopathy appears to predispose brain tumor patients to VTE.[269] In addition, patients with brain tumors are perceived to be at an increased risk for tumor-related intracranial hemorrhage, so the optimal therapy for VTE in patients with brain tumors is unclear.

TABLE 25-5 Drain Management Strategies for Lumbar Drains

TYPE OF DRAIN MANAGEMENT	EXAMPLE OF PHYSICIAN ORDER	NURSING ACTIONS
Drain to a specific level	"Zero to top of mattress and leave drain unclamped."	Check level and zero drainage system routinely
Drain to a specific volume	"Keep lumbar drain output = 20 ml/hour."	Manipulate level of drain up or down to achieve specified volume
Drain at a specific pressure	"Zero to top of mattress. Raise drain to 10 cm H_2O above zero."	Check level and zero routinely; raise drainage system to desired level; system will only drain if ordered pressure exceeded

Data from reference 255.

As a result, many patients with brain tumors are managed with inferior vena caval filters rather than anticoagulation.[272]

♦ Case Study 25-1, Part B

Status Epilepticus

S.B. has been transferred to critical care. After intubation, her follow-up chest x-ray (CXR) showed an area of density in the right middle lobe. Because of her history of smoking, her healthcare team is concerned that this density could represent a neoplasm and she might have a metastatic brain lesion seeded from the lung. The patient is scheduled for a gadolinium-enhanced MRI of the brain and chest to clarify the density noted on the CXR and to look for any brain lesions not visible on her unenhanced CT scan. Because of the high index of suspicion for cancer, S.B. is given a dexamethasone loading dose of 10 mg IV with orders for 4 mg every 6 hours.

The patient remains on a propofol drip with seizure precautions, including padded side rails on the bed. She is sedated without any spontaneous motor activity, but she does withdraw all four extremities to noxious stimuli. Pupils are equal, round, and reactive to light. The earlier noted gaze deviation is no longer present. Her blood pressure has dipped to 104/65 mm Hg. She is in sinus rhythm at a rate of 70 beats/min. Her temperature is 37.8° C and she has been given acetaminophen 650 mg per rectum.

S.B. has now been loaded with phenytoin and is to receive 100 mg IV every 8 hours. The neurologist has ordered an EEG, which shows generalized slowing and no overt seizure activity. The nurse will begin to wean the patient off the propofol while closely observing for any seizure activity. There is a PRN order for lorazepam if any breakthrough seizure activity is noted. She has intermittent compression devices for DVT prophylaxis, and her care providers are discussing the need for an inferior vena caval filter. Her lab values have returned and her blood gases indicate mild metabolic acidosis with a pH of 7.29. Her myoglobin level is slightly elevated but her seizure activity has ceased, so the healthcare team will plan to assess another myoglobin level in 4 hours.

The results of S.B.'s MRIs indicate that the lung nodule is suspicious for cancer, and she will need to undergo a needle biopsy in the future when medically stable. The MRI of the brain demonstrates a 2-cm area of abnormal signal intensity in the left temporal lobe and several smaller areas in the right frontal and left occipital lobes that are suspicious for tumor. She will need a biopsy done on the left temporal brain lesion to determine the pathology and treatment.

Decision point: If you are concerned that S.B. is experiencing nonconvulsive SE, how would you determine if this is happening?

Case continues on page 723

INFECTIONS OF THE CENTRAL NERVOUS SYSTEM

Although the brain is well protected by the bones of the cranium, the meninges, CSF, and the BBB, the CNS is still subject to infections.[129] When the patient with a CNS infection presents in a life-threatening or critical state, admission to a critical care unit will be required. Comprehensive neurologic assessments are a vital component in the care of the patient with a CNS infection. Baseline and ongoing assessments should include LOC, pupillary reactions, motor and sensory function testing, and cranial nerve assessment.

The major classifications of CNS infections include meningitis, encephalitis, and brain abscess. This chapter will address the most common of these infections along with notable high-risk/low-volume populations of current interest.

Meningitis

Meningitis is the inflammation of the pia and arachnoid meninges (defined together as the leptomeninges) that surround the brain and spinal cord.[70] The two most common causes of meningitis, viral and bacterial organisms, will be discussed here. However, it is important to note that meningitis can also be caused by fungi, inflammatory diseases, traumatic injury, and cancer.[182]

Viral Meningitis. Viral meningitis is the most common form of meningitis in the United States, with more than 75,000 cases occurring annually.[265] The true incidence of these infections is difficult to determine because the diagnosis may not be considered, many cases are unreported, or a specific viral etiology is never confirmed.[119] It is typically mild and nonlethal and is usually caused by enteroviruses. Other viruses that can cause viral meningitis include varicella zoster, influenza, mumps, HIV, and herpes simplex type 2.[182] The disease process is usually short-lived and lasts less than 2 weeks.[13]

Enteroviruses are present in mucus, saliva, and feces, so transmission of viral meningitis is generally through fecal-oral contamination or respiratory droplets.[182] The virus then spreads to the CNS. The patient is infectious from 3 days after infection to up to 10 days after symptoms develop. The incubation period is 3 to 7 days.[190]

The term *aseptic meningitis* is often used interchangeably with viral meningitis and refers to patients who have clinical and laboratory evidence for meningeal inflammation with negative routine bacterial cultures.[119] Clinical presentation is generally nonspecific, with signs of meningeal irritation, such as fever, headache, nausea, and vomiting. Occasionally, these are accompanied by photophobia and nuchal rigidity or pain. There is no

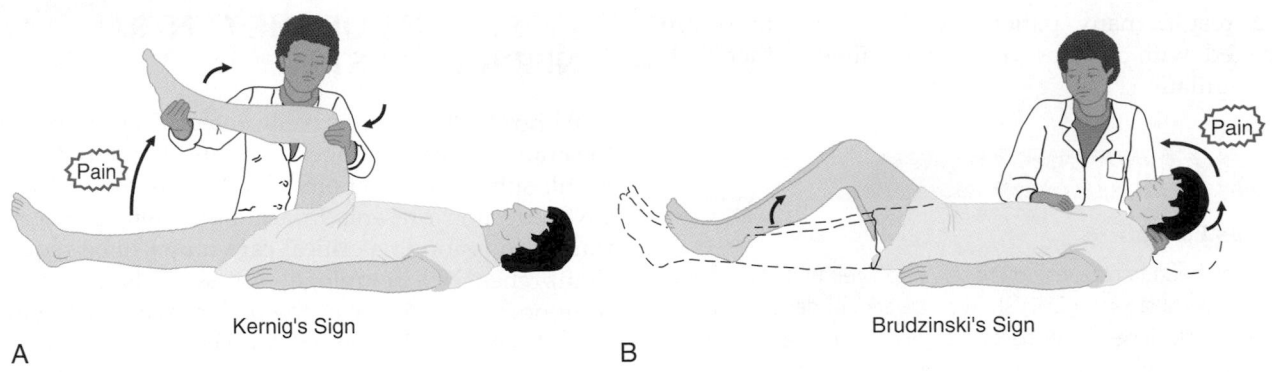

⬍FIGURE 25-9 Clinical assessment for neck pain in meningitis. **A,** Kernig's sign. **B,** Brudzinski's sign.

specific treatment for enteroviral infections, so treatment is aimed at symptomatic and supportive care and most patients recover completely. Acyclovir may be used to treat herpes infections.[265]

Bacterial Meningitis. Bacterial meningitis is also known as acute septic meningitis. It is a neurologic emergency with mortality rates as high as 27%[9,65] and with neurologic sequelae common among survivors.[70,204] There are approximately 1.2 million cases diagnosed and 135,000 deaths annually worldwide.[219] In the United States, the use of vaccines that provide protection for 3 to 5 years or more has dramatically reduced the incidence of *Streptococcus pneumoniae* and *Haemophilus influenzae* forms of bacterial meningitis.[146]

At least 50 kinds of bacteria can cause meningitis.[174] The most common pathogens causing bacterial meningitis in the United States include *Streptococcus pneumoniae* (most common organism in older adults), *Neisseria meningitidis* (causing the characteristic petechial or purpural skin lesions; the most common organisms in children and young adults), group B *Streptococcus, Listeria monocytogenes,* and *Haemophilus influenzae.*[204,287]

The course of the disease and transmission is specific to the pathogen involved. Meningococcal meningitis, caused by *Neisseria meningitidis,* is one of the more familiar forms of meningitis seen in critical care. It is spread through direct contact with respiratory secretions. People at risk include infants and children, young adults, people living in crowded living conditions such as college dormitories, and people exposed to passive and active tobacco smoke.[190]

Clinical symptoms for bacterial and viral meningitis can be similar, so it is imperative to have a high index of suspicion when examining the patient. The classic triad of acute bacterial meningitis consists of high temperature (greater than 38° C), nuchal rigidity, and a change in mental status.[70] The patient may also present with photophobia and a headache that is typically severe and generalized. Kernig's sign and Brudzinski's sign are common tests for nuchal rigidity and meningeal irritation but are positive in only 50% of children and in even fewer adults with bacterial meningitis (Figure 25-9).[210] Seizures occur in 10% of adult patients.[275] Fulminant bacterial meningitis can lead to cerebral infarcts, coma, cerebral edema, and even brain herniation. Systemic complications such as septic shock, pneumonia, and disseminated intravascular coagulation occur in 22% of patients.[194] Other manifestations are specific to the causative organism. Prompt antibiotic therapy is vital to limit mortality[202] and the potentially devastating effects of bacterial meningitis,[9] and it must be specific to the particular infectious pathogen. Although acquisition of a CSF sample for culture is optimal and can quickly determine whether the pathogen is bacterial or viral, a lumbar puncture (LP) cannot always be accomplished in a reasonable time frame (Table 25-6).[265] Blood cultures are often positive and may be the second best choice in order to expedite the administration of antibiotics. A CT scan can and should be done in patients with neurologic symptoms to rule out elevated ICP associated with CNS disease before the LP.[259] This array of tests, which must be completed as quickly as possible, is summarized in recent guidelines with an algorithm to help clarify the steps in the diagnostic process (Figure 25-10).[259]

The role of steroids in the treatment of bacterial meningitis is unclear and controversial. Animal models have indicated that an intense inflammatory response occurs both locally and systemically in bacterial meningitis. This response is enhanced when antibiotics are administered and microbial destruction ensues. Steroids attenuate this inflammatory response.[251] In humans, there have been some studies that indicate that dexamethasone may decrease mortality when administered before the first parenteral dose of an antimicrobial agent.[52] Currently, investigators note decreased mortality or morbidity rates with the use of steroids, and their use in adults with bacterial meningitis is recommended.[259,262]

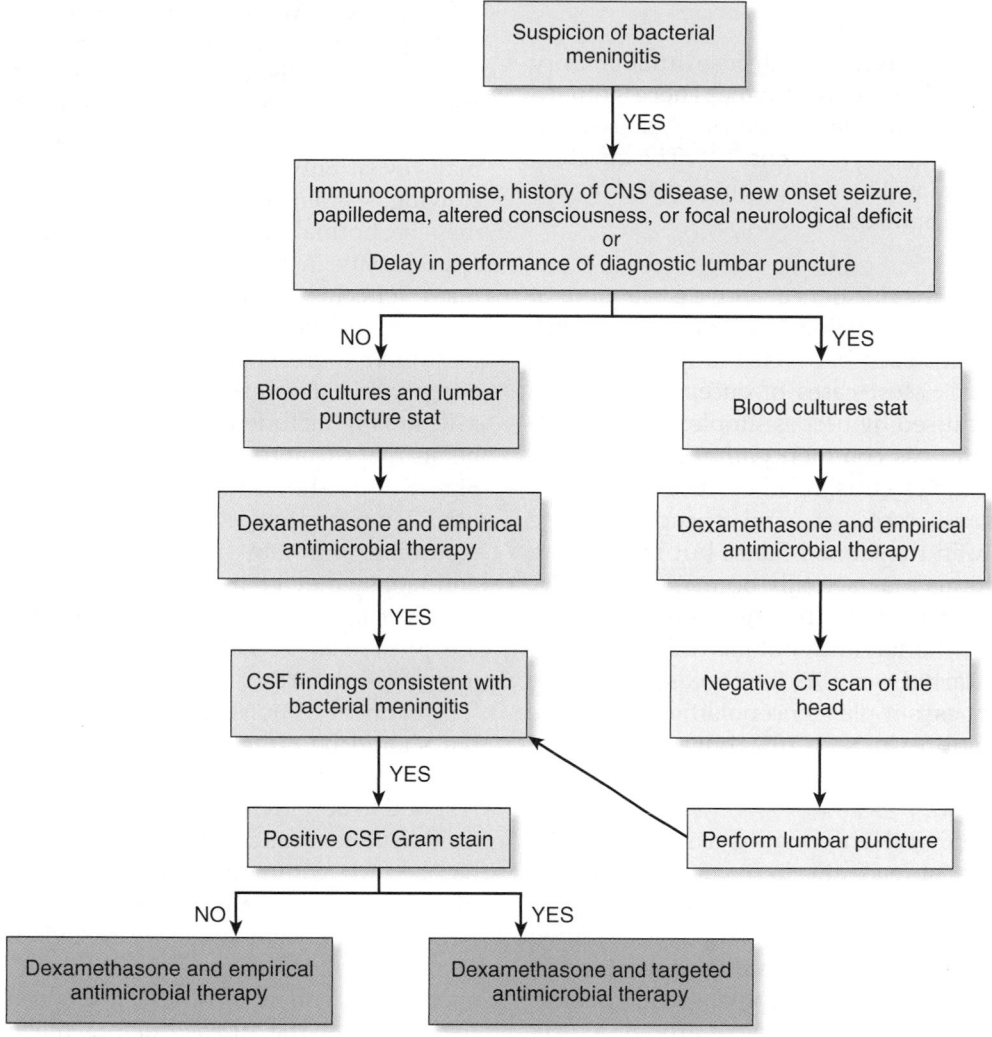

✦FIGURE 25-10 Management algorithm for adults with suspected bacterial meningitis.

TABLE 25-6 Cerebrospinal Fluid Values Diagnostic for Meningitis

PARAMETER	NORMAL CSF	BACTERIAL MENINGITIS	VIRAL MENINGITIS	FUNGAL MENINGITIS
Opening pressure (mm H_2O)	100–180	200–500	≤250	>200
Leukocyte count (white blood cells/mm^3)	0–5	Increased 1000–5000	Increased 50–1000	Increased >20
Neutrophils (%)	0	≥80	<40	
Protein (mg/dl)	18–45	Elevated 100–500	Elevated <200	Elevated >45
Glucose (mg/dl)	45–80; 0.6 times blood glucose level	5–40; <0.3 times blood glucose level	>45	<40

From reference 265.
CSF = Cerebrospinal fluid.

Encephalitis

Encephalitis is an acute, usually diffuse inflammatory process involving the brain parenchyma. There is often a degree of leptomeningeal inflammation such that a combined meningoencephalitis can occur.[42,127] The infection is most commonly caused by a virus but can also be due to bacteria, fungi, or parasites.[265]

Viral Encephalitis. The incidence and distribution of viral encephalitis vary according to geographic regions, with large differences seen between Europe, Asia, and the United States.[127] Most cases of encephalitis in the United States are caused by herpes simplex virus (HSV) types 1 and 2, with less common pathogens including enteroviruses, the rabies virus, or arboviruses.[182]

Several thousand cases of viral encephalitis are reported annually in the United States but many more unreported infections may actually occur.[182] Morbidity and mortality rates vary with the organism, severity of the infection, and whether antiviral medications, when indicated, were started early in the disease process.[42] In untreated herpes simplex encephalitis (HSE), the mortality rate is approximately 70%, but early diagnosis with acyclovir (Zovirax) treatment decreases mortality to 20% to 30%.[273]

Transmission of viral encephalitis varies with the pathogen. HSE is spread through contact with an infected person, rabies is contracted through a bite from a rabid animal, and the arboviruses are transmitted from infected animals to humans through the bite of an infected tick, mosquito, or other blood-sucking insect.[182] The West Nile virus (WNV) is a type of arbovirus usually transmitted by a bite from an infected mosquito.[118] This form of encephalitis is one of several emerging viral infections of the CNS and was only recently initially diagnosed in the United States in 1999. WNV has become more prevalent, with 9862 cases reported in 2003; 560 deaths have occurred over a 5-year period.[182]

Infiltration of the virus into the CNS via the bloodstream or peripheral nerves causes proliferation of polymorphonuclear leukocytes and mononuclear cells. This leads to congestion and swelling of the brain parenchyma, vasculitic lesions, myelin destruction, widespread nerve cell degeneration, necrosis, or hemorrhage.[13] Most viruses are capable of causing either meningitis or encephalitis.[119]

Symptoms of viral encephalitis or meningoencephalitis reflect either focal or diffuse cerebral pathology.[42] Patients present with headache, fever, seizure activity, and nuchal rigidity.[127,129] An altered LOC, ranging from drowsiness to coma, is indicative of the severity of the encephalitis.[42]

Diagnostic testing should include evaluation of CSF, but results may only indicate the presence of inflammation. An increased white blood cell count, elevated protein levels, normal glucose levels, the absence of red blood cells, and negative findings on bacterial cultures are all characteristic of viral CNS infections.[119] An EEG will invariably be abnormal in HSE, though it may reveal only characteristic patterns of generalized slowing.[42] Brain imaging consisting of the simpler CT may be normal initially, but later scans could show hypodensity in the temporal areas, hemorrhage, and mass effect.[13] MRI, especially diffusion-weighted imaging, is the imaging modality of choice[166] and may offer more specific clues as to the cause of the encephalitis. For example, characteristic changes on MRI in HSE include frontotemporal changes and small hemorrhages and lesions in the limbic system.[42] Figure 25-11 shows the MRI of a patient with encephalitis, demonstrating edema in the right temporal lobe. Neuroimaging may not be adequate for diagnosis, and biopsy may be necessary to culture tissue in order to direct appropriate medical therapy. Many patients are prescribed acyclovir empirically, so biopsy is no longer a standard of care.[42]

Treatment options for viral encephalitis are limited but should be targeted to the suspected or identified pathogen when possible. HSE and varicella zoster respond to acyclovir. There is currently no specific antiviral treatment for other forms of viral encephalitis so it has become common medical practice to initiate this pharmaceutical treatment in every patient with suspected viral encephalitis.[42] Acyclovir has been shown to reduce mortality and morbidity in these forms of encephalitis and is most effective when given early in the course of the disease before the patient becomes comatose.[273,274] Patients who have had seizures need to receive anticonvulsants.[127] Surgical removal of necrotic tissue or decompressive craniectomy may be warranted in patients with cerebral edema and impending herniation syndromes.[287] Priorities in treatment focus on symptomatic, supportive, and preventive care.

Brain Abscess

A brain abscess is a focal collection of purulent matter within the brain parenchyma that occurs secondary to an infection, trauma, or surgery.[233] Brain abscesses are relatively rare and account for only 1% of brain lesions in the United States, but the incidence is higher in underdeveloped countries.[13] Approximately 1500 to 2500 cases are diagnosed in the United States each year.[160] Both incidence and mortality rates in the United States from brain abscesses have decreased over the last several decades concurrent with advances in neuroimaging, earlier diagnosis, improved efficacy of antibiotics in preventing and treating brain abscess, and improved surgical techniques.[25,284] Currently,

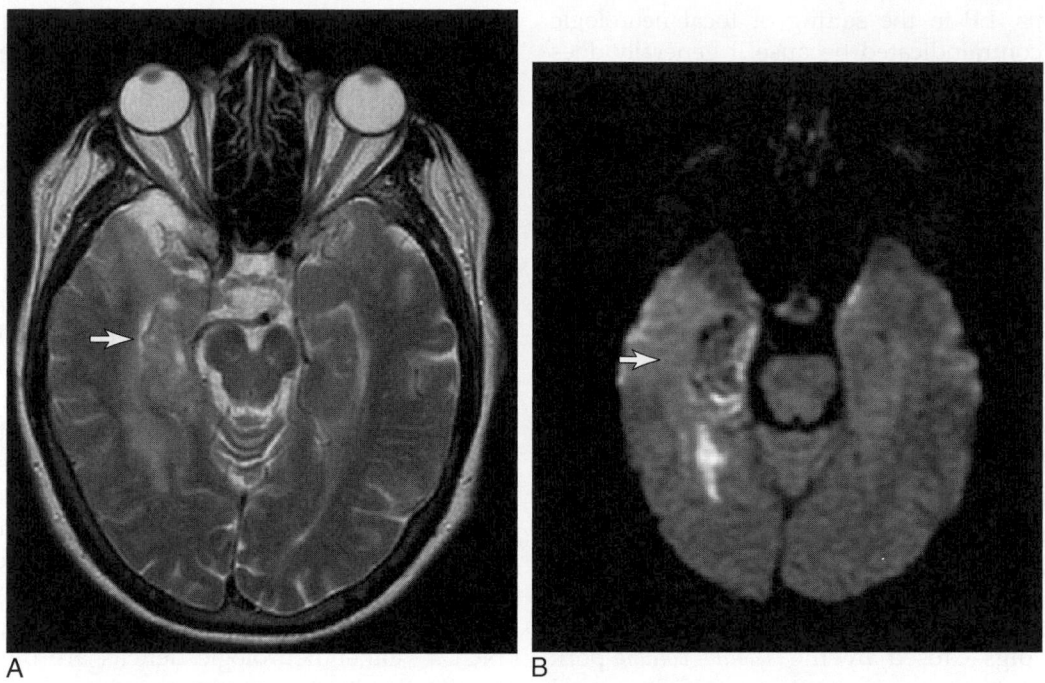

♦FIGURE 25-11 MRI T_2 and diffusion-weighted images of herpes simplex encephalitis in the medial aspect of the right temporal lobe.

mortality rates range from 10% to 30%.[249,284] Several studies have noted that a low Glasgow Coma Scale (GCS) score on admission is associated with a poor prognosis for recovery.[206,249,284] Other factors that might be associated with poor outcome are immunodeficiency and the presence of underlying disease.[284]

Brain abscesses develop through one of three different mechanisms.[144,265] A brain abscess may be associated with a contiguous focus of infection. This mechanism accounts for approximately 40% of brain abscesses and might include direct spread from otitis media, mastoiditis, infection of the frontal or ethmoid sinuses, and dental infection.[286] Another etiology for brain abscesses includes hematogenous spread from a distant infectious source that can arise from bacteremia or parasites seeding into the brain matter. This accounts for 30% of all cerebral abscesses.[265] They are most commonly located in the distribution of the middle cerebral artery.[233] Finally, a brain abscess can be caused by penetrating trauma, skull fracture, or neurosurgical procedures, accounting for approximately 10% of brain abscesses. Twenty percent of brain abscesses are of undetermined cause.[265]

The development and evolution of the abscess and infectious process begin with a stage of "early cerebritis" (days 1 to 3). At this time, inflammatory reactions initiate the formation of edema and CNS necrosis. The "late cerebritis" stage (days 4 to 9) follows, with concomitant escalation of edema and necrosis and formation of pus. The "early capsule stage" (days 10 to 13)

consists of consolidation of a collagen network to separate the necrotic core from the parenchyma. The "late capsule stage" (days 14 and onward) completes the creation of the mature capsular structure.[4,34,144]

The clinical presentation depends upon the location of the abscess and number of lesions, the aggressiveness of the pathogen, the patient's immunologic status, and the degree of intracranial hypertension.[144] Approximately 70% of patients experience headaches.[144] Seizures, usually generalized, are also very common and occur in 25% to 60% of patients.[144,223] Signs and symptoms of a brain abscess can also include fever, nausea/vomiting, altered LOC, and other focal neurologic deficits.[233] These signs may be similar to those of a tumor or space-occupying lesion.

Diagnosis of brain abscess is highly dependent upon neuroimaging. MRI is the diagnostic test of choice, but CT scan with contrast also has a high sensitivity and is easier to obtain.[36,144] The early cerebritis lesion is poorly demarcated and is associated with localized edema that does not enhance following contrast injection. There is evidence of acute inflammation but no tissue necrosis. After several weeks, necrosis and liquefaction occur within the fibrotic capsule. Breakdown of the BBB and the development of the inflammatory capsule are characterized by a thick and diffuse ring enhancement.[233] Stereotactic CT-guided needle aspiration is frequently required to diagnose the infecting pathogen.[36] A comprehensive patient history can help to determine the patient's potential for exposure to certain microorganisms. LP in the setting of focal neurologic symptoms is contraindicated because it generally does not add diagnostic information and it has been associated with brain stem herniation in this patient population.[36,97]

Treatment of brain abscesses is highly dependent upon the specific diagnosis of the infectious pathogen. A combination of antibiotics and surgical excision for drainage may be warranted.[167] The initiation of empiric parenteral antibiotics based on probable pathogens should start as soon as possible and generally follows an extended period of 4 to 8 weeks.[144,232,234] The role of steroids in the treatment of brain abscess is unclear. Most investigators recommend that glucocorticoids are to be used only when substantial mass effect or cerebral edema is present, particularly if the patient is at risk for herniation.[89]

Neurocysticercosis

Cysticercosis is a parasitic systemic infection of humans and pigs caused by the *Taenia solium* pork tapeworm. The term *neurocysticercosis* (NCC) is used when the larva of the tapeworm crosses the BBB and enters the CNS.[81,227]

Systemic infections from this tapeworm affect 50 million people worldwide[227] with 50,000 deaths annually.[59] Endemic areas include significant portions of Central and South America, sub-Saharan Africa, and east and south Asia.[15,231] NCC is the most common parasitic infection of the CNS,[59] and it is the most common cause of acquired epilepsy in these developing countries. Approximately 12% of the admissions to neurologic hospitals in these areas are due to NCC infections.[231] NCC is becoming increasingly common in large metropolitan areas of the United States, with an estimated 1000 cases occurring annually because of immigration of tapeworm carriers.[132,188,227]

Humans usually acquire the *Taenia* tapeworm following the ingestion of improperly cooked infected pork. Living cysticerci (larvae) in the pork attach to the human small intestinal wall and are harbored in that environment. In many cases, the tapeworm remains only in the intestine of its human host.[227] Proglottids of the tapeworm multiply and produce eggs that are passed via the host's feces into the environment. The eggs can survive for months to years there.[227] Wandering pigs subsequently ingest the eggs present in contaminated human stools. Inside the pig intestine, the action of bile and pancreatic enzymes causes the eggs to lose their coats, allowing the oncospheres inside to circulate, penetrate intestinal walls, and localize within the pig musculature as cysticerci, thereby completing the cycle.[39,81,231]

Cysticercosis becomes systemic when humans ingest the *Taenia* eggs (not larva) found in food or water contaminated with infected human feces, or by autoinfection, whereby the eggs are carried into the stomach by reverse peristalsis. The process then mirrors that noted in pigs. Ingested eggs hatch in the intestine, freeing the oncospheres, which invade the intestinal wall and migrate into striated muscle, the brain, liver, and other tissues, where they develop into the cysticerci larva. Cysticerci can survive for years in these human tissues.[227] It is important to realize that human cysticercosis can be acquired by ingesting *Taenia* eggs present in food or water contaminated with the feces of a human tapeworm carrier. Therefore cysticercosis can occur in localities without the presence of pigs and in individuals who do not eat pork.[39,231]

Cysts can travel throughout the body. The most frequent and critical clinical manifestations are caused when the parasites travel across the BBB and lodge in the CNS.[81] Clinical presentation of NCC varies depending on the number, size, and stage of the cysts and the location within the CNS. Seizures are the most common manifestation and occur in up to 70% of patients with NCC.[60] Other neurologic deficits are often focal and localized, with a course that may resemble that of a brain tumor. Headache, intracranial hypertension, motor deficits, and psychiatric symptoms also can occur.[231]

Cysticerci in the brain range from 10 to 50 mm or more and appear to be limited in size by the pressure of adjacent brain matter. They localize near the cerebral cortex or the basal ganglia in areas of rich vascular supply. Cysts also localize in cortical sulci, in the CSF cisterns, or in the ventricles.[231]

Patients in neurologic crisis because of NCC are those with hydrocephalus related to arachnoiditis or ventricular cysts.[68] Cerebral infarctions also occur in response to inflammatory reactions that can occlude the lumen of arterial vessels. In addition, increased ICP occurs in patients with giant cysts or in patients who have intense parenchymal inflammatory responses and edema related to the presence of the parasites.[231]

After entering the CNS, cysticerci go through a predictable maturation process. Signs and symptoms of the disease may not be apparent for months or years.[37] The four stages of NCC evolution begin with the vesicular stage in which vesicles are present with viable cysticerci and clear liquid content with no inflammatory reaction. The infection remains in this stage until overcome by the host's immune system, which destroys the cyst. Next, the colloidal stage occurs, with acute inflammation in which the fluid becomes viscous and turbid and is enclosed by a thick collagen capsule surrounded by edema and gliosis. This stage is identifiable on MRI. The third stage is nodular-granular, characterized by cysticerci that are no longer viable and a cyst filled with coarse mineralized granules. Finally, the disease process enters the calcified stage, in which the parasite remnants appear as a calcified nodule with subsiding edema.[81]

Attention to the particular stage of the lesion is important if surgery is a consideration. Surgery in an early stage could lead to a serious inflammatory reaction by rupture of a cyst and its contents.[227]

The diagnosis of cysticercosis is done through serology testing, and NCC is confirmed via neuroimaging. The serologic enzyme-linked immunoelectrotransfer blot (EITB) assay is used to detect antibodies to *Taenia* antigens, but it is less sensitive in patients with a single brain lesion or when lesions are in the latter stages of development. In addition, a positive response may just indicate the presence of the tapeworm and so will not

definitively diagnosis a brain lesion.[231] In neuroimaging for NCC, MRI is superior to CT scanning because of its ability to recognize the number, location, and evolutionary stages of the cysticerci as well as the presence of any edema (Figure 25-12). CT may be better for visualizing small calcifications. Other diagnostic testing includes stool sampling for *Taenia solium* or ova.[227]

Treatment of neurocysticercosis involves management of the symptoms and of the parasite. Neurologic crises such as increased ICP must be attended to immediately. Hydrocephalus may require a CSF shunting procedure.[231] First-line anti-epileptic drugs are generally

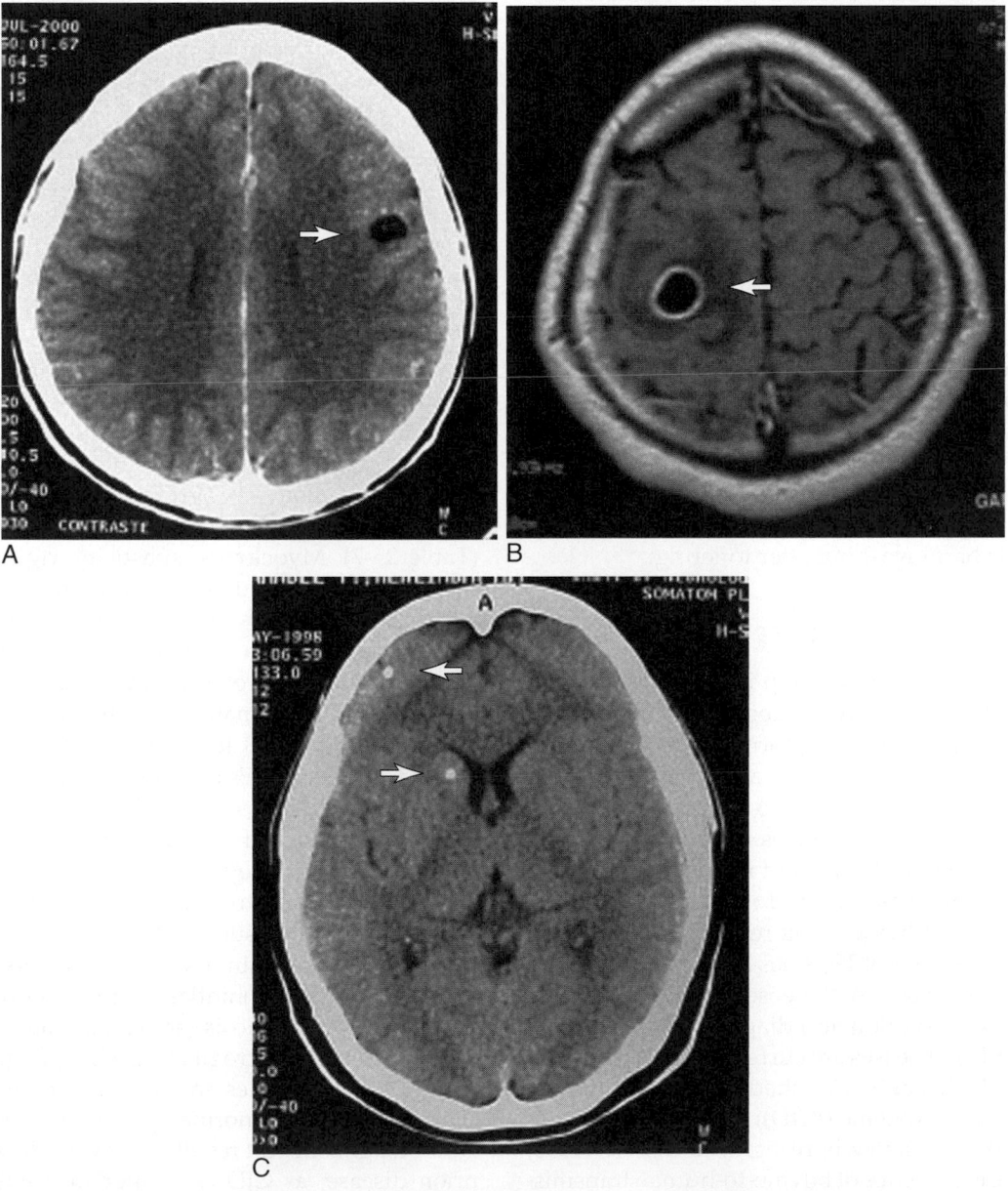

◆FIGURE 25-12 Neurocysticercosis. **A,** Vesicular (living) cysticerci on contrasted CT scan. The scolex (head) is visualized within the cyst as a high-intensity nodule, giving the lesion the classic "hole-with-dot" imaging. **B,** Early signs of inflammation around a cysticercus on MRI. **C,** Calcified (dead) cysticerci normally appear on CT as small, hyperdense nodules without perilesional edema or abnormal enhancement after contrast medium administration. These lesions are usually not visualized by MRI.

effective in controlling seizures.[81] Steroids are controversial but occasionally used to treat perilesional edema or inflammation that occurs at the time of parasite death.[227,231] After the patient is stabilized, antiparasitic (anthelmintic) therapy can be considered.[81]

Anthelmintics are often used but are controversial because of their significant adverse effects, which can include headaches, increased seizure frequency, increased ICP, cerebral infarction, hyperthermia, hypotension, dysrhythmias, and death. Some of these effects are related to the inflammatory reaction created by the dying parasites. Despite the adverse effects associated with anthelmintic use, there is evidence that killing the parasites decreases seizure relapses, shunt failure, disease progression, and even death.[81,82] Drugs of choice are albendazole (Albenza) or praziquantel (Biltricide).[81]

As noted earlier, surgery should be performed after lesions have calcified or at the nodular-calcified stage of NCC. If live cysts are released, severe meningitis may result. Patients who present with a single lesion may benefit most from surgical resection to prevent further complications or symptoms.[231] Ventricular cysts may be amenable to endoscopic removal.[203]

Prevention is key to the control of this disease process but its prevalence in developing countries predisposes to many challenges inherent in creating and maintaining sanitation systems.[81] On an individual basis, the risk of acquiring cysticercosis can be decreased with proper food preparation and thorough cooking of pork. When traveling, especially in endemic areas, it is advisable to ingest food and water only from reliable sources and to observe proper hand washing after toileting.[265]

Creutzfeldt-Jakob Disease

Creutzfeldt-Jakob disease (CJD) is one of a family of rare, progressive, and fatal neurodegenerative disorders known as transmissible spongiform encephalopathies (TSEs) that affect both humans and animals. These devastating diseases are difficult to diagnose, and there are no current treatment strategies. Fortunately, classic CJD, which arises sporadically and is the most common form of human TSE, has occurred in only one case per million people worldwide.[40] More recently, potential for transspecies transfer of TSEs has highlighted the possibility that more cases will be seen by critical care nurses as disease evolution and diagnosis progress.[158]

Five human TSE diseases are currently recognized and include CJD, which can be classified as sporadic (sCJD), familial (fCJD), or iatrogenic (iCJD); variant Creutzfeldt-Jakob disease (vCJD), a newly recognized disease (1996) for which there is evidence of bovine-to-human transmission; Gerstmann-Sträussler-Scheinker syndrome (GSS); fatal familial insomnia (FFI); and kuru.[40]

Animal forms of TSE include bovine spongiform encephalopathy (BSE), scrapie (in sheep and goats),

chronic wasting disease (seen in deer and elk), and transmissible mink encephalopathy. Because of very low incidence, both human and animal TSEs have been unfamiliar and relatively nonthreatening for much of the public population. Recent events regarding BSE have changed that perception. In the 1980s the United Kingdom experienced an outbreak of BSE, commonly referred to as "mad cow disease." Scientific scrutiny of this particular outbreak provided strong evidence for the possibility that BSE was transmitted across species to humans as vCJD through the ingestion of BSE-contaminated cattle products.[22,113] Suddenly, humans were threatened by a fatal illness of what used to be considered only a bovine disease. There is continued concern that other animal prion diseases could also cross species and become transmissible to humans.[158]

Prions, cellular *proteinaceous infectious* particles, are the agents responsible for the TSEs. Prions are found naturally in humans and appear to be involved with neuronal development and prevention of cell death.[156] Mutation of the normal prion, which may have a genetic predisposition in certain people,[113,158] leads to development of the disease process. Accumulation of mutated prions in neurologic tissue leads to cell death and results in the formation of the characteristic vacuoles that give the brain a classic spongiform appearance.[268]

The time interval from initial exposure to clinical presentation may be months or years.[113] However, when neurologic changes are noted, the typical clinical picture of CJD is of a rapidly progressive dementia over a period of days to weeks in the patient who is 60 to 80 years of age (Table 25-7). Myoclonus, spasticity, rigidity, or tremor may be present. Seizures are common and cortical blindness may occur as a result of occipital involvement. Patients frequently are residents of the critical care unit for treatment of neurologic sequelae and while diagnosis is pending. Unfortunately, death is imminent and usually occurs within 3 to 12 months.[38] Interventions for individuals with TSEs center on supportive care.

Definitive diagnosis of CJD is through neuropathologic examination of the brain tissue at autopsy. Brain biopsies can be done to detect the presence of CJD but care must be taken to collect the sample from the exact site of infected tissue or the result may be a false negative.[74] The brain tissue of patients with TSE is characterized by noninflammatory neurodegeneration (loss of neurons), gliosis (activation and proliferation of astrocytes and microglial cells), spongiform change (microscopic vacuoles in the brain parenchyma), and accumulation of abnormal prions in brain plaques.[158] Other diagnostic test results may vary depending on the prion disease, as CJD can differ markedly from vCJD (see Table 25-7). MRI scanning for various forms of CJD may be helpful as a diagnostic tool (Figure 25-13).[158,241]

Transmission to humans appears most probable in either iCJD or vCJD. Iatrogenic transmission of CJD has

TABLE 25-7   Characteristics of Creutzfeldt-Jakob Disease

	CLASSIC CJD	VARIANT CJD
Occurrence	Recognized since early 1920s Sporadic: 1 case per million population worldwide (risk increases with age: peak incidence 55–65 years of age); in recent years United States has reported fewer than 300 cases/year; this number represents 85% of CJD cases Familial: incidence of CJD is increased 30–100-fold in certain geographic regions including areas of North Africa, Israel, and Slovakia, primarily due to clusters of familial CJD; this represents 15% of CJD cases	First recognized in 1996 As of June 2005 a total of 177 cases of vCJD have been reported in world
Median age at death	68 years	28 years
Median duration of illness	4–5 months	13–14 months
Incubation period	1–30 years depending on site of prion inoculation/exposure	Unknown; 10–15 years, estimate
Clinical signs and symptoms	Dementia; early neurologic signs—myoclonus, cerebellar ataxia, visual problems	Prominent psychiatric/behavioral symptoms; painful dysesthesias; delayed neurologic signs
Diagnostic Criteria	**"Probable" Diagnosis Based on Grouping of Criteria**	
Periodic sharp waves on EEG	Present in 60%–70%	Absent
"Pulvinar sign" on MRI (hyperintensity in posterior thalamus bilaterally)	Not reported; brain atrophy and hyperintensities in basal ganglia or cortex noted in 67%	Present in >75% of cases
CSF 14-3-3 (a protein marker for neuronal injury in CSF)	Positive in >90%; not specific	Positive in 50%; not specific
Biochemical analysis of brain tissue	Variable accumulation of protease-resistant prion protein	Marked accumulation of protease-resistant prion protein
Mode of transmission	Sporadic: spontaneous transformation of normal prion proteins into abnormal prions Familial: patients develop CJD because of inherited mutations of prion protein gene Iatrogenic: related to administration of cadaveric human pituitary hormones; transplantation of dura, cornea, liver; and use of contaminated neurosurgical instruments or stereotactic depth electrodes These routes for transmission have largely been eliminated Etiology unclear; *NOT* related to BSE	Has never been a case that did not have history of exposure within a country where BSE was occurring; believed that people became infected through their consumption of cattle products contaminated with agent of BSE
Treatment	No known treatment; CJD and vCJD invariably fatal, often within 1 year of diagnosis	

Data from references 40, 87, 241, 260, 261.
BSE = Bovine spongiform encephalopathy, CSF = cerebrospinal fluid, CJD = Creutzfeldt-Jakob disease, EEG = electroencephalogram, MRI = magnetic resonance imaging, vCJD = variant Creutzfeldt-Jakob disease.

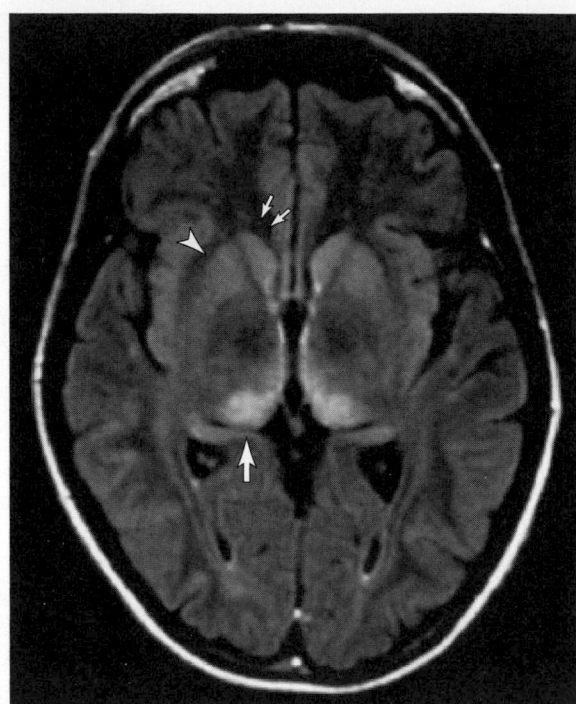

FIGURE 25-13 The pulvinar sign in vCJD MR images of hyperintensity of all deep gray matter nuclei, with the pulvinar *(large arrow)* hyperintense to both the caudate head *(small arrows)* and putamen *(arrowhead)*.

occurred with reuse of contaminated surgical equipment and in human growth hormones from infected cadavers.[87,120] To protect against iatrogenic transmission, universal precautions should always be observed and disposable surgical instruments should be used and then incinerated. The use of hospital protocols can assist staff in following guidelines for handling tissue or instruments that have come into contact with individuals at high risk for CJD. Prions are highly resistant to alcohol, formalin, ionizing radiation, and nucleases, but can be inactivated by use of autoclaving, phenol, detergents, and extremes of pH.[120]

Until recently, it was thought that infected tissue of patients with prion diseases was present only in the CNS. Researchers have now located this infectious process in the lymphoid tissue, tonsils, and appendices of patients with vCJD and in the olfactory mucosa and muscle tissue of those with sCJD.[87,261] There is no evidence that sCJD is transmitted by blood transfusion, but the risk for blood transmission is uncertain and possible in vCJD.[265]

The method of transmission in sCJD is unknown. The search for risk factors has included dietary factors (consumption of animal CNS tissue or vegetarianism), exposure to animals, exposure to blood or uncooked animal products, and occupational exposures, but none of these has been shown to alter the risk of sCJD. There has been only one documented conjugal pair of cases, and there is no evidence of transplacental infection.[120]

Awareness of potential routes of transmission has changed healthcare practices, but individuals with known exposure in the past should still remain vigilant for signs or symptoms of the disease.

As described earlier, transmission between species does appear likely in vCJD, and prevention of exposure to BSE is critical. A dramatic decline in BSE in the U.K. has followed the institution of governmental restrictions on bovine feeding practices and the importation of cattle, sheep, goats, and related products from all European countries.[40]

Research on the treatment of TSEs has focused on the inhibition of the accumulation of mutated prions, but results have not been encouraging. Immunotherapy against prion diseases using antibodies has had some success in vitro and in mice.[159] Development of a simple test to detect prion infection is crucial in any effort to reduce the risk of transmission and to allow for the timely initiation of treatment.[158]

Ventriculostomy-Related Infections

The final category of CNS infections in this chapter addresses a nosocomial issue. External ventricular drains (EVDs), otherwise known as ventriculostomy catheters, are used to temporarily drain CSF or to monitor ICP.[32,153] The catheter is inserted into one of the lateral ventricles of the brain using aseptic technique. Insertion of the catheter takes place in either the patient's room or the operating suite, the device is left in place for days to weeks, and the system is occasionally opened for CSF sampling or instillation of antibiotics.[193,240] Occasionally, this indwelling catheter leads to an infectious process in the brain.

Despite the need for EVD placement in some patients, there has always been a concern for potential infection because of the invasive nature of the catheter, being placed through brain parenchyma into the ventricle. This concern could potentially limit the use of EVDs in patients who might otherwise benefit from them. It is estimated that the infection rate for EVDs is approximately 10%. However, the analysis of these statistics is confounded by the patient population itself, which tends to have potentially infectious preexisting brain diagnoses (e.g., craniotomy, skull fracture, intraventricular hemorrhage).[153]

In an effort to define the nature of these infections and create a plan for prevention, investigators have studied various groups of patients, different protocols for antibiotic administration, and individualized plans for duration of monitoring.[153] The differences in study methodologies make it difficult to make standardized recommendations for the care of this patient population. In addition, there are different types of equipment and varying definitions of infection, colonization, and contamination. Nonetheless, some common risk factors associated with EVD infection have emerged and are listed in Box 25-3. Healthcare practitioners should be aware of and minimize the patient's exposure to these factors when possible.

In general, most studies defined an infection as a positive CSF culture obtained from the catheter or a LP. Various bacteria were cited as the offending pathogen, with some studies noting predominance of gram-positive cocci[242] and others reporting gram-negative bacilli,[154] but a broad range of bacteria has been isolated in many studies and no single agent has been consistently associated with these infections.[153]

Treatment of the EVD infection with antibiotics is targeted to the specific pathogen. However, the efficacy of IV antibiotics is questionable because of limited penetration into the CSF through the BBB. Some clinicians administer antibiotics directly into the ventriculostomy catheter to treat the infection.[193] Because of the challenges in treatment, prevention of infection is optimal. The use of prophylactic antibiotics has been shown to decrease the incidence of EVD infections, but it can also predispose the patient to a more resistant organism if infections should occur.[200] Critical care nurses can assist the healthcare team and advocate for the patient by working to minimize the risk factors for EVD infection.

NEUROMUSCULAR DISORDERS

Patients with chronic neuromuscular disorders occasionally experience exacerbations related to their disease process that may require admission to critical care. There are also some neuromuscular disorders that arise acutely and need management in critical care. This section will cover several of these topics.

Myasthenia Gravis

Myasthenia gravis (MG) is an acquired autoimmune neuromuscular disease characterized by varying degrees of weakness of the voluntary skeletal muscles of the body. The hallmark of MG is muscle weakness that is exacerbated by periods of activity and improves

after rest. This chronic disease process occurs to varying degrees in different individuals. LOC and sensory functioning are not impacted.[58] Likewise, smooth and cardiac muscle groups are not affected by the disease.[187] Many patients with MG experience periodic exacerbations of severe muscle weakness termed *myasthenic crises* that might bring the individual into critical care for respiratory failure, ventilatory support, and medication management.[20]

It is estimated that 20 out of every 100,000 persons in the United States has MG.[179,187] This number has increased slightly in recent years probably because of longer life spans and improved diagnostic capabilities. With current treatment modalities, MG patients have a near-normal life expectancy.[187,253,254] A female-to-male predominance exists with a 3:2 ratio.[187] MG can occur at any age, but incidence peaks in the third decade of life (usually women) and then again in the sixth and seventh decades (primarily men).[183,253]

MG is caused by an immune-mediated defect in the postsynaptic membrane of the neuromuscular junction (Figure 25-14). During nerve-to-muscle conduction, an impulse originates in the brain, travels down through nerve tissue, and reaches the synapse between the nerve and muscle known as the neuromuscular junction. In a normal synapse, acetylcholine (ACh) is released from the nerve ending, travels across the junction, and binds to receptors on the muscle fiber. When enough receptors are activated, the muscle contracts.

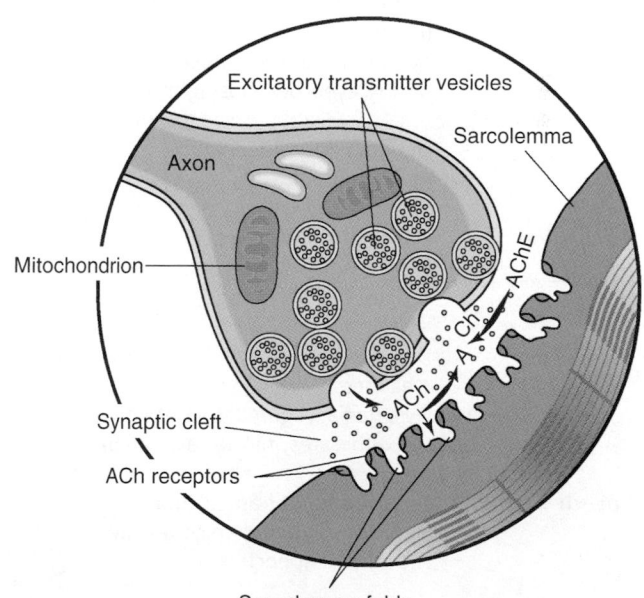

⬆FIGURE 25-14 Normal neuromuscular junction. Acetylcholine (ACh) released from the nerve initiates muscle contraction, and acetylcholinesterase (AChE) breaks down ACh, limiting the duration of contraction. In myasthenia gravis, a widened synaptic cleft and a reduced number of ACh receptors disrupt normal transmission of impulses and lengthen duration of contraction.

The patient with MG develops autoantibodies that block or destroy the ACh receptor sites. Patients become symptomatic once the number of ACh receptors is reduced to about 30% of normal.[187]

The thymus gland is associated with MG, but the relationship is unclear. Thymic abnormalities, either hyperplasia or thymoma, have been noted in up to 75% of patients with MG.[187] It is theorized that certain cells within the thymus may be the source of the autoantigen that destroys the ACh receptors. Another hypothesis suggests that there could be an infectious agent that resembles the ACh receptor and triggers an immune response in MG patients.[253]

Patients with MG may present with weakness of any voluntary muscle, but there are muscle groups typically associated with the disease process (Table 25-8). A standardized classification system based on severity of disease describes symptoms that may begin solely with ocular muscle weakness; progress through weakness of the limbs and the bulbar muscles of breathing, swallowing, and speech; and finally result in a generalized MG, which describes severe weakness requiring intubation for airway preservation.[117]

MG is diagnosed by a clinical examination and a history of fatigue after activity of the hallmark muscle groups. The serology test for the presence of antibodies to the ACh receptor site is considered a diagnostic gold standard because it is highly specific for MG and is positive in 90% of patients with generalized disease;[253] antibodies may not be present in patients with only ocular forms of the disease.[58,183]

Two different electrophysiologic tests are often used for MG diagnosis. Repetitive nerve stimulation will demonstrate a progressive reduction in muscle action potential. Single-fiber electromyography, the most sensitive test in MG, assesses the action potentials generated by closely adjacent muscle fibers of the same motor unit.[253] Another test for MG is the edrophonium (Tensilon) test. Edrophonium is a drug that blocks the breakdown of ACh and temporarily increases the levels of ACh at the neuromuscular junction, which will briefly relieve weakness symptoms.[183] This test is associated with an infrequent but serious potential for bradycardia or hypotension, so it is generally used only when the need for diagnosis is urgent such as when a definitive diagnosis is needed in a rapidly failing patient in critical care.[253]

Fortunately for those patients with MG, medications are now available to treat this disorder and so most patients are able to live relatively normal lives. Acetylcholinesterase inhibitors slow the rate of ACh metabolism and temporarily improve neuromuscular transmission and muscle strength. Pyridostigmine (Mestinon) is the most widely used of this family of drugs and is generally the initial treatment of choice for MG. Neostigmine (Prostigmin) is also used but has more unfavorable gastrointestinal side effects.[222] It is critical that patients with MG receive their medications in a timely, scheduled manner. If a dose is late, weakness of the muscles of swallowing may make it difficult to administer.[183,253] Most patients tolerate acetylcholinesterase inhibitors well but they may require additional treatment strategies to minimize MG symptomatology.[253]

Corticosteroids, which improve MG in the vast majority of patients, are usually reserved for MG patients with moderate or severe disease because of the potential for side effects with long-term use.[253] Immunosuppressive drugs may also be used to suppress the production of abnormal antibodies. This class of drugs includes azathioprine, cyclophosphamide, cyclosporine, methotrexate, and mycophenolate mofetil. The immunosuppressives may take weeks or months to reach effectiveness, so they may be started concurrently with steroids.[253] Plasma exchange therapy, which decreases the number of circulating ACh antibodies and improves muscle strength, is used most frequently during times of myasthenic crisis or preoperatively before thymectomy, but is also used on a chronic basis as needed.[222,253]

TABLE 25-8 Muscle Groups Affected in Myasthenia Gravis

INVOLVED MUSCLE GROUP	RESULTANT DEFICIT
Facial	Facial droop Blank facial expression; inability to frown or smile; inability to tightly close eyelids or puff out cheeks; weakness in raising eyebrow, closing mouth
Extraocular	Diplopia; loss of conjugate gaze Asymmetric ptosis
Mastication	Difficulty chewing food Weak and slow tongue movements Fatigue during eating
Swallowing	Decreased pharyngeal and palatal weakness Dysphagia; regurgitation of liquid through nares; risk for aspiration
Speech	Dysarthria; poor articulation Dysphonia/altered voice quality; hypernasal speech
Musculoskeletal system	Altered muscle strength and functional ability in proximal upper and lower extremities Weakness of muscles of respiration; shortness of breath, shallow respirations, inability to cough effectively

Data from references 58, 187, 253.

As noted earlier, disorders of the thymus are common in patients with MG, affecting approximately 75% of individuals.[253] Thymectomy reduces symptoms and may ameliorate the disease in some individuals through an unclear influence on the immune system,[183] but a total resection of the thymus is technically difficult and residual tissue limits the effectiveness of this intervention.[58] Depending upon the extent of the thymectomy, the approach, and patient comorbidities, MG patients may require postoperative care in critical care for observation and recovery.

Myasthenic Crisis. Patients with MG are susceptible to acute exacerbations in their disease process. Crisis episodes typically occur in 12% to 16% of MG patients within 2 to 3 years after diagnosis,[20,254] but it is possible to see myasthenic crisis in the patient who has not yet been diagnosed. These acute episodes are often predictable and follow exposure to certain triggers (Box 25-4). Infections are associated with 30% to 40% of crises, most commonly a respiratory tract infection.[254] Physical stress and certain medications are also associated with MG crisis.[20,25,58]

Myasthenic crisis can be life threatening because of impaired swallowing and respiratory failure.[20,222] The muscles that control swallowing weaken to the point that swallowing restrictions are necessary to avoid the risk of aspiration. Artificial means of feeding may be needed. In addition, the muscles that control breathing weaken such that ventilation is no longer adequate and the patient requires a mechanical ventilator. Median duration of hospitalization for myasthenic crisis is approximately 1 month, with the patient spending about half this time intubated.[254] When treated aggressively, myasthenic crisis is associated with a good outcome.[178]

The reversal of any triggering agents or events should be initiated immediately. Treatment of infection should be aggressive. MG crisis can be fatal in a minority of cases but tends to be associated with medical comorbidities.[254]

The respiratory status of MG patients needs to be closely monitored. The susceptible muscle groups include those involved in respiration (diaphragm, intercostals, scalene, sternocleidomastoid) but also the upper airway muscles.[121] Vital capacity, tidal volume, negative inspiratory force, and positive expiratory force should be monitored.[20] Controversy exists regarding the exact timing for intubation in this patient population, but most practitioners monitor various respiratory parameters for worsening trends and advocate for conservative early intubation.[20] Regardless of respiratory measurements, if the patient exhibits a wet, gurgling, or stridorous voice, intubation for airway protection may be required.[168] When patients are free of crisis triggers and are getting stronger on examination, evaluation for weaning can begin.[254]

Treatment options for the patient in myasthenic crisis include plasmapheresis or IV immunoglobulin G (IVIG). Plasmapheresis is generally considered the first-line treatment because it produces rapid improvement in 75% of MG patients with severe weakness,[168] but it has not been shown to decrease the duration of the crisis or the morbidity or mortality associated with it.[71] IVIG may be as effective as plasmapheresis; there is no current evidence supporting one strategy over the other.[155] The clinical improvement noted with plasmapheresis or IVIG may be transitory, so there must be plans for other long-term treatment options such as corticosteroids or immunosuppressants[90] to carry the patient through the recovery period.

Guillain-Barré Syndrome

Guillain-Barré syndrome (GBS), also referred to as acute inflammatory demyelinating polyneuropathy (AIDP), is a grouping of autoimmune syndromes characterized by progressive muscle weakness usually associated with an escalating phase, a plateau period,

---

Box 25-4

Triggers for Myasthenic Crisis

1. Infection (especially respiratory tract)
2. Changes in medications
3. Aspiration
4. Physical or emotional stress
5. Specific medications:

Do Not Use in Myasthenia Gravis Patients:
- D-Penicillamine
- Interferon botulinum toxin

May Be Associated With Myasthenic Crisis:
- Antidysrhythmic agents
  a. Quinidine
  b. Procainamide hydrochloride
  c. Verapamil
- Antibiotics
  a. Aminoglycosides
  b. Ciprofloxacin
  c. Quinine derivatives (quinolones)
  d. Ampicillin
  e. Erythromycin
- Anti-hypertensive agents
  a. Beta blockers
  b. Calcium channel blockers
- Magnesium-containing compounds
  a. Magnesium sulfate and citrate
- Neuromuscular blocking agents
  a. Succinylcholine chloride
  b. Curare derivatives
- Other
  a. Phenytoin
- Lithium

Data from references 20, 58, 281.

and then followed by spontaneous remission.[92] The annual incidence of GBS is approximately 1 to 4 cases per 100,000 persons[107,207] and occurs at all ages and in both sexes.[92] Severity of the disease process is predictive of outcome, and current mortality rates are as high as 20%, primarily in patients requiring mechanical ventilation.[44,72] Since the incidence of polio has greatly decreased, GBS is now the most common cause of acute flaccid paralysis in healthy people.[211]

GBS is considered a syndrome rather than a disease because it is not clear that a specific disease-causing agent is involved. The cause of this syndrome is unknown, but it is generally believed to be an autoimmune response to a bacterial or viral infection. Approximately two thirds of patients report a respiratory tract or gastrointestinal infection 1 to 3 weeks before the onset of the clinical manifestations of neuropathy.[197] GBS has followed and been associated with infection by *Campylobacter jejuni,* cytomegalovirus, and Epstein-Barr virus.[115] Influenza vaccines have also been associated with GBS such that the current risk is estimated to be 1 to 2 cases per 1 million persons immunized.[135,186]

GBS affects both the motor and the sensory pathways of the peripheral nervous system.[278] Characteristic peripheral and cranial nerve damage can be either that of a demyelinating process or that of an acute axonal degeneration.[186] The latter could explain residual deficits in some patients.[285]

The typical clinical presentation for GBS is a rapidly evolving symmetric paralysis in the extremities, more commonly affecting the legs than the arms.[278] Although tingling and dysesthesias occur in the extremities, motor findings are by far the more prevalent.[186,278] Many patients experience motor deficits that ascend from the toes and legs into the arms, muscles of respiration, and cranial nerves in a matter of hours or days.[61] In addition to weakness and diminished or absent reflexes, there are also signs of autonomic dysfunction in 50% of patients. Box 25-5 lists the clinical features of GBS.[110,285]

All patients must be monitored for unpredictably rapid deterioration because up to 30% of patients will require mechanical ventilation at some point.[92,109,155] Factors associated with the need for mechanical ventilation include rapid disease progression, bulbar dysfunction (dysarthria, dysphagia, or impairment of the gag reflex), bilateral facial weakness, or dysautonomia.[137] Determining criteria for the need for intubation and mechanical ventilation include a vital capacity less than 15 ml/kg and an inability to protect the airway.[212] The progressive period of the disease can last from days up to 4 weeks.[114]

After acute progression of the illness, a plateau phase occurs lasting for several weeks in which there is stabilization but little change.[186] During the acute escalating phase and even the plateau period of GBS, admission

---

Box 25-5

Clinical Features of Guillain-Barré Syndrome

1. Progressive ascending symmetric weakness of the limbs
   - Involvement of proximal and distal muscles
   - Depressed or absent reflexes
   - Involvement of cranial nerves (facial nerves most commonly involved)
2. Numbness and tingling in the hands and feet
   - Mild sensory symptoms or signs
3. Respiratory failure
4. Pain
   - Back, shoulder girdle, and posterior thighs
5. Autonomic dysfunction
   - Cardiac dysrhythmias (tachycardia, bradycardia, asystole)
   - Orthostatic hypotension
   - Paralytic ileus
   - Bladder dysfunction
   - Abnormal sweating
6. Progression to peak disability in 4 weeks

Data from references 110, 211, 285.

---

to critical care may be necessary. Patients might require airway protection, intubation, and mechanical ventilation as noted previously, but, in addition, the potential for neuropathic autonomic dysfunction and hemodynamic instability warrants monitoring and action by critical care staff.[92] Cardiac monitoring for dysrhythmias may be required. Other areas of concern for nurses include pain management, prevention of VTE, nutritional adequacy, and psychological support.[92]

After the plateau, the subsequent recovery period may be as little as a few weeks or as long as several years.[186] About 30% of those with GBS still have a residual weakness after 3 years.[181] Causes of death include acute respiratory distress syndrome, sepsis, pulmonary emboli, and unexplained cardiac arrest. Factors associated with a poorer outcome include older age, severe and rapidly progressive disease, prolonged mechanical ventilation (longer than 1 month), persistent abnormal findings on electromyography, and preexisting pulmonary disease.[138]

Diagnosis of GBS relies heavily on the clinical examination and patient history. CSF will appear normal initially but after 7 to 10 days will show increased levels of protein without an increase in the number of white blood cells.[211,285] Electrophysiologic studies for nerve conduction and muscle contraction are used to determine the existence of any slowing or a block in conduction.[2]

Treatment options for acute GBS are limited. The American Academy of Neurology practice parameter recommendations for GBS treatment are listed in Box 25-6.[108] Both plasmapheresis and IVIG are effective in hastening motor recovery, but there does not appear to be any

Box 25-6

American Academy of Neurology Recommendations for the Treatment of Guillain-Barré Syndrome

- Plasma exchange is recommended for adults with GBS who are unable to walk unaided and who start treatment within 4 weeks of the onset of neuropathic symptoms.
- Plasma exchange should also be considered for ambulatory patients examined within 2 weeks of the onset of symptoms.
- IVIG is recommended for adult patients with GBS who are unable to walk unaided and who start treatment within 2 or possibly 4 weeks of the onset of symptoms.
- The effects of plasma exchange and IVIG are equivalent.
- Corticosteroids are not recommended for the management of GBS.
- Sequential treatment with plasma exchange followed by IVIG, or immunoadsorption followed by IVIG, is not recommended for patients with GBS.
- Plasma exchange and IVIG are options for children with severe GBS.

Data from reference 108.
GBS = Guillain-Barré syndrome, IVIG = intravenous immunoglobulin G.

additional clinical improvement when both modalities are used.[196] Nursing management is multidimensional and team-focused for support of the patient and family. Priorities of care include monitoring and maintaining adequate respiratory and cardiovascular status, avoiding the complications of immobility, promoting adequate nutritional support (see the Nutrition box on p. 720), providing pain management (Box 25-7), relieving anxiety, maintaining

Box 25-7

Pain Management in the Critically Ill Neuroscience Patient

It is common for neuroscience patients to have an altered level of consciousness or impaired cognition. Because the most reliable and valid indicator of pain is the patient's self-report, these patients may experience difficulty when communicating their degree of pain. Many hospitals and critical care units use a variety of different pain scales to assist patients in quantifying and describing their pain, but these scales generally rely on the patient's ability to communicate with the care provider.

For many neuroscience patients, nurses must rely on scales that measure the following:[93]

Pain-Related Behavior
- Movement—restlessness
- Facial expressions and vocalizations—grimacing, crying
- Posturing—evidence of guarding or splinting

*Physiologic Indicators**
- Increased heart rate
- Increased blood pressure
- Increased respiratory rate

*The absence of these indicators does not indicate the absence of pain.[191]

Nurses should also consider the many possible pain generators for the critically ill patient. Sources of acute pain are usually the most obvious and include surgical incisions and traumatic injuries. Also remember chronic pain conditions[93] and consider which procedures will cause critically ill patients pain (e.g., suctioning, placement or removal of tubes, turning, dressing changes).[191]

Recommendations include the following:[248]
- Pain assessment and response to therapy should be performed regularly using a scale appropriate to the patient population and systematically documented.
- Patients who cannot communicate should be assessed through subjective observation of pain-related behaviors and physiologic indicators and the change in these parameters following analgesic therapy.
- Sedation of agitated critically ill patients should be initiated only after providing adequate analgesia and treating reversible physiologic causes.
- Sleep promotion should include optimization of the environment and nonpharmacologic methods to promote relaxation with adjunctive use of hypnotics.

Nonpharmacologic Interventions for the Management of Pain
- Proper positioning
- Stabilization of fractures
- Elimination of irritating physical stimulation (e.g., proper positioning of ventilator tubing)
- Heat or cold therapy
- Titrating environmental stimulation
- Relaxation
- Music therapy
- Massage

Pharmacologic Therapies for the Management of Pain
- Opioids
- Nonsteroidal antiinflammatory drugs (NSAIDs)
- Neuropathic pain agents
- Acetaminophen
- Sleep aids

communication, and providing emotional support and patient/family teaching.[102,109]

Critical Illness Polyneuropathy/Myopathy

Critical care nurses have long recognized that patients under their care developed generalized weakness syndromes when experiencing a severe illness in critical care. Until the mid-1980s, this weakness was attributed to starvation-induced or disuse atrophy. However, it is now clear that the function of peripheral nerves, neuromuscular junctions, and skeletal muscles all can be adversely affected in critically ill patients through a variety of mechanisms.[90,136,155,173]

A classification system for these acquired nerve and muscle disorders has not been specifically established.

Because patients have been noted to experience both neuropathic and myopathic changes and they are frequently found in combination,[95] it has been suggested to refer to this syndrome as critical illness polyneuropathy/myopathy (CIP/M).[90] It is estimated that between 25% and 50% of patients in medical and surgical critical care units experience CIP/M.[90] In one study, of the patients who were mechanically ventilated for 5 to 7 days, 50% to 100% were noted to have an axonal polyneuropathy on routine electrophysiologic testing.[56] It has been associated with prolonged mechanical ventilation and prolonged lengths of intensive care and hospital stays.[83] One study estimated that the development of this motor weakness was associated with an additional $66,000 in additional charges per patient (1996 dollars).[213]

◆ NUTRITION

Nutritional Care of the Critically Ill Neuroscience Patient

Neuroscience patients in critical care are challenged to receive adequate and appropriate nutrition for a myriad of reasons. The critical care nurse must be aware of these special needs.

- Some neuroscience populations (e.g., traumatic brain injury) are associated with hypermetabolic and hypercatabolic states, predisposing these patients to the potential for malnutrition.[277]

Risk of Aspiration

- An altered level of consciousness (LOC) is noted in many neuroscience patients. Patients with a reduced LOC are at high risk for aspiration and should not be fed orally until the LOC has improved.[94,248]
- Many critically ill neuroscience patients require both enteral feedings for nutritional support and the use of mechanical ventilation with artificial airways.
  - Artificial airways add to the risk of aspiration. Endotracheal cuff pressures should be maintained at 20 to 25 cm H_2O.[215]
  - Guidelines to prevent aspiration in patients receiving enteral feedings recommend elevation of the head of the bed (HOB) to an angle of 30 to 45 degrees.[246]
- Traditional nursing practice for the care of many neuroscience patients is to establish routine elevation of the HOB to 30 degrees. However, recent literature suggests that some ischemic stroke patients and those requiring higher cerebral perfusion pressures may benefit from lower HOB positions, possibly even flat positioning, to promote an increase in blood flow to ischemic brain tissue.[69,282] Head of

bed positioning for cerebral perfusion may conflict with that needed for safe administration of enteral feedings.

Medications Commonly Prescribed in the Neuroscience Population Influence Nutritional Needs

- Phenytoin has been shown to interact with enteral feedings, and there are many reports and studies showing dramatic decreases in phenytoin serum concentrations when co-administered with enteral feedings. These decreased phenytoin concentrations may increase the risk of seizures. There is no standardized intervention recommended to overcome this problem.[11] There does not seem to be any benefit in interrupting nasogastric feeding for 2 hours before and 2 hours after the administration of phenytoin.[170]
- Steroids are given to many patient populations (e.g., brain tumors, central nervous system infections, Guillain-Barré syndrome to decrease inflammation and edema).[89]
- Propofol is the drug of choice when given for sustained sedation in the neuroscience patient because of its rapid onset and short duration of action once discontinued.[248] It has been used to reduce elevated increased intracranial pressure and may decrease cerebral blood flow and metabolism.[124] Practitioners can temporarily stop the infusion, perform a neurologic assessment, and restart the infusion, all within a short time frame. Propofol is prepared in a phospholipid preparation that should be counted as nutritional intake. When used over an extended time or at high doses, the lipid preparation can lead to hypertriglyceridemia.[214] Triglycerides should be monitored during drip infusion.

CIP/M is characterized by symmetric limb muscle weakness and atrophy. Sparing of the cranial nerves is frequently noted. Deep tendon reflexes are reduced or absent and there is often some sensory loss to light touch and pinprick in peripheral nerves.[31,90] This phenomenon can be common in the intensive care unit, and nursing staff should have a high index of suspicion for its occurrence.

CIP/M occurs most often in patients with sepsis or organ failure,[53,57,77] and it is a presumed manifestation of the systemic inflammatory response syndrome.[136,280] Hyperglycemia has been associated with this syndrome in several studies.[57,264] CIP/M may also be associated with the use of corticosteroids and neuromuscular blocking agents.[57,83] Patients of increased age[77] and female gender[57] may also be at higher risk.

Most episodes of CIP/M present 7 or more days after the onset of the critical illness although it may occur as soon as 2 days after the diagnosis of sepsis.[252] Involvement of the phrenic nerve in combination with intercostal muscle weakness contributes to respiratory insufficiency and difficulty weaning patients from mechanical ventilation.[90]

Nerve conduction studies and electromyography can confirm the presence of a neuromuscular disorder that is not necessarily apparent from clinical examination.[55] Biopsy and autopsy specimens show degeneration of axons with little or no associated inflammation or demyelination, consistent with a denervation atrophy.[136]

No specific treatment is known to have been proven to be effective against this polyneuropathy or myopathy. Intensive insulin therapy and serum glucose control have been shown to decrease the risk of CIP/M.[136,264,280] Aggressive efforts in preventing and treating sepsis will likely also reduce the incidence of this syndrome.[55] The benefit of physical therapy is unknown but may be minimal, especially in the early stages of recovery.[95] Even in patients who have experienced only mild to moderate nerve injury, recovery of muscle strength can take weeks to months. Electrodiagnostic testing may demonstrate residual nerve dysfunction several years after the critical illness episode.[73]

THERAPEUTIC HYPOTHERMIA AFTER CARDIAC ARREST

Most critical care nurses are familiar with the scenario of the patient who survives an episode of cardiac arrest only to be left with a devastating neurologic disability as a result of widespread cerebral hypoxia. Until recently, there were no interventions available to alter the course of this neurologic sequela. In 2002 two landmark studies were published that investigated the use of controlled hypothermia in patients who experience cardiac arrest

because of ventricular fibrillation and have subsequent return of spontaneous circulation, but remain unconscious. When these patients were cooled to 32° to 34° C for 12 to 24 hours, they had improved neurologic outcome.[24,111] Nurses who care for patients who have undergone coronary artery bypass surgery are familiar with the concept of controlled moderate hypothermia to protect the brain against global ischemia. The exact mechanism for this effect is not clear but it is thought that hypothermia reduces cerebral oxygen consumption although many multifactorial mechanisms are probably involved.[111]

The International Liaison Committee on Resuscitation (ILCOR)[112] issued an advisory statement in 2003 with the recommendation that unconscious adult patients with spontaneous circulation after out-of-hospital arrest should be cooled to 32° to 34° C for 12 to 24 hours when the initial rhythm was ventricular fibrillation. In addition, such cooling may also be beneficial for other rhythms or in-hospital cardiac arrest. Although these statements seem straightforward, the actual patient care involved in carrying out this recommendation can be challenging. Hospitals that have adopted the use of controlled therapeutic hypothermia should have established protocols to ensure standardized and comprehensive treatment for all patients.

Initially, patients who meet criteria to enter the hypothermia protocol need to be identified. The patient who is unconscious and has spontaneous circulation restored will then need to be intubated (if not already done), sedated, and medicated to control shivering. Shivering during cooling leads to warming and will increase overall oxygen consumption.[112] Nursing care involves ensuring that the hypothermia protocol is followed and that complications of hypothermia are avoided. Complications in this patient population might include cardiac dysrhythmias, coagulopathy/bleeding, infection, seizures, and pressure ulcers.[104,111]

Cooling the patient can be accomplished by many methods although none yet have combined efficacy and ease of use. Depending on the choice of the practitioners in the facility, the patient may be cooled by lowering the room temperature; using icepacks in specified body areas, cooling blankets above and below the patient,[112] or special head or body wraps;[91] infusing chilled IV saline;[23] and using intravascular cooling catheters.[1] Hypothermia is typically induced as soon as possible although the treatment appears to be successful even if delayed for 4 to 6 hours.[24] The optimal rate of cooling has not been determined but study protocols have noted that the goal temperature was reached in 2 to 16 hours.[24,111] Core body temperature is measured by bladder or pulmonary artery catheter. Laboratory values should be monitored for electrolyte imbalances, potential infectious situations, and coagulopathies. The patient is kept sedated without shivering for 18 to 24 hours and then is passively allowed to rewarm.[112]

DETERMINATION OF DEATH BY NEUROLOGIC CRITERIA

Care of the critically ill, by its very nature, will involve end-of-life decisions for some patients. Traditional notions for the lay public on the determination of death are related to cessation of the heartbeat. The advent of cardiopulmonary support systems that can help to maintain, at least temporarily, adequate perfusion to other body systems despite the lack of apparent brain activity has created confusion regarding the timing of and ultimately the determination of death. Even the use of the term *life support* implies that active withdrawal of the same is what determines the point of death. Lack of clarity regarding these issues has necessitated the establishment of criteria to determine brain death in the context of a beating heart.

Brain death is defined as irreversible cessation of all functions of the entire brain, including the brain stem,[205] and must be diagnosed by a physician. In brain death, irreversibility is determined when the etiology of coma sufficient to account for loss of brain functions is established, the possibility of recovery of brain function is excluded, and the cessation of all brain functions persists for a period of observation or therapy.[239] Table 25-9 outlines confirmatory tests of brain death.

Clinically, there are prerequisites that must be met for brain death determination. This includes evidence of an acute CNS event compatible with death found either clinically or with neuroimaging techniques. In the clinical neurologic assessment of brain death, repeat clinical evaluation of cardinal findings in brain death is recommended. Most experts recommend an interval of 6 hours between assessments.[238] In 1968 the Harvard Ad Hoc Committee on Brain Death published a report describing the clinical characteristics of "irreversible coma."[96] These criteria are still used today in diagnosing brain death and consist of the following:

- *Coma or Unresponsiveness.* The patient shows total unawareness of external stimuli and unresponsiveness to painful stimuli. Spontaneous voluntary motor activity, shivering, seizure activity, and involuntary decerebrate or decorticate posturing are all absent in brain death because they require some degree of cerebral activity.[239] However, patients may exhibit spontaneous motor activity as a result of intact spinal pathways even in brain death.[101] Because this motor activity is the result of spinal reflexes, it is not cerebrally modulated and does not indicate brain activity. These responses are typically in younger persons and can consist of flexion/withdrawal of extremities or movement of the torso or neck.[276] Any motor activity in the patient who is brain dead can be very disconcerting to both staff and family and requires a knowledgeable and compassionate nursing approach.

TABLE 25-9 Brain Stem Reflexes and Brain Death Criteria

BRAIN STEM REFLEX	BRAIN DEATH CRITERIA
Pupillary signs	Pupils may be round, oval, or irregularly shaped. Most pupils are midposition, 4–6 mm in diameter, although variations from 4–9 mm are compatible with brain death. Pupillary light reflex is absent. Precautions: Various drugs such as atropine and opiates can influence pupil size, making it difficult to determine reactivity. Topical administration of drugs and ocular trauma may influence both pupil size and reactivity. Preexisting ocular abnormalities may also complicate pupillary assessment. See the Research Utilization box on p. 723.
Ocular movements	Both oculocephalic (doll's eyes) and vestibulo-ocular (caloric test) reflexes are absent in brain death. Precautions: Contraindications to testing for oculocephalic reflexes include suspected fracture or instability of cervical spine. Contraindications to testing of vestibulo-ocular reflexes include impaired integrity of tympanic membranes. The vestibulo-ocular reflex can be diminished by some medications (sedatives, aminoglycosides, tricyclic antidepressants, anticholinergics, and antiseizure agents) as well as facial trauma involving auditory canal and petrous bone.
Facial sensory and motor responses	Corneal reflexes are absent in brain death—test with cotton-tipped swab. Jaw reflexes are absent—look for grimace to painful stimuli. Precautions: Severe facial trauma can inhibit interpretation of facial brain stem reflexes.
Pharyngeal and tracheal reflexes	Gag reflex is absent in brain death—evaluate by stimulating posterior of pharynx with a tongue blade. Cough reflex is absent—test by using bronchial suctioning.

Data from reference 239.

- *Absence of Brain Stem Reflexes.* Brain stem reflexes are the clinical indication of brain stem function. The loss of brain stem functioning is incompatible with life. All brain stem reflexes will be absent in brain death.[101] Table 25-9 lists brain stem reflex assessment techniques and indicators for brain death criteria.[238] The Research Utilization box on p. 723 provides information on clinical research with use of a pupillometer for assessment of pupillary function.

Pupillometer for Objective Measurement of Pupil Size and Velocity

NEW TECHNOLOGY

Automated pupillometer.

CLINICAL ISSUE

Pupil size and reactivity have long been part of the standard neurologic examination in patients with an altered level of consciousness or any type of brain dysfunction. Critical care practitioners recognize that manual pupillary examination is highly subjective and susceptible to interexaminer variability.

SUMMARY

This study examined the interexaminer variability measured in manual pupillary examinations as compared with a portable automated pupillometer. Twenty patients were examined by two groups of three examiners using both the manual examination with a penlight or similar light source and a portable automated pupillometer capable of measuring pupil size and reaction. Pupil size and reactivity were compared. The study found that results with the automated pupillometer were more accurate and reliable among examiners than the manual examinations in measuring pupil size and reactivity.

APPLICATION

Automated pupillometry may be useful in providing critical care nurses with a precise, objective, and reliable measurement of pupil size and reactivity. The pupillometer is currently available for purchase and use.

NEED FOR FURTHER STUDY

Further research using the pupillometer needs to be carried out in larger studies comparing patients with more varied diagnoses including brain injuries and situations involving increased ICP.

Meeker, M., et al. (2005). Pupil examination: validity and clinical utility of an automated pupillometer. *J Neurosci Nurs,* 37(1), 34–40.

- *Apnea.* Loss of brain stem function definitively results in loss of centrally controlled breathing, with resultant apnea. Apnea testing is based upon the theory that an elevated partial pressure of arterial carbon dioxide ($PaCO_2$) level will stimulate the respiratory drive in the patient with intact brain stem function. Advisory guidelines for determination of death based on clinical and research data recommend achieving $PaCO_2$ levels of greater than 60 mm Hg for maximal stimulation of brain stem

respiratory centers.[172] Target $PaCO_2$ levels may be higher in patients with chronic hypercapnia. Hospitals typically have protocols for apnea testing that include hyperoxygenating before testing along with supplemental oxygen given during the test to guard against hypoxia and potential cardiac dysrhythmias and hypotension.[239]

In addition to the above-noted clinical criteria, all potentially reversible confounding factors for coma must be excluded. These factors include use of neuromuscular blocking agents, severe electrolyte imbalance, severe acid-base abnormalities, and severe metabolic or endocrine disturbances. Brain death criteria can still be met in patients who have been on barbiturate therapy if levels are subtherapeutic.[276] The patient's core body temperature must be greater than or equal to 32° C,[99] and healthcare providers must confirm the absence of drug intoxication or poisoning.[239]

As with many other processes that exist in hospitals, protocols can help to define and expedite care plans. In this instance, a protocol in place for the diagnosis of brain death can aid practitioners in the decision-making process and help in describing the process to family members, who are under considerable stress and can benefit from clear direction and support.

Case Study 25-1, Part C

Status Epilepticus

Several hours after being weaned from propofol, S.B. gradually started to move all extremities and regain consciousness. She followed commands intermittently, and wrist restraints were required to keep her from removing her endotracheal tube. She was "bucking" the ventilator and her ventilations were not synchronized with the machine. S.B.'s blood pressure increased as she became more agitated and rose to 175/110 mm Hg with a heart rate of 115 beats/min in a sinus tachycardia. Her pupils were equal, round, and midline at 4 mm and she occasionally tracked to request.

Suddenly, S.B. stopped moving and lay still. Her nurse called to her but the patient was no longer following any verbal commands. Her left arm and leg withdrew to noxious stimuli but her right arm and leg exhibited extensor posturing. Upon pupil examination, it was noted that her left pupil was now 7 mm and sluggishly reactive while the right pupil was 3 mm and also sluggishly reactive. Blood pressure is 130/100 mm Hg but S.B.'s heart rate has dropped to 50 beats/min and she is in a junctional rhythm.

Decision point: What is happening to S.B.?

Decision point: What steps should the nurse take?

Decision point: What treatment plan for the next 24 hours might the nurse anticipate?

MULTIDISCIPLINARY PLAN OF CARE FOR NEUROSCIENCE PATIENTS

PROBLEM	INTERVENTION	RATIONALE	EXPECTED OUTCOME	COMMENTS
Impaired airway	Consider patients at risk for impaired airway: Altered LOC Altered motor or sensory function, especially involving bulbar muscles Use of sedation, anxiolytics, or chemical paralysis Excessive respiratory secretions compromising respiratory effort Advanced age Position patient to open airway: HOB up and midline Assess swallowing ability: attempt to feed or administer oral meds only when patient awake and alert Initiate use of artificial airway as needed Use oral airway or nasal trumpet as needed Intubation or mechanical ventilation as needed Have suction equipment available and use for control of secretions	Early identification of patients at risk for impaired airway allows for timely intervention and crisis avoidance. Patient positioning and attention to level of alertness will promote airway maintenance and reduce risk of aspiration. Artificial airways are used for airway control and optimization of respiratory status.	Airway remains patent. Patients at risk for altered airway will be identified and addressed early. Patient will not aspirate.	Nasal airway and nasogastric tube contraindicated in patients with basilar skull trauma or surgery.
Respiratory failure	Consider patients at risk: Decreased/altered LOC Weakness in muscles of breathing Monitor respiratory status and implement individualized plan of care to address: Assess respiratory rate and effort; watch for irregular neuroventilatory patterns, sonorous respirations, stridor Respiratory secretions LOC O₂ sat ABGs Incentive spirometry or other respiratory measures	Identification and early action for neuroscience patients with respiratory failure in the critical care unit can decrease episodes of aspiration, atelectasis, and pneumonia.	Patients at risk for respiratory failure are identified and treated early, minimizing secondary hypoxic insult to brain.	

PROBLEM	INTERVENTION	RATIONALE	EXPECTED OUTCOME	COMMENTS
Injury to self	Consider patients at risk for injury to self: Altered LOC, related to disease process, medications Altered motor or sensory function Presence of equipment Unfamiliar routine and environment Control patient environment: Remove tubes, lines, equipment from patient access and discontinue as soon as possible Restrain, use sitter, or involve family as needed for patient safety Install padded side rails with suction and oxygenation equipment available for seizure precautions Provide emotional support; medications as indicated Helmet for patients with craniectomy/bone flap removal Fall risk assessment and prevention: Keep patient bed in low position Call light and basic needs available at all times Maintain toileting schedule Promote adequate sleep Provide mobility opportunities Provide frequent reorientation as appropriate	Early identification of patients at risk allows for prevention of injury or expedient treatment. Prevent dislodgement of tubes by patient and decrease risk of injury. Fall risk assessment triggers implementation of hospital programs to prevent injury from falls.	Patients will be injury-free.	
Knowledge deficit	Consider patients/family at risk: New or complex diagnosis Learning disability related to cognitive status, memory deficit, altered LOC, disease process Educate patient and family: Assess ability to learn and current knowledge base Give information on diagnosis, prognosis, medications, treatment plan Explain hospital policies and procedures for patient safety Involve family in plan of care Provide multiple types of materials to allow for individual differences and learning at another time when less stressed	Involving patients in education and plan of care encourages participation and empowers them to take responsibility for own care.	Patients report increased knowledge.	

Table continues on page 726

PROBLEM	INTERVENTION	RATIONALE	EXPECTED OUTCOME	COMMENTS
Deep vein thrombosis (DVT) prevention	Assess patients for risk factors: Bed rest, decreased mobility, lower extremity weakness/paralysis, altered LOC Hypercoagulable states (e.g., cancer) Presence of intravascular catheters (e.g., central venous line) Monitor extremities for DVT in patients at high risk Implement action steps to prevent DVT: Anticoagulant therapy, compression stockings, as ordered Encourage out-of-bed activity and leg exercises as appropriate	Prevention of DVT improves outcome and decreases recovery time.	Patient will not experience DVT.	
Anxiety/ emotional support	Consider patients at risk: New diagnosis Altered LOC Lack of social support system Encourage calm environment: Decrease stimuli Limit visitors as necessary Reorient patient as appropriate Administer neuro-related medications in a timely manner to optimize neuro functioning (e.g., anticholinesterase medications for myasthenia gravis) Administer anxiolytics/sedatives as needed and appropriate	Decreasing anxiety leads to improved coping and improved ability for patient to participate in plan for recovery.	Anxiety levels will be minimal and action will be taken to decrease anxiety when level is elevated.	

ABG = Arterial blood gas, HOB = head of bed, LOC = level of consciousness, O$_2$ = oxygen.

MULTIDISCIPLINARY PLAN OF CARE

The critical care of a neuroscience patient is a team effort that must address every body system and encompass not only patient but also family social and psychological well-being. The Multidisciplinary Plan of Care on pp. 724-726 presents aspects of care for this patient population.

CONCLUSIONS

Critical care nurses work with many diverse populations of patients with neurologic symptomatology. Advanced knowledge and proficiency are necessary to determine whether the neurologic picture of the patient reflects true CNS involvement, neurologic manifestations of a systemic process, or a combination of both. Nurses are uniquely qualified and positioned to provide expert care to neuroscience patients with either common or rare diagnoses. As technology advances, neuroscience promises to be an area of great expansion and challenge.

REFERENCES

1. Al-Senani, F. M., et al. (2004). A prospective, multicenter pilot study to evaluate the feasibility and safety of using the CoolGard System and ICY catheter following cardiac arrest. *Resuscitation*, *62*, 143–150.
2. Al-Shekhlee, A., et al. (2005). New criteria for early electrodiagnosis of acute inflammatory demyelinating polyneuropathy. *Muscle Nerve*, *32*(1), 66–72.
3. Alldredge, B., et al. (1995). Evaluation of out-of-hospital therapy for status epilepticus. *Epilepsia*, *36*(suppl 4), 44–48.
4. Amar, A. P. G. S., & Apuzzo, M. L. J. (2000). Treatment of central nervous system infections: a neurosurgical perspective. *Neuroimaging Clin North Am*, *10*(2), 445–459.
5. American Association of Neuroscience Nurses. (2004). *Guide to the care of the patient with seizures* (2nd ed.). Chicago: American Association of Neuroscience Nurses.
6. American Cancer Society. (2006, March 10). *What are the key statistics for brain and spinal cord tumors in adults?* www.cancer.org.
7. Aminoff, M. J., & Simon, R. P. (1980). Status epilepticus; causes, clinical features and consequences in 98 patients. *Am J Med*, *69*, 657–665.
8. Arnold, S. M., & Patchell, R. A. (2001). Diagnosis and management of brain metastases. *Hematol Oncol Clin North Am*, *15*, 6–21.
9. Aronin, S. I., Peduzzi, P., & Quagliarello, V. J. (1998). Community-acquired bacterial meningitis: risk stratification for adverse clinical outcome and effect of antibiotic timing. *Ann Intern Med*, *129*(11), 862–869.
10. Arrer, E., et al. (2002). Trace protein as a marker for cerebrospinal fluid rhinorrhea. *Clin Chem*, *48*(16), 939–941.
11. Au Yeung, S. C., & Ensom, M. H. (2000). Phenytoin and enteral feedings: does evidence support an interaction? *Ann Pharmaco Ther*, *34*(7–8), 896–905.
12. Barclay, L. (2005, June 28). *fMRI evaluation may aid management of seizure disorder*. Medscape from WebMD. www.medscape.com.

13. Barker, E. (2002). Central nervous system infections. In E. Barker (Ed.), *Neuroscience nursing: a spectrum of care* (2nd ed., pp 131–167). St Louis: Mosby.
14. Barker, E. (2002). Cranial surgery. In E. Barker (Ed.), *Neuroscience nursing: a spectrum of care* (2nd ed., pp 303–349). St Louis: Mosby.
15. Barker, E. (2002). Infectious and autoimmune processes. In E. Barker (Ed.), *Neuroscience nursing: a spectrum of care* (2nd ed., pp 664–667). St Louis: Mosby.
16. Barker, E. (2002). Management of seizures and epilepsy. In E. Barker (Ed.), *Neuroscience nursing: a spectrum of care* (2nd ed.). St Louis: Mosby.
17. Barker, E. (2002). Metabolic disorders. In E. Barker (Ed.), *Neuroscience nursing: a spectrum of care* (2nd ed., pp 195–215). St Louis: Mosby.
18. Barker, E., & Chao, P. W. (2002). Neurodiagnostic & laboratory studies. In E. Barker (Ed.), *Neuroscience nursing: a spectrum of care* (2nd ed., pp 99–128). St Louis: Mosby.
19. Batchelor, T., & DeAngelis, L. M. (1996). Medical management of cerebral metastases. *Neurosurg Clin North Am*, *7*, 435–453.
20. Bedlack, R. S., & Sanders, D. B. (2000). How to handle myasthenic crisis; essential steps in patient care. *Postgrad Med*, *107*(4), 211–222.
21. Behin, A., et al. (2003). Primary brain tumours in adults. *Lancet*, *361*, 323–331.
22. Belay, E. D., et al. (2005). Variant Creutzfeldt-Jakob disease death, United States. *Emerg Infect Dis*, *11*(9), 1351–1354.
23. Bernard, S. A., et al. (2003). Induced hypothermia using large volume, ice-cold intravenous fluid in comatose survivors of out-of-hospital cardiac arrest: a preliminary report. *Resuscitation*, *56*, 9–13.
24. Bernard, S. A., et al. (2002). Treatment of comatose survivors of out-of-hospital cardiac arrest with induced hypothermia. *N Engl J Med*, *346*, 557–563.
25. Bernardini, G. L. (2004). Diagnosis and management of brain abscess and subdural empyema. *Curr Neurol Neurosci Rep*, *4*, 448–456.
26. Bethel, S. A. (1999). Use of lumbar cerebrospinal fluid drainage in thoracoabdominal aortic aneurysm repairs. *J Vasc Nurs*, *17*(3), 53–58.
27. Bittencourt, P. R. M., et al. (1990). High-dose praziquantel for neurocysticercosis: efficacy and tolerability. *Eur Neurol*, *30*, 229–234.
28. Bleck, T. P. (1999). Management approaches to prolonged seizures and status epilepticus. *Epilepsia*, *40*(suppl 1), S59–S63.
29. Bleck, T. P. (2005). Refractory statue epilepticus. *Curr Opin Crit Care*, *11*, 117–120.
30. Bohan, E. M. (2002). Brain tumors. In E. Barker (Ed.), *Neuroscience nursing: a spectrum of care* (2nd ed., pp 269–301). St Louis: Mosby.
31. Bolton, C. (1994). The polyneuropathy of critical illness. *Intensive Care Med*, *9*, 132–136.
32. Bota, D. P., et al. (2005). Ventriculostomy-related infections in critically ill patients: a 6-year experience. *J Neurosurg*, *103*, 468–472.
33. Brem, S., & Panattil, J. G. (2005). An era of rapid advancement: diagnosis and treatment of metastatic brain cancer. *Neurosurgery*, *57*, S4-5–S4-9.
34. Britt, R. H., & Enzmann, D. R. (1983). Clinical stages of human brain abscess on serial CT scans after contrast infusion: computerized tomographic, neuropathological and clinical correlations. *J Neurosurg*, *55*, 972–989.
35. Buelow, J. M., et al. (2004). Epilepsy. In M. K. Bader & L. R. Littlejohns (Eds.), *AANN core curriculum for neuroscience nursing*. St Louis: Saunders.
36. Calfee, D. P., & Wispelwey, B. (2000). Brain abscess. *Semin Neurol*, *20*(3), 353–360.
37. Cameron, M., & Durack, D. (1997). Helminthic infections. In W. M. Scheld, R. J. Whitley & D. T. Durack (Eds.), *Infections*

of the central nervous system (2nd ed., pp 845–878). Philadelphia: Lippincott-Raven.

38. Cashman, N. R. (1997). A prion primer. *Can Med Assoc J, 157*(10), 1381–1385.

39. Centers for Disease Control and Prevention, Division of Parasitic Diseases. (2004, May 5). *Cysticercosis.* www.dpd.cdc.gov.

40. Centers for Disease Control and Prevention. (2005, June 29). *Prion diseases.* www.cdc.gov.

41. Chapman, M. G., Smith, M., & Hirsch, N. P. (2001). Status epilepticus. *Anaesthesia, 56*, 648–659.

42. Chaudhuri, A., & Kennedy, P. G. E. (2002). Diagnosis and treatment of viral encephalitis. *Postgrad Med, 78*, 575–583.

43. Chernoff, D., & Stark, P. (2004, Sept 27). *Principles of magnetic resonance imaging.* UpToDate Online 13.2. www.utdol.com.

44. Chio, A., et al. (2003). Guillain-Barre syndrome: a prospective, population-based incidence and outcome survey. *Neurology, 60*, 1146–1150.

45. Chu, K., et al. (2001). Diffusion-weighted magnetic resonance imaging in nonconvulsive status epilepticus. *Arch Neurol, 58*, 993–998.

46. Claassen, J., et al. (2002). Predictors of functional disability and mortality after status epilepticus. *Neurology, 58*, 139–142.

47. Cock, H. R., & Schapira, A. H. (2002). A comparison of lorazepam and diazepam as initial therapy in convulsive status epilepticus. *QJM, 95*, 225–231.

48. Cohen-Gadol, A. A., Stoffman, M. R., & Spencer, D. D. (2003). Emerging surgical and radiotherapeutic techniques for treating epilepsy. *Curr Opin Neurol, 16*, 213–219.

49. Corona, T., et al. (1996). Single-day praziquantel therapy for neurocysticercosis. *N Engl J Med, 334*, 125–130.

50. Coulter, D. A., & DeLorenzo, R. J. (1999). Basic mechanisms of status epilepticus. *Adv Neurol, 79*, 725–733.

51. Davis, A. E., et al. (2004). Neurodiagnostic tests. In M. K. Bader & L. R. Littlejohns (Eds.), *AANN core curriculum for neuroscience nursing* (pp 174–189). St Louis: Saunders.

52. de Gans, J., & van de Beek, D. (2002). Dexamethasone in adults with bacterial meningitis. *N Engl J Med, 347*, 1549–1556.

53. De Jonghe, B., et al. (2002). Paresis acquired in the intensive care unit: a prospective multicenter study. *JAMA, 288*(22), 2859–2867.

54. DeAngelis, L. M. (2001). Brain tumors. *N Engl J Med, 344*, 114–123.

55. Deem, S., Lee, C. M., & Curtis, J. R. (2003). Update in nonpulmonary critical care: acquired neuromuscular disorders in the intensive care unit. *Am J Respir Crit Care Med, 168*, 735–739.

56. DeJonghe, B., et al. (1998). Acquired neuromuscular disorders in critically ill patients: a systematic review. *Intensive Care Med, 24*, 1242–1250.

57. DeJonghe, B., et al. (2002). Paresis acquired in the intensive care unit: a prospective multicenter study. *JAMA, 288*, 2859–2863.

58. Del Bene, M., & Polak, M. (2002). Neuromuscular & autoimmune disorders. In E. Barker (Ed.), *Neuroscience nursing: a spectrum of care* (2nd ed., pp 685–718). St Louis: Mosby.

59. Del Brutto, O. H. (2005). Neurocysticercosis. *Semin Neurol, 25*(3), 243–251.

60. Del Brutto, O. H., et al. (1992). Epilepsy due to neurocysticercosis: analysis of 203 patients. *Neurology, 42*, 389–392.

61. DeLisser, H. M. (2005, Jan 3). *Guillain-Barre syndrome in adults.* UpToDate Online 13.2.www.utdol.com.

62. DeLorenzo, R. J., et al. (1996). A prospective, population-based epidemiologic study of status epilepticus in Richmond, Virginia. *Neurology, 46*, 1029–1035.

63. DeLorenzo, R. J., et al. (1999). Comparison of status epilepticus with prolonged seizure episodes lasting from 10 to 29 minutes. *Epilepsia, 40*, 164–169.

64. DeVroom, H. L., et al. (2004). Nervous system tumors. In M. K. Bader & L. Littlejohns (Eds.), *AANN core curriculum for neuroscience nursing.* St Louis: Saunders.

65. Durand, M. L., et al. (1993). Acute bacterial meningitis in adults: a review of 493 episodes. *N Engl J Med, 328*, 21–28.

66. During, M. J., & Spencer, D. D. (1993). Extracellular hippocampal glutamate and spontaneous seizure in the conscious human brain. *Lancet, 341*, 1607–1610.

67. Engel, J., et al. (2003). Practice parameter: temporal lobe and localized neocortical resections for epilepsy. Report of the Quality Standards Subcommittee of the American Academy of Neurology, in Association with the American Epilepsy Society and the American Association of Neurological Surgeons. *Neurology, 60*, 538–547.

68. Estanol, B., et al. (1983). Mechanisms of hydrocephalus in cerebral cysticercosis: implications for therapy. *Neurosurgery, 13*, 119–123.

69. Fan, J. (2004). Effect of backrest position on intracranial pressure and cerebral perfusion pressure in individuals with brain injury: a systematic review. *J Neurosci Nurs, 36*(5), 278–289.

70. Fekete, T., & Quagliarello, V. (2005, Jan 7). *Clinical features and diagnosis of acute bacterial meningitis in adults.* UpToDate Online 13.2. www.utdol.com.

71. Fink, M. E. (1993). Treatment of the critically ill patient with myasthenia gravis. In A. H. Ropper (Ed.), *Neurological and neurosurgical intensive care* (3rd ed., pp 351–362). New York: Raven.

72. Fletcher, D. D., et al. (2000). Long-term outcome in patients with Guillain-Barre syndrome requiring mechanical ventilation. *Neurology, 54*, 2311–2315.

73. Fletcher, S. N., et al. (2003). Persistent neuromuscular and neurophysiologic abnormalities in long-term survivors of prolonged critical illness. *Crit Care Med, 31*, 1012–1014.

74. Fontenot, A. B. (2003). The fundamentals of variant Creutzfeldt-Jakob disease. *J Neurosci Nurs, 35*(6), 327–331.

75. Fountain, N. B. (2000). Status epilepticus: risk factors and complications. *Epilepsia, 41*, S23–S30.

76. Gaitainis, J. N., & Drislane, F. W. (2003). Status epilepticus: a review of different syndromes, their current evaluation, and treatment. *Neurologist, 9*, 61–76.

77. Gamacho-Montero, J., et al. (2001). Critical illness polyneuropathy: risk factors and clinical consequences. A cohort study in septic patients. *Intensive Care Med, 27*, 1288–1296.

78. Gandhi, D. (2004). Computed tomography and magnetic resonance angiography in cervicocranial vascular disease. *J Neuro-Ophthalmol, 24*(4), 306–314.

79. Garcia, H. H., & Del Brutto, O. H. (2003). Imaging findings in neurocysticercosis. *Acta Tropica, 87*, 71–78.

80. Garcia, H. H., et al. (1997). Albendazole therapy for neurocysticercosis: a prospective double-blind trial comparing 7 versus 14 days of treatment. *Neurology, 48*, 1421–1427.

81. Garcia, H. H., Gonzalez, A. E., & Gilman, R. H. (2003). Diagnosis, treatment and control of *Taenia solium* cysticercosis. *Curr Opin Infectious Dis, 16*, 411–419.

82. Garcia, H. H., et al. (2004). A trial of antiparasitic treatment to reduce the rate of seizures due to cerebral cysticercosis. *N Engl J Med, 350*, 249–258.

83. Garnacho-Montero, J., et al. (2005). Effect of critical illness polyneuropathy on the withdrawal from mechanical ventilation and the length of stay in septic patients. *Crit Care Med, 33*(2), 349–354.

84. Gilbert, K. L. (2000). Evaluation of an algorithm for treatment of status epilepticus in adult patients undergoing video/EEG monitoring. *J Neurosci Nurs, 32*, 101–107.

85. Gilbert, T., Wagner, M., & Halukurike, V. (2001). Use of bispectral electroencephalogram monitoring to assess neurologic status in unsedated, critically ill patients. *Crit Care Med, 29*, 1996–2000.

86. Glantz, M. J., et al. (2000). Practice parameter: anticonvulsant prophylaxis in patients with newly diagnosed brain tumors: report of the Quality Standards Subcommittee of the American Academy of Neurology. *Neurology, 54,* 1886–1893.

87. Glatzel, J., et al. (2005). Human prion diseases. *Arch Neurol, 62,* 545–552.

88. Goldenberg, I., & Matetzky, S. (2005). Nephropathy induced by contrast media: pathogenesis, risk factors and preventive strategies. *Can Med Assoc J, 172*(11), 1461–1471.

89. Gomes, J. A., et al. (2005). Glucocorticoid therapy in neurologic critical care. *Crit Care Med, 33*(6), 1214–1224.

90. Green, D. M. (2005). Weakness in the ICU: Guillain-Barre syndrome, myasthenia gravis, and critical illness polyneuropathy/myopathy. *Neurologist, 11*(6), 338–347.

91. Hachimi-Idrissi, S., et al. (2001). Mild hypothermia induced by a helmet device: a clinical feasibility study. *Resuscitation, 51,* 275–281.

92. Hahn, A. F. (1998). The Guillain-Barre syndrome. *Lancet, 352,* 635–640.

93. Hamill-Ruth, R. J., & Marohn, M. L. (1999). Evaluation of pain in the critically ill patient. *Crit Care Clin, 15*(1), 36–54.

94. Hammond, C. A. S., & Goldstein, L. B. (2006). Cough and aspiration of food and liquids due to oral-pharyngeal dysphagia. *Chest, 129,* 154–168.

95. Hansen-Flaschen, J. (2005, April 13). *Neuromuscular disorders of critical illness.* UpToDate Online 13.2. www.utdol.com.

96. Harvard Medical School Ad Hoc Committee. (1968). Report of the Ad Hoc Committee of the Harvard Medical School to Examine the Definition of Brain Death. *JAMA, 205,* 337–340.

97. Heilpern, K. L., & Lorber, B. (1996). Focal intracranial infections. *Infect Dis Clin North Am, 10,* 879–890.

98. Heit, J. A., et al. (2000). Risk factors for deep vein thrombosis and pulmonary embolism: a population-based case-control study. *Arch Intern Med, 160,* 809–815.

99. Henneman, E. A., & Karras, G. E. (2004). Determining brain death in adults: a guideline for use in critical care. *Crit Care Nurs, 24*(5), 50–56.

100. Hickey, J. V. (2003). Brain tumors. In J. V. Hickey (Ed.), *The clinical practice of neurological and neurosurgical nursing* (5th ed., pp 483–508). Philadelphia: Lippincott Williams & Wilkins.

101. Hickey, J. V. (2003). Ethical perspectives and end-of-life care. In J. V. Hickey (Ed.), *The clinical practice of neurological and neurosurgical nursing* (5th ed., pp 31–42). Philadelphia: Lippincott Williams & Wilkins.

102. Hickey, J. V. (2003). Neurodegenerative diseases. In J. V. Hickey (Ed.), *The clinical practice of neurological and neurosurgical nursing* (5th ed., pp 661–692). Philadelphia: Lippincott Williams & Wilkins.

103. Hickey, J. V. (2003). Seizures and epilepsy. In J. V. Hickey (Ed.), *The clinical practice of neurological and neurosurgical nursing* (5th ed., pp 619–640). Philadelphia: Lippincott Williams & Wilkins.

104. Hickey, J. V., & Hock, N. H. (2003). Stroke and other cerebrovascular diseases. In J. V. Hickey (Ed.), *The clinical practice of neurological and neurosurgical nursing* (5th ed., pp 559–602). Philadelphia: Lippincott Williams & Wilkins.

105. Hilbish, C. (2003). Bispectral index monitoring in the neurointensive care unit. *J Neurosci Nurs, 35*(6), 336–338.

106. Hudak, C. M., & Gallo, B. M. (1997). Quick review of neurodiagnostic testing. *Am J Nurs, 97*(7), 16CC–16FF.

107. Hughes, R. A. C., & Rees, J. H. (1997). Clinical and epidemiological features of Guillain-Barre syndrome. *J Infect Dis, 176*(suppl 2), S92–S98.

108. Hughes, R. A. C., et al. (2003). Practice parameter; immunotherapy for Guillain-Barre syndrome; report of the Quality Standards Subcommittee of the American Academy of Neurology. *Neurology, 61,* 736–740.

109. Hughes, R. A. C., et al. (2005). Supportive care for patients with Guillain-Barre syndrome. *Arch Neurol, 62,* 1194–1198.

110. Hund, E. F., et al. (1993). Intensive care management and treatment of severe Guillain-Barre syndrome. *Crit Care Med, 21,* 433–439.

111. Hypothermia After Cardiac Arrest Study Group. (2002). Mild therapeutic hypothermia to improve the neurologic outcome after cardiac arrest. *N Engl J Med, 346,* 549–556.

112. International Liaison Committee on Resuscitation. (2003). Therapeutic hypothermia after cardiac arrest; ILCOR advisory statement. *Circulation, 108,* 118–121.

113. Irani, D. N. (2003). The classic and variant forms of Creutzfeldt-Jakob disease. *Semin Clin Neuropsychiatry, 8*(1), 71–79.

114. Italian Guillain-Barre Study Group. (1996). The prognosis and main prognostic indicators of Guillain-Barre syndrome: a multicentre prospective study of 297 patients. *Brain, 119,* 2053–2061.

115. Jacobs, B. C., et al. (1998). The spectrum of antecedent infections in Guillain-Barre syndrome: a case-control study. *Neurology, 51,* 1110–1115.

116. Jane, J. A., et al. (2005). Perspectives on endoscopic transsphenoidal surgery. *Neurosurg Focus, 19*(6), 1–10.

117. Jaretzki, A., et al. (2000). Myasthenia gravis: recommendations for clinical research standards. *Neurology, 55*(1), 16–23.

118. Jeha, L. E., et al. (2003). West Nile virus infection: a new acute paralytic illness. *Neurology, 61,* 55–59.

119. Johnson, R. P., & Gluckman, S. J. (2005, March 4). *Overview of viral infections of the central nervous system.* UpToDate Online 13.2. www.utdol.com.

120. Johnson, R. T., & Gibbs, C. J. (1998). Creutzfeldt-Jakob disease and related transmissible spongiform encephalopathies. *N Engl J Med, 339,* 1994–2004.

121. Juel, V. C. (2004). Myasthenia gravis: management of myasthenic crisis and perioperative care. *Semin Neurol, 24*(1), 75–81.

122. Kaal, E. C. A., & Vecht, C. J. (2004). The management of brain edema in brain tumors. *Curr Opin Oncol, 16,* 593–600.

123. Kapur, J., & Macdonald, R. L. (1997). Rapid seizure-induced reduction of benzodiazepine and Zn sensitivity of hippocampal dentate granule cell GABA receptors. *J Neurosci, 17,* 7532–7540.

124. Kelly, D. F., et al. (1999). Propofol in the treatment of moderate and severe head injury: a randomized, prospective double-blinded pilot trial. *J Neurosurg, 90,* 1042–1052.

125. Kelso, A. R., & Cock, H. R. (2004). Advances in epilepsy. *Brit Med Bull, 72,* 135–148.

126. Kemper, E. M., et al. (2004). Modulation of the blood-brain barrier in oncology: therapeutic opportunities for the treatment of brain tumours. *Cancer Treatment Rev, 30,* 415–423.

127. Kennedy, P. G. E. (2004). Viral encephalitis: causes, differential diagnosis, and management. *J Neurol Neurosurg Psychiatry, 75* (suppl 1), i10–i15.

128. Khoshbin, S. (2003, March 6). *Clinical neurophysiology.* UpToDate Online 13.2. www.utdol.com.

129. King, D. S. (1999). Central nervous system infections; basic concepts. *Nurs Clin North Am, 34*(3), 761–771.

130. Klos, K. J., & O'Neill, P. (2004). Brain metastases. *Neurologist, 10*(1), 31–46.

131. Koehler, P. J. (1995). Use of corticosteroids in neuro-oncology. *Anticancer Drugs, 6,* 19–25.

132. Kossoff, E. H. (2005, April 15). *Neurocysticercosis.* www.emedicine.com.

133. Krishnamurthy, K. B., & Drislane, F. W. (1999). Depth of EEG suppression and outcome in barbiturate anesthetic treatment for refractory status epilepticus. *Epilepsia, 40,* 759–762.

134. Kumar, M. A., et al. (2005). The syndrome of irreversible acidosis after prolonged propofol infusion. *Neurocrit Care, 3*(3), 257–259.

135. Lasky, T., et al. (1998). The Guillain-Barre syndrome and the 1992–1993 and 1993–1994 influenza vaccines. *N Engl J Med, 339*, 1797–1803.

136. Latronico, N., Peli, E., & Botteri, M. (2005). Critical illness myopathy and neuropathy. *Curr Opin Crit Care, 11*, 126–130.

137. Lawn, N. D., et al. (2001). Anticipating mechanical ventilation in Guillain-Barre syndrome. *Arch Neurol, 58*, 893–898.

138. Lawn, N. D., & Wijdicks, E. F. (1999). Fatal Guillain-Barré syndrome. *Neurology, 52*, 635–640.

139. Lee, T., et al. (2004). Transnasal endoscopic repair of cerebrospinal fluid rhinorrhea and skull base defect: ten-year experience. *Laryngoscope, 114*, 1475–1481.

140. Lemke, D. M. (2004). Epidemiology, diagnosis, and treatment of patients with metastatic cancer and high-grade gliomas of the central nervous system. *J Infusion Nurs, 27*(4), 263–269.

141. Lin, J., & Bonventre, J. V. (2005). Prevention of radiocontrast nephropathy. *Curr Opin Nephrol Hypertens, 14*, 105–110.

142. Lindenbaum, Y., Kissel, J. T., & Mendell, J. R. (2001). Treatment approaches for Guillain-Barre syndrome and chronic inflammatory demyelinating polyradiculoneuropathy. *Neurol Clin, 19*, 187–204.

143. Lindstrom, D. R., et al. (2004). Management of cerebrospinal fluid rhinorrhea: the Medical College of Wisconsin experience. *Laryngoscope, 114*(6), 969–974.

144. Livraghi, S., Melancia, J. P., & Antunes, J. L. (2003). The management of brain abscesses. *Technical Standards Neurosurg, 28*, 285–313.

145. Logroscino, G., et al. (1997). Short-term mortality after a first episode of status epilepticus. *Epilepsia, 38*, 1344–1349.

146. Lohsl, C., & Spader, C. (2005, Aug 29). Meningitis: a new vaccine brings hope for old fears. *NurseWeek*, 16–17.

147. Lothman, E. (1990). The biochemical basis and pathophysiology of status epilepticus. *Neurology, 40*(suppl 2), 13–23.

148. Louis, D. N., & Stemmer-Rachamimov, A. O. (2000). Pathology and classification. In M. Bernstein & M. S. Berger (Eds.), *Neuro-oncology: the essentials*. New York: Thieme.

149. Lowenstein, D. H. (2005). Treatment options for status epilepticus. *Curr Opin Pharmacol, 5*, 334–339.

150. Lowenstein, D. H., & Alldredge, B. K. (1998). Status epilepticus. *N Engl J Med, 338*(14), 970–976.

151. Lowenstein, D. H., & Aminoff, M. J. (1992). Clinical and EEG features of status epilepticus in comatose patients. *Neurology, 42*, 100–104.

152. Lowenstein, D. H., Bleck, T., & Macdonald, R. L. (1999). It's time to revise the definition of status epilepticus. *Epilepsia, 40*, 120–122.

153. Lozier, A. P., et al. (2002). Ventriculostomy-related infections: a critical review of the literature. *Neurosurgery, 51*, 170–182.

154. Lyke, K. E., et al. (2001). Ventriculitis complicating use of intraventricular catheters in adult neurosurgical patients. *Clin Infect Dis, 33*, 2028–2034.

155. MacDuff, A., & Grant, I. S. (2003). Critical care management of neuromuscular disease, including long-term ventilation. *Curr Opin Crit Care, 9*, 106–112.

156. MacKnight, C. (2001). Clinical implications of bovine spongiform encephalopathy. *Clin Infect Dis, 32*, 1721–1730.

157. Maddox, T. G. (2002). Adverse reactions to contrast material: recognition, prevention, and treatment. *Am Fam Physician, 66*(7), 1229–1234.

158. Mallucci, G., & Collinge, J. (2004). Update on Creutzfeldt-Jakob disease. *Curr Opin Neurol, 17*, 641–647.

159. Mallucci, G., et al. (2003). Depleting neuronal PrP in prion infection prevents disease and reverses spongiosis. *Science, 302*, 871–874.

160. Mamelak, A. N., et al. (1995). Improved management of multiple brain abscesses: a combined surgical and medical approach. *Neurosurgery, 36*, 76–85.

161. Manno, E. M. (2003). New management strategies in the treatment of status epilepticus. *Mayo Clin Proc, 78*, 508–518.

162. Mao, V. H., et al. (2000). Endoscopic repair of cerebrospinal fluid rhinorrhea. *Otolaryngol—Head Neck Surg, 122*(1), 56–60.

163. March, K., Wellwood, J., & Arbour, R. (2004). Technology. In M. K. Bader & L. R. Littlejohns (Eds.), *AANN core curriculum for neuroscience nursing* (4th ed., pp 199–226). St Louis: Saunders.

164. Marik, P. E., & Varon, J. (2004). The management of status epilepticus. *Chest, 126*, 582–591.

165. Markand, O. N. (2003). Pearls, perils, and pitfalls in the use of the electroencephalogram. *Semin Neurol, 23*(1), 7–46.

166. Maschke, M., et al. (2004). Update of neuroimaging in infectious central nervous system disease. *Curr Opin Neurol, 17*, 475–480.

167. Mathisen, G. E., & Johnson, J. P. (1997). Brain abscess. *Clin Infect Dis, 25*, 763–768.

168. Mayer, S. (1997). Intensive care of the myasthenic patient. *Neurology, 48*(suppl 5), 70S–75S.

169. Mayer, S. A., et al. (2002). Refractory status epilepticus. *Arch Neurol, 59*, 205–210.

170. McLeod, S., et al. (2000). A comparison of the effects of two schedules of enteral phenytoin administration of serum phenytoin levels. *Austral J Neurosci, 13*(2), 5–12.

171. McNamara, J. O. (2001). Drugs effective in the therapy of the epilepsies. In J. G. Hardman, L. E. Limbird & A. G. Gilman (Eds.), *Goodman and Gilman's the pharmacologic basis of therapeutics* (10th ed., pp 521–547). New York: McGraw-Hill.

172. Medical Consultants on the Diagnosis of Death to the President's Commission for the Study of Ethical Problems in Medicine and Biobehavioral Research. (1981). Guidelines for the determination of death. *JAMA, 246*, 2184–2186.

173. Meeker, M., et al. (2005). Pupil examination: validity and clinical utility of an automated pupillometer. *J Neurosci Nurs, 37*(1), 34–40.

174. Meningitis Research Foundation. (2004, Sept 28). *Bacterial meningitis*. www.meningitis.org.

175. Merten, G. J., et al. (2004). *JAMA, 291*, 2328–2334.

176. Mitchell, W. G. (1996). Status epilepticus and acute repetitive seizures in children, adolescents, and young adults; etiology, outcome, and treatment. *Epilepsia, 37*(suppl 1), S74–S80.

177. Murthy, J. M., & Jayashree, N. T. (2004). Continuous EEG monitoring in the evaluation of non-convulsive seizures and status epilepticus. *Neurol India, 52*(4), 430–435.

178. Murthy, J. M. K., et al. (2005). Myasthenic crisis: clinical features, complications and mortality. *Neurol India, 53*(1), 37–40.

179. Myasthenia Gravis Foundation of America, I. (2001). *Facts about autoimmune myasthenia gravis for patients and families.*

180. National Brain Tumor Foundation. (2004). *Diagnosis*. www.braintumor.org/patient_info.

181. National Institute of Neurological Disorders and Stroke. (2005, July 8). *Guillain-Barre syndrome fact sheet*. www.ninds.nih.gov.

182. National Institute of Neurological Disorders and Stroke. (2005, June 10). *Meningitis and encephalitis fact sheet*. www.ninds.nih.gov.

183. National Institute of Neurological Disorders and Stroke. (2005, March 31). *Myasthenia gravis fact sheet*. www.ninds.nih.gov.

184. National Institute of Neurological Disorders and Stroke. (2005, April 22). *Neurological diagnostic tests and procedures*. www.ninds.nih.gov.

185. Nawaz, S., et al. (1998). Clinical risk associated with contrast angiography in metformin treated patients: a clinical review. *Clin Radiol, 53*(5), 342–344.

186. Newswanger, D. L., & Warren, C. R. (2004). Guillain-Barré syndrome. *Am Fam Physician, 69*, 2405–2410.

187. Newton, E. (2001, Dec 10). *Myasthenia gravis*. eMedicine. www.emedicine.com.

188. Ong, S., et al. (2002). Neurocysticercosis in radiographically imaged seizure patients in U.S. emergency departments. *Emerg Infect Dis, 8*, 608–613.

189. Pardridge, W. M. (2002). Targeting neurotherapeutic agents through the blood-brain barrier. *Arch Neurol, 59*, 35–40.

190. Parini, S. M. (2002). The meningitis mind-bender. *Nurs Management, 33*(8), 21–26.

191. Pasero, C., & McCaffery, M. (2002). Pain in the critically ill. *Am J Nurs, 102*(1), 59–60.

192. Peterson, K. (2001). Brain tumors. *Neurol Clin, 19*(4), 887–902.

193. Pfausler, B., et al. (2003). Treatment of staphylococcal ventriculitis associated with external cerebrospinal fluid drains: a prospective randomized trial of intravenous compared with intraventricular vancomycin therapy. *J Neurosurg, 98*, 1040–1044.

194. Pfister, H., Feiden, W., & Einhaupl, K. (1993). Spectrum of complications during bacterial meningitis in adults: results of a prospective clinical study. *Arch Neurol, 50*, 575–581.

195. Piscatelli, N., Schiff, D., & Batchelor, T. (2003, Sept 22). *Classification of brain tumors*. UpToDate Online 13.2. www.utdol.com.

196. Plasma Exchange/Sandoglobulin Guillain-Barré Trial Group. (1997). Randomised trial of plasma exchange, intravenous immunoglobulin and combined treatments in Guillain-Barre syndrome. *Lancet, 349*, 225–230.

197. Polak, M., et al. (2004). Neuromuscular disorders of the nervous system. In M. K. Bader & L. R. Littlejohns (Eds.), *AANN core curriculum for neuroscience nursing* (4th ed., pp 757–780). St Louis: Saunders.

198. Polednak, A. P. (1996). Interpretation of secular increases in incidence rates for primary brain tumors in Connecticut adults, 1965–1988. *Neuroepidemiology, 15*, 51.

199. Polk, C., et al. (2004). Perioperative surgical considerations. In M. K. Bader & L. Littlejohns (Eds.), *AANN core curriculum for neuroscience nursing* (4th ed., pp 227–245). St Louis: Saunders.

200. Poon, W. S., Ng, S., & Wai, S. (1998). CSF antibiotic prophylaxis for neurosurgical patients with ventriculostomy: a randomised study. *Acta Neurochir Suppl, 71*, 91–93.

201. Prather, S. H., et al. (2003). Caring for the patient undergoing transsphenoidal surgery in the acute care setting: an alternative to critical care. *J Neurosci Nurs, 35*(5), 270–275.

202. Proulx, N., et al. (2005). Delays in the administration of antibiotics are associated with mortality from adult acute bacterial meningitis. *Q J Med, 98*, 291–298.

203. Psarros, T. G., Krumerman, J., & Coimbra, C. (2003). Endoscopic management of supratentorial ventricular neurocysticercosis: case series and review of the literature. *Minimally Invasive Neurosurg, 46*(6), 331–334.

204. Quagliarello, V., & Scheld, W. M. (1997). Treatment of bacterial meningitis. *N Engl J Med, 336*, 708–716.

205. Quality Standards Subcommittee of the American Academy of Neurology. (1995). Practice parameters for determining brain death in adults. *Neurology, 45*, 1012–1014.

206. Qureshi, H. U., et al. (2002). Predictors of mortality in brain abscess. *J Pakistan Med Assoc, 52*(3), 111–116.

207. Rees, J. H., et al. (1998). Epidemiological study of Guillain-Barre syndrome in south east England. *J Neurol Neurosurg Psychiatry, 64*, 74–77.

208. Rihal, C. S., et al. (2002). Incidence and prognostic importance of acute renal failure after percutaneous coronary intervention. *Circulation, 105*, 2259–2264.

209. Rogers, D. O. (2003). Cerebrovascular complications in cancer patients. *Neurol Clin, 21*(1), 167–192.

210. Roos, K., & Tunkel, A. (1997). Acute bacterial meningitis in children and adults. In W. M. Scheld & D. T. Durack (Eds.), *Infections of the central nervous system* (2nd ed., pp 335–402). Philadelphia: Lippincott-Raven.

211. Ropper, A. H. (1992). The Guillain-Barre syndrome. *N Engl J Med, 326*, 1130–1135.

212. Ropper, A. H., & Kehne, S. M. (1985). Guillain-Barre syndrome: management of respiratory failure. *Neurology, 35*, 1662–1665.

213. Rudis, M. I., et al. (1996). Economic impact of prolonged motor weakness complicating neuromuscular blockade in the intensive care unit. *Crit Care Med, 24*(10), 1749–1756.

214. Sanchez-Izquierdo-Riera, J. A., et al. (1998). Propofol versus midazolam: safety and efficacy for sedating the severe trauma patient. *Anesth Analg, 86*, 1219–1224.

215. Sanko, J. S. (2004). Aspiration assessment and prevention in critically ill enterally fed patients. *Gastroenterol Nurs, 27*(6), 279–285.

216. Sater, R. A., & Rostami, A. (1998). Treatment of Guillain-Barré syndrome with intravenous immunoglobulin. *Neurology, 51* (6 suppl 5), S9–S15.

217. Schabet, M. (1999). Epidemiology of primary CNS lymphoma. *J Neurooncol, 43*, 199.

218. Schacter, S. C. (2005, May 5). *Overview of the management of epilepsy in adults*. UpToDate Online 13.2. www.utdol.com.

219. Scheld, W. M., et al. (2002). Pathophysiology of bacterial meningitis: mechanism(s) of neuronal injury. *J Infect Dis, 186*(suppl 2), S225–S232.

220. Schlosser, R. J., & Bolger, W. E. (2002). Nasal cerebrospinal fluid leaks. *J Otolaryngol, 31*(suppl 1), S28–S37.

221. Schumacher, G. E., et al. (1991). Test performance characteristics of the serum phenytoin concentration (SPC): the relationship between SPC and patient response. *Ther Drug Monit, 13*, 318–324.

222. Schwendimann, R. N., Burton, E., & Minagar, A. (2005). Management of myasthenia gravis. *Am J Therapeutics, 12*, 262–268.

223. Seydoux, C., & Francioli, P. (1992). Bacterial brain abscesses: factors influencing mortality and sequelae. *Clin Infect Dis, 15*, 394–398.

224. Sheth, R. D. (2002). Epilepsy surgery; presurgical evaluation. *Neurol Clin N Am, 20*, 1195–1215.

225. Sheth, R. D., & Gidal, B. E. (1998). Refractory status epilepticus: response to ketamine. *Neurology, 51*, 1765–1766.

226. Shorvon, S. (2001). The management of status epilepticus. *J Neurol Neurosurg Psychiatry, 70*, II22–II27.

227. Shulman, D. L., et al. (2002). Neurocysticercosis: nursing perspectives. *J Neurosci Nurs, 34*, 237–241.

228. Sills, A. K. (2005). Current treatment approaches to surgery for brain metastases. *Neurosurgery, 57*(5), S4-24–S24-32.

229. Simon, R. P. (1985). Physiologic consequences of status epilepticus. *Epilepsia, 26*(suppl 1), S58–S66.

230. Singer, I., Oster, J. R., & Fishman, L. (1997). The management of diabetes insipidus in adults. *Arch Intern Med, 157*(12), 1293–1301.

231. Sotelo, J., & Del Brutto, O. H. (2002). Review of neurocysticercosis. *Neurosurg Focus, 12*, 1–7.

232. Southwick, F. S. (2003, Sept 11). *Brain abscess*. UpToDate Online 13.2. www.utdol.com.

233. Southwick, F. S. (2005, Nov 30). *Pathogenesis, clinical manifestations, and diagnosis of brain abscess*. UpToDate Online 14.1. www.utdol.com.

234. Southwick, F. S. (2005, Dec 21). *Treatment and prognosis of brain abscess*. UpToDate Online 14.1. www.utdol.com.

235. Stecker, M. M. (2005, May 5). *Management of status epilepticus in adults*. UpToDate Online 13.2. www.utdol.com.

236. Stecker, M. M., Kramer, T. H., Raps, E. C., et al. (1998). Treatment of refractory status epilepticus with propofol: clinical and pharmacokinetic findings. *Epilepsia, 39*, 18–26.

237. Sullivan, J. (2005). Lumbar subarachnoid catheter insertion (assist) for cerebral spinal fluid pressure monitoring and drainage. In D. J. L. M. Wiegand & K. K. Carlson (Eds.), *AACN procedure manual for critical care* (5th ed., pp 748–755). St Louis: Elsevier Saunders.

238. Sullivan, J., Seem, D. L., & Chabalewski, F. (1999). Determining brain death. *Crit Care Nurs, 19*, 37–46.

239. Sullivan, J., & Severance-Lossin, L. (2005). Determination of death. In D. J. L.-M. Weigand & K. K. Carlson (Eds.), *AACN procedure manual for critical care* (5th ed., pp 1174–1182). St Louis: Elsevier Saunders.

240. Sullivan, J., & Severance-Lossin, L. (2005). Intraventricular catheter insertion (assist), monitoring, care, troubleshooting, and removal. In D. J. L.-M. Wiegand & K. K. Carlson (Eds.), *AACN procedure manual for critical care* (5th ed., pp 730–737). St Louis: Elsevier Saunders.

241. Summers, D. M., et al. (2004). The pulvinar sign in variant Creutzfeldt-Jakob disease. *Arch Neurol, 61*, 446–447.

242. Sundberg, G., Nordstrom, D. H., & Soderstrom, S. (1988). Complications due to prolonged ventricular fluid pressure recording. *Brit J Neurosurg, 2*, 485–495.

243. Sunshine, J. (2004). CT, MR imaging, and MR angiography in the evaluation of patients with acute stroke. *J Vasc Interv Radiol, 15*, S47–S55.

244. Surawicz, T. S., et al. (1999). Descriptive epidemiology of primary brain and CNS tumors: results from the Central Brain Tumor Registry of the United States, 1990–1994. *Neurooncol, 1*, 14.

245. Suresh, T. N., et al. (2001). Intracranial haemorrhage resulting from unsuspected choriocarcinoma metastasis. *Neurol India, 49* (3), 231–236.

246. Tablan, O. C., et al. (2004). Guidelines for preventing healthcare-associated pneumonia, 2003. *Morb Mortal Weekly Rep, 53*(RR-3), 1–36.

247. Takayanagui, O. M., & Jardim, E. (1992). Therapy for neurocysticercosis. Comparison between albendazole and praziquantel. *Arch Neurol, 49*, 290–294.

248. Task Force of the American College of Critical Care Medicine of the Society of Critical Care Medicine et al. (2002). Clinical practice guidelines for the sustained use of sedatives and analgesics in the critically ill adult. *Am J Health Syst Pharm, 59*, 150–178.

249. Tattevin, P., et al. (2003). Bacterial brain abscesses: a retrospective study of 94 patients admitted to an intensive care unit (1980 to 1999). *Am J Med, 115*, 143–148.

250. Tatum, W. O., Alavi, A., & Stecker, M. M. (1994). Technetium-99m-HMPAO SPECT in partial status epilepticus. *J Nucl Med, 35*, 1087–1094.

251. Tauber, M. G., Khayam-Bashi, H., & Sande, M. A. (1985). Effects of ampicillin and glucocorticoids on brain water content, cerebrospinal fluid pressure, and cerebrospinal fluid lactate levels in experimental pneumococcal meningitis. *J Infect Dis, 151*, 28–34.

252. Tennila, A., et al. (2000). Early signs of critical illness polyneuropathy in ICU patients with systemic inflammatory response syndrome or sepsis. *Intensive Care Med, 26*, 1360–1363.

253. Thanvi, B. R., & Lo, T. C. N. (2004). Update on myasthenia gravis. *Postgrad Med J, 80*, 690–700.

254. Thomas, C., et al. (1997). Myasthenic crisis: clinical features, mortality, complications and risk factors for prolonged intubation. *Neurology, 48*(5), 1253–1260.

255. Thompson, H. (1998). *Lumbar drain management*. Chicago: American Association of Neuroscience Nurses.

256. Towne, A. R., et al. (1994). Determinants of mortality in status epilepticus. *Epilepsia, 35*, 27–34.

257. Treiman, D. M., et al. (1998). A comparison of four treatments for generalized convulsive status epilepticus: Veterans Affairs Status Epilepticus Cooperative Study Group. *N Engl J Med, 339*, 792–798.

258. Treiman, D. M., Meyers, P. D., Walton, N. Y., et al. (1996). Status epilepticus. *Baillieres Clin Neurol, 5*, 821–839.

259. Tunkel, A. R., et al. (2004). Practice guidelines for the management of bacterial meningitis. *Clin Infect Dis, 39*, 1267–1284.

260. Tyler, K. L., & Anderson, C. A. (2005, May 11). *Creutzfeldt-Jakob disease*. UpToDate. www.utdol.com.

261. Tyler, K. L., & Anderson, C. A. (2005, April 22). *Variant Creutzfeldt-Jakob disease*. UpToDate. www.utdol.com.

262. Van de Beek, D., et al. (2004). Steroids in adults with acute bacterial meningitis: a systematic review. *Lancet: Infect Dis, 4*, 139–143.

263. van den Bent, M. J. (2001). The diagnosis and management of brain metastases. *Curr Opin Neurol, 14*, 717–723.

264. van den Burghe, G. H., et al. (2001). Intensive insulin therapy in the surgical intensive care unit. *N Engl J Med, 345*, 1359–1362.

265. Vandemark, M. V., et al. (2004). Infectious and autoimmune processes. In M. K. Bader & L. R. Littlejohns (Eds.), *AANN core curriculum for neuroscience nursing* (4th ed., pp 619–672). St Louis: Saunders.

266. Vecht, C. J., et al. (1994). Dose-effect relationship of dexamethasone on Karnofsky performance in metastatic brain tumors: a randomized study of doses of 4, 8, and 16 mg per day. *Neurology, 44*, 675–680.

267. Vespa, P. M., et al. (1999). Increased incidence and impact of nonconvulsive and convulsive seizures after traumatic brain injury as detected by continuous electroencephalographic monitoring. *J Neurosurg, 91*, 750–760.

268. Wallace, M. (1998). Creutzfeldt-Jakob disease: assessment and management update. *J Gerontol Nurs, 25*, 17–24.

269. Walsh, D. C., & Kakkar, A. K. (2001). Thromboembolism in brain tumors. *Curr Opin Pulm Med, 7*, 326–331.

270. Warwick, J. M. (2004). Imaging of brain function using SPECT. *Metab Brain Dis, 19*, 113–123.

271. Waterhouse, E. J., & DeLorenzo, R. J. (2001). Status epilepticus in older patients: epidemiology and treatment options. *Drugs Aging, 18*, 133–142.

272. Wen, P. Y., & Marks, P. W. (2002). Medical management of patients with brain tumors. *Curr Opin Oncol, 14*, 299–307.

273. Whitley, R. J. (1990). Viral encephalitis. *N Engl J Med, 323*, 242–250.

274. Whitley, R. J., & Gnann, J. W. (2002). Viral encephalitis: familiar infections and emerging pathogens. *Lancet, 359*, 507–514.

275. Wijdicks, E. (2000). Acute bacterial infections of the central nervous system. In E. Wijdicks (Ed.), *Neurologic catastrophes in the emergency department* (pp 183–194). Boston: Butterworth Heinemann.

276. Wijdicks, E. F. M. (2001). The diagnosis of brain death. *New Engl J Med, 344*(16), 1215–1221.

277. Wilson, R. F., Dente, C., & Tyburski, J. G. (2001). The nutritional management of patients with head injuries. *Neurol Res, 23*(2–3), 121–128.

278. Winer, J. B. (2002). Treatment of Guillain-Barre syndrome. *Q J Med, 95*, 717–721.

279. Wintermark, M., et al. (2005). Comparative overview of brain perfusion imaging techniques. *Stroke, 36*, e83–e99.

280. Witt, N. J., et al. (1991). Peripheral nerve function in sepsis and multiple organ failure. *Chest, 99*, 176–181.

281. Wittbrodt, E. T. (1997). Drugs and myasthenia gravis; an update. *Arch Intern Med, 157*, 399–408.

282. Wojner, A. W., El-Mitwalli, A., & Alexandrov, A. V. (2002). Effect of head positioning on intracranial blood flow velocities in acute ischemic stroke: a pilot study. *Crit Care Nurs Q, 24*(4), 57–66.

283. Working Group on Status Epilepticus. (1993). Treatment of convulsive status epilepticus: recommendations of the Epilepsy

Foundation of America's working group on status epilepticus. *JAMA, 270,* 854–859.

284. Xiao, F., et al. (2005). Brain abscess: clinical experience and analysis of prognostic factors. *Surg Neurol, 63,* 442–450.

285. Yamamoto, L., & Texas, V. (2004). Guillain-Barre syndrome versus electrolyte imbalances; comorbidities that complicate the neurologic examination. *Top Emerg Med, 26*(3), 186–200.

286. Yen, P. T., Chan, S. T., & Huang, T. S. (1995). Brain abscess: with special reference to otolaryngologic sources of infection. *Otolaryngol—Head Neck Surg, 113,* 15–20.

287. Ziai, W. C., & Geocadin, R. G. (2001). Central nervous system infections; a critical care approach. *Curr Neurol Neurosci Rep, 1,* 577–586.

UNIT 6

GASTROINTESTINAL

CHAPTER 26 Gastrointestinal Bleeding

Michael W. Day

Bleeding into the gastrointestinal (GI) tract is a common problem found in critically ill patients; it has many sources. The bleeding may be caused by primary pathophysiology in the GI tract (e.g., gastric or peptic ulcers) or, less commonly, develop secondary to pathology outside of the GI tract (e.g., ovarian cancer perforating into the bowel). The source of the bleeding may be simple, short-term, and self-limiting (e.g., Mallory-Weiss tear at the esophagogastric junction caused by repeated retching). GI bleeding may also represent a life-threatening hemorrhage (e.g., ruptured esophageal varix). Several different causes of GI bleeding may be found in the same patient. Whatever the causes, GI bleeding can have a negative impact on the patient's mortality and morbidity.

Although GI bleeding is rarely the cause for a hospitalization, it does carry a mortality rate of approximately 10% in patients hospitalized for its treatment.[22] Although the mortality rate is significant, patients rarely die from the GI bleed; instead, a comorbidity, organ system dysfunction, or sepsis is usually the cause of death. The mortality rate associated with upper GI bleeding is about 4% in young patients but may be as high as 15% in older adult patients.[4]

Sources of GI bleeding can be characterized as either upper gastrointestinal (i.e., esophagus, stomach, and duodenum) or lower gastrointestinal (i.e., jejunum, ileum, colon, and rectum). The division between the upper and lower GI tract is considered the ligament of Treitz, which separates the duodenum and jejunum. Upper GI bleeding is more common[23] and is usually caused by peptic ulcers or esophageal and gastric varices. Bleeding from the lower GI tract represents about 20% of GI bleeds.[4]

Patients at the highest risk for GI bleeding usually have some pathology in the GI system. Some of these sources of bleeding may not cause large blood loss until they are significantly advanced (e.g., colon cancer). Other sources of bleeding (e.g., esophageal varices) are usually heralded by some identifiable history (e.g., history of chronic, excessive alcohol use) or symptoms (e.g., diarrhea with inflammatory bowel disease). However, one group of critically ill patients may develop GI bleeding in response to their medical condition—the stress ulcer. Stress ulcer formation has been well documented in the critically ill; a number of methods have been used over the years to prevent its occurrence, including antacids to histamine-2 blockade. The advent of proton pump inhibitors (PPI) has added a significant tool in the prevention of stress ulcers and is more effective than histamine-2 blockade.[2]

APPLIED PHYSIOLOGY AND PATHOPHYSIOLOGY

The primary functions of the GI tract include absorption of nutrients (primarily small bowel) and water (large bowel), elimination of waste (as stool),[18] and immunity (gut-associated lymphatic tissue [GALT]).[44] To support the multiple functions of the GI tract, it is richly supplied with blood vessels along its entire length and is therefore subject to many sources of bleeding.

Upper GI bleeding may be caused by a variety of disease processes. It may be as simple as a Mallory-Weiss tear of the esophagus or as complex as varices of the esophagus or stomach, or even cancer. However, upper GI bleeding is often caused by acid disease processes occurring in the esophagus (gastroesophageal reflux disease [GERD]), the stomach (gastritis, erosions, and ulcer formation), or the duodenum (ulcer formation).

A Mallory-Weiss tear is a laceration of the gastroesophageal junction mucosa that occurs with violent retching or vomiting. It is most often self-limiting, but occasionally requires intervention, such as endoscopy, for simple repair.

On the other hand, esophageal and gastric varices usually represent a complex life-threatening condition. Esophageal and gastric varices are caused by the same pathology—liver disease, which increases the back pressure into the portal vein, resulting in dilation of the veins that drain from the esophagus, stomach, and the entire GI tract. Chapter 27 provides more comprehensive information about liver dysfunction and failure. When varices develop, they enlarge at a rate of 4% to 10% a year, increasing the likelihood that they will begin to bleed over time.[15] Like all veins, the veins in the esophagus and stomach are meant to be a low-pressure system, draining through the portal vein and into the liver. Damage to the liver's blood vessels by a variety of diseases (such as chronic alcohol ingestion, chemical exposure, and hepatitis) increases resistance to the flow of blood into the portal vein (Figure 26-1). This increased resistance causes back pressure transmitted into the esophagus and gastric veins, causing dilation. Over time, if the pressure becomes too great, the veins will leak or burst, dumping blood directly into the esophagus or stomach, which occurs in approximately 20% of patients with cirrhosis.[35] The stomach usually reacts to large amounts of blood by reversing peristalsis, causing vomiting.

With acid disease processes, several types of injury may occur. Normally, the lower esophageal sphincter (LES) relaxes approximately 1 to 2 hours after eating. Chyme, the semi-fluid mass of partially digested food, may be occasionally refluxed up into the esophagus by the peristalsis of the stomach. However, the acid in the chyme is usually neutralized by saliva and cleared back into the stomach by peristalsis, often within a couple of minutes. In the case of GERD, patients tend to have reduced LES pressures. Coupled with increased abdominal pressure (e.g., coughing, lifting, bending forward) or a recumbent position after eating, it is much more likely the chyme will be refluxed into the esophagus. A number of structural abnormalities of the esophagogastric junction (e.g., hiatal hernia or incompetent esophagogastric sphincter) may also be present and contribute to the formation of GERD.[20] Over time, the esophagus, subjected to repeated exposure to the stomach acids, develops an erosive esophagitis that can progress into ulcers and may potentially bleed.[17]

When food enters the stomach, it is subjected to acids and pepsin, converting it into the semi-fluid chyme by breaking down food fibers and protein, respectively. The secretion of the stomach acids is inhibited by prostaglandins. Normally, the mucosal barrier of the stomach protects the gastric mucosa from the digestive actions of both pepsin and acid, as the chyme is digested. Gastritis is caused by any mechanism interfering with this normal process. One example of such a mechanism is seen with the ingestion of nonsteroidal antiinflammatory drugs (NSAIDs), which inhibit prostaglandins. This inhibition, in turn, allows for increased acid formation, gut inflammation, and an increased risk of bleeding.[24] Another chemical causing chronic inflammation is ethanol (alcohol). As the gastritis continues, the same processes described previously may lead to gastric ulcer formation. A common example is the pathogen *Helicobacter pylori*, which adheres to the mucosal-secreting cells in the stomach, causing a chronic gastritis that can lead to gastric mucosal atrophy.[3,17,34,49]

As seen with gastritis, *H. pylori* is also a major cause of duodenal ulcers. A number of additional factors affecting acid and pepsin formation and control are also implicated in the formation of duodenal ulcers, which are more common than gastric ulcers. A duodenal ulcer may heal spontaneously, but will usually recur over time. If the ulcer is large enough to erode into the base of the duodenum, blood vessels are likely to be breached, allowing blood to enter the GI tract, where it may flow retrograde into the stomach to be vomited or passed in the stool (Figure 26-2).

A type of ulcer common to critically ill patients is the stress ulcer.[31] Stress ulcers are caused by the hypoperfusion and ischemia of the GI tract inherent with multisystem trauma, hemorrhage (from a source other than the GI tract), and sepsis. In addition, stress ulcers have been related to emotional distress. Most stress ulcers form in the stomach or duodenum. The term *Cushing's ulcer* has been applied to stress ulcers found in patients with brain surgery or head trauma. The term *Curling's ulcer* has been applied to stress ulcers found in patients suffering from major burn injuries. Regardless of the cause, the result is an ulcer eroding into the base of the GI tract, opening a blood vessel and allowing free flow of blood into the gut (Figure 26-3).[34]

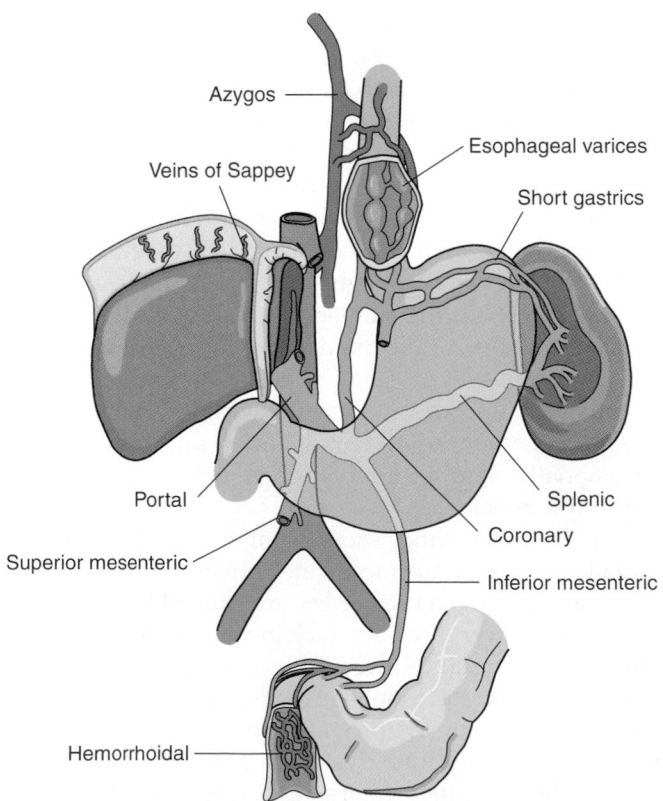

Azygos

Veins of Sappey

Esophageal varices

Short gastrics

Portal

Splenic

Superior mesenteric

Coronary

Inferior mesenteric

Hemorrhoidal

⬆FIGURE 26-1 Varices related to portal hypertension.

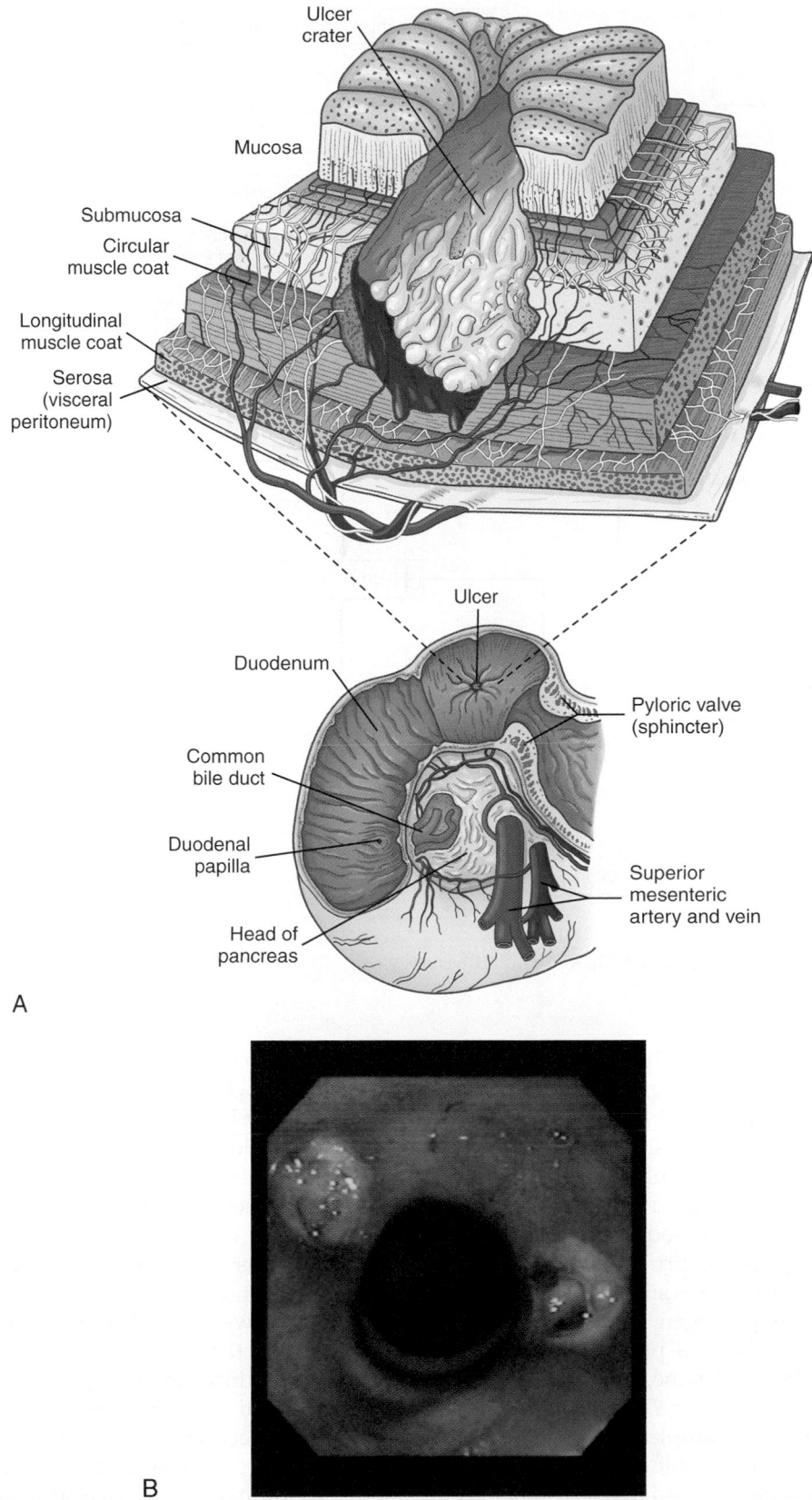

FIGURE 26-2 Duodenal ulcer. **A,** Deep ulceration in the duodenal wall extending as a crater through the entire mucosa and into the muscle layers. **B,** Duodenal ulcer. Visualized on endoscopy.

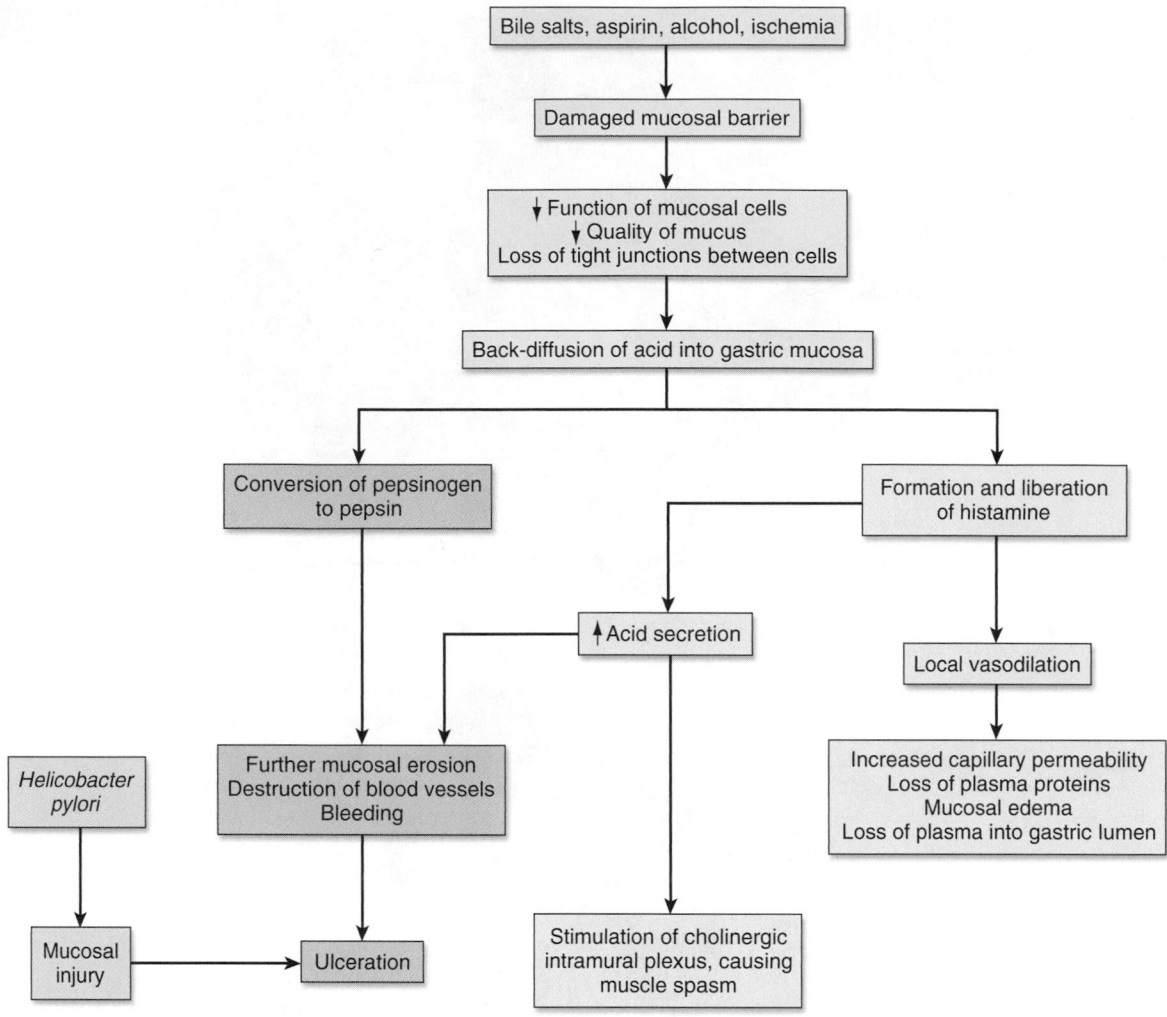

◆FIGURE 26-3 Pathophysiology of gastric ulcer formation.

Cancers of the upper GI tract may cause small amounts of blood loss but usually present with other symptoms before significant blood loss occurs. Patients with cancers of the esophagus and stomach usually have symptoms that mimic GERD and ulcer disease, with an added feature of significantly rapid weight loss.

As with upper GI bleeding, blood loss in the lower GI tract is caused by many disease processes. The bleeding may be caused by chronic diseases such as ulcerative colitis. Unfortunately, a new pathogen, *Escherichia coli* 0157: H7, has emerged. It produces a potent cytotoxin that causes damage to the large intestine, leading to a rapidly evolving bloody diarrhea.[7] Lower GI bleeding may also be caused by something as simple as internal hemorrhoids in the rectum from chronic straining to have a bowel movement or as complex and lethal as a colorectal cancer.

Mucosal angiodysplasia, a degenerative or congenital arteriovenous malformation of the GI vasculature, is the most common cause of lower GI bleeding[48,51,54] and may be confused with bleeding from a diverticulum.[54] The source of such bleeding may be very difficult to identify because of its location (i.e., middle of the jejunum), small size, and the small volume and subacute nature of the bleeding (rather than massive and acute).[54]

In chronic disease of the lower GI tract, such as Crohn's disease (also known as regional enteritis) and ulcerative colitis, the colon is the usual source of bleeding. The small bowel is implicated in lower GI bleeding in about 10% of the cases.[31] Crohn's disease is caused by an idiopathic inflammatory process that may affect the GI tract from the mouth to the anus. It is commonly confined to the ileocecal area, where the ileum merges into the colon, and the colon itself. The disease causes fissures, both longitudinal and transverse, to develop and usually involves the entire intestinal wall in the affected tissue. The fissures, caused by the continuing inflammation, create a "cobblestone" appearance, with areas of edema.

Ulcerative colitis, also an idiopathic inflammatory disease, is confined to the mucosal surface of the lower GI tract, usually of the distal colon (sigmoid and rectum). The inflammation affects just the mucosal surface and usually does not penetrate through the intestinal wall. However, when severe, it can cause ulcerations, abscesses, and perforations that may produce large, bloody diarrheal stools.

Even though *E. coli* 0157:H7 has been recognized as a significant pathogen since 1982, it still accounts for an estimated 73,000 cases of infection and 61 deaths per year in the United States.[7] It is typically associated with eating undercooked beef but can also be spread by person-to-person contact from poor hand washing. The bacteria cause an inflammatory process in the colon that leads to sloughing of tissue in a bloody, mucoid diarrhea. The disease process is usually self-limiting, if the patient is relatively healthy. However, the young (younger than 5 years of age) and older adults or those with comorbidities are at significantly greater risk for developing a more serious disease, hemolytic uremic syndrome, which causes massive red blood cell destruction and acute renal failure.[7]

An additional cause of lower GI bleeding is diverticular disease. Diverticula, multiple small pouches in the colon, are found in about 5% to 10% of the population but are usually asymptomatic, a disease referred to as diverticulosis.[34] When the diverticula become filled with stool and develop inflammation, they may cause pain and bleeding, referred to as diverticulitis.[34] An additional source of lower GI bleeding is hemorrhoids. While GI bleeding related to esophageal and gastric varices is widely recognized, hemorrhoids may also be dilated from portal hypertension and are also subject to leakage and rupture, although much less frequently. In addition, hemorrhoids may simply be caused by chronic straining to have a bowel movement and may be of little consequence, other than the associated pain.

PREVENTION

Prevention of GI bleeding usually focuses on the underlying pathology, rather than the bleeding itself. Examples of prevention strategies would include colorectal screening for occult blood and use of proton pump inhibitors (PPIs) by critically ill patients.[33] Additionally, patients with a known personal or family history or risk for a specific disease may be routinely assessed with endoscopy to catch the disease state early, such as in colon cancer.[30]

Another cause of GI bleeding is GERD, which has been the focus of many studies and can be prevented by several medications. Reflux acid diseases have been treated with antacids and histamine-2 blockers, and, most currently, PPIs have emerged as the treatment of choice.[27] In addition, new therapies, such as gastrin vaccine and gamma-aminobutyric acid (GABA) agonists, are on the horizon that may add new dimensions of treatment.[37]

The ubiquitous use of NSAIDs has had a major impact on the development of upper GI bleeding, with their use being responsible for as many as 10% of upper GI bleeds.[24] These drugs are also recognized to be associated with lower GI pathology (i.e., gut inflammation and bleeding).[24] While the cyclooxygenase 2 (COX-2) inhibitors provided a significant decrease in the incidence of GI bleeding when compared to NSAIDs,[49] the increased number of cardiovascular deaths related to COX-2 inhibitors has rendered this advantage over NSAIDs a moot point. Even low-dose aspirin taken for its cardioprotective effect promotes an increased incidence of GI bleeding, with 10% to 15% of hospital admissions for GI bleeding associated with long-term, low-dose aspirin use.[49] Despite current recommendations to substitute clopidogrel for aspirin in patients with aspirin-induced gastric bleeding, clopidogrel (Plavix) had a higher bleeding rate when compared to aspirin with esomeprazole (Nexium), a PPI.[8] Goldstein, Huang, Amer, et al. also found that adding a PPI for patients taking NSAIDs significantly decreased the incidence of bleeding episodes.[11] Medications used to treat gastrointestinal bleeding are outlined in the Medication table on p. 742.

Helicobacter pylori is identified as a significant cause of both gastric and duodenal ulcers, but because it is so prevalent, general preventive therapy is not likely to have an effect on ulcer formation in the general population. However, eradication of *H. pylori* should be considered if a patient has additional risk factors (e.g., chronic NSAID usage or a history of ulcers).[49]

With esophageal and gastric varices, prevention is directed to stopping both the initial and subsequent bleeding episodes. Surgical shunting of blood away from the liver (portocaval shunts) has been effective in preventing the initial bleeding episode, but this procedure is associated with greater operative mortality and increased encephalopathy.[34] Although endoscopic banding may prevent bleeding, there are not enough data to recommend this procedure for all patients. Beta blockade has been shown to substantially decrease both the risk of bleeding and the number of bleeding-related deaths, by allowing alpha-adrenergic constriction of the mesenteric arterioles, reducing portal venous flow.[29,46] However, beta blockers must be taken continually or the varices will rebleed.[1] Long-acting nitrates, which cause systemic vasodilation, may be useful for those unable to tolerate beta blockade or

MEDICATIONS USED IN GASTROINTESTINAL BLEEDING

MEDICATION	ACTIONS	DOSAGE	SPECIAL CONSIDERATIONS
Esomeprazole (Nexium)	Proton pump inhibitor; reduces gastric acid secretion	20–40 mg PO per day for 4–8 weeks; maintenance dose of 20 mg PO per day	Should not be taken more than 6 months No more than 20 mg/day in patient with severe hepatic failure Give 1 hr before meals
Isosorbide mononitrate (Imdur)	Decreases blood pressure and subsequent gastrointestinal intravascular pressure	20 mg twice a day with approximately 7 hr between doses; 30–120 mg of extended-release tablets once a day	*Significant* hypotension possible if used with sildenafil, tadalafil, or vardenafil May cause postural hypotension

Propranolol (Inderal)	Decreases blood pressure and subsequent gastrointestinal intravascular pressure	Initially, 80 mg PO divided into two doses or one extended-release form
		Maintenance dose of 120–240 mg daily or 120–160 mg of extended-release form
			Use with caution in patients receiving:
			    Calcium channel blockers
			    Cardiac glycosides
			Avoid with haloperidol
			Contraindicated in patients with bronchial asthma, or with heart rates less than 60 beats/min

Omeprazole (Prilosec)	Proton pump inhibitor; blocks formation of gastric acid by competitive binding of secretory surface of gastric parietal cells	20–40 mg daily for most conditions; doses of 120 mg tid given in patients with pathologic hypersecretory conditions (e.g., Zollinger-Ellison syndrome)	Avoid giving with medications requiring low gastric pH (e.g., ampicillin, iron, ketoconazole) because poor absorption may occur
Octreotide (Sandostatin)	Decreases both splanchnic blood flow and portal vein pressure, allowing coagulation to take place	25–50 mcg/hr continuous IV infusion for up to 5 days	May cause bradycardia; dysrhythmias; glucose, fluid, and electrolyte imbalances
Vasopressin (Pitressin)	Decreases bleeding from varices by systemic vasoconstriction, which also decreases splanchnic blood flow and portal vein pressure	0.4 unit/min continuous IV infusion up to 1 unit/min	May cause hypertension and myocardial ischemia

those who do not respond to it.[15] Isosorbide mononitrate, when compared to propranolol, was equally effective in decreasing bleeding events and mortality, but had a worse long-term survival rate.[15] Various combinations of therapy have been studied, and a variety of findings were produced. Sarin et al. found that in patients with noncirrhosis varices, band ligation was more effective than a combination of beta blockade and nitrates in preventing the initial bleeding episode.[40] Two additional studies confirmed that band ligation was more effective than beta blockade in patients with cirrhosis.[19,28] Adding beta blockade to band ligation provides no additional decrease in bleeding episodes, but does decrease the recurrence of the varices.[41] On the other hand, one study using endoscopy to prevent an initial bleeding episode had to be stopped prematurely because of a significant (60%) bleeding rate, identified by the authors as being iatrogenic.[47] These considerations are discussed in the Research Utilization box on p. 743.

♦ RESEARCH UTILIZATION

Use of Beta-Blocker Therapy in Patients With Cirrhosis

CLINICAL ISSUE

The authors provide a detailed analysis of the literature regarding beta-blocker therapy in patients with cirrhosis.

SUMMARY

The authors provide a detailed description of the effects of this class of medications on portal hypertension, the usual causative agent of gastric and esophageal variceal bleeding. The authors cite multiple studies that have demonstrated the efficacy of beta blockers in reducing portal hypertension and thus decreasing both the incidence and the severity of gastric and esophageal variceal bleeding. In addition, the authors outline the complications associated with such therapy, including medication side effects that contribute to a significant failure rate.

APPLICATION

The authors conclude with recommendations for current therapy using various beta blockers.

NEED FOR FURTHER STUDY

Future studies are needed to evaluate some of the newer beta blockers and determine how they may be used to prevent variceal bleeding.

Talwalkar, J. A., & Kamath, P. S. (2004). An evidence medicine approach to beta-blocker therapy in patients with cirrhosis. *Am J Med, 116*, 759–766.

For patients with established cirrhosis, endoscopic evaluation for the varices is warranted to determine their size and assess the risk for bleeding, as large varices are amendable to beta blockade that prevents the initial bleeding episode. In addition, large varices can be ligated before they bleed, making this technique particularly important and useful in preventing the initial bleeding episode,[15] which may carry a significant mortality risk.

ASSESSMENT

Physical Assessment Findings

Patients with GI bleeding often present without pain. The initial assessment should focus on the ABCs of airway, breathing, and circulation. Establishing a baseline regarding hemodynamic stability, including the standard vital signs of heart rate, blood pressure, respiratory rate, pulse oximetry, temperature, and level of consciousness, must be accomplished as soon as possible and may be helpful in determining the amount of blood lost.[22] If the patient is able to tolerate changes in position, orthostatic changes in blood pressure and heart rate may provide additional information. Frequent reassessments of the previously listed vital signs are important to determine significant changes and to establish a trend. Other assessments (see Chapter 40) may provide additional information. As noted above, pain is often not present with GI bleeding.[53] However, the abdomen may exhibit rigidity (increased abdominal wall muscle tone) or guarding (spasm of abdominal wall muscles, detected on palpation), or both, if there is peritoneal irritation caused by a perforation of the GI tract. Whereas both rigidity and guarding may indicate the need for immediate surgical evaluation, bleeding confined to the interior of the GI tract will not usually cause such symptoms. In addition, older adults are less likely to exhibit rigidity or guarding, as a result of decreased muscle tone and changes in the sympathetic nervous system seen with aging.

GI bleeding may initially present in many ways (Figure 26-4). The bleeding may be found with a guaiac test of gastric contents or stool that reveals trace amounts of blood or as frank bright red vomitus or the passage of bright red bloody stool. Blood loss identified by guaiac testing requires a loss of more than 10 ml/day;[31] guaiac-positive stools may be found up to 2 weeks after the bleeding has stopped.[53] An underappreciated subtlety of guaiac testing is that the cards for testing vomitus and stool are separate and distinct and CANNOT be used interchangeably. Bleeding from either the upper or the lower GI tract may also be significant and represent a life-threatening episode. Bright red blood in vomit is referred to as *hematemesis.* Hematemesis that is consistent in appearance with coffee grounds indicates that the blood has been in the stomach for a significant length of time, where the digestive enzymes have partially digested it. When hematemesis has occurred, placement of a nasogastric (NG) tube for aspiration and warmed isotonic solution lavage may be helpful in initially identifying the level of bleeding and clearing the stomach of blood, but this procedure has not been shown to stop the bleeding.[53] The fear of placing an NG tube in a patient with possible esophageal varices is unwarranted.[35]

When bright red blood comes from the rectum, it is referred to as *hematochezia.* Maroon, semi-liquid stools usually represent a bleeding site that is in the proximal

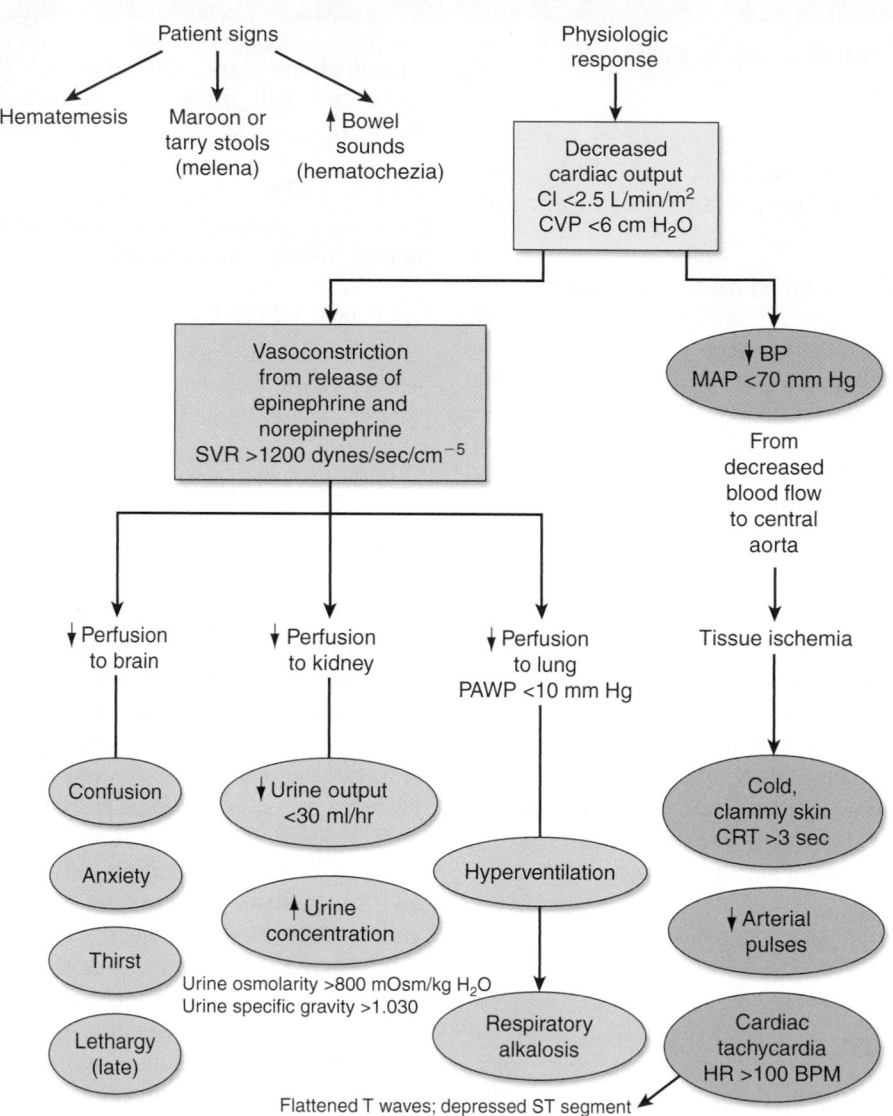

♦FIGURE 26-4 Presentation of gastrointestinal bleeding. BP = Blood pressure, CI = cardiac index, CRT = capillary refill time, CVP = central venous pressure, HR = heart rate, MAP = mean arterial pressure, PAWP = pulmonary artery wedge pressure, SVR = systemic vascular resistance.

colon (ascending or transverse). Blood loss may take the form of melena, which is stool that is black and tarry, with a very distinct odor. Melena represents blood in the GI tract that has been altered by the intestinal juices, usually from the upper GI tract. In fact, for many experienced critical care nurses, the distinctive odor of maroon stools, or melena, is the first indication of GI bleeding (Table 26-1).

Bleeding into and from the GI tract may be subtle and insidious, causing an iron-deficiency anemia over time. Of greater concern is the rapid loss of significant amounts of blood from any source. Hypovolemia caused by the blood loss may be compensated for a

time, but eventually, if the bleeding is not stopped, the patient will begin to display signs of hypovolemic shock.

An additional component of GI bleeding is the effect of the blood on the GI tract itself. Blood from the GI tract may range in color and consistency from bright red and liquid, to maroon and semi-liquid, to black and tarry. The transitions in color and consistency are dictated by the length of time the blood is exposed to the digestive enzymes. In addition, the presence of blood within the GI tract will usually increase peristalsis, sometimes dramatically, resulting in diarrhea and incontinence of stool. If the source of the bleeding is in the upper GI tract,

TABLE 26-1 Presentations of Gastrointestinal Bleeding

PRESENTATION	DEFINITION
Acute bleeding	
Hematemesis	Bloody vomitus; either fresh, bright red blood or dark, grainy digested blood with "coffee grounds" appearance
Melena	Black, sticky, tarry, foul-smelling stools caused by digestion of blood in gastrointestinal tract
Hematochezia	Fresh, bright red blood passed from rectum
Occult bleeding	Trace amounts of blood in normal-appearing stools or gastric secretions; detectable only with guaiac test

Data from reference 17.

it will often cause vomiting. However, if the blood passes into, or originates in, the lower GI tract, its high osmotic load will cause its rapid passage, resulting in diarrhea or incontinence of stool.

The patient with GI bleeding may be completely asymptomatic or may be in hypovolemic shock from massive bleeding. While the symptoms and physical assessment findings may suggest the type of disease process, they should always be confirmed with diagnostic studies. If pain is present, it is usually related to the underlying pathology. Upper GI bleeding caused by GERD or ulcers is often manifested by chronic indigestion, which usually increases in intensity over time, before the initial bleeding episode. The upper abdominal pain associated with GERD typically occurs shortly after eating and may be increased by overeating, coughing, or assuming a recumbent position immediately after eating. The pain associated with gastric and duodenal ulcers is quite similar, being intermittent in nature, located in the upper abdomen, and relieved by antacids. However, the pain of gastric ulcers may occur immediately after eating, whereas the pain of duodenal ulcers usually begins when the stomach has emptied or at night and then resolves by morning.[17]

Patients with Crohn's disease typically have little pain, but the chronic inflammation of a section of the colon may produce some regional tenderness. The pain of ulcerative colitis, on the other hand, may range from vague discomfort to a cramping pain that is continuous. Infections with *E. coli* 0157:H7 are not usually associated with pain, even though the patient may experience abdominal cramping. Patients with colorectal cancer

may have pain, but it is usually a late sign.[34] Hemorrhoids usually cause pain only during bowel movements with the passage of stool across the inflamed tissues.

If blood is deposited into the stomach from any source, it will usually result in nausea, retching, and vomiting. With varices, the bleeding may be insidious over a prolonged time or the varix may rupture, causing a rapid loss of blood into the stomach, which represents a true emergency. Because the blood from a ruptured varix is venous, it typically is dark red. However, even though the source of the bleeding is venous, the back pressure from the portal hypertension can rapidly exsanguinate the patient. Bleeding from gastric or duodenal ulcers may be subtle and insidious as well, but may also become life-threatening if the ulcer penetrates into the blood vessels that are laced throughout the mucosal and muscular walls of stomach and duodenum.[17]

As with bleeding from the upper GI tract, bleeding from the colon or rectum may be subtle or massive. Minor bleeding may be found with Crohn's disease, but the seemingly small amounts of blood loss may lead to significant anemia, over time. Bleeding is more prevalent with ulcerative colitis, especially with severe disease. Bleeding with colorectal cancer may also range from the subtle to the massive, especially in advanced cases (Figure 26-5). Bleeding from diverticulitis usually stops spontaneously, but the site may rebleed 20% to 30% of the time.[53] Blood from the ascending and transverse colon is usually dark red in color, whereas bleeding from the descending colon and rectum is bright red and usually on the surface of the stool, rather than mixed into it. Typically, the more bright red the blood, the more distal the bleeding source in the colon. Although hemorrhoids may cause bleeding, they usually do not represent a significant threat to the patient unless they are caused by portal hypertension.

Laboratory Findings

The traditional use of measurement of hematocrit and hemoglobin levels may not provide an adequate evaluation of the scope of the blood loss, because red blood cells (RBCs) and plasma are lost in equal proportion.[4] Additionally, with volume resuscitation, the hematocrit and hemoglobin levels will usually begin to decrease. Coagulation studies will allow the establishment of a baseline and provide data to track trends over time. Typing and cross-matching of the patient's blood to banked blood provides for the rapid transfusion of blood, should it be needed.[22] Blood urea nitrogen (BUN) levels may be elevated because of the digestion and absorption of the protein in the blood as it passes through the small intestine, usually within

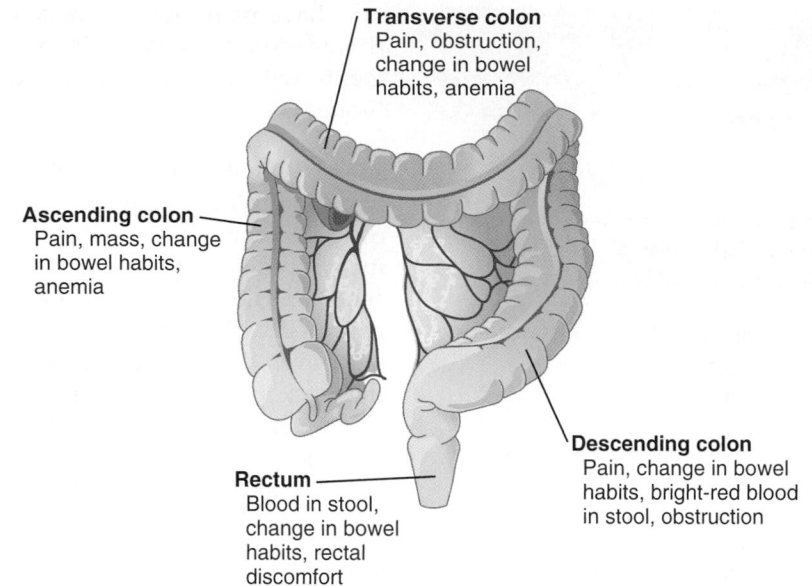

Transverse colon
Pain, obstruction, change in bowel habits, anemia

Ascending colon
Pain, mass, change in bowel habits, anemia

Descending colon
Pain, change in bowel habits, bright-red blood in stool, obstruction

Rectum
Blood in stool, change in bowel habits, rectal discomfort

✦**FIGURE 26-5** Signs and symptoms of colorectal cancer by location of primary lesion.

24 hours.[34] However, this same phenomenon does not occur with bleeding originating in the colon, because digestion does not occur in the colon.[34]

Identification of an *H. pylori* infection can be determined either by invasive tests to sample the gut flora or by noninvasive tests (e.g., serologic, saliva, stool, or urine tests) to determine the presence of an IgG antibody specific to *H. pylori*. A urea breath test can determine the presence of *H. pylori* with a sensitivity and specificity of greater than 90%.[49]

Radiology Findings

Flat-plate abdominal x-rays are used to identify the presence of as little as 5 ml of free air in the peritoneal space.[51] Such a finding indicates that a perforation of the stomach or small bowel has occurred. However, the flat-plate abdominal x-ray cannot detect or differentiate between blood and other types of fluid in the gut or the peritoneal space.

Radiology studies using barium have had a long history in identifying and quantifying GI disease. In the case of GI bleeding, such studies may be able to identify the source (such as a gastric or duodenal ulcer) and are safer and less invasive than endoscopy. Enteroclysis, filling the small bowl with contrast medium through a catheter advanced nasally or orally into the duodenum or jejunum, can provide an effective evaluation of bleeding in the small bowel.[51]

Computed tomography (CT) and magnetic resonance imaging (MRI) are used with intravenous contrast (angiography) to identify sources of GI bleeding that may be difficult to identify by other means. This is particularly true with bleeding that has defied location by endoscopy. A unique aspect of CT is the use of digital reconstruction of the interior lumen of the GI tracts, although a high false-positive rate prevents it from becoming a general screening tool.[31] CT is more likely to be used because there are usually less restrictions associated with a CT compared to an MRI (scanning speed, issues with ferrous metals, confined patient space).

Angiography, using radiopaque contrast media and fluoroscopy, may be very useful in identifying obscure or unidentifiable sources of GI bleeding.[12] However, a bleeding rate of greater than 0.5 ml per minute must be present before identification of an arterial bleeding site with angiography can be accomplished.[53] In addition to traditional fluoroscopy, both CT and MRI may also be used as a platform for angiography. Scintigraphy, the use of radionuclide contrast media and imagery, may also be used to identify a bleeding source and can identify bleeding sources with rates as low as 0.1 ml per minute.[53]

Diagnostic Evaluations

Although a bleeding lesion may be found with contrast studies, some method of treatment must then be undertaken; this is where endoscopy has come to the forefront of assessing and treating GI bleeding.[51] Endoscopy offers the opportunity to directly visualize the lesion, remove samples for biopsy and study, and deliver therapy directly to the lesion.

Endoscopy is used when the patient presents with signs and symptoms indicating pathology that could be evaluated or treated, such as GI bleeding. It may also be used when other studies (e.g., contrast studies) are unable to identify the cause of the bleeding. The endoscope may be introduced into the upper GI tract through the mouth (esophagogastroduodenoscopy [EGD]) or into the colon (colonoscopy).

EGD provides rapid and effective assessment and treatment of upper GI bleeding sources in the vast majority of cases. As stated by Pasricha and Zuckerman (p. 791)[31], "Endoscopy is mandatory in all patients with significant upper gastrointestinal bleeding, with the rare exception being the terminally ill patient in whom the outcome is unlikely to be affected." EGD not only can provide assessment and treatment but also can help predict the incidence of rebleeding. EGD should be considered whenever there is active upper GI bleeding. Although some clinicians prefer gastric lavage, via a naso- or orogastric tube, before the endoscopy to increase visibility, others believe that it may produce artifact; the practice remains controversial.[31] While gastric lavage may be helpful in clearing the stomach of blood, it has not been proven to stop bleeding and, if iced, may actually prolong the bleeding and increase clotting time.[53] Should lavage be considered, it is important to use warmed normal saline or lactated Ringer's solution to prevent both hypothermia and the potentially significant loss of electrolytes in the lavage solution. Tap water may be used for the lavage, but its low osmolality may draw electrolytes out of the circulatory system into the stomach, where they are removed when the lavage solution is withdrawn from the stomach.

Care must be taken to ensure the patient's safety during the procedure. For patients who are actively bleeding, endoscopy should be completed in critical care or the emergency department, where emergency intubation and respiratory management can be quickly accomplished, if needed. For those patients with relatively slow or inactive GI bleeding who are hemodynamically stable, the procedure may be performed in an endoscopy suite.

Endoscopy for lower GI bleeding is less straightforward. Patients with active bleeding and hematochezia or melena should have an EGD completed initially to eliminate the upper GI tract as the source of the bleeding. Traditionally, colonoscopy has been used only after an adequate bowel preparation. However, some clinicians complete the test without bowel preparation in an early attempt to locate the source of active bleeding, often with guidance from angiography or scintigraphy for an approximation of the bleeding location.[12,51]

Capsule endoscopy, the use of a small video capsule that is swallowed and passes through the entire GI tract, is emerging as the most effective method of assessing the distal small bowel, which is beyond the reach of endoscopes. As it moves through the small bowel, the device transmits two images per second to a receiver carried by the patient as he or she goes about the daily routine. The process usually takes about 4 hours to complete. The quality of the video picture rivals that of traditional endoscopes.[50] While some recommend integration of the devices into current diagnostic algorithms,[14] others suggest that further comparative research is required before the routine use of these unique devices should change practice.[32]

MULTIDISCIPLINARY PLAN OF CARE

As shown in Figure 26-6 and in the Multidisciplinary Plan of Care on pp. 748-749, the initial treatment of GI bleeding will depend on several factors, including the amount and time frame of the blood loss, the patient's response to the loss, and any underlying medical conditions, including comorbidities. In addition, the amount of blood initially lost is an indication of the possibility of rebleeding after treatment, with large blood losses more likely to rebleed than small blood losses.[31] The prime consideration in an acutely ill patient with a GI bleed is to establish hemodynamic stability as quickly as possible.[4,12,53] Typically, significant blood loss will result in hypovolemic shock; treatment for hypovolemic shock is well documented in Chapter 40. Blood transfusions may be required to establish hemodynamic stability and increase the hematocrit level to a value in the 30% to 34% range, but overtransfusion may lead to rebound portal hypertension in patients with cirrhosis, causing further bleeding.[15] The use of recombinant clotting factor VIIa has been studied and shown to be effective in decreasing acute bleeding treatment failures in patients with significant liver disease.[5]

If massive hematemesis is present and the patient's airway is unable to be protected, endotracheal intubation should be rapidly accomplished.[15,42,53] When the bleeding is massive, a limited endoscopic evaluation may help pinpoint the source of the bleeding and facilitate further treatment, including surgical intervention. A naso- or orogastric tube may be needed to clear blood from the bleeding site before endoscopy, but should not be used in an attempt to stop the bleeding by lavage.[53] Once the patient has been stabilized and the source of the bleeding identified, definitive treatment to stop the bleeding can be initiated.

With its widespread utilization, endoscopy has evolved as the preeminent treatment of GI bleeding.[53] Endoscopy, either as an EGD or as a colonoscopy, uses similar methods to stop GI bleeding in both the upper and the lower GI tract.[53] However, there are some differences, based on the anatomy and the pathophysiology involved. There are several endoscopic methods

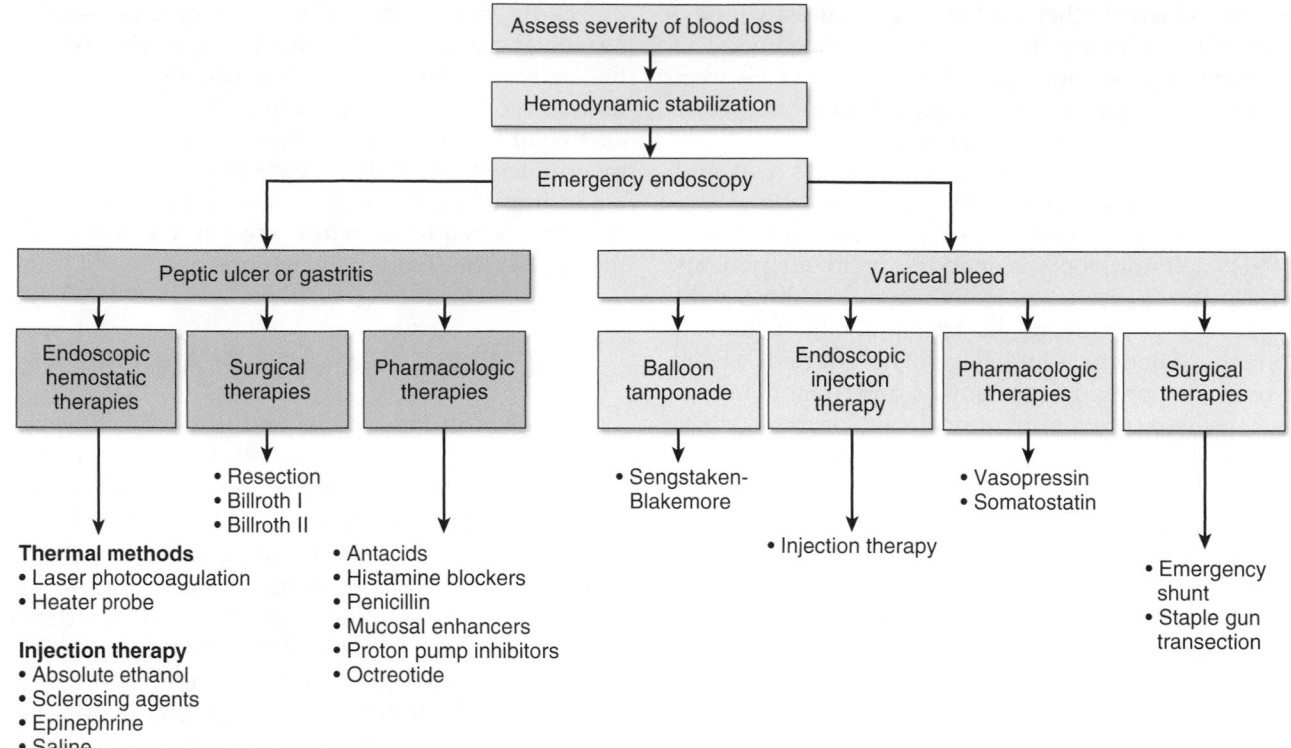

FIGURE 26-6 Algorithm for guiding treatment of gastrointestinal bleeding.

MULTIDISCIPLINARY PLAN OF CARE FOR PATIENTS WITH GI BLEEDING

PROBLEM	INTERVENTION	RATIONALE	EXPECTED OUTCOME
Prevention	Deliver various medications (e.g., proton pump inhibitors) appropriately (dose, times)	Significantly decreases bleeding episodes	Gastric and stool samples remain guaiac negative. No episodes of frank bleeding
Compromised airway	Endotracheal intubation with decrease in level of consciousness or massive hematemesis	Preserves airway patency and allows effective oxygenation and ventilation. Significantly decreases possibility of aspiration of gastric contents	Oxygen saturation higher than 90% and arterial blood gases indicate effective oxygenation (Sao_2 >90%) and ventilation ($Paco_2$ between 35 and 45 mm Hg)
Hypovolemia	Administer crystalloids and blood products	Maintains systemic perfusion	Blood pressure higher than 90 mm Hg
Active GI bleeding	Insert and maintain a nasogastric tube. Perform/assist with endoscopic therapies	Evacuates blood from stomach and allows for lavage, as needed. Usually provides definitive treatment of acute bleeding episodes	No repeat of bleeding episodes

PROBLEM	INTERVENTION	RATIONALE	EXPECTED OUTCOME
Adjunctive therapies	Deliver various medications (e.g., octreotide, proton pump inhibitors) appropriately (dose, times) Insert and maintain balloon tamponade therapy	Significantly decreases bleeding episodes and increases effectiveness of endoscopic therapies Provides temporary hemostasis pending endoscopy	No repeat episodes of frank bleeding
Continued bleeding	Prepare for immediate transport to operative suite	Recurrent bleeding episodes usually indicate need for surgical intervention	Safely delivered to operative suite

$Paco_2$ = Partial pressure of arterial carbon dioxide, Sao_2 = arterial saturation of oxygen.

employed to stop bleeding. Injections of various substances (alcohol, epinephrine, saline, various sclerosants) into the bleeding site will cause scarring or vasoconstriction, stopping the bleeding. Coagulation of the bleeding area or vessel with a laser or thermal probe is also effective. Isolation of the bleeding varix can be accomplished with various mechanical devices (clips, bands) that occlude the blood flow into the bleeding site.[4] Typically, clips resemble simple staples while bands resemble small rubber bands. Both types of devices are secured at the base of the varix, occluding its blood supply. Some clinicians will utilize a combination of these methods.[53] One study found that outcomes using epinephrine injection and thermal coagulation compared to ligation with clips were not significantly different in treating bleeding varices.[39] However, another study found that although both sclerotherapy and band ligation were equally effective in stopping the bleeding, band ligation was superior with respect to cost, speed of achieving hemostasis, recurrence of bleeding, and complications.[52] Adding omeprazole (Prilosec) to endoscopic therapy significantly decreased rebleeding episodes.[45] Bacterial infection can be a significant complication of endoscopy, and Hou et al. (2004) demonstrated that antibiotic prophylaxis significantly decreases both infection and rebleeding in patients with esophageal varices.[16] A reference for assisting with endoscopy is found in the *AACN Procedure Manual for Critical Care*.[6]

Bleeding from a Mallory-Weiss tear is usually self-limiting; 80% to 90% of patients will stop bleeding spontaneously.[53] Occasionally patients will require endoscopic procedures to stop the bleeding, using injection or coagulation therapies, with angiography and embolic therapy being reserved for those patients who rebleed.

While esophageal and gastric varices may be treated endoscopically with both injection and coagulation therapies, medications such as octreotide (Sandostatin) and vasopressin (Pitressin) may be used before the endoscopy in an attempt to slow the bleeding and allow endoscopic therapies to be pursued.[4,35] Octreotide decreases the amount of both splanchnic blood flow and portal vein pressure, allowing coagulation to take place. Octreotide is administered intravenously with an initial bolus of 25 to 100 mcg, followed by a continuous infusion of 25 to 50 mcg per hour. Because it controls bleeding in approximately 85% of bleeding varices, octreotide should be considered early in the course of treatment.[35] Vasopressin decreases bleeding from varices by systemic vasoconstriction, which also decreases splanchnic blood flow and portal vein pressure. Intravenous dosages start at 0.4 unit per minute, increasing to no more than 1 unit per minute, to control bleeding. However, because it exerts its effects systematically, vasopressin can cause hypertension and may induce myocardial ischemia and peripheral vasoconstriction. The hypertension associated with vasopressin may be treated with the addition of intravenous nitroglycerin to keep the systolic blood pressure between 90 and 100 mm Hg. The nitroglycerin decreases the systemic hypertension associated with vasopressin without affecting the splanchnic blood flow and pressure, and is more effective than vasopressin alone. While still used in some institutions, vasopressin has largely been replaced by octreotide because of the former's side effects.[15] Although both medications are useful, they perform "stop gap" therapy to allow endoscopy to be performed.[35]

Endoscopy has been established as the treatment of choice for bleeding esophageal varices, using both sclerosing agents (solutions injected into the bleeding sites that cause thrombosis and obliteration) and thermal coagulation modalities.[35] The addition of octreotide to sclerotherapy has demonstrated an increased control of bleeding.[15] In addition, endoscopy allows the use of ligation or banding of the varices, which strangulates the defect, allowing it to slough off in time (Figure 26-7). Banding with small "O" rings has evolved as the premier method of treatment of esophageal varices[35] because of its quick application and lower complication rates compared to sclerotherapy, which may cause transmural damage to the esophagus. Once the acute episode of bleeding is successfully treated, repeated endoscopy procedures are performed to obliterate all of the existing varices, significantly preventing rebleeding episodes. An additional benefit of banding is the rapidity with which the varices can be treated, limiting the number of procedures the patient must endure.[35]

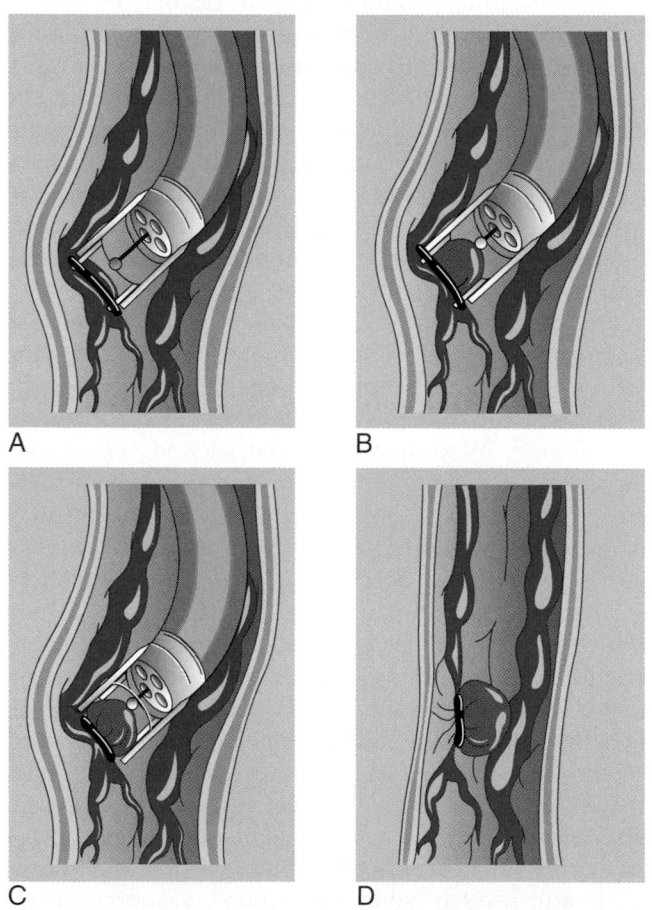

♦FIGURE 26-7 Endoscopic variceal ligation technique. **A,** The endoscope, with an attached ligating device, is brought into contact with the varix just above the gastroesophageal junction. **B,** Suction is applied, pulling the varix-containing mucosa into the dead space created at the end of the endoscope. **C,** A tripwire is pulled, releasing the band around the aspirate tissue. **D,** Ligation is completed.

Gastric varices usually bleed less often than esophageal varices, but the blood loss is often greater.[35] While banding and various modes of sclerotherapy are appropriate, use of a tissue adhesive (various forms of cyanoacrylate) that activates when it comes into contact with blood may be a safe alternative.[13,36] However, there are multiple reports of significant adverse events associated with this therapy, including embolization and vessel wall ulceration.[21,38] Because the success rate of endoscopic treatment of gastric varices is limited, with an associated significant rebleeding rate, other modes of therapy may be indicated to decrease the pressure being exerted on the gastric venous complex, including the transjugular intrahepatic portosystemic shunt (TIPS) procedure (see Chapter 27).

A type of device that has become less common but still may have a place in caring for patients bleeding from esophageal or gastric varices is balloon tamponade therapy. The devices, which consist of combinations of esophageal and gastric balloons (Sengstaken-Blakemore and Minnesota tubes), are also equipped with various suction ports to allow evacuation of blood from the esophagus or stomach (Figure 26-8). The devices are effective in stopping the bleeding episode, but rely on mechanical compression. Therefore, if the tubes are removed prematurely, the bleeding may resume. They are typically employed when there are no endoscopic therapies readily available. In addition, they are technically difficult to safely maintain and have many complication potentials. A reference for using the devices is found in the *AACN Procedure Manual for Critical Care.*[10]

Gastric and duodenal ulcers are also typically treated with injection or coagulation endoscopy. While ligation with a clip may be used for ulcers, Lin et al.[26] found that injection sclerotherapy and thermal coagulation usually produce better outcomes; Shimoda et al. found that both techniques were equally effective.[43] However, stress ulcers are much less likely to be successfully treated with endoscopy.[53] Because of the impact of *H. pylori* on the formation of ulcers, a treatment regimen may involve PPI to decrease acid production and antibiotics to eliminate the pathogen. Selective therapy to eradicate *H. pylori* is more effective for duodenal ulcers than gastric ulcers. Eradication of *H. pylori* is cost-effective for gastric ulcers over 2 years and for duodenal ulcers over 1 year, when compared to other types of therapies.[49] Arkkila et al. found that eradicating *H. pylori* significantly increased healing rates and decreased recurrence of ulcer formation.[2] The use of high-dose, intravenous omeprazole has been proven to be cost-effective in reducing the incidence of rebleeding in postendoscopic treatment for ulcers.[25]

Colonoscopy uses the same techniques to stop bleeding in the lower GI tract.[53] While hematochezia

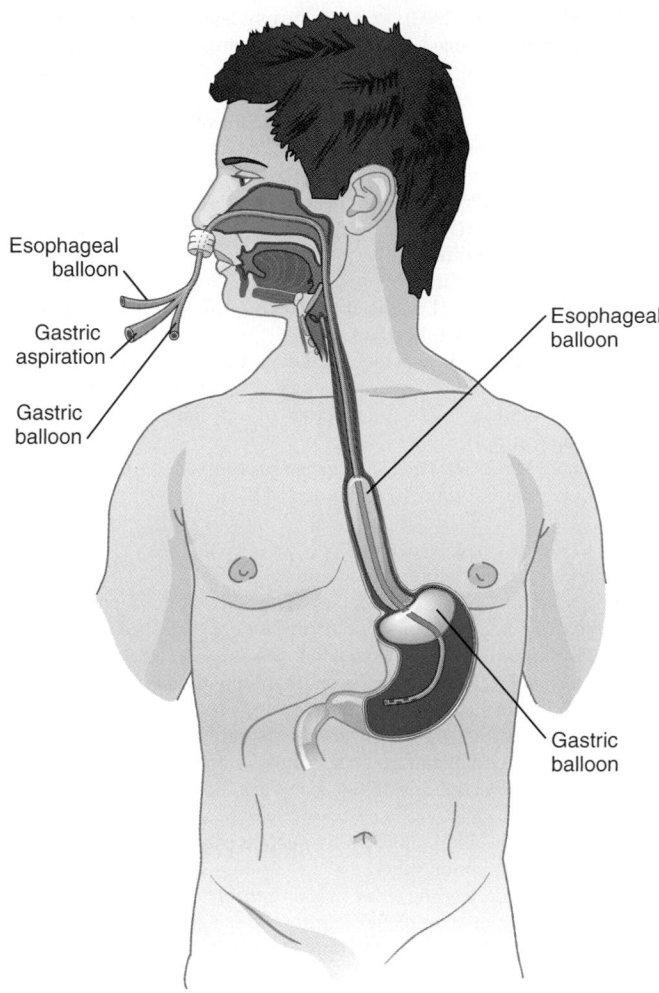

Esophageal
balloon

Gastric
aspiration

Gastric
balloon

Esophageal
balloon

Gastric
balloon

◆FIGURE 26-8 Balloon tamponade therapy: Sengstaken-Blakemore tube in place with both the esophageal and gastric balloons inflated.

hemodynamically unstable, rapid surgical intervention may be the most effective treatment. As part of the surgical approach, endoscopy may also be used interoperatively to assist in identifying the source of the bleed.[53] The surgical techniques will vary depending upon the source of the bleeding. "Over-sewing" of various ulcers, often combined with selective vagotomy, is a standard therapy, with removal of the offending portion and anastomosis of the surgical wounds. A vagotomy will sever portions of the vagus nerve where it enters the stomach, decreasing acid production, which is partially controlled by the vagus nerve. One exception to the surgical approach is stress ulcers, simply because they are often scattered throughout the gastric mucosa and, as such, do not lend themselves to surgical removal. Stress ulcers will rebleed approximately 50% of the time after surgery.[31] Therefore prevention is certainly the preferable alternative.

CONCLUSIONS

Gastrointestinal bleeding is a significant cause of both mortality and morbidity in the critical care setting. These are some of the most challenging patients that critical care nurses care for, involving resuscitation, diagnostics, and therapy to stop the bleeding. Often the pathology may be effectively prevented from causing the bleeding in the first place. Depending on the source of the bleeding, multiple modes of therapy are appropriate for stopping the source of the bleeding and preventing its recurrence. Understanding the pathophysiology and various treatments provides a more complete understanding of the nurse's role in providing care for these complex patients.

usually indicates bleeding from the lower GI tract, approximately 10% of the time the source is found in the upper GI tract,[4] necessitating an endoscopic evaluation of the upper GI tract[53] as well as the colon. If colonoscopy is unable to locate and coagulate the bleeding site, it may be able to isolate the specific section of the colon that is the source of the blood, allowing the surgeon a more focused surgical approach.[4,53]

Some bleeding sites (e.g., diverticula, angiodysplasia) may be more appropriately treated with angiotherapy, using intra-arterial vasopressin to cause vasospasm, usually in much smaller doses than used systemically. Additionally, angiography may be used to deploy coils or Gelfoam into the vessel at the bleeding site, causing the development of a thrombosis.[53]

Those patients who do not respond to medical, endoscopic, or radiologic invasive therapies may require surgical intervention. When a patient remains

REFERENCES

1. Abraczinskas, D. R., et al. (2001). Propranolol for the prevention of first esophageal variceal hemorrhage: a lifetime commitment? *Hepatology, 34*, 1096–1102.
2. Arkkila, P. E., et al. (2003). Eradication of *Helicobacter pylori* improves the healing rate and reduces the relapse rate of nonbleeding ulcers in patients with bleeding peptic ulcer. *Am J Gastroenterol, 98*, 2149–2156.
3. Behrman, S. W. (2005). Management of complicated peptic ulcer disease. *Arch Surg, 140*, 201–208.
4. Bjorkman, D. J. (2004). Gastrointestinal hemorrhage and occult gastrointestinal bleeding. In L. Goldman & D. Ausiello (Eds.), *Cecil textbook of medicine* (22nd ed.). Philadelphia: Saunders.
5. Bosch, J., et al. (2004). Recombinant factor VIIa for upper gastrointestinal bleeding in patients with cirrhosis: a randomized, double-blind trial. *Gastroenterology, 127*, 1123–1130.
6. Carlson, K. K. (2005). Scleral endoscopic therapy. In D. J. L. M. Wiegand & K. K. Carlson (Eds.), *AACN procedure manual for critical care* (5th ed.). St Louis: Saunders.

7. Centers for Disease Control and Prevention (CDC). (2004). *Escherichia coli 0157:H7*. Atlanta, Ga: Centers for Disease Control and Prevention. www.cdc.gov/ncidod/dbmd/diseaseinfo/escherichiacoli_g.htm.

8. Chan, F. K., et al. (2005). Clopidogrel versus aspirin and esomeprazole to prevent recurrent ulcer bleeding. *N Engl J Med, 352,* 238–244.

9. Conrad, S. A., et al. (2005). Randomized, double-blind comparison of immediate-release omeprazole oral suspension versus intravenous cimetidine for the prevention of upper gastrointestinal bleeding in critically ill patients. *Crit Care Med, 33,* 760–765.

10. Day, M. W. (2005). Esophagogastric tamponade tube. In D. J. L. M. Wiegand & K. K. Carlson (Eds.), *AACN procedure manual for critical care* (5th ed.). St Louis: Saunders.

11. Goldstein, J. L., Huang, B., Amer, F., et al. (2004). Ulcer recurrence in high-risk patients receiving nonsteroidal anti-inflammatory drugs plus low-dose aspirin: results of a post HOC subanalysis. *Clin Ther, 26,* 1637–1643.

12. Green, B. T., & Rockey, D. C. (2003). Acute gastrointestinal bleeding. *Semin Gastrointest Dis, 14*(2), 44–65.

13. Greenwald, B. D., et al. (2003). N-2-Butyl-cyanoacrylate for bleeding gastric varices: a United States pilot study and cost analysis. *Am J Gastroenterol, 98,* 1982–1988.

14. Hartmann, D., Schilling, D., Bolz, G., et al. (2004). Capsule endoscopy, technical impact, benefits and limitations. *Langenbeck's Arch Surg, 389,* 225–233.

15. Hegab, A. M., & Luketic, V. A. (2001). Bleeding esophageal varices. *Postgrad Med, 109*(2), 75–7681–86, 89.

16. Hou, M. C., et al. (2004). Antibiotic prophylaxis after endoscopic therapy prevents rebleeding in acute variceal hemorrhage: a randomized trial. *Hepatology, 39,* 746–753.

17. Huether, S. E. (2002a). Alterations of digestive function. In K. L. McCance & S. E. Huether (Eds.), *Pathophysiology: the biological basis for disease in adults and children* (4th ed.). St Louis: Mosby.

18. Huether, S. E. (2002b). Structure and function of the digestive system. In K. L. McCance & S. E. Huether (Eds.), *Pathophysiology: the biological basis for disease in adults and children* (4th ed.). St Louis: Mosby.

19. Jutabha, R., et al. (2005). Randomized study comparing banding and propranolol to prevent initial variceal hemorrhage in cirrhotics with high-risk esophageal varices. *J Gastroenterol, 128,* 870–881.

20. Kahrilas, P. J., & Lee, T. J. (2005). Pathophysiology of gastroesophageal reflux disease. *Thoracic Surg Clin, 15,* 323–333.

21. Kok, K., et al. (2004). Distal embolization and local vessel wall ulceration after gastric variceal obliteration with N-butyl-2-cyanoacrylate: a case report and review of the literature. *Endoscopy, 36,* 442–446.

22. Krumberger, J. M. (2005). How to manage an acute upper GI bleed. *RN, 68*(3), 34–39.

23. Laine, L. (2001). Gastrointestinal bleeding. In E. Braunwald et al. (Eds.), *Harrison's principles of internal medicine* (15th ed.). New York: McGraw-Hill.

24. Lanas, A. (2005). Gastrointestinal injury from NSAID therapy. *Postgrad Med, 117*(6), 23–28, 31.

25. Lee, K. K., et al. (2003). Cost-effectiveness analysis of high-dose omeprazole infusion as adjuvant therapy to endoscopic treatment of bleeding peptic ulcer. *Gastrointest Endosc, 57*(2), 160–164.

26. Lin, H. J., Perng, C. L., Sun, I. C., et al. (2003). Endoscopic haemoclip versus heater probe thermocoagulation plus hypertonic saline-epinephrine injection for peptic ulcer bleeding. *Digestive Liver Dis, 35,* 898–902.

27. Locke, G. R. (2005). Current medical management of gastroesophageal reflux disease. *Thoracic Surg Clin, 15,* 369–375.

28. Lui, H. F., et al. (2002). Primary prophylaxis of variceal hemorrhage: a randomized controlled trial comparing band ligation, propranolol, and isosorbide mononitrate. *Gastroenterology, 123,* 735–744.

29. Merkel, C., et al. (2004). A placebo-controlled clinical trial of nadolol in the prophylaxis of growth of small esophageal varices in cirrhosis. *Gastroenterology, 127,* 476–484.

30. Pasricha, P. J. (2004). Gastrointestinal endoscopy. In L. Goldman & D. Ausiello (Eds.), *Cecil textbook of medicine* (22nd ed.). Philadelphia: Saunders.

31. Pasricha, P. J., & Zuckerman, G. R. (2004). Stress ulcer syndrome. In L. Goldman & D. Ausiello (Eds.), *Cecil textbook of medicine* (22nd ed.). Philadelphia: Saunders.

32. Pennazio, M. (2004). Small-bowel endoscopy. *Endoscopy, 36,* 32–41.

33. Pisegna, J. R. (2002). Pharmacology of acid suppression in the hospital setting: focus on proton pump inhibition. *Crit Care Med, 30*(6 suppl), S356–S361.

34. Porth, C. M. (2002). *Pathophysiology: concepts of altered health states.* Philadelphia: Lippincott Williams & Wilkins.

35. Prakash, C., & Zuckerman, G. R. (2004). Variceal bleeding. In L. Goldman & D. Ausiello (Eds.), *Cecil textbook of medicine* (22nd ed.). Philadelphia: Saunders.

36. Rengstorff, D. S., & Binmoeller, K. F. (2004). A pilot study of 2-octyl cyanoacrylate injection for treatment of gastric fundal varices in humans. *Gastrointest Endosc, 59,* 553–558.

37. Richter, J. E. (2005). New investigational therapies for gastroesophageal reflux disease. *Thoracic Surg Clin, 15,* 377–384.

38. Rickman, O. B., Utz, J. P., Aughenbaugh, G. L., et al. (2004). Pulmonary embolization of 2-octyl cyanoacrylate after endoscopic injection therapy for gastric variceal bleeding. *Mayo Clin Proc, 79,* 1455–1458.

39. Saltzman, J. R., et al. (2005). Prospective trial of endoscopic clips versus combination therapy in upper GI bleeding (PROTECCT—UGI bleeding). *Am J Gastroenterol, 100,* 1503–1508.

40. Sarin, S. K., et al. (2005a). Endoscopic variceal ligation plus propranolol versus endoscopic variceal ligation alone in primary prophylaxis of variceal bleeding. *Am J Gastroenterol, 100,* 805–807.

41. Sarin, S. K., et al. (2005b). Evaluation of endoscopic variceal ligation (EVL) versus propranolol plus isosorbide mononitrate/nadolol (ISMN) in the prevention of variceal rebleeding: comparison of cirrhotic and noncirrhotic patients. *Dig Dis Sci, 50,* 1538–1547.

42. Scott, J. M. (2005). Endotracheal intubation. In D. J. L. M. Wiegand & K. K. Carlson (Eds.), *AACN procedure manual for critical care* (5th ed.). St Louis: Saunders.

43. Shimoda, R., et al. (2003). Evaluation of endoscopic hemostasis with metallic hemoclips for bleeding gastric ulcer: comparison with endoscopic injection of absolute ethanol in a prospective, randomized study. *Am J Gastroenterol, 98,* 2198–2202.

44. Spahn, T. W., & Kucharzik, T. (2004). Modulating the intestinal immune system: the role of lymphotoxin and GALT organs. *Gut, 53,* 456–465.

45. Sung, J. J., et al. (2003). The effect of endoscopic therapy in patients receiving omeprazole for bleeding ulcers with nonbleeding visible vessels or adherent clots: a randomized comparison. *Ann Intern Med, 139,* 237–243.

46. Talwalkar, J. A., & Kamath, P. S. (2004). An evidence-based medicine approach to beta-blocker therapy in patients with cirrhosis. *Am J Med, 116,* 759–766.

47. Triantos, C., et al. (2005). Primary prophylaxis of variceal bleeding in cirrhotics unable to take beta-blockers: a randomized trial of ligation. *Aliment Pharmacol Ther, 15,* 1435–1443.

48. Van Gossum, A. (2001). Obscure digestive bleeding. *Best Pract Res Clin Gastroenterol, 15,* 155–174.

49. Vaira, D., et al. (2005). Peptic ulcer and *Helicobacter pylori*: update on testing and treatment. *Postgrad Med, 117*(6), 17–21, 24–31.

50. Wikipedia. (2005). *Capsule camera*. http://en.wikipedia.org/wiki/Capsule_camera.

51. Wittich, G. R. (2004). Diagnostic imaging procedures in gastroenterology. In L. Goldman & D. Ausiello (Eds.), *Cecil textbook of medicine* (22nd ed.). Philadelphia: Saunders.

52. Zargar, S. A., et al. (2005). Endoscopic ligation vs. sclerotherapy in adults with extrahepatic portal venous obstruction: a prospective randomized study. *Gastrointest Endosc, 61*(1), 58–66.

53. Zuckerman, G. R., & Lotsoff, D. S. (2004). Upper and lower gastrointestinal bleeding: principles of diagnosis and management. In R. S. Irwin & J. M. Rippe (Eds.), *Intensive care medicine* (5th ed.). Philadelphia: Lippincott Williams & Wilkins.

CHAPTER 27 Liver Dysfunction and Failure

Rhonda K. Martin and Tarek Hassanein

The liver is the largest internal organ of the human body, weighing 1200 to 1500 g and performing more than 8000 defined functions.[5] The complexity of the liver's role means that alterations in function can cause a myriad of multisystem problems, whether the alteration is related to acute or chronic liver disease or to multisystem organ dysfunction.

Liver dysfunction is usually defined clinically by the presence of jaundice, ascites, or hepatic encephalopathy, evident by an increase in the levels of liver injury enzymes (aspartate transaminase [AST]/alanine transaminase [ALT]), total or direct bilirubin, and the international normalized ratio (INR).[33]

ACUTE LIVER FAILURE

Acute liver failure, or ALF (formerly known as fulminant liver failure), is defined by the occurrence of jaundice and any degree of mental alteration (e.g., hepatic encephalopathy) in a patient without preexisting liver disease who has had an illness of less than 26 weeks' duration.[43] It is a clinical syndrome caused by massive hepatic necrosis leading to the development of severe hepatic failure. The onset of jaundice usually precedes the onset of encephalopathy in these cases. Paradoxically, the shorter the period from the onset of jaundice to hepatic coma, the better the prognosis.[29]

There are approximately 2000 cases of ALF in the United States each year. ALF often affects young adults, and carries a high morbidity and mortality rate. The most common cause of ALF has changed in recent years. In 1969 the most frequent cause of ALF was hepatitis B.[36] In 2000 the most common causes had changed to acetaminophen toxicity (39%) and other drug reactions (13%). Other sources include hepatitis D (as a co-infection with hepatitis B), autoimmune liver disease, shock or hypoperfusion, Wilson's disease (a dysfunction of copper metabolism), and mushroom poisoning, usually with *Amanita phalloides*. In 2000 a total of 73% of ALF patients were women.[36] Current short-term survival is less than 15%, but survival after transplant is greater than 67%.[29]

These cases are often devastating to patients and families because of the rapid onset, progression to coma and death, or urgent need for liver transplantation. Close relatives need to be informed of the potentially poor prognosis and possible need for transplant, and kept involved in the decision-making process. ALF patients should be referred and transferred to a transplant facility early in the presentation because they often deteriorate rapidly and require specialized intensive care, urgent transplant evaluation and listing, and possibly hepatic and renal extracorporeal support therapy.

ACUTE-ON-CHRONIC LIVER DYSFUNCTION AND FAILURE

Chronic liver disease is a disease state of greater than 6 months' duration. Acute-on-chronic liver failure occurs in patients who have an underlying advanced cirrhosis and experience an additional derangement (e.g., infection, bleeding, primary disease exacerbation, secondary disease) causing acute liver decompensation.[5]

The risk factors for chronic liver disease vary according to the type and cause of disease. For instance, viral hepatitis and parasitic liver disease risk factors are related mostly to infectious exposure risks, and nonalcoholic fatty liver disease and steatohepatitis are related to nutrition, obesity, and dyslipidemia.[20] Table 27-1 lists risk factors for the most common diseases associated with acute-on-chronic liver dysfunction/failure.

The incidence of liver disease in the United States is on the rise, but because the onset of many types of liver disease is insidious, with a latent period between onset and clinical detection, the true incidence and prevalence may not be known.[54] The incidence of newly diagnosed liver disease is estimated at 72.3 per 100,000 population.[54] The most common chronic liver disease is hepatitis C, followed by alcoholic liver disease, nonalcoholic fatty liver disease, and hepatitis B.[53] The prevalence of hepatitis C in the United States is estimated at 4 million cases, or approximately 1.8% of the population. Chronic liver disease and cirrhosis are the eleventh most prevalent causes of death in the United States overall, ranked

TABLE 27-1 Risk Factors for Common Liver Diseases

LIVER DISEASE	RISK FACTORS
Drug-induced liver disease	Age, female, poor nutrition, underlying liver disease, drug interactions
Fatty liver disease	Obesity, diabetes mellitus, lipid disorders
Hepatic abscess	Lower socioeconomic status in endemic areas, institutionalized patients, homosexual behavior, travelers
Hepatitis A	Fecal-oral transmission: daycare centers, contaminated food, infected mollusks; travel to endemic hepatitis A virus (HAV) areas; anal-oral sex
Hepatitis B	High-risk sexual behavior (unprotected sex, multiple partners, homosexual partners), intravenous drug use, hemodialysis, healthcare workers, vertical transmission during pregnancy
Hepatitis C	Blood-borne transmission: transfusions, tattoos, intravenous drug use
Hepatocellular carcinoma	Cirrhosis, chronic hepatitis B or C, α_1-antitrypsin disease, exposure to carcinogens
Hereditary hemachromatosis	Family history of disease, Caucasian, alcohol use
Primary biliary cirrhosis	Female, Hispanic, family history of disease
Primary sclerosing cholangitis	Irritable bowel disease, male, age 40–60, family history of disease

Data from reference 20.

Box 27-1

Classification of Hepatic Diseases

CHOLESTATIC
- Primary
  - Primary biliary cirrhosis
- Secondary
  - Biliary cirrhosis
  - Congenital conditions (e.g., biliary atresia)
  - Drug-induced cholestasis
  - Sclerosing cholangitis

HEPATOCELLULAR
- Alcohol (Laënnec's cirrhosis)
- Autoimmune hepatitis
- Cryptogenic (cause unknown)
- Hepatitis
  - Infectious: bacterial, viral, parasitic
  - Drug-induced: NSAIDs, halothane, sulfonamides, ketoconazole, phenytoin, INH, rifampin, carbon tetrachloride, poisonous mushrooms
- Ischemia
- Vascular congestion (e.g., Budd-Chiari syndrome)

METABOLIC
- Hemachromatosis
- Pregnancy (acute fatty liver; Hemolysis, Elevated Liver enzymes, and Low Platelet count [HELLP] syndrome)
- Wilson's disease

TUMORS
- Hepatoblastoma
- Primary hepatocellular carcinoma
- Secondary tumors (e.g., lymphomas, metastasis)

Disease prevention involves specific diagnoses and includes decreased alcohol intake, avoidance of hepatotoxic substances, including acetaminophen, weight control, limiting exposure to infectious diseases, and vaccination against hepatitis A and B. The incidence of hepatitis A has declined markedly in the United States from 9.1 cases per 100,000 in 1992 to 2.6 cases per 100,000 in 2003. This is attributed to implementation of routine hepatitis A vaccinations in children.[36] Currently, there is no vaccination available for hepatitis C.

APPLIED PHYSIOLOGY

The liver is situated in the right upper quadrant of the abdomen, from the fifth rib to the manubrium. It is divided into two major lobes, which are further subdivided into eight functional segments (Figure 27-1).

seventh for ages 35 to 44 and fourth for ages 45 to 54 years; viral hepatitis is the tenth leading cause of death in this age-group.[43] Liver diseases can be classified into four major categories: hepatocellular diseases affecting the liver parenchyma, cholestatic diseases affecting the biliary ducts, metabolic diseases, and tumors. Specific diseases are listed in Box 27-1.

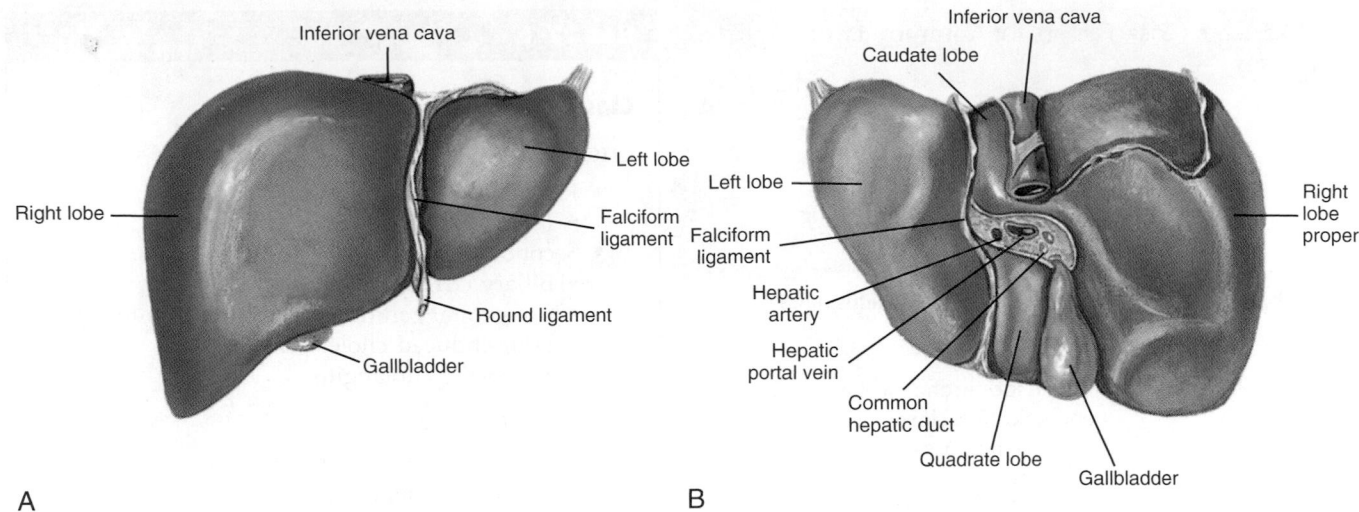

♦FIGURE 27-1 Gross structure of the liver. **A,** Anterior view. **B,** Posterior view.

The liver has a dual circulation much like the lungs. The portal vein brings blood directly from the mesenteric circulation to the parenchyma for processing, while the hepatic artery supplies the organ with oxygenated blood. Venous outflow is via the hepatic veins into the inferior vena cava.[5]

The functional unit of the liver is the lobule (Figure 27-2). Blood enters the lobule via the portal tract, flowing over plates of hepatocytes for processing. It empties into the central vein, which progresses to the hepatic veins. Bile canaliculi run countercurrent to blood flow in the lobule, eventually gathering and forming the hepatic ducts and common bile duct. Bile moves to the gallbladder via the cystic duct for storage and concentration. The cystic duct branches off the common bile duct, which delivers bile to the duodenum through the sphincter of Oddi.[5,14]

The liver has tremendous functional reserve, maintaining homeostasis with only 20% of viable parenchyma. Its main functions are metabolic, excretory, detoxification, and immunologic, and include detoxification of toxins and drugs, breakdown of bilirubin and production of bile acids, production and deamination of proteins, fat metabolism, glucose and acid-base maintenance, excretion of drugs and hormones, and metabolism and storage of metals and vitamins.[5,16] Hepatic tests can be classified into four major groups (Table 27-2).

Cirrhosis

It has been said that if the patient lives long enough, all causes of chronic liver disease lead to cirrhosis.[23] Cirrhosis is the end result of chronic, ongoing liver disease. It begins with fibrosis, which is the healing process that mitigates with chronic liver injury.[22] The hepatic

stellate cells, parenchymal liver cells thought to regulate intrahepatic blood flow, have been implicated in the formation of collagen and fibrin in the presence of liver damage. These fibrin fibers contract over time, causing shrinking and hardening of the liver and distortion of the architecture of the lobules. This impairs blood flow through the liver, causing portal hypertension, splenomegaly, ascites, and variceal bleeding. Manifestations of cirrhosis can be detected by using abdominal ultrasound, computed tomography, or magnetic resonance imaging. Early stages and progression of cirrhosis are confirmed by liver biopsy.[46,48]

The severity and prognosis of liver failure resulting from cirrhosis are assessed using the Child-Turcotte-Pugh scoring system (Table 27-3). Cirrhosis can be considered compensated or decompensated. Compensated or stable cirrhosis is defined by biopsy-proven cirrhosis in a patient who has never had signs of decompensation (e.g., variceal hemorrhage, ascites, encephalopathy). Conversely, cirrhotic patients who experience any of these complications are described as having decompensated cirrhosis. The onset of decompensation is associated with higher mortality.[22,33,43] Disease severity and mortality risk in patients with alcoholic hepatitis may be estimated by using a discriminant function formula (Maddrey score), calculated as follows:

$$\text{Discriminant function} = 4.6 \times [(\text{prothrombin time} - \text{control PT} + (\text{serum bilirubin level})]$$

where PT refers to the prothrombin time and the bilirubin concentration is measured in units of milligrams per deciliter.[52] A value greater than 32 mg/dl is associated with a high short-term mortality, and has been used to determine the need for specific treatment in patients with severe alcoholic hepatitis.

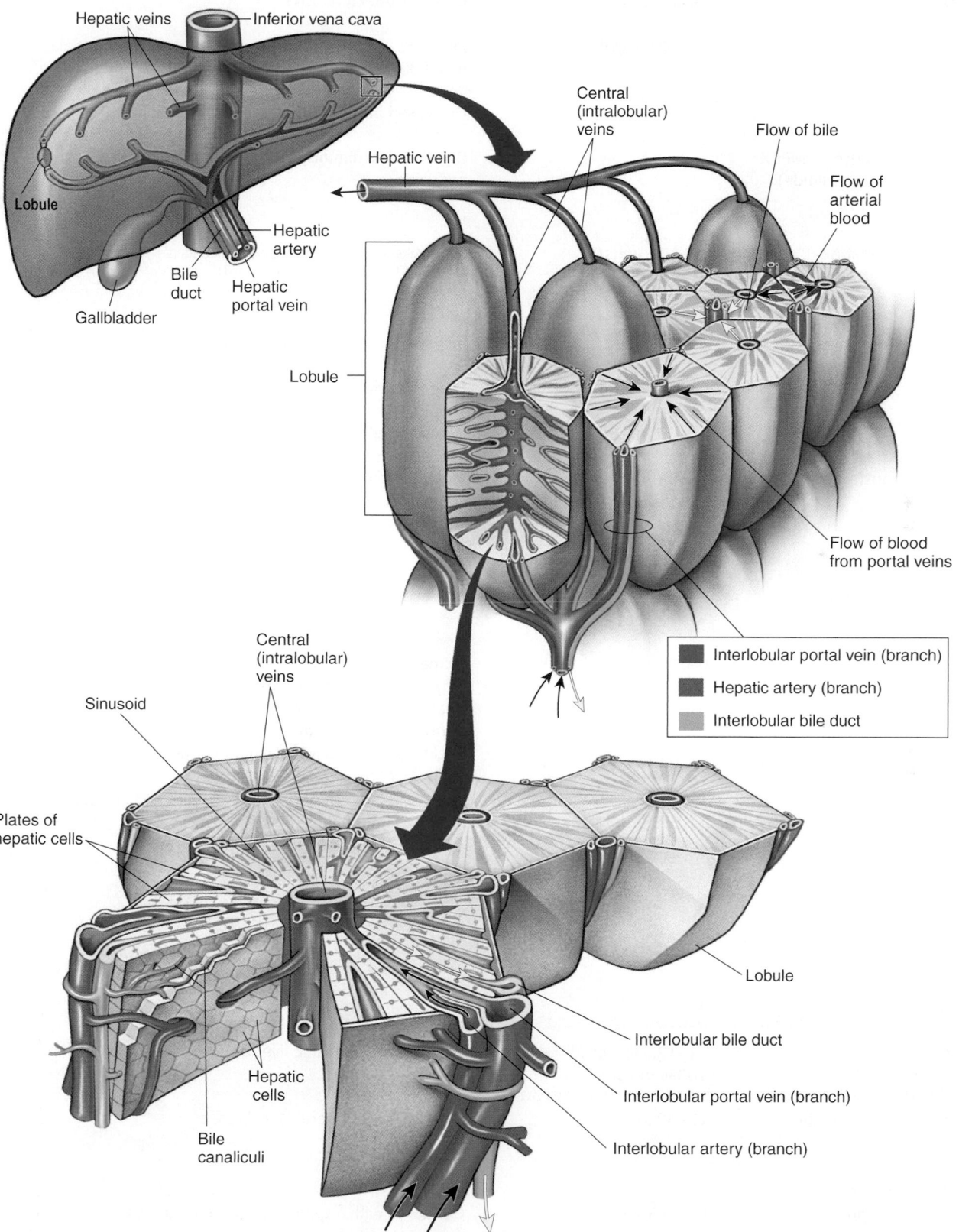

FIGURE 27-2 Structure of the lobule, the functional unit of the liver.

TABLE 27-2 Liver Function Tests

CLEARANCE	NORMAL VALUES	CLINICAL IMPLICATIONS
Ammonia	10–80 mcg/dl	Increases with hepatocellular dysfunction as ammonia metabolism is decreased
Galactose clearance		Decreased in diminished hepatic function
Lidocaine clearance to MEGX (monoethylglycinexylidide)		Decreased in diminished hepatic function, decreased hepatic perfusion
Cholestasis		
Alkaline phosphatase	30–120 units/L	Increases in obstruction and cirrhosis
Bilirubin		
Indirect (unconjugated)	0.2–0.8 mg/dl	Increases with lysis of red blood cells
Direct (conjugated)	0.1–0.3 mg/dl	Increases with hepatocellular injury or obstruction
Total	0.3–1.0 mg/dl	Increases with biliary obstruction
γ-Glutamyltransferase (GGT)	8–38 units/L; females younger than 45: 5–27 units/L	Most sensitive liver enzyme in detecting obstruction, cholangitis, or cholecystitis Can be used to detect chronic alcohol ingestion
Liver Injury		
Alanine aminotransaminase (ALT)	4–36 units/L	Increases in hepatocellular injury
Aspartate aminotransaminase (AST)	0–35 units/L	Increases in hepatocellular injury May rise to 20 times normal in acute hepatitis In acute extrahepatic obstruction, quickly rises to 10 times normal; falls as swiftly In cirrhosis, degree of elevation correlated to degree of inflammation
Lactate dehydrogenase (LDH) LHD isoenzyme 4: most liver specific	100–190 units/L	Increases in hepatitis
Synthetic Function		
Clotting Function Tests		
INR	1	
Prothrombin time	11–12.5 sec or 85%–100% of control	Increases with chronic liver disease, vitamin K deficiency
Partial thromboplastin time	25–40 sec	Increases with severe liver disease
Protein Studies		
Total serum protein	6.4–8.3 g/dl	Decreases with hepatocellular injury, cirrhosis
Serum albumin	3.5–5 g/dl	Decreases in cirrhosis, liver disease, viral hepatitis, ascites
Serum globulin	2.3–3.4 g/dl	Decreases in cirrhosis, liver disease, viral hepatitis; can increase in autoimmune hepatitis

TABLE 27-3 Child-Turcotte-Pugh System for Scoring the Severity and Prognosis of Liver Failure Caused by Cirrhosis

CLINICAL AND BIOCHEMICAL MEASUREMENTS	Points Scored for Increasing Abnormality		
	1	2	3
Encephalopathy (grade)	None	1 and 2	3 and 4
Ascites	Absent	Slight	Moderate
Bilirubin (mg/dl)	1–1.9	2–2.9	>3
Albumin (g/dl)	>3.5	2.8–3.5	<2.8
Prothrombin time (sec prolonged)	1–4	4–6	>6
For primary biliary cirrhosis: bilirubin (mg/dl)	1–4	4–10	>10
CHILD GRADE	**Total Score**		
A	5–6		
B	7–9		
C	≥10		

From reference 39a.

Hepatic Encephalopathy

Hepatic encephalopathy (HE) is defined as a disturbance in central nervous system function resulting from hepatic insufficiency. These disturbances are usually exhibited clinically as interruption of nerve impulse transmission, and cognitive and behavioral changes.[8,37] These changes are staged from 0 to 4 (Box 27-2). The pathophysiology of hepatic encephalopathy is incompletely understood. There is evidence that ammonia plays a key role in HE. Ammonia is produced in the gut by urease activity of bacteria on nitrogenous waste products, and from deamination of glutamine in the small bowel. Ammonia levels often do not correlate with levels of HE; patients with minimally elevated venous ammonia levels in ALF can be comatose, while patients with chronic liver disease and ammonia levels higher than 100 mg/dl will exhibit minimal signs of HE.[8] Serum ammonia levels are best measured in arterial blood samples, before passage through the liver, and the sample should be processed immediately.[5] Other substances recognized in the development of HE are octopamines, phenol, mercaptans, and intrinsic benzodiazepines.[13,49] It is believed that these substances in part induce gamma-aminobutyric acid (GABA) pathways, which downregulate nerve impulse transmission. This downregulation is characterized by altered nerve transmission, which is exhibited as asterixis, hippus

(asterixis or jerking contraction of the pupils), decreased or absent deep tendon reflexes, or absent gag and corneal reflexes.[8,33] Deposition of manganese in the central nervous system has also been implicated in neurologic dysfunction in chronic liver disease, as it deposits in basal ganglia and induces extrapyramidal symptoms.[45]

Box 27-2

West Haven Criteria of Altered Mental State

Stage 0: Lack of detectable changes in personality or behavior; asterixis absent.
Stage 1: Trivial lack of awareness; shortened attention span; impaired addition or subtraction skills; hypersomnia, insomnia, or inversion of sleep pattern; euphoria or depression; asterixis is detectable.
Stage 2: Lethargy or apathy; disorientation; inappropriate behavior; slurred speech; obvious asterixis.
Stage 3: Gross disorientation; bizarre behavior; semistuporous to stupor; asterixis is generally absent.
Stage 4: Coma.

Patients with chronic liver disease can have induction or worsening of HE by precipitating factors. These factors include infection, bleeding, fluid and electrolyte imbalances, medications, hypoxia, and primary or secondary disease exacerbation. Many medications are key factors in triggering HE, and include sedatives, narcotics, and diuretics. Alterations in hepatic, splanchnic, or systemic circulation can shunt blood from the hepatic parenchyma, bypassing the liver and preventing the processing of toxins, leading to HE.[8,35] Causes of this include thrombosis, spontaneous or surgical portosystemic shunt, and placement of a transjugular intrahepatic portosystemic shunt (TIPS).[14,22] The development of overt HE is usually seen in patients who are Childs Class B or C, and carries an overall poor prognosis without transplantation.[37]

The role of nursing in detecting and managing hepatic encephalopathy cannot be overemphasized. The nurse needs to be alert to changes in mental status, and rapidly implement appropriate treatments, including administering medications, providing for patient safety, preventing aspiration, placing nasogastric or enteral feeding tubes, and arranging for elective intubation to protect the airway. Patient and family education and support about HE and treatment are essential. Patients often become afraid or confused with encephalopathy and require reorientation, direction with activities of daily living (ADLs), and empathy. It is important to also screen for depression.[37]

Treatment of HE is based on several areas. The most important aspect of management is to treat the precipitating factors or conditions. Dietary education is considered first-line management for HE. Protein converts to urea and ammonia, which can increase ammonia levels; however, the catabolic state of liver disease increases the need for protein for immune system and organ maintenance. Dietary protein is usually restricted for the first 24 hours and then reintroduced with moderate protein restriction, usually 1 to 1.5 g of protein per kilogram per day, or 60 to 80 g per day.[38,41] Vegetable and dairy proteins are preferred to animal sources, as they provide a higher calorie to nitrogen ratio and more nonabsorbable fiber, increasing colonic acidification and decreasing ammonia-producing bacteria. Oral and enteral formulas that have high levels of branched-chain amino acids are also preferred, as higher serum levels of branched-chain amino acids to aromatic amino acids can improve HE.[38,41,42] Zinc is a cofactor for urea cycle enzymes and promotes clearance of ammonia. Oral zinc replacement is recommended in zinc-deficient or malnourished patients.[42]

The effects of sedatives and narcotics are prolonged in liver disease and can worsen HE. Sedation of these patients should be avoided; if agitation is unmanageable, short-acting benzodiazepines or propofol (Diprivan) should be used, and can be reversed with flumazenil (Romazicon), if necessary.[8,43] Naloxone (Narcan) should be given if narcotic use is suspected as a precipitator of HE.[8]

The mainstays of treating hepatic encephalopathy remain correction of the precipitating factors and use of nonabsorbable disaccharides and antibiotics. The most commonly used medication is lactulose, a nonabsorbable disaccharide. It works by acidifying the colon, encouraging diffusion of ammonia from the blood into the gut. The cathartic effect of lactulose also encourages expulsion of ammonia ions. It can be given orally or via nasogastric tube, or as a retention enema when diluted with water. The goal for dosing is to produce two to three bowel movements per day.[8,35] Use of lactulose can increase abdominal distention, fluid and electrolyte loss through diarrhea, and hypernatremia. If these occur, lactulose dosing should be decreased or discontinued. Polyethylene glycol (GoLYTELY) and oral mannitol (Osmitrol) are also used for bowel cleansing if lactulose is inadequate.

Enteral antibiotics are used to treat HE in place of, or in conjunction with, lactulose. These work by decreasing the number of gut flora and reducing the activity of glutaminase in intestinal villi. Neomycin is most frequently used. Although gastrointestinal (GI) absorption is poor, it does occur, and the absorbed drug can be nephrotoxic and ototoxic. Neomycin is not recommended in patients with renal dysfunction. Metronidazole (Flagyl) has been shown to improve resistant HE.[8,33] Rifaximin (Xifaxan), a nonabsorbable antibiotic, is also a safe and well-tolerated treatment.[8,35] Flumazenil and bromocriptine (Parlodel) exert their neurologic effects directly on the brain. Flumazenil is recommended for stage 3 or 4 encephalopathy, or suspected benzodiazepine use. A large, multicenter trial reported no incidence of seizures with flumazenil in liver disease patients.[8,24] Bromocriptine can be used in cases unresponsive to other therapies.[13] If a spontaneous or surgical portosystemic shunt or TIPS is present, occlusion with placement of vascular coils can be considered when all other treatment options have failed and portal hypertension is controlled.[10,39]

Portal Hypertension. Portal hypertension (PHTN) can be caused by any condition that impairs portal blood flow. The types of PHTN are classified in relation to where the cause of increased pressure occurs in relation to the sinusoids of the lobule.[47] Presinusoidal PHTN occurs before the sinusoids, usually in the portal vein and its branches, and includes portal vein thrombosis (usually from tumors or masses) and cavernous vein transformation. Sinusoidal PHTN occurs within the liver parenchyma, with increased intrahepatic resistance. This is seen with cirrhosis, schistosomiasis (a parasitic disease), and sarcoidosis. Postsinusoidal PHTN occurs primarily in the hepatic veins and branches and includes Budd-Chiari syndrome (a coagulopathic disorder causing hepatic vein thrombosis and resistance to blood outflow), venoocclusive disease of the hepatic veins or inferior vena cava, and severe congestive heart failure.[8,47]

Progression of cirrhosis or severe necrosis of the liver promotes resistance to blood flow through the liver. In turn, the myelofibroblasts and stellate cells within the liver sinusoids cause vasoconstriction within the sinusoids in response to systemic vasoconstrictors, such as endothelin-1 and angiotensin II, leading to an increase in portal resistance. Blood backs up under pressure in the portal, splenic, and mesenteric circulation, causing portal hypertension.[5,27] This in turn results in portosystemic shunts, esophageal and gastric varices, hemorrhoids, caput medusae (enlarged, engorged umbilical and abdominal veins), and ascites.[22]

As portal pressure builds, the spleen enlarges. Splenomegaly from portal hypertension causes sequestration of blood cells, particularly platelets, and leads to anemia, leukopenia, and thrombocytopenia.[5]

The effects of portal hypertension can be debilitating and life-threatening. The most severe complications of PHTN are ascites, spontaneous bacterial peritonitis, hepatic encephalopathy, hepatorenal syndrome, varices, and gastrointestinal (GI) bleeding.

Ascites. Ascites is the most common major complication of cirrhosis and is seen in some cases of ALF.[27] It is the accumulation of fluid and protein in the peritoneal space with resulting abdominal distention. This maldistribution of fluid and oncotic molecules increases the amount of total body water, and is associated with dilution of serum sodium and decreased intravascular volume.[17,12]

Ascites is most commonly caused by portal hypertension, although up to 20% of cases can have nonhepatic causes (e.g., carcinoma, peritoneal tuberculosis, heart failure[22,46]). Communication of fluid from the abdominal compartment into the negative pleural space causes hepatic hydrothorax, with hypoxia, orthopnea, atelectasis, and possible pneumonia. Hepatic hydrothorax occurs in 5% of all patients with cirrhosis and 12% of all patients with decompensated cirrhosis. This is most commonly seen on the right side.[18,28]

The mainstay of treatment of ascites includes limiting sodium intake to 2 g/day, restricting fluid intake, using diuretics, and educating the patient regarding compliance with restrictions and the plan of care.[46] Diuretics include potassium-sparing diuretics, which are aldosterone antagonists that exert their effect on the collecting tubules. This treatment is effective in liver disease because these patients do not completely metabolize intrinsic aldosterone, resulting in sodium and water retention. It is used in combination with loop diuretics, which help control the hyperkalemia seen with aldosterone antagonists and are synergistic in producing diuresis.[46,47] Diuretics are very effective when serum creatinine level is less than 1.5 mg/dl and renal function is intact. Large-volume paracentesis rapidly removes the abdominal fluid via a percutaneous needle or trocar and is used for patients with respiratory distress related to abdominal distention. Albumin 25% is used as a volume expander and infused at 6 to 8 g/L of fluid removed to prevent the hemodynamic and renal instability associated with large fluid shifts.[12,48] In cases of massive ascites resistant to diuretics, renal impairment, and hepatic hydrothorax, a TIPS is used to help control ascites and improve intravascular volume to promote kidney function (Figure 27-3). The TIPS helps to reestablish blood flow from the portal to the hepatic circulation by means of a vascular stent placed between branches of the portal and hepatic veins through the liver parenchyma. The stent is placed under fluoroscopy by the interventional radiologist.[9,14] The stent can become occluded, initially by thrombus or over time by epithelialization of the lumen. TIPS patency is monitored by periodically performing abdominal Doppler ultrasonography. Immediate complications of TIPS placement include hemorrhage, infection, congestive heart failure from increased preload, renal dysfunction from contrast dye, and hepatic encephalopathy from increased shunting of blood past the liver parenchyma.[14] Nursing care post-TIPS includes frequent physical assessment for worsening hepatic encephalopathy (altered mental status, asterixis, increased serum ammonia concentration); bleeding (abdominal distention, tenderness or rebound tenderness indicative of intra-abdominal bleeding and peritoneal irritation, increased heart rate with decreased blood pressure, increased pulse pressure, decreased hematocrit); fever; chills; signs and symptoms of congestive heart failure or renal failure (including shortness of breath, rales, decreased oxygen saturation, jugular venous distention, decreased urine output, increased creatinine level); and worsening hepatic function (increased INR, increased bilirubin level).[14]

Systemic Hemodynamics. Patients with liver disease are in a constant state of systemic inflammatory response syndrome (see Chapter 42). This manifests with low mean arterial pressure and peripheral vascular resistance. These systemic changes are related to a number of factors including accumulation of vasoactive peptides and cytokines, such as tumor necrosis factor-alpha and interleukins 1 and 6.[11] The formation of ascites also creates fluid shifts with a decrease in intravascular volume, further lowering blood pressure and filling

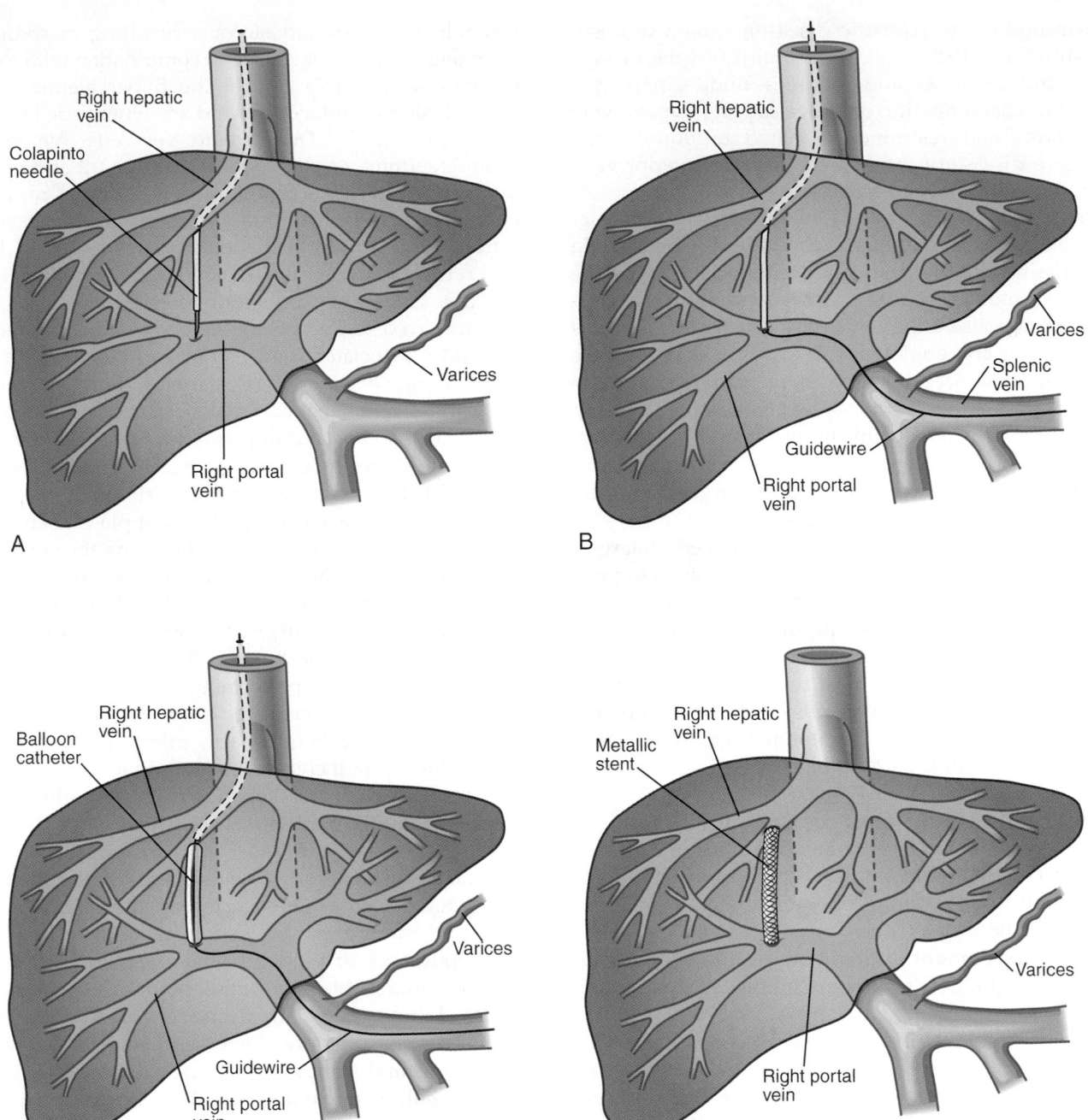

♦FIGURE 27-3 Transjugular intrahepatic portosystemic shunt (TIPS) to help control ascites. **A,** A sheathed transjugular needle is advanced out of a hepatic vein into an intrahepatic branch of the portal vein. **B,** A guidewire is threaded through the needle into the splenic vein. **C,** The parenchymal liver tract between the hepatic and portal veins is ligated using a balloon angioplasty catheter. **D,** A metallic stent is deployed with the shunt tract.

pressures. Patients with liver failure at times require hemodynamic monitoring with a central venous pressure (CVP) line or pulmonary artery catheter. Fluid boluses with normal saline, albumin, or blood products help to normalize the CVP to 8 to 10 mm Hg, and alpha-adrenergic agents (e.g., midodrine [ProAmatine], phenylephrine [Neo-Synephrine]) are useful in maintaining mean arterial blood pressure at 60 to 70 mm Hg.[43]

Glucose, Acid-Base, and Electrolyte Imbalances. Metabolic derangements are common in acute and chronic liver failure. Acidosis can be caused by an increase in serum lactate levels from reduced conversion in the diseased liver or by respiratory compromise from abdominal distention, ascites, hepatic hydrothorax, or depressed respiratory rate.[43] Respiratory alkalosis is associated with the tachypnea and hypocapnia of worsening encephalopathy. Metabolic alkalosis may develop following administration of citrated blood products, as the citrate converts in part to bicarbonate.[43] Serum magnesium, phosphorus, and potassium levels are frequently low from poor intake and the use of diuretics and may require replacement throughout the hospital course.[14] Hyponatremia is usually dilutional in nature and should NOT be corrected rapidly, as this can result in demyelinating syndromes (e.g., central pontine and oncotic myelinolysis, seizures). Because lactate conversion is impaired, the infusion of lactated Ringer's solution is discouraged in liver dysfunction.[5,43]

Serum glucose levels tend to elevate in early ALF or in chronic liver failure patients who are in stress states (e.g., infection, bleeding). Hypoglycemia is seen in severe liver failure, as glucose generation and regulation are lost.[5,43] Fingerstick glucose results need to be monitored frequently, usually every 1 to 4 hours. Dextrose 10% infusions or enteral feedings are given to maintain glucose levels.

Malnutrition. All liver disease patients tend to present in a hypercatabolic state, with varying degrees of protein energy malnutrition (the highest caloric and protein requirements are in patients with acute alcoholic hepatitis and sepsis). Consultation with a nutritionist is imperative to improve and maintain nutritional balance, especially in the presence of renal dysfunction.[41] Enteral feedings should be initiated early to provide substrate, prevent stress ulcers, and maintain gut integrity. Special care must be exercised to prevent aspiration, including keeping the head of the bed elevated, monitoring tube feeding residuals, observing for abdominal distention, and using duodenal or jejunal feeding tubes. Multivitamin, thiamine, and folate supplements are required to replenish depleted stores. The usual dose of thiamine is 100 mg daily, and of folate 1 mg daily. All vitamins can be given enterally or intravenously.[41,42] Expanded nutritional information is provided in the Nutrition box at right.

Coagulopathy. Coagulopathy is a potentially life-threatening complication of liver failure. Causes are multifactorial, with derangements of both clot formation and degradation. Synthesis of clotting factors by the liver is decreased, along with absorption and utilization of vitamin K. The decrease in hepatic production of

---

◆ NUTRITION

Considerations for Nutrition

Patients with chronic and acute liver disease have varying degrees of nutritional deficiencies, which is referred to as *protein energy malnutrition (PEM)*. Traditionally, protein was restricted in patients with hepatic encephalopathy to prevent generation of ammonia. However, because of varying degrees of protein deficiency and hypermetabolism, PEM and protein requirement may be high even in these patients. The highest protein and caloric requirements are for patients with acute alcoholic hepatitis, who conversely usually have the poorest baseline nutritional status. Malabsorption, particularly from medications causing high gut motility (e.g., lactulose, neomycin), can also increase PEM.

CALORIES

- Patients with liver dysfunction have PEM until proven otherwise.
- Provide a nutrition consult to assess baseline and daily nutritional status.

PROTEIN

- Consider protein restriction only for severe (stage 3 or 4) encephalopathy, usually 60–80 g/day.
- Aim for maximum tolerable protein intake, usually 1.2 g/day (range 1–1.5 g/day).
- Give branched-chain amino acid formulas for patients with stage 3 or 4 hepatic encephalopathy.

FLUID

- Enforce fluid restriction for patients with hyponatremia (1000–1500 ml/day) and ascites.

ELECTROLYTES

- Aim for sodium restriction of 2 g/day for patients with ascites and edema.
- Provide frequent glucose monitoring, with glucose and insulin administration.

VITAMINS AND MINERALS

- Supplement with zinc, folic acid, thiamine, and multivitamins.
- Evaluate for fat-soluble vitamin deficiencies (A, D, E, K), and supplement as needed.

SPECIAL CONSIDERATIONS

- Consider total parenteral nutrition only in patients with prolonged (>4 days) poor intake who cannot tolerate enteral feedings.

Data from references 38, 41, 42.

antithrombolytics can also result in accelerated clot destruction. GI bleeding accelerates the utilization of clotting factors as well.[5,21]

It is important not to overhydrate patients, with maintenance of central venous pressure at 8 to 10 mm Hg and mean arterial pressure at 60 to 70 mm Hg, especially in those patients with varices.[16] Transfusions rates should be monitored carefully. Targeted blood replacement therapy involves replacing those factors that are proven deficient or needed to control bleeding.[21,30] Red blood cells are generally given to keep the hematocrit at 25% to 30%. Platelets are generally not transfused unless levels are below 10,000/mm^3 with no evidence of bleeding, or at or below 50,000/mm^3 if there is active bleeding or before invasive procedures.[33] Fresh frozen plasma (FFP) or frozen plasma (FP) is administered if the INR is greater than 1.5 in the presence of bleeding or before invasive procedures. Cryoprecipitate is given if the fibrinogen level is less than 100 mg/dl (see Chapter 36). If the INR is not corrected with 2 to 4 units of FFP, factor VIIa administration is considered. Factor VIIa is a clotting factor that is poorly produced in liver failure, and is volatile and found in inadequate amounts in banked blood products. It is given as an IV bolus and can rapidly correct the INR to normal range without the fluid load of FFP. Factor VIIa is scarce and expensive, and can induce antibody formation with repeated doses.[43,44]

Gastrointestinal Bleeding. Bleeding from esophagogastric varices accounts for one third of all deaths of patients with cirrhosis. Up to 90% of all cirrhotic patients will experience a GI bleed.[21]

The formation of portal hypertension increases the pressure in the veins of the GI tract. As a result of this increased pressure, a system of collateral circulation develops (Figure 27-4). This collateral circulation connects with systemic veins to shunt a portion of the portal venous blood back into systemic circulation, bypassing the liver and lowering portal pressure. Even with this shunting, under continued high pressures, the thin venous walls weaken and develop pouches, with loss of competence of the venous valves, creating varices (particularly in the esophagus and stomach) and internal and external hemorrhoids. The varices can rupture, causing life-threatening GI bleeding. The veins of the gastric lining can also become engorged and friable, causing portal hypertensive gastropathy.[27]

Nonspecific beta antagonists or blockers (e.g., propranolol [Inderal], atenolol [Tenormin]), are used chronically to decrease portal pressure and prevent bleeding, and have been proven to prevent rebleeding.[1] Nitrates can be added to decrease portal pressure if the patient's blood pressure is stable enough to tolerate the additional drug.[1,24]

Esophagogastroduodenoscopy (EGD) is performed to examine the upper GI tract and manage bleeding. Bleeding is controlled by variceal banding. This is accomplished by placing rubber bands at the base of the varix under direct endoscopic visualization. Endoscopic sclerotherapy, in which a sclerosing agent such as ethanol is injected directly into the varix to induce thrombosis, is also used to control bleeding.[6,24,25] Banding is preferred over sclerotherapy because it results in less incidence of recurrent bleeding. The TIPS is used as a second-line therapy in patients who have failed pharmacologic therapy and endoscopic intervention.[6] After liver transplantation, portal pressures usually normalize with disappearance of varices.[11]

A temporary method for a massive or continued GI bleed is the gastroesophageal compression tube (Chapter 26). These tubes are more commonly know as Sengstaken-Blakemore or Minnesota tubes, and are most helpful in controlling bleeding gastric varices, which are not normally amenable to banding or sclerotherapy. These tubes should only be used for 24 to 48 hours.[21] Esophageal rupture and pneumomediastinum are the most serious complications from using these tubes. If GI bleeding is recurrent after variceal banding/sclerotherapy or is uncontrolled, a TIPS or surgical portosystemic shunt can be done emergently to decrease portal pressure.[6,9]

Hemorrhoid rupture is less common than esophageal and gastric variceal bleeding, but more difficult to control. Medical treatment is the same as for esophageal varices. Colonoscopy can be performed to localize bleeding and allow for application of fibrin. For variceal bleeding uncontrolled by all conventional measures, selective embolization of the involved vessels via vascular catheters by the interventional radiologist can be considered.[6,9]

The nurse must be alert to signs and symptoms of GI bleeding. These include increased pulse pressure, decreased blood pressure and CVP or wedge pressure, falling hematocrit, abdominal distention, blood or coffee ground material in the nasogastric tube, or emesis, melena, or hematochezia. Nasogastric tubes should be inserted with minimal trauma and placed to low intermittent suction to prevent erosions to the gastric mucosa. Rectal tubes and trumpets should be avoided to prevent hemorrhoidal bleeding, which is difficult to control. Treatment includes octreotide (Sandostatin) infusion to decrease portal pressure, with gastric protective agents.[1] Lactulose or other cathartics and nonabsorbable antibiotics are used to decrease the protein load from breakdown of blood in the gut and prevent worsening of hepatic encephalopathy. Blood component therapy should be targeted to volume

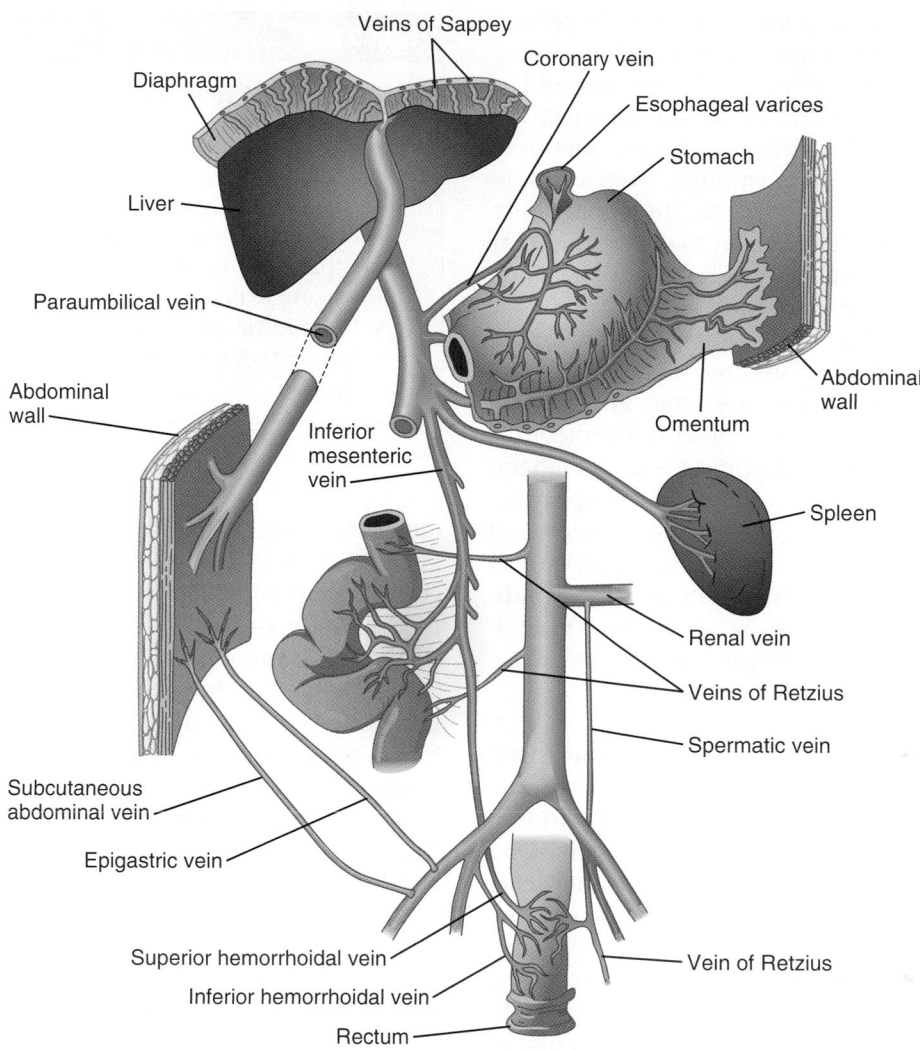

◆FIGURE 27-4 Collateral circulation in the liver.

replacement without overhydration. The usual target central venous pressure range is 8 to 10 mm Hg. Prophylactic antibiotics are used to prevent gram-negative infection after GI bleeding and interventional procedures.[1]

Infection. All patients with liver dysfunction are at risk for bacterial or fungal infection. This is due in part to the loss of Kupffer cell function within the hepatic sinusoids. These cells phagocytize gram-negative bacteria leaked from the gut; loss of function results in gram-negative bacteremia.[46] Malnutrition and increase in toxins cause general immune system suppression, increasing the likelihood of infection.[38] The presence of ascites predisposes the patient to spontaneous bacterial peritonitis (SBP). This is defined as a polymorphic neutrophil (PMN) count of greater than 250 mm^3 in ascitic fluid.[46] Treatment of SBP includes intravenous antibiotics and albumin, which reduces the incidence of renal

dysfunction.[48] For patients not prescribed prophylactic antibiotics or antifungals, infection surveillance (including blood, sputum, and urine cultures; chest x-ray) is recommended.[33,46] Infection must be detected and treated aggressively, as it can cause acute-on-chronic liver failure, exacerbate hepatic encephalopathy, precipitate hepatorenal syndrome type 1, and prevent the patient from receiving a transplant or cause complications after transplant.[11] Prophylactic antibiotics and antifungals should be considered, especially for pretransplant patients. Aminoglycosides are poorly metabolized in liver failure patients and are hepatotoxic and nephrotoxic; they should not be used in patients with liver failure.[46]

Hepatopulmonary Syndrome and Portopulmonary Hypertension. The lung vasculature is affected in liver disease, in that microdilation of capillary channels can occur, causing hepatopulmonary syndrome, or arterial constriction can result in portopulmonary hypertension.[19,33] Hepatopulmonary syndrome occurs in approximately 10% to 15% of patients with cirrhosis and is defined by intrapulmonary dilation and abnormal alveolar gas exchange. Symptoms include hypoxia that does not improve with oxygen administration, dyspnea, clubbing of digits, and cyanosis. Oxygenation sometimes improves with laying the patient flat to perfuse alveolar beds. Treatment is symptomatic. The syndrome often reverses over time after liver transplantation.[11]

Portopulmonary hypertension (PPH) is defined by a mean pulmonary artery pressure of greater than 25 mm Hg with a normal pulmonary artery wedge pressure. It is estimated to occur in up to 4% of all cirrhotics.[19] Symptoms include fatigue, dyspnea, and peripheral edema. Treatment for PPH is the same as that for primary pulmonary hypertension—prostaglandins, epoprostenol (Flolan), and treprostinil (Remodulin) infusions, or oral bosentan (Tracleer). Liver transplantation is contraindicated in moderate to severe cases because of high mortality from cardiopulmonary complications, particularly during anesthesia induction.[11]

Hepatorenal Syndrome. Hepatorenal syndrome (HRS) occurs in acute and chronic liver disease. It is characterized by abnormal renal function, splanchnic arterial vasodilation, and alterations in intrinsic renal blood flow.[10] There are two types. Type 1 has a rapid onset and progression and is usually triggered by bacterial infections. Most patients die within 2 weeks of onset of type 1 HRS if not treated. Type 2 is characterized by a slow, steady reduction in renal function with resistance to diuretics. The diagnosis of HRS is one of exclusion, focused on eliminating other causes of renal dysfunction (Box 27-3). Liver failure patients, particularly with ascites, tend to have low intravascular volume and SVR, which promotes prerenal azotemia and lowered urine output. Fluid bolus with normal saline or albumin tends to restore urine output in these cases.[9,10] If the patient is fluid resuscitated, with adequate mean arterial pressure (MAP) and no evidence of renal disease, sepsis, or use of nephrotoxic drugs, they are characterized as having HRS. Patients with HRS should be managed by monitoring urine output, weight, blood pressure and hemodynamic parameters, and levels of blood urea nitrogen, creatinine and electrolytes, and urine sodium and urea.

Treatment of HRS focuses on redirecting internal and external renal blood flow. The kidneys maintain intrinsic blood flow by producing prostaglandins, which cause renal vasodilation. Prostaglandin inhibitors, such as nonsteroidal antiinflammatory drugs, should not be given to liver failure patients.[10,43] A combination of midodrine (a peripheral vasoconstrictor), octreotide (a splanchnic vasoconstrictor), and albumin

---

> **Box 27-3**
>
> ### Criteria for Diagnosing Hepatorenal Syndrome
>
> - Creatinine level greater than 1.5 mg/dl or 24-hr creatinine clearance less than 40 ml/min
> - Absence of shock, infection, or fluid losses
> - No improvement after diuretic withdrawal and expansion of plasma volume with 1.5 L IV plasma expansion
> - Proteinuria less than 500 mg/day
> - No evidence of renal parenchymal or obstructive disease

From reference 4a.

(an oncotic agent) has been used to successfully treat HRS.[4] Terlipressin (a potent splenic vasoconstrictor), and albumin infusions are currently the standard treatment for hepatorenal syndrome type 1 worldwide; however, terlipressin is not available yet in the United States.[40] Dialytic therapy may be required as support until infection subsides or as a bridge to transplantation. The preferred mode of dialysis is continuous renal replacement therapy or extended daily dialysis rather than intermittent hemodialysis.[16] This prevents the hypotension and worsening cerebral edema seen with hemodialysis, and provides for real-time fluid and electrolyte regulation.[16,43] Studies have shown that extracorporeal albumin dialysis (ECAD) has shown efficacy in improving patients with HRS type 1.[49] HRS usually reverses with liver transplantation.[10,11]

Cerebral Edema and Herniation. Cerebral edema is realized as the most serious complication of liver failure. Indeed, any patient with stage 3 or 4 hepatic encephalopathy should be treated as a cerebral edema patient. The pathologic mechanisms are not fully understood, but are believed to be linked to edema of astrocytes in the brain and loss of cerebral blood flow autoregulation.[53] Recent studies show that an arterial ammonia level of greater than 200 mg/dl is associated with increased risk of cerebral herniation.[13] Noncontrast head computed tomography (CT) scan usually shows a generalized tightness of the brain with no shift in the ventricles. Intracranial pressure (ICP) monitoring is performed in some centers, with a goal to keep the ICP less than 20 to 25 mm Hg and a cerebral perfusion pressure (CPP) of 50 to 60 mm Hg. Patients should be positioned with the head of bed elevated 30 degrees, with the patient's head midline. The environment should be kept quiet and nonstimulating. Mannitol is effective in reducing ICP in ALF and can be used if renal function is adequate and serum osmolality is less than 320 mOsm/L.[43,53] Hyperventilation to reduce partial pressure of arterial carbon dioxide ($Paco_2$) to 25 to 30 mm Hg has been shown to quickly lower ICP, but the effects are short-lived, and the treatment is not recommended.[33] Seizures can occur, especially in the presence of electrolyte derangements. Phenytoin is the drug of choice for seizures over other agents that are hepatically or renally excreted.[43] Cisatracurium besylate (Nimbex) is preferred if neuromuscular blockade and paralysis are required, as it is metabolized through an acid-base pathway that is independent of the kidneys and liver. Propofol is the preferred sedative agent as it is reversible with flumazenil and better tolerated hemodynamically.[43]

Recent studies have demonstrated the effectiveness of moderate hypothermia (32° C to 33° C) in reducing ICP and stabilizing cerebral metabolism, as discussed in the Research Utilization box below.[27,51] This treatment should be implemented for patients with ALF and stages 3 to 4 HE by using ice packs or cooling blankets, decreasing the room temperature, cooling the ventilator humidifier, or employing commercially available regional cooling systems.

treatment modality. The method is widely available, simple, and inexpensive.

NEED FOR FURTHER STUDY

Additional multicenter studies with larger numbers of patients are needed to (1) examine the effects of mild hypothermia (34° to 35° C) versus moderate hypothermia on intracranial hypotension in ALF, (2) evaluate the optimal length of time for hypothermia in ALF, and (3) examine the possible complications of hypothermia treatment in ALF, including exacerbation of coagulopathies, immune system suppression, infection, sepsis, and multisystem organ dysfunction.

Jalan, R., et al. (2004). Moderate hypothermia in patients with acute liver failure and uncontrolled intracranial hypertension. *Gastroenterology, 127,* 1338–1346.

◆ RESEARCH UTILIZATION

Intracranial Pressure

CLINICAL ISSUE

Approximately 20% of patients with acute liver failure die from increased intracranial pressure (ICP) and cerebral herniation. Treatment options for increased ICP in acute liver failure are limited, and many patients have uncontrolled intracranial hypertension unresponsive to conventional therapy.

SUMMARY

In this single-center study, 14 patients with ALF and intracranial pressure not controlled by conventional therapy (2 doses of mannitol, removal of 500 ml of plasma fluid by venovenous hemofiltration) were cooled to a temperature of 33.1° ± 0.5° C from the time of enrollment until liver transplant, spontaneous recovery, or death. A reduction in ICP was noted within the first hour of treatment in all patients and sustained for 24 hours. Of the eight patients who had pupillary changes before treatment, seven had normalized pupillary reactions. Of the seven patients treated with hypothermia for more than 24 hours, five experienced increases in ICP that responded to treatment with mannitol. Of the 14 patients, 13 were successfully bridged to liver transplantation.

APPLICATION

With the limited number of modalities available for controlling intracranial hypertension in ALF, moderate hypothermia is currently recommended as a

◆ Case Study 27-1

Alcohol, Hepatitis, and the Liver

J.C. is a 52-year-old Caucasian male with history of end-stage liver disease secondary to alcoholic (Laënnec's) cirrhosis and hepatitis C. He presented in the emergency department with hematemesis. His assessment findings and laboratory values were as follows: alert, oriented to person, place, time, and purpose; anxious. His skin was pale and diaphoretic, with deep skin/scleral icterus and spider angiomas on the trunk. Abdominal ascites with fluid wave, caput medusae, diffuse tenderness to palpation with no rebound tenderness were present along with edema of the lower extremities. Vital signs included temperature: 100° F; heart rate: 62 beats/min; respiratory rate: 26 breaths/min; blood pressure: 80/40 mm Hg; output: 10 ml/hr. Laboratory values revealed glucose: 280 mg/dl; blood urea nitrogen: 57 mg/dl; creatinine: 3.6 mg/dl; sodium: 121 mEq/L; potassium: 6.9 mEq/L; bicarbonate: 16 mEq/L; magnesium: 1.3 mEq/L; phosphorus: 2.2 mEq/L; ammonia: 67 mcg/dl; AST: 65 mg u/L; ALT: 230 u/L; bilirubin: direct 6.5 mg/dl, total 10 mg/dl; white blood cell count: 14.2/mm³; hemoglobin: 6.3 g%; hematocrit: 20 g/dl; platelets: 45,000/mm³; and international normalized ratio (INR): 2.6. His abdominal ultrasound with Doppler study demonstrated a small, echogenic liver consistent with cirrhosis. There was decreased flow in the right portal vein. The kidneys demonstrated normal blood flow with no hydronephrosis or echogenicity.

Decision point: What type of liver failure does the patient have?

Decision point: What other tests would be helpful in this case?

MULTIDISCIPLINARY PLAN OF CARE

The liver failure patient is one of the most complex and challenging patients seen in critical care. Meticulous care coordinated among many disciplines is required for a positive patient outcome. The critical care nurse is the key factor in providing and coordinating this care, as described in the Multidisciplinary Plan of Care below and on p. 769. The coordinated management of acute liver failure patients in particular should be started at presentation at community hospitals and carried through to transfer to a tertiary liver center. This helps to ensure the patient's condition is optimized throughout the continuum of care. Box 27-4 is an example of a treatment protocol for referring hospitals and interfacility transport.

MULTIDISCIPLINARY PLAN OF CARE FOR PATIENTS WITH LIVER DYSFUNCTION/FAILURE

PROBLEM	INTERVENTION	RATIONALE	EXPECTED OUTCOME	COMMENTS
Risk for alterations in mental status	Assess mental status using Glasgow Coma Scale and hepatic encephalopathy (HE) scoring scale every 1–2 hours	Early detection and intervention will prevent worsening of encephalopathy and cerebral edema	Patient will not have progression of hepatic encephalopathy OR HE will be detected and treated early	
Risk for bleeding	Monitor line and wound sites, drainage tubes for bleeding Monitor for nasogastric bleeding and melena/bloody stools Assess abdomen for distention, rebound tenderness Monitor vital signs, hemodynamic parameters for changes Monitor complete blood cell count (CBC), coagulation studies every 8–12 hours	Early detection will prevent anemia, hemorrhage, and hemodynamic instability	Patient will have a stable hematology profile with no hemodynamic instability Bleeding will be detected and treated early	
Risk for hemodynamic instability	Monitor vital signs, hemodynamic parameters for changes, especially fever, decreased blood pressure, decreased filling pressures Monitor intake and output Monitor cardiac rhythm, especially for flattened T waves, prolonged QT interval, torsades de pointes	Early detection and intervention may prevent further organ compromise and complications	Patient will have stable vital signs and hemodynamic parameters	Serum glucose
Risk for electrolyte imbalances	Monitor laboratory values: Serum electrolytes Phosphorus, magnesium, albumin, and lactate Serum glucose Monitor fingerstick glucose results Replace glucose, albumin, and electrolytes as needed	Prevent glucose and electrolyte imbalances	Patient will be euglycemic with stable laboratory values	

PROBLEM	INTERVENTION	RATIONALE	EXPECTED OUTCOME	COMMENTS
Risk for infection	Monitor vital signs, line site, wounds, and abdomen for signs of infection Evaluate gag reflex and ability to protect airway Administer antibiotics/antifungals	Early detection of infection and timely treatment Prevention of aspiration	Patient will have no evidence of infection *OR* Infection will be detected and treated early	
Risk for hypoxia	Assess oxygen saturation, arterial blood gases (ABGs) Assess breath sounds Monitor fluid status	Early detection and intervention may prevent further hypoxia and organ damage	Patient will have stable ABGs and oxygen saturation	
Risk for cerebral edema	Assess patient with Glasgow Coma Scale Monitor intracranial pressure/cerebral perfusion pressure (ICP/CPP) Administer mannitol Implement and maintain hypothermia	Prevention of cerebral edema and herniation	Patient will have no evidence of cerebral herniation	

Risk for malnutrition	Assess creatinine, albumin values at least daily
	Assess protein and caloric requirements and intake:
	  Required daily intake per nutritionist
	  Calorie count
	Administer vitamins:
	  multivitamin, thiamine, folate
	Monitor weights
		Prevention of malnourishment and starvation state	Patient will have adequate nutritional balance	

REFERRAL/LISTING FOR LIVER TRANSPLANTATION

Liver transplantation remains the mainstay of treatment for many patients with liver failure. Chronic liver disease patients should be referred for transplantation when they develop evidence of synthetic dysfunction (low albumin level, elevated PT/PTT), experience their first complication of decompensation (ascites, variceal bleeding, hepatic encephalopathy), are diagnosed with hepatocellular tumors, or develop malnutrition.[11,32] All cases of acute liver failure should be referred for transplant evaluation and listing in an expedient manner.

The Model for End-Stage Liver Disease (MELD) score, originally used to predict 90-day mortality in patients with chronic liver disease, is now used by the United Network for Organ Sharing (UNOS) to prioritize and list patients with chronic liver disease for transplant in the United States. Implemented in 2002, the score is a logarithmic calculation based on three laboratory values: total bilirubin level, INR, and creatinine level. The calculation produces a numerical score. Patients with a MELD score of 30 or more have a higher risk of mortality. Status 1 on the UNOS transplant list is not associated with the MELD score and is reserved for patients with acute liver failure with a predicted life expectancy of less than 7 days.[11,55] These patients have the highest priority for receiving organs. Patients with renal failure may require simultaneous listing for liver and kidney transplant.[11,55]

Financial considerations are unavoidably linked to the transplant evaluation process.[37] Initial screening for funding for transplant is usually done by the transplant referral center, along with the initial psychosocial screening.

Box 27-4

Acute Liver Failure Transport Protocol Example

UCSD MEDICAL CENTER

THE LIVER CENTER/CENTER FOR TRANSPLANTATION, TREATMENT PROTOCOL

Management of Fulminant and Acute Hepatic Failure for Outside Medical Facilities and for Interfacility Transport Outside Medical Facility.

1. Contact the hepatologist on call at UCSDMC by contacting the page operator at _____. After the case is reviewed and discussed with the referring physician, the hepatologist will contact the Hillcrest Transfer Center to initiate transfer to UCSDMC Hillcrest.

2. If drug overdose is suspected:
   - a. Contact the Poison Control Center
   - b. Draw acetaminophen levels
   - c. For acetaminophen toxicity, continue *N*-acetyl cysteine PO or IV until AST/ALT are normalized.

3. Send the following tests: comprehensive drug screen, blood alcohol level, comprehensive metabolic panel (SMAC 22), magnesium, complete blood count with differential, PT/TPP, INR, fibrinogen, blood cultures, urinalysis, urine culture, chest x-ray; urine electrolytes, total protein, and urea.

4. Place 2 large-bore peripheral IV catheters, preferably in the antecubital space. AVOID CENTRAL LINE PLACEMENT. If a central line catheter is needed, correct the INR to 1.5 or less, and use the femoral or internal jugular veins. DO NOT use the subclavian sites, as this can result in a life-threatening pneumothorax or hemothorax.

5. IT IS VITAL THAT THESE PATIENTS BE COOLED TO A TEMPERATURE OF 32–34° C. This has been shown to decrease cerebral edema in liver failure. Treat the patient as you would a head injury patient:

   - Place cooling blankets above and below the patient.
   - Place ice packs over the liver, in the femoral and antecubital spaces, and over the internal jugular veins.
   - Keep the head of the bed elevated at a 45-degree angle. Do not flex the knees.
   - Keep the head midline.
   - Maintain a quiet, non-stimulating environment.

6. Sedate the patient with propofol as needed for agitation.

7. For stage 3 or 4 hepatic encephalopathy, intubate the patient.

8. DO not overhydrate the patient; use normal saline, blood products, or albumin for volume expansion. Do not use lactated Ringer's solution.

Interfacility Transportation.

1. Maintain cerebral edema precautions and moderate hypothermia throughout transport.
   - Place cooling blankets above and below the patient.
   - Place ice packs over the liver, in the femoral and antecubital spaces, and over the internal jugular veins.
   - Keep the head of the bed elevated at a 45-degree angle. Do not flex the knees.
   - Keep the head midline.

2. Do NOT use lactated Ringer's for fluid replacement. Do NOT overhydrate the patient.

3. Bring ALL test results, chart notes, and digitalized images with the patient.

4. Call the UCSD Hillcrest Transfer Center for any questions regarding transport or clinical management, at telephone _____. They will connect you with the hepatologist on call.

LIVER SUPPORT DEVICES

There remains an obvious need to support liver disease patients with devices as a bridge to liver transplant, or ideally to regeneration and recovery of native organ function. The development and availability of liver support devices (LSDs), however, have lagged behind other artificial organ support devices, such as renal dialysis, ventilators, membrane oxygenators, and ventricular support devices. This is related to the complexity of liver functions and the difficulty in developing technology to mimic these functions. The ideal liver support device must be able to regulate fluid, electrolyte, glucose, and acid-base balance, and provide clearance of circulating ammonia, false neurotransmitters (such as GABA), cytokines, and other hepatic toxins (particularly those that are protein-bound, such as bilirubin). The device should also synthesize critical molecules and orchestrate all these functions to preserve homeostasis and allow for hepatic regeneration. There should also be no complications from the therapy.[26]

Depending on whether or not cellular components are used, liver support devices can be classified as nonbiologic. Nonbiologic support devices use noncellular technologies to mimic certain aspects of liver function. The technologies utilize special filter membranes and resins, charcoal, or albumin in the dialysate to remove larger molecular weight or protein-bound substances that are not removed by conventional dialysis methods.[18,26]

Conventional dialytic therapies are also used in part for liver support. These modalities are particularly useful in patients experiencing renal dysfunction often seen with liver disease. Continuous renal replacement therapies (CRRTs) are routinely used for fluid, glucose, electrolyte, and acid-base regulation, and removal of small to middle-weight molecules, including some cytokines. Plasmapheresis and therapeutic plasma exchange (TPE) involves the removal of toxins by plasma removal and replacement. Previous studies showed no advantage to using this technique.[7,16] There are more recent case reports of successfully using TPE with CRRT to bridge patients to transplantation.[7] None of these nonbiologic methods provide synthesis of critical substances.

Biologic LSD devices employ isolated liver cells in bioreactors to mimic liver function. Other detoxifying components, such as charcoal and resin columns, are sometimes added to the system. These devices have the advantage of providing some synthetic function and toxin clearance that is comparable to native liver function. Several types are being developed worldwide; three are in active development in the United States with clinical trials in process.

Controlled trials of devices are needed, but are difficult to design and fund. Ongoing funding for research and development is required to bring an LSD to market, but infusion of funds often parallels the stock market and general economy. Safety remains a concern, particularly transmission of disease from the bioreactor hepatocytes. The profession needs to actively focus on specific areas of LSD development and research and sequence these activities logically to best utilize time and resources. The Acute Liver Failure Group, formed in 2003 by 24 U.S. centers and funded by the National Institutes of Health, will examine the role and development of liver support devices as part of its overall goal.[24] As clinical trials are completed, it is anticipated that both modalities will have a place in treating liver failure, with the less expensive nonbiologic LSDs used for less sick patients, and the more costly and complicated biologic LSDs reserved for more critical patients with less liver function.[50] Besides LSDs, other modalities in development include implantable "constructed" livers of hepatocytes grown on an artificial matrix, hepatocyte transplantation, and transgenic xenografts harvested from genetically altered animals to resemble human livers.[26,50]

◆ Case Study 27-2

A Diagnosis

S.M. is a 19-year-old African female who presented in the emergency department of a small community hospital with her mother. S.M. has complained of difficulty concentrating and tremors for 2 weeks. Three days ago she complained of nausea, vomiting, edema, and jaundice. Her mother states that S.M. has been moody and depressed, and on the day of admission had hallucinations and became violent toward family members. Her physical findings included being responsive to commands, flailing all extremities, and yelling one or two incomprehensible words. There was no asterixis. Her deep tendon reflexes were reduced to +1/4. She had a minimal gag reflex, and sluggish pupillary response at 4 mm bilaterally. Her skin was warm and flushed, with scleral icterus. Her abdomen was flat with minimal bowel sounds. Her liver border was palpated at 5 cm below costal margin. She was anuric. Her vital signs included temperature: 99.2° F, pulse was 110 beats/min; respiratory rate: 34 breaths/min; and blood pressure: 125/80 mm Hg. Her laboratory values revealed glucose: 63 mg/dl; BUN: 76 mg/dl; creatinine: 3.6 mg/dl; sodium: 148 mEq/L; potassium: 5.0 mEq/L; bicarbonate: 13 mEq/L; magnesium: 1.5 mEq/L; ammonia: 145 mcg/dl; AST: 5400 u/L; ALT: 4900 u/L; bilirubin: direct 2.1 mg/dl, total 4.5 mg/dl; white blood cell count: 10.0/mm³; hemoglobin: 13.5 g%; hematocrit: 42%; platelets: 145,000/mm³; and ratio INR 4.0.

Decision point: Based on the onset of symptoms and clinical data, what type of liver failure does the patient have?

Decision point: What is your initial treatment plan for this patient?

CONCLUSIONS

The complexity of liver dysfunction and disease and the multisystemic effects it creates make the nursing management of these patients one of the most challenging in critical care. Multidisciplinary planning and care coordination and timely referral for transplant are essential in producing optimal patient outcomes.

REFERENCES

1. Abraldes, J. G., Dell'Era, A., & Bosch, J. (2004). Medical management of variceal bleeding in patients with cirrhosis. *Can J Gastroenterol, 18,* 109–113.

2. Akriviadis, E., et al. (2000). Pentoxifylline improves short-term survival in severe acute alcoholic hepatitis: a double-blind, placebo-controlled trial. *Gastroenterology, 119*, 1637–1648.

3. Allen, J., Hassanein, T., & Bhatia, S. (2001). Advances in bioartificial liver devices. *Hepatology, 34*(3), 447–455.

4. Angeli, P., et al. (1999). Reversal of type 1 hepatorenal syndrome with the administration of midodrine and octreotide. *Hepatology, 29*, 1660–1670.

4a. Arroyo, V., et al. (1996). Definition and diagnosis of refractory ascites and hepatorenal syndrome in cirrhosis. *Hepatology, 23* (11), 164–176.

5. Bacon, B. R. (2000). Liver anatomy and physiology. In B. R. Bacon & A. M. Bisceglie (Eds.), *Liver disease: diagnosis and management.* New York: Churchill Livingstone.

6. Baille, J. (2005). Endoscopic variceal therapy. New York: AASLD/AHPBA Surgical Forum.

7. Biancofiore, G., Bindi, L., et al. (2003). Combined twice-daily plasma exchange and continuous veno-venous hemodiafiltration for bridging severe acute liver failure. *Transpl Proc, 35*(8), 3011–3014.

8. Blei, A. T., & Cordoba, J. (2005). Hepatic encephalopathy. *Am J Gastroenterol, 96*, 1868–1876.

9. Boyer, T., & Jaskal, Z. (2005). The role of transjugular intrahepatic protosystemic shunt in the management of portal hypertension. *Hepatology, 41*(2), 1–15.

10. Cardenas, A., Uriz, J., Gines, P., et al. (2000). Hepatorenal syndrome. *Liver Transplant, 6*, S63–S71.

11. Carithers, R. L. (2004). AASLD practice guideline: liver practice guideline: liver transplantation. *Liver Transplant, 1*, 122–135.

12. Choudhury, J., & Sanyal, A. (2003). Treatment of ascites. *Curr Treat Options Gastroenterol, 6*(6), 481–491.

13. Clemmesen, J. O., Larsen, F. S., Kondrup, J., et al. (1999). Cerebral herniation in patients with acute liver failure is correlated with arterial ammonia concentration. *Hepatology, 29*, 648–653.

14. Conn, H., Palmaz, J., et al. (2000). *TIPS: transjugular intrahepatic portosystemic shunts.* New York: Igaku-Shoin.

15. D'Amico, G., et al. (2005). Uncovered transjugular intrahepatic portosystemic shunt for refractory ascites: a meta-analysis. *Gastroenterology, 129*, 1282–1293.

16. Davenport, A., Will, E. J., & Davidson, A. (1993). Improved cardiovascular stability during continuous modes of renal replacement therapy in critically ill patients with acute hepatic and renal failure. *Crit Care Med, 21*, 328–338.

17. Deasy, J. (2005). Evaluating abnormal liver tests. *Clin Rev, 15*(9), 29–34.

18. Demetriou, A., Brown, R., Busuttil, R., et al. (2004). Prospective, randomized controlled trial of a bioartificial liver in treating acute liver failure. *Ann Surg, 239*(5), 667–670.

19. Fallon, M. (2001). Hepatopulmonary and portopulmonary hypertension, AASLD Annual Meeting, Dallas, Tex.

20. Friedman, L. S., & Keefe, E. (1998). *Handbook of liver disease.* New York: Churchill Livingstone.

21. Grace, N. (1997). ACG treatment guideline: diagnosis and treatment of gastrointestinal bleeding secondary to portal hypertension. *Am J Gastroenterol, 92*, 1081–1091.

22. Gines, P., Quintero, E., Arroyo, V., et al. (1987). Compensated cirrhosis: natural history and prognostic factors. *Hepatology, 7*, 12–18.

23. Hassanein, T. (1995). Personal communication.

24. Hassanein, T. (2004). Personal communication.

25. Haynes, G., et al. (2003). Albumin administration—what is the evidence of clinical benefit? A systematic review of randomized controlled trials. *Eur J Anaesthesiol, 20*(10), 771–793.

26. Huges, R., & Williams, R. (1996). Use of bioartificial and artificial liver support devices. *Semin Liver Disease, 16*(4), 435–444.

27. Jalan, R., et al. (2004). Moderate hypothermia in patients with acute liver failure and uncontrolled intracranial hypertension. *Gastroenterology, 127*, 1338–1346.

28. Jones, E. G. (2001). Hepatic hydrothorax: a retrospective case study. *J Am Acad Nurse Pract, 13*(5), 209–222.

29. Lee, W. M. (2003). *Acute liver failure in the United States.* Available at Thiemeconnect.com.

30. Lubel, J., & Angus, P. (2005). Modern management of portal hypertension. *Intern Med J, 35*, 45–49.

31. Maddrey, W. C., et al. (1978). Corticosteroid therapy of alcoholic hepatitis. *Gastroenterology, 75*, 193–199.

32. Maddrey, W., Schiff, E., & Sorrell, M. (2001). *Transplantation of the liver.* Philadelphia: Lippincott Williams & Wilkins.

33. Marreno, J., Martinez, F., & Hyzy, R. (2003). Advances in critical care hepatology. *Am J Respir Crit Care Med, 168*, 1421–1426.

34. Mas, A., Rodes, J., Sunyer, L., et al. (2003). Comparison of rifaximin and lactitol in the treatment of acute hepatic encephalopathy: results of a randomized, double-blind, double-dummy, controlled clinical trial. *J Hepatol, 38*, 51–58.

35. Massa, P., Vallerino, E., & Dodero, M. (1993). Treatment of hepatic encephalopathy with rifaximin: double-blind, double-dummy study versus lactulose. *Eur J Clin Res, 4*, 7–18.

36. (2005). *National Vital Statistics Rep, 53*(17), 1–2.

37. Nunes, F. A., Olthoff, K. M., & Lucey, M. R. (2000). Liver transplantation: indications, pre-transplant evaluation, and short-term post-transplant management. In B. R. Bacon & A. M. Bisceglie (Eds.), *Liver disease: diagnosis and management.* New York: Churchill Livingstone.

38. Nutritional status in cirrhosis. (2004). Italiane Multicentre Cooperative Project on Nutrition in Liver Cirrhosis. *J Hepatol, 21*, 317–325.

39. Ochs, A. (2005). Transjugular intrahepatic portosystemic shunt. *Dig Dis, 23*(1), 56–64.

39a. O'Grady, J., (2000). *Comprehensive clinical hepatology,* New York: Mosby.

40. Ortega, R., et al. (2002). Terlipressin therapy with and without albumin for patients with hepatorenal syndrome: results of a prospective, nonrandomized study. *Hepatology, 36* (4), 941–948.

41. Patton, K. M., & Aranda-Michel, J. (2002). Nutritional aspects in liver disease and liver transplantation. *Nutr Clin Pract, 17*, 332–340.

42. Plauth, M., Merli, M., Kondrup, J., et al. (1997). ESPEN guidelines for nutrition in liver disease and transplantation. *Clin Nutr, 16*, 43–55.

43. Polson, J., & Lee, W. (2005). AASLD position paper: the position paper: the management of acute liver failure. *Hepatology, 41*, 1179–1197.

44. Romero-Castro, R., et al. (2004). Recombinant-activated factor VII as hemostatic therapy in eight cases of severe hemorrhage from esophageal varices. *Clin Gastroenterol Hepatol, 2*(1), 78–84.

45. Rose, C., Butterworth, R. F., Zayed, J., et al. (2002). Manganese deposition in basal ganglia structures results from both portal-systemic shunting and liver dysfunction. *Gastroenterology, 117*, 640–644.

46. Runyon, B. (2004). Management of adult patients with ascites caused by cirrhosis. *Hepatology, 27*(1), 264–272.

47. Sanyal, A., & Shah, V. (2005). *Portal hypertension: pathobiology, evaluation, and treatment.* Totowa, NJ: Humana.

48. Sort, P., Navasa, M., Arroyao, V., et al. (1999). Effect of intravenous albumin on renal impairment and mortality in patient with cirrhosis and spontaneous bacterial peritonitis. *N Engl J Med, 34*, 403–409.

49. Stange, J., Hassanein, T., et al. (2002). The Molecular Adsorbent Recycling System as a liver support system based on albumin dialysis: a summary of preclinical investigations, prospective,

randomized, controlled clinical trial and clinical experience from 19 centers. *Artificial Organs, 26*(2), 1525–1594.

50. Stuart, S. (2002). Liver assist devices: proof of life. *Start-Up*, March, 19–28.

51. Swingman, C., et al. (2004). Selective alterations of brain osmolytes in acute liver failure: protective effect of mild hypothermia. *Brain Res, 999*, 118–123.

52. Tilg, H., & Kayser, A. (2005). *Management of acute alcoholic hepatitis*. Available at http://www.easl.ch/PGC/Tilg.pdf.

53. Tofteng, F., & Larsen, F. S. (2004). Management of patients with fulminant hepatic failure and brain edema. *Metabolic Brain Dis, 19*, 207–214.

54. Wasley, A., & Samandari, T. (2005). Incidence of hepatitis A in the United States in the era of vaccination. *JAMA, 294*(2), 246–248.

55. Wiesner, R. H. (2004). MELD/PELD and the allocation of deceased donor livers for Status 1 recipients with acute fulminant hepatic failure, primary nonfunction, hepatic artery thrombosis, and acute Wilson's disease. *Liver Transplant, 10*, S17–S22.

Eleanor Fitzpatrick

Acute pancreatitis is an acute inflammatory condition within the pancreas caused by the premature activation of pancreatic enzymes and the digestion of the gland by its own enzymes. In the normal pancreas, these enzymes are transported via the pancreatic duct into the duodenum, where they are activated and used for digestion of carbohydrates, fats, and proteins (Figure 28-1). In acute pancreatitis, the intracellular proteases are activated before transport. Acute pancreatitis ranges in severity from a mild glandular form of edema to severe hemorrhagic or infected pancreatic necrosis with multiple organ dysfunction syndrome (MODS). The disease affects not only the pancreas but also surrounding structures and remote organ systems. Acute pancreatitis is self-limiting in approximately 80% of cases; however, the fulminant, severe form of the disorder results in high mortality rates and requires complex management techniques.[36]

DEFINITION

Acute pancreatitis is a disorder of the exocrine pancreas. The function of the exocrine pancreas consists of synthesis and secretion of digestive enzymes into the small intestine to catalyze the hydrolysis and digestion of carbohydrates, proteins, and fats.[16] Many of the enzymes are proteases synthesized as proenzymes (zymogens) and require proteolytic activation by cleavage of their propeptides.[16] The enzymes amylase, trypsin, lipase, and others are secreted in their inactive form, becoming active upon entrance to the duodenum. Acute pancreatitis is an inflammatory condition of the pancreas initiated by injury to the acinar cells of the exocrine pancreas, resulting in premature activation and release of damaging enzymes. The enzymes and the subsequent release of other inflammatory chemicals cause destruction within the pancreas itself (autodigestion) as well as the surrounding tissues and distant organ systems. The Atlanta International Symposium on Pancreatitis defined the mild form of the disease as parenchymal interstitial edema

with rapid recovery. Severe acute pancreatitis includes disease states characterized by infection, parenchymal necrosis, hemodynamic compromise, and multiple organ dysfunction requiring intensive management.[6]

The mortality rate in pancreatitis is quite variable; the overall rate ranges from 10% to 15%. Severe acute pancreatitis is associated with a 20% mortality rate, and when infected necrosis ensues, the mortality rate increases to between 40% and 70%.[42,48]

The incidence of acute pancreatitis ranges from 10 to 46 cases per 100,000 per year, accounting for approximately 2% of all hospital admissions. The last decade has shown an increased incidence of acute pancreatitis, perhaps related to a higher sensitivity of diagnostic tests; there may be other yet unknown factors contributing to this increase.[28]

PATIENTS AT RISK

Eighty percent of all episodes of acute pancreatitis are caused by gallstone disease (including biliary sludge and biliary microlithiasis) with migration of stones or excessive alcohol consumption.[40] The remaining 20% of cases are attributable to a multitude of causes, including hyperlipidemias, hypercalcemic states, a variety of medications, infections, trauma, endoscopic retrograde cholangiopancreatography (ERCP), and other etiologies (Box 28-1). In approximately 10% to 20% of those with pancreatitis, no cause is ever identified; this is termed idiopathic disease.[35]

Some persons at risk for developing acute pancreatitis may be able to prevent its occurrence or recurrence. However, many etiologies of this disorder (e.g., gallstone formation and prescribed medication use) may impede implementing preventive strategies. Those who use alcohol in excess may prevent pancreatitis by limiting intake of this substance. Some lipid disorders may be controlled by diet and medications. Prophylaxis or rapid treatment for some infections may prevent the subsequent development of acute pancreatitis.

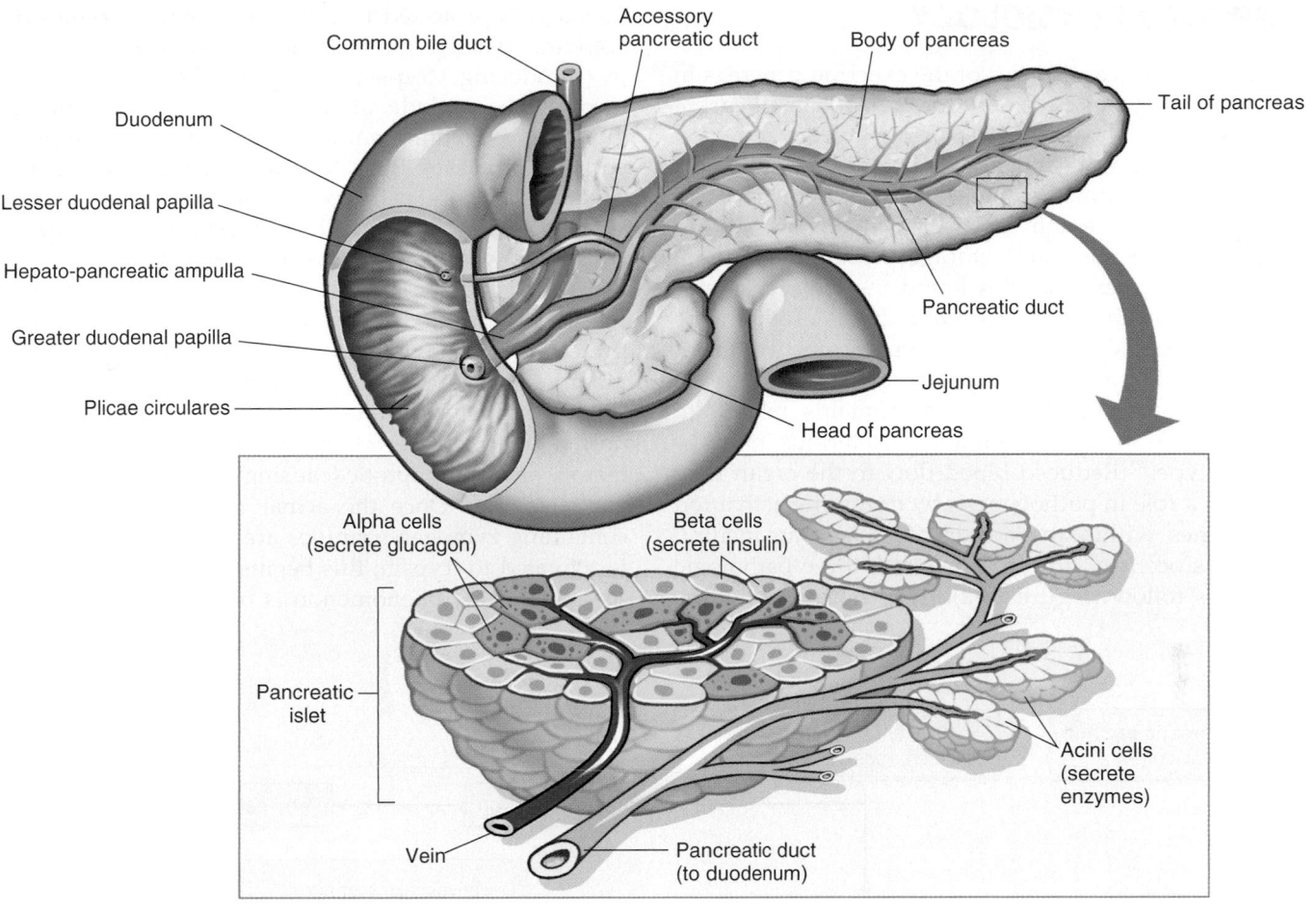

FIGURE 28-1 The normal pancreas.

Box 28-1

Etiologies of Acute Pancreatitis Biliary Disease

- Gallstones
- Biliary sludge
- Microlithiasis
- Alcohol
- Drugs
  - Thiazide diuretics
  - Acetaminophen
  - Oral contraceptives
  - L-Asparaginase
  - Furosemide
  - Sulfonamides
  - Azathioprine
  - Tetracycline
- Lipid abnormalities
  - Hypertriglyceridemia
- Hypercalcemia
- Surgery (particularly gastric or biliary)
- Trauma
- Infectious agents
  - Viruses (hepatitis, mumps, coxsackie, rubella)
  - Bacteria (*Legionella, Mycoplasma pneumoniae, Campylobacter*)
- Pregnancy—second and third trimesters
- Hereditary
- Idiopathic

APPLIED PHYSIOLOGY

Pancreatitis is a disorder of the exocrine pancreas in which the enzymes necessary for metabolism of carbohydrates, fats, and protein are prematurely activated by events within the acinar cells before their transport into the duodenum. In homeostasis, trypsinogen and other proteases remain in an inactive state during synthesis, transport, and storage within membrane-confined zymogen granules found in acinar cells and after secretion into the pancreatic duct.[16] Though the exact pathophysiology of this premature activation of the pancreatic proteases trypsin and phospholipase A is unknown, the likely cause remains related to events within the acinar cell after deleterious injury to this cell type.[28] Reduced blood flow to the organ may also play a role in pathogenesis by triggering activation of enzymes within the acinar cell. Once an inciting insult has occurred to the acinar cell, three pathologic responses follow (Figure 28-2). In its normal state, the

pancreas is protected from its proteolytic enzymes by secreting inactive proenzymes (zymogens) and also by producing trypsin inhibitor. Other protective mechanisms include an acidic pH within zymogen granules, preventing enzymatic activity, and the presence of proteases that degrade other already active proteases. Theoretically, premature activation of trypsinogen when acinar cell homeostasis is disrupted could overwhelm protective mechanisms and lead to damage of the zymogen-confining membrane and the release of activated proteases.[16] When these inherent protective mechanisms are overwhelmed, the acute inflammatory process is initiated by enzyme-induced tissue destruction. Intracellular zymogens are activated, normal pancreatic secretion is inhibited, and proinflammatory and proapoptotic (causing cell death) mediators are released.[31] Once the acinar cell and proenzyme-containing zymogen granules are injured, trypsinogen is activated to trypsin; this begins the autodigestion of the gland. This phenomenon is believed to be related

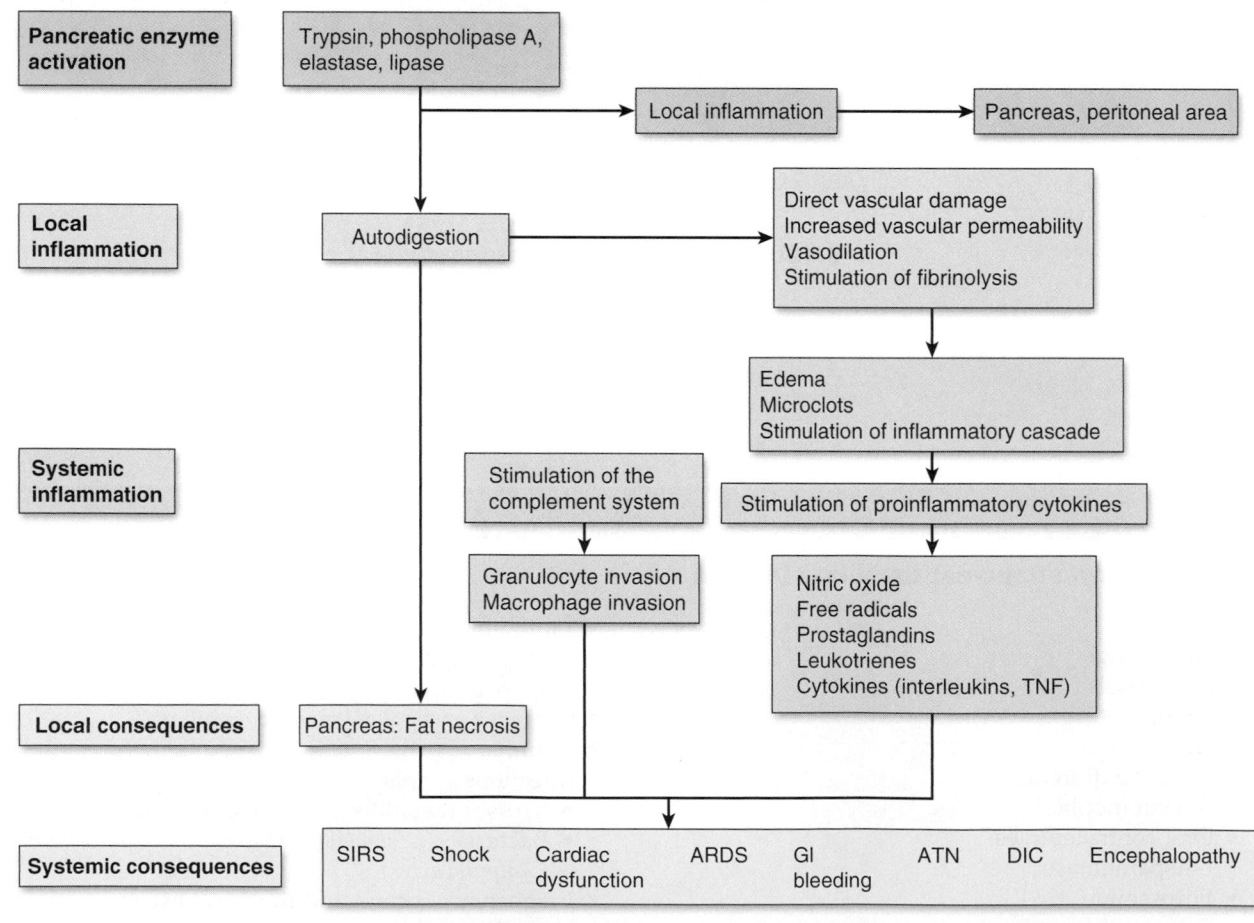

♦FIGURE 28-2 Pancreatic acinar cell injury.

to the acinar cell damage then affecting lysosomes and zymogen granules within the cell itself, causing inappropriate fusion of these two intracellular structures and the subsequent premature activation of trypsinogen.[20] This triggers a cascade effect, leading to the activation of other pancreatic enzymes. Zymogen activation and autodigestion result in a local inflammatory response. The inflammatory mediators are released into the general circulation and result in cytokine-mediated systemic leukocyte activation.[36] The severe inflammation results in early glandular edema that may contribute to diminished blood flow to the organ. The vascular insult within the pancreas continues with the onset of vascular thrombosis and vasospasm, causing the release of oxygen free radicals, contributing to further apoptosis (pancreatic cell death).[31] The inflammatory process may extend to peripancreatic tissues and to the systemic circulation. Another important mechanism in the pathogenesis of acute pancreatitis is obstruction of the pancreatic duct and impaired bile flow with interstitial collection of lipase, which can initiate local inflammation.[20]

Acute pancreatitis has been classified into two main categories—mild and severe. This classification system was developed in 1992 at the International Symposium on Acute Pancreatitis in Atlanta, Georgia.[6] The Atlanta classification categorizes pancreatitis without parenchymal necrosis as interstitial or edematous pancreatitis—the mild form. Those patients categorized with severe acute pancreatitis meet one of the following criteria: organ failure with either shock, pulmonary insufficiency, renal failure, or gastrointestinal bleeding; local complications (e.g., necrosis, pseudocyst, or abscess); at least three of Ranson's criteria (Box 28-2); or at least eight of the Acute Physiology and Chronic Health Evaluation II (APACHE II) criteria (Chapter 3).[40]

The intense inflammation and edema caused by the release of activated enzymes and digestion of the pancreas by these enzymes are responsible for the primary symptom of pancreatitis—abdominal pain. Abdominal pain occurs as a presenting symptom in 95% of those with acute pancreatitis.[35] This pain is commonly described as midepigastric, deep, constant, and excruciating, and may radiate to the dorsal regions of the back. Pain receptors in the retroperitoneum are also stimulated by the resultant cell death and necrosis that ensues from the destructive active intracellular enzyme activity of trypsinogen, phospholipase A, and elastase. Finally, patients may present with pain related to the obstruction of the pancreatic duct from a migrating gallstone. Abdominal distention, nausea, vomiting, and paralytic ileus are seen in many patients with acute pancreatitis. This is related to the effects of the copious amounts of

---

Box 28-2

Ranson's Criteria for Predicting the Severity of Acute Pancreatitis at Admission or on Diagnosis

- Age greater than 55 years (greater than 70 years)*
- Leukocyte count greater than $16,000/mm^3$ (greater than $18,000/mm^3$)
- Serum glucose level greater than 200 mg/dl (greater than 220 mg/dl)
- Serum LDH greater than 350 units/L (greater than 400 units/L)
- Serum AST greater than 250 units/L

DURING INITIAL 48 HOURS

- Decrease in hematocrit greater than 10%
- Increase in BUN greater than 5 mg/dl (greater than 2 mg/dl)
- Total serum calcium level greater than 8 mg/dl
- Base deficit greater than 4 mEq/L (greater than 5 mEq/L)
- Estimated fluid sequestration greater than 6 L (greater than 4 L)
- Partial pressure of arterial oxygen less than 60 mm Hg

Adapted from reference 5a.
*Criteria values for nonalcoholic acute pancreatitis differing from those in alcohol-related disease are in parentheses.
AST = Aspartate transaminase, BUN = blood urea nitrogen, LDH = lactate dehydrogenase.
For correlation between number of positive criteria and related mortality, see Box 28-3 on p. 779.

---

retroperitoneal fluid and the local inflammatory processes suppressing the action of intestinal peristalsis.

Hallmarks of acute pancreatitis include its effect on local as well as distant structures. Acute pancreatitis may progress from a local to a systemic disorder. Complement is activated in response to the action of trypsin, attracting macrophages and polymorphonuclear leukocytes to the damaged pancreas and pancreatic bed. Progressive inflammation and increasing vascular permeability result with local necrosis of the gland.[20] The damaged capillary membrane, now hyperpermeable, allows large amounts of protein-rich fluid to escape into the interstitium and retroperitoneal space. Fluid losses are extreme, with up to 6 liters or more becoming sequestered in pancreatic and peripancreatic edema.[9] This is the genesis of the hemodynamic instability seen in acute pancreatitis, causing hypotension, tachycardia, and signs of decreased perfusion to vital organ systems (decreasing urine output, altered level of consciousness) as well as decreased filling pressures (e.g., central venous pressure or pulmonary artery wedge pressure [PAWP]). The highly permeable capillary membrane is also responsible for losses of electrolytes, especially calcium. This leads to calcium combining with the free fatty acids present in the locale from fat necrosis. This process, known as saponification, causes the deposition of calcium soaps.[20] Hypocalcemia can be severe and is identifiable clinically by neuromuscular changes including Trousseau's sign (carpopedal spasm with inflation of a blood pressure cuff) and Chvostek's sign (muscle spasm with tap on the facial nerve) as well as muscular tetany and seizures.

Cardiovascular compromise may also result from the damaging effects of the enzymes, particularly elastase. This enzyme has a direct effect on the structural integrity of blood vessels, leaving patients at risk for developing thrombosis or, in rare cases, hemorrhage. Changes in the arterial wall are secondary to contact with proteolytic enzymes and other products of pancreatic injury. Arteries in close proximity to an inflamed or infected site may be the only risk factor for the formation of an arterial injury or pseudoaneurysm, which may rupture and cause spontaneous hemorrhage.[47]

Intracellular pancreatic enzymes and cytokines released from damaged pancreatic cells begin to autodigest structures surrounding the pancreas within the pancreatic bed. Peripancreatic fat is digested by lipase.

Tachypnea and dyspnea are also seen in severe acute pancreatitis as a result of splinting from the presence of subdiaphragmatic inflammation. These symptoms also arise when patients are experiencing pain and may be hypoventilating, thus precipitating the development of atelectasis and potentially pneumonia. Pleural effusions, especially left sided, can develop with the migration of large amounts of retroperitoneal fluid into the thoracic cavity via lymphatic channels.[7] Patients with pleural effusions may present with basilar crackles.

Necrotic tissue and areas of hemorrhage within the pancreas and its surrounding tissue provide an excellent medium for bacterial infection, especially with organisms from an inflamed biliary tree and permeable colonic sources. Any infectious process in this area increases the morbidity and mortality associated with severe acute pancreatitis. These processes may also result in increased pain and the development of fever and an elevated white blood cell count.

Rare physical findings include ecchymosis of the groin, flank, and thigh (Grey Turner's sign) related to retroperitoneal bleeding into the fascia in hemorrhagic acute pancreatitis. This bleeding may also cause the development of the uncommon Cullen's sign of periumbilical ecchymosis. Neither of these signs is specific to the diagnosis of acute pancreatitis.

◆ Case Study 28-1, Part A

Assessment and Management of Acute Pancreatitis

44-year-old J.D. developed severe, sharp, excruciating mid-epigastric pain, radiating to his mid back. The pain was not alleviated with position changes. He also began vomiting large amounts of bilious fluid. After several hours, he notified his wife, who brought him to the emergency department. He was still in severe pain when seen; a rapid assessment was performed. J.D.'s medical history is significant for hypertension controlled with hydrochlorothiazide (Microzide). J.D.'s heart rate was 138 beats/min and regular, blood pressure 80/44 mm Hg, respiratory rate 32 breaths/min and regular, and temperature of 100° F. J.D. was noted to have abdominal tenderness, distention, and decreased bowel sounds; he had continued to have intermittent nausea but no further vomiting. He remained hypotensive, so lactated Ringer's solution was administered at 150 ml/hr. His respiratory status was monitored closely as his breath sounds were somewhat decreased with few bibasilar crackles. His oxygen saturation by pulse oximetry (SpO_2) was 90%, and he was administered oxygen at 2 L/min. STAT laboratory results showed an elevated serum amylase level of 775 units/L, lipase level of 1290 units/L, white blood cell (WBC) count of 18,000/mm³, ionized calcium level of 3.2 mg/dl, and potassium level of 3.0 mEq/L. He was given 9.3 mEq of intravenous calcium gluconate over 1 hour and 40 mEq of potassium chloride over 4 hours. An ultrasound of the abdomen was performed, revealing two large gallstones and retroperitoneal fluid. A CT scan confirmed the suspected diagnosis of acute pancreatitis likely related to gallstone disease. Given his hemodynamic and pulmonary status, he was admitted to the critical care unit.

Decision point: What risk factors does J.D. have for the development of acute pancreatitis?

Decision point: What were the physical assessment findings with which J.D. presented to the emergency department? What is the rationale for the development of each?

Case continues on page 783

ASSESSMENT OF SEVERITY AND EARLY RISK STRATIFICATION

The clinical course of pancreatitis can vary widely, from the mild transitory form to severe, necrotizing disease with local and systemic complications. As such, determining the severity of the disease process is a critical element of the management strategy for this disease. There has been much effort placed in the attempt to identify objective predictive markers to grade the severity of pancreatitis early in the course of the disease, even at the time of admission to the hospital.[36] Using this information, clinicians can best guide the timing and aggressiveness of interventions as well as the most appropriate placement of patients within the hospital according to their acuity. Two commonly used grading systems are Ranson's criteria (despite its limitations, including the inability to fully gauge severity until after 48 hours) (see Box 28-2) and the APACHE II system. They use clinical assessment parameters and biochemical measurements to determine the severity of acute pancreatitis.[15] It is important to quickly identify on admission those 20% of patients who will develop the most severe disease with complications. These are the individuals who might benefit most from early critical care management.[28]

The Modified Glasgow scoring system and the Acute Physiology and Chronic Health Evaluation II and III are two additional methods for risk stratification. The CT grading system of Balthazar is also widely used (Table 28-1). All grading systems have some limitations.[4,7,24] Varied criteria can be used to aid the clinician in identifying severity and thus anticipating the course of the disease and its outcomes. Clinical criteria, serum markers, and radiographic features are several of the methods used for early risk stratification.

Ranson's criteria and the Modified Glasgow system rely on a collection of clinical and biochemical variables measured upon patient presentation and within

the first 48 hours of admission (see Box 28-2).[7] These assessments may be useful in identifying patients most at risk who require intensive interventions. Three or more Ranson indicators present initially or within 48 hours correlate with severe acute pancreatitis related to signs of organ failure and likely critical illness. The mortality associated with the number of Ranson's criteria is presented in Box 28-3. The Modified Glasgow criteria are collected upon patient presentation, daily, and at any time within 48 hours after hospital admission/diagnosis. In this system, each of the following is worth 1 point: age over 55, an arterial partial pressure of oxygen tension (PaO_2) less than 60 mm Hg, a blood glucose level higher than 182 mg/dl, a blood urea nitrogen level higher than 46 mg/dl, a serum calcium level lower than 8 mg/dl, a white blood cell count greater than 15,000/mm^3, a serum glutamic-oxaloacetic transaminase level higher than 100 units/L, a serum lactate dehydrogenase level higher than 600 units/L, and an albumin level lower than 3.2 mg/dl. A score higher than 3 within 48 hours indicates severe disease.[7,12] Because data collection in both the Ranson and the Modified Glasgow grading systems is not completed before the 48-hour mark, a high index of suspicion by the clinician is vital when monitoring these patients in order to identify when changes may be heralding the onset of complications. The APACHE II score can be used at the 24-hour mark and daily thereafter and can be applied to predict the onset of complications and the potential for increased mortality. Those patients who develop extrapancreatic complications such as respiratory or renal dysfunction or those who have pancreatic necrosis on contrast-enhanced CT will likely experience the most severe course of the disease.[4,24,28]

LABORATORY FINDINGS

As the cells of the pancreas are destroyed, the enzymes amylase and lipase are released into the circulation during an acute attack. Measurement of amylase

TABLE 28-1 Computed Tomography Severity Index

CHARACTERISTIC	CT SEVERITY INDEX (CTSI)
Level of Inflammation	
Normal pancreas	0
Focal or diffuse enlargement	1
Peripancreatic inflammation	2
Single collection of fluid	3
Multiple fluid collections or gas	4
Pancreatic Necrosis	
None	0
Less than 30% necrosis	2
30%–50% necrosis	4
More than 50% necrosis	6

Data from reference 4. Used with permission.

Box 28-3

Ranson's Criteria and Related Mortality

Number of Positive Criteria

0–2	<5% mortality
3–4	20% mortality
5–6	40% mortality
7 or more	100% mortality

From reference 15a.

and lipase levels is used for the confirmation of the diagnosis of acute pancreatitis. Serum enzyme levels, typically greater than three times normal, are seen to increase within 6 to 12 hours. The half-life of elevated amylase is shorter than that of lipase, and clearance of amylase is affected by impaired renal function and intravascular fluid status. Because it persists longer after the onset of the attack and because the pancreas is the only source of lipase, estimation of serum lipase levels has somewhat more superior sensitivity and specificity and greater accuracy than lipase.[44] Isoamylase levels specific to pancreatic injury are measured in some laboratories and are more indicative of the disease. Urine amylase levels may also be elevated and remain so for several days. Serum lipase level is a reliable marker of acute pancreatitis. It remains elevated for a longer period and has a sensitivity and specificity for the disease that approaches 90%.[37] Neither serum amylase nor serum lipase levels correlate to the severity of the disease.

White blood cell count may be elevated because of the inflammatory process or resultant infection. Derangements in serum glucose levels are common as beta cells of the pancreas, which produce insulin, are also damaged by the inflammatory process. Liver function tests may be mildly elevated, especially bilirubin levels and transaminases, if the acute pancreatitis is related to a biliary cause such as gallstone disease.

A history of fasting triglyceride levels higher than 1000 mg/dl or a persistent elevation after the acute inflammatory process has resolved may be seen if hypertriglyceridemia is the cause of acute pancreatitis.[40] Many enzymes and serum markers are released by damaged pancreatic cells when they are injured in severe acute pancreatitis. These levels have been tested for their ability to provide prognostic information in the setting of acute pancreatitis. Research is ongoing in an effort to identify a serum marker accurate in its predictive value for the severity of pancreatitis. Two promising laboratory tests are C-reactive protein (CRP) and urinary trypsinogen activation peptide (uTAP). CRP is a marker of inflammation and is elevated in acute pancreatitis. This test is readily available and inexpensive, with an 86% sensitivity within 48 hours of presentation of symptoms. A CRP value of 150 mg/L may be the point of differentiation between mild and severe acute pancreatitis.[35] Pancreatic zymogen destruction and activation of trypsinogen are key occurrences in acute pancreatitis. In an effort to determine the severity of the disease, trypsinogen activation peptide (TAP) has been studied. uTAP concentrations have provided good prognostic information related to the severity of acute pancreatitis. This is a manual test with limited stability, thus preventing its widespread use. More clinically applicable testing of uTAP is in development.[28,34] Though not yet clinically applicable, several other serum markers may hold diagnostic promise. They are procalcitonin, interleukin-6, and neutrophilic elastase.[28,35]

RADIOLOGY FINDINGS

Contrast-enhanced CT scanning is the most extensively studied diagnostic intervention for the identification of acute pancreatitis, staging of its severity, and detection of complications.[35] Dynamic CT carries an 87% sensitivity for diagnosis of this disorder.[28] This level of sensitivity allows for the differentiation of severe acute pancreatitis from many other conditions that may present with abdominal pain and elevated levels of pancreatic enzymes. Of note is the ability of this diagnostic modality to delineate local complications such as peripancreatic necrosis with or without infection.[40] Grading systems for the severity of acute pancreatitis have been developed using CT imaging alone to determine risk stratification of the disease.[3,28] The computed tomography severity index (CTSI) quantifies the presence and amount of pancreatic necrosis and extent of inflammation, and it has shown promise in predicting outcomes in acute pancreatitis (see Table 28-1).[3,4,44]

Plain radiographic films of the chest and abdomen are two initial diagnostic interventions used to identify abnormalities responsible for the onset of abdominal pain and other presenting symptoms. The chest x-ray may reveal the presence of pleural effusion, particularly left-sided, often associated with acute pancreatitis.

Abdominal ultrasonography can be used to detect gallstones although bowel gas from pancreatitis-related ileus may limit its accuracy. Ultrasound is, however, a routine element of the evaluation process for acute pancreatitis. It provides important information regarding the pancreas and biliary structures and does so quickly and efficiently as it is readily available.[35,40] Magnetic resonance imaging (MRI) and magnetic resonance cholangiopancreatography (MRCP) with gadolinium provide information about the pancreas similar to that obtained with CT scanning, but provide more valuable information regarding the biliary tree. This technology has great future potential but is currently reserved for individuals in whom contrast-enhanced CT is contraindicated or when a mild form of the disease is suspected.[35] MRI and MRCP as well as esophageal ultrasound (EUS) have the capability of detecting small bile duct stones; however, they are not routinely used.[40]

COMPLICATIONS OF ACUTE PANCREATITIS

Cardiopulmonary Complications

The injury to the pancreas alone is not responsible for the morbidity and mortality of acute pancreatitis. It is in fact the systemic and local complications that ensue which can threaten the course and patient outcomes of this devastating disease entity (Figure 28-3). In addition to the regional pancreatic inflammation related to the local complications, a systemic response to the activated neutrophils and complement products in the area occurs and is linked to distant organ dysfunction.[5] This response is in part related to the absorption of activated enzymes and inflammatory mediators from the retroperitoneum.

The first weeks after the onset of symptoms in acute pancreatitis are marked by systemic inflammatory response syndrome (SIRS).[47] Release of proinflammatory mediators is thought to contribute to the pathogenesis of SIRS-related multisystem complications involving injury to the heart, lungs, kidneys, and other organs.[18]

Another factor integral to the development of MODS is microvascular endothelial cell injury with systemic capillary leak, which occurs in association with the release of inflammatory mediators, bradykinin, and histamine.[5] Cardiovascular complications of severe pancreatitis often mimic septic shock even though no infection, in fact no organism, exists.[20] Hypovolemic shock is one complication caused by the capillary damage related to the action of enzymes and vasoactive substances. Bleeding, a rare complication, can develop as a consequence of the erosion of local blood vessels by elastase and other enzymes. Progressive and uncontrolled vasodilation occurs, prompted by the kinin released from damaged acinar cells; this contributes to the severity of the shock state. Those patients whose assessment and management include the use of a pulmonary artery catheter (PAC) will exhibit a decreased systemic vascular resistance. Cardiac output will be increased in response to the massive fluid sequestration and other factors. Theorized myocardial depressant factors (MDFs) of tumor necrosis factor (TNF), interleukin-1B, and nitrous oxide released in sepsis may also contribute to the development of cardiovascular complications.[21] Dysrhythmias are also frequently seen. They may arise from the severe electrolyte abnormalities seen in acute pancreatitis as well as to the presence of MDFs and the depressed contractile response of the myocardium in acute sepsis.

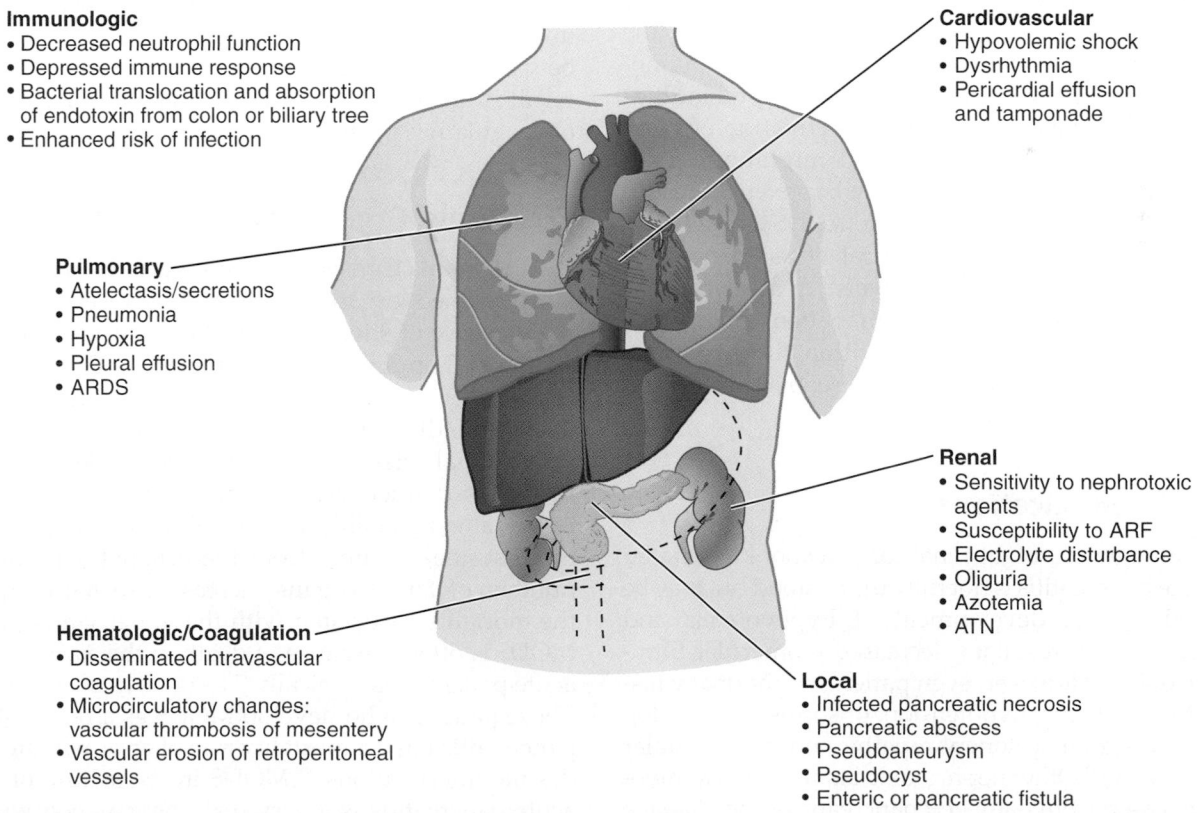

Immunologic
- Decreased neutrophil function
- Depressed immune response
- Bacterial translocation and absorption of endotoxin from colon or biliary tree
- Enhanced risk of infection

Pulmonary
- Atelectasis/secretions
- Pneumonia
- Hypoxia
- Pleural effusion
- ARDS

Hematologic/Coagulation
- Disseminated intravascular coagulation
- Microcirculatory changes: vascular thrombosis of mesentery
- Vascular erosion of retroperitoneal vessels

Cardiovascular
- Hypovolemic shock
- Dysrhythmia
- Pericardial effusion and tamponade

Renal
- Sensitivity to nephrotoxic agents
- Susceptibility to ARF
- Electrolyte disturbance
- Oliguria
- Azotemia
- ATN

Local
- Infected pancreatic necrosis
- Pancreatic abscess
- Pseudoaneurysm
- Pseudocyst
- Enteric or pancreatic fistula

◆**FIGURE 28-3** Local and systemic complications of acute pancreatitis. ARDS = Acute respiratory distress syndrome, ARF = acute renal failure, ATN = acute tubular necrosis. From Alspach, J (2001). *AACN's Instructor Resource Manual for the Core Curriculum*, handout 5–36. Philadelphia: Saunders. Used with permission.

Pulmonary Complications

The pulmonary complications associated with acute pancreatitis are many, ranging from mild hypoxemia to life-threatening acute lung injury. Hypoxia can arise from atelectasis associated with the hypoventilation seen with abdominal pain and distention and from diaphragmatic elevation caused by the large amounts of retroperitoneal fluid. Pleural effusions, common on the left side, result from the movement of peripancreatic fluid through lymphatic channels into the pleural space. This results in a reduced vital capacity, negatively impacting normal ventilation.

Pancreatitis-associated lung injury is complex and not fully understood. The underlying mechanisms associated with the development of acute lung injury (ALI) in pancreatitis are many and include the release of inflammatory mediators (e.g., neutrophils, cytokines, chemokines, adhesion molecules).[32] Vasoactive substances and cytokines absorbed at the site of pancreatic injury are transported to other organ systems. These biochemicals, including phospholipase A and free fatty acids, incite injury to the lung, disturbing and ultimately destroying the alveolar capillary membrane, increasing capillary permeability. Migrating neutrophils, long implicated as mediators of ALI and acute respiratory distress syndrome (ARDS), release toxic products of elastase and collagenase at the site of the damaged alveoli.[32] Pancreatic elastase activates pulmonary TNF, which also contributes to neutrophil infiltration and pulmonary vascular leak. Activation of these processes results in interstitial fluid migration within the lungs and worsening, refractory hypoxemia, resulting in ARDS. Hypoxemia related to ARDS as well as to atelectasis, pneumonia, and pleural effusion must be readily identified and aggressively treated because these are all significant factors in patient outcomes.[5] Up to 60% of deaths occurring within the first week after the onset of severe acute pancreatitis are caused by pulmonary complications.[22]

Renal Complications

The pathogenesis of the renal complications associated with acute pancreatitis is not fully understood but may be explained by the development of hypovolemia and hypotension with resultant decreased glomerular filtration rate (GFR). However, even patients without any history of hypovolemia, hypotension, or sepsis can develop membranous glomerulonephropathy and acute tubular necrosis (ATN).[5] Other nephrotoxic insults, such as myoglobin released from damaged pancreatic tissue, damage the distal renal tubules and may contribute to the onset of ATN and acute renal failure. The development of acute renal failure (ARF) occurs in approximately 20% of patients and is a poor prognostic indicator, increasing the mortality rate to more than 80%.[22,25]

Gastrointestinal Complications

Gastrointestinal complications may also arise from the inherent cardiovascular instability. Decreased perfusion to the gastrointestinal tract may contribute to adynamic ileus. The local inflammatory process in the retroperitoneum can have a direct negative impact on gastrointestinal structures. Patients can develop splenic vein thrombosis, which precipitates esophageal and gastric varices with the potential for rupture. Weakened mesenteric and splenic vessels, altered by damaging proteases, can form a pseudoaneurysm that also can rupture and cause dangerous hemorrhage.[20]

Hematologic and Coagulation Derangements

Pervasive microvascular endothelial cell injury takes a toll on normal coagulation. Microcirculatory injury with vascular thrombosis can adversely affect the mesenteric circulation with resultant visceral ischemia. The onset of disseminated intravascular coagulation in acute pancreatitis may be in response to exaggerated microvascular clotting from enzyme-related injury or be caused by the development of severe sepsis. The result is uncontrolled microvascular clotting, depletion of coagulation proteins, and bleeding.

Multiple Organ Dysfunction Syndrome

The Atlanta Consensus Conference on Acute Pancreatitis defined organ failure in this disease entity as the presence of shock (systolic blood pressure less than 90 mm Hg), pulmonary insufficiency (PaO_2 less than 60 mm Hg), renal failure (creatinine level greater than 2 mg/dl after initial volume resuscitation), or gastrointestinal bleeding (greater than 500 ml/24 hr).[6] MODS is defined as a syndrome of progressive but potentially reversible organ failure involving two or more systems remote from the original insult. As the number of failed organs increases, so naturally does the mortality associated with the underlying disease.[25] MODS is often the cause of death in the early course of acute pancreatitis, typically 7 to 14 days after diagnosis. Those patients who develop MODS as a result of acute pancreatitis have a mortality rate of approximately 50% despite interventions.[35] MODS in the setting of severe acute pancreatitis is a very real phenomenon with few confirmed management strategies except for prevention, when possible, early identification, and intensive supportive care.

Local and Systemic Infectious Complications

Infectious complications are the bane of management of acute pancreatitis, frequently worsening the clinical course.[22] Those with severe acute pancreatitis are at increased risk for infection because of the use of invasive venous and arterial catheters in the assessment and management of this disease. Episodic hyperglycemia associated with pancreatitis is also a risk factor for infection. Translocation of gut bacteria from an unused or underused intestinal mucosa can result in sepsis or abscess formation. Absorption of endotoxin from an inflamed adjacent colon or biliary system can also yield similar infectious sequelae. Late deterioration in organ function occurs during the second to third week after the onset of symptoms. This phase is marked by the secondary infection of areas of pancreatic or peripancreatic necrosis. The development of pancreatic necrosis resulting from local vessel destruction and thrombosis is commonly recognized within 4 days of the onset of symptoms. It is seen in 20% of patients with acute pancreatitis and is defined as greater than 30% of nonenhancement on contrast-enhanced CT.[41] Once necrotic, this area either can be sterile or can become secondarily infected. Infection of this type is a potentially life-threatening cause of sepsis in acute pancreatitis.[47] Infected pancreatic necrosis is the development of a diffuse area of nonviable pancreatic parenchyma that is secondarily infected, most commonly with *Escherichia coli, Bacteroides, Staphylococcus,* or *Candida albicans.*[41] Fever, leukocytosis, and abdominal pain are the hallmarks of the complication. The extensive tissue damage and loss associated with infected pancreatic necrosis also carry the potential of additional complications including intestinal or pancreatic fistula formation and bleeding from other retroperitoneal structures.[41] The majority of patients with severe early organ dysfunction have been identified as also having pancreatic necrosis on CT scan.[8,41]

Pancreatic abscess, a walled-off intra-abdominal collection of pus and debris, is a late local complication of acute pancreatitis, often taking 4 to 6 weeks to develop. Signs and symptoms include increased abdominal tenderness, fever, and leukocytosis. This abscess commonly develops following the infection of an area of pancreatic necrosis. With rapid intervention (i.e., percutaneous drainage or surgical excision and lavage), this complication can be well controlled, limiting adverse patient outcomes.[22,44]

Pancreatic pseudocysts are collections of pancreatic secretions and cellular debris enclosed by a wall of fibrous or granulation tissue that does not have a layer of epithelial cells in its lining. They develop as a result of an active protease-weakened capsular structure and persistent pancreatic ductal leak. Pseudocysts form in approximately 5% of all cases of acute pancreatitis.[42] They may take up to 6 weeks to become mature. Pseudocysts may cause increased abdominal discomfort, rupture, become infected, or become so large that they obstruct the intestine or genitourinary system; therefore they must be monitored closely via ultrasound or CT scan and be drained by percutaneous, surgical, or endoscopic methods when they become complicated.[22,44]

◆ Case Study 28-1, Part B

Assessment and Management of Acute Pancreatitis

J.D. was admitted to surgical critical care. He rapidly decompensated with unstable vital signs and became hypotensive and tachycardic; his urine output was less than 30 ml/hr. A CT scan revealed pancreatic necrosis and retroperitoneal inflammation with large retroperitoneal fluid sequestration. His SpO_2 was 88% on supplemental oxygen; arterial blood gas showed a PaO_2 of 54 mm Hg; he was tachypneic and complained of shortness of breath. His chest x-ray continued to show pleural effusion as well as atelectasis.

Decision point: What complications is J.D. likely experiencing?

Decision point: What interventions are required for J.D.?

Case continues on page 787

MULTIDISCIPLINARY PLAN OF CARE

The clinical course of acute pancreatitis varies from mild disease to the severe, necrotizing form. Those patients with the mild form (80% of cases) will require intravenous therapy and optimal pain management.[47] Those with severe acute pancreatitis (20% of cases) may benefit from intensive monitoring given the potential for progressive organ dysfunction or local complication.[33] Scoring systems are available to identify those who will progress to the severe form of the disease and are advantageous but cannot replace the assessment and interventions of skilled clinicians. In fact, the supportive care provided in critical care is vital to improving patient outcomes as no specific evidence-based interventions have been identified to treat severe acute pancreatitis.

Inflammation is the hallmark of severe acute pancreatitis. Early in the course of the disease, there is an extravasation of protein-rich intravascular fluid into the peritoneal cavity, resulting in hemoconcentration.[41] Monitoring of the hematocrit (Hct) is important in identifying those at risk for this hemoconcentration before altered perfusion becomes apparent. Hct levels also provide a framework by which practitioners can assess the effectiveness of interventions aimed at restoring normal intravascular fluid status. Maintaining adequate intravascular volume may be considered the most essential therapeutic goal in the management of acute pancreatitis. Patients with acute pancreatitis can sequester enormous amounts of fluid not only into the retroperitoneal space and the intraperitoneal cavity but also into the gut and the pleural cavity. These marked intravascular fluid losses mandate that volume deficits be estimated and replenished. Adequate fluid resuscitation may require 5 to 10 liters of crystalloid or colloidal fluids in 24 hours during the first days after admission.[28] Early vigorous intravenous hydration via at least large-bore peripheral intravenous access is critical to restore circulating volume. Central venous access (CVC lines) or the use of PACs not only provide access for rapid infusion of intravenous fluids and blood but also provide critical clinical data needed to manage the hemodynamically unstable adult or the patient with co-existent cardiopulmonary disease who requires massive volume resuscitation. To estimate the required fluid resuscitation requirements, central venous pressure (CVP) should be monitored closely together with hourly urine excretion and daily Hct measurements. CVP should be raised to approximately 8 to 12 mm Hg, urine output should be maintained at 0.5 ml/kg/hr, and Hct should be maintained at 30%.[28,44] In those patients whose course is complicated by sepsis or the SIRS response, the resuscitation strategy should involve administration of intravenous fluid targeted to a PAWP of 12 to 15 mm Hg for maximal benefit.[17] This target PAWP is a realistic goal for most patients with acute pancreatitis.[39] In an effort to meet these end points and provide the needed amount of fluid, the minimal requirements must be calculated and retroperitoneal losses estimated in the first 24 to 48 hours. The known or estimated retroperitoneal losses must be added to the maintenance fluid needs to correct potentially life-threatening deficits. Maintenance fluid requirements calculated for a 24-hour period use the following weight-based formula: For the first 10 kg of body weight, the fluid needs are 100 ml/kg/day. For the second 10 kg of weight, add 50 ml/kg/day; 20 ml/kg/day is added for every kilogram more than 20 kg. The sum is then divided by 24 to determine the hourly rate.[23] For example, a 70-kg person should receive 250 to 300 ml/hr of balanced salt solution when maintenance needs are calculated and retroperitoneal losses considered.[41] Monitoring the clinical response to volume resuscitation is also accomplished by accurate hourly intake and output measurements. Urinary output of 0.5 ml/kg/hr should be achieved when volume infusion is adequate, in the

absence of renal complications. Vigorous intravenous hydration may improve vascular supply and pancreatic perfusion and prevent the development of necrosis and other complications. The intravascular hypovolemia that accompanies acute pancreatitis subsequently leads to diminished pancreatic blood flow. Preventing further pancreatic ischemia by aggressive volume resuscitation may thwart further activation and release of inflammatory mediators.[41] Aggressive fluid resuscitation may also reduce the risk of developing acute renal failure.

Patients with pancreatic necrosis of either the sterile or the infected variety are at risk for multiorgan complications. Patients with sterile necrosis may be managed medically with supportive care with the use of intravenous hydration and pain management.[26] Once infection develops, the therapeutic approach is directed toward removal of the infected necrotic tissue. Open or laparoscopic surgical approaches (pancreatic necrosectomy) may be required to accomplish this goal.[26] There are less invasive interventions such as percutaneous or endoscopic drainage, but these techniques must be performed at specialized centers, which are currently located in only a few hospitals.[47] Continuous peritoneal lavage via indwelling catheters placed at the time of necrosectomy may also be implemented and maintained for as long as 1 month after the initial procedure. This lavage with closed suction allows for the continued removal of debris, devascularized tissue, and toxins and minimizes systemic absorption of these local toxins. Reexploration of the abdomen is frequently required. Another modality that may be employed after initial necrosectomy is packing of the abdomen, with planned reexploration and intraoperative lavage. For those requiring surgery, the third or fourth week after the onset of symptoms is considered the best timing for debridement and necrosectomy.[47] Because of the massive inflammatory process, a right hemicolectomy may be necessary when the transverse colon is compromised.[35]

Pain management for the patient with acute pancreatitis truly demands a multidisciplinary approach. This primary presenting symptom is most disconcerting to patients and their families. Controlling pain to within acceptable patient limits is perhaps the most important goal for the multidisciplinary healthcare team. In past years the goal of adequate pain relief was accomplished using the narcotic meperidine (Demerol), which causes less stimulation of the sphincter of Oddi than other narcotics. It is now known that all narcotics stimulate this sphincter to some degree and the metabolites of meperidine are toxic, resulting in neuromuscular irritation and, rarely, seizures.[10] Meperidine has a limited role in the management of acute pain as it should be used only for short periods, no more than

48 hours.[1,2] It should be considered for use only in situations in which the patient with acute pain has a documented allergy to other opioids. Further, meperidine is contraindicated in patients with impaired renal function.[1] Morphine does cause smooth muscle contraction around the sphincter. This may result in pain, but morphine and other narcotics (e.g., fentanyl [Sublimaze], hydromorphone [Dilaudid]) have not been shown to adversely affect patient outcomes and are often recommended.[10,12,40] Patient-controlled analgesia may be appropriate for some patients but not for the most critically ill. Patient positioning may alleviate pain when a semi-Fowler's position is used and the patient's legs are positioned toward the chest. Maintaining nothing by mouth (NPO) status is thought to prevent/decrease pain because of avoidance of pancreatic stimulation. The presence of nausea, vomiting, abdominal distention, and ileus also contributes to the need for remaining NPO until the acute inflammatory process resolves.

The treatment of acute pancreatitis remains symptom-focused and supportive, with no specific medications currently available.[47] Despite many prospective, randomized controlled studies, few medications have been shown to be effective in the management of this disease. One category of medications found to be effective in the management of some patients with pancreatitis is antibiotics. Antibiotics are not indicated for patients with a mild form of the disease. They are, however, indicated for patients with documented infection, including cholangitis, infected pancreatic necrosis, or pseudocyst. Antibiotic choice should be based upon culture and sensitivity results. However, the use of antibiotics remains controversial in patients with severe acute pancreatitis and documented necrosis but without infection.[13,33] Many studies with varied antibiotics have been performed, but definitive use of antibiotics in this setting remains controversial. Some believe prophylaxis against infection is not necessary in the setting of sterile necrosis.[13] Other experts hold the opinion that antibiotic prophylaxis is indicated to reduce the likelihood of infected pancreatic necrosis. Broad-spectrum antibiotics with good penetration into the pancreatic tissue are often recommended.[31] Most practitioners agree that limiting prophylaxis with antibiotics to only 7 to 14 days may decrease the occurrence of other secondary infections.[44] There is no justification for antimicrobial prophylaxis in patients without necrosis, given the relatively low incidence of infectious complications in this setting.[33]

Patients with acute pancreatitis are at nutritional risk because of protein losses, an extreme catabolic state, and lack of oral intake. Severe acute pancreatitis is associated with tryptic autodigestion of the pancreas, protein catabolism, metabolic instability, and increased nutritional requirements. Total parenteral nutrition (TPN) has traditionally been used to provide nutritional support because it avoids stimulation of the exocrine pancreas. (See the Nutrition box on p. 786.) It is known, however, that TPN may increase metabolic and septic complications. Recent clinical studies, summarized in the Research Utilization box on p. 786, have shown that enteral nutrition (EN) is safer and less expensive when compared to TPN.[19,27,29] Most patients with acute pancreatitis can tolerate jejunal feeding with elemental formulas.[19,27,29,38] The jejunal route can be achieved by the insertion of a nasojejunal tube beyond the ligament of Treitz or by surgical placement of a jejunal catheter. TPN should be reserved for patients who cannot tolerate enteral nutrition or who experience an exacerbation of their disease with enteral feedings.[19] As an example, the patient with an adynamic ileus would not be a candidate for enteral nutrition. Though it is known that EN may not meet all of the nutritional requirements of patients with acute pancreatitis because of feeding interruptions for studies, positioning, and diagnostic testing and also because of high residuals in the stomach as well as other causes, it is still the most effective nutritional intervention.[19,27,29,38] EN should be considered as primary therapy in severe acute pancreatitis. It not only provides needed protein and calorie nutrition but also limits increases in gut permeability, thus reducing the septic potential of bacterial translocation. Evidence-based data also exist indicating that EN can diminish disease severity in severe acute pancreatitis, reduce the incidence of complications (e.g., central line sepsis), and shorten the length of hospitalization.[29] The protein intake goal for any patient with acute pancreatitis is 1.5 g/kg/day. There is a nutritional requirement for essential fats, and some of the energy should be supplied enterally or parenterally as lipids. It is safe to provide lipids either enterally or parenterally in most patients if serum triglyceride levels remain less than 400 mg/dl.[19] Patients are monitored during their nutritional therapy for acute-phase protein levels and quantitative urine urea nitrogen levels to assess the impact of either enteral or parenteral nutrition on preventing protein/calorie malnutrition.

In the management of acute pancreatitis, ERCP is usually reserved for those with evidence of biliary obstruction (e.g., jaundice) or cholangitis and a persistently elevated serum bilirubin level (greater than 5 mg/dl). In these patients, early ERCP with sphincterotomy and stone extraction is indicated. If ERCP cannot be performed because it is not available or because of extreme technical difficulty, alternative methods of biliary drainage should be considered.[33]

The development of a pancreatic pseudocyst, one of the local complications of acute pancreatitis, may

▲ NUTRITION

Nutrition for the Pancreatitis Patient With Mild Pancreatitis	Severe Pancreatitis
• Nothing by mouth • Intravenous fluids • When pain resolves, begin clear liquid diet with gradual advancement; assess for changes in condition (e.g., pain, nausea, vomiting, rising amylase and lipase levels) once oral feeding begins	• Nothing by mouth • Enteral nutrition with elemental formula, preferably via jejunal route, beginning at 20 ml/hr and advancing to goal over 24–48 hr • In patients in whom enteral access cannot be achieved or who cannot tolerate enteral feeding, TPN with carbohydrates, protein, and lipids (if triglycerides <400 mg/dl) • Protein requirements via enteral or parenteral route = 1.5 g/kg/day

resolve spontaneously but may become infected, cause urinary or gastrointestinal obstruction, or rupture, releasing toxic enzymes and inflammatory cytokines. It may contain several liters of exudate. It is generally agreed that early in the development of the pseudocyst, manipulation or drainage should not be attempted unless complications ensue.[22] Once the encapsulation has matured, it can be drained endoscopically, percutaneously, or, in some cases, surgically.

Intra-abdominal abscesses may occur late in the course of acute pancreatitis and be responsible for a delayed septic state. Such abscesses can be percutaneously drained and the infection treated with appropriate antibiotics. Surgical debridement and lavage may be required if the abscess is not amenable to percutaneous drainage.

Systemic complications of acute pancreatitis include pulmonary, cardiovascular, renal, and gastrointestinal sequelae. Intensive assessment for early signs of the onset of these abnormalities is a critical part of the multidisciplinary plan of care. Pulmonary complications may be manifested by worsening hypoxemia and respiratory distress with radiographic changes. The prevention and management of atelectasis and pneumonia include vigorous pulmonary toilet, incentive spirometry, turning, positioning, and close scrutiny of continuous pulse oximetry and arterial blood gas results. The goal

▲ RESEARCH UTILIZATION

A Comparison of Enteral Nutrition and Total Parenteral Nutrition

CLINICAL ISSUE

For many years the mainstay of nutrition in the management of severe acute pancreatitis was parenteral nutrition with total parenteral nutrition (TPN). Enteral nutrition (EN) had been considered contraindicated in this population. Nasojejunal feedings with tubes placed distal to the ligament of Treitz have recently been studied extensively and found to be safe and cost-effective; in fact, they are recommended to meet the nutritional requirements and to prevent complications in acute pancreatitis. Clinically, however, it is difficult to place tubes via the nose to this location. This study seeks to compare nasogastric feedings to nasojejunal feedings.

SUMMARY

This study randomized 50 consecutive patients with severe acute pancreatitis to either nasogastric (NG) or nasojejunal (NJ) feedings through a small-bore feeding tube. The two groups were compared by means of APACHE II scores, serum C-reactive protein (CRP) levels, pain patterns by visual analog scale (VAS) score, and analgesic requirements. Complications were monitored as well as total length of hospital and ICU stays. No

significant difference was found in APACHE scores, CRP levels, pain scores, or analgesic needs. Overall mortality was 24.5% with 5 deaths in the NG group and 7 in the NJ group.

APPLICATION

EN has become the gold standard for management of nutritional requirements in severe acute pancreatitis. It not only prevents protein/calorie malnutrition but also may prevent problems commonly associated with central venous catheter use for TPN as well as ameliorating other inflammatory complications. Clinically, however, the proper placement of nasojejunal tube remains challenging. This study provides information indicating that the more easily placed NG tube may in fact provide some of the same advantages and provide a practical therapeutic approach to the early nutritional management of patients with severe acute pancreatitis.

NEED FOR FURTHER STUDY

Future investigation is necessary to evaluate NG/NJ feedings as a viable and efficacious intervention in the management of acute pancreatitis.

Eatlock, F. C., Chong, P., Menezes, N., et al. (2005). A randomized study of early nasogastric versus nasojejunal feeding in severe acute pancreatitis. *Am J Gastroenterol, 100*(2), 432–439.

for these interventions is to maintain the Pa_{O_2} greater than 70 mm Hg and arterial oxygen saturation greater than 93%. If severe, pleural effusion may be managed by thoracentesis or chest tube placement. The development of pulmonary emboli is thwarted by prophylaxis of deep vein thrombosis by the use of antithrombotic compression sleeves or stockings and subcutaneous heparin unless the patient is actively bleeding (Chapter 9). Noninvasive positive pressure ventilation may be used to treat some of respiratory abnormalities associated with acute pancreatitis.[14] Respiratory failure in severe acute pancreatitis may be related to the development of one or more of these complications or to the occurrence of ARDS. Respiratory failure associated with acute pancreatitis is managed with intubation and mechanical ventilation, often using the lung protective strategies of low tidal volume and high respiratory rate or high-frequency jet ventilation (oscillation) with permissive hypercapnia.[43] Other ventilatory interventions include positive end-expiratory pressure (PEEP) with levels of fraction of inspired oxygen (Fi_{O_2}) adequate to achieve a Pa_{O_2} of greater than 60 mm Hg. Barotrauma and oxygen toxicity are always a concern in the management of pancreatitis-related ARDS. Placing the patient in the prone position has also shown some benefit, especially if initiated early in the course of the syndrome;[27,43] research is ongoing regarding patient outcomes using this strategy.

Patients with acute pancreatitis are at risk for the onset of cardiovascular complications (e.g., dysrhythmias, hypovolemic or septic shock). Electrolyte (e.g., calcium, magnesium, and potassium) and glucose derangements also occur frequently and are problematic. Patients must be closely monitored for the early development of these potentially life-threatening disorders. Cardiac monitoring, careful control of intake and output, monitoring of CVP and PA pressures, and maintenance of aggressive volume resuscitation are all key in prevention of these complications. In addition, serum electrolytes and glucose levels must be frequently assessed in an effort to correct any deficiency. Low total levels of calcium (less than 8 mg/dl) not only are a negative prognostic sign but also precipitate dysrhythmias and so must be effectively managed. It is most accurate, when evaluating for hypocalcemia, to measure the ionized or unbound level of calcium. This is the physiologically active form of calcium. Losses of potassium and magnesium into retroperitoneal exudates also mandate frequent serum determinations and replacement to maintain levels within the normal range. The members of the healthcare team also must monitor for the development of clinical signs and symptoms related to electrolyte abnormalities (e.g., cardiac abnormalities and muscular tetany). Chapter 31 provides more detailed information on electrolyte abnormalities. Persistent dysrhythmias not eradicated

by aggressive electrolyte replacement may require the use of dysrhythmic medications. The shock state may necessitate the use of vasoactive medications when volume resuscitation alone does not correct the hemodynamic instability. Overall, the use of inotropes and vasoactive substances should be considered only after intravascular volume has been optimized.[14]

◆ Case Study 28-1, Part C

Assessment and Management of Acute Pancreatitis

Four days after admission, J.D. remained intubated and ventilated but experienced worsening oxygenation and a chest x-ray revealing fluffy white infiltrates. Ten days after admission, J.D. developed fever, elevated WBC count, and increased abdominal pain.

Decision point: What complications have now occurred in J.D.'s course?

Decision point: What interventions do you anticipate for the problems previously identified for J.D.?

Decision point: What is J.D.'s current complication and how should it be treated?

Elevated glucose levels have been associated with increased morbidity and mortality rates in critical care. Intensive glucose control with continuous intravenous insulin infusion has been shown in randomized, controlled studies to reduce morbidity and mortality and improve patient outcomes.[45] Hyperglycemia is a common entity in acute pancreatitis and demands close scrutiny and protocol-driven management to maintain blood glucose levels at or less than 110 mg/dl.[11,45] This strategy is also effective in the prevention and management of sepsis and septic shock. The use of antibiotics is also indicated when an infectious source is identified and may also be useful prophylactically. Fluid therapy and vasopressors are part of the mainstay of treatment for the patient with septic shock. Newer therapies such as the intravenous infusion of recombinant human activated protein C have also been used effectively to manage sepsis and septic shock.[30] Recombinant human activated protein C must be used with caution in this population, however, because of the potential for retroperitoneal bleeding.[31]

Bleeding, though a rare complication, must be closely monitored because of the potential for disruption in the gastrointestinal mucosa and for development of disseminated intravascular coagulation (DIC). Nurses need to monitor for bruising and bleeding, especially at venipuncture sites and other breaks in skin continuity. Stools are assessed closely for the presence of gross or occult blood. Intravenous and arterial punctures should be minimized. Small-bore needles are used as necessary, and pressure is applied to the site to prevent bleeding. Coagulation studies are monitored closely for abnormalities, and coagulation proteins are replaced as needed. Shock caused by a hemorrhagic event whatever its cause, is treated aggressively with intravenous fluids, blood, and blood products as necessary (Chapter 40). The end points of resuscitation include normalization of the patient's blood pressure and pulse and indices of end-organ perfusion (e.g., mentation, urine output, skin perfusion).[14] If central access is in place or inserted, filling pressures are monitored with the goal of volume resuscitation to normalize these parameters.

The renal and gastrointestinal complications of acute pancreatitis may occur because of decreased blood flow to these organs associated with hemodynamic instability. Local inflammation may also play a role in the onset of these disorders.[20] When preventive measures such as aggressive volume resuscitation fail and acute renal failure develops, patients may require management with hemodialysis. The patient with persistent hemodynamic compromise is treated with renal replacement therapy, commonly in the form of continuous veno-venous hemodialysis (CVVHD). An adynamic ileus may develop related to decreased intestinal motility and is managed with nasogastric suction and continued NPO status.

Patients with acute pancreatitis can develop gastrointestinal bleeding (Chapter 26) from many sources. Upper gastrointestinal bleeding related to peptic ulcer formation can be effectively prevented by the use of histamine antagonists.[28] Identification of the bleeding site and hemodynamic stabilization of the patient with a life-threatening hemorrhage of the gastrointestinal tract are of critical importance. Bleeding sites may be diagnosed and eradicated by endoscopic methods such as bipolar or laser coagulation. Angiography may be needed to identify a source of bleeding; it also facilitates interventions such as angiographic embolization.[47] Surgery may be required to repair/remove a bleeding site if nonsurgical methods prove unsuccessful. While diagnosis and definitive management are under way, aggressive volume resuscitation continues. Recurrent gastrointestinal bleeding or gastrointestinal perforation will require surgical correction.

There have been attempts to control the inflammatory response in patients with severe acute pancreatitis. This uncontrolled inflammation is believed responsible for the massive physiologic response and the multitude of complications. The role of many inflammatory mediators in acute pancreatitis has been investigated in hopes of identifying an antiinflammatory therapy, but there has been limited success and few human studies.[18,47] Currently, most experts agree that there is no compelling evidence to support the use of immune-modulating therapies such as anti-TNF and lexipafant.[47] Other medications trialed, but without evidence of effectiveness in the treatment of severe acute pancreatitis, include somatostatin, cimetidine (Tagamet), and calcitonin (Miacalcin).[10,33]

MULTIDISCIPLINARY PLAN OF CARE: SUPPORTIVE INTERVENTIONS AND ELIMINATING THE CAUSE OF ACUTE PANCREATITIS

PROBLEM	INTERVENTION	RATIONALE	EXPECTED OUTCOME
Volume depletion caused by retroperitoneal losses from capillary leak	Administer balanced salt solution or colloid or packed red blood cells to maintain Hct of 30% Use central venous catheter for rapid fluid administration and monitoring of CVP PAC used for cases complicated by cardiopulmonary diseases or complications Monitor urine output every hour	Protects against hemodynamic compromise and organ hypoperfusion Third spacing of fluid can have life-threatening results	Normal clinical parameters of heart rate less than 100 beats/min, MAP greater than 70 mm Hg, urine output greater than 0.5 ml/kg/hr, CVP of 8–12 mm Hg, PAWP of 12–15 mm Hg
Abdominal pain related to retroperitoneal inflammation, fluid sequestration, and premature activation of locally released proteases	Maintain NPO status Nasogastric tube indicated only for those with paralytic ileus, nausea/vomiting	Prevents stimulation/secretion by pancreas and amelioration of inflammatory response	Patient reports reduced pain on a 10-point pain assessment scale or nonverbal indicators reveal signs of pain relief

PROBLEM	INTERVENTION	RATIONALE	EXPECTED OUTCOME
	Semi-Fowler's position	Controls migration of enzymes	
	Intravenous narcotic analgesia via bolus dosing or patient-controlled route Avoid meperidine because of extreme side effects and toxic metabolites	All narcotics increase pressure at sphincter of Oddi but use of morphine, hydromorphone, etc. has not worsened course of disease or outcomes	
Electrolyte imbalance caused by retroperitoneal losses and decreased intake	Vigorous calcium replacement to maintain serum ionized calcium >4.5 mg/dl Intensive glucose control, maintaining levels between 80 and 110 mg/dl Potassium and magnesium replacements	Electrolyte and glucose derangements result in severe complications and increased mortality and morbidity	Normal serum calcium, potassium, magnesium, glucose levels; no dysrhythmias; no tetany
Altered nutrition: less than patient requirements related to reduced intake, NPO status, abdominal pain, nausea and vomiting related to possible ileus	For those with complicated, severe acute pancreatitis, enteral nutrition via a feeding tube placed below ligament of Treitz Parenteral nutrition for those who fail enteral trial or who have ileus	Meets calorie and nutritional needs while preventing bacterial translocation and central venous catheter-related complications	No weight loss, normal levels of acute-phase proteins, reduced septic episodes
	Avoid use of fats in TPN if triglyceride level elevated	Excessive triglyceride levels stimulate pancreatic activity	
Infected pancreatic necrosis	Antibiotic administration based on organisms cultured and tested Surgical debridement (necrosectomy) and postoperative lavage or planned staged re-laparotomy Radiologic and endoscopic drainage	Controls septic source and prevents further absorption of activated enzymes and inflammatory mediators Shown to prevent progression and to decrease mortality	No septic episodes, amelioration of inflammatory response
Pancreatic pseudocyst	Monitor size and effects to identify complication No intervention unless complicated Once matured, endoscopic, percutaneous, or surgical drainage	Cyst should be mature (over weeks to months) before intervention Some small pseudocysts resolve spontaneously	No related complications Uneventful drainage
Hemorrhage	Replace fluid volume losses due to bleeding with crystalloid and blood to reestablish pre-hemorrhage cardiovascular status Diagnosis by endoscopy, selective angiography Endoscopic control of bleeding, angiographic embolization, or surgical repair Monitor for DIC and treat symptomatically	Prevents hemodynamic collapse	Cessation of bleeding Normal Hct Normal clinical parameters of HR less than 100 beats/min, MAP greater than 70 mm Hg, urine output greater than 0.5 ml/kg/hr, CVP of 8–12 mm Hg, PAWP of 12–15 mm Hg

Table continues on page 790

PROBLEM	INTERVENTION	RATIONALE	EXPECTED OUTCOME
Respiratory compromise related to atelectasis, pneumonia, pleural effusion, or ARDS	Continuous monitoring of oxygen saturation Chest radiograph and blood gas analysis if hypoxemia is suspected Supplemental oxygen, intubation with mechanical ventilation for ventilatory failure or refractive hypoxia Use of lung protective strategies with ARDS	Improves respiratory status and prevents total cardiopulmonary collapse related to untreated respiratory failure	Pao_2 greater than 60 mm Hg Pco_2 may be elevated slightly above normal Improving radiograph, improving oxygenation while lessening Fio_2 levels as tolerated Eventual extubation with no oxygen requirements
Renal dysfunction related to oliguria, azotemia, ATN, ARF	Volume resuscitation Monitor intake and output, creatinine Renal replacement therapy (CVVHD)	Provides support for renal system until inflammatory process resolves and renal function improves	Urine output greater than 0.5 ml/kg/hr Creatinine less than 2 mg/dl
Potential for infection related to bacterial invasion of retroperitoneal exudates and systemic absorption	Monitor for fever Monitor WBC Abdominal assessment Monitor for other signs of infection or inflammation	Rapid identification of infectious source	WBC $<10,000/mm^3$ No fever Absence of other signs of infection
	CT scan if suspect intra-abdominal infection	Diagnostic accuracy	
	Organism-specific antibiotics Percutaneous or surgical removal of infectious collections	Eradicates organism	
Patient and family education	Multidisciplinary teaching related to disease and its causes, treatments, and complications Education related to avoidance of alcohol if etiology	Providing information may decrease anxiety	Decrease fears and anxiety Prevent recurrence

ATN= Acute tubular necrosis, ARDS = Acute respiratory distress syndrome, ARF = acute renal failure, CT = computed tomography, CVP = central venous pressure, CVVHD = continuous veno-venous hemodialysis, Fio_2 = fraction of inspired oxygen, Hct = hematocrit, HR = heart rate, MAP = mean arterial pressure, NPO = nothing by mouth, PAC = pulmonary artery catheter, Pao_2 = partial pressure of arterial oxygen tension, $Paco_2$ = partial pressure of arterial carbon dioxide, PAWP = pulmonary artery wedge pressure, TPN = total parenteral nutrition, WBC = white blood cell count.

Though most elements of the Multidisciplinary Plan of Care on pp. 788-790 are aimed at supportive interventions, perhaps the most vital tactic in caring for the patient with severe acute pancreatitis is to effectively eliminate the cause whenever possible. The management of this disease and the myriad of complications with which it presents is quite complex. A multidisciplinary approach is critical for successful treatment and optimal patient outcomes.

management in an effort to reduce organ involvement and potential dysfunction. Intensive assessment and monitoring are necessary for the identification of adverse events so that interventions might commence rapidly.

It is necessary to keep in mind that there are few effective remedies for the physiologic impact acute pancreatitis brings to bear on the human host. Further research is required to explore new medications, new management strategies for the complications, and new methods to improve patient outcomes.

CONCLUSIONS

Once the diagnosis of severe acute pancreatitis has been made, thus begins the need for expert, evidence-based

REFERENCES

1. AHCPR. (1992). *Acute pain management in adults: operative or medical procedures or trauma*. U.S. Department of Health and Human Services Pub No. AHCPR 92–0019.

2. American Pain Society (APS). (1992). *Principles of analgesic use in the treatment of acute pain and cancer pain* (3rd ed.). Skokie, Ill: The Society.

3. Balthazar, E. J. (2002). Complications of acute pancreatitis: clinical and CT evaluation. *Rad Clin North Am, 40*(6), 1211–1227.

4. Balthazar, E. J. (1990). Acute pancreatitis: value of CT in establishing prognosis. *Radiology, 174*(2), 331–336.

5. Bentrem, D. J., & Joehl, R. J. (2003). Pancreas: healing response in critical illness. *Crit Care Med, 31*(8 suppl), S582–S589.

5a. Blarney, S. L., Imrie, C. A., O'Neill, J., et al. (1984). Prognostic factors in acute pancreatitis. *Gut, 25,* 1340–1346.

6. Bradley, E. L. (1993). A clinically based classification system for acute pancreatitis: summary of the International Symposium on Acute Pancreatitis, Atlanta, Sept 11–13, 1992. *Arch Surg, 128*(5), 586–590.

7. Burton, F. R. (2005). Diagnosis and risk stratification in acute pancreatitis. In C. E. Forsmark (Ed.), *Pancreatitis and its complications.* Totowa, NJ: Humana.

8. Buter, A., et al. (2002). Dynamic nature of early dysfunction determines outcome in acute pancreatitis. *Brit J Surg, 89*(3), 298–302.

9. Carey, L. C. (1979). Extra-abdominal manifestations of acute pancreatitis. *Surgery, 86*(2), 337–342.

10. Chari, S. T., & Vege, S. S. (2005). *Treatment of pancreatitis,* 2005. www.UptoDate.com.

11. Clement, S., Braithwaite, S. S., et al. (2004). Management of diabetes & hyperglycemia in hospitals. *Diabetes Care, 27*(2), 553–591.

12. Despins, L., Kivlahan, C., & Cox, K. R. (2005). Acute pancreatitis: diagnosis and treatment of a potentially fatal condition. *AJN, 105*(11), 54–57.

13. Dragonov, P. (2005). Treatment of severe pancreatitis. In C. E. Forsmark (Ed.), *Pancreatitis and its complications.* Totowa, NJ: Humana.

14. Fink, M. P., Abraham, E., Vincent, J. L., et al. (2005). *Textbook of critical care* (5th ed.). Philadelphia: Elsevier Saunders.

15. Gavaghan, M. (2002). The pancreas—hermit of the abdomen. *AORN J, 75*(6), 1109–1138.

15a. Glazer, G., & Ranson, J. H. C. (1988). (Eds.), *Acute pancreatitis: experimental and clinical aspects of pathogenesis and management.* Philadelphia: Saunders.

16. Halangk, W. (2005). Early events in acute pancreatitis. *Clin Lab Med, 25*(1), 1–15.

17. Hollenberg, S. M., Ahrens, T. S., et al. (2004). Practice parameters for hemodynamic support of sepsis in adult patients: 2004 update. *Crit Care Med, 32*(9), 1928–1948.

18. Johnson, C., et al. (2001). Double-blind, randomized, placebo-controlled study of a platelet activating factor antagonist, lexipafant, in the treatment and prevention of organ failure in predicted severe acute pancreatitis. *Gut, 48*(1), 62–69.

19. Kaushik, N., & O'Keefe, J. D. (2004). Severe acute pancreatitis: nutritional management in the intensive care unit. *Nutr Clin Pract, 19*(1), 25–30.

20. Khokar, A. S., & Seidner, D. L. (2004). The pathophysiology of pancreatitis. *Nutr Clin Pract, 19*(1), 5–15.

21. Krishnagopalan, S., Dumar, A., & Parillo, J. E. (2002). Myocardial dysfunction in the patient with sepsis. *Curr Opin Crit Care, 8*(5), 376–388.

22. Law, N. M., & Freeman, M. L. (2003). Emergency complications of acute and chronic pancreatitis. *Gastroenterol Clin North Am, 32*(4), 1169–1194.

23. LeFor, A. T., & Gomella, L. G. (2006). *Surgery on call* (4th ed.). New York: Lange Medical Books/McGraw-Hill.

24. Liu, T. H., et al. (2003). Acute pancreatitis in intensive care unit patients: value of clinical and radiologic prognosticators at predicting clinical course and outcomes. *Crit Care Med, 31*(4), 1026–1030.

25. Livingston, D. H., & Dietch, E. A. (1995). Multisystem organ failure: a common problem in surgical intensive care unit patients. *Ann Med, 27*(1), 13–20.

26. Malangoni, M. A., & Martin, A. S. (2005). Outcomes of severe acute pancreatitis. *Am J Surg, 189*(3), 273–277.

27. Marik, P. E., & Zaloga, G. P. (2004). Meta-analysis of parenteral nutrition versus enteral nutrition in patients with acute pancreatitis. *BMJ, 328*(7453), 1407–1412.

28. Mayerle, J., Simon, P., & Lerch, M. M. (2004). Medical treatment of acute pancreatitis. *Gastroenterol Clin North Am, 33*(4), 855–869.

29. McClave, S. A. (2004). Defining the new gold standard for nutrition support in acute pancreatitis. *Nutr Clin Pract, 19*(1), 1–3.

30. McKinley, M. (2005). Shock and sepsis. In M. L. Sole, D. G. Klein & M. J. Moseley (Eds.), *Introduction to critical care nursing* (4th ed.). Philadelphia: Elsevier Saunders.

31. Nagar, A. B., & Gorelik, F. S. (2005). Epidemiology and pathophysiology of acute pancreatitis. In C. E. Forsmark (Ed.), *Pancreatitis and its complications.* Totowa, NJ: Humana.

32. Napolitano, L. M. (2002). Pulmonary consequences of acute pancreatitis: critical role of the neutrophil. *Crit Care Med, 30*(9), 2158–2159.

33. Nathens, A. B., et al. (2004). Management of the critically ill patient with severe acute pancreatitis. *Crit Care Med, 32*(12), 2524–2536.

34. Neoptolemos, J. P., Kemppainen, E. A., et al. (2000). Early prediction of severity in acute pancreatitis by urinary trypsinogen activation peptide: a multi-centre study. *Lancet, 355*(9219), 1955–1960.

35. Orbuch, M. (2004). Optimizing outcomes in acute pancreatitis. *Clin Fam Pract, 6*(3), 607–629.

36. Papachristou, G. I., & Whitcomb, D. C. (2004). Predictors of severity and necrosis in acute pancreatitis. *Gastroenterol Clin North Am, 33*(4), 871–890.

37. Proctor, D. D. (2003). Critical issues in digestive diseases. *Clin Chest Med, 24*(4), 623–632.

38. Raimondo, M., & Scolopio, J. S. (2005). What route to feed patients with severe acute pancreatitis: vein, jejunum or stomach? *Am J Gastroenterol, 100*(2), 440–441.

39. Robinson, L. (2005). Gastrointestinal alterations. In M. L. Sole, D. G. Klein & M. J. Mosely (Eds.), *Introduction to critical care nursing.* Philadelphia: Elsevier Saunders.

40. Swaroop, V. S., Chari, S. T., & Clain, J. E. (2004). Severe acute pancreatitis. *JAMA, 129*(23), 2865–2868.

41. Tenner, S. (2004). Initial management of acute pancreatitis: critical issues during the first 72 hours. *Am J Gastroenterol, 99*(12), 2489–2494.

42. Toruli, J. (2002). Working party report: guidelines for the management of acute pancreatitis. *J Gastroenterol Hepatol, 17*(suppl), 15–39.

43. Udobi, K. F., & Childs, E. W. (2004). Sepsis/acute respiratory distress syndrome. *Clin Fam Pract, 6*(1), 315–322.

44. UK Working Party on Acute Pancreatitis. (2005). UK guidelines for the management of acute pancreatitis. *Gut, 54*(suppl III), iii1–iii9.

45. Van den Berghe, G. (2001). Intensive insulin therapy in critically ill patients. *N Engl J Med, 345*(19), 1359–1367.

46. Ward, N. S. (2002). Effects of prone position ventilation in ARDS: an evidence based review of the literature. *Crit Care Clin, 18*(1), 35–44.

47. Werner, J., et al. (2005). Management of acute pancreatitis: from surgery to interventional intensive care. *Gut, 54*(3), 426–436.

48. Yousaf, M., McCallion, K., & Diamond, T. (2003). Management of severe acute pancreatitis. *Brit J Surg, 90*(4), 407–420.

CHAPTER 29

The Gut in Critical Illness

Andrea P. Marshall

During episodes of critical illness the gastrointestinal (GI) system often becomes compromised. Physiologic changes (e.g., the shunting of blood from the GI tract to the vital organs) result in hypoperfusion and decreased tissue oxygenation and function. Consequently, changes to normal gut physiology (e.g., digestion, absorption, immunity, and protection) may occur; this may further compromise the critically ill patient. Assessment of GI perfusion in the critically ill patient is a useful strategy to monitor for signs of hypoperfusion or adequacy of resuscitation.

This chapter will explore three key issues related to the gut in critical illness: assessment of the adequacy of gut perfusion using gastric tonometry; prevention of stress-related mucosal disease; and the assessment and management of intra-abdominal hypertension and abdominal compartment syndrome.

NORMAL GASTROINTESTINAL PHYSIOLOGY

The physiology of the GI system is most commonly associated with its role in digestion and absorption of nutrients (e.g., amino acids, lipids, vitamins, minerals, and water). However, during critical illness, normal GI physiology responsible for digestion and absorption of nutrients may be altered. For example, the primary function of the stomach is to produce gastric acid and pepsin. While gastric acid production is commonly thought to increase in critical illness, most critically ill patients do not hypersecrete gastric acid.[37] Rather, gastric acid secretion is often diminished in the critically ill, with an increase in gastric pH observed even when gastric acid secretion is not pharmacologically inhibited.[61,137]

The small bowel also plays an important part in the digestion and absorption of nutrients. Mechanical digestion together with the chemical digestion of carbohydrates, amino acids, lipids, and nucleic acids is essential for breaking down the nutrients into a form absorbable by the small intestine.[49,148] The processes of diffusion, facilitated diffusion, osmosis, and active transport in the small intestine are responsible for the absorption of

90% of all nutrients.[148] The remaining 10% of nutrients are absorbed in the large intestine. The ability of the small intestine to absorb these nutrients can be impaired during critical illness;[49] however, most critically ill patients appear to be able to tolerate enteral nutrition, making the clinical significance of impaired absorption unclear.

While the digestion and absorption of nutrients is an important aspect of normal GI physiology, its role in immunity and protection is of equal importance to the critically ill patient. The GI tract has a variety of mechanisms in place that prevent the movement of substances (other than nutrients, water, and electrolytes) across the gut wall (Table 29-1). In the setting of critical illness, where GI hypoperfusion may be present, these mechanisms normally protecting the body against movement of bacteria across the gut wall may be diminished.

ALTERATIONS TO NORMAL GASTROINTESTINAL PHYSIOLOGY IN CRITICAL ILLNESS

Alterations to normal GI physiology in critical illness primarily relate to hypoperfusion and decreased oxygenation in this highly metabolic area. Previously, GI dysfunction in critical illness was described in relation to clinical presentations that became symptomatic as a result of well-established GI ischemia[55] (Box 29-1). Consequently, a focus on the prevention and early detection of GI ischemia has become vital in minimizing ischemia-related gut dysfunction in the critically ill.

Gastrointestinal Mucosal Hypoperfusion

Adequate oxygenation is necessary to maintain normal structure and function in all body tissues. Regional oxygen delivery is influenced by alterations in global oxygen delivery and oxygen consumption;[15] however, GI hypoxia may also be present despite normal oxygen delivery and consumption.[40]

The GI system is particularly susceptible to alterations in regional blood flow and oxygen delivery (Box 29-2). The ability of the GI system to undergo intense

TABLE 29-1 Protective Mechanisms of the Gastrointestinal System

MECHANISM	ACTION
Epithelial cell shedding	Limits bacterial adhesion
Gut-associated lymphoid tissue	Provides immune tolerance against food antigens and normal intestinal flora
Hydrochloric acid secretion	Increases gastric acidity and destroys bacteria
Kupffer cells	Liver tissue macrophages for destroying foreign substances
Motility	Propels bacteria through GI tract
Mucin production	Prevents adhesion of bacteria to wall of GI tract
Zona occludens	Prevents bacteria from moving across wall of GI tract

Box 29-1

Gastrointestinal Dysfunction in Critical Illness

- Acalculous cholecystitis
- Gallbladder perforation
- Gastrointestinal perforation
- Gastrointestinal stress bleeding
- Intolerance of enteral feeds
- Ileus
- Ischemic enterocolitis
- Mechanical obstruction
- Pancreatitis

Data from reference 87.

Box 29-2

Causes of Tissue Hypoxia Within the Gastrointestinal System

- Countercurrent oxygen exchange from vessels within the villi
- Higher critical tissue oxygen delivery concentration than the rest of the body
- "Plasma skimming" causes a decreased hematocrit of blood supplying the villi
- Redistribution of blood to vital organs may persist even when normal systemic hemodynamics have been reestablished
- Splanchnic vasoconstriction is proportionally greater than other vascular beds

Data from reference 75.

vasoconstriction and to shunt blood to the central circulation[40] results in a regional decrease in blood flow and oxygen delivery while nonspecific measurements of total body oxygen delivery remain unchanged. During shock states, decreased blood flow because of vasoconstriction occurs in this region first and is restored last, following successful resuscitation.[150] In shock states, the gut attempts to maintain adequate cellular oxygenation by increasing the amount of oxygen extracted from the blood. This increase in oxygen extraction may prevent serious compromise of tissue oxygenation even in the presence of reduced oxygen delivery.[1] Despite the ability of the gut to increase oxygen extraction in the setting of reduced oxygen delivery, the GI system remains susceptible to hypoxia, particularly if oxygen consumption is limited by oxygen delivery.[54]

The anatomic arrangement of the GI blood vessels may also contribute to mucosal hypoxia (Figure 29-1). Within the mucosa a series of finger-like projections called villi are formed. These villi vastly increase the epithelial surface area available for digestion and absorption. The blood vessel arrangement in each villus consists of a central arteriole and venous capillaries situated approximately 20 μm apart. Blood flows through these vessels in opposite directions and, coupled with their close proximity, facilitates the diffusion of oxygen and other small molecules between the blood vessels,[20] resulting in a decrease in oxygen delivery to the villus tip.

In low-flow states, the slow transit time leads to stasis and competitive extraction at lower levels of the villus, producing hypoxia at the villus tip. Furthermore, reductions in arterial blood pressure cause the precapillary sphincters to relax. The relaxation of these sphincters promotes blood flow to more capillaries, increasing the number of perfused capillaries and the size of the vascular bed. The combination of low blood pressure and a larger vascular bed also slows blood flow through the villi, ultimately contributing to hypoxia and ischemia at the villus tip.[55]

During the period of ischemia and hypoxia, byproducts of anaerobic metabolism, known as oxygen free radicals, are also generated. With successful resuscitation of the GI tract, blood flow and oxygen delivery are restored to the area and simultaneously, oxygen free radicals are liberated. These oxygen free radicals contribute to microvascular and mucosal changes characteristic of ischemia and reperfusion of the gut mucosa.[54]

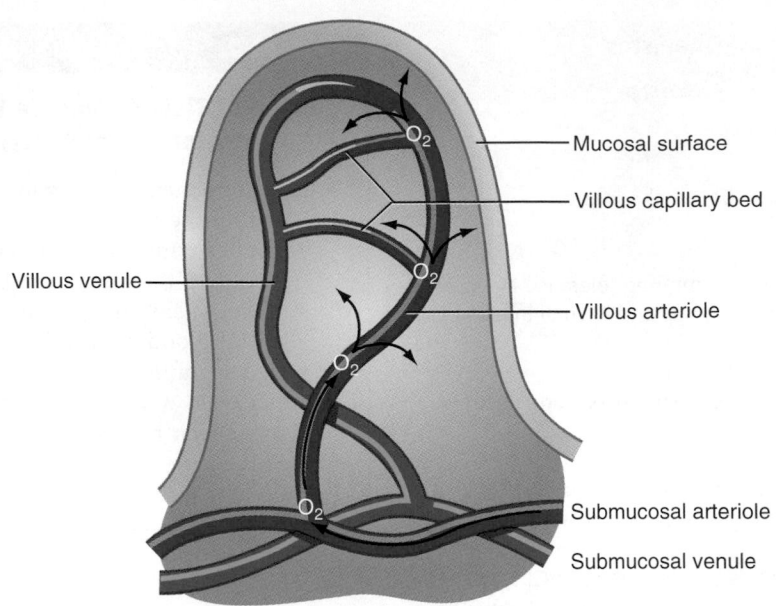

Mucosal surface

Villous capillary bed

Villous venule

Villous arteriole

Submucosal arteriole

Submucosal venule

⬍FIGURE 29-1 Blood supply to the GI mucosa villus.

Consequences of Gastrointestinal Hypoperfusion. The consequences of GI hypoperfusion are significant and include the following:

- Disruption of the physical barrier to pathogens
- Disruption of chemical control of bacterial overgrowth
- Decreased peristalsis
- Reduced immunologic activities of gut-associated lymphoid tissue

In healthy individuals, all of these mechanisms work efficiently to contain bacteria within the GI tract. However, during critical illness reduced oxygenation may contribute to decreased cellular function and failure of these protective mechanisms. Consequently, bacterial proliferation and translocation from the GI tract to the systemic circulation may occur.[66]

Disruption of the Physical Barrier to Pathogens. The mucosal lining of the entire GI tract creates a physical barrier to bacterial invasion. The mucosa is composed of epithelial cells produced and replaced approximately every 3 to 5 days.[113] This constant shedding means that pathogens have little chance to colonize and invade the GI tract because they are shed simultaneously with the epithelial cells. The epithelial cells are also highly metabolic, consuming large amounts of oxygen, and consequently are susceptible to reduced oxygen delivery and changes in vascular flow.[126] Reductions in mucosal oxygen delivery may therefore lead to mucosal atrophy and

epithelial cell death, reducing the ability of the epithelial cells to provide a mechanical barrier to pathogens.

The junctions between epithelial cells also provide a barrier to microorganisms. Intermediate junctions (zonula adherens) function primarily in cell-cell adhesion[113] while the tight junctions (zonula occludens) limit the movement of bacteria and toxins across the gut wall.[153] The impaired mucosal perfusion and mucosal atrophy associated with critical illness may increase the permeability of the tight junctions and permit the movement of pathogens across the mucosal barrier.[32]

Mucus cells also line the surface of the GI mucosa, and, when stimulated by food or irritation, the mucosal surface cells secrete large quantities of a very thick, alkaline mucus. In the stomach, a mucus layer approximately 1 mm thick is formed, coating the wall of the stomach and protecting it against autodigestion.[113] Further protection is provided by the glycoproteins contained within the mucus that prevent bacteria from adhering to and colonizing the mucosal wall.[29]

Disruption of Chemical Control of Bacterial Overgrowth. Parietal cells in the stomach produce hydrochloric acid and keep the intragastric environment relatively acidic, with a pH of approximately 3.0. An acidic pH has bactericidal and bacteriostatic properties,[63] thus limiting overgrowth in the stomach. This inhibition of bacterial growth by hydrochloric acid production may not be an effective mechanism in the critically ill because hydrochloric acid production within the stomach has been noted to decrease as a consequence of critical illness.[17,49] Changes in gastric pH associated with critical illness may facilitate bacterial proliferation within the stomach.

The secretion of bicarbonate in the small intestine provides further protection for the epithelium. The binding of bicarbonate ions with hydrogen ions to form water and carbon dioxide (CO_2) prevents hydrogen ions from damaging the duodenal wall.[75] Although this is a relatively efficient system, some hydrogen ions still reach the mucosal layer and the bicarbonate in the microvasculature is needed to neutralize them. In normal physiologic states, as the number of hydrogen ions increases, there is a proportional increase in mucosal blood flow, supplying more bicarbonate ions.[75] However, in critical illness, often associated with a low-flow state within the gut, bicarbonate ion production may be limited, reducing the effectiveness of this protective mechanism and allowing damage to the gut mucosa to occur.

Farther down the GI tract, normal gut flora, capable of surviving in the more alkaline environment of the lower gut, attaches to the mucosal cells of the colon, preventing colonization of unwanted pathogens.[113] Antibiotic therapy, commonly used in the management of critical illness, may reduce the population of normal gut flora and provide opportunities for pathogenic overgrowth.[126]

Bile salts may also provide protection against bacteria by breaking down the liposaccharide portion of the endotoxin[78] and thereby detoxifying gram-negative bacteria in the gut. The deconjugation of bile salts into secondary bile acids also inhibits the proliferation of pathogens and may destroy their cell walls.[44] However, normal gut flora is required for the deconjugation of bile acids to secondary bile acids; therefore a reduction in the number of normal gut flora, such as may occur secondary to antibiotic therapy, may inhibit this protective mechanism.

Reduced Immunologic Activities of Gut-Associated Lymphoid Tissue. Protection against bacterial invasion is also provided by gut-associated lymphoid tissue,[93] one of the largest immune organs in the body.[113] When this lymphoid tissue is exposed to antigens it has the ability to mount cell-mediated and humoral-mediated immune responses,[113] which have a cytotoxic effect on the bacteria.[29] Thus the immunologic function of the GI system is important in maintaining regional and global protection against the invasion of bacteria. However, in critical illness, reduced oxygen and nutrient supply could impede the ability of the gut to function as an immunologic

organ and thus the GI system's ability to protect the body against bacteria is diminished.

The various physical, chemical, and immunologic barriers provide the initial defense against bacterial invasion. Should bacteria and their by-products cross the gut barrier and enter the systemic circulation, the reticuloendothelial system, made up of Kupffer cells in the liver and spleen, provides a back-up defense. In the event that pathogens cross the gut barrier and enter the systemic circulation, they will drain from the extensive vasculature supplying the GI tract and into the portal vein.[148] The blood is then directed to the liver. As it enters the liver, it comes into contact with the extensive reticuloendothelial system, where the pathogens are destroyed through phagocytosis by the Kupffer cells.[90] However, alterations in regional blood flow in critical illness result in a shunting of blood to the central circulation and a decrease in hepatic blood flow. Consequently, pathogens and debris that enter the intestinal circulation may not reach the Kupffer cells and systemic bacteremia may result.

The blood vessels of the GI system are part of a more extensive system called the splanchnic circulation, which includes blood flow through the liver, spleen, and pancreas. The structure of the splanchnic circulation, is such that blood passes through the gut, spleen, and pancreas before entering the liver by way of the portal vein. Consequently, the changes in GI perfusion have the capacity to impact hepatic perfusion, oxygenation, and function. In approximately 50% of critically ill patients, ischemic hepatitis or "shock liver" occurs and is evidenced by jaundice, the elevation of liver function test values, or overt hepatic dysfunction.[139] Ischemic hepatitis can vary from a mild elevation of serum aminotransferase and bilirubin levels in septic patients to an acute elevation following hemodynamic shock. Ischemic hepatic injury influences morbidity and mortality but remains underdiagnosed,[139] likely because the clinical signs become apparent long after hypoperfusion has occurred. Physiologic changes contributing to ischemic hepatitis include alterations to the portal and arterial blood supply as well as the hepatic microcirculation.[139] The degree to which the liver is damaged is directly related to the severity and duration of hypoperfusion; both anoxic and reperfusion injury can damage hepatocytes and the vascular endothelium.

The liver plays an important role in the inflammatory process. Kupffer cells—tissue macrophages in the liver—normally detoxify substances that may trigger systemic inflammation and produce proteins and antiproteases that control the inflammatory response. However, in the setting of splanchnic hypoperfusion, liver dysfunction may occur and these processes may be inhibited.

GASTRIC TONOMETRY

The GI system is complex in its structure and function. Its role in the digestion and absorption of nutrients is well understood, and its ability to protect the body against the invasion of organisms is increasingly being appreciated. In the critically ill, the role of the gut has become an area of interest because of its susceptibility to ischemia and hypoxia that may be linked to alterations in GI structure and function, which in turn contributes to the development of multiple organ dysfunction syndrome (MODS).

Gastric tonometry has been developed as a minimally invasive method of monitoring perfusion, and possibly oxygenation, of the GI tract and splanchnic organs. Monitoring of perfusion and oxygenation in the GI region is important because changes in GI blood flow may occur in the absence of systemic hemodynamic disturbances;[42,72] such changes provide an earlier warning of hypoperfusion than conventional assessments of perfusion (e.g., arterial blood pressure). Hypoperfusion contributes to decreased oxygen delivery within the highly metabolic splanchnic region, with the longer-term consequences being the development of GI dysfunction and MODS.[104] The ability of gastric tonometry to provide real-time and specific monitoring of gastric perfusion makes it a useful tool for monitoring patients at risk of splanchnic hypoperfusion.[31] Early attention to gastric hypoperfusion may prevent the development of MODS and improve outcomes for critically ill patients,[42,48] although data suggesting an improvement in outcome based on treatment guided by tonometrically derived variables are lacking.[48]

Historical Development

The concept of monitoring GI regional CO_2 levels was described in the literature as early as 1926,[91] at which time diffusion was identified as the fundamental physiologic principle underlying the effective development of gastric tonometry. Subsequent studies using early tonometers[9] were able to demonstrate increases in the levels of gastric partial pressure of carbon dioxide (PCO_2) in overtly "shocked" patients. However, measurement of PCO_2 in the gastric luminal fluid remained problematic.[30] The search for a solution to these problems led to refinement of the existing aspiration-based process and the development of CO_2-permeable silicone tubes.[70] The ongoing recognition of the impact of critical illness on the GI tract[50] led to the development of the modern gastric tonometer (Tonometrics catheter, Datex-Ohmeda, Madison, Wisc), which is produced commercially and licensed for use worldwide (Figure 29-2).

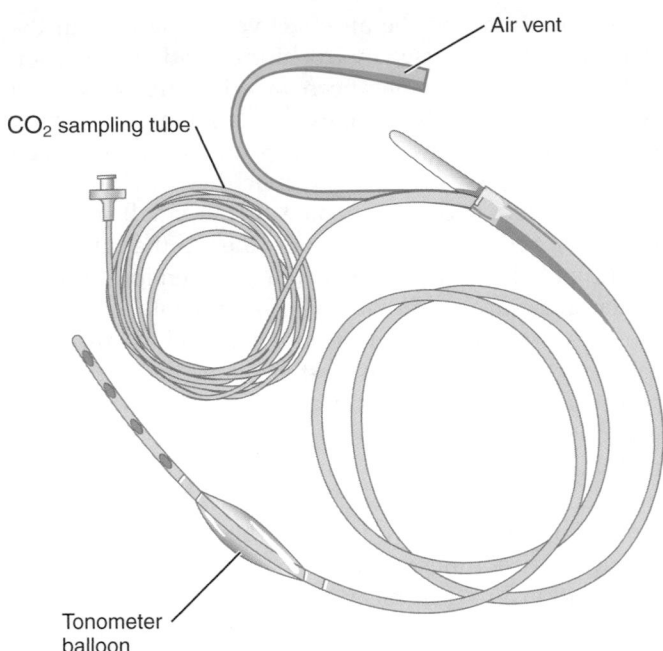

◆FIGURE 29-2   The gastric tonometer. CO_2 = Carbon dioxide.

Principles of Gastric Tonometry

The principle of diffusion, which governs gas movement and the equilibration of the partial pressure of gases between two liquids that are separated by a semipermeable membrane, is used as the basis for tonometric measurements.[52] The PCO_2 of the surrounding tissues and the PCO_2 of the lumen of an associated hollow visceral organ are maintained in a state of equilibrium.[30] Therefore the PCO_2 in the GI mucosa ($PiCO_2$) is the same as the PCO_2 in the gastric lumen.[26]

Theoretically, the CO_2 produced by the GI mucosa during cellular activity should move from an area of higher partial pressure (mucosa) to an area of lower partial pressure (gastric lumen). Because the tonometer balloon is permeable to CO_2 and is situated in the gastric lumen, the gas diffuses from the gastric lumen into the balloon until equilibrium is reached.[86] Simply, the measurement of gastric intramucosal CO_2 concentration is achieved by the sampling of fluid or air from a CO_2-permeable balloon, which forms part of the gastric tonometer.

Physiologic Underpinnings of Gastric Tonometry

Gastric tonometry is designed to monitor splanchnic perfusion because a reduction in blood flow to this area is thought to be an *early* indicator of the development of shock. It is in patients who are susceptible to covert shock that the use of gastric tonometry will have its greatest success. The ability to monitor the adequacy of splanchnic perfusion allows clinicians to observe the early development of shock that would otherwise be undetected by monitoring global measurements of perfusion and oxygenation (e.g., hypotension, decreased cardiac output, and increased lactate levels[11]). The physiologic underpinnings of gastric tonometry include the links between tissue oxygen delivery, cellular utilization of oxygen, and CO_2 production described earlier in this chapter.

Physiologic Influences on the Measurement of Carbon Dioxide Within the Tonometer Balloon

Tonometric measurements can be influenced by physiologic changes that may occur in the critically ill; an appreciation of these circumstances is necessary in order to evaluate tonometric measurements within the clinical context of individual patients. Under normal conditions, the P_{CO_2} in regional tissues such as the GI tract should approximate the partial pressure of CO_2 in the arterial blood;[13] however, pathologic conditions may cause changes in regional CO_2 levels to occur. Furthermore, any increase in arterial CO_2 concentration will be reflected by an increase in regional CO_2 concentration (i.e., when a patient has a preexisting elevated arterial CO_2 concentration).

The high diffusibility of CO_2 may also influence its measurement regionally.[7] For example, in the setting of anemia or reduced oxygen uptake in the lung, tissue perfusion may be adequate but tissue oxygen delivery reduced. In such circumstances, anaerobically generated CO_2 may be flushed from the tissue into the venous blood, thus lowering regional CO_2 values and masking the increased production.[133] Conversely, if a reduction in blood flow is present then the regional CO_2 level may increase even though aerobic metabolism and normal CO_2 production exist.[120]

During anaerobic metabolism an increase in regional CO_2 concentration may occur secondary to an overall increase in hydrogen ion production and the buffering of these ions with bicarbonate ions.[14,120] While it is commonly assumed that an increase in hydrogen ion concentration results from lactic acid formation during anaerobic metabolism, the necessary dissociation occurs only when the tissue pH is less than 6.0.[41] The increase in hydrogen ion production is more likely the result of the rapid rate of adenosine triphosphate (ATP) breakdown in comparison to ATP regeneration.[14] So, in the setting of acute local metabolic acidosis, an increase in tissue CO_2 concentration may

reflect buffering of hydrogen ions rather than the increased production of lactic acid.

Regional acidosis may also occur during ischemia; however, the acidosis is not entirely explained by reduced blood flow. When a mathematical gas exchange model of CO_2 is used, it is demonstrated that the changes in tissue P_{CO_2} secondary to reduced blood flow are minimal when compared to the CO_2 produced when hydrogen ions are buffered with bicarbonate.[52] Nevertheless, the increase in P_{CO_2} as a consequence of reduced blood flow has been demonstrated in canine models.[131,157]

Any increase in tissue CO_2 levels is influenced by complex physiologic processes, making it difficult to state conclusively that increases in regional CO_2 concentration occur primarily as a result of decreased regional tissue perfusion or oxygenation. Rather, this increase in regional CO_2 concentration should be viewed as an index of tissue hypoperfusion as opposed to an *absolute* indicator of tissue hypoxia.[102]

Clinical Evaluation of Tonometrically Derived Measurements

Gastric tonometry only directly measures one variable—the partial pressure of CO_2 in the GI mucosa.[13,94] The accuracy of measuring the partial pressure of CO_2 within the tonometer balloon (Pt_{CO_2}) has been established; data indicate that it closely matches the direct measurement of the intramucosal partial pressure of CO_2[33,105] by the mass spectrometer.[26]

Current data suggest a Pt_{CO_2} of less than 50 mm Hg is acceptable;[146] however, a comparison of baseline GI CO_2 values obtained during several research studies[5,53,73,76] demonstrates some variation in values measured. As few studies on gastric tonometry have been performed in healthy adult patients, there are no values widely accepted as normal for GI CO_2 levels derived by a gastric tonometer;[59,121] it has been recommended that each institution establish its own reference values.[39,122] It is also important to note that changes from the baseline reading for a P_{CO_2} level are as important as the maintenance of readings within a predetermined range. Furthermore, there can be several clinical explanations for changes to the Pt_{CO_2}, highlighting the need for nurses to consider tonometric measurements within the clinical context of the patient.

Catheter Position. Interpretation of regional CO_2 values can be confounded by the disparity between values obtained in different parts of the GI tract.[53,103] In fact, it has been suggested that monitoring P_{CO_2} in the gastric mucosa may not necessarily reflect conditions in the segments of bowel most at risk for ischemia—namely, the small bowel and the proximal portion of the colon—that rely on the superior mesenteric artery for their blood supply.[7,152] It has also been suggested following demonstration that the levels of P_{CO_2} vary in different sections of the GI system and that the small bowel may be more sensitive to hypoperfusion, suggesting that monitoring this regional area of the GI tract may provide an earlier indicator of gut hypoperfusion.[118] The varying P_{CO_2} levels within the GI tract suggest that migration of the gastric tonometer from the lumen of the stomach into other areas of the intestine may produce fluctuating P_{CO_2} levels that may be unrelated to changes in splanchnic perfusion. Despite the disparity in measurements detectable in different areas of the bowel, the P_{CO_2} level still increases in all areas when decreased GI perfusion occurs.[103,152] In clinical practice, the monitoring of measurement trends is valuable; it is essential that nurses regularly verify the position of the gastric tonometer, either through clinical assessment or by radiograph, after insertion and regularly during the monitoring period.

Increased Pt_{CO_2} Unrelated to Gastrointestinal Hypoperfusion.

The concept of increased CO_2 concentration through the buffering of hydrochloric acid by bicarbonate in the stomach, and its influence on intramucosal pH (pHi), has been examined in vitro.[2,43] These studies demonstrate that the buffering of hydrogen ions with bicarbonate may contribute to an increase in measured Pt_{CO_2} that cannot necessarily be attributed to intestinal ischemia but that these increases in Pt_{CO_2} can be prevented by the administration of histamine-2 receptor antagonists[2] (Figure 29-3).

The use of histamine-2 receptor blockade as a method of preventing the back-diffusion of CO_2, and thus measurement error, has been examined in healthy volunteers.[59,107] The titration of hydrogen ions and bicarbonate may increase intraluminal production of CO_2, and the administration of histamine-2 receptor antagonists may eliminate these errors in measurement. However, the presence of GI dysfunction and reduced gastric acid secretion that may be present in critical illness[49] make it difficult to determine whether histamine-2 receptor antagonists would be useful when tonometry is used in the critically ill.[2,5,88,149]

The lack of consensus regarding the routine use of histamine-2 receptor blockade during tonometry results in variability in clinical practice; however, this should not significantly interfere with patient assessment and management if nurses consider measurement trends and the patient's clinical presentation when evaluating tonometric measurements.

Calculated Tonometric Variables.

While GI CO_2 level is the only value directly obtained from the use of gastric tonometry, gastric intramucosal pH (pHi) continues to be the variable most reported in the literature as the measure of regional tissue perfusion.[56] pHi is a calculated variable and involves the use of both the directly measured variable Pt_{CO_2} and the indirectly measured variable bicarbonate concentration.

The calculation of pHi is reliant on two key assumptions: that the CO_2 concentration measured by the tonometer will approximate the CO_2 concentration of the GI mucosa and that the bicarbonate concentration measured in arterial blood will be the same as the bicarbonate concentration in the mucosa. In 1982 Fiddian-Green et al.[43] proposed that the Pt_{CO_2} and the arterial bicarbonate concentration value be used in a modified Henderson-Hasselbalch equation to calculate the pHi (Figure 29-4).

The use of these values to calculate gastric pHi was intended to provide an indication of gastric mucosal acidity. This was based on the assumption that during reduced perfusion to the gastric tissues, anaerobic metabolism would occur and subsequently produce an increased amount of CO_2 that would be measured by the gastric tonometer.[101] Consequently, increased CO_2 concentration, when applied to the Henderson-Hasselbalch equation, would result in a decrease in the calculated pHi. However, the notion of a calculated intramucosal pHi has slowly lost favor following closer examination of the assumptions underpinning its calculation. To calculate gastric pHi using a modified Henderson-Hasselbalch equation, the arterial bicarbonate level is required. However, the assumption that the arterial bicarbonate level equals the mucosal

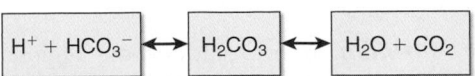

♦FIGURE 29-3 The production of carbon dioxide as a result of the buffering of hydrogen by bicarbonate. CO_2 = Carbon dioxide, H^+ = hydrogen ion, HCO_3^- = bicarbonate, H_2CO_3 carbonic acid, H_2O = water.

$$pHi = 6.1 + \log_{10}\left[\frac{HCO_3^-}{Pico_{2(ss)} \times 0.03}\right]$$

6.1 = pK for the HCO_3^-/CO_2 system in plasma at 37°C

0.03 = Solubility of CO_2 in plasma at 37°C

♦FIGURE 29-4 The modified Henderson-Hasselbalch equation for calculating pHi. HCO_3^- = Bicarbonate, pHi = intramucosal pH, $Pico_2$ = partial pressure of intramucosal carbon dioxide.

bicarbonate level may not always be upheld as bicarbonate does not readily diffuse across cellular membranes.[7] Consequently, the equilibration between cellular, mucosal, and arterial bicarbonate levels may be difficult to achieve. For example, although tissue bicarbonate concentration may approximate the bicarbonate concentration in arterial blood in stable physiologic conditions,[50] this might not hold true during periods of mucosal hypoperfusion.[143] Reduced blood flow may also cause discrepancies between mucosal and arterial bicarbonate values.[7] These possible discrepancies between arterial and mucosal bicarbonate levels may influence calculated measurements such as pHi, and hence clinicians are now more commonly assessing $PtCO_2$ values rather than calculated pHi measurements.

Systemic acid-base abnormalities, which are common in critically ill patients, also influence the calculation of pHi, decreasing the specificity of the calculation.[127,132] For example, patients with acute renal failure commonly develop systemic metabolic acidosis. Likewise, systemic metabolic alkalosis or administration of bicarbonate can directly influence the calculated pHi.[16] Consequently, any patient with metabolic derangements influencing the arterial pH would have a similar change in GI pH. While changes to the calculation of pHi have been suggested,[97] this strategy has not been embraced because of the increased use of other assessable variables, for example, the difference between the arterial and mucosal PCO_2 measurements (CO_2 gap).[133]

Regional CO_2 concentration is directly influenced by arterial CO_2[16] concentration, and in patients with normal systemic arterial CO_2 values, misinterpretation of the regional CO_2 level should not occur. However, critically ill patients often also exhibit respiratory dysfunction, producing abnormal arterial CO_2 values that may change acutely. When the CO_2 gap is calculated, the influences of respiratory and metabolic acid-base abnormalities are eliminated. Thus the CO_2 gap may be a more specific marker of GI mucosal blood flow than pHi or $PtCO_2$. The CO_2 gap could then be used as the measure of mucosal perfusion instead of the calculated pHi value.[57,151]

Despite the demonstrable superiority of using the CO_2 gap to evaluate mucosal blood flow, a normal CO_2 gap in healthy or critically ill patients has yet to be clearly described in the literature. Under normal conditions, there should be no difference between the regional and arterial CO_2 values. Critically ill patients, however, may frequently experience alterations in regional blood flow that may influence the $PtCO_2$, or may experience alterations in CO_2 removal, which would result in an increased $PaCO_2$. Several studies have addressed the issue of an acceptable CO_2 gap; the recommended values are listed in Table 29-2.

TABLE 29-2 Recommended Values for Carbon Dioxide Gap (mm Hg)

RECOMMENDED CO_2 GAP	POPULATION IN WHICH CO_2 GAP WAS DETERMINED
9.5	19 healthy volunteers[147]
Less than 20	35 clinically stable surgical[110] patients
Less than 7.5	16 multiple-injured patients[109]

CO_2 = Carbon dioxide.

Influence of Enteral Feeding. Enteral nutrition is the preferred method of nutritional support in critical illness[65,135,154] and is thought to have a role in improving GI blood flow.[68] However, concurrent monitoring and feeding of the gut in critical illness does not occur because of the belief that enteral nutrition will influence the measurement of PCO_2.[16]

An increase in $PtCO_2$ appears to occur during intragastric enteral feeding[84] but not during post-pyloric enteral feeding.[76] While post-pyloric feeding is suggested as the preferred route for enteral nutrition administration in patients with GI monitoring,[76] it has also been suggested that enteral feeding can be withheld for a minimum of 1 hour before obtaining $PtCO_2$ measurements when patients are fed into the stomach.[84]

Furthermore, a sustained increase in $PtCO_2$ following enteral feeding is not observed and the $PtCO_2$ appears to stabilize after 24 hours of enteral feeding.[85] It is possible that the initial increase in $PtCO_2$ is related to a reversal of GI mucosal vasoconstriction[55] and increased gastric mucosal blood flow associated with the administration of enteral feeding.[89] Ongoing administration of enteral feeding solution may maintain improved gastric mucosal blood flow, preventing the buildup of CO_2 in the mucosal vasculature. This may explain why, in the absence of illness-related crises, the $PtCO_2$ values appear to stabilize after the initial administration of enteral feeding.

Because there are few data examining the influence of enteral nutrition on tonometric measurements, it is likely that the convention of withholding enteral feeding is practiced. However, if the presence of enteral feeding is believed to influence tonometric measurements, it is reasonable for nurses to also be actively emptying the stomach by aspirating gastric contents through the tonometer.[26] The impact of withholding feedings or aspiration of gastric contents is an important consideration for nurses evaluating the nutritional intake of the critically ill.

TECHNICAL LIMITATIONS OF GASTRIC TONOMETRY

While gastric tonometry is used in many clinical areas, its widespread adoption has not occurred. This may be due in part to the technical limitations and potential for procedural error associated with using this device. However, ongoing work in this area has resulted in technological advances in the measurement of $Ptco_2$ that have assisted in overcoming both technical limitations and procedural error. Nevertheless, it is imperative that nurses have a clear understanding of the technical limitations and potential for measurement error as many clinical areas continue to obtain tonometric measurements manually.

Procedural Errors

Technical limitations have been primarily associated with the use of normal saline (NS) as the tonometric medium to determine $Ptco_2$ and analysis of $Ptco_2$ by certain blood gas analyzers. There is additional concern about procedural error that may occur during sampling from the device. These issues have been well identified in the literature,[16] and the recognition of their impact on the measurement and interpretation of tonometric measurements has led to considerable improvements in this technology.

Operator Error. Initial methods of measuring $Ptco_2$ using the Tonometrics catheter (Datex-Ohmeda, Madison, Wisc) were time consuming and cumbersome.[38] Operator error has also been identified as a contributor to incorrect determination of the $Ptco_2$,[25] suggesting the need for trained personnel to collect data.[38] Technological developments have led to the use of automated sample collection with the use of intermittent air tonometry and, consequently, many, if not all, of these procedural errors have been eliminated.[101]

Normal Saline as the Tonometric Medium. A further limitation of gastric tonometry using NS as the tonometric medium results from the poor stability of CO_2 in unbuffered NS.[16] If air is accidentally introduced into the sample, CO_2 may diffuse out of the NS, resulting in a lowered $Ptco_2$ value. Therefore the NS must be handled in an anaerobic fashion and quickly analyzed to prevent degassing of the sample.[101]

The use of NS in gastric tonometry has limitations specifically related to its use as a medium in which to sample CO_2. First, NS has no buffering ability so CO_2 is readily lost from the solution.[16] An uncapped sample of NS at room temperature will lose CO_2 rapidly, so it is recommended that once the NS is aspirated, the CO_2 level be quickly determined in the blood gas

analyzer. Anaerobic sampling of the $Ptco_2$ may improve the stability of CO_2, and if the sample is also placed on ice, CO_2 levels may remain stable for up to 20 minutes.[101]

To improve the stability of tonometrically measured CO_2, alternative tonometric solutions have been investigated. Several studies[71,122,145] have demonstrated an improvement in precision and bias when solutions other than saline are used within the tonometer balloon. However, the introduction of air tonometry has largely superseded their use in the clinical and research settings.

Measurement of $Ptco_2$ Using Arterial Blood Gas Machines. The use of arterial blood gas analyzers to measure the Pco_2 level of NS instilled into the tonometer balloon has also been associated with a degree of measurement error. This may be a consequence of the calibration of blood gas analyzers, which are designed to measure the Pco_2 in blood only. To minimize the bias when using NS as the tonometric solution, it is recommended that the same blood gas analyzer be used consistently, that the instrument bias be determined, and that the institution establish its own reference values for use clinically.[122] The bias created by the measurement of CO_2 concentration in NS by blood gas analyzers is eliminated with the use of intermittent, automated air tonometry (Tonocap TC-200, Datex-Ohmeda, Madison, Wisc).

Semi-Continuous Measurement of $Ptco_2$

The difficulties with using NS as a tonometric medium have only recently seen air tonometry explored as an alternative, and often preferred, tonometric medium. The process of air tonometry was introduced with the development of the Tonocap TC-200 and the tonometry module, E-TONO (Datex-Ohmeda, Madison, Wisc). These devices allow for semi-continuous monitoring of intramucosal CO_2 level using air as a tonometer medium (Figure 29-5).

Studies clearly demonstrate that air tonometry is equal or superior to NS tonometry.[24,147] Air tonometry provides more rapid $Ptco_2$ results than does NS tonometry and eliminates procedural error associated with the manual sampling of the NS. Furthermore, avoiding the use of arterial blood gas analyzers to determine $Ptco_2$ can help improve the correlation between mucosal CO_2 level and $Ptco_2$.

Gastric tonometry is predominantly used for the monitoring of splanchnic perfusion, and perhaps oxygenation, in an area of the body first to be affected in the presence of covert shock. Although not widely used, tonometry has the potential to provide nurses with a much earlier warning of hemodynamic

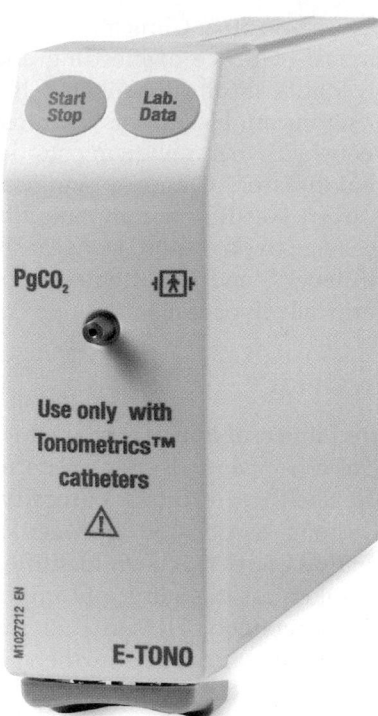

♦FIGURE 29-5 The tonometry module, E-TONO.

compromise than the traditional assessments. The use of gastric tonometry in the assessment of the critically ill patient will likely be debated for some time, contributing to the slow incorporation of this technology in clinical practice. Furthermore, ongoing technological advances, such as the development of sublingual capnometry, may supplant gastric tonometry as a method of evaluating tissue oxygenation in the critically ill, as explained in the Research Utilization box below. Nevertheless, the physiologic underpinnings of this technology are valuable to consider within the context of any critically ill patient and provide nurses with a sound foundation for considering the role of oxygen delivery and the effect of shock on the GI tract during episodes of critical illness.

♦ RESEARCH UTILIZATION

Sublingual Capnometry and Tissue Oxygenation

CLINICAL ISSUE

Organ dysfunction continues to be a significant problem for patients with life-threatening illnesses; it is well established that circulatory failure causes tissue hypoxia and hypercapnia. There has been a decade of research and clinical use of gastric tonometry that measures intramucosal P_{CO_2} as a marker for splanchnic hypoperfusion. Gastric tonometry is invasive, affected by support strategies such as enteral feeding, and requires specialized equipment. Consequently, its use has not become widespread in clinical practice. Further development of this monitoring strategy led to refinement of the measurement of gastric P_{CO_2} and the development of alternative methods of measuring tissue hypercapnia, such as sublingual capnometry.

SUMMARY

This study sought to determine the prognostic value of sublingual P_{CO_2} ($P_{SL}CO_2$), lactate concentration, and mixed venous oxygen saturation in hemodynamically unstable intensive care patients. Oxyhemodynamic variables, arterial lactate concentration, and $P_{SL}CO_2$ were measured in 54 unselected sequential intensive care patients. Measurements were obtained at insertion of the pulmonary artery catheter and then 4 and 8 hours thereafter. Data analysis showed that the most sensitive marker for tissue perfusion was the difference between $P_{SL}CO_2$ and Pa_{CO_2} in hemodynamically unstable critically ill patients. A $P_{SL}CO_2$ difference of greater than 25 mm Hg was the best discriminator of outcome. In both survivors and nonsurvivors, initiation of treatment led to a decrease in both the $P_{SL}CO_2$ and the $P_{SL}CO_2$ difference while arterial lactate and mixed venous oxygen saturation remained unchanged.

APPLICATION

The predictive value of $P_{SL}CO_2$ as a single measure is very good (area under the curve, 0.75); however, the use of a single prognostic variable for individual patients requires a predictive power of nearly 100% (area under the curve, 1.00) to eliminate false-positive predictions. However, in terms of guiding clinical practice, the authors have described a useful method of early detection of tissue hypoperfusion and evaluation of existing treatment.

NEED FOR FURTHER STUDY

While sublingual capnometry may provide a useful method of monitoring tissue oxygenation that overcomes some of the limitations of gastric tonometry, this technology has yet to be widely evaluated in a variety of clinical settings and patient populations. Future studies need to examine the cost-benefit relationship of this technology as well as address its limitations in clinical use and develop strategies for the automatic calculation of $P_{SL}CO_2$ difference.

Marik, P. E., & Bankov, A. (2003). Sublingual capnometry versus traditional markers of tissue oxygenation in critically ill patients. *Crit Care Med, 31,* 818–822.

STRESS-RELATED MUCOSAL DISEASE IN CRITICALLY ILL PATIENTS

In the early 1930s an association between central nervous system injury and gastroduodenal disease became apparent;[27] some years later, endoscopic studies in patients with severe cutaneous burns[28] showed similar results. It is now commonly accepted that the physiologic stress associated with critical illness contributes to the development of stress-related mucosal disease.

Prevalence

Stress-related mucosal disease is common in the critically ill and is associated with an increase in morbidity and mortality.[34] The prevalence of this problem in the critically ill depends on how stress-related mucosal disease is defined. The definition is an important consideration when evaluating research in this area. In endoscopic studies, the prevalence of mucosal injury is between 75% and 100%;[28,111] it is suggested that this injury occurs rapidly. Occult bleeding is defined as a positive guaiac test of stools or gastric aspirates. When this clinical end point is used, the prevalence of stress-related mucosal disease is estimated to be 15% to 50%. Clinically, overt bleeding is defined as clinical evidence of bleeding and occurs in approximately 5% of critically ill patients.[36] It is suggested that clinically significant bleeding is the most important end point to consider when reviewing studies on stress-related mucosal disease.[34] Clinically significant bleeding is defined as overt bleeding accompanied by hemodynamic changes (e.g., hypotension, tachycardia, or a drop in hemoglobin level[22]) and is estimated to occur in less than 3.5% of critically ill patients.[22,114]

Pathophysiology

Stress-related mucosal injury is characterized by diffuse superficial erosions or deeper, more focal lesions that are more likely to result in clinically important bleeding. A strong association between physiologic stress and mucosal injury has been identified, although the pathophysiology of this clinically important problem is not fully understood.[36] It is thought that the cause of stress-related mucosal disease in the critically ill is related to a number of factors and results from an imbalance between protective mechanisms and factors that promote mucosal injury (Table 29-3).

TABLE 29-3 Factors Contributing to Stress-Related Mucosal Disease

Protective Mechanisms	Mucosal prostaglandins	Protect mucosa by stimulating blood flow, mucus and bicarbonate production[58] Stimulate epithelial cell growth and repair
	Mucosal bicarbonate barrier	Forms a physical barrier to acid and pepsin, preventing injury to epithelium[6]
	Epithelial restitution and regeneration	Epithelial cells rapidly regenerate but process is highly metabolic and may be impaired by physiologic stress[6]
	Mucosal blood flow	Helps remove acid from mucosa, supplies bicarbonate and oxygen to mucosal epithelial cells[35]
	Cell membrane and tight junctions	Tight junctions between mucosal epithelial cells prevent back-diffusion of hydrogen ions[47]
Factors Promoting Injury	Acid	Acid is a key issue in pathogenesis of stress-related mucosal injury; however, not all critically ill patients hypersecrete acid[47,137] However, small amounts of acid may still cause injury; prevention of acid secretion has led to a reduction in injury[22]
	Pepsin	May cause direct injury to mucosa[128,129] Facilitates lysis of clots[36]
	Mucosal hypoperfusion	Reduced mucosal blood flow results in reduced oxygen and nutrient delivery, making epithelial cells susceptible to injury[47] Contributes to mucosal acid-base imbalances Results in formation of free radicals

Reperfusion injury	Nitric oxide, which causes vasodilation and hyperemia, is released during hypoperfusion and results in an increase in cell-damaging cytokines[156]
Intramucosal acid-base balance	Mucus layer protects epithelium and traps bicarbonate ions that neutralize acid; thus decrease in bicarbonate secretion results in intramucosal acidosis and local injury[6]
Systemic acidosis	Results in increased intramucosal acidity[35]
Free oxygen radicals	Generated as a result of tissue hypoxia, free oxygen radicals cause oxidative injury to mucosa[108]
Bile salts	Bile salts reflux from duodenum into stomach and may have a role in stress-related damage although exact mechanism is uncertain[124]
Helicobacter pylori	Conflicting results about role of *Helicobacter pylori* as a cause of stress-induced mucosal disease in critically ill[125,130]

Risk Factors

The risk of developing stress-related mucosal disease is not the same for all critically ill patients. A number of factors are associated with the risk of stress-related mucosal disease (Box 29-3). Patients with multiple risk factors are particularly susceptible.

Two independent risk factors have been identified and include mechanical ventilation for longer than 48 hours and coagulopathy. In a prospective multicenter study, risk factors for clinically important bleeding associated with stress-related mucosal disease were examined in patients admitted to intensive care. Patients with respiratory failure that required mechanical ventilation for longer than 48 hours were 16 times more likely to develop stress-related mucosal disease (odds ratio 15.6) while patients with a coagulopathy, demonstrated by a platelet count of less than 50,000/mm³, an

international normalized ratio of greater than 1.5, or a partial thromboplastin time of greater than 2.0 times the control value, were 4 times more likely (odds ratio 4.3).[23] Interestingly, the data in this study showed that of the 847 patients with risk factors, only 31 (3.7%) experienced clinically important bleeding, and of the 1405 patients without risk factors, only 2 (0.1%) experienced clinically important bleeding.

While the prevalence of clinically important bleeding is low for critically ill patients, even for those with risk factors, it remains a clinical concern because of the associated increased mortality rate. Peura and Johnson[111] found that patients with stress-related mucosal bleeding had a mortality rate of 57% compared to those without risk factors who had a mortality rate of 24%. Similarly, Cook et al.[23] found increased mortality associated with stress-related mucosal disease (48.5% vs. 9.1%). Clearly, it is important to identify patients at risk for the development of stress-related mucosal bleeding so that appropriate treatment strategies can be initiated and so that those who are not at risk are not exposed to unnecessary prophylaxis.

STRESS-RELATED MUCOSAL DISEASE: PROPHYLAXIS

When considering the pathophysiology of stress-related mucosal disease, it is clear that GI ischemia contributes to the development of injury. Adequate regional resuscitation plays an important role in preventing this complication of critical illness. Likewise, acid secretion is an important factor, even though many critically ill patients hyposecrete gastric acid.[36] Consequently, therapy is often initiated to maintain the gastric pH greater than 4. Medications used in the prophylaxis of stress-related mucosal disease are highlighted in the Medication table on pp. 804-805.

Box 29-3

Risk Factors Associated With the Development of Stress-Related Mucosal Bleeding

- Coagulopathy
- CNS injury/surgery
- Hepatic failure
- Multiple organ dysfunction syndrome
- Mechanical ventilation longer than 48 hours
- Multiple trauma
- Organ transplantation
- Shock
- Severe sepsis
- Severe burns (greater than 30% of body surface area)
- Renal failure

Data from reference 34.

MEDICATIONS USED TO MINIMIZE STRESS-RELATED MUCOSAL INJURY

MEDICATION	ACTION	DOSAGE	SPECIAL CONSIDERATIONS
Antacids	Weak bases that readily combine with hydrochloric acid, neutralizing it	Aluminum hydroxide magnesium carbonate (Maalox): 10–20 ml PO 3–4 times daily between meals and at bedtime	Aluminum-containing antacids may bind with other drugs (e.g., warfarin, digoxin)
Histamine-2 receptor blockers	Competitive inhibitor of histamine-2 receptor, which, when stimulated, leads to acid production	Cimetidine (Tagamet): 800 mg PO at bedtime, or 400 mg PO morning and at bedtime, or 200 mg PO 3 times daily and 400 mg PO at bedtime; 300 mg IV every 6–8 hr; should not exceed 2400 mg/day	Cimetidine may slow metabolism of other drugs, thereby enhancing their effects
Ranitidine (Zantac)		300 mg PO taken as single dose or 150 mg taken twice daily; 50 mg IV (e.g., 2 ml diluted in 20 ml of 0.9% sodium chloride and given as slow injection over not less than 5 min), may be repeated every 6–8 hr; or as IV infusion of 25 mg/hr for 2 hr; infusion may be repeated at 6–8-hr intervals Can give as continuous infusion at 6.25 mg/hr	Dosage should be reduced if renal failure is present
Nizatidine (Axid)		150 mg PO twice daily or 300 mg PO daily	
Famotidine (Pepcid)		20 mg dose IV over period of no less than 2 min and subsequently by repeated injection or by infusion of 20 mg over a 30-min period every 12 hr	
Proton pump inhibitors	Proton pump inhibitors stop production of hydrogen ions in parietal cells, thereby blocking hydrochloric acid secretion		In animal models, high-dose and long-term use of proton pump inhibitors produces hypochlorhydria, which reflexively leads to increase in gastrin production and hyperplasia of parietal cells Long-term use in humans is contraindicated until further long-term safety data can be established
Lansoprazole (Prevacid)		15–30 mg PO daily	
Omeprazole (Prilosec)		20–40 mg PO daily	

MEDICATION	ACTION	DOSAGE	SPECIAL CONSIDERATIONS
Pantoprazole (Protonix)		40 mg PO daily; IV 20–40 mg daily	
Sucralfate (Carafate)	In presence of acid, sucralfate polymerizes to form thick pastelike substance that adheres to gastric mucosa, protecting it from acid	1 g PO 4 times daily (before meals and bedtime) for up to 8 weeks	Sucralfate needs an acidic environment to work so should not be taken with meals or antacids. Use caution in renal impairment due to risk of aluminum accumulation and toxicity

Antacids

Antacids directly neutralize gastric acid and have been shown to be effective in reducing significant stress-related bleeding.[6] One of the disadvantages of this therapy is the time-intensive nature of administering antacids every 1 to 2 hours. Furthermore, antacids can contribute to further complications (e.g., aluminum toxicity, hypophosphatemia, diarrhea, or hypermagnesemia). These factors have led to their infrequent use within the critical care setting.

Histamine-2 Receptor Antagonists

Histamine-2 receptor antagonists are commonly used in the critically ill to inhibit the production of gastric acid, which is achieved by the drug's binding to the histamine-2 receptor on the basement membrane of the parietal cell.[34] However, gastric acid secretion may also occur through stimulation of the acetylcholine or gastrin receptors present in parietal cells;[116] therefore complete blocking of gastric acid production does not occur when histamine-2 receptor antagonists are used. A further limitation of histamine-2 receptor antagonists is the development of tolerance that may occur within 72 hours of administration.[95] Nevertheless, this pharmacologic strategy to prevent stress-related mucosal disease remains commonplace in critical care.[136]

Bolus parenteral administration of this drug is most common in the critically ill, although it is suggested that continuous infusion of histamine-2 receptor antagonists may be more effective in suppressing gastric acid.[60] The decrease in gastric acidity as a result of histamine-2 receptor antagonist use was viewed as beneficial from the perspective of preventing stress-related mucosal disease. However, concern existed in relation to changes in gastric pH that could lead to bacterial overgrowth in the stomach, microaspiration, and consequently an increase in the incidence of nosocomial pneumonia,[96] a finding that was not evident in a larger randomized controlled trial comparing sucralfate with ranitidine in mechanically ventilated patients.[22]

Proton Pump Inhibitors

Proton pump inhibitors (PPIs) have been available for clinical use for over a decade and have a greater ability to maintain an increased intragastric pH than histamine-2 receptor antagonists.[138] These drugs work by irreversibly binding to the proton pump, effectively blocking all three receptors responsible for gastric acid secretion by the parietal cell.[34] Available PPIs include omeprazole (Prilosec), lansoprazole (Prevacid), and pantoprazole (Protonix).

The widespread use of PPIs in critical care has been limited by the fact that intravenous preparations of PPIs only became available in the United States in 2001. While PPIs can be given through a nasogastric tube, doing so requires mixing with a liquid solution containing sodium bicarbonate to protect the drug from gastric acid.[116] An additional consideration is the delayed gastric emptying that may occur in the critically ill, thereby limiting the bioavailability of the drug.

Clinical evaluation of the efficacy of PPIs is somewhat limited; few studies have specifically studied the prophylactic use of PPIs for stress-related mucosal diseases.[12] Two initial studies[18,112] showed that clinically significant GI bleeding did not occur in patients treated with the PPI omeprazole. However, these studies did not have a comparison group, used an open label design, and were limited by sample size.[18] A subsequent randomized controlled trial demonstrated a reduction in clinically important bleeding in patients receiving omeprazole (6%)[77] compared to patients who received ranitidine (Zantac) (31%). However, this study too was limited by sample size, lack of blinding, and a higher proportion of at-risk patients in the ranitidine group.[18] Given the recency of intravenous PPI availability, further research examining the efficacy of these preparations is expected.

Sucralfate

Sucralfate (Carafate) provides protection against stress-related mucosal disease through a number of mechanisms. Sucralfate provides a protective barrier on the surface gastric epithelium, stimulates mucus and bicarbonate secretion, stimulates epithelial renewal, improves mucosal blood flow, and enhances prostaglandin release.[34] Given orally or via a nasogastric tube, sucralfate is well tolerated but appears to be less effective than histamine-2 receptor antagonists in decreasing clinically significant bleeding.[22] Earlier reports comparing sucralfate with ranitidine showed a decrease in the development of pneumonia in those patients receiving sucralfate; however, these findings were not supported in a subsequent Level I randomized controlled trial.[22]

Enteral Nutrition

It is thought that the presence of enteral feeding solution results in an increase in intragastric pH, thereby minimizing acid injury. Several studies have demonstrated a lower incidence of stress-related bleeding in mechanically ventilated[115] and burn patients,[100] while others were unable to show a significant effect on increasing gastric pH.[10]

Critical illness and the associated hypoperfusion can contribute to the development of stress-related mucosal disease. Consequently, monitoring and prophylactic treatment are important in minimizing the clinically important bleeding associated with an increased mortality rate.

ABDOMINAL COMPARTMENT SYNDROME

Abdominal compartment syndrome (ACS) is being recognized more frequently in critically ill patients. The torso is considered a single compartment.[99] When the intra-abdominal pressure (IAP) rises in this closed anatomic space, blood flow may be reduced and tissue viability threatened.[134] ACS is potentially fatal. Consequently, it is imperative that all clinicians be aware of

the underlying physiologic changes, assessment, and management in at-risk patients.

The term *ACS* is used to describe a combination of increased intra-abdominal pressure and organ dysfunction.[74] Clear operational definitions of IAP are lacking. It is not always clear whether the mean, median, or maximal IAP pressures are measured and reported. It is, however, the trend for the maximal IAP to be normally used in clinical decision making regarding treatment.[80] When a persistently high IAP is observed, the term *intra-abdominal hypertension* (IAH) is used.

Etiology

For some time, many clinicians have come to associate the development of ACS with surgical patients; however, it is evident ACS can and does occur in a variety of patient populations.[99] Factors associated with IAH include body mass index, fluid resuscitation, multiple transfusions, total sepsis-related organ failure (SOFA) score, and respiratory, renal, and coagulation SOFA subscores. However, only blood transfusion and the rate of fluid resuscitation are significantly correlated with IAH.[82] Independent risk factors for the development of IAH included abdominal surgery, fluid resuscitation, ileus, and liver dysfunction.[83] These are, of course, important factors to consider when identifying at-risk patients.

Pathophysiology

Increased IAP results from an increase in pressure within the confined anatomic space of the abdominal cavity. This increase in pressure may result from causes such as intraperitoneal bleeding, peritonitis, ascites, or distention of the gas-filled bowel. Clinical data show that increases in IAP result in physiologic changes in vital organ function.[98] Early detection of increases in IAP is difficult; however, these increases are not believed to be clinically significant. However, sustained IAP or the development of IAH affects regional blood flow and impairs tissue perfusion, which may result in MODS.[106] The pathophysiologic consequences occur as a direct result of increased pressure within the abdominal cavity, resulting in vascular compression, direct compression of the organs, and elevation of the diaphragm.[45] Because of these physiologic changes, it is critical to remember that intracardiac pressures may be falsely elevated because of the increased IAP. Consequently, caution should be exercised when instituting clinical management on the basis of an elevation of intracardiac pressure.[123] A summary of the physiologic changes associated with ACS is provided in Table 29-4.

TABLE 29-4 Physiologic Changes Associated With Abdominal Compartment Syndrome

SYSTEM	PHYSIOLOGIC EFFECTS
Respiratory	Cephalad deviation of diaphragm leads to decreased lung and chest wall compliance[62] Peak inspiratory pressures increase[99] Functional residual volume and lung capacity are reduced, resulting in ventilation/perfusion mismatching Hypoxia and hypercarbia may result, necessitating mechanical ventilation Pulmonary vascular resistance increases[3]
Cardiovascular	Inferior vena cava and portal vein compression results in decreased venous return Decreased left ventricular compliance[98] Artificially increased right atrial pressure, pulmonary artery occlusion pressure[123] Decreased cardiac index[92] Elevated systemic vascular resistance from arteriolar vasoconstriction and increased IAP[3]
Renal	Oliguria (IAP 15–20 mm Hg)[142] Anuria (IAP greater than 30 mm Hg) May be a consequence of decreased cardiac output, compression of renal vessels, increased renal vascular resistance, or redistribution of blood flow to renal medulla[62]
Gastrointestinal	Decreased splanchnic perfusion and tissue hypoxia Increased gastrointestinal mucosal acidosis[64] Reduced hepatic blood flow[99] Abnormalities in normal gut mucosal barrier function, which may permit bacterial translocation[3] Decreased abdominal wall blood flow[98] Increased pressure on esophageal varices may result in bleeding[81]
Neurologic	Increased intracranial pressure because of impaired venous return[8]

IAP = Intra-abdominal pressure.

Measurement of Intra-Abdominal Pressure

Clinical assessment of the abdomen is not a sensitive or accurate technique for detecting increased IAP.[69] Measurement of pressure within the bladder has been validated as closely approximating IAP[46] and has evolved as the gold standard for IAP measurement.[80] This technique can, however, be influenced by the measurement technique. For example, air bubbles in the system and changes in transducer positions may influence pressure measurement, with wide variations in IAP being noted.[117] There is also little consistency in the amount of fluid used to prime the bladder; this may result in overestimates of IAP.[51]

There are a variety of techniques for measuring IAP described in the literature[80] including bladder measurement techniques and manometry. Manometry techniques are proving to be rapid and cost-effective; however, they have not been validated and are consequently not used routinely in clinical assessment.[80] For this reason, the bladder measurement technique is the primary method use to obtain IAP measurement.

The procedures for IAP measurement techniques (described below) may differ; however, the clinical considerations for performing measurements are similar and outlined in Table 29-5.

Bladder Measurement of Intra-Abdominal Pressure. The original technique described by Kron et al.[74] involves the disrupting of the sterile closed urinary drainage system. Under sterile conditions, the indwelling urinary catheter is disconnected and 50 to 100 ml of NS injected. The bladder is then clamped distal to the collection port. A manometer or transducer is connected using a 16-gauge needle for each individual measurement. This technique is time consuming and involves multiple manipulations of a normally closed, sterile system. Techniques using fluid-filled pressure monitoring systems are also prone to artifact that may distort the IAP pressure waveform. Measurement error may occur if the correct technique for leveling the transducer (at the symphysis pubis) is not followed. The original technique devised by Kron[74] was revised by adding two stopcocks—the first with a 60-ml syringe attached and the second with a disposable

TABLE 29-5 Pitfalls in Intra-Abdominal Pressure Measurement

PITFALL	CAUSE
Bladder measurement techniques (the gold standard) are not uniform	Recommendations for normal saline instillation into bladder vary (0–250 ml)
Changes in patient position	IAP can be influenced by changing patient's position
Difficulty validating IAP measurements	Bladder IAP measurements are compared to direct measurements obtained under anesthesia; uncertain whether comparisons between paralyzed, anesthetized patients and general critical care population can be made
Distortions of pressure signal	Over- or underdamping of dynamic response of measurement system
Over- or underestimation of IAP	Malpositioning of transducer Air bubbles in system
Uncertainty about complete bladder emptying	Ideally bladder should be completely emptied before IAP measurement

IAP = Intra-abdominal pressure.

transducer. An 18-gauge intravenous catheter was inserted into the aspiration port of the indwelling catheter and the needle removed. This catheter was then attached to the saline-filled pressure tubing. This technique is safer (needleless) and reduces the time for measurements; however, kinking of the catheter and leaking from the catheter insertion site can be problematic (Figure 29-6).

Refinements of this technique have been implemented to simplify the procedure and limit the number of manipulations.[80] The revised closed system repeated measurement technique employs a ramp of three stopcocks inserted into the drainage tubing of the urinary collection bag. A standard infusing set, together with a 1-L bag of NS, is attached to the first stopcock. A 60-ml syringe is connected to the second stopcock, and the pressure transducer is connected to the third stopcock. The pressure transducer is leveled at the symphysis pubis and the system is flushed with NS (Figure 29-7). This technique has the advantage of reducing repeated opening of the sterile system. IAP measurements consume only about 2 minutes of nursing time.

Continuous measurements can also be made using a three-way urinary catheter, with IAP being measured through the irrigation port.[4] This technique is reliable with IAP over a wide range of pressures and is a simple technique to use. Further simplifying the measurement of IAP is the introduction of commercially prepared intra-abdominal pressure monitoring kits, which may further reduce nursing time and eliminate some of the problems associated with IAP monitoring.

Gastric Measurement of Intra-Abdominal Pressure.
Trauma, peritoneal adhesions, pelvic hematomas or fractures, abdominal packing, or a neurogenic bladder may cause overestimation of IAP measurements.[80] In these circumstances, or if the patient does not have an indwelling urinary catheter, the stomach can be used to measure IAP. A standard nasogastric tube or a gastrostomy tube can be used with 50 to 100 ml of NS instilled into the stomach.[99] This technique may interfere with nasogastric feeding and possibly increase the risk of aspiration in some patients. The use of a gastric tonometer has been described and demonstrates good correlation between intravesical methods and gastric tonometer.[141]

Similarly, an esophageal balloon catheter can be inserted into the stomach, the end of which is connected to a standard three-way stopcock and pressure transducer (Figure 29-8). The air is removed from the balloon and 1 to 2 ml of air is reintroduced. The balloon is then connected to a "dry" transducer system. This system allows for continuous measurement and is less time consuming than the tonometer method. However, air is reabsorbed after a couple of hours, necessitating frequent recalibration of the device. Failure to recalibrate the device or fluctuations in the reinstilled volume may result in inaccurate measurement of IAP.[80]

The importance of monitoring IAP in at-risk patients has led to the development of an IAP catheter. This device is similar to a nasogastric tube and has an air pouch at the tip. The pressure transducer, hardware, and device for filling the air pouch are all contained

Transducer
To bedside monitor

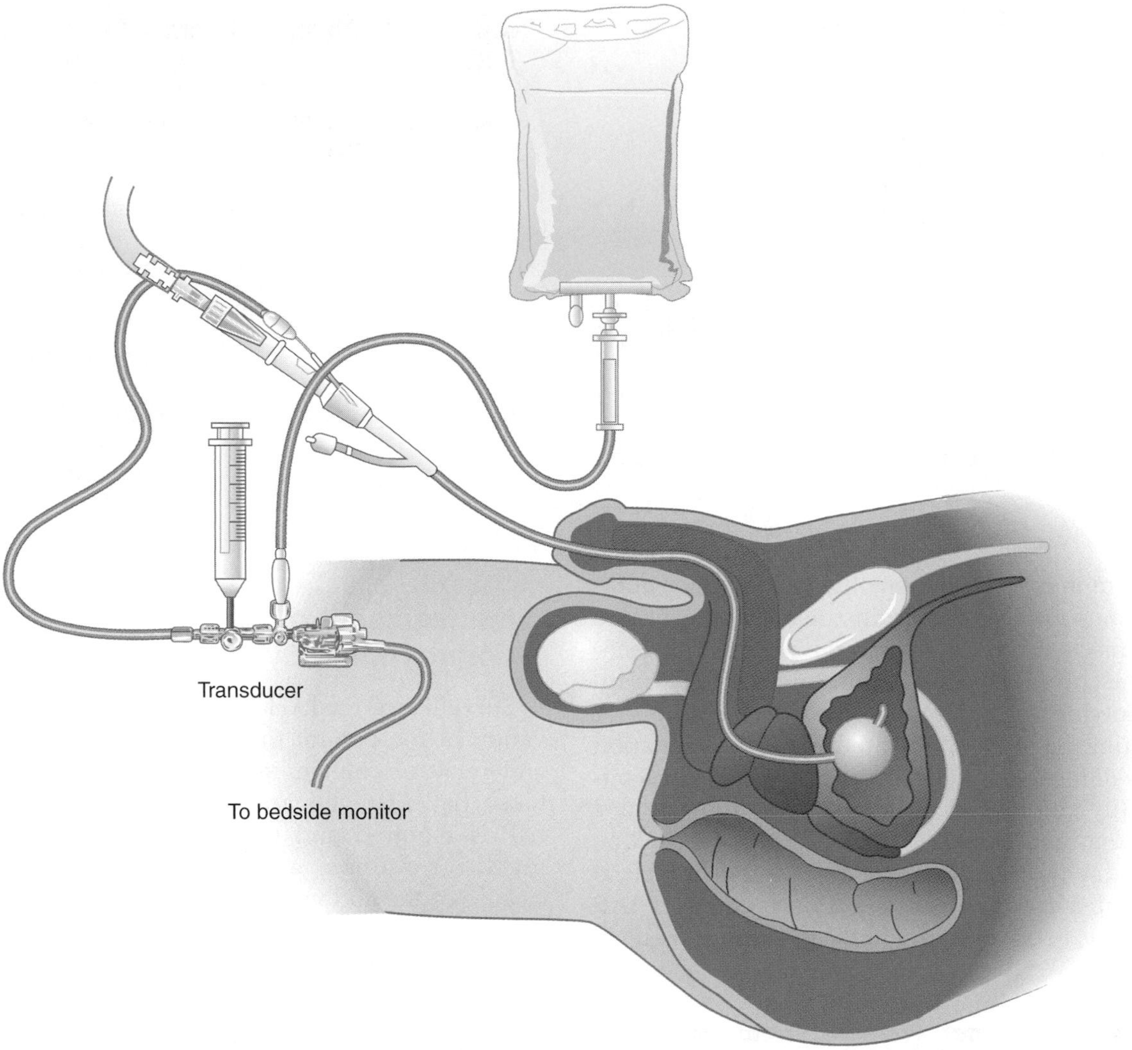

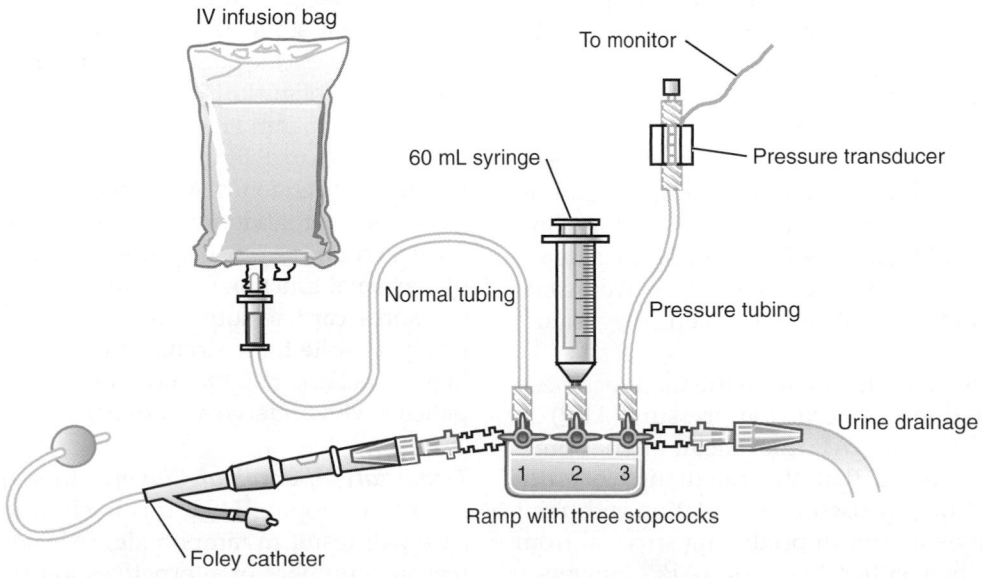

FIGURE 29-6 The closed system single measurement technique.

IV infusion bag
To monitor
60 mL syringe
Pressure transducer
Normal tubing
Pressure tubing
Urine drainage
1 2 3
Ramp with three stopcocks
Foley catheter

FIGURE 29-7 Revised closed system technique for measurement of intra-abdominal pressure.

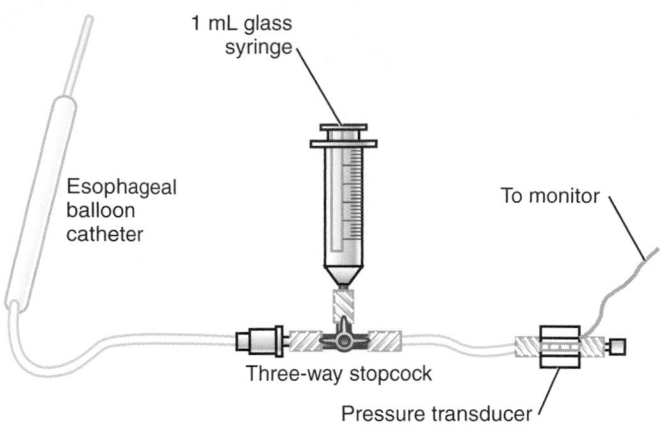

♦FIGURE 29-8   IAP measurement with an esophageal balloon.

TABLE 29-6   Abdominal Compartment Grading System

GRADE	BLADDER PRESSURE (mm Hg)	MANAGEMENT
I	10–15	Maintain normovolemia
II	16–25	Fluid resuscitation
III	26–35	Abdominal decompression
IV	Greater than 35	Abdominal decompression with reexploration

Data from reference 62.

in the IAP monitor. Every hour the IAP monitor automatically performs a zero adjustment of the device and then injects 0.1 ml of air into the pouch. This technique is fast, reproducible, accurate, and fully automated, allowing for continuous measurement of IAP. Initial results have demonstrated a good correlation between IAP measurements obtained through this continuous fully-automated technique and the standard intravesical measurements.[79] This technique would be most suited where continuous monitoring of IAP is required. Further work may see this method of IAP measurement used both in clinical settings and in clinical trials.

Normal Intra-Abdominal Pressure. In the spontaneously breathing patient, IAP is normally either atmospheric or subatmospheric. Mechanical ventilation, however, causes the IAP to increase near end-inspiration. After abdominal surgery, IAP may be increased slightly; no serious consequences were noted in surgical patients whose IAP remained less than 13 mm Hg.[74] However, it has been noted that an IAP as low as 10 mm Hg can result in changes in end-organ function.[81] The inconsistencies in defining increased IAP and IAH lead to further confusion regarding the assessment of this clinically important problem. As IAP cannot be considered outside the clinical context of the patient, an abdominal compartment grading system has been suggested[62] (Table 29-6).

Because IAP is variable among patients, it has been suggested that abdominal perfusion pressure (APP) be calculated by subtracting IAP from mean arterial pressure (MAP). It appears that the calculation of APP may be a more clinically useful resuscitation end point and is statistically superior in predicting survival from IAH and ACS than either MAP or IAP;[19] however, further well-designed research is needed in this area.

Management of Abdominal Compartment Syndrome

Surveillance for IAH and ACS requires close observation of the patient to identify potential risk factors and relevant changes to physiologic parameters. For those patients who are at risk, close monitoring of IAP is required and preemptive measures are instituted. For example, a decision may be made to delay closure of the abdomen or to use an alternative means of abdominal content coverage. For the nonsurgical patient, optimal resuscitation may be important in preventing IAH; overresuscitation needs to be avoided.[3]

Abdominal Decompression. Decompressive laparotomy may be indicated in some patients with IAH. In Table 29-6, suggested parameters for IAH and associated management strategies are provided. Many other clinicians will assess the patient for signs of physiologic deterioration (e.g., oliguria, hypotension, and acidosis) plus IAP in excess of 25 mm Hg and will use these clinical assessment findings to determine the optimal timing for abdominal decompression.[62] At present, there are no absolute guidelines for abdominal decompression.[98] However, early decompression has been associated with reversal of abnormal function (e.g., improvement in peak airway pressures, cardiac output, and urinary output). Unfortunately, despite these dramatic improvements in physiologic function, a 50% mortality rate may remain in patients who undergo abdominal decompression.[140]

Temporary Abdominal Closure. In surgical patients at risk of developing IAH, it is likely primary fascial closure will result in tamponade, IAH, and ACS. For this reason, a number of alternatives to primary fascial closure have been investigated. General principles of this strategy include providing a tension-free and watertight coverage of the abdominal contents to prevent fluid loss and evisceration.[3] Delayed closure of the abdomen presents a number of challenges for the clinician:

- Mechanical containment of the abdominal contents
- Removal of exudate
- Measurement of third-space fluid losses
- Infection control

Prosthetic Mesh. Temporary closure of the abdomen can be achieved in a variety of ways. Nonabsorbable prosthetic mesh may be used. Data suggest that this may be a successful strategy in reducing the incidence of IAH in some patients.[21,64] However, the use of mesh closure is associated with an increased rate of enterocutaneous fistula formation.[144]

The Bogota Bag. The Bogota bag, constructed from a sterilized 3-L genitourinary irrigation bag, is another alternative method of temporary closure and protection of the abdominal contents. The use of this bag provides a transparent, watertight seal, allowing the underlying bowel to be regularly assessed.[144] Limitations of this device include trauma to the abdominal wall when securing the bag and the inability to actively remove exudate.

The Wittmann Patch. The Wittmann patch is an artificial burr closure of the abdomen and uses a Velcro-like device to reduce the gap between the wound edges. The device is sutured to the free fascial edges, allowing two prosthetic sheets to be joined along the midline, achieving wound closure.[155] Like the Bogota bag, this technique exposes the fascial edges to further trauma.

Topical Negative Pressure. Topical negative pressure is a new technique that avoids trauma to the fascia or skin. This technique is described in Figure 29-9. The use of topical negative pressure allows for multiple procedures, control of exudate, and a decrease in intra-abdominal pressure; minimizes fascial trauma;

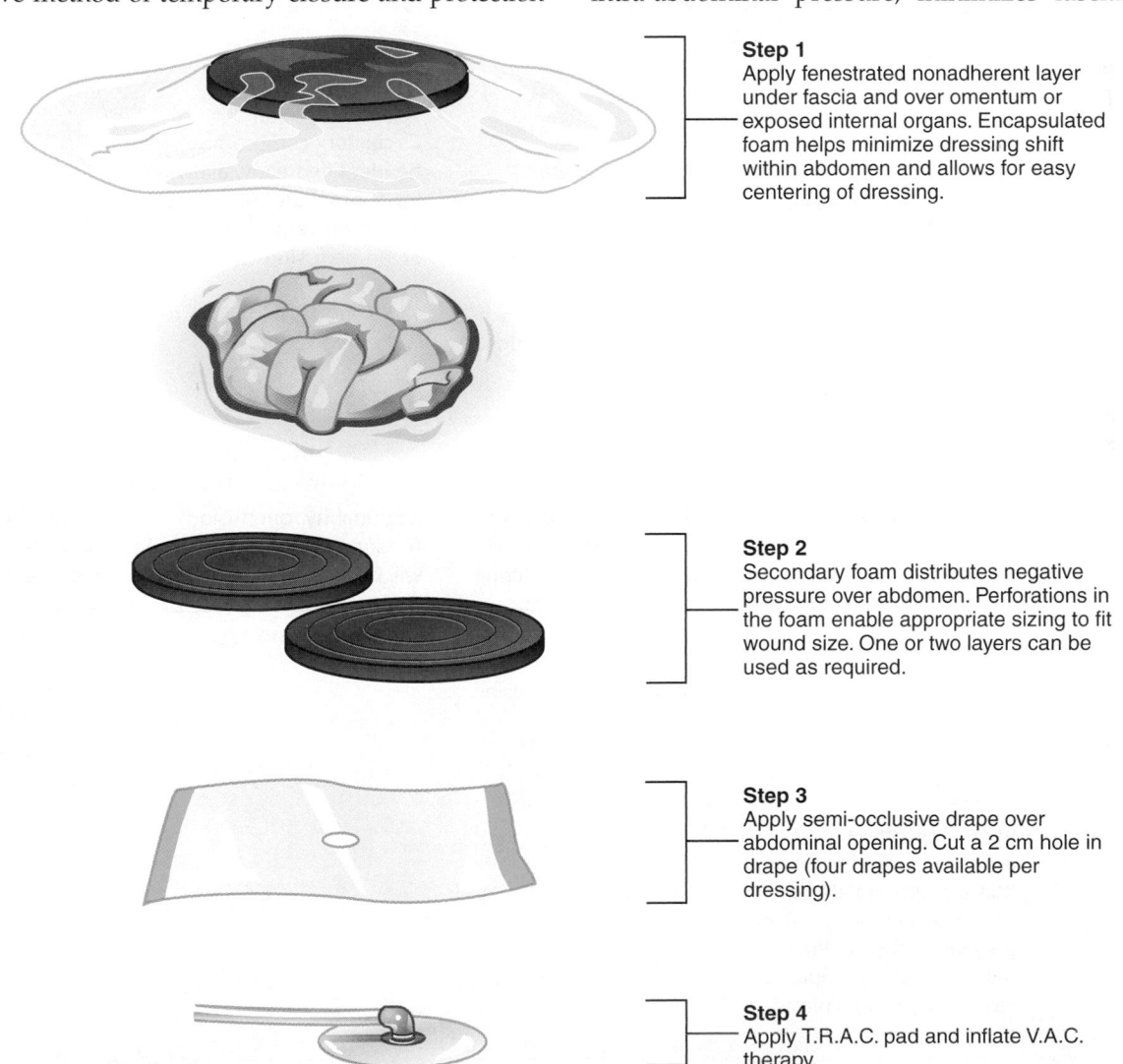

Step 1
Apply fenestrated nonadherent layer under fascia and over omentum or exposed internal organs. Encapsulated foam helps minimize dressing shift within abdomen and allows for easy centering of dressing.

Step 2
Secondary foam distributes negative pressure over abdomen. Perforations in the foam enable appropriate sizing to fit wound size. One or two layers can be used as required.

Step 3
Apply semi-occlusive drape over abdominal opening. Cut a 2 cm hole in drape (four drapes available per dressing).

Step 4
Apply T.R.A.C. pad and inflate V.A.C. therapy.

⬍FIGURE 29-9 Applying topical negative pressure using the vacuum-assisted closure abdominal dressing system.

and reduces the frequency of dressing changes.[67] The negative pressure created by this device is useful in reducing IAP by decreasing edema and facilitating evacuation of intra-abdominal fluid. As a consequence, blood flow to the wound is increased and the exposure to pathogens is minimized.[67] Whichever technique is used to manage the open abdomen, the key issues in patient management include infection control, fluid balance, and minimization of iatrogenic tissue injury.

Many critically ill patients are at risk for the development of increased IAP and ACS. The increase in mortality associated with the development of ACS warrants close monitoring of IAP, particularly in at-risk patients, so that early intervention can be instituted and complications associated with ACS minimized.

MULTIDISCIPLINARY PLAN OF CARE

With the exception of providing nutritional support, the primary goal of GI management in the critically ill centers on ensuring adequate GI perfusion and minimizing the physiologic consequences of hypoperfusion, such as the development of stress-related mucosal disease. Critically ill patients at risk for increased intra-abdominal pressure will benefit from monitoring of intra-abdominal pressures, and in some cases abdominal decompression may be warranted. A multidisciplinary approach to the management of GI system dysfunction in the critically ill is required and is outlined in the Multidisciplinary Plan of Care below and on p. 813.

MULTIDISCIPLINARY PLAN OF CARE

PROBLEM	INTERVENTION	RATIONALE	EXPECTED OUTCOME	SPECIAL CONSIDERATIONS
Risk of development of GI mucosal hypoperfusion	Assess adequacy of resuscitation including BP, MAP, HR, urine output, neurologic status.	These global assessments are important and can clearly indicate need for more direct and aggressive resuscitation. However, these parameters do not reflect regional perfusion and may be within acceptable limits even with mucosal hypoperfusion.	Circulatory compromise will be identified early, allowing for appropriate treatment and improvement in end-organ perfusion.	
	For most accurate assessment of GI hypoperfusion, monitor GI mucosal CO_2 levels using gastric tonometry.	The gut is the first area in body to undergo vasoconstriction during shock; thus gastric tonometry will provide an early indicator of GI mucosal hypoperfusion.	Regional hypoperfusion (or successful resuscitation) will be identified earlier than is possible through use of global assessment parameters.	Calculated tonometric measurements (such as CO_2 gap) take into account any systemic increases/decreases in CO_2 level.
	Implement strategies to improve tissue oxygenation that are appropriate to patient's clinical presentation (e.g., fluid resuscitation, inotropic or vasoactive agents, blood products).			

PROBLEM	INTERVENTION	RATIONALE	EXPECTED OUTCOME	SPECIAL CONSIDERATIONS
Risk of development of stress-related mucosal disease	Ensure adequacy of resuscitation by assessing BP, MAP, HR, urine output, neurologic status, and gastric mucosal CO_2 using tonometry.	Mucosal hypoperfusion is a risk factor for development of stress-related mucosal disease.	Clinically significant bleeding will be avoided.	
	Assess for risk factors for stress-related mucosal disease: Mechanical ventilation longer than 48 hr Coagulopathy Shock Severe sepsis CNS injury/surgery Severe burns (>30% BSA) MODS Renal failure Hepatic failure Multiple trauma Organ transplantation	Assessing for risk factors can ensure that early prophylactic treatment is instituted.		
	Consider implementation of pharmacologic agents that protect against stress-related mucosal disease.			
Risk of development of intra-abdominal hypertension	Monitor IAP in patients who are at risk: Abdominal surgery Fluid resuscitation Ileus Liver dysfunction	Identification of persistently increased IAP will result in timely treatment and prevention of further complications.	Treatment will be initiated before abdominal compartment syndrome develops.	It is important to consider medical and surgical patients as being at risk for development of IAH.
Abdominal decompression is required	If possible, visually monitor bowel and assess for changes in perfusion.	This allows for early identification of compromised blood flow to gut.		
	Monitor fluid loss from open wound.	Considerable fluid loss may result from an open abdominal wound and contribute to fluid imbalance.		
	Maintain sterile technique in wound management.			

BP = Blood pressure, BSA = body surface area, CNS = central nervous system, CO_2 = carbon dioxide, GI = gastrointestinal, HR = heat rate, IAP = intra-abdominal pressure, IAH = intra-abdominal hypertension, MAP = mean arterial pressure, MODS = multiple organ dysfunction syndrome.

REFERENCES

1. Antonsson, J. B., et al. (1995). Changes in gut intramucosal pH and gut oxygen extraction ratio in a porcine model of peritonitis and hemorrhage. *Crit Care Med, 23*(11), 1872–1881.

2. Baigorri, F., Calvet, X., & Duarte, M. (1994). Effect of ranitidine treatment in gastric intramucosal pH determination in critical patients. *Intensive Care Med, 20*, S2.

3. Bailey, J., & Shapiro, M. J. (2000). Abdominal compartment syndrome. *Crit Care, 4*, 23–29.

4. Balogh, Z., et al. (2004). Continuous intra-abdominal pressure measurement technique. *Am J Surg, 188*, 679–685.

5. Bams, J. L., et al. (1998). Reliable gastric tonometry after coronary artery surgery: need for acid secretion suppression despite transient failure of acid secretion. *Intensive Care Med, 24*, 1139–1143.

6. Beejay, U., & Wolfe, M. M. (2000). Acute gastrointestinal bleeding in the intensive care unit: a gastroenterologist's perspective. *Gastroenterol Clin North Am, 29*, 309–336.

7. Benjamin, E., & Oropello, J. M. (1996). Does gastric tonometry work? No. *Crit Care Clin, 12*(3), 587–601.

8. Bloomfield, G. L., et al. (1997). A proposed relationship between increased intra-abdominal, intrathoracic, & intracranial pressure. *Crit Care Med, 25*, 496–503.

9. Boda, D., & Muranyi, L. (1959). "Gastrotonometry": an aid to the control of ventilation during artificial respiration. *Lancet, 273*, 181–182.

10. Bonten, M. J. M., et al. (1996). Intermittent enteral feeding: the influence on respiratory and digestive tract colonization in mechanically ventilated intensive-care-unit patients. *Am J Resp Crit Care Med, 154*, 394–399.

11. Boyd, O., et al. (1993). Comparison of clinical information gained from routine blood-gas analysis and from gastric tonometry for intramural pH. *Lancet, 341*, 142–145.

12. Brett, S. (2005). Science review: the use of proton pump inhibitors for gastric acid suppression in critical illness. *Crit Care, 19*(1), 45–50.

13. Brinkmann, A., et al. (1998). Monitoring the hepato-splanchnic region in the critically ill patient. *Intensive Care Med, 24*, 542–556.

14. Brown, S. D., & Gutierrez, G. (1997). Does gastric tonometry work? Yes. *Crit Care Clin, 12*(3), 569–585.

15. Buckley, S., & Kudsk, K. A. (1998). Metabolic response to critical illness and injury. *AACN Clin Issues, 5*(4), 443–449.

16. Calvet, X., Baigorri, F., & Artigas, A. (1995). Gastric intramucosal pH determination: limitations of the technique. In M. R. Pinsky, J. F. Dhainaut & A. Artigas (Eds.), *The splanchnic circulation: no longer a silent partner.* Berlin: Springer.

17. Calvet, X., et al. (1995). Effect of ranitidine in gastric intramucosal pH determinations in critically ill patients. *Am J Resp Crit Care Med, 151*(4), A334.

18. Cash, B. D. (2002). Evidence-based medicine as it applies to acid suppression in the hospitalized patient. *Crit Care Med, 30*(6 suppl), S373–S378.

19. Cheatham, M. L., et al. (2000). Abdominal perfusion pressure: a superior parameter in the assessment of intra-abdominal hypertension. *J Traum Inj Infect Crit Care, 49*(4), 621.

20. Cholley, B., & Payen, D. (1996). Regulation of gut perfusion. In J. L. Rombeau & J. Takala (Eds.), *Gut dysfunction in critical illness.* Berlin: Springer.

21. Ciresi, D. L., Cali, R. F., & Senagore, A. J. (1999). Abdominal closure using nonabsorbable mesh after massive resuscitation prevents abdominal compartment syndrome and gastrointestinal fistula. *Am Surg, 65*, 720–724.

22. Cook, D., et al. (1998). A comparison of sucralfate and ranitidine for the prevention of upper gastrointestinal bleeding in patients requiring mechanical ventilation. *N Engl J Med, 338*, 791–797.

23. Cook, D. J., Fuller, H. D., & Guyatt, G. H. (1994). Risk factors for gastrointestinal bleeding in critically ill patients. *N Engl J Med, 330*, 377–381.

24. Creteru, J., et al. (1997). Monitoring gastric mucosal carbon dioxide pressure using gas tonometry. *Anesthesiology, 87*(3), 504–510.

25. Crispin, C., et al. (1995). How consistently do RNs perform the procedure of collecting specimens for measurement of gastric pHi and CO_2? *Intensive Crit Care Nurs, 11*, 123–125.

26. Cunningham, J. A., et al. (1987). Extraluminal and intraluminal PCO_2 levels in the ischemic intestines of rats. *Curr Surg, 44*, 229–232.

27. Cushing, H. (1932). Peptic ulcers and the interbrain. *Surg Gynecol Obstet, 55*, 1–34.

28. Czaja, A. J., McAlhany, J. C., & Pruitt, B.-A. J. (1974). Acute gastroduodenal disease after thermal injury. An endoscopic evaluation of incidence and natural history. *N Engl J Med, 291*, 925–929.

29. Dark, D. S., & Pingleton, S. K. (1993). Nutrition and nutritional support in critically ill patients. *J Intensive Care Med, 8*, 16–33.

30. Dawson, A. M., Trenchard, D., & Guz, A. (1965). Small bowel tonometry assessment of small gut mucosal oxygen tension in dog and man. *Nature, 206*, 943–944.

31. de Souza, R. L., et al. (2001). Assessment of splanchnic perfusion with gastric tonometry in the immediate postoperative period of cardiac surgery in children. *Arquivos Brasileiros Cardiologia, 77*(6), 509–519.

32. Deitch, E. A. (1994). Bacterial translocation: the influence of dietary variables. *Gut,* (suppl 1), S23–S27.

33. Desai, V., et al. (1993). Gastric intramural Pco_2 during peritonitis and shock. *Chest, 104*, 1254–1258.

34. Duerksen, D. R. (2003). Stress-related mucosal disease in critically ill patients. *Best Pract Res Clin Gastroenterol, 17*(3), 327–344.

35. Durham, R. M., & Shapiro, M. J. (1991). Stress gastritis revisited. *Surg Clin North Am, 71*, 791–810.

36. Fennerty, M. B. (2002). Pathophysiology of the upper gastrointestinal tract in the critically ill patient: rationale of the therapeutic benefits of acid suppression. *Crit Care Med, 30*(6 suppl), S351–S355.

37. Fennerty, M. B. (2004). Rationale for the therapeutic benefits of acid-suppression therapy in the critically ill patient. *Medscape Gastroenterol, 6*(3).

38. Ferguson, A. P. (1996). Gastric tonometry: evaluating tissue oxygenation. *Crit Care Nurse, 16*(6), 48–55.

39. Fiddian-Green, R. G. (1992). Tonometry: theory and applications. *Intensive Care World, 9*(2), 60–65.

40. Fiddian-Green, R. G. (1993). Associations between intramucosal acidosis in the gut and organ failure. *Crit Care Med, 21*(2), S103–S107.

41. Fiddian-Green, R. G. (1995). Gastric intramucosal pH, tissue oxygenation and acid-base balance. *Br J Anaesthesiol, 74*, 591–606.

42. Fiddian-Green, R. G., et al. (1993). Goals for the resuscitation of shock. *Crit Care Med, 21*(2), S25–S30.

43. Fiddian-Green, R. G., Pittenger, G., & Whitehouse, W. M. (1982). Back-diffusion of CO_2 and its influence on the intramural pH in gastric mucosa. *J Surg Res, 33*, 39–48.

44. Flock, M. H., et al. (1972). The effect of bile acids on intestinal microflora. *Am J Clin Nutr, 25*, 1418–1426.

45. Fritsch, D. E., & Steinmann, R. A. (2000). Managing trauma patients with abdominal compartment syndrome. *Crit Care Nurse, 20*(6), 48–59.

46. Fusco, M. A., Martin, S., & Chang, M. C. (2001). Estimation of intra-abdominal pressure by bladder pressure measurement: validity and methodology. *J Trauma, 50*(2), 297–302.

47. Goldin, G. F., & Peura, D. A. (1996). Stress-related mucosal damage. What to do or not to do. *Gastrointest Endosc Clin North Am, 6*, 505–526.

48. Gomersall, C. D. E., et al. (2000). Resuscitation of critically ill patients based on the results of gastric tonometry. *Crit Care Med, 28*, 607–614.

49. Groeneveld, A. B. J. (1996). Gastrointestinal exocrine failure in critical illness. In J. L. Rombeau & J. Takala (Eds.), *Gut dysfunction in critical illness*. Berlin: Springer.

50. Grum, C. M., et al. (1984). Adequacy of tissue oxygenation in intact dog intestine. *J Appl Physiol, 56*, 1065–1069.

51. Gudmundsson, F. F., et al. (2002). Comparison of different methods for measuring intraabdominal pressure. *Intensive Care Med, 28*, 509–514.

52. Gutierrez, G., & Brown, S. D. (1995). Gastric tonometry: a new monitoring modality in the intensive care unit. *J Intensive Care Med, 10*, 34–44.

53. Guzman, J. A., Lacoma, F. J., & Kruse, J. A. (1998). Gastric and esophageal intramucosal P_{CO_2} (P_{iCO_2}) during endotoxemia. *Chest, 113*(4), 1078–1083.

54. Haglund, U. (1993). Intestinal mucosal blood flow and oxygenation in sepsis. *Br J Intensive Care*, 49–54.

55. Haglund, U. (1994). Gut ischaemia. *Gut,* (suppl 1), S73–S76.

56. Hamilton, M. A., & Mythen, M. G. (2001). Gastric tonometry: where do we stand? *Curr Opin Crit Care, 7*(2), 122–127.

57. Hamilton-Davies, C., et al. (1997). Comparison of commonly used clinical indicators of hypovolaemia with gastrointestinal tonometry. *Intensive Care Med, 23*, 276–281.

58. Hawkey, C. J., & Rampton, D. S. (1985). Prostaglandins and the gastrointestinal mucosa: are they important in its function, disease, or treatment? *Gastroenterology, 89*, 1162–1188.

59. Heard, S. O., et al. (1991). Gastric tonometry in healthy volunteers: effect of ranitidine on calculated intramural pH. *Crit Care Med, 19*(2), 271–274.

60. Heiselman, D. E., Hulisz, D. T., & Fricker, R. (1995). Randomized comparison of gastric pH control with intermittent and continuous intravenous infusion of famotidine in ICU patients. *Am J Gastroenterol, 90*, 277–279.

61. Higgins, D., Mythen, M. G., & Webb, A. R. (1994). Low intramucosal pH is associated with failure to acidify the gastric lumen in response to pentagastrin. *Intensive Care Med, 20*, 105–108.

62. Hunter, J. D., & Damani, Z. (2004). Intra-abdominal hypertension and the abdominal compartment syndrome. *Anaesthesia, 59*, 899–907.

63. Husebye, E. (2005). The pathogenesis of gastrointestinal bacterial overgrowth. *Chemotherapy, 51*(suppl 1), 1–22.

64. Ivatury, R. R., et al. (1998). Intra-abdominal hypertension after life-threatening penetrating abdominal trauma: prophylaxis, incidence and clinical relevance to gastric mucosal pH and abdominal compartment syndrome. *J Trauma, 44*, 1016–1021.

65. Jeejeebhoy, K. (2005). Enteral feeding. *Curr Opin Clin Nutr Metab Care, 21*(2), 187–191.

66. Johnson, D., & Mayers, I. (2001). Multiple organ dysfunction syndrome: a narrative review. *Can J Anaesth, 48*(5), 502–509.

67. Kaplan, M. (2004). Managing the open abdomen. *Ostomy Wound Manage, 50*(suppl 1A), C2–C8.

68. Kazamias, P., et al. (1998). Influence of enteral nutrition-induced splanchnic hyperemia on the septic origin of splanchnic ischaemia. *World J Surg, 22*(1), 6–11.

69. Kirkpatrick, A. W., et al. (2000). Is clinical examination an accurate indicator of raised intra-abdominal pressure in critically injured patients? *Can J Surg, 43*(3), 207–211.

70. Kivisaari, J., & Niinikoski, J. (1973). Use of Silastic tube and capillary sampling technic in the measurement of tissue PO_2 and P_{CO_2}. *Am J Surg, 125*, 623–627.

71. Knichwitz, G., et al. (1996). Gastric tonometry: precision and reliability are improved by a phosphate buffered solution. *Crit Care Med, 24*(3), 512–516.

72. Koivisto, T., et al. (2001). Gastric tonometry after subarachnoid haemorrhage. *Intensive Care Med, 27*(10), 1614–1621.

73. Kolkman, J. J., et al. (1999). Increased gastric P_{CO_2} during exercise is indicative of gastric ischaemia: a tonometric study. *Gut, 44*, 163–167.

74. Kron, I. L., Harman, P. K., & Nolan, S. P. (1984). The measurement of intra-abdominal pressure as a criterion for abdominal re-exploration. *Ann Surg, 199*, 28–30.

75. Lash O'Neill, P. (1996). Gastrointestinal system: target organ and source of multiple organ dysfunction syndrome. In V. Huddleston Secor. (Ed.), *Multiple organ dysfunction and failure: pathophysiology and clinical implications*. St Louis: Mosby.

76. Levy, B., et al. (1998). Gastric versus duodenal feeding and gastric tonometric measurements. *Crit Care Med, 26*(12), 1991–1994.

77. Levy, M., et al. (1997). Comparison of omeprazole and ranitidine for stress ulcer prophylaxis. *Dig Dis Sci, 42*(6), 1255–1259.

78. Lord, L. M., & Sax, H. C. (1994). The role of the gut in critical illness. *AACN Clin Issues, 5*(4), 450–458.

79. Malbrain, M. L. N. G. (2003). Validation of a novel fully automated continuous method to measure intra-abdominal pressure (IAP). *Intensive Care Med, 29*(suppl 1), S73.

80. Malbrain, M. L. N. G. (2004). Different techniques to measure intra-abdominal pressure (IAP): time for critical re-appraisal. *Intensive Care Med, 30*, 357–371.

81. Malbrain, M. L. N. G. (2004). Is it wise not to think about intra-abdominal hypertension in the ICU? *Curr Opin Crit Care, 10*, 132–145.

82. Malbrain, M. L. N. G. (2004). Prevalence of intra-abdominal hypertension in critically ill patients: a multi centre epidemiological study. *Intensive Care Med, 30*, 822–829.

83. Malbrain, M. L. N. G., et al. (2005). Incidence and prognosis of intraabdominal hypertension in a mixed population of critically ill patients: a multiple-center epidemiological study. *Crit Care Med, 33*(2), 315–322.

84. Marik, P. E., & Lorenzana, A. (1996). The effect of tube feeding on the measurement of gastric intramucosal pH. *Crit Care Med, 24*(9), 1498–1500.

85. Marshall, A., & West, S. (2003). Gastric tonometry and enteral nutrition: a possible conflict in critical care nursing practice. *Am J Crit Care, 12*(4), 349–356.

86. Marshall, A. P., & West, S. H. (2004). Gastric tonometry and monitoring gastrointestinal perfusion: using research to support nursing practice. *Nurs Crit Care, 9*(3), 123–133.

87. Marshall, J. C. (1996). *Clinical markers of gastrointestinal dysfunction*. Berlin: Springer-Verlag.

88. Maynard, N., et al. (1994). Influence of intravenous ranitidine on gastric intramucosal pH in critically ill patients. *Crit Care Med, 22*, A79.

89. Maynard, N., et al. (1995). Increasing splanchnic blood flow in the critically ill. *Chest, 108*, 1648–1654.

90. Maynard, N. D. (1993). *Splanchnic ischaemia in the critically ill*. London: London University Press.

91. McIver, M. A., Redfield, A. C., & Benedict, E. B. (1926). Gaseous exchange between the blood and the lumen of the stomach and intestines. *Am J Physiol, 76*, 92–111.

92. McNelis, J., Marini, C. P., & Simms, H. H. (2003). Abdominal compartment syndrome: clinical manifestations and predictive factors. *Curr Opin Crit Care, 9*, 133–136.

93. McVay, L. D. (1996). Immunology of the gut. In J. L. Rombeau & J. Takala (Eds.), *Gut dysfunction in critical illness*. Berlin: Springer.

94. Meisner, F. G., Habler, O. P., Kemming, G. I., et al. (2001). Changes in $P(i)CO_2$ reflect splanchnic mucosal ischaemia more reliably than changes in pHi during haemorrhagic shock. *Langenbecks Arch Surg, 386*(5), 333–338.

95. Merki, H., & Wilder-Smith, C. H. (1994). Do continuous infusions of omeprazole and ranitidine retain their effect with prolonged dosing? *Gastroenterology, 106,* 60–64.

96. Metz, D. C. (2005). Preventing the gastrointestinal consequences of stress-related mucosal disease. *Curr Med Res Opin, 21*(1), 11–18.

97. Michagin, G., Jensen, P. J., & Klint-Andersen, P. (1996). The accuracy of gastric tonometry: a matter of mathematical thinking. *Intensive Care Med, 22*(11), 1273.

98. Moore, A. F. K., et al. (2004). Intra-abdominal hypertension and the abdominal compartment syndrome. *Brit J Surg, 91,* 1102–1110.

99. Morken, J., & West, M. A. (2001). Abdominal compartment syndrome in the intensive care unit. *Curr Opin Crit Care, 7,* 268–274.

100. Moscona, R., et al. (1985). Prevention of gastrointestinal bleeding in burns: the effects of cimetidine or antacids combined with early enteral feeding. *Burns Incl Therm Inj, 12,* 65–67.

101. Mythen, M., & Faehnrich, J. (1996). Monitoring gut perfusion. In J. L. Rombeau & J Takala (Eds.), *Gut dysfunction in critical illness.* Berlin: Springer.

102. Mythen, M. G., & Webb, A. R. (1996). Perioperative plasma volume expansion reduces the incidence of gut mucosal hypoperfusion during cardiac surgery. *Arch Surg, 130,* 423–429.

103. N'Fonoyim, J. M., Benjamin, E., & Silverstein, J. H. (1992). Discrepancies between gastric and sigmoid tonometry in hemorrhagic shock. *Circ Shock, 37,* A33.

104. Nieuwenhuijzen, G. A., Deitch, E. A., & Goris, R. J. A. (1996). The relationship between gut-derived bacteria and the development of the multiple organ dysfunction syndrome. *J Anat, 189,* 537–548.

105. Nok, M., et al. (1993). Comparison of gastric wall Pco_2 during hemorrhagic shock. *Circ Shock, 40,* 194–199.

106. Oda, J., et al. (2002). Amplified cytokine response and lung injury by sequential hemorrhagic shock and abdominal compartment syndrome in a laboratory model of ischemia-reperfusion. *J Trauma, 52,* 625–632.

107. Parviainen, I., et al. (1996). Effect of nasogastric suction and ranitidine on the calculated gastric intramucosal pH. *Intensive Care Med, 22,* 319–323.

108. Perry, M. A., et al. (1986). Role of oxygen radicals in ischemia-induced lesions in the cat stomach. *Gastroenterology, 90*(2), 362–367.

109. Pestel, G., et al. (1999a). Intramucosal Pco_2 monitoring using gas tonometry in multiple injured patients. *Crit Care Med, 27*(1), A119.

110. Pestel, G., et al. (1999b). Tolerance limit of the gastric-arterial CO_2-difference (GADCO$_2$) in a clinical setting. *Crit Care Med, 27*(1), A120.

111. Peura, D. A., & Johnson, L. F. (1985). Cimetidine for prevention and treatment of gastroduodenal mucosal lesions in patients in an intensive care unit. *Ann Intern Med, 103,* 173–177.

112. Phillips, J., et al. (1996). A prospective study of simplified omeprazole suspension for the prophylaxis of stress-related mucosal damage. *Crit Care Med, 24*(11), 1793–1800.

113. Phillips, M. C., & Olson, L. R. (1993). The immunologic role of the gastrointestinal tract. *Crit Care Nurs Clin North Am, 5*(1), 107–120.

114. Pimentel, M., et al. (2000). Clinically significant gastrointestinal bleeding in critically ill patients in an era of prophylaxis. *Am J Gastroenterol, 95,* 2801–2806.

115. Pingleton, S., & Hadzima, S. K. (1983). Enteral alimentation and gastrointestinal bleeding in mechanically ventilated patients. *Crit Care Med, 11*(1), 13–16.

116. Pisegna, J. R. (2002). Pharmacology of acid suppression in the hospital setting: focus on proton pump inhibition. *Crit Care Med, 30*(6 suppl), S356–S361.

117. Pouliart, N., & Huyghens, L. (2002). An observational study on intraabdominal pressure in 125 critically ill patients. *Crit Care, 6*(suppl 1), S3.

118. Puyana, J. C., et al. (2000). Directly measured tissue pH is an earlier indicator of splanchnic acidosis than tonometric parameters during hemorrhagic shock in swine. *Crit Care Med, 28*(7), 2557–2562.

119. Raff, T., Germann, G., & Hartmann, B. (1997). The value of early enteral nutrition in the prophylaxis of stress ulceration in the severely burned patient. *Burns, 23,* 313–318.

120. Rasmussen, I., & Haglund, U. (1992). Early ischemia in experimental fecal peritonitis. *Circ Shock, 38,* 22–28.

121. Reinoso-Barbero, R., et al. (1998). Reference values of gastric intramucosal pH in children. *Paediatr Anaesth, 8,* 135–138.

122. Riddington, D., et al. (1994). Measuring carbon dioxide tension in saline and alternative solutions: quantification of bias and precision in two blood gas analyzers. *Crit Care Med, 22*(1), 96–100.

123. Ridings, P. C., et al. (1995). Cardiopulmonary effects of raised intra-abdominal pressure before and after intravascular volume expansion. *J Trauma, 39,* 1072–1075.

124. Ritchie, W.-P. J., & Mercer, D. (1991). Mediators of bile acid-induced alterations in gastric mucosal blood flow. *Am J Surg, 161,* 126–130.

125. Robertson, M. S., Cade, J. F., & Clancy, R. L. (1999). *Helicobacter pylori* infection in intensive care: increased prevalence and a new nosocomial infection. *Crit Care Med, 27,* 1276–1280.

126. Romito, R. A. (1995). Early administration of enteral nutrients in critically ill patients. *AACN Clin Issues, 6*(2), 242–256.

127. Russell, J. A. (1997). Gastric tonometry: does it work? *Intensive Care Med, 23,* 3–6.

128. Samloff, I. M. (1989). Peptic ulcer: the many proteinases of aggression. *Gastroenterology, 96,* 586–595.

129. Schiessel, R., Feil, W., & Wenzl, E. (1990). Mechanisms of stress ulceration and implications for treatment. *Gastroenterol Clin North Am, 19,* 101–120.

130. Schilling, D., et al. (2000). Low seroprevalence of *Helicobacter pylori* infection in patients with stress ulcer bleeding—a prospective evaluation of patients on a cardiosurgical intensive care unit. *Intensive Care Med, 26*(12), 1832–1836.

131. Schlichtig, R., & Bowles, S. A. (1992). Decreasing intestinal interstitial pH reflects metabolic acidosis during flow stagnation. *Am Rev Resp Dis, 145,* A792.

132. Schlichtig, R., & Bowles, S. A. (1994). Distinguishing between aerobic and anaerobic appearance of dissolved CO_2 in intestine during low flow. *J Appl Physiol, 76,* 2443–2451.

133. Schlichtig, R., Mehta, N., & Gayowski, T. J. P. (1996). Tissue-arterial Pco_2 difference is a better marker of ischemia than intramural pH (pHi) or arterial pH-pHi difference. *J Crit Care, 11*(2), 51–56.

134. Shein, M., et al. (1995). The abdominal compartment syndrome: the physiological and clinical consequences of elevated intra-abdominal pressure. *J Am Coll Surg, 180,* 745–753.

135. Simpson, F., & Doig, G. (2004). Parenteral vs. enteral nutrition in the critically ill patient: a meta-analysis of trials using the intention to treat principle. *Intensive Care Med, 31*(1), 12–23.

136. Spirt, M. J. (2003). Acid suppression in critically ill patients: what does the evidence support? *Pharmacotherapy, 23*(10, part 2), 87S–93S.

137. Stannard, V. A., et al. (1988). Gastric exocrine "failure" in critically ill patients: incidence and associated features. *Br Med J, 296,* 155–156.

138. Steinberg, K. P. (2002). Stress-related mucosal disease in the critically ill patient: risk factors and strategies to prevent stress-

related bleeding in the intensive care unit. *Crit Care Med, 30* (6 suppl), S362–S364.

139. Strassburg, C. P. (2003). Gastrointestinal disorders of the critically ill. Shock liver. *Best Pract Res Clin Gastroenterol, 17*(3), 369–381.

140. Sugrue, M., & D'Amour, S. (2001). Review of publications identifying outcomes after decompression in patients with ACS. *J Trauma, 51,* 419.

141. Sugrue, M., et al. (1994). Intra-abdominal pressure measurement using a modified nasogastric tube: description and validation of a new technique. *Intensive Care Med, 20,* 588–590.

142. Sugrue, M., et al. (1999). Intra-abdominal hypertension is an independent cause of postoperative renal impairment. *Arch Surg, 134,* 1082–1085.

143. Sun, S., Weil, M. H., & Tang, W. (1992). Gastric intramural bicarbonate: limitations of the tonometry method. *Crit Care Med, 20,* S66.

144. Swan, M. C., & Banwell, P. E. (2005). The open abdomen: aetiology, classification and current management strategies. *J Wound Care, 14*(1), 7–11.

145. Takala, J., et al. (1994). Saline P_{CO_2} is an important source of error in the assessment of gastric intramucosal pH. *Crit Care Med, 22*(11), 1877–1879.

146. Takala, J. (2001). *Gastrointestinal tonometry.* Helsinki, Finland: Datex Ohmeda.

147. Taylor, D. E., et al. (1997). Measurement of gastric mucosal carbon dioxide tension by saline and air tonometry. *J Crit Care, 12*(4), 208–213.

148. Tortora, G. J., & Grabowski, S. R. (2003). *Principles of anatomy and physiology.* Hoboken, NJ: John Wiley and Sons.

149. Tzelepis, G., et al. (1996). Comparison of gastric air tonometry with standard saline tonometry. *Intensive Care Med, 22,* 1239–1243.

150. Vallet, B., Neviere, R., & Chagnon, J.-L. (1996). Gastrointestinal mucosal ischaemia. In J. L. Rombeau & J. Takala (Eds.), *Gut dysfunction in critical illness.* Berlin: Springer.

151. Vincent, J.-L, & Creteur, J. (1998). Gastric mucosal pH is definitely obsolete—please tell us more about gastric mucosal pCO_2. *Crit Care Med, 26*(9), 1479–1481.

152. Walley, K. R., et al. (1998). Small bowel tonometry is more accurate than gastric tonometry in detecting gut ischaemia. *J Appl Physiol, 85*(5), 1770–1777.

153. Wells, C. L., & Erlandsen, S. L. (1996). Bacterial translocation: intestinal epithelial permeability. In J. L. Rombeau & J. Takala (Eds.), *Gut dysfunction in critical illness.* Berlin: Springer.

154. Wernerman, J. (2005). Guidelines for nutritional support in intensive care unit patients: a critical analysis. *Curr Opin Clin Nutr Metab Care, 8*(2), 171–175.

155. Wittmann, D. H., et al. (1993). A burr-like device to facilitate temporary abdominal closure in planned multiple laparotomies. *Eur J Surg, 159,* 75–79.

156. Yasue, N., & Guth, P. H. (1988). Role of exogenous acid and retransfusion in hemorrhagic shock-induced gastric lesions in the rat. *Gastroenterology, 94,* 1135–1143.

157. Zhang, H., & Vincent, J.-L. (1993). Arteriovenous differences in P_{CO_2} and pH are good indicators of critical hypoperfusion. *Am Rev Resp Dis, 148,* 867–871.

CHAPTER 30

Liver, Kidney, and Pancreas Transplantation

Patricia Radovich

There are more than 102,000 people awaiting organ transplantation; 75,000 are waiting for a kidney transplant, more than 4100 are waiting for a pancreas or kidney-pancreas transplant, and more than 17,000 individuals are awaiting liver transplantation. Patients wait from 2 to 5 years for a transplant unless they have suffered acute liver failure, and the current wait in that situation is approximately 27 days.[47] Transplantation has come a long way since the first organ transplant and is a dynamic and continually evolving area of practice. Patients with end-stage disease awaiting transplantation present the clinical challenge of maintaining the patient with multisystem dysfunction until transplantation. The process of transplantation is a complex intermixture of the patient disease, the timing of transplantation, and the quality of organ received. With the shortage of deceased donor organs and increase in deaths on the waiting lists, there has been in increase in the use of marginal donors.[28] In the immediate post-transplantation setting, the resumption of organ function, prevention of the complications from pretransplant organ damage, and prevention of infection dominate the nursing care of the transplant patient.

LIVER RECIPIENT BEFORE TRANSPLANT

Liver transplantation has become a routine procedure with excellent outcomes.[47] Liver transplant recipients before transplantation usually are in the hospital either in acute care or in critical care, although in some circumstances, patients are at home. Patients on the United Network for Organ Sharing (UNOS) waiting list for liver transplant receive organs based upon the Model for End-Stage Liver Disease (MELD) score except in the case of acute liver failure. Patients with acute liver failure receive a listing status of 1, the highest listing, due to the estimated life span of less than 72 hours. In patients with chronic liver disease the MELD score is a logarithmic calculation based on three laboratory values: total bilirubin level, international normalized ratio (INR), and creatinine level.[47] Patients must have a minimum score of fifteen before they can receive a transplant.

The etiology of liver recipients' liver disease is varied, and recipients may suffer from a variety of organ system dysfunctions as a result of their liver failure before transplantation that will carry over into their postoperative course and influence their progress to recovery.[45]

The varied etiologies of liver disease are listed in Box 30-1. The recurrence of liver disease after transplantation can be immediate or can occur after several years, as in the patient with biliary liver disease.

Patients awaiting liver transplant may suffer from encephalopathy; as their condition worsens, this alteration in consciousness may progress from personality changes and lethargy to coma, potentially refractory to medical management. In addition, the development of hepatorenal syndrome affects both their fluid balance and their ability to eliminate toxins cleared by the renal system. As the liver dysfunction worsens, a systemic problem with coagulopathy occurs, making the patient susceptible to bleeding and therefore an increased risk of intracranial hemorrhage. The portal hypertension increases and—coupled with coagulopathy—increases the risk of gastrointestinal hemorrhage. These complications, coupled with the severe malnutrition of liver disease, create a complex patient with neurologic, cardiovascular, pulmonary, gastrointestinal, gastrourinary, and immune system dysfunction. It is this composite patient who proceeds to the operating room and returns to the critical care unit. Chapter 27 provides more comprehensive information about liver failure.

Psychologically these patients go into the transplant with very different perspectives. Patients with acute hepatic failure may find their postoperative course a terrifying experience as often they have lapsed into coma before the awareness of a need for transplantation occurred. Patients with chronic liver failure experience both elation and guilt after transplantation as they recall their extreme disability before the transplant but also deal with the awareness that, in most cases, someone died for them to receive their transplant.[45]

Etiology of Liver Disease

ACUTE

- Drug induced (acetaminophen, herbal supplements, prescription medication)
- Viral hepatitis (hepatitis A, B, or D)
- Autoimmune disease
- Iatrogenic

CIRRHOSIS

- Alcoholic liver disease
- Autoimmune disease
- Viral hepatitis (hepatitis B and C)
- Biliary atresia
- Primary biliary cirrhosis
- Primary sclerosing cholangitis
- Nonalcoholic fatty liver disease
- Cryptogenic
- Budd-Chiari syndrome
- Wilson's disease
- Hemochromatosis
- Glycogen storage disease
- α_1-Antitrypsin deficiency
- Urea cycle defects
- Primary hereditary oxalosis

LIVER TRANSPLANTATION

Types of Liver Donors

In the past, liver transplantation was performed using organs only from deceased organ donors. With the increase in individuals awaiting liver transplantation and the rising number of deaths while waiting, today's liver transplants may come from two sources: living and deceased. Living liver donation was initially developed for pediatric recipients; it is now offered in adult liver transplant programs. This process allows a patient to receive a transplant while in optimal physical condition without severe decompensation. However, this procedure, a low-risk operation in the pediatric population, has become a high-risk procedure in the adult population. In some cases, the donor is more susceptible to complications than the recipient because the donor is losing 60% of a functioning liver, whereas the recipient is gaining 60% of a fully functional liver in place of a dysfunctional liver.[13] The recipient of a partial liver transplant may have more complications than one who has received a whole organ, due to the large number of anastomoses that are required and the fact that the liver is less than 100% in volume. Those receiving the whole organ may be considerably more ill at the time of surgery because of progressive liver dysfunction and the severity of their disease process[13] (Figure 30-1).

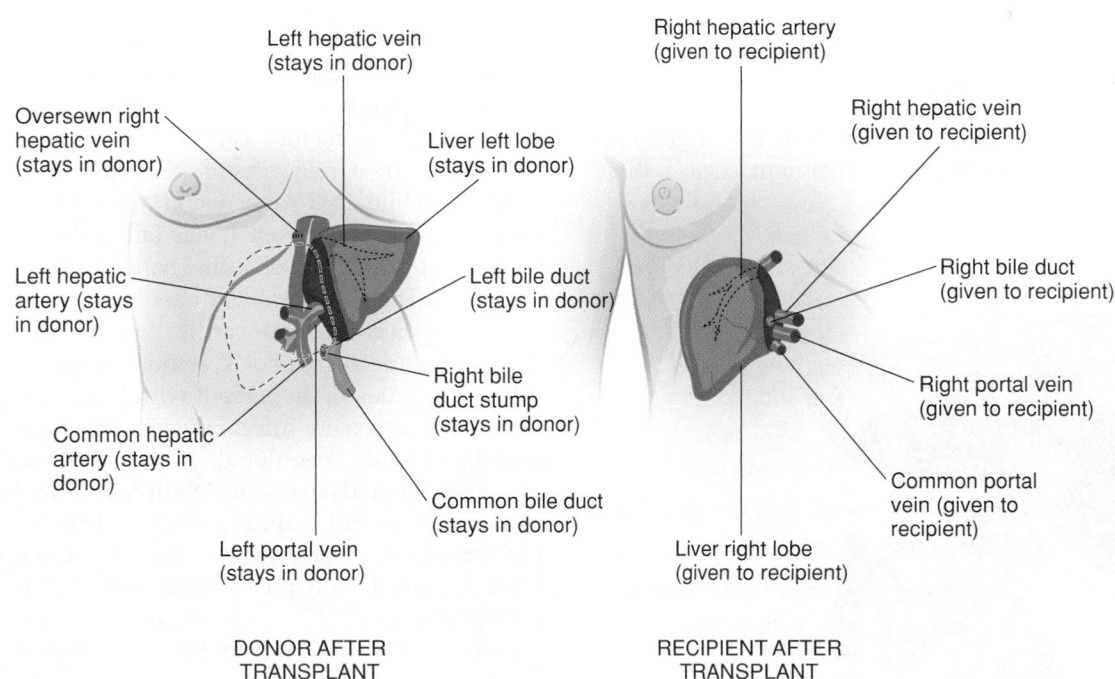

DONOR AFTER TRANSPLANT

RECIPIENT AFTER TRANSPLANT

⬆FIGURE 30-1 Liver transplantation—portion taken from donor and portion transplanted to recipient.

The deceased donor process can involve the use of a whole organ or a split liver. In a split liver transplant, the donated organ is divided into two grafts. One portion of the split liver, usually the left lobe, goes to a child and the right lobe to an adult; however, it is also possible a small-size adult might benefit from a left-lobe procedure.[46] The whole-organ donation provides an entire liver to a patient awaiting liver transplantation. Those receiving a whole-organ are the most severely ill patients with a high MELD score, who have decompensated and have multisystem dysfunction. It is these patients who, upon arrival in critical care, can present a challenge to the critical care nurse (Figure 30-2).

The transplant team determines which procedure is best for the recipient by using the MELD score along with the patient's anatomic structure. The MELD model predicts liver disease severity and has been shown to be useful in predicting mortality in patients with compensated and decompensated cirrhosis.[47]

Preoperative Care

Before liver transplantation, the hospitalized patient may be malnourished and require close neurologic observation for progressive encephalopathy or, in acute liver failure, risk of herniation. These patients may also require mechanical ventilation and monitoring for fluid and electrolyte imbalances because of progressive renal dysfunction. Liver failure patients are also at risk for the development of infections with prolonged hospitalization.[25,33,38]

Postoperative Care

Individual variability characterizes the immediate postoperative care of the liver recipient. One patient

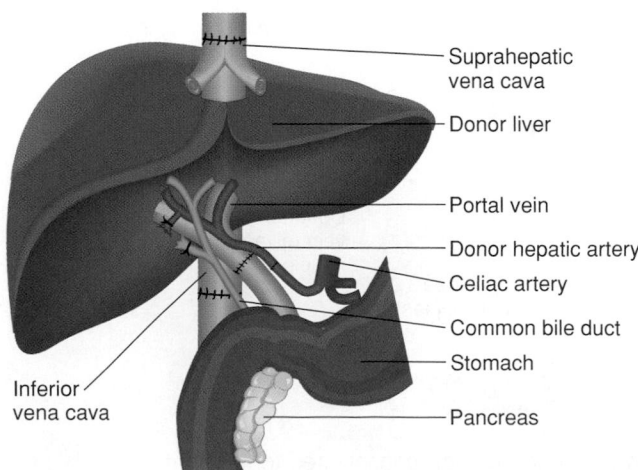

♦FIGURE 30-2 Suture lines following liver transplantation.

Labels on figure:
- Suprahepatic vena cava
- Donor liver
- Portal vein
- Donor hepatic artery
- Celiac artery
- Common bile duct
- Stomach
- Pancreas
- Inferior vena cava

may have an uncomplicated surgery, remain hospitalized for 5 to 7 days, and be discharged. Another patient may have a difficult operation, multiple transfusions, and long operative time; have a prolonged stay in critical or acute care; transfer to rehabilitation; require close outpatient supervision; and have frequent readmissions for complications.

The postoperative patient arriving in critical care will be on a ventilator, have a pulmonary artery catheter (PAC) arterial line, and often have another central venous line or dialysis catheter on the opposite side of the PAC. The patient will have three abdominal drains: a nasogastric tube, Foley catheter, and on occasion a T-tube. An arterial blood gas, comprehensive metabolic panel, lactate, complete blood count, and prothrombin time (PT) and INR should be obtained within 1 hour of arrival in critical care. Admission routines would also include assessing ventilation and neurologic function as well as determining if the drains are to suction or bulb, depending upon the surgical orders.[17,33]

Primary Graft Nonfunction

Survival of the liver transplant patient depends upon early graft function. In the immediate postoperative period, graft function is a concern as development of primary nonfunction (PNF) occurs in up to 3% of grafts.[30] Graft injury (where the liver is damaged) within the first 3 days is most often caused by PNF or hepatic artery thrombosis.[17] PNF can result from an unstable donor, preexisting disease in the donor, inadequate or overly long organ preservation, an imperfect recipient operation, or a perioperative immunologic reaction. These factors can occur in combination or separately. In a majority of PNF, the liver produces little or no bile after reperfusion, preexisting coagulopathy worsens, and lactate levels fail to decrease or even increase. Postoperatively, the patient usually remains comatose. The preoperative hyperdynamic state demonstrated by an elevated cardiac output/cardiac index (CO/CI) and decreased systemic vascular resistance (SVR) continues in the patient with impaired graft function. PNF adversely affects every organ system and is associated with coagulopathy, persistent coma, hypoglycemia, hemodynamic instability, and acidosis. If the situation does not improve within 24 to 36 hours, the patient's only chance for survival is retransplantation. Overall, this is the most lethal complication of liver transplantation.[30,31,41,48] It is important in the first hours after transplant to recognize PNF as compared to reperfusion injury.

In reperfusion injury, liver function tests, specifically the transaminases (i.e., aspartate transaminase [AST] and alanine transaminase [ALT]), are elevated for 24 to 48 hours, reflecting preservation injury (injury resulting from the liver's being out of the body and stored in cold solution until transplantation). The bilirubin level also rises. Depending upon the severity of preservation injury or amount of steatosis (fat) in the new liver, this elevation may persist for several weeks. More critically ill patients with severe elevation of the liver tests before transplantation may have a decrease in their total bilirubin level after transplantation, but

it may take weeks before it normalizes completely. The PT and INR should begin to normalize within the first few hours after transplantation; the patient's level of consciousness should improve within approximately 12 hours following surgery.[27,34] If the laboratory tests do not show normalization, there is concern for PNF (Figure 30-3).

Primary poor function is a less severe form of PNF. Liver test elevations are usually lower as the synthetic

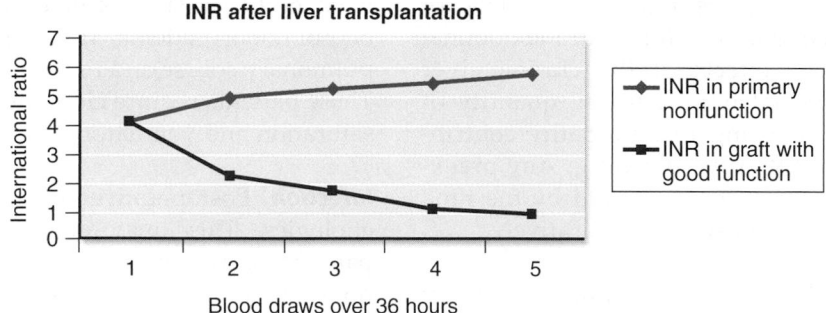

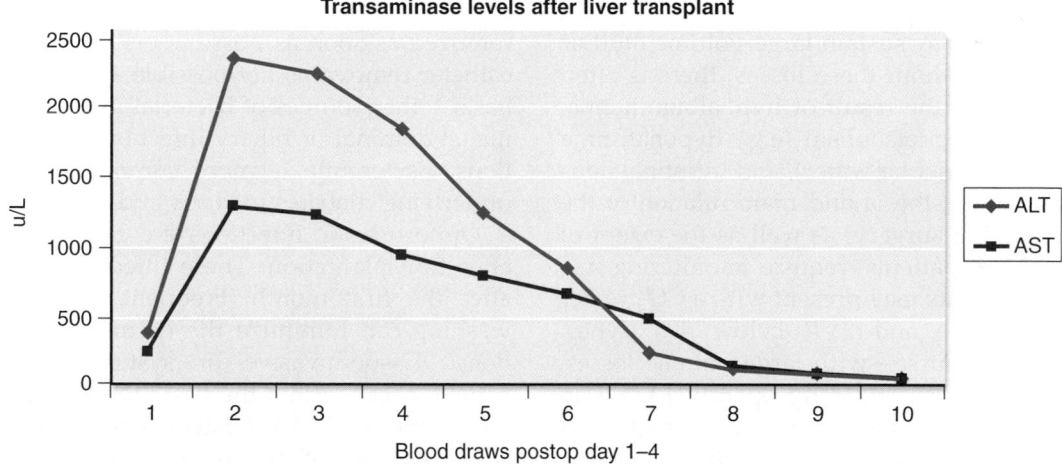

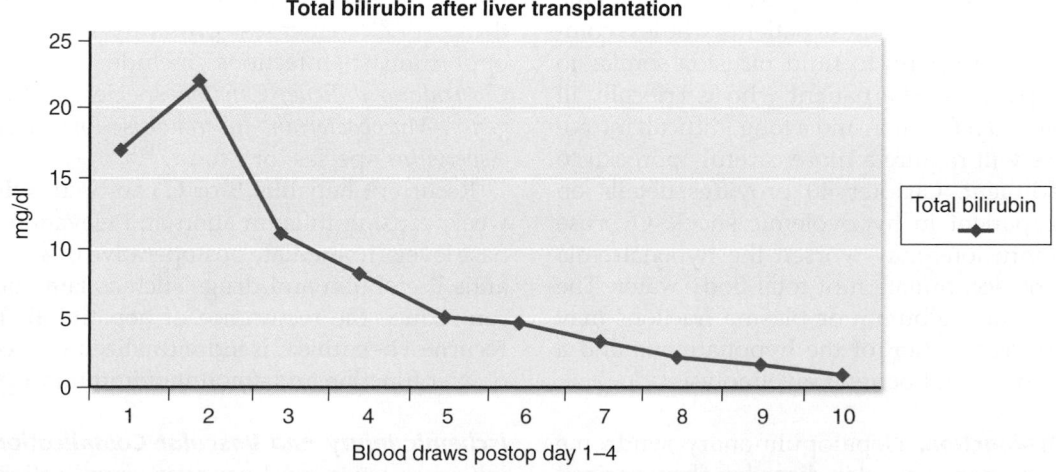

◆FIGURE 30-3 Laboratory value testing after liver transplantation.

function is partially preserved. These patients may continue to have some coagulopathy but it is less severe. Because of the poor liver function, portal hypertension may continue, resulting in postoperative ascites. The treatment of this condition is mainly supportive; most grafts will eventually recover, although some patients may require retransplantation.[17,48]

Postoperative Bleeding. Postoperative bleeding is a potential early complication following liver transplantation. The literature suggests that 10% to 15% of patients require reoperation for intra-abdominal hemorrhage.[17,37,48] The effects of the chronic liver disease, severity of portal hypertension, quantity of transfusions, and preexisting coagulopathy contribute to the risk of postoperative bleeding. Any preexisting coagulopathy should be corrected by the time the patient reaches critical care postoperatively.[1]

Hemodynamic Instability. Hemodynamic instability may exist before the transplant and continue in the early postoperative period because of the hyperdynamic circulatory status of these patients. Patients undergoing liver transplantation may sustain large-volume fluid or blood losses. Even without these losses, there is often fluid sequestration as the result of hypoalbuminemia, alterations in sodium metabolism (e.g., hyponatremia from too much intravascular water), and intestinal ileus caused by general anesthesia and manipulation of the intestinal tract during surgery, as well as the extent of the surgery. These patients require monitoring via a PAC. Initially, patients may present with a CO greater than 12 liters/minute and SVR below 400 dynes. The intra-operative course—with large volume losses, transfusion requirements, and long operative times in addition to preoperative malnutrition, abnormal renal function, and ascites volume—increases the risk for the development of inadequate vascular volume. Low filling pressures, falling CO, and increasing SVR will reflect the volume and cardiac status of these patients. The less complicated cases will respond to fluid infusion similar to other surgical patients. The patient who is critically ill with multisystem dysfunction and a long, difficult intraoperative course will require a more careful approach to volume replacement. Chapter 40 provides details on caring for the patient in hypovolemic shock. Overuse of crystalloid infusions may worsen the hyponatremia and increase the accumulation of total body water. The infusion of too much albumin or plasma fractions may result in the overcorrection of the hyponatremia and a significant risk of central pontine myelinolysis.[25,33,34]

Pulmonary Dysfunction. Hepatopulmonary syndrome (HPS) is a pulmonary vascular disorder characterized by chronic liver disease, intrapulmonary vascular dilation, and arterial hypoxemia. The degree of hypoxemia varies with each patient, with little correlation to either the severity or the cause of the underlying liver disease. Patients will have resolution of this condition after transplantation, usually over days to weeks.[44] The patient without HPS and with an uncomplicated liver transplant requiring few transfusions and a shorter surgical time will usually be extubated within 12 to 24 hours of the surgical procedure. Patients with more complicated surgeries, or with preexisting pulmonary conditions such as atelectasis, severe malnutrition, or pulmonary edema, may have a more complicated pulmonary course and remain intubated for 3 to 4 days. These patients require close monitoring of their oxygen saturation and ventilatory status.

Infection. Postoperative infections have a variety of etiologies. They may occur because of nosocomial pathogens, as a result of reactivation of latent infections, or from opportunistic infections. Early infections are primarily bacterial. Late-occurring infections are fungal or viral. The bacterial infections may be the result of indwelling catheters; catheters should be removed as soon as possible or, for patients in whom catheter removal is not possible, changed on a regular basis. Other sources of bacterial infection are pneumonia, abdominal or biliary infections, and wound infections. Bacteremia is more common in patients with underlying diabetes mellitus and malnutrition.

Opportunistic infections are rare in the first week after transplantation. These infections tend to appear after the first month. Frequent and thorough hand washing can minimize the occurrence of these infections. Tissue-invasive or systemic viral infections usually occur within the first month and include cytomegalovirus (CMV), Epstein-Barr virus (EBV), herpes simplex virus (HSV), varicella-zoster virus (VZV), and adenovirus. These may present as fever, malaise, nausea, vomiting, diarrhea, leukopenia, and failure to thrive. VZV emerges primarily as shingles. Other opportunistic infections include *Nocardia asteroides*, *Clostridium difficile*, *Candida* species, *Listeria monocytogenes*, *Mycobacterium tuberculosis*, *Pneumocystis jiroveci*, *Aspergillus* species, or *Mucor*.[10,17,32]

Recurrent hepatitis B or C can occur within the first week, causing inflammation and elevation of transaminase levels. Immediate postoperative treatment with hepatitis B globulin and drugs such as lamivudine (Epivir) can reduce the recurrence of hepatitis B. Treatment of recurrent hepatitis C is individualized with consideration of liver function and amount of immunosuppression.

Ischemic Injury and Vascular Complications. Ischemic injury, rejection, and vascular complications are a concern in the postoperative period. While hepatic artery thrombosis (HAT) can occur early or late in the recovery period,[34] this complication occurs in 5% of patients and can be due to cold ischemia, anastomotic problems, or rejection. It results in ischemia and is the second leading cause of graft failure in the immediate postoperative period.[17] HAT may cause necrosis of the bile ducts and the operative anastomosis, leading to delayed bile leak in 7 days to 2 months after the transplant. Ultrasound evaluation of liver anastomosis and flow is usually performed within the first few hours after the patient arrives in critical care.

The thrombosis of the hepatic artery can lead to bilomas (i.e., collection of bile outside the bile ducts) and bacteremia, resulting from abscess formation and at times leading to sepsis. Often these patients will respond to antibiotics. These symptoms may present as subtle changes, with the abnormality in hepatic arterial flow noted upon ultrasound evaluation of the artery. The development of HAT may result in the loss of portions or the entire liver graft because of necrosis in the first few days to 2 weeks after transplantation.

Diagnosis of HAT usually causes a rapid increase in transaminase levels, but there can also be subtle elevations. Changes in the volume, color, or character of the bile can indicate a hepatic artery problem. Ultrasound evaluation of the liver within the first 24 hours can assist with the early diagnosis of this complication. Hepatic artery stenosis without thrombosis can occur in the first 100 days after transplant, leading to graft dysfunction and the need for balloon angioplasty or surgical revision. The outcome of the transplant can be compromised, depending upon the length of time the liver lacks the hepatic artery blood supply. In some cases, retransplantation may be necessary if revision is unable to be accomplished or graft failure continues.[17,48]

Portal Vein Thrombosis. Portal vein thrombosis (PVT) occurs less frequently, only 1% to 13% of recipients, than hepatic artery thrombosis. The risk factors for PVT include portal vein thrombosis before transplant, previous portal vein surgery or manipulation, or a hypercoagulable state. The signs of this complication are the development of portal hypertension, ascites, edema, encephalopathy, and elevated liver function tests. This complication may be seen in the first month after transplantation. An ultrasound in the first few hours of transplant can diagnose reduced flow in the portal vein. If the thrombus develops after the first month, complications of portal hypertension—encephalopathy, variceal hemorrhage, multiorgan failure—will be seen.[38,43]

Outflow Obstruction. Outflow tract obstruction occurs because of restriction of blood flow through the hepatic

veins.[33,43] The clinical presentation of the outflow obstruction depends upon the type of outflow anastomosis and the location of the obstruction. If the obstruction is at the inferior vena cava when the transplant is performed with the standard surgical technique, the patient will have normal hepatic function, edema of the lower extremities, and the development of lumbar collaterals. If the obstruction is at the suprahepatic cava when either the standard surgical technique or the piggyback surgical technique is performed, the recipient can have the full manifestation of Budd-Chiari syndrome. Budd-Chiari syndrome occurs with obstruction of the hepatic vein. This obstruction of the hepatic vein prevents blood from leaving the liver and returning to the heart. The symptoms of this are ascites, abdominal pain, and elevation of liver function tests. Outflow tract obstruction can lead to hemorrhage because of an anastomotic leak or bleeding from collateral vessels. This usually is recognized within 24 hours of the initial surgery. Venous congestion or Budd-Chiari syndrome occurs in 1% to 3% of transplants and may present up to 1 month post-transplant with jaundice, ascites, gastrointestinal (GI) bleeding, hepatomegaly, and coagulopathy.[17,38,43]

Biliary Complications. Biliary complications occur in 10% to 20% of all liver transplant recipients.[20] Eighty percent of all biliary complications occur within the first 6 months after transplantation, the majority within the first 3 months.[20] Clinical presentation of this complication may be subtle. Noninvasive examinations may not detect small obstructions or leaks.[20] Complications of the biliary system can be due to technical complications of the anastomosis or ischemic injury related to compromised arterial blood supply, preservation injury, rejection, or ascending infection, where microorganisms from the duodenum are translocated into the bile ducts because of obstruction and bile stasis.[17] Bile leaks within the first few days after transplantation are usually the result of disruption of the surgical anastomosis. Late bile leaks are usually due to ischemic injury or removal of T-tubes. With the reduction in use of T-tubes, this complication is seen less frequently.[35] Recipients of split livers (partial grafts or reduced-size grafts) can have bile leakage from the cut surface, the cystic duct remnant, unrecognized accessory ducts, or choledochoenteric anastomoses. Pain in the right upper quadrant, fever, and leukocytosis may be included in the presentation.[31]

Biliary strictures may be anastomotic or ischemic; the mechanism of injury is the same as that for a biliary leak. Biliary strictures evolve over time and present after the first month post-transplantation. The patient may present with jaundice, cholangitis, or asymptomatic elevation of liver function tests, specifically the alkaline phosphatase and bilirubin levels.[17] Ultrasound may not identify the biliary tract problem, and an endoscopic retrograde cholangiopancreatography (ERCP) may be needed to identify, place internal biliary stents that bypass the biliary stricture or leak, and decompress biliary blockages. In 14% of cases, the patient will need to return to the operating room for a revision and choledochojejunostomy to Roux limb (Roux-en-Y).[9] Patients who have had Roux-en-Y procedures will need a percutaneous cholangiography if they have further problems with their bile ducts.[9]

Diagnostic Testing. Evaluation of the patient for vascular or biliary complications requires that the patient undergo ultrasound within the first 12 hours of the postoperative period. This test is usually done at the patient's bedside. If there is persistent dysfunction, magnetic resonance imaging (MRI) can be performed in conjunction with magnetic resonance angiography (MRA) and magnetic resonance cholangiopancreatography (MRCP) to evaluate the vessels and bile ducts. A liver biopsy may also be performed either percutaneously at the bedside or by the transjugular method in interventional radiology to provide histologic information on inflammation caused by rejection, recurrent disease, reperfusion injury, or outflow obstruction.[17,25,38]

Renal Failure and Electrolyte Abnormalities. Patients with advanced liver disease can develop hepatorenal syndrome before liver transplantation. Hepatorenal syndrome is characterized by acute renal failure, increased urine: plasma osmolality, low urinary sodium level, and the absence of pathologic changes in the kidney (the tubular function remains intact). The renal failure seen in HRS should resolve after liver transplantation. These patients are at increased risk after transplantation for delayed return of renal function, creating continued fluid and electrolyte imbalances, and may require the use of renal replacement therapy until renal function returns.[36] The use of calcineurin inhibitors for immunosuppression will also need to be adjusted during this time to prevent worsening of the renal function because of nephrotoxicity. Approximately 14% of these recipients may go on to develop chronic renal failure.[36] Renal failure is defined by a glomerular filtration rate of less than 30 ml/min per $1.73\,m^2$ body surface area and a creatinine level greater than 1.6 mg/dl.[36]

Malnutrition. Pretransplantation nutrition is challenging in liver failure patients. More than 80% of liver transplant patients exhibit moderate to severe malnutrition in the face of enteral and parenteral supplementation.[25] It is the patient's liver function in the postoperative period that determines the level of metabolic stress and nutritional needs. If the allograft function is good, the immediate postoperative hypermetabolism is short. However, if the postoperative course includes delayed graft function, the patient may be volume overloaded and intolerant of enteral feedings. These patients may require parenteral nutrition to provide adequate calories and protein and to correct metabolic abnormalities while minimizing sodium and water accumulation.[25] During the acute post-transplantation period, adequate nutrition is crucial to help prevent infection, promote wound healing, support metabolic demands, replenish lost stores, and mediate the immune response.[25] See the Nutrition box below.

▲ NUTRITION

Nutrition for Organ Transplant Recipients

- **Calories:** 130% to 150% of calculated basal energy expenditure. The upper range of calories is recommended for underweight patients and the lower range for overweight patients.
- **Protein:** 1.5 to 2.0 g/kg. Protein catabolic rate is increased because of surgical stress and high-dose corticosteroids. Adequate amounts of protein are required for wound healing and prevention of infection.
- **Carbohydrate:** 50% to 70% of nonprotein calories. Serum glucose levels may be increased because of medications, metabolic stress, or infection.
- **Fluid:** 1 ml/calorie. Adjust on the basis of output.
- **Electrolytes:** Individualize.
- **Vitamins and minerals:** Individualize.
- **Special considerations:** Some patients may have been receiving total parenteral nutrition or enteral feedings before transplant. Once the gut is functional after surgery, determination of the adequacy of oral intake can be obtained. If the oral intake is inadequate, the patient may receive tube feedings in addition to the enteral intake. If there is a delay in the return of gut function after surgery, total parenteral nutrition should be instituted if it has not already been and then reevaluated upon the return of gut function. If renal function is delayed, enteral or total parenteral nutrition formulas can be concentrated.

Modified from reference 19.

Rejection. Rejection in the liver transplant patient can occur in the early days to weeks after transplantation. Hyperacute rejection occurs within minutes to days posttransplant and is extremely rare. Acute rejection is the more common form of rejection seen in liver transplantation. It occurs within the first 6 months of transplantation, and between 60% and 80% of liver transplant recipients will have at least one rejection episode.[24,34] Graft injury, evidenced by elevated liver function tests between 3 and 14 days after transplantation, can be due to acute cellular rejection. This form of rejection is T-cell mediated and causes tissue destruction. In chronic rejection, there is intimal hyperplasia of small and medium-sized arteries, resulting in progressive ischemia in the transplanted organ. This leads to loss of the bile ducts, ductopenic rejection, and cholestasis, which over time may lead to retransplantation.[24,34] While patients with both acute and chronic rejection may remain asymptomatic, some patients may present with symptoms of a nonspecific nature, with complaints of malaise, decreased appetite, right upper quadrant pain, jaundice, and low-grade fever. The first laboratory tests that will show elevations identifying rejection are the alkaline phosphatase and gamma-glutamyltransferase (GGT) levels, followed by an elevation of the rest of the liver function tests.

Treatment of rejection usually begins with boluses of corticosteroids. The addition of mycophenolate mofetil (CellCept) to the medication regimen and changing to tacrolimus (Prograf) from cyclosporine (Gengraf) have also been recommended.[39,49] A total of 10% to 15% of acute rejection episodes will not respond to steroids; antilymphocytic agents (muromonab-CD3 [OKT3], antilymphocyte globulin (ALG) [Atgam], antithymocyte globulin (ATG) [Thymoglobulin]) or anti-interleukin-2 receptor antibodies are used to address rejection in these cases.[34,45] While ATG is more commonly used and may cause fever and chills, OKT3 is a monoclonal antibody that can cause some patients to develop pulmonary edema and severe flulike symptoms. Patients receiving this medication should have a chest x-ray immediately before drug administration and premedication with medications such as methylprednisolone (Medrol), acetaminophen (Tylenol), and an antihistamine.[34,45] Commonly used immunosuppressant medications are shown in the Medication table below and on p. 826.

MEDICATIONS USED AFTER LIVER, KIDNEY, OR PANCREAS TRANSPLANT

MEDICATION	ACTIONS	DOSAGE	SPECIAL CONSIDERATIONS
Cyclosporine (Neoral, Gengraf, Sandimmune)	Inhibition of T lymphocytes through suppression of interleukin-2 production and release	IV: 5–6 mg/kg 12 hr before transplant Maintenance: 2–10 mg/kg/day in divided doses PO: 10–18 mg/kg 4–12 hr before transplant Maintenance: 5–15 mg/kg/day in divided doses, tapered to 3–10 mg/kg/day	Monitor serum concentrations Monitor for nephrotoxicity (25%–37% incidence); hepatotoxicity (4%–7% incidence); usually responsive to dose reduction. May cause hypertension, tremors, confusion, seizures, hyperkalemia, hypomagnesemia, hemolytic-uremic syndrome, hyperlipidemia. Multiple drug, food, and herbal interactions. Brands are not bioequivalent and should not be used interchangeably. Oral dose will depend on formulation.
Tacrolimus (Prograf)	Inhibition of T lymphocytes through suppression of interleukin-2 production	Liver transplant: PO: 0.1–0.15 mg/kg/day divided into two doses given every 12 hrs IV: 0.03–0.05 mg/kg/day as continuous infusion Renal transplant: IV: 0.03–0.05 mg/kg/day as continuous infusion	Monitor serum concentrations. Monitor for nephrotoxicity and glucose intolerance. May cause hypertension, tremors, confusion, seizures, hyperkalemia hemolytic-uremic syndrome, hyperlipidemia.

Table continues on page 826

MEDICATION	ACTIONS	DOSAGE	SPECIAL CONSIDERATIONS
		PO: 0.2 mg/kg/day in 2 divided doses 12 hr apart	
Sirolimus (Rapamycin)	Inhibition of activation and proliferation of T lymphocytes by IL-2, IL-4, and IL-5	PO: 6 mg loading dose. Maintenance: 2–5 mg/day. Doses adjusted based on 24 hour trough levels.	Not recommended for use 30 days post liver transplant due to hepatic artery thrombosis. Monitor serum concentrations. Monitor CBC, renal function tests, and lipids. May cause hypertension and hyperlipidemia, bone marrow suppression, hemolytic-uremic syndrome.
Mycophenolate mofetil (CellCept)	Inhibits inosine monophosphate dehydrogenase in purine synthesis pathway, thereby inhibiting T and B lymphocytes	Renal: 1 g twice daily IV/PO. Liver: 1 g twice daily IV; 1.5 g twice daily PO.	Compatible only with D_5W infusions. May cause bone marrow suppression, diarrhea, and vomiting. Monitor CBC, LFTs. Blood levels may be monitored.
Azathioprine (Imuran)	Interferes with DNA and RNA synthesis and inhibition, differentiation, and proliferation of both T and B lymphocytes	Renal transplant: IV/PO: 2–5 mg/kg/day on day of transplant; 1–3 mg/kg/day as maintenance.	May cause bone marrow suppression, hepatotoxicity, nausea and vomiting. Monitor CBC and LFTs.
Methyl-prednisolone (Solu-Medrol)	Suppression of migration of leukocytes; inhibits lymphokine-mediated amplification of macrophages and lymphocytes	PO: 4–100 mg/day. Dose will depend on degree of immunosuppression required. IV: 100–250 mg intraoperative, then dose tapered per physician order until PO initiated. Liver: bolus of 250–500 mg IV q 24 hours × 3 for rejection.	Monitor for hyperglycemia, hypokalemia, fluid retention, hypertension, impaired wound healing, myopathy, osteoporosis, gastric ulcers, sleep disturbances, and psychosis.
Prednisone	Suppression of migration of leukocytes; inhibits lymphokine-mediated amplification of macrophages and lymphocytes	PO: 4–48 mg/day. Dose will depend on degree of immunosuppression required. Dose will depend on time since transplant, rejection history, infection history.	Monitor for same adverse effects as for methylprednisolone.

CBC = Complete blood cell count, LFTs = liver function tests.

Drug Metabolism. The metabolism of medications during the recovery from liver transplantation depends upon the degree to which the new liver functions normally. If the new liver is significantly compromised by ischemia, infection, recurrent disease, or rejection, more complex management is required. Drug toxicities may develop in the early postoperative period in the patient with delayed return of liver function and ongoing or developing renal impairment. Cyclosporine and tacrolimus may cause dose-related cholestasis and nephrotoxicity and are readily reversed with dose reduction. In addition, tacrolimus or cyclosporine activity may be inhibited by or may inhibit the metabolism of other medications. Some medications (e.g., aminoglycosides, erythromycin, ketoconazole) work synergistically with tacrolimus and cyclosporine to cause nephrotoxicity. Other medications (e.g., azithromycin [Zithromax], verapamil [Calan], fluconazole [Diflucan], erythromycin, cimetidine [Tagamet]) increase tacrolimus or cyclosporine levels, resulting in toxicity.[34,39] Some medications (e. g., phenytoin [Dilantin], rifampin [Rifadin], certain herbs) decrease tacrolimus or cyclosporine efficacy and have the potential to increase the risk of rejection.[39] Posttransplant impairment of synthesis of bile acids, reduced biliary secretion, and altered intestinal absorption may all predispose the recipient to TPN cholestasis. In the immediate postoperative period, reduced hepatic function can also result in altered metabolism of narcotics and sedatives. The dosing of these medications needs to be carefully monitored to prevent alterations in mentation.

Assessment of the Liver Transplant Patient

Assessment of the neurologic system is a priority in the liver transplant recipient who is prone to neurologic abnormalities. These abnormalities can range from profound coma to transient peripheral neuropathy. Alterations in mental status occur in 10% to 30% of recipients.[17] The patient who remains in a persistent coma may be symptomatic of primary nonfunction of the graft. Patients who are alert after surgery may still demonstrate the effects of their pretransplant encephalopathy, sleep deprivation and disorientation, or posttransplant immunosuppression (steroids, tacrolimus). Steroids can cause psychosis, mood swings, increased irritability, and severe depression. Tacrolimus can cause headaches, peripheral neuropathy, paresthesia, and tremors.[17] Seizures occurring post-transplantation are due to metabolic and electrolyte anomalies such as hyponatremia, or toxicity from tacrolimus or cyclosporine. They can also be the result of an intracranial event (e.g., stroke).[17]

Any change in level of consciousness should be evaluated by a head CT or MRI. Treatment of seizures is complicated by the fact that most antiseizure medications interfere with the metabolism of cyclosporine, tacrolimus, and sirolimus. Gabapentin (Neurontin) and levetiracetam (Keppra) are the only antiseizure medications that do not require hepatic metabolism or influence the plasma levels of immunosuppressive drugs. Intracranial hemorrhage can occur spontaneously in the setting of coagulopathies, thrombocytopenia, and hypertension. Cerebral edema is common in patients who have undergone liver transplant for acute hepatic failure. The hyperammonemia of acute hepatic failure leads to swelling of the astrocytes and increased water content of the brain. This leads to increased cerebral edema and intracranial pressure and in some cases, herniation.[26,45]

It is important to assess drains for types and amounts of drainage to ensure that postoperative bleeding, reduced bile production, and biliary leaks are identified early.[45] Monitoring of liver function tests, coagulation studies, and acid-base balance is also important. If the graft is not functioning (PNF), coagulopathies will persist, lactic acid will accumulate (leading to metabolic acidosis), and liver function tests will not begin to normalize. Liver function tests will be increased in the first few hours after transplantation, but after the first 24 hours they should begin moving toward normal. The liver function stabilization process will take several days, with the bilirubin lagging behind the AST and ALT.[45]

Liver transplant recipients frequently have some renal dysfunction along with electrolyte and acid-base disturbances before transplantation. After transplantation they have significant increases in total body sodium and water content and receive high doses of corticosteroids during the procedure, along with large volumes of blood products and crystalloid solutions. Many of the patients will have a mild metabolic acidosis on arrival to the critical care unit from lactic acid accumulation, which results from decreased tissue perfusion during the procedure as well as the large volume of blood transfusions. This period of acidosis is transient; the patients develop metabolic alkalosis from corticosteroids and the use of diuretics, producing a hypochloremic, hypokalemic alkalosis. In addition, nasogastric hydrogen ion losses and citrate in blood products contribute to a developing alkalosis. In the immediate postoperative period, the development of alkalosis and hypocalcemia can occur secondary to blood component therapy and the conversion of the citrate anticoagulant in the new liver to bicarbonate. Once the allograft begins to function well, electrolyte replacement can begin. The use of H_2 blockers and the resumption of gastric function will reduce the hydrogen ion loss.[17] The critical care nurse must monitor the comprehensive metabolic panels for alterations in liver function tests, electrolyte abnormalities, and renal function.

Oliguria is common in the early recovery phase and usually resolves within 24 hours. Many patients will have abnormal renal function preoperatively because of low serum albumin levels, diuretic use, and frequent paracentesis, resulting in low intravascular volumes and decreased renal perfusion. Patients may also suffer from HRS, which will not resolve spontaneously post-transplantation, but more gradually as the liver function improves. Postoperative oliguria may develop as a result of intraoperative blood and body fluid losses. Fluid administration and fluid shifts occurring postoperatively will resolve this condition. Administration of tacrolimus and cyclosporine doses is adjusted based upon serum creatinine levels. Accurate intake and output in conjunction with hemodynamic monitoring via a PAC is important for maintaining the patient's fluid balance.[17]

The assessment of the liver transplant patient focuses on a systemic evaluation of each organ system with integration of the laboratory values, preexisting conditions, and effects of interventions. The integration of organ systems and the effects of dysfunction on other body systems are also key to optimal patient outcomes in transplantation. Any malaise, pain or tenderness over the liver area, development of jaundice, or elevation of liver function tests is of concern.

Liver and Kidney Transplantation

Approximately 20% of patients undergoing a liver transplantation will have significant preoperative kidney dysfunction of an intrinsic cause (e.g., glomerulonephritis, polycystic kidney disease) and require a kidney transplant in addition to the liver transplant.[23] In these cases, the patient may be managed one of two ways. The liver transplant is done first; the patient is sent to critical care for stabilization and liver function determination. Approximately 4 to 5 hours later the patient is returned to the operating room, the kidney transplant performed, and the patient sent back to critical care, where monitoring of both organs will occur. The second approach would have the patient remaining in the operating room, receiving intraoperative dialysis, and then have the kidney transplantation. The patient returns to critical care upon completion of both transplants. The liver transplant gives a form of immunologic protection to the other transplanted organ, with the liver allograft enhancing the development and absorption of antibodies that would lead to rejection.[23]

MULTIDISCIPLINARY PLAN OF CARE

The primary goal in the immediate postoperative course is to ensure optimal graft function; if the graft is not functioning, the cause should be identified as early as possible. Secondary goals in the treatment of these patients are the prevention of infection and improvement in organ function of other organs affected by the liver failure. In addition to the transplant surgeon, the intensivist, the hepatologist, the respiratory therapist, the critical care nurse, the nutritionist, the radiologist, and pharmacists are all crucial to the provision of information and the development and implementation of a plan of care for the liver transplant patient. The Research Utilization box at right

examines the stress experienced by transplant patients. The Multidisciplinary Plan of Care on pp. 829-831 illustrates how the collaboration of all team members helps ensure optimal outcomes for these complex patients.

◆ RESEARCH UTILIZATION

Liver Transplant Recipients' Experiences: Stress-Inducing Factors

CLINICAL ISSUE

The purpose of this study was the identification of potentially stress-generating factors related to critical care stay from the viewpoints both of patients undergoing liver transplantation or elective major abdominal surgery and of their caregivers to identify differences and similarities that may help optimize patient care.

SUMMARY

The intensive care unit (ICU) Environmental Stressor Scale questionnaire was administered to 104 liver transplant recipients, 103 major abdominal surgery patients, 35 nurses, and 21 physicians. The ICU staff was asked to complete the questionnaire on the basis of their perception of patient stressors. Both patient groups identified the following major stressors: being unable to sleep, being in pain, having tubes in nose/mouth, missing husband/wife, and seeing family and friends only a few minutes a day. The healthcare providers correctly identified the most stressing factors for the patients, but gave them higher scores. The qualitative evaluations of potentially stress-inducing critical care situations were substantially the same in the two patient groups, but the transplant recipients seemed to feel them more acutely. Although the caregivers identified the most discomfiting situations, they overestimated the degree of stress these situations cause.

APPLICATION

The staff of critical care should be educated about and seek to understand and reduce (even by means of simple interventions) the particular causes of psychophysical stress felt by their patients.

NEED FOR FURTHER STUDY

Future studies need to identify the effects of stress-generating factors not only on other surgical populations but also on patients admitted to the intensive care environment for nonsurgical diagnosis.

Biancofiore, G., et al. (2005). Stress-inducing factors in ICUs: what liver transplant recipients experience and what caregivers perceive. *Liver Transplant, 8,* 967–972.

MULTIDISCIPLINARY PLAN OF CARE FOR LIVER, KIDNEY, AND PANCREAS TRANSPLANT PATIENTS

PROBLEM	INTERVENTION	RATIONALE	EXPECTED OUTCOME
Risk for development of graft failure	Increased monitoring of patients who present with: • Prolonged ischemia time • Prolonged operating room time • Patients who do not awaken postoperatively Monitor the following: Neurologic status (hourly) Laboratory values immediately postoperatively and when ordered: Basic electrolytes PT/INR AST/ALT Alkaline phosphatase Total bilirubin Lactate Random blood glucose Drain output Abdominal ultrasound results Changes in hemodynamic status especially CO/CI and SVR	Early identification of patients allows for early intervention by transplant team (possibly return to operating room or relisting for retransplant).	Patients at risk for primary nonfunction will be identified early. Patients at risk for continued ATN or pancreatic dysfunction will be identified early.
Risk for infection	Careful aseptic technique when doing dressing changes, line changes, etc. Monitor vital signs for changes: Elevated temperature Increase in HR Increase in CO/CI Decrease in SVR Decrease in BP Monitor laboratory values: WBC Platelet count Culture results Ensure staff and visitors wash hands before entering room and wear masks Discontinue unneeded IV lines Monitor IV lines and wounds for signs of infection Administer any antibiotics or antiviral medications as ordered	Prevention of contamination of immunocompromised patients by healthcare team. Early identification of infection will allow team to initiate early culture and treatment plan.	Patients will not develop infection; if infection does develop, it will be identified early.

Table continues on page 830

PROBLEM	INTERVENTION	RATIONALE	EXPECTED OUTCOME
	Monitor vital signs for changes that would indicate volume loss Monitor laboratory values: Hemoglobin/hematocrit Platelets	Early identification and treatment of volume loss may prevent further organ dysfunction.	Early identification and initiation of treatment will occur.
Risk of volume depletion	Monitor intake and output every 12 hours Monitor vital signs hourly for hypovolemic patterns (i.e., tachycardia, narrowed pulse pressure) Monitor patient for nausea, dizziness, orthostatic hypotension	Transplanted kidneys can have high-volume dysfunction, creating hypovolemic state. Pancreatic transplants can have hyperglycemia if there is rejection, leading to large volume losses from osmotic diuresis.	Euvolemia will be maintained.
Risk of volume overload	Monitor vital signs/filling pressures every hour and as needed Monitor urine output every 1 hr and as needed Monitor breath sounds Monitor changes in respiratory patterns Administer diuretics as ordered Renal replacement therapy as needed	Patients with renal dysfunction may not be able to accommodate volume shifts that occur with major surgery, multiple transfusions, and potential delayed kidney function.	Hemodynamic stability will be maintained.
Risk of rejection	Administer immunosuppressive medications as ordered Monitor laboratory values within first hour and then as ordered: AST/ALT Alkaline phosphatase Total bilirubin GTT Creatinine Urine amylase if bladder drainage Random blood glucose (hyperglycemia) Monitor vital signs for increased temperature	First few months after transplantation are when the risk of rejection is the highest.	If rejection occurs, prompt identification will allow for prompt treatment.

PROBLEM	INTERVENTION	RATIONALE	EXPECTED OUTCOME
Risk of malnutrition	Obtain nutritional consult Monitor caloric intake Weigh daily Maintain tube feeding/total parenteral nutrition until oral intake can sustain caloric needs	The liver transplant patient is very malnourished before transplantation. The caloric needs of all patients post-transplantation are increased, and optimizing their nutritional intake is important to good outcomes.	With optimal nutrition, wound healing, mobilization, and ventilation will be improved.
Risk of hypertension	Monitor blood pressure every 1 hr and as needed Administer antihypertensive medications promptly Monitor central venous pressure/pulmonary artery pressure every hour and as needed	Because of postoperative stressors, pain, shivering, anxiety, fluid overload, tacrolimus or cyclosporine therapy, and renal dysfunction, patient may develop hypertension, which may increase risk for venous congestion in newly transplanted liver, dehiscence of arterial anastomosis, and intracranial bleed.	Control of blood pressure and fluid volume will minimize postoperative complications.
Risk of alterations in levels of consciousness	Monitor neurologic status Monitor liver function by evaluating laboratory data Monitor effects of immunosuppressive therapy	Encephalopathy that existed before liver transplant may require time to fully resolve. Immunosuppressive therapy can cause alterations in perceptions and behaviors.	Normal neurologic functioning will be observed and side effects of immunosuppressive therapy will be minimized.

ALT = Alanine transaminase, AST = aspartate transaminase, ATN = acute tubular necrosis, BP = blood pressure, CI = cardiac index, CO = cardiac output, GTT = glucose tolerance test, HR = heart rate, INR = international normalized ratio, SVR = systemic vascular resistance, PT = prothrombin time.

CONCLUSIONS

The care of the liver transplant patient presents the critical care team with one of the more complex and challenging endeavors. Early recognition of complications and communication of these findings allow for prompt intervention and progress toward optimal outcomes for these patients.

RENAL TRANSPLANTATION

Patients at Risk

Renal transplantation offers a potential to return to a healthy life. It has many advantages over dialysis, the primary one being an improved quality of life. With the improvements in tissue typing, immunosuppression, and postoperative treatment, the patient and graft survival rates continue to increase.[6] Today there are more than 75,000 patients waiting for a kidney transplant and more than 4100 awaiting a kidney-pancreas transplant.[47] In 2006, there were 17,000 kidney transplants and 924 kidney-pancreas transplants performed in the United States.[47] The main causes of the renal failure leading to transplantation are diabetes mellitus, hypertension, and glomerulonephritis. The patients awaiting kidney transplantation are at increased risk for cardiovascular, pulmonary, and neurologic complications in addition to an increased risk of infection because of their immunocompromised state.[6] Currently, most patients undergoing kidney transplantation do not require admission to critical care unless they have comorbidities increasing their postoperative risk or intraoperative problems develop that require close monitoring. The most common complication requiring a kidney transplantation patient to be admitted to critical care is respiratory distress.[42]

Kidney transplant patients may receive their organs from non–heart-beating donors (the heart has arrested and the donor is declared deceased according to circulatory-respiratory criteria), from deceased donors (brain death determination has been made), or from living donors.[7] The surgery is usually 3 hours in duration. The donated kidney is implanted in the right or left lower quadrant of the recipient, determined by the anatomy of the donated kidney, through a hockey stick–shaped incision extending from the iliac crest to the symphysis pubis (Figure 30-4).

Postoperative Care

The complications occurring most often following kidney transplantation are urologic complications; hemodynamic instability; hypertension; fluid, electrolyte, or

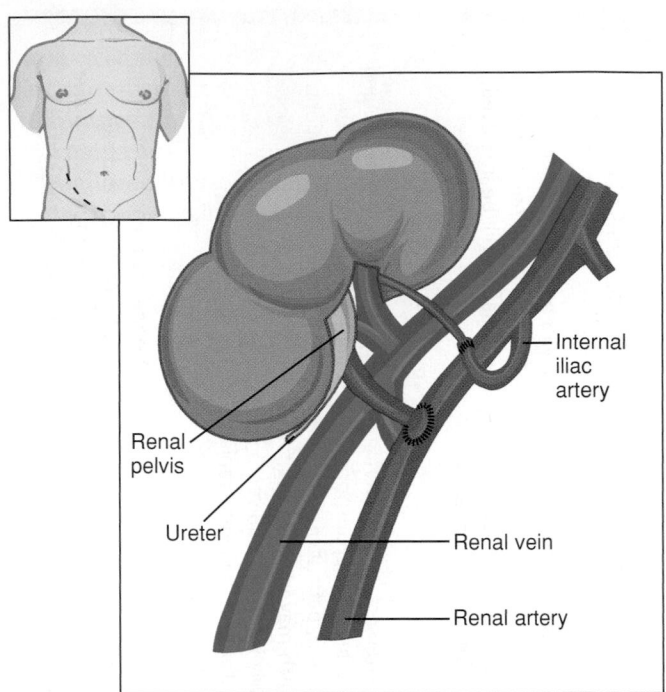

♦FIGURE 30-4 Standard lower-quadrant incision for renal allograft.

acid-base imbalances; and ongoing renal dysfunction. Infection, pancytopenia, recurrent renal disease, and hyperlipidemia may also develop in weeks to months after the transplant.[6,7]

Urologic and Vascular Complications. Urologic complications are more common (1% to 3%) when wound healing is impaired.[7,18] These complications can include the development of a lymphocele (a pocket of lymph accumulation); compression of the iliac vein, causing ipsilateral leg swelling; hematoma, leading to pain; infection; and ureteral stenosis or occlusion. Ureteral obstruction can be diagnosed by hydronephrosis visualized on ultrasound. It may be the result of blood clots, poor implantation, ureteral sloughing, or ureteral kinking. Symptoms may be pain over the transplanted kidney or lower abdominal pain, decreased urine output, and increased blood urea nitrogen (BUN) and serum creatinine levels.[7,18] Stenting or surgical repair may be required to reduce the obstruction.

Urine leaks from the anastomotic site may occur in the early postoperative period or at the onset of post-transplant diuresis. They may be the result of technical problems (e.g., a non-watertight reimplantation of the ureter) or develop from ureteral sloughing secondary to disruption of ureteral blood flow or a tight ureteral stenosis. Urine leaks are characterized by decreased urine output with increasing serum creatinine level and severe pain. This can also be indicative of rejection.

An ultrasound should be performed to determine if there is a surgical problem and if a biopsy is necessary. If the symptoms are due to a urologic complication, reinsertion of the Foley catheter is required, and the patient is returned to the operating room for reexploration.[18]

Pseudoaneurysms secondary to infection, arterial thrombus, or venous thrombosis require early identification in order to preserve the organ. Arterial or venous thrombus can occur as early as the first 2 to 3 days after transplantation and is characterized by decreased urine output, swelling, and pain. Late renal arterial stenosis leading to hypertension and graft dysfunction may require dilation and stenting or surgical intervention.[6]

Postoperative bleeding may occur when the small vessels in the renal hilum have increased perfusion. The bleeding of these vessels may not have been apparent intraoperatively secondary to vasospasm of these small vessels.[18] Renal ultrasound with Doppler is performed in the first 24 hours postoperatively to provide early identification of these problems.

Hemodynamic Instability. Prolonged cold ischemic time can result in delayed function of the transplanted kidney, leading to intravascular volume problems. These patients can be volume overloaded before dialysis has been restarted postoperatively if oliguria or anuria is present. Volume depletion may occur in the patient with high-output renal failure, requiring close monitoring of central venous pressure (CVP), blood pressure (BP), and heart rate.[5–7]

Hypertension. About 60% to 80% of kidney transplant recipients have multifactorial etiology of their hypertension.[6,21–23] Some of the etiologies include the effects of retained native kidneys, parenchymal disease of the transplanted organ, effects of immunotherapy, renal artery stenosis, and weight gain.[7] Preoperative hypertension is rarely cured by kidney transplantation and may continue to be a problem in the postoperative care of the kidney transplant patient. Cardiovascular death, as a result of myocardial infarction, stroke, or complications of peripheral vascular disease, is the most common cause of death in renal transplant patients.[6,21–23]

Electrolyte and Acid-Base Imbalances. Electrolyte imbalances of hyperkalemia, hyperphosphatemia, and hyponatremia exist before kidney transplantation. Patients are dialyzed before surgery to minimize the impact of these imbalances during the intraoperative period. In the postoperative period, these electrolyte imbalances may continue or can be exacerbated by the transplant. Surgical tissue destruction coupled with the impaired renal function leads to further hyperkalemia, a frequent postoperative complication. Hyponatremia can also occur with the excessive administration of hypotonic fluids in the presence of renal impairment. Hypomagnesemia is a manifestation of high-output acute tubular necrosis, and hypophosphatemia results when the glomerular filtration rate (GFR) suddenly normalizes in patients with preexisting hyperparathyroidism, which is common in patients with renal disease. In addition to these imbalances, the impaired renal excretion of hydrogen ion after surgery can lead to metabolic acidosis. Close monitoring of electrolytes and acid base is essential in the early postoperative days.[5,6,18,23]

Renal Dysfunction. Patients receiving deceased donor kidneys with preservation times of greater than 24 hours may experience delayed graft function. Renal dysfunction in the postoperative period is characterized as anuria (less than 50 ml/24 hour) or oliguria (less than 400 ml/24 hour) and is the result of acute tubular necrosis (ATN). However, urine leak, ureteral obstruction, and vascular thrombosis must be ruled out. The period of ATN can last from several days to weeks, with gradually improving kidney function. These patients are at high risk for developing fluid overload in the immediate postoperative period. Most patients can be supported by dialysis until their urine output increases and their serum creatinine and BUN levels begin to normalize.[7]

Polyuria is commonly observed after living related kidney donation and is the result of osmotic diuresis in the face of rapidly normalizing GFR. In some renal transplant patients, the development of ATN creates a renal concentration deficit that results in increased urine output with azotemia. These patients are at high risk of dehydration unless their volume status is carefully monitored and maintained.

Delayed graft function can result in the need for dialysis in the first few weeks after transplantation. Ischemic ATN occurs in 10% to 40% of patients and carries with it the increased risk of acute rejection.[6] In renal transplant patients, the development of acute renal failure after initial graft function has been established can be caused by a variety of complications (Box 30-2).

Rejection. Rejection is always a risk in transplantation as the body recognizes the transplanted kidney as non-self. Hyperacute rejection is mediated by preformed antibodies and can occur immediately following the vascular anastomosis or days later (delayed hyperacute rejection). This condition is characterized by necrosis of parenchymal tissue, resulting in a toxic state that progresses to disseminated intravascular coagulation. There is an abrupt decrease in renal function, with rapidly increasing serum creatinine level, fever, malaise, graft tenderness, and oliguria. This condition often leads to graft loss even with antirejection treatment.[5,6,14]

Box 30-2

Etiologies of Renal Failure After Initial Graft Function

- Volume depletion
- Arterial thrombosis
- Venous thrombosis
- Anastomotic stricture
- Obstruction by perinephric fluid (hematoma or lymphocele)
- Drug-induced nephrotoxicity
- Allergic interstitial nephritis
- Hemolytic-uremic syndrome

Acute cellular rejection can occur within the first 6 months after transplantation and may not be manifested as an elevated serum creatinine level.[5,6,14] It is instead characterized by fever, chills, myalgias, and arthralgias and reversed with immunosuppressive treatment.

Chronic rejection or chronic allograft nephropathy occurs most commonly after the first 6 months posttransplant. This condition is characterized by a slow decrease in the GFR with a slow increase in the serum creatinine level accompanied by proteinuria and a worsening of the patient's systemic hypertension. It can be due to inadequate immunosuppression or non-immunosuppressive factors. The non-immunosuppression factors include hypertension, hyperlipidemia, nephrotoxicity, viral infections, ischemia and reperfusion injury, or the use of herbal supplements. Some patients may develop frank nephrotic syndrome (syndrome of massive protienuria) with edema, hypoalbuminemia, and hyperlipidemia.[5,6,14]

Infection. Infection in the kidney transplant patient is a significant concern because of the higher amounts of immunosuppression received, the alteration in the body's normal defenses because of surgery, and the impact of end-stage renal disease. Comorbidities of diabetes mellitus, lupus, malnutrition, and increased age may compound the effects of the immune response.[7] The common infections in the first month are bacterial and fungal wound infections, urinary tract infections, nosocomial pneumonitis, and line-associated bacteremias and fungemias.[6] Viral infections, especially those of cytomegalovirus, Epstein-Barr, herpes simplex, and varicella-zoster, may be reactivated in the transplant patient because of the pharmacologic immunosuppression and donor recipient mismatching.[7] Infection with parvovirus or human polyomavirus BKV (BK virus) may also occur and can lead to graft dysfunction and potential graft loss.[15,29]

KIDNEY-PANCREAS OR PANCREAS-ONLY TRANSPLANTATION

Patients at Risk

Pancreatic transplantation is a method of physiologically controlling glucose metabolism. Currently, there are approximately 1700 patients awaiting pancreas-only transplants and more than 2400 awaiting kidney-pancreas transplants. In 2004 there were 604 pancreas-only transplants and 880 kidney-pancreas transplants.[47] Pancreatic transplantation can occur in one of three ways: pancreas alone; pancreas simultaneously transplanted with a kidney; or pancreas transplanted after an earlier kidney transplant. The majority of recipients for a pancreatic transplant have type 1 diabetes mellitus. Select type 2 diabetes patients who are insulin dependent and have diabetic nephropathy may be considered. Recipients of a pancreatic transplant are sent to critical care for 24 hours to ensure glycemic control and monitor for the development of pancreatitis or rejection. The pancreas is a very immunogenic organ: the risk of rejection is higher than that for other organs.[23,40]

The pancreas transplant can be performed with either bowel (enteric) or bladder drainage (Figure 30-5). Enteric drainage has distinct advantages over bladder drainage and is therefore more frequently used today. The use of enteric drainage has eliminated the complications of acidosis and dehydration as well as many of the urologic complications. There are, however, increased risks for abdominal complications with enteric drainage, such as peritonitis. In patients receiving a pancreas transplant

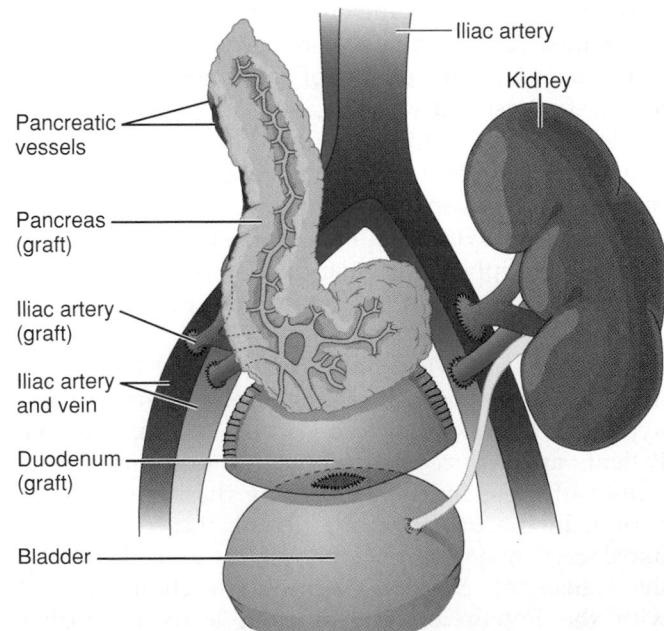

⬥FIGURE 30-5 Simultaneous kidney-pancreas transplant.

after a kidney transplant, enteric drainage is preferred because it allows for better monitoring of the pancreas graft independent of the kidney transplant.[12,16,40]

Postoperative Complications

Postoperative complications of pancreatic transplantation include vascular complications, acidosis and dehydration, rejection infection, hematuria, glycemic control, pancreatitis, and urethritis.

Vascular Complications. Vascular thrombosis occurs in 3% to 10% of transplanted organs.[23] It is a very early complication, occurring within 48 hours of transplantation. The thrombosis is usually in the pancreas portal vein. The cause is believed to be associated with reperfusion pancreatitis and the relatively low-flow state of the transplanted pancreas. Anticoagulation is the treatment for this condition. In patients who receive a simultaneous kidney-pancreas transplant, if the anticoagulation is ineffective, splenic vein thrombosis can occur. Recipients who receive a pancreas alone are at risk for thrombosis of the transplanted organ and necrosis if the anticoagulation is ineffective.[23]

Acidosis and Dehydration. In patients with a bladder-drained pancreas, bicarbonate and water secretions are not reabsorbed in the distal intestine but instead are washed out of the bladder with the urine. Without replacement of the lost water and bicarbonate, these patients develop severe metabolic acidosis and dehydration with orthostatic hypotension. Serum bicarbonate levels less than 10 mmol/L and potassium levels greater than 6 mmol/L can develop. As a result of these conditions, patients are at an increased risk for electrocardiographic changes and dysrhythmias. These conditions do not occur in patients with enteric drainage.[2,7,8]

Immunosuppression. Management of immunosuppression is critical to long-term outcomes after transplantation. Intense immunosuppression prevents rejection, but increases the risk of infection and malignancy and may contribute to dysfunction of other organ systems. Weak immunosuppression decreases the risk of infection and malignancy, but increases the risk of rejection and subsequent transplanted organ dysfunction. Consequently, appropriate immunosuppression (see the Medication table on pp. 825-826) requires careful attention and close monitoring and is always individualized.

Rejection. Early detection of graft rejection is a challenge. In recipients with simultaneous kidney-pancreas transplant, kidney dysfunction has been used as a monitor of both kidney and pancreas rejection. In bladder-drained pancreas transplants, monitoring of the urinary amylase level provides information on the function of the pancreatic graft. With more enteric drainage transplants being performed, hyperglycemia can be a sign of rejection. The use of radionuclide pancreas examinations and in some cases pancreatic biopsies also can provide information for timely diagnosis and treatment of rejection.[8]

Infection. The most common infection in the pancreas transplant patient with bladder drainage is urinary tract infections, which occur in more than 35% of patients.[40] The risk of infection is increased because of diabetes, recent urinary tract surgery, an indwelling Foley catheter, immunosuppression therapy, and an increase in the urine pH from the pancreatic bicarbonate secretions. Recurrent urinary tract infections may also develop. Common organisms are *Staphylococcus, Enterococcus, Pseudomonas,* and *Candida;* thus the risk for septicemia is high.[6,7]

Hematuria. Hematuria occurs in 10% to 15% of bladder-drained pancreatic recipients.[40] It is usually a result of ischemia-reperfusion injury to the duodenal mucosa or to a bleeding vessel on the suture line that is aggravated by the anticoagulation protocols. The hematuria may occur for 1 to 2 weeks or more. Hematuria is usually self-limiting; the main concern is prevention of urethral obstruction from blood clots.

Glycemic Control. In the first few days to weeks after pancreatic transplantation there is a dramatic improvement in glucose control; however, hyperglycemia may occur as a result of the steroids used for immunosuppression. This usually responds to dose reduction. Occasionally, the hyperglycemia is due to delayed graft function. When hyperglycemia presents suddenly, it may be the result of pancreas graft thrombosis and requires an ultrasound evaluation. If the thrombosis occurs early or there is associated graft pain and fever, the patient may return to the operating room for reexploration.[6]

Pancreatitis. Almost all patients will have some degree of pancreatitis (see Chapter 28). Temporary elevation of serum amylase levels for 48 to 96 hours after transplantation is common. These episodes are usually transient and mild.[23] Allograft pancreatitis may be caused by reperfusion injury, donor instability, increased age of the donor, or increased ischemic time or rejection. In patients with enteric drainage, the development of a bowel obstruction can lead to pancreatitis. Patients with bladder drainage can develop reflux pancreatitis. This may be the result of urinary retention and reflux to the pancreas via the duodenal cuff as a result of diabetic bladder dysfunction, bladder outlet obstruction, or a urinary tract infection (UTI), resulting in loss of bladder tone, reflux, and microbial irrigation. In the absence of retention, obstruction, or UTI, it may be caused by disruption of bladder filling pressures (bladder nerves sense when the bladder is full, usually about 300 to 500 ml of urine).[6,7,23]

Urethritis. Many patients who receive bladder-drained grafts suffer from urologic complications secondary to altered urinary pH causing mucosal injury secondary to pancreatic digestive enzymes. They are at increased risk for developing urethral strictures and cystitis with inflammation and hemorrhage. In worse cases, they can develop ureteral disruption. Female recipients are at risk for developing excoriating lesions of the perineum after a vaginal yeast infection; 9% to 28% will develop gross hematuria, anastomotic leaks, graft pancreatitis, rejection, thrombosis, or CMV duodenitis. Approximately 20% of bladder drainage recipients will require enteric conversion.[6,7]

Assessment

Nursing assessment of the kidney or kidney-pancreas transplant patient focuses on fluid and electrolyte management and prevention of infection. In addition, for those patients who received a pancreas transplant, glycemic monitoring is crucial. Accurate intake and output measurement and monitoring CVP pressures are key to maintaining fluid hemostasis. Evaluation and notification of the healthcare team of any electrolyte or glucose abnormalities and attention to electrolyte balance correction will minimize these patients' risk of complications. Assessment of vital signs, skin temperature, and wound integrity for early signs of infection can prevent the development of more serious infections and sepsis.

MULTIDISCIPLINARY PLAN OF CARE

The primary goal in caring for the kidney or kidney-pancreas transplant patient is to maintain fluid, electrolyte, and glucose balance and to prevent infection. In addition to the physicians, the advanced-practice nurses, the critical care nurse, the pharmacist, and the dietitian are crucial to the development and implementation of a plan of care for these patients. The collaboration of these team members results in a comprehensive plan of care such as the one shown in the Multidisciplinary Plan of Care on pp. 829-831.

HOSPITALIZATIONS FOR NONTRANSPLANT CONCERNS

With the number of transplants being performed annually in the United States increasing and the survival rates continuing to increase, critical care teams are more likely to see patients admitted with complications from their transplant or for non–transplant-related causes such as motor vehicle accidents or myocardial infarctions. Transplant patients are lifelong immunocompromised patients because of their regimen of immunosuppressive medications. Inadequate immunosuppression can lead to rejection, whereas too much immunosuppression can lead to increased risk of infection. Their immunosuppressive regimen also puts them at increased risk for the development of malignant disease. The malignant diseases include cancer of the skin, lips, and cervix and lymphomas. It is important to note that regardless of the reason the patient is admitted, the transplant team should be notified to evaluate the immunosuppression regimen and provide consultation on the role the transplant is playing in the current reason for hospitalization.

CONCLUSIONS

The complexity of postoperative care is increased in transplant patients. Their special needs require attention to detail and identification of the nuances that can indicate the development of a complication that would place both the patient and the transplanted organ at risk.

REFERENCES

1. Abecassis, M., et al. (2000). Liver transplantation. In F. P. Stuart, M. Abecassis, & D. B. Kaufman (Eds.), *Organ transplantation.* Georgetown, Tex: Landes Bioscience.
2. Adame, M., et al. (2004). A prospective comparison of bladder versus enteric drainage in vascularized transplantation. *Transplant Proc, 36,* 1524–1525.
3. Baccarani, U., et al. (2001). Percutaneous mechanical fragmentation and stent placement for the treatment of early posttransplantation portal vein thrombosis. *Transplantation, 72,* 1572–1574.
4. Bakthavatsalam, R., et al. (2001). Rescue of acute portal vein thrombosis after liver transplantation using a cavoportal shunt at re-transplantation. *Am J Transplant, 1,* 284–287.
5. Barone, C. P., Martin-Watson, A. I., & Barone, G. W. (2004). The postoperative care of the adult renal transplant recipient. *MedSurg Nurs, 13,* 296–303.
6. Bartucci, M. R., & Hricik, D. E. (2002). Kidney transplantation. In S. Cupples (Ed.), *Solid organ transplantation.* New York: Springer.
7. Bartucci, M. R. (1999). Kidney transplantation: state of the art. *AACN Clin Issues, 10,* 153–163.
8. Boggi, U., et al. (2005). Ninety-five percent insulin independence rate 3 years after pancreas transplantation along with portoenteric drainage. *Transplant Proc, 37,* 1274–1277.
9. Branch, M. S., & Clavien, P. (2001). Biliary complications following liver transplantation. In P. G. Killenberg (Ed.), *Medical care of the liver transplant patient* (2nd ed.). Malden, Mass: Blackwell.
10. Chiu, L. M., Domagala, B. M., & Park, J. M. (2004). Management of opportunistic infections in solid-organ transplantation. *Prog Transplant, 14,* 114–129.

11. Concepcion, C., et al. (2003). Effects of orthotopic liver transplantation on vasoactive systems and renal function in patients with advanced liver cirrhosis. *Digest Dis Sci, 48,* 179–186.

12. Conway, P., et al. (1998). Simultaneous kidney pancreas transplantation: patient issues and nursing interventions. *ANNA J, 25,* 455–460.

13. Curran, C. (2005). Adult-to-adult living donor liver transplantation: history, current practice, and implications for the future. *Prog Transplant, 15,* 36–42.

14. Danovitch, G. M. (2001). Immunosuppressive medications and protocols for kidney transplantation. In G. M. Danovitch (Ed.), *Handbook of kidney transplantation.* Philadelphia: Lippincott Williams & Wilkins.

15. deBruyn, G., & Limaye, A. P. (2004). BK virus-associated nephropathy in kidney transplant recipients. *Rev Med Virol, 14,* 193–205.

16. Dimercurio, B., Henry, L., & Kirk, A. D. (2002). Simultaneous kidney-pancreas transplantation. In S. Cupples (Ed.), *Solid organ transplantation.* New York: Springer.

17. Everson, G. T., & Kam, I. (2001). Immediate postoperative care. In W. C. Maddrey, E. R. Schiff, & M. F. Sorrell (Eds.), *Transplantation of the liver.* Philadelphia: Lippincott Williams & Wilkins.

18. Gritach, H. A., & Rosenthal, J. T. (2001). The transplant operation and its surgical complications. In G. M. Danovitch (Ed.), *Handbook of kidney transplantation* (3rd ed.). Philadelphia: Lippincott Williams & Wilkins.

19. Hasse, J. M. (2001). Nutrition assessment and support of organ transplant recipients. *JPEN/J Parenter Enteral Nutr, 25,* 120–132.

20. Jagannath, S., & Kalloo, A. N. (2002). Biliary complications after liver transplantation. *Curr Treat Options Gastroenterol, 5,* 101–112.

21. Jardin, A. G. (2005). Assessing the relative risk of cardiovascular disease among renal transplant patients receiving tacrolimus or cyclosporine. *Transplant Int, 18,* 379–384.

22. Kaufman, D. B., et al. (2004). Immunosuppression: practice and trends. *Am J Transplant, 9*(suppl), 38–53.

23. Kaufman, D. B. (2003). Kidney transplantation. In F. P. Stuart, M. Abecassis, & D. B. Kaufman (Eds.), *Organ transplantation.* Georgetown, Tex: Landes Bioscience.

24. Lilly, L. B., Ding, J., & Levy, G. A. (2001). The immunology of hepatic allograft rejection. In W. C. Maddrey, E. R. Schiff, & M. F. Sorrell (Eds.), *Transplantation of the liver.* Philadelphia: Lippincott Williams & Wilkins.

25. Lowell, J. A., & Shaw, B. W. (2001). Critical care of liver transplant recipients. In W. C. Maddrey, E. R. Schiff, & M. F. Sorrell (Eds.), *Transplantation of the liver.* Philadelphia: Lippincott Williams & Wilkins.

26. Lowell, J. A., & Shaw, B. W., Jr. (2001). Critical care of liver transplant recipients: selected topics. In W. C. Maddrey, E. R. Schiff, & M. F. Sorrell (Eds.), *Transplantation of the liver.* Philadelphia: Lippincott Williams & Wilkins.

27. Manzarbeitia, C. (2005). Liver transplantation. In P. Tushar, et al. (Ed.), *Emedicine.* www.emedicine.com.

28. Merritt, W. T. (2005). Issues affecting liver transplantation. *Best Pract Res Clin Anaesthesiol, 19,* 17–34.

29. Moudgil, A. (2001). Association of parvovirus B19 infection with idiopathic collapsing glomerulopathy. *Kidney Int, 59,* 2126–2133.

30. Neuberger, J. (2000). Liver transplantation. *J Hepatol, 32,* 198–207.

31. Oh, C. K., et al. (2004). Independent predictors for primary nonfunction after liver transplantation. *Yonsei Med J, 45,* 1155–1161.

32. Paya, C. V. (2002). Prevention of fungal infection in transplantation. *Transplant Infect Dis, 4*(suppl 3), 46–51.

33. Penko, M. E., & Tirbasco, D. (1999). An overview of liver transplantation. *AACN Clin Issues, 10,* 176–184.

34. Pirsch, J. D., & Douglas, M. J. (2002). Liver transplantation. In S. Cupples (Ed.), *Solid organ transplantation.* New York: Springer.

35. Qian, Y. B., et al. (2004). Risk factors for biliary complications after liver transplantation. *Arch Surg, 139,* 1101–1105.

36. Randhawa, P. S., & Shapiro, R. (2005). Chronic renal failure after liver transplantation. *Am J Transplant, 5,* 967–968.

37. Roberts, J. P., et al. (2003). Liver and intestine transplantation. *Am J Transplant, 3*(suppl), 78–90.

38. Russ, P. D., et al. (2004). Liver transplantation, complications. *Emedicine.* www.emedicine.com.

39. Speeg, K. V., Halff, G. A., & Schenker, S. (2001). In W. C. Maddrey, E. R. Schiff, & M. F. Sorrell (Eds.), *Transplantation of the liver.* Philadelphia: Lippincott Williams & Wilkins.

40. Steen, D. C. (1999). The current state of pancreas transplantation. *AACN Clin Issues, 10,* 164–175.

41. Stieber, A. C., Makowka, L., & Starzl, T. E. (1992). In T. E. Starzl, R. Shapiro, & R. L. Simmons (Eds.), *Atlas of organ transplantation.* New York: Gower Medical Publishing.

42. Subhash, H. S., et al. (2002). Characteristics, survival, and prognostic factors of renal transplant recipients requiring admission to medical intensive care unit. *Indian J Crit Care Med, 6,* 96–99.

43. Suhocki, P., Chari, R., & Clavien, P. (2001). Vascular aspects of liver transplantation. In P. G. Killenberg (Ed.), *Medical care of the liver transplant patient* (2nd ed.). Malden, Mass: Blackwell.

44. Swanson, R. L., Wiesner, R. H., & Krowka, M. (2005). Natural history of hepatopulmonary syndrome: impact of liver transplantation. *Hepatology, 41,* 1122–1129.

45. Tart, J., & Gentile, J. (2001). Recovery following liver transplant. In P. G. Killenberg (Ed.), *Medical care of the liver transplant patient* (2nd ed.). Malden, Mass: Blackwell.

46. University of Southern California Liver Newsletter. (2005). www.surgery.usc.edu/divisions/hep.

47. UNOS Statistics. (2006). *OPTN: organ procurement and transplantation network.* www.unos.org.

48. Wang, Z. F., & Liu, C. (2004). Liver retransplantation: indications and outcomes. *Hepatobiliary Pancreat Dis Int, 3,* 175–178.

49. Wiesner, R. H., et al. (2005). Mycophenolate mofetil combination therapy improves long-term outcome after liver transplantation in patients with and without hepatitis C. *Liver Transplant, 11,* 750–759.

UNIT 7 RENAL

CHAPTER 31

Electrolyte Emergencies

Michael W. Day and Rhonda S. Milam

Electrolyte imbalances impact both the mortality and morbidity of critically ill patients and can present a range of issues that often require the efforts of a multidisciplinary team. Electrolyte imbalances may present as simple routine therapy and intervention addressed every day (e.g., intravenous [IV] potassium boluses). Typically, electrolyte imbalances are the result of an underlying disease, but may also be caused by a patient's behaviors (e.g., a patient with a psychiatric disorder who drinks 10 gallons of water in less than 24 hours). Electrolyte imbalances may be iatrogenic, as seen with the excessive use of diuretics or prolonged bedrest. Electrolyte imbalances may present as a minor problem or represent a life-threatening emergency, requiring immediate treatment.

The electrolyte imbalances most commonly seen in the critical care setting are those involving potassium, sodium, and calcium. Phosphorus and magnesium imbalances are less commonly discussed in nursing literature. As a result, there may be less general knowledge regarding the importance of these electrolytes in body functions, the assessment and cause of their abnormalities, and an understanding of the appropriate therapy.

While laboratory-derived serum electrolyte values are usually used as the reference points for these imbalances, it needs to be understood that these values must be assessed in the context of the patient's disease process, along with a physical examination and an understanding of the patient's comorbidities and current treatments. Electrolyte reference values will differ from reference to reference and from institution to institution, depending upon the method of analysis used.[31] In the clinical setting, it is important to understand and have access to the specific institution's reference values, often printed on laboratory readouts.

An additional issue for consideration is that different parts of the world use different units of measurement. Countries that use Système Internationale (SI) units of measurement convey electrolyte concentrations in terms of a millimole (mmol), which is equal to one-thousandth of the molecular weight of the electrolyte in question. Healthcare institutions in the United States typically report some electrolyte concentrations (potassium and sodium) in terms of milliequivalents per liter (mEq/L),

which is equal to the atomic weight of an electrolyte, in milligrams, divided by its valence. Calcium, magnesium, and phosphorus are usually reported in milligrams per deciliter (mg/dl). For those electrolytes that are measured in mEq/L, a simple conversion to mmol/L units is found by dividing the mEq/L by the chemical's valence (mmol/L = mEq/L divided by the valence). However, a significant amount of confusion exists when comparing the remaining electrolytes (calcium, magnesium, and phosphorus) because they are measured in milligrams per deciliter (mg/dl) in the United States and millimoles per liter (mmol/L) with the SI system.[24] For clarity, it must be noted not only that the reference measurement is different (mg vs. mmol) but also that the reference volumes for each are different (mg/*dl* vs. mmol/*L*). For ease of reference and to avoid confusion on the part of the reader of this chapter, both measurement systems will be displayed when discussing the various electrolyte levels. The electrolyte levels used as both "normal" and excessively high and low "panic" levels in this chapter are derived from Jacobs, DeMott, and Oxley and are specific to the adult patient (Table 31-1).[15] It is important to note that the "panic" levels from this source are often significantly beyond the "normal" upper and lower limits. If an electrolyte level is outside the "normal" range but has not reached the "panic" limit, it needs to be critically evaluated in the context of the patient's condition and may require emergency treatment to prevent patient harm.

The most effective prevention for electrolyte imbalances is to maintain adequate nutrition. In a normal, healthy state, adults seldom need any electrolyte supplementation. However, as noted above, electrolyte abnormalities may be caused in a normally healthy patient by patient behaviors or by therapies designed to treat a specific disease.

APPLIED PHYSIOLOGY

Electrolytes are found throughout the body in bone, muscle, and cartilage, bound to protein, and in intracellular and extracellular fluid as "free" or "ionized"

TABLE 31-1 Normal Adult Serum Levels of Electrolytes

ELECTROLYTE	U.S. UNITS	SYSTÈME INTERNATIONALE (SI) UNITS
Potassium	3.5-5.5 mEq/L	3.5-5.5 mmol/L
Sodium	135-145 mEq/L	135-145 mmol/L
Calcium		
Serum	8.6-10 mg/dl	2.15-2.50 mmol/L
Ionized	4.64-5.28 mg/dl	1.16-1.32 mmol/L
Magnesium	1.5-2.3 mg/dl	0.62-0.95 mmol/L
Phosphorus	2.5-4.5 mg/dl	0.81-1.45 mmol/L

Data from reference 15.

TABLE 31-2 Distribution of Electrolytes in Body Compartments

	EXTRACELLULAR FLUID (ECF) (mEq/L)	INTRACELLULAR FLUID (ICF) (mEq/L)
Potassium	5	156
Sodium	142	10
Calcium	5	4
Magnesium	2	26
Phosphate	2	40-95

electrolytes in the blood's serum. Electrolytes are either positively charged ions, referred to as cations, or negatively charge ions, referred to as anions. Each electrolyte charge is shown by a superscript "+" or "−" after the chemical symbol (e.g., K^+ for potassium and Na^+ for sodium).[14] Measurements of electrolytes are done using the patient's blood serum or plasma (values for serum and plasma are essentially interchangeable).[24] Serum electrolyte measurements are the basis for diagnosing and treating electrolyte imbalances. Electrolytes are actively shifted back and forth between the intracellular fluid (ICF) and extracellular fluid (ECF) by the various mechanisms of the cellular membrane. The shifting of

electrolytes creates electrical potentials that occur at the cellular level, allowing each cell to complete its specific function. The relative distribution of the various electrolytes in both intracellular and extracellular fluids is displayed in Table 31-2. Electrolyte concentrations are also affected by the acid-base balance; this issue is addressed in Chapter 32. Each electrolyte is regulated by specific pathways within the body; each has specific roles in maintaining homeostasis.[24]

MULTIDISCIPLINARY PLAN OF CARE

The ideal means of treating electrolyte imbalances is prevention. If a patient has mild electrolyte disturbances, either high or low, the initial treatment is to seek out and address the causes of the imbalances. The intent of electrolyte imbalance treatment is to prevent harm to the patient, without necessarily returning the electrolyte to a "normal" level.[24] Treatment should always be focused on the patient, never on the lab value itself.

POTASSIUM

Applied Physiology

Potassium (K^+) is the major intracellular electrolyte. Approximately 98% of the body's total potassium is normally stored inside the cells, and 2% is maintained in the ECF. This is referred to as the potassium gradient.[5] This gradient regulates the electrical membrane potential of both muscle and nerve cells, affecting the excitability of both types of cells, and contributes to contractions of skeletal, smooth, and cardiac muscles.[14] The most life-threatening issue related to potassium imbalance occurs in cardiac conduction and contraction. Extremes of potassium cause significant conduction defects and dysrhythmias. A low serum potassium level will decrease the resting potential of a cell; thus the cell will require a greater stimulus to reach the threshold potential, resulting in decreased contractile force of the heart and delayed conduction, causing widened QRS complexes and bradycardia. With an elevated serum potassium level, the resting potential of a cell will be increased, requiring less stimulus to reach the threshold potential of the cell, making it more likely the patient will develop ventricular dysrhythmias. In addition, the rate of repolarization is increased with high serum potassium levels and decreased with low serum potassium levels. Because of its importance in a variety of systems, even small changes in serum potassium concentrations may produce significant changes in cellular functioning.[5,31]

Potassium is important for maintenance of the osmotic gradient within cells, maintenance of acid-base balance, and concentration of urine by the kidney. Potassium is an important component in energy metabolism, including the conversion of carbohydrates to energy, amino acids into protein, and glucose into glycogen.[31]

Dietary intake is the normal source of potassium, which may be absent in a hospitalized patient receiving nothing by mouth (NPO), if also receiving no supplemental nutrition. Potassium's excretion is primarily regulated by the kidneys. However, because the kidneys may take several hours to excrete a significant load of potassium, it can shift back and forth between the ECF and ICF quite rapidly, temporarily normalizing serum potassium levels.

In the kidney, potassium is initially freely filtered out of the blood as it passes through the glomerulus. Potassium is selectively reabsorbed from the filtrate in the proximal tubule and loop of Henle and may, depending on serum levels, be secreted into the filtrate in the distal and collecting tubules and eliminated in the urine. This mechanism allows the body to very closely regulate potassium levels, based on the ECF concentration. Aldosterone plays an important role in regulating both potassium and sodium concentrations. Aldosterone causes the kidneys to retain sodium at the expense of potassium, which is then lost into the urine. Renal regulation of potassium is also significantly affected by the hydrogen ion concentration (acid)[31] (see Chapter 32).

Shifts of potassium between the ICF and ECF are caused by a number of factors. Epinephrine and insulin, from both endogenous and exogenous sources, cause a shift of potassium from the ECF to the ICF. Epinephrine causes the shift to occur as a response to stress, pain, or any process stimulating the sympathetic nervous system "fight or flight" response. Insulin causes the shift of potassium into the cells to sequester the high potassium loads that may occur with the ingestion of a meal. Conditions that cause an increased extracellular osmolality, such as diabetic ketoacidosis (DKA), will cause water to shift out of the cells, creating an artificial increase in the ICF potassium level, which then moves into the ECF by diffusion. In an acidotic state, excess hydrogen ions (H^+) enter the cells and force the potassium into the ECF, increasing the serum levels of potassium. In an alkalotic state, this process is reversed, pulling potassium into the cells, decreasing the serum levels. Both of these processes are in response to the cell's attempt to maintain electrical neutrality. The body has a tremendous ability to adapt to increased intake of potassium, over time. This process, known as potassium adaption, occurs as the potassium intake increases, causing an increase in renal excretion of potassium.[14] However, in certain clinical situations, especially when the shifts occur rapidly, the increased intake of potassium can produce changes in the potassium levels that are lethal.[31]

Laboratory Findings. As noted in Table 31-1, a normal potassium value is 3.5 to 5.5 mEq/L (3.5 to 5.5 mmol/L). The correct technique in drawing the potassium blood sample is important to ensure accurate results. If the patient squeezes the fist during a venous blood draw, the muscular contraction can liberate potassium from the muscles, falsely elevating the potassium level. In addition, the use of a tourniquet should be avoided, if possible.[15] Because hemolysis of red blood cells will liberate potassium and falsely elevate the serum level, it is imperative to make every effort to prevent hemolysis from occurring. Hemolysis can occur with something as simple as shaking the blood-filled tube or sending the sample through a pneumatic tube system.[24]

Hyperkalemia

Figure 31-1 provides an algorithm for diagnosing the cause of hyperkalemia. Because potassium is efficiently excreted by the kidneys, it is unusual for hyperkalemia to occur when renal function is normal. When the kidneys are damaged, acutely with acute tubular necrosis (ATN) or in a more chronic condition such as chronic renal failure, there is a loss of ability to filter and excrete potassium and hyperkalemia occurs, with the level increasing above 5.5 mEq/L (5.5 mmol/L). If renal function is even partly compromised from a variety of sources (e.g., nonsteroidal antiinflammatory drugs [NSAIDs], hypotension, hypoxia, hypovolemia, sepsis, advanced age), the patient is at an increased risk for hyperkalemia, especially when supplemental potassium is given. Close observation of laboratory results is necessary to identify problems early.

A number of medications can cause an elevated potassium level. Two common classes of drugs given to patients with hypertension and heart disease (angiotensin-converting enzyme [ACE] inhibitors and angiotensin receptor blockers [ARBs]) are implicated in hyperkalemia, especially when diabetes, congestive heart failure, or decreased renal function is also present.[27,29] The use of spironolactone (Aldactone), a potassium-sparing diuretic used in the treatment of hypertension and congestive heart failure, inhibits potassium secretion into the filtrate of the distal renal tubule.[24] Subcutaneous heparin, 5000 units twice a day, can increase potassium levels by up to 1.7 mEq/L (1.7 mmol/L) over a period of 3 days.[29] There are also a number of herbal supplements that have substantial amounts of potassium (noni juice, alfalfa, dandelion, horsetail, and nettle). Digitalis-like substances that may exacerbate hyperkalemia are found in such herbal remedies as chan su, milkweed, lily of the valley, Siberian

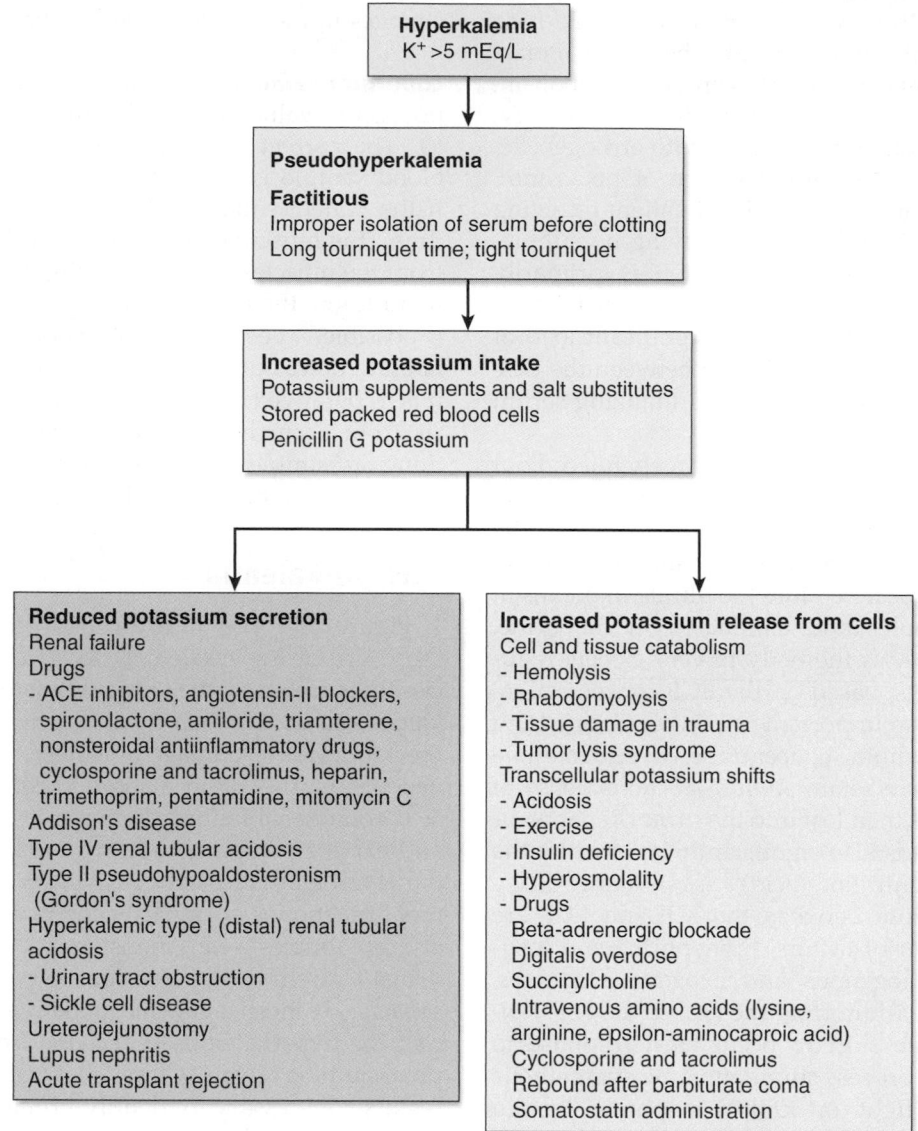

Hyperkalemia
K⁺ >5 mEq/L

Pseudohyperkalemia

Factitious
Improper isolation of serum before clotting
Long tourniquet time; tight tourniquet

Increased potassium intake
Potassium supplements and salt substitutes
Stored packed red blood cells
Penicillin G potassium

Reduced potassium secretion
Renal failure
Drugs
- ACE inhibitors, angiotensin-II blockers,
  spironolactone, amiloride, triamterene,
  nonsteroidal antiinflammatory drugs,
  cyclosporine and tacrolimus, heparin,
  trimethoprim, pentamidine, mitomycin C
Addison's disease
Type IV renal tubular acidosis
Type II pseudohypoaldosteronism
 (Gordon's syndrome)
Hyperkalemic type I (distal) renal tubular
acidosis
- Urinary tract obstruction
- Sickle cell disease
Ureterojejunostomy
Lupus nephritis
Acute transplant rejection

Increased potassium release from cells
Cell and tissue catabolism
- Hemolysis
- Rhabdomyolysis
- Tissue damage in trauma
- Tumor lysis syndrome
Transcellular potassium shifts
- Acidosis
- Exercise
- Insulin deficiency
- Hyperosmolality
- Drugs
  Beta-adrenergic blockade
  Digitalis overdose
  Succinylcholine
  Intravenous amino acids (lysine,
  arginine, epsilon-aminocaproic acid)
  Cyclosporine and tacrolimus
  Rebound after barbiturate coma
  Somatostatin administration

⬍**FIGURE 31-1** Algorithm for diagnosing the cause of hyperkalemia. K⁺ = Potassium.

ginseng, and hawthorn berries.[27] The risk factors for hyperkalemia tend to be cumulative, increasing the likelihood for hyperkalemia when more factors are present. Within the critical care setting, renal insufficiency or failure, coupled with the delivery of exogenous potassium, is a common cause of hyperkalemia.[5,14,31]

Elevated potassium levels are also seen with respiratory or metabolic acidosis, again from a variety of respiratory or metabolic sources (e.g., hypoventilation, lactic acid accumulation, certain drug overdoses, or DKA). As the pH decreases, the accumulating hydrogen ions are shifted into the ICF, driving the potassium into the ECF and increasing serum levels (see Chapter 32).

Since potassium is available mostly in the ICF, any mechanism that causes significant muscle damage

(e.g., crush injuries, burns, damage to large muscle groups) will cause the release of potassium from the damaged tissue.[14] In addition, such injuries also release excessive amounts of myoglobin, which then obstruct the glomerulus, preventing potassium from being filtered from the blood. This process is referred to as rhabdomyolysis and, even in the face of normal baseline renal function, such sudden increases in potassium levels may drive the ECF level into the abnormally high range.[24]

There are additional causes of hyperkalemia. The excessive use of potassium-containing salt substitutes, a common dietary recommendation for cardiac patients to decrease sodium consumption, may produce hyperkalemia, especially if large amounts of the salt substitute are consumed quickly.[15,29] Addison's disease, and the resultant decrease in aldosterone production, can cause a decrease in the amount of potassium excreted by the kidney, raising the potassium level. Again, it must be noted that significant increases in potassium levels are usually the result of some decrease in renal function with a concomitant increase of potassium in the ECF.

As noted previously, potassium has a significant impact on the action potential of cells. This is especially important in the cardiac system, where both the conduction system and the myocardium itself rely on potassium. As the potassium level increases, the cells will depolarize more rapidly from their resting potential. If the potassium continues to increase, the resting potential will exceed the threshold potential and the cells will not be able to repolarize. This phenomenon is frequently seen in the characteristic electrocardiograph (ECG) changes that reflect both hyperkalemia and hypokalemia (Figure 31-2 and Table 31-3). As the potassium level increases, the T wave becomes tall and peaked, with a shortened QT interval. If the potassium level continues to increase, the PR interval will

TABLE 31-3 Electrocardiographic Findings Associated With Disturbances in Serum Electrolyte Levels	
ELECTROLYTE ABNORMALITY	**ELECTROCARDIOGRAPHIC FINDINGS**
Hypokalemia	Decreased T-wave amplitude T-wave inversion ST segment depression Prominent U wave Prolongation of QT (U) interval Ventricular tachycardia Torsades de pointes
Hyperkalemia	
Mild	Large-amplitude T waves "Peaked" or "tented" T waves
Moderate	PR interval prolongation Decreased P-wave amplitude, disappearance QRS complex widening Conduction blocks with escape beats
Severe	Sine wave pattern Ventricular fibrillation Asystole
Hypocalcemia	Prolongation of QTc interval Ventricular dysrhythmias Torsades de pointes
Hypercalcemia	Shortening of QTc interval Bradydysrhythmias
Hypomagnesemia or **hypermagnesemia**	No unique ECG abnormalities, but often associated with calcium abnormalities

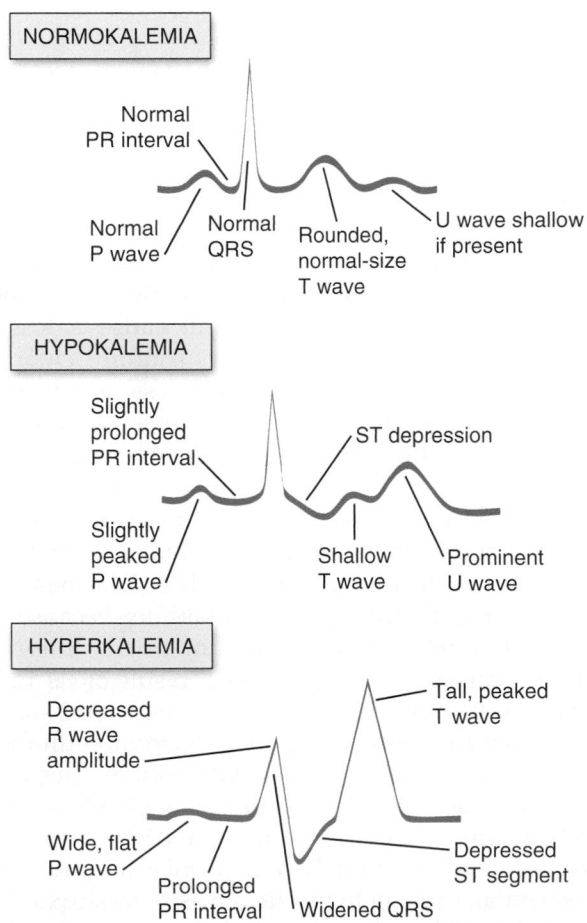

FIGURE 31-2 ECG changes with potassium imbalances.

become prolonged, the QRS complex will widen, and the ST segment will become depressed, often with a bradycardia.[5,31] Because of the importance of potassium in neuromuscular conduction and contraction, elevated potassium levels will interfere with these functions within the heart.

Physical Assessment Findings. In hyperkalemia, commonly seen symptoms include nausea, vomiting, abdominal cramps, diarrhea, weakness and dizziness, muscle cramps, hypotension, paresthesias (typically the first sign),[14,24] and ascending paralysis. In addition, the ECG changes described previously may be the first indication of the abnormality.[5,31]

Laboratory Findings. When potassium levels increase to greater than 5.5 mEq/L (>5.5 mmol/L), the nurse will need to assess for contributing factors. These factors include the following: the presence of potassium in IV solutions, parenteral nutrition (PN), and medications; the existence of acidosis; decreasing renal function; the use of medications that could increase potassium levels (spironolactone, ACE inhibitors, ARBs).[15] The patient's condition will also need to be assessed to determine if the patient is exhibiting signs and symptoms of hyperkalemia and the potassium level is likely to continue to rise. If the patient is exhibiting signs and symptoms of hyperkalemia, immediate treatment will need to be initiated. A potassium level of greater than 6.5 mEq/L (>6.5 mmol/L) is considered a "panic" level.[15]

Treatment. When hyperkalemia is noted, the first step is to reduce potassium intake, eliminating any potassium supplementation (and any medication that potentially increases potassium levels, e.g., spironolactone, ACE inhibitors, ARBs).[5]

The American Heart Association's Advanced Cardiac Life Support for Experienced Providers (ACLS-EP) uses a staggered approach to treating hyperkalemia. "Mild hyperkalemia" (5 to 6 mEq/L [5 to 6 mmol/L]) is treated by removing potassium from the body by a number of means, including furosemide (Lasix), 1 mg/kg slow IV push; sodium polystyrene sulfonate (Kayexalate), 15 to 30 g, per mouth or nasogastric tube or per rectum (PR); or dialysis, depending upon the patient's history and condition.[5] Sodium polystyrene sulfonate is a resin that exchanges sodium for potassium in the gut, increasing the sodium concentration in the ECF. It should be used with caution in patients with congestive heart failure or with concurrent hypernatremia. In addition, if given per rectum, it must be retained for more than 30 to 60 minutes to create effective ion exchange, which can be a challenge for the patient and the critical care nurse.[24,36]

ACLS-EP defines "moderate" hyperkalemia as potassium levels from 6 to 7 mEq/L (6 to 7 mmol/L) and recommends therapies that are designed to create a temporary shift of potassium from the ECF into the ICF, thus temporarily decreasing the serum potassium levels. This shift may be accomplished by one of three different medications. Sodium bicarbonate, up to 1 mEq/kg, is given over 5 minutes, creating a temporary alkalosis. A combination of glucose (25 g of a 50% solution) and regular insulin (10 units) given over 15 to 30 minutes drives potassium into the ICF. Nebulized albuterol, 5 to 20 mg, may be given over 15 minutes.[5]

When a severe potassium elevation (>7 mEq/L [>7 mmol/L]) or a widened QRS complex or other potassium-induced ECG changes are found, immediate steps must be taken to counteract the effects of potassium on the cardiac conduction system. The initial emergency treatment is to give 5 to 20 ml of 10% calcium chloride over 2 to 5 minutes. Calcium chloride is then followed by sodium bicarbonate or IV insulin and glucose, as noted previously, to shift the potassium from the ECF to the ICF. Follow-up treatment removes potassium from the body and includes diuretics, exchange resins, or renal replacement. Renal replacement is the treatment of choice with hyperkalemia associated with renal failure.[5,24] The medication table on p. 847 summarizes the treatment of hyperkalemia.

Hypokalemia

Applied Physiology and Pathophysiology. Hypokalemia (<3.5 mEq/L [<3.5 mmol/L]) may be caused by a number of problems. Figure 31-3 provides an algorithm to use in diagnosing the causes of hypokalemia. While a lack of dietary intake is a possible source of the problem, hypokalemia is typically confined to those patients who do not consume adequate amounts of protein, fruits, and vegetables.[46] The groups at risk for inadequate intake include older adults, patients with chronic alcohol abuse, and those with eating disorders.[14] In addition, though it is not clear how the relationship occurs, hypokalemia can also be caused by hypomagnesemia.[24]

A change in the blood pH can have a profound effect on potassium levels. A decrease in the hydrogen ion concentration will cause an increase in the pH, a state of alkalosis, that drives the potassium into the ICF, decreasing the serum potassium levels (see Chapter 32).[14]

The body may lose potassium from both the gastrointestinal (GI) and renal systems. Vomiting, diarrhea, and gastrointestinal suctioning will cause a loss of potassium, but, more importantly, sodium, chloride, and hydrogen ions are also lost. The loss of both fluid and sodium further activates the renin-angiotensin-aldosterone system, which causes the kidneys to increase potassium excretion because of sodium retention, decreasing the serum potassium levels. The loss of hydrogen ions may create an alkalotic state, driving the potassium in the ECF into the ICF. Diarrhea may also cause significant losses of potassium because the considerable amounts of potassium in the intestinal contents will not be absorbed as a result of its rapid transit through the gut.[14,24] Potassium is reabsorbed in the distal tubules of the kidneys. Common diuretics (thiazides, furosemide, bumetanide [Bumex], osmotic diuretics) cause an increase in secretion of sodium, which in turn increases the tubular urine flow. This increased tubular urine flow then inhibits potassium reabsorption, causing hypokalemia as potassium is lost in the urine. This is the rationale for potassium supplementation in many patients taking diuretics. The use of

TREATMENTS FOR HYPERKALEMIA

TREATMENT	DOSE	ROUTE	TIME TO ONSET	DURATION OF EFFECT	MECHANISM OF ACTION AND EFFECTS
Calcium chloride, calcium gluconate*†	1-2 g (10-20 ml of 10% solution)	Intravenous over 5-10 min	1-2 min	10-30 min	Antagonizes cardiac conduction abnormalities
Sodium bicarbonate*	50-100 mEq	Intravenous over 2-5 min	30 min	2-6 hr	Increases serum pH; redistributes potassium into cells
Insulin (regular)* (with dextrose)	5-10 units	Intravenous with 50 ml of 50% dextrose injection	15-45 min	2-6 hr	Redistributes potassium into cells
Dextrose 50%	50 ml (25 g)	Intravenous over 5 min	30 min	2-6 hr	Increases insulin release; redistributes potassium into cells; prevents hypoglycemia when insulin is given
Dextrose 10%	1000 ml (100 g)	Intravenous over 1-2 hr	30 min	2-6 hr	Increases insulin release; redistributes potassium into cells; prevents hypoglycemia when given with insulin
Furosemide	20-40 mg	Intravenous	5-15 min	4-6 hr	Increases renal potassium loss
Sodium polystyrene sulfonate‡	15-60 g	Oral or rectal	1 hr	4-6 hr	Resin exchanges sodium for potassium; increases fecal potassium elimination
Albuterol	10-20 mg	Nebulized over 10 min	30 min	1-2 hr	Stimulates sodium-potassium pump; redistributes potassium into cells
Hemodialysis	2-4 hr	Not applicable	Immediate	Variable	Removes potassium from plasma

*First-line therapies in hyperkalemic emergencies.
†Repeat dose in 5 minutes if abnormal electrocardiogram persists. Calcium chloride may also be used, but calcium gluconate is preferred over calcium chloride for peripheral venous administration because it causes less venous irritation. Calcium chloride (1000 mg = 13.6 mEq calcium) provides three times more calcium than calcium gluconate (1 g = 4.56 mEq calcium).
‡Can be used to treat acute hyperkalemia, but the effects may not be seen for several hours. Removes 0.5-1 mEq of potassium per 1 g of sodium polystyrene sulfonate.

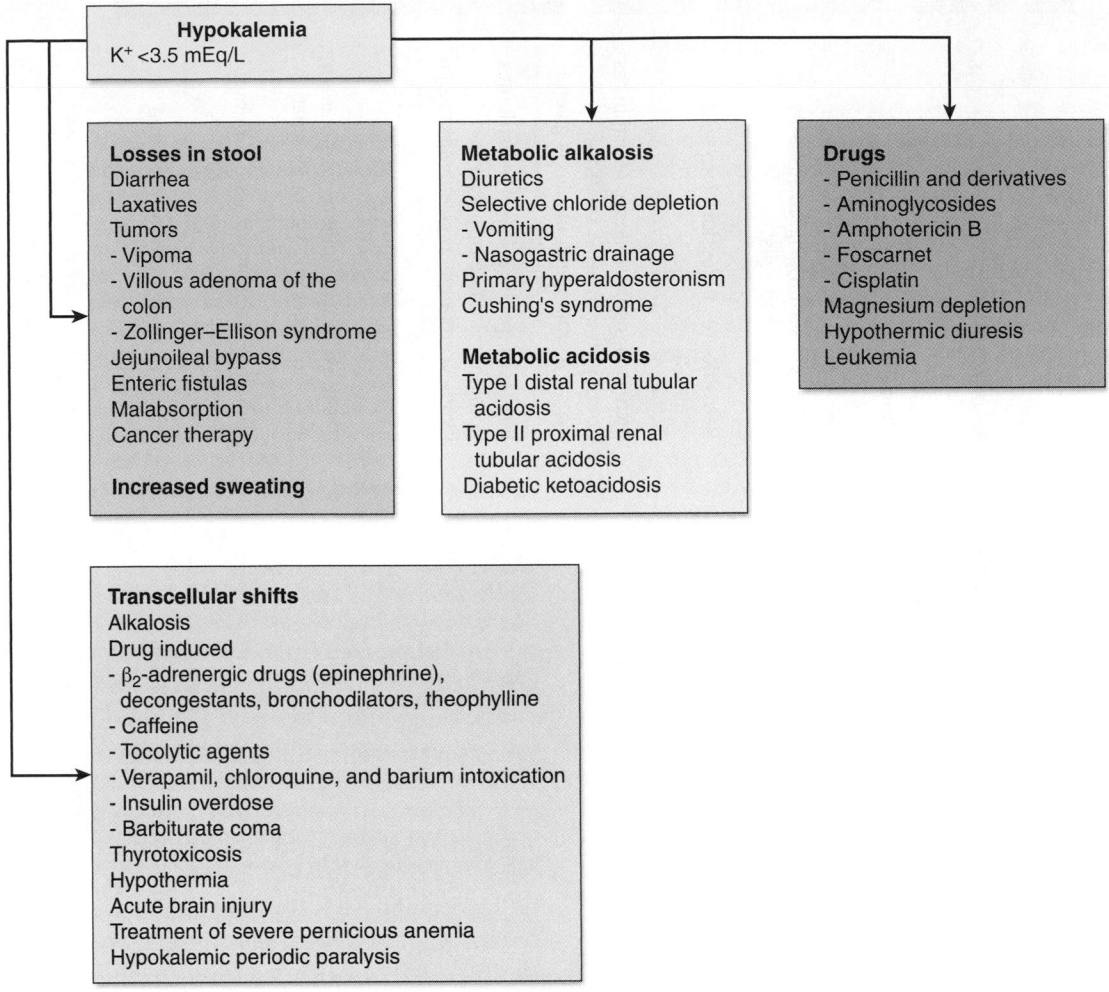

Hypokalemia
K^+ <3.5 mEq/L

Losses in stool
Diarrhea
Laxatives
Tumors
- Vipoma
- Villous adenoma of the
  colon
- Zollinger–Ellison syndrome
Jejunoileal bypass
Enteric fistulas
Malabsorption
Cancer therapy

Increased sweating

Metabolic alkalosis
Diuretics
Selective chloride depletion
- Vomiting
- Nasogastric drainage
Primary hyperaldosteronism
Cushing's syndrome

Metabolic acidosis
Type I distal renal tubular
  acidosis
Type II proximal renal
  tubular acidosis
Diabetic ketoacidosis

Drugs
- Penicillin and derivatives
- Aminoglycosides
- Amphotericin B
- Foscarnet
- Cisplatin
Magnesium depletion
Hypothermic diuresis
Leukemia

Transcellular shifts
Alkalosis
Drug induced
- β_2-adrenergic drugs (epinephrine),
  decongestants, bronchodilators, theophylline
- Caffeine
- Tocolytic agents
- Verapamil, chloroquine, and barium intoxication
- Insulin overdose
- Barbiturate coma
Thyrotoxicosis
Hypothermia
Acute brain injury
Treatment of severe pernicious anemia
Hypokalemic periodic paralysis

FIGURE 31-3 Algorithm for diagnosing the causes of hypokalemia. K^+ = Potassium; β, beta.

loop and osmotic diuretics is the most common cause of hypokalemia.[31] Hypokalemia is found in more than 20% of hospitalized patients and may be present in 40% of patients taking thiazide diuretics.[11] Another medication implicated in hypokalemia is the common bronchodilating agent albuterol. Two treatments within 1 hour can decrease the serum potassium level by up to 1 mEq/L (1 mmol/L).[11] Hypokalemia may be caused by the release of aldosterone, which, in turn, may be caused by primary aldosteronism or secondary aldosteronism, resulting from such clinical conditions as renal artery stenosis, congestive heart failure, or the administration of glucocorticoids.[5]

When a diabetic patient experiences DKA or hyperosmolar hyperglycemic state (HHS), the excess hydrogen ions cause a significant shift of potassium from the ICF to the ECF, increasing the serum potassium level. Potassium is lost in the significant diuresis that occurs early with hyperglycemia. This is one of the hallmarks of DKA and HHS. When DKA and HHS

are treated with fluids, the acidosis is reversed and the potassium in the ECF shifts into the ICF, causing a clinically significant lowering of the ECF potassium level. Insulin exacerbates this process because it facilitates the passage of both glucose and potassium into the ICF.[3]

When the potassium level in the ECF is low, the ECG is adversely affected. The PR interval becomes prolonged and the ST segment depressed. The T wave becomes flattened and the U wave may become noticeable. While ECG changes associated with hypokalemia are not usually life-threatening, when associated with digitalis toxicity they can cause lethal ventricular dysrhythmias, particularly in patients with preexisting cardiac dysfunction.[11] Potassium and digitalis compete for the same binding sites of the sodium-potassium pump on the cellular membrane. If there is less potassium to bind to the sites, digitalis will bind to the sites and exert an exaggerated effect, such as profound bradycardia.[14]

Physical Assessment Findings. The symptoms related to hypokalemia include neuromuscular irritability, with muscular weakness or fatigue (usually of the large muscle groups of the legs or arms), muscle cramps or tenderness, paresthesias, and paralysis (seen with severe hypokalemia). The patient may have GI symptoms such as anorexia, nausea (with or without vomiting), abdominal distention, and paralytic ileus (seen with severe hypokalemia).[14,31] The abdominal complaints may hinder the patient from consuming normal nutrition, causing a further decrease in potassium levels.[31] In addition, the ECG changes may be the first indication of the abnormality (see Table 31-3).[5,11,31]

Laboratory Findings. As with hyperkalemia, when the potassium level decreases below 3.5 mEq/L (<3.5 mmol/L), the nurse must investigate the reasons for the losses. GI losses include vomiting, diarrhea, and GI suctioning, and the presence of alkalosis should be assessed. A careful review of medications that could cause the hypokalemia includes thiazides, furosemide, bumetanide, osmotic diuretics, and albuterol.[14] A potassium level of less than 2.5 mEq/L (<2.5 mmol/L) is considered a "panic" level.[15]

Treatment. Hypokalemia is initially treated by identifying and correcting losses of potassium. A careful review of GI losses is in order, as significant amounts of potassium may be lost with vomiting, GI suctioning, or diarrhea. Medications should be evaluated for their potential for decreasing serum potassium levels (e.g., diuretics, insulin, albuterol, amphotericin B). In addition, as alkalosis will shift potassium into the cells, patients with coexisting hypokalemia and alkalosis will usually need less potassium replacement, especially if the alkalosis is being corrected, because as homeostasis is achieved, potassium will reenter the ECF.[5] Chapter 32 provides a complete discussion of the impact of pH on potassium levels.

Oral replacement therapy is the preferred method of treating hypokalemia; however, when the patient's condition is unstable, IV replacement may be needed.[24] When using the oral route to replace potassium, 40 to 100 mEq may be given daily. It is preferably given with meals and usually not more than 20 mEq at any one time to prevent nausea and vomiting.[24,36] When delivering IV potassium for replacement in a stable patient, the usual dose is no more than 10 to 20 mEq per hour. If the potassium concentration is greater than 20 mEq/L, use a central IV line to prevent burning of peripheral veins. When a patient is suffering from life-threatening hypokalemia (paralysis, impaired respiratory function, or unstable cardiac dysrhythmias), a rapid central IV infusion of potassium chloride (2 mEq/min over 10 minutes) followed by a slower infusion of 1 mEq/min

over 10 minutes, for a total dose of 30 mEq, may be considered.[5] Institution protocols may prohibit a nurse from doing this, and a physician may be required to administer the dose.

SODIUM

Applied Physiology and Pathophysiology

As noted in Table 31-2, sodium is the most abundant cation in the ECF, accounting for approximately 90% to 95% of the total ECF cation load. Because it is the most abundant electrolyte in the ECF, it has a major impact on water balance by its influence on osmolarity, the concentration of an osmotically active substance within a solution. Simply put, where sodium goes, water tends to follow, helping to maintain the water balance in the various compartments of the body. Sodium also interacts with both potassium and calcium to regulate the propagation of nerve impulses and muscular contractions. Sodium is involved in transportation of materials across the cellular membranes, various cellular functions, cellular metabolism, and acid-base balance.[1,14]

The normal serum sodium concentration is 135 to 145 mEq/L (135 to 145 mmol/L) and is maintained by renal function, which, in turn, is influenced by multiple factors. The average Western diet is very high in sodium, usually about 5 to 6 grams per day, much more than the modest 500 mg/day the body requires.[14] Sodium is freely filtered from the blood in the glomerulus of the kidney, with the resultant renal filtrate being exceptionally high in sodium. As the filtrate travels through the distal tubules of the kidney, sodium is selectively reabsorbed, depending on the sodium concentration in the blood, as regulated by the macula densa of the glomerulus. The resorption of sodium is significantly impacted by activation of the renin-angiotensin-aldosterone system. When the ECF sodium level or renal perfusion is decreased or the potassium level increases, aldosterone increases the resorption of sodium and decreases the resorption of potassium in the distal tubules. In addition to the effects of aldosterone, angiotensin II, the end product of the renin-angiotensin system, also causes a systemic vasoconstriction, increasing renal perfusion and increasing the reabsorption of sodium and excretion of potassium in the urine.

Natriuretic hormones (atrial natriuretic peptide [ANP], brain natriuretic peptide [BNP], and urodilatin from the kidney) decrease blood pressure and cause both sodium and water to be excreted, thus decreasing blood pressure.[14] ANP, produced and secreted in the atria, is released with increased atrial stretch. BNP is secreted and stored in the ventricles and is released in response to increases in ventricular filling pressures. BNP was first identified in porcine brains, hence the name "brain" natriuretic peptide. Urodilatin is produced in the tubules of the kidneys and is secreted in response to increased blood pressure.

Because of the intimate relationship between sodium and water, changes in the sodium concentration (the amount of sodium for a given amount of water) will also result in changes in the serum osmolality (concentration of a solution expressed in milliosmoles of solute particles per kilogram of solute [mOsm/kg]).[31]

This is of particular importance during treatment, as too rapid correction of sodium concentrations may cause increased cellular edema, which can be devastating within the brain.

Hypernatremia

Hypernatremia (>145 mEq/L [>145 mmol/L]) occurs when the concentration of sodium is increased in relation to the amount of fluid in the ECF. While hypernatremia is often associated with hypovolemia, it is important to remember that hypernatremia can occur in the setting of hypovolemia, euvolemia, or hypervolemia[45] (Figure 31-4). The major effect of increased sodium concentration is to create an osmotic gradient, pulling water from the ICF into the ECF, a process that may create a significant cellular dehydration, and subsequent dysfunction of individual cells, organs, and systems. Hypernatremia is caused by two processes: (1) net water loss or (2) net sodium gain.[1]

Net water losses are further divided into "pure" water losses and losses of hypotonic fluid. With "pure" water losses, the body loses significant amounts of free water and insignificant amounts of sodium. Examples of this type of loss include unreplaced large insensible losses over a short period of time, such as is seen with high body temperatures, unconditioned exercise, or inadequate water intake (hypodipsia). "Pure" water losses may also be caused by diabetes insipidus, which in turn can have two separate etiologies: neurogenic and nephrogenic. *Neurogenic* diabetes insipidus results from an inadequate release of antidiuretic hormone (ADH) from the posterior lobe of the pituitary gland,

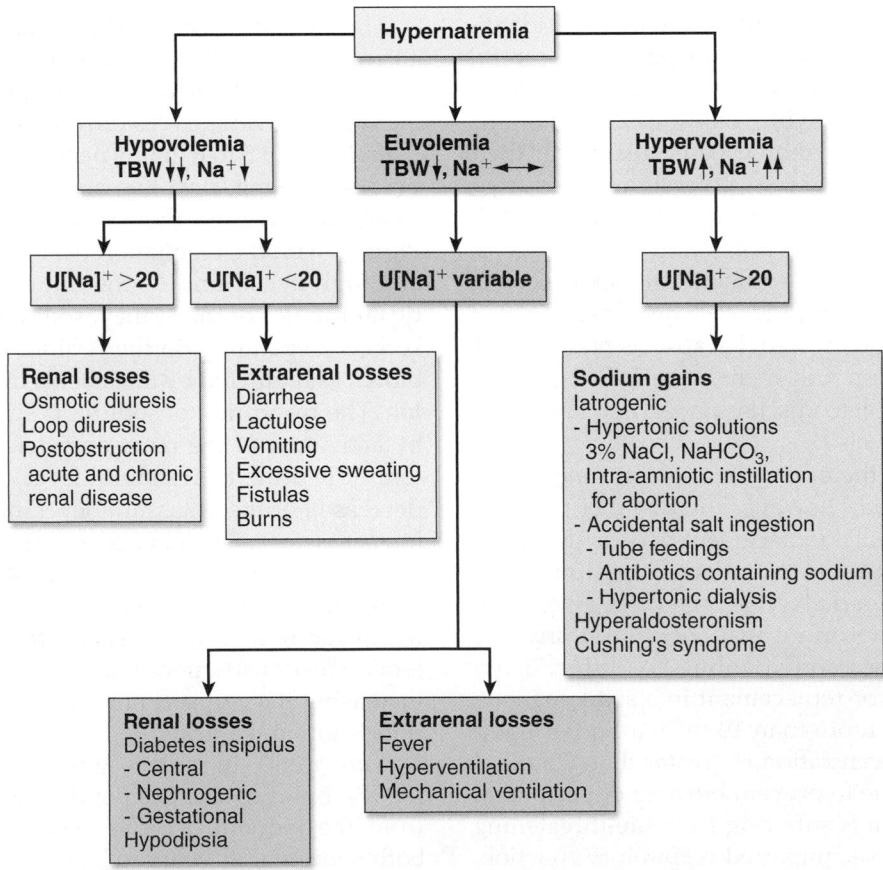

✦**FIGURE 31-4** Algorithm for diagnosing the causes of hypernatremia. Na^+ = Sodium, NaCl = sodium chloride, $NaHCO_3$ = sodium bicarbonate, TBW = total body water, U = urinary.

from a variety of causes. With *nephrogenic* diabetes insipidus, there are adequate amounts of ADH, but the tubules of the kidneys, due to inherited or acquired abnormalities, cannot respond to ADH to reabsorb water. The end result of either form of diabetes insipidus is a significant loss of water in the urine, increasing the serum sodium concentration.[1]

Hypernatremia is also caused by hypotonic fluid loss; while both sodium and water are lost, the proportion of water loss is greater, creating a net loss of water. Most commonly, this process occurs via the kidneys, often with the use of various diuretics. Another renal cause of hypotonic fluid loss is the osmotic diuresis that occurs with mannitol administration or hyperglycemia. Serum osmotic pressure draws fluid from the ICF into the ECF. As the blood volume increases, filtration pressure increases and sodium is resorbed. The net result is the loss of more water than sodium into the urine, creating hypernatremia. Hypotonic fluid loss also occurs in the GI tract with vomiting, diarrhea, GI suctioning, or enterocutaneous fistulas, or with the use of osmotic agents in the GI tract, such as lactulose. Significant burns can also cause hypotonic fluid loss.[1]

Hypernatremia may be caused by a net gain of sodium. While this can be seen with seawater ingestion and the ingestion of excessive amounts of sodium chloride, it is much more commonly associated with iatrogenic causes. Such causes include hypertonic enteral (EN) or parenteral nutrition (PN) and hypertonic solutions delivered to the patient in the form of IV solutions, enemas, emetics, or dialysis. Hypernatremia may also be caused by primary hyperaldosteronism, which increases the release of aldosterone, causing the kidneys to reabsorb more sodium than water. Cushing's syndrome, a condition of excessive glucocorticoid steroid production, also causes the retention of sodium, leading to hypernatremia.[1]

Physical Assessment Findings. The physical assessment of a patient with sodium imbalances may yield conflicting findings. Often similar findings occur with both hypernatremia and hyponatremia. It is *imperative* that the physical assessment findings be correlated with both various laboratory tests and the patient's history.

The signs and symptoms associated with hypernatremia are more commonly seen with sudden or large shifts in the sodium concentration and are manifested by the loss of fluid from the ICF to the ECF as the body attempts to decrease sodium concentration in the ECF. The dehydration will cause weight loss, requiring significant attention to daily weights. Thirst, if the patient can express it, is often the first sign of hypernatremia. Older, bed-bound, and mentally challenged patients are at increased risk because of their inability to express thirst or acquire fluids in response to thirst. Dehydration becomes more clinically evident, with dry mucous membranes and sclera. Salivation decreases, making it difficult to swallow. As the central nervous system (CNS) cells become dehydrated, the patient may complain of headache or exhibit restlessness and agitation. If the hypernatremia occurs quickly, the cell crenation and brain shrinkage can cause rupture of blood vessels and hemorrhage.[1] Reflexes will be decreased, and as the hypernatremia worsens, the patient may slip into a coma or develop seizures.[31]

Laboratory Findings. When the serum sodium concentration is greater than 145 mEq/L (>145 mmol/L), there should be an investigation of why it is elevated to possibly prevent further increase. A serum sodium concentration of greater than 150 mEq/L (>150 mmol/L) is considered a "panic" level.[15]

Treatment. A thorough evaluation of the patient is mandatory before elevated serum sodium concentration is treated, to ensure appropriate treatment of the cause. The cause of the sodium imbalance must be addressed while treating the hypernatremia.[1] If the patient is hemodynamically unstable, fluid resuscitation with 0.9% NaCl is appropriate until the patient is stable. At this point, the sodium imbalance may be addressed. If the issue is water loss, then "free water" is delivered to the patient in the form of 5% dextrose (D_5W), often in combination with hypotonic sodium chloride (0.2% to 0.45% NaCl).[1] The treatment course is usually extended over 48 hours to prevent too rapid a correction of the serum sodium level. If the sodium level is corrected too quickly with rapid administration of free water, the blood-brain barrier will prevent the equalization of fluid in cerebral tissue, which may cause significant cerebral edema (Figure 31-5).[24] If hypernatremia is being caused by excess sodium being delivered to the patient, in the form of IV fluids, medications, or enteral or parenteral feedings, they must be stopped and modified to decrease the sodium loads. Vasopressin may be used to treat hypernatremia associated with diabetes insipidus, but must be used with caution because of excess water retention and a rebound hyponatremia.[24]

Hyponatremia

Hyponatremia (<135 mEq/L [<135 mmol/L]) occurs when the concentration of sodium is decreased in relation to the amount of fluid in the ECF. It represents one of the most confusing of the electrolyte disorders, because a patient with hyponatremia may present with a low, normal, or even elevated intravascular or extracellular

♦FIGURE 31-5 Impact of hypernatremia on the brain.

volume (Figure 31-6). Indeed, some of the same pathologies that cause hypernatremia can also cause hyponatremia, such as vomiting, diarrhea, or diuretic use.[1,2] Hyponatremia may be caused by mechanisms that cause the body to lose more sodium than water. Examples include renal losses, such as seen with diuretics, osmotic diuresis (e.g., mannitol, hyperglycemia, or the presence of ketones), and the effects of Addison's disease (adrenocortical insufficiency). The loss of more sodium than water can also occur with vomiting, diarrhea, or excessive sweating or when fluid is sequestered in the ECF away from the vascular system ("third spaced"), such as found in burns, pancreatitis, or muscle trauma.[2]

Hyponatremia may also be caused by processes that increase the amount of water in the ECF. If the ECF water volume increases without a concomitant increase in the sodium levels, the sodium concentration will decrease, causing hyponatremia. This is sometimes referred to as a "dilutional" or hypovolemic hyponatremia. Examples include congestive heart failure, liver disease, acute or chronic renal failure, or even pregnancy.[2]

A patient with normal circulating fluid volumes may also have hyponatremia. For example, thiazide diuretics tend to cause the excretion of more sodium than water. Over time, this can create a hyponatremic state. Hypothyroidism and adrenocortical insufficiency cause more sodium than water to be excreted by the kidneys (see Chapter 35).[2]

Syndrome of inappropriate antidiuretic hormone (SIADH) may also cause hyponatremia. ADH normally is released from the posterior pituitary gland in response to decreased circulating blood volume, causing the kidneys to reabsorb water, increasing the ECF. In SIADH, the normal negative feedback system is disrupted and ADH continues to be secreted. As water is continually reabsorbed, a dilutional hyponatremia develops. SIADH is caused by stress, pain, lung cancers, head trauma, or multiple medications (see Chapter 35).[24,31]

It is worth mentioning that a patient suffering from DKA or HHS may have a relative hyponatremia that may actually mask normal or even high sodium levels.[3,15] As blood glucose elevates osmotic pressure in the intravascular spaces, the high glucose levels seen in both DKA and HHS exert an osmotic effect, diluting the sodium. In order to maintain normal osmotic pressure, sodium is secreted by the tubules in an effort to decrease osmotic pressure. This dilution of the ECF and secretion of sodium may cause an artificial hyponatremia, when,

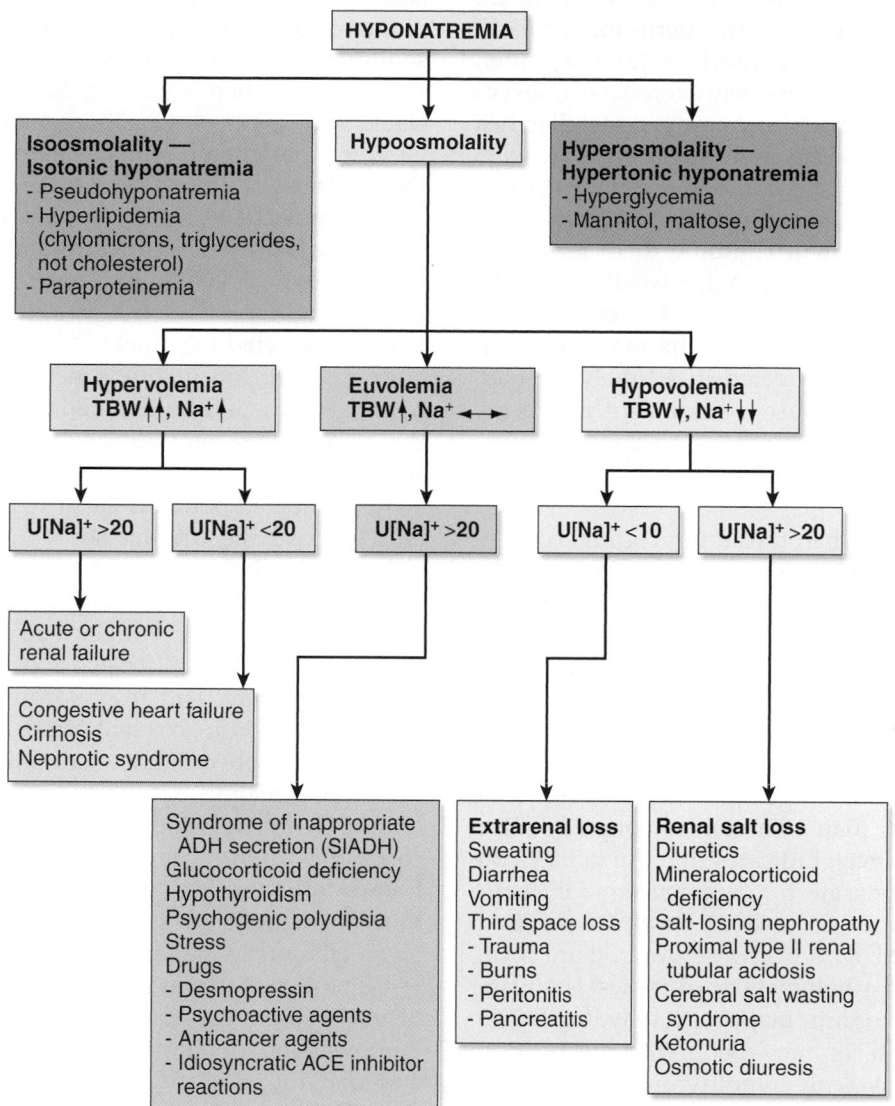

◆FIGURE 31-6 Algorithm for diagnosing the causes of hyponatremia. Na^+ = Sodium, TBW = total body water, U = urinary.

in fact, the sodium level may be normal or even elevated. A simple formula can provide accurate information regarding the true serum sodium level. For every 100 mg/dl the blood glucose level is above 100, add 1.6 mEq or mmol to the measured sodium level to obtain the *corrected* sodium level (Box 31-1). The *corrected* sodium calculation is required to deliver the appropriate fluid for resuscitation of patients in both DKA and HHS (see Chapter 34).[3]

Physical Assessment Findings. As with hypernatremia, the signs and symptoms of hyponatremia are more commonly seen with sudden or large shifts in the sodium concentration. The decreased sodium concentration in the ECF will cause water to collect in the ICF, leading

---

Box 31-1

Sample Serum Sodium Level Calculation

For example, if the glucose level was 924 mg/dl and the measured serum sodium level was 128 mEq/L (128 mmol/L), the *corrected* sodium level would be 140.8 mEq/L (140.8 mmol/L), a normal sodium level.

$$924 - 100 = 824 \text{ (difference for glucose above 100)}$$

$$8 \text{ per } 100$$

$$8 \times 1.6 = 12.8$$

$$128 + 12.8 = 140.8 \text{ (corrected sodium)}$$

to cellular edema. The patient will exhibit significant pitting edema, in the legs or on the sternum. The early signs of fatigue, muscle cramps, and weakness are often seen in patients who are excessively exercising. Coexisting nausea, vomiting, abdominal cramps, and diarrhea may also be present. As the water content of the CNS cells increases, dysfunction becomes more evident; signs include headache and lethargy. If the hyponatremia continues, the CNS edema will continue to increase and symptoms will evolve to gross motor weakness, disorientation, confusion, and decreased deep tendon reflexes. Ultimately, seizures and coma may occur.[31] If the sodium level is not corrected in a timely manner, the cerebral edema will cause a significant rise in the intracranial pressure and may cause an uncal or transtentorial herniation of the temporal lobe.[15]

Laboratory Findings. When the serum sodium concentration is decreased below 135 mEq/L (<135 mmol/L), an investigation of why it is low should be instituted, which may prevent its further decline. A serum sodium concentration of less than 125 mEq/L (<125 mmol/L) is considered a "panic" level.[15]

Additional laboratory tests that are helpful with a differential diagnosis in hyponatremia include urine sodium and blood urea nitrogen (BUN). A random urine sodium level of less than 10 mmol/L, coupled with a low serum sodium level, indicates that the kidneys are attempting to compensate for hyponatremia by reabsorbing sodium. A urine sodium level greater than 10 mmol/L, coupled with a low serum sodium level, indicates that some pathology (e.g., diuretics) is causing the kidneys to lose sodium inappropriately. In SIADH, the urine sodium level may be greater than 20 to 40 mmol/L, whereas with hypothyroidism the urine sodium level may be greater than 40 mmol/L. Calculating the fractional excretion of sodium (FENa) assists the nurse in assessing the cause of sodium loss. The fractional excretion of sodium is expressed by the formula:

$$FENa = \{[\text{urine Na} \div \text{urine Cr}] \times [\text{serum Cr} \div \text{serum Na}]\} \times 100$$

with the result being a percentage. A FENa of less than 1%, coupled with hyponatremia, usually indicates that the kidneys are attempting to compensate for hyponatremia by reabsorbing sodium.[15]

Treatment. The initial treatment for hyponatremia in a patient with normal or increased ECF volume is almost always water restriction. Loop diuretics (e.g., furosemide) may be added to the treatment to increase the amount of ECF volume excreted in the urine. Replacing lost sodium may also be a key component of treatment. If the patient can tolerate oral intake, replacement may be accomplished with a diet high in sodium. If the patient is unable to eat but has a functioning GI system, the sodium may be delivered by GI tubes (nasal, oral, or percutaneous). When a patient has hyponatremia associated with hypovolemia or cannot take sodium via the GI tract, parenteral replacement with normal saline (NS) or lactated Ringer's solution is appropriate. It may be necessary to use *small* amounts of hypertonic (3% to 5%) saline if the patient is symptomatic and is normovolemic or hypervolemic. Extreme caution must be exercised using hypertonic saline, as sodium concentration may be corrected too quickly.[2,24]

The use of the methods noted previously to treat hyponatremia will be dictated by the patient's condition, symptoms, and duration of the hyponatremia. According to Metheny (p. 67), "The goal of therapy in symptomatic hyponatremia is to reduce brain water and increase the plasma sodium concentration level only to the point necessary to maintain normal respiration and keep the patient free of seizures and alert, and at the same time prevent osmotic demyelination."[24] If the hyponatremia has existed for more than 48 hours, the CNS will have had an opportunity to accommodate to the low sodium concentration. If the sodium level is corrected too quickly, water will be drawn from the brain, creating dehydration and cerebral damage (Figure 31-7).[2,31] While there are multiple formulas for correcting sodium level and the appropriate time frames to be used,[2,24] the guiding principle should be to treat the patient's symptoms rather than to reach a given laboratory value.

When hyponatremia is caused by SIADH, treatment of the underlying cause must also be addressed. The treatment of hyponatremia begins with water restriction and loop diuretics, advancing to thoughtful administration of hypertonic saline (3% to 5%) as the patient's condition dictates.[24] Still in the experimental stage, the use of vasopressin receptor antagonists has been found to selectively increase water excretion by the kidneys while promoting sodium retention. Wong et al. studied the use of vasopressin receptor antagonists in patients with cirrhosis, congestive heart failure (CHF), and SIADH[49] while Gheorghiade et al. studied its effects in patients with CHF.[13] Both groups found that water excretion increased, as did serum sodium levels, thus correcting hyponatremia in both groups of patients.

CALCIUM

Applied Physiology and Pathophysiology

Most of the calcium in the body (99%) is stored in the bones and teeth; serum calcium (also referred to as "total" calcium) represents the remaining 1% and

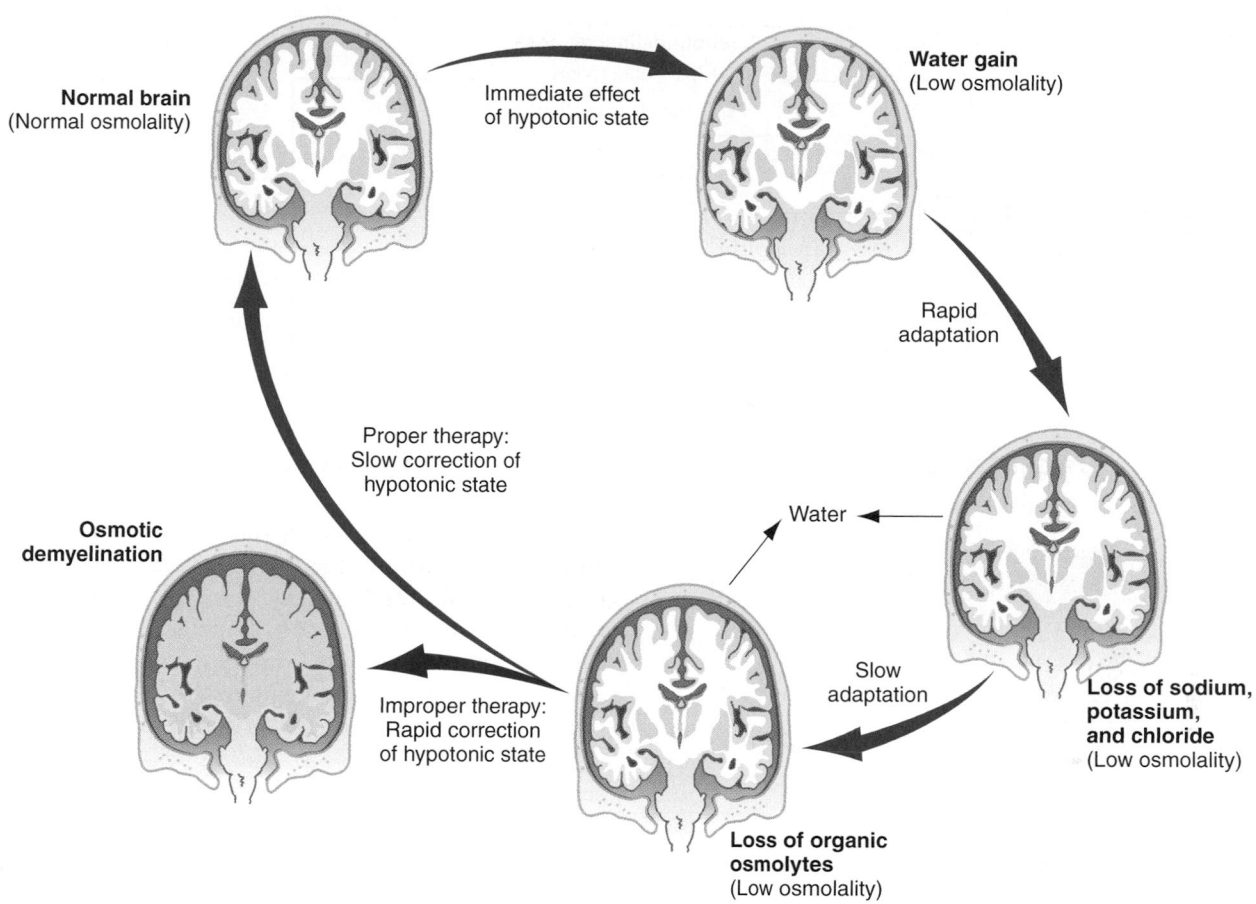

♦FIGURE 31-7 Impact of hyponatremia on the brain.

is divided into three distinct components. Approximately 10% of serum calcium is in a "complexed" form bound to another electrolyte and not available for the cells to use as an electrolyte. Another 47% is bound to protein, but this amount may vary with both the amount of protein in the blood and the blood's pH. Like "complexed" calcium, protein-bound calcium does not function as an electrolyte but is readily available to influence the ionized calcium level. The remaining 43% of serum calcium is free or ionized calcium that does act as an electrolyte. However, as noted previously, the levels of protein-bound calcium may fluctuate with the pH, which in turn will affect the ionized calcium level. If the pH is increased (alkalosis), the increase in protein-bound calcium will cause a decrease in ionized calcium and vice versa. It is therefore important, when caring for a hypoalbuminemic patient, to make a correction to the calcium level to account for the additional calcium that will be unbound to protein. This correction can be made using the following formula:

Serum calcium concentration $+ \ (0.8 \ \times$

$$[4 - \text{serum albumin concentration}])$$

Even though the proportions of protein-bound and ionized calcium may change with the pH, the total serum calcium concentration does not change.*

A large variety of body functions are dependent upon calcium, including muscle contraction, contractility of the heart and blood vessels, platelet aggregation, and coagulation.[5] Calcium is important in nerve transmission and cardiac contraction, relaxation, and automaticity.[8,24] As it is a major extracellular cation, it is usually actively "pumped" out of the cells, along with sodium. Calcium also makes the cellular membrane more impervious to elevated potassium and magnesium levels.[5]

Calcium levels in the body are regulated by the parathyroid glands (Figure 31-8). There are usually four parathyroid glands, which are located on the posterior aspect of the thyroid gland (Figure 31-9). The number of parathyroid glands may normally vary from as few as two to as many as six. The parathyroid gland manufactures and secretes parathyroid hormone (PTH), in response to the ionized calcium level. When the ionized calcium level decreases, PTH is released,

*References 5, 8, 15, 24, and 50.

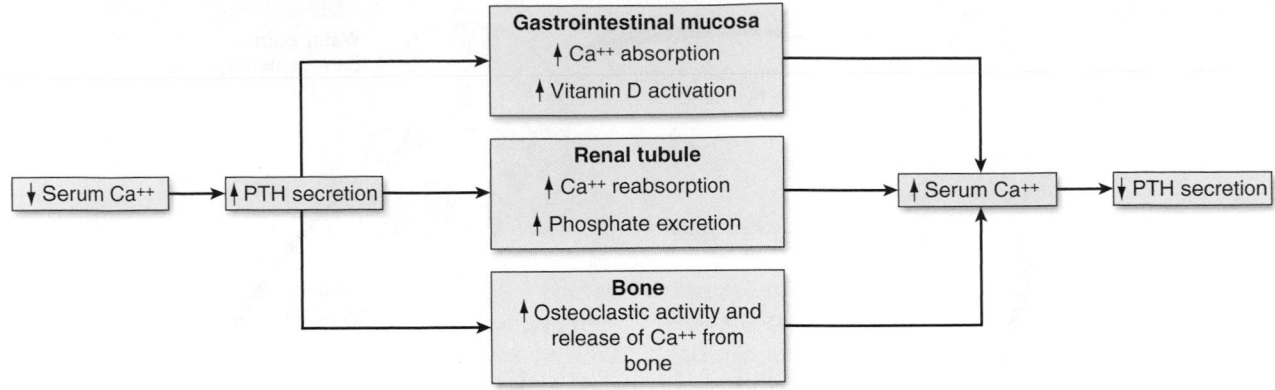

♣FIGURE 31-8 Calcium homeostasis. Ca^{++} = Calcium, PTH = parathyroid hormone.

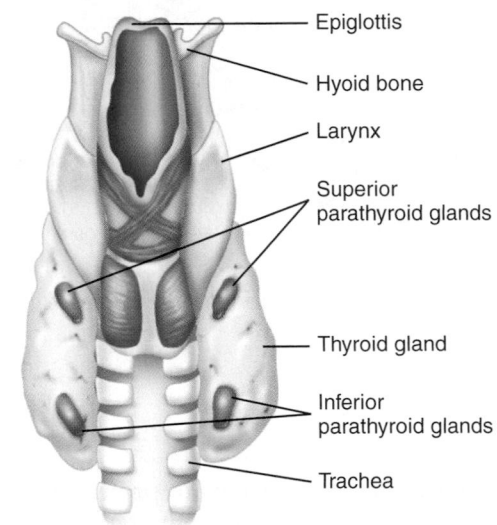

- Epiglottis
- Hyoid bone
- Larynx
- Superior parathyroid glands
- Thyroid gland
- Inferior parathyroid glands
- Trachea

♣FIGURE 31-9 Thyroid and parathyroid glands.

causing the ionized calcium levels to increase by several mechanisms. As calcium is stored primarily in bone, PTH will cause the release of calcium from bone and reabsorption of calcium, into the ionized form, by decreasing calcitonin level. Calcitonin, a hormone secreted by the thyroid gland, is responsible for the deposition of calcium in bone; a decrease in its concentration will liberate calcium from bone, increasing the ionized calcium level.[5] In the kidneys, PTH increases the amount of calcium reabsorbed from filtrate in the proximal and distal tubules, while at the same time decreasing the amount of phosphorus reabsorbed. This selective resorption of calcium and excretion of phosphorus allows for an increase in the ionized calcium level, without increasing the phosphorus levels. When the phosphorus is reabsorbed at the same rate as calcium, chelation of calcium and phosphorus will occur

and it may be deposited in soft tissue.[31] PTH also will stimulate the kidneys to synthesize 1,25-dihydroxyvitamin D (vitamin D$_3$, the active form of vitamin D, which is also known as calcitriol), which, in turn, increases calcium uptake from the GI tract.* Increases in the ionized calcium levels will create negative feedback to the parathyroid gland, to decrease the secretion of PTH.[31,50]

Hypercalcemia

The most common causes of hypercalcemia are cancers and hyperparathyroidism,[5,24] both of which liberate calcium from bone. As many as 20% of patients with cancer have hypercalcemia.[50] While the mechanism is not entirely clear, it is known that some cancers secrete a parathyroid-like substance that would cause hypercalcemia. Hypercalcemia is also caused by prolonged immobilization, muscle weakness, or paralysis preventing weight bearing. Excessive ingestion of milk products or calcium-containing antacids may also cause hypercalcemia. Women who ingest large amounts of calcium in an effort to prevent osteoporosis may develop hypercalcemia.[8,31,50]

Physical Assessment Findings. Calcium is important in neuromuscular and cardiovascular activity; signs and symptoms will typically be seen in these areas.[31] Hypercalcemia (>10 mg/dl [>2.50 mmol/L]) will usually result in decreased neuromuscular activity, resulting in muscular weakness, loss of muscle tone, and lethargy. Hypercalcemia may cause changes in behavior ranging from subtle changes in personality to stupor or coma. The patient may experience nausea or vomiting, anorexia, and constipation. Cardiovascular effects include shortening of the QTc interval, hypertension, and atrioventricular (AV) blocks, all of which may be potentiated by digitalis toxicity and can lead

*References 5, 8, 30, 31, and 50.

to cardiac arrest (see Table 31-3).[5,24] High levels of calcium in the urinary filtrate may interfere with the ability of ADH to cause the kidney to concentrate urine, leading to a significant diuresis. Chronic excessive calcium in the urine may cause the deposition of renal calculi in the tubules or collecting system.[31,50]

Laboratory Findings. Hypercalcemia is defined as serum calcium level greater than 10 mg/dl (>2.50 mmol/L). Panic levels are considered greater than 14 mg/dl (>3.50 mmol/L).[15] A prolonged blood draw with an excessively tight tourniquet can falsely elevate the calcium levels, as can elevated levels of protein or albumin.[31]

Treatment. Hypercalcemia is initially treated with rehydration and increased urinary loss of calcium through forced diuresis with fluids and loop diuretics. Typically, 500 ml of NS is "bolused" and then the patient is assessed for response. This pattern is repeated until the patient is stable. The fluid challenge may be coupled with furosemide (1 mg/kg).[5] Thiazide diuretics are contraindicated as they may increase calcium reabsorption. Steroids are effective in treating hypercalcemia by inhibiting the effects of vitamin D, increasing the renal excretion of calcium, and decreasing the uptake of calcium from the GI tract.[6] A relatively new class of drugs, bisphosphonates (pamidronate [Aredia], etidronate [Didronel]), help lower calcium levels and have been used extensively in various types of cancers[8,24] and chronic renal disease patients. A third bisphosphonate given orally, clodronate (Bonefos), is available in Europe but is not currently available in the United States.[8] However, researchers have recently begun to use this class of drugs to increase bone density and decrease serum calcium levels in hemiplegic stroke patients[39] and patients immobilized with hip fractures.[40] If a patient does not tolerate the bisphosphonates, plicamycin (an antibiotic used in oncology) may be considered, but it has significant side effects and is less effective.[24] Other drugs that are sometimes used to decrease liberation of calcium from bones include calcitonin (Miacalcin) and glucocorticoids.[5,6,31] If the patient has preexisting heart failure or renal failure, renal replacement is needed to remove the excess calcium.[5] If the patient is suffering from primary hyperparathyroidism, surgical excision of the glands is indicated.[8]

Hypocalcemia

Hypocalcemia is much less common than hypercalcemia[5] and is the result of one of three different mechanisms: increased renal losses, binding of ionized calcium to protein, or decreased PTH. Phosphate and calcium maintain an inverse relationship (when one increases, the other decreases and vice versa). Elevated phosphate levels are often found in patients with renal insufficiency and failure. When phosphate levels increase because of renal failure, calcium levels are often decreased. Other factors influencing calcium balance include magnesium, vitamin D, and inflammatory mediators. As magnesium levels decrease, the release of PTH and its action on bone, liberating calcium, are suppressed. Magnesium deficiency needs to be corrected before the calcium levels can be normalized. Excessive vitamin D will also suppress the secretion of PTH.[8,31,50] There are increasing data to suggest that inflammatory mediators may "down regulate" PTH, decreasing the calcium level.[9] Another author suggests that hospitalized older adults are at risk for vitamin D deficiency, which can also cause hypocalcemia.[20]

Hypocalcemia may be incorrectly identified when the total serum calcium level is found to be low (<8.6 mg/dl [<2.15 mmol/L]) in combination with hypoproteinemia. Because of the amount of calcium that is protein-bound (47%), the amount of protein (primarily albumin) in the serum will impact the total serum calcium level. If the total calcium level is determined to be below normal limits, an ionized calcium level must be measured to determine the true amount of the active calcium electrolyte. Various references use a variety of formulas to calculate the effect of low protein (or albumin) levels on the amount of ionized calcium. However, the only truly effective way to determine the amount of ionized calcium is to actually measure it.[20,24] Hypocalcemia may also be caused by acute pancreatitis; the saponification of fats and calcium in the retroperitoneum effectively removes the calcium from the circulation.[24,31] The delivery of large amounts of banked blood, especially over a short time, may cause hypocalcemia because the citrate used to preserve banked blood combines with the ionized calcium and eliminates it from the stores of active electrolytes. Citrate is metabolized by the liver, so any disease process (e.g., shock, liver disease, sepsis) that decreases liver function may increase the levels of citrate,[14,50] which will combine with more calcium. Recent data indicate that propofol (Diprivan) decreases calcium levels and increases PTH levels, but it is unclear if there is any clinical relevance to these changes.[6]

Physical Assessment Findings. Hypocalcemia typically causes increased neuromuscular activity and negative effects on the cardiovascular system. Increased neuromuscular activity causes a decrease in the excitation threshold and is characterized by numbness and tingling, particularly around the mouth and in the hands and feet. Muscle spasms and tetany of the hands, feet, and face may be seen or elicited during an assessment. Chvostek's sign (twitching of the lip, nose, or face in response to a repeated tapping of the facial nerve just

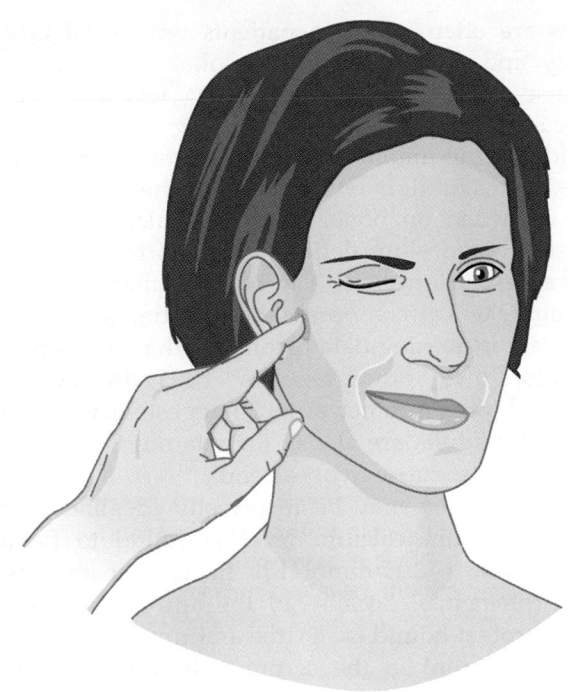

♦FIGURE 31-10 Chvostek's sign.

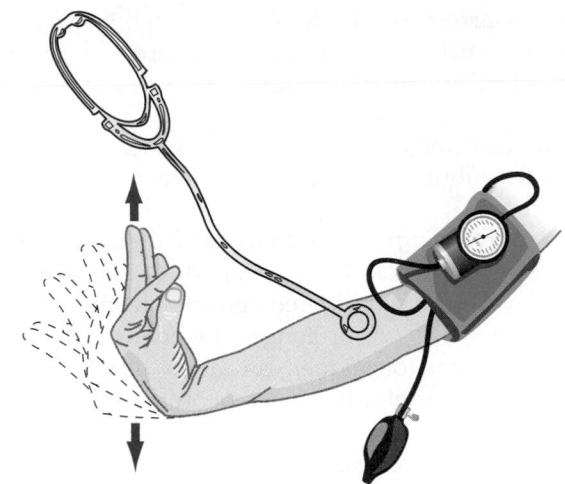

♦FIGURE 31-11 Trousseau's sign.

TABLE 31-5 Calcium Supplements

CALCIUM SALT	ELEMENTAL CALCIUM (mEq/g)	ELEMENTAL CALCIUM (%)	ELEMENTAL CALCIUM PROVIDED BY 1 G OF SALT (mg)
Calcium chloride	13.6	27	270
Calcium gluconate	4.56	9	90

below the zygomatic arch, anterior to the ear) or Trousseau's sign (a forceful flexion of the fingers and hand when a blood pressure cuff is inflated above the systolic pressure and held for 3 minutes) are both indicators of tetany (Figures 31-10 and 31-11).[8,50] Hyperreflexia is also found.[14] The cardiovascular effects of hypocalcemia are significant and can include hypotension, increased QT interval (which may lead to ventricular dysrhythmias including ventricular tachycardia and torsades de pointes),[5] decreased cardiac output, and decreased response to medications that utilize calcium, including digitalis, dopamine (Intropin), and norepinephrine (Levophed) (see Table 31-3).[31]

Laboratory Findings. Hypocalcemia is defined as a serum calcium level less than 8.6 mg/dl (<2.50 mmol/L). Panic levels are equal to or less than 6 mg/dl (≤1.50 mmol/L).[15] When low serum calcium levels are found, an ionized calcium MUST be measured before the delivery of calcium (gluconate or chloride). The normal range of ionized calcium is 4.64 to 5.28 mg/dl (1.16 to 1.32 mmol/L), with a panic value of <2.8 mg/dl (<0.7 mmol/L).[15]

Treatment. The treatment for hypocalcemia appears relatively straightforward: administer calcium. However, different calcium preparations supply different amounts of calcium (Table 31-5). Calcium chloride has three times as much elemental calcium as calcium gluconate. Calcium chloride is 27% elemental calcium,

calcium gluconate only 9%. If the patient is relatively stable and able to tolerate oral intake, calcium in the form of either citrate or carbonate can be given.[8] When treating hypocalcemia in the critical care setting, IV calcium, in the form of calcium gluconate or chloride, is given slowly when the patient is symptomatic or has significantly low calcium levels.[8,31,50] While some authorities recommend calcium gluconate because it is less irritating than calcium chloride,[5,24] it is about one third the concentration of calcium chloride (0.465 mEq/L vs. 1.4 mEq/L).[34,35] If calcium chloride is given, it should be delivered into the largest available vein and via a central vein, if possible. If the patient's condition allows the extra fluid, calcium is ideally mixed with a compatible IV solution and should not be delivered in the same IV line at the same time as bicarbonate or phosphorus, as it will form a precipitate.[24,50] Whenever hypocalcemia is found, magnesium levels should be evaluated and corrected if low.[8]

MAGNESIUM

Applied Physiology and Pathophysiology

Magnesium is necessary for multiple functions essential to maintain life. Among these are nerve conduction; membrane stabilization; cardiovascular tone; movement of sodium, potassium, and calcium in and out of cells; and cellular metabolism of energy.[31,43] Magnesium is the fourth most abundant cation in the body and the second most abundant intracellular cation. About 50% of magnesium is stored in bone and 39% to 49% is stored in the intracellular space.[31] Only about 1% to 2% of body magnesium is available in the ECF and about 0.3% is available in serum. About one third to one half of serum magnesium is bound to protein or chelated to salts, and about one half is ionized.[3,22]

Magnesium is absorbed mostly in the jejunum and ileum, both by passive diffusion and by active transport. The kidneys play the largest role in maintaining magnesium balance. Renal excretion drops to very low levels when magnesium needs to be conserved and increases tremendously when serum magnesium levels rise, thus maintaining a strict balance. The thick ascending loop of Henle is where most of the magnesium filtered by the glomeruli is reabsorbed. Loop diuretics and thiazides impede reabsorption, causing increased urinary magnesium losses.[16,31]

While magnesium concentration in the serum is very low, it is important in more than 300 enzyme reactions. It is required for the metabolism of carbohydrates, protein, and fat; for genetic transcription and replication; and for all reactions involving adenosine triphosphate (ATP), including the functioning of the sodium-potassium pump, membrane stabilization, nerve conduction, and neuromuscular function.[43]

Laboratory Values. Normal ranges for magnesium are 1.5 to 2.3 mg/dl (0.62 to 0.95 mmol/L) as shown in Table 31-3. Serum magnesium levels are poor indicators of body magnesium status. Like potassium, hemolysis will elevate serum magnesium levels as intracellular levels are more than 16 times higher than ECF levels.[22] In addition, any other process that results in cell breakdown and release of intracellular contents will raise serum magnesium levels, possibly masking a deficiency. Examples of this are catabolism and rhabdomyolysis. Acidemia results in redistribution of magnesium from ICF to ECF, raising serum magnesium levels.[38] Alkalosis has the opposite effect, lowering serum magnesium levels.[22]

Hypermagnesemia

Serum magnesium levels above the normal range occur in 5.7% to 9.3% of hospitalized patients.[47,48] However, because magnesium levels are not part of most routine laboratory panels, hypermagnesemia is often missed. In one study, researchers assessed the magnesium levels of all of the blood samples delivered to a laboratory for routine electrolyte analysis ($n = 1033$) and found magnesium abnormalities in 546 of the samples. They also found that 87% (52/59) of patients with hypermagnesemia did not have a physician request for a magnesium level.[47]

The patients at greatest risk for hypermagnesemia are those with renal insufficiency or failure, especially with iatrogenic magnesium supplementation. As creatinine clearance falls below 30 ml/min, slightly increased magnesium levels are commonly seen and patients are usually asymptomatic. Symptomatic hypermagnesemia occurs rarely without magnesium supplementation.[12] Even with good renal function, excessive magnesium supplementation can be life-threatening. Case reports have demonstrated hypermagnesemia in patients with normal renal function from oral or rectal Epsom salts;[26,42] medication errors in IV repletion of magnesium deficiency;[44] oral intake of magnesium hydroxide, magnesium carbonate, or magnesium citrate from common antacid or laxative formulas;[23,24] and the use of magnesium to decrease labor contractions.

Physical Assessment Findings. Hypermagnesemia primarily affects the central nervous and cardiovascular systems.[22] Mild hypermagnesemia is usually asymptomatic. Signs and symptoms of hypermagnesemia begin as levels rise above 4.9 mg/dl (>2 mmol/L) when deep tendon reflexes become diminished. As magnesium levels further increase, severe vasodilation and hypotension may be seen. When magnesium levels rise above 9.7 mg/dl (>4 mmol/L), changes in the cardiac conduction system and neuromuscular paralysis may lead to respiratory failure and cardiac arrest.[5] As long as deep tendon reflexes are present, respiratory paralysis is not likely.[22] ECG changes may include increased PR and QT intervals, increased QRS duration, and complete AV block, and may progress to asystole (see Table 31-3).[4] Hypocalcemia often accompanies high magnesium levels and worsens symptoms.[4]

Laboratory Findings. Mild hypermagnesemia is usually asymptomatic. Early signs do not usually appear until magnesium levels rise above 4.9 mg/dl (>2.01 mmol/L). However, there is considerable variability in the literature regarding the relationship between elevated magnesium levels and the onset of signs and symptoms.

Treatment. Since most cases of life-threatening hypermagnesemia are iatrogenic, prevention is key. Generally avoid giving any medication containing magnesium to patients with renal failure. If magnesium must be given, the patient should be closely monitored for hypermagnesemia and the supplementation stopped, as needed.[4,5]

If hypermagnesemia is identified, the first step in treatment is to discontinue any magnesium supplementation. Often, this is all that is required to correct mild to moderate hypermagnesemia in patients with good renal function. In more severely hypermagnesemic patients, there are two additional mainstays of treatment. The first is to remove magnesium from the body. When renal function is sufficient, renal magnesium excretion can be induced by giving normal saline and furosemide. Monitor for potassium and calcium deficits and correct as needed. Renal replacement must be used to remove magnesium when renal function is impaired. The second mainstay of treatment for moderate to severe hypermagnesemia is to antagonize the effect of magnesium by giving intravenous calcium as chloride or gluconate.[4,5]

Hypomagnesemia

Hypomagnesemia is clinically much more common than hypermagnesemia. Magnesium depletion may have severe consequences for patients and often goes unrecognized.[47] The incidence of hypomagnesemia in hospitalized patients is 11% to 26% in the general medical population,[19,48] 61% in postoperative patients admitted to critical care,[10] and 20% in general medical patients admitted to critical care.[32] Patients with other electrolyte disturbances, such as low potassium, sodium, phosphorus, and calcium levels, are at higher risk of hypomagnesemia, because of the interactions of magnesium with other electrolytes.[3,33,47,48]

Low magnesium levels are usually caused by poor intake, increased renal or GI excretion, or acute shifts between the ICF and ECF. Hypomagnesemia from poor intake is seen in alcoholism, in protein-calorie malnutrition, and in patients receiving magnesium-free parenteral nutrition. Excess GI magnesium losses occur in short-bowel syndrome, steatorrhea, chronic diarrhea, and gastrointestinal suctioning. Increased renal magnesium losses are commonly seen in patients with uncontrolled diabetes and patients with renal tubular disorders. Ketoacidosis from starvation or diabetes increases renal magnesium loss.[3] Multiple medications may lead to hypomagnesemia, including thiazides, loop diuretics, aminoglycosides, cyclosporine, cisplatin, and amphotericin B. Magnesium may shift from the ECF to the ICF when insulin and dextrose are given, especially in the presence of metabolic alkalosis. "Hungry bone syndrome" following parathyroidectomy may cause low serum levels as the magnesium is deposited in newly formed bone.[41]

Hypocalcemia and hypokalemia typically accompany magnesium deficiency. Renal potassium conservation is impaired in hypomagnesemia, resulting in refractory hypokalemia. Thus magnesium deficiency must be suspected when hypokalemia does not correct despite supplementation.[22,31]

Physical Assessment Findings. Low magnesium levels often cause no symptoms. When symptoms are present, they mainly involve the neurologic and cardiovascular systems. Hypocalcemia, hypokalemia, and metabolic alkalosis often accompany magnesium deficiency, so signs and symptoms may overlap.[16] The most common symptoms include muscle twitches, cramps, hyperactive deep tendon reflexes, vertigo, or ataxia. Chvostek's or Trousseau's sign or paresthesias may be present. Other symptoms may include mental status changes, dysphagia, nystagmus, tetany, new-onset hyperglycemia, or seizures (see Figures 31-10 and 31-11).[5,22,31] The clinician may suspect hypomagnesemia when low potassium levels do not respond to supplementation and when other electrolyte abnormalities such as hyponatremia and hypocalcemia are present.[4]

Cardiovascular symptoms include tachycardia, ventricular dysrhythmias, especially torsades de pointes, and worsening signs of digitalis toxicity. ECG changes that occur include ST depression, T-wave inversion, prolonged QT interval, widened QRS complex, shortened PR interval, and flattening or inversion of P waves in the precordial leads (see Table 31-3). Treatment-resistant ventricular fibrillation (VF) or other dysrhythmias suggest magnesium deficiency.[4,5,31]

Laboratory Findings. Low serum magnesium levels indicate a deficiency. However, normal levels do not rule *out* deficiency. Low magnesium levels may be seen in hypoproteinemia since 20% of serum magnesium is protein-bound.[3] Even when serum magnesium levels are normal, a high index of suspicion for deficiency should be maintained for patients with high risk.

Treatment. Treatment of magnesium deficiency depends on whether symptoms are present and also on their severity. Mild or asymptomatic hypomagnesemia may be treated with oral or enteral magnesium salts such as magnesium sulfate or magnesium oxide. Keep in mind that the major side effect of oral or enteral magnesium salts is diarrhea.

Moderate to severe symptomatic hypomagnesemia is treated with intravenous magnesium sulfate 1 to 2 g.[5] Additional doses may be needed in patients with severe hypomagnesemia manifesting as seizures or torsades de pointes.

Calcium salts (gluconate and chloride), usually 1 g of gluconate, are also given because hypomagnesemic patients are also hypocalcemic.[4] Because correction of a total body magnesium deficiency may take days to weeks of therapy,[5] additional magnesium to replace the total body deficit can be given as 6 g in daily intravenous fluid over 3 to 7 days.[5]

In patients with renal insufficiency, magnesium must be given cautiously. If during infusion deep tendon reflexes decrease or disappear, or if hypotension develops, stop the infusion and measure the magnesium level.[22]

PHOSPHORUS

Applied Physiology and Pathophysiology

Phosphorus, a nonmetallic chemical element, is crucial to all body functions. In any discussion of how phosphorus functions in the body, it is important to have an understanding of terms to prevent misconceptions or confusion. Phosphorus, the chemical element, is never found alone in the body; it is always combined with other elements, usually in the form of inorganic phosphates (abbreviated as HPO_4^{2-} and $H_2PO_4^-$).[46] While some authorities may use the terms interchangeably, in the context of this chapter, the word "phosphorus" will be used when discussing the laboratory value and the word "phosphate" will be used when discussing how phosphorus is utilized in body functions.

Phosphate is the essential energy source for cellular function in the body and the maintenance of life. When ATP is cleaved to adenosine diphosphate (ADP), a phosphate molecule is liberated, creating energy for the cell. This process is crucial to electrolyte transport (sodium, potassium, calcium) across cellular membranes; nerve conduction; red blood cell function; muscular contractions; metabolism of carbohydrates, protein, and fats;[24,28] and in virtually every enzyme system.[46] Phosphate is important as a building block of cellular membranes and is responsible for many intracellular functions, including mitochondrial function[24,28,50] and leukocytosis.[28]

The vast majority of phosphate is found in the bone and is inextricably linked with calcium metabolism; phosphorus and calcium are inversely related to each other (if one increases, the other decreases).[14] Phosphates in the blood circulate either protein-bound (12%), complexed with other minerals (33%), or in an ionized form. A normal diet provides more than adequate amounts of phosphate. The kidneys are responsible for elimination of 90% of phosphate and will retain phosphate as needed by the body, by reabsorbing it in the renal tubules in response to plasma phosphate levels.[24,28,46]

Phosphate (and calcium) levels are regulated by PTH, vitamin D, and calcitonin. These three substances interact to control absorption from the GI tract, deposition and resorption from bone, and excretion and resorption by the kidneys. PTH, secreted in response to hypocalcemia, decreases the circulating or serum phosphate level by increasing its excretion from the kidneys. Vitamin D increases phosphate uptake from the GI tract, and calcitonin decreases phosphate excretion from the kidneys.[14,28,50]

Hyperphosphatemia

The incidence of hyperphosphatemia is most commonly seen in the setting of renal insufficiency and failure. Because the kidneys are efficient in eliminating phosphate, levels do not usually increase until the kidneys have lost more than 75% of their function.[15] Phosphate levels may also increase because of tumor lysis (resulting from chemotherapy for cancer), large muscle trauma (crush injuries), and heatstroke. Hyperphosphatemia may also be caused by the excessive use of phosphate-containing enemas or laxatives, even with normal kidney function. If a renal failure patient ingests excessive amounts of vitamin D, hyperphosphatemia may occur. Excessive phosphate combines with calcium to form an insoluble compound called calcium phosphate, which may be deposited throughout the body, especially the kidneys, heart, lungs, cornea, and skin. While rare, it is a serious complication in patients suffering from end-stage renal failure and inadequate control of their phosphate levels.[9,24,50]

Physical Assessment Findings. Elevated phosphate combines with ionized calcium and decreases the calcium level, with the major signs and symptoms seen with hyperphosphatemia related to the low calcium concentration. Hypocalcemia typically causes increased neuromuscular activity and negative effects on the cardiovascular system. The increased neuromuscular activity is caused by the decrease in the excitation threshold and is exhibited by numbness and tingling, particularly around the mouth and in the hands and feet. Muscle spasm, to the point of tetany, of the hands, feet, and face may be seen or even elicited during an assessment. Chvostek's sign and Trousseau's sign are both indicators of tetany. Hyperreflexia is also found (see Figures 31-10 and 31-11).[24] The cardiovascular effects of hypocalcemia are significant and can include hypotension, increased QT interval (which may lead to ventricular dysrhythmias including ventricular tachycardia and torsades de pointes),[5] decreased cardiac output, and decreased response to medications that act through calcium, including digitalis, dopamine, and norepinephrine.[31,50]

Laboratory Findings. Phosphates are the chemically active forms of phosphorus that the body uses for energy. However, laboratory values are expressed in terms of phosphorus.[24]

Hyperphosphatemia is defined as phosphorus levels greater than 4.5 mg/dl (>1.45 mmol/L). Because the effects of hyperphosphatemia are long term and do not have a significant impact on patient survival, there is no "panic" level.[15]

Treatment. The main treatments of hyperphosphatemia are decreasing the intake of phosphates and binding phosphates in the gut using a variety of agents (aluminum hydroxide, calcium acetate, lanthanum, sevelamer). All of the above agents work in the GI tract and are NOT available IV. If a patient has reasonable renal function, a saline IV may increase phosphate excretion.[24] Continuous renal replacement therapy (CRRT) can cause hypophosphatemia.[46]

Hypophosphatemia

Hypophosphatemia is a significant issue for critically ill patients. Hypophosphatemia can occur because of a depletion of body stores or a shift of phosphates from the ECF into the ICF.[24] Depletion of body stores occurs with excessive alcohol use. While there is some relation to the inadequate diets of most patients with chronic alcoholism, hypophosphatemia has been found in chronic alcoholism patients with normal diets, leading to speculation that some other mechanism is also involved. Medications used to bind phosphorus in the GI tract can cause a significant hypophosphatemia when used to excess. Extensive thermal burns may cause hypophosphatemia. It usually occurs a number of days after the initial injury and is thought to be related to the forced diuresis that results from fluid resuscitation.[24,28,50] In addition, hypophosphatemia is a common occurrence in patients receiving CRRT.[46] Hospitalized older adults are at risk for vitamin D deficiency, which can also cause hypophosphatemia.[20]

A shift of phosphate from the ECF to the ICF is a significant cause of hypophosphatemia and can occur in a variety of settings. Patients may have several of these causes simultaneously in the critical care setting. Epinephrine has been implicated in causing a decrease in phosphate levels in patients,[17,18] but its mechanism is unclear. Respiratory alkalosis, caused by overventilation, can cause a shift of phosphorus into the cells with a resultant decrease in the phosphorus level by up to 0.5 mg/dl (0.16 mmol/L). Patients suffering from DKA and HHS can excrete significant amounts of phosphate in the urine and still have normal serum phosphorus levels. The treatment of both of these diabetic emergencies with insulin and fluids will drive phosphate from the ECF into the ICF, potentially creating a significant hypophosphatemia (see Chapter 34).[24]

A significant cause of hypophosphatemia is known as "refeeding syndrome," which occurs when a malnourished patient is started on either PN or EN. A malnourished patient will have a depleted ICF phosphate level, while the ECF level will remain relatively normal. When the patient begins to receive nutrition, even in modest amounts, the increased levels of glucose and insulin, from either the PN formula or the patient's pancreas, cause a significant shift of phosphates from the ECF into the ICF. This shift dramatically decreases the ECF phosphate level and puts the patient at risk for hypophosphatemia. This usually occurs from 24 to 72 hours after the feedings start and is more common in PN than EN.[21,24,28]

The effects of hypophosphatemia are significant and wide ranging and are the result of a decrease in the levels of ATP and 2,3-diphosphoglycerate (2,3-DPG), an enzyme that is necessary for the release of oxygen from red blood cells. Low ATP and 2,3-DPG levels cause red blood cells to be more fragile, therefore more likely to hemolyze, and less able to release oxygen to peripheral tissues.[28] Both factors are implicated in significant tissue hypoxia. Because of the low phosphate levels, muscular strength will decrease and the muscles may even begin to disintegrate, causing an increase in creatinine phosphokinase (CPK) level and rhabdomyolysis. This muscle weakness and destruction is also implicated in respiratory failure, and especially in the failure of mechanically ventilated patients who are unable to be weaned because of muscle fatigue. The respiratory muscle failure, coupled with the tissue hypoxia, can have a profoundly negative effect on the patient who is being weaned. The heart is also susceptible to hypophosphatemia-induced decreases in contractility. Hypophosphatemia may even cause a cardiomyopathy that can be reversed with phosphate repletion. In addition, hypophosphatemia is associated with a decreased response to both inotropic and vasoactive medications.[24,28]

Physical Assessment Findings. The major assessment findings in hypophosphatemia are seen as muscular weakness, changes in mental status (increased irritability, weakness, numbness, lack of coordination, confusion, seizures, coma), hypoxia, and potential difficulty in maintaining cardiac output or blood pressure, even with supportive medications.[14,15,24]

Laboratory Findings. When the phosphorus level drops below 2.5 mg/dl (<0.81 mmol/L) hypophosphatemia exists. When the phosphorus level drops below 1.5 mg/dl (<0.49 mmol/L), severe hypophosphatemia exists. A "panic" level is considered below 1 mg/dl (<0.32 mmol/L).[15]

Treatment. The initial treatment of hypophosphatemia is to treat the causes, if possible. If the patient has a functioning GI tract, oral or enteral replacement with a variety of phosphate products is appropriate. The ability of the patient to tolerate such products may be limited by nausea or diarrhea. If the patient is unable to tolerate the oral or enteral replacement or if the hypophosphatemia is significant (<1 mg/dl [<0.32 mmol/L]), SLOW replenishment via IV may be utilized, using any number of published dosing schemes. If the replenishment is too rapid, hypocalcemia may occur. The key to replenishment of phosphates is that it must be done over a period of days to allow equilibrium to occur between the ECF and the ICF.[24,46]

CONCLUSIONS

Electrolyte imbalances represent some of the most complex medical emergencies faced by critical care nurses. The physiologic processes of potassium, sodium, calcium, magnesium, and phosphorus are interlinked and may present a confusing picture. However, an in-depth knowledge of the pathophysiology can prepare the critical care nurse with the methods of assessment, identification, and treatment that can sometimes dramatically influence their patients' lives.

REFERENCES

1. Adrogué, H. J., & Madias, N. E. (2000a). Hypernatremia. *N Engl J Med, 342*, 1493–1499.
2. Adrogué, H. J., & Madias, N. E. (2000b). Hyponatremia. *N Engl J Med, 342*, 1581–1589.
3. Alfrey, A. C. (2003). Normal and abnormal magnesium metabolism. In R. W. Schrier (Ed.), *Renal and electrolyte disorders* (6th ed.). Philadelphia: Lippincott Williams & Wilkins.
3a. American Diabetes Association. (2004). Hyperglycemic crises in diabetes. *Diab Care, 27*(suppl 1), S94–S102.
4. American Heart Association. (2000). Part 8: Advanced challenges in resuscitation. Section 1: Life-threatening electrolyte abnormalities. *Resuscitation, 46*, 253–259.
5. American Heart Association. (2003). *ACLS for experienced providers.* Dallas: Author.
6. Ariyan, C. E., & Sosa, J. A. (2004). Assessment and management of patients with abnormal calcium. *Crit Care Med, 34*(suppl), S146–S154.
7. Batcheller, J. (1994). Syndrome of inappropriate antidiuretic hormone secretion. *Crit Care Nurs Clin North Am, 6*, 687–692.
8. Bushinsky, D. A., & Monk, R. D. (1998). Calcium. *Lancet, 352*, 306–311.
9. Carlstedt, F., & Lind, L. (2001). Hypocalcemic syndromes. *Crit Care Clin, 17*, 139–153.
10. Chernow, B., et al. (1989). Hypomagnesemia in patients in post-operative intensive care. *Chest, 95*, 391–397.
11. Cohn, J. N., et al. (2000). New guidelines for potassium replacement in clinical practice. *Arch Intern Med, 160*, 2429–2436.
12. Gibbs, M. A., Wolfson, A. B., & Tayal, V. S. (2002). Electrolyte disturbances. In J. A. Marx (Ed.), *Rosen's emergency medicine: concepts and clinical practice* (Vol 2, 5th ed.). St Louis: Mosby.
13. Gheorghiade, M., et al. (2003). Vasopressin V2-receptor blockade with tolvaptan in patients with chronic heart failure: results from a double-blind, randomized trial. *Circulation, 107*, 2690–2696.
14. Huether, S. E. (2002). The cellular environment: fluids and electrolytes, acids and bases. In K. L. McCance & S. E. Huether (Eds.), *Pathophysiology: the biological basis for disease in adults and children* (4th ed.). St Louis: Mosby.
15. Jacobs, D. S., DeMott, W. R., & Oxley, D. K. (2004). *Lexi-Comp's laboratory test handbook* (3rd ed.). Cleveland, OH: Lexi-Comp.
16. Kapoor, M., & Chan, G. Z. (2001). Fluid and electrolyte abnormalities. *Crit Care Clin, 17*, 503–529.
17. Kjeldsen, S. E., et al. (1988). Decreased serum phosphate in essential hypertension: related to increased sympathetic tone. *Am J Hypertens, 1*(4 Pt 1), 403–409.
18. Kjeldsen, S. E., et al. (1986). Serum phosphate and sympathetic tone in mild essential hypertension. *Acta Med Scand Suppl, 714*, 119–123.
19. Lum, G. (1992). Hypomagnesemia in acute and chronic care patient populations. *Am J Clin Pathol, 97*, 827–830.
20. Lyman, D. (2005). Undiagnosed vitamin D deficiency in the hospitalized patient. *Am Fam Pract, 71*, 299–304.
21. Marinella, M. A. (2003). The refeeding syndrome and hypophosphatemia. *Nutr Rev, 61*, 320–323.
22. Matz, R. (1993). Magnesium: deficiencies and therapeutic uses. *Hosp Pract (Off Ed).*, Apr 30; *28*(4A), 79–82, 85–87, 91–92.
23. McLaughlin, S. A., & McKinney, P. E. (1998). Antacid-induced hypermagnesemia in a patient with normal renal function and bowel obstruction. *Ann Pharmacother, 32*, 312–315.
24. Metheny, N. M. (2000). *Fluid and electrolyte balance: nursing considerations.* Philadelphia: Lippincott Williams & Wilkins.
25. Myers, J. S. (2001). Oncologic emergencies. In S. E. Otto (Ed.), *Oncology nursing* (pp. 498–581). St Louis: Mosby.
26. Nordt, S. P., et al. (1996). Hypermagnesemia following an acute ingestion of Epsom salt in a patient with normal renal function. *J Toxicol Clin Toxicol, 34*, 735–739.
27. Palmer, B. F. (2004). Managing hyperkalemia caused by inhibitors of the renin-angiotensin-aldosterone system. *N Engl J Med, 351*, 585–592.
28. Peppers, M. P., Geheb, M., & Desai, T. (1991). Hypophosphatemia and hyperphosphatemia. *Crit Care Clin, 7*, 201–214.
29. Perazella, M. A. (2000). Drug-induced hyperkalemia: old culprits and new offenders. *Am J Med, 109*, 307–314.
30. Piano, M. R., & Huether, S. E. (2002). Mechanisms of hormonal regulation. In K. L. McCance & S. E. Huether (Eds.), *Pathophysiology: the biological basis for disease in adults and children* (4th ed.). St Louis: Mosby.
31. Porth, C. M. (2004). *Essentials of pathophysiology.* Philadelphia: Lippincott Williams & Wilkins.
32. Reinhart, R. A., & Desbiens, N. A. (1985). Hypomagnesemia in patients entering the ICU. *Crit Care Med, 13*, 506–507.
33. Rubeiz, G. J., Thill-Baharozian, M., Hardie, D., et al. (1993). Association of hypomagnesemia and mortality in acutely ill medical patients. *Crit Care Med, 21*, 203–209.
34. RXlist.com. (2005a). *Calcium chloride.* www.rxlist.com/cgi/generic3/calciumcl.htm.
35. RXlist.com. (2005b). *Calcium gluconate.* www.rxlist.com/cgi/generic3/calciumgluc.htm.
36. RXlist.com. (2005c). *Kayexelate.* www.rxlist.com/cgi/generic2/kayexalate.htm.
37. Rxlist.com. (2005d). *K-dur.* www.rxlist.com/cgi/generic/kclsr_ids.htm.

38. Salem, M., Munoz, R., & Chernow, B. (1991). Hypomagnesemia in critical illness: a common and clinically important problem. *Crit Care Clin*, *7*, 225–252.

39. Sato, Y., et al. (2000). Beneficial effect of intermittent cyclical etidronate therapy in hemiplegic patients following an acute stroke. *J Bone Miner Res*, *15*, 2487–2494.

40. Sato, Y., et al. (2004). Beneficial effect of etidronate therapy in immobilized hip fracture patients. *Am J Phys Med Rehabil*, *83*, 298–303.

41. Stern, J. M. (2005). Oncology fluid and electrolyte disorders. *Support Line*, *27*(3), 19–27.

42. Tofil, N. M., Benner, K. W., & Winkler, M. K. (2005). Fatal hypermagnesemia caused by an Epsom salt enema: a case illustration. *South Med J*, *98*, 253–256.

43. Toto, K. H., & Yucha, C. B. (1994). Magnesium: homeostasis, imbalances and therapeutic uses. *Crit Care Nurs Clin North Am*, *6*, 767–783.

44. Vissers, R. J., & Purssell, R. (1996). Iatrogenic magnesium overdose: two case reports. *J Emerg Med*, *14*, 187–191.

45. Weiss-Guillet, E., Takala, J., & Jakob, S. (2003). Diagnosis and management of electrolyte emergencies. *Best Practice Res Clin Endocrinol Metabolism*, *17*, 623–651.

46. Whitemire, S. J. (2003). Fluids, electrolytes and acid-base balance. In L. E. Matarese & M. M. Gottschlich (Eds.), *Contemporary nutrition support practice* (2nd ed.). Philadelphia: Saunders.

47. Whang, R., & Ryder, K. W. (1990). Frequency of hypomagnesemia and hypermagnesemia: requested vs. routine. *JAMA*, *263*, 3063–3064.

48. Wong, E. T., et al. (1983). A high prevalence of hypomagnesemia and hypermagnesemia in hospitalized patients. *Am J Clin Pathol*, *79*, 348–352.

49. Wong, F., et al. (2003). A vasopressin receptor antagonist (VPA-985) improves serum sodium concentration in patients with hyponatremia: a multicenter, randomized, placebo-controlled trial. *Hepatology*, *37*, 182–191.

50. Yucha, C. B., & Toto, K. H. (1994). Calcium and phosphorus derangements. *Crit Care Nurs Clin North Am*, *6*, 747–766.

CHAPTER 32

Complex Acid-Base Disorders and Associated Electrolyte Imbalances

Kathleen H. Toto

Acid-base and electrolyte imbalances are common in acutely ill patients. They frequently complicate critical illness and are often the central focus of emergency therapy. Acid-base disorders can be as simple as a compensated respiratory acidosis or as complex as a triple disorder, such as metabolic acidosis combined with a metabolic and respiratory alkalosis. In the acutely ill adult, mixed acid-base disorders are also common. Differentiating between a compensated acid-base disorder and a mixed disorder can be challenging. Additionally, both alkalosis and acidosis are often accompanied by multiple electrolyte imbalances, complicating both the clinical presentation and the treatment. This chapter will review acid-base physiology and discuss a systematic approach to diagnosing simple and mixed acid-base disturbances utilizing advanced arterial blood gas (ABG) interpretation methods and the anion gap. The etiology, clinical manifestations, associated electrolyte imbalances, and treatment of metabolic acidosis, metabolic alkalosis, respiratory acidosis, and respiratory alkalosis will be reviewed. The three steps used to distinguish a simple compensated acid-base disorder from a complex, mixed acid-base disorder will be reviewed. Case studies will be discussed to illustrate salient aspects of caring for acutely ill patients with acid-base and electrolyte emergencies.

PATIENTS AT RISK

Critically ill patients are at particular risk for acid-base and electrolyte disorders, including patients with acute renal failure, volume depletion, acute respiratory distress, chronic obstructive pulmonary disease (COPD), shock, and especially those with multiple organ dysfunction syndrome.

ACID-BASE PHYSIOLOGY

Acid-base balance is maintained through complex interactions between cellular, renal, pulmonary, cardiovascular, gastrointestinal (GI), and hepatic systems.

Disruptions in any one of these systems can result in an acid-base imbalance with severe adverse consequences. The arterial pH is the primary indicator of acid-base balance and is a reflection of hydrogen ion (H^+) concentration in the blood. Under normal circumstances, the pH is maintained within the range of 7.35 to 7.45. The arterial pH is affected by the interplay of acids (substances able to give up H^+ ions) and bases (substances able to accept H^+ ions). As the H^+ concentration in the blood increases, the pH decreases. Conversely, as the H^+ concentration in the blood decreases, the pH increases. Maintaining the H^+ concentration and pH within normal limits is, in part, controlled by the carbonic acid-bicarbonate buffer system, as represented by the formula:

$$H^+ + HCO_3^- \rightleftharpoons H_2CO_3 \rightleftharpoons H_2O + CO_2$$

When the blood H^+ concentration increases, bicarbonate (HCO_3^-) combines with the excess acid to form carbonic acid (H_2CO_3), which then dissociates into water (H_2O) and carbon dioxide (CO_2). Excess CO_2 can be excreted via the lungs. Conversely, if base (HCO_3^-) levels increase, the carbonic acid-bicarbonate buffer system will buffer the excess base.

Aside from the carbonic acid-bicarbonate buffer system, sodium phosphate ($NaHPO_4$), hemoglobin (Hgb), and serum proteins (albumin) also function as buffers. Serum proteins can act as either acids or bases by releasing or binding H^+ as needed. Hgb, a protein in red blood cells, also buffers acids in a similar fashion to serum proteins and can carry CO_2. These buffer systems are linked to renal and pulmonary mechanisms and work to maintain the ratio of acid to bicarbonate at 20:1. As long as this ratio is maintained, the pH will remain within normal limits.

Definitions and Normal Values

The primary parameters important in acid-base assessment include the acids, H^+ and partial pressure of arterial carbon dioxide ($PaCO_2$), and the base HCO_3^-. Diagnosing acid-base imbalances at the bedside begins with assessing serum chemistries and the arterial blood gas (Table 32-1).

Acidemia is defined as a decrease in the blood pH below 7.35, whereas *acidosis* is a physiologic process characterized by a primary decrease in HCO_3^- level (metabolic acidosis) or a primary increase in $Paco_2$ (respiratory acidosis). The terms *acidosis* and *acidemia* are not interchangeable because the presence of an acidosis is not always associated with acidemia. For example, a patient with COPD may have a respiratory acidosis characterized by a primary increase in the $Paco_2$. However, the patient may not be acidemic if a concurrent metabolic alkalosis (primary increase in HCO_3^- level) is present, which could occur in the COPD patient receiving loop diuretics. In this situation, there is a mixed or complex acid-base disorder—respiratory acidosis and metabolic alkalosis—that could present with a normal pH.

Conversely, alkalemia is defined as an increase in the blood pH above 7.45, whereas alkalosis is a physiologic process characterized by a primary increase in HCO_3^- level (metabolic alkalosis) or a primary decrease in the $Paco_2$ (respiratory alkalosis). A patient can have a physiologic process resulting in an alkalosis in the absence of alkalemia.

Understanding Compensation

Acid-base disorders are caused by primary changes in the excretion of $Paco_2$ (respiratory disorders) or changes in plasma HCO_3^- level (metabolic disorders).

TABLE 32-1 Labs Used in Acid-Base Assessment: Normal Values

Arterial Blood Gas	
pH	7.35–7.45
$Paco_2$	35–45 mm Hg
HCO_3^-	24–28 mEq/L
Serum Chemistries	
Na^+	135–145 mEq/L
K^+	3.5–5 mEq/L
Cl^-	95–105 mEq/L
Total CO_2*	26–32 mEq/L

*The total CO_2 concentration in the chemistry panel is a reflection of HCO_3^- ion concentration and is substituted for HCO_3^- in the anion gap formula.
Cl = Chloride, HCO_3^- = bicarbonate, K^+ = potassium, Na^+ = sodium, $Paco_2$ = partial pressure of arterial carbon dioxide.

A primary disorder means that the changes in $Paco_2$ or HCO_3^- are due to a metabolic or respiratory disorder and are *not* secondary to a pH change (compensation). Under normal circumstances, all deviations from normal in acid-base balance trigger compensatory mechanisms that tend to return blood pH toward the normal level as illustrated by the following equation:

$$H^+ = 24 \times Paco_2 \text{(respiratory component)}$$

$$HCO_3^- \text{(renal/metabolic component)}$$

As shown in the above equation, it is important to emphasize that the H^+ ion concentration is determined by the ratio of the $Paco_2$ to HCO_3^- concentration, not the absolute values. Thus H^+ concentration is directly proportional to $Paco_2$ and inversely proportional to HCO_3^- concentration. Metabolic acid-base disorders result in deviations in HCO_3^- from normal, whereas respiratory acid-base disorders are due to deviations in $Paco_2$ from normal. Consider the following: under normal circumstances $Paco_2$, HCO_3^- concentration, and H^+ ion concentration are as follows:

$$(H^+ = 40 \text{ nmol/L}) = 24 \times (Paco_2 = 40 \text{ mm Hg})$$

$$(HCO_3^- = 24 \text{ mEq/L})$$

In metabolic acidosis, the H^+ concentration is increased because the denominator on the right side (bicarbonate concentration) is reduced. As the acidosis develops, causing the $Paco_2$ to fall, the H^+ concentration returns toward normal because the ratio is partially restored to the normal level. For example, if a patient suddenly develops lactic acidosis, causing the HCO_3^- level to decrease to 12 mEq/L (half of normal), the immediate effect is for the H^+ level to increase proportionately to 80 nmol/L (double); the pH would fall from 7.40 to 7.10. However, compensation, if normal, will occur, stimulating an increase in minute ventilation, resulting in a decrease in $Paco_2$ to 22 mm Hg. The net effect is that the increase in H^+ concentration is limited to 60 nmol/L and blood pH only falls to 7.22, instead of 7.10.

Conversely, the compensatory mechanism for a metabolic alkalosis (a primary increase in plasma HCO_3^- concentration) is a decrease in minute ventilation, resulting in an increase in $Paco_2$. This increase in $Paco_2$ acts to move the blood pH toward normal. Remember, in general, these compensatory mechanisms *do not* return the blood pH completely to the normal range of 7.35 to 7.45 but rather toward the normal range.[8,19]

Application of Acid-Base Principles

The assessment and diagnosis of acid-base disorders require a systematic approach beginning with interpretation of the ABG and serum chemistries and calculation of the anion gap. Evaluation of the anion gap is critical in acid-base assessment because it may be the only clue to the presence of a metabolic acidosis in the setting of a mixed acid-base disorder where the pH is normal.

The Anion Gap

The extracellular fluid is normally electroneutral, meaning that the sum of anions (negative ions) is equal to the sum of cations (positive ions) (Figure 32-1).

The primary measured anions in the plasma include chloride (Cl^-) and HCO_3^-; the primary cation is sodium (Na^+). The smaller quantities of anions not included in the anion gap formula include albumin, sulfate, phosphate, and others. The smaller quantities of cations not included in the formula include potassium (K^+), calcium (Ca^{++}), magnesium (Mg^{++}), and others. The ions not included in the anion gap formula are termed "unmeasured ions." The anion gap is calculated using the values in the serum chemistry panel as follows:

$$\text{Anion gap} = Na^+ - (Cl^- + HCO_3^-)$$

Because the unmeasured ions are not all included in the formula, there is a normal difference or "gap" ranging from approximately 9 to 16 mEq/L; the normal range may vary depending on the individual laboratory. If this gap is increased, it signifies the presence of additional unmeasured ions in the plasma. The addition of H^+, an acid, is buffered by HCO_3^-, a base, causing an increase in the anion gap, signifying the presence of a metabolic acidosis. When calculating the anion gap using the serum chemistry panel, it is important to remember that the HCO_3^- concentration

is represented as total CO_2 concentration on the chemistry panel. The total CO_2 concentration is a combination of HCO_3^- concentration, dissolved CO_2 concentration, and H_2CO_3 concentration, the most predominant of which is HCO_3 concentration. Typically, the plasma total CO_2 concentration is approximately 1 mEq greater than the arterial HCO_3^- concentration. Therefore for practical purposes, the total CO_2 concentration on the chemistry panel is substituted for HCO_3^- concentration in the anion gap formula. The total CO_2 concentration on the serum chemistry panel represents a base and should not be confused with the Pa_{CO_2} on the ABG, a reflection of respiratory acid. Box 32-1 demonstrates calculation of the anion gap.

In the example, the anion gap of 25 mEq/L is greater than the expected gap of 9 to 16 mEq/L and signifies the presence of a metabolic acidosis. The anion gap can be slightly elevated in a respiratory or metabolic alkalosis because of changes in protein-hydrogen buffering. However, if the anion gap is greater than 20 mEq/L, a metabolic acidosis is present.[19]

A systematic approach to the interpretation of the ABG and anion gap is essential to accurately diagnose acid-base disorders. This becomes particularly important in the setting of mixed acid-base disorders (two or more primary disorders occurring simultaneously). For example, a patient with a respiratory alkalosis and a metabolic acidosis may have a normal arterial pH despite a low HCO_3^- level and a low Pa_{CO_2} (lower than that which would occur with compensation for the metabolic acidosis). Systematic assessment of the ABG and the anion gap will allow for the diagnosis and treatment of these complex acid-base disorders, which might otherwise be overlooked, and is outlined in Box 32-2.

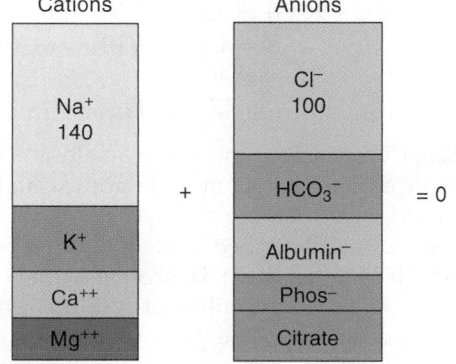

♦FIGURE 32-1 The anion gap. Ca^{++} = Calcium, Cl^- = chloride, HCO_3^- = bicarbonate, K^+ = potassium, Mg^{++} = magnesium, Na^+ = sodium, Phos = phosphate.

Box 32-1

Calculation of the Anion Gap

Serum Chemistries
$Na^+ = 140$ mEq/L
$K^+ = 5$ mEq/L
$Cl^- = 100$ mEq/L
$CO_2 = 15$ mEq/L
Anion gap calculation: $Na^+ - (Cl^- + HCO_3^-)$
$$= 140 - (100 + 15)$$
$$= 140 - 115$$
$$= 25 \text{ mEq/L}$$

Cl^- = Chloride, Na^+ = sodium, K^+ = potassium.

Box 32-2

Three-Step Approach to Diagnosing Simple and Mixed Acid-Base Disorders

STEP 1: USING THE ARTERIAL BLOOD GAS, IDENTIFY THE MOST APPARENT DISORDER

1. Look at the pH first.
   a. If the pH is less than 7.35, acidemia is present and may be due to a metabolic or respiratory disorder:
      - If the HCO_3^- concentration is low, metabolic acidosis is present.
      - If the Pa_{CO_2} is high, respiratory acidosis is present.
   b. If the pH is greater than 7.45, alkalemia is present and may be due to either a metabolic or a respiratory disorder.
      - If the HCO_3^- concentration is high, metabolic alkalosis is present.
      - If the Pa_{CO_2} is low, respiratory alkalosis is present.
      NOTE: If the pH is normal and either the HCO_3^- or the Pa_{CO_2} (or both) is abnormal, at least two acid-base disorders are present: a mixed acid-base disorder. This situation should not be misinterpreted as compensation of a primary disorder because the pH is not normalized even with full compensation. To identify one of the acid-base disturbances present, start by picking the HCO_3^- or Pa_{CO_2} value that is most abnormal.

Example:

ABG values: pH = 7.40, Pa_{CO_2} = 60 mm Hg,
HCO_3^- = 36 mEq/L

In this example the pH is normal and both the HCO_3^- and the Pa_{CO_2} values are abnormal; a mixed acid-base disorder is present. The Pa_{CO_2} is elevated; a respiratory acidosis is present. The HCO_3^- level is elevated; a metabolic alkalosis is also present. The interpretation of this disorder is a primary respiratory acidosis and a primary metabolic alkalosis, a mixed acid-base disorder. Use the formulas below in Step 2 to confirm the interpretation.

STEP 2: APPLY FORMULAS TO DETERMINE IF COMPENSATION IS PRESENT OR IF THERE IS A MIXED ACID-BASE DISORDER

1. If a metabolic acidosis is present, use the following formula to calculate what the predicted Pa_{CO_2} would be if compensated:

$$Pa_{CO_2} = (1.5 \times HCO_3^-) + 8$$

Example:

pH = 7.30, Pa_{CO_2} = 30 mm Hg, HCO_3^- = 14 mEq/L
Predicted Pa_{CO_2} = (1.5 × 14) + 8
= 21 + 8
= 29 mm Hg

Interpretation: Compensated metabolic acidosis. The predicted Pa_{CO_2} approximates (within 2 mm Hg) the measured Pa_{CO_2}.

Shortcut: When fully compensated, the Pa_{CO_2} closely approximates the last two digits of the blood pH within the range of 7.10 to 7.40. This rule-of-thumb applies only to metabolic acidosis and does *not* apply for a pH outside of this range. If the Pa_{CO_2} does not approximate the last two digits of the pH, a mixed acid-base disturbance should be considered. In the example above, avoid the math and quickly interpret this as a compensated metabolic acidosis because the digits to the right of the pH decimal point = 30 and the Pa_{CO_2} = 30 mm Hg.

Determining a Mixed Acid-Base Disorder
If the measured Pa_{CO_2} on the ABG does not approximate the predicted Pa_{CO_2}, calculated using the equation above, there is a mixed acid-base disorder. Consider the following example:

$$pH = 7.15, Pa_{CO_2} = 45 \text{ mm Hg}, HCO_3^- = 15 \text{ mEq/L}$$

The pH is low and the HCO_3^- is low; this is a metabolic acidosis. To determine if it is compensated, the predicted Pa_{CO_2} can be calculated using the formula above *or* the "shortcut" can be used. In this example, the measured Pa_{CO_2} of 45 mm Hg does *not* approximate the predicted Pa_{CO_2} of 15 mm Hg; it is much higher than expected. In this example, both a primary metabolic acidosis and a primary respiratory acidosis are present, a mixed disorder.

2. If there is a *metabolic alkalosis*, use the following formula to calculate what the predicted Pa_{CO_2} would be if compensated:
   Predicted Pa_{CO_2} = 40 + 0.7 × (measured HCO_3^- − normal HCO_3^-)

Example:
pH = 7.49, Pa_{CO_2} = 48 mm Hg, HCO_3^- = 36 mEq/L

Predicted $PaCO_2$ = 40 + 0.7(36 − 26)
= 40 + 0.7(10)
= 40 + 7
= 47 mm Hg

Interpretation: Compensated metabolic alkalosis. The calculated predicted Pa_{CO_2} of 47 mm Hg approximates the measured Pa_{CO_2} of 48 mm Hg.

NOTE: The shortcut described in Step 1 cannot be used to determine if compensation is present with a metabolic alkalosis. The shortcut only works in the setting of a metabolic acidosis when the pH is between 7.10 and 7.40.

3. If a *respiratory acidosis* is present, use the following rules to determine what the predicted HCO_3^- concentration would be if compensated:

Acute respiratory acidosis:
 HCO_3^- concentration increases by up to 1 mEq for every 10 mm Hg increase in Pa_{CO_2}

Chronic respiratory acidosis:
 HCO_3^- concentration increases by up to 3.5 mEq for every 10 mm Hg increase in Pa_{CO_2}

4. If there is a *respiratory alkalosis,* use the following rules to determine what the predicted HCO_3^- concentration would be if compensated:[19]

Acute respiratory alkalosis:
 HCO_3^- concentration decreases by up to 2 mEq for every 10 mm Hg decrease in Pa_{CO_2}

Chronic respiratory alkalosis:
 HCO_3^- concentration decreases by up to 5 mEq for every 10 mm Hg decrease in Pa_{CO_2}

If the measured values do not approximate the predicted values using the formulas and rules in Step 2, a mixed acid-base balance is present.

Data from reference 19.
ABG = Arterial blood gas, Cl^- = chloride, HCO_3^- = bicarbonate, Na^+ = sodium, Pa_{CO_2} = partial pressure of arterial carbon dioxide.

STEP 3: CALCULATE THE ANION GAP

Calculation of the anion gap is the third step in diagnosing an acid-base disorder and is important in determining the presence of mixed imbalances as well as differentiating an elevated anion gap metabolic acidosis from a non-elevated anion gap metabolic acidosis.

The anion gap is calculated using the serum chemistry panel as follows:

$$Anion\ gap = Na^+ - (Cl^- + HCO_3^-)$$

When calculating the anion gap using the serum chemistry panel, it is important to remember that the HCO_3^- concentration on the chemistry panel is represented as total CO_2 concentration. The normal range for the anion gap is approximately 9 to 16 mEq/L.

PRIMARY ACID-BASE DISORDERS

Metabolic Acidosis

Metabolic acidosis is characterized by physiologic processes resulting in a decrease in the plasma bicarbonate concentration, whereas acidemia is defined as an arterial pH less than 7.35. There are three general mechanisms responsible for a metabolic acidosis:

- Increased acid production (e.g., ketoacidosis, lactic acidosis)
- Decreased acid excretion (e.g., renal failure)
- Bicarbonate loss (e.g., diarrhea, GI fistula)

Using the Anion Gap to Diagnose a Metabolic Acidosis.
The anion gap is a helpful tool in determining the presence and etiology of a metabolic acidosis. The anion gap helps to differentiate a metabolic acidosis due to the loss of bicarbonate versus the addition or accumulation of acid. In addition, the detection of an elevated anion gap in the setting of a normal pH will help to unmask mixed acid-base disorders.

The normal range for the anion gap is approximately 9 to 16 mEq/L. In a metabolic acidosis caused by the addition or accumulation of acid in the plasma (e.g., lactic acidosis, ketoacidosis, renal failure), there will be an increase in the anion gap. If the metabolic acidosis is due to the loss of bicarbonate (e.g., diarrhea, GI fistula), the anion gap will remain within normal limits despite the presence of a metabolic acidosis (Figure 32-2). Box 32-3 lists causes of metabolic acidosis differentiated by the anion gap.

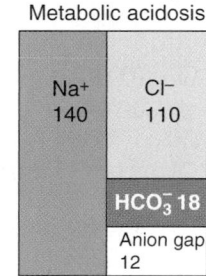

FIGURE 32-2 Metabolic acidosis: high vs. normal anion gap. Cl^- = Chloride, HCO_3^- = bicarbonate, Na^+ = sodium.

Box 32-3

Causes of Metabolic Acidosis

Elevated Anion Gap* (Gain of Acid)	Non–Anion Gap (HCO_3^- Loss)
Ketoacidosis	Gastrointestinal bicarbonate loss
Uremia (renal failure)	Diarrhea
Salicylate intoxication	Pancreatic or biliary fistula
Starvation ketosis	Ileostomy
Methanol	Small bowel drains
Alcoholic ketosis	Ureterosigmoidostomy
Unmeasured osmoles: ethylene glycol, paraldehyde	Anion exchange resin: cholestyramine
Lactic acidosis	Renal tubular acidosis

*The mnemonic KUSSMAUL can be used to help remember the causes of a metabolic acidosis associated with an elevated anion gap.

◆ Case Study 32-1, Part A

Metabolic Acidosis

C.S. is a 27-year-old male admitted to the emergency department (ED) after a motor vehicle collision. He had been trapped in his vehicle for over 6 hours before being found and extricated by paramedics. He sustained crush injuries to his upper and lower extremities as well as blunt abdominal trauma. His vital signs include blood pressure (BP): 80/palpable, heart rate (HR): 138 beats/min (sinus tachycardia), and respirations: 34 breaths/min. Physical exam revealed that his pupils were equal and reactive to light (PEARL); he was difficult to arouse. He was in a sinus tachycardia; S_1, S_2 were clear. His lungs were clear and his abdomen was distended and diffusely tender with decreased bowel sounds. His upper and lower extremities were lacerated, discolored, and swollen.

Laboratory Values:

Serum Chemistries	Arterial Blood Gas	Enzymes
Na^+: 140 mEq/L	pH: 7.15	CK: 3159 units/L
K^+: 6.9 mEq/L	$Paco_2$: 16 mm Hg	CK-MB: negative
Cl^-: 100 mEq/L	Pao_2: 90 mm Hg	LDH: 2550 units/L
CO_2: 8 mEq/L	HCO_3^-: 6 mEq/L	
Creatinine: 2.5 mg/dl	Saturation: 97%	
BUN: 16 mg/dl		
Glucose: 140 mg/dl		
Ca^{++}: 6 mg/dl		
Ionized Ca^{++}: 4.8 mg/dl		
Albumin: 4.5 mg/dl		
Phosphorus: 10.8 mg/dl		
Mg^{++}: 2 mEq/L		

Decision Point: Diagnose and determine the etiology of the acid-base disorder.

Case continues on page 875

Causes of Metabolic Acidosis

Causes of metabolic acidosis are differentiated by those disorders associated with an elevated anion gap (greater than 20 mEq/L) and those associated with no significant elevation in the anion gap (less than 20 mEq/L). In the critical care setting, there are four common causes of an elevated anion gap metabolic acidosis: lactic acidosis, ketoacidosis, renal failure (uremia), and ingestion of toxins. The most common cause of a *non*–anion gap metabolic acidosis is GI bicarbonate loss from diarrhea (see Box 32-3).

Elevated Anion Gap Metabolic Acidosis

Lactic Acidosis. Lactic acidosis is a common cause of metabolic acidosis in the critically ill patient. Lactic acidosis is typically the result of tissue hypoxia associated with inadequate perfusion or severe hypoxia. When tissues receive inadequate blood flow or oxygen delivery, they convert from aerobic to anaerobic metabolism, resulting in the production of lactic acid. Common conditions causing lactic acidosis include cardiogenic shock, hypovolemic shock, septic shock, mesenteric ischemia, acute respiratory failure, severe anemia, carbon monoxide poisoning, and metformin.[20] In the critically ill patient, lactic acidosis is often accompanied by acute renal failure caused by renal hypoperfusion. The metabolic acidosis in this situation can be quite severe and is compounded by reduced renal clearance of lactic acid as well as other acids.[10]

Ketoacidosis. Ketoacidosis occurs when cells are unable to use glucose as an energy source for metabolism and convert to the metabolism of fatty acids, which produces ketoacids (beta-hydroxybutyrate and acetoacetate). There are three causes of ketoacidosis: diabetic ketoacidosis (DKA), alcohol ingestion, and starvation. DKA typically occurs in the type 1 diabetes patient who has inadequate insulin for a given level of physiologic stress, resulting in hyperglycemia with a blood glucose level that is typically greater than 300 mg/dl.[8] DKA can occur from omission of insulin therapy, new-onset type 1 diabetes, or a physiologic stress raising the blood glucose level (e.g., infection, acute myocardial infarction, trauma, surgery, pregnancy). When there is inadequate insulin in the setting of hyperglycemia, cellular starvation occurs and metabolism converts from utilization of glucose to the breakdown of fatty acids; the end product of fatty acid metabolism is ketoacids.

Alcoholic ketoacidosis is due to excessive alcohol ingestion and is often associated with starvation. Both alcoholic and starvation ketoacidosis are associated with hypoglycemia and decreased hepatic production of glucose. In this state of hypoglycemia, the pancreas releases less insulin and cells must convert to metabolism of fatty acids for energy. As in DKA, the metabolism of these fatty acids produces ketoacids. Unlike DKA, starvation and alcoholic ketoacidosis are characterized by blood glucose levels less than 150 mg/dl.[8] In all three states of ketoacidosis—DKA, alcoholic, and starvation—the buildup of ketoacids in the plasma reduces the plasma bicarbonate level and results in a metabolic acidosis associated with a high anion gap.

Renal Failure. In both acute and chronic renal failure, there is a reduction in the glomerular filtration rate and a decreased ability of the kidneys to clear acids from the plasma. As a result, H^+ accumulates in the plasma, lowering the plasma HCO_3^- concentration, causing a metabolic acidosis. In the critically ill patient, the presence of renal failure often perpetuates or worsens other causes of metabolic acidosis because of limited clearance of acids in the setting of overproduction of acids. Examples of concomitant causes of metabolic acidosis in a critically ill patient include septic shock with ischemic acute tubular necrosis, DKA with dehydration and prerenal acute renal failure, and trauma with rhabdomyolysis and nephrotoxic acute tubular necrosis.

Ingestion of Toxins. The ingestion of various acid-producing substances can cause a metabolic acidosis. These substances include salicylate (aspirin), ethylene glycol (antifreeze and organic solvents), methanol (wood alcohol), and paraldehyde (sedative). Ingestion of these substances may be seen in suicide attempts or accidental overdose. Typically, the ingested substance is not an acid but is metabolized into an acid (methanol, ethylene glycol).[20] This increase in acid production lowers the plasma bicarbonate level and results in a high anion gap metabolic acidosis. Additionally, concurrent tissue hypoperfusion and lactic acidosis often contribute to metabolic acidosis in these patients.

Non–Anion Gap Metabolic Acidosis. A non–anion gap metabolic acidosis is due to a loss of bicarbonate from either the kidney or the GI tract. The most common cause of this type of metabolic acidosis in the acutely ill patient is diarrhea. Diarrhea causes a loss of bicarbonate and an increase in chloride concentration, leading to metabolic acidosis with a normal anion gap. A less common cause of a non–anion gap metabolic acidosis is renal tubular acidosis (RTA).

Gastrointestinal Bicarbonate Loss. The loss of bicarbonate from the GI tract results in an increase in H^+ and chloride concentrations. Moderate to severe diarrhea is the most common cause of a non–anion gap metabolic acidosis and is often associated with volume depletion that may cause a concomitant lactic acidosis if volume depletion is severe.[23] Other causes of GI bicarbonate loss that can cause a non–anion gap metabolic acidosis include ileostomies, small bowel drains, and pancreatic drains or fistulas.

Renal Tubular Acidosis. RTA, also called type II RTA, is relatively uncommon in the acute care setting. RTA is characterized by an impairment of the renal tubules' ability to reabsorb HCO_3^- and excrete H^+, resulting in a metabolic acidosis not associated with an increase in the anion gap.[20]

Manifestations of Metabolic Acidosis

Metabolic acidosis affects many organ systems and is often associated with intercurrent electrolyte imbalances. The life-threatening effects of a severe metabolic acidosis, a pH less than 7.2, are manifested in many body systems and are most prominent in the cardiovascular, metabolic, and neurologic systems (Box 32-4).

Box 32-4

Manifestations of Severe Metabolic Acidosis (pH Less Than 7.2)

CARDIOVASCULAR
- Decreased cardiac contractility
- Increased pulmonary vascular resistance leading to pulmonary edema
- Arteriolar vasodilation (hypotension and decreased systemic vascular resistance)
- Decreased responsiveness to catecholamines (endogenous and exogenous)
- Decreased ventricular fibrillation threshold

NEUROLOGIC
- Altered mental status: obtundation, coma
- Increased intracranial pressure (cerebral vasodilation)

RESPIRATORY
- Hyperventilation
- Decreased respiratory muscle strength leading to fatigue requiring intubation

METABOLIC
- Catabolism
- Insulin resistance
- Increased metabolic demands

ELECTROLYTE IMBALANCES
- Hyperkalemia
- Increased ionized calcium level

ABDOMINAL
- Nausea, vomiting, abdominal pain

Data from references 1, 16, 20.

Electrolyte Imbalances Associated With Metabolic Acidosis

Hyperkalemia. (Serum K^+ level greater than 5 mEq/L). Hyperkalemia is commonly seen with metabolic acidosis. In the setting of metabolic acidosis, H^+ moves into the cells in an attempt to reduce plasma acid concentrations. To maintain electrical neutrality, potassium moves out of the cell, which can cause hyperkalemia (Figure 32-3). In the critically ill patient, hyperkalemia and metabolic acidosis are often compounded by comorbidities (e.g., acute renal failure, tissue catabolism). These factors play an important role in contributing to the ongoing hyperkalemia associated with metabolic acidosis.

Ionized Calcium Increase. (Greater than 5 mg/dl or 1.32 mmol/L). An increase in the ionized calcium level can also occur in the setting of a metabolic acidosis. Calcium circulates in the plasma in three forms: free or unbound (ionized); protein bound; and complexed to anions such as phosphate, lactate, citrate, and bicarbonate. Although the total calcium level is more commonly measured, the ionized calcium level is the physiologically active form of calcium in the body and a more important indicator of the clinical severity of calcium imbalances. Changes in plasma H^+ concentration will affect the ionized calcium level through a change in protein binding. For example, in the setting of a metabolic acidosis, proteins act as a buffer by binding H^+ and maintain electrical neutrality by releasing calcium, thereby increasing ionized calcium levels (see Figure 32-3). Conversely, in the setting of a metabolic alkalosis, proteins release H^+ and bind calcium, resulting in a decrease in ionized calcium levels. It is important to remember that the total calcium concentration will not be affected by these shifts; the patient may develop signs and symptoms of hypocalcemia in the setting of a normal total calcium concentration. An ionized calcium level must be obtained to more accurately assess the effect of pH on changes in the ionized calcium level. For each 0.1 unit decrease in the pH, the ionized calcium level will increase by 0.2 mg/dl.[4] In summary, pH and ionized calcium concentration tend to be inversely related.

Treatment of Metabolic Acidosis

There are three steps in the management of metabolic acidosis. These include the identification of the cause, determination of compensation, and implementation of appropriate interventions. The first priority should *always* be aimed at identifying and correcting the primary disorder (Table 32-2).

In DKA, the metabolic acidosis is corrected by the administration of intravenous insulin. Providing insulin to these patients converts metabolism from fatty acids back to glucose, thereby stopping ketoacid production. Additionally, hydration is important to improve renal perfusion and promote excretion of ketoacids.

In patients with acute renal failure, treating metabolic acidosis can be challenging, especially if the patient is volume expanded. Administration of sodium bicarbonate to the oliguric, volume-overloaded patient with acute renal failure can be catastrophic because of the high sodium load that could result in pulmonary edema. In these patients, metabolic acidosis is best treated with renal replacement therapy (RRT).[20]

The metabolic acidosis associated with salicylate intoxication is treated with alkalinization of the blood and the urine, using intravenous sodium bicarbonate.

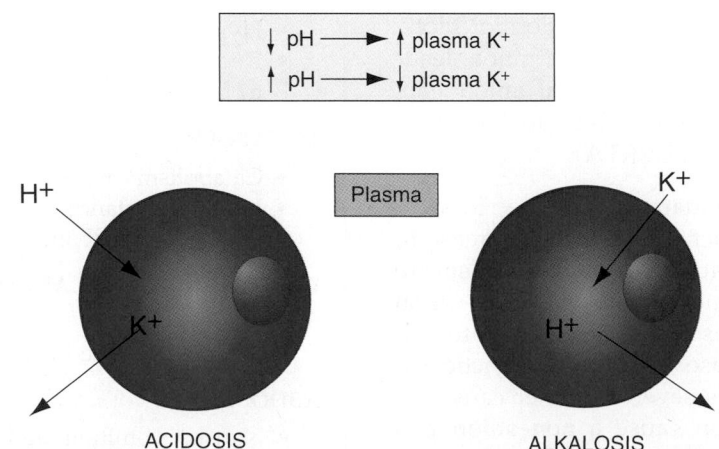

▼FIGURE 32-3 Effect of pH on transcellular shifting of K^+ and hydrogen. H^+ = Hydrogen, K^+ = potassium.

TABLE 32-2 Treatment of the Underlying Cause of Elevated Anion Gap Acidosis

DISORDER	TREATMENT
Diabetic ketoacidosis	Insulin, saline
Acute renal failure	Dialysis
Salicylate intoxication	Diuresis, alkalinization of urine, dialysis
Starvation ketosis	Refeeding (glucose and thiamine), electrolyte replacement
Methanol	Ethanol infusion, dialysis
Alcoholic ketoacidosis	Glucose, thiamine, saline, electrolyte replacement
Ethylene glycol	Ethanol infusion, dialysis
Lactic acidosis	Correct underlying cause

Increasing the blood pH in this setting reduces the diffusion of salicylate into the central nervous system (CNS), where it is toxic; additionally, alkalinization of the urine improves renal excretion of salicylate.[20] However, fluid overload can occur with sodium bicarbonate; therefore it should be administered cautiously to those at risk (patients with underlying heart or renal disease and advanced age). For these patients, salicylate intoxication can be treated with RRT.

Starvation and alcoholic ketosis are characterized by hypoglycemia and low insulin levels. These disorders are treated by restoring caloric intake with glucose, which stimulates insulin release and suppresses ketogenesis.[8] It is also important to replace thiamine, electrolytes, and volume in these malnourished patients.[20]

Methanol and ethylene glycol poisonings often occur as a result of a suicide attempt or accidental ingestion. Ethylene glycol is the organic solvent in antifreeze. Ingestions of both of these poisons are associated with CNS disturbances and severe anion gap metabolic acidosis. Both methanol and ethylene glycol intoxication are treated by inhibiting the generation of toxic metabolites that occurs as alcohol dehydrogenase metabolizes these poisons. This is accomplished by administering intravenous or oral ethanol. Ethanol has a greater affinity for alcohol dehydrogenase than methanol and ethylene glycol. When ethanol is administered in the setting of methanol or ethylene glycol poisoning, alcohol dehydrogenase will preferentially metabolize ethanol, thereby decreasing generation of toxic metabolites from methanol and ethylene glycol.[20] RRT is also an effective treatment for clearing methanol and ethylene glycol from the blood in patients with large ingestions or severe metabolic acidosis.[1]

Lactic acidosis is probably one of the most challenging types of metabolic acidosis to treat in the acutely ill adult. It typically occurs with septic, cardiogenic, or hypovolemic shock and is associated with hemodynamic compromise, hypoperfusion, and tissue hypoxia. To stop the production of lactic acid, perfusion to tissues must be restored by treating the underlying cause. If the metabolic acidosis is severe (pH less than 7.20), there is decreased responsiveness to both endogenous and exogenous catecholamines, which means that vasopressors and positive inotropes are not effective at improving hemodynamics and restoring perfusion in these patients. Additionally, acute renal failure often accompanies these various types of shock, complicating the metabolic acidosis by reducing renal acid clearance. RRT may be needed to correct metabolic acidosis in patients with severe lactic acidosis and renal failure.

After treating the underlying cause, the second step in treating a metabolic acidosis is to confirm the presence of respiratory compensation. If the $Paco_2$ is higher than that predicted using the formulas previously discussed (see Box 32-2), a respiratory acidosis is also present. In the setting of a metabolic acidosis combined with a respiratory acidosis (mixed disorder), there is compensation failure and the acidemia can be severe. In this situation, the pH can be improved by supporting ventilation.[6] In the patient who is already on a ventilator, increasing the minute ventilation (increased tidal volume or respiratory rate) will create an artificial respiratory compensatory response by decreasing the $Paco_2$ and raising blood pH. If the patient is not on a ventilator and is demonstrating signs of respiratory fatigue (i.e., restlessness, tachypnea, shallow respirations), intubation should be considered to support ventilation and decrease the $Paco_2$.[14,22]

Bicarbonate Therapy. The third consideration in the treatment of a metabolic acidosis is whether or not to administer sodium bicarbonate. The administration of bicarbonate to correct metabolic acidosis is controversial. Before giving bicarbonate, every effort should be made to correct the underlying process causing the acidosis and support ventilation and respiratory compensation. In the setting of a severe metabolic acidosis (pH less than 6.90 to 7.10 and HCO_3^- level less than 8 to 10 mEq/L), bicarbonate may be administered.[24] The goal of administering bicarbonate in metabolic acidosis is to prevent or reverse the detrimental consequences of severe acidemia on the cardiovascular system, restore hemodynamic stability, and allow for additional time to treat the underlying cause. However, there are no controlled studies demonstrating the benefit (improved survival) of bicarbonate administration in patients with diabetic ketoacidosis or lactic acidosis.[16] Additionally, there are many detrimental side effects of bicarbonate, including volume overload, hyperosmolality, "overshoot" metabolic alkalosis, and a decrease in oxygen release from Hgb.[16]

Sodium Bicarbonate. Intravenous sodium bicarbonate is most commonly used for the treatment of a severe metabolic acidosis when indicated. Sodium bicarbonate contains 50 mEq of HCO_3^- and 50 mEq of Na^+. It should be administered via a continuous intravenous infusion. Bolus dosing should be avoided except in emergent situations.[1] The bicarbonate infusion should be continued until the pH reaches approximately 7.20. If treatment continues until the pH is normal or near normal, there is a risk of rebound alkalosis. This occurs as organic acids (e.g., lactic acid, ketoacids) are converted to HCO_3^- by the liver, causing the pH to drift even higher after the infusion of sodium bicarbonate is discontinued.

The appropriate dose of sodium bicarbonate required to correct a patient's serum HCO_3^- level can be estimated using the base deficit formula, shown below. An example is illustrated in Box 32-5.

$$HCO_3^- \text{ deficit} = 0.5 \times \text{body weight (kg)} \times (\text{desired } HCO_3^- - \text{measured } HCO_3^-)$$

However, in critically ill patients many ongoing processes will perpetuate or compensate for the metabolic acidosis and can make it difficult to predict the base deficit accurately. Therefore repeated measurements of the arterial blood gas and serum electrolytes (to calculate the anion gap) must be performed in order to guide therapy.

Side Effects of Sodium Bicarbonate. Side effects of sodium bicarbonate are serious and include hypernatremia, hyperosmolality, overshoot alkalosis, volume overload, and rapid drop in the ionized calcium level. Sodium bicarbonate should be administered very cautiously in patients with heart failure and renal failure because of a limited ability to excrete sodium and the potential to worsen volume overload. Intermittent dialysis or continuous renal replacement therapy using a bicarbonate-based buffer, versus an acetate- or lactate-based buffer, can be used in the treatment of metabolic acidosis in this specialized population.[13]

Nursing Considerations When Preparing a Sodium Bicarbonate Infusion. Sodium bicarbonate is extremely concentrated and caution must be taken when preparing a bicarbonate infusion to avoid administration of a hypertonic fluid. Sodium bicarbonate vials (50 ml) should be added to a *hypotonic* solution (e.g., D_5W or 0.45% normal saline [NS]). Mixing sodium bicarbonate in an isotonic solution (e.g., 0.9% NS) will result in a hypertonic solution that could cause acute hypernatremia and fluid shifts in the brain. Consider the different sodium concentrations of the IV bicarbonate solutions listed in Table 32-3. The administration of the IV bicarbonate solution in example 1 could cause acute hypernatremia and a hyperosmolar state, resulting in fluid shifts from the intracellular space into the extracellular space. In the brain, this can result in rapid shrinking of brain volume, altered mental status, and even coma. Administration of the solution in example 2 would be similar to 0.45% NS, a hypotonic solution that could have adverse effects on lowering the serum sodium concentration. Example 3 would be the preferred IV bicarbonate solution because it is isotonic and will not cause acute changes in the serum sodium level or serum osmolality. Example 3 yields an isotonic solution with 150 mEq of bicarbonate replacement.

Alternative Treatments of Metabolic Acidosis. Because of the adverse effects of sodium bicarbonate administration, other forms of base have evolved as alternative treatments for metabolic acidosis.

THAM (tris-hydroxymethyl-aminomethane) is a sodium-free compound that buffers protons. Administration of THAM does not result in CO_2 generation, as seen with sodium bicarbonate, and therefore THAM does not lower intracellular pH.[16] THAM has been used successfully to reduce the severity of acidemia in the setting of permissive hypercapnia without increasing Pa_{CO_2} generation.[25] However, THAM has not been widely used because it is eliminated by the kidneys and is only effective if it is excreted.[16] This limits the use of THAM to patients with normal renal function.

Box 32-5

Calculating the Base Deficit

Base deficit formula:

$$HCO_3^- \text{ deficit} = 0.5 \times \text{body weight (kg)} \times (\text{desired } HCO_3^- - \text{measured } HCO_3^-)$$

Example: Calculating the base deficit

Patient weight = 70 kg

Measured HCO_3^- = 12 mEq/L

Desired HCO_3^- = 26 mEq/L

$$
\begin{aligned}
HCO_3^- \text{ deficit} &= 0.5 \times 70 \times (26 - 12) \\
&= 0.5 \times 70 \times 14 \\
&= 0.5 \times 980 \\
&= 490 \text{ mEq/L } NaHCO_3
\end{aligned}
$$

TABLE 32-3 Preparation of a Sodium Bicarbonate Infusion

SOLUTION	VOLUME	Na$^+$ CONCENTRATION	HCO$_3^-$ CONCENTRATION
NaHCO$_3$	50 mL	50 mEq	50 mEq
D$_5$W	1 L	0 mEq	0 mEq/L
0.45% NS	1 L	0 mEq	77 mEq/L
0.9% NS	1 L	0 mEq	154 mEq/L

Examples of Sodium Concentration in NaHCO$_3$ Drips With Various IV Fluids

Example 1: Two vials of NaHCO$_3$ (100 ml) in 1 L of NS will yield a Na$^+$ solution of 230 mEq/L (Hypertonic)

Example 2: Two vials of NaHCO$_3$ (100 ml) in 1 L of D$_5$W will yield a Na$^+$ solution of 90 mEq/L (Hypotonic solution: similar to 0.45% saline)

Example 3: Three vials of NaHCO$_3$ (150 ml) in 1 L of D$_5$W will yield a Na$^+$ solution of 130 mEq/L (Isotonic solution)

HCO$_3^-$ = Bicarbonate, Na$^+$ = sodium, NaHCO$_3$ = sodium bicarbonate, NS = normal saline.

Additional side effects of THAM include hyperkalemia, hepatotoxicity, and respiratory depression.

Carbicarb is another alternative base that has been used to treat metabolic acidosis. It is a mixture of sodium bicarbonate and sodium carbonate that generates less CO$_2$ than sodium bicarbonate. Similar to THAM, it has some benefit over sodium bicarbonate because it does not lower intracellular pH. Small clinical trials in patients with mild metabolic acidosis have shown Carbicarb to be effective, but there are no published studies using Carbicarb in humans to treat severe metabolic acidosis.[16]

RRT is an effective treatment for metabolic acidosis, especially in patients with renal failure or certain intoxications (e.g., ethylene glycol, salicylate). Clinically, it is difficult and may be deleterious to administer large quantities of bicarbonate by bolus or continuous infusion because of the risk of volume overload, pulmonary edema, hypernatremia, and hyperosmolality. However, with RRT, large quantities of base can be delivered, volume status can be normalized, and electrolyte imbalances can be treated. Various types of RRT can be used to treat acid-base and electrolyte disorders in the acutely ill adult, including hemodialysis and continuous renal replacement therapies (CRRT). For treating metabolic acidosis, the use of bicarbonate as a source of base in the dialysate is recommended over the other bicarbonate precursors (lactate or acetate) because of the potential detrimental effects if these acids accumulate before being metabolized.[16]

◆ Case Study 32-1, Part B

Metabolic Acidosis

A 12-lead electrocardiogram (ECG) is obtained and shows sinus tachycardia with PR = 0.22 ms, flattened P waves, QRS = 0.14 ms, tall peaked T waves.

The patient is intubated, put on a ventilator, and hyperventilated. A Foley catheter and two central lines are placed and the following medications administered: sodium bicarbonate 2 vials IV, insulin 10 units IV, D$_{50}$ 1 ampule IV, calcium gluconate 10% 10 ml IV.

The central venous pressure (CVP) is measured at 2 cm H$_2$O. IV NS is administered "wide open," and despite volume replacement the CVP does not increase. A bicarbonate infusion was ordered as follows: NS 1 L + 3 vials sodium bicarbonate at 150 ml/hr. Shortly after the bicarbonate drip is started, the patient begins to have tetany. Nephrology is consulted for emergency dialysis.

Decision point: What are the manifestations of metabolic acidosis?

Decision point: What are the electrolyte imbalances associated with metabolic acidosis in this case?

Decision point: Was it appropriate to treat the metabolic acidosis with NaHCO$_3$?

Decision point: Was the bicarbonate drip preparation ordered correctly?

Decision point: Why did the patient have tetany?

Treatment of a *non–anion gap* metabolic acidosis resulting from GI bicarbonate losses (e.g., diarrhea, fistula) is aimed at stopping diarrhea, restoring volume status, and replacing bicarbonate losses.

METABOLIC ALKALOSIS

Metabolic alkalosis is a common acid-base disorder seen in the critical care setting.[26] It can be defined as a physiologic process that can cause alkalemia if not corrected, whereas alkalemia is defined as an increase in the blood pH greater than 7.45. Metabolic alkalosis

is due to a primary increase in plasma bicarbonate concentrations, resulting in an increase in blood pH. Severe alkalemia (blood pH greater than 7.60) can be life-threatening because of its effect on cerebral and myocardial perfusion.

Causes of Metabolic Alkalosis

Metabolic alkalosis is usually due to loss of acid combined with chloride loss. In the hospitalized patient, metabolic alkalosis most commonly results from either diuretics causing renal loss of acid (ammonium chloride) or prolonged nasogastric (NG)

◆ Case Study 32-2, Part A

Metabolic Alkalosis

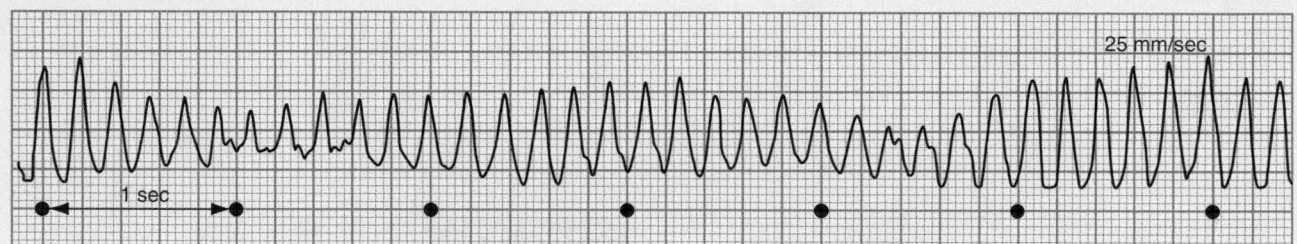

25 mm/sec

1 sec

P.G., a 57-year-old, morbidly obese female, was singing in her church choir when she experienced a syncopal episode. She was brought to the ED by her family. While waiting to be seen, she experienced another syncopal episode and was found to be pulseless. CPR was started; the patient was put on a monitor and found to be in the above rhythm.

She was defibrillated and converted to sinus rhythm. Within minutes her rhythm returned to polymorphic ventricular tachycardia (torsades de pointes) requiring defibrillation. She continued in sinus rhythm with intervals of torsades and then developed ventricular fibrillation that converted to sinus rhythm after three countershocks. She was given magnesium sulfate 2 g IVP and lidocaine 200 mg IVP and started on a lidocaine drip at 3 mg/min. She has a history of hypertension.

History of Present Illness:

The patient complained of lower abdominal pain and anorexia for 3 days. She also had intermittent episodes of vomiting for the last 2 days. In addition, she noticed numbness and tingling around her mouth and in her fingertips for the last day. Despite feeling ill, she continued to take her "blood pressure medication," hydrochlorothiazide (Microzide) 50 mg a day. Her vital signs were HR: 98 beats/min, BP: 102/66 mm Hg, and respirations: 16 breaths/min. Temperature was 38.4° C.

Physical exam revealed her PEARL; she was alert and oriented. She was in a normal sinus rhythm, with a normal S_1, S_2, and no S_3; her neck veins were flat. Her lungs were clear and her abdomen rounded, nontender to palpation with positive bowel tones. Her extremities were cool and dry, peripheral pulses palpable, and no pedal edema.

Laboratory Values:

Serum Chemistries	Arterial Blood Gas
Na^+: 131 mEq/L	pH: 7.56
K^+: 2.3 mEq/L	$Paco_2$: 60 mm Hg
Cl^-: 70 mEq/L	Pao_2: 63 mm Hg
CO_2: 55 mEq/L	HCO_3^-: 54 mEq/L
Glucose: 162 mg/dl	Saturation: 93%
Creatinine: 1.9 mg/dl	
BUN: 41 mg/dl	
Ca^{++}: 8 mg/dl	
Ionized Ca^{++}: 3.1 mg/dl	
Phosphorus=: 2 mg/dl	
Mg^{++}: 1.5 mg/dl	
Albumin: 4.2 mg/dl	

Decision point: Interpret the blood gas and calculate the anion gap.

Case continues on page 878

suctioning or vomiting causing GI loss of acid (hydrochloric acid).[11] In these situations, metabolic alkalosis is typically associated with hypochloremia and volume depletion, also termed a *contraction alkalosis* (Box 32-6).

In states of volume depletion, the kidney will respond by reabsorbing sodium and water. Renal reabsorption of sodium can occur as either sodium chloride or sodium bicarbonate. In most states of metabolic alkalosis, there is a preexisting chloride deficiency, so the kidney must reabsorb sodium bicarbonate instead of sodium chloride, thus maintaining and perpetuating the metabolic alkalosis that was originally due to acid loss. This type of metabolic alkalosis usually responds to chloride administration (sodium chloride or potassium chloride) and is referred to as *chloride-responsive* metabolic alkalosis.

A less common cause of metabolic alkalosis is termed *chloride-resistant* metabolic alkalosis. In the acutely ill patient, this can occur with administration of substrates such as lactate, citrate, or acetate. Lactate is a component in the intravenous solution lactated Ringer's and in dialysate solutions. Citrate is an anticoagulant and preservative used in the preparation of packed red blood cell transfusions and RRT. Acetate is a component commonly added to parenteral nutrition and dialysate. When given in sufficient quantities, these substrates can generate or perpetuate a metabolic alkalosis as the liver converts them to bicarbonate.

Another cause of chloride-resistant metabolic alkalosis can be seen with "overshoot" treatment of a metabolic acidosis. In DKA, as well as lactic acidosis, if sodium bicarbonate is administered to the point of normalizing or near-normalizing the pH, an "overshoot" alkalosis will develop. This occurs as the liver continues to metabolize lactate and ketoacids and convert them to bicarbonate, resulting in a late-onset metabolic alkalosis.

Manifestations of Metabolic Alkalosis

Metabolic alkalosis can compromise myocardial and cerebral perfusion by causing arteriolar constriction. Additionally, metabolic alkalosis causes respiratory depression and decreased tissue oxygenation and is associated with numerous electrolyte imbalances (Box 32-7).

Electrolyte Imbalances Associated With Metabolic Alkalosis

Electrolyte imbalances are common with metabolic alkalosis. In part, this is due to the volume and electrolyte depletion occurring with diuretics and vomiting or

---

Box 32-7

Manifestations of Severe Metabolic Alkalosis (pH Greater Than 7.6)

CARDIOVASCULAR

- Arteriolar constriction
- Decreased coronary blood flow, leading to angina, acute MI in patients with coronary artery disease
- Predisposition to refractory supraventricular dysrhythmias:
  - Multifocal atrial tachycardia, paroxysmal supraventricular tachycardia and ventricular dysrhythmias: monomorphic and polymorphic ventricular tachycardia, long QT interval, and ventricular fibrillation

NEUROLOGIC

- Decreased cerebral blood flow
- Paresthesias, tetany, seizures (secondary to decreased ionized calcium)
- Lethargy, delirium, stupor

RESPIRATORY

- Hypoventilation leading to hypercapnia and hypoxemia
- Failure to wean from ventilator

ELECTROLYTE IMBALANCES

- Hypokalemia
- Decreased ionized calcium
- Hypomagnesemia (associated imbalance)
- Hypophosphatemia (associated imbalance)

METABOLIC

- Decreased oxygen delivery at tissue level
- Stimulation of organic acid production

Data from references 8 and 20.

Box 32-6

Causes of Metabolic Alkalosis

Chloride Responsive	Chloride Resistant
Vomiting	Administration of bicarbonate
NG suction	precursors
Diuretic therapy	Lactate
Loop diuretics	Citrate
Thiazides	Acetate
	Potassium depletion
	Hyper-reninemic states
	Primary hyperaldosteronism

with NG suctioning. Additionally, metabolic alkalosis causes electrolyte imbalances because of transcellular shifts of electrolytes and changes in protein binding of some electrolytes, especially calcium.

Hypokalemia. (Serum potassium level less than 3.5 mEq/L). Hypokalemia is common in metabolic alkalosis because of renal and GI losses of potassium (diuretics, vomiting, or diarrhea). Hypokalemia also occurs as a result of transcellular shifts of extracellular potassium into the cell in exchange for hydrogen. H^+ moves out of the cell in an attempt to correct the alkalosis and potassium moves into the cell to maintain electrical neutrality (see Figure 32-3).

Low Ionized Calcium. (Ionized calcium level less than 4 mg/dl or 1.16 mmol/L.) Calcium-protein binding is influenced by plasma pH. In alkalemic states, H^+ ions are released from protein. This exposes negatively charged sites that bind ionized calcium, thus reducing the plasma ionized calcium concentration (Figure 32-4). The clinical significance of this phenomenon is that in an alkalemic state, there is a reduction in the ionized calcium level and the patient may develop manifestations of hypocalcemia such as paresthesias, tetany, and seizures, despite a normal total calcium level.

Hypophosphatemia. (Serum phosphorus level less than 2.8 mg/dl) and **hypomagnesemia** (serum magnesium level less than 1.5 mEq/L). Low phosphorus and low magnesium levels typically accompany metabolic alkalosis. However, metabolic alkalosis is not a primary cause of these electrolyte imbalances as it is with hypokalemia and low ionized calcium concentration.

Because metabolic alkalosis is commonly associated with diuresis or vomiting/NG suction, there can be excessive renal or GI losses of both phosphorus and magnesium. Hypomagnesemia potentiates the neuromuscular manifestations of low ionized calcium level, including tetany and seizures. Additionally, hypomagnesemia in the setting of metabolic alkalosis potentiates the arrhythmogenic effects of hypokalemia, including both supraventricular and ventricular dysrhythmias.

Case Study 32-2, Part B

Metabolic Alkalosis

A 12-lead ECG showed normal sinus rhythm with a ventricular rate of 99 beats/min, PR interval = 0.16 ms, QRS = 0.56 ms, QT = 0.44 ms, QTc = 0.56 ms.

The patient received the following intravenous fluids and electrolyte replacement in the ED:

1 L NS + KCl 60 mEq IV at 125 ml/hr; KCl 60 mEq PO; $MgSO_4$ 6 g in normal saline 500 ml IV over 3 hours.

The patient was transferred to critical care. Her electrolyte replacement, in divided doses, over the next 48 hours was as follows: KCl: 420 mEq; phosphate: 2 g; $MgSO_4$: 10 g.

Decision point: What is the most likely etiology of the metabolic alkalosis?

Decision point: What are the manifestations of metabolic alkalosis in this case?

Decision point: What are the electrolyte imbalances associated with metabolic alkalosis in this case?

Case continues on page 879

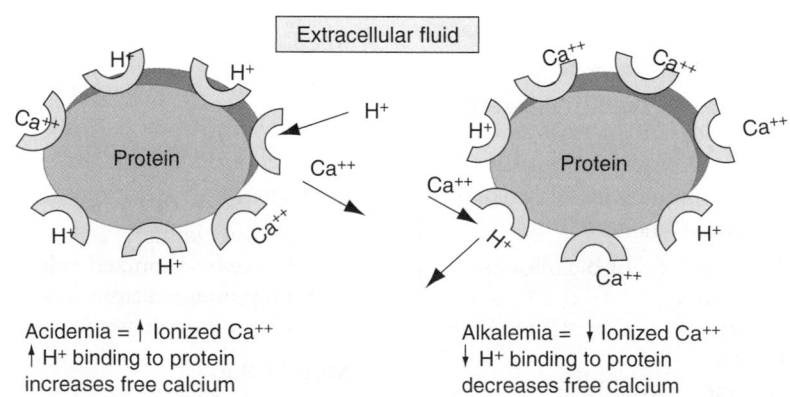

Acidemia = ↑ Ionized Ca^{++}
↑ H^+ binding to protein increases free calcium

Alkalemia = ↓ Ionized Ca^{++}
↓ H^+ binding to protein decreases free calcium

⬍FIGURE 32-4 Effect of pH on ionized calcium. Ca^{++} = Calcium, H^+ = hydrogen.

Treatment of Metabolic Alkalosis

Alveolar hypoventilation is the compensatory respiratory response to metabolic alkalosis, increasing the $Paco_2$, thereby decreasing blood pH. However, in most patients, this compensation is limited to a rise in $Paco_2$ to 55 to 60 mm Hg because an accompanying hypoxemia (partial pressure of arterial oxygen tension [Pao_2] less than 50 mm Hg) will stimulate ventilation.[8]

In the volume-depleted patient with chloride-responsive metabolic alkalosis, every effort should be made to stop the processes responsible for causing the metabolic alkalosis. The cause of vomiting should be determined and treated, NG suctioning should be discontinued if possible, an H_2 blocker to reduce gastric acid production should be administered, and the diuretic dose should be decreased if possible or a potassium-sparing diuretic should be considered.

These patients need replacement of volume with NS. Additionally, chloride must be replaced in the form of sodium chloride or potassium chloride. Remember that the most common causes of metabolic alkalosis in the acutely ill adult are vomiting/NG suctioning with loss of hydrochloric acid and diuresis with loss of ammonium chloride. In these volume-depleted, chloride-deficient patients, the kidney is reabsorbing sodium but because there is a chloride deficiency, sodium is reabsorbed as sodium bicarbonate. This renal reabsorption of sodium bicarbonate perpetuates the existing metabolic alkalosis. Replacing chloride is a critical part of correcting metabolic alkalosis. As chloride stores are replenished, the kidney will reabsorb sodium chloride and excrete bicarbonate.

Concurrent electrolyte imbalances are common in the setting of a metabolic alkalosis and treatment often includes replacement of chloride, potassium, phosphate, and magnesium. Patients with cardiac and renal dysfunction present challenges to correcting metabolic alkalosis because administration of sodium chloride may cause volume overload and administration of potassium chloride may result in hyperkalemia.

Patients Requiring Aggressive Treatment of Metabolic Alkalosis.

Alkalemia reduces respiratory drive. Patients with COPD pending intubation or failure to wean/extubate should be closely monitored for respiratory failure. Aggressive treatment of metabolic alkalosis in these patients will improve respiratory drive. Alkalemia also causes arteriolar vasoconstriction. Patients with coronary artery disease and acute myocardial infarction should be closely monitored for the development of ischemia. Aggressive correction of metabolic alkalosis will improve coronary blood flow by promoting arteriolar vasodilation.[7] In the patient with cerebral dysfunction, aggressive correction of metabolic alkalosis will improve cerebral blood flow by promoting arteriolar vasodilation.

If alkalemia is still severe despite attempts to correct the underlying disorder, the diuretic acetazolamide (Diamox) 250 to 375 mg once or twice a day may be administered to enhance renal HCO_3^- excretion.[2] This may be useful in the patient who is volume overloaded and cannot tolerate a saline infusion to correct alkalosis. Infusion of intravenous hydrochloric acid as a 0.1 to 0.2 N solution (100 to 200 mmol of hydrogen per liter) at a rate of 0.1 to 0.2 mmol/kg/hr has been used for many years to aggressively treat severe metabolic alkalosis.[2,3] However, a serious side effect of hydrochloric acid administration is tissue necrosis, should extravasation occur. Even when administered through a central line, extravasation into the chest wall can occur and can be fatal.[3] Precursors of hydrochloric acid, such as ammonium chloride, may also be used to treat a metabolic alkalosis but also have deleterious side effects including elevation of serum ammonia levels and tissue necrosis.[2,20] Hydrochloric acid infusions and ammonium chloride are rarely given, not only because of their serious side effects but also because their onset of action is not fast enough to prevent life-threatening complications of severe metabolic alkalosis.[20]

The treatment of chloride-resistant metabolic alkalosis and volume expansion is focused on removal of the underlying cause of the persistent mineralocorticoid activity. If this is not possible, administration of potassium-sparing diuretics (amiloride [Midamor] or spironolactone [Aldactone]) to block the action of mineralocorticoids in the kidney that are promoting renal H^+ loss may be effective in these patients.[20]

▲ Case Study 32-2, Part C

Metabolic Alkalosis

The labs 48 hours after admission were as follows:

Serum Chemistries	Arterial Blood Gas
Na^+: 138 mEq/L	pH: 7.45
K^+: 3.8 mEq/L	$Paco_2$: 41 mm Hg
Cl^-: 102 mEq/L	Pao_2: 92 mm Hg
CO_2: 28 mEq/L	HCO_3^-: 27 mEq/L
Glucose: 133 mg/dl	Saturation: 97%
Creatinine: 1.2 mg/dl	
BUN: 12 mg/dl	
Ca^{++}: 8.6 mg/dl	
Ionized Ca^{++}: 4.3 mg/dl	
Phosphorus$^=$: 3.1 mg/dl	
Mg^{++}: 2.2 mEq/L	

P.G.'s abdominal complaints were considered a symptom of *Escherichia coli* bacteremia and pyelonephritis. She was treated with antibiotics and discharged to home 5 days after admission.

Decision point: How should the metabolic alkalosis and electrolyte imbalances be treated?

RESPIRATORY ACIDOSIS

Respiratory acidosis is a clinical disorder characterized by alveolar hypoventilation resulting in hypercapnia ($Paco_2$ greater than 45 mm Hg) and acidemia (arterial pH less than 7.35). CO_2 is a metabolic waste product eliminated by the lungs. If the lungs fail to eliminate CO_2, it will accumulate in the blood, causing acidemia. Hypercapnia is always the result of inadequate ventilation. Hypoxemia typically accompanies respiratory acidosis because of hypoventilation.

Causes of Respiratory Acidosis

Respiratory acidosis should be differentiated between acute and chronic causes of hypoventilation (Box 32-8).

Compensation in Respiratory Acidosis. The initial clinical approach to the patient with a respiratory acidosis is to determine whether the disorder is acute or chronic, or if it is acute *on* chronic. For example, a patient with stable chronic COPD or asthma can have an acute exacerbation with an increase in $Paco_2$ above the baseline. The compensatory mechanism for an increase in $Paco_2$ is to increase the plasma bicarbonate concentration. In an acute respiratory acidosis, the carbonic acid-bicarbonate buffer system is ineffective because the CO_2 produced in the buffering reaction cannot be eliminated as a result of the existing respiratory disorder.[8] However, non-bicarbonate buffers (e.g., protein, phosphate, Hgb) can effectively absorb the excess H^+. This response occurs within hours of the onset of an acute respiratory acidosis but produces only minimal compensation. In an acute respiratory acidosis, the compensatory response will only increase the HCO_3^- level by up to 1 mEq for every 10 mm Hg increase in the $Paco_2$.[19]

The definitive compensatory response for a persistent respiratory acidosis is in the kidneys but will take 3 to 5 days to complete.[8,14] The renal response to a respiratory acidosis is to increase the production and reabsorption of bicarbonate and to increase the production and excretion of the acid ammonium.[14] Renal compensation to a chronic respiratory acidosis will increase the HCO_3^- level by up to 3.5 mEq for every 10 mm Hg increase in the $Paco_2$.[19]

Manifestations of Respiratory Acidosis

The clinical manifestations of an acute respiratory acidosis are seen primarily in the neurologic system and can be attributed to vasodilation causing an increase in cerebral blood flow and also to a decrease in the pH of the cerebral spinal fluid.[14] Hypoxemia invariably accompanies an acute respiratory acidosis and may dominate the clinical presentation with signs and symptoms of acute respiratory distress (e.g., tachypnea, restlessness).[14] With chronic respiratory acidosis, symptoms are less common, since renal compensation has had time to return the pH toward normal (Box 32-9).

Treatment of Respiratory Acidosis

The most important aspect of treating respiratory acidosis, as with all acid-base disorders, is to diagnose and treat the underlying cause. Initially, supplemental

---

Box 32-8

Causes of Respiratory Acidosis

Acute Hypoventilation	Chronic Hypoventilation
Disorders Affecting Gas Exchange	
ARDS	Asthma/COPD
Acute lung injury	Interstitial lung disease
Pulmonary emboli	Pulmonary fibrosis
Asthma/COPD exacerbation	
Pulmonary edema	
Pneumothorax or hemothorax	
Inadequate mechanical ventilation	
Respiratory Muscle Weakness	
Neuromuscular blockade	Neuromuscular disorders
Hypophosphatemia and hypokalemia	Multiple sclerosis
Acute spinal cord injury: C3, C4, C5	Guillain-Barré
Diaphragmatic paralysis secondary to trauma	Amyotrophic lateral sclerosis
Decreased Respiratory Drive	
Drugs inhibiting respiratory drive	
Narcotics	Pickwickian syndrome
Anesthetics	Primary hypoventilation
Sedatives	Central sleep apnea
Excessive oxygen therapy in COPD	
Metabolic alkalosis	
Cerebral trauma	
Myxedema coma (hypothyroidism)	
Airway Obstruction	
Foreign body	
Laryngospasm	

Data from references 8 and 26.
ARDS = Acute respiratory distress syndrome, COPD = chronic obstructive pulmonary disease.

Box 32-9

Manifestations of Acute Respiratory Acidosis

NEUROLOGIC

- Increased cerebral blood flow
- Headache, blurred vision
- Restlessness, anxiety
- Tremors, asterixis
- Somnolence (carbon dioxide narcosis)
- Stupor, coma

CARDIOVASCULAR

- Peripheral vasodilation and hypotension
- Dysrhythmias

PULMONARY

- Accompanying hypoxemia

---

oxygen should be administered to treat accompanying hypoxemia. In patients with COPD exacerbation, supplemental oxygen should be administered cautiously because hypoxemia, versus hypercapnia, stimulates their respiratory drive.

Reversal of a high $Paco_2$ will always require an increase in alveolar ventilation. This is accomplished by controlling the underlying disease. For example, asthma should be treated with bronchodilators and steroids, narcotic oversedation can be reversed with naloxone (Narcan), and a chest tube should be inserted to treat a pneumothorax or hemothorax. In some instances, endotracheal intubation and mechanical ventilation will be necessary for management of symptomatic or progressive hypercapnia, severe hypoxemia, or depression of the respiratory center. Mechanical support of ventilation can be used until the underlying disease process causing the respiratory acidosis can be reversed. For example, pneumonia with severe hypoxemia and hypercapnia will require treatment with antibiotics, whereas treatment of pulmonary edema will include aggressive diuresis. The decision to intubate and mechanically ventilate the patient is based on clinical judgment and is dependent on many factors such as reversibility of illness, severity of illness, and patient fatigue.[8]

RESPIRATORY ALKALOSIS

Respiratory alkalosis is a clinical disorder characterized by hypocapnia ($Paco_2 < 35$ mm Hg) and alkalemia (pH > 7.45). Respiratory alkalosis occurs as a result of increased elimination of CO_2 beyond what would normally be produced as a metabolic waste product. Respiratory alkalosis is always due to hyperventilation.

Causes of Respiratory Alkalosis

Respiration is regulated by two sets of chemoreceptors: central chemoreceptors located in the respiratory center in the brain stem and peripheral chemoreceptors located in the carotid and aortic arteries. The central chemoreceptors are stimulated by a drop in the cerebrospinal fluid pH, which typically occurs from an increase in $Paco_2$ or metabolic acidosis. The peripheral chemoreceptors are stimulated primarily by hypoxemia. When the Pao_2 falls below 60 mm Hg, the peripheral chemoreceptors signal an increase in ventilation to improve hypoxemia; this results in a drop in the $Paco_2$.[8] The hyperventilation that characterizes respiratory alkalosis typically results from stimulation of these chemoreceptors in the setting of hypoxemia and metabolic acidosis. Many nonphysiologic stimuli can also cause hyperventilation, including direct stimulation of the respiratory center, mechanical ventilation, and pulmonary disease (Box 32-10).

Box 32-10

Causes of Respiratory Alkalosis

HYPOXEMIA (Pao_2 less than 60 mm Hg)

- Asthma
- Chronic obstructive pulmonary disease
- Heart failure
- High-altitude residence
- Hypotension
- Pneumonia
- Pulmonary edema
- Pulmonary emboli
- Severe anemia

CARDIOPULMONARY DISEASE (INDEPENDENT OF HYPOXEMIA)

- Heart failure
- Mitral valve disease
- Pulmonary hypertension

DIRECT STIMULATION OF RESPIRATORY CENTER

- Anxiety or pain
- Gram-negative sepsis
- Hepatic failure
- Neurologic disorders (stroke, tumors)
- Pregnancy (caused by progesterone)
- Rapid correction of metabolic acidosis with sodium bicarbonate
- Salicylate intoxication

HYPERVENTILATION

- Anxiety attacks, psychogenic conditions
- Mechanical ventilation (high rate or tidal volume settings)

Data from references 8 and 14.

Compensation in Respiratory Alkalosis. There are two components in the compensatory response to a respiratory alkalosis: an acute response and a chronic response. The initial buffering response to an acute respiratory alkalosis is to move H^+ ions out of the cell buffers (proteins, phosphate, and hemoglobin) into the extracellular space. This cellular response occurs within minutes of the onset of an acute respiratory alkalosis but does not dramatically increase the pH. The compensatory response to an acute respiratory alkalosis will only decrease plasma HCO_3^- levels by up to 2 mEq for every 10 mm Hg rise in the $Paco_2$.[19]

In the presence of a persistent or chronic respiratory alkalosis, a more powerful renal compensatory response will take 2 to 3 days to achieve maximum compensation. The kidneys decrease renal H^+ ion and ammonium excretion, thereby retaining more acid, reducing plasma HCO_3^- levels and lowering the pH toward normal. In a chronic respiratory alkalosis, the plasma HCO_3^- level will decrease by up to 5 mEq for every 10 mm Hg decrease in the $Paco_2$.[19] The renal response to persistent respiratory alkalosis is much greater than the cellular compensatory response seen with an acute respiratory alkalosis.

Manifestations of Respiratory Alkalosis

The symptoms of an acute respiratory alkalosis are primarily due to increased irritability of the central and peripheral nervous systems. Alkalosis impairs cerebral function, increases membrane excitability, and reduces cerebral and coronary blood flow by causing arteriolar vasoconstriction. Similar to metabolic alkalosis, there are many electrolyte imbalances associated with respiratory alkalosis, including a low ionized calcium level, hypokalemia, and hypophosphatemia (Box 32-11).

Electrolyte imbalances associated with acute respiratory alkalosis can occur rapidly in response to an increased pH and are due to transcellular electrolyte shifts. As hydrogen moves out of the cell to lower the pH, potassium will move into the cell, resulting in hypokalemia. Additionally, phosphate moves rapidly into the cell and can reduce the serum phosphate levels to as low as 0.5 to 1.5 mg/dl.[8] The ionized calcium level also falls, as free calcium binds to proteins in exchange for hydrogen release (see Figure 32-4).

Treatment of Respiratory Alkalosis

The treatment of respiratory alkalosis, similar to the treatment of the previously discussed acid-base disorders, should be directed at correction of the underlying disorder causing the hyperventilation. For example, a patient being mechanically ventilated with high

---

Box 32-11

Manifestations of Acute Respiratory Alkalosis

NEUROLOGIC

- Reduced cerebral blood flow
- Light-headedness
- Altered level of consciousness
- Paresthesias (circumoral and peripheral)
- Hyperreflexia and tetany
- Seizures

CARDIOVASCULAR

- Reduced coronary artery blood flow
- Refractory supraventricular and ventricular dysrhythmias

PULMONARY

- Pulmonary vasculature vasodilation

ELECTROLYTE IMBALANCES

- Low ionized calcium
- Hypokalemia
- Hypophosphatemia (rapid onset)
- Low serum bicarbonate (compensatory)

---

minute volumes should have the tidal volume or the rate settings reduced. In conscious patients with symptomatic alkalemia, rebreathing into a paper bag will increase the pH by increasing the $Paco_2$ in the inspired air. There is no rationale for sedation or administering respiratory depressants in the treatment of respiratory alkalosis.

MIXED ACID-BASE DISORDERS

A mixed acid-base disorder is defined as two or more primary acid-base disorders that occur simultaneously. These disorders may "mask" each other and can be diagnosed only with a thorough evaluation of acid-base status. For example, a patient with acute decompensated heart failure, hypotension, and pulmonary edema who is receiving high-dose diuretics can have a triple acid-base disorder as follows: metabolic acidosis secondary to hypotension causing hypoperfusion, resulting in a lactic acidosis; metabolic alkalosis secondary to diuretics causing renal acid loss; and respiratory acidosis resulting from pulmonary edema with $Paco_2$ retention. In this scenario, it is possible that the patient could have a relatively normal pH because of the offsetting effects of alkalosis and acidosis.

▲ Case Study 32-3, Part A

Mixed Acid-Base Disorders

C.L., a 52-year-old Hispanic female, presents to the emergency department with a 2-day history of abdominal pain, distention, nausea, vomiting, weakness, and dizziness. She has been unable to keep liquids or solids down. She has no significant medical history. An abdominal x-ray done in the ED is consistent with a small bowel obstruction. Vital signs included BP: 70/56 mm Hg, HR: 112 beats/min (sinus tachycardia), respirations: 24 breaths/min (shallow), and temperature: 38.2° C. Physical exam revealed her to be alert and oriented. She has no S_1, S_2, no murmurs or gallops; jugular venous distention not visible. Her lungs were clear to auscultation. Her abdomen was distended and diffusely tender. Extremities were cool and dry; no pedal edema was noted.

Laboratory Values:

Serum Chemistries	Arterial Blood Gas
Na^+: 131 mEq/L	pH: 7.41
K^+: 2.7 mEq/L	$Paco_2$: 50 mm Hg
Cl^-: 70 mEq/L	Pao_2: 58 mm Hg
CO_2: 28 mEq/L	HCO_3^-: 28 mEq/L
Glucose: 196 mg/dl	Saturation: 93%
Creatinine: 2.4 mg/dl	
BUN: 42 mg/dl	
Ca^{++}: 8.6 mg/dl	
Phosphorus$^=$: 1.2 mg/dl	
Mg^{++}: 1.6 mEq/L	

Decision point: Assess the acid-base status of this patient using the steps in Box 32-2.

Decision point: What are the associated electrolyte imbalances and their cause?

Decision point: How should the acid-base disorders be treated?

Case continues above, right

Mixed acid-base disorders can also present with grossly abnormal changes in pH when the primary disorders block compensation for each other.[14] For example, a patient with a respiratory acidosis caused by acute respiratory distress syndrome (ARDS) *and* a metabolic acidosis caused by acute renal failure could present with a life-threatening acidemia. In this example, the presence of a primary respiratory acidosis prevents a compensatory hypocapnia in the setting of a primary metabolic acidosis. Additionally, the presence of a primary metabolic acidosis caused by renal failure renders the kidneys unable to generate a compensatory increase in the plasma bicarbonate level in the setting of a primary respiratory acidosis.

▲ Case Study 32-3, Part B

Mixed Acid-Base Disorders

Three hours after admission, the patient has received a total of 3 L of IV NS, 60 mEq of IV KCl, and 40 mmol of IV potassium phosphate. She has a nasogastric tube in place connected to low wall suction. Her vital signs were BP: 92/60 mm Hg, HR: 96 beats/min, and respirations: 26 breaths/min (shallow).

Laboratory Values:

Serum Chemistries	Arterial Blood Gas
Na^+: 132 mEq/L	pH: 7.31
K^+: 3.2 mEq/L	$Paco_2$: 69 mm Hg
Cl^-: 82 mEq/L	Pao_2: 32 mm Hg
CO_2: 27 mEq/L	HCO_3^-: 27 mEq/L
Creatinine: 2.0 mg/dl	Saturation: 89%
BUN: 31 mg/dl	
Ca^{++}: 8.7 mg/dl	
Phosphorus$^=$: 1.8 mg/dl	

Decision point: Interpret the acid-base status after initial treatment.

Case continues below

A systematic approach to diagnosing simple and mixed acid-base disorders (see Box 32-2) is critical to identifying the presence of mixed imbalances. Table 32-4 provides examples of common mixed acid-base disorders seen in the critical care setting. There are many possibilities and combinations of mixed acid-base disorders; however, the two primary acute respiratory acid-base disorders—respiratory acidosis and respiratory alkalosis— cannot coexist.[14]

▲ Case Study 32-3, Part C

Mixed Acid-Base Disorders

The patient is intubated, mechanically ventilated, and sent to the operating room for correction of the small bowel obstruction. During surgery, she receives additional intravenous fluids and electrolyte replacement (NS, KCl, potassium phosphate). One week later, before discharge her labs are as follows:

Serum Chemistries	Arterial Blood Gas
Na^+: 141 mEq/L	pH: 7.42
K^+: 4.8 mEq/L	$Paco_2$: 37 mm Hg
Cl^-: 100 mEq/L	Pao_2: 92 mm Hg
CO_2: 29 mEq/L	HCO_3^-: 28 mEq/L
BUN: 10 mg/dl	Saturation: 91%
Creatinine: 0.6 mg/dl	
Ca^{++}: 8.6 mg/dl	
Phosphorus$^=$: 2.8 mg/dl	

Decision point: Interpret the acid-base and electrolyte status of this patient before discharge.

TABLE 32-4 Common Causes of Mixed Acid-Base Disorders in the Acutely Ill Adult

ACID-BASE DISORDERS	EXAMPLE	CLINICAL FEATURES
Metabolic acidosis and Respiratory acidosis	Acute renal failure with pulmonary edema	High anion gap acidosis and hypoventilation with $Paco_2$ retention
Metabolic acidosis and Respiratory alkalosis	Salicylate intoxication Sepsis with severe liver disease	High anion gap acidosis with respiratory stimulation and hyperventilation with $Paco_2$ loss
Metabolic acidosis and Metabolic alkalosis	Diabetic ketoacidosis with vomiting Heart failure patient receiving high-dose loop diuretics	Ketoacidosis with gastrointestinal hydrochloric acid loss Lactic acidosis with high anion gap and excessive renal acid loss secondary to diuretics
Respiratory acidosis and Metabolic alkalosis	ARDS with permissive hypercapnia and gastric suction COPD patient receiving high-dose loop diuretics	Hypoventilation with retention of $Paco_2$ and gastrointestinal hydrochloric acid loss
Respiratory alkalosis and Metabolic alkalosis	Hyperventilation in neurosurgical patient receiving loop diuretics	High minute volume settings on ventilator with $Paco_2$ loss and excessive renal acid loss secondary to diuretics
Metabolic alkalosis, Metabolic acidosis and Respiratory alkalosis	Protracted vomiting with hypovolemic shock in patient with a neurologic disorder causing hyperventilation	Loss of hydrochloric acid with vomiting, high lactic acid level from shock causing drop in HCO_3^-, low $Paco_2$ from hyperventilation Patient could present with normal pH despite triple acid-base disorder
Metabolic acidosis, Metabolic alkalosis, and Respiratory acidosis	Cardiogenic shock with pulmonary edema in patient receiving high-dose diuretics	Lactic acidosis caused by shock, retention of $Paco_2$ because of pulmonary edema and poor gas exchange, renal acid loss secondary to diuretics

Data from reference 14.
ARDS = Acute respiratory distress syndrome, COPD = chronic obstructive pulmonary disease, HCO_3^- = bicarbonate, $Paco_2$ = partial pressure of arterial carbon dioxide.

CONCLUSIONS

Acid-base and electrolyte imbalances are extremely common in the acutely ill adult. Extreme aberrations in the blood pH can cause life-threatening hemodynamic derangements and organ dysfunction, especially when the acid-base derangement is acute. Successful treatment of acid-base imbalances is contingent upon an accurate diagnosis, which becomes challenging in the setting of mixed acid-base disorders. It is critically important to assess acid-base status with a systematic approach to ensure recognition of all acid-base disorders that may be present, even in the setting of a normal pH.

REFERENCES

1. Androgue, H. J., & Madias, N. E. (1998). Management of life-threatening acid-base disorders, Pt 1. *N Engl J Med, 338*(1), 26–34.
2. Androgue, H. J., & Madias, N. E. (1998). Management of life-threatening acid-base disorders, Pt 2. *N Engl J Med, 338*(2), 107–111.
3. Buchanan, I. B., et al. (2005). Chest wall necrosis and death secondary to hydrochloric acid infusion for metabolic alkalosis. *Southern Med J, 98*(8), 822–824.
4. Bushinsky, D., & Monk, R. (1998). Calcium. *Lancet, 352,* 306–311.
5. Chonghaile, M., Higgins, B., & Laffey, J. (2005). Permissive hypercapnia: role in protective ventilatory strategies. *Curr Opin Crit Care, 11,* 56–62.
6. Daniel, S. R., et al. (2004). Uncompensated metabolic acidosis: an under-recognized risk factor for subsequent intubation requirement. *J Trauma, 57*(5), 993–997.

7. Fangio, P., et al. (2004). Coronary spasm in a 59-year-old woman with hyperventilation. *Can J Anesthesia, 51,* 850–851.

8. Faubel, S., & Topf, J. (1999). *The fluid, electrolyte and acid-base companion.* San Diego: Alert and Oriented Publishing.

9. Gazmuri, R. J. (1999). Buffer treatment for cardiac resuscitation: putting the cart before the horse? *Crit Care Med, 27*(5), 875–876.

10. Gutierrez, G., & Wulf, M. (2005). Lactic acidosis in sepsis: another commentary. *Crit Care Med, 33*(10), 2420–2422.

11. Halperin, M., & Goldstein, M. (1999). *Fluid, electrolyte, and acid-base physiology; a problem-based approach* (3rd ed.). Philadelphia: Saunders.

12. Hardern, R. D., & Quinn, N. D. (2003). Emergency management of diabetic ketoacidosis in adults. *Emerg Med J, 20,* 210–213.

13. Heering, P., et al. (1999). Acid-base balance and substitution fluid during continuous hemofiltration. *Kidney Int, 56,* S37–S40.

14. Kaehny, W. D. (2003). Pathogenesis and management of respiratory and mixed acid-base disorders. In R. W. Schrier (Ed.). *Renal and electrolyte disorders* (6th ed.). Philadelphia: Lippincott Williams & Wilkins.

15. Kellum, J. A. (2005). Determinants of plasma acid-base balance. *Crit Care Clin Crit Care Nephrol, 21*(2), 329–346.

16. Kraut, J., & Kurtz, I. (2006). Controversies in the treatment of acute metabolic acidosis. *Nephrol Self-Assessment Program, 5*(1), 1–9.

17. Machata, A. M., et al. (2005). Rare but dangerous adverse effects of propofol and thiopental in intensive care. *J Trauma Injury Infect Crit Care, 58*(3), 643–645.

18. Mikhail, J. (1999). Resuscitation end points in trauma. *AACN Clin Issues, 10*(1), 10–21.

19. Preston, R. A. (2002). *Acid-base, fluids, and electrolytes; made ridiculously simple.* Miami: MedMaster.

20. Shapiro, J. I., & Kaehny, W. D. (2003). Pathogenesis and management of metabolic acidosis and metabolic alkalosis. In R. W. Schrier (Ed.). *Renal and electrolyte disorders* (6th ed.). Philadelphia: Lippincott Williams & Wilkins.

21. Sterns, R., & Palmer, B. (2006). Fluid, electrolyte, and acid-base disturbances. *Nephrology Self-Assessment Program, 5*(1), 10–54.

22. Subashini, D., et al. (2004). Uncompensated metabolic acidosis: an under recognized risk factor for subsequent intubation requirement. *J Trauma, 57*(5), 993–997.

23. Szaflarski, N. L., & Hanson, W. (1997). Metabolic acidosis. *AACN Clin Issues: Adv Practice Acute Crit Care, 8*(3), 481–496.

24. Viallon, A., et al. (1999). Does bicarbonate therapy improve management of severe diabetic ketoacidosis? *Crit Care Med, 27*(12), 2690–2693.

25. Weber, T., et al. (2000). Tromethamine buffer modifies the depressant effect of permissive hypercapnia on myocardial contractility in patients with acute respiratory distress syndrome. *Am J Respir Crit Care Med, 162,* 1361–1365.

26. Webster, N. R., & Kulkarni, V. (1999). Metabolic alkalosis in the critically ill. *Crit Rev Clin Lab Sci, 36*(5), 497–510.

CHAPTER 33

Acute Renal Failure

Robert Rothwell and Karen K. Carlson

Acute renal failure (ARF) is the most common renal disorder seen in critically ill patients and has the potential to negatively impact all other body systems. Between 5% and 20% of critically ill patients will develop ARF, often accompanied by multiple organ dysfunction syndrome (MODS).[8,13] This number increases in patients who develop sepsis; the incidence of ARF is 19% in moderate sepsis, 23% in severe sepsis, and 51% in septic shock when blood cultures are positive.[53,56] Despite many advances in the care and outcomes of critically ill patients, mortality in ARF patients remains near 50%[35,45] and as high as 70%[30] to 90%[13] in the septic or MODS patient. This mortality is nearly identical to the mortality seen in these patients 20 years ago.[11] Even if the renal insufficiency is mild (manifested by a lowered glomerular filtration rate [GFR]), not requiring any type of renal replacement, ARF continues to negatively contribute to overall patient outcomes and increases risk of mortality by 50%.[34]

Given the negative impact of renal insufficiency on mortality, even in its mild forms, efforts to prevent ARF are imperative. While not always preventable, those patients who present at increased risk and deserve additional prophylactic attention have been well described in the literature. Advanced age, preexisting renal insufficiency (even mild elevation in creatinine level), diabetes, hypertension, and heart failure have long been recognized to place patients admitted to critical care at higher risk for the development of ARF.[2,48] Risk further increases with pathologic stressors such as hypotension or sepsis.[43,48,59] When the patient's plan of care requires diagnostic procedures or certain treatment modalities (e.g., medications, surgery, nonsurgical interventions, and cardiopulmonary resuscitation [CPR]), risk increases further.

It is estimated that 5% to 25% of postsurgical patients develop ARF with or without the need for renal replacement.[2,20,37] These studies found age, elevated preoperative creatinine level, diabetes, decreased cardiac ejection fraction, increased body weight, heart failure, presence of carotid bruit, duration of cardiopulmonary bypass, and previous revascularization increased patient risk for the development of ARF.

It has long been recognized that a leading cause of nosocomial ARF is contrast-induced nephropathy (CIN)[26] with preexisting elevation in serum creatinine level being the most important risk factor.[36] While the pathophysiology is not fully understood, the insult is thought to be multifactorial. Contrast may transiently decrease left ventricular (LV) function and cardiac output (CO), renal blood flow, and GFR, suggesting hypersensitivity or a direct (tubule) nephrotoxic impact, particularly to the proximal tubular cells.

Critically ill patients often have a host of conditions increasing their risk for the development of renal failure. Patients are older, having lowered renal reserves, and may have hypertension, diabetes, cardiac disease, hepatitis C, or human immunodeficiency virus. Additionally, as patients age, those with chronic renal insufficiency who are maintained on dialytic therapy as part of their lifestyle may be admitted with an acute nonrenal crisis that requires continued renal replacement during their critical care stay.

In summary, while advanced age, diabetes, and elevated preoperative creatinine level appear to be the best predictors of the development of postoperative/postprocedural renal failure and increased length of stay and mortality, many other factors play a role. All patients admitted to critical care should be viewed as having the potential to develop renal dysfunction.

PREVENTION OF RENAL FAILURE

Whenever possible, prophylactic intervention should be instituted in patients identified to be at risk for the development of ARF. Prevention of ARF includes identifying patients at risk, avoiding nephrotoxic substances, and providing careful assessment and monitoring of the following:

Fluid balance (especially in patients presenting with signs of hypovolemia or who are bring treated with diuretics)
Hemodynamics
Renal function (including decreased urine output and the use of appropriate types and doses of

MEDICATIONS USED TO PREVENT OR TREAT ACUTE RENAL FAILURE

MEDICATION	ACTIONS	DOSAGE	SPECIAL CONSIDERATIONS
Acetylcysteine (Mucomyst)	Is a scavenger of oxygen free radicals; free radicals can overwhelm and deplete endogenous antioxidants, which are cytoprotective	600 mg PO twice a day the day before and after procedure[60] **or** 150 mg/kg in 500 ml of NS over 30 min; follow with 50 mg/kg in 500 ml of NS over 4 hr	Give loading dose immediately before contrast media
$NaHCO_3^-$ infusion	Reduces injury by alkalinizing urine, helping to decrease formation of free radicals	154 mEq/L $NaHCO_3$ in D_5W; infuse at 3 ml/kg/hr before radiocontrast injection, and 1 ml/kg/hr for 6 hr after contrast	Hold diuretics[44]
Loop diuretics: furosemide (Lasix), bumetanide (Bumex)	Increase GFR, increasing tubular flow to prevent cast formation and obstruction of tubules	Furosemide by IV injection; bumetanide, edecrin by continuous infusion Doses depend on response	Should only be given after adequate fluid loading is ensured These have been shown to have no effect on delaying RRT or on morbidity or mortality
Mannitol (Osmitrol)	Osmotic diuresis	12.5–25 g slow IV push	Causes less electrolyte imbalance than loop diuretics, but may cause volume expansion that can exacerbate congestive heart failure

GFR = Glomerular filtration rate, NS = normal saline, $NaHCO_3$ = sodium bicarbonate, RRT = renal replacement therapy.

◆ Case Study 33-1, Part A

Risk Factors for Developing Acute Renal Failure

While working in his garden, 75-year-old R.F. complained to his wife about increasing back pain. He was encouraged by his wife to rest. Several hours later when she tried to wake him, he was unarousable. She called 911; he was taken to the ED. His vital signs on admission were BP: 70/52 mm Hg and heart rate: 136 beats/min with frequent premature ventricular contractions. His skin was pale, cool, and clammy, and neck veins were flat. His medical history was unremarkable. A central line was placed and NS run wide open. He was sent for an urgent CT scan, where it was revealed that he had a leaking abdominal aneurysm. He was taken to the operating room, and after successful resection of his aneurysm he was transferred to critical care.

Decision Point: At this point, what are R.F.'s risk factors for developing ARF?

Decision Point: What measure would you expect to carry out in the immediate postoperative period to help prevent ARF?

Case continues on page 893

medications, especially those used during contrast studies and for pre-, intra-, and postprocedural end-organ protection).[41]

The target outcomes for intervention would include preservation of existing renal function, prevention of the complications associated with ARF, and avoidance of the need for chronic renal replacement.[64] The Medication table above presents the details of interventions to attempt to prevent renal failure.

DEFINITION

There is no universally accepted definition for ARF. It is, however, commonly described as the abrupt reduction in the GFR. The GFR, a clinical assessment tool used to measure renal function, is the volume of plasma cleared of a given substance in a minute. Normal GFR in adults is 125 milliliters (ml)/minute or 180 liters (L)/day.[22] Any decrease in GFR leads to the retention of nitrogenous waste products (azotemia) and the associated inability of the body to maintain normal fluid and electrolyte homeostasis.[15] As a more useful definition for the clinical setting, ARF is described as a decrease in GFR of 50%, a doubling of serum creatinine level, or an absolute increase in creatinine level of 0.5 mg/dl or greater above a certain cutoff point (e.g., 2 to 3.5 mg/dl).[51]

In 2004 the Acute Dialysis Quality Initiative Group proposed a new classification scheme for acute renal failure.[5,28] As described in Table 33-1, using the RIFLE acronym, a patient's renal function is classified, based on the GFR, serum creatinine level, and urine output, into three levels of renal dysfunction or two potential renal clinical outcomes. Optimistically, use of these classifications, subject to more study, will help standardize the study and subsequent discussion about ARF, for both prevention and treatment purposes. As well, recovery from ARF should be evaluated relative to the definition used to describe the renal function. Using the RIFLE criteria, Bellomo[4] suggested that complete recovery has occurred if patients return to their baseline classification; partial recovery has occurred if there is a persistent positive change in the patients' classification without the persistent need for renal replacement therapy (RRT).

In addition, in 2005 the Acute Kidney Injury Network published consensus recommendations encouraging a shift in the thought from ARF to acute kidney injury. These recommendations follow through on further developed discussions surrounding the thought that there is a continuum of renal dysfunction that may eventually result in failure. This continuum is potentially reversible. Use of this new terminology is similar to the way MODS has replaced the multiple organ failure terminology.

APPLIED PATHOPHYSIOLOGY

TYPES OF RENAL FAILURE

The etiologies of ARF are commonly cataloged into three broad categories, each associated with the location of the dysfunction. Physiologically, normal renal function is the sum of adequate filtration of the blood, renal tubule processing of the filtrate, and elimination of the final urine product. Therefore renal failure (dysfunction) can occur secondary to a reduction in renal blood flow that prohibits adequate filtration (i.e., prerenal); to an inflammatory, ischemic, or nephrotoxic injury to the tubules (i.e., intrarenal); or from obstruction of elimination (i.e., postrenal). The multiple causes of each type ARF are most easily understood when related to the underlying pathophysiology. Diagnosis of the type of renal failure is imperative so that appropriate interventions can be instituted without delay.

TABLE 33-1 Classification Scheme for Acute Renal Failure (ARF)*

LEVELS OF RENAL DYSFUNCTION	GFR CRITERIA	SERUM CREATININE CRITERIA	URINE OUTPUT CRITERIA
Risk of renal dysfunction	GFR decreased by >25%	Serum creatinine increased by 1.5 times baseline	Urine output of <0.5 ml/kg/hr for 6 hr
Injury to kidney	GFR decreased by >50%	Serum creatinine increased by 2 times baseline	Urine output of <0.5 ml/kg/hr for 12 hr
Failure of kidney function	GFR decreased by >75%	Serum creatinine increased by 3 times baseline or >4 mg/dl	Urine output of <0.3 ml/kg/hr for 24 hr or anuria for 12 hr
Clinical Outcomes			
Loss of kidney function	Persistent ARF: complete loss of kidney function for >4 weeks: need for renal replacement for >4 weeks		
End-stage kidney disease	End-stage kidney disease for >3 months: need for dialysis for >3 months		

From reference 4.
*If the patient demonstrates criteria from more than one classification, the criteria that demonstrate the more severe classification should be used.
ARF = Acute renal failure, GFR = glomerular filtration rate.

This diagnosis will be made using patient history and physical assessment findings along with pertinent laboratory and radiologic findings.

Prerenal Renal Failure

Prerenal renal failure is caused by any clinical condition resulting in decreased renal perfusion. It accounts for 40% of nosocomial renal failure.[51] Common etiologies of prerenal renal failure in the critically ill are listed in Box 33-1. No matter which clinical situation is responsible for the decrease in renal blood flow, the pathophysiologic consequences are the same. The decrease in renal perfusion decreases afferent arteriole pressure, leading to a decreased GFR. In response to this decreased GFR, while there is no

actual damage to the glomerular filtration or nephron function, the kidney is unable to function normally; this type of renal failure is deemed to be prerenal renal failure.

The kidneys normally receive between 20% and 25% of the CO (i.e., the renal fraction) or approximately 1200 ml/minute. While renal oxygen consumption is high, normal renal blood flow is in excess of that required for simple renal metabolic requirements, reinforcing that high flow is necessary for urine formation and other renal functions. Likewise, the design of the interrelatedness of the renal vasculature and renal tubules is reflective of the interdependence between blood supply and renal function.

Blood flow to the kidney is normally protected through autoregulation. The primary purpose of autoregulation is to maintain constant renal blood flow, which provides for precise control of renal excretion of water and other solutes.[22] Autoregulation occurs in both the efferent and afferent arterioles by influencing the degree of vascular tone (i.e., vasoconstriction or vasodilation). In response to changes in arterial pressure or renal tubular flow, via autoregulation, these arterioles vasoconstrict or vasodilate as needed to maintain normal renal blood flow. Unfortunately, this mechanism is only functional with an arterial pressure of 80 to 170 mm Hg.[22] When arterial pressure falls below 80 mm Hg, autoregulation is seriously impaired; the vessels are maximally vasodilated.

In addition, normal compensatory mechanisms are stimulated whenever low pressure or perfusion is sensed by the kidney. Activation of the renin-angiotensin-aldosterone system (see Chapter 12) results in peripheral and glomerular vasoconstriction via adrenergic stimulation by angiotensin II (further decreasing renal perfusion) and an increase in sodium and water reabsorption as the manifestation of the activity of both angiotensin II and aldosterone. The aldosterone-induced sodium reabsorption results in a low urine sodium level and low fractional excretion of sodium (FENa) (Table 33-2).

Urine sodium values less than 20 mEq/L are most often associated with volume depletion severe enough to compromise renal blood flow. This suggests that tubular function is still intact, conserving sodium appropriately. A urine sodium value greater than 40 mEq/L suggests that tubular function is impaired, as seen in intrarenal and chronic renal failure (CRF). FENa can be a useful measurement to evaluate renal tubular function. It assesses the ratio of the amount of sodium in the urine to the amount of sodium filtered by the kidney. Normally, less than 1% of sodium is excreted because kidneys with normal function reabsorb 99% of all filtered sodium. When the FENa is greater then 1%, it is suggestive of tubular dysfunction.

Box 33-1

Causes of Prerenal Renal Failure

HYPOVOLEMIA

- Hemorrhage
- Gastrointestinal losses: vomiting, diarrhea, nasogastric loss
- Burns
- Diaphoresis
- Overdiuresis
- Movement into interstitial space (edema, ascites)
- Hypovolemic shock

DECREASED CARDIAC OUTPUT

- Myocardial infarction
- Tamponade
- Cardiac dysrhythmias
- Heart failure
- Pulmonary embolism
- Tension pneumothorax

DECREASED SYSTEMIC VASCULAR RESISTANCE

- Anaphylaxis
- Sepsis
- Multiple organ dysfunction syndrome
- Overuse of antihypertensive medications
- Neurogenic shock
- Septic shock

MEDICATIONS

- Loop diuretics
- Angiotensin-converting enzyme inhibitors
- Prostaglandin inhibitors
- Chemotherapeutic agents
- Vasoactive medications (e.g., epinephrine, norepinephrine)

TABLE 33-2 Differential Laboratory Diagnosis of Renal Dysfunction

	NORMAL	PRERENAL	INTRARENAL	POSTRENAL
Urine volume	1–1.5 L/day	<400 ml/day	<400 ml/day	Variable
Urine specific gravity	1.010–1.020	1.020 or greater	Fixed (1.010 or less)	Fixed (1.010 or less)
Urine osmolality	500–850 mOsm/L	>500 mOsm/L	<350 mOsm/L	≤350 mOsm/L
Serum BUN	10–20 mg/dl	>25 mg/dl	>25 mg/dl	<25 mg/dl
Serum creatinine	0.6–1.2 mg/dl	Normal to slightly elevated	>1.2 mg/dl	>1.2 mg/dl
Serum BUN: creatinine ratio	10:1	20:1 or greater	(10–15):1; both elevated but ratio remains constant	(10–15):1; both elevated but ratio remains constant
Urine sodium		<20 mEq/L	>40 mEq/L	>40 mEq/L
FENa		<1%	>1%*	>1%

*When the patient is not under the influence of diuretics.
BUN = Blood urea nitrogen, FENa = fractional excretion of sodium.

Under the influence of antidiuretic hormone (ADH), also stimulated by low renal perfusion, and aldosterone, more water is reabsorbed, leading to decreased urine production (oliguria) and increased urine concentration (increased urine specific gravity and osmolality).

Urea is easily filtered and actively reabsorbed much more readily than creatinine primarily because of urea's smaller molecular size and affinity to movement with water. Serum blood urea nitrogen (BUN) levels elevate while, for a time, serum creatinine levels remain relatively normal. This is demonstrated by one of the hallmark signs of prerenal failure, a BUN:creatinine ratio of 10–15:1.

Renal blood flow is also influenced by the sympathetic nervous system (SNS), hormones, and medications. SNS influence is vasoconstrictive in nature; anything that stimulates the SNS (e.g., hypotension) will cause renal vasculature vasoconstriction. Hormonal influences include the renin-angiotensin-aldosterone system and ADH, already discussed. Renal prostaglandins (i.e., PGE_2, PGI_2) modulate the impact of vasoactive substances on the kidney. While renal prostaglandins do not have a major influence on the GFR in normal circumstances, they are thought to temper the renal vasoconstrictive effects of the SNS, especially on the afferent arterioles. This opposition to vasoconstriction helps prevent excess reduction of renal blood flow.

Certain pharmacologic interventions (e.g., epinephrine or norepinephrine) cause renal vasoconstriction. Renal prostaglandin inhibitors (e.g., aspirin and other nonsteroidal antiinflammatory drugs) may cause significant reductions in renal blood flow under stressful situations (e.g., volume depletion or surgery).[22] While long held to be true in clinical practice, there is no compelling evidence that dopamine has any positive influence on renal function.[3,18] This is explained in the Research Utilization box below.

▲ RESEARCH UTILIZATION

The Use of Renal (Low) Dose Dopamine in the Critical Care Unit

CLINICAL ISSUE

The use of renal (low) dose dopamine in the critical care unit has been a routine part of practice since the early 1960s. This low-dose (1–3 mcg/kg/min) dopamine was believed to increase renal blood flow and the elimination of sodium, leading to an improvement in renal function. Despite a lack of controlled trials that demonstrated a positive effect on renal function, widespread use persists.

SUMMARY

This study analyzed 61 trials, published over nearly the past 40 years. It contains an excellent table that summarizes the included trials. The analysis of these studies shows that low-dose dopamine demonstrated no effect on mortality, on the need for renal replacement, or on adverse events. However, caution is advised when interpreting the impact of dopamine on adverse effects as many studies included in the analysis did not capture adverse effect data. Clinically, urine output did improve on the first day of therapy; improvements in serum creatinine levels and creatinine clearance were clinically insignificant. No significant changes were seen following day 1.

APPLICATION

Given that dopamine does increase urine output, albeit briefly, and may not cause adverse effects, use of low (renal) dose dopamine will remain controversial. It is important for clinicians to be aware that there is no demonstrated beneficial effect on renal function.

NEED FOR FURTHER STUDY

Future studies are needed to identify the effect of dopamine on adverse effects.

Friedrich, J. O., et al. (2005). Meta-analysis: low dose dopamine increases urine output but does not prevent renal dysfunction or death. *Ann Intern Med, 142*, 510–524.

Intrarenal Renal Failure

When there is inflammatory, nephrotoxic, or ischemic injury directly to the nephron, the renal failure is described as intrarenal (intrinsic) renal failure. Intrinsic insults to the kidneys result in renal cellular damage, to the vasculature, glomerulus, tubules, or interstitium, ultimately resulting in functional problems. A healthy glomerulus prevents filtration of plasma proteins and cellular elements; when the glomerulus has been damaged, proteins and cellular debris can enter the renal tubules and lead to obstruction of the lumen. Common causes of intrarenal failure are listed in Box 33-2.

The major cause of intrarenal failure is acute tubular necrosis (ATN), caused by ischemic or nephrotoxic insults to the kidney.[33] In critical care, 35% to 50% of all ATN is associated with sepsis.[8,12,24,35] ATN following surgery is responsible for 20% to 25% of all nosocomial ARF; many of these patients also had prerenal factors involved.[10]

Inflammatory (e.g., glomerulonephritis) and immune disorders (e.g., systemic lupus erythematosus, poststreptococcal infections) can also cause intrarenal failure. With these disorders, the GFR is decreased because of immune-related hemodynamic changes as well as physical structural damage. Intrarenal renal failure may be the sequelae of infectious or infiltrative diseases

Box 33-2

Etiologies of Intrarenal Renal Failure

INFLAMMATORY

- Post-streptococcal glomerulonephritis
- Membranous glomerulonephritis
- Membranoproliferative glomerulonephritis (from antigen-antibody complexes, cryoglobulins)
- Interstitial nephritis
- Acute pyelonephritis
- Allergic nephritis
- Hypercalcemia
- Uric acid nephropathy
- Myeloma of the kidney
- Rhabdomyolysis (trauma, seizures, prolonged coma, muscle disease)
- Myoglobin
- Transfusion reaction

ISCHEMIC

- Uncorrected hypoperfusion
- Renal artery thrombosis
- Shock

NEPHROTOXIC

- Medications: aminoglycoside antibiotics, anesthetic agents
- Radiographic contrast dyes
- Pesticides
- Fungicides
- Heavy metals
- Organic solvents

OBSTRUCTIVE

- Renal thrombosis
- Nephrolithiasis
- Sickle cell disease
- Trauma/crush injuries

(e.g., sarcoidosis, cancers such as lymphoma or leukemia) as well as some medications. While there is neither tubule nor glomerular damage, interstitial nephritis is characterized by inflammatory cell infiltrates in the renal interstitium, and a decrease in the GFR. Approximately 5% to 20% of acute intrarenal failure is caused by these types of problems.[35,51]

As discussed earlier, the kidneys are highly metabolic, receive a large portion of the CO, and are therefore extremely vulnerable to ischemic or toxic injury. In ischemic or nephrotoxic injury, there is damage to both the vasculature and the tubules. Tubular injury is most common. Nephrotic ischemic injury is the most common cause of intrarenal failure and presents as ATN. With less oxygen available, there is decreased

ATP production, and therefore wastes and toxins accumulate in the cell. In the tubules, an increase in intracellular calcium level leads to necrosis and apoptosis, with relocation of the sodium, potassium, and adenosinetriphosphatase (ATPase) from the basement membrane. This relocation interferes with normal sodium transport, increasing distal delivery of sodium chloride, causing swelling of cells and activation of tubular glomerular feedback, ultimately decreasing GFR. If ischemia worsens, nitric oxide is produced, causing cellular damage and lysis of tubular cells. Cast formation, tubular obstruction, and tubular destruction result, causing back leak of the glomerular filtrate, which leads to interstitial edema and further decreases GFR. Cumulatively, these mechanisms contribute to the decreased renal function observed in ATN.[31]

ATN also results in vascular endothelium injury. The damaged endothelium responds in an exaggerated fashion to vasodilators released as part of the stress response (e.g., bradykinin and acetylcholine). This response, along with the loss of autoregulation, exacerbates the effects of the ischemia.

Given the large blood flow through the kidney, it is by nature susceptible to damage as toxic substances are filtered. The kidney's great reabsorptive and concentrating abilities lead to the delivery of large amounts of toxins to the tubular epithelial cells. When presented with a nephrotoxin, the generation of toxic metabolites as well as the high energy consumption requirement, coupled with marginal oxygen delivery, further increase the susceptibility of the kidney to damage.

Postrenal Renal Failure

If the dysfunction of the kidney is related to obstruction of the renal flow structures after the nephron, the renal failure is termed *postrenal renal failure*. In response to the obstruction of urine flow, the ureters and renal pelvis dilate (visible on ultrasound or computed tomography [CT] scan), and intratubular pressure may increase until it exceeds glomerular filtration pressure; glomerular filtration is decreased. Filtration may cease entirely in response to a complete obstruction, while a partial obstruction will decrease filtration. As with any decrease to the GFR, initially the tubules will respond by increasing reabsorption of sodium and water, leaving the urine volume low, the urine sodium level high, and the urine concentration high. Given time, sodium and water reabsorption decrease as the tubules become damaged. Permanent renal damage can occur if the obstruction is not addressed: the extent of that damage is determined by the location, duration, and degree of obstruction. Common etiologies of postrenal renal failure in the critically ill are listed in Box 33-3.

ASSESSMENT

Assessment findings of the prerenal failure patient correlate with the cause of the decreased flow to the kidneys. If the underlying problem is hypovolemia or decreased peripheral vascular resistance, the patient will appear to be hypovolemic (Box 33-3). If the hypovolemia is serious, the patient may manifest signs of hypovolemic shock (Chapter 40). If the cause is related to a decreased vascular resistance, the patient will also exhibit signs and symptoms similar to those seen with hypovolemia because the patient will be experiencing a relative hypovolemia. If the decreased perfusion is secondary to decreased CO, the patient's presentation will be different (Table 33-3). Pertinent laboratory findings seen in renal failure, including the laboratory differentiation between prerenal and intrarenal failure, are outlined in Table 33-2. Application of assessment findings aids in accurate diagnosis of the cause of decreased renal blood flow and will therefore aid in appropriate treatment.

The physical assessment findings in the intrarenal failure patient differ dependent upon the underlying cause of the problem. When the injury is ischemic in nature, secondary to prolonged decreased perfusion, the patient may initially present with findings of hypovolemia or decreased CO (see Table 33-3). As renal

Box 33-3

Etiologies of Postrenal Renal Failure

TUBULAR OBSTRUCTION
- Polycystic kidney
- Uric acid crystals

URETERAL OBSTRUCTION
- Tumors
- Strictures
- Fibrosis

BLADDER OBSTRUCTION
- Prostatic hypertrophy
- Tumors
- Calculi
- Blood clots
- Neurogenic causes
- Anticholinergic medications

URETHRAL OBSTRUCTION
- Calculi
- Strictures
- Stenosis
- Catheter obstruction

TABLE 33-3 Assessment Findings in Prerenal Renal Failure

FLUID DEFICIT/DECREASED PERIPHERAL VASCULAR RESISTANCE	DECREASED CARDIAC OUTPUT
Oliguria	Oliguria
Tachycardia	Tachycardia
Hypotension	Hypotension
Dry mucous membranes	
Decreased PAP, PAWP, RAP	Elevated PAP, PAWP, RAP
Flat neck veins	Distended neck veins
Lethargy	
Coma	

PAP = Pulmonary artery pressure, PAWP = pulmonary artery wedge pressure, RAP = right atrial pressure.

dysfunction is established, patient presentation will reveal the manifestations of the lack of renal function (see Table 33-2).

Once tubular dysfunction is established, sodium reabsorption is hindered. Urine sodium level and FENa are increased. The concentrating ability of the kidney is impaired, resulting in lower osmolality and lower specific gravity of the urine.

♦ **Case Study 33-1, Part B**

Determining Renal Status and Treatment Priorities

R.F. was admitted to critical care with an arterial pressure of 94/42 mm Hg, CVP 3 mm Hg, PAWP 5 mm Hg, cardiac index (CI) 1.6, venous oxygen saturation (SVo$_2$) 55%. His arterial blood gas was pH 7.35, Paco$_2$ 35 mm Hg, Pao$_2$ 66 mm Hg, and HCO$_3^-$ 17 mEq/L on 100% Fio$_2$. He received 7 units of red blood cells and 13 L of crystalloid intraoperatively. He has a swollen, tense abdomen with retention sutures on the incision and a urine output of 5 ml/hr with BUN 45 mg/dl and creatinine 1.7 mg/dl, despite running fluids. The anesthetist reports that the aortic cross-clamp time was prolonged, and the aneurysm was proximal to the renal arteries, necessitating grafting of both renal arteries.

Decision Point: What is the patient's current renal status, and what are your treatment priorities?

Two days later R.F. is weaned off the ventilator. His renal function has deteriorated, despite aggressive efforts at

providing adequate renal blood flow. His creatinine is 3.5 mg/dl, BUN 65 mg/dl; the patient is anuric, with urine output essentially nil for the past 24 hours. The urinalysis shows a sodium level >20 mEq/L, FENa of 3%, and casts. A diuretic trial of mannitol 25 g was ordered, to which there is no response. Furosemide (Lasix) 100 mg IV was ordered to be followed by 500 mg hydrochlorothiazide (Hydro-DIURIL) IV. There was no response to the diuretics, so the physician orders a renal CT with contrast to look for perioperative renal artery thrombus. The patient remains oliguric, requiring fluid for BP support.

Decision Point: What are your treatment priorities?

Case continues on page 909

Uremic Complications

The exposure of the body to the uremic compounds in ARF is completely different when compared with CRF patients. The impact of the accumulation of uremic waste products in the CRF patient is well known. However, there are limited data available describing uremic toxicity in the setting of ARF. Instead of accumulation of retention compounds over months or even years, exposure to retention compounds in ARF patients lasts for a period of days or weeks. While it is apparent that patients in ARF are affected by their uremic states, knowledge of uremic toxicity in CRF patients cannot be completely applied to patients with ARF,[24] given that ARF patients have had only hours' or days' exposure to urea, creatinine, and a host of other accumulated compounds.[63]

Cardiovascular Manifestations

The cardiovascular manifestations of ARF can almost all be linked to the volume status of the patient. For example, hypertension is a common finding in these patients related to their volume overload and increased peripheral vascular resistance. Since renal perfusion is often low, the renin-angiotensin-aldosterone system is activated, increasing sodium and water retention as well as causing peripheral vasoconstriction under the influence of angiotensin II.

CO is often high for similar reasons but may decrease over time as fluid shifts to the interstitial space, causing peripheral or pulmonary edema, ascites, or intra-abdominal hypertension. As well, CO is also compromised by the metabolic acidosis, hypertension, anemia, and electrolyte abnormalities seen in ARF.

ARF patients may develop heart failure or have their preexisting heart failure exacerbated by ARF. Dysrhythmias are common, again related to the acidosis, hyperkalemia, hypermagnesemia, and hypocalcemia.

Over time, uremic pericarditis may develop. Usually aseptic, the pericardial sac becomes inflamed and fluid develops as a response to the uremic toxins. Clinically, patients will present with pain, fever, and pericardial friction rub, which may occur before the pain and disappear with the accumulation of fluid. As well, these patients will be tachycardic and hypotensive and have a narrowed pulse pressure and a paradoxical pulse.

Respiratory Manifestations

For an already ischemic kidney, hypoxemia presents an added renal risk. Fluid volume overload can lead to pulmonary congestion, pleural effusions, or intra-abdominal hypertension, all of which decrease gas exchange in the untreated ARF patient. The ARF patient also experiences interstitial edema caused by dysregulation of the inflammatory cascade and increased vascular permeability (capillary leak), which can lead to lung perfusion dysregulation, fluid shifts, capillary leak, and pulmonary edema. Over time, urea retention products contribute to inflammation and additional capillary leak in the pulmonary bed. These may all contribute to the development of pulmonary edema, causing the patient to present with shortness of breath and frothy sputum along with rales and rhonchi. These patients may have normal cardiac filling pressures related to the previously described loss of capillary integrity and fluid leak. The common finding of hypoalbuminemia in ARF patients only adds to the fluid leak because these patients have decreased colloid oncotic pressure; therefore fluid is not held in the vascular space but instead is allowed to move interstitially more easily.

The kidney is a highly metabolic organ and in addition to the constant vigilance of the critical care nurse, current monitoring and therapeutic technology make hypoxemia easy to anticipate but not always easily treatable. Even brief interruptions in oxygenation can worsen any ischemic intrarenal damage. Both arterial and central venous oxygen saturation should be monitored, giving the nurse advance warning of any hypoxemic threat to the patient. Episodes of low CO leading to hypotension, frequently seen in the ARF patient, must be responded to quickly in order to preserve oxygen delivery to the kidneys and prevent further intrarenal damage and worsening metabolic acidosis (lactic acidosis).

Hematologic Manifestations

The ARF patient will become anemic, a finding seen as early as 10 days after the onset of renal dysfunction. This anemia decreases the blood's oxygen-carrying capacity, which may further compromise cardiac and pulmonary stability.

Not only do critically ill ARF patients have a number of factors that contribute to bone marrow suppression, but also they experience bleeding, hemodilution, decreased red blood cell survival, gastrointestinal (GI) bleeding, perioperative blood loss, and intravascular hemolysis, all of which contribute to their anemic state. Additionally, their anemia is worsened by acidosis, uremic toxins, and decreased or absent erythropoietin production. Without adequate erythropoietin, there is decreased synthesis and increased breakdown of red blood cells.

In the untreated ARF patient, uremia also causes increased fragility of the membrane of the red blood cells and hence decreases red blood cell half-life. Additionally, uremic coagulopathy interferes with coagulation and leads to increased blood loss. Because many critical care patients have concomitant cardiac and pulmonary disease, anemia may be catastrophic. Since it takes weeks for synthetic erythropoietin to become effective, transfusion may be the best option to increase hemoglobin value in the ARF patient.

The risk of infection in ARF is increased because of leukocyte dysfunction. The leukocyte count may rise, but the ability of the leukocyte to combat infection is impaired. Normal inflammatory responses are also blunted. Therefore the nurse should continually assess for signs of infection, which occurs in up to 70% of ARF patients and accounts for the cause of death in as many as 40% of ARF patients.[25] Infection control interventions would include using strict aseptic technique, minimizing invasive line manipulation, providing frequent mouth and pulmonary care, minimizing use of vascular catheters, removing indwelling catheters where possible, and monitoring the blood cell counts and patient temperature diligently (see Chapter 9).

Gastrointestinal Manifestations

The patient's nutrition will be affected as the result of uremia-mediated gastritis, which can result in anorexia, nausea, dyspepsia, vomiting, diarrhea or constipation, and gastric ulceration. There is evidence that ARF itself may be caused by the inflammatory cascade. Since the inflammatory response is seldom localized to one organ system, but also affects other organ systems, the kidney is caught up in the flood of inflammatory mediators. Unable to excrete these factors, the kidney cannot compensate for the resultant acidosis, contributing to the inflammatory response. Acidosis leads to increased nitric oxide levels (a vasodilator) and lowers blood pressure (BP) or may cause shock, as well as exacerbating lung and GI injury, hindering the natural GI barrier function of preventing bacterial translocation (see Chapter 30).[25]

ARF patients do have a tendency toward GI bleeding. The kidney plays a role in the inactivation and removal of GI hormones. As renal function is lost, plasma gastrin and gastric ammonia levels rise. This can lead to gastritis and the development of ulcerations. With the development of acute, erosive ulcerations, both the upper and lower GI tract may be affected. The risk for GI bleeding can be exacerbated once RRT is begun as a consequence of the anticoagulation used.

Neurologic Manifestations

Uremic toxins decrease cerebral blood flow and can compromise cerebral oxygen utilization. Neurologic changes observed in the ARF patient are directly related to the rate at which renal dysfunction develops, and these patients usually respond favorably to RRT. Mental status abnormalities should be considered warning signs indicating the patient with ARF needs to be started on RRT. There is central nervous system depression from accumulation of waste products, mainly urea and other retention products. The patient may become depressed, apathetic, and obtunded. RRT is limited in its ability to prevent the central nervous system effects of uremia. These patients may manifest changes in consciousness, showing alterations in psychomotor skills, thinking, memory, speech, perception, and emotion. Signs of neurologic alteration often proceed more rapidly in the ARF patient than the CRF patient.

INTERVENTIONS

Patients in renal failure must be managed collaboratively by the entire healthcare team. Unfortunately, much of the care of the patient in ARF is supportive, rather than curative. This collaboration must begin with the early recognition of those patients who might be at risk for the development of renal failure. While the interventions used in the renal failure patient have changed over the past few years, there remains a focus on primary recognition of the potential for renal failure as well as the early institution of RRT to assist in the prevention of the development of complications from the uremia associated with ARF.

In prerenal failure, target outcomes would include accurate cause identification and intervention, restoration of renal blood flow, preservation of existing renal function, prevention of the complications associated with ARF (and the associated prolonged length of stay), and avoidance of the need for chronic RRT.[64] When caring for a patient in prerenal renal failure, interventions must be tailored to the cause of the hypoperfusion. If the problem is volume related, then volume should be aggressively replaced. If the patient is

in cardiac failure (see Chapter 12), interventions may include antidysrhythmic medications, positive inotropic agents, preload and afterload manipulations, and, in some situations, application of the intra-aortic balloon pump. If the problem is a decreased systemic vascular resistance, vasoconstrictors should be administered. Once intrarenal failure is established, because of the widespread systemic effects of ARF, there are a variety of clinical challenges for the critical care team, including fluid balance, electrolyte balance, acid-base balance, prevention and treatment of infection, prevention of further kidney damage, minimization of the effects of the developing uremia, and establishment of adequate nutrition.

Because prevention of ARF is of utmost importance, the restoration of adequate circulating blood volume takes precedence over other interventions in the oliguric patient. Anticipatory interventions, such as additional fluid and elective diuresis when a renal insult is a possibility (e.g., radiologic imaging using contrast dyes), should also be implemented.

In the situation of exposure to radiocontrast dyes, if the patient has diabetes, is elderly or dehydrated, or has even slight elevation in creatinine level, additional IV fluid should be administered, as shown in the Multidisciplinary Plan of Care on pp. 896-899. The team pharmacist should also be consulted for modifying drug doses and anticipating the effect of radiocontrast dye. These steps are crucial in preventing CIN in many critically ill patients.

Fluid Balance

Fluid balance in the patient with compromised renal function is on a continuum, making maintenance of fluid homeostasis a challenge. Renal perfusion must be maintained while not placing the patient at risk for the complications of fluid overload. Initially, patients may present with a fluid volume deficit. Any patient who has experienced a fluid loss and is at risk for fluid volume deficit is also a candidate for the development of prerenal failure. If the insult is too great or the healthcare team is unable to adequately intervene in the prerenal patient, renal dysfunction may progress.

Typically, patients with renal dysfunction will not have a maintenance IV in place. Efforts to manage fluid balance often begin with placing a pulmonary artery catheter (PAC) and measuring cardiac filling pressures in order to establish a clear picture of the patient's fluid status. If the patient demonstrates orthostatic hypotension, or has a central venous pressure (CVP) less than 4 mm Hg or a pulmonary artery wedge pressure (PAWP) less than 8 mm Hg, a crystalloid fluid challenge may be done with normal saline (NS) as a 1000-ml bolus over 30 minutes. NS is the fluid of choice as

MULTIDISCIPLINARY PLAN OF CARE FOR THE PATIENT WITH ACUTE RENAL FAILURE

PROBLEM	INTERVENTION	RATIONALE	EXPECTED OUTCOME	COMMENTS
Risk for development of renal failure	Careful consideration of patients who present with: • Advanced age • Preexisting renal insufficiency (any elevation in creatinine) • Diabetes • Hypertension • Heart failure	Early identification of patients allows for appropriate prophylactic intervention, especially in preparation for diagnostic testing or surgery.	Patients at risk for renal failure will be identified early.	
	Monitor vital signs, hemodynamic parameters, and renal function tests: • BP, MAP, HR • CVP, PAP, PAWP, SVR • UO • Specific gravity • BUN • Creatinine • Urine sodium • FENa	Good assessment provides data needed to develop a plan of care.	Early change in renal perfusion and renal function will be identified.	
	For most accurate monitoring of fluid status, institute hemodynamic monitoring with a PA or CVP catheter.			
	Avoid nephrotoxins (e.g., aspirin, nonsteroidal antiinflammatory agents, aminoglycosides, cyclosporine).	Renal damage will be prevented.		
Potential for contrast-induced nephropathy	If possible, withhold diuretics, angiotensin-converting enzyme inhibitors, angiotensin receptor blockers, nonsteroidal antiinflammatory agents, and other nephrotoxins for 24 hr before procedure.[46]			
	Institute preprocedural hydration: • 100–150 ml of 0.45% or 0.9% NS[46] for 3–5 hr before procedure[57] and at least 6 hr following procedure	Well-hydrated kidneys are at lower risk for development of renal failure.	Achieve a urine output of 150 ml/hr following procedure.	

PROBLEM	INTERVENTION	RATIONALE	EXPECTED OUTCOME	COMMENTS
	• Alternatively, 1 ml/kg/hr of 0.45% or 0.9% NS 12 hours before and after procedure[46] If patient is at risk for heart failure or volume overload, PA catheterization is suggested.[56]			
	For procedures involving contrast: • Consider low dose of a lower osmolar contrast agent[5] • Avoid repeated dose of contrast in a short time (less than 48 hr)	Use of lower osmolar contrast is reasonable to minimize risk of development of renal failure.[5]		
	For high-risk patients, infuse isotonic bicarbonate solution 3 ml/kg/hr as long before procedure as possible, followed by 1 ml/kg/hr for at least 6 hr postprocedure.[45]	Alkalinizing urine helps minimize formation of free radicals after use of radiocontrast.	Creatinine level will not increase for 48 hr following procedure.[45]	
	Consider prophylactic use of acetylcysteine PO or IV (see Medication table, p. 887).	Acetylcysteine is a scavenger of oxygen free radicals. Free radicals can overwhelm and deplete endogenous antioxidants, which are cytoprotective.	Likelihood of contrast-induced renal failure will be reduced.	
Fluid volume deficit	Institute fluid challenge: Administer 500–1000 ml of IV NS solution over 20–30 min. Evaluate urine output and hemodynamic parameters, if available. Repeat as needed.	A fluid challenge is given to sufficiently increase intravascular volume with goal of increasing renal perfusion. NS has an intravascular half-life of only 20–30 min so fluids must be given quickly. An improvement in hemodynamics and urine output suggests patient has fluid deficit and could benefit from additional fluid.	Hemodynamics and renal perfusion will be improved: • CVP 8–12 mm Hg (12–15 mm Hg in mechanically ventilated patients) • MAP ≥65 mm Hg • UO ≥0.5 ml/kg/hr If no urine production, verify urinary catheter patent, then stop fluid challenge.	There is controversy surrounding the best fluids and methods to use when attempting to increase renal perfusion (see references 27, 32, 52, 57, 65).
Fluid volume overload	Restrict fluids as needed. Provide meticulous intake and output (include insensible losses) measurements.	Track fluid balance to detect fluid weight gain (1 L = 2.2 kg).		

Table continues on page 898

MULTIDISCIPLINARY PLAN OF CARE FOR THE PATIENT WITH ACUTE RENAL FAILURE—cont'd

PROBLEM	INTERVENTION	RATIONALE	EXPECTED OUTCOME	COMMENTS
	Take daily weights.	Avoid overhydration.	Weight should remain relatively constant. A small weight loss (0.2–0.3 kg/day) may be explained by normal catabolism.	Daily weight remains the gold standard for tracking fluid balance. Weight should remain within a narrow range while in ARF.
	Calculate daily fluid needs, considering replenishment of insensible losses. Monitor filling pressures.	Helps to ensure adequate hydration and CO.	Weight gain may indicate fluid movement into interstitial or intracellular space.	For filling pressures, the patient should have a central venous pressure line at minimum, preferably a pulmonary artery catheter because ARF has myocardial depression effects.
	Administer diuretics as ordered (see Medication table, p. 887). Institute RRTs as indicated.			RRTs may remove water. Fluids may be needed to support BP during dialysis or continuous RRT.
Altered pharmacokinetics because of loss of renal function	Keep pharmacist informed of current GFR, creatinine, and BUN. Ensure all medications are dosed based on current renal status.	Doses might need to be increased while patient is on renal replacement, or decreased between filtration runs to avoid toxicity.	Nephrotoxicity caused by polypharmacy will be minimized by good communication of current renal status and replacement therapy with team pharmacist.	
Increased catabolic state because of ARF	Administer nutrition as prescribed, working collaboratively with nutritionist (see Nutrition box on p. 910). Monitor prealbumin, albumin, and transferrin (if available).	Diet, whether enteral or parenteral, must provide ample calories to maintain positive nitrogen balance, but minimize additional solute or nitrogen load. Follow recommended formulas for carbohydrates, fats, and protein in diet to maintain patient in anabolic state.	Patient will maintain visceral protein stores. Tube-feeding formula will minimize excess carbon dioxide production in mechanically ventilated renal failure patient. Enteral route is safer.	Energy supplied by consuming the body's own protein stores is far less than that required to synthesize new protein.

PROBLEM	INTERVENTION	RATIONALE	EXPECTED OUTCOME	COMMENTS
Increased risk of infection	Use aseptic technique with all indwelling catheters. Remove all catheters as soon as feasible. Provide excellent oral and pulmonary care. Administer antibiotics as prescribed. Assist with insertion and protect security and asepsis of access catheter for RRT, using full barrier mode.	Uremic patient is at increased risk of infection. Any break in skin or mucosa is a greater threat to uremic patient because of effect of uremic toxins on neutrophils.	Patient will not develop catheter-related bloodstream infection or urinary tract infection.	Indwelling urinary catheter should be discontinued in all anuric patients and considered in all oliguric patients.
Risk for poor oxygenation	Continuously monitor arterial oxygen venous saturation. Provide supplemental oxygen as needed, and recommend mechanical ventilator adjustments PRN.	Kidney needs adequate perfusion, which may be lost with low BP or during hypoxemic episodes.	Arterial and venous saturations will be maintained in normal range.	Monitor serial blood gases.
Metabolic acidosis	Monitor labs for acid-base balance. Reduce dietary protein if not on RRT.	Acidemia may cause myocardial depression, dysrhythmias, and hypotension.	pH will be maintained in normal range.	Maintain HCO_3^- level >15 mEq/L when possible.
Hyperkalemia	Monitor electrolytes. Implement conservative measures to decrease potassium (Chapter 31). Institute RRT when necessary.	One of the most typical complications of ARF is hyperkalemia, which can cause lethal dysrhythmias.	Patient will remain normokalemic.	Interventions will moderate electrolyte disorder until RRT can be started. Refractory hyperkalemia is one of the reasons to begin RRT.

ARF = Acute renal failure, BP = blood pressure, BUN = blood urea nitrogen, CO_2 = cardiac output, CVP = central venous pressure, FENa = fractional excretion of sodium, HCO_3^- = bicarbonate, HR = heart rate, MAP = mean arterial pressure, NS = normal saline, PA = pulmonary artery, $\bar{P}AP$ = pulmonary artery pressure, PAWP = pulmonary artery wedge pressure, RRT = renal replacement therapy, SVR = systemic vascular resistance, UO = urine output.

it is the most isotonic fluid without adding potentially dangerous electrolytes (e.g., potassium, calcium as found in lactated Ringer's [LR]) to the vascular space. Hypotonic IV solutions, such as D_5W or half normal saline, will redistribute quickly into the intracellular space, and therefore will not increase the intravascular volume to support perfusion of the kidney.

Volume expanders, such as plasma or hetastarch, may be given, but must be used cautiously, preferably by experienced clinicians using monitored cardiac filling pressures, since colloids can worsen pulmonary edema, especially if the patient has acute lung injury. Colloids may redistribute and take additional water from the circulatory space into the interstitial space, thus worsening a pulmonary insult.

If there is no response to the fluid challenge, shown by increasing filling pressures or the presence of urine within 30 minutes, CO is measured, if possible, and additional fluid is administered until the CVP reaches 6 to 8 mm Hg and the PAWP reaches 12 to 15 mm Hg. If the CO is still low and there is no urine response, the fluids should be given until the CVP reaches 10 to 12 mm Hg and the PAWP is close to 20 mm Hg. If the CO and arterial pressure remain low, an appropriate vasopressor may be considered to increase CO (see Chapter 41). If lack of urine production continues, prerenal failure has been ruled out; the cause is intrarenal.[38] At this point, the administration of diuretics could be considered.

As described previously, intrarenal failure results in loss of the kidneys' ability to form and concentrate urine. Management of this stage of renal failure becomes critical as the patient will likely become oliguric. As renal function deteriorates, fluid overload often becomes more of an issue. While there is no evidence that diuretics decrease the incidence of ARF, morbidity and mortality, or length of hospital stay,[5] or alter the need for dialysis, diuretics may convert oliguric to nonoliguric ARF, which while comforting to clinicians, does little for the patient.[9] The diuretics chosen should be planned with as little risk to the fragile patient as possible. If they are ineffective, residual problems may develop.

Fluid overload is a common finding in ARF as the kidneys are incapable of clearing fluids. This may manifest in heart failure, pulmonary edema, and cerebral edema. The occurrence of these disorders in the patient with ARF strongly suggests a fluid volume excess and needs be treated aggressively. If fluid overload does not respond to diuretics, uncontrollable fluid overload is commonly the finding that causes the healthcare team to determine that renal replacement is necessary. While ARF patients may show normal cardiac filling pressures with a modest weight gain, they may still develop pulmonary edema. This may occur as a result of inadequately treated uremia, which while previously thought

to cause a capillary leak syndrome, more recently has been demonstrated to represent imbalance in hydrostatic and oncotic fluid pressures, leading to pulmonary infiltrates.

Caution should be applied to the use of daily weights as the gold standard of fluid balance. The catabolic ARF patient, not receiving an adequate daily diet whether enteral or parenteral, may lose weight at the rate of ½ pound per day. The critical care nurse, in collaboration with the nutritionist, should estimate daily visceral weight loss in the patient who is receiving inadequate daily calories. With that additional information, the actual net weight change can be calculated.[21]

In the past, nonoliguric renal failure had been thought to have a better outcome than oliguric renal failure. As a result, diuretics were often used to try to convert oliguric to nonoliguric ARF. Unfortunately, diuretics have not been shown to be beneficial and may lead to a worse outcome.[9] Therefore it is reasonable for the nurse to question an order for diuretics in the oliguric patient.

Mannitol (Osmitrol) is often used to promote osmotic diuresis; it causes less electrolyte disturbances than other diuretics while still promoting urine formation. It inhibits sodium reabsorption and increases plasma osmolality, thereby causing extra fluid to move into the intravascular space from the interstitial and intracellular spaces. If mannitol proves ineffective, it should not be repeated as it can cause fluid overload and intracellular dehydration. Loop diuretics, such as furosemide (Lasix), ethacrynic acid (Edecrin), or bumetanide (Bumex), diminish sodium reabsorption in the loop of Henle, facilitating both water and sodium excretion. It is important to remember, however, that loop diuretics are nephrotoxic and may enhance the nephrotoxicity of other substances.

In an attempt to improve urine output, in some healthcare facilities dopamine (Intropin) may be tried; however, there are several studies that have shown no utility to the use of "renal dose dopamine."[3,9,14,18] While dopamine does not enhance renal function via direct renal vasculature vasodilation, as once believed, it still may be of use in the ARF patient when used at the higher cardiac doses to increase heart rate and contractility, thereby increasing renal blood flow.

Dopamine can be used to increase CO after circulating volume has been established. If the infusion rate required causes tachycardia, dopamine should be stopped and other inotropic agents such as dobutamine (Dobutrex) or milrinone (Primacor) considered. Higher doses of dopamine mimic sympathetic nervous system activation, causing renal vasoconstriction, which leads to sodium and water retention, just the opposite of what is needed to promote urine formation.

While less likely to occur before the institution of renal replacement in ARF, the patient may develop a fluid volume deficit, despite the kidneys' poor filtering abilities. This can occur from GI bleeding, diarrhea, or vomiting. In these cases, the sodium level will likely be unchanged; fluid replacement is required and should match the composition of the fluid lost.[21]

Alterations in Electrolyte Balance

Sodium retention frequently occurs as a result of loss of excretion capability. Hyponatremia can also develop as a result of fluid repletion with hypotonic solutions. It is exacerbated by impaired free water clearance and causes cell swelling, leading to neurologic symptoms from headache to confusion to coma.[25] The more acute the onset of hyponatremia, the more likely the patient will experience serious signs and symptoms, including seizures (see Chapter 31).

Hyperkalemia is also a common complication of ARF. Since hyperkalemia is a prevalent disorder, it is important to be well-informed in its management. Treatment should strive to obtain potassium levels of ≤6.5 mEq/L to avoid the risk of cardiac arrhythmias, which may range from peaked T waves to cardiac arrest. Refer to Chapter 31 for additional information on hyperkalemia. If the potassium level is higher than 6.5 mEq/L and cannot be lowered using conservative interventions, renal replacement should be considered.

A key to solving these recurrent problems is to make serial assessments and evaluations in patients at risk for ARF, which includes those critically ill patients with risk factors listed earlier this chapter. Routine evaluations of electrolyte values will guide replacement at correct rates, thus avoiding iatrogenic electrolyte imbalance. It is also important to remember that cardiac stability in ARF patients may be enhanced by addressing their electrolyte abnormalities aggressively.

Metabolic Acidosis

The kidneys play a key role in preservation of acid-base balance. When renal function is decreased, there is accumulation of organic anions such as phosphate and other unmeasured anions.[58] There is also decreased production of bicarbonate via the decreased proximal tubule reabsorption and regeneration. Because these patients are also hypoalbuminemic, they have less protein buffering capacity; all these factors lead to metabolic acidosis. Additionally, many patients have other etiologies of acidosis coexistent with the renally mediated acidosis. These might include lactic acidosis or shock, respiratory acidosis induced by permissive hypercapnia ventilation in acute lung injury, or, less frequently, ketoacidosis. Therefore mild to moderate metabolic acidosis is often found in patients with ARF.[21,58]

The first defense against the metabolic acidosis of ARF is dietary restriction of protein, liberalized as soon as the patient is started on RRT. The acidosis of ARF can be moderated with bicarbonate infusion (HCO_3^-) as needed, but if the HCO_3^- concentration is less than 15 mEq/L and refractory to other interventions such as bicarbonate infusion, renal replacement should be initiated.[7] As with electrolyte abnormalities, it is important to remember that aggressively treating ARF patients' acidosis may be part of the key to addressing their cardiac instability.

RENAL REPLACEMENT

Renal replacement, delivered through a variety of means, is a process by which fluid and waste products are filtered through a semipermeable membrane to assist in elimination from the body. It may be done with or without the addition of a dialysate solution (patient-specific and prepared by prescription to include fluid, glucose, and electrolytes). The decision to implement RRT is usually based on one of the following issues: volume overload unresponsive to diuretics or fluid restriction, unmanageable hyperkalemia, unrelenting metabolic acidosis, or symptomatic or rapidly progressing uremia (i.e., altered mental status, GI bleeding, or pericarditis with pericardial effusion).

Although there have been recommendations in the literature as early as 1960 that renal replacement be started earlier rather than later, there is no clear consensus on the best method; an optimal, clearly defined starting point; or an optimal dose of renal replacement. Studies conducted decades ago[17,29,50,61] showed reduced morbidity and mortality with early initiation of renal replacement; more current studies[6,19] have not shown similar results, perhaps a reflection of the more complex patient presenting with renal failure. The therapy chosen and dose used must be individually tailored to the patient's specific situation.

RRT is classified as either intermittent or continuous (Figure 33-1). Most commonly, one of four types of renal placement is employed for critically ill patients with ARF: peritoneal dialysis (PD), hemodialysis (HD), sustained low-efficiency dialysis (SLED)/extended daily dialysis (EDD), or continuous renal replacement therapy (CRRT), of which there are a number of variations. The four types have advantages and disadvantages and vary in their effectiveness, need for anticoagulation, complications, and the time, access, and technical support required. Of these types, the latter three are used most frequently in critical care.

Peritoneal Dialysis

Utilizing the peritoneal membrane as the semipermeable membrane, PD is the least frequently used type

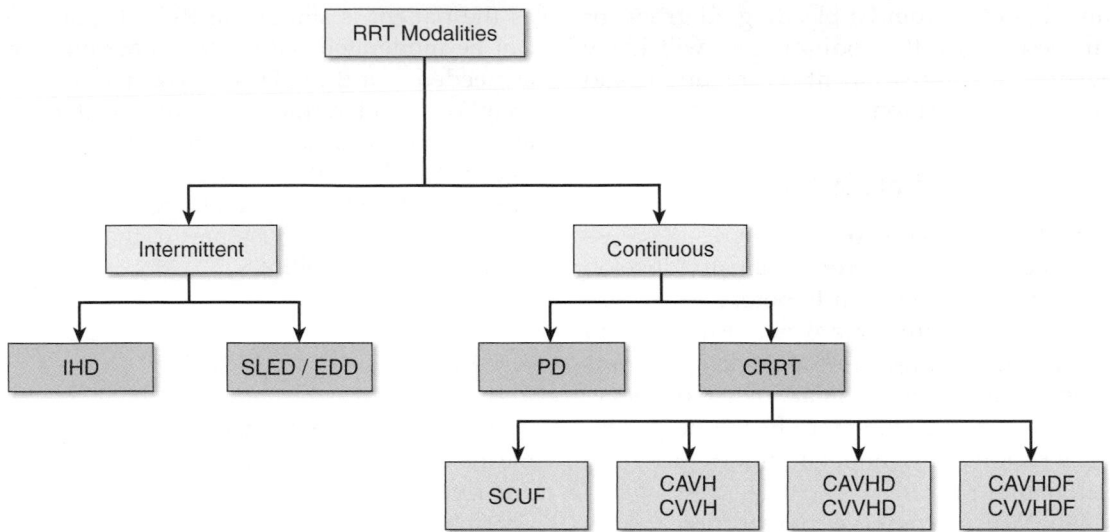

⬍FIGURE 33-1 Modalities of renal replacement therapy (RRT). CAVH = Continuous arteriovenous hemofiltration, CAVHD = continuous arteriovenous hemodialysis, CAVHDF = continuous arteriovenous hemodiafiltration, CRRT = continuous renal replacement therapy, CVVH = continuous venovenous hemofiltration, CVVHD = continuous venovenous hemodialysis, CVVHDF = continuous venovenous hemodiafiltration, EDD = extended daily dialysis, IHD = intermittent hemodialysis, PD = peritoneal dialysis, SCUF = slow continuous ultrafiltration, SLED = sustained low-efficiency dialysis.

of renal replacement in critical care. The dialysate fluid is infused through a catheter into the peritoneal cavity, where it dwells for a prescribed period of time (from 1 hour up to 6 hours) and is then drained. Through osmosis, diffusion, and filtration via the concentration gradients established by the composition of the dialysate (e.g., higher glucose concentration enhances water elimination), excess water, electrolytes, and waste products move into the dialysate and are removed from the body when the infusate is drained. This process is repeated throughout treatment. Patients are at risk for the development of peritonitis, protein loss into the dialysate, and hyperglycemia.

While PD may be effective, the process of fluid and waste elimination is not as efficient as it is in other types of renal replacement; therefore PD is not often the first choice of renal replacement in critical care. However, it does offer several advantages over other methods. Because fluid movement is slower, patients with cardiovascular instability are not subject to the effects of rapid fluid shifts, making PD more tolerable. Critically ill patients with serious dysrhythmias or hypotension can have effective renal replacement.[1,54] PD is also considered a safer option in patients with cerebral edema. As an additional benefit, patients undergoing PD do not require anticoagulation, so those at risk for bleeding may be candidates. It may also be used in selected healthcare facilities, such as those without access to advanced technology, and in certain patient populations, such as pediatric patients. It may also be used in

critical care to maintain a patient with CRF who has been on PD at home.

Hemodialysis

HD is an extremely effective method of removing fluid and waste products. It involves the movement of the patient's blood through a semipermeable membrane housed in a specialized dialysis filter. It requires a large central vascular access catheter to be in place. Once the dialysis machine is primed with the patient's blood, the dialysate fluid is run through the filter in the opposite direction of the blood. This countercurrent flow produces an increased concentration gradient, making the filter more efficient in fluid and solute removal. Additionally, by the addition of positive hydrostatic pressure to the blood compartment and negative hydrostatic pressure to the dialysate compartment, fluid removal can be determined and enhanced (ultrafiltration).

Possibly the greatest advantage of HD is its efficiency. Fluids, wastes, and electrolytes can be effectively removed within a 3- to 4-hour window of time on a daily or every other day schedule. This may be especially important in those patients with toxic potassium levels or fluid overload progressing to pulmonary edema. However, large fluid shifts and the required anticoagulation can make HD unsuitable for some critically ill patients.

Because HD can cause rapid fluid shifts, hypotension, and dysrhythmias, the HD patient must be monitored carefully, especially during the initiation of the HD treatment. This is crucial in the critically ill adult with comorbidities complicating their ATN, such as recent myocardial infarction, septic shock, or adult respiratory distress syndrome. The filter must be anticoagulated, presenting the potential for bleeding in these patients.

Critical care nurses do not routinely perform HD as it is very technical and complex: it is more often done by specially trained HD nurses. The *AACN Procedure Manual for Critical Care*[39] is an excellent reference for those seeking more information about the details of the dialysis procedure itself. Even so, the critical care nurse does remain responsible for the ongoing nursing care. During HD, the nurse must be prepared to quickly adjust vasopressors or add fluid in the form of crystalloid or albumin to prevent severe BP drops. An already damaged kidney is extremely susceptible to further damage during hypotensive episodes, so these should be scrupulously minimized for any hope of renal recovery.[23,51] The patient may begin bleeding from surgical sites, skin breakdown, the oral cavity, or airways. Frequent coagulation studies are done to guard against inadvertent systemic anticoagulation.

A hybrid of traditional HD is currently being employed by some institutions. SLED and EDD are both slower dialysis therapies. The patient is dialyzed using a conventional dialysis machine but utilizing modification of blood and dialysate flow speeds.[49] These methods combine the advantages of both HD and CRRT, providing for hemodynamic stability but achieving enhanced water and solute removal.

Continuous Renal Replacement Therapies

CRRT is an additional means by which fluids, wastes, and electrolytes, as well as other small to medium size particles, can be removed from the body via ultrafiltration and dialysis in patients with ARF. There are a number of different procedures available; the most appropriate for the patient's situation should be selected. The following options are available: slow, continuous ultrafiltration (SCUF) (Figure 33-2); continuous arteriovenous hemofiltration (CAVH)—fluid removal and fluid replacement (Figure 33-3); continuous arteriovenous hemodialysis (CAVHD)—fluid and solute removal with dialysate (Figure 33-4); continuous arteriovenous hemodiafiltration (CAVHDF)—fluid replacement with dialysate (Figure 33-5); continuous venovenous hemofiltration (CVVH)—fluid removal and fluid replacement (Figure 33-6); continuous venovenous hemodialysis (CVVHD)—fluid and solute removal with dialysate (Figure 33-7); and continuous venovenous hemodiafiltration (CVVHDF)—fluid replacement

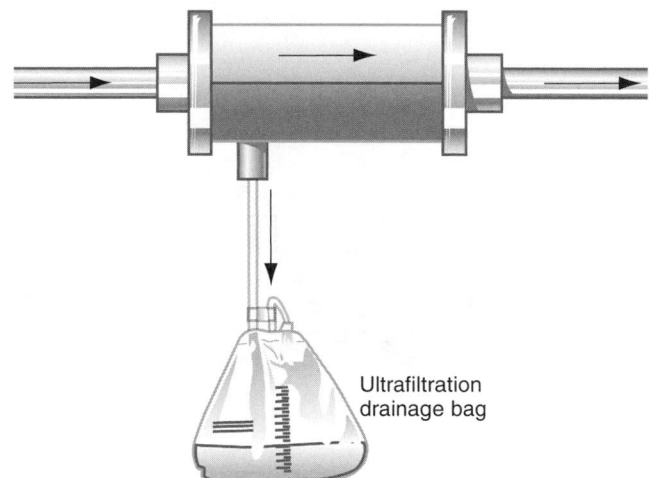

♦FIGURE 33-2 Slow, continuous ultrafiltration (SCUF): fluid removal, no fluid replacement.

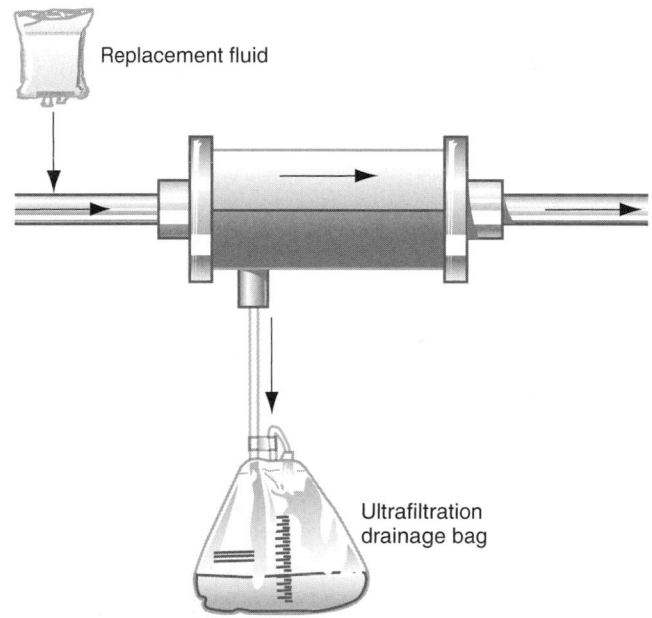

♦FIGURE 33-3 Continuous arteriovenous hemofiltration (CAVH): fluid removal and fluid replacement.

with dialysate (Figure 33-8). Table 33-4 provides comprehensive information about the different types of CRRT, including the principles of fluid and solute movement employed, access needed, indications for use, advantages and disadvantages, and complications.

CRRT is generally thought to be able to achieve similar water and solute removal as HD but with less hemodynamic instability. Fluid removal is continuous and slow as compared to the 1- to 4-L removal during a 3- to 4-hour HD treatment. In addition, because fluid removal is slower, the drop in serum osmolality seen

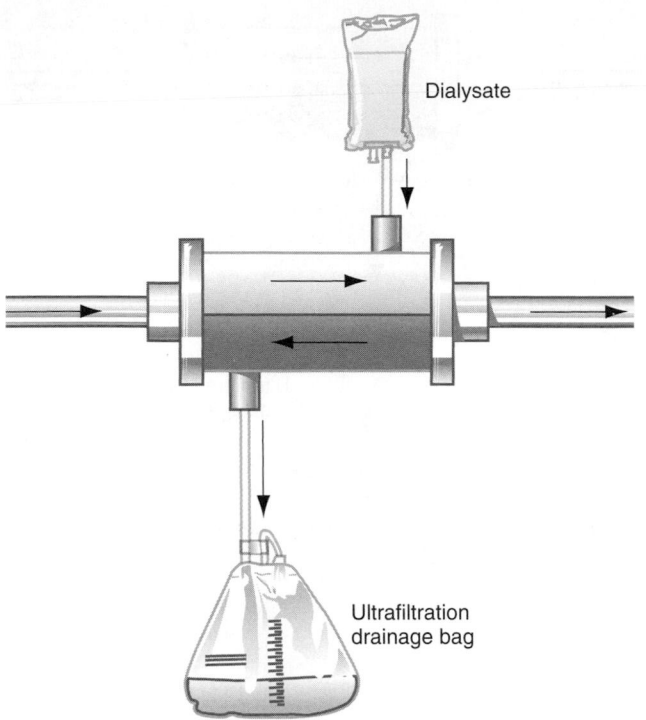

FIGURE 33-4 Continuous arteriovenous hemodialysis (CAVHD): fluid and solute removal with dialysate.

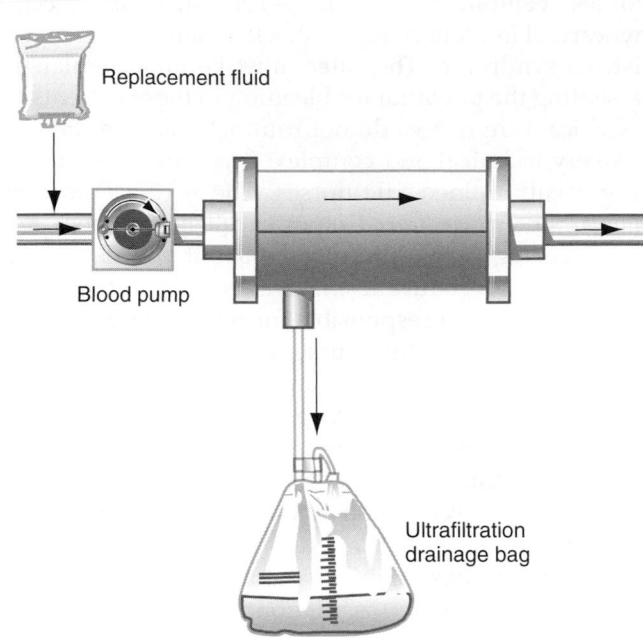

FIGURE 33-6 Continuous venovenous hemofiltration (CVVH): fluid removal with fluid replacement.

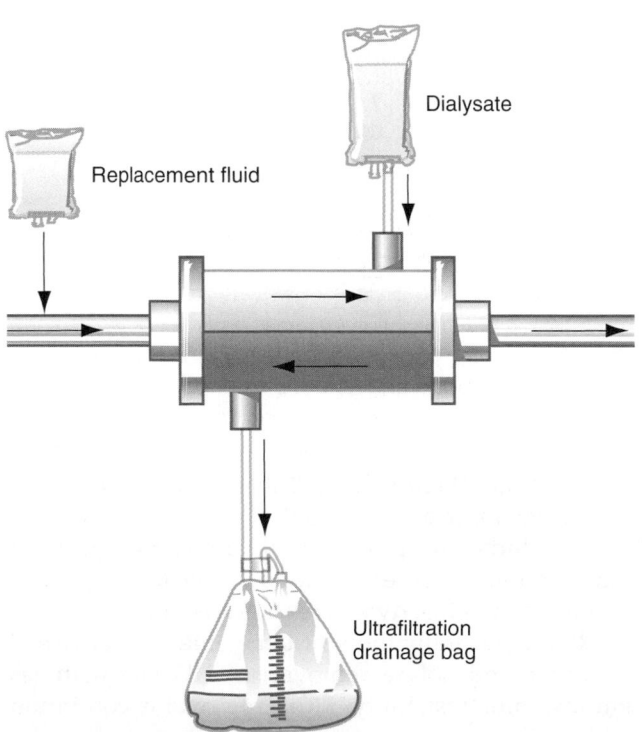

FIGURE 33-5 Continuous arteriovenous hemodiafiltration (CAVHDF): fluid replacement with dialysate.

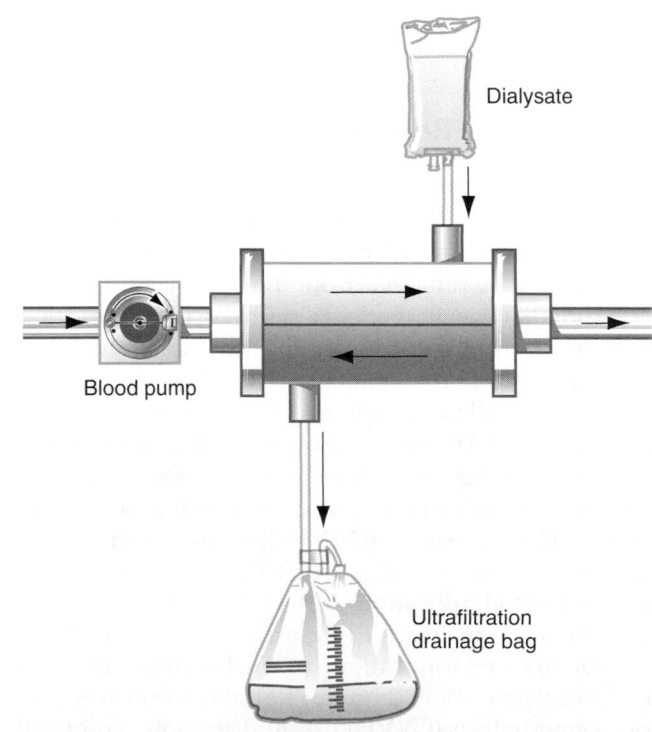

FIGURE 33-7 Continuous venovenous hemodialysis (CVVHD): fluid and solute removal with dialysate.

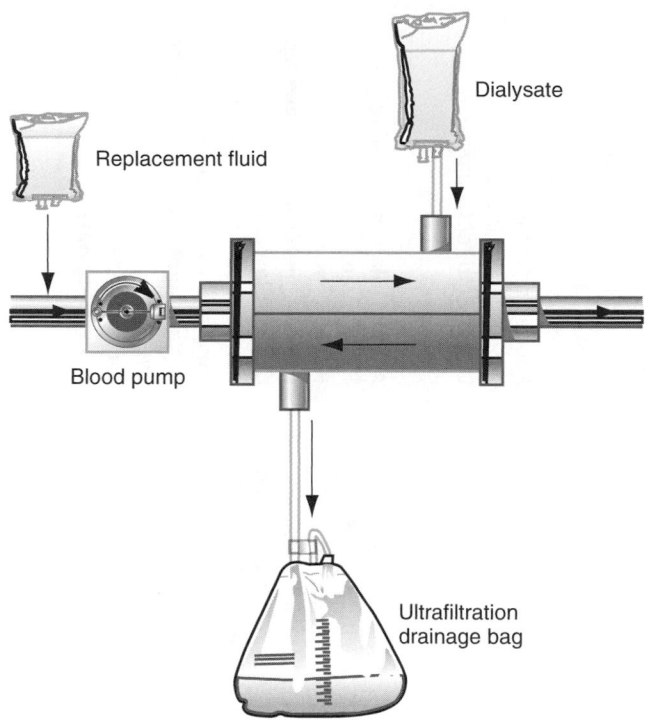

♦FIGURE 33-8 Continuous venovenous hemodiafiltration (CVVHDF): fluid replacement with dialysate.

with HD that encourages the movement of water into the extracelluar space does not occur.[47] Interestingly, a recent survey of nephrologists reported that 52% of them used CRRT for non-ARF reasons, such as fluid control, heart failure, acute respiratory distress syndrome, and sepsis.[55]

All of the CRRT machines use a highly permeable biocompatible filter similar to those used in HD. These consist of hollow fibers or sheets of biofilter in a plastic case. The filter material, pore size, and affinity to water/solute removal determine the efficiency of the filter and the amount/rate of material removed.

While the descriptions of the various CRRT methods are simplistic, the automatic, or integrated, CRRT machines contain all the necessary pumps and scales or flow monitors to measure effluent amounts with a computerized control module to monitor and coordinate operations. Although several arteriovenous options have been listed, arterial pressure sources are rarely used today since there has been a 15% to 20% morbidity associated with arterial cannulation with large-bore dialysis catheters.[5] Therefore blood is usually pumped from the vascular access through the filter. The access required for renal replacement will usually be a large-bore Y-catheter inserted in the central vein. Vascular access is critical to the success of any type of CRRT. The lumen size, catheter patency, and catheter positioning must be adequate to ensure that ordered blood flow

can be achieved. Placement should be checked to ensure that there is no overlap with any other vascular access catheter. The same infection control standards that are outlined in Chapter 9 should be maintained to prevent catheter-associated infection.

As the blood flows slowly through the hemofilter, which can lead to premature clotting, the blood needs to be anticoagulated and diluted. There are additional rotor pumps to provide heparin, citrate, or other anticoagulants and replacement fluid to prevent clotting of the hemofilter. The hemofilters are highly permeable to water and electrolytes and other small solutes such as bicarbonate, creatinine, and urea nitrogen, but are relatively impermeable to plasma proteins and blood cellular components. The potential for loss of large amounts of fluid exists, and serum osmolality can greatly increase, placing the patient at risk for dehydration. Therefore replacement IV solutions are used in varying amounts depending upon the patient's net hourly fluid loss. The effluent also contains large amounts of bicarbonate. Losing large amounts of bicarbonate can worsen the patient's metabolic acidosis. Consequently, the replacement fluid often has a high bicarbonate content; it is not merely a maintenance fluid such as NS or LR, which contains only the precursor to bicarbonate.

Many patients in the United States are currently receiving dialytic CRRT. This involves using dialysate solution as in HD through the filter, countercurrent to the flow of blood. As in HD, concentration gradients are established to aid in removal of solutes while helping avoid acid-base, electrolyte, and blood glucose imbalance. The concentration gradients allow faster removal of solutes, without necessarily increasing fluid losses to the filter. In addition, some institutions are using hybrid RRT in place of CRRT setups. These include SLED and EDD and use standard HD machines. Practice is usually collaborative between nephrology and critical care nurses.

The benefits of CRRT are many (Box 33-4); it is surprising that CRRT is used more frequently in other countries than in the United States, which uses CRRT in only about 10% to 20% of cases of ARF. Even with the stated physiologic benefits of CRRT, the ubiquitous acceptance and use have been limited for several reasons. Continuous therapy requires the involvement of trained nursing and medical staff 24 hours a day. Depending on unit resources, some critical care units may not be able to provide such a level of support. Additionally, if CRRT is used only 5 to 10 times per year, the cost of maintaining a trained staff may be unjustified, and expertise hard to maintain. Depending on the organization of patient care, CRRT may be more expensive than intermittent HD. Finally, the issues of continuous circuit anticoagulation and potential risk of bleeding continue as major concerns.[5] In order for a CRRT team

TABLE 33-4 Continuous Renal Replacement Therapies

MODE	PRINCIPLES INVOLVED	ACCESS	PUMP ASSISTED	INDICATIONS	ADVANTAGES	COMPLICATIONS AND DISADVANTAGES*
Ultrafiltration Therapies						
SCUF (slow, continuous ultrafiltration)	Ultrafiltration Convection	Arteriovenous Venovenous	No Yes	Diuretic-resistant, volume-overloaded, hemodynamically unstable patient who cannot tolerate rapid fluid shifts	Continuous, gradual treatment (fewer high and low extremes)	**Anticoagulation, bleeding** **Hypotension** **Hypothermia** **Access complications (bleeding, clotting, infection)** **Requires strict monitoring of fluid and electrolyte replacement to avoid deficits or overload** **Air embolism** **ICU setting only** **Requires 1:1 nurse-to-patient ratio** Prolonged, large-bore arterial cannulation required Ideally need MAP of 60 mm Hg to drive extracorporeal circuit Poor control of azotemia, may need dialysis Minimal solute clearance Poor emergent treatment of hyperkalemia/acidosis Loss of limb (distal arterial ischemia)
CAVH (continuous arteriovenous hemofiltration)	Ultrafiltration Convection	Arteriovenous	No	Diuretic-resistant, volume-overloaded, hemodynamically unstable patient who cannot tolerate rapid fluid shifts Parenteral or enteral alimentation in volume-overloaded patient	Continuous, gradual treatment (fewer high and low extremes) High rate of fluid removal/replacement allows flexibility in fluid balance	**Anticoagulation, bleeding** **Hypotension** **Hypothermia** **Access complications (bleeding, clotting, infection)** **Requires strict monitoring of fluid and electrolyte replacement to avoid deficits or overload** **Air embolism** **ICU setting only**

MODE	PRINCIPLES INVOLVED	ACCESS	PUMP ASSISTED	INDICATIONS	ADVANTAGES	COMPLICATIONS AND DISADVANTAGES*
						Requires 1:1 nurse-to-patient ratio Prolonged, large-bore arterial cannulation required Ideally need MAP of 60 mm Hg to drive extracorporeal circuit Poor control of azotemia, may need dialysis Poor emergent treatment of hyperkalemia/acidosis Loss of limb (distal arterial ischemia)
CVVH (continuous venovenous hemofiltration)	Ultrafiltration Diffusion Solute removal	Venovenous	Yes	Diuretic-resistant, hemodynamically unstable, volume-overloaded patient who cannot tolerate rapid fluid shifts Parenteral or enteral alimentation in volume-overloaded patient	Precise fluid control Can be done in patient with low MAP Ease of initiation Large volume of parenteral nutrition may be administered No arterial cannulation Better solute clearance than CAVH	**Anticoagulation, bleeding** **Hypotension** **Hypothermia** **Access complications (bleeding, clotting, infection)** **Requires strict monitoring of fluid and electrolyte replacement to avoid deficits or overload** **Air embolism** **ICU setting only** **Requires 1:1 nurse-to-patient ratio** Waste product removal not as effective as CVVHDF Requires special pump to augment blood flow through extracorporeal circuit Requires training of ICU nurses in use of pump

Table continues on page 908

Table 33-4 Continuous Renal Replacement Therapies—cont'd

MODE	PRINCIPLES INVOLVED	ACCESS	PUMP ASSISTED	INDICATIONS	ADVANTAGES	COMPLICATIONS AND DISADVANTAGES*
Dialysis Therapies						
CAVHD (continuous arteriovenous hemodialysis) CAVHDF (continuous arteriovenous hemodiafiltration)	Ultrafiltration Diffusion Solute removal Convection	Arteriovenous	No	Volume-overloaded, hemodynamically unstable patient with azotemia or uremia Catabolic acute renal failure Electrolyte imbalances and acidosis Parenteral and enteral alimentation in volume-overloaded, catabolic patient	Precise fluid control Ease of initiation Large volume of parenteral nutrition may be administered	**Same as CAVH** **Hyperglycemia** Hypernatremia Hypophosphatemia
CVVHD (continuous venovenous hemodialysis) CVVHDF (continuous venovenous hemodiafiltration)	Ultrafiltration Diffusion Solute removal	Venovenous	Yes	Volume-overloaded, hemodynamically unstable patient with azotemia or uremia Catabolic acute renal failure Electrolyte imbalances and acidosis Parenteral and enteral alimentation in volume-overloaded, catabolic patient	No arterial cannulation Precise fluid control Ease of initiation Large volume of parenteral nutrition may be administered Better solute clearance than CAVHDF Can be done in patient with low MAP	**Same as CVVH** **Hyperglycemia** Hypernatremia Hypophosphatemia

Modified from Giuliano, K., and Pysznik, E. (1998). Renal replacement therapy in critical care: implementation of a unit-based CVVH program. *Crit Care Nurs, 18,* 40-45.
*Complications and disadvantages appearing in boldface are common to CAVH, CAVHD, CVVH, and CVVHDF.
ICU = Intensive care unit, MAP = mean arterial pressure.

Box 33-4

Benefits of Continuous Renal Replacement Therapies

- Continuous control of fluid status
- Hemodynamic stability
- Control of acid-base status
- Ability to provide protein-rich nutritional support while achieving excellent uremic control
- Control of electrolyte balance
- Control of phosphate and calcium balance
- Prevention of rapid shifts in intracerebral water
- Minimal risk of infection
- High level of biocompatibility

to be successful, care must be collaborative between the critical care staff and physicians, nutritionist, pharmacists, and, in many cases, nephrologists.

Drug Therapy During Renal Replacement. Consultation with the team pharmacist is necessary throughout the care of the ARF patient. Before RRT, medication dosing must be tailored according to the patient's renal function. During RRT, the pharmacist is invaluable in making necessary adjustments in drug therapy. Many drugs that cleared via the kidneys are even more greatly affected by renal replacement. There are few studies of the actual percentages of drug removal during CRRT, so the nurse will have to estimate with the pharmacist's help which drugs are more greatly affected and thus need to have either a substitute drug administered or an increase in dosage provided. For example, if midazolam (Ativan) is being used for sedation and the patient becomes awake or agitated during filtration, propofol (Diprivan) could be substituted if increasing the midazolam does not keep the patient adequately sedated. The GFR is more important than absolute serum creatinine level in adjusting dosages. These data should be monitored by the nurse so that the team can track drug dosing and effect between and during RRT. The intrinsic renal function, including the phase of the function, must be considered when making medication decisions regarding patient care.

If vasopressors or inotropic agents are used during RRT, the BP must be carefully monitored and the nurse prepared to increase the infusion rate or supplement with fluid bolus to achieve satisfactory perfusion pressure. Additionally, it is important to remember that a portion of the catecholamine infusion can be removed with CRRT, so the need for increased infusion rates during CRRT should not be unexpected.

Case Study 33-1, Part C

Continuing Treatment Priorities

Despite all efforts, R.F.'s renal status deteriorates to acute tubular nephropathy. He has been fluid replenished to CVP 14 mm Hg, PAWP 17 mm Hg, and CI 2, with his BP hovering in the 90s/50s. His urine output is zero; creatinine 7.9 mg/dl, and BUN 80 mg/dl; pH 7.22, $Paco_2$ 32 mm Hg, HCO_3^- 16 mEq/L, and K^+ 7.5 mEq/L, despite treatment with sodium polystyrene (Kayexalate). He is somnolent because of his increased BUN. Informed consent must be obtained for renal replacement.

Decision Point: What are your treatment priorities?

After 7 days of CRRT, the patient's renal function improves; his creatinine declines to 3.2 mg/dl, BUN 42 mg/dl, K^+ 5 mEq/L, and pH 7.38.

Decision Point: What could you do to monitor the urine production without reinserting the Foley catheter since you want to minimize the patient's risk of infection after his renal insult?

NUTRITION IN ACUTE RENAL FAILURE WITH RENAL REPLACEMENT THERAPY

General nutrition in critical care is discussed in Chapter 6. In the ARF patient, the goal is to minimize catabolism and prevent malnutrition. Adequate calories need to be provided but fluid, potassium, sodium, and protein restricted until the patient begins RRT.

The current standard is to start nutrition as early as possible. If the patient is unable to eat, the nurse should recommend feeding tube placement unless contraindicated. If the patient cannot be fed by enteral means, then parenteral feeding should be started as soon as possible, again to maintain the patient in an anabolic state, to maximize tissue healing, and to stop tissue breakdown. The Nutrition box on p. 910 offers a summary of nutrition support recommendations for adult CRRT patients.

Once on RRT, the patient has more specific nutritional needs resulting from the increased loss of proteins via the filtration process. The critical care nurse should be aware of these unique nutritional requirements and ensure that the patient's nutritional needs during RRT are met. The ARF patient is acutely hypermetabolic and catabolic, with worsening azotemia from tissue breakdown. The team dietitian will recommend either enteral or parenteral nutrition that contains adequate protein, carbohydrates, and fats to provide an energy source that will spare tissue breakdown. Enteral nutrition is recommended, if

♦ NUTRITION

Nutrition Support Recommendations for Adult Continuous Renal Replacement Therapy Patients

- Protein, fluid, and electrolyte restrictions are not necessary during CRRT.
- Protein requirements during CRRT have ranged between 1.5 and 2.5 g/kg reference weight.
- Indirect calorimetry, where possible, is recommended to identify caloric needs of CRRT patients. Caloric delivery should provide 100%–130% of resting energy expenditure.
- Otherwise, energy needs can be predicted using 25–35 calories/kg reference weight.
- Although the enteral route is preferred for nutrition support, PN may be indicated in the presence of gastrointestinal dysfunction or hemodynamic instability.
- Water-soluble vitamin supplementation is necessary for patients treated with CRRT.
- Standard multivitamin and trace element levels are appropriate with PN.
- Uninterrupted CRRT leads to a dramatic decline in serum magnesium, potassium, and phosphorus levels secondary to intracellular shifting and increased losses with ultrafiltration. Anticipation of these abnormalities can yield appropriate supplementation and electrolyte repletion.
- The safest approach to treat severe hyperglycemia in CRRT patients is through the use of a continuous regular insulin infusion.[62]
- The nutrition regimen should be based on the changes that occur in the patient's clinical and metabolic status.

possible. It is essential to provide adequate protein with all the essential amino acids in order to preserve the body's visceral protein stores. CRF patients require special protein-limited diets to decrease the rate of accumulation of waste products that must be cleared by dialysis. Typically, patients can receive hemodialysis no more than two to three times weekly, whereas in critical care the patient may be maintained on CRRT or have daily HD. Thus there is no need to limit protein intake in these patients because the patient can be dialyzed or ultrafiltered easily in critical care. ARF patients become rapidly and deeply catabolic if undernourished.

Many ARF patients develop glucose intolerance and insulin resistance despite normal basal levels of insulin. There may even be an exaggerated response to intravenous glucose administration. The ARF patient seems to have a poor peripheral utilization at the tissue level.[40] Adverse effects of hyperglycemia include fluid and electrolyte imbalance, increased susceptibility to infection, and decreased function of neutrophils and leukocytes, making the patient more susceptible to infection and poor wound healing. When added to the effect on the immune system of ARF, hyperglycemia exacerbates the risk and the severity of infection in these critically ill patients.[66] Because the kidneys clear insulin, the requirement for insulin may be markedly reduced in diabetic patients in ARF. The critical care nurse must be mindful of this higher basal level of insulin during the episode of renal failure and make adjustments in controlling blood glucose level in order to avoid severe hypoglycemia in these patients.

Because the ARF patient develops insulin resistance, frequent measurements of blood glucose level and treatment with insulin are necessary. It is often easier to use continuous insulin infusion since the patient is on CRRT. In addition, because the ARF patient is highly susceptible to infection, tight glycemic control should be enforced.[62]

MULTIDISCIPLINARY PLAN OF CARE

The primary goal, once a patient develops any type of renal failure, is to reestablish homeostasis as quickly as possible. The underlying cause should be identified and eliminated if possible. In addition to the physician, advanced practice nurse, and critical care staff nurse team, the pharmacist and dietitian are crucial to the development and implementation of a plan of care for the patient with ARF.

Prevention of ARF must be a priority and begins with early identification of those patients at risk. When patients are identified as at risk for ARF, the critical care nurse should institute interventions as needed to ameliorate the risk of ARF (see the Multidisciplinary Plan of Care on pp. 896-899). In prerenal situations, every effort should be made promptly to restore adequate perfusion so that the renal function does not become further impaired. If the insult is one of an intrarenal nature, interventions should be instituted to address the patient's fluid overload and electrolyte imbalances, including the following: ensuring adequate oxygenation; preventing or treating infection; providing adequate, early nutrition; preventing further nephrotoxicity by monitoring and modifying medication administration; and treating the patient's acid-base abnormalities. When appropriate, renal replacement therapies should be instituted. While the critical care nurse is usually not directly responsible for RRT, the nurse will maintain responsibility for the overall care of these patients, including any complications that arise during therapy.

CONCLUSIONS

Caring for patients with acute renal failure is challenging for the critical care team and must begin with a focus on prevention. Because of their position at the bedside, the importance of critical care nurses to the difficult tasks of identification of patients at risk as well as recognizing and treating the common causes of renal failure cannot be overstated. There is much controversy over best practice in the care of renal failure; the long-term effects of ARF are unclear. As with other organs, progressive renal disease after severe ARF is common.

REFERENCES

1. Amerling, R., et al. (2004). Continuous flow peritoneal dialysis: current perspectives. *Contrib Nephrol, 140,* 294–304.
2. Antunes, P. E., et al. (2004). Renal dysfunction after myocardial revascularization. *Eur J Cardiothorac Surg, 25,* 597–604.
3. Australian and New Zealand Intensive Care Society (ANZICS) Clinical Trials Group. (2000). Low-dose dopamine in patients with early renal dysfunction: a placebo-controlled randomized trial. *Lancet, 356,* 2139–2143.
4. Bellomo, R., et al. (2004). Acute renal failure—definition, outcome measure, animal models, fluid therapy and information technology needs: the Second International Consensus Conference of the Acute Dialysis Quality Initiative (ADQI) Group. *Crit Care, 8,* R204–R212.
5. Bellomo, R., D'Intini, V., & Ronco, C. (2005). Renal replacement therapy in the ICU. In M. P. Fink, et al. (Eds.), *Textbook of critical care* (5th ed., pp 1151–1158). Philadelphia: Saunders.
6. Bouman, C. S. C., et al. (2002). Effects of early high-volume continuous venovenous hemofiltration on survival and recovery of renal function in intensive care patients with acute renal failure: a prospective, randomized trial. *Crit Care Med, 30,* 2205–2211.
7. Brady, H. R., Clarkson, M. R., & Lieberthal, W. (2004). Acute renal failure. In B. M. Brenner (Ed.), *Brenner & Rector's the kidney* (Vol 1, 7th ed., pp 1215–1292). Philadelphia: Saunders.
8. Brivet, F. G., et al. (1996). Acute renal failure in intensive care units—causes, outcomes, and prognostic factors of hospital mortality; a prospective, multicenter trial. French Study Group on Acute Renal Failure. *Crit Care Med, 24*(2), 192–198.
9. Cantarovich, F., et al. (2004). High dose furosemide for established ARF: a prospective randomized, double-blind, placebo-controlled, multicenter trial. *Am J Kidney Dis, 44,* 4029.
10. Carmichael, P., & Carmichael, A. R. (2003). Acute renal failure in the surgical setting. *Aust NZ J Surg, 73,* 144–153.
11. Clermont, G., et al. (2002). Renal failure in the ICU: comparison of the impact of acute renal failure and chronic renal failure. *Kidney Int, 62,* 986–996.
12. Cole, I., et al. (2000). A prospective multi-center study of the epidemiology, management, and outcome of severe renal failure in a "closed" system. *Am J Respir Crit Care Med, 162,* 191–196.
13. DeMendonca, A., et al. (2000). Acute renal failure in the ICU: risk factors & outcomes evaluated by the SOFA score. *Intensive Care Med, 26,* 915–921.
14. Denton, M. D., Chertow, G. M., & Brady, H. R. (1996). "Renal dose" dopamine for the treatment of acute renal failure: scientific rationale, experimental studies and clinical trials. *Kidney Int, 50,* 4–14.
15. Edelstein, C. L., & Schrier, R. W. (2003). Acute renal failure: pathogenesis, diagnosis, and management. In R. W. Schrier (Ed.), *Renal and electrolyte disorders* (6th ed., pp 401–455). Philadelphia: Lippincott Williams & Wilkins.
16. Fang, L. S., et al. (1980). Low fractional excretion of sodium with contrast media-induced acute renal failure. *Arch Intern Med, 140,* 531–533.
17. Fischer, R. P., et al. (1966). Early dialysis in the treatment of acute renal failure. *Surg Gynecol Obstet, 123,* 1019–1023.
18. Friedrich, J. O., et al. (2005). Meta-analysis: low dose dopamine increases urine output but does not prevent renal dysfunction or death. *Ann Intern Med, 142,* 510–524.
19. Gillum, D. M., et al. (1986). The role of intensive dialysis in acute renal failure. *Clin Nephrol, 25,* 249–255.
20. Godet, G. (1997). Risk factors for acute postoperative renal failure in thoracic or thoracoabdominal aortic surgery: a prospective study. *Anesth Analg, 85,* 1227–1232.
21. Greenberg, A., & Palevsky, P. M. (2001). Disturbances in fluid, electrolyte and acid-base balance. In S. G. Massry & R. J. Glasscock (Eds.), *Textbook of nephrology* (4th ed.). Philadelphia: Lippincott Williams & Wilkins.
22. Guyton, A. C., & Hall, J. E. (2000). *Textbook of medical physiology.* Philadelphia: Saunders.
23. Hladunewich, M., & Rosenthal, M. H. (2000). Pathophysiology and management of renal insufficiency in the perioperative and critically ill patient. *Anesthesiol Clin North Am, 18*(4), 773–789.
24. Hoste, E. A., et al. (2003). Acute renal failure in patients with sepsis in a surgical ICU: predictive factors, incidence, comorbidity, and outcome. *J Am Soc Nephrol, 14,* 1022–1030.
25. Hoste, E. A. J., & De Waele, J. J. (2005). Physiologic consequences of acute renal failure on the critically ill. *Crit Care Clin, 21,* 251–260.
26. Hou, S. H., et al. (1983). Hospital acquired renal insufficiency: a prospective study. *Am J Med, 74,* 243–248.
27. Jakob, S. M. (2004). Prevention of acute renal failure—fluid repletion and colloids. *Int J Artif Organs, 27,* 1043–1048.
28. Kellum, J. A., et al. (2005). Consensus development in acute renal failure: the Acute Dialysis Quality Initiative. *Curr Opin Crit Care, 11*(6), 527–532.
29. Kleinknecht, D., et al. (1972). Uremic and non-uremic complications in acute renal failure: evaluation of early and frequent dialysis on prognosis. *Kidney Int, 1,* 190–196.
30. Klenzak, J., & Himmelfarb, J. (2005). Sepsis and the kidney. *Crit Care Clin, 21,* 211–222.
31. Kribben, A., Edelstein, C. L., & Schrier, R. W. (1999). Pathophysiology of acute renal failure. *J Nephrol, 12*(suppl 2), S142–S151.
32. Lameire, N. (2005). The pathophysiology of acute renal failure. *Crit Care Clin, 21,* 197–210.
33. Lameire, N., Van Biesen, W., & Vanholder, R. (2005). Acute renal failure. *Lancet, 365,* 417–430.
34. Levy, E. M., Viscoli, C. M., & Horowitz, R. I. (1996). The effect of acute renal failure on mortality: a cohort analysis. *JAMA, 275,* 1489–1494.
35. Liano, F., et al. (1998). The spectrum of acute renal failure in the intensive care unit compared to that seen in other settings. *Kidney Int Suppl, 66,* S16–S24.
36. Maeder, M., et al. (2005). Contrast nephropathy: review focusing on prevention. *J Am College Cardiol, 44,* 1763–1771.
37. Mangano, C. M., et al. (1998). Renal dysfunction after myocardial revascularization: risk factors, adverse outcomes, and hospital resource utilization. The Multicenter Study of Perioperative Research Group. *Ann Intern Med, 128,* 194–203.
38. Marino, P. C. (1998). *The ICU book* (2nd ed.). Baltimore: Williams & Wilkins.
39. Martin, R. (2005). Continuous renal replacement therapies. In D. L. M. Wiegand & K. K. Carlson (Eds.), *AACN procedure manual for critical care.* Philadelphia: Saunders.

40. Massry, S. G., & Smogorzewski, M. (2001). Metabolic and endocrine abnormalities in acute renal failure. In S. G. Massry & R. J. Glasscock (Eds.), *Textbook of nephrology* (4th ed.). Philadelphia: Lippincott Williams & Wilkins.

41. McCullough, P. A., & Soman, S. S. (2005). Contrast-induced nephropathy. *Crit Care Clin, 21,* 261–280.

42. Mehta, R. L., Pascual, M. T., Soroko, S., and Chertow, G. M. (2002). Diuretics, mortality and nonrecovery of renal function in acute renal failure. *JAMA, 288,* 2547–2553.

43. Menashe, P. I., Ross, S. A., & Gottlieb, J. E. (1988). Acquired renal insufficiency in critically ill patients. *Crit Care Med, 16,* 1106–1109.

44. Merten, G. J., et al. (2004). Prevention of contrast induced nephropathy with sodium bicarbonate: a randomized controlled trial. *JAMA, 291,* 2328–2334.

45. Metcalfe, W., et al. (2002). Acute renal failure requiring renal replacement therapy: incidence and outcome. *QJM, 95,* 579–583.

46. Mueller, C., et al. (2002). Prevention of contrast media-associated nephropathy: randomized comparison of 2 hydration regiments in 1620 patients undergoing coronary angioplasty. *Arch Intern Med, 162,* 329–336.

47. Murray, P., & Hall, J. (2000). Renal replacement therapy for acute renal failure. *Am J Respir Crit Care Med, 162,* 777–781.

48. Nash, K., Hafeez, A., & Hou, S. (2002). Hospital-acquired renal insufficiency. *Am J Kidney Dis, 39,* 930–936.

49. O'Reilly, P., & Tolwani, A. (2005). Renal replacement therapy III: IHD, CRRT, SLED. *Crit Care Clin, 21,* 367–378.

50. Parsons, F. M., et al. (1961). Optimum time for dialysis in acute reversible renal failure: description and value of improved dialyzer with large surface area. *Lancet, 1,* 129–134.

51. Poole, B. D., & Schrier, R. W. (2005). Acute renal failure. In M. P. Fink, et al. (Eds.), *Textbook of critical care* (5th ed.). Philadelphia: Saunders.

52. Ragaller, M. J. R., Hermann, T., & Koch, T. (2001). Volume replacement in the critically ill patient with acute renal failure. *J Am Soc Nephrol, 12*(2, suppl 17), S33–S39.

53. Rangel-Frausto, M. S., et al. (1995). The natural history of the systemic inflammatory response syndrome (SIRS): a prospective study. *JAMA, 273,* 117–123.

54. Rao, P., Passadakis, P., & Oreopoulos, D. G. (2003). Peritoneal dialysis in acute renal failure. *Perit Dial Int, 23*(4), 320–322.

55. Ricci, Z., et al. (2006). Practice patterns in the management of acute renal failure in the critically ill patient: an international survey. *Nephrol Dial Trans, 21*(3), 690–696.

56. Riedemann, N. C., Guo, R. F., & Ward, P. A. (2003). The enigma of sepsis. *J Clin Invest, 112,* 460–467.

57. Roberts, I., et al. (2004). Colloids versus crystalloids for fluids resuscitation in critically ill patients. *Cochrane Database Syst Rev, Oct, 18*(4), CD000567.

58. Rocktaeschel, J., Morimatsu, H., Uchino, S., et al. (2003). Acid-base status of critically ill patients with acute renal failure: analysis based on Stewart-Figg methodology. *Crit Care, 7,* R60–R66.

59. Schrier, R. W., & Wang, W. (2004). Acute renal failure and sepsis. *N Engl J Med, 351,* 159–169.

60. Tepel, M., & Zidek, W. (2002). Acetylcysteine and contrast media nephropathy. *Curr Opin Nephrol Hypertens, 11*(5), 503–506.

61. Teschan, P. E., et al. (1960). Prophylactic hemodialysis in the treatment of acute renal failure. *Ann Intern Med, 53,* 992–1016.

62. Van den Berghe, G., Wouters, P., Weekers, F., et al. (2001). Intensive insulin therapy in critically ill patients. *N Engl J Med, 345,* 1359–1367.

63. Vanholder, R., De Smet, R., Glorieux, G., et al. (2003). Review of uremic toxins: classification, concentration, and inter-individual variability. *Kidney Int, 65,* 1934–1943.

64. Venkatataman, R. (2005). Prevention of acute renal failure. *Crit Care Clin, 21,* 281–289.

65. Vercueil, A., Grocott, M. P., & Mythen, M. G. (2005). Physiology, pharmacology, and rationale for colloid administration for the maintenance of effective hemodynamic stability in critically ill patients. *Transfus Med Rev, 19,* 93–109.

66. Wooley, J. A., Btaiche, I. F., & Good, K. L. (2005). Metabolic and nutritional aspects of acute renal failure in critically ill patients requiring CRRT. *Nutr Clin Pract, 20,* 176–191.

UNIT *8*

ENDOCRINE

CHAPTER 34

Glycemic Control

Carol S. Manchester and Mary Fran Tracy

Diabetes mellitus (DM) is a chronic disorder of metabolism characterized by hyperglycemia. The disease state is associated with major abnormalities in the metabolism of carbohydrates, proteins, and fats. With increasing duration and severity of hyperglycemia, specific complications develop related to microvascular, macrovascular, and neurologic physiologic alterations in multiorgan systems.

Recently, the U.S. Centers for Disease Control and Prevention released new statistics describing diabetes in America. It is estimated that 20.8 million Americans, or 7% of the U.S. population, have this disease. Of those, 14.6 million people are diagnosed and 6.2 million people remain undiagnosed.[11,29] An estimated 41 million Americans have prediabetes, defined as impaired fasting glucose (IFG) level or impaired glucose tolerance (IGT). Diabetes is the sixth leading cause of death, and causes adults to have heart disease death rates two to four times higher than adults without DM. The incidence of cerebrovascular accidents (CVAs) is two to four times greater in persons with diabetes. Seventy-three percent of adults with diabetes have hypertension, and it is the leading cause of new cases of blindness, kidney failure, and nontraumatic lower extremity amputations. Approximately 60% to 70% of people with diabetes have mild to severe peripheral or autonomic neuropathies. Dental disease, complications of pregnancy, and susceptibility to infection are all sequelae of hyperglycemia.[10,28] The total cost of diabetes care in the United States in 2002 was $132 billion. Of this, $92 billion was spent on direct medical costs and $40 billion was spent on indirect costs, such as disability, work loss, and premature mortality.[9,68,69]

For years, attention to diabetes management has centered on ambulatory care. The reports of the Diabetes Control and Complications Trial (DCCT)[31] and the United Kingdom Prospective Study Group (UKPDS)[62,63] demonstrated that glycemic control does, in fact, reduce the risks and complications of retinopathy, neuropathy, and nephropathy in this population. These results provided the impetus for enhanced glycemic control and diabetes self-management over the past decade. However, evidence that glycemic control was of value

in the acute care setting was essentially non-existent until 1999.* In 2004 the American College of Endocrinology[13] released a position statement on inpatient diabetes and metabolic control stating, "As the result of recent clinical trials and focused research efforts, it is now apparent that new approaches and intensified efforts at metabolic regulation may improve short-, intermediate-, and long-term outcomes in patients with diabetes in the hospital for therapeutic procedures and for treatment of the complications of this illness."

When the acute complications of diabetes—including diabetic ketoacidosis (DKA), hyperosmolar hyperglycemic nonketotic syndrome (HHNS), and moderate to severe hypoglycemia—occur, they usually result in a hospital admission.[7] It is estimated that individuals with hyperglycemia have a 50% increased risk of hospitalization within their lifetime and a 20% increased risk of postoperative complications, including myocardial infarctions (MI) and CVAs.[15,21,65] The incidence of hospitalization increases with age, duration of diabetes, and the presence of diabetes-related complications. The actual prevalence of diabetes in hospitalized patients is not known because diabetes is not typically the principal diagnosis.[47] Thirty-eight percent of patients were found to have a DRG code related to DM; however, the National Hospital Discharge Survey Database 2000 demonstrated that only 8% of all patients with a code for diabetes had it as the principal diagnosis.[30] "Discharge diagnosis codes may underestimate the true prevalence of diabetes in hospitalized patients by as much as 40%."[30]

In acute and critical care, the state of hyperglycemia has become a key variable in the quest to understand and enhance quality care and clinical outcomes. An elevation in blood glucose level and altered peripheral uptake and utilization of insulin are well documented in critically ill patients.[64] Van den Berghe[64,65] has reported that intensive insulin therapy via intravenous insulin infusion to maintain a blood glucose level at less than or equal to 110 mg/dl substantially reduced mortality in the intensive care unit, in-hospital mortality, and morbidity among critically ill patients in surgical

---

*References 21, 37, 38, 49, 51, 65, 67.

◆ **RESEARCH UTILIZATION**

Hyperglycemia With Insulin Resistance

CLINICAL ISSUE

Hyperglycemia with insulin resistance is an issue with many critically ill patients, for both those with and those without diabetes. It is thought that poor control of glucose levels can lead to complications, including septicemia, polyneuropathy, and death. The authors conducted a prospective, randomized controlled study to compare the outcomes of critically ill patients who received intensive management of blood glucose levels with those receiving conventional glucose management.

SUMMARY

A total of 1548 mechanically ventilated patients admitted to the surgical ICU between Feb 2000 and Jan 2001 were enrolled in the study. Subjects were randomly assigned to receive either the intensive insulin therapy protocol (glucose target of 80–100 mg/dl) or the conventional insulin therapy protocol (glucose target of 180–200 mg/dl) in an effort to manage blood glucose levels during the critical care stay. Enteral or parenteral feedings were initiated within 24 hours of critical care admission, and insulin doses were adjusted based on strict algorithms. The primary outcome measure was death in critical care. Additional measures included death during the hospital stay; number of critical care days or readmissions; need for ventilatory support, renal replacement therapy, or vasoactive medications; polyneuropathy; inflammation markers; bloodstream infections; and need for transfusions. The study groups were similar with regard to demographic and clinical (including acuity scores) characteristics on study enrollment, and no significant differences were found in preexisting diabetes or elevated glucose levels, diagnosis of renal failure, or type of cardiac surgery on admission to the ICU. Nearly 99% of the intensive treatment group received insulin administration as compared to only 39% of the conventional treatment group.

APPLICATION

Maintaining glucose levels consistently less than 110 mg/dl resulted in a significant decrease in morbidity and mortality, both in critical care units (32% reduction) and in hospital patients, regardless of history of diabetes. Fewer intensive treatment group patients required prolonged renal replacement therapy and mechanical ventilation or had episodes of septicemia. There was also a significant reduction in critical care length of stay, though not in hospital length of stay. Nursing plays a key role in aggressively managing glucose levels in this high-risk and complex population.

NEED FOR FURTHER STUDY

Future studies are needed to continue to define nursing's role in managing glucose levels.

Van den Berghe, G., et al. (2001). Intensive insulin therapy in critically ill patients. *N Engl J Med, 345*, 1359–1367.

---

critical care.[64] This is further addressed in the Research Utilization box above. Malmberg et al. have also reported that intensive insulin treatment reduced long-term mortality in diabetic patients with an acute MI, despite significantly high admission levels of blood glucose and hemoglobin A_{1c}.[49] These studies have motivated clinicians in direct hospital care to shift the paradigm from focusing only on prevention of hypoglycemia while treating the chief complaint and disorder to providing actual glycemic management.[42,43]

PATIENTS AT RISK

Individuals at risk in the acute care environment include patients diagnosed with DM; patients with stress-induced hyperglycemia, sepsis, multisystem failure, or obesity; and patients administered large doses of exogenous steroids or other pharmacologic agents that alter glucose metabolism. This very well can account for nearly all critically ill patients. Risk of complications while hospitalized is determined by the diagnosis of diabetes before admission, the age at diagnosis and duration of the disease, the presence and severity of secondary complications of diabetes, and the degree of glycemic control achieved before admission as demonstrated by the A_{1c} value. Typically, individuals who have had diabetes for more than 10 years, who were diagnosed as a child, or who have a glycosylated hemoglobin A_{1c} (HbA$_{1c}$) level greater than 7% are at increased risk. Additionally, all critically ill patients are at risk from lack of detection and management of hyperglycemia. Levetan et al.[46] found that in a study of 1034 adults consecutively admitted to an inner-city teaching hospital, chart review showed that 13% had blood glucose levels greater than 200 mg/dl. Of these, 36% remained undiagnosed at the time of discharge, despite frequent documentation of hyperglycemia in progress notes.[42,46,47]

DEFINITION

DM is a group of metabolic diseases characterized by hyperglycemia resulting from defects in insulin secretion, insulin action, or both.[2] Hyperglycemia can be related to DM or can exist independently of the presence of the disease. The following criteria are included in the diagnosis of DM: a fasting plasma glucose level greater than or equal to 126 mg/dl; symptoms of diabetes plus a random plasma glucose measurement greater than or equal to 200 mg/dl; or a 2-hour post-load (75 g of anhydrous glucose dissolved in water) glucose level greater than or equal to 200 mg/dl during an oral glucose tolerance test. Hyperglycemia in the absence of diabetes can be determined by any elevation of plasma glucose level above the normal range of 70 to 100 mg/dl. Prediabetes, a name that encompasses impaired glucose tolerance (IGT) and impaired fasting glucose (IFG), is now diagnosed as a fasting plasma glucose value of 100 to 125 mg/dl.[2]

CLASSIFICATION OF DIABETES MELLITUS

There are several types of DM and hyperglycemia. Type 1 diabetes is an autoimmune disease resulting in an absolute deficiency of insulin. The hormone insulin is produced by the beta cells located within the islets of Langerhans in the pancreas. These cells are destroyed over a variable period of time. Type 1 DM comprises 5% to 10% of those with the diagnosis of diabetes.[2] In type 1, it is possible for an individual to have additional autoimmune disorders, including Graves' disease, Hashimoto's thyroiditis, Addison's disease, celiac sprue, vitiligo, autoimmune hepatitis, myasthenia gravis, and pernicious anemia.[2,17,55] The autoimmune destruction of beta cells can be determined by the presence of specific antibodies such as insulin autoantibodies, islet cell antibodies, autoantibodies to islet tyrosine phosphatase markers, and glutamic acid decarboxylase autoantibodies.[65] Also, serum C-peptide and insulin levels can demonstrate the presence of endogenous insulin. The normal range for C-peptide is 0.78 to 1.89 ng/ml. This value diminishes as beta cell destruction continues. Serum insulin levels are based on normal insulin production. The average individual who is not pregnant or obese produces 0.5 to 0.7 unit of insulin/kg/day. Type 1 diabetes can present as diabetic ketoacidosis. It occurs primarily in children and youth, yet it can occur also in adulthood and is life-threatening if untreated. Latent autoimmune diabetes or type 1½ is a category of diabetes currently being researched and explored.[32]

Type 2 DM accounts for 90% of all individuals with this disease.[2] Of the individuals with type 2, 80% have "diabesity." This is representative of the dual epidemic in the United States of type 2 diabetes and obesity.[3] A state of insulin resistance, type 2 diabetes is hallmarked by a defect of the peripheral receptors and altered insulin secretory function.[2] Individuals with type 2 DM frequently have normal to elevated insulin levels initially, but over time will have diminished insulin secretion. Initially, fasting blood glucose levels may be within normal range, but postprandial levels are elevated.[3] Metabolic acidosis is not commonly associated with this form of diabetes, although it can occur. Type 2 diabetes occurs more commonly in the adult, yet the incidence of the disease in children has increased over the last decade with the rise of childhood obesity and sedentary lifestyles in today's youth.[53] The focus in type 2 diabetes today is prevention and delay of onset of the disease.[5]

Gestational diabetes mellitus (GDM) occurs during pregnancy. It is defined as "any degree of glucose intolerance with onset or first recognition during pregnancy."[2] The prevalence of GDM is estimated at approximately 14% of all pregnancies in the United States. Of all pregnancies complicated by diabetes, 90% are attributed to GDM and only 10% are attributed to preexisting primary DM in the patient.

Prediabetes is a condition in which the fasting plasma glucose level is between 100 and 125 mg/dl.[2] Individuals falling into this category are at high risk for developing type 2 DM. Typically, individuals demonstrate characteristics of the metabolic syndrome such as central adiposity, hyperglycemia, hyperlipidemia, hypertension, and, in females, polycystic ovary syndrome. It is estimated that 50% of all individuals with prediabetes will develop type 2 diabetes in their lifetime.

The last classification of diabetes mellitus encompasses all other reasons and causes of hyperglycemia. Included in this category are those with genetic defects, diseases of the exocrine pancreas (e.g., pancreatitis, neoplasia, cystic fibrosis, hemochromatosis), endocrinopathies (e.g., acromegaly, Cushing's disease, somatostatinoma), chemically induced hyperglycemia (secondary to glucocorticoids, immunosuppressants, estrogens, loop diuretics), and stress-induced hyperglycemia (e.g., surgery, trauma, infection).[2] Hyperglycemia in acute care in the nondiabetic individual falls into this category.

PHYSIOLOGY OF GLUCOSE METABOLISM

Euglycemia is achieved through the actions of pancreatic islet cell hormones. Glucagon, the antagonist to insulin, is produced by the alpha cells within the islets of Langerhans. Insulin and amylin are produced by the beta cells, and somatostatin is produced by the delta cells. It is the careful balance of glucose entering and leaving the bloodstream related to the action of these hormones that maintains glucose homeostasis[14,55] (Figure 34-1).

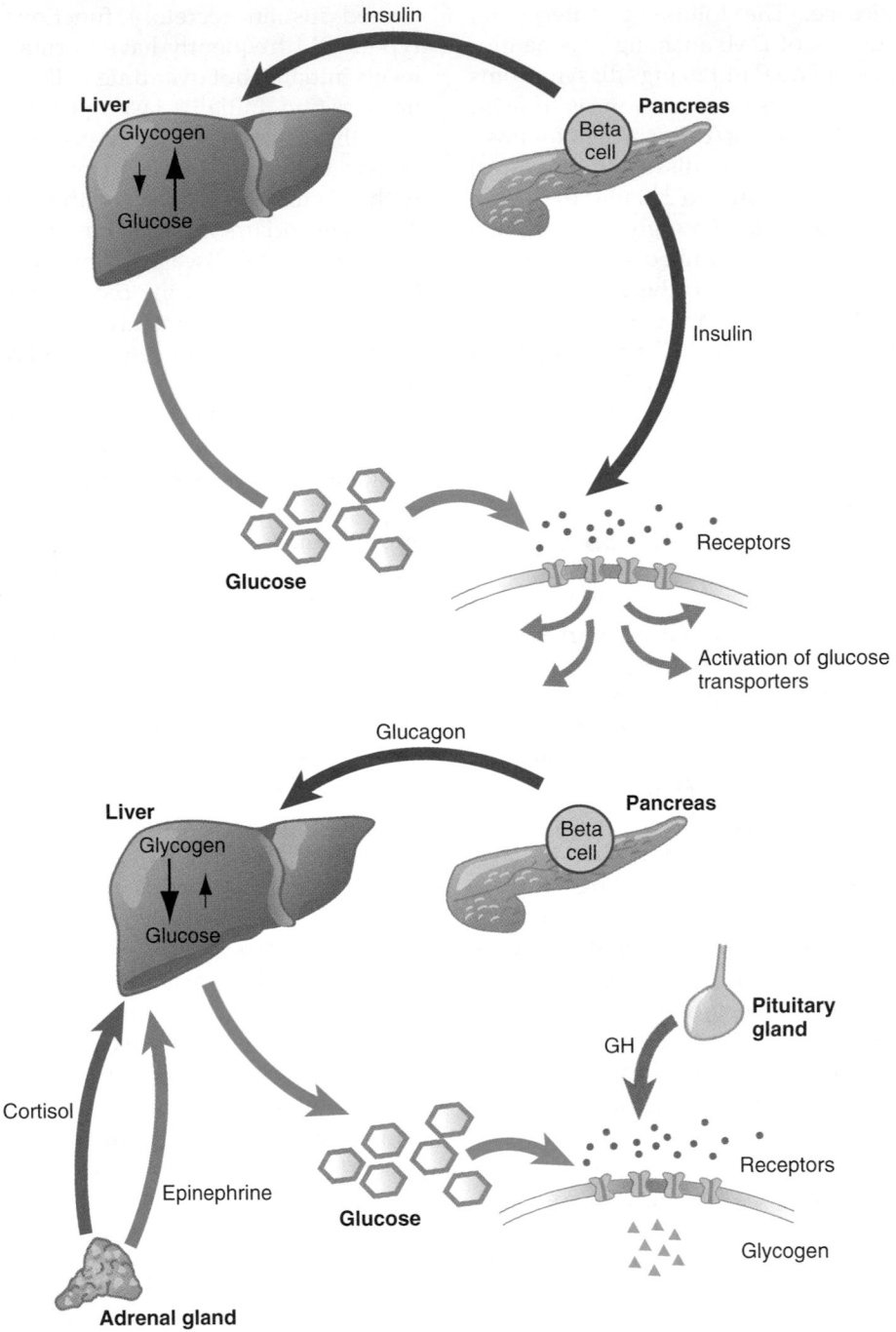

FIGURE 34-1 Regulation of serum glucose concentration.

Regulation of insulin begins with the autonomic nervous system. Pancreatic islet cells are innervated with parasympathetic and sympathetic nerves. The parasympathetic nerves extend via the vagus nerve. It is thought that these nerves play a significant role in insulin secretion that occurs at the sight and smell of food. Sympathetic nerves are employed and stimulated at times of acute stress. Thus stress-induced hyperglycemia is a phase of inhibited insulin secretion and stimulated glucagon secretion, resulting in a state of insulin resistance and a rise in blood glucose level. There are also neuropeptides that are located within the islet nerve terminals. Vasoactive intestinal peptide, cholecystokinin, galanin, and neuropeptide Y have been identified as playing a role in the transfer of glucose from the intestines, kidneys, and liver to insulin-dependent tissues or insulin-independent tissues.

Functions of the Pancreatic Hormones

Insulin's chief role is to allow glucose to move from the blood into insulin-sensitive tissues (muscle and fat) to provide fuel and allow for the storage of energy. Insulin promotes glycogenesis while inhibiting lipolysis, keto-genesis, gluconeogenesis, glycogenolysis, and glycemia. Thus the storage of proteins and fats is also promoted. This is depicted in Figure 34-2. Identified in 1987, amylin is a second beta cell hormone that assists in the regulation of blood glucose level.[14] Amylin is released along with insulin, but functions differently. The main role of amylin is to alter the flow of glucose into the bloodstream during the postprandial phase by delaying gastric emptying, decreasing glucagon secretion from the alpha cells, and minimizing the post-meal glucose spike.[14] Glucagon increases blood glucose concentrations. This is accomplished by promoting gluconeogenesis, glycogenolysis in the liver and skeletal muscle, lipolysis, and proteolysis. Somatostatin acts as an inhibitor to the secretion of both insulin and glucagon.

The hormones cannot function properly without cell receptors. Insulin and glucagon must be able to bind to the receptor in order for glucose to be transported. Specific glucose transporters have been identified and are named GLUT-1 through GLUT-5. GLUT-4 is specific to muscle and fat, and it is this transporter that allows for glucose transport after insulin has bound to the receptor.[55]

Under normal conditions, the pancreatic islets secrete insulin continuously to maintain euglycemia. This continuous insulin secretion regulates glucose levels through gluconeogenesis and glycogenolysis in the liver and kidney, as well as elevations in blood glucose concentration that are the result of counter-regulatory hormone release, including glucagon, cortisol, cate chol-amines, and growth hormone. Additional boluses or bursts of insulin are secreted in response to meals in order to prevent postprandial glucose excursions. The amount of insulin secreted is regulated by arterial glucose concentrations and is maintained between 70 and 100 mg/dl.

Recently, incretin hormones, or glucagon-like peptide-1 (GLP-1), have been determined to be naturally occurring, insulin-releasing hormonal factors secreted by the intestine to facilitate metabolic homeostasis in response to food ingestion.[33] For further information, see the Medication table on p. 920. GLP-1 receptor (GLP-1R) agonists activate the beta cell GLP-1R, increasing the ability of the pancreas to release insulin in response to ingested glucose. GLP-1 inhibits excessive postprandial glucagon release, and it assists in regulating nutrient absorption. Gastric peristalsis is slowed, increasing digestion and facilitating nutrient absorption as the food moves from the stomach into the small intestine. This action helps reduce or avoid gastric dumping. All of this contributes to a decrease in postprandial glucose peaks.

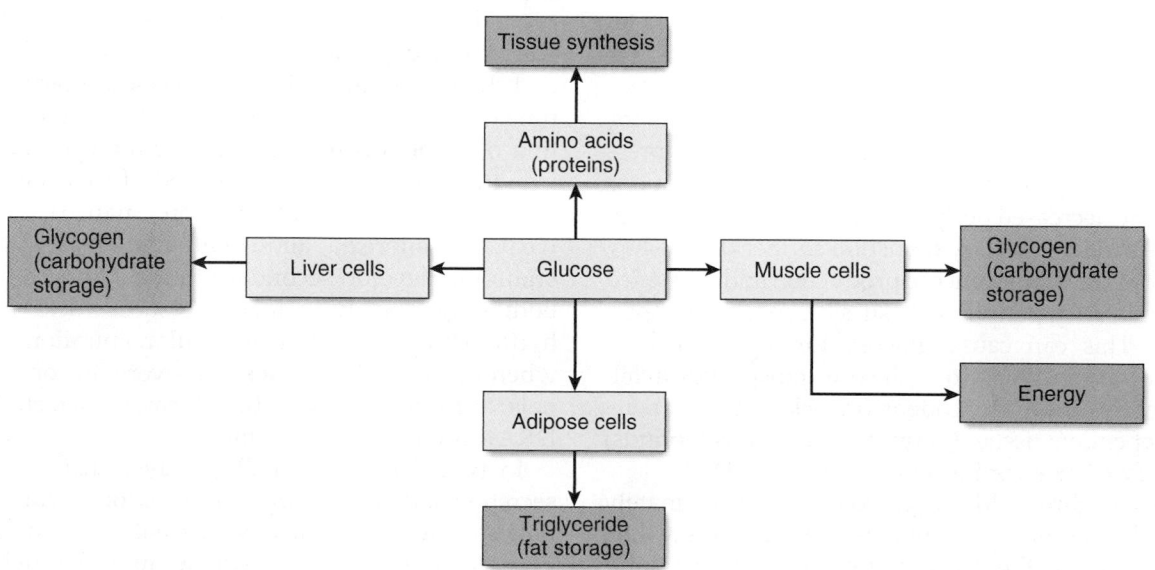

⬥FIGURE 34-2   Normal metabolism of glucose in the presence of sufficient insulin.

INCRETIN HORMONES

MEDICATION	ACTIONS	DOSAGE	SPECIAL CONSIDERATIONS
Pramlintide (Symlin)	Adjunct therapy in type 1 and type 2 patients who have less than optimal postprandial glycemic control	Type 1: initial dose 15 mcg; titrate by 15 mcg up to 30–60 mcg as needed Type 2: initial dose 60 mcg; can use up to 120 mcg as needed Subcutaneous administration with mealtime insulin; 2 inches apart from insulin injection	Dose must be held if NPO or eating less than 30 g of CHO Contraindicated in gastroparesis Nausea is a common side effect. Do not titrate until nausea has been absent for 3 days. Decrease insulin (preprandial, short, or rapid-acting) by 50% during start of pramlintide. If $HbA_{1c} > 9\%$, pramlintide should not be used.
Exenatide (Byetta)	Adjunct therapy to improve glycemic control in type 2 patients on metformin, a sulfonylurea, or a combination of both	Initiate at 5 mcg subcutaneously twice daily: after one month, can titrate to 10 mcg twice daily if needed Administer with meals	Contraindicated in type 1 DM, severe renal impairment, severe gastrointestinal disease Contraceptives and antibiotics should be taken 1 hr before injection Dose must be held if NPO or eating less than 30 g of CHO

CHO = Carbohydrate, DM = diabetes mellitus, NPO = nothing by mouth.

PATHOPHYSIOLOGY OF DIABETES MELLITUS AND HYPERGLYCEMIA

Glucose homeostasis requires an individual to have normal insulin secretion and normal sensitivity to insulin. Regardless of the cause of hyperglycemia, altered insulin secretion or altered insulin sensitivity leading to insulin resistance results in pathogenesis.

In type 1 DM, the autoimmune beta cell destruction reduces beta cell mass by 80% to 90% by the time metabolic decompensation occurs.[17,55] The insulin secretion is insufficient at this point to regulate hepatic glucose production. Initially, postprandial hyperglycemia occurs, demonstrating the inability of the body to suppress hepatic glucose production during meal absorption, as well as some decreased peripheral glucose uptake and utilization. As the availability of insulin further diminishes, increased basal hepatic glucose production and decreased glucose uptake by peripheral tissues cause fasting hyperglycemia. This can cause glucose toxicity, a state of hyperglycemia in which the glucose transporters available on both insulin-dependent (muscle, fat) and non–insulin-dependent tissues (brain, red blood cells, wounds) are severely reduced or inactivated[17] (Figure 34-3).

The renal threshold of glucose is approximately 180 mg/dl.[17] When blood glucose reaches this value, the kidney begins the process of osmotic diuresis, and glucosuria results. It is important to note that the normal aging process actually increases renal threshold and pregnancy decreases renal threshold. Thus an older adult may not display glucosuria until the blood glucose level reaches 300 mg/dl, and in a pregnant woman glucosuria may occur at 120 mg/dl.[17] Polyuria and polydipsia are the classic symptoms of hyperglycemia. Without available insulin, the cells are effectively starving and not being nourished. To compensate, lipolysis and proteolysis occur, resulting in weight loss, and polyphagia develops. Glucagon, growth hormone, epinephrine, and cortisol levels increase, contributing to hepatic glucose production, lipolysis, ketogenesis, and proteolysis. With osmotic diuresis, the skin becomes warm and dry; rubor can be detected on the cheeks; and changes occur in vision. This is secondary to the volume depletion of the vitreous humor and the accumulation of sorbitol behind the lens of the eye, causing the lens to temporarily change shape. If this state persists without adequate intervention, nausea, vomiting, weakness, anorexia, and eventual abdominal pain and cramping develop secondary to the presence of ketone bodies, specifically acetone, acetoacetic acid, and beta-hydroxybutyric acid. Kussmaul respirations develop when the metabolic acidosis is severe. In some individuals, a fruity odor to the breath can be detected. This is DKA, and it is life threatening.

In type 2 diabetes mellitus, dysfunction of insulin secretion and of the peripheral receptors occurs. Individuals secrete insulin at low, normal, or high rates, but the secretion of the hormone may be delayed or altered in response to a glucose load. This typically results in postprandial hyperglycemia. The receptors resist allowing insulin to bind to the site, and do not allow glucose to enter the cell for utilization or storage.

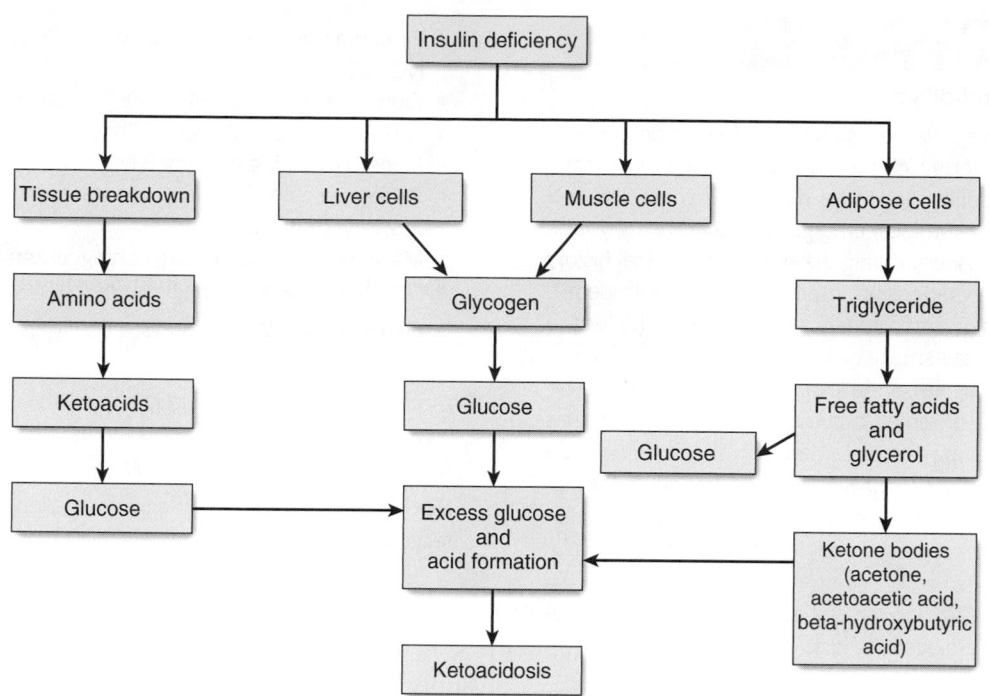

⬍FIGURE 34-3 Untreated diabetic ketoacidosis.

Glycogenolysis occurs, further raising the blood glucose concentrations, and peripheral uptake of glucose is diminished.

A less common form of type 2 diabetes in children is called maturity-onset diabetes of the young. This is actually an autosomal dominant form of DM in which a mutation of the enzyme glucokinase occurs, resulting in abnormal glucose sensing by the beta cells and impaired insulin secretion.[55] Symptoms of this form of type 2 DM include fatigue, dry skin, and a wound that will not heal. Frequently, individuals with this disease remain undiagnosed until an event occurs, such as cellulitis, myocardial infarction (MI), or cholecystitis, causing the need for one to seek medical attention. However, all symptoms of type 1 DM may be present, depending on the severity of the disease.

ACUTE COMPLICATIONS OF DIABETES MELLITUS

Diabetic Ketoacidosis

DKA is a serious, life-threatening condition caused by a profound insulin deficiency and an elevation of counter-regulatory hormones, leading to increased hepatic and renal glucose production and impaired glucose utilization in peripheral tissues. As a result,

free fatty acids and ketone bodies are released into the bloodstream, causing ketonemia and metabolic acidosis[6,17,36,66] characterized by hyperglycemia, ketosis, dehydration, and electrolyte imbalance. This acute complication is primarily found in type 1 patients, but it can occur in patients with type 2 DM as well. The mortality rate for DKA is less than 5% in experienced centers[6] but is reported as high as 10%.[35]

Causes or Precipitating Factors of Diabetic Ketoacidosis

The onset of type 1 DM can present as DKA simultaneously when an individual is discovering the presence of an illness. Infection is the most common trigger for DKA.[6] Other triggers include stress, CVA, MI, alcohol abuse, pancreatitis, trauma, drugs, anorexia or bulimia, the deliberate or inadvertent omission of insulin, mismanagement of glucose levels when ill, pregnancy, and ambulatory continuous subcutaneous insulin infusion pump malfunction.

The signs and symptoms of DKA occur within a short period of time. Excess caloric intake over the amount of insulin available (either omission of insulin, undertreatment, or an absolute lack of produced usable insulin) or excess production from counter-regulatory sources can result in DKA within 24 hours. The signs and symptoms previously stated for hyperglycemia

Case Study 34-1, Part A

Abnormal Metabolism

L.W. is a 38-year-old Native American male with an 8-month history of angina for which he had not sought medical care. He was playing softball when he developed chest pain and was transported to the local emergency department by family, losing consciousness during the transport. Medical history is significant for hypertension, morbid obesity, dyslipidemia, and a family history of coronary artery disease. He was a ½- to 1-pack-per-day smoker.

A coronary angiogram at the local hospital showed a 100% occlusion of his proximal circumflex artery. A stent was placed, and development of cardiogenic shock required an intra-aortic balloon pump (IABP). He was intubated for pulmonary edema and transferred to a university medical center for evaluation of potential need for further left ventricular assistance.

On admission, L.W. had signs of acute renal failure, respiratory failure, and cardiogenic shock.

Assessment on Admission:

- Blood pressure 90/50 mm Hg
- Pulmonary artery pressure 42/30 mm Hg
- Right atrial pressure 10 mm Hg
- Oxygen saturation by pulse oximetry 94%
- Lungs: diffuse basilar crackles; no cyanosis
- Heart: S_1, S_2, normal sinus rhythm
- Abdomen: soft with no bowel sounds auscultated
- Extremities: cool, peripheral pulses weak; no edema

Labs on Admission:

Potassium = 2.9 mEq/L
Chloride = 103 mEq/L
BUN = 38 mg/dl
Creatinine = 2.03 mg/dl

Glucose = 358 mg/dl	Arterial blood gas
HbA$_{1c}$ = 7.8%	pH = 7.3
Calcium = 7.4 mg/dl	Paco$_2$ = 46 mm Hg
Phosphorus = 3.7 mg/dl	Pao$_2$ = 86 mm Hg
Magnesium = 2 mg/dl	Bicarbonate = 16 mEq/L
Albumin = 3.4 g/dl	

BUN = Blood urea nitrogen, Paco$_2$ = partial pressure of arterial carbon dioxide, Pao$_2$ = partial pressure of arterial oxygen tension.

Medications on Admission to Critical Care:

- Dopamine (Intropin)—titrate to keep mean arterial pressure greater than 65 mm Hg—infusing between 3 and 10 mcg/kg/min
- Furosemide (Lasix)—20 mg/hr IV
- Heparin—800 units/hr IV infusion
- Propofol (Diprivan)—20 mcg/kg/min IV
- Norepinephrine (Levophed)—0.03 mcg/kg/min IV
- Clopidogrel (Plavix)—75 mg NG daily

- Pantoprazole sodium sesquihydrate (Protonix)—40 mg NG daily
- Ciprofloxacin (Cipro)—400 mg IV every 24 hr
- Vancomycin—2 g IV every 12 hr
- Piperacillin—4.5 g IV every 8 hr
- Potassium chloride to correct potassium levels—20 mEq IV every 1 hr × 2
- Magnesium sulfate to correct magnesium levels—2 g IV
- Morphine sulfate—4 mg IV every 4 hr as needed for pain

Decision point: What risks for underlying diabetes did the patient exhibit?

Decision point: How quickly should the patient's glucose level be corrected and what are the risks associated with correcting the glucose level too quickly?

Decision point: What additional challenges are present related to maintaining glycemic control?

Case continues on page 926

apply to DKA. If left untreated, altered mental status or sensorium and coma are signs of ensuing death. Table 34-1 identifies laboratory values seen in DKA.

The treatment of DKA is focused on fluid replacement, continuous intravenous insulin therapy, and electrolyte stabilization. It is important to remember that when replacing fluid following such a significant diuresis, electrolytes are significantly depleted. As insulin is administered, potassium is driven from the bloodstream into the cell. This results in a drop in serum potassium level. As fluid is replaced and the amount of insulin administered plateaus, potassium will reenter the blood space and can result in hyperkalemia. Electrocardiogram monitoring is necessary in moderate to severe DKA to monitor for T wave alterations or the appearance of a U wave, alerting staff to cardiac irritability.

The administration of intravenous insulin requires hourly blood glucose monitoring until stable, which is defined as within the target range for 4 consecutive hours.[6,35] When the blood glucose level stabilizes, monitoring every 2 hours is appropriate. A return to hourly testing is indicated if the glucose concentration fluctuates outside of the designated target range. The titration of insulin can be done per standardized protocols* or by 0.5-unit increments to maintain blood glucose levels within a specified target range. The goal is to have the glucose level decrease by 50 to 70 mg/dl/hr.[6,35] When the blood glucose level reaches 250 mg/dl, a dextrose source must be administered.[6,35] Glycemic targets for individuals being treated for DKA are individually established on the basis of one's insulin

---

*References 21, 37, 38, 39, 43, 46, 48, 58.

TABLE 34-1 Laboratory Values for DKA and HHNS

LABORATORY VALUES	MILD DKA	MODERATE DKA	SEVERE DKA	HHNS
Glucose	>250 mg/dl	>250 mg/dl	>250 mg/dl	>600 mg/dl
Sodium	Variable	Variable	Variable	Normal or high
Potassium	Variable	Variable	Variable	Variable
Venous pH	7.25–7.30	7–7.24	<7	>7.3
Bicarbonate	15–18 mEq/L	10 to <15 mEq/L	<10 mEq/L	>15 mEq/L
Serum beta-hydroxybutyric acid	Positive	Positive	Positive	Small
Serum osmolality	Variable	Variable	Variable	>320 mOsm/kg
Anion gap	>10	>12	>12	Variable
BUN/creatinine	Elevated	Elevated	Elevated	Elevated
Amylase	Increased	Increased	Increased	May increase
Hematocrit	Increased	Increased	Increased	Increased
Liver functions	May increase	May increase	May increase	May increase

BUN = Blood urea nitrogen, DKA = diabetic ketoacidosis, HHNS = hyperosmolar hyperglycemic nonketotic syndrome.

TABLE 34-2 Target Blood Glucose Values

LOCATION	PREPRANDIAL	1-HOUR POSTPRANDIAL	MAXIMAL GLUCOSE	GLYCOSYLATED HEMOGLOBIN A$_{1C}$
Intensive care unit	80–110 mg/dl		110 mg/dl	
Acute care: NPO	80–110 mg/dl		110 mg/dl	
Acute care: fed state	90–130 mg/dl		<180 mg/dl	
Prelabor	80–100 mg/dl	120 mg/dl		
Labor and delivery			100 mg/dl	
Outpatient	90–130 mg/dl		<180 mg/dl	<7%

NPO = Nothing by mouth.

sensitivity factor, age, and weight, and can range from as high as 200 mg/dl for a neonate to as low as 80 to 110 mg/dl for an intensely managed individual.[6,13,35] A summary of recommended glycemic targets in the acute care setting can be found in Table 34-2.

As the glycemic target is achieved and the ketosis has cleared, usually over a 24-hour time period, the insulin regimen must shift from intravenous insulin to basal/bolus subcutaneous management.[4,17,21,35, 36,42,43,46,58] Basal insulin is the insulin delivered that will stabilize blood glucose levels for 24 hours. Thus intermediate- and long-acting insulins noted in the Medication table below are basal insulins. NPH, given twice daily (in the morning and at bedtime) for true basal coverage, is the only intermediate-acting insulin

available in the United States. Glargine, a long-acting insulin, is peakless and is administered once a day. On occasion, it is given twice a day if a large volume of the drug (greater than 100 units) is being given at one time. Detemir, a new twice-a-day insulin with long action, became available in the United States in 2006. It has special properties in that it binds to albumin, increasing the predictability of action. However, in patients with renal or hepatic impairment, a decreased clearance of the insulin is seen as the impairment worsens. The first subcutaneous injection of basal insulin as the patient is transitioned from IV to subcutaneous administration must be administered 2 hours before the discontinuation of the infusion.[6,21,43,66]

INSULIN PREPARATIONS: ONSET, PEAK, AND DURATION*

INSULIN PREPARATION	ONSET OF ACTION	PEAK DURATION	EFFECTIVE DURATION	MAXIMUM DURATION
Human				
Rapid-Acting Insulin Analogs				
Lispro (Humalog)	0.2–0.5 min	0.5–1.5 hr	3–4 hr	4–6 hr
Aspart (NovoLog)	0.2–0.5 min	0.5–1.5 hr	3–4 hr	4–6 hr
Glulisine (Apidra)	0.2–0.5 min	0.5–1.5 hr	3–4 hr	4–6 hr
Short-Acting Insulin				
(Regular)	0.5–1 hr	2–3 hr	3–6 hr	6–8 hr
Intermediate-Acting Insulin				
(NPH)	2–4 hr	6–10 hr	10–16 hr	14–18 hr
Long-Acting Insulin Analogs				
Glargine (Lantus)	1.1 hr	None	24 hr	24 hr
Detemir (Levemir)	3–4 hr	6–8 hr	6–23 hr	23 hr
Premixed Fixed Combinations				
Humulin and Novolin 70/30; Humulin 50/50	Peak as NPH and regular			
Humalog mix 75/25	0.2–0.5 min	Dual peak	10–16 hr	14–18 hr
NovoLog mix 70/30	0.2–0.5 min	Dual peak	10–16 hr	14–18 hr
Animal				
Short-Acting Insulin				
(Regular)	0.5–2 hr	3–4 hr	4–6 hr	6–10 hr
Intermediate-Acting Insulin				
(NPH)	4–6 hr	8–14 hr	16–20 hr	20–24 hr

*Note: There are many variables that can affect the absorption rates of subcutaneous insulin injections. This timetable is a guideline to aid in predicting an individual's response to insulin.

Bolus insulin includes rapid- and short-acting insulin. Rapid-acting insulin is used for prandial coverage and correction of abnormally elevated blood glucose levels. Because the duration of rapid-acting insulin is 3 to 4 hours, this type of insulin medication works extremely well for carbohydrate (CHO) counting,[3] for adjustment of insulin to CHO ratios, and for the purpose of correcting an abnormally elevated blood glucose level. Aspart, lispro, and glulisine are the available rapid-acting analogs. Regular insulin is short-acting insulin. Because it can be given every 6 hours, regular insulin is appropriate for glucose level correction when an individual is receiving nothing by mouth (NPO), is receiving continuous total parenteral nutrition, or is receiving a continuous enteral feed. It is also beneficial in combination with the intermediate-acting insulin NPH to maintain euglycemia overnight when the patient is receiving cycled nocturnal feedings and steroid bursts, because this insulin combination peaks simultaneously with peak corticosteroid levels in the bloodstream. Regular insulin should not be utilized in the fed state for correction.[16] The action time of regular insulin is 4 to 6 hours, which is beyond the administration times of regular insulin before meals and at bedtime. Therefore it can accumulate or "stack," creating the potential for hypoglycemia later in the day. The exception to this rule is the individual who is a "grazer"—a person who "nibbles" and eats throughout the day without actual meal patterns.

In the fed state, the consistent CHO meal plan is the standard diabetes diet today. The Nutrition box at right provides a summary of nutrition recommendations in hyperglycemia. CHOs are the chief source of immediate fuel and are responsible for the post-load peak glucose spike, typically at the 2-hour postprandial mark. By providing consistent amounts of CHOs throughout the day at meals, and snacks only if desired, wide glycemic excursions are reduced and targets can be achieved. In patients with type 1 DM and many with type 2 diabetes, it is beneficial to match rapid-acting insulin to CHO intake, to maintain targets. As previously mentioned, this is accomplished by providing an insulin-to-CHO ratio that is a set number of units of rapid-acting insulin for a set number of CHO grams or units. In the hospital setting, insulin is given immediately during or after the meal to ensure that the patient will indeed consume the CHO units provided on the meal tray.

The identification of precipitating factors is critical to the successful treatment of DKA as interventions must be initiated to treat underlying infections or comorbid conditions.[6,17,66] Ongoing assessment, intervention, and monitoring are critical. Observing and assessing for indications of fluid overload secondary to the fluid replacement, respiratory distress secondary

◆ NUTRITION

Nutrition Recommendations in Hyperglycemia

Nutrition Source	Type 1 and Type 2 Diabetes Mellitus and Hyperglycemia
Calories	Maintain metabolic requirements
Meal plan	Consistent carbohydrate
Carbohydrates	60%–70% of total calories
Proteins	15%–20% of total calories; modify if impaired renal function
Fats	10% of total calories; cholesterol less than 300 mg/day
Fiber	Variety of fiber-containing foods
Electrolytes	No added salt; if hypertensive, 2 g sodium; if renal impairment, potassium restriction
Fluids	Restrict only if indicated
Vitamins and minerals	Folate, calcium, zinc, chromium, magnesium
Total parenteral nutrition	25–35 kcal/kg body weight
Enteral feedings	Standard formula of 50% carbohydrate or low carbohydrate of 33%–40%
Supplements	Moderate carbohydrate with fiber to reduce postsupplement glucose spike

to the metabolic acidosis, cerebral edema secondary to the rapidity of glucose level decrease and rehydration, and hypoglycemia must be the standard of practice.

Patient and family education are extremely important following an acute DKA event. Preventing future episodes can occur only if the individual understands the reasons for the DKA event and is instructed in its management, including how to appropriately manage and problem-solve changes in glucose level related to illness; how to compensate for increased insulin requirements with the utilization of a subcutaneous insulin correction scale with rapid-acting insulin; and when it is necessary to call for assistance. Also, the availability of medications and tools for self-management, including a glucose meter, test strips, lancets, ketone sticks, and adequate nutritional supplements, is crucial. Follow-up care and education should be established before discharge.

◆ Case Study 34-1, Part B

Abnormal Metabolism

The continuous insulin infusion protocol was initiated because L.W.'s glucose level was 358 mg/dl, and blood glucose levels were tracked hourly as outlined below.

Hour of Infusion	Blood Glucose (mg/dl)	Insulin Infusion (units/hr)
1	358	Insulin bolus of 10 units Infusion started at 4 units/hr
2	301	Infusion increased to 6 units/hr
3	260	Infusion increased to 8 units/hr
4	199	Infusion increased to 9 units/hr
5	145	Infusion increased to 10 units/hr
6	99	Infusion maintained at 10 units/hr
7	88	Infusion decreased to 9 units/hr

Chemistry panels were followed as the glucose level normalized and other systems stabilized. Results were as follows:

- Sodium = 139 mEq/L
- Potassium = 3.5 mEq/L
- Chloride = 105 mEq/L
- BUN = 57 mg/dl
- Creatinine = 5.17 mg/dl
- Calcium = 7.8 mg/dl
- Magnesium = 2.7 mg/dl

The insulin infusion was titrated in 0.5- to 1-unit increments to successfully maintain glucose levels between 80 and 110 mg/dl. The IABP remained in place and cardiac status stabilized. Norepinephrine was weaned off. A small-bore feeding tube was placed post-pylorus and enteral feedings started. Because creatinine and BUN levels were rising, a nephrology consult was obtained and a catheter was placed for dialysis to treat the acute renal failure.

Decision point: What electrolyte shifts should you expect as the insulin infusion is initiated?

Decision point: Should the insulin infusion be transitioned to a subcutaneous regimen on initiation of enteral feedings?

Case continues on page 936

HYPEROSMOLAR HYPERGLYCEMIC NONKETOTIC SYNDROME

HHNS is a syndrome with four primary features: severe hyperglycemia, absence of ketosis, profound dehydration, and neurologic manifestations (Figure 34-4). HHNS evolves over several days to several weeks, occurring most often in type 2 DM patients and in older adults. In HHNS, insulin availability is insufficient to facilitate glucose utilization and uptake at peripheral sites, resulting in hyperglycemia. Although it can occur, there is limited lipolysis and ketogenesis. Massive osmotic diuresis is the hallmark of HHNS, with significant volume depletion and electrolyte loss. If this is untreated, death can occur.[6,55,66]

The chief precipitating factors for HHNS are infection, especially pneumonia and urinary tract infections; myocardial ischemia; gastrointestinal bleed; arterial thrombosis; stress; severe gastroenteritis; drugs including thiazide and loop diuretics; hemodialysis and peritoneal dialysis; and hypertonic feedings, such as prolonged parenteral nutrition or high-protein or gastric tube feedings. Because this is more commonly associated with older adults, many individuals who develop HHNS have dementia or altered mentation. There can be a delay in the identification of HHNS as the abnormal mental state masks the neurologic changes associated with the syndrome. Residents of long-term care facilities are at increased risk for the development of HHNS.[6]

The symptoms associated with HHNS are polydipsia, polyuria, polyphagia, weakness, dehydration, weight loss, and blurred vision. Gastrointestinal symptoms, such as nausea, vomiting, abdominal pain, and cramping, are much milder in HHNS as compared to DKA. Physical findings include altered skin turgor, tachycardia, hypotension, alteration in mental status, focal neurologic signs (such as hemisensory deficits, hemiparesis, aphasia), and seizures. See Table 34-1 for a list of laboratory values common in HHNS.

As in DKA, the primary treatment for HHNS is fluid replacement, insulin therapy, and electrolyte replacement. Initial treatment of fluid therapy is for intravascular and extravascular volume expansion, and increasing renal perfusion. Hemodynamic monitoring, measurement of intake and output, and physical examination are measures to determine adequacy of fluid replacement.[6] Individuals who have cardiac or renal comorbidities must be monitored carefully during fluid resuscitation to avoid overload. Electrolytes, particularly potassium, magnesium, and phosphorus, are replaced as necessary, and monitoring is done every 2 hours until stable. When the blood glucose level reaches 300 mg/dl, it is important that some dextrose (typically as dextrose 5% with 0.45% NaCl) be administered to offer some caloric source and to avoid hypoglycemia. The amount is dependent on the patient's age and comorbid conditions.

As in DKA, intravenous insulin infusions are the standard of practice. Intravenous insulin is given as regular insulin in a 1:1 concentration (1 unit of U-100 regular human insulin to 1 ml of normal saline). IV insulin

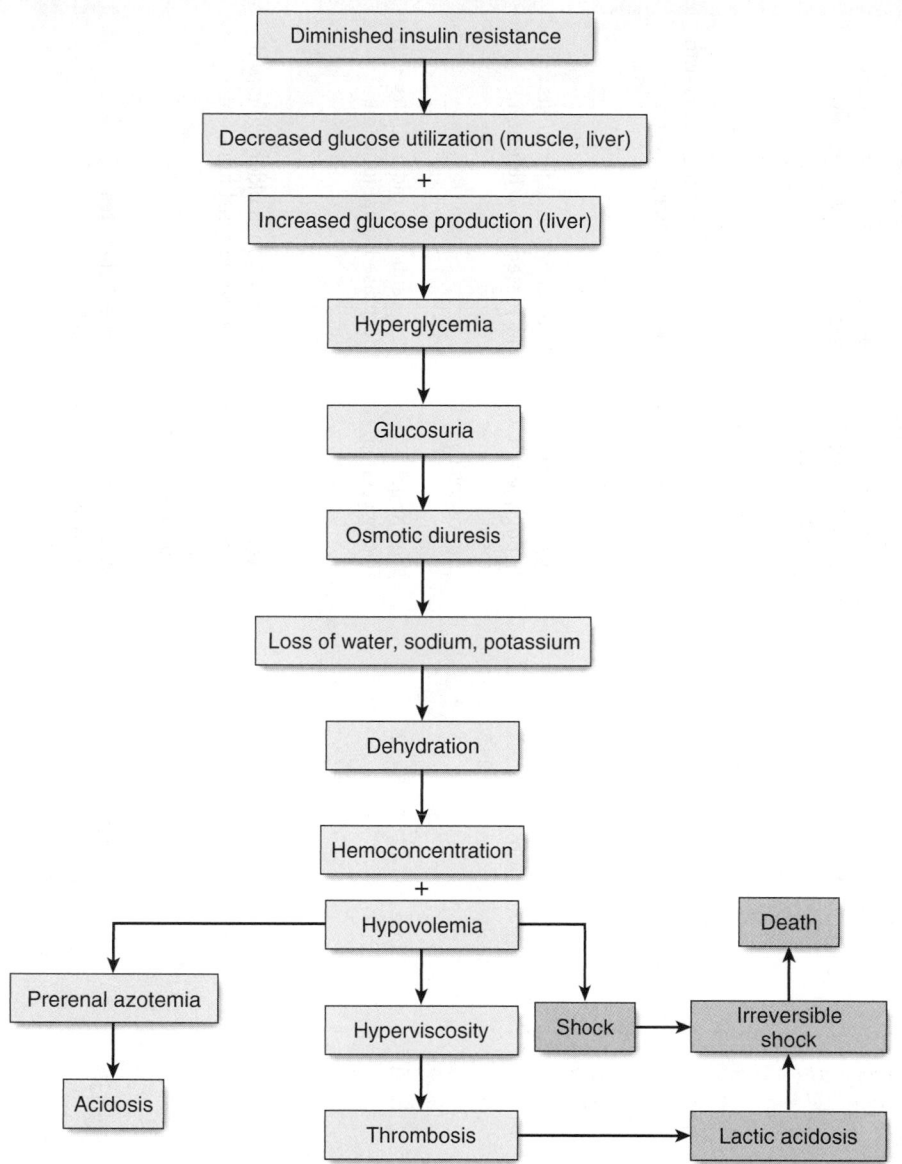

♦FIGURE 34-4   Pathophysiology of hyperosmolar hyperglycemic nonketotic syndrome.

should be continued until the HHNS is resolved as demonstrated by corrected laboratory values and the individual's ability to tolerate oral food and fluids. Once this occurs, insulin should be transitioned to basal/bolus subcutaneous management.[21,42,43] The first dose of basal insulin should be administered 2 hours before the discontinuation of the insulin infusion. Rapid-acting insulin (such as aspart, lispro, or glulisine) should be administered to cover prandial intake or as correction.

Oral diabetes agents are not able to maintain euglycemia in an acute crisis.[21,43] If appropriate, they can be reinstituted closer to discharge to determine effectiveness. A list of oral diabetes agents is provided in the Medication table on pp. 928-931.

Nutrition goals are the provision of energy for basic metabolic requirements, calories for reasonable weight, maintenance of euglycemia, maintenance of normal blood pressure, and maintenance of lipid profile within

ORAL DIABETES AGENTS

CLASS/ACTION	GENERIC (TRADE NAME)	DOSE SIZE	DOSE/DAY (in mg)	DOSE INTERVAL	PEAK (hr) DURATION (hr)	SIDE EFFECTS	CONTRAINDICATIONS
Sulfonylurea/ secretagogue; beta cell	Glyburide (Micronase, DiaBeta)	2.5, 5 mg	1.25–20	1–2 times daily with meals	4 ——— 12–24	Weight gain, hypoglycemia, gastrointestinal (GI) upset, photosensitivity	Use caution in older adults with decreased renal function.
Sulfonylurea/ secretagogue; beta cell	Micronized glyburide (Glynase PresTab)	1.5, 3, 6 mg	0.75–12	1–2 times daily with meals	2 ——— 12–24	Weight gain, hypoglycemia, GI upset, photosensitivity	Use caution in older adults with decreased renal function.
Sulfonylurea/ secretagogue; beta cell	Glipizide (Glucotrol)	5, 10 mg	2.5–40	1–3 times daily 30 min before meals	1–3 ——— 12–24	Weight gain, hypoglycemia, GI upset, photosensitivity	Use caution in older adults with decreased renal function.
Sulfonylurea/ secretagogue; beta cell	Glipizide-GITS (Glucotrol XL)	2.5, 5, 10 mg	2.5–20	1 time daily with meal	6–12 ——— 24	Weight gain, hypoglycemia, GI upset, photosensitivity	Use caution in older adults with decreased renal function.
Sulfonylurea/ secretagogue; beta cell	Glimepiride (Amaryl)	1, 2, 4 mg	1–8	1 time daily with meal	2–3 ——— 24	Weight gain, hypoglycemia, GI upset, photosensitivity	Use caution in older adults with decreased renal function.
Meglitinide/ secretagogue; beta cell	Repaglinide (Prandin)	0.5, 1, 2 mg	0.5–16	1–4 times daily, 1–30 min before meals	1 ——— 4–6	Weight gain, hypoglycemia, GI upset, photosensitivity	Type 1 diabetes DKA
Meglitinide/ secretagogue; beta cell	Nateglinide (Starlix)	60, 120 mg	180–360	1–3 times daily, 1–30 minutes before meals	0.3 ——— 4	Weight gain, hypoglycemia	Type 1 diabetes DKA

CLASS/ACTION	GENERIC (TRADE NAME)	DOSE SIZE	DOSE/DAY (in mg)	DOSE INTERVAL	PEAK (hr) / DURATION (hr)	SIDE EFFECTS	CONTRAINDICATIONS
Thiazolidinedione/ sensitizer; receptor	Rosiglitazone (Avandia)	2, 4, 8 mg	4–8	1–2 times daily	n/a __ days-weeks	Edema, weight gain, increased ovulation in premenopausal women	Do not give if ALT is greater than 2.5 times ULN. Monitor LFTs every 2 months for first 12 months of therapy. Evaluate for previous MI, CAD, HF, aortic or mitral valve disease. Use cautiously in Class I or II NYHA HF; do not use in Class III or IV NYHA HF. Monitor weight.
Thiazolidinedione/ sensitizer; receptor	Pioglitazone (Actos)	15, 30, 45 mg	15–45	1 time daily	n/a __ days-weeks	Edema, weight gain, increased ovulation in premenopausal women	Do not give if ALT is greater than 2.5 times ULN. Monitor LFTs every 2 months for first 12 months of therapy. Evaluate for previous MI, CAD, HF, aortic or mitral valve disease. Use cautiously in Class I or II NYHA HF; do not use in Class III or IV NYHA HF. Monitor weight.
Biguanide/ sensitizer; liver, receptor	Metformin (Glucophage; Riomet oral solution 100 mg/ml)	500, 850, 1000 mg	1000–2550	1–3 times daily with meals	2–3 __ 12–18	Nausea, diarrhea, abdominal pain, possible resumption of ovulation in premenopausal anovulatory women	Lactic acidosis is a rare side effect if renal, hepatic, or cardiac disease or dysfunction is present. Caution patients against excessive alcohol intake with hepatic impairment. **Discontinue metformin at time of or before radiologic studies involving IV iodinated contrast materials. Withhold metformin for 48 hr after procedure and restart only after renal function has been reevaluated and determined to be normal.** Do not give if creatinine greater than 1.4 mg/dl in females; greater than 1.5 mg/dl in males.

Table continues on page 930

ORAL DIABETES AGENTS—cont'd

CLASS/ACTION	GENERIC (TRADE NAME)	DOSE SIZE	DOSE/DAY (in mg)	DOSE INTERVAL	PEAK (hr) DURATION (hr)	SIDE EFFECTS	CONTRAINDICATIONS
Biguanide/sensitizer; liver, receptor	Metformin extended release (Glucophage XR)	500, 750 mg	1000–2000	1 time daily with evening meal	4–8 — 24	Nausea, diarrhea, abdominal pain, possible resumption of ovulation in premenopausal anovulatory women	Lactic acidosis is a rare side effect if renal, hepatic, or cardiac disease or dysfunction is present. Caution patients against excessive alcohol intake with hepatic impairment. **Discontinue metformin at time of or before radiologic studies involving IV iodinated contrast materials. Withhold metformin for 48 hours after procedure and restart only after renal function has been reevaluated and determined to be normal.** Do not give if creatinine greater than 1.4 mg/dl in females; greater than 1.5 mg/dl in males.
Alpha-glucosidase inhibitor/delays digestion and absorption of CHO; small intestine	Acarbose (Precose)	25, 50, 100 mg	150–300	1–3 times daily at start of each meal	n/a — 2–3	Diarrhea, flatulence, abdominal discomfort	**Do not give if creatinine greater than 2 mg/dl or creatinine clearance less than 25 ml/min.** Use cautiously with inflammatory bowel disease, colonic ulceration, or obstructive bowel disorders. Do not give if cirrhosis of liver is present.

CLASS/ACTION	GENERIC (TRADE NAME)	DOSE SIZE	DOSE/DAY (in mg)	DOSE INTERVAL	PEAK (hr) DURATION (hr)	SIDE EFFECTS	CONTRAINDICATIONS
Alpha-glucosidase inhibitor/delay digestion and absorption of CHO; small intestine	Miglitol (Glyset)	25, 50, 100 mg	150–300 mg	1–3 times daily at the start of each meal	n/a 2–3	Diarrhea, flatulence, abdominal discomfort	**Do not give if creatinine greater than 2 mg/dl or creatinine clearance less than 25 mL/min.** Use cautiously with inflammatory bowel disease, colonic ulceration, or obstructive bowel disorders. Do not give if cirrhosis of the liver is present.
Fixed combinations	Glyburide and metformin (Glucovance)	1.25/250, 2.5/500, 5/500 mg	2.5/500–20/2000	1–2 times daily with meals	See above See above	See above	See above
Fixed combinations	Glipizide and metformin (Metaglip)	2.5/250, 2.5/500, 5/500 mg	2.5/500–10/2000	1–2 times daily with meals	See above See above	See above	See above
Fixed combinations	Rosiglitazone and metformin (Avandamet)	1/500, 2/250, 2/500, 4/500, 2/1000, 4/1000 mg	1/500–8/2000	1–2 times daily with meals	See above See above	See above	See above

ALT = Alanine aminotransferase, CHO = carbohydrate, CAD = coronary artery disease, DKA = diabetic ketoacidosis, GI = gastrointestinal, HF = heart failure, LFT = liver function test, MI = myocardial infarction, NYHA = New York Heart Association, ULN = upper limits of normal.

normal limits. Individualizing the plan to encourage compliance and satisfaction by the client is also important. A consistent CHO meal plan is standard. However, because 80% of individuals with type 2 diabetes are obese,[2,17] counting fat grams to achieve overall caloric reduction has been successful. Within the hospital setting, it is important to note that multiple nutrition-related issues affect glycemic control and can result in hypoglycemia: people who are ill frequently have a decreased appetite; meal trays may be delayed from the kitchen; the timing of meals is inconsistent because of tests, procedures, and rounds; inconsistent CHO content alters glycemia; physical activity is decreased from the well state; and glucose monitoring may not be timely.[57] Thus the nurse must work closely with the patient and the dietitian to optimize consistency and stabilize glucose level.

Blood glucose monitoring is done routinely at the bedside. Point-of-care testing is critical and should be done every 4 or every 6 hours when the patient is NPO and hourly when the patient is receiving an IV infusion of insulin; fasting, preprandial, and bedtime glucose monitoring should occur when the patient is being fed. There are also situations where obtaining 2-hour postprandial blood glucose levels is required; this is to determine the adequacy of the insulin to CHO ratio prescribed. Nocturnal values are also helpful between 0200 and 0300 to identify hypoglycemia.

All precipitating factors must be identified and treated. Ongoing observation and assessment of mentation and neurologic checks are necessary. Obtaining information from a relative or care facility regarding baseline mental status can be quite helpful in determining alterations the patient is experiencing.

In an effort to prevent a recurrence of HHNS, patient, family, and facility staff education might be indicated. Adjustment of the patient's medical regimen as indicated and follow-up care are extremely important.

HYPOGLYCEMIA

Iatrogenic hypoglycemia occurs in people with type 1 and type 2 diabetes who are treated with insulins, incretin hormones, or sulfonylureas (see the Medication tables on pp. 920, 924, and 928-931). According to Cryer,[25] hypoglycemia is the critical limiting factor in the glycemic management of diabetes in both the short term and long term. This was evident in the Diabetes Control and Complications Trial,[31] which found that intensive glycemic management to target glucose levels reduced long-term sequelae of DM with one risk—the frequency of hypoglycemia increased.

Hypoglycemia is a low plasma glucose concentration below or equal to the lower limit of normal, which is 70 mg/dl. It is accompanied by symptoms that are relieved when the plasma glucose level is raised.[12] In the past, hypoglycemia has been categorized as mild (60 to 70 mg/dl), moderate (46 to 59 mg/dl), and severe (less than or equal to 45 mg/dl). More recently, the American Diabetes Association Workgroup on Hypoglycemia identified severe hypoglycemia as "an event requiring assistance of another person to actively administer CHO, glucagons, or other resuscitative actions."[12] They also documented symptomatic hypoglycemia as an event during which typical symptoms of hypoglycemia are accompanied by a measured plasma glucose concentration less than or equal to 70 mg/dl, and asymptomatic hypoglycemia as an event not accompanied by typical symptoms of hypoglycemia but with a measured plasma glucose concentration less than or equal to 70 mg/dl.[12] The problem is compounded by excess insulin or a secretagogue (a beta cell stimulating oral hypoglycemia agent) available in the bloodstream, physical activity, caloric intake, drug interactions, alcohol, altered insulin sensitivity, gastroparesis, and renal insufficiency.[24,25]

The physiologic mechanism of counter-regulation (regulation of plasma glucose levels) is impaired in diabetes. Insulin levels do not decrease, glucagon levels do not increase, and epinephrine levels are increased because of a lower glycemic threshold for epinephrine secretion.[12] Hypoglycemic unawareness or a loss of the warning symptoms of hypoglycemia can develop 5 years after diagnosis of DM.[17,25]

The signs and symptoms of hypoglycemia can be divided into two categories. First, adrenergic symptoms are seen from excessive secretion of counter-regulatory hormones, such as epinephrine, which increases the liver's glucose production and inhibits glucose utilization, and glucagon, which stimulates the release of glycogen from the liver. Growth hormone and cortisol have minimal action in an acute hypoglycemic event.[55] Diaphoresis, tremors, tachycardia, hypotension, anxiety, hunger, pallor, circumoral tingling, and increased respirations are early warning signs of a low blood glucose level. Neuroglycopenic symptoms develop when there is an inadequate supply of glucose to the central nervous system. Dizziness, headache, clouding of vision, blunted mental activity, loss of fine motor skills, confusion, slurred speech, irritability, abnormal behavior, numbness, fatigue, seizures, and loss of consciousness are associated with severe hypoglycemia; this can be fatal. In neonates and children under the age of 2, hypoglycemia has been associated with impaired learning and brain development.[25,35]

The treatment of hypoglycemia in acute care needs to be consistent. Standardized protocols or order sets enable the care provider to respond in a timely manner with appropriate intervention. Oral CHOs should be the first choice for treatment in an alert patient who is able to swallow and eat. One carbohydrate unit or 15 g of CHO will raise blood glucose concentration 30 to 45 mg/dl. The rule of 15 is often instituted and also taught to patients: administer 15 g of CHO and recheck blood glucose level in 15 minutes. Administer an additional 15 g of CHO and recheck every 15 minutes until the glucose level is greater than 100 mg/dl. When a patient is semiconscious or unconscious, glucagon can be administered subcutaneously or intramuscularly, or 50% dextrose can be given intravenously. It is important to note that glucagon can cause severe nausea and vomiting. Therefore the patient should be placed in the side-lying position so that aspiration does not occur during administration. Prevention of hypoglycemia and its severity is warranted. However, it must not be achieved at the expense of glycemic control. Thus careful management of insulin and oral agents, nutrition, intravenous fluids, pharmacologic therapy, and conditions that can predispose an individual to hypoglycemia must be assessed and evaluated regularly.[21,43,59]

HYPERGLYCEMIA

Regardless of whether an individual is known to have diabetes, hyperglycemia has been associated with poor clinical outcomes and increased mortality and morbidity over the past decade.* The connection between hyperglycemia and less than optimal clinical outcomes has been studied extensively. Findings have demonstrated associations with immune function, the inflammatory process, vascular alterations, and neuronal damage.†

Individuals with hyperglycemia have decreased host resistance and immunosuppression.[22] There are multiple studies that have identified phagocytic dysfunction in the presence of hyperglycemia.[21,40,70] A reduction in T-cell populations for both CD-4 and CD-8 subsets has also been reported. Bacterial, viral, and fungal growth have increased in clients with blood glucose levels greater than 200 mg/dl.[22,40] It appears that any patient with an elevated blood glucose level is at increased risk for infection.[21,70] This holds

particular importance for postoperative patients and those with nonhealing or deep wounds.

The largest volume of research has been conducted in the cardiovascular population. In this population, it is apparent that elevated blood glucose levels are associated with ischemia, infarction, and reduced coronary collateral blood flow.[21] Platelet aggregation and "sticky" red blood cells increase thrombus formation. This increases the risk of a pulmonary embolism, a deep vein thrombosis, a clotted IV access line, or a major thrombotic event. Catecholamine alterations and elevations in blood pressure are also found in hyperglycemia.[18,20] Inflammatory markers such as free radicals, cytokines, and nitric oxide can be found in the presence of hyperglycemia.[56] These are associated with acute MI and the severity of cardiac dysfunction that results. Endothelial cell dysfunction is linked to increased cellular adhesion, increased cell permeability, inflammation, and thrombosis.[56,60] It is thought that hyperglycemia has a direct effect on endothelial cell function by causing chemical inactivation of nitric oxide.[27] With this information, it is apparent why 50% of individuals with known diabetes have cardiovascular disease.[10,28]

Cerebral ischemia also can occur from hyperglycemia. Clement et al.[21] summarize findings associated with increased mortality, length of stay, and severity in acute stroke. Less than optimal outcomes are the result of increased tissue acidosis and lactate levels found with increased blood glucose concentrations, the effects of stress, and the release of insulin counter-regulatory hormones.[19,21]

Stress-induced hyperglycemia is the result of an increased release of counter-regulatory hormones. When these are released, catabolism is increased, hepatic gluconeogenesis occurs, and lipolysis begins. Serum glucose, free fatty acids, ketones, and lactate are by-products of this cycle. As the glucose concentration rises, insulin secretion is hindered by glucose toxicity. This cycle cannot be stopped without treatment interventions to achieve euglycemia.[46]

The treatment for acute hyperglycemia includes all modalities that assist in maintaining near-euglycemia. Selection of appropriate fluids, nutrition, insulin (or incretins and orals), and concomitant pharmacologic agents and also treatment for comorbid conditions are essential to achieve good outcomes.[1,26] The physician, advanced practice nurse, staff nurse, pharmacist, dietitian, social worker, care coordinator, and educator are essential members of the healthcare team. If possible, a coordinated plan of care must be developed with the patient's input as well in order to achieve optimal outcomes. The Multidisciplinary Plan of Care on pp. 934-936 addresses acute hyperglycemia in the adult.

---

*References 13, 21, 22, 27, 34, 40, 44, 46, 52, 56, 61, 64, 65, 67.
†References 15, 18, 19, 20, 23, 27, 49, 50, 54.

MULTIDISCIPLINARY PLAN OF CARE FOR PATIENTS WITH DISORDERS OF GLYCEMIC CONTROL

PROBLEM	INTERVENTION	RATIONALE	EXPECTED OUTCOME
Hyperglycemia	Initial IV bolus of regular insulin at 0.15 units/kg. Continuous IV insulin infusion of regular insulin at 0.1 unit/kg/hr. If blood glucose does not fall by 50 mg/dl in hour 1, infusion rate is doubled every hour until steady glucose decline of 50–75 mg/dl achieved. Monitor blood glucose hourly until stable; within target range for 4 consecutive hours; then change to every-2-hr monitoring. Monitor B-HOB every 4 hr until clear × 2; a minimum of 24 hr.	This steady provision of insulin decreases plasma glucose by 50–75 mg/dl/hr. Continuous infusion allows peripheral receptors to become saturated with insulin, eventually achieving level at which glucose is allowed to enter cell.	Glucose values decrease by 50–75 mg/dl/hr. Achieve target glucose range of 80–110 mg/dl.
Maintenance of euglycemia	Transition from IV insulin to subcutaneous insulin: Calculate TDD based on 0.4–1 unit/kg/24 hr. Compare this to total 24-hr insulin intake divided by 24. 50% of TDD is basal insulin and 50% is bolus or prandial insulin. Administer first dose of subcutaneous insulin 2 hr before discontinuation of infusion. Monitor blood glucose at time of first subcutaneous injection, time of IV discontinuation, 2 hr later, and then fasting, preprandial, and bedtime values; may consider postprandial and nocturnal testing for clinical data only to assess adequacy of TDD.	As glucose is stabilized and patient is able to eat, transition to basal/bolus insulin management is necessary. By providing basal and bolus insulin, normal pancreatic physiology is closely achieved.	Glucose values are maintained at 90–130 mg/dl fasting and less than 180 mg/dl peak postprandial. 100–140 mg/dl is an adequate bedtime blood glucose level.
Volume depletion	Provide initial assessment: For hypovolemic shock, administer NS or plasma expander. For mild hypotension: if Na$^+$ high or normal, give 0.45% NS at 4–14 ml/kg/hr; if Na$^+$ low, give NS at 4–14 ml/kg/hr. When serum glucose reaches 250 mg/dl in DKA or stress-induced or 300 mg/dl in HHNS, change IV fluid to 5% dextrose with 0.45% NaCl at 150–250 ml/hr, monitoring for fluid overload. Monitor serum and urine osmolality.	Osmotic diuresis occurs when glucose level remains greater than renal threshold and body decompensates to clear glucose and ketone bodies. Profound fluid loss is associated with this. Fluid replacement is to expand intravascular and extravascular volume and restore renal perfusion.	BP stabilized with diastolic greater than or equal to 70 mm Hg and systolic greater than or equal to 100 mm Hg and less than 130 mm Hg. Tachycardia is resolved. Skin turgor and mucous membranes improve. Lungs are clear to auscultation. Mental status is stable. Neurologic checks are stable and within normal limits. Induced change in serum osmolality should not exceed 3 mOsm/kg/hr.

PROBLEM	INTERVENTION	RATIONALE	EXPECTED OUTCOME
Potassium alterations	If initial K^+ is less than 3.3 mEq/L, insulin should be held and 40 mEq of K^+ given per hour until greater than or equal to 3.3 mEq/L. If initial K^+ is greater than or equal to 5 mEq/L, do not administer K^+ and check value every 2 hr. If initial K^+ is greater than or equal to 3.3 mEq/L but less than 5 mEq/L, give 20–30 mEq K^+ in each liter of IV fluid to maintain K^+ at 4–5 mEq/L.	Osmotic diuresis causes depletion of total body potassium. Insulin administration affects electrical activity of potassium, requiring careful administration of insulin with hypokalemia.	Potassium stabilizes between 4 and 5 mEq/L. No cardiac irritability No U waves or altered T waves. No respiratory muscle weakness.
Alteration in acid-base, magnesium, phosphorus, bicarbonate, and other electrolytes	If pH is less than 6.9, give $NaHCO_3$ 100 mmol; dilute in 400 ml H_2O and infuse at 200 ml/hr. If pH is 6.9–7, give 50 mmol diluted in 200 ml H_2O and infuse at 200ml/hr; repeat HCO_3^- infusion every 2 hr until pH greater than 7. Serum Na^+ should be corrected for hyperglycemia at 100 mg/dl. For glucose greater than 100 mg/dl, add 1.6 mEq/L to sodium value to obtain corrected serum sodium. Evaluate electrolytes, BUN, creatinine, and glucose every 2 hr until within normal limits, then every 4 hr, then daily.	Osmotic diuresis is accompanied by electrolyte depletion. DKA is characterized by metabolic acidosis, accompanied by decrease in pH. To stabilize moderate to severe acidosis, administration of bicarbonate is indicated. Magnesium and phosphorus should be replaced if indicated.	pH is greater than 7. $NaHCO_3$ is within normal limits. Magnesium and phosphorus are within normal limits.
Nausea and vomiting in DKA	Place nasogastric tube. Maintain NPO status until ketosis has cleared.	In acute illness with nausea and vomiting secondary to ketosis, prevention of aspiration is necessary. Also, nasogastric tube will allow for more careful I&O monitoring.	Nasogastric tube is removed when nausea and vomiting have subsided, bowel tones are audible, and ketosis has cleared.
Airway maintenance	Intubation may be required in severe metabolic acidosis.	Volume depletion, metabolic acidosis, respiratory muscle weakness can require need for intubation and airway protection.	Respiratory rate of 16–20 breaths/min unassisted is achieved.
Nutrition/caloric requirements	Maintain NPO status until ketosis has fully cleared. When able to tolerate clear liquids, start consistent CHO meal plan. Need for TPN and enteral tube feedings can be determined on an individual basis.	Nausea, vomiting, abdominal discomfort, and cramping will subside when ketosis clears. Caloric and nutrient loss accompanies osmotic diuresis. It is critical to provide maintenance or additional energy requirements for metabolic function.	Consistent CHO meal plan is ordered. Insulin: CHO ratio is provided for rapid-acting insulin analog to bolus for meals. CHO units consumed are recorded.

Table continues on page 936

PROBLEM	INTERVENTION	RATIONALE	EXPECTED OUTCOME
Education	Diabetes self-management education and tools for behavior modification must be provided.	Prevention of recurring events requires thorough assessment of patient's knowledge, cognitive ability, visual ability, dexterity, and coping and problem-solving ability.	Provide documentation of knowledge and skill assessment. Provide documentation of diabetes patient education.
Discharge planning	Adequate access to necessary medications, durable medical equipment, and follow-up care must be assessed and determined.	Successful self-management of hyperglycemia is dependent upon access to necessary items for managing DM. It has been demonstrated that individuals engaged with their healthcare team have enhanced motivation and compliance with self-care.	All necessary prescriptions are written and determination of individual's ability to fill them assessed. Follow-up instructions, appointments, and interaction established. Support group resources provided.

Data from references 1, 6, 13, 17, 21, and 35.
B-HOB = Beta-hydroxybutyric acid, BP = blood pressure, BUN = blood urea nitrogen, CHO = carbohydrate, DKA = diabetic ketoacidosis, DM = diabetes mellitus, HCO_3^- = bicarbonate, HHNS = hyperosmolar hyperglycemic nonketotic syndrome, I&O = intake and output, IV = intravenous, K^+ = potassium, Na^+ = sodium, $NaHCO_3$ = sodium bicarbonate, NPO = nothing by mouth, NS = normal saline, TDD = total daily dose, TPN = total parenteral nutrition.

◆ Case Study 34-1, Part C

Abnormal Metabolism

At 72 hours after admission, L.W.'s cardiac status was stable enough to warrant discontinuing the IABP. L.W. was successfully extubated and dopamine was discontinued. He started to take food orally on a high consistent CHO diet, and the insulin drip was transitioned to a basal/bolus program as outlined below. L.W. had been continuing to receive approximately 5 units/hr of continuous insulin infusion to maintain his glucose level between 80 and 110 mg/dl.

- Basal insulin dosing: Glargine 60 units subcutaneously every morning
- Prandial insulin: Aspart 2.5 units; 1 CHO unit for each meal
- Correction insulin:
  - Aspart 2 units for every 30 mg/dl above a target blood glucose level
  - Blood glucose level of 110 mg/dl; based on premeal blood glucose measurement
  - Aspart 1 unit for every 30 mg/dl above 200 mg/dl at bedtime

The first dose of 60 units of glargine was given while the insulin drip was still infusing. Two hours after the first dose, the infusion was discontinued.

L.W.'s first meal after transitioning to subcutaneous dosing consisted of 8 ounces of skim milk, 2 pieces of toast, ½ cup of oatmeal, 4 ounces of apple juice, and 1 poached egg, equaling 5 CHO units (15 g of CHOs = 1 carb unit).

His preprandial glucose level was 180 mg/dl. Therefore after he finished his meal, the nurse gave him a total of 18.5 units of aspart—12.5 units for the CHO meal coverage and an additional 6 units to correct for the preprandial glucose level.

L.W. was transferred out of critical care to the progressive care unit. As he continued to stabilize and prognosis was determined, education was required for long-term care of what was identified as previously undiagnosed type 2 diabetes.

Decision point: Why is the insulin infusion continued another 2 hours after the initial dose of glargine?

Decision point: Identify interventions to avoid hypoglycemic episodes.

Decision point: Describe the educational requirements for L.W. as he prepares to be discharged home.

Conclusions. Glycemic management in the hospitalized patient directly impacts the clinical outcomes of patients with DM or hyperglycemia. It is imperative that members of the healthcare team are diligent in the assessment, intervention, and evaluation of all variables that affect serum glucose concentrations in an effort to achieve optimal glycemic control.

REFERENCES

1. American Diabetes Association. (2005). Standards of medical care in diabetes. *Diabetes Care, 28*(suppl 1), S4–S36.
2. American Diabetes Association. (2005). Diagnosis and classification of diabetes mellitus. *Diabetes Care, 28*(suppl 1), S37–S42.
3. American Diabetes Association. (2001). Postprandial blood glucose. *Diabetes Spectrum, 14*, 71–74.
4. American Diabetes Association. (2004). Insulin administration. *Diabetes Care, 27*(suppl 1), S105–S109.
5. American Diabetes Association. (2004). Prevention or delay of type 2 diabetes. *Diabetes Care, 27*(suppl 1), S47–S54.
6. American Diabetes Association. (2004). Hyperglycemic crises in diabetes. *Diabetes Care, 27*(suppl 1), S94–S102.
7. American Diabetes Association. (2004). Hospital admission guidelines for diabetes. *Diabetes Care, 27*(suppl 1), S103.
8. American Diabetes Association. (2004). Nutrition principles and recommendations in diabetes. *Diabetes Care, 27*(suppl 1), S36–S46.
9. American Diabetes Association. (2004). Economic costs of diabetes in the U.S. in 2002. *Diabetes Care, 26*(3), 917–932.
10. American Diabetes Association. (2002). *National fact sheet.*
11. American Diabetes Association. (2005). *Diabetes facts.*
12. American Diabetes Association Workgroup on Hypoglycemia. (2005). Defining and reporting hypoglycemia in diabetes. *Diabetes Care, 28*(5), 1245–1249.
13. American College of Endocrinology. (2004). Position statement on inpatient diabetes and metabolic control. *Endocr Pract, 10*(1), 77–82.
14. Amylin Pharmaceuticals, Inc. (1998). Beta-cell dysfunction in diabetes: the roles of amylin and insulin. *Monograph*, 1–24.
15. Aviles-Santa, L., & Raskin, P. (1998). Surgery and anesthesia. In H. Lebovitz (Ed.), *Therapy for diabetes mellitus and related disorders* (3rd ed.). Alexandria, Va: The American Diabetes Association.
16. Baldwin, D., et al. (2005). Eliminating inpatient sliding scale insulin: a reeducation project with medical house staff. *Diabetes Care, 28*(5), 1008–1011.
17. Bode, B. Ed. (2004). *Medical management of type 1 diabetes*, (4th ed.), Alexandria, Va: American Diabetes Association.
18. Capes, S. E., Malmberg, K., & Gerstein, H. C. (2000). Stress hyperglycemia and increased risk of death after myocardial infarction in patients with and without diabetes: a systematic overview. *Lancet, 355*, 773–778.
19. Capes, S. E., et al. (2001). Stress hyperglycemia and prognosis of stroke in nondiabetic and diabetic patients: a systematic overview. *Stroke, 32*, 2426–2432.
20. Chaudhuri, A. (2002). Vascular reactivity in diabetes mellitus. *Curr Diab Rep, 2*, 305–310.
21. Clement, S., et al. (2004). Management of diabetes and hyperglycemia in hospitals. *Diabetes Care, 27*(2), 553–591.
22. Coursin, D. B. (2004). Perioperative diabetic and hyperglycemic management issues. *Crit Care Med, 32*(suppl 1), S116–S125.
23. CREATE-ECLA Trial Group Investigators. (2005). Effect of glucose-insulin-potassium infusion on mortality in patients with acute ST-segment elevation myocardial infarction. *JAMA, 293*(4), 437–446.
24. Cryer, P. E. (2002). Negotiating the barrier of hypoglycemia in diabetes. *Diabetes Spectrum, 15*, 20–27.
25. Cryer, P. E. (2003). Hypoglycemia in diabetes. *Diabetes Care, 26*, 1902–1912.
26. Dagogo-Jack, S., George, M., Alberti, D., et al. (2002). Management of diabetes mellitus in surgical patients. *Diabetes Spectrum, 15*(1), 44–48.
27. Dandona, P. (2002). Endothelium, inflammation, and diabetes. *Curr Diab Rep, 2*, 311–315.
28. Department of Health and Human Services, Centers for Disease Control and Prevention. (2003). *National diabetes fact sheet.*
29. Department of Health and Human Services, Centers for Disease Control and Prevention. (2005). *National diabetes fact sheet.*
30. Department of Health and Human Services, Centers for Disease Control and Prevention. (2003). *National hospital discharge survey database, 2000.*
31. Diabetes Control and Complications Trial Research Group. (1993). The effect of intensive treatment of diabetes on the development and progression of long-term complications in insulin-dependent diabetes mellitus. *N Engl J Med, 329*, 977–986.
32. DiMario et al. (2001). Autoimmune diabetes not requiring insulin at diagnosis (latent autoimmune diabetes of the adult). *Diabetes Care, 24*(8), 1460–1467.
33. Drucker, D. (2005). Incretin mimetics in the treatment of type 2 diabetes. *CADRE Curr Diab Prac, 4*(1), 1–3.
34. Finney, S. J. (2003). Glucose control and mortality in critically ill patients. *JAMA, 290*, 2041–2047.
35. Franz, M., Ed. (2003). *A core curriculum for diabetes education, diabetes management therapies.* Chicago, Ill: The American Association of Diabetes Educators.
36. Freeland, B. S. (2003). Diabetic ketoacidosis. *Diabetes Educator, 29* (1), 384–395.
37. Furnary, A. P. (1999). Continuous intravenous insulin infusion reduces the incidence of deep sternal wound infection in diabetic patients after cardiac surgical procedures. *Ann Thoracic Surg, 67*, 353–362.
38. Furnary, A. P., et al. (2003). Continuous insulin infusion reduces mortality in patients with diabetes undergoing coronary artery bypass grafting. *J Thoracic Cardiovasc Surg, 125*, 1007–1021.
39. Goldberg, P., Roussel, M., & Inzucchi, S. (2005). Clinical results of an updated insulin infusion protocol in critically ill patients. *Diabetes Spectrum, 18*(1), 188–191.
40. Golden, S. H., et al. (1999). Perioperative glycemic control and the risk of infectious complications in a cohort of adults with diabetes. *Diabetes Care, 22*, 1408–1414.
41. Havel, P. J. (2004). A scientific review: the role of chromium in insulin resistance. *Diabetes Educator, Suppl 2004*, 2–14.
42. Hirsch, I. (2002). *Insulin in the hospital setting.* New York: Adelphi.
43. Hirsch, I., Braithwaite, S., & Verderese, C. (2005). *Practical management of inpatient hyperglycemia.* Lakeville, Conn: Hilliard Publishing.
44. Hirsch, I. (2003). The burden of diabetes. *Diabetes Care, 26*, 1613–1614.
45. Kaufman, F. (2005). *Diabesity: the obesity-diabetes epidemic threatens America and what we must do to stop it.* New York: Bantam Dell.
46. Levetan, C. S. (2000). Hospital management of diabetes. *Endocrinol Metab Clin North Am, 29*, 745–770.
47. Levetan, C. S., et al. (1998). Unrecognized diabetes among hospitalized patients. *Diabetes Care, 21*, 246–249.
48. Levetan, C. S. (1995). Impact of endocrine and diabetes team consultation on hospital length of stay for patients with diabetes. *Am J Med, 99*, 22–28.
49. Malmberg, K., et al. (1997). Prospective randomized study of intensive insulin treatment on long-term survival after acute myocardial infarction in patients with diabetes (DIGAMI study). *Brit Med J, 314*, 1512–1515.
50. Malmberg, K., et al. (1999). Glycometabolic state at admission: important risk marker of mortality in conventionally treated patients with diabetes mellitus acute myocardial infarction. *Circulation, 99*(20), 2626–2632.
51. Malmberg, K., et al. (1995). Randomized trial of insulin-glucose infusion followed by subcutaneous insulin treatment in diabetic

patients with acute myocardial infarction (DIGAMI study): effects on mortality at 1 year. *J Am Coll Cardiol, 26,* 57–65.

52. McGuire, D., et al. (2004). Association of diabetes mellitus and glycemic control strategies with clinical outcomes after acute coronary syndromes. *Am Heart J, 147*(2), 246–252.

53. Mokdad, A., et al. (1999). The spread of the obesity epidemic in the United States, 1991–1998. *JAMA, 282,* 1519–1522.

54. Najarian, J., et al. (2005). Improving outcomes for diabetic patients undergoing vascular surgery. *Diabetes Spectrum, 18*(1), 53–60.

55. Niewoehner, C., Ed. (1998). *Endocrine pathophysiology,* (Chapter 8: Pancreatic islet hormones, diabetes mellitus and hypoglycemia). Madison, Conn: Fence Creek Publishing.

56. Port, S., et al. (2005). Blood glucose: a strong risk factor for mortality in nondiabetic patients with cardiovascular disease. *Am Heart J, 149*(8), 209–214.

57. Swift, C., & Boucher, J. (2005). Nutrition care for hospitalized individuals with diabetes. *Diabetes Spectrum, 18*(1), 31–38.

58. Thompson, C., et al. (2005). Hyperglycemia in the hospital. *Diabetes Spectrum, 18*(1), 20–27.

59. Tomky, D. (2005). Detection, prevention, and treatment of hypoglycemia in the hospital. *Diabetes Spectrum, 18*(1), 39–43.

60. Trovati, M., & Anfossi, G. (2002). Mechanisms involved in platelet hyperactivation and platelet-endothelium interrelationships in diabetes mellitus. *Curr Diab Rep, 2,* 316–322.

61. Trence, D. L. (2003). The rationale and management of hyperglycemia for inpatients with cardiovascular disease: time for change. *J Clin Endocrinol Metab, 88,* 2430–2437.

62. United Kingdom Prospective Diabetes Study Group (UKPDS). (1998). Intensive blood glucose control with sulfonylureas or insulin compared with conventional treatment and risk of complications in patients with type 2 diabetes. *Lancet, 352,* 837–853.

63. United Kingdom Prospective Diabetes Study Group (UKPDS). (1998). Intensive blood glucose control with metformin on complications in overweight patients with type 2 diabetes. *Lancet, 352,* 854–865.

64. Van den Berghe, G., et al. (2001). Intensive insulin therapy in critically ill patients. *N Engl J Med, 345,* 1359–1367.

65. Van den Berghe, G., et al. (2003). Outcome benefit of intensive insulin therapy in the critically ill: insulin dose versus glycemic control. *Crit Care Med, 31*(2), 359–366.

66. Umpierrez, G. (2002). Diabetic ketoacidosis and hyperglycemic hyperosmolar syndrome. *Diabetes Spectrum, 15,* 28–36.

67. Umpierrez, G., et al. (2002). Hyperglycemia: an independent marker of in-hospital mortality in patients with undiagnosed diabetes. *J Clin Endocrinol Metab, 87*(3), 978–982.

68. Yassin, A. S., et al. (2002). Disability and its economic impact among adults with diabetes. *J Occup Environ Med, 44,* 136–142.

69. Zhang, M. M., et al. (2004). Application of economic analysis to diabetes and diabetes care. *Ann Intern Med, 140*(11), 972–977.

70. Zerr, K. J., et al. (1997). Glucose control lowers the risk of wound infection in diabetics after open heart operations. *Ann Thoracic Surg, 63,* 356–361.

CHAPTER 35 Pituitary, Thyroid, and Adrenal Disorders

Diane Byrum and Peggy L. Kirkwood

Almost every cell and organ in the body is influenced by the endocrine system, which plays a vital role in maintaining homeostasis. Hormones are chemical substances released from endocrine glands that transfer information and instructions regulating the function of the specific target gland or tissue. Hormones are secreted in minimal amounts in response to a need, producing either a local or a global effect (e.g., cortisol affects every cell in the body).[14] To serve as a reservoir for acute changes,[14] many hormones are transported in the vascular system bound to plasma proteins. Although many different hormones circulate throughout the bloodstream, each one affects only the cells that are genetically programmed to receive and respond to its message. Hormone levels are influenced by factors such as stress, infection, and changes in fluid balance.[7,10,14]

The endocrine system is regulated by feedback in much the same way that a thermostat regulates the temperature in a room. For instance, when a signal is sent from the hypothalamus to the pituitary gland in the form of a "releasing hormone," the pituitary gland secretes a "stimulating (or tropic) hormone" into the circulation. The tropic hormone signals the target gland to secrete its own specific hormone. As the level of hormone rises in the circulation, the hypothalamus and pituitary gland stop the secretion of releasing and stimulating hormones. This slows secretion from the target gland. Hormones maintain homeostatic balance as a result of this interactive negative feedback system, which utilizes other hormones, blood, chemicals, and the nervous system (Figure 35-1).[14]

When the endocrine system is out of control, many local and systemic responses can be manifested as changes in energy metabolism, fluid and electrolyte imbalances, and disruption of homeostasis. Many common disorders are either deficiencies or excesses of hormones. Excesses or deficiencies are either primary (related to the target gland or organ response to the hormone) or secondary (related to defects in secretion of the releasing/inhibiting hormone or tropic hormone).[7,58] However, hormone-resistant states and iatrogenic causes also play a role in endocrine disorders.[10,11] Additionally, aging can lead to endocrine function

abnormalities, including changes in levels of hormones secreted, response by the target gland or organ, metabolism of the hormone, or decreased biological activity (Figure 35-2).[29] Understanding and integrating knowledge of the endocrine system's intricate relationship to all cells will help critical care nurses make clinical decisions related to the care of patients with endocrine disorders.[2,29,52,55,62]

APPLIED PATHOPHYSIOLOGY

Via the autonomic nervous system, the sympathetic nervous system and endocrine system are coordinated through activities of the anterior hypothalamus, the anterior and posterior pituitary glands, the thyroid gland, and the adrenal medulla and cortex (Figure 35-3). As a starting place to understand the outcomes of stimulation of these various organs, the hypothalamus is connected to the posterior pituitary via nerve tracts. Of interest to critical care clinicians, antidiuretic hormone (ADH) [arginine vasopressin (AVP)] is produced and stored in the hypothalamus but is released by the posterior pituitary in response to increases in serum osmolality (greater than 290 mOsm/L), thirst, or decreases in the circulating volume.[33] ADH regulates the amount of body water through its action on the distal tubules and collecting ducts of the nephron, normally impermeable to water.[11,14,26,52] The actions of ADH occur in the cortical and medullary collecting ducts of the kidney through the vasopressin receptor V2. AVP binds to V2 receptors and mediates the antidiuretic response by activating aquaporin 2 (AQP2) water channels. Activation of AQP2 results in increased permeability of this normally water-tight membrane. Driven by the osmotic gradient of sodium, water is reabsorbed into the vascular bed, producing concentrated urine.[30,33] In response to decreasing osmolality (less than 275 mOsm/L), via the negative feedback loop, the release of ADH is inhibited.[33] In addition, stimulation or inhibition of ADH is impacted by a number of medications and situations commonly seen in critical care.[11,14]

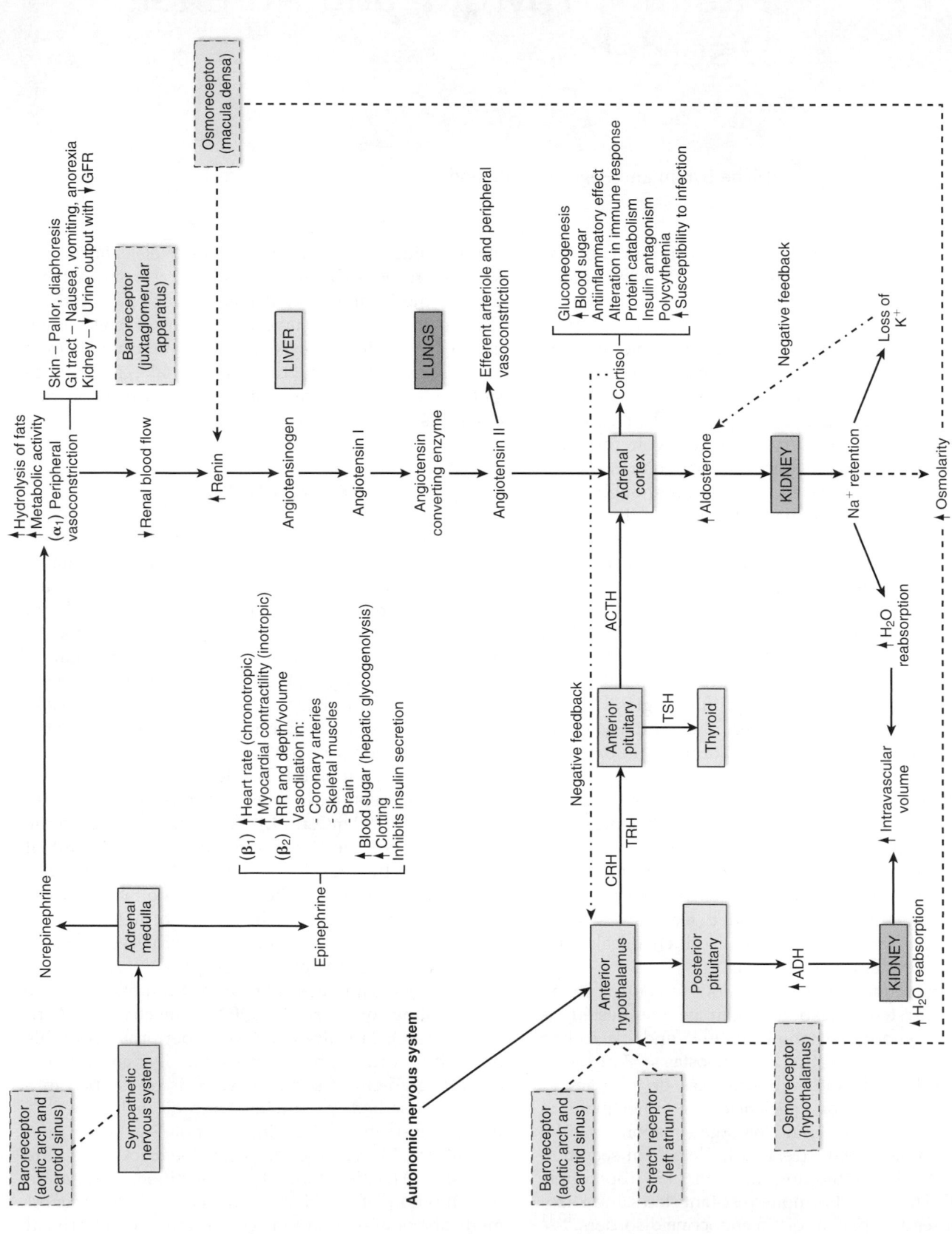

◆FIGURE 35-1 Hormonal maintenance of homeostasis. α = Alpha, ACTH = adrenocorticotropic hormone, β = beta, CRH = corticotropin-releasing hormone, GFR = glomerular filtration rate, K⁺ = potassium, Na⁺ = sodium, TRH = thyroid-releasing hormone, TSH = thyroid-stimulating hormone.

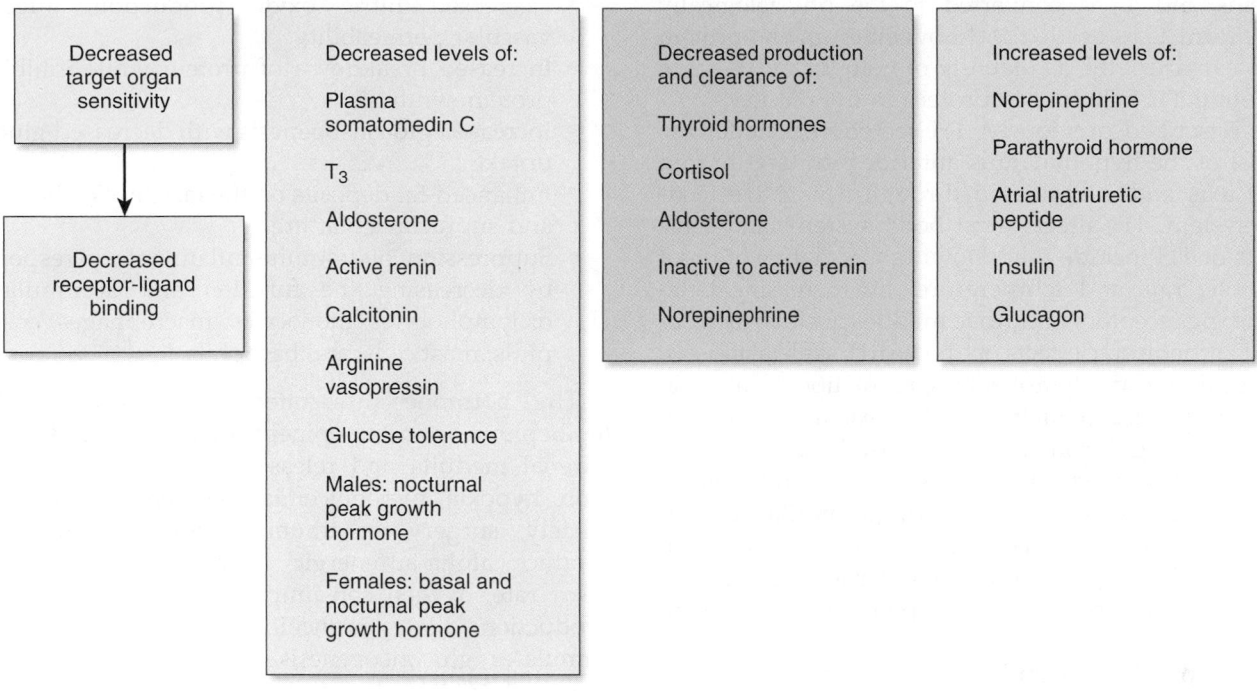

✦FIGURE 35-2 Changes in the endocrine system associated with aging.

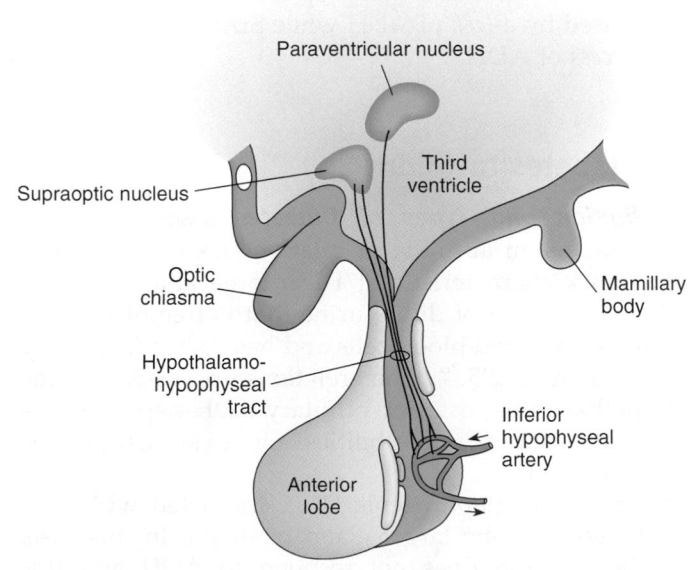

✦FIGURE 35-3 Mechanisms of endocrine control: Hypothalamus connection and influence of posterior pituitary.

The hypothalamus is connected to the anterior pituitary through a capillary system that allows secretion of thyrotropin-releasing hormone (TRH) directly into the blood supply to the anterior pituitary. TRH, a releasing factor, is synthesized and stored in the hypothalamus and is secreted in response to decreased levels of T_4 (thyroxine) or T_3 (triiodothyronine), exposure to cold, catecholamines, and arginine vasopressin release.[24] The response to TRH release is bimodal: first, it stimulates the anterior pituitary gland to release thyrotropin-stimulating hormone (TSH); and second, it increases hormone synthesis.[24] TRH and TSH release is inhibited by increased T_3 and T_4 levels, glucocorticoids, chronic illness, somatostatin, and pituitary tumors.[24,31]

Both T_3 and T_4 contain 59% to 65% of the iodine in the body.[24] In order for T_3 and T_4 to be synthesized by the follicular cells of the thyroid gland, iodide must be oxidized into iodine; therefore the ability of the thyroid gland to autoregulate is directly influenced by the availability of iodide.[24] Ninety percent of total thyroid hormone (TH) is the physiologically inactive form T_4 and 10% is the physiologically active form T_3. Once secreted into the bloodstream, T_3 and T_4 are bound to proteins and T_4 is converted to the physiologically active form T_3 as needed.[24,31] Low albumin and protein levels can affect the availability of both T_4 and T_3 since 99% of all TH is bound to protein in the plasma.[43]

As described previously, TH secretion is under the control of the hypothalamus-anterior pituitary-thyroid gland axis and is regulated through a negative feedback system. TH affects most body systems and cells. Effects of TH include the following: regulation of basal metabolic rate and temperature, by increasing beta-adrenergic receptors in cardiac muscle (positive inotropic and chronotropic effects on the heart), skeletal muscle, adipose tissue, and lymphocytes; regulation of catecholamine sensitivity; regulation of hypoxic and hypercapnic drive; regulation of the 2,3-diphosphoglycerate content in red blood cells, which assists with release of oxygen to the tissues; regulation of gut motility; regulation of bone turnover; regulation of muscle contraction and relaxation; regulation of cholesterol synthesis; and regulation of hormone and pharmacologic agent turnover.[24]

The two adrenal glands sit atop each kidney. Each gland consists of two distinct areas: the cortex or outer layer and the medulla or inner layer.[8,9,20] The adrenal medulla secretes catecholamines (epinephrine and norepinephrine), which stimulate the sympathetic nervous system alpha and beta receptors. The adrenal cortex secretes glucocorticoids, such as cortisol, in response to adrenocorticotropic hormone (ACTH).[10,14] In addition, mineralocorticoids (e.g., aldosterone) are also secreted indirectly from the adrenal cortex in response to increased potassium levels, activation of the renin-angiotensin system, or decreased plasma volume.[8,20]

The adrenal glands are under the control of the hypothalamus-anterior pituitary axis and the sympathetic nervous system. The body sends a signal to the hypothalamus via the central nervous system in response to a stressor such as pain, hypotension, hypoglycemia, hypoxemia, trauma, or cytokine discharge.[38,39,54] Based on the interpretation of this message by the hypothalamus, corticotropin-releasing hormone (CRH) is either secreted or inhibited. If secreted, CRH travels to the anterior pituitary via the rich blood supply connection, where ACTH is secreted. ACTH travels to the adrenal gland, where it acts to secrete cortisol directly or aldosterone indirectly. When glucocorticoids are released from the cortex, the following actions occur:

- Increased sodium/water retention with potassium excretion
- Synthesis of sodium-potassium-adenosine triphosphatase, which effects synthesis of catecholamines and catecholamine receptors, producing a positive inotropic effect

- Decreased nitric oxide production, affecting vascular permeability
- Increased breakdown of protein while inhibiting protein synthesis
- Increased gluconeogenesis with decreased glucose uptake
- Enhanced fat deposits on the face, neck, abdomen, and supraclavicular area
- Suppression of immune-inflammatory responses by decreasing the function and accumulation of lymphocytes, monocytes, macrophages, eosinophils, mast cells, and basophils.[5,39,40,54]

The hormones associated with fight or flight (epinephrine and norepinephrine) are stored in the adrenal medulla and released in response to stress, pain, hypoxia, hypoglycemia, hypotension, fluid loss, anxiety, surgery, or trauma. These catecholamines produce alpha-adrenergic activity, which increases heart rate, oxygen consumption, and carbon dioxide production; dilates bronchioles; slows digestion; and stimulates gluconeogenesis and lipolysis as energy sources.[9,14,29,32,62] In response to increased serum cortisol levels, the hypothalamus inhibits CRH from being released and the negative feedback mechanism is able to keep cortisol levels within a narrow range.[8,9,32,52]

DISORDERS OF ANTIDIURETIC HORMONE

There are two disorders of ADH: diabetes insipidus (DI) and syndrome of inappropriate ADH (SIADH). DI is caused by a *lack* of ADH while SIADH is caused by an *excess* of ADH.

Diabetes Insipidus

Definition and Types of Diabetes Insipidus. DI is defined as an absolute or relative lack of ADH. The hallmark characteristic of DI is large amounts (2 to 20 liters a day) of dilute urine that is free of protein, glucose, and red blood cells and has a specific gravity less than 1.005.[26] The relationship between the hypothalamus-posterior pituitary-ADH-nephron axis presents several possibilities for dysfunction (see Figure 35-2):

- Primary or nephrogenic DI is associated with dysfunction of the target gland or organ. In this case, the nephron does not respond to ADH and this results in an inability to concentrate urine. Nephrogenic DI is usually due to chronic renal disease, hypokalemia, hypercalcemia, and medications such as lithium and demeclocycline (Declomycin), as well as disease processes that damage the interstitium of the nephron.[3,14] In nephrogenic DI, levels of circulating AVP can be either normal or increased.

- Neurogenic (central) DI results from a lack of production of ADH in the hypothalamus, an inability to store ADH in the pituitary, or a malfunction of the osmoreceptors. This type is known as secondary DI or hypothalamic-pituitary dysfunction. Neurogenic DI is distinguished from other causes of DI by decreased levels of plasma AVP.[3,14]

- Psychogenic DI is an obsessive-compulsive disorder in which the patient ingests large amounts of water, thereby essentially turning off ADH secretion.[31]

- Gestagenic DI occurs during pregnancy. This form of DI leads to an increased breakdown of AVP related to increased levels of circulating vasopressinase, an enzyme responsible for the breakdown of AVP.[63]

Patients at Risk. Neurogenic DI is the most common dysfunction seen in patients with damage to the hypothalamus/posterior pituitary area as a result of head trauma or neurosurgery.[1,7,14] If only the posterior pituitary is damaged, ADH can still be manufactured and secreted from the hypothalamus.[7,14] Typically, the presentation for central DI is triphasic:

- Phase 1, the polyuric phase, is a transient form of DI. Polyuria lasts 4 to 5 days; there is total lack of AVP.
- Phase 2, the antidiuretic phase, is 5 to 6 days of normal ADH release from stored ADH in the hypothalamus.
- Phase 3, the permanent phase, is when polyuria resumes after the storage of ADH is exhausted.[1]

Approximately 20% of all DI is related to non–tumor-related brain surgery, 9% is related to removal or manipulation of the pituitary gland, 16% is related to traumatic brain injury (TBI), 25% is related to removal of brain tumors, and 30% is idiopathic.[10] In addition, certain drugs, such as alcohol, phenytoin (Dilantin), and alpha-adrenergic agents, can inhibit the secretion of AVP. Additionally, since many surgical, trauma, or critically ill patients are being sedated or mechanically ventilated, limiting their natural ability to ingest water, prompt diagnosis and treatment of DI is imperative to prevent severe dehydration and cardiovascular collapse.[7,14,58] Mortality is rare as long as prompt diagnosis is made and free water is replaced.

Clinical Presentation. The clinical presentation of DI consists of copious amounts (2 to 20 L per day) of dilute, colorless urine with urine osmolality 50 to 100 mOsm/L, specific gravity 1.005 or less, and urine output greater than 200 ml/hour for 2 consecutive hours in a patient with known risk factors.[26] Plasma osmolality will be greater than 285 mOsm/L and serum sodium level will be greater than 147 mEq/L related to loss of free water, while retaining sodium.[1] In addition, signs and symptoms of hypovolemia and dehydration will be present such as tachycardia, hypotension, and increased blood urea nitrogen (BUN) and creatinine levels.[14,58]

Diagnostic Evaluation. To diagnose DI, specific laboratory tests should include serum and urine osmolality, serum ADH levels, serum sodium level, and urine specific gravity. There are two diagnostic tests that differentiate neurogenic from nephrogenic DI.[4,7] The water deprivation test can be used in a non-critically ill patient to differentiate AVP deficiency from other types of polyuria. However, because this test can take up to 18 hours to complete, it is rarely used for critically ill patients.[3,7]

The most definitive test is a vasopressin replacement test, which replaces aqueous vasopressin either nasally, IV, or intramuscularly. Measurements of urinary output and urine osmolality are collected before exogenous vasopressin replacement. The urinary output and urine osmolality are measured every 30 minutes for 2 hours. Neurogenic DI is diagnosed if urine output and osmolality decrease after administration of exogenous vasopressin, signaling a problem with the hypothalamus-pituitary axis (HPA). Nephrogenic DI is diagnosed when there is no decrease in urine output and osmolality following administration of exogenous vasopressin, signaling a decreased response in the collecting duct of the kidney tubules.[4,7,10,18]

Multidisciplinary Plan of Care. Collaborative management of the patient with DI should include rehydration with hypotonic (0.45% normal saline) solutions to replace free water, as outlined in the Medication table on p. 944. Exogenous vasopressin replacement should be administered to prevent dehydration and hypovolemic shock. As summarized in the Multidisciplinary Plan of Care on pp. 944-945, patients with DI should have continuous monitoring of intake and output, weight, and vital signs, as well as monitoring of laboratory values such as serum sodium, serum osmolality, and urine specific gravity. DI can transiently resolve only to reappear or become permanent.[1,4,7,14]

MEDICATIONS USED IN DIABETES INSIPIDUS AND SYNDROME OF INAPPROPRIATE ANTIDIURETIC HORMONE

MEDICATIONS	ACTIONS	DOSAGES	SPECIAL CONSIDERATIONS
Diabetes Insipidus			
Desmopressin (DDAVP) (Neurogenic DI)	Acts on renal tubules to promote sodium and water reabsorption[58]	Nasal: 0.1–0.4 ml metered dose or calibrated plastic catheter 5–20 mcg (0.05–0.2 ml) IV or subcutaneously: 0.5–1 ml daily divided doses PO: 0.05 to 0.8 mg daily in divided doses	Lithium and demeclocycline diminish ADH effects while fludrocortisone and glucocorticoid steroids enhance ADH response[18,26,47]
Vasopressin (Neurogenic DI)	Acts on renal tubules to promote sodium and water reabsorption	IM/subcutaneously: 5–10 units 2–4 times/day as needed IM/subcutaneously: 2.5–5 units every 2–3 days for chronic therapy	Hypersensitivity Anaphylaxis
Lypressin (Neurogenic DI)	Acts on renal tubules to promote sodium and water reabsorption[58]	Nasal: 5–20 units 3 or 7 times per day	Titrate to urinary output
SIADH			
Demeclocycline (Declomycin) (Nephrogenic)	Interferes with action of ADH renal collecting duct[46,58]	150 mg PO 4 times a day or 300 mg twice a day	Effect may take 1 week (not indicated in emergency management) Hypersensitivity to tetracyclines Nephrotoxic—monitor BUN/creatinine[3,17] May cause photosensitivity
Furosemide (Lasix) (Nephrogenic)	Elicits a loss of free water by inhibition of sodium and chloride reabsorption in ascending loop of Henle and distal tubule	40 mg IV initially—may increase to 80 mg IV if insufficient response	Ototoxicity, photosensitivity

Data from references 3, 4, 14, 17, 18, 26, 46, 47, 58.
ADH = Antidiuretic hormone, BUN = blood urea nitrogen, DI = diabetes insipidus, SIADH = syndrome of inappropriate antidiuretic hormone.

MULTIDISCIPLINARY PLAN OF CARE FOR THE PATIENT WITH DIABETES INSIPIDUS

PROBLEM	INTERVENTION	RATIONALE	EXPECTED OUTCOME	SPECIAL CONSIDERATIONS
Risk for development of DI	Careful consideration of patients who present with: *Neurogenic* • Traumatic brain injury • Brain tumors • Hypophysectomy • Aneurysms	Early identification of patients allows for appropriate prophylactic intervention, especially in preparation for diagnostic testing or surgery.	Patients at risk for DI will be identified early.	With severe TBI, the incidence of DI increases related to increased edema and pressure on hypothalamus-pituitary. Patients with

PROBLEM	INTERVENTION	RATIONALE	EXPECTED OUTCOME	SPECIAL CONSIDERATIONS
	• Thrombus • Neurologic infection • Metastatic tumors: breast, lung, leukemia *Nephrogenic* • Chronic renal failure • Hypokalemia or hypercalcemia • Medications (lithium, demeclocycline, clonidine) • Infiltrative/inflammatory renal disease			hypophysectomy require life-long ADH replacement. Patient and family education is necessary as well as Medic-Alert bracelet.[1,14,26] Nephrogenic DI is primarily related to end-stage renal disease; prognosis is poor.
Assess for signs and symptoms of hypotension	Monitor vital signs, hemodynamic parameters, and ADH secretion/response: • BP, MAP, HR • CVP, PAP, PAWP, SVR • Urine output • Urine specific gravity • BUN • Creatinine • Urine sodium • Urine osmolality • Serum osmolality • Serum sodium • Electrolytes • Serum ADH	Monitor for 7–10 days postneurosurgical procedures/traumatic brain injury because DI can appear to resolve, then reappear.[1,2]	Early/late changes in ADH secretion and renal response to ADH will be identified.	Fluid status is monitored most accurately using hemodynamic monitoring with a pulmonary artery or central venous pressure catheter.
Fluid volume deficit related to DI	ADH and hypotonic water replacement See Medication table (p. 944) Hypotonic water replacement 0.45% NS to replace urinary output; replace urinary output ml for ml [58]	Aqueous vasopressin assists to decrease free water elimination. Hypotonic solutions replace free water to prevent hypovolemia and dehydration.[63,64]	Patient will exhibit: • Decreased serum osmolality • Decreased serum sodium • Increased urine osmolality • Decreased urine output • Tachycardia/hypotension resolved • PAWP/CVP within normal limits	Replacement dose is based on severity of DI. Adverse effects include headache, nausea, diarrhea, and edema. Can precipitate chest pain. Effects decreased by lithium, alcohol, Declomycin, heparin, and large amounts of epinephrine.
Free water deficit as a result of insufficient ADH and polyuria	Replace free water (see above) Low sodium and protein diet/tube feedings (see Nutrition box on p. 947)	Sodium adds to hypernatremia, increasing osmolality. Protein breakdown adds to osmolality.[58]	Water deficit resolves.	

Data from references 1, 2, 4, 14, 26, 30, 58, 63, 64.
ADH = Antidiuretic hormone, BP = blood pressure, BUN = blood urea nitrogen, CVP = central venous pressure, DI = diabetes insipidus, HR = heart rate, MAP = mean arterial pressure, NS = normal sodium, PAP = pulmonary artery pressure, PAWP = pulmonary artery wedge pressure, SVR = systemic vascular resistance, TBI = traumatic brain injury.

◆ Case Study 35-1

Diabetes Insipidus

L.C., a 19-year-old female, arrives in the emergency department following a motor vehicle accident in which her car ran down a 20-foot embankment. She was awake at the scene with a strong odor of alcohol present. She was not wearing a seat belt and was thrown from the driver's seat into the passenger's seat, striking her head.

Paramedics noted a large laceration above her right eyebrow with blood present in her nose and ear. Two large-bore IVs were started with 9% normal saline (NS) infusing at 100 ml/hr, and spinal precautions were instituted. Her Glasgow Coma Scale (GCS) score on the scene as well as en route was 10–12, but she became progressively more combative.

On arrival to the emergency department her assessment shows the following: GCS = 6; blood pressure (BP) = 90/50 mm Hg; heart rate (HR) = 128 beats/min; shallow respirations; lacerations and bruising to her flank, mid-back area, sternum, chest, and ribs. CT scan reveals a depressed skull fracture in the right temporal area, several small hematomas, multiple rib fractures, and pulmonary and renal contusions on the right. The decision is made to intubate and she is placed on fraction of inspired oxygen (FiO_2) = 40%, synchronized intermittent mandatory ventilation (SIMV) = 15. She is transferred to a critical care bed.

Decision point: What are L.C.'s risk factor(s) for the development of DI?

Upon arrival to the critical care unit, BP remains 80–90 mm Hg systolic despite 6 L of 0.9% NS. Pulse rate ranges from 112 to 130 beats/min and the GCS is 6–8.

Laboratory Values

CBC	Chemistries	Other
Hgb 18 g/dl	Na^+ 140 mEq/L	Blood alcohol greater
Hct 43%	K^+ 4.9 mEq/L	than 100 mg/dl
WBC	Cl^- 98 mEq/L	Lactate level 1.1 mmol/L
10,000/μl	HCO_3^- 24 mEq/L	Base deficit 8 mmol/L
Platelets	BUN 18 mg/dl	Plasma osmolality
198,000/μl	Creatinine	280 mOsm/L
	0.7 mg/dl	Urine specific gravity
	Total calcium	1.025
	9 mg/dl	Urine osmolality
	Mg^{++} 1.5 mEq/L	654 mOsm/L
	PO_4^{2-} 4 mg/dl	Urinalysis: moderate
		amount of RBCs
		ABGs: pH 7.48, $PaCO_2$
		35 mm Hg, PaO_2 95
		mm Hg, HCO_3^- 24 mEq/L,
		O_2 saturation 95%

Urine output during the first 6 hours was the following: 11 PM = 90 ml; 12 PM = 120 ml; 1 AM = 190 ml; 2 AM = 280 ml; 3 AM = 430 ml; 4 AM = 580 ml. L.C. has repeat diagnostic laboratory values for the following: serum Na^+ = 150 mEq/L, plasma osmolality = 307 mOsm/L, urine specific gravity = 1.005, Hct = 35%, Hgb = 12 mg/dl, lactate level = 4 mmol/L, base deficit = 4 mmol/L. ABGs: pH = 7.28, $PaCO_2$ = 49 mm Hg, PaO_2 = 89 mm Hg, HCO_3^- = 18 mEq/L, O_2 saturation = 88%.

At 3 AM the physician orders vasopressin 0.25 ml four times a day, change IV fluids to 0.45% NS, replacing urine output ml for ml, and serum sodium, serum osmolality every day for 3 days.

Decision point: Explain the results of the initial CBC, chemistries, and other tests.

Decision point: Explain the laboratory values 6 hours after admission to critical care.

Decision point: Explain the physician's orders.

L.C.'s Hct and Hgb stabilized. Within the next 2 days, her serum Na^+, serum osmolality, and specific gravity and urine output returned to normal. She developed acute respiratory distress syndrome related to rib fractures and lung contusion, which resolved by hospital day 10. L.C. experienced no other episodes of DI.

ABGs = Arterial blood gases, BUN = blood urea nitrogen, Cl^- = chloride, HCO_3^- = bicarbonate, Hct = hematocrit, Hgb = hemoglobin, K^+ = potassium, Na^+ = sodium, Mg^{++} = magnesium, O_2 = oxygen, PaO_2 = partial pressure of arterial oxygen tension, $PaCO_2$ = partial pressure of arterial carbon dioxide, PO_4^{2-} = phosphate, RBC = red blood cells.

Syndrome of Inappropriate Antidiuretic Hormone

Definition and Types of Syndrome of Inappropriate Antidiuretic Hormone. SIADH is defined as inappropriate retention of free water leading to dilutional hyponatremia related to excess ADH.[3,64] The patient retains excess water in relationship to sodium. Serum sodium level is less than 134 mEq/L, and serum osmolality is less than 275 mOsm/L. Urine osmolality increases, with urine sodium levels greater than 40 mmol/L and urine specific gravity 1.030.[46,47] The increased intravascular fluid leads to an increase in the glomerular filtration rate and increased atrial natriuretic peptide release, contributing to the excretion of sodium.[7] Occasionally, the excess water accumulates in the intracellular space rather than the intravascular space, causing some patients to remain euvolemic or become only slightly volume-overloaded.[46,47]

Other underlying disease processes causing hyponatremia must be ruled out before SIADH can be confirmed. Adrenal insufficiency and hypothyroidism should be assessed with measurements of random serum cortisol and thyroid-stimulating hormone (TSH) levels.[26,64] In addition, nephrotic syndrome, acute renal failure, hepatic failure, and cardiac failure should be eliminated as possible diagnoses; all of these can lead to hyponatremia and increased extracellular fluid volume.[64]

SIADH can manifest as four osmoregulatory defects:

- Type A SIADH (approximately 20% of all cases) is caused by a (malignant or nonmalignant) tumor that secretes erratic amounts of ADH-like substances.[7,10,31,58]
- Type B SIADH (approximately 35% of all cases) results from reset osmostat occurring in chronic debilitating illness, such as encephalitis, HIV, malnutrition, quadriplegia, and psychosis, as well as in pregnancy.[46,47,58] The osmoreceptors are reset to secrete ADH at lower serum osmolalities (250 to 260 mOsm/L)[64] or the osmoreceptors are overly sensitive to serum osmolality changes.[7,58]
- Type C SIADH (approximately 35% of all cases) is associated with temporary dysfunction of the osmoreceptors, which causes ADH to leak, and selective loss of suppression causes continued secretion even though osmolality is low.[46,47,58]
- Type D SIADH (approximately 10% of all cases) is related to increased sensitivity of ADH in the nephron.[7,58]

Patients at Risk. Patients presenting with neurologic trauma, hemorrhage, meningitis, encephalitis, and neurologic effects of alcohol withdrawal are at risk for the development of SIADH.[17,42,58] In addition, oat cell or small cell carcinomas of the lung produce a paraneoplastic syndrome in which ADH-like substances are found in the tumor cells. These ADH-like substances have the ability to synthesize, store, and secrete ADH and are found in 60% of patients with small cell carcinomas.[42] Slow tumor growth over time can lead to a gradual increase in water retention and hyponatremia.[42] In addition, other tumors of the duodenum, pancreas, brain, prostate, and thymus, as well as leukemia, lymphoma, and Hodgkin's disease, can produce ADH-like substances.[7,26] Nonmalignant pulmonary disease processes that may lead to SIADH hyponatremia include viral/bacterial pneumonias and tuberculosis.[42,64] Medications associated with SIADH include chlorpropamide (Diabinese), chemotherapeutic agents, nonsteroidal antiinflammatory drugs, thiazide diuretics, angiotensin-converting enzyme inhibitors, narcotics, nicotine replacement therapy, and selective serotonin reuptake inhibitors (SSRIs).[17,19,63] Studies indicate increases in SIADH in older adult women taking SSRIs, especially in the first few weeks of treatment.[63] Additionally, nicotine replacement therapy has been shown to enhance release of ADH, increasing the risk for the development of SIADH.[19] In critically ill patients, nicotine patches are often used to decrease the agitation associated with nicotine withdrawal. Sodium levels should be monitored in these critically ill patients receiving nicotine replacements.[19] Other common causes include

anesthesia, pain, anxiety, stress response (from trauma, surgery, burns, or sepsis), hypoxemia, hypotension, and positive-pressure ventilation.[46]

Clinical Presentation. The clinical presentation of SIADH relates to hyponatremia and relative water intoxication as well as neurologic and gastrointestinal manifestations such as personality changes, headache, confusion, abdominal cramps, nausea, and vomiting.[3,7,26,31,46] Nutritional recommendations for patients with pituitary, thyroid, and adrenal disorders are given in the Nutrition box below.

♦ NUTRITION

Nutritional Care for the Patient With Pituitary, Thyroid, or Adrenal Disorders

Disease Process	Nutritional Considerations

Diabetes insipidus	Parenteral hyperalimentation
	  Can lead to hyperglycemia
	  Tight glucose control is needed to prevent additional free water loss
	Enteral tube feedings
	  Can pull water into gastrointestinal tract
	  Addition of free water to hypertonic tube feedings to prevent diarrhea[3,30,46,58]

Syndrome of inappropriate antidiuretic hormone	Hyponatremia
	  IV replacement 0.09% normal saline
	  3% sodium chloride if serum sodium level less than 120 mEq/L[63,64]

Thyroid storm	During acute phase, support hypermetabolic state to prevent loss of lean body mass and protein[23,46]

Myxedema coma	Motility of gastrointestinal tract decreases
	  Withhold food early in treatment
	Hyponatremia
	  0.09% normal saline should be replaced slowly with caution
	  3% sodium chloride if serum sodium level less than 120 mEq/L[12,34]

Adrenal insufficiency	Hypoglycemia common
	  Replace glucose based on blood glucose level
	  2–4 ml/kg of 25% dextrose, D_5W continuous infusion to prevent further hypoglycemia[13,38]

Data from references 3, 12, 13, 30, 34, 38, 44, 58, 63, 64.

Subtle signs and symptoms include inability to concentrate, weakness, fatigue, dyspnea on exertion, anorexia, loss of taste, and increased thirst.[26] SIADH can occur slowly over time, allowing the brain cells to adjust, masking the neurologic symptoms.[3] If hyponatremia occurs rapidly, it can lead to seizures, coma, and a 50% chance of death.[3]

Diagnostic Evaluation. Hyponatremia can be caused by many underlying disease processes. Therefore differential diagnoses should be considered and ruled out before a diagnosis of SIADH is made. A series of preliminary lab studies would include serum and urine osmolality, urine specific gravity, urine sodium calculation of fractional excretion of sodium, serum electrolytes, glucose, urea, creatinine, BUN, total proteins, triglycerides, uric acid, TSH, plasma cortisol, and ADH levels.[46,47,63] Chest x-ray and head computed tomography (CT) scan may be helpful to rule out carcinomas, lung disease, or cerebral edema.[42]

Multidisciplinary Plan of Care. Collaborative management of the patient with SIADH should include restriction of fluids to 1000 to 1500 ml/day and institution of measures to alleviate thirst/dry mouth by providing oral care, chilled beverages, and hard candy (if conscious).[3,14] Patients who have severe hyponatremia (less than 115 mEq/L) should be treated with 3% sodium chloride by calculating deficit (Chapter 31) and replacing sodium to increase the serum sodium level no more than 1 to 2 mEq/L per hour over the first 2 to 4 hours, decreasing to 0.5 to 1.9 mEq/L per hour as the serum sodium level approaches 120 mEq/L. Sodium must be replaced slowly to prevent the brain cells from shrinking, which could lead to a complication known as osmotic demyelination syndrome or central pontine myelinosis.[7,64]

In addition, medications can be used to reduce the secretion of ADH or block the effects (see the Medication table on p. 944).[7,14] Demeclocycline and lithium decrease the kidneys' response to ADH, while furosemide (Lasix) a loop diuretic, helps to diurese excess water and raises the serum sodium level.[14,58] Potassium, magnesium, and phosphorus levels need to be monitored to prevent electrolyte imbalances.[14,64]

Conclusions. Early recognition of SIADH can be difficult, as the major presenting symptom is hyponatremia. Hyponatremia has a myriad of causes, which must be ruled out before making the diagnosis of SIADH. Once the diagnosis is made, early treatment focused on slowly replacing sodium and reducing intravascular volume should be instituted. Treatment of patients with SIADH is outlined in the Multidisciplinary Plan of Care below and on p. 949.

MULTIDISCIPLINARY PLAN OF CARE FOR THE PATIENT WITH SYNDROME OF INAPPROPRIATE ANTIDIURETIC HORMONE

PROBLEM	INTERVENTION	RATIONALE	EXPECTED OUTCOME	SPECIAL CONSIDERATIONS
Risk for development of SIADH	Careful consideration of patients who present with: *Neurogenic* • Traumatic brain injury • Brain tumors • Aneurysms • Thrombus • Neurologic infections • Metastatic tumors: lung, duodenum, pancreas, prostate, thymus, leukemia, lymphoma, Hodgkin's • Pulmonary: viral/ bacteria pneumonia, tuberculosis	Early identification of patients allows for appropriate prophylactic intervention, especially in preparation for diagnostic testing or surgery.	Patients at risk for SIADH will be identified early.	All patients with bronchogenic carcinoma should be monitored judiciously for hyponatremia and SIADH. Most critically ill patients are at increased risk for development of SIADH related to hypotension, hypoxemia, anxiety, pain, and positive pressure mechanical ventilation.[1,14]

PROBLEM	INTERVENTION	RATIONALE	EXPECTED OUTCOME	SPECIAL CONSIDERATIONS
	Nephrogenic • Chronic renal failure • Medications (chemotherapeutic agents, nicotine replacement, SSRIs) • Infiltrative/ inflammatory renal disease			
	Monitor: • BP • HR • Urine output • Specific gravity • BUN/creatinine • Urine sodium • Urine osmolality • Serum osmolality • Serum sodium • Electrolytes: potassium chloride bicarbonate • Serum ADH • FENa • TSH • Cortisol • Glucose • Total proteins • ABGs Serial neurologic exams for conscious patients[47]	TSH level will provide information about thyroid disorders, primarily hypothyroidism, that lead to hyponatremia. Normal cortisol and potassium levels rule out adrenal insufficiency. Normal glucose level rules out hyperglycemia as a cause. Normal total proteins assist to rule out liver disease. Serial neurologic exams assist with early detection of mental status changes, the most common symptom of SIADH in conscious patients.[1,14,33,46]		Monitoring of hemodynamic parameters in SIADH would not provide useful information since SIADH is a euvolemia hyponatremia in which the extra volume is intracellular, not intravascular. If a pulmonary artery catheter is in place, an elevated CVP and PAWP would assist in ruling out SIADH. Early changes related to neurologic status can be detected for the conscious patient. For the unconscious patient, serial serum sodium and monitoring of other lab values assist in correction of SIADH.
Potential for seizures	Decrease production of free water and increase excretion of free water by interfering with ADH-tubule interaction See Medication table on p. 944 Restrict free water intake PO usually 500–1000 ml/ day Stop all hypotonic solutions Replace sodium loss	Restriction or discontinuation of all hypotonic fluids limits the free water intake. For extremely low serum sodium levels or symptomatic hyponatremia, 3% sodium chloride can be used with caution. Do not increase sodium levels greater than 1–2 mEq/L per hour or 12 mEq/day.	Patient will exhibit: Increased serum osmolality Decreased serum sodium Decreased serum ADH Decreased urine osmolality Increased urine output	

Data from references 1, 3, 4, 14, 19, 26, 33, 46, 47, 64.
ADH = Antidiuretic hormone, ABGs = arterial blood gases, ADH = antidiuretic hormone, BP = blood pressure, BUN = blood urea nitrogen, CVP = central venous pressure, FENa = fractional excretion of sodium, HCO_3^- = bicarbonate, HR = heart rate, NS = normal saline, PAWP = pulmonary artery wedge pressure, PO = by mouth, SIADH = syndrome of inappropriate antidiuretic hormone, SSRIs = selective serotonin reuptake inhibitors, TSH = thyroid-stimulating hormone.

◆ Case Study 35-2

SIADH

R.D., a 67-year-old female, is brought to the emergency department after her family reported she fell down four steps, breaking her ankle. She was confused and combative on arrival. Her history includes controlled hypertension, asthma, recent diagnosis of depression, ventricular pacemaker, mitral valve replacement, and history of cigarette smoking 1–2 packs per day times 45 years. Her family reports R.D. stopped smoking 3 weeks ago and has been using "one of those patches." Her medications include hydrochlorothiazide (Microzide) 25 mg/day, albuterol (Proventil) 2 puffs every 4 hours, warfarin (Coumadin) 3 mg every other day, paroxetine (Paxil) 20 mg/day (started 2 months earlier); a 21-mg nicotine transdermal patch is found on her left arm.

R.D. continues to be confused but is not combative. Pulse oximetry reveals 91% saturation; she has expiratory wheezes throughout her lung fields. A left ankle fracture is confirmed by x-ray and chest x-ray reveals left pulmonary contusion. Vitals signs: pulse 112 beats/min, BP 160/90 mm Hg, respiratory rate 28 breaths/min, temperature 99.3° F. She is placed on 40% aerosol mask, and D_5W 0.45% NS is started at 100 ml/hr.

CBC Results and Laboratory Values

CBC Results	Laboratory Values
WBCs 8800/mm^3	Na$^+$ 129 mEq/L
RBCs 4.2 μl	K$^+$ 3.9 mEq/L
Hgb 12.8 g/dl	Cl$^-$ 100 mEq/L
Hct 39%	Glucose 138 mg/dl
	BUN 18 mg/dl
	Creatinine 1.1 mg/dl
	Serum osmolality 282 mOsm/L

The decision is made to take R.D. to the operating room to fix her ankle.

Decision point: What other disease processes must be ruled out before SIADH can be confirmed?

Following surgical repair to her ankle, R.D. is admitted to critical care because of her pulmonary contusion, asthma history, and failure to wean and extubate in the recovery room.

Decision point: What risk factors does R.D. have for the development of SIADH?

During the next 24 hours, her urinary output decreased to 200 ml, despite two doses of furosemide 40 mg IV and increasing IV fluid to 125 ml/hr. Morning lab values were as follows: Na$^+$ = 112 mEq/L, K$^+$ = 3.3 mEq/L, Cl$^-$ = 87 mEq/L, glucose = 102 mg/dl, Hct = 30 μl, Hgb = 10 μl, BUN = 9 mg/dl, creatinine = 0.9 mg/dl, serum osmolality = 258 mOsm/L, urine osmolality = 880 mOsm/L, urine specific gravity = 1.030.

Decision point: What additional information leads to the diagnosis of SIADH?

The physician orders demeclocycline 250 mg four times per day, fluid restriction of 1000 ml/day, discontinue IV fluids, draw serum Na$^+$ every 1 hr, 0.3% NS IV to replace calculated sodium deficit.[14,26,64]

Decision point: Why is the sodium deficit calculated, and why is it important to replace sodium slowly?

Decision point: Explain the rest of the physician's orders as they relate to the treatment of SIADH.

In R.D., the diagnosis of SIADH is made secondary to polysubstance administration (thiazide diuretics, SSRI, nicotine replacement), asthma, administration of hypotonic IV solutions, and stress response related to her ankle fracture and surgery. Her hyponatremia is corrected over the next few days. Before discharge, the acute care nurse practitioner adjusts R.D.'s medications to prevent subsequent episodes of SIADH.

THYROID GLAND DISORDERS

The conditions associated with thyroid dysfunction include hyperthyroidism, which can lead to the life-threatening disorder thyroid storm (thyrotoxicosis); and hypothyroidism, which can lead to the life-threatening disorder myxedema coma.

Hyperthyroidism (Thyrotoxicosis/ Thyroid Storm)

Hyperthyroidism results from increased levels of circulating TH. The major systemic effects associated with hyperthyroidism are increased metabolic activity, intolerance to heat, and stimulation of the sympathetic nervous system.[37,44,53,59] The most common causes of hyperthyroidism are Graves' disease, resulting from an autoimmune toxic goiter, and multinodular goiter, seen commonly in the older adult population. Other causes include an inappropriate secretion of TSH from pituitary neoplasms secreting TSH-like substances as well as non-neoplastic pituitary secretion of TSH.[37,53] As with all disorders of HPA relationships, there are two distinct mechanisms of thyroid dysfunction. Primary disorders, in which TSH levels are increased, are related to the thyroid gland-target organ/tissue response, and secondary disorders, in which TSH levels are decreased, are associated with problems in the axis.[23,24]

Although hyperthyroidism is a relatively common disorder, thyroid storm, a life-threatening exacerbation of hyperthyroidism, is rare. Thyroid storm has a 20% to 30% mortality rate even with prompt treatment and is more common in women (10%) than men (2%), with a peak age of occurrence at 20 to 49 years.[53,56] Because of the long half-lives of T_3 (22 hours) and T_4, a thyroid storm can last for a considerable period of time.[23,24,37]

Patients at Risk. Any patient with preexisting hyperthyroidism[53] or undiagnosed hyperthyroidism is at risk. In older adults, hyperthyroidism can be mimicked by other underlying disease processes or expected age-related changes.[53] Often the elderly patient will present with nervousness, palpitations, tremors, fatigue, and depression. Many older patients are already being treated with beta-adrenergic blockers for hypertension, medications that can effectively conceal any tachycardia and tremors.[53] Older adult patients are at increased risk whenever their thyroid hormone replacement medication is increased or changed. This is related to decreased metabolism of the drug and increased half-life of the drug in older people; in addition, different brands may have different levels of thyroid hormone.[53]

Thyroid storm is an exaggerated form of hyperthyroidism and has a variety of triggers. Medications placing the patient at risk include nonsteroidal antiinflammatory drugs, salicylates, tricyclic antidepressants, insulin, thiazide diuretics, amiodarone (Cordarone),[37,41,53] chronic steroid therapy, and fludrocortisone agents.[16,23,44,53,56] Additional triggers that pose a risk include noncompliance with anti-thyroid medications, infection, trauma, surgical procedures (Table 35-1),[22] alcohol abuse, pregnancy, radioactive iodine therapy, diabetic ketoacidosis, and both physical and emotional stress.[16,23,44,53,56] The overall mortality rate is 10% to 20%; however, with prompt diagnosis and treatment, the prognosis is good.[23]

Clinical Presentation. The hallmark signs of thyroid storm are fever, tachycardia, tremors, intolerance to heat, sweating, nausea, vomiting, and diarrhea.[56] Less common findings include weight loss with increased appetite,

TABLE 35-1 Surgical Considerations for Endocrine Disorders

ENDOCRINE DISORDER	PREOPERATIVE CONSIDERATIONS	POSTOPERATIVE CONSIDERATIONS
Hyperthyroidism (thyroid storm)	Establish euthyroid if possible If euthyroid not possible: • Beta blocker to decrease SNS response to surgery, block conversion to T_3 • Propylthiouracil—blocks TH synthesis • Glucocorticoids—block release and conversion of TH • Drugs have shortened half-life related to hypermetabolic state	Related to compromised airway with removal of thyroid gland: • Hematoma, edema, fludrocortisone (obstruction or stridor) • Hypocalcemia (vocal cord tetany, paralysis) • Laryngeal nerve injury (stridor)
Hypothyroidism (myxedema coma)	Assess fluid/electrolyte/hormone status TSH, T_3, T_4 (replace) Cortisol (adrenal insufficiency) Treat hypoglycemia Treat hyponatremia	Hypoventilation: • Blunted baroreceptor responses to hypercarbia and hypoxemia • Muscle weakness • Compromised airway related to large tongue, goiter, obesity Cardiac considerations: • Decreased CO and SV, bradycardia, HF, ECG changes (long QT, T wave inversion) Gastrointestinal considerations: • Delayed gastric emptying (may need NG tube) • Drugs have increased half-lives • Sedatives should be used in small amounts with caution and close observation Emergent surgery considerations: • Aggressive supportive care post-op • Judicious monitoring of response to treatment • T_4 dose daily • Stress-dose steroids every 8 hr • PA catheter Fluids: • Avoid HF and further hyponatremia

Table continues on page 952

Table 35-1 Surgical Considerations for Endocrine Disorders—cont'd

ENDOCRINE DISORDER	PREOPERATIVE CONSIDERATIONS	POSTOPERATIVE CONSIDERATIONS
Adrenal insufficiency	Assess for hypoglycemia and treat Assess for hyperkalemia and treat Steroid coverage is related to operation duration and complexity (lower doses for hernia and higher doses for CABG) Hydrocortisone steroid of choice related to 1:1 glucocorticoid/mineralocorticoid	Monitor for hypoglycemia and treat Monitor for hypotension and treat with fluids (such as NS) Replace steroids as needed

Data from reference 22.
CABG = Coronary artery bypass graft, CO = cardiac output, ECG = electrocardiogram, HF = heart failure, NG = nasogastric tube, NS = normal saline, PA = pulmonary artery, SNS = sympathetic nervous system, SV = stroke volume, TH = thyroid hormone, TSH = thyroid-stimulating hormone, T_3 = triiodothyronine, T_4 = thyroxine.

emotional lability, pulmonary edema, and congestive heart failure.[31] The most common dysrhythmias associated with thyroid storm are supraventricular tachycardias; atrial fibrillation is the most common.[50] Often, in undiagnosed hyperthyroidism, thyroid storm may present as a cerebrovascular accident (CVA), other dysrhythmias (ventricular tachycardia or third-degree block), adrenal insufficiency, coma, jaundice, rhabdomyolysis and acute renal failure, shock, or status epilepticus.[50,56] Sepsis, pheochromocytoma, and malignant hyperthermia have a similar clinical presentation to thyroid storm.[44]

Diagnostic Evaluation. Diagnosis of thyroid storm is based primarily on the presenting clinical assessment and not diagnostic tests. Results of measurements of thyroid levels are useful for the patient who has undiagnosed hyperthyroidism to differentiate primary disease from secondary disease.[24] Thyroid function tests include T_3, T_4, free T_4, T_3 resin uptake, and TSH levels. TSH level is the gold standard used to differentiate primary from secondary thyrotoxicosis.[23,24,43,44] TSH level is decreased in primary disease and increased in secondary disease.[43,44] T_3 and T_4 levels will be elevated in primary disease as well as in thyroid storm because of the increased hypermetabolic state requiring physiologically active T_3. This is a direct result of the amount of T_4 available as well as what is being synthesized.[43]

Multidisciplinary Plan of Care. Collaborative management of the patient with thyroid storm should include early recognition of the condition based on the patient's clinical presentation.[23] Treatment should include medications such as propylthiouracil (PTU) to block peripheral effects of TH. Medications such as iodides and lithium can also be used to inhibit TH release. Propranolol (Inderal) is the first-line drug for the treatment of the beta-adrenergic effects such as tachycardia, hypertension, and tremors.[44] In addition, propranolol prevents conversion of T_4 to T_3, and the effects are seen within 10 minutes of administration. Dexamethasone (Decadron) can be used as a T_4 to T_3 conversion blocker and to assist with stabilization of the cell membrane; however, it can worsen hyperglycemia.[23,44,59] Supplemental oxygen should be given to support the increased oxygen demands of the hypermetabolic state, and hydration is a concern as it relates to loss of fluid from diaphoresis and insensible losses.[23,44,59] For a more in-depth look at thyroid storm medications, see the Medication table below and on p. 953.

MEDICATIONS USED IN THYROID STORM

MEDICATIONS	ACTIONS	DOSAGES	SPECIAL CONSIDERATIONS
Propylthiouracil (PTU)	Inhibits synthesis of TH (organification of iodine) Inhibits peripheral conversion of T_4 to T_3	300–400 mg PO every 4–8 hr	Comatose patients will need NG tube for instillation—only dispensed in an oral preparation
Methimazole (Tapazole)	Inhibits synthesis of TH (organification of iodine)	5–20 mg 3 times a day PO	Comatose patients will need NG or small-bore feeding tube for instillation—only dispensed in an oral preparation[23,59]

MEDICATIONS	ACTIONS	DOSAGES	SPECIAL CONSIDERATIONS
Potassium iodide	Iodides inhibit release of TH by accumulation of colloids and decrease vascularity of gland	5 drops every 6 hr PO **or** Sodium iodide IV 0.25 g IV every 6 hr	Precede administration with thioamides (PTU) to prevent thyroid storm[23,59]
Propranolol (Inderal)	Controls autonomic effects of TH that lead to decreased heart rate, blood pressure, and myocardial oxygen consumption; blocks conversion of T_4 to T_3	10–80 mg PO every 6 hr; maximum dose 120 mg every 6 hr 1–3 mg slow IV, not to exceed 1 mg/min Repeat if needed	First-line drug and may be only drug needed to control thyroid storm[23,37,44,56]
Esmolol (Brevibloc)	Controls autonomic effects of TH that lead to decreased HR, BP, and MVo_2 with shorter duration of action	250–500 mg/kg IV; repeat for desired effect	Hypotension Use with caution in patients with diabetes because can lead to hypoglycemia[59]
Hydrocortisone (Solu-Cortef)	Blocks conversion of T_4 to T_3	100–500 mg IV every 8–12 hr	Use of steroids in thyroid storm has been associated with increased survival[23]

Data from references 23, 27, 37, 44, 56, 59.
BP = Blood pressure, HR = heart rate, MVo_2 = myocardial oxygen consumption, NG = nasogastric, TH = thyroid hormone, T_3 = triiodothyronine, T_4 = thyroxine.

Conclusions. Rapid recognition of patients presenting with thyroid storm is the key to decreasing mortality. If the patient's clinical presentation is consistent with thyroid storm, do not delay treatment to await confirmation of thyroid function tests.[56] Treatment focuses on decreasing thyroid hormone synthesis and secretion, blocking sympathetic nervous system stimulation, and supporting circulation, as described in the Multidisciplinary Plan of Care below and on pp. 954-955.[23,44,59]

MULTIDISCIPLINARY PLAN OF CARE FOR THE PATIENT WITH THYROID STORM

PROBLEM	INTERVENTION	RATIONALE	EXPECTED OUTCOME	SPECIAL CONSIDERATIONS
Risk for development of thyroid storm	Careful consideration of patients who present with underlying thyrotoxicosis and: Trauma Surgery Infection Pregnancy Radioactive iodine therapy Diabetic ketoacidosis Physical/emotional stress Medications: • Salicylates	Early identification of patients allows for appropriate prophylactic interventions, especially in preparation for surgery.	Patients at risk for thyroid storm will be identified early.	Older adults often have symptoms that are masked by underlying disease processes or medications.[14,23,37,44,59] For surgical considerations, see Table 35-1.

Table continues on page 954

PROBLEM	INTERVENTION	RATIONALE	EXPECTED OUTCOME	SPECIAL CONSIDERATIONS
	• NSAIDs • Amiodarone • Chemotherapeutic agents • Thiazide diuretics • Tricyclic antidepressants Alcohol Chronic steroid therapy Noncompliance with anti-thyroid drugs Patients may present in thyroid storm as initial diagnosis when they have undiagnosed thyrotoxicosis[14,59]			
	Assess and monitor vital signs, other physical and physiologic signs and symptoms followed by specific laboratory: Temperature higher than 102° F Heat intolerance Tachycardia Nausea/vomiting/diarrhea Dysrhythmias Tremors Palpitations Oxygen saturations Emotionally labile Laboratory values: • Elevated T_3 • Elevated T_4 • Elevated TSH • CBC with mild leukocytosis	Rapid assessment provides the data needed to develop a further plan of care.		Thyroid storm is diagnosed on clinical presentation. Always begin treatment once the clinical diagnosis is confirmed. Thyroid function tests take several hours to get results.[23,44,59]
Development of thyroid storm	Decrease synthesis of TH Inhibit release of TH (iodides) Block beta-adrenergic effects of TH Block conversion of T_3 to T_4 See Medication table on pp. 952-953 Reduce fever: • Acetaminophen (Tylenol) 325–600 mg every 4 hr PO • Cooling blanket or ice packs	Early treatment decreases risk of death from thyroid storm. PTU and methimazole inhibit synthesis of TH and inhibit peripheral conversion of T_4 to T_3. Iodides inhibit release of TH. Beta-adrenergic blockers are the mainstay to control autonomic effects of TH. In addition they also block conversion of T_4 to T_3.	Thyroid hormone synthesis and levels will return to baseline. Adrenergic effects of TH will be reduced or eliminated. Fever will be reduced or eliminated.	Because of hypermetabolic state, all drug dosages and times will need to be adjusted. Iodine solutions can be given to block release of TH, but only after thiomide solutions (PTU) are given to prevent iodine from being used in TH production. Calcium channel blockers can be used if

PROBLEM	INTERVENTION	RATIONALE	EXPECTED OUTCOME	SPECIAL CONSIDERATIONS
	Destroy the gland: • RAI	Glucocorticoids will block conversion of T_4 to T_3.		beta blockers are ineffective in reducing tachycardia. Glucocorticoids inhibit conversion of T_3 to T_4. Use of steroids has been associated with increased survival. Stress doses are needed to replace accelerated production and increased degradation induced by TH.[59] Salicylates and NSAIDs should not be used as fever reducers as they can cause conversion of T_3 to T_4. For the older adult patient with many potential drug interactions, destruction of the gland with RAI may be a better option.

Data from references 14, 16, 23, 37, 43, 44, 50, 56, 59.
CBC = Complete blood cell count, NSAIDs = nonsteroidal antiinflammatory drugs, PTU = propylthiouracil, RAI = radioactive iodine, TH = thyroid hormone, TSH = thyroid-stimulating hormone, T_3 = triiodothyronine, T_4 = thyroxine.

◆ Case Study 35-3

Thyroid Storm

J.H. is a 38-year-old African-American female. She is admitted to the critical care unit with chief complaints of nervousness, diaphoresis, racing heart, shortness of breath, fatigue, nausea/vomiting, and recent 20-pound weight loss. J.H. has a history of type 1 diabetes, hypertension, and cigarette smoking 1.5 packs per day.

Assessment reveals the following: temperature 102.1° F, pulse 129 beats/min and irregular, sinus rhythm with frequent premature atrial contractions (PACs), BP 188/105 mm Hg, RR 32 breaths/min, O_2 saturation via pulse oximetry 89%. She has visible tremors. She reports she has been taking aspirin 2–3 tablets at least twice a day for the last week for "pounding" headaches. Other medications include Novolin 70/30 10 units subcutaneous every morning with additional Humalog determined by blood glucose level with meals, hydrochlorothiazide 25 mg bid, and albuterol (Proventil) inhaler as needed. She states she has used her albuterol inhaler at least 2–3 times per day in the last week.

As you are continuing your assessment of J.H., the monitor alarms show ventricular tachycardia. J.H. is unconscious, apneic, and pulseless. CPR is begun and she is defibrillated with 200 joules and converts back to normal sinus rhythm (NSR). Pulseless ventricular tachycardia returns and a second shock of 300 joules is delivered with conversion to NSR and a pulse. The physician orders procainamide (Pronestyl) 500 mg bolus followed by a continuous drip. J.H. is conscious, restless, and short of breath. Vital signs: T 102.3° F, BP 200/110 mm Hg, HR 135 beats/min, RR 30 breaths/min, pulse oximetry 88%. She is visibly diaphoretic and complaining of being very "hot."

Additional physician orders include the following: nonrebreather mask 40%; continue procainamide drip; labs: CBC, electrolytes, hemoglobin A_{1c} (HbA$_{1c}$), TSH, T_3, T_4 levels; chest x-ray; IV D_5W 0.45% NS at 100 ml/hr.

Decision point: What assessment parameters led to a diagnosis of hyperthyroidism?

Decision point: What risk factors does J.H. have that would predispose her to thyroid storm?

Decision point: Why did the physician order 40% face mask and TSH, T_4, and T_3?

Initial diagnostic evaluation reveals the following: chest x-ray clear; Hct = 38%, HbA$_{1c}$ = 13 g/dl, WBCs = 12,500/µl, platelets = 250,000/µl; electrolytes: Na$^+$ = 134 mEq/L, K$^+$ = 4.9 mEq/L, Ca^{++} = 13.2 mg/dl; serum glucose = 415 mg/dl; Hgb A$_{1c}$ = 8.6%.

Thyroid levels are now available: TSH 0.05 milliunit/L (normal 0.34–5.00 milliunits/L); T_3 303 ng/dl (normal 90–200 ng/dl); T_4 26.9 ng/dl (normal 5–11.5 ng/dl).

Discuss the results of the thyroid function test.

The physician orders the following: propylthiouracil 200 mg every 4 hr PO; propranolol 40 mg PO every 6 hr; dexamethasone 2 mg every 6 hr IV; acetaminophen 325 mg every 6 hr for temperature over 101° F.

Decision point: Explain the laboratory values.

Decision point: Explain the physician's orders.

Decision point: Why did the physician use procainamide as the dysrhythmic agent for ventricular tachycardia instead of amiodarone?

Decision point: Discuss how aspirin could have precipitated the thyroid storm.

J.H. spent the next 4 days in the critical care unit. Her endocrinologist's acute care nurse practitioner prescribed propylthiouracil 50 mg PO three times a day and explained the importance of medication compliance.

Hypothyroidism and Myxedema Coma

Hypothyroidism is the most common thyroid dysfunction. The different types of hypothyroidism can range from subclinical asymptomatic to severe forms of hypothyroidism with multiple system effects. Hypothyroidism occurs more commonly in older adults, with a 14% to 18% occurrence.[34] As with all other HPA axis dysfunctions, there is a primary and a secondary cause. Primary disorders (95% of all cases) are thyroid gland dysfunction, as occurs commonly in Hashimoto's thyroiditis or in response to antithyroid treatment.[14,31,34] The decreased function of the thyroid gland leads to decreased production of TH and an increase in TSH secretion, leading to formation of a goiter.[23,24,31,44] Less common, secondary causes are from dysfunction in the hypothalamus or pituitary, which results from failure of the pituitary to produce TSH.* In addition to primary and secondary causes, there are iatrogenic causes that include treatment for Graves' disease, thyroidectomy, external iodine ingestion, amiodarone,[41] lithium, interferon, and interleukin-2.[14,24,34,44]

Myxedema coma is an uncommon but life-threatening disorder in which profound hypothyroidism occurs. This causes an inability to regulate temperature, altered mental status, and impaired respiratory function, which eventually leads to a coma.[12,14,23,44] It occurs most commonly in older women who have undiagnosed or subclinical hypothyroidism with exposure to cold, infection, stress of illness, or medications.[34]

***References 9, 14, 23, 24, 43, 44.**

Patients at Risk. Patients at risk for the development of hypothyroidism are older, female, hospitalized patients, and Caucasians with preexisting hypothyroidism.[34] The incidence of hypothyroidism ranges from 0.5% to 6% in younger patients and up to 14% to 18% in older adult patients, with a fivefold to tenfold increased incidence in women more than men.[14,34] If not promptly treated, myxedema coma carries a 50% mortality rate.[34] Even with immediate recognition and treatment, mortality rates are 25%.[34]

Precipitating factors for patients at risk include an infection, exposure to cold, heart failure, trauma, surgical procedures, CVA, gastrointestinal bleed, and carbon dioxide retention. Common medication causes include sedatives, tranquilizers, narcotics, diuretics, amiodarone, lithium, and phenytoin as well as noncompliance with thyroid replacement.*

Clinical Presentation. Confusion with decreased level of consciousness related to reduced blood flow, reduced oxygen delivery, and decreased glucose levels; hypothermia; and unique thick skin changes are present in most patients. The thick skin associated with hypothyroidism and myxedema is a result of accumulation of a mucopolysaccharide substance consisting of hyaluronic acid and chondroitin sulfate bound to protein to form a sticky gel in the interstitial spaces. Water and sodium are drawn into the interstitial space, which leads to a nonpitting edema and intravascular volume loss.[14,28,34] Other common physical findings related to this accumulation of substance in the interstitial spaces are hoarseness and periorbital edema.[34]

Decreased intravascular volume, decreased metabolism, and peripheral vasoconstriction lead to decreased blood flow to the extremities. This inhibits the generation of heat to the hands and feet.[14,34] Physiologic changes related to the cardiac system include decreased blood pressure, heart rate, contractility, and cardiac output as well as slowed conductivity.[14,23,44,49] Nonspecific ST changes and T wave inversion are common. Low-voltage and ventricular dysrhythmias may be noted.[12,34] Pulmonary changes occur as a result of a blunted response in the chemoreceptors that detect hypercarbia and hypoxemia. Hypoventilation is related to muscle weakness. Pleural effusions are common because of sodium and water drawn into the intravascular spaces.[14,22,34,59] Hypoglycemia is common related to the inability to break down carbohydrates, lipids, and protein as an energy source. Lastly, CVA must be ruled out because patients often present unconscious or obtunded.[34,59]

Diagnostic Evaluation. There are several tests that can be ordered to assess thyroid function. TSH level, the

***References 12, 22, 23, 28, 34, 49, 59.**

most sensitive indicator, will be elevated in primary disease states in which the thyroid is dysfunctional. In secondary disease states, TSH level is decreased, representing a dysfunction in the HPA. T_4 and T_3 levels are decreased and unreliable measurements in myxedema coma because most T_4 and T_3 are bound to protein. Reliable assessments are free T_4 (FT_4) and free T_3 (FT_3). Additional lab values include electrolytes (primarily serum sodium), serum glucose, serum osmolality, and arterial blood gases to assess hypoxia and hypercarbia.[12,14,34]

Multidisciplinary Plan of Care. Initial priorities for the patient with myxedema coma should include intubation and mechanical ventilation for correction of hypercapnia and hypoxia and also IV thyroid hormone replacement while awaiting confirmation of myxedema from laboratory tests. Correction of hypothermia should be done with passive rewarming blankets and increased room temperature. In addition, correct hyponatremia of sodium levels less than 120 mEq/L with hypertonic saline in small doses to avoid volume overload. These patients are at increased risk for myocardial ischemia and infarction; close cardiac monitoring is imperative.*

---

*References 12, 14, 23, 28, 44, 49.

◆ Case Study 35-4

Myxedema Coma

A.H. is a 74-year-old Caucasian female found in the backyard of her home by a neighbor. She was unresponsive and cold to the touch. The outside temperature was 45° F. The neighbor does not know much about A.H.'s medical history. Assessment reveals the following: an obese white female; nonpitting edema noted in her hands and feet; enlarged tongue; sparse gray hair; abdominal distention with absent bowel sounds; bradycardia, rate of 45 beats/min, with T wave inversion; temperature of 93° F rectally; BP 90/50 mm Hg; respirations 10 breaths/min, shallow, with diminished breath sounds; pulse oximetry 75%.

Decision point: What clinical symptoms would lead you to a diagnosis of myxedema coma?

The decision is made to intubate emergently. Intubation is difficult because of her enlarged tongue. The decision is made to perform rapid-sequence intubation with succinylcholine. She is placed on a ventilator with the following settings: tidal volume (Vt) 800 ml, rate 20, Fio_2 50%. The physician orders the following: stat chest x-ray, ABGs, CBC, electrolytes, glucose, BUN, serum creatinine, urinalysis, free T_4, TSH, cortisol level, blood, urine, sputum cultures, and

toxicology screen. IV D_5NS at 100 ml/hr, levothyroxine IV 300 mcg.

Decision point: Explain the physician's orders.

Laboratory results reveal the following: CBC: Hgb = 9 g/dl, Hct = 34%, WBC = 18,000/mm³; ABGs, $Paco_2$ = 6 mm Hg, Pao_2 = 45 mm Hg (initial, before intubation); ABGs now, $Paco_2$ = 48 mm Hg, Pao_2 = 93 mm Hg; glucose = 78 mg/dl; Na^+ = 124 mEq/L; K^+ = 4.9 mEq/L; cortisol = 10 mcg/dl (normal 4–25 mcg/dl); TSH = 39.9 microunits/L (normal 0.4–4.6 microunits/L); free T_4 less than 0.03 ng/dl (normal 1.0–2.3 ng/dl); BUN = 50 mg/dl; creatinine = 2.1 mg/dl; BUN/creatinine ratio = 25:1; urinalysis, dark yellow, cloudy, foul-smelling, greater than 4 WBCs and WBC casts. Chest x-ray reveals scattered atelectasis. The physician orders hydrocortisone IV 100 mg and levofloxacin (Levaquin) 500 mg IV.

Decision point: Explain why the physician ordered hydrocortisone, and why you would give it.

Decision point: Explain how the ventilator settings improved the ABGs.

Decision point: Explain how the laboratory values verify the diagnosis of myxedema.

Decision point: What prompted the physician to order levofloxacin before culture results?

Conclusions. Early recognition of patients presenting with myxedema coma is the key to decreasing mortality as this dysfunction affects every body system. Immediate and aggressive management consisting of multiple treatments is imperative to survival. As illustrated by the Multidisciplinary Plan of Care on pp. 958-959, treatment focuses on replacing thyroid hormone, restoring sympathetic nervous system stimulation, and supporting circulation and oxygenation.

ADRENAL INSUFFIENCY IN CRITICAL ILLNESS

Definition of Adrenal Insufficiency

Addison's disease is defined as hypofunction of the adrenal gland, while adrenal insufficiency (AI) is defined as an absolute lack of cortisol or relative lack of cortisol, which occurs in critical illness.[14,35,39,40,54] The normal stress response is activated in the face of pain, hypotension, hypoglycemia, hypoxemia, trauma, or cytokine discharge.[35,39,40,54] The normal cortisol levels are diurnal, peaking around 8:00 AM with the lowest levels occurring at 4:00 PM.[8,14,32] Critically ill patients in stressed states can have consistently high levels of serum cortisol, from 2 to 10 times normal, with loss of diurnal differences.[39,40]

MULTIDISCIPLINARY PLAN OF CARE FOR THE PATIENT WITH MYXEDEMA COMA

PROBLEM	INTERVENTION	RATIONALE	EXPECTED OUTCOME	SPECIAL CONSIDERATIONS
Risk for development of myxedema coma	Careful consideration of patients who present with underlying hypothyroidism and: Trauma Surgery Infection Exposure to cold Physical/emotional stress Heart failure Stroke Gastrointestinal bleeding Hypercarbia Medications: • Sedatives • Tranquilizers • Narcotics • Diuretics • Phenytoin (Dilantin) • Lithium • Amiodarone (Cordarone) Noncompliance with thyroid drugs Patients may present in myxedema coma as initial diagnosis when they have undiagnosed or subclinical hypothyroidism	Early identification of patients allows for appropriate prophylactic intervention.	Patients at risk for myxedema coma will be identified early.	Older adult patients are at increased risk for subclinical hypothyroidism and subsequently myxedema coma.[28,34,53]
	Assess and monitor vital signs and other physical and physiologic signs and symptoms followed by specific laboratory values: Temperature lower than 95° F Bradycardia less than 30 beats/min Hypoventilation Seizures Ileus Confusion Skin: nonpitting edema, especially periorbital, hands, and feet 12-lead ECG for heart blocks, low voltage, flattened T wave Depression Laboratory values: • Decreased sodium • Decreased serum glucose • Increased cholesterol • Increased CK	Rapid assessment provides data needed to develop a further plan of care. Decreased metabolism leads to decreased temperature. Heart is profoundly depressed related to decreased production of myocyte contractile protein and enzymes. While lungs are not typically affected, there is respiratory muscle dysfunction with depressed respiratory drive and increased alveolar-arterial gradient. Fluid accumulations may lead to pleural effusions. Decreased sodium is a result of expanded body water. Increased cholesterol is a	Patient is awake and alert. Vital signs are within normal limits.	Myxedema coma is diagnosed on clinical presentation. Always begin treatment once clinical diagnosis is confirmed. Thyroid function test take several hours to get results.[23,28,44]

PROBLEM	INTERVENTION	RATIONALE	EXPECTED OUTCOME	SPECIAL CONSIDERATIONS
	• ABGs (respiratory failure with Pao_2 less than 50 mm Hg, $Paco_2$ greater than 50 mm Hg, pH lower than 7.35)	result of decreased cholesterol metabolism.		
Patient has increased risk of mortality related to myxedema coma.	Rapid replacement of TH Cortisol replacement if concomitant adrenal insufficiency exists See Medication table on pp. 952-953	Early treatment decreases risk of death from myxedema coma.	Thyroid hormone levels will rise.	Because of hypometabolic state, all drugs, dosages, and times will need to be adjusted for decreased metabolism.[28,34]
	Supportive care	Thyroid replacement is needed to correct hypometabolic state. Because of poor absorption, T_3 and T_4 are replaced IV. Adrenal insufficiency often occurs with myxedema and should be treated with stress doses of cortisol until adrenal function is determined.	Adrenal insufficiency will be corrected.	T_4 is inactive form of TH and provides a stable steady replacement. T_3 is active form of TH and has a short half-life. It is recommended that T_4 and T_3 be administered together. Administer T_3 with caution in patients at risk for dysrhythmias or infarction.[28] If hypotension is unresponsive to prudent fluid replacement, whole blood may be transfused. If still hypotensive, a dopamine drip can be used cautiously. Hypotension can remain resistant until thyroid hormone and cortisol (if needed) are replaced.[23,28,34,59]
	Oxygen: nasal cannula, face mask, BiPAP, or CPAP as needed to correct hypoxia Intubation and mechanical ventilation, if needed Supplemental oxygen is needed	Supplemental oxygen will assist with hypoxia. Mechanical ventilation may be needed to correct hypercarbia and hypoxia. Hypoxia and hypercapnia are common in myxedema related to decreased drive to breathe.	Hypoxemia and hypercarbia will be corrected.	
	IV fluids: 0.9% normal saline 3% normal saline can be administered for severe hyponatremia less than 115 mEq/L	Normal saline will assist to correct hyponatremia. Give cautiously as fluid overload can lead to heart failure because of reduced cardiac function.		
	Warming blankets and central rewarming Temperature monitoring with a rectal probe	True core temperature needs to be determined to monitor rewarming efforts.	Body temperature will return to normal.	Peripheral rewarming with blankets should be conducted with central rewarming to prevent vasodilation.

Data from references 14, 23, 28, 34, 43, 44, 49, 53, 59.
ABGs = Arterial blood gases, BiPap = bi-level positive airway pressure, CPAP = continuous positive airway pressure, CK = creatinine kinase, ECG = electrocardiogram, Pao_2 = partial pressure of arterial oxygen tension, $PaCO_2$ = partial pressure of arterial carbon dioxide, TH = thyroid hormone, T_3 = triiodothyronine, T_4 = thyroxine.

AI can occur as a primary or secondary disorder. Primary disorders are caused by dysfunction of the adrenal gland, while secondary disorders are caused by disorders of the HPA. Primary AI usually affects both glucocorticoids (cortisol) and fludrocortisone (aldosterone). As many as 40% to 65% of all primary AI patients also have hypoaldosteronism, indicated by an increased plasma renin activity in the face of decreased aldosterone levels.[5]

Patients at Risk. The incidence of AI is very rare (less than 0.01%). However, the incidence increases up to 28% for the critically ill, stressed patients.[54] Marik and Zaloga[39] state the incidence may be 30% overall in all critically ill patients and with patients in septic shock the incidence may be as high as 50% to 60%. It is difficult to determine the exact percentage as the underlying disease processes as well as the severity of illness vary widely. Patients with sepsis, systemic inflammatory response syndrome (SIRS), and multiple trauma, as well as complicated surgical patients,[54] are at the greatest risk for AI[5,35,39,40] (Table 35-2). In addition, medications used in the treatment of critically ill patients can lead to AI, such as corticosteroids (secondary AI), ketoconazole (Nizoral) and etomidate (Amidate), rifampin (Xifaxan), and phenytoin (Dilantin) (increased cortisol metabolism). Furthermore, there are many other etiologies for AI: HIV infection; carcinoma of breast, lung, or liver; fungal infections; tuberculosis; acute hemorrhage; and pituitary removal.[35,39,40,54] Critically ill patients with age-related risk include those older than 55; this patient population has threefold greater increases in the incidence of AI than younger patients.[54]

TABLE 35-2 Pituitary, Adrenals, and Thyroid During Sepsis

GLAND/ HORMONE	EFFECTS OF SEPSIS	EFFECTS OF HORMONE REPLACEMENT	CURRENT EVIDENCE-BASED MANAGEMENT
Pituitary/ ADH	Endotoxins in sepsis diminish catecholamine receptor response Vasopressors use catecholamine receptors to stimulate constriction	Vasopressin: • Can reverse diminished response of catecholamine receptors • Causes pulmonary vasoconstriction • Lowers heart rate via baroceptor mediation • Stimulates ACTH release, leading to increased serum cortisol levels	Vasopressin administration 0.04 unit/ min IV infusion can reduce or eliminate need for vasopressors[13]
Adrenal/ cortisol	Inactivation of fludrocortisol Decreased number of or response to fludrocortisol receptors "Catecholamine insensitivity" receptors become less responsive to catecholamines (alpha and beta)[40]	Cortisol can reverse diminished response of catecholamine receptors[40]	Hydrocortisone replacement should be considered for all critically ill patients with serum cortisol level less than 25 mcg/dl or failure to increase cortisol levels greater than or equal to 9 mcg/dl in response to corticotropin stimulation test[38,45] Future research is needed to determine treatment for patients with cortisol levels greater than 25 mcg/dl that do not respond to corticotropin stimulation test[45]
Thyroid/ T_3, T_4	Decreased conversion of T_4 to T_3 Dysfunction of protein binding to TH	Hypothyroxinemia is a strong predictor of mortality; 84% mortality rate noted for an initial T_4 value <3 mg/dl	No substantial evidence to show T_4 replacement improves outcomes[45]

Data from references 13, 38, 40, 45.
ACTH = Adrenocorticotropic hormone, ADH = antidiuretic hormone, TH = thyroid hormone, T_3 = triiodothyronine, T_4 = thyroxine.

Clinical Presentation. The hallmark of AI in the critically ill is refractory, vasopressor-dependent hypotension with increased cardiac output and decreased systemic vascular resistance.[5,13,25,60] The alpha and beta receptors develop SIRS-induced catecholamine insensitivity,[5,25,54] and become less responsive to cortisol even if the serum cortisol level is normal. These desensitized alpha and beta receptors may lead to decreased vascular responsiveness and myocardial depression.[48,54] Early recognition of AI in these patients can eliminate the need for high doses of vasopressors with possible harmful effects.* Other signs and symptoms of AI in critically ill patients include hyponatremia, hyperkalemia, hypercalcemia, hypoglycemia, metabolic acidosis, and eosinophilia. Nonspecific signs include weakness, fatigue, weight loss, unexplained fever, and hyperdynamic circulation usually associated with SIRS or septic shock.[13,38,40,54]

Diagnostic Evaluation. The corticotropin stimulation test is the standard test performed to rule out AI. The cosyntropin ACTH test should be performed early on all patients with a diagnosis of septic shock to recognize those patients in which cortisol replacement would be beneficial.[35,38,39,40,54] If the presumed diagnosis is AI, treatment should begin as soon as the test is completed, before results are reported. However, dexamethasone 2 mg IV can be administered before the corticotropin stimulation test because it does not interfere with the test.[5] The Research Utilization box at right provides an in-depth look at a comparison of adrenal responses under different levels of stress.

A random cortisol level is rarely used to diagnose AI because normal cortisol levels have a diurnal variation.[54] However, Marik and Zaloga[39] concluded that a random serum cortisol measurement could be used in critically ill patients. Critically ill patients not currently being treated with cortisol with random serum cortisol levels less than 25 mcg/dl or greater than 45 mcg/dl have the highest mortality.[39] In addition, other laboratory values should be followed closely, including CBC, electrolytes (sodium, potassium, calcium), BUN, serum creatinine, and serum glucose. Hypoglycemia should be treated with dextrose IV. Thyroid function tests should be performed to rule out thyroid dysfunction or assess concomitant thyroid disorder.[14,23]

Multidisciplinary Plan of Care. If there is a high suspicion of adrenal insufficiency in the critically ill patient and a random serum cortisol measurement is less than 25 mcg/dl, hydrocortisone 100 mg IV should be administered. The response to this treatment should be assessed. If there is clinical improvement, subsequent

---

*References 35, 38, 39, 40, 54, 60.

◆ RESEARCH UTILIZATION

A Comparison of the Adrenal Response of ACTH Stimulation Test in Patients Under Different Levels of Stress

CLINICAL ISSUE

The integrity of the hypothalamus-pituitary axis (HPA) is assessed by stimulation with 250 mcg of a synthetic adrenocorticotropic (ACTH) hormone. The response to this exogenous ACTH is the current standard to assess for adrenal insufficiency, defined as basal cortisol concentrations less than 3.6 mcg/dl or as peak cortisol levels 18–20 mcg/dl 30–60 minutes after ACTH is administered. It has been suggested that a 1-mcg dose could be a more sensitive indicator as it can induce a response similar to acute illness.

SUMMARY

This study sought to compare the adrenal response of the two ACTH stimulation tests in patients under different levels of stress. The study utilized three groups of patients: group A ($n = 20$), ambulatory control; group B ($n = 25$), hospitalized medical patients; and group C ($n = 29$), patients undergoing coronary artery bypass grafting (CABG). The CABG patient was chosen as the stress of surgery is similar to the acute phase of septic shock. All subjects had four consecutive ACTH stimulation tests, and each was randomized to either a 1-mcg or a 250-mcg dose. Group A did not show a difference in response to the 1-mcg versus the 250-mcg dose in cortisol release. Cortisol release was elevated with both doses in groups B and C; however, the 1-mcg dose demonstrated that maximal stimulation is not needed to test the HPA and adrenal reserve. The basal cortisol level for group C was lowest at the time of maximal stress during postextubation.

APPLICATION

The study also identified that increased sensitivity to ACTH can be related to other mechanisms that mediate ACTH release. Pain, fever, and hypovolemia have been identified as factors that lead to increased cortisol levels. This study reveals the physiologically adaptive differences in the HPA related to different levels of stress. In addition, it is proposed that the 1-mcg test could provide a more sensitive indicator of adrenal insufficiency for the patient under moderate or severe stress in critical illness.

NEED FOR FURTHER STUDY

Further studies are needed to compare the two stimulation doses of cortisol (250 mcg or 1 mcg) to determine if the lower dose would provide a more accurate definition of adrenal insufficiency.

Widmer, I., et al. (2005). Cortisol response in relation to severity of stress and illness. *J Clin Endocrinol Metab, 90,* 4579–4586.

IV hydrocortisone doses should be considered.[5,39] Annane et al.[5] found that 28-day mortality and vasopressor-dependent duration were substantially reduced with the administration of hydrocortisone 50 mg IV every 6 hours and fludrocortisone 50 mcg tablet daily. Annane treated all critically ill patients having a random serum cortisol level less than 25 mcg/dl with hydrocortisone 100 mg immediately, and continued the treatment for a few days (100 mg every 8 hours) if the patient showed clinical improvement with the initial dose. Rivers et al.[54] found improved survival and decreased ventilator weaning times in vasopressor-dependent patients treated with hydrocortisone.

Other treatments of AI focus on treatment of hypotension using fluids and vasopressors. In critical illness, ADH stores can become depleted, adding to the hypovolemia. Therefore a continuous drip of arginine vasopressin (0.04 mg/min) may be used to treat hypotension.[14] Serum sodium depletion and serum potassium excess can be normalized by adding an aldosterone replacement, fludrocortisone.[5] In addition, hypoglycemia should be treated with 50% dextrose IV to normalize blood glucose level. A comprehensive plan of care can serve as a guide to the management of AI.

◆ Case Study 35-5

Adrenal Insufficiency

J.W. is a 24-year-old Caucasian male who suffered bilateral lower extremity (BLE) crush injuries in a small rural community. He was taken to a local hospital for stabilization and prepared for transfer. During the 75-minute ambulance transport J.W. had several episodes of hypotension and hypoxemia. He was unconscious upon admission to the trauma center and was taken to the OR immediately for vascular repair of the popliteal and femoral arteries, debridement of BLE, and external fixation.

On day 3, J.W. spikes a fever of 103° F. Blood, urine, and pulmonary bronchial washings are obtained. He developed poor vascular supply and areas of necrosis and was returned to the OR for debridement. After surgery, he is hypotensive (65–70 mm Hg systolic) despite 2 L of NS and three boluses of 250 ml of 3% sodium chloride. The decision is made to start a norepinephrine (Levophed) drip for blood pressure support, and a pulmonary artery catheter is placed. Later that same afternoon, he returns to the operating room for bilateral above-the-knee (AK) amputation. He is mechanically ventilated with Fio$_2$ 60% and continues to be hemodynamically unstable.

Assessment: pulmonary artery catheter readings, CVP = 3 mm Hg, PAP = 15/7 mm Hg, PAWP = 4 mm Hg, SVR = 512 dynes/sec/cm^3, CO = 10 L/min; BP = 92/50 mm Hg; HR = 136 beats/min. His ventilator settings are as follows: mode assist control, rate = 16, Fio$_2$ = 60%, Vt = 900, positive end-expiratory pressure (PEEP) = 15 mm Hg. Laboratory values include ABGs, pH = 7.27, Paco$_2$ = 50 mm Hg, Pao$_2$ = 71 mm Hg; HCO$_3^-$ = 17 mEq/L, O$_2$ saturation = 82%, Na$^+$ = 129 mEq/L, K$^+$ = 5.8 mEq/L, Ca^{++} = 12 mg/dl, serum glucose = 84 mg/dl; Hgb = 10 g/dl, Hct = 30%, WBC = 2000/mm^3, platelets = 75,000/mm^3; creatinine = 2.8 mg/dl, BUN = 30 mg/dl, serum cortisol = 22 mcg/dl (6 PM). He remains hypotensive and unresponsive to fluids. The physician orders vasopressin drip at a continuous rate of 0.04 unit/minute.

Decision point: Discuss events of day 3 that place J.W. at risk for AI.

Decision point: Discuss hemodynamic parameters as they relate to the diagnosis of AI.

Decision point: Discuss ABGs and ventilator settings and what ventilator setting changes are needed.

Decision point: Discuss lab values as they pertain to AI.

Decision point: Discuss the serum cortisol level.

Decision point: Discuss why the physician ordered a vasopressin drip.

The physician writes the following orders: stat chest x-ray, dexamethasone 2 mg IV, and corticotropin stimulation test.

Decision point: Why did the physician order dexamethasone before a corticotropin stimulation test?

Decision point: Explain how a corticotropin stimulation test is performed and why the test was ordered.

Decision point: What would you expect the physician to order for the diagnosis of AI?

On day 5, J.W. was placed on high-frequency oscillating ventilation for worsening respiratory failure related to ventilator-associated pneumonia. On day 7 J.W. expired.

Conclusions. Adrenal insufficiency in the critically ill patient is an emergent situation superposed on an already stressed patient. Adrenal insufficiency as a result of critical illness, especially sepsis and septic shock, requires early identification and management to prevent morbidity and mortality related to persistent catecholamine-resistant shock. The Multidisciplinary Plan of Care on pp. 963-964 summarizes care that focuses on replacing cortisol and correcting hypotension, hyponatremia, and hypoglycemia.

MULTIDISCIPLINARY PLAN OF CARE FOR THE PATIENT WITH ADRENAL INSUFFICIENCY

PROBLEM	INTERVENTION	RATIONALE	EXPECTED OUTCOME	SPECIAL CONSIDERATIONS
Risk for development of AI	Careful consideration of patients who present with: • SIRS • Sepsis, septic shock • Trauma • Complicated surgery • Medications: corticosteroids, ketoconazole, etomidate, rifampin • HIV • Carcinomas: breast, lung, kidney • Fungal infections • Tuberculosis (Addison's disease) • Pituitary removal	Early identification of patients allows for appropriate prophylactic intervention, especially in preparation for diagnostic testing or surgery.	Patients at risk for adrenal insufficiency will be identified early.	All patients with SIRS, sepsis, and septic shock should be considered at increased risk for AI; up to 50%-60% can have occult AI.[39] Patients with hypophysectomy require life-long glucocorticoid and fludrocortisone replacement. Patient and family education is necessary, as is a Medic-Alert bracelet.
	Monitor vital signs, hemodynamic parameters, serum cortisol, and other laboratory values as treatment begins for: • Elevated BP, increased MAP, normal HR • Elevated CVP, normal PAP, elevated PAWP, normal SVR • Adequate urine output • BUN, creatinine • Decreased blood glucose • Electrolytes: normal Na^+, K^+, Ca^{++} • Normal serum cortisol Fluid status is monitored most accurately using hemodynamic monitoring with a pulmonary artery or CVP catheter.	Assessment provides the data needed to develop a further plan of care.	Changes in cortisol secretion and systemic response to cortisol will be identified.[25]	AI can be an insidious secondary disease process that should be suspected in all critically ill patients.[23,39,59,60] Always suspect AI when hypotension is unresponsive to fluid resuscitation and increasing vasopressor therapy.[39] Serial blood glucose levels should be determined to assess increases because steroids increase blood glucose level via breakdown of carbohydrates, fats, proteins.
Refractory hypotension with fluid resuscitation and increasing use of vasopressors	Hydrocortisone replacement: 50–100 mg every 6 hr for 1–2 days, then taper over 7 days[5]	To provide cortisol replacement to improve hypotension and decrease use of vasopressors. To provide aldosterone replacement to assist with correction of hyponatremia and hyperkalemia.	Serum cortisol levels increase. Hypotension improves with cortisol replacement.	Hydrocortisone replacement doses should be no more than 50 mg every 6 hr to 100 mg every 8 hr for short duration (5–7 days) as high replacement doses have been associated with

Table continues on page 964

PROBLEM	INTERVENTION	RATIONALE	EXPECTED OUTCOME	SPECIAL CONSIDERATIONS
		In critical illness, antidiuretic hormone stores can become depleted. This low consistent vasopressin replacement can stabilize BP.		increased morbidity and mortality.[5,39]
Hyponatremia and hyperkalemia as a result of insufficient cortisol	Fluid volume replacement: 0.9% NS (hypertonic saline rarely needed) Assess ECG for hyperkalemia-related changes: tall peaked T waves, PVCs, prolonged QRS Monitor Na$^+$ and electrolyte levels every 6 hr and discontinue as cortisol levels increase and electrolyte imbalances correct	To monitor Na$^+$ and K$^+$ levels to prevent untoward effects of hyponatremia or hyperkalemia.	Serum sodium increases. Serum potassium levels decrease. No ECG changes will occur.	ECG changes detected may not be direct link to hyperkalemia, but as a result of critically ill stressed state of the patient and other concomitant physiologic processes.[23,39,59]

Data from references 5, 14, 23, 25, 39, 59, 60.
AI = Adrenal insufficiency, BP = blood pressure, BUN = blood urea nitrogen, Ca^{++} = calcium, CVP = central venous pressure, ECG = electrocardiogram, HR = heart rate, K$^+$ = potassium, MAP = mean arterial pressure, Na$^+$ = sodium, NS = normal saline, PAP = pulmonary artery pressure, PAWP = pulmonary artery wedge pressure, PVCs = premature ventricular contractions, SIRS = systemic inflammatory response syndrome, SVR = systemic vascular resistance.

REFERENCES

1. Agah, A., et al. (2004). Anterior pituitary dysfunction in survivors of traumatic brain injury. *J Clin Endocrinol Metab, 89*, 4929–4936.

2. Alaca, R., et al. (2002). Anterior hypopituitarism with unusual delayed onset of diabetes insipidus after penetrating head trauma. *Am J Phys Med Rehabil, 81*, 788–791.

3. Albanese, et al. (2001). Management of hyponatremia in patients with cerebral insults. *Arch Dis Child, 85*, 246–251.

4. Amar, A., et al. (2004). Posterior pituitary dysfunction after traumatic brain injury. *J Clin Endocrinol Metab, 89*, 5987–5992.

5. Annane D., et al. (2002). Effect of treatment with low doses of hydrocortisone and fludrocortisone on mortality in patients with septic shock. *JAMA, 288*, 862–871.

6. Arnaldi, G., et al. (2005). Diagnosis and complications of Cushing's syndrome: a consensus statement. *J Clin Endocrinol Metab, 88*, 5593–5602.

7. Aron, D. C., et al. (2004). Hypothalamus & pituitary gland. In F. S. Greenspan & D. G. Gardner (Eds.), *Basic & clinical endocrinology* (7th ed., pp. 106–171). New York: Lange Medical Books.

8. Aron, D. C., et al. (2004). Glucocorticoids & adrenal androgens. In F. S. Greenspan & D. G. Gardner (Eds.), *Basic & clinical endocrinology* (7th ed., pp. 362–408). New York: Lange Medical Books.

9. Batz, B. (2000). Mechanisms of endocrine control. In L. C. Copsted & J. L. Banasik (Eds.), *Pathophysiology: biological and behavioral perspectives* (2nd ed., pp. 880–891). Philadelphia: Saunders.

10. Batz, B. (2000). Alterations in endocrine control. In L. C. Copsted & J. L. Banasik (Eds.), *Pathophysiology: biological and behavioral perspectives* (2nd ed., pp. 884–919). Philadelphia: Saunders.

11. Baxter, J. D., et al. (2004). Introduction to endocrinology. In F. S. Greenspan & D. G. Gardner (Eds.), *Basic & clinical endocrinology* (7th ed., pp. 1–23). New York: Lange Medical Books.

12. Behnia, M., et al. (2000). Management of myxedematous respiratory failure: review of ventilation and weaning. *Am J Med Sci, 320*, 368–373.

13. Brierre, S., et al. (2004). The endocrine system during sepsis. *Am J Med Sci, 328*, 238–247.

14. Byrum, C. D. (2001). The endocrine system. In J. G. Alspach (Ed.), *AACN instructor resource manual for the AACN core curriculum for critical care nursing* (5th ed., pp. 265–293). Philadelphia: Saunders.

15. Cardoso, E., et al. (2003). Spontaneous and cytokine-induced natural killer cytotoxicity in patients with Cushing's disease. *Endocrinologist, 13*, 459–464.

16. Cooper, D. S. (2005). Drug therapy: antithyroid drugs. *N Engl J Med, 352*, 905–917.

17. Dickerson, R. N. (2002). Hyponatremia in neurosurgical patients: syndrome of inappropriate ADH or cerebral salt wasting syndrome? *Hosp Pharm*, 1336–1340.

18. Elovic, E. P. (2003). Anterior pituitary dysfunction after traumatic brain injury. *J Head Trauma Rehabil, 18*, 541–543.

19. Finch, C. K., et al. (2004). Nicotine replacement therapy—associated syndrome of inappropriate antidiuretic hormone. *S Med J, 97*, 322–324.

20. Fitzgerald, P. A., & Gildfien, A. (2004). Adrenal medulla. In F. S. Greenspan & D. G. Gardner (Eds.), *Basic & clinical endocrinology* (7th ed., pp. 106–171). New York: Lange Medical Books.

21. Fresner, Y. T., et al. (2004). Thyroid storm and ventricular tachycardia. *S Med J, 97*, 604–607.

22. Graham, G. T., et al. (2000). Perioperative management of endocrine disorders. *Int Anesth Clin, 38,* 43–58.

23. Gardner, D. G., & Greenspan, F. S. (2004). Endocrine emergencies. In F. S. Greenspan & D. G. Gardner (Eds.), *Basic & clinical endocrinology* (7th ed., pp. 867–873). New York: Lange Medical Books.

24. Greenspan, F. S. (2004). The thyroid gland. In F. S. Greenspan & D. G. Gardner (Eds.), *Basic & clinical endocrinology* (7th ed., pp. 215–256). New York: Lange Medical Books.

25. Hamarahian, A. H., et al. (2004). Measurements of serum free cortisol in critically ill patients. *N Engl J Med, 350,* 1629–1638.

26. Hansberg, A. (2005). Common disorders of the pituitary: hyposecretions versus hypersecretion. *J Infusion Nurs, 28,* 36–44.

27. Hennessey, J. V. (2003). Precise thyroxine dosing: clinical requirements. *Endocrinologist, 13,* 479–487.

28. Hierholzer, K., et al. (1997). Myxedema: pathophysiology and therapy. *Kidney Int Suppl, 51,* S82–S89.

29. Herlihy, B., & Maebius, N. K. (2003). *Human body in health and illness.* St. Louis: Saunders.

30. Iwasaki, Y., & Majzoub, J. A. (1999). Disordered water metabolism: new insights from molecular diagnosis. *Curr Opin Endocrinol Diabet, 6,* 112–118.

31. Jones, R. E. (2002). Alterations in hormonal regulation. In K. L. McCance & S. E. Huether (Eds.), *Pathophysiology: the biological basis for disease in adults and children* (4th ed., pp. 624–666). St. Louis: Mosby.

32. Jones, R. E. (2002). Adrenal insufficiency. In M. T. McDermott (Ed.), *Endocrine secrets* (3rd ed., pp. 255–260). Philadelphia: Hanley and Belfus.

33. Knoers, N. V. (2005). Hyperactive vasopressin receptors and disturbed water metabolism. *N Engl J Med, 352,* 1847–1850.

34. Li, T. M. (2002). Hypothyroidism in elderly people. *Geriatr Nurs, 23,* 88–93.

35. Ligtenberg, J. J. M., & Zijlistra, J. G. (2004). The relative adrenal insufficiency syndrome revisited: which patients will benefit from low-dose steroids? *Curr Opin Crit Care, 10,* 456–460.

36. Liu, H., & Crapo, L. (2005). Update on the diagnosis of Cushing's syndrome. *Endocrinologist, 15,* 165–179.

37. Magner, J. A. (2004). Thyroid-stimulating hormone-mediated hyperthyroidism. *Endocrinologist, 14,* 201–211.

38. Manglik, S., et al. (2003). Glucocorticoid insufficiency in patients who present to the hospital with severe sepsis: a prospective clinical trial. *Crit Care Med, 31,* 1668–1675.

39. Marik, P. E., & Zaloga, G. P. (2002). Adrenal insufficiency in the critically ill: a new look at an old problem. *Crit Care Rev, 1784–1793.*

40. Marik, P. E., & Zaloga, G. P. (2003). Adrenal insufficiency during septic shock. *Crit Care Med, 31,* 141–145.

41. Martino, E., et al. (2001). The effects of amiodarone on the thyroid. *Endocr Rev, 22,* 240–254.

42. Mazzone, P. J., et al. (2003). Endocrine paraneoplastic syndromes in lung cancer. *Curr Opin Pulm Med, 9,* 313–320.

43. McDermott, M. T. (2002). Thyroid testing. In M. T. McDermott (Ed.), *Endocrine secrets* (3rd ed., pp. 269–271). Philadelphia: Hanley and Belfus.

44. McDermott, M. T. (2002). Thyroid emergencies. In M. T. McDermott (Ed.), *Endocrine secrets* (3rd ed., pp. 302–305). Philadelphia: Hanley and Belfus.

45. McDermott, M. T. (2002). Euthyroid sick syndrome. In M. T. McDermott (Ed.), *Endocrine secrets* (3rd ed., pp. 306–307). Philadelphia: Hanley and Belfus.

46. Milionis, H., & Moses, E. (2002). Hyponatremia and SIADH. *Can Med Assoc J, 167,* 450.

47. Milianos, H., et al. (2002). The hyponatremic patient: a systematic approach to laboratory diagnosis. *Can Med Assoc J, 166,* 1056–1062.

48. Minneci, P. C., et al. (2004). Meta-analysis: the effect of steroids on survival and shock during sepsis depends on the dose. *Ann Int Med, 141,* 47–57.

49. O'Connor, C. J., et al. (2003). Severe myxedema coma after cardiopulmonary bypass. *Int Anesthesia Res Soc, 96,* 62–64.

50. Ng Jao, Y. T. F., et al. (2004). Thyroid storm and ventricular tachycardia. *S Med J, 97,* 604–607.

51. Patchier, J., et al. (1999). Brain death and its influence on donor organ quality and outcome after transplantation. *Transplantation, 67,* 343–348.

52. Porterfield, S. P. (2001). *Endocrine physiology* (2nd ed.), St. Louis: Mosby.

53. Rehman, S., et al. (2005). Thyroid disorders in elderly patients. *S Med J, 98,* 543–549.

54. Rivers, E. P., et al. (2001). Adrenal insufficiency in high-risk surgical ICU patients. *Chest, 119,* 889–896.

55. Rosmond, R., & Bjorntorp, P. (2001). Alterations in the hypothalamic-pituitary-adrenal axis in metabolic syndrome. *Endocrinologist, 11,* 491–497.

56. Rufener, S., et al. (2005). Thyroid storm precipitated by infection: an atypical case involving multisystem organ dysfunction. *Endocrinologist, 15,* 111–114.

57. Salim, A., et al. (2005). Aggressive organ donor management significantly increases the number of organs available for transplantation. *J Trauma, 58,* 991–994.

58. Saunders, L. R. (2002). Disorders of water metabolism. In M. T. McDermott (Ed.), *Endocrine secrets* (3rd ed., pp. 208–225). Philadelphia: Hanley and Belfus.

59. Savage, M. W., et al. (2004). Endocrine emergencies. *Postgrad Med J, 80,* 506–515.

60. Schmidt, I. L., et al. (2005). Diagnosis of adrenal insufficiency: evaluation of the corticotrophin-releasing hormone test and basal serum cortisol in comparison to the insulin tolerance test in patients with hypothalamic-pituitary-adrenal disease. *J Clin Endocrinol Metab, 9,* 4193–4198.

61. Sonino, N., et al. (2005). Pharmacological management of Cushing's syndrome: new targets for therapy. *Treat Endocrin, 4,* 87–94.

62. Waugh, A., & Grant, A. (2001). *Anatomy and physiology in health and illness* (9th ed.), Edinburgh: Churchill Livingstone.

63. Yasumasa, I., & Majzoub, J. A. (1999). Disordered water metabolism: new insights from molecular diagnosis. *Curr Opin Endocrinol Diab, 6,* 112–118.

64. Yeates, K. E., et al. (2004). Salt and water: a simple approach to hyponatremia. *Can Med Assoc J, 170,* 363–369.

UNIT **9**

HEMATOLOGIC

CHAPTER 36

Blood Conservation and Blood Component Replacement

Dana M. Kyles

Transfusion practices continue to evolve with rapid progression over the past several decades. While there is a belief that poorer outcomes are associated with higher rates of blood administration and that many blood transfusions are unnecessarily utilized, approximately 14 million blood transfusions do occur in the United States annually.[47] It is estimated that more than 50% of all critical care patients receive at least 1 unit of red blood cells (RBCs) during their hospital stay.[16] In addition, these patients may also receive other blood components to manage coagulopathy or active bleeding.

Anemia is a common problem in critical care. The causes are multifaceted and thought to be a result of frequent iatrogenic phlebotomy, coagulation disorders, sepsis, nutritional deficiencies (i.e., iron, vitamin B_{12}, folic acid), bone marrow suppression, renal failure, impaired erythropoietin response and production, abnormalities in iron metabolism, and other severe illnesses (Table 36-1). The primary causes of anemia are blood loss and abnormal or inadequate production of RBCs. Acute anemia, the consequence of an abrupt reduction in the number of RBCs, may be due to hemolysis or acute, frank hemorrhage as a result of surgical procedures, gastrointestinal (GI) bleeding, or trauma. An additional cause of anemia in critically ill patients is blunted production of endogenous erythropoietin, consistent with anemia related to chronic inflammation.[16,17] While mean serum erythropoietin concentrations are much lower in critically ill patients compared to patients with iron-deficiency anemia,[62] there does not appear to be an association between erythropoietin and hemoglobin (Hgb) levels.

Rapid alterations of serum iron metabolism can contribute to critical care–associated anemia. This is thought to be a result of the heightened inflammatory process, disturbance in iron circulation, decreased serum iron levels, and increased iron storage. Minimum information exists about the reason for altered iron metabolism in the development of iron anemia in critically ill patients.[51] Transferrin, serum iron, and total iron-binding capacity are low in critically ill patients.[17] Serum ferritin levels are normal or elevated. Iron deficiency is a potential cause of blood loss because RBCs require iron for production, growth, and maturation. When there is insufficient iron, less Hgb is produced in the RBCs, resulting in decreased oxygen delivery to the tissues.

Approximately 63% of critically ill patients have Hgb levels below 12 g/dl on admission to critical care.[42] By day 3 in critical care, the percentage of patients with a Hgb level of less than 12 g/dl increases to 95%.[17] Clinical manifestations of mild to moderate anemia are tachycardia, exertional dyspnea, fatigue, and weakness. Severe anemia can cause decreased oxygen delivery to tissues, resulting in anaerobic metabolism and lactate production, myocardial infarction, and ischemic stroke.

To restore and maintain hemostasis, oxygen-carrying capacity, and quality of life for the patient, clinicians must be knowledgeable about component therapy, blood component modifications, adverse effects, blood conservation techniques, and alternatives to transfusion.

CONTROVERSIES IN TRANSFUSION

An RBC transfusion provides immediate improvement of low Hgb levels resulting from deficient RBC production or blood loss. Normal Hgb levels are between 12 and 16 g/dl in women and 13.5 and 18 g/dl in men.[13] The optimal Hgb level in critically ill patients has not been determined. When Hgb levels are reduced, the oxygen-carrying capacity and total oxygen content in the blood decrease. Hgb is intended to rapidly bind oxygen in the lungs and unload it in the tissues.

The normal relationship between Hgb and oxygen unloading is illustrated by the oxyhemoglobin dissociation curve. Oxygen's capability to bind to Hgb is affected by several factors that result in a shifting or reshaping the curve. Hgb function may be altered by a variety of reasons (e.g., pH or 2,3-diphosphoglycerate [DPG] levels). When pH decreases or DPG levels increase, oxygen affinity for Hgb decreases, shifting the dissociation curve to the right, increasing the delivery of oxygen to tissues. The standard curve is also shifted to the right by an increase in temperature or partial pressure of arterial carbon dioxide (Pa_{CO_2}).[46] Alternatively, the curve is shifted to the left by an increased pH or by decreased

TABLE 36-1 Selected Types of Anemias

TYPE OF ANEMIA	DEFINITION/PATHOPHYSIOLOGY
Anemia of chronic inflammatory disease	Chronic disorders with an inflammatory component, such as infection, leading to anemia
Aplastic anemia	Potentially fatal, caused by destruction of bone marrow stem cells and inhibited RBC production; results in pancytopenia and bone marrow hypoplasia
Iron deficiency anemia	Inadequate supply of iron; need for iron is greater than absorption because of impaired gastrointestinal absorption or blood loss from trauma, severe menorrhagia, or gross hematuria
Pregnancy	During pregnancy, plasma volume increases while RBC mass decreases
Sickle cell anemia	Congenital disease causing hemolysis and vascular occlusion because of an abnormal Hgb molecule causing RBC destruction and a sickled shape
Thalassemias	Hereditary hemolytic anemia characterized by defective and impaired Hgb production and impaired RBC synthesis

Hgb = Hemoglobin, RBC = red blood cell.

DPG levels, temperature, or $Paco_2$. A leftward shift increases the affinity of the oxygen for the Hgb, simplifying the mechanism in which Hgb adheres to oxygen, while making it more difficult for oxygen to be released.[46]

Historically, both the literature and clinical practice supported the notion that an RBC transfusion is necessary when the Hgb level is less than 10 g/dl. Such recommendations are based more on tradition than clinical trials and do not take into account the patient's clinical scenario (e.g., whether the patient is experiencing symptoms, the patient's tolerance to the anemia, the underlying pathophysiology). Recent studies recommend the use of restrictive transfusion thresholds in the critically ill patient, suggesting that anemia does not negatively affect short-term mortality.[30,33] A randomized, controlled clinical trial by Hebert et al. suggests a restrictive transfusion threshold appears to be safe

in critically ill patients with cardiovascular disease.[27] Currently, the typical transfusion threshold is a Hgb level of 7 to 8 g/dl,[67] equivalent to a hematocrit (Hct) of 21% to 24%. However, Hgb or Hct levels should not be the only "transfusion triggers" because this may result in unnecessary administration of blood components.[28]

A large number of patients are anemic on admission to critical care or become anemic during their critical care stay.[59] A lack of compelling data has resulted in variable transfusion practices and helps to explain the frequency of transfusion in critical care. A Canadian multicentered, randomized, controlled clinical study by Hebert et al.[26] discovered that transfusion practices significantly vary among physicians and institutions. A European prospective, observational, cross-sectional study by Vincent et al.[69] of 3534 patients supported that anemia was common in critically ill patients; 37% of subjects with a Hgb concentration of less than 10 g/dl received a transfusion during their critical care admission. Approximately 40% of the patients received a transfusion during the critical care stay; the mean pre-transfusion Hgb level was 8.4 g/dl.[69]

Blood components continue to be transfused in critical care despite increasing evidence that blood transfusions may contribute to adverse outcomes (e.g., immunosuppression, transfusion-related acute lung injury (TRALI), organ dysfunction, transmission of infectious diseases [such as hepatitis B or West Nile virus], hemolytic and nonhemolytic transfusion reactions, and alloimmunization).

BLOOD CONSERVATION

At the present time, healthcare professionals are pursuing new alternatives to blood transfusions since many patients, because of religious convictions, medical concerns, or personal preference, are disinclined to receive blood; there are a growing number of alternatives already being instituted to decrease the need for a blood transfusion (e.g., bloodless surgery programs, the use of pharmacologic agents, laser technology or cauterization, and volume expansion). Another important alternative modification would include a universally acceptable, lower transfusion threshold, except in patients with ongoing hemorrhage.

Demand for blood components often exceeds supply because of lack of donors, current U.S. restrictions on the importation of European blood,[70] and the increasing number of transplants and major surgeries requiring massive transfusion. Blood conservation requires vigilant preparation, proactive strategies involving multidisciplinary teams to prevent complications, and careful monitoring of the patient. The primary principles of blood conservation include increasing erythropoiesis, minimizing perioperative and iatrogenic blood loss, and optimizing hemostasis and blood transfusion practices.

Increasing Erythropoiesis

To maintain adequate oxygen delivery to tissues, there must be an adequate number of circulating RBCs. When tissues experience hypoxia, the kidneys and liver respond by producing erythropoietin. Nutrients that play an important role in erythropoiesis include iron, vitamin B_{12}, and folate. Euvolemic, anemic patients with adequate tissue perfusion may benefit from the administration of these nutrients. Others may require pharmacologic intervention with agents such as recombinant human erythropoietin (rHuEPO) to increase erythropoiesis (see the Medication table on pp. 972-973).

Minimizing Perioperative and Iatrogenic Blood Loss

Various techniques can be used during surgery to minimize bleeding and decrease the need for transfusion. Hypotensive anesthesia, also known as controlled hypotension, involves intentionally lowering the patient's blood pressure below normal throughout surgery. This is performed while maintaining perfusion to the heart, lungs, and other organs and tissues. Blood loss is thought to decrease when the patient's blood pressure is low. Other techniques for minimizing blood loss associated with surgery are listed in Table 36-2.

Optimizing Hemostasis and Blood Transfusion Practices

Hemostasis is the method of fibrin formation at the site of vascular injury. This includes the formation of the platelet plug, coagulation activation, cessation of antithrombotic control mechanisms, and fibrin clot degradation, also known as fibrinolysis.

Traditionally, the clotting cascade was described as consisting of an intrinsic and extrinsic pathway. While this classical view of the clotting cascade has been valuable in the interpretation of clotting times, it is considered an in vitro model and may not be physiologically accurate. It has been established that the exposure of tissue factor at the site of injury is the primary physiologic event initiating clotting while subsequent coagulation response occurs on the platelet surface and is regulated by specific receptors.[35]

The critical care nurse caring for a patient undergoing bloodless treatment should be knowledgeable of pharmacologic means and other alternatives to transfusion to prevent and treat anemia.

ALTERNATIVES TO TRANSFUSION

Recombinant Human Erythropoietin

Recombinant human erythropoietin (rHuEPO) is a synthetic growth factor used to supplement the intrinsic hormone normally produced by the kidneys that promotes the formation of RBCs by the bone marrow. Erythropoietin regulates the production of RBCs and initiates the production of Hgb. It has shown to be highly effective in reducing transfusion requirements and increasing Hgb levels in critically ill patients.[18] In the setting of anemia or anticipated anemia, administering erythropoietin prophylactically may decrease the need for blood transfusions.

rHuEPO requires adequate iron stores in order to work effectively. Oral iron will not be sufficient if there is ongoing blood loss. Intravenous (IV) iron supplements, therefore, may be more advantageous. Response to rHuEPO may not be seen until day 3 after therapy begins in iron-depleted patients.

Vitamin K

Bleeding can occur from vitamin K deficiency resulting from poor nutritional status, antibiotic use, infections, or anticoagulants (e.g., warfarin [Coumadin]). Vitamin K assists in the production of calcium-binding coagulation factors II, VII, IX, and X. Although plasma and plasma products can correct factor deficiencies associated with vitamin K deficiency, they should be used only when there is a risk of life-threatening bleeding. According to the *Circular of Information for the Use of Human Blood and Blood Components*,[2] plasma is contraindicated "when coagulopathy can be corrected more effectively with specific therapy, such as vitamin K."

Recombinant Activated Factor VIIa

Recombinant activated factor VII (rFVIIa; NovoSeven; Novo Nordisk A/S, Bagsværd, Denmark) is a hemostatic agent historically used in the United States to treat hemophilia patients with or without inhibitors. In the European Union, it is approved in the treatment of congenital and acquired hemophilia, factor VII deficiency, and Glanzmann thrombasthenia.

rFVIIa has been used in a variety of perioperative and trauma settings for the treatment of massive hemorrhage, acting at the site of injury where tissue factor and collagen are exposed. Most reports of rFVIIa use in trauma are anecdotal. To date there has been one prospective, randomized, double-blind controlled trial of rFVIIa in trauma, conducted by Novo Nordisk A/S13. Overall, there was no significant difference in the outcome measures between the rFVIIa and placebo groups, as explained in the Research Utilization box on pp. 974-975.

PHARMACOLOGIC MEANS TO PREVENT AND TREAT ANEMIA IN CRITICAL CARE

MEDICATION	ACTION	DOSE	SPECIAL CONSIDERATIONS
Aprotinin (Trasylol)	Inhibits fibrinolysis by attaching to plasminogen; prevents it from attaching to the fibrin clot[51]	Cardiopulmonary bypass surgery: 10,000 units IV over 10 min, then loading dose of 1–2 million units over 20–30 min, followed by infusion of 250,000–500,000 units/hr until surgery is complete 1–2 million units are typically added to pump priming fluid as well	Often given during cardiac surgery procedures requiring cardiopulmonary bypass to prevent platelet dysfunction. Potent hemostatic agent that prevents blood loss and preserves platelet function. Naturally occurring serine protease inhibitor Risk of anaphylaxis if patient exposed to products containing aprotinin within previous 12 months
Conjugated estrogens	Exact mechanism unknown although it may include reactivation of platelets and elevated factor VIII and vWF coagulation factors[27]	Abnormal uterine bleeding; 25 mg IV; repeat in 6–12 hr if needed	
Dextran, hetastarch, or pentastarch	Blood volume expander	500–1000 ml IV/day; maximum dose: 1500 ml/day	
Epsilon aminocaproic acid (Amicar)	Inhibits fibrinolysis by attaching to plasminogen; prevents it from attaching to the fibrin clot[51]	Hemorrhage: 4–5 g IV over 1 hr, then 1 g/hr for 8 hr or until hemostasis achieved. Can also give 5 g PO, then 1 g/hr PO for 8 hr or until hemostasis achieved	Promotes clot stability and is useful as adjunctive therapy in hemophilia and some other bleeding disorders[51]
Ferrous sulfate (especially if ferritin levels are decreased)	Hematopoietic agent	Dose depends upon formulation	
Fibrin sealants	The fibrinogen and thrombin in the fibrin sealant combines in the presence of factor XIII and calcium chloride to create a seal or glue[27]		Used in a variety of surgical settings including trauma, neurosurgery, and cardiovascular. Tissue adhesive consisting of human fibrinogen and usually bovine thrombin. Before commercial products available, used "fibrin glue" made in the blood bank from fibrinogen concentrations found in cryoprecipitate.

MEDICATION	ACTION	DOSE	SPECIAL CONSIDERATIONS
Folate	Assists in RBC production	400 mcg daily	Nutritional support Megaloblastic anemia is caused by deficiencies in the B vitamins such as folate, vitamin B_{12}, or both
Recombinant human erythropoietin (rHuEpo)	Regulates erythropoiesis, resulting in higher hemoglobin/hematocrit levels Reduces the need for RBC transfusion	Dosing dependent on indication	Erythropoietin is released into the plasma and binds to the surface of RBCs located in the bone marrow in response to a decrease in tissue oxygenation
Recombinant activated factor VII (rFVIIa) (Novoseven)	Activates coagulation independent of factors VIII and IX Initiates generation of thrombin and fibrin formation Coagulation is activated locally at the site of vascular injury[34,51] RFVIIa binds with tissue factor and activates factors IX and X to their active forms, such as IXa and Xa[34,51]	IV bolus only; give over 2–5 min Hemophilia A or B patients with inhibitors: 90 mcg/kg given every 2 hr until hemostasis is achieved or the treatment has been determined inadequate 35 to 120 mcg/kg in clinical trials For factor VII deficiency, use 15–30 mcg/kg every 4–6 hr until adequate hemostasis is achieved Depending on severity of bleeding, dose and interval may be adjusted	Hemostatic agent used to treat hemophilia A or B patients with or without inhibitors in the United States. Also FDA-approved for treatment of factor VII deficiency Hypersensitivity to mouse, hamster, or bovine protein products
Tranexamic acid	Antifibrinolytic agent that inhibits the activation of plasminogen to plasmin, preventing it from attaching to the fibrin clot[27]	Postoperative hemostasis: 0.5–1g IV given 2–3 times daily for several days after surgery; if further dosing is needed, can use 1–1.5 g PO 3–4 times daily	Promotes clot stability and is useful as adjunctive therapy in hemophilia and some other bleeding disorders[27]
Vitamin B_{12}	Hematopoietic agent	Pernicious anemia: 100 mcg IM daily for 1 week, followed by 100 mcg IM every other day for 7 doses, then every 3–4 days for 2–3 weeks, then monthly	Megaloblastic anemia is caused by deficiencies in the B vitamins such as folate, vitamin B_{12}, or both
Vitamin C	Hematopoietic agent Enhances iron absorption	Dose ranges from 100 mg to 2 g daily depending upon severity of vitamin C deficiency	
Vitamin K (Phytonadione)	Required for the production of specific coagulation factors (factors II, VII, IX and X) in the liver	Hypoprothrombinemia: 2.5–25 mg IV or subcutaneously, repeat in 6–8 hr if needed Can also use 2.5–25 mg PO, repeat in 12–48 hr if needed	Useful as adjunct therapy in the management of hemorrhage Causes of vitamin K deficiency include inadequate dietary intake, poor absorption, and drug interactions (e.g., antibiotics, stroke medications)

Data from references 27, 34, 51, 57.
RBC = Red blood cell, vWF = von Willebrand's factor.

TABLE 36-2 Optimizing Hemostasis and Minimizing Blood Loss

INCREASING ERYTHROPOIESIS	MINIMIZING PERIOPERATIVE AND IATROGENIC BLOOD LOSS	OPTIMIZING HEMOSTASIS AND BLOOD TRANSFUSION PRACTICES
Discontinue medications known to inhibit platelet function (e.g., aspirin, corticosteroids, naproxen [Aleve], clopidogrel [Plavix], ticlopidine [Ticlid], and heparin)	Minimize blood draws by using micro- or pediatric-size blood specimen tubes for laboratory testing Use group blood draws to minimize discard volumes Use smallest recommended discard when drawing samples from lines	For external bleeding, consider use of topical hemostatic agents (e.g., thrombin)
Discontinue herbal replacements that may predispose to bleeding (e.g., dong quai, garlic, ginkgo, ginseng[40])	Apply digital pressure to bleeding sites and institute mechanical occlusion of bleeding vessels by using hemostatic clips or clamps to obstruct blood vessels to minimize bleeding at site of surgery	Discontinue medications that may alter coagulation factor activity
Administer iron, vitamin B$_{12}$, and folate	Consider preoperative autologous donation	Avoid hypothermia (keep patient's temperature greater than 35° C)
	Consider autologous blood cell salvage (autotransfusion)	Apply ice pack after phlebotomy to limit hematoma formation
	Use controlled hypotension: intentionally lowers blood pressure to decrease pressure on blood vessels to minimize bleeding	
	Consider acute normovolemic hemodilution	
	Consider surgical technique (e.g., staged surgeries)	

Data from reference 40.

◆ RESEARCH UTILIZATION

Recombinant Factor VIIa for Bleeding Control in Severely Injured Trauma Patients

CLINICAL ISSUE

Uncontrolled bleeding in trauma associated with coagulopathy is a primary cause of death. Most reports of recombinant factor VIIa (rFVIIa) use in trauma are anecdotal and not based on prospective, randomized, controlled studies. Transfusions are associated with many potential negative patient outcomes and are thought to increase infections and increase hospital length of stay.[15]

SUMMARY

Severely injured trauma patients who required more than 6 units of red blood cells (RBCs) within 4 hours of admission from 32 hospitals throughout Australia, Canada, France, Germany, Israel, Singapore, South Africa, and the United Kingdom were simultaneously randomized to a placebo-controlled, double-blind trial. This study analyzed 301 randomized patients; 143 blunt trauma patients and 134 penetrating trauma patients were randomized separately. Patients with major traumatic brain injury were excluded from the study. Patients who received 6 units of RBCs within a 4-hour window were randomized to receive either three IV injections of rFVIIa (200 mcg/kg initially, followed by 100 mcg/kg at 1 and 3 hours after the first dose) or three injections of placebo in addition to the standard treatment. The first dose was administered after the eighth unit of RBCs if the patient would require additional transfusions.

The primary end point for the study was transfusion requirement. Patients with blunt trauma who received rFVIIa instead of a placebo had a significantly lower number of RBCs transfused (estimated reduction of 2.6

RBC units [p value $= 0.02$]). In addition, the need for massive transfusion, which was defined as greater than 20 units of RBCs, was also reduced by 33% (p value $= 0.03$). Patients with penetrating trauma who received rFVIIa instead of a placebo had a significantly lower number of RBCs transfused (estimated reduction of 1.0 RBC unit [p value $= 0.10$]). The need for massive transfusion was also reduced by 19% (p value $= 0.08$). There was not a significant difference between the two groups in regard to a reduction in fresh frozen plasma, platelets, and cryoprecipitate administration. Secondary end points were mortality and organ failure.

APPLICATION

While there was a trend toward fewer critical complications related to thromboemboli associated with acute respiratory distress syndrome and multiple organ failure in the rFVIIa-treated patients, overall there was no considerable difference in outcome measures between the rFVIIa and placebo groups. There are no firm recommendations for the use of rFVIIa in the exsanguinating trauma patient. Its use should be restricted to those situations in which it is likely to be of maximum benefit, given the excessive cost associated with administering rFVIIa "off-label" or on a "compassionate use" basis.

NEED FOR FURTHER STUDY

There are a variety of patient populations for whom blood transfusions are necessary but undesired or unavailable. More studies are needed to examine the use of nontransfusion alternatives.

Boffard, K. D., et al. (2005). Recombinant factor VIIa as adjunctive therapy for bleeding control in severely injured trauma patients: two parallel randomized, placebo-controlled, double blind clinical trials. *J Trauma, 59*(1), 8–15.

The majority of the published documents have been limited to retrospective case studies and anecdotal reports. However, phase II/III trials of rFVIIa are under way in the United States in such populations as individuals with intracranial hemorrhage.

Administration of rFVIIa has shown to significantly increase the amount of thrombin formation, resulting in fibrin clot formation at the site of vascular injury. As a result of circulating tissue factor and coagulopathy such as that seen in patients with disseminated intravascular coagulation (DIC), rFVIIa may cause thrombosis. However, the overall risk of thrombosis is considered low.[38]

BLOOD COMPONENT REVIEW

The fundamental objective in transfusion therapy is to assist with oxygen delivery to tissues by maintaining the Hgb concentration; the second objective is to maintain hemostatic factor levels to prevent or control bleeding.

Whole blood (WB) is living tissue able to transport electrolytes, proteins, hormones, vitamins, antibodies, heat, and oxygen to the tissues of the body. It can be transfused as WB or as one of its components (Figure 36-1). Up to four blood components can be processed from 1 unit of WB through a series of centrifugation methods. These components include RBCs, plasma, platelets, and cryoprecipitated antihemophilic factor, also known as cryoprecipitate. The plasma can be made into several blood derivatives (e.g., volume expanders, coagulation factor concentrates, and immune globulins).

Blood components may be administered through peripheral IV catheters, intraosseous catheters, portacaths, and most central lines, including peripherally inserted central catheter lines. The size of the lumen catheter should be large enough to allow appropriate flow rates to occur and the component to be transfused within a 4-hour period. Blood components should be transfused through a standard 170- to 260-micrometer filter to remove clots and debris, ideally through an 18-gauge IV catheter. Blood components may be transfused through a smaller gauge IV catheter without a pressure device. If the component is rapidly transfused using a pressure device, hemolysis may occur. To ease the flow of the blood component through the smaller size IV catheter, the component may be diluted with compatible IV fluid if the patient can tolerate the additional volume.

Only IV solutions approved by the Food and Drug Administration (FDA) (e.g., 0.9% normal saline [NS]) may be administered with blood components. Other compatible FDA-approved solutions include Normosol and Plasmalyte. Lactated Ringer's and other solutions that contain calcium should never be infused through the same tubing as blood components. Calcium adheres to citrate (the anticoagulant mixed with the blood components to inhibit clotting during storage) and this leads to hypocalcemia.

Patients rarely need all of the components of WB. Therefore only the necessary portions of WB are transfused to the patient. This treatment is referred to as blood component therapy, allowing several patients to benefit from 1 unit of WB. Exceptional patient and blood management is achieved by giving only the desired or essential components.

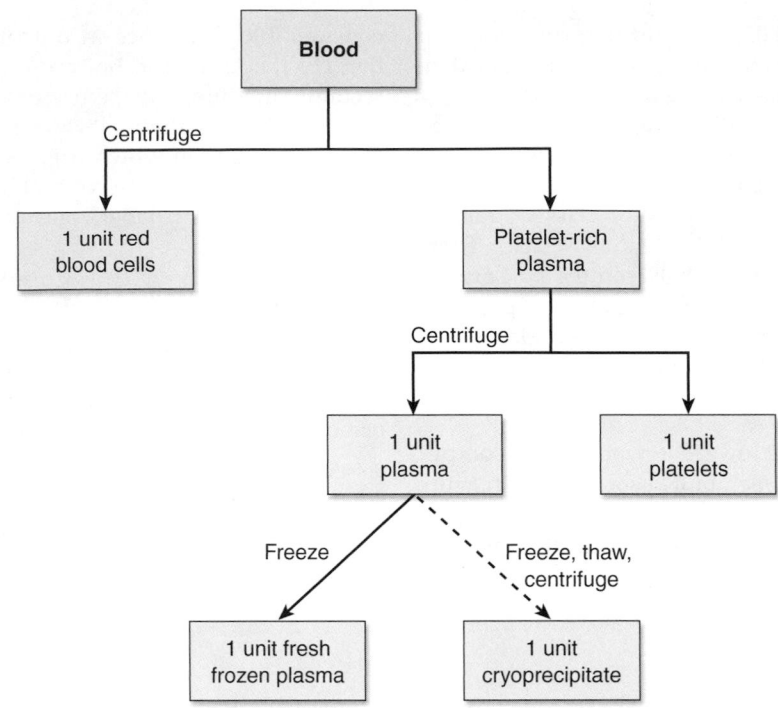

♦FIGURE 36-1 Components made from whole blood.

Whole Blood

Description. WB contains all blood elements (RBCs, white blood cells [WBCs], platelets, and plasma). Each unit of WB contains approximately 500 ml of WB and 70 ml of preservative-anticoagulant. The Hct of a typical unit is 36% to 44%.[26] This component is not ordinarily used because it is not as readily available as RBCs and other blood components. WB is ordinarily used for autologous transfusion or collected to prepare the blood components. It is uncommon to transfuse WB to the general patient population.

Once WB is placed in refrigeration, the platelets are no longer viable. During storage, therapeutic levels of coagulation factors V and VII decrease. A unit of WB must be ABO identical to the recipient (Table 36-3). Table 36-4 lists the proper storage temperature for blood components.

Indications. WB supplies oxygen-carrying capacity and restores blood volume expansion. It may be useful in bleeding patients with symptomatic anemia and a volume deficit in excess of 20% to 30% of their total blood volume. It may be administered to patients who require plasma for clotting factors and have symptomatic anemia or acute bleeding. For most purposes, a unit of WB is therapeutically equivalent to a unit of RBCs and a unit of plasma. WB is transfused regularly in open-heart surgery, pediatric cardiopulmonary bypass, and exchange transfusions in newborn babies with hemolytic disease of the newborn.

TABLE 36-3 Compatibility Chart of ABO Antigens-Antibodies

RECIPIENT'S BLOOD TYPE	ANTIGENS ON RED BLOOD CELL	ANTIBODIES IN PLASMA/SERUM
O	Neither A nor B	Anti-A and anti-B
A	A	Anti-B
B	B	Anti-A
AB	A and B	Neither anti-A nor anti-B

TABLE 36-4 Proper Storage Temperatures for Blood Components

COMPONENT	STORAGE TEMPERATURE
Red blood cells	1°–6° C
Fresh frozen plasma	1°–6° C
Platelets	20°–24° C
Cryoprecipitate	20°–24° C

Data from reference 10.

Red Blood Cells

Description. Each year in the United States, approximately 12 million units of RBCs are transfused.[70] RBCs continually transport oxygen from the lungs to the tissues and are responsible for removing waste (i.e., carbon dioxide [CO_2]). As the blood passes through the body's tissue, Hgb, a protein that binds to oxygen, carries and releases the oxygen to the cells. Hgb contains iron, making it an excellent vehicle for transporting oxygen and CO_2.

RBCs account for approximately 40% of the blood volume. This ratio of RBCs to overall fluid volume is a frequently measured number—the Hct. Bone marrow is continually producing new blood cells. The average life cycle of an RBC is 120 days. After this length of time, RBCs are removed by both the liver and the spleen. The blood itself, however, is recirculated throughout the body. One unit of RBCs is prepared from WB. One unit of RBCs increases the Hgb by 1 g/dl and the Hct by 3% in a non-bleeding, 70-kg patient with an average blood volume.

Once RBCs are separated from a unit of WB, an anticoagulant preservative solution is added to prolong cell life. There are several types of anticoagulant solutions. Optisol, also known as AS-5, is one type of anticoagulant containing mannitol, sodium, adenine, and dextrose. Optisol extends the shelf life of the unit to 42 days. Most units of RBCs have a Hct between 55% and 80%, depending on the anticoagulant used. The average total volume of an RBC unit is 350 ml. One unit of RBCs contains close to 200 ml of RBCs, 100 ml of preservative solution, and approximately 50 ml of plasma. Components should not be placed in staff or patient refrigerators or refrigerators intended for medications. All RBC transfusions must be ABO/Rh compatible with the recipient (Tables 36-3 and 36-5). RBCs do not provide viable platelets, neutrophils, or clinically significant amounts of plasma containing coagulation factors. RBCs should be transfused within 4 hours of removal from refrigeration.

Improvements in cell preservative solutions over the past 15 years have increased the shelf life of RBCs from 21 to 42 days. Rare RBCs (i.e., ones lacking particular antigens) may be stored frozen for up to 10 years. When verifying the RBC label before transfusion, it is important to ensure that the date and time of the unit and the compatibility testing have not expired. If the compatibility testing has expired, the component is considered un-crossmatched and requires a justification form by the primary care provider.

Indications. The major indication for RBC transfusion is symptomatic anemia that has not or will not respond to treatment involving vitamin B_{12}, folic acid, or iron. Transfusion of RBCs should be contingent on clinical presentation rather than arbitrary Hct or Hgb values. Hebert et al. showed that a restrictive RBC transfusion strategy in critically ill patients, maintaining Hgb levels between 7 and 9 g/dl in patients who are not actively bleeding, appeared to be safe in patients with cardiovascular disease. The possible exception to this was patients with acute myocardial infarction and unstable angina.[26] Other considerations include the duration of the anemia, intravascular volume of the recipient, any planned procedures, impending major blood loss, and any preexisting or coexisting medical conditions.

Fresh Frozen Plasma

Description. Fresh frozen plasma (FFP) is prepared from 1 unit of WB by centrifugation or by apheresis collection. It is then frozen and stored at a temperature less than $-30°$ C for up to 1 year. FFP contains normal levels of all clotting factors except platelets. One unit of FFP has a volume of about 200 ml. Table 36-5 describes which blood types of FFP can be transfused with other blood types.

Indications. FFP is indicated when there is a need to replace coagulation factors in association with massive transfusion or DIC, and for the treatment of thrombotic thrombocytopenic purpura. It is also indicated for

TABLE 36-5 Component Compatibility Chart

| RECIPIENT'S BLOOD TYPE | Component to Be Transfused and Permissible Donor Type | | | | |
	WHOLE BLOOD	RED BLOOD CELLS	PLASMA	PLATELETS	CRYOPRECIPITATE
O	O	O	Any type	Any type	Any type
A	A	A or O	A or AB	A or AB	A or AB
B	B	B or O	B or AB	B or AB	B or AB
AB	AB	Any type	AB	AB	AB

reversal of warfarin anticoagulation or when high risk for bleeding is present (e.g., patients with documented coagulation factor deficiencies [such as liver dysfunction]) undergoing an invasive procedure. It should not be transfused as a colloid replacement or a primary volume expander, for nutritional support or replacement, or to promote wound healing. In the absence of an inhibitor (e.g., heparin), hemostasis can be achieved when coagulation factor (e.g., factors VII, X, V) levels are at least 30% of normal and the fibrinogen level is greater than 100 mg/dl.[22] The typical initial dose of FFP is 10 to 20 ml/kg but is dependent upon the patient's clinical response.[11]

Thawed Plasma

Many institutions have started using thawed plasma to minimize wastage of FFP. Thawed plasma is derived from FFP, thawed at 30° to 37° C, and maintained for up to 5 days. Thawed plasma differs from FFP because the factor V and factor VIII levels continue to decrease and, therefore, should not be transfused for replacement of these specific coagulation factors. Some institutions will relabel a unit of FFP as thawed plasma if the component is not transfused within 24 hours of being thawed. Others will label all thawed units of FFP as "thawed plasma" and store them at the appropriate temperature with a 5-day outdate. Thawed plasma should not be transfused in patients requiring replacement of factor V or factor VIII clotting factors. Some facilities may have different or additional criteria used to determine whether patients may receive thawed plasma.

Cryoprecipitate

Description. Cryoprecipitate is obtained when a unit of FFP is slowly thawed at 4° C and centrifuged, producing a component rich in fibrinogen, fibronectin, factor VIII, von Willebrand's factor, and factor XIII. Cryoprecipitate is a source of fibrinogen, used to make fibrin glue, a topical adhesive or hemostatic agent that decreases microvascular bleeding during surgical procedures. It contains concentrated fibrinogen, von Willebrand's factor, factor XIII, and factor VIII. It is available in individual or pooled concentrates and should be considered if the patient is bleeding and the fibrinogen level is less than 100 mg/dl. The American Association of Blood Banks (AABB) *Standards for Blood Banks and Transfusion Services*[1] require each pool of cryoprecipitate to contain a minimum of 150 mg of fibrinogen and 80 units of factor VIII. Cryoprecipitate should be ABO compatible if suspended in plasma during preparation. One unit of cryoprecipitate contains a volume of 10 to 20 ml. Once collected, it can be stored at −18° C for a maximum of 1 year. Cryoprecipitate is later thawed in a 37° C water bath and prepared in individual bags or as a pooled component. Once thawed, it must be kept at room temperature and has an expiration time of 4 hours.

Indications. Cryoprecipitate is indicated for bleeding patients with significant hypofibrinogenemia (less than 100 mg/dl) or those who require an invasive procedure. It has been transfused in uremic patients with platelet dysfunction. The primary indications for cryoprecipitate are the treatment of fibrinogen dysfunction (e.g., patients with DIC) and fibrinogen deficiency (e.g., acute blood loss or liver disease). Effectiveness of cryoprecipitate transfusions is monitored by serum fibrinogen levels and assessment of clinical bleeding.

Platelets

Description. More than 7 million units of platelets are transfused each year in the United States.[70] Platelets are transfused for thrombocytopenia in patients with trauma, major surgical bleeding, platelet dysfunction, and hematologic malignancies. Platelet transfusions should be based on the patient's individual requirements and the cause of the platelet dysfunction or thrombocytopenia. Platelet transfusion practices remain controversial despite studies showing that a threshold of 10,000/μl for prophylactic platelet transfusion is effective in uncomplicated thrombocytopenic patients.[61] To reduce the formation of platelet alloantibodies, it is important to limit the platelet exposure to the recipient.

The plasma of a platelet component should be ABO compatible with the recipient's red blood cells whenever possible. Multiple platelet transfusions can cause platelet refractoriness as a result of platelet alloimmunization—the formation of antibodies usually directed against human leukocyte antigens (HLAs) destroying randomly chosen donor platelets. Table 36-6 compares apheresis platelets with pooled platelets. HLA and platelet-specific alloantibodies are not naturally occurring. The most common causes of HLA alloimmunization are previous blood transfusions and pregnancy. WBCs express HLA Class I antigens and may stimulate HLA antibodies in some patients. For most patients HLA alloimmunization is not associated with clinical problems. However, it can be associated with platelet transfusion refractoriness. Platelets express HLA Class I antigens. Therefore patients who are HLA alloimmunized may rapidly clear transfused platelets, reflective of immune destruction, resulting in an inadequate platelet response called platelet refractoriness.[32] Refractoriness is defined as a consistent failure to achieve expected posttransfusion platelet counts. Refractoriness may be a result of multiple nonimmune conditions often existing in patients who require long-term platelet therapy. To assess the effectiveness, a platelet count should be performed 10 to 60 minutes after the transfusion.[64]

TABLE 36-6 Comparison of Apheresis Platelets With Pooled Platelets

APHERESIS PLATELETS	POOLED PLATELETS
Reduced donor exposure per transfusion	Less risk to donor
Reduced turnaround time and wastage	Lower production costs
Lower WBC content	Reduced plasma exposure to donor
HLA-matched platelets	Increased donor exposure to recipient
5-day shelf life	4-hour expiration once pooled

Apheresis Platelets

Apheresis platelets are obtained from a single donor with the use of an apheresis machine. Centrifugation techniques separate the platelets from the RBCs, WBCs, and most of the plasma. The platelets are kept in a collection bag for later transfusion to a patient. Apheresis platelets generally contain 3×10^{11} platelets or more,[6] depending on collection practices. Apheresis platelets are advantageous compared to pooled platelets because of decreased donor exposures, decreased risk of bacterial contamination, and ease of handling, because the need to pool multiple platelet concentrates is eliminated. Because of recent requirements to test platelets for bacteria, it is also quicker to process apheresis platelets. Apheresis platelets are typically transfused to alloimmunized patients experiencing refractory thrombocytopenia. Platelets not yet pooled are stored for up to 5 days; once platelets are pooled, they must be transfused within 4 hours.

Pooled Platelets

Pooled platelets are from multiple donors and are often ordered as a "sixpack of platelets," indicating 6 pooled units of WB platelet concentrates from six separate donors. Platelet concentrates are prepared from 1 unit of WB by centrifugation and are resuspended in 60 ml of residual plasma. Each unit contains an average of more than 5.5×10^{11} platelets per unit.[7] Platelets that have not been pooled or combined may be stored at room temperature for up to 5 days. There are current methods being studied[54] to prolong the storage time and the method of storage.

Indications. Indications for platelet transfusions are thrombocytopenia, treatment of bleeding, or abnormal platelet function. The etiology of the patient's thrombocytopenia and platelet function should be considered when determining a transfusion threshold. Abnormal platelet function and the cause or severity of bleeding may lower the transfusion threshold. Prophylactic platelet transfusions may be given when the platelet count falls below 10,000/μl in oncology patients with acute leukemia, in hematopoietic stem cell transplant recipients, and in other uncomplicated thrombocytopenic patients. A platelet count greater than 10,000/μl is usually sufficient to prevent spontaneous hemorrhage.

Actively bleeding patients or those who are undergoing a major invasive procedure usually require a platelet count between 50,000 and 100,000/μl to avoid severe bleeding complications. Effectiveness of platelet transfusion is monitored by the serum platelet count.

Platelets contain WBCs and plasma. They are available as pooled platelet concentrates from multiple units of WB platelets or by a single-donor procedure known as platelet pheresis. Platelet concentrates are combined from 4 to 10 donors. A unit of single-donor platelets is usually equivalent to six or more platelet concentrates, the dose commonly ordered for a single platelet transfusion in an adult. Platelet storage is limited to 5 days. A standard size apheresis unit is equivalent to a pool of approximately 4 to 8 single-donor units. The typical dose for an adult recipient is 1 unit of WB platelets/kg. As an example, a 70-kg patient would receive 7 units of WB platelets.

Granulocytes

Description. Granulocytes are collected using an apheresis machine from an ABO- and Rh-compatible donor. They are essential for destruction of bacteria and fungi. Granulocytes should be infused soon after collection because their viability quickly diminishes over time. If this is not possible, storage should be at room temperature for no longer than 24 hours after collection. Granulocytes should not be transfused using a microaggregate or leukocyte reduction filter. Granulocytes should be irradiated to prevent graft-versus-host disease (GVHD) when administered to allogeneic bone marrow transplant (BMT) recipients.

Indications. According to the *AABB Technical Manual*,[6] granulocyte transfusion is controversial but typically administered to patients with the following conditions:

- Severe neutropenia
- Documented infection for 24 to 48 hours not responsive to antibiotics or other therapies
- Bone marrow showing myeloid hypoplasia
- Probable bone marrow function recovery

◆ Case Study 36-1, Part A

Blood Component Modification

D.A., a 19-year-old female, was a restrained driver involved in a high-speed motor vehicle crash in which she was broad-sided on the passenger side. She was intubated at the scene of the accident and taken to the local trauma hospital with right torso trauma. Her systolic blood pressure was 94 mm Hg and her heart rate was 142 beats/min. Her abdomen was large and distended. She had a prolonged capillary refill time, was cold to touch, and appeared pale and mottled. Once admitted, she was taken directly to the operating room (OR). In the OR, a 12-gauge French central line catheter was inserted. At this time, a type and crossmatch was drawn along with coagulation studies, arterial blood gas (ABG), and blood chemistry labs. Her temperature was 35.0° C. External rewarming was initiated by using warm IV fluids to 39.0° C and warm humidified oxygen through the ventilator to keep her core body temperature greater than 35.0° C. A Foley catheter was inserted and an exploratory laporatomy was performed, indicating both liver and splenic lacerations. A splenectomy was performed; the grade IV and V liver lacerations to the right liver lobe were packed using a damage control technique, known as peri-hepatic packing, to control hepatic hemorrhage. Her Hgb level declined to 7 g/dl, equivalent to a Hct of 21%. Her INR was greater than 2.0, PT was greater than 20 seconds, and platelet count declined to 50,000 cells/mm^3. During surgery, D.A. received a total of 10 units of RBCs, 6 units of plasma, and 3 L of IV crystalloid through a blood warmer/rapid infuser. She also received a unit of apheresis platelets. Her urine output was minimal throughout the case. She was transferred to critical care.

D.A.'s vital signs at the time of admission included body temperature 34.6° C, blood pressure 82/56 mm Hg, and heart rate 122–138 beats/min.

A maintenance infusion of NS was started and infused at 150 ml/hr. Emergency hemorrhage panel (EHP) results indicated that the patient was experiencing a coagulopathy. Her INR was 2.6, PT 28.5 seconds, Hct 26%, fibrinogen level 86 mg/dl, and platelet count 82,000 cells/mm^3.

Decision point: What blood components are indicated?

Decision point: Are there other therapies that should be considered at this time?

Case continues on page 988

BLOOD COMPONENT MODIFICATION

Leukocyte Reduction

Leukocyte reduction (LR), also known as leukoreduction, is indicated to decrease occurrence of recurrent febrile nonhemolytic transfusion reactions, to decrease incidence of HLA alloimmunization, and to reduce risk of cytomegalovirus (CMV) infection. LR does not prevent GVHD, nor does it replace the need for irradiation or use of CMV-seronegative components. Most states in this country do not mandate leukoreduction of blood components as standard practice. Washing of RBCs and platelets is not considered a substitute for LR because washing does not remove enough leukocytes to prevent alloimmunization. The majority of WBCs have been removed, eliminating undesirable effects caused by WBCs and their by-products. Components that can be leukocyte-reduced include platelets, RBCs, and WB.

Leukocyte filtration may occur in three scenarios: prestorage, when the component is collected; poststorage, when the component is in the laboratory; or at the bedside, when the unit is transfused. Prestorage leukoreduction seems to have several advantages over bedside leukoreduction. These advantages include a lower incidence of febrile reactions and alloimmunization.[63,65] Leukocyte reduction filters allow RBCs and platelets to pass through the filter while leukocytes are trapped. Manufacturers have modified apheresis machinery to collect platelets with low levels of leukocytes. Additional filtration is unnecessary if this collection method is used.

Indications for Washed Red Blood Cells or Platelets. Before leukocyte reduction filters, washing RBCs was considered the best way to prepare a leukocyte-reduced unit. Today, washing RBCs is not cost-effective, is less efficient, and shortens the availability of units because of an abbreviated shelf life once the component is washed. Washed components are prepared by washing RBCs or platelets with 1 to 2 L of 0.9% NS in an automated cell washer. Washed components remove all but traces of plasma, decrease leukocytes, and remove debris and platelets. Washed RBCs can be considered for patients who have had repeated hypersensitivity reactions to blood components despite prophylactic administration of antihistamines. Washing RBCs or platelets may not reduce the proteins enough to prevent hypersensitivity reactions (e.g., immunoglobulin A [IgA]-deficient patients).

After the components are washed with saline, they are centrifuged and the supernatant removed. Washed RBCs are indicated if the plasma in the component contains antibodies known to be harmful to the recipient or to remove constituents for which the intended recipient is known to have severe side effects. Recipients who are IgA deficient require washed units. RBCs must be transfused within 24 hours of washing because the hermetic seal of the component has been broken. Platelets must be transfused within 4 hours of washing.

Plasma Volume Reduction

Plasma volume reduction occurs when the majority of plasma is removed from platelets and granulocytes after centrifugation. As a result, plasma proteins and cytokines are removed. Volume reduction decreases the component to approximately 100 ml or a specified amount. Plasma volume reduction is indicated in patients who cannot tolerate the full volume of a component or when ABO-incompatible WB platelets are transfused.

Cytomegalovirus-Negative Components

CMV resides on the leukocytes of individuals who have been infected with the virus. The purpose of CMV-negative components is to prevent primary CMV infection in immunocompromised CMV-negative patients at risk of developing serious complications from a primary CMV infection. CMV-negative blood components are indicated for many reasons including CMV-negative bone marrow or organ transplant recipients, even if the marrow or organ donor is also CMV negative; acquired immunodeficiency syndrome (AIDS) or human immunodeficiency virus (HIV)-infected patients; pregnant women; or patients with a congenital immune deficiency. CMV transmission can be prevented by administering CMV-seronegative blood components or LR components. Components that may be CMV negative include RBCs, platelets, WB, and granulocytes. Worldwide, there are a substantial number of CMV-positive carriers with no history of exhibiting the illness. This virus is known to cause CMV-associated pneumonia, myocarditis, retinitis, hepatitis, and gastroenteritis.

Gamma Irradiation

The purpose of irradiating blood components is to prevent transfusion-associated GVHD. Irradiation of WB, granulocytes, RBCs, and platelets inactivates T lymphocytes and prevents them from proliferating and attacking the recipient's tissues as well as altering the genetic material. Irradiated components are indicated for immunocompromised patients (e.g., allogeneic BMT patients). Bone marrow or stem cell transplant candidates requiring transfusion before completing the harvest and patients with congenital or acquired cellular immune deficiencies should also receive irradiated components.[8] Failure to irradiate blood components in these populations can result in GVHD.

Artificial Red Blood Cell Substitutes (Modified Hgb Blood Substitutes, Perfluorochemicals)

Knowledge of the risks associated with transfusion of autologous and allogeneic RBCs and other blood components has increased. These risks include transmission of infectious diseases (e.g., HIV, hepatitis viruses) and bacterial contamination. Through a combination of inclusive and efficient predonation donor screening and testing, the blood supply is safer than ever.

Two major indications for the use of oxygen carriers are acute exsanguination and elective surgery. Characteristics and advantages of blood substitutes include the capability to be universally compatible pre-administration testing, absence of any infectious agents or allergens, ability to be stored without refrigeration, a longer storage life than blood, and ready availability. Possible disadvantages include vasoconstriction because of reduced levels of nitric oxide, gastrointestinal discomfort, and a short time in the patient's circulation (24 to 48 hours).[36]

Currently, there is no FDA-approved blood substitute available on the market. Research in blood substitutes has focused on perfluorocarbons and Hgb substitutes. Blood substitutes attaining advanced clinical trials today are RBC substitutes derived from Hgb.

Hemoglobin-Based Oxygen Carriers

Hemoglobin-based oxygen carriers (HbOCs) represent the largest number of products being developed as blood substitutes. There are three Hgb-based HbOCs that are currently in or have completed phase III trials in the United States. These include Hemopure (HBOC-201, hemoglobin-glutamer 250 [bovine]; Biopure Corp., Cambridge, Mass), PolyHeme (polymerized pyridoxylated hemoglobin; Northfield Laboratories, Chicago, Ill), and Hemolink (hemoglobin-raffimer; Hemosol Incorporated, Toronto, ON, Canada). The Hgb used in these HbOCs is derived from bovine blood, human blood from outdated units, and recombinant technology.

Perfluorochemicals

Unlike HbOCs, perfluorochemicals (PFCs) do not carry oxygen or other gases. Rather, they are outstanding solvents because of their decreased surface tension and intramolecular action.[63] PFCs have essentially unlimited ability to dissolve gases such as oxygen and nitrogen.[66]

CONSIDERATIONS IN BLOOD TRANSFUSION

ABO/Rh Compatibility

Blood is typed according to the presence or absence of antigens on the surface of the RBC and antibodies in the plasma. Plasma contains antibodies to antigens that are not present on the RBC. For example, if the RBC has the A antigen, the plasma will contain the B antibody. Transfusion of ABO-incompatible blood may cause severe intravascular hemolysis.

Rhesus (Rh) System

RBCs contain hundreds of antigens on their surface in addition to the ABO antigen blood group. The Rh system is the most clinically significant non-ABO RBC blood group system (Table 36-7). Approximately 85% of the population is Rh positive and 15% of the population is Rh negative. It is extremely immunogenic and can cause hemolytic disease of the newborn and transfusion reactions. The Rhesus factor or Rh (also known as the D antigen) is present if the D antigen is on the RBC. Un-crossmatched group O RBCs are often used during emergencies until the patient's ABO and Rh type have been determined. Rh-negative RBCs are used for females of childbearing age and pediatric patients (age varies by facility), and Rh-positive group O RBCs are transfused to males and females of non-childbearing age. When group O RBCs are transfused, it is imperative that a pretransfusion specimen be drawn. $Rh_o(D)$ immune globulin (RhoGAM) should be given within 48 hours of giving Rh-positive blood to an Rh-negative woman of childbearing age. Natural occurring D antibodies (anti-D) do not exist unless the patient has been exposed during prior transfusions or pregnancy.

Group O RBCs are not without risk. Unanticipated blood group antibodies can cause fatal transfusion reactions. Many facilities require a physician to complete a justification form documenting the need for the un-crossmatched RBC transfusion.

Autologous Transfusion

There are several categories of autologous transfusion available. These include preoperative (blood is collected and stored until needed), perioperative (acute normovolemic hemodilution [ANH] and cell saver), and postoperative (autotransfusion devices).

Preoperative Autologous Donation

Autologous blood donation is the process of collection, storage, and transfusion of a patient's own blood. There are risks and benefits of preoperative autologous donation. Benefits include preventing some adverse effects (e.g., febrile or allergic transfusion reactions) and providing compatible blood for patients with alloantibodies. Risks include bacterial contamination at the time of donation, potential clerical errors during the collection of the pretransfusion (type and crossmatch) specimen, or possible transfusion of the wrong unit of blood.

These potential complications make it imperative that autologous blood be transfused astutely and only when specifically indicated. It is never reasonable to transfuse an autologous unit simply because it is available or would otherwise be discarded. Similarly, autologous blood should not be transfused to replace iron, to promote wound healing or general well-being, or to normalize the Hgb level.

Perioperative Blood Salvage

In blood salvage techniques, blood shed in the perioperative or postoperative period is collected, processed, and reinfused into the patient. Processing includes filtration or centrifugation and washing before reinfusion.

Acute Normovolemic Hemodilution

ANH is the removal of WB from a patient before a surgical procedure. The WB is replaced with crystalloid IV fluid (e.g., NS) as a substitute to the WB removed. The blood is collected in a standard blood bag containing an anticoagulant and reinfused during surgery, if indicated. The patient must be stable enough to accommodate any potential anemia that the procedure may cause. Collection devices are frequently used to collect the shed blood during surgery and then wash the cells before retransfusion. This procedure is widely used for cardiac, orthopedic, trauma, transplant, and other surgical procedures.

TABLE 36-7 Rh Considerations for Blood Components

PATIENT'S RH TYPE	Rh Considerations for Blood Components				
	WHOLE BLOOD	RED BLOOD CELLS	PLASMA	PLATELETS	CRYOPRECIPITATE
Rh positive	Positive or negative	Positive or negative	Positive or negative	Positive or negative	Irrelevant
Rh negative	Negative	Negative	Positive or negative	Negative	Irrelevant

Postoperative Blood Collection

In postoperative blood collection, washed or unwashed blood is collected from a surgical drain and reinfused to the patient within 6 hours of the collection;[25] 40-micrometer microaggregate filters are used to filter the shed blood before transfusion.

Directed Donor Transfusion

Directed donation is blood that has been donated by a person specified by the patient. Many people elect to have specific individuals (e.g., family members) donate blood for them because they feel that blood from designated individuals is safer than blood donated by anonymous volunteers. However, there is no established medical or scientific evidence that blood from directed donors is advantageous. Therefore the same rigorous donor screening criteria are followed as for regular volunteer blood donors.

Directed donations between blood relatives are gamma-irradiated to prevent transfusion-induced GVHD. Donors must be ABO/Rh compatible with the patient.

Generally, directed donation is discouraged, as there are many risks. For example, blood should not be transfused to a female of childbearing age by her significant other, as it may increase the risk for hemolytic disease of the newborn in mothers receiving blood. Blood donated by a blood relative to another (e.g., between siblings) may cause alloimmunization of potential transplant recipients. Requesting directed donations from family and friends may place the potential donor in an uncomfortable situation, especially if the person does not qualify to donate blood. To prevent being excluded, the potential donor may answer questions untruthfully, unintentionally compromising the safety of the recipient.

Massive Transfusions

Multiple definitions for massive transfusion exist; however, one of the most common is the replacement of one or more blood volumes within 24 hours.[27,69] An adult blood volume is estimated as 70 ml/kg, or approximately 5000 ml, equivalent to 10 or more units of whole blood in a 70-kg adult.

The availability and prompt transfusion of RBCs and blood components are essential to the successful resuscitation of patients who experience acute, massive blood loss. Many institutions have a massive transfusion protocol to ensure prompt availability of blood components and provide guidelines for facilitating timely and adequate replacement of massive blood loss with appropriate blood components. Indications for a massive transfusion include, but are not limited to, the following:

- Significant hemorrhage (e.g., massive upper GI hemorrhage, ruptured aortic aneurysms, and equivalent clinical scenarios)
- Continual hypotension resulting from blood loss exceeding 1500 ml
- Both considerable blood loss and a likelihood that additional considerable blood loss will continue over a short time
- Ongoing blood loss requiring at least 10 units of RBC replacement within 2 hours

The challenge of massive transfusion is that patients may already be in the resuscitation phase before any components besides RBCs are ordered. For some patients, the fibrinogen level is extremely low or becomes low within 30 minutes of arrival into critical care or the emergency department. Although transfusion protocols are not supported by the literature, the purpose of implementing a massive transfusion protocol is to obtain blood components for the patient in a timely manner, to stabilize the coagulation parameters, and to use fewer components before the patient becomes hypothermic or acidotic. Many institutions do use protocols for massive transfusions that incorporate use of a massive transfusion pack (MTP).

An MTP may consist of a variety of components. One example might be an MTP that includes 1 pool of cryoprecipitate, 4 units of plasma, and 1 apheresis platelet pack. Once blood components are transfused, all subsequent blood orders should be based on results of coagulation tests. An example of a massive transfusion protocol is illustrated in Figure 36-2.

After the initial use of the MTP, the blood bank should prepare future blood components for issuance on the basis of pretransfusion laboratory values. It is important to remember that emphasis should be on the patient's clinical presentation and laboratory values, and not on formulas.

Use of Blood Warmers

To minimize the occurrence of dysrhythmias and prevent cardiac arrest associated with massive transfusion, blood warmers are often used for patients who are receiving several rapid transfusions. Blood warmers are not indicated in routine transfusions but should be used when transfusing blood to patients who have cold agglutinins, which are antibodies that react at cold temperatures. Several types of blood warmers are available on the market, including radiant plate and coil warmers and water bath devices.

Some blood warmers have an external pressure device allowing a unit of blood to be transfused within a few minutes. External pressure devices should not exceed 300 mm Hg of pressure and must apply pressure evenly

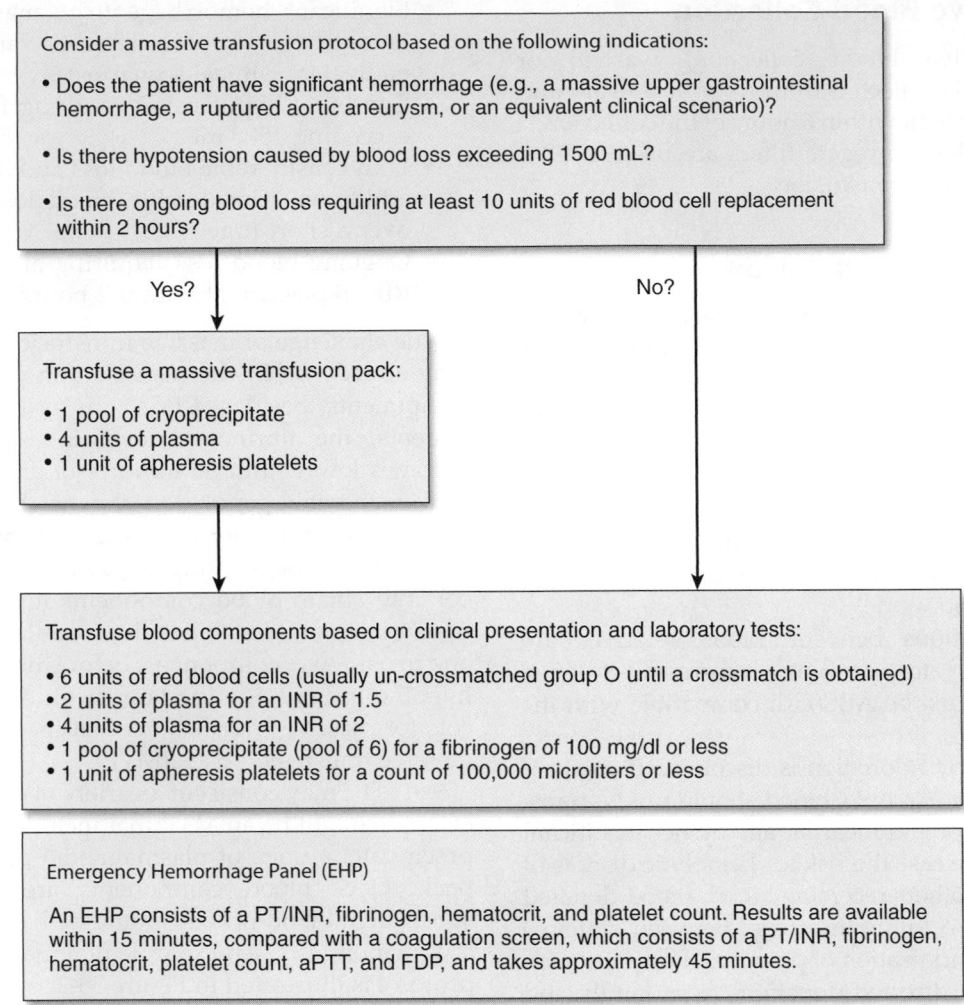

Consider a massive transfusion protocol based on the following indications:

- Does the patient have significant hemorrhage (e.g., a massive upper gastrointestinal hemorrhage, a ruptured aortic aneurysm, or an equivalent clinical scenario)?

- Is there hypotension caused by blood loss exceeding 1500 mL?

- Is there ongoing blood loss requiring at least 10 units of red blood cell replacement within 2 hours?

Yes?   No?

Transfuse a massive transfusion pack:

- 1 pool of cryoprecipitate
- 4 units of plasma
- 1 unit of apheresis platelets

Transfuse blood components based on clinical presentation and laboratory tests:

- 6 units of red blood cells (usually un-crossmatched group O until a crossmatch is obtained)
- 2 units of plasma for an INR of 1.5
- 4 units of plasma for an INR of 2
- 1 pool of cryoprecipitate (pool of 6) for a fibrinogen of 100 mg/dl or less
- 1 unit of apheresis platelets for a count of 100,000 microliters or less

Emergency Hemorrhage Panel (EHP)

An EHP consists of a PT/INR, fibrinogen, hematocrit, and platelet count. Results are available within 15 minutes, compared with a coagulation screen, which consists of a PT/INR, fibrinogen, hematocrit, platelet count, aPTT, and FDP, and takes approximately 45 minutes.

◆FIGURE 36-2 Massive transfusion protocol. aPTT = Activated partial thromboplastin time, FDP = fibrin degradation products, Hct = hematocrit, INR = international normalized ratio, PT = prothrombin time.

over the entire component bag. These should only be used with a large-gauge catheter to prevent hemolysis. Manufacturer instructions should be followed.

ADVERSE EFFECTS RELATED TO TRANSFUSION OF BLOOD COMPONENTS

Transfusion of blood components is considered transplantation of foreign cells and exposes the patient to multiple hazards, including a variety of transfusion reactions, diseases, and inflammatory complications. Transfusions are associated with the potential for negative impact on patient outcomes and are thought to increase infections and hospital length of stay.[15] It is important that clinicians be able to recognize complications and implement immediate interventions, as well as explain the reactions and adverse effects to the patient or the family.

Transfusion of blood components does not come without risk and should not be taken lightly. Any component can cause a reaction. Manifestations of transfusion reactions vary depending on the type of blood component transfused and the clinical condition of the patient receiving the transfusion. Until proven otherwise, any adverse reaction occurring at the time of the transfusion should be considered a transfusion reaction.

Any suspected transfusion reaction or adverse reaction should be reported to the blood bank, because it may be involved in the patient's workup and evaluation. There may also be a reason to quarantine other components donated by the donor in question or other components associated with the unit in question.

Transfusion-Related Acute Bacteremia/Bacterial Contamination

Bacterial contamination of blood components is one cause of transfusion-associated morbidity and mortality. Most deaths[52] related to bacterial contamination of blood components that are reported to the FDA are associated with the transfusion of platelets.[39] Bacterial contamination occurs more often in platelet components, occurring in an estimated 1:1000 to 1:3000 platelet units transfused.[2] When platelets are pooled, the risks increase. Bacteria proliferate depending on the type of component and how it is stored. RBCs have been known to contain *Acinetobacter, Escherichia, Staphylococcus,* and *Pseudomonas* species.[23] Platelets have contained such organisms as *Staphylococcus, Streptococcus, Acinetobacter, Klebsiella,* and *Serratia.*[24] In 2004 the AABB required blood banks to implement strategies to limit bacterial contamination in platelet concentrates and detect growth of bacteria during storage.

Bacteria can be introduced into a donated unit of blood during collection, processing, or pooling, causing sepsis or life-threatening septic shock to the recipient. If the patient experiences severe rigors and high fever (greater than 2° C increase), and severe hypotension, it is important to consider bacterial contamination. Other signs and symptoms include abdominal pain, vomiting, hemoglobinuria, DIC, renal failure, and circulatory collapse, which can occur within minutes of starting the transfusion. Symptoms may occur during or shortly after completion of the transfusion.

Treatment of bacterial contamination includes broad-spectrum antibiotics, vasopressor support in the event of septic shock, and acetaminophen (Tylenol). The implicated unit should be returned to the blood bank so that a Gram stain and culture of the unit can occur. The recipient should also have a Gram stain and culture performed. The blood bank must also be alerted of the possible bacterial contamination so any other donated units associated with the implicated unit can be recalled (Table 36-8).

Transfusion-Associated Graft-Versus-Host Disease

GVHD is a rare complication of a blood transfusion and is associated with an 80% to 90% mortality rate. GVHD is also associated with other transplantations (e.g., BMT). However, its mortality rate associated with BMT is much lower, at 20% to 25%.[25]

Engraftment, the recognition and proliferation of viable donor T lymphocytes present in cellular blood components, can result in transfusion-associated GVHD (TA-GVHD) in a susceptible recipient unable to recognize or destroy them. This generates an immune response against the recipient's antigens. The donor lymphocytes proliferate and injure organs, especially bone marrow, skin, liver, and the gastrointestinal tract. Severely immunocompromised patients (e.g., BMT recipients, Hodgkin's disease) or recipients of directed donations from first-degree relatives are at risk for TA-GVHD. Blood components that contain T cells (e.g., RBCs, WB, platelets, granulocytes) can cause TA-GVHD. Fortunately, TA-GVHD can be prevented by gamma irradiation of cellular blood components.

TA-GVHD usually manifests 2 to 50 days posttransfusion.[71] Signs and symptoms include diarrhea, rash, fever, pancytopenia, elevated levels of hepatic enzymes, and elevated bilirubin levels. Patients have died from overwhelming infection and hematopoietic failure, resulting in more than 90% mortality rate from TA-GVHD.[71]

The diagnosis of TA-GVHD is frequently delayed because symptoms are mild or are attributed to the primary illness. Laboratory tests may show pancytopenia, abnormal liver function tests, and electrolyte abnormalities induced by diarrhea.[40] If the diagnosis is suspected, a biopsy will be taken from the affected skin. A definitive diagnosis is made only if the circulating lymphocytes have a different HLA phenotype from the patient's tissue cells, proving that the circulating lymphocytes came from the donor.[40]

Delayed Hemolytic Transfusion Reaction

A delayed hemolytic transfusion reaction (DHTR) is caused by minor blood group incompatibility such as Rh incompatibility. This amnestic response, which is the heightened level of the immune response that occurs with the second exposure to an antigen, occurs in patients who have been exposed and sensitized to an antigen during a prior transfusion (Rh-positive RBCs transfused to an Rh-negative recipient) or pregnancy. After the exposure occurs, an antibody develops.

DHTRs can take as long as a week or more to present. Signs include extravascular hemolysis, fever, hyperbilirubinemia, decrease in Hct/Hgb levels 3 to 7 days posttransfusion, jaundice, and hemoglobinuria.

A delayed response does not generally activate an acute response, and the patient may be asymptomatic. These reactions may be overlooked because they are usually less severe than an acute hemolytic transfusion reaction. Future transfusions should be avoided until the antibody that caused the reaction can be identified and antigen-negative components become available. Diagnosis is confirmed by a positive indirect antiglobulin test (Coombs' test) (see Table 36-8).

Febrile Nonhemolytic Transfusion Reaction

A febrile nonhemolytic transfusion reaction (FNHTR) is a common reaction, believed to be due to

TABLE 36-8 Adverse Reactions Related to Transfusion of Blood Components

TYPE OF REACTION	CLINICAL PRESENTATION	TREATMENT AND MANAGEMENT	PREVENTION
Acute hemolytic transfusion reaction	Hemoglobinuria Renal failure Dyspnea, tachypnea, hypoxemia Fever (1° C increase in body temperature above baseline) with or without chills Rigors with or without fever Hypotension or hypertension Coagulopathy: diffuse bleeding Severe chest, abdomen, or flank pain Generalized bleeding, DIC Pain at infusion site Urticaria, pruritus, localized edema Hemoglobinuria or anuria Nausea and vomiting Sense of impending doom or anxiety Diaphoresis	Diuretics and additional IV fluids may be administered to increase renal perfusion. Use laboratory tests in investigation. Determine renal function (blood urea nitrogen, creatinine levels). Determine bleeding status (platelet count, PT/INR, aPTT, Hgb/Hct). Determine need for subsequent blood component transfusions. Stop transfusion and send blood bag, administration set, and IV solutions to blood bank.	Rule out clerical error at the time of drawing the blood bank specimen or identifying patient at the time of transfusion. To prevent nonimmune hemolysis, infuse compatible, FDA-approved IV fluids and medications. Pressure devices should not exceed 300 mm Hg. Transfusion through small-bore IV catheters should be avoided when administered via a pressure device.
Febrile nonhemolytic transfusion reactions	Fever Possible rigors Headache Vomiting	To reduce patient's temperature, administer an antipyretic. Provider may request restarting the transfusion at a slower rate. Otherwise, the transfusion may need to be stopped if patient continues to have symptoms. Signs and symptoms may mimic more severe reactions such as AHTR. Use meperidine to prevent or treat rigors. Other medications that may be used are as follows: Aminophylline 6 mg/kg IV loading dose Diphenhydramine (Benadryl) 50–80 mg IM or IV	Leukoreduced components may be warranted. Premedicate with an antipyretic. Administer meperidine to prevent rigors.
Allergic reaction (mild)	Hives Urticaria Pruritus Flushing of skin	Symptoms may subside by slowing rate of transfusion. Administer antihistamine to relieve patient's symptoms or prophylactically if patient experiences recurrent urticarial reactions. Use volume expansion for hypotension or epinephrine (5 ml of a 1:10,000 solution).	Premedicate with antihistamine.

TYPE OF REACTION	CLINICAL PRESENTATION	TREATMENT AND MANAGEMENT	PREVENTION
Allergic reaction (moderate)	Periorbital or perioral edema Wheezes Possible hypotension	Stop the transfusion. Epinephrine may be indicated for severe, persistent urticaria associated with bronchospasm.	When allergic reactions occur despite pretransfusion antihistamine, washed cells may be indicated. Rule out IgA deficiency. If negative, transfuse washed RBCs or platelets.
Allergic reaction (severe), anaphylaxis	Hypotension Respiratory distress Bronchospasms Cough Shock Facial edema Nausea and emesis Absence of fever	May be necessary to administer epinephrine (0.4 ml of 1:1000 solution subcutaneous), steroids, or oxygen as appropriate. Never restart a transfusion when an anaphylactic reaction is suspected or has occurred. Subsequent transfusions may require 0.9% normal saline washed RBCs.	When allergic reactions occur despite pretransfusion antihistamine, washed cells may be indicated. Rule out IgA deficiency. If negative, transfuse washed RBCs or platelets.
Transfusion-related acute lung injury	Severe, progressive dyspnea and decrease in Sa_{O_2} Bilateral pulmonary infiltrates ("white-out") on chest x-rays Noncardiogenic, bilateral pulmonary edema Hypertension or hypotension Tachycardia Fever Chills Wheezes Bronchospasm	Provide supportive care with administration of oxygen, intubation with mechanical ventilation, and blood pressure support. Corticosteroids are not indicated.[52] Diuretics are controversial. Notify blood bank immediately if TRALI is suspected. WBC antibody studies may need to be performed on both patient and blood donor(s).	Institute permanent deferral of donors implicated in TRALI reactions.
Bacterial contamination	Fever increase greater than 2° C (3.5° F) Nausea or vomiting Abdominal cramping Chills, rigors Sudden and severe hypotension Generalized bleeding, DIC Shock Hemoglobinuria Renal failure Dryness and flushing	Inspect component for abnormal color, clotting, or hemolysis. Perform a Gram stain and culture of both patient and implicated unit. Broad-spectrum antibiotics may be indicated.	Inspect unit before administration for discoloration. Blood banks have several methods to detect bacteria (e.g., Gram stain) or to prevent bacterial contamination (e.g., extensive donor screening).

Data from reference 52.
AHTR = Acute hemolytic transfusion reaction, aPTT = activated partial thromboplastin time, DIC = disseminated intravascular coagulation, FDA = Food and Drug Administration, Hct = hematocrit, Hgb = hemoglobin, INR = international normalized ratio, PT = prothrombin time, RBC = red blood cell, Sa_{O_2} = arterial oxygen saturation, TRALI = transfusion-related acute lung injury, WBC = white blood cell.

patient antibodies to leukocyte antigens contained in the donor component. Another theory is that cytokines created during storage of the blood component cause fever and chills in the transfused patients. This type of reaction is more common in patients who have a history of transfusion or pregnancy.[8]

A pretransfusion temperature should be assessed to establish a baseline and allow for evaluation of whether the patient became febrile during or following a transfusion. This will help determine whether the fever was caused by the transfusion or by an underlying condition (e.g., infection or the disease process). If the temperature increases greater than 1° C above baseline early in the transfusion or several hours, typically 1 to 2 hours, after the conclusion of the transfusion, a FNHTR should be considered. Fever is often seen in more life-threatening reactions (e.g., bacterial contamination or acute hemolytic transfusion reactions). Therefore it is important to evaluate the patient and notify the blood bank of such occurrences. The fever will usually respond to antipyretics; meperidine (Demerol) may be useful in treating the rigors. Depending on the severity of the symptoms, the practitioner may request to restart the transfusion at a slower rate. Subsequent transfusions may require premedication with acetaminophen or diphenhydramine (Benadryl). Febrile reactions may be prevented if leukocyte-reduced components are transfused. A patient can still have a FNHTR in the absence of fever if the patient has received prophylactic antipyretics, because these will not suppress the shaking, chills, and discomfort (see Table 36-8).

Allergic Transfusion Reactions

Interaction of a preexisting antibody to a protein or allergen in donor blood may cause an allergic reaction, ranging from mild, to moderate, to severe. This antibody-allergen reaction triggers a cascade of chemical events that affect the respiratory, cardiovascular, and gastrointestinal systems.

Mild Allergic. Mild allergic transfusion reactions are common during and after transfusion. Symptoms include urticaria (hives), pruritus (itching), erythema, and flushing of the skin. Mild reactions respond to IV antihistamines.

Moderate Allergic. Symptoms of moderate allergic reactions include the upper airway and involve laryngeal edema. Wheezing, cyanosis, anxiety, dyspnea, nausea and vomiting, and diarrhea are all signs of moderate allergic reactions. Moderate reactions may respond to IV antihistamines or may require epinephrine (0.4 ml of a 1:1000 solution subcutaneously). Washed RBCs and platelets may be necessary to prevent future allergic reactions.

Severe Allergic. Severe allergic reactions or anaphylactic reactions can cause hypotension, tachycardia, shock, dysrhythmias, and cardiac arrest. Administration of epinephrine (0.4 ml of a 1:1000 solution subcutaneously) and steroids may be necessary. Supportive care with intubation, mechanical ventilation, oxygen, and IV fluids may be indicated. The transfusion should not be restarted if an anaphylactic reaction is suspected or confirmed. Anaphylactic reactions may be associated with anti-IgA antibodies in individuals with IgA deficiency.

◆ Case Study 36-1, Part B

Blood Component Modification

After 36 hours in critical care, D.A. developed several complications, including liver and renal failure, sepsis, heparin-induced thrombocytopenia, and necrosis of her abdominal wall. She grew increasingly hypoxemic, requiring increased amounts of oxygen and positive end-expiratory pressure. Her renal function decreased; her creatinine level was 3.6 mg/dl. She developed increasing intra-abdominal pressures, was hypotensive, and was difficult to ventilate. She was taken immediately to the OR for a second exploratory laparotomy with drainage of the liver laceration and decompression of her abdominal compartment syndrome. During the unpacking of her abdomen, the surgeons noted a severe liver laceration with leakage of bile. A total of 2–2.5 L of old blood, serum, and bile was removed from her abdominal cavity. The surgeons proceeded with the surgery and obtained swabs of the peritoneal fluid for Gram stain and culture. She required 3 units of RBCs perioperatively for a Hct of 23%.

Approximately 10 minutes after leaving the OR, the laboratory began reporting hemolysis in the specimens drawn for postoperative laboratory results. Twelve hours later, the laboratory was still reporting hemolysis. Specimens were then sent for a transfusion reaction evaluation. Over the next 12 hours, the critical care nurses noted decreasing urine output and worsening hypotension requiring increased vasopressor support.

Decision point: What are the complications of an incompatible blood transfusion?

Decision point: What is the nurse's role in assessing for an incompatible blood transfusion?

Case continues on page 990

Nonimmune-Related Hemolysis Transfusion Reaction

Bacterial contamination, accidental freezing of donor units, infusion of incompatible IV fluids either in the donor bag or in the infusion line, incompatible medication administration (no medications should be infused through the same tubing with blood components unless they have been FDA approved), excessive heating (greater than 42° C) of donor units, and pressure devices used for rapid administration can result in nonimmune hemolysis. Nonimmune hemolysis presents with symptoms of hemolysis, yet an antibody screen and direct antiglobulin test (DAT) performed in the laboratory are negative. New-onset hemolysis with a negative DAT fits best with physical/mechanical hemolysis of RBCs. Treatment is focused on the cause of the hemolysis. If physical hemolysis is suspected, a careful analysis of conditions associated with transfusion must be done.

Some patients may tolerate a transfusion with lysed cells without difficulty. Others may experience renal failure, hemoglobinemia, hemoglobinuria, hyperkalemia, hypotension, and other signs of shock. This is usually a diagnosis of exclusion since it mimics hemolytic transfusion reactions, bacterial contamination, and sepsis.

Whenever a transfusion reaction is suspected, the blood bag, tubing, and IV fluids should be sent to the blood bank for evaluation. Care is supportive and may require monitoring of serum potassium level and electrocardiogram signs of hyperkalemia. The patient's kidneys should be well hydrated, yet fluid overload,

particularly in patients with impaired renal or cardiac function, should be avoided.

To prevent lysis it is important to infuse compatible, FDA-approved IV fluids or medications with blood components. IV pumps, warmers, and pressure devices (not to exceed 300 mm Hg) should be well maintained. Transfusion through small-bore catheters should be avoided, especially with pressure devices for infusion. An 18-gauge needle is recommended for adults. Smaller gauge needles (23 gauge or larger) can be used for transfusion in adults but may restrict the flow rate of the transfusion and lengthen the time to infuse a unit (see Table 36-8).

Acute Hemolytic Transfusion Reaction

A hemolytic transfusion reaction is an immunologic or nonimmunologic destruction or rupture of transfused RBCs with the release of intracellular hemoglobin (Figure 36-3). It occurs most commonly from an incompatibility of antigen on the transfused cells with an antibody in the recipient's circulation. Severe hemolytic reactions may occur when as little as 10 ml of ABO-incompatible RBCs are transfused to a recipient.

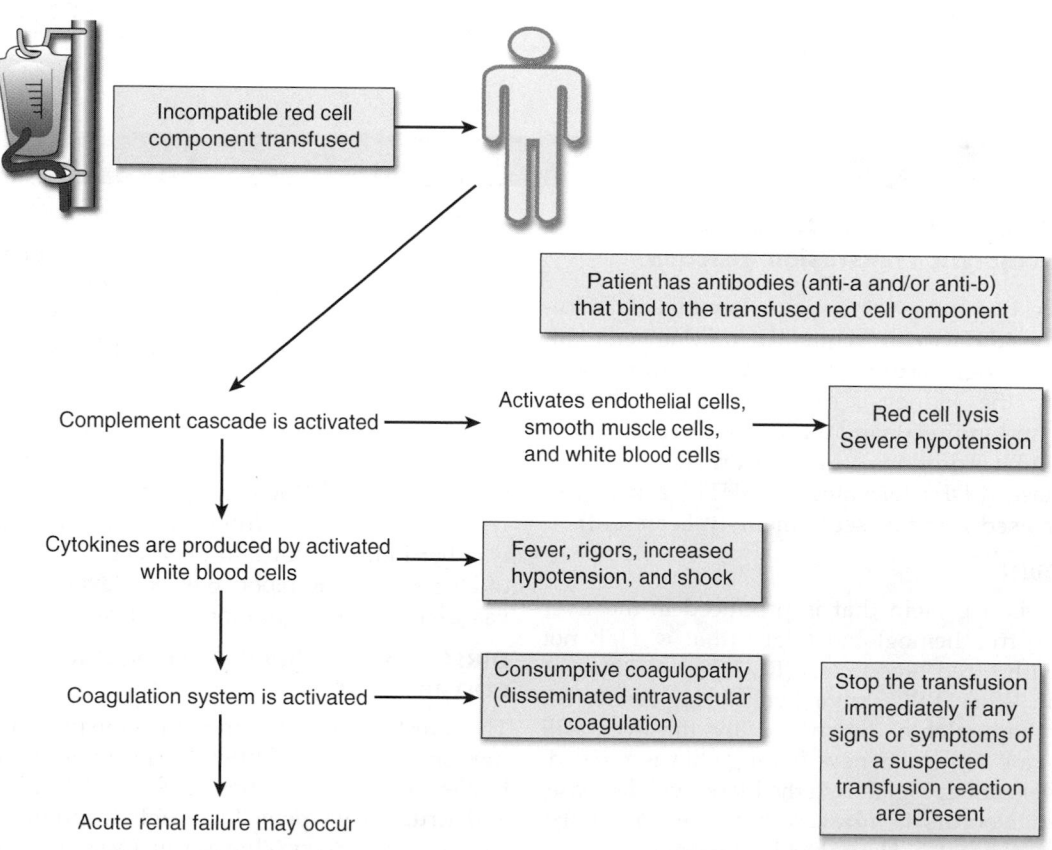

FIGURE 36-3 Pathophysiology of an acute hemolytic transfusion reaction (AHTR).

The blood reacts with the antibodies that exist in the recipient. The antibody and antigen interaction initiates complement activation, coagulation activation, and an inflammatory response related to cytokines.[8] The primary concerns during treatment are optimizing renal perfusion and hemodynamic support with vasopressor agents if the patient becomes hypotensive. If the patient develops coagulopathy, blood component administration may be necessary.

Acute hemolytic transfusion reaction signs and symptoms usually appear within the first 5 to 15 minutes after the transfusion is started, but can happen anytime during the transfusion or afterward, depending on the patient's response. Additional blood components should be avoided until the transfusion reaction investigation is complete, if possible. If the reaction is thought to be caused by the wrong blood type, O-negative RBCs should be transfused if necessary. Diuretics and additional fluids may be administered to increase renal perfusion. Lab testing (blood urea nitrogen, creatinine, platelet count, prothrombin time/international normalized ratio [PT/INR], activated partial thromboplastin time [aPTT], Hgb/Hct) may be ordered to determine renal function, bleeding status, and need for subsequent blood component transfusions.

Clerical errors (e.g., not accurately identifying the patient during collection of the pretransfusion specimen or at the time of administration) are the most common cause of ABO-incompatible transfusions. Vigilance in performing the pretransfusion/compatibility testing (type and crossmatch) and verification by transfusing clinicians according to hospital policies is necessary to prevent a mismatched transfusion. Box 36-1 lists the laboratory tests performed to evaluate for most suspected hemolytic transfusion reactions.

◆ Case Study 36-1, Part C

Blood Component Modification

A thorough transfusion history temporally related to the hemolysis was obtained. The patient received 3 units of RBCs within a few hours before the onset of hemolysis. A clerical check was performed. The antibody screen was repeated and confirmed to be negative. Antiglobulin crossmatch of the 3 units confirmed that they were compatible. A repeat type confirmation on the units confirmed that each unit labeled as group O contained group O RBCs. A visual check of the postreaction blood bank specimen was positive for hemolysis. Hemolysis was not present in the prereaction specimen.

Decision point: What laboratory studies should be obtained at this time?

Decision point: What investigations should be done to assist in determining the cause of her hemolysis?

Box 36-1

Laboratory Investigation Assessment After an Acute Hemolytic Transfusion Reaction

Laboratory testing following an acute hemolytic transfusion reaction (AHTR) will frequently indicate hemoglobinemia or hemoglobinuria (result of free hemoglobin clearance by the kidneys), elevated serum bilirubin levels (total and indirect), and a positive direct antiglobulin test (DAT). Additional tests performed are lactate dehydrogenase (LDH) (elevated in AHTR) and haptoglobin (decreased if intravascular hemolysis present).

HAPTOGLOBIN

Haptoglobin is a protein that is produced in the liver and binds to free hemoglobin (Hgb) (that is, Hgb not contained within red blood cells [RBCs]) in an attempt to remove it. When RBCs are actively being destroyed, the rate of haptoglobin destruction by the liver will exceed the rate at which new haptoglobin is created. Thus the levels of haptoglobin in the blood will decrease, which is what occurs if intravascular or extravascular hemolysis is present.[56] Haptoglobin measures the rate at which RBCs are being destroyed.

LACTATE DEHYDROGENASE

LDH exists in RBCs and is released from damaged cells. LDH is in several tissues such as the heart, liver, and lungs. LDH is as an indicator of acute or chronic tissue damage. LDH level is elevated in intravascular or extravascular hemolysis.[56]

INDIRECT AND TOTAL BILIRUBIN

Bilirubin is a breakdown product of Hgb. When the liver breaks down old RBCs, bilirubin is produced. The liver cannot clear bilirubin from the circulation. The bilirubin is either indirect bilirubin or direct bilirubin. The levels of bilirubin in the blood will be elevated in both intravascular and extravascular hemolysis.[56]

DIRECT ANTIGLOBULIN TEST OR DIRECT COOMBS' TEST

The direct Coombs' test measures the presence of antibodies on the surface of RBCs. It is used to detect autoantibodies and alloantibodies against RBCs. Many diseases and drugs (e.g., penicillin, cephalosporins, streptomycin[9]) can lead to production of these antibodies. These antibodies sometimes destroy RBCs and cause anemia.

OTHER BLOOD-RELATED ISSUES

Red Blood Cell Storage Lesion

The RBC storage lesion is defined as a constellation of biochemical, metabolic, and molecular changes that occurs when RBCs are stored. These changes include a decline in levels of 2,3- DPG and adenosine triphosphate (ATP), resulting in reduced RBC deformability and altered RBC adhesion. These changes eventually result in a limited storage period and permanent damage to the cellular components.[15] In addition, it is thought that leukocytes present in the component may cause RBC lysis. However, there is insufficient evidence to support prestorage leukocyte reduction to improve the quality of the unit and decrease storage lesion.[29]

2,3-Diphosphoglyceric Acid and Adenosine Triphosphate

During storage, levels of DPG decline significantly. The quantity of DPG in the unit of RBCs affects the RBCs' ability to release oxygen to the tissues. When DPG is present, it binds with Hgb so oxygen is available to be utilized by tissues. When it is absent, the open sites on the Hgb molecule bind with oxygen, making it unavailable to the tissues. This causes tissues to scavenge for oxygen from the periphery of the body (hence, the increased affinity for oxygen by Hgb) (left shift of oxyhemoglobin curve).[43]

There is no treatment to increase DPG levels other than to stop hemorrhage so that banked blood is no longer necessary. The restoration of DPG levels following a transfusion of RBCs may take about 12 hours for severely exhausted RBCs to redevelop half of their DPG levels.[29]

ATP levels decrease during storage; however, there are no data to support that this has a direct effect on storage lesion. Instead, it appears to have an effect on intracellular calcium and other mediators, causing cellular dehydration and intracellular hyperkalemia.[7,36] Hyperkalemia may alter cardiac function and cause peaked T waves on the electrocardiogram.[7,36]

Red Blood Cell Deformability

RBCs experience functional and structural changes during storage, making them less able to flow through the microcirculation. This can cause tissue hypoxia, potentially leading to multiple organ dysfunction syndrome (MODS). Berezina et al.[4] examined the influence of storage on RBC rheological properties and found that irreversible changes to the RBC had significantly increased by day 14. These changes consisted of a decrease in cell deformability, pH, and base excess[14] as a result of changes in the membrane phospholipids.[4]

There is evidence that the development of MODS has been associated with transfusion of blood units greater than 14 days old, suggesting that "older" blood is an independent risk factor of MODS.[36,74] Clinical outcomes from transfusing "old" stored blood remain uncertain. A study by Walsh et al.[71] looked at stable, anemic, normovolemic, critically ill patients with established organ failure. In this study, data did not support the idea that older blood is harmful or that fresh blood is beneficial. Some providers support the use of "fresh" blood in specific patient populations (e.g., neonatal or pediatric populations). While a theoretical argument could be made in favor of fresh blood (improved red cell deformability and increased DPG), requesting fresh blood for most patients is not evidence-based. To date, there are varying practices as to when "fresh" blood is indicated.

Red Blood Cell Adhesion

RBC adhesion increases with duration of storage, and prestorage leukoreduction eliminates storage-related adhesion. Transfusion of adhesive RBCs may further compromise tissue blood flow, leading to impaired perfusion and organ dysfunction in the critically ill.

Transfusion-Related Immune Modulation

Since the early 1970s, transfusion of blood components has been associated with immune suppression.[52] Allogeneic transfusions have been associated with poor patient outcomes. Immunomodulatory effects may perhaps be related to the WBCs in blood or storage time of the transfused blood.

Effects of transfusion-related immune modulation (TRIM) include increased postoperative infections, increased tumor recurrence, increased critical care morbidity and mortality, and increased MODS. Leukoreduction will not eliminate TRIM but might diminish its occurrence. Transfusion of allogeneic blood can induce a complex set of effects on the immune system. Prospective clinical studies are required to determine whether leukoreduced blood components are helpful in decreasing the occurrence of TRIM. Some clinical studies suggest that the risk of postoperative infection complications has declined in patients that receive non-leukoreduced components.

Transfusion-Related Acute Lung Injury

For the past 15 to 20 years, TRALI has been recognized as a significant classification of lung injury with an immunological, noncardiogenic basis. In 1983 Popovsky et al. first described noncardiogenic pulmonary edema as a complication related to transfusion treatment.[48] TRALI is defined as noncardiogenic pulmonary edema related to the transfusion of all plasma-containing blood components, including WB, RBCs, plasma, platelets, and cryoprecipitate. It has also occurred after administration of IV immune globulin (IVIg). Before the mid-1980s, the only recognized transfusion reactions involving pulmonary complications included anaphylactic reactions and volume overload. Since 2003 TRALI has been recognized as the leading cause of death related to transfusion in the United States.[48] The mortality from TRALI is 5% to 25%, with the lower rates being more common.[52] TRALI is an underdiagnosed and underreported complication of transfusion. TRALI is often not diagnosed correctly, leading to inappropriate patient treatment.

There are two theories as to the cause of TRALI. The first theory involves donor WBC antibodies, such as Class I and Class II anti-HLA or antigranulocyte antibodies, being transfused to a recipient. WBC antibodies can form from exposure to foreign WBCs in prior transfusions or pregnancies. Antibody strength can decrease or disappear over time. Some patients will continue to make strong antibodies years after their last pregnancy or transfusion. Either these WBC antibodies direct themselves against the recipient's antigens or the recipient's WBC antibodies direct themselves against the donor's WBC antigens. However, this scenario does not consistently cause TRALI.[67] The second theory involves two events. The first event involves recipient pulmonary endothelial activation causing pulmonary sequestration of neutrophils. Following this, a second event occurs causing specific antibodies to be directed against recipient neutrophils in the lungs, resulting in endothelial damage, capillary leak, and TRALI.[67]

Common symptoms associated with TRALI include cough, dyspnea, hypotension or hypertension, tachypnea, and fever (see Table 36-8). Intubated patients with TRALI have copious secretions that collect in the endotracheal tube. TRALI should be considered in all cases of respiratory distress with significant hypoxemia related to a transfusion and should meet the criteria of acute lung injury (ALI) (Box 36-2). Symptoms occur within 6 hours from the start of the transfusion[32] and may include acute respiratory distress, dyspnea, cyanosis, hypoxemia, severe bilateral pulmonary edema without other signs of volume overload, tachycardia, fever (1° to 2° C increase in temperature), chills, and hypotension unresponsive to fluids. TRALI may at first be confined to the lower lung fields. After several hours, it usually involves the entire lung (i.e., whiteout on chest radiograph by interstitial and alveolar infiltrates). While TRALI resolves within 48 to 96 hours from onset,[49] lung injury is often irreversible.

Treatment for TRALI is supportive with administration of oxygen, intubation with mechanical ventilation,

---

Box 36-2

Acute Lung Injury and Adult Respiratory Distress Syndrome Criteria

ALI and ARDS criteria include the following:
- Timing: acute onset of pulmonary insufficiency
- Hypoxemia
- PaO_2/FiO_2 ratio less than 300 mm Hg regardless of PEEP level or oxygen saturation less than 90% on room air
- Bilateral infiltrates consistent with pulmonary edema
- PAWP less than or equal to 18 mm Hg
- No clinical evidence of left atrial hypertension
- Differs from circulatory overload

Mortality rate in ARDS is 35% to 60%.[73]

The National Heart, Lung and Blood Institute Working Group on TRALI revised these criteria to include the following:[67]
- No previous history of ALI before transfusion
- Onset of signs and symptoms should occur within 6 hours of transfusion
- If there is a different ALI risk factor, TRALI should be considered
- If an arterial blood gas is unavailable, oxygen saturation less than or equal to 90% when the patient is on room air

Mortality rate is 5% to 25%.[52]

Data from references 52, 67, and 73.
ALI = Acute lung injury, ARDS = acute respiratory distress syndrome, FiO_2 = fraction of inspired oxygen, PaO_2 = partial pressure of arterial oxygen tension, PAWP = pulmonary artery wedge pressure, PEEP = positive end expiratory pressure, TRALI = transfusion-related acute lung injury.

---

and blood pressure support. Corticosteroids are not indicated,[52] and diuretics, although controversial, may be administered with signs of fluid overload. The blood bank should be notified immediately if TRALI is suspected. Single donors have been traced as the cause of multiple incidents of TRALI and transfusion reactions, so it is critical that such information is communicated to the laboratory. Failure to report to the hospital transfusion service and the blood collection facility may present risk to future recipients. Permanent deferral of donors implicated in TRALI reactions may be necessary.

Post-Transfusion Purpura

Post-transfusion purpura is similar to DHTR except it involves a patient developing an alloantibody in response to a platelet antigen. Recipients will become thrombocytopenic within 5 to 10 days after transfusion. Treatment may include plasmapheresis, used to help decrease the circulating platelet antibody. IVIg—a mixture of proteins containing antibodies, predominantly IgG—has also been proven to be effective as it provides passive, temporary immunity for the body.[11]

Disease Transmission

Risks of Transmission of Transfusion-Related Diseases.
Multiple methods have been utilized to decrease the risk of the transmission of infectious diseases associated with transfusion. Even with strict donor deferral methods, there are many risks associated with transfusion when selecting potential blood donors. The following risks should be considered: hepatitis B and C, HIV and AIDS, human T-cell lymphotropic virus, and other viruses and parasites including *Babesia*, parvovirus, malaria, Chagas' disease, Lyme disease, and West Nile virus. Because of these risks, it is important to transfuse only when necessary and attempt to limit donor exposure.

CONCLUSIONS

Caring for critically ill patients who require transfusion is challenging and multifaceted. Current transfusion practice guidelines and thresholds are controversial. Strategies should be directed toward reducing the transfusion threshold and minimizing blood loss. Concerns about complications related to transfusion have resulted in close examination of conventional transfusion practices in critical care. Future research should be directed toward determining optimal transfusion strategies in a variety of patient populations when blood conservation techniques are not possible.

REFERENCES

1. American Association of Blood Banks 23rd Edition Blood Bank/ Transfusion Service Standards Program Unit. (2004). *Standards for Blood Banks and Transfusion Services* (23rd ed.). Bethesda, Md: American Association of Blood Banks.
2. American Red Cross, America's Blood Centers, American Association of Blood Banks. (2003). *Circular of information for the use of human blood and blood components.* Bethesda, Md: American Association of Blood Banks.
3. Bernard, G. R., et al. (1994). Report of the American-European Consensus Conference on Acute Respiratory Distress Syndrome: definitions, mechanisms, relevant outcomes, and clinical trial coordination. Consensus Committee. *J Crit Care, 9,* 72–81.
4. Berezina, T. L., et al. (2002). Influence of storage on red blood cell rheological properties. *J Surg Res, 102,* 6–12.
5. Bordim, J. O., & Blajchman, M. A. (2002). Transfusion-associated immunomodulation. In T. L. Simon, et al. (Eds.), *Rossi's principles of transfusion medicine* (3rd ed.). Philadelphia: Lippincott Williams & Wilkins.
6. Brecher, M. E. (2002a). Apheresis. In M. E. Brecher, (Ed.), *AABB technical manual* (14th ed.). Bethesda, Md: American Association of Blood Banks.
7. Brecher, M. E. (2002b). Components from whole blood donation. In M. E. Brecher (Ed.), *AABB technical manual* (14th ed.). Bethesda, Md: American Association of Blood Banks.
8. Brecher, M. E. (2002c). Noninfectious complications of blood transfusion. In M. E. Brecher (Ed.), *AABB technical manual* (14th ed.). Bethesda, Md: American Association of Blood Banks.
9. Brecher, M. E. (Ed.). (2002d). The positive DAT and immune-mediated red cell destruction. In M. E. Brecher (Ed.), *AABB technical manual* (14th ed., pp. 439–445). Bethesda, Md: American Association of Blood Banks.
10. Brecher, M. E. (Ed.). (2002e). Components from whole blood donations. In M. E. Brecher (Ed.), *AABB technical manual* (14th ed.). Bethesda, Md: American Association of Blood Banks.
11. Brecher, M. E. (Ed.). (2002f). Blood transfusion practice. In M. E. Brecher (Ed.), *AABB technical manual* (14th ed., pp. 451–483). Bethesda, Md: American Association of Blood Banks.
12. Brecher, M. E. (2002). Appendices. In M. E. Brecher (Ed.), *AABB technical manual* (14th ed.). Bethesda, Md: American Association of Blood Banks.
13. Bufford, K. D., et al. (2005). Recombinant factor VIIa as adjunctive therapy for bleeding control in severely injured trauma patients: two parallel randomized, placebo-controlled, double blind clinical trials. *J Trauma, 59*(1), 8–15.
14. Card, R. T., et al. (1982). Deformability of stored red blood cells. Relationship to degree of packing. *Transfusion, 22,* 96–101.
15. Chin-Yee, I., Arya, N., & d'Almeida, M. S. (1997). The red cell storage lesion and its implications for transfusion. *Transfus Sci, 18,* 447–458.
16. Corwin, H. L. (1999). Blood transfusions in the critically ill patient. *Dis Mon, 45,* 409–426.
17. Corwin, H. L. (2001). Anemia in the critically ill: the role of erythropoietin. *Semin Hematol, 38*(suppl 7), 24–32.
18. Corwin, H. L., et al. (2002). Efficacy of recombinant human erythropoietin in critically ill patients; a randomized controlled trial. *JAMA, 288,* 2827–2835.
19. Corwin, H. L., et al. (2004). The CRIT study: anemia and blood transfusion in the critically ill—current clinical practice in the United States. *Crit Care Med, 32,* 39–52.
20. Dahlbäck, B. (2000). Blood coagulation. *Lancet, 355,* 1627–1632.
21. Friedman, K. D., & Menitove, J. E. (2001). Preparation and clinical use of plasma and plasma fractions. In E. Beutler, et al. (Eds.), *Williams' hematology* (6th ed.). McGraw-Hill: New York.
22. *Further guidance on methods to detect bacterial contamination of platelet concentrates.* (2003). *Association Bulletin #03–12.* Bethesda, Md: American Association of Blood Banks.
23. Goldman, M., & Blajchman, M. A. (1991). Blood product-associated bacterial sepsis. *Transfus Med Rev, 5,* 73–83.
24. Goodnough, L. T. (2005). Alternatives to allogeneic transfusion. In P. L. Mintz (Ed.), *Transfusion therapy: clinical principles and practices* (2nd ed.). Bethesda, Md: AABB Press.
25. Heaton, A., et al. (1989). In vivo regeneration of red cell 2,3–diphosphoglyceric following transfusion of DPG-depleted AS-1, AS-3 and CPDA-1 red cells. *Br J Haematol, 71*(4), 131–136.
26. Hebert, P. C., et al. (1999). A multicenter, randomized, controlled clinical trial of transfusion requirements in critical care. Transfusion Requirements in Critical Care Investigators, Canadian Critical Care Trials Group. *N Engl J Med, 340,* 409–417.
27. Hebert, P. C., et al. (2001). Is a low transfusion threshold safe in critically ill patients with cardiovascular diseases? *Crit Care Med, 29*(2), 227–234.
28. Hill, S., et al. (2002). Transfusion thresholds and other strategies for guiding allogeneic red blood cell transfusion (Cochrane Review). In *The Cochrane Library,* Issue 2. Oxford: Update Software.

29. Hollness, L., et al. (2004). Fatalities caused by TRALI. *Transfus Med Rev, 18,* 184–188.

30. Humphries, J. E., & Ortel, T. L. (2005). Treatment of acquired disorders of hemostasis. In P. L. Mintz (Ed.), *Transfusion therapy: clinical principles and practices* (2nd ed.). Bethesda, Md: AABB Press.

31. Klein, H. G. (2000). The prospects for red-cell substitutes [editorial; comment]. *N Engl J Med, 342,* 1666.

32. Kopko, P. M., et al. (2002). Transfusion-related acute lung injury: report of a clinical look-back investigation. *JAMA, 287,* 1968–1971.

33. LaMuraglia, G. M., et al. (2000). The reduction of the allogeneic transfusion requirement in aortic surgery with a hemoglobin-based solution. *J Vasc Surg, 31,* 299.

34. Lee, J. H. Workshop on Bacterial Contamination of Platelets. CBER, FDA September 24, 1999. www.fda.gov/cber/minutes/workshop-min.htm.

35. Linden, J. V., & Pisciotto, P. T. (1992). Transfusion-associated graft-versus-host disease and blood irradiation. *Transfus Med Rev, 6,* 116.

36. Marik, P. E., & Sibbald, W. J. (1993). Effect of stored-blood transfusion on oxygen delivery in patients with sepsis. *JAMA, 269,* 3024–3029.

37. McGoldrick, M., & Fraser, G. L. (2003). Anemia and epoetin alfa in the intensive care unit. *Hosp Pharm, 38,* 1009–1014.

38. Mitka, M. (2001). FDA wants more restrictions on donated blood. *JAMA, 25,* 286, 408.

39. Mountain, A. (2000). Gene therapy: the first decade. *Trends Biotechnol, 18*(3), 119–128.

40. Muluk, V., & Macpherson, D. S. (2005). Perioperative medication management. UpToDate. www.uptodate.com.

41. Nagel, R. L. (2005). Structure and function of normal human hemoglobins. UpToDate. www.uptodate.com.

42. National Blood Data Resource Center. (2001). Comprehensive report on blood collection and transfusion in the United States. Bethesda, Md: National Data Resource Center.

43. Nester, T. A. (2005). Senior medical technology student case studies and personal conversation, June 15, 2005.

44. NovoSeven Coagulation Factor VIIa (Recombinant) Fact Sheet. (2005). http://press.novonordisk-us.com.

45. Opelz, G., et al. (1973). Effect of blood transfusions on subsequent kidney transplants. *Transplant Proc, 5,* 253–259.

46. Perez, P., et al. for the BACTHEM group and the French Haemovigilance Network. (2001). Determinants of transfusion-associated bacterial contamination: results of the French BACTHEM case-control study. *Transfusion, 41,* 862–872.

47. Piagnerelli, M., & Vincent, J. L. (2004). Role of iron in anemic critically ill patients: it's time to investigate! *Crit Care, 8,* 306–307.

48. Popovsky, M. A., et al. (1983). Transfusion-related acute lung injury associated with passive transfer of antileukocyte antibodies. *Am Rev Respir Dis, 128,* 185–189.

49. Popovsky, M. A., et al. (1992). Transfusion-related acute lung injury: a neglected, serious complication of hemotherapy. *Transfusion, 32,* 589–592.

50. Popovsky, M. (1996). Quality of blood components filtered before storage and at the bedside: implications for transfusion practice. *Transfusion, 36,* 470–474.

51. Popovsky, M. A. (2001). Hemolytic transfusion reactions. In M. A. Popovsky (Ed.), *Transfusion reactions.* Bethesda, Md: AABB Press.

52. Popovsky, M. A. (2001). Transfusion related acute lung injury. In M. A. Popovsky (Ed.), *Transfusion reactions.* Bethesda, MD: AABB Press.

53. Porte, R. J., & Leebeek, F. W. G. (2002). Pharmacologic strategies to decrease transfusion requirements in patients undergoing surgery. *Drugs, 62,* 2193–2211.

54. Rao, M. P., et al. (2002). Blood component use in critically ill patients. *Anaesthesia, 57,* 530–534.

55. Rapaport, S. I., & Rao, L. V. (1995). The tissue factor pathway: How it has become a "prima ballerina." *Thromb Haemost, 74,* 7.

56. Rogiers, P., et al. (1997). Erythropoietin response is blunted in critically ill patients. *Intensive Care Med, 23,* 159–162.

57. Schiffer, C. A., et al. (2001). Platelet transfusion for patients with cancer: clinical practice guidelines of the American Society of Oncology. *J Clin Oncol, 19,* 1519.

58. Silvergleid, A. J. (2005). *Transfusion-associated graft-versus-host disease.* UpToDate. www.uptodate.com.

59. Sirchia, G., Rebulla, P., & Sabbioneda, L. (1995). Preparation of white cell-reduced red cells by filtration: comparison of a bedside filter and two blood bank filter systems. *Transfusion, 35,* 421–426.

60. Slichter, S. (2004). Platelet transfusion: future directions. *Vox Sanguinis, 87,* s2, 47.

61. Spence, R. K., & Mintz, P. L. (Ed.). (2005). *Transfusion in surgery, trauma, and critical care.* In P. L. Mintz (Ed.), *Transfusion therapy: clinical principles and practices* (2nd ed.). Bethesda, Md: AABB Press.

62. Spotnitz, W. D., et al. (Ed.). (2005). Clinical uses of fibrin sealant. In P. L. Mintz (Ed.), *Transfusion therapy: clinical principles and practices* (2nd ed.). Bethesda, Md: AABB Press.

63. Staudinger, T., Locker, G. J., & Frass, M. (1996). Management of acquired coagulation disorders in emergency and intensive-care medicine. *Semin Thromb Hemost, 22,* 93–104.

64. Suzuki, K., et al. (1992). Transfusion-associated graft-versus-host disease in a presumably immunocompetent patient after transfusion of stored packed red cells. *Transfusion, 32,* 358–360.

65. Taylor, R. W., et al. (2002). Impact of allogenic packed red blood cell transfusion on nosocomial infection rates in the critically ill patient. *Crit Care Med, 30,* 102249–102254.

66. Tinmouth, A., & Chin-Yee, I. (2001). The clinical consequences of the red cell storage lesion. *Transfus Med Rev, 15,* 91–107.

67. Toy, P., et al. (2005). Transfusion-related acute lung injury: definition and review. *Crit Care Med, 33,* 721–726.

68. Triulzi, D. J. (2005). Blood components. In D. J. Triulzi (Ed.). *Blood transfusion therapy: a physician's handbook* (8th ed.). Bethesda, Md: AABB Press.

69. Vincent, J. L., et al. (2002). Anemia and blood transfusion in critically ill patients. *JAMA, 288*(12), 1499–1507.

70. Wallace, E. L., et al. (1993). Collection and transfusion of blood and blood components in the United States, 1989. *Transfusion, 33,* 139–144.

71. Walsh, T. S., et al. (2004). Does the storage time of transfused red blood cells influence regional or global indices of tissue oxygenation in anemic critically ill patients? *Crit Care Med, 32,* 364–371.

72. Walsh, T. S. (2004). Red cell requirements for intensive care units adhering to evidence-based transfusion guidelines. *Transfusion, 44,* 1405–1411.

73. Ware, L. B., & Matthay, M. A. (2000). The acute respiratory distress syndrome. *N Engl J Med, 342,* 1334–1349.

74. Zallen, G., et al. (1999). Age of transfused blood is an independent risk factor for postinjury multiple organ failure. *Am J Surg, 178,* 570–572.

CHAPTER 37

Coagulopathies

Diane K. Dressler

Dramatic events in critical care often involve coagulopathies, the disorders of blood coagulation. This chapter will describe normal hemostasis and the multiple disease processes that lead to coagulation abnormalities, along with the recognition and management of these disorders. While the term *coagulopathy* most commonly refers to excessive bleeding, the pathophysiology may also include thrombosis, or inappropriate clotting. Coagulopathy is a threat to every critically ill patient; patients at particular risk include those with sepsis, trauma, burns, and extensive surgery.[3,5] Although some patients have inherited disorders of coagulation, the acquired disorders (e.g., disseminated intravascular coagulation [DIC]) are most likely to complicate critical illness. In addition to covering DIC, this chapter will provide information on the recognition and management of other acquired disorders of coagulation including postoperative coagulopathy, bleeding as a result of anticoagulation, thrombocytopenia, pathologic fibrinolysis, vitamin K deficiency, bleeding associated with failure of specific organ systems, and common thrombotic disorders.

NORMAL HEMOSTASIS AND THE PATHWAYS TO A CLOT

Following an injury, hemostasis is accomplished by the harmonious interaction of three factors: the injured blood vessel wall, the blood platelets, and the plasma coagulation factors. The multiple events in blood clotting begin with spasm of the injured vessel wall and progress through a series of steps that result in clot formation. Vascular spasm is initiated by nervous reflexes in the vessel wall and slows the loss of blood. The spasm is enhanced by the release of thromboxane A_2 from circulating platelets.[15] The degree of spasm is proportional to the amount of trauma, with more spasm occurring with greater injury.[25]

The subsequent hemostatic process entails two major steps identified as primary and secondary hemostasis.

During primary hemostasis, platelet adhesion and aggregation occur, resulting in formation of a platelet plug. Secondary hemostasis involves formation of a fibrin clot (Figure 37-1).[3]

Primary hemostasis is initiated when the injured vessel lining and exposed collagen activate the blood platelets, beginning the processes of platelet adhesion and aggregation. When stimulated, the platelets change their shape from disks to spheres, exposing adhesion molecules that enable the platelets to stick to the surface of the damaged vessel.[37] Platelet adhesion also depends on a protein called von Willebrand factor (vWF) that is produced by the vascular endothelium and circulates attached to factor VIII. The platelet receptors bind to vWF on the injured vessel, enhancing adhesion.[15] Platelets contain mitochondria and enzyme systems that enable them to release adenosine diphosphate (ADP) and synthesize prostaglandins, substances essential in the accumulation of more platelets. The resulting platelet aggregation is self-perpetuating, with continuing release of ADP and thromboxane A_2. Platelet plugs are then formed, stopping the flow of blood from small tears in the vessel. These tiny platelet plugs are important in stopping the flow of blood from injured capillaries and preventing petechiae from forming following the minor bumps and slight trauma associated with normal activities. The key role of platelets cannot be overstated. In addition to their role in both primary and secondary hemostasis, platelets nurture the vascular endothelium, helping maintain its integrity.

Secondary hemostasis is activated and the formation of a fibrin clot begins. When a larger clot is needed, the adhesion and aggregation of platelets are only the beginning of the process. Simultaneously, as platelet plugs form, thromboplastin is released from the injured tissue; attraction of plasma coagulation factors begins. The fibrin complex that eventually makes up the clot is assembled on the platelet surface—yet another step that involves platelets. Glycoprotein IIb/IIIa receptors on the platelet membrane and platelet phospholipids are important components of this process.

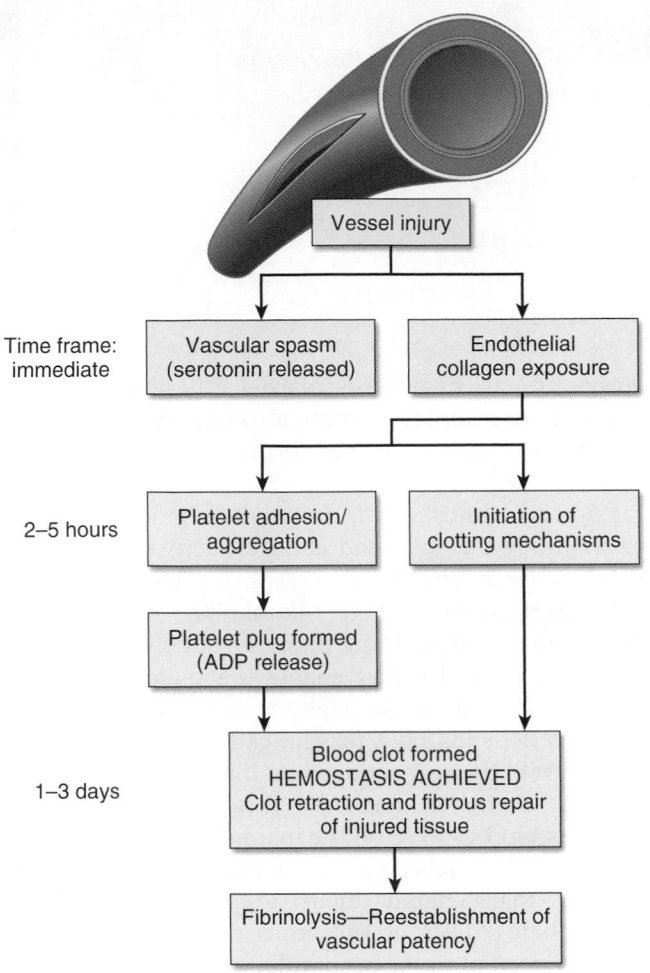

Time frame: immediate

Vessel injury

Vascular spasm (serotonin released)

Endothelial collagen exposure

2–5 hours

Platelet adhesion/ aggregation

Initiation of clotting mechanisms

Platelet plug formed (ADP release)

1–3 days

Blood clot formed
HEMOSTASIS ACHIEVED
Clot retraction and fibrous repair of injured tissue

Fibrinolysis—Reestablishment of vascular patency

◆**FIGURE 37-1** Physiology of coagulation.

There are two known pathways to blood coagulation: the extrinsic and intrinsic pathways (Figure 37-2). Blood clotting is initiated by the extrinsic pathway in response to injury, and is enhanced by the intrinsic pathway.[4] The two pathways are interrelated and necessary for blood coagulation. The overall process involves a series of linked reactions where serine proteases are activated, leading to the subsequent stimulation of a series of factors that culminates in the formation of a fibrin clot. This process is often referred to as the coagulation cascade. The major procoagulant factors are listed in Table 37-1. The liver produces most plasma coagulation factors, including the procoagulant proteins known as fibrinogen, prothrombin, and factors V, VII, IX, X, and XI. These factors circulate through the blood in an inactive form until needed for hemostasis. Some of these factors are referred to by their common names (e.g., prothrombin) while other factors are referred to by roman numerals followed by an "a" once they are activated (e.g., factor VII becomes VIIa). Although there are many factors involved in the coagulation process, rather than

focusing on the exact cascade sequence, it is most important to understand that without adequate factor levels, calcium, and platelet membrane phospholipids, the cascade will be unable to generate an effective clot.

Clotting begins when the extrinsic pathway is activated by trauma to tissues and blood vessels.[3] Tissue trauma results in the release of tissue thromboplastin from endothelial cells. Specific tissues are rich in tissue thromboplastin, including brain, placenta, bone marrow, and mesenteric fat. Injury to these tissues can result in the release of large amounts of tissue thromboplastin and stimulation of appropriate and inappropriate clotting. With any injury, the subsequent interaction of tissue thromboplastin with activated factor VII and calcium is able to activate factor X and the final common pathway. Through the activity of the extrinsic pathway, bleeding from disrupted blood vessels is stopped quickly.[15] The extrinsic pathway in turn stimulates the intrinsic pathway through activation of factor XII (Hageman factor). This initiates a chain reaction where factors XI, IX, VII, and X are activated, a process known to occur more slowly than the extrinsic pathway. The end result is again the activation of the final common pathway.

It is important to note Hageman factor can be activated from damaged endothelium, exposed collagen, injured blood cells, immune reactions, and endotoxin, and is one of the links between the inflammatory process and blood coagulation. Inflammatory mediators released during immune reactions activate both macrophages and the endothelial cells that line blood vessels. This in turn initiates the coagulation process, resulting in the generation of fibrin clots within the blood vessels.[4] It is thought this may be part of the body's attempt to contain pathogens.

In the final common pathway, factor X is activated. Prothrombin is then cleaved to thrombin, a powerful procoagulant considered to be the major enzyme responsible for blood clotting.[14] Thrombin cleaves fibrinogen into fibrin. Through a series of events including factor XIII, the fibrin monomers become fibrin polymers and finally become stable fibrin, forming an actual blood clot. The meshlike clot consists of fibrin strands, red blood cells, and platelets. Clot formation usually occurs within minutes, as reflected by a normal bleeding time. Rapid clot formation is necessary to prevent the platelet plug and clot from washing away from the shear forces of blood flow.[29] After the clot is formed, the mesh retracts, squeezing out the serum, further stabilizing the cross-linked fibrin.

Following the clotting of a blood vessel, the fibrinolytic system is activated by the presence of thrombin and other activated factors in the circulation. The purpose of the fibrinolytic system is to gradually break down the clot and reestablish flow through the vessel. As a clot forms, the proenzyme for fibrinolysis, plasminogen, is incorporated into the clot. Naturally occurring

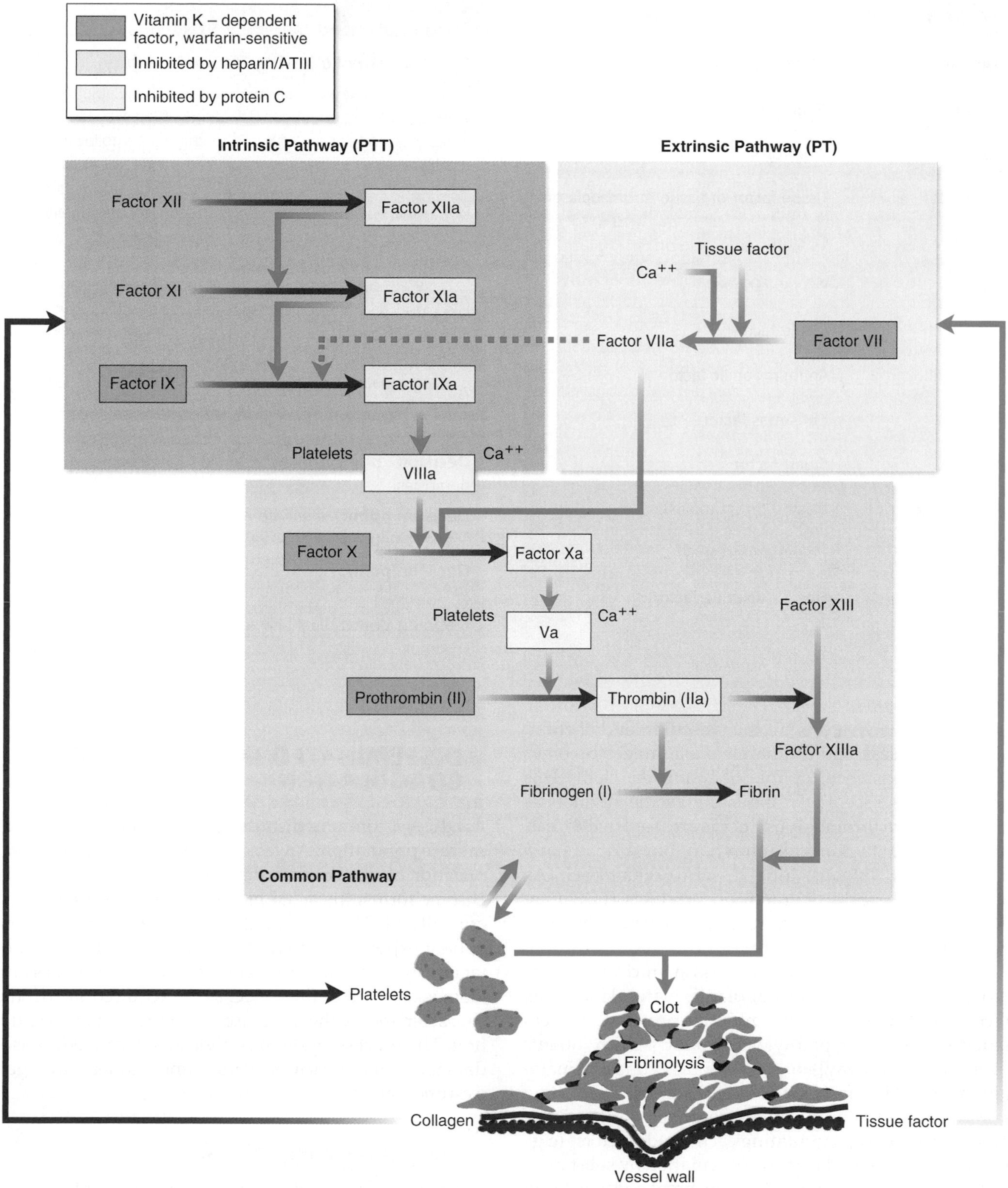

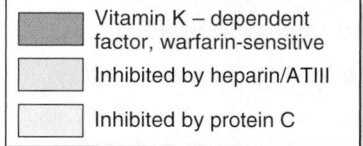

	Vitamin K – dependent factor, warfarin-sensitive
	Inhibited by heparin/ATIII
	Inhibited by protein C

Intrinsic Pathway (PTT)

Factor XII → Factor XIIa

Factor XI → Factor XIa

Factor IX → Factor IXa

Platelets Ca^{++}

VIIIa

Extrinsic Pathway (PT)

Tissue factor

Ca^{++}

Factor VIIa ← Factor VII

Common Pathway

Factor X → Factor Xa

Platelets Ca^{++}

Va

Prothrombin (II) → Thrombin (IIa)

Factor XIII

Factor XIIIa

Fibrinogen (I) → Fibrin

Platelets

Clot

Fibrinolysis

Collagen

Tissue factor

Vessel wall

♦FIGURE 37-2 Coagulation cascade. Ca^{++} = Calcium.

TABLE 37-1 Plasma Procoagulant Factors

FACTOR	COMMON NAME
Factor I	Fibrinogen
Factor II	Prothrombin
Factor III	Tissue factor or tissue thromboplastin
Factor IV	Calcium
Factor V	Proaccelerin
Factor VII	Stable factor
Factor VIII	Antihemophilic factor
Factor IX	Christmas factor
Factor X	Stuart factor
Factor XI	Plasma thromboplastin
Factor XII	Hageman factor
Factor XIII	Fibrin-stabilizing factor

Data from reference 29.

⬦ Case Study 37-1, Part A

Coagulopathy Following Traumatic Injury

B.J. is a 22-year-old male who sustained multiple gunshot wounds to the chest, abdomen, and right leg. He was rushed to surgery, and is now admitted to critical care following thoracotomy, laparotomy, and repair of the right leg wound. He received 4 L of fluid, 4 units of packed RBCs, and 2 units of FFP in the operating room. On admission to critical care, he is sedated and mechanically ventilated. He has almost 200 ml/hr of blood draining from the chest tubes and is noted to have oozing of blood from the abdominal and leg wounds. His blood pressure is labile, and his heart rate ranges from 110 to 120 beats/min. His skin is cool to the touch and urine output is 20 ml/hr.

Coagulopathy is suspected, and a coagulation panel is drawn, including a CBC, PT/INR, aPTT, fibrinogen level, and D-dimer test.

Decision point: What are the two major steps in hemostasis?

Decision point: Where are most of the plasma coagulation factors produced?

Decision point: How is the hemostatic process activated in patients with trauma?

Decision point: What ultimately happens to clots?

Case continues on page 1002

---

plasminogen activators in the vascular endothelium begin the process, and ultimately plasminogen becomes plasmin, a substance capable of lysing the clot.[25] This mechanism is essentially the same as the fibrinolysis achieved when thrombolytic agents are used in the treatment of acute myocardial infarction, but it occurs at a slow rate, allowing the torn vessel to repair itself. As clots dissolve, fibrin degradation products (FDPs) are released into the circulation, and if present in large amounts, act as anticoagulants.

Under normal conditions, there is an intricate balance of procoagulants and anticoagulants. Natural inhibitors of coagulation (e.g., antithrombin III, protein C, protein S, and tissue factor pathway inhibitor [which inhibits the extrinsic pathway]) oppose blood clotting and maintain the blood in a fluid state. If an injury occurs, clotting is initiated and should remain localized to the site of injury. Any extra circulating activated factors (e.g., thrombin) are cleared from the circulation by substances such as antithrombin III. Plasmin breaks down fibrin clots; however, even plasmin is inactivated by antiplasmin, preventing excessive fibrinolysis.[15] This intricate balance may be upset by critical illness, which can destroy or inappropriately stimulate the processes of clotting and fibrinolysis, resulting in coagulopathy.

DISSEMINATED INTRAVASCULAR COAGULATION

DIC is a common disorder of coagulation in the critical care population. Always a secondary process or complication of another disorder, DIC may occur in acute or chronic forms, the acute process seen most often in the critically ill. The process of DIC is unique because the patient experiences hemorrhage and thrombosis simultaneously. The International Society on Thrombosis and Hemostasis has defined DIC as an acquired syndrome characterized by the intravascular activation of coagulation. The process, systemic rather than localized, causes damage to the microvasculature and can lead to organ dysfunction.[22,37]

Pathophysiology of DIC

The main feature of DIC is intravascular clotting. Multiple tiny clots form and are deposited in the microcirculation, where they block perfusion and contribute to multiple organ failure. This extensive clotting is sometimes referred to as a "consumptive coagulopathy" because it depletes the blood of platelets and coagulation factors. Clotting components are utilized much more quickly than the liver and bone marrow can replace them. The overall result is that clots are deposited where they are not needed (in the microvasculature), yet a stable clot cannot form at an injury site. As the process continues, the patient often begins to bleed and may exhibit continuous oozing or frank hemorrhage.

The type of intravascular clotting occurring in DIC differs significantly from physiologic clotting. Clots form in the bloodstream in response to a thrombogenic stimulus that triggers the coagulation cascade (Figure 37-3). The underlying disorder results in damage to body tissues and endothelial injury. This injury triggers systemic activation of coagulation, resulting in unregulated thrombin activity, formation of microvascular thrombi, consumption of platelets and coagulation factors, and abnormal fibrinolysis.[15,23] Initially, fibrinolysis may be suppressed, but later the activation

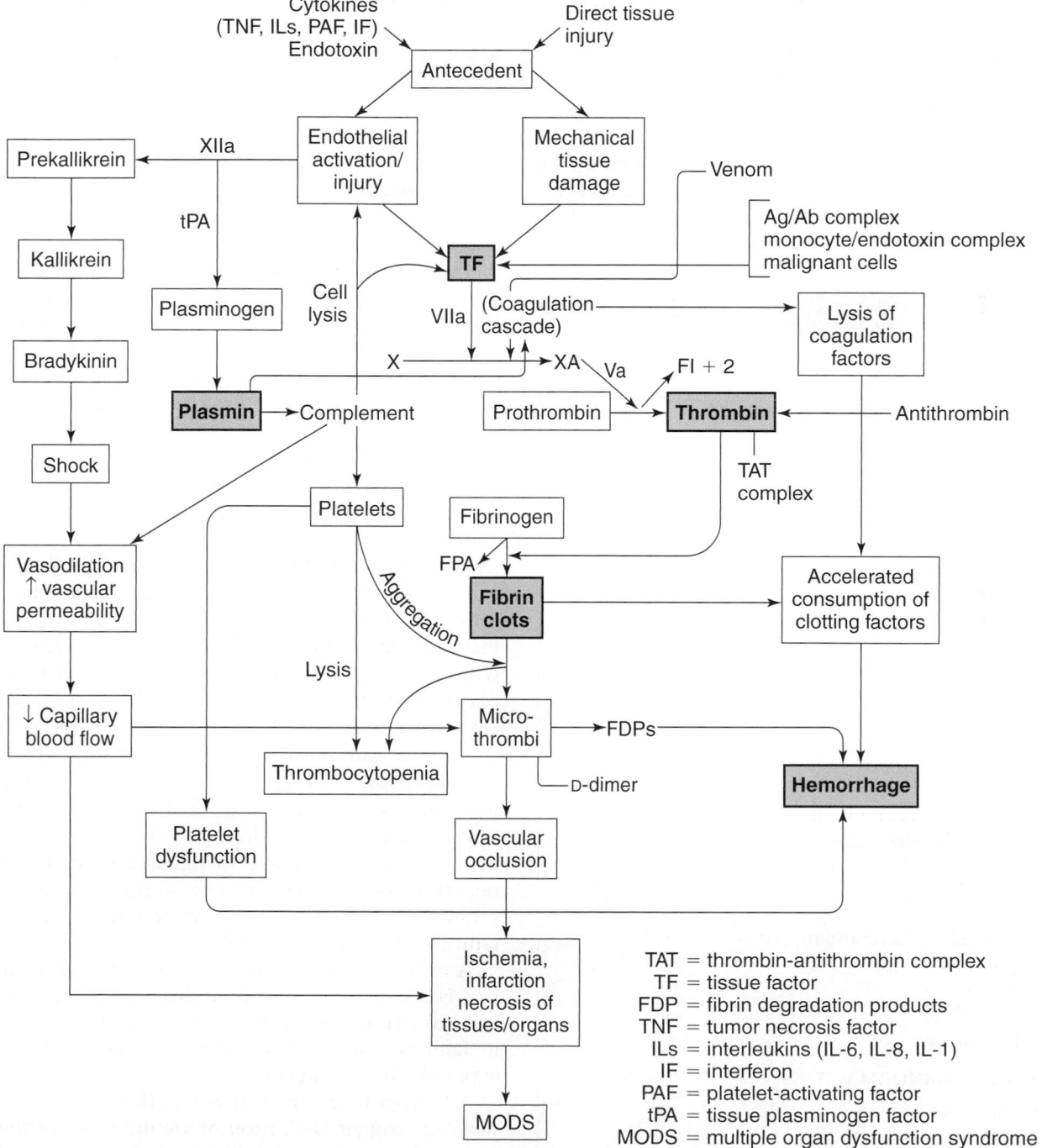

⬥FIGURE 37-3 The pathophysiology of disseminated intravascular coagulation.

of fibrinolysis in turn leads to release of FDPs and D-dimers, a process that may lyse microthrombi while also contributing to more bleeding.

The pathophysiology of DIC is thought to be a physiologic response to the patient's underlying disorder. A critical illness (e.g., major trauma) has an impact on the regulation of coagulation. The cellular elements of the blood, including leukocytes and platelets, are activated; the anticoagulant substances produced by the vascular endothelium are altered.[14] Inflammatory cytokines (e.g., interleukins and tumor necrosis factor) are generated and interfere with antithrombin III, protein C, and other natural anticoagulants.[24] As illness activates the extrinsic and intrinsic pathways, there can be inappropriate stimulation of clotting, fibrinolysis, or both.

Predisposing clinical conditions associated with DIC are multiple, ranging from shock to snakebite (Box 37-1). All types of shock can lead to DIC. Most

---

Box 37-1

Clinical Conditions Associated With Disseminated Intravascular Coagulation

IMMUNOLOGIC REACTIONS

- Transfusion reaction
- Transplant rejection

INFECTION AND SEPSIS

- Gram-negative sepsis
- Gram-positive sepsis
- Viral, protozoal, and fungal sepsis

MALIGNANCY

- Lymphoma
- Leukemia
- Solid tumors

OBSTETRIC COMPLICATIONS

- Amniotic fluid embolus
- Abruptio placentae
- Preeclampsia

TRAUMA

- Extensive traumatic injury
- Thoracic surgery
- Burns
- Snakebite
- Heatstroke

VASCULAR ABNORMALITIES

- Aortic aneurysm
- Vascular malformation

Data from references 2 and 15.

---

commonly, septic shock is implicated when gram-negative bacteremia leads to the release of endotoxin and the subsequent activation of factor XII and the intrinsic pathway. Sepsis from other organisms (e.g., viruses, protozoa, and fungi) is also associated with DIC. Extensive trauma, including the trauma from extensive surgery and burns, may trigger DIC by activating the extrinsic pathway. The mechanisms involved include endothelial damage, release of tissue thromboplastin, and the release of tissue breakdown products (e.g., fat and phospholipid) that can activate clotting.[24]

Systemic cytokine release is also thought to play a major role in trauma patients, as well as those with sepsis.[22] Cytokines damage the vascular endothelium, activating the extrinsic pathway and resulting in the deposition of clots in the microcirculation of major organs.

Complications of trauma, sepsis, and shock add more triggering factors. DIC is enhanced by hypothermia, hypotension, acidosis, and massive transfusion.[3,15] Blood clotting mechanisms are impaired at low body temperature; there is a well-established relationship between the degree of hypothermia and coagulopathy.[20] Hypotension and poor perfusion damage the vascular endothelium and lead to metabolic acidosis. The damaged endothelium may trigger clotting; acidosis may further alter blood coagulation. Massive transfusion can have a dilutional effect on clotting components; administration of stored blood and components may not replace all the lost coagulation factors and platelets.

DIC has long been associated with obstetric problems. Obstetric complications may result in the release of tissue factors into the blood, triggering systemic clotting. Amniotic fluid is known to contain substances that activate coagulation. In addition to the association with amniotic fluid embolus, the leakage of thromboplastin from the placenta has also been implicated in the activation of DIC.[24]

Other diagnoses associated with DIC include immunologic conditions (e.g., organ transplant rejection) and other diverse disorders (e.g., heatstroke). Patients with cancer may also develop DIC because both solid tumors and hematologic malignancies are known to release cytokines, which may precipitate coagulation problems. Metastatic cancer is commonly associated with the chronic form of DIC.

A rare syndrome known as drug-induced hemolytic DIC is associated with certain drugs (e.g., cephalosporins, quinidine, and quinine). This syndrome may lead to fatal hemolysis and thrombosis within days after exposure to these agents.[8]

Although there are many disorders and conditions that may trigger DIC, prompt identification of the disorder is important, because coagulopathy is a predictor of outcome in the critically ill. DIC has been identified as an independent predictor of mortality, especially in patients with sepsis and trauma,[24] adding incentive to timely identification of the clinical and laboratory features of this syndrome.

Clinical Manifestations of DIC

The clinical picture of DIC is quite variable, but can be dramatic, and often presents with bleeding. The bleeding is caused by the continuous consumption of coagulation factors and the fibrinolysis of existing clots. The patient may develop oozing of blood from multiple sites, including incisions and puncture sites. Even sites that are partially healed may begin to bleed as fibrinolysis dissolves preexisting clots. Significant hemorrhagic events such as bleeding from the gastrointestinal (GI) tract, genitourinary tract, and central nervous system are possible.

Patients may develop petechiae, purpura, and large areas of ecchymosis. A peculiar type of skin ischemia, called acrocyanosis, may develop as capillaries become clotted.[17] Acrocyanosis is characterized by gray to purple discoloration of the lips, nose, ears, fingers, and toes. There are sharp irregular areas of demarcation from normal areas of the skin; the patient is at risk for necrosis in the affected areas. The deposition of fibrin in the microvasculature can also lead to multiple organ dysfunction syndrome (MODS). Major organ systems may be affected by microcirculatory clotting, putting the patient at risk of acute renal failure, acute lung injury, hepatic failure, gut failure, and brain dysfunction.

Bleeding and thrombotic/ischemic problems may occur in different tissues and with varying intensity. Clinical manifestations of thrombosis typically result from microcirculatory occlusion. However, in chronic DIC, large thrombi may dominate the clinical picture. It is also important to know that DIC may be detected on a coagulation panel, with abnormal lab results but without any clinical signs of bleeding or thrombosis.[17]

Laboratory Features of DIC

Unlike the inherited disorders of coagulation, acquired disorders may not be diagnosed by a single lab value. DIC is associated with multiple abnormalities in the coagulation mechanism and multiple laboratory indicators of coagulopathy. Many different tests are used to screen for DIC. Table 37-2 lists normal coagulation test values.[25,29,31] The general tests of coagulation are usually elevated in DIC. The prothrombin time/international normalized ratio (PT/INR) measures the integrity of the extrinsic and common pathway.[3] The activated partial thromboplastin time (aPTT) measures the integrity of the intrinsic and

TABLE 37-2 Coagulation Panel Results in Disseminated Intravascular Coagulation

TEST	NORMAL VALUE*
Activated partial thromboplastin time	30–40 sec
D-dimer	Less than 250 ng/ml or less than 250 mcg/L
Fibrin degradation products	Less than 10 mcg/ml
Fibrin monomers	Negative
Fibrinogen	200–400 mg/dl
Hemoglobin	14–18 g/dl
INR	1.0: normal 2.0–3.0: moderate-level anticoagulation 2.5–3.5: high-level anticoagulation
Thrombin time	15 sec
Platelet count	150,000–400,000/mm^3
Red blood cell peripheral smear	Normal

Data from references 25, 29, and 31.
*Values may differ depending on the source.
INR = International normalized ratio.

common pathway.[31] Thrombin time is another general test of coagulation. While all of these values may be elevated in DIC, none of them are diagnostic of the disorder. The Research Utilization box on p. 1002 looks at the value of laboratory parameters as predictors of mortality.

Platelets and fibrinogen levels are typically low in DIC because these factors have been consumed during extensive and inappropriate clotting.[11] There are a number of tests for fibrinolysis that are positive, but not specific, for DIC. FDPs will be elevated. The newer D-dimer test is an accurate enzyme-linked immunosorbent assay (ELISA) that is a more specific indicator of fibrinolysis than other tests. A positive test for fibrin monomers (the unstable form of fibrin) is another indicator of abnormal clotting. It is recognized that FDPs and D-dimers are also elevated in trauma, recent surgery, inflammatory conditions, and thromboembolism.[24] Low levels of plasminogen and α$_2$-antiplasmin are also indicative of excessive fibrinolysis.[23]

The Predictive Value of Laboratory Parameters Following Traumatic Injury

CLINICAL ISSUE

Hemorrhage and coagulopathy are known to contribute to morbidity and mortality following traumatic injury. However, the predictive value of laboratory parameters such as the prothrombin time (PT) and partial thromboplastin time (PTT) is unknown.

SUMMARY

This study analyzed data on more than 7000 patients presenting to a level I trauma center. The prevalence of abnormal PT and PTT levels was 28% and 8%, respectively, in the early post-injury period. A significantly higher number of these patients died. The PT and PTT values were found to be predictors of mortality, whereas other lab values, such as platelet count, were not predictive.

APPLICATION

The incidence of coagulopathy following trauma is high and is a predictor of mortality. Coagulation parameters need to be measured in the early post-injury period, and appropriate interventions implemented.

NEED FOR FURTHER STUDY

Replication of this study in other critical care populations is needed to evaluate the applicability of these results to critical care patients in general.

MacLeod, J.B.A., et al. (2003). Early coagulopathy predicts mortality in trauma. *J Trauma Inj Infec Crit Care, 55*(1), 39–44.

Box 37-2

A Scoring System for the Diagnosis of Disseminated Intravascular Coagulation

Step 1. Analyze risk for DIC. Proceed with assessment if patient has a disorder associated with DIC.

Step 2. Perform screening tests: platelet count, test for fibrinolysis (i.e., FDP or D-dimer), PT/INR, and fibrinogen.

Step 3. Score test results.
- Platelet count: Greater than 100,000 = 0, less than 100,000 = 1, less than 50,000 = 2
- Fibrin-related marker: no increase = 0, moderate increase = 2, strong increase = 3
- PT/INR: normal = 0, above normal = 1, 2× normal = 2
- Fibrinogen: normal = 0, less than normal = 1

Step 4. Calculate score.

If greater than or equal to 5, score is compatible with diagnosis of DIC.

If less than 5, score is suggestive but not affirmative of DIC.

Data from references 24 and 34.

DIC = Disseminated intravascular coagulation, FDP = fibrin degradation product, INR = international normalized ratio, PT = prothrombin time.

A calculation is performed to determine the probability of DIC. Box 37-2 illustrates this calculation using laboratory tests generally available in most institutions.

When analyzing the results of a coagulation panel, there are additional, important considerations. Preexisting conditions (e.g., liver disease, surgery, cancer) may affect factor levels. Monitoring trends may be most important to consider as they indicate whether the coagulopathy is improving or worsening. The diagnosis of DIC and other acquired disorders of coagulation may be difficult, and sometimes a definitive diagnosis cannot be determined.

Management of DIC

Currently there is no definitive treatment for DIC. In a patient with both bleeding and thrombosis, effective management can be challenging. Both blood transfusion and pharmacologic therapy may be prescribed.

In the critically ill patient, the complication of DIC may be a life-threatening situation. A major focus of treatment is addressing the underlying disease process as quickly and aggressively as possible. For example, if the patient is septic, removing the source of infection

Individual factor levels such as factor V and factor VIII are known to be consumed in DIC and may be measured to distinguish DIC from other coagulopathies.[11] Normally the levels of these factors are approximately 100%; depletion of them is indicative of consumption. The complete blood count (CBC) will show a drop in hemoglobin and hematocrit (Hct), reflecting the extent of bleeding. The peripheral blood smear may also show the presence of schistocytes, which are distorted and fragmented red cells, damaged by circulating through partially clotted vessels.

Because there is no single test specific for DIC, the International Society on Thrombosis and Hemostasis has proposed a scoring system for the diagnosis.[24,34] In patients with a condition known to be associated with DIC, the following indicators are scored: platelet count, fibrin-related marker, PT/INR, and fibrinogen level.

Case continues on page 1004

Case Study 37-1, Part B

Risk Factors for the Development of a Coagulopathy

Within a few hours after admission to critical care, B.J.'s blood pressure dropped to 80/60 mm Hg. His heart rate remained at 120 beats/min, and urine output declined to 10 ml/hr. Oozing from surgical wounds and IV sites continued, and the Hct dropped to 25%. Coagulation panel results included the following values: INR, 2.1; aPTT, 44 sec; platelet count, 44,000/mm³; fibrinogen, 80 mg/dl; and D-dimer, 520 ng/dl.

Decision point: What were B.J.'s risk factors for the development of a coagulopathy such as DIC?

Decision point: What nursing interventions can be used to minimize the risk of coagulopathy in the patient with extensive trauma?

Decision point: What signs and symptoms did B.J. exhibit that were suggestive of coagulopathy?

Decision point: What laboratory values were indicative of DIC?

and simultaneously starting antimicrobial treatment are priorities. For some patients, treatment of the underlying problem can lead to improvement within hours; for others DIC may progress in spite of appropriate treatment.[24] Supportive therapy aimed at affected systems may include ventilatory support, fluid replacement, and pharmacologic support. These interventions are key, since hypoxia, hypothermia, hypotension, and acidosis all contribute to continuing coagulopathy.

Transfusion of blood and blood components is often necessary to treat the patient with active bleeding or high risk of bleeding. Administration of red blood cells (RBCs) maintains oxygen-carrying capacity and is necessary for optimizing and maintaining oxygen delivery and utilization, especially in the critically ill. Platelet concentrate may be given for bleeding caused by thrombocytopenia. Fresh frozen plasma (FFP) provides fibrinogen and many other plasma coagulation factors. Cryoprecipitate is given in DIC to replace fibrinogen, factor VIII, and vWF. Vitamin K may be administered to enhance production of clotting components. In addition to the standard blood components, administration of recombinant activated factor VIIa is reported to reduce hemorrhage in trauma patients.[12] This factor is used to treat hemophilia, but in high doses it attaches to activated platelets and enhances the production of a fibrin clot that is resistant to fibrinolysis.[13]

There are always concerns pertaining to blood administration. Known potential adverse effects include

transmission of infection, immune system modulation, alloimmunization with the development of reactive antibodies, and acute lung injury.[36]

In patients with DIC, there has historically been additional concern that transfusion of components may add "fuel to the fire" as the transfused platelets and fibrinogen may be used for more inappropriate clotting; this has never been proven in clinical studies.[24] Regardless of these potential concerns, patients who have severe hemorrhage require transfusion to support end-organ perfusion, maintain oxygen-carrying capacity, and replace lost components. For the actively bleeding patient, a laboratory-guided transfusion protocol provides a guide to therapy.[8] General management guidelines advise close monitoring of Hct, platelet count, INR, aPTT, and fibrinogen levels. DeLoughery describes a specific protocol for the administration of blood and components in coagulopathy.[8] RBCs are given for a hematocrit less than 30%. An INR greater than 1.6 and an abnormal aPTT are indications for 2 to 4 units of FFP. For a fibrinogen level less than 100 mg/dl, 10 units of cryoprecipitate are given. For a platelet count less than 50,000/µl, 6–8 units of random donor platelets are given. Chapter 36 provides more comprehensive information on blood transfusion therapy.

Patients with abnormal lab results but no clinical evidence of bleeding are generally not prescribed blood and components.[24] Patients requiring an invasive procedure may need transfusion to correct laboratory defects.

Pharmacologic therapy may be used to treat DIC. Heparin may be administered with the goal of interrupting the intravascular generation of thrombin and preventing further clotting of the microvasculature.[17] Heparin is most often prescribed for patients with evidence of thromboembolism and extensive fibrin deposition (e.g., acrocyanosis).[24] However, the risk of further bleeding from heparin is a consideration: patients must be closely monitored. The efficacy of heparin in DIC has not been supported in clinical trials.[24]

Recombinant activated protein C is reported to inhibit thrombin generation and microcirculatory clotting, and restore effective fibrinolysis;[1,22] however, the agent has not been tested in patients with a confirmed diagnosis of DIC. New agents known as tissue factor pathway inhibitors (TFPIs) and also antithrombin III concentrate are being evaluated for use in DIC.[3,22] Clinical trials of recombinant TFPIs and antithrombin have been inconclusive regarding the clinical survival benefit afforded by these agents.[21] Additional trials are planned to determine their efficacy in DIC.

In patients fortunate enough to survive DIC, physiologic processes aid in recovery. Plasmin eventually breaks down the fibrin in the microvasculature, restoring circulation. Leukocytes remove deposits of fibrin and complexes, further enhancing the circulation. Over time, the liver and bone marrow replace depleted plasma coagulation factors, platelets, and red blood cells. These processes can enable patients to recover from this serious complication.

◆ Case Study 37-1, Part C

Treatment of the Coagulopathy

During the diagnostic process, B.J. was supported with mechanical ventilation, volume replacement, and dopamine (Intropin) at 5 mcg/kg/min to optimize hemodynamics and tissue perfusion. A hematologist was consulted to aid the diagnosis and treatment of the coagulopathy, and a working diagnosis of DIC was made. Treatment with volume replacement and blood component administration was continued and adjusted according to coagulation panel results and hemodynamic response. B.J. received 4 units of RBCs, 8 units of FFP, and 10 units of cryoprecipitate. Over a 12-hour period, B.J.'s lab work, vital signs, and hemodynamics began to stabilize, the bleeding slowed, and the dopamine was weaned.

Decision point: What is considered to be the most important recommendation for the treatment of DIC?

Decision point: What are the specific therapeutic effects of RBCs, FFP, and cryoprecipitate in the bleeding patient?

Decision point: How is the effectiveness of blood and blood component therapy monitored?

Decision point: What physiologic processes make it possible to recover from DIC?

POSTOPERATIVE COAGULOPATHY

Postoperative bleeding can occur after any surgery. Patients at particular risk include those with presurgical conditions such as hepatic insufficiency or an inherited disorder of coagulation. However, even with preoperative screening of coagulation parameters, it is not always possible to predict which patients will have bleeding problems. Bleeding complications are common following cardiac surgery; this section focuses on those patients.

There are a number of factors that put patients at risk, beginning with the use of cardiopulmonary bypass (CPB).[40] As blood passes through the bypass circuit, contact between blood components and the oxygenator activates coagulation and fibrinolysis. The inflammatory process is also activated by cardiovascular surgery and leads to the release of cytokines and the stimulation of neutrophils, thereby increasing the risk of coagulopathy.[27] CPB decreases both the number and the function

of platelets.[40] Both platelet activation and dysfunction occur; the degree of platelet dysfunction is directly proportional to the duration of bypass and depth of hypothermia.[30] While hypothermia is used routinely to decrease oxygen requirements during surgery, it does contribute to impaired platelet function and postoperative coagulopathy.

Another factor predisposing patients to bleeding is the use of heparin to prevent clotting in the bypass circuit. Heparin is routinely administered while the patient is placed on bypass and is reversed with protamine at the end of the surgery. CPB also enhances fibrinolysis because during the bypass process tissue plasminogen activator is released from endothelial cells. The degree of fibrinolysis also is proportional to the duration of bypass.[40]

There are additional risks for bleeding in the cardiac surgical population. The current liberal use of preoperative anticoagulation is one such risk factor; generally, patients are asked to discontinue anticoagulant medications before surgery. However, stopping platelet inhibitors, glycoprotein inhibitors, and other anticoagulants before urgent procedures is commonly not possible. An additional risk factor is previous thoracic surgery; adhesions from previous operations must be dissected during surgery, significantly increasing the procedural trauma.

It is important to distinguish between coagulopathy and bleeding caused by inadequate hemostasis related to the procedure itself. Patients with coagulopathy will usually have bleeding from multiple sites in addition to excessive chest tube drainage. Patients with inadequate hemostasis will generally have excessive chest tube drainage without bleeding from other sites. In the latter case, reoperation is necessary to identify the site of bleeding and stop the hemorrhage.

Pharmacologic therapy may be used to prevent or treat postoperative coagulopathy. Protamine sulfate (Protamine) may be administered to facilitate reversal of heparin.[27] Aprotinin (Trasylol) is also commonly used in cardiac surgical patients. Aprotinin is a potent protease inhibitor that blocks kallikrein, a mediator that can initiate the coagulation cascade and fibrinolysis.[27] It is administered intravenously during and following cardiac surgery to stabilize clotting and prevent bleeding from excessive fibrinolysis. Dosing protocols vary, but typically a loading dose of 2 million kallikrein inactivator units (KIU) is given, followed by an infusion of 500,000 KIU/hour.[28] Patients who receive aprotinin intraoperatively and postoperatively have been shown to have reduced blood loss and reduced need for blood transfusion.[33] Another agent used to treat postoperative coagulopathy is desmopressin acetate (DDAVP).[27] This agent promotes clotting by increasing plasma levels of factor VIII and vWF, enhancing platelet aggregation. Because platelet dysfunction is known to be a pivotal part of postoperative coagulopathy, administration of platelet concentrate may also be indicated. Serial coagulation panels are done to determine if additional blood products are needed.

BLEEDING RESULTING FROM ANTICOAGULATION

There are many indications for anticoagulation, with most involving actual or potential thrombi and emboli. For example, anticoagulants are an important part of the treatment regimen for patients with acute coronary syndromes, valvular heart disease, atrial fibrillation, and deep venous thrombosis. However, suppression of the normal coagulation pathways carries with it the risk of bleeding. Bleeding may be provoked by

tissue trauma or may be spontaneous and can include bleeding from procedure sites, retroperitoneal hemorrhage, GI bleeding, and intracranial bleeding.

In current clinical practice, the use of anticoagulants has increased.[18] Many diagnostic and treatment protocols, such as those for cardiac catheterization and percutaneous coronary interventions, require the use of anticoagulants. Aside from treatment protocols, many patients receive anticoagulants as part of thromboembolism prevention protocols. For example, a significant number of orthopedic patients receive low molecular weight heparin (LMWH) initially and then transition to warfarin (Coumadin) following joint replacement surgery. Platelet inhibitors, including aspirin, are routinely prescribed for people with cardiovascular disease.

Commonly used anticoagulants are listed in the Medication table below and on pp. 1006-1007. These agents are described briefly, along with the implications for potential bleeding problems.

ANTICOAGULANTS USED IN CRITICAL CARE

DRUG	ACTION	USUAL DOSAGE	SPECIAL CONSIDERATIONS
Argatroban	Inhibits thrombin-mediated fibrin formation	PCI: 25 mcg/kg/min IV; administer bolus of 350 mcg/kg over 3–5 min; check ACT in 5–10 min following bolus If ACT less than 300 sec, give additional bolus of 150 mcg/kg; increase infusion to 30 mcg/kg/min If ACT greater than 450 sec, decrease infusion to 15 mcg/kg/min Once ACT is 300–450 sec, continue with procedure HIT: 2 mcg/kg/min as continuous infusion; adjust dose to aPTT Max dose is 10 mcg/kg/min	Maintain aPTT 1.5–3 times control (not to exceed 100 sec) Start at 0.5 mcg/kg/min in patients with hepatic impairment If initiating warfarin therapy during argatroban infusion, do not use warfarin loading dose
Aspirin	Inhibits cyclooxygenase and platelet aggregation	Suspected MI: 162–325 mg PO immediately with symptoms MI prophylaxis: 75–325 mg PO daily	Risk of GI and postprocedure bleeding Do not coadminister with Aggrenox, which contains aspirin and dipyridamole
Bivalirudin (Angiomax)	Inhibits thrombin-mediated fibrin formation	0.75 mg/kg IV bolus followed by 4-hr infusion at 1.75 mg/kg/hr After 4-hr infusion, administer infusion at 0.2 mg/kg/hr for 20 hr or less as needed	Decrease continuous infusion rate in patients with impaired renal function (CrCl less than 30 ml/min) to 1 mg/kg/hr; no bolus dose reduction is needed Decrease continuous infusion rate to 0.25 mg/kg/hr for hemodialysis patients; no bolus dose reduction is needed

Table continues on page 1006

DRUG	ACTION	USUAL DOSAGE	SPECIAL CONSIDERATIONS
Clopidogrel (Plavix)	Blocks ADP receptors on platelets, preventing binding with fibrinogen	75 mg PO daily	Additive effect with aspirin Patient may receive 300 mg loading dose during PCI
Dipyridamole (Persantine)	Inhibits uptake of adenosine into platelets, reducing aggregation	Prevention: 75–100 mg PO four times daily Diagnostic: 0.142 mg/kg/min IV infused over 4 min; maximum dose 60 mg	Additive effect with aspirin Do not coadminister with Aggrenox, which contains aspirin and dipyridamole
Fondaparinux (Arixtra)	Selective inhibitor of activated factor X	Prophylaxis: 2.5 mg subcutaneous daily for 5–9 days after surgery; first dose 6–8 hr after surgery Treatment: 5 mg daily if weight less than 50 kg; 7.5 mg daily if weight 50–100 kg; 10 mg daily if weight greater than 100 kg	Does not require lab monitoring; used as alternative to enoxaparin Adjust dose in older adults and those with renal impairment Contraindicated if CrCl less than 30 ml/min
Glycoprotein IIb/IIIa receptor inhibitors:	Inhibit binding of platelets with fibrinogen	According to individual agent	Risk of postprocedure bleeding Administer these medications in separate line; no other medications should be added to solution
Abciximab (ReoPro)		MI or PCI: 0.25 mg/kg given 10–60 min before angioplasty or atherectomy, followed by 12-hr infusion of 0.125 mcg/kg/min; maximum 10 mcg/min PCI (unstable angina): 0.25 mg/kg, followed by 18–24-hr infusion of 10 mcg/min; discontinue 1 hr after procedure	Monitor platelet count Risk of immunogenicity since abciximab is a monoclonal antibody; anaphylaxis treatment should be readily available during administration of abciximab
Eptifibatide (Integrillin)		ACS: 180 mcg/kg bolus followed by 2 mcg/kg/min infusion until discharge; maximum dose 15 mg/hr PCI: 180 mcg/kg before PCI; continuous drip of 2 mcg/kg/min and second 180 mcg/kg bolus 10 min after first; continue until discharge or for up to 18–24 hr Maximum infusion = 15 mg/hr	Concurrent aspirin and heparin is recommended Monitor platelet counts. For severe renal insufficiency (CrCl less than 50 ml/min or SCr greater than 2 mg/dl) use same bolus of 180 mcg/kg (maximum 22.6 mg). Decrease infusion to 1 mcg/kg/min (maximum 7.5 mg/hr)
Tirofiban (Aggrastat)		0.4 mcg/kg/min for 30 min; continue at 0.1 mcg/kg/min through procedure and for 12–24 hr following procedure	Monitor platelet count. Heparin can be administered in same line with tirofiban For severe renal insufficiency (CrCl less than 30 ml/min) decrease dose to 0.2 mcg/kg/min for 30 min, then 0.05 mcg/kg/min through procedure and for 12–24 hr following procedure

DRUG	ACTION	USUAL DOSAGE	SPECIAL CONSIDERATIONS
Heparin: Low molecular weight, enoxaparin (Lovenox) dalteparin (Fragmin)	Potentiates antithrombin III, inactivating thrombin and final common pathway	Prophylactic: 30 mg subcutaneously every 12 hr or 40 mg daily Angina, MI: 1 mg/kg subcutaneously every 12 hr or 1.5 mg/kg/day	Monitor platelet count Monitor closely in patients with CrCl less than 30 ml/min; dose adjustment probably required according to clinical situation
Heparin (unfractionated)	Potentiates antithrombin III, inactivating thrombin and final common pathway	Adjusted to target aPTT: Initial: 10,000 units subcutaneously followed by 50–70 units/kg subcutaneously every 4–6 hr Infusion: loading dose 80 units/kg; adjust to aPTT; continuous drip 10–30 units/kg/hr	aPTT testing required, maintain aPTT 1.5–2.5 times control GI bleeding and HIT potential complications Monitor platelet count
Lepirudin (Refludan)	Inhibits thrombin-mediated fibrin formation	0.2–0.4 mg/kg bolus (maximum 44 mg) slowly over 15–20 sec, followed by 0.1–0.15 mg/kg/hr IV infusion for 48 hr or longer (maximum 16.5 mg/hr)	Maintain aPTT 1.5–2.5 times control For renal impairment, decrease initial dose to 0.2 mg/kg Infusion rate for renal impairment: CrCl 45–60 ml/min, use 0.075 mg/kg/hr CrCl 30–44 ml/min, use 0.045 mg/kg/hr CrCl 15–29 ml/min, use 0.0225 mg/kg/hr Contraindicated if CrCl less than 15 ml/min
Warfarin (Coumadin)	Interferes with production of vitamin K–dependent factors	Initial: 5–15 mg PO daily for 2–5 days. Adjust to appropriate target range INR based on clinical situation Daily dosage is patient-specific and highly variable	INR testing required, multiple drug and food interactions

ACS = Acute coronary syndrome, ACT = activated clotting time, ADP = adenosine diphosphate, aPTT = activated partial thromboplastin time, CrCl = creatinine clearance, GI = gastrointestinal, HIT = heparin-induced thrombocytopenia, INR = international normalized ratio, MI = myocardial infarction, PCI = percutaneous coronary intervention, Scr = serum creatinine.

Platelet Inhibitors

Drugs that inhibit platelet activity include aspirin, nonsteroidal antiinflammatory drugs (NSAIDs), thienopyridines, and glycoprotein IIb/IIIa antagonists. Aspirin and NSAIDs inhibit cyclooxygenase and the subsequent production of thromboxane A_2, a necessary step for platelet aggregation (Figure 37-4).[16] Aspirin is the most potent NSAID. Its effects occur within 1 hour, lasting for the duration of the platelet's life span of 5 to 7 days. Aspirin is used to prevent thromboemboli from forming in the arterial system, thereby lowering the risk of cardiovascular events. Patients who have taken aspirin may have postoperative and postprocedure oozing and bleeding; their coagulation panel will show a prolonged bleeding time. These patients may be treated with platelet transfusion or desmopressin.[9]

Clopidogrel (Plavix) is the most commonly used thienopyridine. This oral agent inhibits ADP-induced platelet aggregation and is used to decrease the risk of cardiovascular events. Clopidogrel inhibits platelet aggregation for about 1 week. Treatment for bleeding problems includes platelet transfusion.

The glycoprotein IIb/IIIa inhibitors include the intravenous preparations of abciximab (ReoPro), eptifibatide (Integrillin), and tirofiban (Aggrastat). These agents act on the platelet membrane glycoproteins. They inhibit the final phase of platelet aggregation, preventing the platelets from combining with fibrinogen.[7] Abciximab

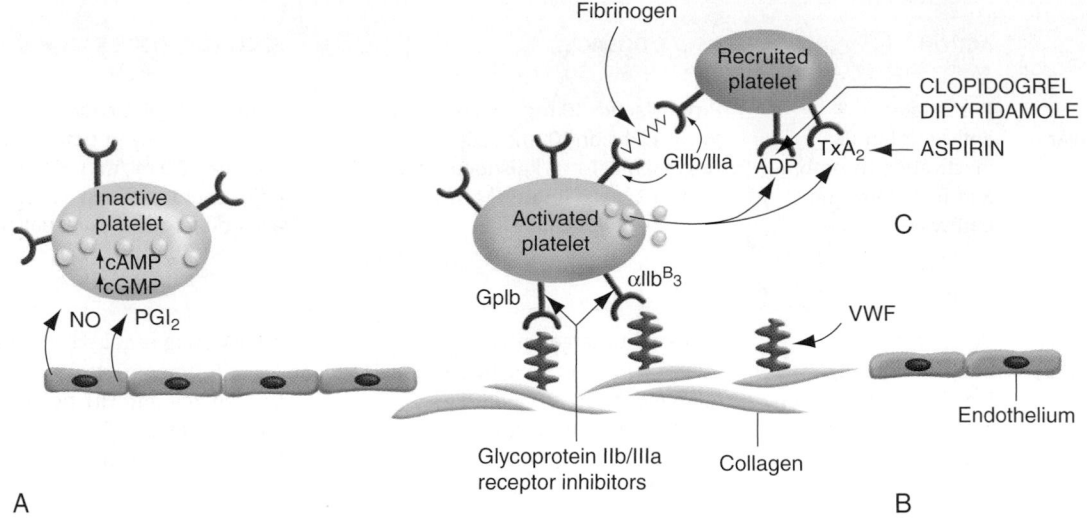

♦FIGURE 37-4 Platelet activation sequence including site of action for platelet-inhibiting medications.

and eptifibatide are commonly used for acute coronary syndromes and coronary interventions. They are associated with better outcomes, but also pose a higher risk of postprocedure bleeding. Treatment for bleeding complications may include transfusion of platelets or blood components containing fibrinogen, depending on the specific glycoprotein inhibitor.[9]

Warfarin

Warfarin is the most commonly used oral anticoagulant. This agent inhibits the production of the vitamin K–dependent coagulation factors in the liver, including prothrombin and factors VII, IX, and X. As shown in Figure 37-5, warfarin inhibits the hemostatic system at multiple sites. The clinical goal is to achieve an INR of 2.0 to 3.0, depending on the indication. In patients who need immediate anticoagulation, heparin is started concomitantly with warfarin while the warfarin dose is adjusted to achieve a therapeutic INR. Warfarin acts slowly, taking days to achieve peak effectiveness, as the body must clear itself of the vitamin K–dependent clotting factors. Unfortunately, it also takes days to reverse the effects. In the event of bleeding complications believed to be associated with warfarin, vitamin K, 5 to 10 mg IV, may be administered, with an expected effect within 4 to 6 hours.[9] If anticoagulation must be reversed quickly, FFP may be administered to restore plasma coagulation factors, enabling normal clotting.[7]

Patients receiving warfarin should be monitored closely for bleeding complications. It is important to note that warfarin interacts with multiple other medications. It is also affected by dietary intake. Foods high in vitamin K (e.g., green leafy vegetables) interfere with the action of the drug. As well, patients whose nutritional

status is poor are at risk of developing a high INR and bleeding problems.

Heparin

Unfractionated heparin (UFH) potentiates antithrombin III, inhibiting both thrombin and factor Xa. The result is inhibition in the final common pathway, preventing the formation of new clots (see Figure 37-5). Heparin has a rapid onset and short half-life. It is used extensively during cardiac procedures and for prevention and treatment of thromboemboli, and is often administered intravenously. Because of its unpredictable response, laboratory testing with aPTT is required; doses may need frequent adjustment. Complications of heparin therapy include bleeding, osteopenia, and heparin-induced thrombocytopenia (HIT).

LMWH is derived from unfractionated heparin through a manufacturing process that alters the molecular structure, leading to smaller molecules. Full-dose LMWH has been shown to be as effective as full-dose UFH for all types of venous thrombosis, prompting recent shifts in treatment protocols.[9] Enoxaparin (Lovenox) and dalteparin (Fragmin) are commonly used forms of LMWH. The action of LMWH is essentially the same as that of unfractionated heparin, but the pharmacodynamics are different.[10] Advantages of LMWH include a more predictable response in comparison to UFH. Because of this, weight-based dosing is used and routine laboratory monitoring is not considered necessary. When indicated, LMWH activity can be measured by anti-factor Xa assay.[9] Dosing is typically a subcutaneous injection, once or twice daily depending on the indication. LMWH is also used in cardiac and other disorders to prevent and treat thromboembolic events.

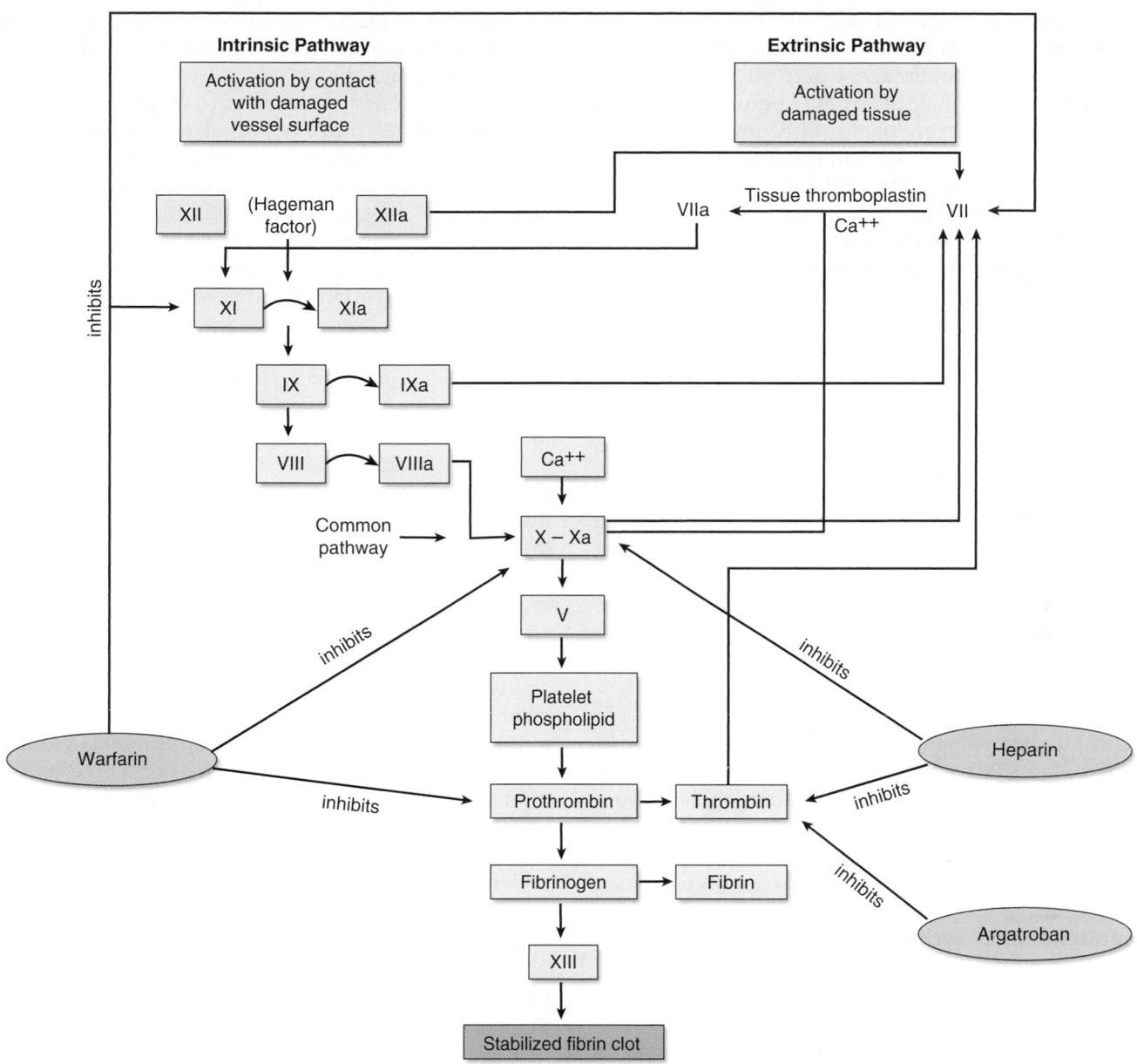

FIGURE 37-5 Coagulation cascade and sites of action of anticoagulant medications. Ca^{++} = Calcium.

Because LMWH is excreted by the kidneys, caution must be used for patients with renal insufficiency.[35] There is a decreased incidence of HIT and osteopenia with LMWH when compared to UFH.[7]

Bleeding is a potential major complication with both UFH and LMWH. The GI tract is the most common site of life-threatening bleeding.[35] Patients receiving these agents need to be closely observed for complications of anticoagulation. Both agents can be reversed by stopping the drug; UFH has a half-life of 30 to 60 minutes, and LMWH several hours. Protamine can be administered if necessary, with the dose calculated according to the timing of the last heparin dose.[9]

Direct Thrombin Inhibitors

The direct thrombin inhibitors are a class of drugs that inhibit thrombin-mediated fibrin formation.[7] These agents include the intravenous preparations of argatroban, lepirudin (Refludan), and bivalirudin (Angiomax), and the oral agent ximelagatran (Exanta).

Argatroban is a synthetic direct thrombin inhibitor used for treatment and prevention of thromboembolic disorders in patients with HIT.[6] Lepirudin, also used for HIT, is a recombinant form of hirudin, a substance isolated from medicinal leeches. The dose of argatroban is adjusted for hepatic insufficiency; lepirudin is adjusted for renal insufficiency. Patients receiving these agents are monitored with aPTT testing, with a goal of 2 to 2.5 times the normal control value. Bivalirudin is a semisynthetic agent derived from hirudin. Because of its short half-life, it may be used instead of heparin during interventional cardiac procedures.[7]

On the horizon, ximelagatran belongs to a new class of oral anticoagulants that inhibit thrombin-mediated activation of coagulation factors and platelets; it may be used in place of warfarin in patients with actual or potential venous thromboembolism and atrial fibrillation. While ximelagatran did not gain FDA approval because of the incidence of liver toxicities, other medications in this class are being developed.[7]

Currently, there is no specific agent routinely used to reverse the effects of direct thrombin inhibitors.[9]

Inhibitors of Factor Xa

Fondaparinux (Arixtra) is a synthetic anticoagulant that selectively inhibits activated factor X. It is administered subcutaneously and is used as an alternative to LMWH to prevent deep venous thrombosis. No laboratory monitoring is required; there is no risk of HIT.[7]

Thrombolytic Agents

Thrombolytic agents such as alteplase (Activase) and reteplase (Retavase) are used in acute myocardial infarction, stroke, and other thromboembolic events. Because these agents pose a significant risk of bleeding, patients should be evaluated for contraindications before these medications are prescribed. Following administration of thrombolytic agents, patients are monitored closely for bleeding complications because bleeding can be serious or even fatal. Bleeding is most commonly due to lysis of hemostatic plugs at the site of vascular procedures (e.g., femoral site). The drug is stopped and a coagulation panel is drawn if signs of bleeding develop. Multiple units of components, including cryoprecipitate, may be prescribed to replace fibrinogen and factor VIII.[9] Chapter 11 provides more comprehensive information on thrombolytic therapy.

THROMBOCYTOPENIA

Thrombocytopenia is the most common platelet disorder seen in critically ill patients[3] and has a variety of causes, including increased destruction of platelets (associated with sepsis), autoimmune disorders, diseases of the liver and spleen, and use of intravascular devices (e.g., intra-aortic balloon pump). Decreased production of thrombocytes by the bone marrow may occur in patients on cytotoxic drugs or those with bone marrow depression from neoplastic disorders.

Thrombocytopenia is also a feature of consumptive coagulopathies (i.e., DIC) and other disorders associated with hemorrhage.

Thrombocytopenia is defined as a platelet count of less than $100,000/mm^3$. A low platelet count does not always lead to bleeding; however, patients with a platelet count of less than $20,000/mm^3$ to $50,000/mm^3$ are often at risk of spontaneous bleeding.[16,31] With this low level, patients may also develop petechiae, ecchymosis, and bleeding mucous membranes or injury sites. There is great variation, however, on how low the platelet count can drop before a patient develops signs. Another consideration, regardless of the platelet count, is whether the platelets are functional. Platelet function can be inhibited by drugs, hypothermia, acidosis, and uremia; platelets of poor quality can lead to bleeding problems. Because there is not a good correlation between the bleeding time and actual bleeding from thrombocytopenia, the test cannot be used to guide therapy.[11]

Treatment of thrombocytopenia often involves treating the underlying cause. Platelet concentrate may be administered to patients with actual or potential hemorrhage. It may also be given to high-risk patients before an invasive procedure. The expected rise in the platelet count depends on platelet consumption, as well as the number of units transfused.[9] When thrombocytopenia is associated with immune system disorders or when it is drug-induced, intravenous immunoglobulin (Ig) may be given.[9,16] In autoimmune disorders, glucocorticoids may be given to suppress antibody formation and help restore circulating platelets. Desmopressin may be administered to patients to enhance vWF and restore platelet function. A bone marrow growth factor (e.g., oprelvekin [Neumega]) may be administered subcutaneously to patients to stimulate platelet production in patients with bone marrow suppression.

HEPARIN-INDUCED THROMBOCYTOPENIA

HIT is a rare but serious complication associated with heparin. It is characterized by a drop in platelet count and the clinical appearance of thromboembolic events. There are two types of HIT.[6] Type I HIT affects 10% to 20% of patients receiving heparin and involves a mild reduction of platelet count 1 to 4 days after starting heparin. It is thought to be due to platelet aggregation and is considered benign.[16] Type II HIT affects 1% to 3% of patients exposed to heparin and is a much more serious condition. It is characterized by a 30% to 50% reduction in platelets and typically occurs 5 to 14 days after heparin is started but can occur earlier if the patient has been previously exposed. It is an immune-mediated process that involves antiplatelet antibodies.[9] The antigens of HIT are not on heparin, but form on platelet factors when they are complexed to heparin. Platelet activation occurs when IgG, heparin, and platelet factor interact to produce procoagulant particles.[38] The resultant clotting abnormality may induce venous or arterial thromboembolism, including pulmonary emboli and thrombosis, affecting the circulation to the upper or lower extremities. Patients with confirmed HIT have up to a 50% risk of having a thrombotic event within 30 days after diagnosis.[17] However, not all patients that develop antibodies will have clinical manifestations of the disorder.[38]

A diagnosis of HIT is suspected when the platelet count drops dramatically in a patient who is receiving heparin or who received heparin within the past few months. HIT should be suspected in a patient with a 50% drop in platelet count, even if the count is still within the normal range.[11] Although no test is 100% specific for HIT, confirmation is made through a platelet aggregation test and serotonin release assay. An ELISA test that detects heparin antibodies is also available.[9] These tests are complex and may take time, so interventions should be started before confirmatory testing results are known.

When HIT is suspected, all forms of heparin should be stopped. Since HIT is an immune reaction, the amount of heparin is not relevant, so even the heparin in IV flushing solutions or priming solutions for blood circuits (e.g., dialysis tubing, arterial lines) must be discontinued. A direct thrombin inhibitor (e.g., IV argatroban or lepirudin) is started to disrupt the generation of thrombi and prevent further compromise to the circulation.[39] Warfarin is not prescribed because it can lead to decreased levels of protein C and exacerbate the thrombosis.[11]

The potential for HIT has important implications for clinical practice. Heparin should be used only when truly needed, and is now avoided for some previously routine uses (e.g., capping peripheral intravenous lines). When heparin is indicated, LMWH may be prescribed because it is less likely to cause HIT.[9,11] Also, patients receiving heparin should be monitored for drops in their platelet count and any clinical indicators of thrombosis.[39] It should be noted that while thrombocytopenia is common in critically ill patients, only a small number are diagnosed with HIT.

PATHOLOGIC FIBRINOLYSIS

Pathologic fibrinolysis is an acute, severe bleeding disorder that can resemble DIC. It can be induced by cardiothoracic surgery, urinary tract surgery, trauma, burns, and cancer of the urinary tract.[17] Extensive tissue damage releases naturally occurring tissue plasminogen activator (tPA). This triggers plasminogen to become plasmin, the substance that lyses fibrin clots. The result is an increase in fibrinolysis and a state similar to that induced by fibrinolytic drugs. In a patient with surgical wounds or trauma, excessive bleeding can result because the patient is unable to form stable clots. The major clinical manifestation of this problem is excessive bleeding from injury sites.

The coagulation panel will show an elevated level of FDPs and D-dimer, indicating excessive fibrinolysis. These findings must be correlated with the patient's history because they are also elevated in trauma, surgery, DIC, or other situations in which clotting and subsequent fibrinolysis occur.

The antifibrinolytic agent aprotinin is commonly used to treat this disorder.[33] Aminocaproic acid (Amicar) is another agent that can be administered orally or intravenously to inhibit fibrinolysis. Both of these agents are contraindicated in DIC.

VITAMIN K DEFICIENCY

Vitamin K is normally obtained from food and from synthesis by intestinal flora. It is absorbed from the GI tract and stored in the liver, where it serves as a cofactor for the production of the prothrombin complex proteins: factors II, VII, IX, X; protein C; and protein S.[17] Body stores of vitamin K are low, and acutely ill patients can become deficient in vitamin K within about 7 to 10 days, making this one of the more common acquired disorders of coagulation. The deficiency is associated with biliary tract surgery, chronic liver disease, inadequate intake, prolonged antibiotic use, and malabsorption syndromes.

The clinical features of vitamin K deficiency include ecchymosis, epistaxis, GI bleeding, and postoperative bleeding. The coagulation panel will show an elevated INR, because without adequate amounts of key coagulation factors clotting time is prolonged. Vitamin K deficiency can be reversed with an oral dose of 10 mg. For patients who are actively bleeding, 5 to 10 mg IV is given over 30 to 60 minutes, with a response expected within 4 to 6 hours.[8] FFP can be administered to provide coagulation factors in an emergency situation.

BLEEDING ASSOCIATED WITH LIVER DISEASE

The liver synthesizes many of the key coagulation components including fibrinogen, factor V, and the vitamin K–dependent factors. In addition, the liver functions in the clearance of substances that participate in feedback loops that control circulating active factors. Patients with liver disease may also have problems with thrombocytopenia and enhanced fibrinolysis, so it is not surprising that patients with hepatic insufficiency are likely to develop bleeding problems. Serious bleeding may follow trauma or surgery in this patient population. Local lesions in the GI tract, such as ulcers or varices, may bleed spontaneously. The risk of bleeding in patients with end-stage liver disease varies and is proportional to the number, severity, and type of clotting factor deficiencies.[19]

The coagulation panel will show many abnormalities in the patient with hepatic insufficiency. The INR is elevated, and factor levels are depleted, but factor levels do not reliably predict bleeding. Some patients may have laboratory evidence of chronic low-grade DIC.[19] Treating this problem involves interventions to treat the underlying liver disease. Other interventions are indicated in patients who are actively bleeding or require surgery or invasive procedures. Transfusion helps temporarily, and FFP supplies coagulation factors. Desmopressin may also be helpful because it raises the level of vWF.[16]

BLEEDING ASSOCIATED WITH UREMIA

Uremia and the associated metabolic abnormalities have an adverse effect on platelet function that places the patient at risk of bleeding. This is a qualitative problem, so the platelet count may be normal but the bleeding time will be prolonged. The bleeding tendency is first treated by interventions that reduce uremia, such as dialysis. Patients also benefit from cryoprecipitate, factor VIII concentrate, and desmopressin to raise plasma levels of vWF and enhance platelet function.[16]

There are additional concerns when heparin is used in patients with renal problems. Because the half-lives of both unfractionated and low molecular weight heparin are decreased in renal insufficiency, the dose is adjusted to avoid bleeding problems.[9]

BLEEDING ASSOCIATED WITH HEAD INJURY

Bleeding problems are a threat to patients with a head injury. Trauma to the brain leads to the release of tissue thromboplastin, triggering the coagulation system soon after the primary injury. The response may lead to a coagulopathy such as DIC.[41] These patients may require transfusion of blood and components.

CIRCULATING INHIBITORS OF COAGULATION

Patients may develop IgG antibodies that interfere with blood coagulation and cause bleeding problems in acute illness. These antibodies may exist naturally in some people, but also can develop in patients with mild factor deficiencies who receive blood products.[17] The antibodies may be referred to as lupus-like inhibitors or antiphospholipid antibodies because they prolong coagulation by binding to platelet phospholipids. The coagulation panel will show a prolonged PT/INR and aPTT. Treatment for bleeding patients may include massive plasma or platelet concentrate infusions. Plasmapheresis may be performed to lower antibody titers.

Lupus anticoagulants and antiphospholipid antibodies have also been associated with the formation of microclots in some patients.[11] A rare disorder known as catastrophic antiphospholipid antibody syndrome can occur, particularly in patients with preexisting autoimmune disorders. MODS can result from the disorder.

THROMBOTIC DISORDERS

In addition to the coagulation disorders associated with bleeding, critically ill patients are known to be at high risk for venous thromboembolism. Some patients have a primary hypercoagulable condition because of abnormalities in the natural factors that prevent blood from clotting such as antithrombin, protein C, and protein S.[32] However, it is more common for critically ill patients to exhibit secondary thrombotic problems as a complication of their diseases and disorders. Patients with many conditions may develop a "hypercoagulable state" that results in the formation of inappropriate blood clots (Box 37-3). Patients at risk for thromboembolic events include those with venous stasis and conditions that alter blood composition to favor coagulation. Included are those with malignancy, pregnancy, and postoperative or post-traumatic states.

Malignancy has long been recognized as a risk factor for thromboembolism and is most common in patients with adenocarcinoma of the GI tract and cancer of the pancreas, lung, and ovary.[32] The tumor growth process is thought to involve the release of hypoxia-induced endothelin and vascular endothelial growth factor, substances that trigger blood coagulation.[2] Mechanical factors (e.g., immobility) increase venous stasis and the risk for thromboembolism.

Pregnancy is associated with increased risk for thrombi for a number of reasons. The placenta releases factors that have procoagulant effects, leading to a hypercoagulable state that peaks in the postpartum period.[32] Venous stasis is increased by pressure on the pelvic veins during pregnancy, and tissue trauma occurs during delivery, adding to the risk.

Following surgery or trauma, patients are at risk of thromboembolism. Tissue factor is released from injured tissue to promote clotting during the acute period, but the activated factors can lead to systemic changes that have procoagulant effects during the recovery period. When this hypercoagulable state is added to endothelial injury and venous stasis, the normal hemostasis process is amplified to include inappropriate clotting in addition to the appropriate clotting at the injury site.

Deep venous thrombosis (DVT) and pulmonary emboli are the most common thromboembolic events in clinical practice.

Deep Venous Thrombosis

Although some patients will develop lower extremity pain, redness, or swelling, the development of DVT can be insidious, with subtle or no early clinical manifestations. Trauma patients have a venous thrombosis rate of almost 60%, and in patients with spinal cord injury the rate is almost 100% without prophylactic measures.[9] Diagnosis usually includes venous ultrasound. D-dimer testing to screen for thrombi may not be as useful in this patient population because acutely ill individuals may have conditions that result in false-positive results.[9]

Current treatment protocols for DVT include LMWH and fondaparinux. Renal clearance of these agents needs to be considered, and doses may require adjustment. LMWH activity does not usually require monitoring, but can be measured by anti-factor Xa assay.[9]

Pulmonary Emboli

Blood clots may embolize from the deep veins into the pulmonary vasculature where they obstruct blood flow to a section or sections of the lungs. Pulmonary emboli vary in number and size, but may become a life-threatening event. Multiple or massive pulmonary emboli can lead to a significant ventilation/perfusion mismatch and circulatory shock.

Clinical manifestations include dyspnea, tachypnea, chest pain, tachycardia, and hemoptysis. Obstruction of pulmonary blood flow leads to hypoxic vasoconstriction, and the patient may develop right ventricular failure in addition to respiratory compromise. Diagnostic techniques include high-resolution helical computed tomography (CT) scan and may also include a chest x-ray, ventilation/perfusion lung scan, and pulmonary angiography.

Treatment protocols include anticoagulation with UFH or LMWH.[9] Thrombolytic therapy may be considered in patients with massive pulmonary emboli accompanied by hypotension and shock. An inferior vena cava filter may be placed to prevent recurrent emboli from reaching the lungs.

Prophylactic measures to prevent thromboembolism include LMWH, intermittent compression devices, and other measures. Currently these measures are recommended for most seriously ill hospitalized patients.[38] Thromboprophylaxis for the acutely ill has received increasing attention and needs to be considered in all patients who do not have contraindications to anticoagulation.

MULTIDISCIPLINARY PLAN OF CARE

The care of patients with coagulopathy requires intensive management by a multidisciplinary team. When coagulopathy is recognized, the team must intervene quickly to prevent hemorrhage that leads to hypovolemic shock, acute anemia, and tissue hypoxia. The team routinely consists of a number of physicians in specialty practice including a hematologist, critical care nurses, pharmacist, respiratory therapists, and others. Laboratory and blood bank personnel are also important team members who support clinical care for these patients. A Multidisciplinary Plan of Care for patients with coagulopathy is outlined on pp. 1014-1016.

MULTIDISCIPLINARY PLAN OF CARE FOR PATIENTS WITH COAGULOPATHIES

PROBLEM	INTERVENTION	RATIONALE	EXPECTED OUTCOMES	SPECIAL CONSIDERATIONS
Risk for fluid volume deficit secondary to blood loss	Assess for clinical signs of bleeding: • Observe all incisions and puncture sites • Check surgical drains frequently • Check mucous membranes • Watch for hematomas, swollen extremities	A comprehensive assessment is done to identify signs of bleeding. Bleeding from multiple sites often indicates coagulopathy.	Early recognition and control of bleeding	Critically ill patients with many diagnoses are at risk for bleeding.
	• Assess abdominal girth • Watch for early signs of shock: increased heart rate, labile BP, low CVP, low urine output • Assess for pain indicative of tissue trauma • Check x-rays for blood, fluid collection	Bleeding may be occult.		
	• Monitor lab results to detect trends in CBC and coagulation studies	Lab results may change before clinical changes occur.		
	• Monitor for acidosis and hypothermia	These contribute to coagulopathy.		
Fluid volume deficit as a result of active bleeding	Monitor laboratory values: • Monitor coagulation panel • Monitor Hgb/Hct			
	Initiate interventions to minimize blood loss: • Apply local measures: pressure to bleeding sites, topical hemostatic agents • Keep patient on bedrest • Stop anticoagulants • Do not disturb clots • Minimize blood discard when drawing from lines	These measures help restore hemostasis.	Prevention of acute anemia and hypovolemic shock	Rapid intervention is needed to prevent serious or even fatal complications from hemorrhage.
	Begin fluid volume replacement: • Initiate crystalloid and colloid IV fluids • Use coagulation panel results to guide transfusion therapy	IV fluids restore preload and maintain cardiac output and tissue perfusion.		See Chapter 36 for more information on blood component therapy.

PROBLEM	INTERVENTION	RATIONALE	EXPECTED OUTCOMES	SPECIAL CONSIDERATIONS
	Begin blood and component transfusion: • Whole blood and red cell mass	Restores volume and oxygen-carrying capacity.		
	• Platelet concentrate	Administered for bleeding caused by thrombocytopenia or qualitative platelet disorders.		
	• Fresh frozen plasma	Contains fibrinogen and many coagulation factors except active platelets.		Administer frozen products as soon as thawed because potency is lost with time.
	• Cryoprecipitate	Contains fibrinogen, factor VIII, vWF.		
	• Albumin	Colloids restore intravascular volume.		Albumin is a blood product.
	• Non-blood plasma expanders: dextran, hetastarch	Plasma expanders may have anticoagulant effect, especially with prolonged use.		Non-blood plasma expanders are available.
	Observe for transfusion reactions	Types of reactions include febrile, hypersensitivity, hemolytic.		
	Observe for complications of massive transfusion	Complications include fluid overload, hypothermia, hyperkalemia, hypocalcemia, and clotting factor depletion.	Fluid overload can lead to HF Hypothermia can contribute to coagulopathy. Other imbalances can contribute to dysrhythmias and circulatory instability	Pretransfusion administration of acetaminophen (Tylenol), diphenhydramine (Benadryl) minimizes febrile reactions.
Risk for injury	Identify patients at risk of coagulopathy: • Detailed patient and family history of bleeding problems	A history of bleeding after dental and other procedures, after injuries, easy bruising, or heavy menses may suggest a potential problem.	Avoid episodes of hemorrhage and tissue injury	Even with the most careful preoperative workup, it is not always possible to identify patients who will have bleeding complications.
	• Detailed medication history including herbals and when anticoagulants started and stopped • Review of preoperative and preprocedure lab work			Prevention of bleeding problems is a combined nursing and medical responsibility.

Table continues on page 1016

PROBLEM	INTERVENTION	RATIONALE	EXPECTED OUTCOMES	SPECIAL CONSIDERATIONS
	Institute bleeding precautions for patients at risk:			
	• Alert staff when invasive procedures are considered	Non-emergency procedures may need to be postponed.		
	• Avoid needle sticks	Even small injuries can lead to hematomas.		
	• Apply pressure to any injury site			
	• Move patient gently with adequate assistance	Skin and soft tissues may be injured easily.		
	• Avoid high cuff inflation pressure with BP readings	Automatic pressure cuffs may cause petechiae and injury.		
	• Provide flotation mattress			
	• Provide gentle mouth care, soft foods, Popsicles	Mucous membranes are easily bruised, and injury may lead to bleeding.		
	• Use pharmacologic agents to prevent GI bleeding	Proton pump inhibitors and H_2-receptor antagonists can prevent GI bleeding in critically ill patients.		
	Provide measures that prevent hypothermia: • Prevent exposure • Eliminate wet linens • Warm IV fluids and blood			
	Provide reassurance to patient and family List all measures used to control bleeding in patient	Bleeding provokes great anxiety.		
Risk for ineffective coping	Inform patient and family of any improvements	Lab values may improve before clinical improvement is obvious.		

BP = Blood pressure, CBC = complete blood cell count, CVP = control venous pressure, Hct = hematocrit, HF = heart failure, Hgb = hemoglobin, GI = gastrointestinal.

CONCLUSIONS

Critically ill individuals may have multiple risk factors for life-threatening complications such as coagulopathy. They need constant monitoring for indicators of bleeding problems, so that the signs are recognized early and interventions are prompt and successful. Critical care nurses play a key role in the assessment and recognition of coagulopathy and in the initiation of appropriate intervention. Prevention of bleeding problems continues to be a priority and is a combined medical and nursing responsibility. Future advances in knowledge of the complexities of blood coagulation will improve the ability to predict and treat coagulation problems, decreasing the incidence of coagulopathy.

REFERENCES

1. Ahrens, T. (2003). Severe sepsis management: are we doing enough? *Crit Care Nurse*, 23(Suppl), 2–15.
2. Aird, W. C. (2005). Coagulopathy. In M. P. Fink, et al. (Ed.), *Textbook of critical care* (5th ed.). Philadelphia: Elsevier.
3. Aird, W. C. (2005). Sepsis and coagulation. *Crit Care Clin*, 21, 417–431.
4. Angerio, A. D., & Fink, D. A. (2002). Thromboembolic disease and cancer: possible new treatments. *Crit Care Nurs Q*, 25(2), 67–73.
5. Brohi, K., et al. (2003). Acute traumatic coagulopathy. *J Trauma Inj Infect Crit Care*, 54(6), 1127–1130.
6. Cleveland, K. W. (2003). Argatroban: a new treatment option for heparin-induced thrombocytopenia. *Crit Care Nurse*, 23(6), 61–69.
7. Deitcher, S. R. (2005). Antiplatelet, anticoagulant, and fibrinolytic therapy. In D. L. Kasper, et al. (Ed.), *Harrison's principles of internal medicine* (16th ed.). New York: McGraw-Hill.
8. DeLoughery, T. G. (2005). Critical care clotting catastrophes. *Crit Care Clin*, 21, 531–562.
9. DeLoughery, T. G. (2005). Venous thromboembolism in the ICU and reversal of bleeding on anticoagulants. *Crit Care Clin*, 21, 497–512.
10. DiDomenica, R. J. (2000). New antithrombotics for the intensive care setting: GP IIb/IIIa inhibitors, low-molecular-weight heparins, and direct thrombin inhibitors. *Crit Care Nurs Q*, 22(4), 61–74.
11. Drews, R. E. (2003). Critical issues in hematology: anemia, thrombocytopenia, coagulopathy, and blood product transfusions in critically ill patients. *Clin Chest Med*, 24, 607–622.
12. Dutton, R. P., et al. (2004). Factor VIIa for correction of traumatic coagulopathy. *J Trauma Inj Infec Crit Care*, 57(4), 709–718.
13. Enomoto, T. M., & Thorborg, P. (2005). Emerging off-label uses for recombinant activated factor VII: grading the evidence. *Crit Care Clin*, 21, 611–632.
14. Esmon, C. T. (2005). Coagulation. In M. P. Fink, et al. (Ed.), *Textbook of critical care* (5th ed.). Philadelphia: Elsevier.
15. Gaspard, K. J. (2005). Disorders of hemostasis. In C. M. Porth (Ed.), *Pathophysiology* (7th ed.). Philadelphia: Lippincott Williams & Wilkins.
16. Hardin, R. I. (2005). Disorders of the platelet and vessel wall. In D. L. Kasper, et al. (Ed.), *Harrison's principles of internal medicine* (16th ed.). New York: McGraw-Hill.
17. Hardin, R. I. (2005). Disorders of coagulation and thrombosis. In D. L. Kasper, et al. (Ed.), *Harrison's principles of internal medicine* (16th ed.). New York: McGraw-Hill.
18. Hollenberg, S. M. (2005). Acute coronary syndromes: management and complications. In M. P. Fink, et al. (Ed.), *Textbook of critical care* (5th ed.). Philadelphia: Elsevier.
19. Kujovich, J. L. (2005). Hemostatic defects in end stage liver disease. *Crit Care Clin*, 21, 563–587.
20. LaPointe, L. A., & Von Rueden, K. T. (2002). Coagulopathies in trauma patients. *AACN Clin Issues*, 13(2), 192–203.
21. LaRosa, S. P., & Opal, S. M. (2005). Tissue factor pathway inhibitor and antithrombin trial results. *Crit Care Clin*, 21, 433–448.
22. Levi, M. (2005). Disseminated intravascular coagulation: what's new? *Crit Care Clin*, 21, 449–467.
23. Levi, M., de Jonge, E., & Meijers, J. (2002). The diagnosis of disseminated intravascular coagulation. *Blood Rev*, 16, 217–223.
24. Levi, M., et al. (2001). Advances in the understanding of the pathogenic pathways of disseminated intravascular coagulation result in more insight in the clinical picture and better management strategies. *Semin Thromb Hemost*, 27(6), 569–575.
25. Lungstrom, N., & Emerson, R. J. (2005). Alterations in hemostasis and blood coagulation. In L. C. Copstead & J. L. Banasik (Eds.), *Pathophysiology* (3rd ed.). St. Louis: Elsevier Saunders.
26. MacLeod, J. B. A., et al. (2003). Early coagulopathy predicts mortality in trauma. *J Trauma Inj Infec Crit Care*, 55(1), 39–44.
27. Munro, N. (2005). Cardiac surgery. In P. G. Morton, et al. (Ed.), *Critical care nursing* (8th ed.). Philadelphia: Lippincott Williams & Wilkins.
28. Niimi, K. S. (2004). Aprotinin dosing: how much is enough? *J Extra-Corporeal Technol*, 36(4), 384–390.
29. Pagana, K. D., & Pagana, T. J. (2005). *Diagnostic and laboratory test reference* (7th ed.). St. Louis: Mosby.
30. Paparella, D., Brister, S. J., & Buchanan, M. R. (2004). Coagulation disorders of cardiopulmonary bypass: a review. *Intensive Care Med*, 30(10), 1873–1881.
31. Rempher, K., & Little, J. (2004). Assessment of red blood cell and coagulation laboratory data. *AACN Clin Issues*, 15(4), 622–637.
32. Schafer, A. I. (2004). Thrombotic disorders. In L. Goldman & D. Ausiello (Eds.), *Cecil textbook of medicine* (22nd ed.). Philadelphia: Saunders.
33. Sedrakyan, A., Treasure, T., & Elefteriades, J. A. (2004). Effect of aprotinin on clinical outcomes in coronary artery bypass surgery: a systemic review and meta-analysis of randomized trials. *J Thorac Cardiovasc Surg*, 128(3), 442–448.
34. Taylor, F. B., et al. (2001). Towards a definition, clinical and laboratory criteria and a scoring system for disseminated intravascular coagulation. *Thromb Haemost*, 86, 1027–1030.
35. Thorevska, N., et al. (2004). Anticoagulation in hospitalized patients with renal insufficiency. *Chest*, 125, 856–863.
36. Vernon, S., & Pfeifer, G. M. (2003). Blood management strategies for critical care patients. *Crit Care Nurse*, 23(6), 34–48.
37. Vincent, J. L., & De Backer, D. (2005). Does disseminated intravascular coagulation lead to multiple organ failure? *Crit Care Clin*, 21, 469–477.
38. Warkentin, T. E., & Cook, D. J. (2005). Heparin, low molecular weight heparin, and heparin-induced thrombocytopenia in the ICU. *Crit Care Clin*, 21, 513–529.
39. Warkentin, T. E., & Greinacher, A. (2004). Heparin-induced thrombocytopenia: recognition, treatment, and prevention: the seventh ACCP conference on antithrombotic and thrombolytic therapy. *Chest*, 126(3 Suppl.), 311S–337S.
40. Whitlock, R., Crowther, M. A., & Ng, H. J. (2005). Bleeding in cardiac surgery: its prevention and treatment—an evidence-based review. *Crit Care Clin*, 21, 589–610.
41. Zink, E. (2005). Head injury. In P. G. Morton, et al. (Ed.), *Critical care nursing* (8th ed.). Philadelphia: Lippincott Williams & Wilkins.

CRITICAL CARE IMMUNOLOGY

CHAPTER 38 Caring for the Immunocompromised Patient

Brenda K. Shelton

Immune compromise is a group of disorders temporarily or permanently affecting different components of the immune system. They may be genetically linked and present at birth, acquired through exposure to specific clinical toxins, or the secondary effect of another disease process. In recent decades, increasing numbers of patients have been admitted to critical care with significant preexisting immune compromise. Medications, nutritional deficits, invasive procedures, chronic illness, and exposure to resistant microbes contribute to immune compromise for most critically ill patients, although intrinsic hematopoietic failure also occurs.

The assessment and management of patients with different immune defects may vary in some aspects, but most clinical care is universal. The admission of immune-incompetent patients to critical care creates unique challenges for critical care practitioners. The experienced critical care nurse serves as a critical link in providing specialized care for these patients. The greatest common risk for morbidity in all immunocompromised patients is development of life-threatening infections; however, their immunologic deficits and subtle clinical presentation may make it difficult to diagnose potentially life-threatening infection. All patients who enter critical care should be assessed for factors that interfere with their normal immune capacity so recognition and appropriate management of their immunocompromised state and infection risk can be instituted. Diagnostic tests and interventions are directed at specific immune defects and the anticipated complications unique to that defect. For example, patients with T-lymphocytic suppression to prevent organ transplant rejection are more prone to viral and opportunistic infections that correlate with the usual functions of the T lymphocyte. These patients are routinely prescribed acyclovir to prevent herpes simplex and trimethoprim sulfamethoxazole for prevention of *Pneumocystis jiroveci*. If immune-supportive interventions are not implemented in time to prevent infection, knowledge of immune deficit and infection history is used to treat the most probable microbe based upon the patient's defined risk factors and probable site of infection. The patient with prolonged granulocytopenia who continues to be febrile despite extensive antibacterial antibiotic coverage is usually treated with antifungal medications with the realization that fungal infection often occurs after granulocytes are suppressed for more than 7 to 10 days.[40]

DEFINITIONS

Immunocompromise is a broad term indicating inadequate white blood cell responses.[38] It may involve the nonspecific immune system or specific immunity. A comparison of the key features of immunologic impairment based on type of physiologic defect is described in Figure 38-1. Nonspecific immune functions include barrier defenses and the actions of complement proteins or granulocytes. The nonspecific immune response is most important in mounting a defense against bacteria and is active in the inflammatory response. The specific immune response is coordinated by B and T lymphocytes and their activated immune chemicals essential for recognition and destruction of viral or opportunistic pathogens. Monocytes have combined specific and nonspecific actions, usually at a tissue level, since monocytes differentiate into tissue macrophages early in their development. Within the term immunocompromise, there are several different types of immune dysfunction.

Granulocytopenia (used interchangeably with neutropenia) is defined as inadequate circulating cells to combat bacterial microbes. The most common granulocytes are the neutrophils. They are the only white blood cell that can be released immaturely (as an immature cell called a band) in response to infection. The presence of a high percentage of bands (greater than 20%) when the total white blood cell count is elevated is indicative of a bacterial infection.

Lymphopenia is defined as a low absolute lymphocyte count (manual count rather than machine averaged). Immune compromise may also be measured by cellular dysfunction rather than number of cells. Individuals who inject unpurified recreational drugs develop impaired T-lymphocytic function even without acquiring an infectious disease such as hepatitis or human immunodeficiency virus.[1,38]

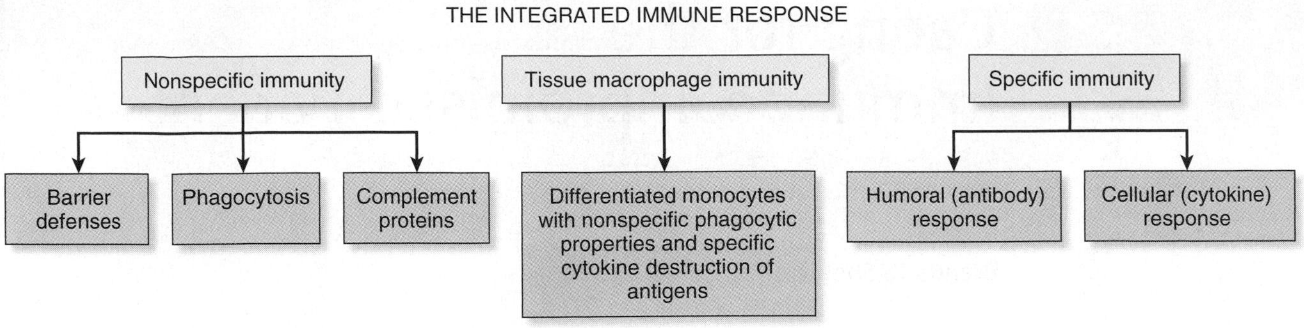

THE INTEGRATED IMMUNE RESPONSE

FIGURE 38-1 Comparison of nonspecific and specific immune function.

PATIENTS AT RISK

Immune compromise can occur as a result of a large variety of health maintenance disorders, comorbid diseases (e.g., diabetes, heart disease), medications, and environmental influences. The degree of compromise and clinical consequences vary according to the specific cells involved and their numbers or severity of dysfunction. In general, patients with granulocytic defects are at greatest risk for bacterial infections; monocyte defects increase the risk for deep-seated organ infections; and

lymphocyte abnormalities result in viral illness, infection with atypical bacteria, or development of malignancy.[38] A detailed listing of patients at risk for common immune defects and the clinical consequences of such disorders are described in Table 38-1.[40] Careful obtainment of a clinical history can aid the critical care nurse in identifying patients with risk factors for immune compromise. Recognition of this risk guides the level of vigilance and specialized therapies to compensate for immune incompetence and propensity for infection.

TABLE 38-1 Characteristics and Risks for Immunocompromised Patient Populations

CHARACTERISTICS	PHYSIOLOGIC MECHANISM OF RISK	POSSIBLE CONSEQUENCES OF RISK FACTOR
Frequent hospitalizations	• Frequent exposure to environmental organisms other than one's own normal environment • Exposure to other people's organisms via staff, equipment, or supplies • Potential exposure to resistant organisms	Hospitalizations are avoided whenever possible to reduce exposure of patient to foreign microbes that are more pathogenic than those in normal living environment. When hospitalizations cannot be avoided, careful separation of patient care items, single patient use items, or thorough cleaning between uses reduces transference of microbes and development of resistant microbes.
Gastrointestinal disease	• Decreased bowel motility allows normal flora to translocate across GI wall to bloodstream • Breaks in mucosal integrity of GI tract predispose patients to microbial transference into bloodstream • Poor circulation to GI tract causes decreased peristalsis and mucosal atrophy; normal flora and intestinal gram-negative organisms can become pathogenic	Maintaining minimal normal GI motility and mucosal integrity reduces amount of infection via GI tract. Using the gut consistently for food and fluid consumption helps maintain normal function. Enteral feeding is always attempted, if at all possible, to enhance GI integrity and function.

CHARACTERISTICS	PHYSIOLOGIC MECHANISM OF RISK	POSSIBLE CONSEQUENCES OF RISK FACTOR
HIV disease	• Viral incorporation into the RNA, then the DNA of immune cells having the CD8+ molecule disrupts normal WBC function and replication, leading to lymphopenia, lymphocyte dysfunction, and macrophage dysfunction • Disruption of these cells leads to many different infections (e.g., unusual bacteria, fungi, opportunistic bacteria, viruses) and lymphoproliferative disorders/ malignancies (e.g., Kaposi's sarcoma, lymphoma)	HIV disease is directly treated with antiretrovirals and immune-reconstituting agents such as interleukin-2. Stabilization of lymphocyte counts reduces risk and incidence of opportunistic infections. When lymphocyte count does drop, prophylactic antimicrobial agents specific to organisms likely to infect these patients are prescribed in a well-defined and protocol-determined manner. Avoidance of activities likely to expose patients to infection and attempts to maintain care in the ambulatory environment may also reduce risk of serious or resistant infections.
Immunosuppressive agents and corticosteroids	• Decreased phagocytic activity • Altered T-cell recognition of pathogens, especially viral • Lack of immune memory to recall antibodies to previously encountered pathogens	Immune-suppressing agents have multiple immune-depressing functions, putting patients at risk for all kinds of infections. Special precautions are implemented and prophylactic antimicrobial agents against common opportunistic organisms may be indicated. These patients also lose immune memory and are candidates for vaccinations, provided that the vaccine does not contain live agents. Patients are taught that they will have blunted inflammatory responses and that subtle symptoms may indicate infections.
Indwelling intravenous catheters	• Indwelling venous or arterial access devices break barrier defenses, with subsequent risk of microbial invasion • Presence of an intravenous device may irritate venous wall and induce inflammatory damage, resulting in a higher risk for microbial invasion	Intravenous catheters breach barrier defenses and increase risk of microbial invasion into the body. Some companies have developed catheters that have been coated or treated with active antimicrobial agents such as silver ions, chlorhexidine, or heparin. Catheters have also been designed with structural variations in an attempt to reduce irritation of veins, thereby minimizing phlebitis and infection (e.g., angled catheter tips, modified catheter anchoring devices). Clinicians must choose the smallest lumen size, least number of lumens, and most appropriate permanence of a device to reduce infection rates. Heightened sterile technique when accessing these devices may also reduce rate of associated infection.
Infants/older adults	• Immature thymus gland in infants increases viral and opportunistic infections • Atrophy of thymus gland in older adults increases viral infection • Decreased antigen-specific immunoglobulins in older adults diminishes immune memory, delayed hypersensitivity reactions	Immature and atrophied immune systems can lead to infection with a variety of organisms from any additional breach in the body's defenses. Frequent, complex, or polymicrobial infections are expected and are guarded against by careful infection prevention techniques and strategies. Recognition of the variety of infectious complications and the potential for their rapid dissemination causes increased vigilance in monitoring and early aggressive interventions for infection. Prophylactic strategies are not usually recommended in these populations, but a low threshold for treatment is implemented.

Table continues on page 1024

Table 38-1   Characteristics and Risks for Immunocompromised Patient Populations—cont'd

CHARACTERISTICS	PHYSIOLOGIC MECHANISM OF RISK	POSSIBLE CONSEQUENCES OF RISK FACTOR
Invasive devices (e.g., Foley catheter, nasogastric tube)	• Altered barrier defenses allow pathogen entry, especially skin organisms	Invasive devices breach barrier defenses and increase risk of microbial invasion into body. Catheters and other invasive devices have been coated with active antimicrobial agents such as silver ions, chlorhexidine, or heparin in an attempt to reduce related infection. Some devices also have structural variations (e.g., altered bluntness of the tip of tracheal suction catheter) that reduce irritation or mucosal injury produced, with the hope of reducing infection rate. Infection monitoring for microbial colonization may also help detect early presence of potential pathogens in high-risk patients.
Malnutrition	• Inadequate WBC count • Reduced neutrophil activity	Altered nutrition increases risk of all infections. Efforts to boost immune-related nutrition deficits may focus on inclusion of glutamine, arginine, and other essential amino acids in nutrient supplements as well as other measures aimed at enhancing nutritional well-being.
Hepatic disease	• Decreased neutrophil count • Decreased phagocytic activity • Lost immunoglobulin production	Hepatic disease increases risk of bacterial infection and rapid dissemination of that infection. Loss of immunoglobulins leads to failed immune memory. Special infection precautions for immunocompromised patients are implemented.
Neutropenia	• Inadequate neutrophils to combat infection	Lack of neutrophils places patient at high risk for bacterial infections that will rapidly disseminate and potentially cause septic shock. Hematopoietic growth factors may be administered as primary or secondary prophylaxis to abrogate the severity (depth of nadir) or longevity of the period of neutropenia.
Pulmonary disease	• Inadequate oxygenation decreases neutrophil activity	Infection risk is increased and can be abrogated by implementing immunocompromised precautions.
Radiation therapy	• Radiation to long bones will interfere with WBC production • Radiation in area of certain endocrine organs can lead to endocrine failure (hypoadrenalism, hypothyroidism) and infection risk • Radiation damage to barrier defenses will predispose patient to invasion by microbes	Destruction of stem cells and existing bone marrow reserve of hematopoietic cells is a common dose-limiting toxicity of radiation therapy involving the long bones, where cells are produced. Destruction of the normal skin and soft tissue barriers is treated with specialized skin care to reduce incidence of infection.
Renal disease	• Decreased neutrophil activity • Decreased immunoglobulin activity	Patients with renal dysfunction are provided extra precautions against bacterial infection, recognizing that they may also show blunted or reduced symptoms of infection. These patients are appropriate candidates for vaccinations against many microorganisms.

CHARACTERISTICS	PHYSIOLOGIC MECHANISM OF RISK	POSSIBLE CONSEQUENCES OF RISK FACTOR
Splenectomy	• Inability to recognize and remove encapsulated bacteria (e.g., streptococci, mycobacteria)	Postsplenectomy, either functional or anatomical, the patient is at risk for specific infections. Vaccination against pneumococci is recommended for these patients. A low threshold of suspicion for streptococci with oropharyngeal or urinary tract symptoms may allow for early antimicrobial therapy.
Surgical procedure/ wounds	• Normal flora may be translocated by surgical procedure • Altered barrier defenses because of surgical entry • Stress of surgery or anesthetic agents may reduce neutrophil activity	Careful surgical preparation of planned surgical site with chlorhexidine scrubs is recommended before many surgical procedures. Shaving involved area remains a debatable practice, with some believing that hair removal reduces risk, and others believing that skin nicks from razor may increase risk of infection. Operating room staff may perform a surgical scrub of site followed by placement of a clear sterile barrier film, which is subsequently cut through for actual procedure. Conscientious postoperative care with fluids, coughing, deep breathing, and early mobility may decrease risk of infection. Being aware of previous colonization or infection before surgery may assist in defining source of fever postoperatively.
Traumatic injuries	• Altered barrier defenses allow pathogen entry • Type of infection dependent upon source and severity of injury (e.g., soil contamination, water contamination, skin flora)	Altered barrier defenses are treated with frequent cleansing, antimicrobial cleansing, covering with sterile dressings to prevent infectious organisms from entering the bloodstream via the open wound. Antimicrobial ointments have not been proven effective. If a wound is thought to be clean and sterile, a clear protective barrier dressing may provide better occlusiveness and guard against microorganism entry.

From reference 40.
GI = Gastrointestinal, HIV = human immunodeficiency virus, WBC = white blood cell count.

For example, patients receiving chemotherapy for any reason would be at risk for the development of immune compromise. In most patients following chemotherapy, the white blood cell count is suppressed for 3 to 10 days.[37] The depth and length of the neutropenia are a reflection of the amount of normal bone marrow reserve. A patient is less likely to have prolonged neutropenia early in the treatment plan unless other risk factors are also present. Risk factors that may prolong the length of neutropenia include older age, viral illness, malnutrition, intravenous drug use, previous chemotherapy, antimicrobials, and antiretrovirals.[11] The experienced critical care nurse should recognize the reversibility of this current medical crisis and consider the patient's health and medication profile to try to predict how long this neutropenia may persist.

Both the presence of tumor and radiation treatment will result in damaged ciliary action, disrupted lymphatic drainage, and altered cough or ability to mobilize secretions. The tumor may also obstruct natural drainage of secretions, causing a postobstructive pneumonia.[23] These risks will not be alleviated after treatment of this specific infectious episode, and should be acknowledged in future treatment plans to reduce the risk of a recurrent infectious episode. This may include the prescription of prophylactic antimicrobial agents or hematopoietic growth factors immediately following administration of the chemotherapy regimen.[8,15]

Many oncology patients receiving frequent chemotherapy have a semi-permanent central venous catheter. Even if there are no current signs of a line-related infection, careful and frequent assessment of the exit site and tunnel should be performed.[8,30,37] Although many tunneled lines are treated with "clean technique" in the home setting, sterile technique should be used for all in-hospital manipulations.[29,30] The microbes that

♦ RESEARCH UTILIZATION

Oral Care in the Intensive Care Unit

CLINICAL ISSUE

The literature demonstrates that colonization of the mouth with respiratory pathogens may contribute to ventilator-associated pneumonia (VAP). Oral care may be an important preventive measure against VAP. Other studies have demonstrated that comprehensive oral care regimens have reduced the incidence of VAP in select populations.

SUMMARY

This survey study asked intensive care unit nurses in the United States to identify the variables influencing their oral care practices and attitudes. A random national sample of 420 intensive care unit directors was asked to participate in a survey of oral care practices and attitudes. Of invited participants, 126 (30%) agreed to participate. Of the accepting institutions, there were 102 represented, with a total of 556 surveys returned. This constituted an 85% response rate among consenting institutions. The data were analyzed by clinical experts to detect the quality of oral care regimen reported by respondents. This was correlated to background characteristics of individual nurses, the work environment, and availability of supplies and implements for oral care. Attitudes were evaluated by opinions assessed on a Likert scale. The variables that predicted the quality of oral care were specialized education about oral care and its benefits, perceived adequate time to perform oral care, assignment of high priority to oral care, and the caregiver's perception of oral care as an unpleasant task to perform.

APPLICATION

Oral care provided to intensive care patients can best be improved by providing staff education on the importance and potential benefits of this practice, having a staffing pattern that supports this practice, and helping all staff perceive this activity as a priority of patient care.

NEED FOR FURTHER STUDY

Studies are needed to evaluate the actual oral care practices of critical care nurses and determine whether these practices alter the oral flora, oral infection rate, or ventilator-associated pneumonia rate. Specific strategies such as different rinses, different flossing instruments, and types of toothbrushes should be evaluated on a more scientific basis.

Furr, L.A. (2004). Factors affecting quality of oral care in intensive care units, *J Adv Nurs, 48*(5), 454–462.

---

produce nosocomial infection are usually more virulent and resistant to antimicrobial therapy.[27,30] Many specific organisms do not easily clear after they have infected a central line (e.g., *Candida, Giardia, Pseudomonas,* and *Staphylococcus*), necessitating removal of the intravenous line from a single episode of infection.[29,30] Research has been inconclusive in identifying specific practices in managing venous access devices that reduce the risk of infection for these patients.[30] More frequent fluid and tubing changes, sterile line accessing, or antimicrobial "lock solutions" may be part of an institutional standard of care, but the benefit of these practices has not been proven.[30,39]

Patients who are receiving broad-spectrum coverage antimicrobials have concomitant destruction of the normal flora that resides in the mouth, gastrointestinal, and genitourinary systems. The overgrowth of nonbacteria, such as the fungus *Candida albicans,* leads to superinfections.[27] This manifests as oral thrush, an erosive rash in skin folds, diarrhea from *Candida,* or fungal urinary tract infections. It is often the bedside nurse who detects these subtle, but potentially fatal infections. Oral care for the immunocompromised patient in order to avoid ventilator-associated pneumonia is discussed in the Research Utilization box above.

♦ Case Study, 38-1, Part A

Evidence-Based Management of the Immunocompromised Patient

S.E. is a 49-year-old diabetic male patient who had a live-donor kidney transplant 8 years ago. Immunosuppressive medications were discontinued 5 years ago, and he has not demonstrated rejection. He most recently presented 3 months ago to the oncology clinic with right axillary lymphadenopathy and dyspnea. Axillary lymph nodes and a 2 × 2-centimeter mass in the right hilar region of the lung were biopsy-positive for follicular lymphoma, a malignancy that affects the antibody-producing B lymphocytes. He received radiation therapy delivered in 7 fractions over 9 days for immediate reduction of the hilar mass obstructing the airway, followed by a multimedication chemotherapy regimen. He has received two cycles of chemotherapy, the last doses given 9 days ago. Today he was admitted from the emergency department for high spiking fevers and hypoxemia. His admission data are as follows:

S.E.'s Admission Findings

Subjective Symptoms

- Headache
- Dyspnea
- Nonproductive cough

Physical Examination

- Vital signs
  - Temperature 39.5°C
  - Pulse rate 134 beats/min with occasional premature atrial contractions
  - Respirations 32 breaths/min
  - Blood pressure 108/42 mm Hg (normally 120–130/ 76–84 mm Hg)
- Breath sounds
  - Faint crackles in bases
  - Diminished in right mid-anterior chest extending into the axilla
- Soft, nontender abdomen with hypoactive bowel sounds
- Oral mucosa is erythematous with ulceration of the buccal mucosa and a white coated tongue
- Semipermanent double-lumen soft Silastic tunneled catheter is noted on the right chest with the tunnel up into the right neck; line is not reddened, swollen, tender, or presenting with exudates

Diagnostic Tests

- Pulse oximetry 86% on room air
- Arterial blood gases
  - pH: 7.31
  - $Paco_2$: 45 mm Hg
  - Pao_2: 58 mm Hg
  - HCO_3^-: 19 mEq/L
- Chest x-ray: slight haziness in right lateral lung, blunted costophrenic angles bilaterally
- Complete blood cell count with WBC differential is pending

Decision point: What does his admission lab work indicate?

Decision point: Given his symptoms, what diagnosis would be made?

Decision point: What are S.E.'s infection risks?

Case continues on page 1030

ASSESSMENT

Physical Findings

When assessing patients who have compromised immune systems, it is essential to be attentive to subtle changes in the patient's baseline assessment. Immune dysfunction blunts normal inflammatory responses, leading to diminished signs and symptoms of infection. The usual white blood cell responses create infectious exudates such as wound drainage or sputum, but these are often not present in immunocompromised patients. Organism-specific lesions may also appear differently in immunocompromised patients. For example, herpes simplex oral lesions usually manifest as a shallow ulcer with a raised red border. This may appear as a flat ulceration without inflammation or border in an immunocompromised patient.[20] A complete physical examination to detect infection includes careful examination of all skin surfaces and orifices where infections are most likely to arise.[15] All suspicious changes in integrity should be cultured for both common and uncommon pathogens.[15]

For many patients, the only symptoms of infection may be fever or pain.[32] If patients are lymphocyte suppressed or receiving corticosteroids, a fever may not even be present.[15] In fact, subnormal temperatures may be equally indicative of infection in the immunocompromised patient, a finding more common in these patients than those with normal immune responses.[39]

Because these patients have such limited protective function, infections rarely remain localized.[39] Because microbial invasion extends systemically, sepsis is often evident. Again, these individuals have reduced symptoms of the severity of infection. Common symptoms such as myalgias or arthralgias occur, but are not accompanied by inflammation.[39] Compensatory tachycardia and a low diastolic blood pressure are common and reflect the degree of vasodilation that accompanies severe sepsis. Surprisingly, these patients do not progress to organ failure as rapidly as individuals with normal inflammatory responses, thought to be related to the lack of white blood cell cytokines that are the etiology of organ failure during sepsis.[33]

An important aspect of assessment in patients with short-term granulocytopenia is the recognition that the absence of symptoms during neutropenia is followed by exacerbated symptoms at the site of infection when the cells begin to repopulate. Patients presenting with infection while neutropenic will develop more severe symptoms and white blood cell infiltration at the site of infection as the bone marrow recovers.[38,40]

Diagnostic Test Results

Physical findings are complemented with diagnostic test results to identify clinical immune suppression disorders. Immune compromise has been referred to as the "silent complication" since the actual absence of cells or cell function is the defined disorder, but it is asymptomatic unless the individual is infected. There are several tests of immunologic function that are important to evaluate the level of immune competence in known at-risk individuals. A summary of diagnostic tests of immune function and the significance of their abnormal results is given in Table 38-2.*

---

*References 3, 7, 9, 37, 38, 40.

TABLE 38-2 Diagnostic Tests of Immune Function

STUDY	DESCRIPTION AND PURPOSE	NORMAL VALUES
WBC count	Measurement of total number of leukocytes. When WBC count is very low, machine counting may be inaccurate and laboratory personnel may hand-count WBCs on slide.	4000–11,000/μl (4–11 × 10^9/L)
WBC differential	Determination of whether each kind of WBC is present in proper proportion; determination of absolute value by multiplying percentage of cell type by total WBC count and dividing by 100. When calculating absolute neutrophil count, both mature neutrophils (segmented neutrophils) and bands are included in calculation. In addition to common WBCs, immature neutrophils, called bands, may be noted as a percentage of total WBC count.	Neutrophils: 50%–70% (0.50–0.70) Neutrophil bands: <20% of total WBC count Eosinophils: 2%–4% (0.02–0.04) Basophils: 0%–2% (0–0.02) Lymphocytes: 20%–40% (0.20–0.40)
Absolute neutrophil count	Calculates number of neutrophils available for combating bacterial infection. Lower than normal values increase risk of infection with typical and atypical bacteria. Severity scoring system for abnormal values is as follows:[9] Grade 1: <2500/mm^3, but >1500/mm^3 Grade 2: >1000/mm^3, but <1500/mm^3 Grade 3: >500/mm^3, but <1000/mm^3 Grade 4: <500/mm^3	>2500/mm^3
Absolute lymphocyte count	Calculates number of lymphocytes available to combat viral and opportunistic infections. Severity scoring system for abnormal values is as follows:[9] Grade 1: 800/mm^3 Grade 2: >500/mm^3, but <800/mm^3 Grade 3: >200/mm^3, but <500/mm^3 Grade 4: <200/mm^3	800–1500 cells/mm^3
Erythrocyte sedimentation rate	Screening tool for serum evidence of the presence of an inflammatory process.	Age- and gender-related normal values may apply; in general, 1–20 mm/hr
Immunoglobin G levels	Of all immunoglobulins, the largest percentage and most universally important is IgG; therefore other specific immunoglobulin levels are not measured.	150–300 mcg/dl
C-reactive protein	While not usually present, it will be detectable in the presence of inflammation or tissue destruction.	Not present
Complement CH_{50}	Total amount of complement components in serum. Can be affected by secondary immune deficiency and autoimmune disorders.	22–55 H_{50} units/ml
Complement C3 level	Amount of C3 in serum. When reduced, can increase risk of sino-pulmonary infections.	85–175 mg/dl
Complement C4 level	Amount of C4 in serum. When reduced, can indicate immune-complex disease.	15–45 mg/dl
C1 inhibitor functional assay	Function of C1 esterase inhibitor that is abnormal may indicate hereditary angioedema.	13.2–24 mg/dl

STUDY	DESCRIPTION AND PURPOSE	NORMAL VALUES
Complement fixation ratio	Immunofluorescence detection of complement complexes indicative of nonspecific immunologic antigen-antibody reactions.	None
HIV antibody test	ELISA test for presence of antibodies to HIV virus can detect reactive antibodies indicative of recent HIV disease.	None
HIV core protein antigen P24	Immunofluorescence detection of core antigen protein of HIV: P24 antigen.	None
HIV envelope glycoprotein GP41	Immunofluorescence detection of envelope protein GP41.	None
HIV cultures	Polymerase chain reaction amplification of viral proteins can be detected early in disease.	Absent
CD4 count (detection of surface marker of some macrophages and some lymphocytes)	CD4 counts are used to monitor progression or response to therapy of anti-HIV therapies. CD4 level is predictive of risk for opportunistic infections, and used as a guide for prescription of prophylactic antimicrobial therapy. Severity scoring system for abnormal values is as follows:[9] Grade 1: >500/mm^3, but less than the lower limit of normal Grade 2: >200/mm^3, but <500/mm^3 Grade 3: >50/mm^3, but <200/mm^3 Grade 4: <50/mm^3	800–1000/mm^3
Antibody panels: hepatitis A, hepatitis B, CMV, RSV	Immunofluorescence detection of antibodies or core antigens to specific viruses.	Absent
Tissue anergy panel	Antigens are injected intradermally, and individuals with normal immune function will activate immunoglobulins, producing a localized "wheal response." Absence of response is indicative of lymphocyte suppression.	Positive wheal reaction to intradermal: tuberculosis, *Candida,* and *Clostridium difficile*
Bone marrow aspirate and biopsy	Technique involves removal of bone marrow through a locally anesthetized site to evaluate status of blood-forming tissue. It is used to diagnose or assess status of hematologic malignancies, to stage some solid tumors (e.g., breast cancer), and for diagnosis of primary bone marrow cell development disorders (e.g., aplastic anemia).	Normal mature cells in adequate numbers, absence of clonal immature cell lines

CMV = Cytomegalovirus, ELISA = enzyme-linked immunosorbent assay, IgG = immunoglobulin G , RSV = respiratory syncytial virus, WBC = white blood cell.

The absolute neutrophil count, lymphocyte counts, and CD4 counts are important diagnostic laboratory tests that demonstrate the severity of deficiency. Many laboratories report these values as percentages of the total count, and individual practitioners must mathematically calculate the "absolute count." The experienced critical care nurse routinely performs this mathematical calculation, shown in Box 38-1, for patients at risk for neutropenia or lymphopenia, interprets the results, and modifies the patient's care as the risk for infection increases.

Grading blood cell deficiency in terms of its severity and risk for infection is a common practice. The National Cancer Therapy Evaluation Program has defined toxicity levels from mild (grade 1), to moderate (grade 2) and severe (grade 3), to life-threatening (grade 4), with death correlating to grade 5.[9] These specific toxicity scales are included within Table 38-2. Lower lymphocyte counts increase the risk of certain common infections, malignancies (e.g., Kaposi's sarcoma, metastatic cervical cancer, malignant lymphoma), and unusual infections (e.g., *Pneumocystis jiroveci*).[3,22,36]

Box 38-1

Calculation of Absolute Neutrophil and Lymphocyte Counts

Percentage of cell multiplied by total WBC = absolute count subtype

0.40 (%neutrophils) × 800 = 320
        Absolute neutrophil count (ANC)
0.40 (%lymphocytes) × 800 = 320
        Absolute lymphocyte count (ALC)

◆ Case Study 38-1, Part B

Evidence-Based Management of the Immunocompromised Patient

S.E. is hypoxemic without white blood cells, but has minimal pulmonary secretions. If his infection has not been adequately treated by the time his white blood cells begin to recover, his respiratory symptoms may worsen as the white blood cells migrate to the site of infection, causing inflammation and altered gas exchange, and he may require urgent mechanical ventilatory support.

Decision point: What interventions should be made at this time?

Decision point: Provide an analysis of his neutropenia at this time.

Case continues on page 1039

MULTIDISCIPLINARY PLAN OF CARE

Prevention of Infection

The general care of patients with immune compromise is supportive and heavily focused on protection from infection. "Immunocompromised patient precautions" are based upon multiple documents published by the Centers for Disease Control,[30,35] the Society of Hospital Infectious Disease,[42] and the National Comprehensive Cancer Network.[15] The precautions may vary somewhat from one institution to another and between different patient populations (granulocyte dysfunction versus lymphocyte dysfunction).

Precautions involve environmental control, personal care routines, and active immune supportive measures. These are summarized in the Multidisciplinary Plan of Care on pp. 1031-1035 and in the following text.*

---

*References 5, 6, 8, 15, 16, 18, 28, 32, 34–37, 40–42.

The Centers for Disease Control and Prevention no longer advocates a category of isolation termed "protective isolation" for patients with immune compromise; however, heightened awareness of their infection risk and separation of these patients from others with infections are still advised.[35,42] In critical care settings, this may include using private rooms normally reserved for patients with resistant infections or wearing protective attire such as gloves and masks because of the highly infectious environment of critical care. When the patient leaves the room for a diagnostic test, the application of a mask on the patient may reduce exposure to environmental molds (e.g., *Aspergillus*) or infectious diseases existing in other people the patient encounters, but is not advocated by all institutions.[19,26] The experienced critical care nurse routinely performs mathematical calculations of absolute counts for patients at risk for neutropenia or lymphopenia, interprets the results, and modifies the patient's care as the risk for infection increases.[7,18,37] Invasive procedures are limited when possible, and some critical care routines may be modified to reduce infections in these high-risk patients. For example, rectal temperature probes and drainage tubes are discouraged because of the chance for perirectal infection if the anal mucosa is damaged.[30] Specific precautions are defined by individual institutions based upon their level of experience and comfort in management of these patients.

Active measures to prevent infection are particularly important for these patients (see the Multidisciplinary Plan of Care on pp. 1031-1035). Healthy living and nonspecific immune support (such as adequate sleep and nutritional support) as well as avoidance of infection risks (such as invasive procedures) are implemented to avoid infection until immune function is restored. *Immune nutrition* is a new term used to imply a base nutrition aimed at supporting the growth and activity of white blood cells. Diets high in protein and vitamins and low in complex carbohydrates and sugar are generally recommended. The addition of nutritional supplements such as arginine and glutamine is thought to target immune function, but not yet supported by a large body of evidence.[24] Although it is unclear whether exposure to food pathogens can induce infection in immune-compromised patients, a low-microbial diet has been advocated in the literature and is summarized in the Nutrition box on p. 1036.[28,41,44] A lack of research evidence to support this specialized diet has led to inconsistency in practice. New information is available that demonstrates the importance of using the gastrointestinal tract, even for small amounts of feeding, as a means to maintain gastrointestinal mucosal integrity.[17] This is thought to reduce translocation of bacteria from the GI tract into the bloodstream.

MULTIDISCIPLINARY PLAN OF CARE FOR THE IMMUNOCOMPROMISED PATIENT

PROBLEM	INTERVENTION	RATIONALE	EXPECTED OUTCOME
Risk for development of infection from environmental exposures	• Single-patient rooms • Conscientious hand hygiene by all healthcare providers and visitors • Single-use patient care items	• Decrease exposure to potential pathogens.	• Absence of nosocomial infection
	• Place mask on patient when leaving room if directed by institutional immunocompromised precautions[42]	• Airborne organisms can easily cause infection in immunocompromised host. Masks prevent breathing in airborne organisms.	• Absence of respiratory tract infection
	• No fresh flowers or plants	• Standing water and soil harbor microorganisms that can become airborne and cause infection.	• Absence of exposure
	• Patient wears a high-filtration mask when transported to and from hospital or outside enclosed unit as directed by institutional immunocompromised precautions and presence of construction[35]	• Airborne risks are common in hospital environment from other sick persons or environmental contaminants. The high-filtration mask is geared to eliminate exposure to molds.	• Absence of infection
	• Set up construction barriers when performing ceiling or wall repairs in hospital	• Protect against environmental airborne contaminants known to reside in walls, ceilings, ventilation systems.	• Absence of infection with nosocomial organisms known to be associated with construction
Risk for development of infection from host risk factors	• Daily personal hygiene with an antibacterial soap	• Skin flora or contaminants can transmit across breached barriers to cause localized or systemic infections.	• Water-based organisms such as *Pseudomonas* or *Legionella* do not infect wounds or open lesions

Table continues on page 1032

PROBLEM	INTERVENTION	RATIONALE	EXPECTED OUTCOME
	• Assess oral cavity every shift, noting presence of erythema, ulcerations, pseudomembrane (milky opaque white area indicative of dead mucous membrane occurring before sloughing of tissue), oral pain, dry mouth	• A focused oral assessment on a routine basis will detect the earliest changes that may be indicative of oral infection. Dry mouth predisposes to *Candida*.	• Absence of oral infection
	• Oral care inclusive of brushing and rinsing at least three times a day • If not intubated and normally part of patient's routine to floss, this practice should be continued even if mild to moderate bleeding risks are present • If normal oral care cannot be performed, frequent and vigorous rinsing with sterile water, saline, or bicarbonate solution (1 Tbsp/1 L) can reduce oral organisms • At-risk patients should also receive prophylactic topical antifungal or antiviral agents • It is unclear whether chlorhexidine rinses improve oral health; although it may reduce risk of candidal infection and oral infection in general, there has been a link between its use and development of resistant gram- negative microbes	• Thorough oral care has been shown to reduce number of oral organisms that can later act as respiratory pathogens, causing nosocomial pneumonia. If regular oral care regimens cannot be performed, even vigorous rinsing reduces number of flora in mouth. • Prophylactic topical oral antimicrobials can reduce incidence of superinfections such as *Candida* (thrush) or oral herpes.	
	• Evaluate nutritional status and optimize nutritional support • Using GI tract for nutritional support may have additive effect of maintaining mucosal integrity and reducing bacterial translocation into peritoneum • In patients who are eating, receiving oral antimicrobial agents or a low-microbial diet may reduce risk of GI infection	• Altered nutrition increases the risk of acquiring infection.	• Maintenance of nutritional parameters such as albumin levels, tissue antigen responses, white blood cell counts

PROBLEM	INTERVENTION	RATIONALE	EXPECTED OUTCOME
	• Monitor nutritional parameters	• Detect abnormalities and facilitate early intervention.	
	• Administer prophylactic antimicrobial therapy targeted for specific patient risk groups	• Defined high-risk populations such as HIV infected, prolonged granulocytopenia, preexisting infection risks (e.g., history of rheumatic heart disease) may warrant prophylactic antimicrobial therapy.	• Absence of common infections in patients with defined risks
Risk for development of infection from invasive procedures or surgery	• Avoid invasive procedures whenever possible • Noninvasive interventions may be equally effective in some instances; for instance, a venous pH closely correlates to an arterial pH and may be drawn to reduce need for arterial blood gases in some patients	• Reduce risk for infection while maintaining equivalent standards of care.	• Few infections related to invasive procedures
	• Limit use of large-bore and multilumen percutaneously inserted intravenous lines when possible • Consider tunneled catheters such as Hickman catheters that have lower risk of infection	• There are well-defined characteristics of invasive catheters that increase risk for infection, such as large bore, multilumen, femorally placed, multiple operators for insertion or care, nearby draining wounds or excrement.	• Line-related infections reduced
	• When invasive procedures or surgery is necessary, prophylactic antimicrobial agents are ordered: administer immediately before or at start of procedure	• Prophylactic antimicrobials have been shown to reduce infection risk related to specific invasive procedures such as gastrointestinal surgery.	• Procedure-related infections below average in immune-compromised patient group

Table continues on page 1034

PROBLEM	INTERVENTION	RATIONALE	EXPECTED OUTCOME
	• Avoid insertion of tubes or drains that can further impair barrier defenses unless other options are not available; for instance, rectal temperature, rectal tubes, and suppositories should be avoided when possible	• Reduces injury to mucosal barrier defenses.	• Less infection
Risk for infection with resistant microbes	• Ensure antimicrobial medications are given on time, over the time prescribed, and for the full course of therapy	• Reduces the risk for development of resistant microbes.	• Absence of infection with resistant microbes
	• Most immunocompromised patients are ordered broad-spectrum antimicrobial therapy even before culture results are available • If cultures become positive, therapy should be modified to be specific to microbe • Nurse should monitor culture results and report evidence of infections	• Prompt, targeted therapy for culture results decreases exposure to excessive potent antimicrobial agents that can lead to resistance.	
Evidence of infection	• Culture all possible sites of infection using proper technique for each location • Expect that reculturing will not be performed until antimicrobial therapy has been in place at least 72 hours, or patient's condition changes dramatically	• Infections in immunocompromised patient may be subtle and not in an obvious location. Careful technique and thorough culturing of potential sites maximize culture yield.	
	• Chest x-ray to assess for symptoms of infection is helpful when respiratory symptoms are present, but not thought to contribute to diagnosis of infection in absence of respiratory symptoms	• Chest x-rays are rarely abnormal in patients without respiratory symptoms because the x-ray lags behind clinical symptoms by approximately 24 hours.	
	• Administer antimicrobial therapy as ordered • Monitor antimicrobial therapy blood levels as ordered or indicated	• Optimizes the clinical effects of the agents.	

PROBLEM	INTERVENTION	RATIONALE	EXPECTED OUTCOME
	• Contain infectious exudates with occlusive dressings changed when soiled or at least every 72 hours, preventing spread of microbes to other parts of body	• Prevents the spread of infection.	
Evidence of temperature dysregulation (hypothermia or hyperthermia) from infection	• Monitor temperature by most accurate means possible	• Axillary and tympanic temperatures are often associated with user variations. Oral temperature may be inaccurate in patients who are mouth breathing. Rectal temperatures should be avoided when possible because of the risk for infection. Bladder temperatures are considered similar to rectal in accuracy.	• Afebrile
	• Check temperature frequently, especially with any other suspicious symptoms such as mental status changes or oliguria	• Temperature may be the only early indication of infection in the immunocompromised patient. Patients with other potential symptoms of sepsis should have their temperature checked frequently with a low threshold for culturing.	
	• Report subnormal temperatures as well as temperatures ≥38.3° C orally or 37.3° C core	• Low temperatures are equally likely to indicate infection and may have a higher association with gram-negative organisms or septicemia.	

GI = Gastrointestinal, HIV = human immunodeficiency virus, WBC = white blood cell count.

▲ NUTRITION

Considerations for Nutrition in Immunocompromised Patients

GENERAL GUIDELINES

Calories
- Balanced calories from a variety of healthy food choices are encouraged.
- No specific calorie limitations exist.

Protein
- Protein intake is encouraged to enhance tissue maintenance and repair.
- Healthy protein nutrition can reduce the risk for infection.

Fluids
- Fluids are generally encouraged. Improved hydration can enhance natural clearance of microbes via excretions such as sputum or urine.

Electrolytes
- Patients may experience hypophosphatemia when lymphocyte depleted because lymphocytes contain high amounts of phosphorus.

Vitamins and Minerals
- Supplemental vitamins and minerals are encouraged to enhance tissue maintenance and repair.
- Selenium is thought to enhance hematopoietic cell development, and adequate quantities may improve blood cell growth.
- Zinc is thought to reduce the risk of infection through enhancement of immune competence.

SPECIAL CONSIDERATIONS

Food substances to avoid:
- Fermented, unpasteurized drinks
- Cultured yogurt, buttermilk, sourdough
- Fermented hard and soft cheeses such as blue cheese
- Raw or partially cooked eggs
- Raw or partially cooked meat

Food substances to consume cautiously after careful cleaning or evaluation for contamination:
- Salads
- Uncooked fresh fruit or vegetables
- Fresh shell nuts
- Cheese without mold

Food substances that can be consumed freely:
- Fully cooked meats
- Fully cooked fruits or vegetables
- Processed breads and cereals

Vaccinations to prevent common infections such as meningitis and pneumococcus are recommended for patients with special risk factors, provided that the vaccine does not contain live organisms.[2,25,30] Organ transplant recipients should receive vaccination against influenza, pneumococcus, and meningitis.[2] Patients with surgical (e.g., treatment for traumatic injury or chronic leukemia) or functional splenectomy (e.g., infarcted spleen with sickle cell crisis) should always receive a pneumococcal vaccine because this is an important organism normally removed by splenic macrophages.[14] Other immunocompromised patients who may be candidates for specific vaccinations include the following: older adults, intravenous drug users, human immunodeficiency virus (HIV)-infected individuals, and those with renal or hepatic impairment.[3,15,42] In situations in which the immune compromise is related to a reversible etiology, the priority is to eliminate the causative agent and provide symptomatic support until the disorder is reversed.[15] This may be the objective when immune compromise is due to medications that can be discontinued, or disease that can be stabilized. For example, if immune compromise is related to infection with HIV, antiretroviral therapy may restore lymphocyte counts and reduce the severity of immune compromise.[3,22]

In patients who are at particular risk for defined microorganisms, prophylactic antimicrobial therapy may be employed. Prophylactic antimicrobial agents are approved for routine use in patients with prolonged neutropenia or HIV infection, or in recipients of immunosuppressant agents for autoimmune disease or to prevent rejection after organ transplant.* The regimen prescribed will be based on host variables, the type of immune defect, and anticipated infectious organisms. For example, the prophylactic regimen for HIV-infected individuals is well defined. Once the CD4 count is below 500/ mm^3, pneumocystis prophylaxis with trimethoprim-sulfamethoxazole is started. When the CD4 count further decreases below 200/mm^3, antimycobacterial therapy is initiated, and as the count drops below 50/mm^3, agents against cytomegalovirus are prescribed.[3,22,36]

Enhancement of Immune Function

As outlined in the Medication table on p. 1037, specific interventions to enhance immunologic function may be indicated for patients who are at high risk for life-threatening infections. The specific type of immune support will depend upon the identified deficit. Bone marrow growth factors, also called colony-simulating factors, support bone marrow regrowth after chemotherapy so that the depth and length of neutropenia are diminished, reducing the risk of infection.[6,11,15,37] These are usually administered approximately 24 hours after the last dose of chemotherapy. These agents are available as a single, every 3- to 4-week injection or daily injections that start

---

*References 3, 15, 22, 30, 36, 42.

IMMUNE SUPPORT THERAPIES

GROWTH FACTOR	INDICATIONS	DOSE	NURSING CONSIDERATIONS
Hematopoietic Factors/Growth Colony-Stimulating Factors			

Granulocyte colony-stimulating factor (GCSF, filgrastim, pegfilgrastim)	• Chemotherapy-induced neutropenia
	• Antiretroviral-induced neutropenia
	• Under investigation:
	  • Sepsis in children
	  • Autoimmune neutropenia
	  • Neutropenia of chronic illness
		Filgrastim: single daily dose of 5–20 mcg/kg IV or subcutaneously every day for up to 2 weeks based upon post-chemotherapy nadir; administer slowly subcutaneously over 1 min; administer over 30 min IV
		Pegfilgrastim: single one-time dose of 6-mg IV or subcutaneous dose once per chemotherapy cycle, and no more frequently than every 21 days
			• Should not be used 24 hr before to 24 hr after administration of antineoplastic chemotherapy; same-day administration of pegfilgrastim is currently under investigation.
			• In daily dosing agent, therapy should be continued within this 2-week time frame until WBC count reaches 10,000 cells/mm³.
			• Hypersensitivity reactions may occur. Administer slowly, observing for rash, hives, or respiratory distress.
			• Monitor total WBC count and differential.
			• Prepare patient for possible adverse effects: fever, bone pain, and redness at injection site.
			• Advise patients how to manage adverse effects with over-the-counter medications such as acetaminophen.

Granulocyte macrophage colony-stimulating factor (sargramostim, IL-3)	• Post–hematopoietic stem cell transplant • Chemotherapy-induced neutropenia	Single daily dose of 250 mcg/m²; administer IV over 2 hr	• Should not be used 24 hr before to 24 hr after administration of antineoplastic chemotherapy.
Immune Globulin Replacement			

Intravenous immune globulin (Gammagard, Gammar-IV, Iveegam, Sandoglobulin, Venoglobulin-S)	• Primary immunodeficiency syndromes
	• Immune thrombocytopenia
	• Chronic lymphocytic leukemia
	• Immune reconstitution after hematopoietic stem cell transplantation
	• Specific products indicated for defined viral infections (e.g., cytomegalovirus, respiratory syncytial virus)
	Under investigation for:
	  • Chronic disease-related IgG deficiency
	  • Sino-pulmonary infections
		Single dose of 100–200 mg/kg IV
		May be given for 3–5 consecutive days
		IV dosing and duration of therapy are variable according to clinical situation.
		Also available in a subcutaneous formulation for primary immunodeficiency syndromes.
			• Retest IgG levels after administration (should be >300 mg/dl).
			• Reconstitution or dilution is required for all products.
			• Determine special requirements for each specific product: may require a 15-micrometer filter; some may only be administered centrally; some are contraindicated in patients with renal dysfunction.
			• Hypersensitivity may occur. Administer by slow titration (increasing rate every 15–30 min over a 1–2 hr period) with frequent observation and assessment of vital signs and respiratory function.

IgG = Immunoglobulin G, WBC = white blood cell.

the day after chemotherapy and are given for approximately 10 days, or until the blood count begins to return to normal.[37] If immunoglobulin (Ig) deficiency (IgG levels less than 300 mg/dl) is present, intravenous immunoglobulin is available as replacement therapy.[15,42] Intravenous immunoglobulin infusions are administered slowly, with careful monitoring for hypersensitivity reactions. When lymphocyte activity is altered, there are no clear treatments. The experienced critical care nurse can recognize patients who are candidates for immune replacement therapies and the specific nursing care required during administration of these agents.

Treatment of Infection

When infections occur in patients with immune compromise, the list of possible pathogens is extensive and challenging to anticipate. When symptoms of infection are present, broad-spectrum bactericidal antibiotics aimed to target both gram-positive and gram-negative organisms are prescribed.[15] Unlike other patients with infections, antimicrobials are initiated at the first sign of infection rather than after the return of positive cultures.[15] These patients have been reported to progress from infection to septic shock in mere hours without comprehensive antimicrobial therapy. This often dictates administration of agents normally requiring approval from the appropriate infectious disease authority.[32] Efficient standing order sets or automated approval processes for management of these patients exist in many institutions.[26] An experienced critical care nurse should be familiar with these policies and facilitate administration of appropriate antimicrobial therapy within 2 hours of the onset of symptoms.[37] Antimicrobials administered in the setting of immune compromise may require higher doses for a longer time.[15] Sometimes multiple antibiotics are administered simultaneously to cover the same microbe.[32]

Patients who develop severe, refractory infections and remain immune compromised have little chance of fully recovering. Granulocyte transfusions can temporarily combat severe microbial infections, but their infusion is associated with a high incidence of hypersensitivity reactions.[15,21] Guidelines for administration of granulocyte transfusions are included in Box 38-2.[21,37]

Box 38-2

Administration of Granulocyte Transfusions

SELECTION OF CANDIDATES

- Refractory infection
- Presumed fungal infection
- Persistent and refractory granulocytopenia

ADMINISTRATION GUIDELINES

- Cell preparation
  - Granulocytes must be gamma irradiated before administration.
  - Blood bank requires several hours to prepare granulocytes.
- Before starting the infusion
  - Obtain baseline vital signs, oxygen saturation, and breath sounds. Notify the physician of any abnormalities.
  - Premedicate routinely with diphenhydramine (Benadryl) 25–50 mg and acetaminophen (Tylenol) 650 mg.
  - Some patients may also require hydrocortisone (Solu-Cortef) 100 mg before transfusion.
  - Administer premedications 15 to 30 minutes before beginning transfusion.
  - Prime standard blood tubing without additional filters with normal saline.
- During infusion
  - Administer granulocytes by gravity only. Infusion pumps may damage the cells.

- Transfusion must begin within 30 minutes of arrival on unit, and infused at a rate of 1×10^{10} cells per 30 minutes, not to exceed 500 ml/hr.
- Gently agitate bottom of bag every 15 minutes to ensure mixing of cells suspended in plasma. Cells settling in the bottom of bag may infuse too quickly, resulting in bolus effect.
- Ongoing assessments of vital signs and breath sounds are performed frequently during the infusion.

NURSING IMPLICATIONS

- Reactions are common and may range from a mild to moderate rash and hives to severe hypersensitivity reaction with severe respiratory distress.
- WBCs should migrate to the site of infection, and the patient may demonstrate symptoms reflecting WBC infiltration (e.g., dyspnea, crackles in the presence of pneumonia).
- Have emergency equipment, oxygen delivery system, and suction available.
- For rigors during transfusion, administer meperidine (Demerol) 10 mg IV every 5 minutes up to a total dose of 50 mg. Alternative drugs for rigors may be morphine in 0.5-mg increments or small doses of benzodiazepines.
- Avoid infusion of amphotericin or other blood products within 6 hours of WBC transfusion if at all possible.

Adapted from reference 37.

Oral infection is a common occurrence among immunocompromised patients. Before administration of antimicrobial therapy, a culture of one of the oral ulcerations is performed and sent for bacteria, mycology, and virology evaluation. Although the lesions do not appear infected, immunocompromised patients often do not display traditional symptoms of infection. Additionally, lesion appearance may be atypical for well-known organisms, and the open lesions may actually be herpetic infection, not simply a result of chemotherapy. Oral ulcerations in granulocytopenic patients may appear to be nonspecifically erythematous, yet culture positive for fungus or virus. This is particularly concerning in patients who have had previous immunosuppression therapy (such as renal transplant patients) and then are administered long-term lymphocyte suppression after the transplant, predisposing them to herpes simplex infection.

The most common infections in patients with lymphocyte suppression are herpes simplex reactivation and *Pneumocystis jiroveci*.[42] Checking herpes antibody titers is part of the routine care for long-term immunosuppressed patients such as those who have had a transplant. Although this patient population may be initially herpes simplex antibody negative, it may be advisable to recheck antibody titers. If they are now positive, acyclovir prophylaxis to prevent reactivation

Case Study 38-1, Part C

Evidence-Based Management of the Immunocompromised Patient

S.E. has multiple risks for infection and is currently experiencing a clinically significant infection. The length and severity of his neutropenia can be abrogated by administration of hematopoietic growth factors after chemotherapy doses during subsequent cycles, but hematopoietic growth factors are not normally introduced once the WBC count is already reduced unless life-threatening infection is present. S.E.'s current clinical condition may warrant its use, but it is unclear whether it will shorten the neutropenic period or will aid in recovery from infection.[11] These agents are more strongly recommended in patients with neutropenia and invasive fungal infection or refractory gram-negative infection.[11,15] The growth factor will encourage rapid return of the white blood cell count, reducing the risk of future infections. Because the oncology team is not caring for S.E. during this episode of infection, the critical care nurse must ensure a complete discharge summary and communication with the oncology team so that these prophylactic growth factors are ordered with the next cycle of chemotherapy.

Decision point: What prophylactic steps would be taken to decrease S.E.'s risk for future infection?

Decision point: Specifically, what interventions should be made to prevent oral infections?

Box 38-3

Nursing Practice Pearls of Immunocompromised Care

1. Have a high index of suspicion.
   Immunocompromise is NOT just found in patients with hematologic or immune disorders.
2. Be a detective.
   Immunocompromised patients do NOT exhibit the usual common signs and symptoms of infection, and subtle symptoms should not be overlooked.
3. Beware—The patient may get worse before getting better.
   The return of immune function often heralds symptom exacerbation. As white blood cell and other supportive immune function returns to normal in patients with temporary deficits, the white blood cell response causes "white out" that leads to symptom exacerbation.
4. Look at and culture every opening or potential opening.
   Immune-compromised patients can be colonized with large quantities of normal non-pathogenic flora, or resistant microbes. These can become the source of infection. Keep a broad view of possible infectious organisms— uncommon and resistant microbes may be the culprits.
5. Proactively prevent infection in every aspect of your care.
   Realize that the smallest infractions in infection control technique can cause life-threatening infection, and take special care to protect your patient.
6. Learn which antimicrobial agents target specific microbes and understand your patient's unique infection risks.
   Your understanding of how the risk factors for infection dictate antimicrobial agent choices during early signs of infection can help the multidisciplinary team be comprehensive in its consideration of therapy choices.
7. Think of creative options.
   Be the advocate to explore additional risks for infection or avenues for treatment such as IgG replenishment or granulocyte transfusions.

may be initiated. Antimicrobial prophylaxis against other opportunistic organisms such as *P. jiroveci* may also be administered.

CONCLUSIONS

Patients with compromised immune systems are cared for in critical care far more frequently than credited in the literature. Although hematologic and immunologic disorders comprise some of these patients, it is often a more subtle state of compromise from medical-surgical disorders or therapies that affects patients. The role of the critical care nurse in recognizing high-risk patients and implementing heightened surveillance cannot be underestimated. Preventive and proactive management of the immune system dysfunction before the onset of infection is a key to successful recovery for many patients. Extra infection prevention strategies can be taken for granted, but unless conscientious attention is paid to everyday elements of care, serious infection threatens the lives of these patients. A number of strategies aimed at this specialized care can be incorporated into routine intensive care nursing orientations. Key pearls of care for immunocompromised patients that can be shared quickly with nurses working in the intensive care unit are included in Box 38-3.

REFERENCES

1. Alonzo, N. C., & Bayer, B. M. (2002). Opioids, immunology, and host defenses of intravenous drug abusers. *Infect Dis Clin North Am, 16*(3), 553–569.
2. Ballout, A., et al. (2005). Vaccinations for adult solid organ transplant recipient: current recommendations. *Transplant Proc, 37*(6), 2826–2827.
3. Bartlett, J. G. (2005). *The Johns Hopkins Hospital 2004–2005 guide to care of patients with HIV infection.* Philadelphia: Lippincott Williams & Wilkins.
4. Binkley, C. (2004). Survey of oral care practices in US intensive care units. *Am J Infect Control, 32,* 161–169.
5. Brennan, M. T., et al. (2004). The role of oral microbial colonization in ventilator-associated pneumonia. *Oral Surg Oral Med Oral Pathol Oral Radiol Endod, 98*(6), 665–672.
6. Buchsel, P. C., et al. (2002). Granulocyte macrophage colony-stimulating factor: current practice and novel approaches. *Clin J Oncol Nurs, 6*(4), 198–205.
7. Cagan, D., Franco, M., & Vasquez, D. (2002). The ABCs of low blood count. *Clin J Oncol Nurs, 6*(1), 34–37.
8. Camp-Sorrell, D. (2005). Myelosuppression. In J. K. Itano & K. N. Taoka (Eds.), *Core curriculum for oncology nursing* (4th ed., pp. 259–274). Philadelphia: Elsevier.
9. Cancer Evaluation Program. (2006) *Common terminology criteria for adverse events, v. 3.0 (CTCAE).* Bethesda, Md: DCTD, NCI, NIH, DHHS, http://ctep.cancer.gov.
10. Choi, Y. W., et al. (2004). Effects of radiation therapy on the lungs: radiologic appearances and differential diagnosis. *Radiographics, 24*(4), 985–987, discussion 998.
11. Crawford, J., et al. (2005). *NCCN practice guidelines. Myeloid growth factors, v.2.2005.* Jenkintown, Pa: National Comprehensive Cancer Network, www.nccn.org.
12. Deutchle, T., et al. (2005). Nasal cytologies—impact of sampling method, repeated sampling and interobserver variability. *Rhinology, 43*(3), 215–220.
13. Eggimann, P., Wolff, M., & Garbina, J. (2005). Oral nystatin as antifungal prophylaxis in critically ill patients: an old SDD tool to be renewed? *Intensive Care Med, 31,* 1466–1468.
14. El-Alfy, S. E., & El-Sayed, M. H. (2004). Overwhelming postsplenectomy infection: is quality of patient knowledge enough for prevention? *Hematol J, 5*(1), 77–80.
15. Freifeld, A. G., et al. (2003). *NCCN practice guidelines for fever and neutropenia, v.1.2005.* Jenkintown, Pa: National Comprehensive Cancer Network, 2005, www.nccn.org.
16. Furr, L. A. (2004). Factors affecting quality of oral care in intensive care units. *J Adv Nurs, 48*(5), 454–462.
17. Griffiths, R. D., & Bongers, T. (2005). Nutrition support for patients in the intensive care unit. *Postgrad Med J, 81*(960), 629–636.
18. Guinan, J. L., McGuckin, M., & Nowell, P. C. (2003). Management of health-care–associated infections in the oncology patient. *Oncology, 17*(3), 415–420; discussion 423–426.
19. Hahn, T., Cummings, K. M., & Michale, K. (2002). Efficacy of high-efficiency particulate air filtration in preventing aspergillosis in immunocompromised patients with hematologic malignancies. *Infect Control Hosp Epidemiol, 23,* 525–531.
20. Herget, G. W., et al. (2005). Generalized herpes simplex virus infection in an immunocompromised patient—report of a case and review of the literature. *Path Res Prac, 201*(2), 123–129.
21. Hubel, K., et al. (2002). Granulocyte transfusion therapy for infections in candidates and recipients of HPC transplantation: a comparative analysis of feasibility and outcome for community donors versus related donors. *Transfusion, 42*(11), 1414–1421.
22. Kaplan, J. E., et al. (2002). Guidelines for preventing opportunistic infections among HIV-infected persons—2002. Recommendations of the U.S. Public Health Service and the Infectious Diseases Society of America. *MMWR Recomm Rep, 51*(RR-8), 1–52.
23. Kocak, Z., et al. (2005). Challenges in defining radiation pneumonitis in patients with lung cancer. *Int J Radiat Oncol Biol Phys, 62*(3), 635–638.
24. Koretz, R. L. (2003). Immunonutrition: can you be what you eat? *Curr Opin Gastroenterol, 19*(2), 134–139.
25. Machado, C. M. (2005). Reimmunization after hematopoietic stem cell transplantation. *ExpRev Vaccines, 4*(2), 219–228.
26. Mayhill, C. G. (2004). *Hospital epidemiology and infection control.* Philadelphia: Lippincott Williams & Wilkins.
27. Mims, C. A., Nash, A., & Stephen, J. (2001). *Mims' pathogenesis of infectious disease* (5th ed.). San Diego: Academic Press.
28. Moody, K., Charlson, M. E., & Finlay, J. (2002). The neutropenic diet: what's the evidence? *J Pediatr Hematol Oncol, 24*(9), 717–721.
29. Moran, A. B., & Camp-Sorrell, D. (2002). Maintenance of venous access devices in patients with neutropenia. *Clin J Oncol Nurs, 6,* 126–130.
30. O'Grady, N., et al. (2002). Centers for Disease Control and Prevention: Guidelines for the prevention of intravascular catheter-related infections. *MMWR Recomm Rep, 51*(RR-10), 1–29.
31. O'Reilly, M. (2003). Oral care of the critically ill: a review of the literature and guidelines for practice. *Aust Crit Care, 16*(3), 101–110.
32. Pizzo, P. A. (1999). Current concepts: fever in immunocompromised patients. *N Engl J Med, 341*(12), 893–900.
33. Regazzoni, C. J., et al. (2003). Neutropenia and the development of the systemic inflammatory response syndrome. *Intensive Care Med, 29*(1), 135–138.
34. Schleder, B. J. (2003). Taking charge of ventilator-associated pneumonia. *Nurs Manage, 34*(8), 27–33.

35. Sehulster, L., & Chinn, R. Y. (2003). Guidelines for environmental infection control in health-care facilities. Recommendations of CDC and the Healthcare Infection Control Practices Advisory Committee (HICPAC). *MMWR Recommen Rep, 52*(RR-10), 1–42.

36. Sepkowitz, K. A. (2002). Opportunistic infections in patients with and patients without acquired immunodeficiency syndrome. *Clin Infect Dis, 34*(9), 1098–1107.

37. Shane, K. A., & Shelton, B. K. (2004). Bone marrow suppression. In B. K. Shelton, C. R. Ziegfeld & M. M. Olsen (Eds.), *Manual of cancer nursing*. Philadelphia: Lippincott Williams & Wilkins.

38. Shelton, B. K. (2001). Hematological and immune disorders. In M. L. Sole, M. L. Lamborn & J. C. Hartshorn (Eds.), *Introduction to critical care nursing* (3rd ed.). Philadelphia: Saunders.

39. Shelton, B. K. (2003). Evidence-based care for the neutropenic patient with leukemia. *Semin Oncol Nurs, 19*(2), 133–141.

40. Shelton, B. K. (2005). Infections. In C. H. Yarbro, M. H. Frogge & M. Goodman (Eds.), *Cancer nursing principles and practice* (6th ed., pp. 698–722). Boston: Jones & Bartlett Publishers.

41. Smith, L. H., & Besser, S. G. (2000). Dietary restrictions for patients with neutropenia: a survey of institutional practices. *Oncol Nurs Forum, 27*(3), 515–520.

42. Sullivan, K. M., et al. (2001). Preventing opportunistic infections after hematopoietic stem cell transplantation: the Centers for Disease Control and Prevention, Infectious Diseases Society of America, and American Society for Blood and Marrow Transplantation Practice guidelines and beyond. *Hematology Am Soc Hematol Educ Program*, 392–421.

43. Taylor, A. L., Marcus, R., & Bradley, J. A. (2005). Post-transplant lymphoproliferative disorders (PTLD) after solid organ transplantation. *Crit Rev Oncol Hematol, 56*(1), 155–167.

44. Wilson, B. J. (2002). Dietary recommendations for neutropenic patients. *Semin Oncol Nurs, 18*(1), 44–49.

CHAPTER 39

Bone Marrow Transplantation

Carol E. Jacoby and Christine Smith Schulman

The first successful human hematopoietic stem cell transplantation (HSCT) using bone marrow occurred in 1968.[2] Since then, the field of HSCT, commonly referred to as bone marrow transplantation (BMT), has expanded rapidly. Major advances have occurred since the late 1980s, when immunosuppressant agents such as cyclosporine (Gengraf, Neoral) were discovered and the ability to extract stem cells directly from the peripheral blood (apheresis) was developed.[2,61] Hematopoietic stem cell transplants are done using bone marrow, peripheral blood stem cells (PBSCs), and umbilical cord blood. The three major types of stem cell transplants are autologous (self), allogeneic (non-self), and syngeneic (identical twin). Even though both the field and the terminology of transplant are rapidly evolving, currently patients and transplant centers are commonly referred to as BMT, regardless of the type of cells received.

Care of the BMT patient requires a specially trained staff; most care is accomplished on the BMT wards. However, because of the complexity of the patients and the high risk of life-threatening complications, the patient may need support in critical care. During the transplant process, patients may have prolonged periods of neutropenia, setting the stage for life-threatening septic events requiring vasopressor support. In addition, patients will have periods of time when they are thrombocytopenic and are at high risk of bleeding.[11] Essentially every system is at risk during the transplant process; admission to critical care may be necessary following cardiovascular, infectious, renal, gastrointestinal, and respiratory events related to BMT.[38]

Care of the critically ill BMT patient is often stressful for critical care staff because of a lack of familiarity with the transplant process and the aggressive oncologic interventions. This chapter reviews the information regarding the BMT process, long-term prognosis, expected complications, and symptom management important to the critical care nurse when providing care for these complex patients.

AUTOLOGOUS STEM CELL TRANSPLANTATION

Autologous stem cell transplant (auto) is used to treat a variety of malignant disorders. Some of the most common diseases currently being treated with transplant are listed in Box 39-1. This type of transplant involves collecting marrow or PBSCs from the patient before myeloablative therapy and infusing them back into the person from whom the stem cells originated.[11] Autologous stem cell transplants are primarily done to rescue someone from the toxic effects of myeloablative chemotherapy that was specifically designed for disease eradication or a prolonged remission state.[3]

It is not common to see an autologous stem cell transplant for acute leukemia; however, age of the patient, comorbid conditions, toxicity of the myeloablative regimen, and lack of a suitable allogeneic donor are some of the reasons an autologous PBSC may be utilized. When a patient is diagnosed with leukemia, the chromosomes are analyzed for the multiple known chromosomal abnormalities commonly seen in leukemia. These abnormalities have been divided into good, moderate, and poor prognostic indicators.[78] A patient with good or moderate chromosomal abnormalities may have a prolonged period of remission or, rarely, a potential cure from an autologous stem cell transplant.[16]

ALLOGENEIC STEM CELL TRANSPLANTATION

When the stem cells originate from another person, the transplant is called an allogeneic (allo) stem cell transplant. The goal of the allogeneic stem cell transplant is treatment of the underlying malignancy and replacement of the malfunctioning immune system. Most allogeneic transplants are used to treat diseases of the bone marrow, the most common of which are listed in Box 39-2. An allogeneic stem cell transplant originates from a donor that has human leukocyte antigen

---

Box 39-1

Common Diseases Treated With Autologous Stem Cell Transplantation

LYMPHOPROLIFERATIVE DISORDERS

Chronic lymphocytic lymphoma
Hodgkin's disease (HD)
Multiple myeloma (MM)
Non-Hodgkin's lymphoma (NHL)

SOLID TUMORS

Breast cancer
Ewing's sarcoma (pediatric patients)
Neuroblastoma (pediatric patients)
Renal cell carcinoma
Testicular cancer

LEUKEMIA

Acute lymphoblastic leukemia (ALL)
Acute myelogenous leukemia (AML)
Chronic myeloid leukemia (CML)

Data from references 80 and 92.

Box 39-2

Common Diseases Treated With Allogeneic Stem Cell Transplants

LEUKEMIA

Acute lymphoblastic leukemia (ALL)
Acute myelogenous leukemia (AML)
Chronic lymphocytic lymphoma
Chronic myeloid leukemia (CML)
Hodgkin's disease (HD)
Multiple myeloma (MM)
Non-Hodgkin's lymphoma (NHL)

HEMATOLOGIC DISORDERS

Aplastic anemia (AA)
Myelodysplastic syndrome (MDS)
Sickle cell anemia
Beta-thalassemia

IMMUNODEFICIENCIES

Severe combined immunodeficiencies
Wiskott-Aldrich syndrome

Data from references 80 and 92.

(HLA) compatibility with the recipient.[4] These stem cells come from a sibling and are usually denoted as an allo, or they can come from an unrelated donor and are denoted by multiple names such as matched unrelated donor (MUD) stem cell transplants. Full siblings are tested first before a search for an unrelated donor is initiated in the International Bone Marrow Transplant Registry (IBMTR).[52]

The final type of stem cell transplant is technically an allogeneic transplant, but functions more like an autologous stem cell transplant. This transplant, known as a syngeneic stem cell transplant, occurs when the stem cells originate from an HLA identical twin. In this scenario, the immune systems of the donor and recipient are identical and donor stem cells will not see the recipient's body as a foreign entity. Immunosuppressive medications are not required; therefore a syngeneic stem cell transplant is associated with fewer complications.[4] However, it is also associated with much lower cure rates of the underlying disease because of the loss of the graft-versus-host disease (GVHD) effect.[13]

Compatibility between donor and recipient is essential to minimize the potential of GVHD, graft rejection, and graft failure.[4] GVHD is a pathologic condition in which the donor cells recognize that the patient (recipient) is not self and attack the cells and tissues of the patient. The incidence of GVHD is extremely varied, ranging from 16% to 66% in related matched donors to as high as 70% to 90% in unrelated or related transplants with HLA mismatches.[58] It is difficult to interpret this information because multiple factors, including compatibility issues, influence the incidence of GVHD. In clinical practice, it is possible to perform a transplant without a 100% HLA match with the donor; however, as the number of mismatches increase, the risk of graft rejection and GVHD rises.[38] GVHD is discussed in greater detail later in this chapter. Transplants can be done from siblings or parents that match only half of the alleles usually required for a transplant. These transplants, known as haplo-allogeneic stem cell transplants, are associated with a significantly higher percentage of severe GVHD and graft rejection.[47]

PRETRANSPLANT CONSIDERATIONS

Recipient Evaluation and Preparation

A thorough evaluation of the patient (recipient) before transplant is essential to determine the patient's ability to withstand the rigors of transplantation. The pretransplant workup is essentially the same for an autologous and allogeneic PBSC transplant. Physical examination is performed with special attention to neurologic, pulmonary, cardiovascular, and skin integrity assessment. A complete medical history must be obtained with a particular focus on previous treatment for the patient's cancer or hematologic disorder. Information is obtained regarding response to treatment, duration of remissions, and current status of disease.[89] The patient must demonstrate that he/she has a treatment-responsive disease in order to be considered for a transplant.[36] Treatment-responsive disease means that, when applicable, the patient has shown that the malignancy responds to chemotherapy (e.g., in the case of lymphoma, there is a greater than 50% reduction in tumor size seen on computed tomography [CT] scan; in the case of leukemia, there must be either a significant reduction in leukemia or no leukemia at the time of transplant).[36,69]

The patient must meet certain physical criteria to be eligible for a stem cell transplant. First, an evaluation of the patient's ability to manage activities of daily living is performed. Many transplant centers use the Eastern Cooperative Oncology Group (ECOG) scale to evaluate the performance status (Table 39-1).[89] Each transplant center has specific standards for this evaluation, but precise criteria must also be met.[89] For example, a patient must score a performance status of 0 to 2 on the ECOG scale to be eligible for a stem cell transplant.[89]

The patient must also pass a number of clinical tests within 1 month of the planned transplant. The patient must demonstrate an adequate left ventricular ejection fraction of at least 40% to 50% and pulmonary function tests that are more than 50% of the predicted value for the patient's age, height, and weight. These tests include forced vital capacity, forced expiratory volume in 1 second (FEV_1), and diffusing capacity.[89] Multiple laboratory studies are evaluated, including liver function tests and creatinine clearance.[36] Complete restaging of the patient's underlying disease is done within 1 month before the transplant. This could be accomplished using CT scans, positron-emission tomography scans, and bone marrow biopsies and aspirates. Finally, some centers also choose to require dental, nutritional, or neuropsychiatric evaluations.[89]

Many centers request a gynecologic evaluation for female patients. In addition, premenopausal females must undergo a pregnancy test immediately before starting the preparative regimen.[89] Many centers require that menstruating female patients receive hormone therapy for suppression of menses because menstrual blood loss when the patient is thrombocytopenic can be significant. At these centers, the patient will usually remain on menses suppression until the platelet count has stabilized without requiring platelet support.[7]

A complete social work evaluation is usually required.[89] One important function this provides is identification of the patient's primary caregiver and assistance in relocation when necessary. The patient and the caregiver are usually required to be within 30 minutes of the transplant center for a required length of time after the transplant; this requirement can be significantly extended if complications occur.[48]

TABLE 39-1 Eastern Cooperative Oncology Group Performance Status

GRADE	ECOG PERFORMANCE STATUS
0	Fully active, able to carry on all predisease performance without restriction
1	Restricted in physically strenuous activity but ambulatory and able to carry out work of a light or sedentary nature, e.g., light housework, office work
2	Ambulatory and capable of all self-care but unable to carry out any work activities; ambulatory more than 50% of waking hours
3	Capable of only limited self-care; confined to bed or chair more than 50% of waking hours
4	Completely disabled; cannot carry on any self-care; totally confined to bed or chair
5	Dead

ECOG = Eastern Cooperative Oncology Group.

Case Study 39-1, Part A

A Diagnosis of Acute Myelogenous Leukemia

J.H. is a 30-year-old female college student in her usual state of good health when she sought medical attention at the student health facility for flu-like symptoms for 2 to 3 weeks. Her specific complaints were cough, sore throat, runny nose, occipital lymphadenopathy, and fatigue. A CBC was drawn that was markedly abnormal. Her WBC was 77,000/mm³, Hct 30.4%, and platelet count 38,000/mm³. Other lab values were unremarkable except for a lactate dehydrogenase (LDH) of 719 units/L. Her past medical history was noncontributory, and her family history was notable for a paternal grandfather with myeloma and a paternal aunt with breast cancer. She has two full siblings. There was no history of smoking, illegal drug abuse, or alcohol abuse. She had no allergies to medicines and did not take any medications regularly except for acetaminophen or ibuprofen for infrequent headaches. She was admitted to the hospital for further evaluation because a hematologic malignancy was suspected. A bone marrow biopsy and aspirate showed acute myelogenous leukemia (AML).

The patient was treated with standard chemotherapy for her disease, which she tolerated well. During her 1-month stay in the hospital, the patient had minimal (grade 1) mucositis and neutropenic fevers. Her hospital course was otherwise unremarkable. A repeat bone marrow biopsy showed remission was achieved. She went on to receive further chemotherapy without significant complications. After her last round of chemotherapy, she underwent apheresis to collect autologous stem cells.

After initial diagnosis, the patient's siblings were evaluated for HLA compatibility. Unfortunately, neither was found to be a match and a search for an unrelated donor was started while the patient underwent consolidation (additional chemotherapy to put the patient in remission or minimal disease state before transplant). The patient was initially diagnosed in November and was admitted to the hospital in July of the following year for her matched unrelated stem cell transplant.

Decision point: Why did the patient with AML have her stem cells collected for an autologous PBSC transplant?

Decision point: Why were the parents or other family members not checked to see if they were a match before going to the unrelated donor?

Case continues on page 1052

Box 39-3

Preparative and Reduced-Intensity Regimens

COMMON PREPARATIVE REGIMENS

- Myeloablative regimens
- Cyclophosphamide (Cytoxan)/total body irradiation (Cy/TBI)
- Busulfan (Myleran)/cyclophosphamide (Cytoxan) (Bu/Cy); busulfan (Myleran)/melphalan (Alkeran)/thiotepa (Thioplex)/(BuMelt)
- Busulfan (Myleran)/etoposide (VePesid, VP-16)/ara-C (cytarabine)/melphalan (Alkeran) (BEAM)
- Busulfan (Myleran)/etoposide (VePesid, VP-16) (Bu/VP-16)
- High-dose melphalan (Alkeran)

REDUCED-INTENSITY REGIMENS

- Fludarabine (Fludara)/TBI (Flu/TBI)
- Busulfan (Myleran)/fludarabine (Fludara)/TBI (Bu/Flu/TBI)

Conditioning Regimen

The goals of the conditioning phase of the BMT are to treat the underlying disease and to prepare the patient for receiving the transplant.[46] The conditioning regimen eradicates disease and creates space in the bone marrow for the newly transplanted cells. The type of conditioning regimen is determined by the disease being treated, the age of the patient, and whether the transplant is allogeneic or autologous.[18] In the case of allogeneic transplant, the conditioning regimen is also immunosuppressive to allow engraftment of the donated cells. Autologous transplantation does not require immunosuppressive therapy. The conditioning regimen may be chemotherapy alone or in combination with total body irradiation (TBI).[18] Multiple conditioning regimens have been developed as a result of controlled clinical trial investigation; a list of common conditioning regimens is found in Box 39-3.

Conditioning regimens are varied and range from 2 to 8 days.[18] Although great strides have been made in controlling side effects/toxicities of chemotherapy and/or radiation, there can still be significant complications during the conditioning regimen and afterward. Aggressive symptom management for physical side effects and psychosocial support are essential during this period.[46] The terms *side effects* and *toxicities* are used interchangeably when discussing the effects of the preparative regimen.

For the average patient, the effect of the conditioning regimen on the bone marrow occurs within days.

Pancytopenia (leukopenia, anemia, and thrombocytopenia) usually occurs within 2 to 6 days of completion of the conditioning regimen.[18] The patient must be closely monitored for drug toxicities during this time, which may persist even after engraftment occurs.[46] Each chemotherapy agent is associated with specific toxicities. Common manifestations of toxicities include fever, mucositis, nausea, vomiting, skin changes, diarrhea, and bleeding. Specific chemotherapeutic agents and their toxicities are included in the Medication table on p. 1046.

All patients become pancytopenic and require varying degrees of blood product support.[18] Risk factors associated with reversible cytopenia after transplantation include preparative chemotherapy, bacterial and viral infection, septicemia, and GVHD.[8] Because allogeneic stem cell transplants require myeloablative conditioning regimens, they are associated with significant side effects.[8] When determining the maximum amount of chemotherapy that a patient can receive, the dosage is often limited by the effects on the marrow. When the patient's bone marrow is damaged beyond its ability to repair itself or requires a protracted amount of time to repair, the chemotherapy is considered myeloablative. Without rescue of the stem cells from either the patient (autologous) or the donor (allogeneic), the patient would die from marrow failure attributable to prolonged neutropenia, anemia, and thrombocytopenia.[25]

Many research studies are currently under way to evaluate transplant outcomes utilizing less toxic conditioning regimens, known as reduced-intensity transplants, mini-transplants, and midi-transplants. For these transplants, it is imperative that the patient be in

CHEMOTHERAPY AGENTS COMMONLY USED IN BONE MARROW TRANSPLANT PREPARATIVE REGIMENS

DRUG	CLASSIFICATION	METABOLISM	TOXICITY
Busulfan (Busulfex)	Alkylating agent	Liver	Myelosuppression Nausea/vomiting Mucositis Hyperpigmentation of skin Hepatotoxicity
Cytarabine (ara-C)	Antimetabolite	Liver, plasma	Myelosuppression Nausea/vomiting Erythema of skin Painful hand-foot syndrome (rare) Cerebral ataxia Lethargy Pulmonary complications Erythema of skin Alopecia
Cyclophosphamide (Cytoxan)	Alkylating agent	Liver	Myelosuppression Hemorrhagic cystitis Dysuria Alopecia Nausea/vomiting Hypersensitivity reaction with rhinitis Cardiac toxicity
Etoposide (VePesid, VP-16)	Topoisomerase II inhibitor	Liver	Myelosuppression Nausea/vomiting, anorexia Alopecia Mucositis Diarrhea
Fludarabine (Fludara)	Antimetabolite	Nucleoside transport system	Myelosuppression Immunosuppression Nausea/vomiting (mild) Fever
Melphalan (Alkeran)	Alkylating agent	Blood	Myelosuppression Mucositis
Thiotepa (Thioplex)	Alkylating agent	Urine	Myelosuppression Nausea/vomiting, anorexia

remission or have a low tumor burden because the conditioning regimen is based more on immunosuppression and emptying marrow space than on disease control.[8] The common goal of these more conservative regimens is to minimize the stress to the patient without compromising eradication of the disease. These regimens are more geared toward preparing the marrow site rather than treating the disease and use the new immune system to abolish the underlying malignancy. The ability of the new immune system to treat the underlying malignancy is commonly referred to as *graft-versus-tumor effect* and occurs in allogeneic stem cell transplants.[34]

Donor Evaluation

Compatibility between donor and recipient is essential to minimize the potential of GVHD, graft rejection, and graft failure. The primary criterion for suitable donor identification in allogeneic transplants is HLA compatibility. The set of genes that determines an individual's HLA type is known as the major histocompatibility complex and is found on human chromosome 6.[42] Blood type and Rh factor are not criteria for determining eligibility of a donor. Other factors taken into consideration are the age of the donor, gender, parity, and history of infectious diseases.[42] There is no age limit in the evaluation of a donor, but consideration of underlying health issues is essential. The donor must be able to undergo either a surgical procedure (bone marrow harvest) or apheresis with colony-stimulating therapy for collection of peripheral stem cells. Any person with a history of a hematologic malignancy is not a candidate to become a donor.[89] Other required tests include screening for infectious disease. Donors are screened for multiple viruses such as human immunodeficiency virus (HIV), cytomegalovirus (CMV), herpes simplex virus (HSV), varicella-zoster virus (VZV), Epstein-Barr virus (EBV), hepatitis (A, B, C), and syphilis (by rapid plasma reagin). A past exposure to a virus does not necessarily prohibit the person from becoming a donor, but the recipient must be informed of the risk of possible disease transmission. Some centers will use donors with active hepatitis C, depending on the viral load. The only current absolute contraindication is HIV.[89]

Stem Cell Harvesting, Mobilization, and Collection

The three sources for stem cells include peripheral blood, bone marrow, and umbilical cord blood. It is unclear if there is a distinct advantage of one source over the other. Presently, a stage III multicenter randomized clinical trial by the Blood and Marrow Transplant Clinical Trials Network is evaluating if there is survival benefit for peripheral blood versus bone marrow as the source of hematopoietic stem cells. This study compares colony-stimulating factor–mobilized peripheral stem cell transplants to bone marrow transplants in HLA-matched unrelated donors.[27] This is an important study because existing data are only retrospective.

CD-34+ antigen is a marker located on the surface of stem cells. When collecting stem cells, each center has a defined goal of the number of CD-34+ cells per kilogram of recipient weight. The absolute minimal requirement for optimal engraftment is unknown.[18] If the collection is for autologous stem cell transplant, the cells are immediately cryopreserved with dimethyl sulfoxide (DMSO) solution and stored in liquid nitrogen until the recipient is ready for infusion.[33] Cells collected for allogeneic transplant are transported to the location of the recipient as quickly as possible following harvest, often across long distances if the unrelated donor is from another country.

Apheresis of Peripheral Blood. PBSCs are collected from the blood by a process known as apheresis,[4] which is usually performed in an inpatient or outpatient apheresis clinic. Apheresis is accomplished by removing whole blood from the donor's IV line and passing it through a centrifuge where the stem cells are removed. The remainder of the person's blood is then returned through a second IV line. The donor undergoes apheresis once daily until an adequate number of cells for transplantation are collected. Most healthy donors can have enough stem cells collected in one or two sessions.[61]

Because stem cells are not overly abundant in the peripheral blood, colony-stimulating factors such as granulocyte colony-stimulating factor (G-CSF) or granulocytic macrophage colony-stimulating factor must be given before collection to drive the hematopoietic stem cells into the peripheral circulation. This process is called mobilization.[61] For autologous collection, the stem cells are usually collected following a round of chemotherapy used for both mobilization and tumor reduction. In allogeneic collection, for siblings and matched unrelated donors, growth factors alone are used for mobilization. Growth factors are given daily by subcutaneous injection for 5 days before the collection occurs.[6]

There are instances when collection of stem cells can be difficult. This occurs most often in patients who have been exposed to multiple previous chemotherapy regimens. Investigational drugs are currently being studied to promote the mobilization of stem cells into the peripheral blood to enhance collection.[44]

Harvesting of Bone Marrow. Collection of stem cells from the bone marrow is accomplished by a bone marrow harvest performed in the operating room using general anesthesia. The procedure usually takes 1 to 2 hours; the donor may require hospitalization overnight for observation. Approximately 1 to 1.5 L of marrow is removed, depending on the percentage of stem cells in the collection and the body weight of the recipient.[33] Marrow collected from the harvest is processed to remove fat and bone particles in the cell processing lab and then transported to the recipient's location. The donor may experience pain at the harvest site; pain management is required. Occasionally, the donor may need a blood transfusion after donation, but often the patient can regenerate the blood withdrawn and requires only iron supplementation.[33]

Collection of Umbilical Cord Blood. Parents must be approached before delivery for permission to collect umbilical blood for donation. Immediately after delivery, the umbilical cord and the placenta are drained of blood into a special bag or into syringes provided by the umbilical cord storage facility. After transportation to the storage facility, the product is frozen using the same process as with autologous stem cell collection.[63] Because the number of stem cells is limited, the recipient of the umbilical cord stem cell transplant is usually a child or a smaller adult.[4]

TRANSPLANTATION AND ENGRAFTMENT

Bone marrow infusions and stem cell infusions are performed by specially trained BMT nursing staff. Dedicated BMT centers have policies and procedures for infusion procedures and typically require the presence of a bone marrow transplant physician, physician assistant, or nurse practitioner during all or part of the stem cell infusion. The actual infusion of stem cells is a relatively simple procedure.

Autologous stem cells are thawed immediately before infusion. Patients are premedicated with medications such as acetaminophen (Tylenol), diphenhydramine (Benadryl), and hydrocortisone (Solu-Cortef) to prevent allergic reactions or anaphylaxis. Patients are also prehydrated to maintain renal perfusion. Dopamine (Intropin) is readily available at the bedside in the event of hypotension during the autologous stem cell infusion.[33] Cells are infused into a central venous catheter over 15 to 60 minutes, depending on the total volume of the product. The transplant is performed on the BMT ward per institution protocols. Some centers require bedside cardiac monitoring while others do not. Vital signs, including heart rate, blood pressure, respiratory rate, and pulse oximetry, are monitored closely throughout the infusion. Temperature is generally recorded as with all blood product infusions.[33]

Patients are closely monitored for complications that occur immediately following the transfusion. Following large-volume stem cell infusions, pulmonary edema or volume overload can occur; respiratory rate and oxygen saturation should be closely monitored along with assessment for jugular venous distention, dyspnea, cough, and adventitious lung sounds.[66] Patients are at risk for an acute hemolytic transfusion reaction if they are receiving stem cells from an ABO-mismatched donor and require close monitoring for symptoms suggestive of this adverse reaction (Chapter 36).[33] Other side effects can include dry cough, flushing, nausea/vomiting, hypotension, bradycardia, and heart block. In rare circumstances, severe reactions of anaphylaxis and flash pulmonary edema have been reported.[53] Most of these side effects can be attributed to the DMSO used in the cryopreservation process. Other common side effects from DMSO include garlic-like taste and odor.[30] Although in some centers this is washed out to minimize

the potential side effects, the transplant nurse must be aware of these potential severe adverse events.

As with any blood product, the patient may experience infusion-related reactions, which can occur following both autologous and allogeneic transplantation. Signs of infusion-related reaction include headache, nausea/vomiting, abdominal cramping, bradycardia, fever, flushing, and hypertension.[29] Life-threatening reactions may result in temporarily stopping the infusion, stabilizing the patient, and possibly transferring the patient to a critical care unit. Once the patient is stabilized, the remainder of the stem cells are infused. Without infusion of an appropriate quantity of stem cells, the patient could experience significant delay in engraftment or even failure to engraft. Patients who experience failure to engraft, or significant delay in engraftment, have a 70% to 80% mortality rate because of the prolonged time the patient is pancytopenic.[46]

After the day of transplant (day 0), the patient will begin to experience effects of the conditioning regimen, including pancytopenia.[46] During the immediate posttransplant period, the patient is monitored closely with daily laboratory analysis (including complete blood cell count [CBC], electrolytes, blood urea nitrogen, creatinine, and liver function panel), vital sign monitoring, and physical assessment. All transplant patients are closely observed for signs of infection, bleeding, neurologic changes, and cardiovascular and respiratory compromise.[46]

Stem cells migrate to the marrow within 24 hours of infusion to begin the recovery of marrow function. Recovery of marrow function is called engraftment.[46] Initial signs of engraftment are improvement in CBC and, more specifically, the white blood cell (WBC) count starts to rise.[46] In a study of lymphoma patients, the median time to see early evidence of engraftment is 11 days after infusion of peripheral stem cells and 14 days after infusion of marrow.[54] Factors influencing engraftment include the dose of stem cells infused, source of stem cells, underlying disease (particularly in autologous transplant), posttransplant immunosuppressive therapy, and splenomegaly.[8]

Although patients have an absolute neutrophil count (ANC) of zero, they are very vulnerable to infections.[24] Toxicities of the conditioning regimens are also a concern, and require close assessment and intervention. The patient usually remains hospitalized during this time, although there is a growing trend to perform autologous stem cell transplants in the outpatient setting as much as possible. Reduced-intensity transplants are usually done on an outpatient basis unless there is a complication. Most of these patients need to be seen on a daily basis and are required to live within 30 minutes of the transplant facility. A decrease in hospital days was demonstrated when the conditioning regimens and transplant were performed in the ambulatory setting. However, this practice did not prevent admission to the hospital when complications occurred.[34]

Engraftment usually occurs approximately 9 to 14 days after infusion of stem cells.[54] In general, the WBC count increases over several days until the patient achieves a normal white blood cell count. Growth factors (e.g., G-CSF) are commonly used in myeloablative stem cell transplants to hasten white blood cell recovery.[8] Because the effect of the conditioning regimen on the WBC count can be quite subtle in reduced-intensity transplants, growth factors are not typically used for these transplants. At times it is difficult to absolutely determine the time of engraftment.[34] For myeloablative stem cell transplants, engraftment is easily determined because patients have a negligible WBC count for several days. Typically, the WBCs are the first to rise, followed days to weeks later by the red blood cells (RBCs) and the platelets.[8] The allogeneic patient will often still require blood product support after discharge from the hospital.[46]

PSYCHOSOCIAL IMPLICATIONS

Psychosocial support of the patient and the designated caregiver is essential throughout the entire transplant course. The experience of transplant, the extensive hospital course, and also the side effects of multiple medication regimens can be emotionally challenging and exhausting for the patient with a profound effect on the family and other support systems.[32] Inpatient and outpatient support and intervention from a dedicated BMT social worker are necessary.[51] Many centers offer prehospitalization information and/or classes to prepare the patient and caregiver for the transplant and provide them with written material and notebooks. Support groups are often available for the entire transplant process to enhance coping skills of the patients and caregivers.[75]

In the past, isolation from family and friends was an issue. However, patients are no longer placed in isolation, and are allowed visitors. Visitors are restricted only if they show signs of illness. Caregivers stay with the patient during hospitalization and assist with primary care needs; they are encouraged to participate in educational instruction sessions, particularly those related to discharge preparation.[32] Despite vigorous efforts to engage caregivers in discharge education, caregivers often do not remember all that was taught. Provision of written discharge materials and contact information is essential in the event of questions and emergencies.[48]

If the BMT patient should require critical care, it is important that the family maintain contact with the BMT social worker who has worked with them throughout the hospital and pretransplant period for ongoing support.[48] Critical care visiting hour restrictions and routines may limit caregivers' ability to be with their loved ones; this can be quite difficult as they are routinely encouraged to stay with the patient as much as possible during the transplant hospitalization. The critical care nurse should acknowledge the active participation of the family member in the patient's care and adjust visiting policies as needed.

The long-term prognosis for BMT patients when they require critical care intervention varies. If the patient requires intubation and has multisystem organ dysfunction, the mortality rate is very high. Statistics vary from institution to institution; however, the increases in survival are believed to be related to advances in care and an improved pretransplant selection bias. This topic is discussed in the Research Utilization box below.[64]

◆ RESEARCH UTILIZATION

Evaluation of Survival of Hematopoietic Stem Cell Transplant Patients Who Required Critical Care

STUDY METHOD

This study was a retrospective multicenter analysis.

CLINICAL ISSUE

Historically, hematopoietic stem cell transplant (HSCT) patients who require transfer to the critical care unit have done poorly. However, the trends are changing and continued examination of what type of complications require transfer to the critical care unit and their outcome is imperative to help guide decisions in transferring patients.

SUMMARY

This study evaluated the survival rates of HSCT patients who required transfer to the critical care unit between 1997 and 2003. This included both patients during the engraftment period (<30-days posttransplant) and after engraftment. Two hundred and nine patients were evaluated and survival rates from critical care through a 1-year survival were compared. Multiple factors were evaluated. It was found that mechanical ventilation, hyperbilirubinemia, and active graft-versus-host disease were independent predictors of mortality. Also noted was that patients who were admitted during the engraftment period had an improved survival rate as compared to patients admitted with late complications of HSCT.

Continues on page 1050

◆ RESEARCH UTILIZATION—CONT'D

APPLICATION

The study showed that survival rates for HSCT patients admitted to the critical care unit were improving and that aggressive care is justified. Also shown was poor outcome for patients with late complications of HSCT who required mechanical ventilation.

NEED FOR FURTHER STUDY

This study shows that survival is improving in the HSCT patient who requires critical care unit care. Further evaluation in larger studies would be beneficial in helping to determine more predictors of outcome in these patients.

Pene, F., et al. (2006). Outcome of critically ill allogeneic hematopoietic stem-cell transplantation recipients: a reappraisal of indications for organ failure supports. *J Clin Oncol, 24*(4), 643–649.

Frequent discussions with patients and families are needed throughout the transplant course and as complications and life-threatening events occur. Discussion concerning advance directives should occur before hospitalization for every transplant patient. Many patients embark on the transplant process with a high level of hope and initially want everything done to achieve remission of their disease. Typical BMT patients are young to middle-aged adults with young families who desire aggressive intervention. However, the transplant process is a high-risk procedure and the patient and family must be informed of the considerable risks and mortality.[48] When patients require critical care admission, it is important for the critical care nurse to ensure the advance directives are addressed in the patient's care plan, as illustrated in the sample Multidisciplinary Plan of Care below. Conversations and decisions can be difficult because even though the patient may be cancer free from the conditioning and transplant process, the patient may be suffering from the sometimes irreversible effects of toxicities or complications.[46]

MULTIDISCIPLINARY PLAN OF CARE FOR PATIENTS UNDERGOING BONE MARROW TRANSPLANTATION

PROBLEM	INTERVENTION	RATIONALE	EXPECTED OUTCOME	COMMENTS
Impaired airway: respiratory failure	Identify HSCT patients at risk for impaired airway: • Excessive respiratory secretions compromising respiratory effort related to grade 4 mucositis • Altered level of consciousness because of medications (analgesics, anxiolytics) or neurologic event (CVA, intracranial bleed) Monitor respiratory status: • Monitor RR and oxygen saturation every 1–2 hours as indicated by clinical condition Provide airway control: • Elevate HOB • Swallowing evaluation, if indicated • Have suction available at bedside • Assist with intubation and support mechanical ventilation, as needed Provide pulmonary care: • Encourage ambulation if appropriate • Encourage incentive spirometry • Assess patient's ability to clear airway	Identification of patients at risk for airway compromise is essential to prevent possible complications. Secretion control in the patient with severe mucositis is essential to minimize risk of aspiration.	Patient will have appropriate control of airway. Patient will avoid aspiration. Protection of airway will occur before patient is in respiratory distress.	Pain management is essential in mucositis patients. Management of secretions is also imperative; can be either copious from poor ability to swallow or thick and tenacious from poorly functioning saliva glands.

PROBLEM	INTERVENTION	RATIONALE	EXPECTED OUTCOME	COMMENTS
Increased risk of infection	Monitor patients for early signs of infection: • Temperature check every 4 hours • Notify team of first temperature of 100.4° F immediately • Follow standing orders for neutropenic fevers • Monitor skin for changes consistent with infection • Monitor central line insertion site and change dressings according to protocol • Protect patient from any visitors who appear infected	Early identification of patients with infection affects survival of neutropenic immunosuppressed patients.	Patient will have immediate intervention when infection is suspected. Team will be notified immediately. Antibiotics will be initiated within 1 hour of first fever in neutropenic patient.	Staff or visitors with contagious infections should not interact with patient.
Risk of bleeding	Monitor thrombocytopenic patients for signs of bleeding: • Test stools for occult blood • Neuro checks every shift and as indicated by clinical condition; notify team of change in level of consciousness immediately • Minimize invasive procedures, e.g., needle sticks, intramuscular injections, insertion of tubes • Avoid anticoagulation in patient with platelet count less than 50,000/mm^3	Early intervention of thrombocytopenic patient who has hemorrhage will improve outcomes.	Patients at risk for bleeding will be identified and appropriate interventions will be initiated.	
Knowledge deficit of plan of care	Identify patients at risk: • Newly diagnosed patient • Learning deficit Educate patient and family: • Neutropenic precautions • Bleeding precautions • Infection risks • Provide written material when appropriate	Education of patients and family members increases compliance with interventions.	Increased knowledge and understanding of treatment plan will result in effective coping and compliance with care.	
Impaired oral mucosa	Identify patients at risk: • Patients with preparative regimens that make them at risk for mucositis • Patients unable to perform adequate oral care • Patients unable to take in adequate oral fluids or nutrition due to pain issues Monitor patient by: • Documenting pain level with vital signs • Assessing oral mucosa every 4 hours and documenting interventions	Identification of patients with mucositis is imperative for providing adequate pain management and symptom control. Also important to assist in identifying patients potentially at risk for nutritional issues.	Patient will have adequate pain control of oral discomfort. Patient will have access to topical therapy and saline rinses for oral cavity. Patient will be offered appropriate food sources during periods of mucositis.	

Table continues on page 1052

PROBLEM	INTERVENTION	RATIONALE	EXPECTED OUTCOME	COMMENTS
	• Providing interventions for pain control, topical versus systemic pain management • Offering food supplements or soft foods			
Anxiety/ emotional support	Identify patients at risk: • Newly diagnosed patient • Post-BMT procedure patient • Lack of support system Support patient: • Allow caregiver to remain with patient when possible • Involve caregiver in plan of care • Assure patient and family that BMT guidelines are being followed and BMT team involved in care	Decreasing anxiety promotes improved ability to cope with complications. Allowing caregivers to continue to participate in care will decrease their anxiety.	Anxiety related to need for critical care unit stay will be minimized. Psychological interventions will be initiated when anxiety level assessed as increased.	

Data from references 1 and 45.
BMT = Bone marrow transplant, CVA = cerebrovascular accident, HOB = head of bed, HSCT = hematopoietic stem cell transplant, RR = respiratory rate.

The transplant team is also vulnerable to burnout and a feeling of hopelessness. Care of the complex bone marrow transplant patient and the degree of emotional support needed by this patient population take a toll on staff. Many are not aware of the effects of this burden and experience burnout, resulting in absenteeism, a lack of passion, and loss of interest in their jobs.[48] BMT team members do not often have the opportunity to express grief following patient death. Many patients die after they have been discharged from the hospital from relapse or complications from GVHD or sepsis. It is crucial for critical care staff to notify the BMT team of patient deaths so that they may participate in memorial services if they desire. Formalized bereavement programs assist BMT and critical care staff in dealing with the loss of their patients. Encouraging patients who have recovered from a critical care unit stay to later visit the unit can be beneficial both to the staff and to the patient.[48]

◆ Case Study 39-1, Part B

A Diagnosis of Acute Myelogenous Leukemia

The preparative regimen for the patient's MUD PBSC transplant was TBI and cyclophosphamide. The patient did well through the preparative regimen. By day +5 following the transplant, the patient had grade 3 mucositis. This required a PCA pump for pain management and initiation of TPN. When steroids were added on day +7 per protocol for GVHD prophylaxis, the patient became hyperglycemic and required insulin therapy. On day +8 she also developed her first neutropenic fever, and imipenem (Primaxin) was started according to protocol. Within 36 hours, the patient became tachycardic and hypotensive. Despite aggressive fluid resuscitation of 2 liters of IV fluid, her mean arterial pressure remained less than 50 mm Hg, requiring critical care admission for further fluid resuscitation and vasopressor support. At the time of transfer, the patient's blood cultures were repeated as well as her CXR. Because of her severe mucositis and continued fever, vancomycin (Vanocin) was added to give her better gram-positive coverage. The CXR done on admission to the critical care unit was without evidence of pneumonia, but admission blood cultures showed gram-positive streptococci in clusters.

Decision point: Why was vancomycin added before culture results were obtained?

Decision point: What other types of infections would the patient be at risk for acquiring?

Decision point: What special considerations related to her transplant need to be in place for this patient during critical care resuscitation?

Case continues on page 1061

COMPLICATIONS OF TRANSPLANT

There are multiple complications that are common in stem cell transplant patients. They are exposed to many toxic agents and experience significant damage to their immune systems while going through the transplant process, making them susceptible to life-threatening complications that frequently require transfer to critical care. Every attempt is made to keep these patients on the BMT ward; however, GVHD, infection, excessive bleeding, and metabolic and neurologic complications are common and require the expertise of the critical care team.

Graft-Versus-Host Disease

GVHD, unique to allogeneic HSCT, occurs when the infused donor stem cells recognize the recipient as foreign tissue. There are two forms of GVHD: acute GVHD (aGVHD) and chronic GVHD (cGVHD). There is a 9% to 50% incidence of GVHD in allogeneic stem cell transplants, with a higher incidence in MUD stem cell transplants.[22] In general terms, aGVHD occurs within the first 100 days of transplant and cGVHD occurs after the 100-day mark.[23] This is an arbitrary timeline; the clinical presentation is the determining factor. GVHD is a serious complication, with mortality rates as high as 50% directly or indirectly related to GVHD.[85] Risk factors other than histoincompatibility include gender mismatch, donor parity, age of the donor, posttransplant viral infections, and use of donor lymphocyte infusions posttransplant.[21]

Surprisingly, effects of GVHD can also have a positive feature. In retrospective data analysis of allogeneic transplant leukemia patients (e.g., chronic myeloid leukemia in chronic phase and acute myeloid leukemia/acute lymphoblastic leukemia transplanted in first remission), the IBMTR noted a statistically significant decrease in relapse of patients who experienced GVHD.[21] This was attributed to the graft-versus-leukemia (GVL) effect, in which immunocompetent donor cells recognize and eliminate the malignant cells.[60] In contrast, there is a high incidence of relapse in autologous transplanted patients because the transplanted cells originate from the donor, and thus GVL cannot occur.[21]

Because of the high mortality with GVHD, all allogeneic stem cell transplant patients are placed on GVHD prophylaxis.[31] Without any immunosuppressive therapy, all patients would die from GVHD. Each center has protocols for prophylaxis, with the most common approach to use a p-glycoprotein inhibitor (cyclosporine or tacrolimus [Prograf, FK-506]) and methotrexate (Folex, Rheumatrex). Many centers also add a third line of immunosuppression with steroids (prednisone). Over time, the immunosuppressive therapy is tapered off as tolerated over months.[20] During this time, the patient is assessed frequently for the flare-ups of GVHD.[21]

aGVHD occurs within the first 100 days posttransplant and can involve the skin, liver, or GI system. It must be treated aggressively as it is often life threatening.[21] A standard grading scale is used to determine the grade of skin, gut, and liver involvement (Table 39-2). aGVHD may involve only one system, but often presents with involvement of more than one system. In general, the more systems affected, the higher the level of aGVHD. The overall grade is determined by another scale, which combines the three body systems (Table 39-3). Grades 3 and 4 GVHD can be very hard to control with immunosuppressive medicines and at times are not reversible.[31] Because of the high doses of immunosuppressive medications required to treat this disease, the patient has a much higher risk of infectious complications and a significant increase in mortality.[40]

Skin aGVHD presents as a rash that ranges from mild erythema involving the neck, ears, and palms of hands/soles of feet to epidermal necrolysis resembling a third-degree burn.[41] Diagnosis is done by clinical presentation and a skin biopsy. Early intervention is imperative. If the clinical suspicion for aGVHD is high, topical steroid therapy is initiated while awaiting biopsy results; if presentation is severe, systemic steroid therapy is required.[73]

TABLE 39-2 Clinical Staging of Acute Graft-Versus-Host Disease

STAGE	SKIN	LIVER (BILIRUBIN)	GUT
+	Maculopapular rash on <25% of body surface	2–3 mg/dl	Diarrhea 500–1000 ml/day or persistent nausea
++	Maculopapular rash on 25%–50% of body surface	3–6 mg/dl	Diarrhea 1000–1500 ml/day
+++	Generalized erythroderma	6–15 mg/dl	Diarrhea >1500 ml/day
++++	Desquamation and bullae	>15 mg/dl	Pain with or without ileus

Data from reference 72.

TABLE 39-3 Clinical Grading of Acute Graft-Versus-Host Disease*

	Stage			
OVERALL GRADE	SKIN	LIVER	GUT	FUNCTIONAL IMPAIRMENT
0 (None)	0	0	0	0
1 (Mild)	+ to ++	0	0	0
2 (Moderate)	+ to +++	+	+	+
3 (Severe)	++ to +++	++ to +++	++ to +++	++
4 (Life threatening)	++ to ++++	++ to ++++	++ to ++++	+++

Data from reference 72.
*Chronic graft-versus-host disease has manifestations similar to those of systemic progressive sclerosis, systemic lupus erythematosus, lichen planus, Sjögren's syndrome, eosinophilic fasciitis, rheumatoid arthritis, and primary biliary cirrhosis. Median day of diagnosis in human leukocyte antigen (HLA)-identical sibling recipients is 201 days after transplant; it is earlier (159 and 133 days, respectively) in HLA-nonidentical related and unrelated donor marrow recipients. Staging and classification help predict prognosis.

Gut aGVHD manifests with nausea, vomiting, or diarrhea. The diagnosis is made from clinical presentation, but biopsy via endoscopy is important to rule out an infectious etiology. The symptoms are usually not subtle and can be very difficult to control. Patients with gut aGVHD can have 2 to 5 L of stool daily;[42] therefore aggressive fluid repletion and electrolyte management are extremely important. If the symptoms are severe, the patient requires hospitalization and total parenteral nutrition (TPN) support is often necessary. Medications may need to be given intravenously until the symptoms are under control. Use of oral medications should be minimized because of stimulation of the gastrointestinal tract in addition to poor absorption.[41]

Liver aGVHD is noted almost exclusively by lab changes as jaundice is the only clinical finding. Elevated levels of bilirubin in the blood, with or without elevated levels of transaminases or alkaline phosphatase, is the typical lab value noted; diagnosis is made through a liver biopsy.[31] This is often a risky procedure, depending on the patient's coagulation studies and platelet requirements. A transjugular liver biopsy is often the preferred method of obtaining a biopsy to minimize blood loss.[41] The procedure is not without risk, however, so is done only if clinically necessary. If biopsy-proven GVHD exists in another system, the liver biopsy is often deferred.[31]

Medical management of aGVHD can be very difficult. The first line of treatment is aggressive steroid therapy, with starting doses ranging from 1 to 10 mg/kg/day, as shown in the Medication table below and on p. 1055. Prednisone is used if the patient can take medications orally; methylprednisolone is substituted if malabsorption is a risk factor. If the patient does not respond to therapy within 1 week, the patient is considered a nonresponder and attempts are made at using other immunosuppressive agents, but none have shown significant clinical benefit.[31] Grade 2–4 (overall) GVHD is associated with a high mortality rate.[21]

MEDICATIONS COMMONLY USED IN CARE OF THE HSCT PATIENT

DRUG	ACTION	INDICATION AND USUAL DOSAGE	SPECIAL CONSIDERATIONS
GVHD Prophylaxis Corticosteroids (methylprednisolone, prednisone)	See Chapter 18	*GVHD prophylaxis:* Variable: typical starting dose 0.5 mg/kg/day; can be split between 2 doses *GVHD treatment:* Variable: typical starting dose 1–10 mg/kg/day[31]	See Chapter 18

DRUG	ACTION	INDICATION AND USUAL DOSAGE	SPECIAL CONSIDERATIONS
Cyclosporine (Gengraf, Neoral)	See Chapter 18	Starting dose usually 3–5 mg/kg IV twice daily, then titrated for desirable trough[21] Converted to oral dosing when patient able to take PO meds	See Chapter 18
Tacrolimus (Prograf, FK 506)	See Chapter 18	Starting dose is 0.03–0.05 IV bid, titrated for desirable trough[21] Converted to oral dosing when patient able to take PO meds	See Chapter 18
Methotrexate (Folex, Rheumatrex)	Inhibits conversion of folic acid to tetrahydrofolic acid; inhibits precursors to DNA, RNA, and cellular proteins[67,88]	15 mg/m^2 IVP on day +1, 10 mg/m^2 IVP on day +3 and day +6, may also have final dose on day +10[21]	Dose to be adjusted for severe mucositis, renal or liver insufficiency[21] Effects reversed by leucovorin if necessary[67]
Growth Factors Filgrastim (Neupogen, G-CSF)	Stimulates production of neutrophils in bone marrow[88]	5 mcg/kg/day subcutaneous or IV[88] For stem cell mobilization: 10 mcg/kg/day subcutaneously[88]	Monitor for bone pain
Sargramostim (Leukine, GM-CSF)	Stimulates production of monocytes and macrophages; also induces production of cytokines[88]	250 mcg/m^2/day IV or subcutaneously[88]	Monitor for fevers, fatigue, myalgia, arthralgia, headache[88]

Data from references 21, 31, 67, and 88.
DNA = Deoxyribonucleic acid, G-CSF = granulocyte colony-stimulating factor, GM-CSF = granulocyte macrophage colony-stimulating factor, GVHD = graft-versus-host disease, RNA = ribonucleic acid.

cGVHD usually occurs in patients who have had aGVHD, although it may occur without aGVHD.[43] cGVHD occurs at least 100 days after transplantation and may occur many years after transplant.[85] Because GVHD is associated with graft-versus-disease effect, cGVHD is believed to be one of the most important factors in long-term disease-free survival. This comes at a cost, however, because GVHD has immunosuppressive qualities and requires long-term immunosuppressive therapy, putting the patient at high risk for increased mortality from infection.[95]

Like aGVHD, cGVHD can affect the skin, gut, or liver (Table 39-4). The symptoms and screening studies, however, are different from the acute phase (Table 39-5). For example, skin changes are usually lichen planus (shiny reddish-purple flat bumps[6]) and the cutaneous presentation of scleroderma. The skin also shows evidence of epidermal hypertrophy and atrophic dermis.[41] Liver cGVHD is associated with elevated levels of alkaline phosphatase with or without transaminase. Gut cGVHD symptoms include nausea, vomiting, and diarrhea, although the presentation may be much more subtle than in aGVHD. Anorexia, progressive weight loss, and dysphagia may also be present. Alterations in the oral mucosa range from mild lichen planus on the buccal membranes to ulceration.[95] Biopsy is recommended for diagnosis of GVHD because even though it is more common to have only one body system involved, cGVHD can be present in multiple organs at the same time. Other forms of cGVHD involve the lungs, vagina, eyes (sicca syndrome), and kidneys (nephritic syndrome).[41]

Treatment decisions for cGVHD are based on severity of involvement and whether one organ or multiple organ systems are affected.[59] First-line medications

TABLE 39-4 Clinicopathologic Classification of Chronic Graft-Versus-Host Disease*

CLASSIFICATION	CLINICOPATHOLOGY
Limited	**Either or both of the following:** Localized skin involvement Hepatic dysfunction because of chronic GVHD
Extensive	**Either of the following:** Generalized skin involvement Localized skin involvement or hepatic dysfunction because of chronic GVHD **Plus one of the following:** Liver histology showing chronic aggressive hepatitis, bridging necrosis, or cirrhosis Involvement of eye (Schirmer's test with <5-mm wetting) Involvement of minor salivary glands or oral mucosa demonstrated on labial biopsy Involvement of any other target organ

Data from reference 9.
*Different screening studies have been used to help in diagnosis and staging of chronic GVHD.
GVHD = Graft-versus-host disease.

TABLE 39-5 Screening Studies for Graft-Versus-Host Disease

ORGAN OR SYSTEM	CLINICAL FINDINGS	SCREENING STUDIES
Dermal	Dyspigmentation Xerosis Erythema Scleroderma Onychodystrophy Alopecia	Skin biopsy (3-mm punch biopsy from back and forearm areas)
Oral	Lichen planus Xerostomia	Oral biopsy from lower lip
Ocular	Sicca Keratitis	#1 Schirmer's test
Hepatic	Jaundice	Alkaline phosphatase AST Bilirubin
Pulmonary	Obstructive/restrictive lung disease	Pulmonary function studies Arterial blood gas
Vaginal	Sicca Atrophy	Gynecologic evaluation
Nutritional	Protein and calorie deficiency	Weight Muscle/fat store measurement
Clinical performance	Contractures Debility	Karnofsky score Lansky play index

Data from reference 58.
AST = Aspartate aminotransferase.

used for cGVHD are the same as those for aGVHD. P-glycoprotein inhibitors and steroid therapy are commonly used, and mycophenolate (CellCept) is often added. Extracorporeal photopheresis (ECP) is often tried if the disease is extensive. ECP is a pheresis procedure that exposes a percentage of the lymphocytes to methoxypsoralen. These lymphocytes then undergo ultraviolet irradiation. This process has been shown to decrease the immune activity of the lymphocytes after being returned to the central circulation. The exact method by which this procedure improves cGVHD is not known.[10] ECP appears to be most effective in skin cGVHD, but is sometimes tried with other types of cGVHD.[31]

Infection

Infection is a very common posttransplant complication and is due to multiple factors including underlying disease, host flora, and pretreatment infections.[17]

The patient is at the highest risk for bacterial and fungal infections when neutrophils are at their lowest concentration. Neutropenia can occur at varying times during the stem cell transplant course, but is always present during a myeloablative transplant before engraftment and can last for several days to weeks.[24] Assessment of the patient for neutropenia requires

calculation of an ANC. Neutropenia occurs when the ANC drops below 1500 mm^3 (Box 39-4).[28] Risk factors for neutropenia are listed in Box 39-5. Sepsis is a common reason for admission of the BMT patient to critical care and is associated with a high mortality rate.[64] The conditioning regimen results in the absence of WBCs, including granulocytes, monocytes/macrophages, and lymphocytes, making the patient vulnerable to infection. Immunosuppressive therapy, necessary to prevent and to treat GVHD, also contributes to patient susceptibility to infection.[76] In addition, the patient faces different infectious risks depending on whether the patient is in the preengraftment, postengraftment, or late postengraftment phase of the transplant course.[17]

During the preengraftment stage (i.e., the time from the conditioning regimen until the time of engraftment), major infection risk factors are bacterial infections from

Box 39-4

Absolute Neutrophil Count Calculation

To calculate an ANC, a CBC with a differential is needed.

ANC FORMULA

Add the percentage of polymorphonuclear cells (or neutrophils) and the bands (or segs) together; then multiply by the total number of WBCs.

For example, CBC with WBC of 3200/mm^3, neutrophils 28%, bands 2%:

$$28 + 2 = 30\% \times 3.2 = \text{ANC of } 1000 \text{ mm}^3$$

Data from reference 88.
ANC = Absolute neutrophil count, CBC = complete blood cell count, WBC = white blood cells.

Box 39-5

Neutropenia Risk

- Mild neutropenia: ANC falls between 1800 and 1000/mm^3
- Moderate neutropenia: ANC falls between 500 and 1000/mm^3
- Severe neutropenia: ANC falls below 500/mm^3

Data from reference 28.
ANC = Absolute neutrophil count.

mucositis and breaks in the skin barrier from central lines. The most common bacteria seen are coagulase-negative staphylococci, *Staphylococcus aureus*, *Viridans streptococci*, *Pseudomonas aeruginosa*, Enterobacteriaceae, and *Stenotrophomonas maltophilia*. In addition, the patient is at risk from fungal infections such as *Candida albicans*, *Candida glabrata*, and *Candida krusei*. Other fungal infections can come from mold such as *Aspergillus*, *Fusarium*, and Zygomycetes. Viral infections can also become an issue; the most common seen during this time period are herpes simplex virus as well as common community respiratory viruses.[76]

During the postengraftment time (i.e., up to 3 months after the transplant), the patient remains at risk for the same type of bacterial and fungal infections as during the preengraftment period. In addition, the patient becomes vulnerable to an increasing array of viral infections: cytomegalovirus, human herpesvirus (6, 7, and 8), adenovirus, enteric viruses, and respiratory viruses. Parasitic infections, including *Pneumocystis jiroveci* pneumonia (fomerly known as *Pneumocystis carinii*)[83] and toxoplasmosis, are also of concern. Finally, the patient is at risk for mycobacterium infections, although acute infections are rare and reactivation is much more common.[24,76]

During the late postengraftment stage (i.e., more than 3 months after the transplant), the patient continues to have the same risks as during the other times, but can also have other viral infections such as varicella-zoster virus and Epstein-Barr virus. The risk to the patient is directly linked to chronic GVHD and the requirement of lengthy immunosuppressive therapy.[76]

Transplant centers use protocols for antimicrobial prophylaxis to decrease infectious risks to the BMT patient.[35] Most patients receive a broad-spectrum oral antibiotic, such as a fluoroquinolone, for both gut decontamination and gram-negative prophylaxis. In addition, they are started on an antiviral agent such as acyclovir (Zovirax) and an antifungal agent such as fluconazole (Diflucan), itraconazole (Sporanox) solution, or voriconazole (Vfend). The antiviral and antifungal prophylaxis will continue until the patient either is weaned to low doses or is no longer prescribed immunosuppressive agents. The broad-spectrum oral antibiotic is continued until the first fever spike or until engraftment, when the ANC rises above 1000 mm^3. Lastly, the patient will be given *Pneumocystis jiroveci* prophylaxis with trimethoprim-sulfamethoxazole (Bactrim, Septra); for patients who are allergic to the sulfa component of this drug, dapsone may be given. It is important to note that trimethoprim-sulfamethoxazole itself can be immunosuppressive; therefore neutropenic patients may be changed to monthly IV doses of pentamidine (Pentam 300).[35]

Recognition of first fever (38° C or 100.4° F) during neutropenia requires immediate intervention. During the time of neutropenia, the patient's response to infection is blunted and finding a source can be difficult; therefore testing of all potential infectious sites is imperative.[91] A full fever workup can include blood cultures, urine cultures, chest x-ray (CXR), and throat and stool cultures. Broad-spectrum intravenous antibiotics to cover gram-negative and gram-positive organisms are instituted immediately. Also it is critical to provide coverage based on the transplant center's experience and pathogen history.[17] Most BMT centers have a standard of initiation of antibiotics within 1 hour after fever spike, relying on preprinted order sets that allow the BMT nurse to initiate immediate interventions.[86] If fever continues for several days despite broad-spectrum antibacterial agents, fungal infection should be presumed and antifungal therapy should be broadened.[8] Common sites of infection in neutropenic patients include skin and mucous membranes, respiratory tract, urinary tract, and indwelling devices (e.g., catheter, venous access devices). Rectal tubes and rectal thermometers and suppositories are strictly avoided in this patient population.[94]

Anemia

Anemia may be due to bleeding from thrombocytopenia and ongoing blood loss, but the primary cause of underlying anemia is temporary cessation of marrow production of RBCs following the conditioning regimen.[65] The average RBC survives approximately 120 days;[5] the need for replacement is due to the long life span and slower production rate of RBCs. Most stem cell transplant patients require support with transfusions of packed RBCs, and standing orders for transfusions for hemoglobin levels less than 8 g/dl or hematocrit (Hct) levels less than 24% are common, although this varies slightly among institutions.[46] Patients may receive more aggressive transfusion support should they become symptomatic from anemia with severe fatigue, shortness of breath, or hypotension.[46]

Blood products should be irradiated, leukoreduced, and CMV negative. Blood products are irradiated to prevent transfusion-associated GVHD, a rare phenomenon that occurs most often in HSCT patients. Irradiation kills the donor's lymphocytes that drive the GVHD response.[90] In addition, donor leukocytes can cause the patient to become alloimmunized. When this occurs, the patient does not have an appropriate rise in the platelet count following platelet transfusions, resulting in the need for multiple platelet transfusions.[29]

Because anemia can be quite prolonged in the transplant patient, agents such as erythrocyte colony-stimulating factors are sometimes initiated in the postengraftment period to stimulate production of RBCs.[46] During long-term followup, it is important that these patients be closely monitored for hemolysis or autoimmune hemolytic anemia because both of these complications are associated with several of the immunosuppressive agents commonly used.[57]

Thrombocytopenia

Thrombocytopenia is defined as a low platelet count.[65] A normal platelet count is 150,000 to 400,000 cells/mm[3]. The average life span of a platelet is 9 to 10 days.[87] Thrombocytopenia can occur up to 7 to 10 days after the conditioning regimen, but often occurs more rapidly. In particular, thrombocytopenia can last for several months following allogeneic stem cell transplant.[46]

The patient is supported with single-donor pheresed platelet products.[29] Although the risk of bleeding increases substantially when the platelet count falls below 50,000 cells/mm[3], many BMT centers typically do not transfuse the patient unless the platelet count falls below 10,000 cells/mm[3] or has symptoms of bleeding.[29] This is adjusted to a higher threshold if the patient has had a previous issue with bleeding. The thrombocytopenic patient needs to be watched carefully for new onset of headaches or any other neurologic deficit because they may be early signs of intracranial hemorrhage.[62] Invasive procedures need to be supported aggressively with platelet transfusions to minimize risk of bleeding. Such procedures should be done only if absolutely necessary, and the patient must be monitored closely for signs of blood loss and hemorrhagic shock.[62] Box 39-6 outlines care of the thrombocytopenic patient.

Mucositis

Mucositis is the breakdown of epithelial cells following administration of chemotherapy.[20] This can occur from the oral cavity all the way through the intestines to the anus and is a common complication following the preparative regimen for a stem cell transplant. It is much more common with the myeloablative regimens; the worst mucositis usually develops in patients exposed to total body irradiation. Oral mucositis occurs in about 40% of patients receiving chemotherapy. This percentage is higher (up to 100%) for myeloablative stem cell transplants because of the aggressive chemotherapy regimens, exposure to TBI, and prolonged neutropenic state before engraftment.[12] Mucositis should be evaluated daily by the practitioner. Stringent oral care, nutritional support, and pain management are imperative.[12]

One of the most common scales for evaluating mucositis is from the World Health Organization (Table 39-6). Symptoms of mucositis include change in taste and

---

Box 39-6

Management of Thrombocytopenia*

- Assess for fall risk.
- Maintain and reinforce bleeding precautions (no toothbrush, gentle nose blowing only, no use of weights, no running).
- Avoid the use of straight-edge razors; use electric razors to remove unwanted hair.
- Do not use tourniquets.
- Minimize invasive procedures, e.g., needle sticks, injections, enemas, or suppositories.
- Avoid sexual intercourse if platelet count is <50,000/mm[3].
- Avoid use of tampons.
- Avoid having dental care until platelet counts normalize.
- Use toothettes for oral care; avoid use of toothbrushes and dental floss when thrombocytopenic.
- Suppress menses.

Data from reference 55.
*For patients with platelet counts of <50,000 cells/mm[3].

TABLE 39-6 World Health Organization Rating Scale of Mucositis

GRADE	SYMPTOM
0	No symptoms
1	Soreness and erythema
2	Erythema, ulcers; can eat solid food
3	Ulcers; requires liquid diet only
4	No possible alimentation

Data from reference 93.

ability to swallow, pain when swallowing or talking, hoarseness, edema of the oral mucosa and tongue, mucosal ulcerations, and xerostomia (changes in the oral moisture, amount and quality of secretions, and oral ulcerations).[12]

Nursing interventions include oral assessment every 4 hours using the evaluation tool preferred by the institution. Careful documentation of mucositis using a consistent evaluation tool is essential for consistency and continuity of care for the patient. Resolution of the symptoms usually does not occur until around the time of engraftment.[12]

Once mucositis has occurred, the treatment is symptomatic. The patient is encouraged to continue with frequent oral normal saline rinses. Aggressive pain management is necessary for comfort and to ensure compliance with oral care interventions. Pain management begins with topical therapy that coats and numbs the oral cavity along with oral pain medication. Often the mucositis will progress and the patient will require patient-controlled analgesia (PCA) with morphine (Duramorph), hydromorphone (Dilaudid), or fentanyl (Duragesic).[12]

Nutritional Issues

Frequently, these patients require nutritional support during their hospital stay because mucositis makes it too painful for the patient to eat and swallow or because of intractable nausea and vomiting from the effects of the chemotherapy throughout the gastrointestinal tract.[74] TPN is the usual method of nutritional support because a feeding tube places the patient at unnecessary risk from both infection and bleeding. In addition, absorption is poor because of the mucositis.[12] Close monitoring of the patient's blood glucose level is imperative, especially if the patient is receiving steroid

therapy for immunosuppression. Electrolyte management can be difficult and can require daily monitoring. The Nutrition box below describes this further.

◆ NUTRITION

Nutritional Care of the Hematopoietic Stem Cell Patient

Hematopoietic stem cell transplant (HSCT) patients have unique nutritional needs throughout their transplant. These are magnified when the patient requires transfer to the critical care unit.

- Increased metabolic needs:
  Because of the side effects of chemotherapy and radiation therapy, the patient already has increased metabolic needs. In addition, fever, infection, and graft-versus-host disease (GVHD) can also exacerbate nutritional deficit.
- Decreased intake:
  Multiple factors, such as mucositis, nausea, and vomiting, prevent the HSCT patient from intake of adequate nutrition.
- Poor absorption:
  Diarrhea refractory to therapy can occur with chemotherapy, radiation, and GVHD. The diarrhea can be severe, leading to loss of nutrients and electrolytes and making absorption of nutrition questionable.

NUTRITION SUPPLEMENTATION

Parenteral Nutrition
  HSCT: During engraftment phase—Initiation of parenteral nutrition is often done early to try to manage high caloric needs. Close observation of electrolyte and fluid management is essential. The patient has multiple medications that can cause electrolyte management difficulties. Steroid therapy is commonly used for GVHD prophylaxis and can cause significant hyperglycemia. Aggressive management, including an insulin drip if indicated, is appropriate. Cyclosporine can cause hyperglycemia, hypokalemia, and hypomagnesemia. Enteral feedings are contraindicated because of the infectious risk of duodenal feeding tube placement and concern for poor absorption.
  GVHD: For patients with GVHD of the gut, parenteral nutrition is exclusively used in the acute phase. The patient is unable to absorb nutrients from the gastrointestinal tract in the early stages. Diarrhea is often severe, causing increased issues with fluid and electrolyte management.

Continues on page 1060

Enteral Feeding

HSCT: Late complications—When the patient is admitted to the critical care unit for late complications such as infection or pulmonary/cardiac issues, enteral feedings are often appropriate and the desired approach to meet nutritional needs. Diarrhea volume must be followed closely as the patient is always a candidate to develop GVHD.

GVHD: When the gut GVHD has improved, enteral feedings are often used to stimulate regeneration. This is not meant to meet the nutritional needs, but is often used as a supplement to parenteral nutrition.

Data from references 13, 14, 45, and 68.

Veno-Occlusive Disease of the Liver

Veno-occlusive disease (VOD) of the liver is a potentially fatal disease occurring in 5% to 54% of BMT patients[56] as a complication of the conditioning regimen. This process is now also called sinusoidal obstruction syndrome (SOS).[50] It usually develops within 2 weeks after transplantation. The risk increases in patients with preexisting liver disease or underlying infection or liver abnormalities.[26] VOD/SOS occurs when fibrous material accumulates and destroys the fine venules in the liver, leading to portal hypertension, liver congestion, and liver destruction. Clinical manifestations usually begin within 1 to 3 weeks of the transplantation and are characterized by hyperbilirubinemia, ascites with rapid weight gain, right upper quadrant pain, and jaundice.[50] If mild, the liver can heal and resume normal function, usually within 14 days. When severe, VOD/SOS may also cause coagulopathy, hepatic encephalopathy, hepatorenal syndrome, and multiorgan failure in severe cases.[26]

Unfortunately, there is no clear effective therapy for reversing VOD/SOS and, therefore, care is largely supportive. There continues to be a great deal of study in this area to develop innovative therapies. Current modalities being studied are alteplase defibrotide (Activase), antithrombin (Thrombate III), prostaglandin E_1, antioxidants, and transjugular intrahepatic portosystemic stent shunt.[26]

Pulmonary Complications

Acute pulmonary complications develop in 40% to 60% of patients after HSCT.[79] Pulmonary complications, which can arise from infectious as well as noninfectious causes, can lead to transfer of the BMT patient to critical care. Infectious causes are commonly bacterial, fungal, or viral in nature; however, parasitic infections (e.g., *Pneumocystis jiroveci*) can also occur.[94]

There are multiple noninfectious causes of pulmonary complications. Pulmonary edema, both cardiogenic and noncardiogenic, can originate from many causative factors including acute and chronic cardiac toxicity from certain chemotherapy agents and total body irradiation.[84] Aspiration can occur, especially in patients with severe mucositis, because of difficulty handling oral secretions and the need for opiate analgesia.[12] There is also risk of diffuse alveolar hemorrhage, an entity that is poorly understood but associated with poor survival rates, especially if ventilatory support is required.[49] Idiopathic interstitial pneumonitis (idiopathic pneumonia syndrome, [IPS]) can occur rapidly after transplantation or present months later and is associated with a high mortality rate. IPS is widespread alveolar injury in the absence of active infection. The symptoms are dyspnea, nonproductive cough, hypoxemia, and fever. Radiographic changes are diffuse, but nonspecific.[79] Treatment is supportive, although steroid therapy is a possible treatment modality. Most patients do recover, but if the patient progresses to the point of requiring intubation and ventilation, the mortality is more than 90%.[56]

Another possible lung complication is engraftment syndrome, occurring around the time of engraftment. Usually seen when the WBC count rises very quickly, the patient experiences progressive respiratory difficulty with noted weight gain.[74] It is frequently associated with a skin rash. Diagnosis is made after ruling out any infectious etiology of respiratory changes. Aggressive support is imperative and often requires intubation and mechanical ventilation. Treatment is supportive and the condition usually responds to high-dose steroid therapy.[79]

Chronic pulmonary complications can also occur, and as with acute pulmonary complications, the causes are both infectious and noninfectious.[77] The danger from infectious causes is directly related to the length of time immunosuppressive medications are required.[94]

Noninfectious causes of chronic pulmonary complications are more often associated with allogeneic stem cell transplants, specifically bronchiolitis obliterans (BO). BO is an obstructive airway disease; it is a form of chronic GVHD that can be mild or quite debilitating.[15] It is usually irreversible and is associated with decreased pulmonary function tests, especially FEV_1. Diagnosis is done either by tissue testing through a surgical procedure (lung biopsy) or according to the clinical presentation and specific CT scan changes. In the early stages, changes in tissue samples show tissue with fibropurulent exudates including lymphocytes, neutrophils, and macrophages. In later stages, tissue samples show severe epithelial damage and the bronchioles can be completely occluded by connective tissue.[15] Treatment is mainly supportive as no therapy has been shown to be particularly effective. Both oral and inhaled forms of steroid therapy have been studied, with variable results.[59]

Relapse of Primary Disease

Relapse of the patient's primary disease after an HSCT is associated with an extremely high mortality rate that is dependent on multiple factors, such as underlying disease, type of stem cell transplant (auto versus allo), age of patient, and extent of complications. Mortality following relapse can be greater than 80%.[4,39] The first line of therapy is to quickly withdraw immunosuppressive therapy, thus encouraging the new immune system to work against the malignancy. Unfortunately, this puts the patient at high risk for severe GVHD.[77] If the patient does not have onset of GVHD, administration of donor lymphocytes may be considered to stimulate GVHD in the patient. While GVHD can be an effective method of controlling disease, it takes time and often the rapidity of the relapse requires more aggressive intervention.

Frequently, additional chemotherapy must be given before the donor lymphocyte infusion to get the primary disease under control. This treatment option can be considered only if the patient is more than 100 days after myeloablative treatment because undue toxicity risk must be avoided.[81]

Patients can be considered for a second HSCT. If the first transplant was an autologous stem cell transplant, patients can then be considered for an allogeneic stem cell transplant. If the relapsed patient had an allogeneic stem cell transplant, it is very rare that a second would be considered.[82]

CONCLUSIONS

Patients experiencing BMT provide multiple challenges to the health care team during all phases of the transplant process. While the majority of these patients are managed in specialized BMT units, occasionally complications during both pretransplant and posttransplant care require admission to critical care. It is important that the critical care nurse understand the BMT transplant procedure, as well as the unique problems these patients encounter, in order to plan, provide, and coordinate the complicated care these patients, and their families, require.

⬧ Case Study 39-1, Part C

A Diagnosis of Acute Myelogenous Leukemia

Final identification revealed a coagulase-negative staph bacteremia. Fever dissipated within 48 hours of initiation of vancomycin therapy. The patient was successfully weaned off vasopressors after 36 hours of antibiotic therapy and fluid resuscitation. She received single-donor pheresed platelets for a platelet count of 27,000/mm³ and 2 units of irradiated, leukoreduced, and CMV-negative packed RBCs for an Hct of 19%. Her mucositis remained quite painful and PCA analgesia continued. The BMT nutritionist adjusted her TPN support to better meet her ongoing nutritional needs until she was able to tolerate oral intake. Imipenem was continued until the patient had an ANC of >1000 mm³ (day 13 after transplant). At that time the imipenem was stopped and vancomycin was continued for 14 days of therapy. The patient was transferred out of the critical care unit after 4 days, and she received care in the BMT unit until she was discharged home 10 days later.

Decision point: Once she is stable following her critical care resuscitation, what care considerations related to her BMT need to be addressed?

Decision point: Are patients ever admitted to the critical care unit for GVHD?

Decision point: How can the critical care nurse best support the patient and family during this unexpected complication?

REFERENCES

1. Alspach, J. G. (1998). *Core curriculum for critical care nursing* (5th ed.). Annapolis, Md: Saunders.
2. American Cancer Society. *Introduction.* www.cancer.org/docroot/ETO/content?eto_1_4X_bone_marrow_stem_cell_introduction.
3. American Cancer Society. *Introduction.* www.cancer.org/docroot/ETO/content/ETO_1_4X_Types_of_Stem_Cell_Transplants.asp?sitearea=ETO.
4. American Cancer Society. *Introduction.* www.cancer.gov/cancertopics/factsheet/Therapy/bone-marrow-transplant.
5. American Cancer Society. *What are the possible side effects of chemotherapy?* www.cancer.org/docroot/ETO/content/ETO_1_4X_What_Are_The_Side_Effects_of_Chemotherapy.asp?sitearea=ETO.
6. American Osteopathic College of Dermatology. www.aocd.org/skin/dermatologic_diseases/lichen_planus.html.
7. Amsterdam, A. et al. (2004). Treatment of menorrhagia in women undergoing hematopoietic stem cell transplantation. *Bone Marrow Transpl, 34,* 363–366.
8. Appelbaum, R. D. (2003). The current status of hematopoietic cell transplantation. *Ann Rev Med, 54,* 491–512.
9. Atkinson, K. et al. (1989). Consensus among bone marrow transplanters for diagnosis, grading and treatment of chronic graft-versus-host disease: Committee of the International Bone Marrow Transplant Registry. *Bone Marrow Transpl, 4,* 247–254.
10. Atkinson, K. (2000). Chronic graft-versus-host disease. In K. Atkinson (Ed.), *Clinical bone marrow and blood stem cell transplantation.* Cambridge, U.K.: Cambridge University Press.

11. Baltic, T., & Bakitas, M. (2005). Principles of bone marrow and hematopoietic cell transplantation. In C. H. Yarbro et al. (Eds.), *Cancer nursing.* Sudbury, Mass: Jones and Bartlett.

12. Beck, S. L. (2004). Mucositis. In C. H. Yarbro (Ed.), *Cancer symptom management* (3rd ed.). Sudbury, Mass: Jones and Bartlett.

13. Bergerson, S. L. (1998). Nutritional support in bone marrow transplant recipients. In R. K. Burt et al. (Eds.), *Bone marrow transplantation.* Georgetown, Tex: Landes Bioscience.

14. Bergerson, S. L. (1998). Transfusions. In R. K. Burt et al. (Eds.), *Bone marrow transplantation.* Georgetown, Tex: Landes Bioscience.

15. *Bronchiolitis obliterans.* http://path.upmc.edu/divisions/pulm-path/bron02.htm.

16. Burt, R. et al. (1998). Acute myeloid leukemia—AML. In R. K. Burt et al. (Eds.), *Bone marrow transplantation.* Georgetown, Tex: Landes Bioscience.

17. Burt, R., & Walsh, T. (1998). Infection prophylaxis in bone marrow transplant recipients—myths, legends and microbes. In R. K. Burt et al. (Eds.), *Bone marrow transplantation.* Georgetown, Tex: Landes Bioscience.

18. Burt, R., & Wilson, W. H. (1998). Conditioning (preparative) regimens. In R. K. Burt et al. (Eds.), *Bone marrow transplantation.* Georgetown, Tex: Landes Bioscience.

19. Cancer Information Network. http://patient.cancerconsultants.com/stemcell_treatment.aspx?id=944.

20. Cancer Supportive Care. www.cancersupportivecare.com/mucositis.html.

21. Chao, N. J. (1998). Graft versus host disease. In R. K. Burt et al. (Eds.), *Bone marrow transplantation.* Georgetown, Tex: Landes Bioscience.

22. Chao, N. J. (2004). Prevention and treatment of acute graft-versus-host disease: recommendations. *UpToDate 14.1.* www.utdol.com/utd/content/topic.do?topicKey=hcell_tr/5229&view=print.

23. Chao, N. J. (2005). Clinical manifestations and diagnosis of chronic graft-versus-host disease. *UpToDate14.1.* www.utdol.com/utd/content/topic.do?topicKey=hcell_tr/6824&view=print.

24. Chawla, R. et al. (Jan 30, 2006). Infections after bone marrow transplantation. www.emedicine.com/ped/topic2850.htm.

25. Chen, J., Law, P., & Ball, E. D. (2000). Failure of engraftment. In E. D. Ball (Ed.), *Hematopoietic stem cell therapy.* New York: Churchill Livingstone.

26. Cheng, D., Laing, F., & Bringham, R. A. D. *Hepatic venoocclusive disease.* http://brighamrad.harvard.edu/Cases/bwh/hcache/192/full.html.

27. *Clinical Trials.com. A phase III randomized, multicenter trial comparing G-CSF mobilized peripheral blood stem cell with marrow transplantation from HLA compatible unrelated donors* .www.clinicaltrials.gov/ct/show/NCT00275678?order=1.

28. Clinician's Ultimate Reference. www.globalrph.com/anc.htm.

29. Cottler-Fox, M. (1998). Transfusions. In R. K. Burt et al. (Eds.), *Bone marrow transplantation.* Georgetown, Tex: Landes Bioscience.

30. Cottler-Fox, M. (1998). Marrow processing and cryopreservation. In R. K. Burt et al. (Eds.), *Bone marrow transplantation.* Georgetown, Tex: Landes Bioscience.

31. Couriel, D. et al. (2004). Acute graft-versus-host disease: pathophysiology, clinical manifestations, and management. *Blood, 101* (9), 1936–1946.

32. Cutler, C. (2004). Bone marrow transplant. In T. A. Stern (Ed.), *Facing cancer. A complete guide for people with cancer, their families and caregivers.* New York: McGraw-Hill.

33. Demko, S. (1998). Transplantation procedures. In R. K. Burt et al. (Eds.), *Bone marrow transplantation.* Georgetown, Tex: Landes Bioscience.

34. Djulbegovic, B. et al. (2003). Nonmyeloablative allogeneic stem cell transplantation for hematologic malignancies: a systematic

review. *Cancer Control, 10*(1), 17–41. www.medscape.com/viewarticle/449119_print.

35. Dykewics, C. A. (2001). Summary of the guidelines for preventing opportunistic infections among hematopoietic stem cell transplant recipients. *Clin Infect Dis, 33,* 139–144.

36. Evidence-based Reviews, American Society of Blood and Marrow Transplantation. (2004). *Biology of Blood and Marrow Transplantation.* www.asbmt.org/policystat/policy.html.

37. Finkielman, J. D. et al. (2004). Mortality rate and length of stay of patients admitted to the intensive care unit in July. *Crit Care Med, 32*(5), 1161–1165.

38. Flomenberg, N. et al. (2004). Impact of HLA class I and class II high resolution matching on outcomes of unrelated donor bone marrow transplantation: HLA-C mismatching is associated with a strong adverse effect on transplant outcome. *Blood, 104*(7), 1923–1930.

39. Giralt, S. A., & Champlin, R. E. (2000). Relapse after hematopoietic stem cell transplantation: mechanisms and treatment. In E. D. Ball (Ed.), *Hematopoietic stem cell therapy.* New York: Churchill Livingstone.

40. *Graft versus host disease. Indiana Blood and Marrow Transplantation.* www.ibmtindy.com/faq/graft.htm.

41. Grokera, H., Haznedaroglu, I. C., & Chao, N. J. (2001). Acute graft-vs-host disease: pathobiology and management. *Exper Hematol, 29*(3), 259–277.

42. Hensel, N. (1998). MHC and bone marrow transplantation. In R. K. Burt et al. (Eds.), *Bone marrow transplantation.* Georgetown, Tex: Landes Bioscience.

43. Higman, M. A., & Vogelsang, G. B. (2004). Chronic graft-versus-host disease: review. *Br J Haematol, 125*(5), 435–454.

44. Hype and Hope. www.hypeandhope.com/wt/page/index/it_1126030323.

45. Itano, J., & Taoka, K. N. (2005). *Core curriculum for oncology nursing.* (4th ed., pp 29–52, 259–316, 809–827). St Louis: Elsevier.

46. Jones, R. J., Shpall, E., & Champlin, R. (2006). Bone marrow transplantation. In D. W. Kufe et al. (Eds.), *Cancer medicine* (pp. 879–897). Hamilton, Ontario: BC Decker.

47. Kato, S. et al. (2000). Allogeneic hematopoietic transplantation of CD34+ selected cells from an HLA haplo-identical related donor. A long-term follow-up of 135 patients and a comparison of stem cell source between the bone marrow and the peripheral blood. *Bone Marrow Transplant, 26*(12), 1281–1290.

48. Kennedy, V. N. (1993). The role of social work in bone marrow transplantation. *J Psychosocial Oncol, 11*(1), 103–118.

49. Kotloff, R. M., Ahya, V. N., & Crawford, A. S. (2004). Pulmonary complications of solid organ and hematopoietic stem cell transplantation. *Am J Respir Crit Care Med, 170,* 22–48.

50. Kumar, S. et al. (2003). Hepatic veno-occlusive disease (sinusoidal obstruction syndrome) after hematopoietic stem cell transplantation. *Mayo Clin Proc, 78*(5), 589–598.

51. Lee, S. J. et al. (2005). Routine screening for psychosocial distress following hematopoietic stem cell transplantation. *Bone Marrow Transplant, 35*(1), 77–83.

52. Leitman, S., & Stroneck, D. (2005). Magic matches: unrelated-donor transplants facilitated by the National Marrow Donor program. *ASHI Quarterly.* www.ashi-hla.org/publicationfiles/ASHI_Quarterly/29_4_2005/ 5_magic_matches.pdf.

53. Leukemia/BMT Program of BC. www.vch.ca/bmt/public/treatment/bmt_day.html.

54. Lewis, A. (2005). Autologous stem cells derived from the peripheral blood compared to standard bone marrow transplant; time to engraftment: a systematic review. *Int J Nurs Studies, 42,* 589–596.

55. London Health Sciences Centre.www.lrcc.on.ca/cancer-and-treatment/managing-side-effects-lowplatelets.xml.

56. Long, G. D. (1998). Regimen related toxicity—first 30 days. In R. K. Burt et al. (Eds.), *Bone marrow transplantation* (pp 507–509). Georgetown, Tex: Landes Bioscience.

57. Mach-Pascual, S., Samii, K., & Beris, P. (1996). Microangiopathic hemolytic anemia complicating FK506 (tacrolimus) therapy. *Am J Hematol, 52*(4), 310–312.

58. Mandanas, R. (2002). Graft versus host disease. *EMedicine*. www.emedicine.com/med/topic926.htm.2002.

59. Marcellus, D. C., & Vogelsang, G. B. (2000). Chronic graft-vs-host disease. In E. D. Ball (Ed.), *Hematopoietic stem cell therapy*. New York: Churchill Livingstone.

60. Mavroudis, P. A. (1998). Graft versus leukemia effect of allogeneic BMT. In R. K. Burt et al. (Eds.), *Bone marrow transplantation*. Georgetown, Tex: Landes Bioscience.

61. McLeod, B. C. et al. (1997). *Apheresis: principles and practice* pp 223–250). Chicago: AABB Press.

62. *Medline Plus*. www.nlm.nih.gov/medlineplus/ency/article/000 796.htm.

63. Moise, K. J. (2005). Umbilical cord stem cells. *Obstet Gynecol, 106* (6), 1393–1407.

64. Naeem, N. et al. (2006). Transfer of the hematopoietic stem cell transplant patient to the intensive care unit: does it really matter? *Bone Marrow Transplant, 37*(2), 119–133.

65. National Cancer Institute.www.cancer.gov/templates/db_alpha. aspx?expand=M.

66. Ng, T. M. et al. (2006). Contemporary issues in the pharmacologic management of acute heart failure. *Crit Care Ref, 22*(2), 199–219.

67. *Nursing 2001 drug handbook* (21st ed.). Springhouse, Pa: Springhouse Corp.

68. *Nutritional issues in cancer care* (pp 253–264). (2005). Pittsburgh, Pa: Oncology Nursing Society.

69. Oblan, D. J. (2000). Evaluation of patients before hematopoietic stem cell transplantation. In E. D. Ball (Ed.), *Hematopoietic stem cell therapy*. New York: Churchill Livingstone.

70. Oken, M. M., et al. (1982). Toxicity and response criteria of the Eastern Cooperative Oncology Group. *Am J Clin Oncol, 5*, 649–655.

71. Pene, F., et al. (2006). Outcome of critically ill allogeneic hematopoietic stem-cell transplantation recipients: a reappraisal of indications for organ failure supports. *J Clin Oncol, 24*(4), 643–649.

72. Przepiorka, D., et al. (1995). Consensus conference on acute GVHD grading. *Bone Marrow Transplant, 15*, 825–828.

73. Przepiorka, D., & Cleary, K. (2000). Therapy of acute graft-vs-host disease. In E. D. Ball (Ed.), *Hematopoietic stem cell therapy*. New York: Churchill Livingstone.

74. Reitz-Anderson, L. (2005). Complications of hematopoietic cell transplantation. In C. H. Yarbro et al. (Eds.), *Cancer nursing*. Sudbury, Mass: Jones and Bartlett.

75. Ryst, E. (2004). The impact of cancer on the family. In T. A. Stern (Ed.), *Facing cancer. A complete guide for people with cancer, their families and caregivers*. New York: McGraw-Hill.

76. Sable, C. A., & Donowits, G. R. (1994). Infections in bone marrow transplant recipients. *Clin Infect Dis, 18*(3), 273–284.

77. Shannon, J. B. (Ed.), (2000). *Transplant source book* (pp. 184–206). Detroit: Omnigraphics.

78. Slovak, M. L., & Murata-Collins, J. L. (2000). Cytogenetic aspects of hematopoietic stem cell transplantation. In K. Atkinson (Ed.), *Clinical bone marrow and blood stem cell transplantation*. Cambridge, U.K.: Cambridge University Press.

79. Soubani, A. O., Miller, K. B., & Hassoun, P. M. (1996). Pulmonary complications of bone marrow transplantation. *Chest, 109*, 1066–1077.

80. St. Jude's Children's Research Hospital. www.stjude.org/stemcell-trans/0,2527,419_4890,00.html.

81. Stewart, F. M. (1998). Patient and donor evaluation. In R. K. Burt et al. (Eds.), *Bone marrow transplantation*. Georgetown, Tex: Landes Bioscience.

82. Stewart, F. M. (1998). Relapse after bone marrow transplantation. In R. K. Burt et al. (Eds.), *Bone marrow transplantation*. Georgetown, Tex: Landes Bioscience.

83. Stringer, J. R. et al. (2002). A new name *(Pneumocystis jiroveci)* for Pneumocystis from Humans. *CDC, 9*(8), www.cdc.gov/ncidod/EID/vol8no9/_ftn1#_ftn1.

84. *The Adult Marrow and Blood Transplantation Program*. www.healthcare.uiowa.edu/InternalMedicine/Patients/BoneMarrow/Healthpro/Pulmonary/Interstitial.htm.

85. Vogelsang, G. (2001). How I treat chronic graft versus host disease. *Blood, 97*, 1196–1201.

86. White, N. et al. (2005). Protocols for managing chemotherapy-induced neutropenia in clinical oncology practices. *Cancer Nurs, 28*(1), 62–69.

87. Wikipedia, the Free Encyclopedia. en.wikipedia.org/wiki/Platelet.

88. Wilkes, G. M., & Barton-Burke, M. (2004). *Oncology nursing drug handbook*. Sudbury, Mass: Jones and Barlett.

89. William, L. A., & McCarthy, P. L. (1998). Patient and donor evaluation. In R. K. Burt et al. (Eds.), *Bone marrow transplantation*. Georgetown, Tex: Landes Bioscience.

90. Williamson, L. M., & Warwick, R. M. (1995). Transfusion associated graft versus host disease and its prevention. *Blood, 9*, 251–261.

91. Witt, M. D., & Chu, L. A. (2002). Infections in the critically ill. In R. S. Bangard et al. (Eds.), *Current critical care diagnosis and treatment* (2nd ed.). New York: Lang.

92. *Women's Health Information*. www.womenshealth.co.uk/diseases_treated.html.

93. World Health Organization. (1979). *Handbook for reporting results of cancer treatment* (pp 15–22). Geneva, Switzerland: WHO.

94. Wujcik, D. (2004). Infection. In C. H. Yarbro (Ed.), *Cancer symptom management* (3rd ed.). Sudbury, Mass: Jones and Bartlett.

95. Young, L. (2003). *A family perspective on a program for bone marrow transplantation of adults*. Madison, Wisc: Policy Institute for Family Impact Seminars.

MULTISYSTEM DISORDERS

CHAPTER 40

Shock and End Points of Resuscitation

John J. Gallagher

Shock was described by Samuel D. Gross in the 1870s as the "rude unhinging of the machinery of life." Although dramatically descriptive, it does not describe the true physiologic basis of this devastating condition. Shock, simply defined, is a state of inadequate tissue perfusion resulting in inadequate oxygen delivery and/or utilization by the cell.[51] As a result, alteration of cellular energy production, from the normal and efficient aerobic pathway to the less efficient anaerobic pathway, causes cellular acidosis and the accumulation of the cellular waste product, lactic acid.[51,103,109,117] The inability to correct or reverse shock results in increasing oxygen debt, worsening tissue acidosis, organ system dysfunction, and eventually, death.[103,105,109] Key to preventing these unfortunate outcomes is the ability to rapidly recognize and treat the patient in shock before a refractory shock state is established.*

The purpose of this chapter is to provide an advanced working knowledge of shock and its treatment through detailed discussion of altered cellular oxygen delivery and consumption associated with various shock types and stages. General shock resuscitation strategies are addressed, along with global and regional end points used to guide the resuscitation process.

APPLIED PHYSIOLOGY OF CELLULAR METABOLISM

Normal cellular function is dependent on sufficient amounts of oxygen reaching the cell mitochondria for use in the production of adenosine triphosphate (ATP).[51,103,117] Four steps have been described in this process. First, oxygen is taken into the lungs to the pulmonary capillaries. Second, oxygen must diffuse into the blood. Third, oxygen must be transported through blood flow to the tissues and cells and, finally, it must diffuse into the cell and mitochondria to be used.[51] Under normal circumstances, through the aerobic metabolic pathway, oxygen along with nutrient substrates is converted through glycolysis to pyruvate. Pyruvate is, in turn,

converted to acetyl coenzyme A (CoA). Through the tricarboxylic acid (Krebs) cycle, CoA is converted to hydrogen then oxidized to water, generating 38 moles of high-energy ATP to facilitate normal cellular function.[51,103,109]

In shock states the reduced delivery of oxygen to the cell, or inability of the mitochondria to use the oxygen delivered, results in the less efficient anaerobic pathway. In the absence of adequate oxygen, pyruvate is converted to lactic acid rather than CoA, generating only 2 moles of ATP.[25,28,51,103,109] This amount of ATP is insufficient to support normal cellular metabolism; cellular acidosis will result. Key to preventing or reversing this undesirable event is optimization of cellular oxygen delivery and consumption.

OXYGEN DELIVERY, CONSUMPTION, AND EXTRACTION

As described, the delivery of oxygen to the tissues and cells is multifactorial. Normal oxygen delivery (DO_2) is approximately 1000 ml/min; when indexed to body surface area (DO_2I), 600 ml/min. Oxygen delivery (index) is determined by the product of the cardiac index (CI) and the arterial oxygen content (CaO_2)* (Table 40-1 outlines common tissue oxygen indices). Though simply stated, multiple factors in each of these components determine the effectiveness of the delivery process.

Cardiac output (CO) is the product of the heart rate (HR) and stroke volume (SV). The SV is further determined by the preload, afterload, and contractility of the ventricle.[28] CaO_2 is primarily a product of the hemoglobin (Hgb) concentration and arterial oxygen saturation (SaO_2). DO_2 may be compromised if one or more of these components is negatively affected and will result in a reduction of oxygen delivery to the cells below the critical threshold required for normal cellular oxygen consumption (Figure 40-1). For example, any reduction in CO, associated alterations in HR, myocardial damage (contractility), hypovolemia (preload), or vascular outflow obstruction (afterload) will compromise oxygen

---

*References 51, 80, 103, 105, 106, 113.

*References 15, 28, 51, 80, 103, 109.

TABLE 40-1 Normal Values and Formulas for Tissue Oxygenation Indices

TISSUE OXYGEN VARIABLE-NORMAL VALUES	FORMULA
Arterial oxygen content 17–20 ml/dl	Cao_2 $Cao_2 = (0.0031 \times Pao_2) + [1.34\,Hgb \times (Sao_2/100)]$
Venous oxygen content 12–15 ml/dl	Cvo_2 $Cvo_2 = (0.0031 \times Pvo_2) + [1.34\,Hgb \times (Svo_2/100)]$
Arterial oxygen saturation 95%-100%	Sao_2 $Sao_2 = [Hbo_2/(Hgb + Hbo_2)] \times 100$
Oxygen delivery 950–1150 ml/min	Do_2 $Do_2 = CO \times Cao_2 \times 10$
Oxygen delivery index 550–600 ml/min/m²	Do_2I $Do_2I = Do_2/BSA$
Oxygen consumption 195–285 ml/min	Vo_2 $Vo_2 = CO \times (Cao_2 - Cvo_2) \times 10$
Oxygen consumption index 120–140 ml/min/m²	Vo_2I $Vo_2I = Vo_2/BSA$
Mixed venous oxygen saturation 65%-80%	Svo_2 $Svo_2 = Sao_2 - [Vo_2/(CO \times 1.34\,Hgb \times 10)]$
Central venous oxygen saturation 60%-80%	$Scvo_2$

BSA = Body surface area, Cao_2 = arterial oxygen content, CO = cardiac output, Cvo_2 = venous oxygen content, Do_2 = oxygen delivery, Do_2I = oxygen delivery index, Hgb = hemoglobin, Hbo_2 = deoxyhemoglobin, Pao_2 = partial pressure of arterial oxygen tension, Pvo_2 = partial pressure of venous oxygen, Sao_2 = arterial oxygen saturation, $Scvo_2$ = central venous oxygen saturation, Svo_2 = mixed venous oxygen saturation, Vo_2 = oxygen consumption, Vo_2I = oxygen consumption index.

delivery.[15,28,58,61] Pulmonary injury/pathology may affect delivery of oxygen to the blood, whereas conditions reducing Hgb concentration (e.g., hemorrhagic shock) will negatively affect Cao_2.

OXYGEN CONSUMPTION

Under normal conditions, Do_2 to the tissues far exceeds the oxygen consumption (Vo_2) requirements of the cells (Figure 40-2). Cellular oxygen consumption requirements are approximately 250 ml/min, or 125 ml/min/m² when indexed to body surface area (Vo_2I). This translates into an oxygen extraction rate of 25%, or one quarter of the Do_2I. The approximate 75% difference between Do_2I and Vo_2I is a buffer, allowing for modest decreases in Do_2 as well as increases in cellular consumption based on changing metabolic needs.* Vo_2I is the product of the CI and the difference in the arterial and venous oxygen content ($Ca-Vo_2$). Clinically $Ca-Vo_2$ is substituted by Sao_2–mixed venous oxygen saturation (Svo_2) as shown below.

$$Vo_2I = CI(Hgb \times 1.34 \times [Sao_2 - Svo_2]) \times 10$$

Conditions increasing cellular metabolism (e.g., fever, pain, agitation, shivering) will increase the Vo_2I, requiring a higher percentage of oxygen extraction. Conversely, alleviation of these conditions may reduce cellular oxygen requirements.[28,58]

OXYGEN DELIVERY DEPENDENCE AND OXYGEN DEBT

Under normal circumstances the delivery of oxygen to the cells far exceeds the cellular metabolic needs. In circumstances in which delivery is severely compromised (i.e., shock), delivery of oxygen to the tissues may fall below a critical threshold (Figure 40-3). Below

*References 15, 51, 80, 103, 109, 117.

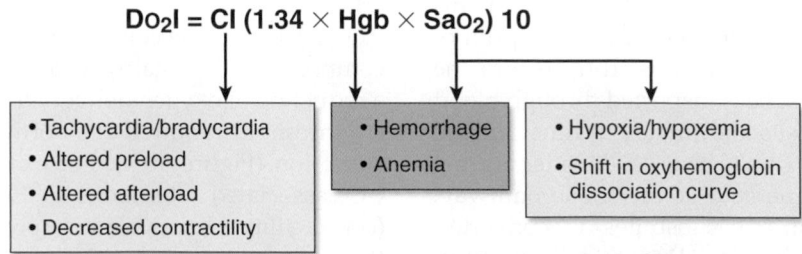

♦FIGURE 40-1 Factors affecting oxygen delivery. Do_2I = Oxygen delivery index, CI = cardiac index, Hgb = hemoglobin, Sao_2 = arterial oxygen saturation.

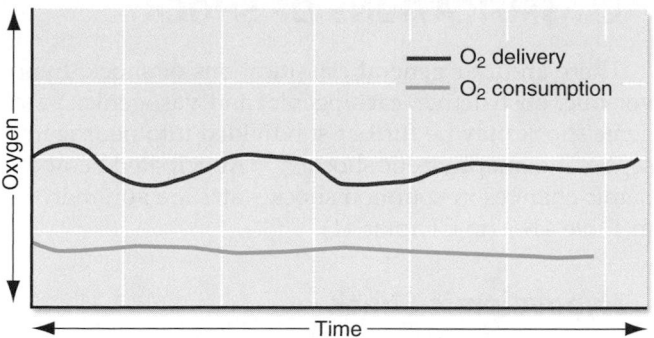

FIGURE 40-2 Normal relationship between oxygen delivery and consumption: Under normal conditions, oxygen delivery to the tissues far exceeds the oxygen consumption requirements of the cells.

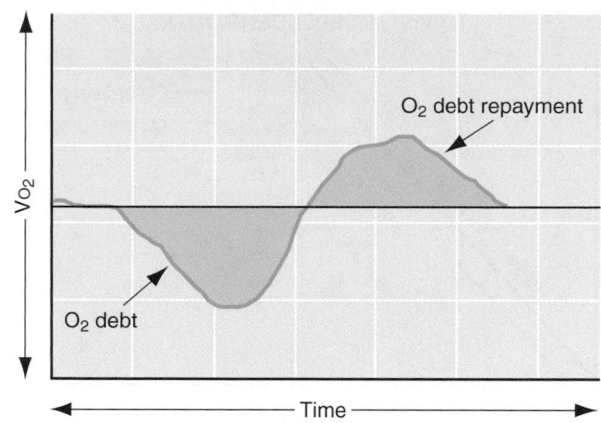

FIGURE 40-4 Oxygen debt: The condition of supply dependency, if persistent, will result in conversion to anaerobic metabolism and a state of oxygen debt at the cellular level. Additional cellular compromise may occur when the cell is unable to utilize available oxygen. Vo_2 = Oxygen consumption.

this critical delivery (Do_2I) threshold, Vo_2I becomes "dependent" on oxygen delivery. Consequently, the cell cannot compensate for the decrease in oxygen delivery by extracting more oxygen to meet its metabolic needs; additional oxygen is not available.* This condition of "supply dependency," if persistent, will result in conversion to anaerobic metabolism and a state of oxygen debt at the cellular level (Figure 40-4).[90] Additional cellular compromise may result when the cell is unable to use available oxygen (e.g., mitochondrial dysfunction associated with sepsis). The duration of the underlying conditions and extent to which the oxygen debt increases, negatively affect organ dysfunction and mortality. Restoration of optimal oxygen delivery to the

---

*References 12, 15, 28, 51, 105, 106.

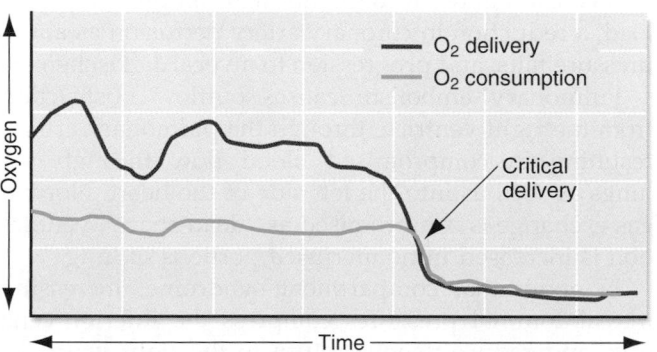

FIGURE 40-3 Onset of oxygen delivery dependency: In circumstances where delivery is severely compromised (i.e., shock), delivery of oxygen to the tissues may fall below a critical threshold. Below this critical delivery threshold, oxygen consumption becomes dependent on oxygen delivery.

tissues in an effort to reverse this process is the primary goal of any resuscitation efforts.

Clinical assessment of the relationship between Do_2I and Vo_2I, the onset of supply dependency, and the reversal of this state are a matter of continual debate.[64,80,105,106,109] In the 1980s, several studies demonstrated a relationship between the calculated measurement of Do_2 and consumption in animal and human subjects. This included the relationship to oxygen delivery–dependent consumption. Interventions improving Do_2I were noted to result in parallel improvements in Vo_2I, as long as a state of supply dependency existed. The resolution of the supply dependency state was felt to exist once Vo_2I levels plateaued while Do_2I continued to rise.[105,106] However, a continually increasing Vo_2I without plateau in parallel to therapeutically increasing Do_2I levels was felt to demonstrate persistent cellular oxygen debt and ongoing need for resuscitation (Figure 40-5). Based on these initial research findings, efforts to drive Do_2I to supernormal levels of greater than 600 ml/min/m^2 and to increase Vo_2I level in excess of 170 ml/min/m^2 were proposed to reverse supply dependency and improve survival.[106]

Many of these initial conclusions were based on an observed parallel relationship between the mathematically calculated values for Do_2I and Vo_2I. Subsequent research has not consistently found evidence of the supply-dependent relationship described in earlier studies. Although differences in methodology among studies may account for some of these differences, the concept of "mathematical coupling error" has been proposed as a possible reason for the observed

Vo$_2$I IS DEPENDENT ON Do$_2$I

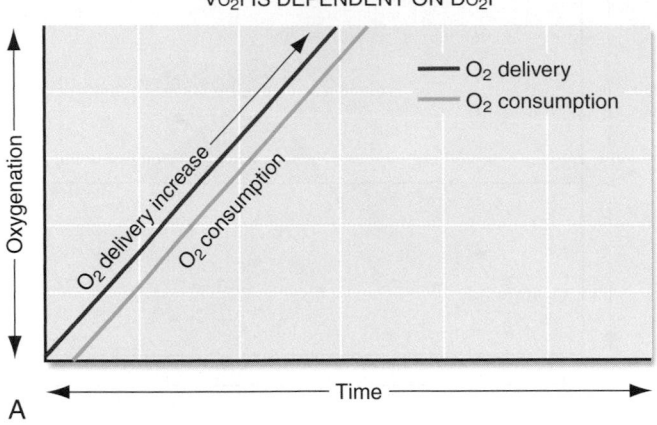

Vo$_2$I IS INDEPENDENT OF Do$_2$I

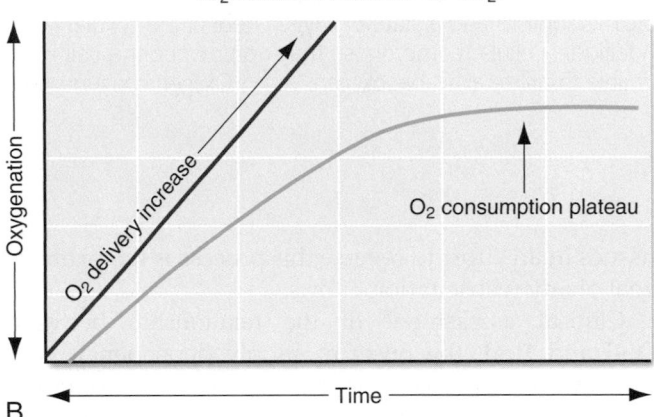

✦FIGURE 40-5 Response of oxygen consumption (Vo$_2$I) to increased oxygen delivery in **(A)** supply-dependent and **(B)** supply-independent states.

relationship between Do$_2$I and Vo$_2$I.[103,109] Mathematical coupling is a phenomenon occurring when two formulas share common variables used in their calculation. Both Do$_2$I and Vo$_2$I formulas use CI, Hgb, and oxygen saturation. These may result in the appearance of a relationship between the calculated values of Do$_2$I and Vo$_2$I that does not exist. Further, any errors in the measurement of the variables used in the calculation (i.e., CI), will result in erroneous calculation of both Do$_2$I and Vo$_2$I. Caution also must be exercised when using biological variables from the same patient, because relationships or coupling of variables may exist. In an effort to control for coupling errors, Vo$_2$I may be measured by indirect calorimetry rather than be derived mathematically.[51,109] By using calorimetry to calculate Vo$_2$I, previously observed relationships between calculated Do$_2$I and Vo$_2$I as well as supply dependency were not observed. The clinical usefulness of these parameters as end points of resuscitation will be discussed.

CLASSIFICATIONS OF SHOCK

There are four general classifications of shock: hypovolemic, obstructive, cardiogenic, and vasogenic. Vasogenic shock may be further subdivided into neurogenic, septic, and anaphylactic shock.[28, 61] Anticipated hemodynamic changes in common shock states are summarized in Table 41–2 (in Chapter 41).

Hypovolemic Shock

Hypovolemic shock, the most prevalent form of hypoperfusion, occurs when the vascular system loses blood or fluid either externally or internally, leading to a fall in perfusion pressure. Though the most common cause of hypovolemic shock is hemorrhage, any condition resulting in volume loss from the vascular space can cause hypovolemia.[61] Hemorrhagic shock is described in four stages, summarized in Table 40-2.[4] Conditions that lead to hypovolemic shock are listed in Box 41–2 (in Chapter 41).

Obstructive Shock

Obstructive shock results from a mechanical obstruction to blood flow and a resultant reduction in CO. When intravascular volume is sufficient, conditions prevent normal circulation of the blood volume. Conditions resulting in obstructive shock include tension pneumothorax, pericardial tamponade, pulmonary embolus, superior vena cava syndrome, and abdominal compartment syndrome.[4,28] A tension pneumothorax causes an increase in intrathoracic pressure, resulting in compression of the heart and vena cava. Venous return to the heart is compromised, reducing preload and CO.

In cardiac tamponade a collection of fluid within the unyielding pericardial sac compresses the myocardium, preventing adequate filling of the heart chambers. These events result in reduced CO through compromised preload, a reduction in coronary artery perfusion as aortic pressure falls, and progression to myocardial ischemia.

Pulmonary embolism causes outflow obstruction from the right ventricle through the pulmonary artery, resulting in compromised blood flow through the lungs as well as into the left side of the heart. Normal gas exchange is compromised as "dead space" ventilation is increased in nonperfused portions of lung.

In abdominal compartment syndrome, increasing intraabdominal pressures compress the inferior vena cava and reduce venous return to the right ventricle, compromising preload. Compression of the descending aorta increases afterload and left ventricular workload, further compromising CO.

Lastly, superior vena cava syndrome (SVCS) results from obstruction to the superior vena cava, resulting in

TABLE 40-2 Classification of Hemorrhagic Shock

PARAMETER	CLASS 1	CLASS 2	CLASS 3	CLASS 4
Blood loss (%)	15%	15%-30%	30%-40%	More than 40%
Blood loss (ml)	Up to 750	750–1500	1500–2000	More than 2000
Mental status	Slightly anxious	Mildly anxious	Anxious/confused	Confused/lethargic
Pulse rate	Less than 100	Greater than 100	Greater than 120	Greater than 140
Blood pressure	Normal	Normal	Decreased	Decreased
Pulse pressure	Normal/increased	Decreased	Decreased	Decreased
Respiratory rate	14–20	20–30	30–40	Greater than 35
Urinary output (ml/hr)	>30	20–30	5–15	Negligible
Fluid replacement Crystalloid: blood loss 3 ml:1 ml	Crystalloid	Crystalloid	Crystalloid/blood	Crystalloid/blood

From reference 4.

reduced blood return to the right ventricle, reduced preload, and reduced CO. The cause of SVCS is mechanical obstruction of the vena caval lumen or external compression of the vessel.

Cardiogenic Shock

Cardiogenic shock occurs when the heart is unable to pump enough blood to meet the body's demand for oxygen. The number one cause of cardiogenic shock is myocardial infarction (see Box 41–1 in Chapter 41). This condition may result from significant muscle ischemia associated with acute coronary syndrome as well as structural damage from traumatic injury to the heart muscle, valves, or coronary arteries. Chronic conditions (e.g., congestive heart failure, valvular pathology) also may result in this cardiogenic shock.

Vasogenic Shock

Though significantly different in etiology, the vasogenic types of shock similarly result in impaired or reduced systemic vascular resistance (SVR) with maldistribution of blood flow and altered organ perfusion. Although intravascular volume remains normal, a functional hypovolemia occurs as a result of increased vascular capacitance from reduction in SVR.

Neurogenic Shock

Neurogenic shock is most often the result of spinal cord injury (SCI) above the level of T1, which results in unopposed parasympathetic innervation.[61,65] This leads to system vasodilation and hypotension due to loss of sympathetic tone. Unlike other types of shock, compensatory tachycardia does not occur because of parasympathetic predominance. Rather, bradycardia is present, along with warm skin temperature and normal or flushed skin color.[4,11,28,65,108] In the absence of coexisting hypovolemia, volume resuscitation is not indicated.

A condition frequently confused with neurogenic shock is spinal shock. Spinal shock, also associated with SCI, results in the loss of sensory, motor, or reflex function below the level of the injury. Spinal shock may last from days to weeks after the injury. Return of key reflexes (i.e., bulbocavernous reflex, deep tendon reflexes) signifies the end of spinal shock.

Septic Shock

Septic shock is the result of infection overwhelming host defenses. Sepsis is the number one cause of death in noncoronary critical care units, with approximately 750,000 cases annually.[32] The critically ill and injured as well as immunocompromised patients are most at risk. Septic shock results from severe sepsis and is manifested by hypotension refractory to fluid resuscitation with associated tissue perfusion deficits.

These perfusion deficits are related to maldistribution of blood flow, vasodilation, and depression of myocardial contractility.[15,66] In addition, there is leakage of intravascular fluid volume as the result of mediator-damaged capillaries, resulting in a hypovolemic component to septic shock. At the mitochondrial level is an inability to extract and use oxygen in a normal fashion. This is seen even in the presence of adequate oxygen delivery, an aspect of sepsis still poorly understood.[66] A more detailed description of sepsis and septic shock is found in Chapter 41.

Anaphylactic Shock

Anaphylaxis is a clinical syndrome representing a severe systemic allergic reaction after exposure to a specific antigen in a previously exposed individual. The release of mast cells and basophil mediators is responsible for the systemic physiologic response seen in anaphylaxis. Anaphylactic shock is defined by the presence of cardiovascular collapse and associated airway compromise as the result of anaphylaxis.[28,33,43]

Causative agents of anaphylactic reactions that may lead to shock are mediated by immunoglobulin E (IgE). These include insect stings, medications, peanuts and tree nuts, latex, shellfish, fish, milk, eggs, and wheat. Anaphylactoid reactions related to non–IgE-mediated responses are associated with triggers such as nonsteroidal antiinflammatory drugs, diagnostic contrast agents, and opiates.[43]

The diagnosis of anaphylaxis and anaphylactic shock is based on the clinical observation of a severe and rapidly occurring allergic reaction with the presence of hemodynamic instability. Hemodynamic instability differentiates anaphylactic shock from anaphylaxis. This instability is caused by antigen-antibody–mediated vasodilation and redistribution of blood volume, as well as capillary permeability and loss of fluid volume into the interstitial space (angioedema). Although symptoms usually present rapidly, onset may be delayed for as long as 1 hour after exposure (Box 40-1). Resolution may begin as treatment is instituted, but can take up to 24 hours. An important and problematic aspect of these reactions is the potential for a second-phase reaction between 1 and 38 hours after the first (10 hours on average). This biphasic reaction pattern may be less severe, equally severe, or more severe than the first.[43]

Once life-threatening conditions have been treated and stability achieved, an effort to find the cause of reaction is essential. If not readily apparent, the patient must undergo testing in order to determine the cause of the reaction so future reactions may be avoided.

Box 40-1

Clinical Features of Anaphylaxis

NEUROLOGIC
- Anxiety
- Dizziness
- Weakness
- Syncope
- Seizures

RESPIRATORY
- Nasal congestion/sneezing
- Hoarseness
- Stridor
- Oropharyngeal/laryngeal edema
- Brochospasm
- Cough
- Tachypnea
- Cyanosis
- Respiratory arrest

CARDIOVASCULAR
- Tachycardia
- Hypotension
- Dysrhythmias
- Myocardial ischemia/infarction
- Cardiac arrest

GASTROINTESTINAL
- Nausea/vomiting
- Abdominal pain
- Diarrhea

SKIN
- Flushing
- Angioedema
- Urticaria
- Rash/erythema
- Pruritus

Data from reference 43.

GENERAL PHASES OF SHOCK

The initial onset of shock is a cellular phenomenon; therefore, detection through traditional clinical assessment may be difficult, especially when strong compensatory mechanisms are intact. Uninterrupted shock occurs in a predictable pattern, moving from an initial compensatory stage through progressive or uncompensated shock and eventually to a refractory stage and death. Although overlap exists between the stages, defined pathophysiologic findings are attributed to each stage as shock progresses.[28] Within each classification of shock, each of these stages exists; however, the phases are most often associated with the model of hypovolemic shock. No matter what the precipitating event, the initial pathophysiology of all types of shock is similar.

Compensatory Phase

The initial, or compensatory, phase is characterized by mechanisms designed to restore homeostasis. Compensatory mechanisms are aimed at preserving vital organ perfusion at the expense of integumentary and splanchnic perfusion. Whether the inciting event is a volume (hypovolemic), a pump (cardiogenic), or a resistance (vasogenic) problem, perceived loss of vascular volume inhibits afferent discharge of baroreceptors in the aortic arch and carotid sinus, stimulating sympathetic nervous system output, causing the release of catecholamines to increase HR, contractility, and ultimately CO.

Patients enter the compensatory phase of shock after the initial insult. These compensatory changes, via activation of the sympathetic nervous system, occur in an effort to maintain normal homeostasis in the face of, and primarily affect, the cardiovascular system under neurohumoral control. This is mediated through stimulation of hormones primarily from the adrenal cortex and medulla (i.e., norepinephrine, epinephrine).[28,61]

Activation of the anterior pituitary occurs with release of adrenocorticotropic hormone as well as endorphins, thyroid-stimulating hormone, and growth hormone. The posterior pituitary secretes antidiuretic hormone (ADH), stimulating the reabsorption of water from the kidneys. Activation of the renin-angiotensin-aldosterone system stimulates the release of aldosterone from the adrenal cortex, increasing sodium and water reabsorption. Cortisol is also secreted to increase mobilization of glucose and stimulate protein catabolism.[28,61]

The overall purpose of this response is to improve tissue perfusion and support cellular metabolism through four mechanisms. First, CO is improved via the increases in HR and contractility. Second, blood flow is increased to central, essential organs as the result of the peripheral vasoconstriction. Third, plasma volume is increased by the retention of sodium and water and the shifting fluid from the interstitium into the vascular space, which occurs more slowly over 6 to 12 hours. Finally, glyconeogenesis and increased catabolism are designed to provide substrate availability for cell metabolism.[28,51]

Early clinical findings in the compensatory phase of shock are subtle and easily missed without methodic assessment. Early findings associated with the initial release of epinephrine and norepinephrine include the onset of anxiety and restlessness along with pallor and a decrease in peripheral skin temperature. A slight increase in HR, progressing to tachycardia, is designed to compensate for initial reductions in SV in order to preserve CO and is a hallmark sign of tissue hypoperfusion. Therefore, normal blood pressure (BP) may be maintained for some time and is not a reliable indicator of shock in this phase. Later, arterial pulse pressure narrows as diastolic pressure increases in the face of reduced systolic pressure. Additionally, increases in HR and contractility will increase myocardial oxygen consumption.

Efforts to restore vascular volume mediated through aldosterone and ADH result in renal conservation of water and reduction in urinary output (UO) to less than 0.5 to 1.0 ml/kg.[28] This may not be apparent without the presence of a urinary catheter. Hypoperfusion of the splanchnic organs in this phase of shock results in ischemic injury to the mucosal layer of the intestine.[18,37,49,74,79] This has been linked to translocation of bacteria from the intestine to the circulation, with potential to initiate systemic inflammatory response and sepsis.

Reversal of shock in this phase usually results in favorable outcomes. The most important intervention is reversal of the primary cause (detailed interventions are discussed later).

Decompensated Phase

Progression of shock beyond the compensatory phase results in exhaustion of compensatory mechanisms.[4,15,51] Worsening of signs and symptoms associated with hypoperfusion manifest, along with hypotension. Hypotension is a hallmark clinical finding signaling the transition from the compensatory to decompensated shock phase. On the cellular level, impaired mitochondrial function occurs. Metabolic acidosis, reflecting onset of anaerobic metabolism, is clinically detectable through serum lactate and base deficit. In addition, failure of the sodium-potassium pump results in cellular swelling with impairment of substrate diffusion necessary for normal function. In septic shock, progression from the hyperdynamic state or "warm phase" to the hypodynamic or "cold phase" of shock exemplifies the progression from compensation to decompensation.[15,28,66]

During the compensatory phase of shock, perfusion to integumentary and splanchnic organs was initially shunted to preserve core organ function, resulting in ischemia of the intestinal mucosal layer. Perfusion to core organs such as the brain, heart, kidneys, and liver now becomes significantly compromised. Clinical manifestations include altered level of consciousness, progressive hypotension, hypothermia, coagulopathy, and anuria.[28]

Irreversible Shock Phase

Failure to reverse the progression of shock through either physiologic compensatory mechanisms or resuscitative measures results in further deterioration to irreversible or refractory shock. During this phase, ongoing hypoperfusion results in irreversible cellular and organ damage. Arterioles and venules passively dilate, and cellular and capillary permeability results in fluid shift to the interstitial space with impairment of oxygen delivery to the cell. Mitochondrial dysfunction and failure of the sodium-potassium pump result in osmotic cellular swelling and death. Organ dysfunction and failure is marked by increasing lactate levels and worsening base deficit. Application of vasopressor agents may be necessary as exhaustion of endogenous catecholamine stores occurs. These measures may result in artificial improvement of hemodynamic values, but they do little to improve perfusion or function of organ systems suffering irreversible damage and necrosis.[18,28] The hallmark of this phase is predictable progression of organ system dysfunction, and eventually death.

RESUSCITATION MEASURES IN SHOCK

Regardless of the type of shock, the overall goal of treatment is the restoration and maintenance of oxygen delivery to the tissues. Key to this process is a systematic approach to patient assessment, with priority therapeutic interventions based on this assessment. Programs such Advanced Trauma Life Support,[4] Advanced Trauma Care for Nurses,[108] and Advanced Cardiac Life Support[5] from the American Heart Association are designed to instruct clinicians in resuscitation.

Initial Evaluation

Initial priorities in the management of shock are guided by a primary assessment to detect immediate life-threatening issues with interventions based on these findings. This process should be employed regardless of the type of shock or the setting. A modified application of the ABC—airway, breathing, circulation—approach to assessment and intervention advocated in the instructional programs is applicable to all types of shock. All strategies are aimed at improving Do_2 and are discussed in more detail and illustrated in Figure 40-6.

Airway and Breathing. Initial evaluation in shock requires priority evaluation of the airway with intervention, as necessary. Although not all patients require airway intervention, close assessment for progressive

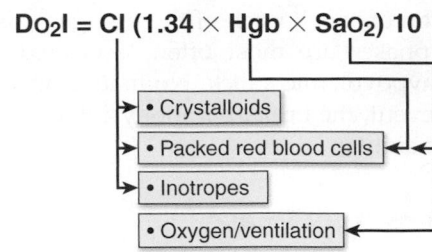

⇧FIGURE 40-6 Interventions augmenting oxygen delivery. Do_2I = Oxygen delivery index, CI = cardiac index, Hgb = hemoglobin, Sao_2 = arterial oxygen saturation.

changes in level of consciousness and inability to maintain a natural airway must be observed. However, in the case of progressing shock, a proactive approach to gaining airway control is preferred over waiting until the patient decompensates. Definitive airway control is best accomplished by insertion of a cuffed endotracheal tube by a practitioner experienced in endotracheal intubations.[4,108] When anatomic or situational conditions (e.g., facial trauma) prevent intubation, insertion of a surgical airway is the preferable alternative.

Initial assessment of adequate respiratory function involves standard physical assessment principles. In addition to observation of respiratory rate and pattern and the presence and quality of breath sounds, adjuncts such as pulse oximetry and end-tidal carbon dioxide (CO_2) monitoring may be used.[3] Arterial blood gases should be obtained to provide initial information about pulmonary gas exchange as well as information related to presence of acid-base abnormalities. All patients should receive high-flow oxygen (100%) immediately, whether or not airway management is required. Oxygen therapy may be adjusted once adequate tissue oxygenation has been established.[4,108]

In patients requiring airway support, mechanical ventilation also may be required. The duration of mechanical ventilation and the ventilation strategies employed are determined by a number of patient-specific factors. In patients in whom shock may be rapidly reversed or conditions reversed (e.g., operative repair of traumatic injury), ventilation may be required only for a short time. Conversely, the need for ongoing resuscitation or the presence of complications (e.g., pneumonia, acute lung injury or sepsis) may prolong the need for ventilation. Additionally, the application of specialized lung-protective ventilation modes and strategies may be indicated based on the patient's needs. Detailed discussion of these strategies is found in Chapter 20.

Circulation. Assessment and management interventions in the circulatory component are probably most often associated with the resuscitation of shock. Broadly, these encompass the restoration and augmentation of vascular volume (preload),* as well as optimizing systemic vascular resistance (afterload) and myocardial contractility.[17,28,109] Each of these tasks, though simply stated, encompasses various strategies based on the type of shock and the individual needs of the patient.

Fluid Resuscitation

Fluid Delivery and Warming Mechanisms. In patients with a hypovolemic component of their shock state, reliable vascular access with the ability to deliver large volumes of fluid quickly is essential.[4,61,86,108,110] In initial resuscitation, large-bore peripheral venous access is required.[4,108] Central access may be reserved for those patients with anticipated ongoing resuscitation and monitoring needs as well as those situations in which peripheral access is unobtainable.[4]

Equally important is the need to maintain normothermia in shock. Resuscitation with large quantities of fluid and banked blood products places the patient at risk for the development of hypothermia and associated coagulopathy. The presence of preexisting acidosis along with these factors has been well described in hemorrhagic shock patients as the "Triad of Death."[25,61,86] Prevention, rather than treatment, is essential in reducing complications and associated mortality. Warming is discussed in Chapter 7.

All shock states, no matter what their etiology, result in a decreased venous return, or a decreased preload. Regardless of whether fluid is lost in the form of hemorrhage, as fluid shifts from the vascular to interstitial space, or expansion of the intravascular capacity, because of vasodilation, preload augmentation with fluids must precede the use of vasopressor agents to increase vascular tone.[4,28,95,108]

Isotonic Crystalloids. Isotonic crystalloid solutions, used in the resuscitation of shock, distribute into the extracellular fluid space. Approximately 25% remain in the intravascular space, whereas 75% will accumulate in the interstitial space. These solutions include isotonic saline solution (0.9% normal saline [NS]) and balanced salt solutions (i.e., lactated Ringer's [LR]). Crystalloid solutions have the advantage of being inexpensive and readily available in the clinical setting while providing adequate volume expansion in most situations.[15,38,99,120]

The volume of crystalloid required depends on the type of shock state. In hypovolemic shock related to

hemorrhage, each milliliter of blood loss may require up to 3 ml of crystalloid solution to replace blood volume (3:1 ratio).[4,61,108] Although this may be effective in early compensatory shock, it is of limited value in ongoing hemorrhage because crystalloid solutions have no ability to carry oxygen. In such situations, administration of packed red blood cells (PRBCs) is required and should be considered after the administration of approximately 2 L of crystalloid without improvement in hemodynamic stability.[4,108]

In septic shock, capillary permeability and fluid shifts from intravascular to interstitial space create a relative hypovolemia. Although the patient appears edematous and volume overloaded, there is inadequate vascular volume, further compounding the problem of maldistribution of blood flow common in septic shock. These patients may require the administration of up to 10 L or more of crystalloid to adequately restore the vascular volume.[8,15,28,32,53] Similar capillary permeability may occur in anaphylactic shock as a result of histamine release. Short-term volume resuscitation may be necessary to compensate for this fluid shift that occurs along with the coexisting vasodilation.[36]

Two shock types in which volume resuscitation is not routinely indicated are cardiogenic and neurogenic shock. In cardiogenic shock, myocardial contractility is compromised. Strategies are aimed at preload and afterload reduction to reduce unnecessary cardiac workload and oxygen requirements. Administration of fluid would be harmful unless clear evidence of hypovolemia is present or cardiogenic shock is caused by right ventricular infarction. In neurogenic shock, vasodilation is responsible for a condition of relative hypovolemia. The use of alpha adrenergic agents (e.g., phenylephrine [Neo-Synephrine]) is aimed at restoring vascular tone and is the preferred treatment strategy unless hypovolemia coexists.[8,15,28,53] Indiscriminate use of fluid in neurogenic shock will produce volume overload once vascular tone is restored, resulting in neurogenic pulmonary edema.

Isotonic crystalloid solutions are the mainstay of fluid resuscitation in shock. Because these solutions approximate the osmolality of body fluid, they minimize initial fluid shift from the vascular space. LR offers the advantage of a closer physiologic electrolyte balance. NS is the only solution that can be administered in the same IV line as blood products.[61] Both are readily available and inexpensive compared with other resuscitants. It is important to recognize the limitations of isotonic crystalloid solutions based on electrolyte composition. Caution must be exercised with the administration of large volumes of these solutions, specifically NS, because of the risk of developing hyperchloremic metabolic acidosis when using large volumes for resuscitation.[16,62,86,103] Additionally some

---

*References 4, 15, 17, 61, 73, 86, 95.

data implicate NS as the cause of neutrophil sequestration and activation when used in large volumes during fluid resuscitation that may contribute to initiating an inflammatory response.[48]

Hypertonic Crystalloids. Hypertonic saline solution (HSS) has been advocated for a number of resuscitation situations based on several desirable characteristics.[38] First, the administration of HSS is associated with an immediate mobilization of fluids from the intracellular space to the extracellular compartments, specifically the intravascular space. Additionally, it is associated with increased myocardial contractility, reductions in endothelial tissue edema, reduction in blood viscosity due to hemodilution, and improvement in microcirculation. Further modulation of immune response also has been described by noted reduction of neutrophil sequestration and priming in the lungs, prevention of CD11 activation by lipopolysaccharides, and expression and release of elastase, cytokines, free radicals, and adhesion molecules responsible for cellular damage.*

As a resuscitant in shock states, HSS is most often defined as a concentration of 7.5%, either alone or in combination with dextran. In hypovolemic shock, it is clear that use of HSS results in lower fluid volume requirements.[38] This effect is not only related to the fluid shifts from intracellular to extracellular compartments, but also an observed improvement in myocardial contractility, precapillary vasodilation, venoconstriction, and decrease in pulmonary vascular resistance. Patients with coexisting head injury and shock may benefit from these effects because HSS used in this population has been associated with increased cerebral perfusion pressure, decreased intracranial pressure, and reductions in cerebral edema.[38,48,86] Immunomodulatory effects include lower levels of inflammatory cytokines such as tumor necrosis factor (TNF-α) and interleukin 6 (IL-6). These mediators are associated with the occurrence of acute respiratory distress syndrome (ARDS) and multiple organ dysfunction syndrome (MODS) as well as significant mortality in these populations.[48,85]

Similar benefits to those described have been noted in investigations using HSS in sepsis.[88,118] This is not surprising, given the fact both hemorrhagic shock and sepsis are associated with systemic inflammatory response and hypovolemia. It is important to recognize that although theoretic and some physiologic benefits exist, a survival benefit has not been recognized in the majority of studies involving HSS.[38] Potential disadvantages to HSS include fluid volume overload associated with fluid shifts from the intracellular and interstitial space and hypernatremia.

Colloid Solutions

Colloids consist of plasma protein fractions as well as synthetic solutions including hydroethyl starch (hetastarch), dextran, and combination solutions of colloids and crystalloids.[38,99,112,120] Colloids are composed of larger molecules, allowing them to remain in the vascular space for longer periods while having the additional benefit of augmenting vascular fluid volume through osmotic pull from the interstitial and intracellular spaces.

Theoretically, these qualities should make colloid solutions a desirable alternative to crystalloid solutions in shock resuscitation. However, in the face of capillary leak associated with immune system activation, leakage of albumin into the interstitial space may result in undesirable fluid shift out of the vascular space. Though a number of colloid solutions are available, for the purpose of clinical relevance, only albumin and hydroethyl starch solutions are discussed further.

Albumin. Five percent (5%) albumin solution is the most commonly used albumin concentration for fluid volume resuscitation. Infusion of 1 L of 5% albumin will increase the intravascular volume by 500 to 1000 ml.[15] Though impressive, the use of albumin as a resuscitation solution has failed to show outcome benefit over less expensive and more readily available crystalloid solutions. Further, there have been conflicting data questioning the safety of albumin.[99]

In the recent multicenter, randomized control Saline versus Albumin Fluid Evaluation (SAFE) study discussed in the Research Utilization box on p. 1077,[112] a 4% albumin solution was compared with NS for fluid resuscitation; 28-day mortality was measured in patients admitted to critical care who required volume resuscitation. Both medical and surgical patients were included with subgroups for trauma, severe sepsis, and ARDS. Although there was no increased mortality risk for patients treated with albumin, there was no reported clinical advantage to the routine use of albumin over crystalloid. Mortality findings of the SAFE trial are in contrast to a previous meta-analysis of the Cochrane Injuries Group Albumin Review,[99] which reported a 6% increase in absolute risk of death with albumin use over crystalloid. However, analysis of current research data does not support the routine use of colloids over crystalloid solutions as a resuscitation fluid in shock.[99] Although recent data suggest that albumin use may not be harmful, it is hard to justify given the significant expense of albumin compared with crystalloid and other synthetic colloids.

---

*References 38, 48, 88, 95, 99, 103.

◆ RESEARCH UTILIZATION

Optimal Choice of Resuscitation Fluid in the Critically Ill

CLINICAL ISSUE

The optimal choice of resuscitation fluid in the critically ill is constantly debated. Whether this decision affects patient outcome is the most important question. Whereas crystalloid solutions remain the cornerstone of early volume resuscitation therapy, the colloid albumin has been used based on its theoretic benefit of remaining in the vascular space longer. Scientific data have not supported the use of albumin as a resuscitant and in fact provided evidence that albumin use may increase mortality, calling into question its safety.

SUMMARY

This multicenter, randomized, double-blind trial was conducted in a heterogeneous population of 6997 critically ill patients. The study was conducted in 16 academic tertiary hospitals in Australia and New Zealand. The investigational group of 3497 patients received albumin (4%), and the control group of 3500 patients received normal saline. There was no significant difference in mortality (28 days); new single organ system failure; days in the intensive care unit, on mechanical ventilation or on renal replacement therapy; or length of hospital stay. The study provides detailed information of subgroups. This is the largest prospective trial comparing albumin to crystalloid.

APPLICATIONS

This trial does not support previous evidence (mainly by meta-analysis) that mortality is increased with albumin use. Given the significant cost of albumin compared with crystalloid, and lack of evidence of superiority of albumin in general resuscitation, there is not sufficient evidence to recommend its general use.

NEED FOR FURTHER STUDY

Further study of larger subgroups is needed for reliable outcome data. Additionally, comparison with other synthetic colloids may be valuable.

The SAFE Study Investigators (2004). A comparison of albumin and saline for fluid resuscitation in the intensive care unit. *N Engl J Med*, 350, 2247–2256.

Hydroxyethyl Starch Solutions. Hydroxyethyl starch solution is a synthetic colloid composed of 6% hydroxyethyl starch and sodium chloride. The theoretic benefits of using hydroxyethyl starch are similar to those associated with albumin. Additionally, hydroxyethyl starch, though more expensive than crystalloids, is less expensive than albumin.

Although beneficial in sustaining intravascular volume, hydroxyethyl starch solutions possess several undesirable characteristics, most notably the potential for coagulopathy through inhibition of fibrin clot formation through its inhibitory effect on platelets and plasmatic functions. Acute renal failure also has been associated with the use of hydroxyethyl starch, as has a reduction in measured intramucosal pH (pHi).[86,118] Hyperchloremic acidosis also may occur with hydroxyethyl starch use.[15,86] Third-generation hydroxyethyl starch solutions such as Hextend, a 6% hydroxyethyl starch combined with a buffered salt solution, are purported to reduce these undesirable side effects, specifically coagulation abnormalities. There are limited data to support this claim until more trials have been conducted.[15,86]

Combined Agents. Review of the literature reveals a number of trials evaluating the use of combination agents in shock resuscitation. These include colloids combined with HSS, colloid combined with isotonic solutions, and modified gelatin solutions. Some benefits may exist in using these agents, but there is insufficient evidence to support general use in shock resuscitation and no outcome benefit to date.[45,99,112]

Blood Products and Substitutes. A discussion of resuscitation would be incomplete without mention of transfusion therapy. Although crystalloid and colloid solutions are key components of fluid resuscitation, they lack the ability to carry oxygen and provide components necessary to support normal coagulation function (see Chapter 36 for detailed discussion of transfusion therapy).

Currently, the most developed type of blood substitute applicable for use in the resuscitation of shock is Hgb-based oxygen carriers. Many are undergoing phase III clinical trials, but are not available for clinical use at this time (see Chapter 36 for more information on blood substitutes).[61,85,86]

NUTRITIONAL SUPPORT IN SHOCK

The approach to nutritional support for patients in shock is multifactorial and includes the underlying cause of shock and any underlying organ dysfunction.[107,115] The timing of initiating nutritional support and method of delivery also are important.

There is little argument that critically ill patients require nutritional support. This is especially true of patients in shock who enter a catabolic state related to the hypermetabolic state of the underlying illness (Chapter 6 provides comprehensive information about nutrition in the critical ill patient). As important as how much and what to feed is when to feed. Patients in shock undergoing active resuscitation should have nutritional support measures delayed until hemodynamic stability has been achieved. There are no current scientific data to support the implementation of nutritional support in patients with conditions resulting in decreased intestinal perfusion.[7,107] Further, no data can be found to support the use of parenteral nutrition in patients who are in shock. In addition to the compensatory redistribution of blood flow away from the intestine to the central organs associated with shock, the use of vasopressor agents further decreases already compromised perfusion.[18,107] Although enteral nutrition may be beneficial in maintaining intestinal mucosal integrity, the intestinal shock state may result in inadequate perfusion to accommodate normal digestive function and may further stress already compromised tissue oxygenation at the gut level.[18,107]

In the presence of adequate gut function, enteral feeding is preferred over parenteral nutrition.[7,47,107] Enteral feeding helps to maintain the intestinal mucosal barrier, is associated with better wound healing and lower infection rates, and is less costly than parenteral nutrition. If not contraindicated, enteral nutrition should begin within 24 hours. In patients in whom enteral nutrition is contraindicated, parenteral nutrition may be considered. Patients who are well nourished at baseline may be able to forgo initiation of parenteral nutrition support if it is anticipated they will tolerate enteral support in 7 to 10 days.[115] This may not be reasonable, however, in patients with hypermetabolic shock conditions such as burns or sepsis in which immediate support is required to meet significant metabolic needs and long-term nutritional support is anticipated.[7,47,69,115] See Chapter 6 for a more detailed discussion on nutritional support.

END POINTS OF RESUSCITATION

The resuscitation process is a continuum across the phases of care from initial resuscitation on admission, through surgery and into critical care. Throughout this process, the patient must be constantly evaluated in light of clinical parameters that indicate resolution or worsening shock. Developing an understanding of these parameters, or "end points of resuscitation," is essential to effectively monitor the critically ill or injured patient in shock.

The goal of shock resuscitation is to restore oxygen delivery to the cells to support normal metabolic function. Determining when resuscitation is complete requires ongoing evaluation of physiologic markers or "end points" of resuscitation. These are clinical measures reflecting either global and/or regional changes

or improvements in tissue perfusion and oxygenation. A clear understanding of the benefits and limitations of these end points is essential in order to improve clinical utility during resuscitation.[103,113]

Regardless of the type of shock, resuscitation efforts are guided by end points assisting in determining the success of therapeutic interventions. However, these measurements vary in complexity and usefulness, depending on the severity of shock and level of resuscitation. For example, the patient in uncompensated hypovolemic shock with tachycardia, hypotension, and oliguria clearly requires resuscitative intervention. As resuscitation successfully progresses, resolution of these conditions is expected. In this case, basic end points, HR, BP and UO, are adequate to signal physiologic improvement. However, the end points do not speak to the adequacy of global oxygen delivery to the tissues and the reversal of compensated or covert levels of shock.* Determination of success at these levels requires the use of more sophisticated laboratory markers and application of both invasive and noninvasive monitoring devices to measure global and regional tissue oxygenation. Although no one end point is superior in all situations, systematic evaluation of multiple end points can assist in fine-tuning resuscitation efforts. In this section, specific end points are discussed, proceeding from basic clinical assessment to more complex lab data and information obtained from physiologic monitoring devices. Additionally, a model of evaluating global indicators before progressing to regional or local indicators is used (Figure 40-7).

As noted, the assessment of routine vital signs provides an initial indication of physiologic improvement during resuscitation efforts. Increase in HR is an early compensatory effort to improve CO as part of the stress response mediated by the catecholamine release from the adrenal glands. Further efforts to increase CO by improving SV are achieved through renal conservation of fluid under the influence of ADH and aldosterone.[28,61]

Under many circumstances, tachycardia may be a reliable indicator to the onset of a compensatory response to shock.[4,103,108] However, there are several disadvantages to using this parameter. Patients may be unable to develop a tachycardic compensatory response, or may develop tachycardia for reasons other than a compensatory response to shock.

Those in the first category may include patients with cardiac conduction disturbances, history of heart transplant, older adult patients, and those on medications (e.g., beta blockers) that preclude compensatory increases in HR. Patients in neurogenic shock from high spinal cord injury present with bradycardia as a result of

*References 12, 37, 49, 79, 86, 95, 103, 113.

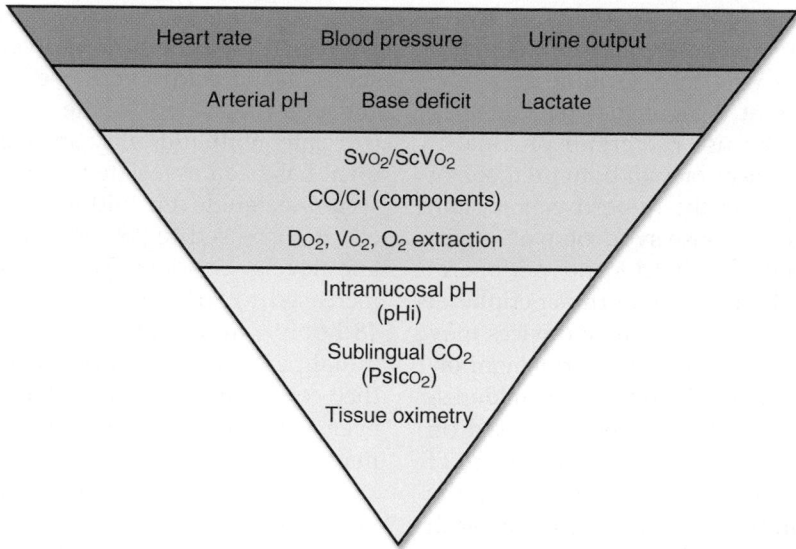

♦FIGURE 40-7 Progression of resuscitation end points from global to tissue specific.

lost sympathetic control and unopposed parasympathetic influence.[4,28,65,108] This occurs even in the presence of coexisting hypovolemia that would normally trigger a tachycardic response in a patient without a spinal cord injury. Additionally, well-conditioned patients (i.e., athletes or young adults) with lower resting HRs may not become profoundly tachycardic, because they are able to compensate by increasing SV to improve CO.

Patients in the second category may be tachycardic as a result of conditions other than shock. These include hypoxia as well as other physiologic triggers of the stress response including pain, anxiety, and delirium. Damage to the myocardium in blunt cardiac injury or the presence of preexisting conduction disturbances may also preclude usefulness of HR as a resuscitation end point. Finally, the presence of fever and influence of cytokines released as a result of systemic inflammatory response and sepsis result in persistent tachycardia independent of a compensatory response.

Blood Pressure

BP, similar to HR, is a common parameter used to gauge hemodynamic stability and guide resuscitative efforts. In shock states, change in BP is a late finding, reflecting that compensatory mechanisms are already beginning to fail.[3,28,103,108] Consequently, BP is not a useful parameter for early detection of shock. Furthermore, the presence of a "normal" BP does not guarantee the adequacy of perfusion at the cellular level.

Despite these issues, resuscitation efforts aimed at restoring adequate BP are appropriate as long as these limitations are considered. Initial efforts to improve BP

may include administration of volume expanders in the face of suspected hypovolemia and the use of vasodilatory or vasopressor agents.[4,12,15,28,32] The BP end points for resuscitation must be individualized for each patient and determined in conjunction with other parameters more fully reflective of improved function at the end-organ level. A systolic BP of 100 mm Hg may be adequate to achieve organ perfusion in a healthy individual, whereas a higher pressure may be necessary in those with preexisting hypertension. Emphasis on maintaining improvements in mean arterial pressure (MAP), to greater than 60 mm Hg, may be more appropriate than a target systolic pressure.[15] Most important, it must be remembered that BP is a measurement of vascular tone, not perfusion. Inadequate organ perfusion may exist even in the presence of a "normal" BP.

An important aspect of using BP as an end point is the method by which it is measured. These may be grouped into two types. Measurement of arterial pressure is accomplished through placement of a radial or femoral arterial line and allows for assessment of pressure on a continuous, real-time basis. It is considered the gold standard for BP monitoring.[9,28] The second method determines BP through the measurement of arterial blood flow.[9] This is accomplished manually through direct auscultation of Korotkoff sounds by use of a stethoscope/Doppler, or through the use of an automated noninvasive oscillometric device. Although both methods measure BP, measurement is accomplished in different ways. Arterial lines directly measure *pressure*; auscultatory methods determine pressure through the measurement of *flow*. Because of this difference, comparative BPs evaluated via the two methods in the same patient may yield different results.[9,28] Therefore correlation of measurements obtained between the two methods is not an appropriate way to determine accuracy. Additionally, it is important to note that the presence of pathophysiology and the use of certain pharmacologic agents may affect the accuracy of both methods of measurement. For example, in the hyperdynamic state of systemic inflammatory response syndrome or sepsis, the presence of abnormally high CO and peripheral vasodilation will result in higher than normal peripheral blood flow.[9] Because of this, auscultatory devices may overestimate the BP in relation to direct arterial monitoring. Conversely, the direct arterial method may underestimate or overestimate true arterial pressure based on the site of catheter insertion as well as the influence of pharmacologic agents. These scenarios highlight the importance of understanding the limitations of each method of monitoring as well as the use of BP in general as an end point of resuscitation.

Urine Output

The use of UO as an end point of resuscitation is based on the assumption that reductions or improvements in renal perfusion will subsequently result in like changes in UO. In adults, the production of 1 to 2 ml/kg of urine per hour has been the accepted end point to reflect adequate end-organ perfusion. As noted, UO decreases in shock states as part of the compensatory response geared to restore vascular volume, under the influence of ADH and aldosterone. This assumes that normal renal function is present. However, in patients in whom normal renal function is reduced or even absent, this end point is not reliable.[28,103,122] Such conditions may result in the presence of preexisting oliguria or anuria (i.e., chronic renal failure). Conversely, adequate UO despite perfusion abnormalities may exist when the kidneys are unable to concentrate urine. This may be observed in older adult populations as well as in the presence of renal failure or conditions such as diabetes insipidus. Further, the influence of medications affecting renal blood flow or those that induce artificial diuresis must be considered when using UO as a parameter to evaluate the adequacy of resuscitation.

In uncompensated shock, the use of HR, BP, and UO may be appropriate end points in light of the limitations discussed. However, further evaluation of additional end points reflective of global tissue oxygenation is critical to determine if adequate tissue perfusion is present.

Serum Lactate Levels

Lactic acid is a by-product of anaerobic metabolism. In addition to increased lactate production in shock states, lactic acid levels may exceed the liver's excretory ability. In normal conditions, lactate levels are less than 2 mmol/L; however, in the presence of shock, lactic acid levels rise.[31,95,103] As a resuscitation end point, elevated lactate levels have been shown to correlate with mortality in shock states. Patient survival has been associated with the ability to normalize serum lactate levels within 24 hours. Mortality significantly increased to 25% for those who normalized lactate levels between 24 and 48 hours, and further increased to 86% for those who did not normalize by 48 hours.[1] In a study by Manikis and colleagues, the initial peak in lactate levels as well as the duration further correlated in the development of MODS.[72] However, it is important to discuss several conditions that may limit the usefulness of lactate levels

Lactate is efficiently metabolized in the patients with normal liver function. Metabolism may be further augmented in hyperdynamic states as perfusion to the liver is increased. Because of this, the lactic acid level may not rise in the presence of shock until hepatic perfusion becomes significantly compromised.[1,25] Additionally, some organs such as the heart use lactate as an energy source. This consumption may further be the cause of lactate levels not rising significantly. In contrast, certain conditions may result in elevated lactate levels and are not reflective of hypoperfusion. These include the presence of liver disease in which lactate clearance may be impaired, as well as acute alcohol intoxication.[41] There are insufficient data to support the use of an absolute lactate value or range of values as an end point of resuscitation. Improvement in survival using lactate as an end point also has not been shown.[1,25,72] With this in mind, evaluation of trended lactate levels may be most helpful in guiding the need for more aggressive resuscitation measures.

Arterial Base Deficit

Arterial base deficit is another indicator of anaerobic metabolism that may be used to guide resuscitation. Obtained as part of the arterial blood gas panel, arterial base deficit is reflective of serum bicarbonate utilization in an attempt to buffer acidosis. It is directly calculated by the blood gas analyzer from the pH, partial pressure of arterial oxygen tension ($Paco_2$), and serum bicarbonate (HCO_3^-). Resuscitation measures used in successful restoration of tissue perfusion and cellular oxygenation should produce a reduction in base deficit as acidosis resolves. Davis and associates classified base deficit abnormalities into mild, moderate, and severe. A mild base deficit is seen at levels between 2 and 5 mmol/L, moderate between 6 and 14 mmol/L, and severe base deficit at greater than 14 mmol/L.[30,122] Further study revealed a base deficit level of greater than 6 mmol/L was associated with severe injury in most patients;

however, patients older than 55 years of age were more likely to have a normal base deficit than younger patients when the Injury Severity Score (ISS) was greater than 16.[30]

In trauma patients, increasing base deficit is was associated with ongoing blood loss.[42,98,114] Significant base deficits were also associated with lower BPs on admission and significant resuscitation fluid volume requirements.[114] Similar to other end points, base deficit is most helpful in determining the effectiveness of resuscitation measures when trended. Patients who fail to improve their base deficit levels were found to have impaired oxygen consumption and extraction profiles as well as a greater tendency to develop MODS and death. In trauma patients, the positive predictive value of base deficit in determination of outcome is improved when combined with ISS, low Glasgow Coma Scale (GCS) score, hypothermia, and ongoing blood requirements.[42,98,113]

As with any end point, caution must be used in interpreting values in light of preexisting patient conditions and disease states. Elevations in base deficit unrelated to shock may be found. These include alcohol intoxication, hyperchloremic acidosis, and preexisting renal failure. Although alcohol intoxication results in elevation of base deficit independent of shock, base deficit levels greater than 4 to 6 mmol/L should be considered significant.[29,40,41,123] Findings by Dunne and colleagues noted both base deficit and lactate levels retain predictive outcome accuracy in patients using alcohol as well as other drugs.[41] Hyperchloremic acidosis is associated with the administration of large volumes of resuscitation fluids (NS and to a lesser degree, LR).[62] This phenomenon occurs as the chloride portion of these balanced salt solutions raises serum chloride more rapidly than serum sodium concentrations. This results in hyperchloremia, favoring a shift toward hydrochloric acid in the balance with sodium hydroxide, causing pH to fall.[62] Brill and co-workers noted that base deficit is not predictive of mortality when altered as a result of hyperchloremic acidosis.[16]

Monitoring Technology

Patients who fail to respond in a predictable fashion to resuscitation measures may require additional monitoring in the form of a pulmonary artery catheter (PAC), oximetric central venous catheter, or transesophageal Doppler. Traditionally these devices have provided information helpful in resuscitation such as right-sided heart pressures and calculated CO. More sophisticated devices provide oximetric capability to measure the Svo_2 as well as continuous CO. More recently, continuous measurement of right ventricular end-diastolic volume index (RVEDVI) has been made possible and more accurately estimates right ventricular

preload during volume resuscitation. The esophageal Doppler offers the advantage of being less invasive than a PAC. When placed in the esophagus, information is obtained about descending aortic blood flow (Figure 40-8). Hemodynamic variables (CO, preload, afterload, contractility) can be calculated by interpreting the Doppler waveforms.[27,90,104,116] Disadvantages to this approach include inability to obtain oximetry from the device and the need for continual esophageal placement for ongoing monitoring. These parameters may be useful in helping the clinician achieve resuscitation goals and are discussed in more detail later.

Oxygen Monitoring

Much of the information obtained from the PAC may be used to calculate Do_2I. Normal Do_2I of 500 to 600 ml/min/m^2 provides four times the amount of oxygen required to sustain normal Vo_2 at the tissue level. Increased oxygen demands by the tissues are met primarily by increasing the rate of oxygen extraction (ERo_2) from the delivery surplus.[28,51,105] As mentioned, the theory of oxygen delivery dependence in shock was based on the observed relationship between calculated values of Do_2I and Vo_2I by several researchers during resuscitation. Subsequent research in this area has not supported these initial proposals.[80,109,117]

First, the observed improvement in mortality associated with patients who achieved higher CO and Do_2 during resuscitation may be more of a marker of physiologic reserve in that patient group. The inability to

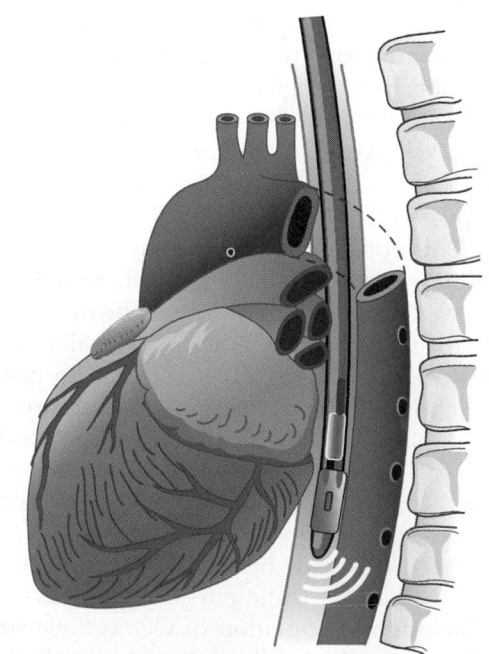

⬧FIGURE 40-8 Esophageal Doppler monitor probe.

achieve improvement may indicate lack of this reserve and a tendency to untoward outcome. Unfortunately there is insufficient evidence that exogenous application of measures to increase Do_2 improves survival.[64,80]

Second, initial findings of supply dependency demonstrated by a relationship between mathematically derived values of Do_2 and Vo_2 have not been consistently found in other studies.[64,80] This is especially true when calculated Do_2 is compared with indirect calorimetry measurements of Vo_2 using metabolic monitors rather than the calculated value. The influence of mathematical coupling from shared variables, such as CO (index), Hgb, and oxygen saturation, used in both the Do_2I and Vo_2I equations has been discussed.[117]

In addition to limitations, more recent studies have called into question the benefit of aggressively resuscitating to achieve supranormal levels of delivery and consumption. This is primarily based on inability to reproduce the benefits initially observed and evidence that supranormal strategies may be associated with higher mortality and complications such as abdominal compartment syndrome.[71,117] McKinley and associates[80] described no advantage to resuscitating beyond physiologic Do_2I and Vo_2I targets. This may be in part related to the physiologic stress caused by aggressive volume resuscitation, administration of blood products, and use of pharmacologic agents. Based on these more recent data, it is recommended that resuscitation efforts be aimed at achieving but not exceeding physiologic targets. Such goals include a Do_2I of 500 ml/min/m^2, while targeting a Vo_2I that meets the metabolic needs of the patient. Normal Vo_2I is 120 to 130 ml/min/m^2. This may increase as metabolic needs increase in conditions of pain, agitation, fever, and any condition resulting in systemic inflammatory response. A "normal" Vo_2I in these conditions may range from 180 to 260 ml/min/m^2, as Vo_2I may rise 50% to 100% above normal.[28]

The rate of oxygen extraction is represented by the Vo_2I/Do_2I ratio (ERo_2). In normal conditions, the ERo_2 is approximately 20% to 25% of the circulating Do_2I.[28,109] This normal percentage may be deceiving, as Do_2I declines proportionally to Vo_2I, maintaining a 20% to 25% ERo_2. Although ERo_2 may be normal, delivery and consumption are not. In critical illness the extraction rate may increase in response to metabolic demands (early sepsis) or decrease as cells are unable to use available oxygen because of mitochondrial dysfunction associated with late sepsis or refractory shock. Therefore the resuscitation goal should be aimed at achieving physiologic Do_2I as early as possible, in order to prevent the onset of organ dysfunction and failure.[15,60,80,103,109] Therapeutic efforts to increase oxygen delivery include manipulation of CO and elevation of arterial oxygen content. Efforts to achieve these goals include controlling extremes in HR, augmenting

preload and contractility, and optimizing afterload. Arterial oxygen content may be improved through the delivery of supplemental oxygen and by raising Hgb levels in an effort to increase oxygen saturation. Further efforts to limit unnecessary oxygen consumption through the treatment of pain, agitation, fever, or other underlying causes will help to achieve this goal.[57,58]

Mixed Venous Oxygen Saturation

The aforementioned assessment of the balance between Do_2 and Vo_2 is accomplished in the acute care setting by measurement of Svo_2[15,28,58,103] and more recently, measurement of central venous oxygen saturation ($Scvo_2$).[32,97] Svo_2 is measured in the pulmonary artery through the use of a fiberoptic PAC and recorded in percentage of Hgb saturated with oxygen. Normal Svo_2 is between 60% and 80%, reflecting the saturation of mixed arterial blood after tissue extraction of oxygen from the blood when it has circulated through the body. $Scvo_2$ measurement has been proposed as an alternative to Svo_2. $Scvo_2$ is approximately 5% higher than Svo_2 owing to the fact it is measured proximal to the right heart, where maximal extraction of oxygen from the blood has yet to occur. $Scvo_2$ is measured through the use of an oximetric multilumen[58] catheter placed into the superior vena cava. This device may be placed more quickly in environments such as the emergency department, where PAC placement may not be feasible. Additionally, complications associated with PAC may be avoided. Limitations of the device include inability to measure parameters such as CO, pulmonary artery wedge pressures, and RVEDVI. In addition, the catheter lumens are not large enough to accommodate rapid volume infusions required for some resuscitation scenarios (e.g., trauma). The device has found favorable application in early goal-directed therapy of the septic patient. Resuscitation efforts are directed to early optimization of $Scvo_2$.

Regardless of method, the measurement of Svo_2 or $Scvo_2$ provides information about the balance between oxygen delivered and consumed. A change in Svo_2 of 10% or more warrants closer evaluation. Assessment as to whether the change is related to an alteration in Do_2I or in Vo_2I is necessary.[58] Some examples of these situations are included in Box 41-4. Once cause is established, efforts aimed at improving supply and limiting unnecessary demand may be targeted.[58]

Hemodynamic Indices

To achieve desired end points of resuscitation, hemodynamic parameters (targets) contributing to Do_2I must be optimized. These targets must be individualized for each patient, but are primarily focused on improving the CI component of the oxygen delivery equation, specifically heart rate and ventricular SV (the effect of heart rate has been discussed in detail). Efforts to improve SV are more complex. They include the manipulation of cardiac preload, afterload, and contractility. The relationship among these parameters is illustrated in Figure 40-9.

Preload

Preload is blood volume in the ventricles prior to systole. Based on the principles of Starling's law, preload may be manipulated by increasing the volume into the ventricle to increase stretch of the myocardial fibers.[21,22,67,73] This will result in increased recoil of these fibers during systole, increasing cardiac SV. Limitation to this approach occurs with overstretch of the myocardial fibers, resulting in a decreasing SV and CO. This is represented by the plateau portion of the Starling curve.[73] Traditional markers to evaluate preload include central venous pressure (CVP), pulmonary artery pressure (PAP), and pulmonary artery wedge pressure (PAWP). The main limitation of these parameters is that they are measurements of pressure rather than actual volume.[67,101,103]

Measurements of pressure have traditionally been used as a surrogate for volume, which is not feasible through standard hemodynamic monitoring devices at the bedside. The assumed relationship is that increasing pressures are reflective of increased preload volume. Conversely, low pressures reflect low volume.[2,67] This relationship does not exist in the presence of certain cardiovascular pathology or other circumstances adversely affecting intrathoracic pressure. Such things may include valvular disease, decreased myocardial

compliance, changes in chest wall compliance, abdominal compartment syndrome, and therapeutic strategies such as positive-pressure ventilation and positive end-expiratory pressure (PEEP). These conditions may result in hemodynamic pressure changes that are not necessarily reflective of volume.[19-22]

Right Ventricular End-Diastolic Volume Index

Recent development of PACs with the ability to measure ejection fraction allow for the calculation of continuous right heart end-diastolic volume index (RVEDVI) and provide an additional parameter to evaluate preload. RVEDVI is calculated using the right ventricular ejection fraction (RVEF).[2,67,101] RVEF is computed by the continuous computer evaluation of the thermodilution curve used to calculate CO. RVEF is then divided by the SV index (SVI) to determine end-diastolic volume (index). End-systolic volume index (ESVI) may be determined by subtracting the SVI from the EDVI.[2,67,101] (Table 40-3 summarizes normal volumetric parameters.)

It has been suggested that RVEDVI should replace traditional preload markers such as CVP and PAWP.[17,19-22,67,101] These suggestions are based on the limitations of these traditional parameters as noted above and recent research data showing superiority of RVEDVI as a marker for volume resuscitation. Studies have noted that RVEDVI was correlated better than PAWP with improvements in CI.[17,19-22,34-36,101] Another study noted that RVEDVI was not prone to influences of intrathoracic pressure associated with positive-pressure ventilation and PEEP.[36] Suggested targets for RVEDVI based on current research range from $100 \, \text{ml/m}^2$ to greater than $120 \, \text{ml/m}^2$ while evaluating ejection

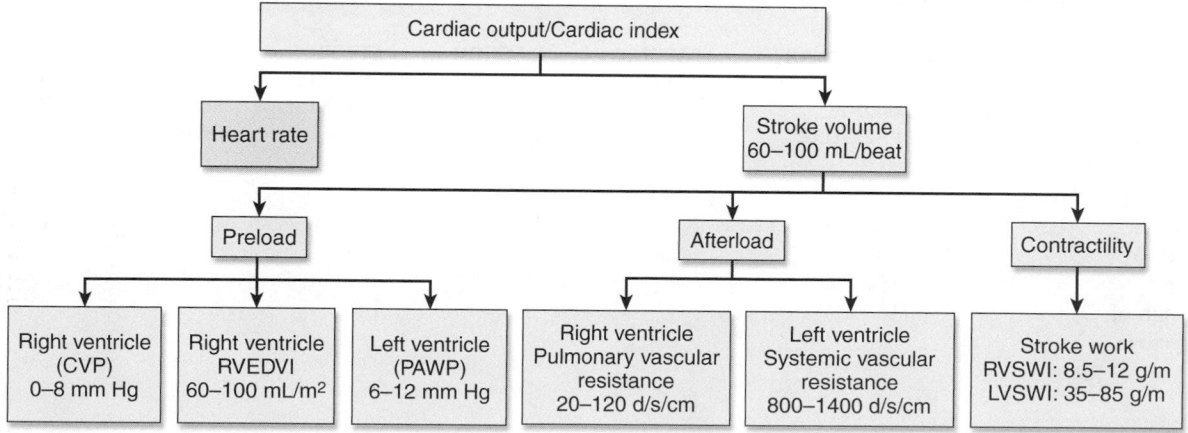

♦**FIGURE 40-9** Relationship of hemodynamic parameters. CVP = Central venous pressure, RVEDVI = right ventricular end-diastolic volume index, PAWP = pulmonary artery wedge pressure, RVSWI = right ventricular stroke work index, LVSWI = left ventricular stroke work index.

TABLE 40-3 Normal Volumetric Parameters

VOLUMETRIC PARAMETERS	NORMAL VALUES
Stroke volume (SV)	60–100 ml/beat
Stroke volume index (SVI)	35–60 ml/m²
Right ventricular end-diastolic volume (RVEDV)	100–160 ml/beat
Right ventricular end-diastolic volume index (RVEDVI)	60–100 ml/m²
Right ventricular end-systolic volume (RVESV)	50–100 ml/beat
Right ventricular end-systolic volume index (RVESVI)	30–60 ml/m²
Right ventricular ejection fraction (RVEF)	40%-60%

Data from references 28 and 67.

fraction (EF), SVI, ESVI, and CI.* In hypovolemia, augmentation of vascular volume should result in increasing RVEDVI and subsequent improvements in EF, SVI, and CI based on the Starling curve.[73] Overshooting the curve can be appreciated as RVEDVI continues to increase without improvement in EF or a noted decrease in EF and SVI.[67] Table 40-4 illustrates the change in RVEDVI and its components when fluid resuscitation is initiated.

*References 17, 19–22, 35, 36, 101.

Caution must be exercised in using RVEDVI in certain patient conditions. These include any patient in whom thermodilution CO measurement may be considered inaccurate. Conditions such as regurgitant flow or septal defect affecting the accuracy of the thermodilution method may also affect the accuracy of the RVEDVI calculation.[67]

Afterload

Defined as resistance to blood-volume ejection from the ventricle, afterload is calculated as systemic vascular resistance (SVR) for the left side of the heart and pulmonary vascular resistance for the right side.[28] Limitations to the calculation of these parameters are related to the mathematical calculation and potential coupling errors of these indices, based on other measured parameters. Manipulation of afterload in shock is dependent on the type of shock and characteristics. For example, in conditions of abnormally low afterload that result from the vasodilation of neurogenic shock or septic shock, the use of vasopressor agents may be necessary.[28] Conversely, the patient in cardiogenic shock may require afterload-reduction measures such as vasodilators and balloon counterpulsation to improve CO.[15,28]

Contractility

Contractility is the force of myocardial contraction. Myocardial contractility is somewhat affected by preload as discussed in the context of Starling's law.[21,22,65] In addition to the manipulation of preload, the use of inotropic agents to improve contractility will improve SV and CO. Some of these agents have associated afterload-reducing properties as well, which

TABLE 40-4 Right Ventricular End-Diastolic Response to Volume Resuscitation

CHANGE IN BASELINE PARAMETERS AFTER 2 L OF FLUID	CENTRAL VENOUS PRESSURE	PULMONARY ARTERY WEDGE PRESSURE	CARDIAC INDEX	EJECTION FRACTION	STROKE VOLUME INDEX	END-DIASTOLIC VOLUME INDEX	END-SYSTOLIC VOLUME
Optimal response	↑	↑	↑	↑	↑	↑	↓ ↔
Overstretch of Starling curve	↑	↑	↓	↓	↓	↑	↑
Poor myocardial compliance	↑	↑	↓	↓	↓	↓ ↔	↑

Data from references 2, 19–23, 28, 34–36, 67, 73.
↑ = Increase, ↓ = decrease, ↔ = no change.

must be considered in the face of preexisting hypotension. Calculated indices of right and left ventricular stroke work indices (RVSWI, LVSWI) provide some information about the degree of ventricular energy output.[21,22,28,94] Stroke work indices describe the work the respective ventricles perform and may be helpful in determining poor cardiac function. Ventricular stroke work index is the product of change in pressure and change in volume. It may be calculated for both the right and left ventricles as follows:

$$LVSWI = (MAP - PAWP) \times (SVI) \times (0.0136)$$
Normal range: 43 to 61 g/m^2

$$RVSWI = (Mean\ PAP - CVP) \times (SVI) \times (0.0136)$$
Normal range: 7 to 12 g/m^2

In most shock states ventricular stroke work index is decreased. This may be due to reduction in SVI as a result of hypovolemia, increased vascular resistance, or decrease in contractility.[21]

End-Tidal Carbon Dioxide

Capnography is the measurement of exhaled CO_2. Devices used to measure exhaled CO_2 fall into two categories: colorimetric and photometric detectors. Colorimetric detectors demonstrate a reaction (color change) in the presence of CO_2. They do not quantify CO_2, they only detect its presence. Their application has been primarily to detect successful airway placement into the trachea during endotracheal intubation. Photometric measurement devices measure the presence and quantity of the CO_2 molecule, allowing for quantification of CO_2 levels and display of the CO_2 waveform.[3]

Measurement of CO_2 has many clinical applications including guidance of resuscitation. The partial pressure of end-tidal CO_2 (PET_{CO_2}) correlates with the partial pressure of arterial CO_2 (Pa_{CO_2}) levels in the absence of alveolar capillary diffusion abnormalities. Normally the Pa_{CO_2}-PET_{CO_2} gradient is less than 5 mm Hg. In conditions of reduced or absent pulmonary blood flow, such as shock and cardiac, PET_{CO_2} is reduced or absent.[2,39,59]

Several studies noted a reduction in PET_{CO_2} that correlated with reductions in CO associated with several shock states including hemorrhagic, cardiogenic, and septic shock.[39,59] Additional studies have shown that PET_{CO_2} correlates well with return of spontaneous circulation and increased effectiveness of cardiac compressions. Levine and colleagues noted that PET_{CO_2} levels lower than 10 mm Hg after 20 minutes of resuscitation correlated with 100% mortality in patients suffering out-of-hospital arrest.[68]

◆ Case Study 40-1, Part A

Resuscitating an Unstable Patient With Traumatic Injury

J.T. is a 32-year-old male unrestrained driver who struck a cement bridge support at high speed. On arrival of emergency medical services, he is found to be unresponsive with a best GCS score of 6 (eyes: 1, verbal: 1, motor: 4), labored respirations at 30 per minute, weak radial pulses of 130 beats per minute (bpm), and a palpable BP of 84 mm Hg. He has sustained a large laceration to the forehead, crepitus is noted over the left chest, and an obvious deformity of the left femur is present. After an hour-long extrication, he arrives to the trauma resuscitation area. Before arrival he was intubated, underwent needle decompression of the left chest for a suspected tension pneumothorax, and received 2 L of lactated Ringer's through two 14-gauge IV catheters placed by the prehospital team. Despite these interventions, his heart rate is 140 bpm and his blood pressure has not improved. During primary assessment and intervention, his airway placement is reconfirmed by measurement of end-tidal CO_2 and auscultation of breath sounds. He undergoes placement of a left 36 French chest tube for 500 ml of blood and insertion of a large-bore central line. In addition to continued infusion of warmed isotonic crystalloid solution (LR), warmed, non–type-specific O-negative PRBCs are initiated via the rapid infuser unit. A focused abdominal sonogram for trauma exam is completed to reveal large amounts of fluid in the pelvis and around the liver. Based on these findings, and continued hemodynamic instability, J.T. is taken to the operating room for emergent laparotomy.

After 2 hours in the operating room, he arrives at the critical care unit having undergone staged (damage control) laparotomy. His injuries included ruptured spleen, multiple liver lacerations, and transsection of the colon. He received 5 L of lactated Ringer's, 10 units of PRBCs, 8 units of fresh frozen plasma, and 6 units of platelets. His estimated blood loss was 4 L. His UO during the case was only 100 ml. Intraoperatively, a continuous cardiac output, end-diastolic volume PAC and arterial line were placed. His hemodynamic data are outlined as follows:

Case continues on page 1086

Arterial Blood Gases		Laboratory Tests		Hemodynamic Profile	
pH	7.20	Hgb	9	Temp	35° C
PaCO$_2$	36	Hct	28	HR	122 bpm
PaO$_2$	90	Platelets	200	BP	100/50 mm Hg
HCO$_3^-$	12	PT	16 sec	CVP	8 mm Hg
BE/BD	−11	WBC	18	PAP	25/8 mm Hg
SaO$_2$	93%	Glucose	180 mg/dl	PAWP	6 mm Hg
Vent settings		BUN	20 mg/dl	SvO$_2$	62%
Vt	600	Cr	0.8 mg/dl	RVEDVI	68 ml/m^2
Mode/rate	A/C 14	Na$^+$	136 mg/dl	RVESVI	38 ml/m^2
FiO$_2$	1	K$^+$	3.7 mg/dl	RVEF	20%
PEEP	+5	Cl$^-$	118 mg/dl	RVSWI	3
Static comp.	0.045	CO$_2$	26 mg/dl	LVSWI	25
		Ca^{++}	7 mg/dl	CO/CI	6.2 L/min/3.5 L/min/m^2
		Lactate	8 mg/dl	SVI	30 ml/beat/min
				SVR	1600 dynes
				PVR	120 dynes
				CXR	Large left pulmonary contusion and multiple L rib fractures

BE/BD = Base excess/base deficit, BUN = blood urea nitrogen, Ca^{++} = calcium, Cl = chloride, Cr = creatinine, CXR = chest x-ray, FiO$_2$ = fraction of inspired oxygen, Hct = hematocrit, K$^+$ = potassium, Na$^+$ = sodium, PIP = peak inspiratory pressure, PT = prothrombin time, Temp = temperature, UO = urine output, Vt = tidal volume, WBC = white blood cell.

As the critical care team takes over the care of this patient, the priority of care must focus on the continued resuscitation from shock that began in the prehospital phase of care.

Decision point: What parameters indicated incomplete resuscitation?

Decision point: What types of fluids should have been used?

Decision point: What types of treatment might be expected in the immediate postoperative period?

Case continues on page 1094

REGIONAL RESUSCITATION END POINTS

Global resuscitation end points reflect a general picture of tissue oxygenation. Although they provide a summary view of balance between delivery and demand, they do not provide information specific to individual organ systems, especially in circumstances in which maldistribution of blood flow may be present such as septic shock.

Certain organ systems such as the gastrointestinal tract, may be inadequately perfused despite the presence of normal global end points.[37,44,49,74,97] Hypoperfusion occurs as physiologic compensatory mechanisms favor central circulation over "less essential" organ systems such as the gastrointestinal and integumentary systems. During resuscitation, perfusion to these systems may be restored last or not at all.[14,28,100] It is clear that resuscitation cannot be considered complete until all organ beds are adequately perfused. Regional monitoring can allow such determination, and has been the focus of much clinical research.

Intramucosal pH

The gastrointestinal system, more specifically the intestine itself, is highly susceptible to hypoperfusion in the compensatory stages of shock. The innermost layer of the intestine, the mucosa, is most susceptible because it receives oxygen and nutrients by diffusion from the intestinal villi.[32,62,67,86] Deprivation of adequate perfusion for as little as an hour may result in mucosal damage and intestinal permeability. These circumstances occur despite the presence of normal global parameters, and the condition has been termed "covert compensated shock."[14,44,49,100]

The use of intestinal pHi has been studied clinically since the 1980s. It is calculated using the partial pressure of CO_2 from the intestinal lumen measured through the use of device called a tonometer, placed in the stomach or intestine. This technique was first demonstrated in 1964 by Bergofsky, using the urinary bladder and gallbladder. Fiddian-Green and associates later used tonometry in the stomach.[44] Specifics on use and limitations of pHi as a monitoring tool are covered in Chapter 29.

A normal pHi value is clinically defined as greater than 7.35. Less than 7.35 is considered intramucosal acidosis.* Gys and co-workers noted a pHi less than 7.32 to correlate with short-term mortality.[50]

The clinical reliability of pHi as a predictor of outcome has been demonstrated by a number of studies over the past decade. In 1991, Doglio and colleagues demonstrated that patients who presented with a low pHi (less than 7.35) and maintained this acidotic state after 12 hours had an 87% mortality rate. Conversely, those who arrived with normal pHi on admission and maintained this state had a 27% mortality rate.[37] Patients who arrived acidotic and improved by 12 hours had lower mortality than those presenting with normal pH who became acidotic. Both Gutierrez and associates[49] and Maynard and colleagues[79] demonstrated a statistically significant predictive value of pHi to predict outcome. Global measurements of oxygen delivery, consumption and extraction, however, did not consistently discriminate between survivors and nonsurvivors. In later studies conducted by Ivatury and co-workers in injured patients, intramucosal acidosis was consistently associated with poor outcome. The first study found that the presence of intramucosal acidosis was present in 80% of the nonsurvivors, with 75% of the patients with multiple organ failure having a low pHi.[55] A later study with similar methodology noted that only 7% of patients with pHi greater than 7.30 at 24 hours developed multiple organ dysfunction, whereas 75% of patients who failed to normalize pHi by 24 hours experienced multiple organ failure.[56]

Although clinically significant acidosis can be detected, the ability to correct intramucosal acidosis by augmenting global delivery parameters has not proven consistently effective. Interventions to attempt this have included volume augmentation, the administration of packed red blood cells, and use of vasopressors as well as mesenteric vasodilators.[83] Future research must focus on strategies to successfully resuscitate the splanchnic organ system.

Sublingual Capnometry

Sublingual capnometry was first proposed in 1998 as a more clinically acceptable alternative to gastric tonometry. The tongue is the most proximal portion of the GI tract, sharing similar circulation and neuronal control as the esophagus and stomach.[89,119] It was theorized that measurement of the partial pressure of sublingual CO_2 ($PslCO_2$) could provide the similar clinical value to pHi obtained through gastric tonometry.[14,75,76]

The sublingual capnometry device consists of an electronic computer device that analyzes the concentration of CO_2, a fiberoptic probe, and a disposable sensor. The probe/sensor is placed in the sublingual pocket in contact with the sublingual mucosa (Figure 40-10). CO_2 diffuses into the sensor into a contained fluorescent dye. The intensity of the dye solution is directly affected by the intensity of CO_2 from the tissue. The CO_2 dissolves to carbonic anhydrase and pH decreases. The change in pH is detected and quantified by the electronic computer device in 2 minutes.[89]

Although technically simpler to perform than gastric tonometry, some limitations of the device still exist. Current sublingual capnometry devices are designed for intermittent measurements of $PslCO_2$; therefore, repeat measures must be taken over time to trend changes in patient condition. In addition, any conditions limiting access to the oral cavity may prevent use of the device. These include oral trauma, surgical fixation of the jaw, and patient combativeness.

Several research studies have shown promising support for the use of sublingual capnometry. In 1999, Weil and colleagues[119] demonstrated the positive predictive value of $PslCO_2$ in detecting circulatory shock when comparing healthy volunteers with a group of critically ill patients with different subsets of clinical conditions. A $PslCO_2$ of greater than 70 mm Hg has a strong positive predictive value for diagnosis of shock. Several studies support the interchangeable use of $PslCO_2$ with gastric CO_2 values obtained through gastric tonometry.[77-77,92,119] Rackow and associates[93] studied the use of $PslCO_2$ in patients with cardiac failure. $PslCO_2$ correlated well with intramucosal CO_2 ($PiCO_2$) levels and lactate concentrations. The gradient between $PslCO_2$ and $PaCO_2$ was described as greater in nonsurvivors than survivors, but sample size was not large

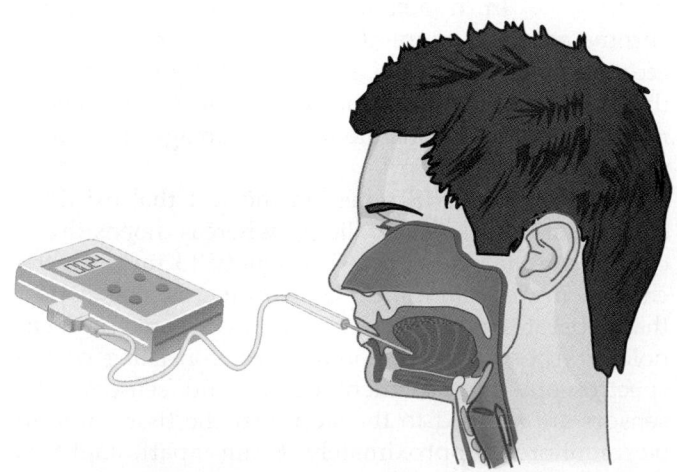

♦FIGURE 40-10 Sublingual capnometry.

---

enough to predict outcomes. Marik, during a clinical validation study in 2001, noted similar findings.[75] In 2003, Marik and co-workers noted that a $PslCO_2$-$PaCO_2$ gradient of greater than 25 mm Hg was predictive of negative outcome. Further, the gradient was responsive to resuscitative efforts, showing promise as potential resuscitation end point.[76,77]

Initial studies support sublingual capnometry as an alternative to gastric tonometry for determining the mucosal CO_2.[14,75–77,92,119] Further research with larger sample sizes in homogeneous clinical conditions is still needed to confirm predictive ability and to determine its clinical usefulness in guiding resuscitation efforts.

Near-Infrared Spectroscopy

An ideal end point for resuscitation is one that can continuously measure the adequacy of oxygenation at the cellular level, reflecting function at the mitochondrial level. Near-infrared spectroscopy (NIS) is based on the Beer-Lambert law, stating that light transmission through a solution with a dissolved solute decreases as concentration of the solute increases. In humans, three compounds change spectra when oxygenated: cytochrome aa3, myoglobin, and Hgb.[24] This change in spectra is used to determine the presence of oxygen binding on these substances and is the basis for current pulse oximetry devices. Unlike other technologies used to assess oxygenation, NIS can assess both the presence of oxyhemoglobin and the degree to which the cellular component cytochrome aa3 has been oxidized. Cytochrome aa3 is a copper molecule responsible for cellular oxygen use an indicator of cellular oxygen consumption. Cytochrome aa3 is the final receptor in the oxygen transport chain. In a healthy cellular environment, the oxyhemoglobin and redox state (oxidation-reduction) is tightly coupled.[24,86,103] In hypoxemia at the cell level, cytochrome aa3 is uncoupled from Hgb and remains in a reduced state. This state is reflective of mitochondrial dysfunction and may indicate the release of oxygen-radical species responsible for cell damage and multiple organ dysfunction.*

Operationally, NIS relies on the fact that oxidized cytochrome aa3 reflects light, whereas nonoxidized cytochrome aa3 does not. The ability to measure the change in reflectance in cytochrome is one aspect that separates NIS from conventional oximetric technology. The device is noninvasive, consisting of the spectroscopy measurement device and sensors. The sensors are applied to the skin over the tissue area to be monitored approximately 6 mm apart. Light is

passed through the tissue between the probes and determines Hgb saturation and cytochrome aa3 oxidation.[24,26,103,111]

Significant and promising research has been conducted in laboratory hemorrhage models as well as compartment syndrome simulation. Several investigators have also evaluated this technology in human subjects such as trauma patients in shock.[26,111] Summary findings of these investigations reveal consistent correlation with gastric tonometry and systemic oxygen delivery parameters in hemorrhagic shock models. Additionally, uncoupling of cytochrome aa3 has been described in patients who go on to develop multiple organ dysfunction and failure. In compartment syndrome, NIS accurately reflects changes in muscle tissue oxygenation even in the presence of hypotension. Further, normalization of oxygenation to the tissues has been detected after fasciotomy.[26,111,122]

NIS also has been used to measure pH by analyzing the spectral changes in the imidazole ring of the histidine residue within Hgb. NIS has been used to continuously measure small-bowel pH in a hemorrhage model because it represented an accurate alternative to gastric tonometry.[24] In this application, the ability to monitor continuously offers an advantage over the intermittent gastric tonometry method to measure resuscitation progress.[24,26,111] Though currently not in widespread use, this may change as additional research comes to support clinical application in a variety of shock states.

MULTIDISCIPLINARY PLAN OF CARE

Resuscitation of the patient in shock requires a well-orchestrated team approach. Key to successful patient outcome is the application of an organized and systematic approach to care. These priorities are outlined in the Multidisciplinary Plan of Care on pp. 1089-1093. Commonly used medications are presented in the Medication table on pp. 1116-1121 in Chapter 41. After management of immediate life-threatening issues, interventions to optimize nutritional support and prevent complications are key to reducing morbidity and mortality associated with critical illness. These goals are best achieved through the combined talents of a multidisciplinary critical care team, to which the advanced practice nurse contributes unique knowledge and skills.

Treatment strategies for hypovolemic shock are aimed at maintaining cardiopulmonary function and restoring intravascular volume through volume replacement, while providing definitive treatment for the underlying cause of the shock state.[4,61,108,113]

---

*References 24, 26, 103, 111, 122.

MULTIDISCIPLINARY PLAN OF CARE FOR RESUSCITATION OF THE PATIENT IN SHOCK

PROBLEM	INTERVENTION	RATIONALE	EXPECTED OUTCOME	SPECIAL CONSIDERATIONS
Inadequate ventilation and oxygenation	Assess and establish control of patient's airway. Provide a definitive airway.	Provides controlled airway for oxygenation and ventilation; reduces chance of aspiration.	Patent airway.	A definitive airway is a cuffed airway in the trachea: • Endotracheal tube • Surgical cricothyrotomy • Tracheostomy
	Assess respiratory effort and general appearance for evidence of compromise. • Rate • Pattern Use of accessory muscles Skin color Diagnostic studies: • Arterial blood gas • Pulse oximetry • End-tidal CO_2	Provides an indication of respiratory compromise, allowing early intervention.	Early compromise in ventilation is determined and corrected.	
	Provide high-flow oxygen in all shock states (100%)	Increases oxygen delivery to the circulatory system, improves oxygen delivery.	Oxygen delivery to the circulatory system is achieved and tissue hypoxemia is avoided	
	Initiate mechanical ventilation for indications of respiratory failure.	Improves compromised ventilation.	Restoration of normal ventilation.	
	Correct conditions impairing normal ventilation such as tension pneumothorax, open pneumothorax or hemothorax	Improves compromised ventilation and relieves obstructive causes of shock.	Restoration of normal ventilation and resolution of obstructive component of shock.	
Risk or presence of actual or relative hypovolemia	Consider patients at risk for shock resulting from hypovolemia: • Hemorrhage • Burns • Sepsis • Anaphylaxis • Pancreatitis	Identification allows for anticipation and early treatment.	Evidence of hypovolemia is detected early and treated.	

Table continues on page 1090

PROBLEM	INTERVENTION	RATIONALE	EXPECTED OUTCOME	SPECIAL CONSIDERATIONS
	• Ascites • Ileus • Aortic aneurysm • Vomiting/diarrhea • Fever Assess for indicators of hypovolemia: • Mental status changes • Tachycardia • Skin color & temp • BP (narrow pulse pressure) and MAP • Decreased UO Assess additional invasive hemodynamic parameters if available: • CVP, PAP, PAWP • CI, SV, EF, EDVI • SVR, PVR • RVSWI, LVSWI			
	Initiate volume replacement with isotonic crystalloid solutions unless other resuscitants are indicated based on patient condition • Lactated Ringer's solution • Normal saline solution (0.9%) **Others as indicated** • Packed red blood cells for hemorrhage or anemia below clinical threshold • Synthetic colloids (hetastarch) • Hypertonic saline solution • Fractionated blood products (FFP, platelets)	Evidence supports the use of crystalloid solution for initial resuscitation unless conditions dictate use of other solutions.	Targeted end points are achieved.	
	Monitor the patient during volume resuscitation for improvement or deterioration in above assessment parameters.	Ongoing monitoring of vital signs, hemodynamic parameters, and targeted end points of resuscitation indicate patient response to resuscitation efforts.		

PROBLEM	INTERVENTION	RATIONALE	EXPECTED OUTCOME	SPECIAL CONSIDERATIONS
	Establish and target global and regional resuscitation end points to include: Global • BD • LA • $Svo_2/Scvo_2$ • Do_2I, Vo_2I • $PETCO_2$ Regional • Gastric pHi • Sublingual carbon dioxide • Tissue spectroscopy			
	Anticipate and assess for complications related to volume resuscitation: • Circulatory overload • Hyperchloremic acidosis • Transfusion-related acute lung injury • Intraabdominal hypertension/abdominal compartment syndrome	Complications related to volume resuscitation may be treated early, preventing further patient morbidity.	Complications related to volume resuscitation are avoided or detected early and treated.	
Alterations in vascular tone (low resistance) causing maldistribution of blood flow and reduced tissue perfusion	Consider patients at risk for shock related to decreased vascular tone: Vasogenic types • Neurogenic shock • Anaphylaxis • Septic shock Assess and monitor parameters above to identify the presence of shock.	Patients in certain shock states or phases of shock may experience alterations in vascular tone, resulting in maldistribution of blood flow.	Normal vascular tone is restored and organ perfusion is optimized as evidenced by normal CI, SVR, LA, and BD.	
	Initiate volume resuscitation first where hypovolemia coexists with altered vascular tone. Initiate vasopressor agents as indicated based on desired physiologic effects (see the Medication table on pp. 1116-1121 in Ch 41).	In coexisting hypovolemia, volume resuscitation aimed at filling the depleted vascular space takes priority over initiation of vasopressors.		
	Monitor patient for improvement in hemodynamic parameters and targeted end points.	Ongoing monitoring of vital signs, hemodynamic parameters, and targeted end points of resuscitation will indicate patient response to resuscitation efforts.		

Table continues on page 1092

PROBLEM	INTERVENTION	RATIONALE	EXPECTED OUTCOME	SPECIAL CONSIDERATIONS
	Monitor for complications related to vasopressor agents including: • Dysrhythmias • Organ/tissue hypoperfusion • Tissue necrosis	May indicate the need to change agents. Complications may be detected and treated.	No complications relate to therapy.	
Reductions in cardiac output related to altered myocardial contractility	Identify patients at risk for shock related to alterations in myocardial contractility due to myocardial damage or the influence of depressant factors: • Cardiogenic • Septic shock *Consider in other shock types in the presence of normovolemia and normal vascular tone.* Evaluate previously discussed parameters and end points. Focus evaluation: • Svo_2, $Scvo_2$ • CI, SV, EF, RVEDVI, Do_2I, Vo_2I • RVSWI, LVSWI • SVR, PVR	Patients may be at risk for altered contractility related to myocardial damage or inflammatory cytokines.	CO is optimized through improvements in contractility and afterload reduction.	
	Initiate inotropic agents to improve contractility (see Table 41–10). Initiate afterload reduction measures as indicated: • Vasodilators • Intraaortic balloon counterpulsation • Ventricular assist device	These strategies improve CO by improving pump function and reducing ventricular outflow resistance (improved ventricular/arterial coupling)		
Alteration in nutrition related to hypermetabolism and decreased nutritional intake	Assess baseline nutritional status through formal evaluation by clinical nutritional support service.	Baseline assessment of nutritional status will determine nutritional status and anticipated nutritional requirements.	Nutritional support is provided to meet metabolic requirements.	

PROBLEM	INTERVENTION	RATIONALE	EXPECTED OUTCOME	SPECIAL CONSIDERATIONS
	Initiate nutritional support by enteral route as early as possible after resolution of shock unless contraindicated by GI injury or pathology.	The intestine is the route of choice for nutritional support in the absence of compromised gut perfusion or integrity. It is associated with lower infection complications and may prevent the translocation of pathologic bacteria from the intestine.		
	Initiate total parenteral nutrition in patients in whom enteral nutrition is contraindicated.			
Patient is at risk for complications related to shock and treatment interventions	Assess for the onset of complications related to shock and treatment interventions: • Organ dysfunction • ALI/ARDS • Hepatic/GI • Renal Hematologic: • Intraabdominal hypertension/compartment syndrome Infections: • Ventilator-associated pneumonia • Bloodstream infections • Urinary tract infections	Persistent shock states result in decreased organ perfusion, cellular death, organ dysfunction and failure. Organ dysfunction should be anticipated and supported. Infections related to invasive treatments may occur. Evidence-based strategies to prevent complications should be initiated.	Organ function is maintained Infection complications are prevented	

ALI = Acute lung injury, ARDS = acute respiratory distress syndrome, BD = base deficit, BP = blood pressure, CI = cardiac index, CO = cardiac output, CVP = central venous pressure, Do_2I = oxygen delivery index, EDVI = end-diastolic volume index, EF = ejection fraction, FFP = fresh frozen plasma, GI = gastrointestinal, LA = lactic acid, LVSWI = left ventricular stroke work index, MAP = mean arterial pressure, PAP = pulmonary artery pressure, PAWP = pulmonary artery wedge pressure, pHi = intramucosal pH, PVR = pulmonary vascular resistance, RVSWI = right ventricular stroke work index, $Scvo_2$ = central venous oxygen saturation, SV = stroke volume, Svo_2 = mixed venous oxygen saturation, SVR = systemic vascular resistance, UO = urinary output, Vo_2I = oxygen consumption index.

▲ Case Study 40-1, Part B

Treating Septic Shock

Forty-eight hours later, J.T. is noted to be febrile (temp 38.5° C), with a WBC count of 20,000. Blood and urine cultures have been sent along with bronchoalveolar lavage fluid for culture. He has been taken back to the operating room twice for abdominal washout. His abdomen remains "open" with a vacuum closure system in place. He is noted to have a worsening oxygenation profile (Pao_2/Fio_2 ratio), decreased static lung compliance, worsening renal function, elevated liver profile, and climbing glucose levels. Over the past 24 hours he has required 6 L of LR and 1 L of hetastarch to maintain BP. His RVEDVI reveals adequate preload, and SVI and EF are improved. Despite fluids, his MAP was less than 60 mm Hg. The decision was made to initiate norepinephrine at 2 mcg/min and titrate to achieve a MAP greater than 60 mm Hg. After 1 hour, norepinephrine (Levophed) was titrated to 10 mcg/min and a decision was made to add vasopressin at 0.04 unit/min. The current profile for this patient is below:

Arterial Blood Gases		Laboratory Tests		Hemodynamic Profile	
pH	7.32	Hgb	8.5	Temp	38.5° C
$Paco_2$	34	Hct	26	HR	128 bpm
Pao_2	75	Platelets	120	BP	110/50 mm Hg
HCO_3^-	20	PT	16 sec	CVP	6 mm Hg
BE/BD	−3	WBC	20	PAP	25/12 mm Hg
Sao_2	90%	Glucose	220 mg/dl	PAWP	10 mm Hg
Vent settings		BUN	30 mg/dl	Svo_2	78%
Vt	700	Cr	2.1 mg/dl	RVEDVI	135 ml/m²
Mode/rate	A/C16	Na^+	132 mg/dl	RVESVI	66 ml/m²
Fio_2	1	K^+	4.8 mg/dl	RVEF	55%
PEEP	+12	Cl^-	118 mg/dl	RVSWI	9 g/M/m²
PIP	50 cm	CO_2	26 mg/dl	LVSWI	53 g/M/m²
Static comp.	0.025	Ca^{++}	8 mg/dl	CO/CI	11 L/m/6 L/m/m²
Pao_2/Fio_2 ratio	75	Mg^{++}	2.2 mg/dl	SVI	65 ml/beat/m²
		Lactate	3.1 mg/dl	SVR	580 dynes
				PVR	50 dynes
				SV	60 ml/m²
				CXR	Bilateral white infiltrates

Mg^{++} = Magnesium.

Decision point: What physiologic and global parameters suggest that this patient is in septic shock?

Decision point: What are the priorities of care for this patient?

Decision point: Which vasopressors are most appropriate for the patient in shock?

COMPLICATIONS OF SHOCK

The complications associated with shock are related to either hypoxic organ system injury from perfusion deficits or the side effects of resuscitation efforts. The degree of organ system dysfunction and failure is directly related to the duration and severity of shock. Inability to reverse the shock state in a timely manner will result in organ failure, even in systems unrelated to the initial insult. This includes neurologic injury, myocardial ischemia, ARDS, acute tubular necrosis/renal failure, hepatic failure, hematologic failure (such as disseminated intravascular coagulation), and intestinal ischemia.

Treatment-related complications include those of volume resuscitation, use of vasopressors, and reperfusion injury as circulation is restored. Intraabdominal hypertension and secondary abdominal compartment syndrome, for example, result as crystalloid solutions shift from the intravascular to interstitial space, increasing intestinal edema within the peritoneal cavity.[71,81,121] This results in pressure on pulmonary, cardiovascular and renal structures, impairing normal function. Vasopressors employed to improve vascular tone and organ

♦ Case Study 40-1, Part C

Evaluating Organ-Specific Parameters

On hospital day 5, J.T. is hypotensive, oliguric, and edematous, with the following profile. Blood and sputum cultures reveal gram-negative bacteria, and antibiotic therapy is tailored to the specific organism. He is noted to be bleeding from his invasive line and drain sites. He has received 8 L of crystalloid over a 12-hour period. His vasopressor requirements include norepinephrine at 12 mcg/min and vasopressin at a physiologic replacement dose of 0.04 mcg/min.

Phenylephrine is added at 40 mcg/min, and BP improves to a mean of 65 mm Hg. Dobutamine is initiated to improve myocardial contractility after BP improves with vasopressors. Continuous renal replacement therapy is initiated in light of deteriorated renal function, metabolic acidosis, and hemodynamic instability. The ventilator mode is changed to airway pressure release ventilation as a lung protective strategy.

Arterial Blood Gases		Laboratory Tests		Hemodynamic Profile	
pH	7.28	Hgb	9.2	Temp	36° C
$Paco_2$	34	Hct	27	HR	115 bpm
Pao_2	68	Platelets	50	BP	84/40 mm Hg (MAP 54)
HCO_3^-	17	PT	20 sec	CVP	6 mm Hg
BE/BD	−6	WBC	25	PAP	20/10 mm Hg
Sao_2	90%	Glucose	230 mg/dl	PCWP	6 mm Hg
Vent settings		BUN	30 mg/dl	Svo_2	89%
IP (PEEP high)	35 cm H_2O	Cr	3 mg/dl	RVEDVI	150 ml/m²
Mode/rate	APRV	Na^+	130 mg/dl	RVESI	105 ml/m²
Fio_2	1	K^+	5.5 mg/dl	RVEF	40%
PEEP low	0 cm H_2O	Cl^-	118 mg/dl	RVSWI	5 g/M/m²
Release	0.9 sec	CO_2	26 mg/dl	LVSWI	29 g/M/m²
Pao_2/Fio_2 ratio	68	Ca^{++}	6 mg/dl	CO/CI	4 L/m/2.2 L/m/m²
		Mg^{++}	1.6 mg/dl	SVR	400 dynes
		Lactate	5 mg/dl	PVR	50 dynes
				SVI	45 ml/beat/m²
				CXR	Bilateral white infiltrates

APRV= Airway pressure-release ventilation.

Over the next 48 hours, there are improvements in BP, and vasopressors are tapered off. The patient's oxygen requirements progressively decrease and he weans from mechanical ventilation over the next week. He is successfully extubated on hospital day 20.

Decision point: Why are organ-specific parameters more informative than physiologic or global parameters?

Decision point: What are three likely complications for someone who has been in uncompensated shock? What laboratory or clinical findings correlate with these complications?

perfusion may ultimately reduce end-organ perfusion as blood is shunted away from some tissue beds. Ischemic injury and necrotic limbs may be an unintentional but realistic effect of these agents.[28]

Infections associated with preexisting patient medical conditions, current illness, and iatrogenesis are an all too common occurrence in critical care. These include ventilator-associated pneumonia, catheter-related bloodstream infection, urinary tract infections, and wound infections. Reductions in tissue perfusion related to shock, medications, and nutritional deficit place the patient at risk for developing nosocomial pressure ulcers. Active effort to reduce potentially preventable

complications through application of evidence-based guidelines is the role of the advanced practice nurse. Through these efforts is achieved the ultimate goal of creating "safe passage" for the patient through the critical care environment.

CONCLUSIONS

The process of shock resuscitation is complex. All efforts are aimed at reversing tissue hypoxia and preserving organ function to optimize chances of patient survival. It requires a team approach, in which each member contributes unique knowledge and skill. Monitoring the progression of resuscitation requires continual evaluation of multiple end points. Progression of monitoring from simple to complex parameters, some requiring invasive monitoring devices, has been the current practice in critical care. As technology and knowledge advance, there is hope that more sensitive end points will emerge, requiring less-invasive technology. As the main coordinator of patient care, clinical expert, consultant, educator, and researcher, the experienced staff nurse is in a key position to advance knowledge, influence care, and, most important, contribute to a positive outcome for the patient in shock.

REFERENCES

1. Abramson, D. (1993). Lactate clearances and survival following injury. *J Trauma, 35,* 584–589.
2. Adams, K. L. (2004). Hemodynamic assessment: the physiologic basis for turning data into clinical information. *AACN Clin Issues, 15*(4), 534–546.
3. Ahrens, T., & Sona, C. (2003). Capnography application in acute and critical care. *AACN Clin Issues, 14*(2), 123–132.
4. American College of Surgeons Committee on Trauma. (2004). Shock. In *Advanced trauma life support for doctors (ATLS),* Vol. 7. Chicago: The American College of Surgeons.
5. American Heart Association (2004). *ACLS Provider Manual.* Texas: Dallas.
6. Ashby, D. T., Stone, G. W., & Moses, J. W. (2003). Cardiogenic shock in acute myocardial infarction. *Catheter Cardiovasc Interv, 59,* 34–43.
7. Baudouin, S. V., & Evans, T. W. (2003). Nutritional support in critical care. *Clin Chest Med, 24,* 633–644.
8. Beale, R. J., et al. (2004). Vasopressor and inotropic support in septic shock: an evidence-based review. *Crit Care Med, 32*(11 Suppl.): S455–S465.
9. McGhee, B. H., & Bridges, E. J. (2002). Monitoring arterial blood pressure: what you may not know. *Crit Care Nurse, 22*(2), 60–78.
10. Berthold, B., et al. (2004). Comparison of esophageal Doppler, pulse contour analysis, and real-time pulmonary artery thermodilution for the continuous measurement of cardiac output. *J Cardiothorac Vasc Anesth, 18*(2), 185–189.
11. Bilello, J. F., et al. (2003). Cervical spinal cord injury and the need for cardiovascular intervention. *Arch Surg, 138,* 1127–1129.
12. Bilkovski, R. N., Rivers, E. P., & Horst, H. M. (2004). Targeted resuscitation strategies after injury. *Curr Opin Crit Care, 10,* 529–538.
13. Bishop, M. H., et al. (1995). Prospective, randomized trial of survivor values of cardiac index, oxygen delivery, and oxygen consumption as resuscitation endpoints in severe trauma. *J Trauma, 38,* 780–787.
14. Boswell, S. A., & Scalea, T. M. (2003). Sublingual capnometry: an alternative to gastric tonometry for the management of shock resuscitation. *AACN Clin Issues, 14*(2), 176–184.
15. Bridges, E. J., & Dukes, S. (2005). Cardiovascular aspects of septic shock: pathophysiology, monitoring and treatment. *Crit Care Nurse, 25*(2), 14–42.
16. Brill, S. A. (2002). Base deficit does not predict mortality when it is secondary to hyperchloremic acidosis. *Shock, 17,* 459–462.
17. Burger, W. (2001). Influence of right ventricular pre and afterload on right ventricular ejection fraction and preload recruitable stroke work relation. *Clin Physiol, 21*(1), 85–92.
18. Ceppa, E. P. (2003). Mesenteric hemodynamic response to circulatory shock. *Curr Opin Crit Care, 9,* 127–132.
19. Chang, M. C. (1996). Preload assessment in trauma patients during large volume resuscitation. *Arch Surg, 131*(7), 728–731.
20. Chang, M. C. (1997). Cardiac preload, splanchnic perfusion, and their relationship during resuscitation in the trauma patients. *J Trauma, 42*(4), 577–582.
21. Chang, M. C. (1998). Redefining cardiovascular performance during resuscitation; ventricular stroke work, power, and the pressure-volume diagram. *J Trauma, 45*(3), 470–478.
22. Chang, M. C., et al. (2002). Improving ventricular-arterial coupling during resuscitation from shock: effects on cardiovascular function and systemic perfusion. *J Trauma, 53*(4), 679–685.
23. Cheatham, M. L., et al. (1999). Preload assessment in patients with and open abdomen. *J Trauma, 46*(1), 16–22.
24. Cohn, S. M., Crookes, B. A., & Proctor, K. G. (2003). Near-infrared spectroscopy in resuscitation. *J Trauma, 54*(5 Suppl.), 199–202.
25. Criddle, L. M., Eldredge, D. H., & Walker, J. (2005). Variables predicting trauma patient survival following massive transfusion. *J Emerg Nurs, 31*(3), 236–242.
26. Crookes, B. A., et al. (2005). Can near infrared spectroscopy identify the severity of shock in trauma patients? *J Trauma, 58* (4), 806–813.
27. Dark, P. M., & Singer, M. (2004). The validity of trans-esophageal Doppler ultrasonography as a measure if cardiac output in critically ill adults. *Intensive Care Med, 30,* 2060–2066.
28. Darovic, G. O. (2002). *Hemodynamic monitoring: invasive and noninvasive clinical applications* (3rd ed.). Philadelphia: Saunders.
29. Davis, J. W. (1997). Effect of alcohol on the utility of base deficit in trauma. *J Trauma, 43,* 507–510.
30. Davis, J. W., et al. (1998). Base deficit in the elderly: a marker of severe injury and death. *J Trauma, 45,* 873–877.
31. DeBacker, D. L. (2003). Lactic acidosis. *Intensive Care Med, 29,* 699–702.
32. Dellinger, P. R. (2004). The surviving sepsis campaign guidelines for the management of severe sepsis and septic shock: background, recommendations, and discussion from an evidence-based review. *Crit Care Med, 32*(11), S445–S595.
33. Dewachter, P., et al. (2005). Anaphylactic shock. *Anesthesiology, 103*(1), 40–44.
34. Diebel, L. N., et al. (1992). End-diastolic volume. A better indicator of preload in the critically ill (comment). *Arch Surg, 127*(7), 817–822.
35. Diebel, L., et al. (1994). End-diastolic volume versus pulmonary artery wedge pressure in evaluating cardiac preload in trauma patients. *J Trauma, 37*(6), 950–955.
36. Diebel, L. N., Myers, T., & Dulchavsky, S. (1997). Effects of increasing airway pressure and PEEP on the assessment of cardiac preload. *J Trauma, 42*(4), 585–590.
37. Doglio, G. R., et al. (1994). Gastric mucosal pH as a prognostic index of mortality in critically ill patients. *Crit Care Med, 19,* 1037–1040.
38. Dolich, M. O., & Cohn, S. M. (1999). Solutions for volume resuscitation in trauma patients. *Curr Opin Crit Care, 5*(6), 523–528.
39. Dubin, A., et al. (2000). End-tidal CO_2 pressure determinants during hemorrhagic shock. *Intensive Care Med, 26,* 1619–1623.
40. Dunham, C. M. (2000). Base deficit level indicating major injury is increased with ethanol. *J Emerg Med, 18,* 165–171.
41. Dunne, J. R., et al. (2002). Lactate and base deficit in trauma: does alcohol or drug use impair their predictive accuracy? *J Trauma, 58*(5), 959–966.
42. Eachempati, S. R., et al. (2002). Factors associated with mortality in patients with penetrating abdominal vascular trauma. *J Surg Res, 108,* 222–226.
43. Ellis, A. K., & Day, J. H. (2003). Diagnosis and management of anaphylaxis. *CMAJ, 169*(4), 307–312.

44. Fiddian-Green, R. C. (1987). Predictive value of stomach wall pH for complications after cardiac operations: comparison with other monitoring. *Crit Care Med, 15*, 153–156.

45. Fink, M. P. (2003). Ringer's ethyl pyruvate solution: a novel resuscitation fluid for the treatment of hemorrhagic shock. *J Trauma, 54*(5 Suppl.), 141–143.

46. Fleming, A., et al. (1992). Prospective trial of supranormal values as goals of resuscitation in severe trauma. *Arch Surg, 127*, 1175–1181.

47. Griffiths, R. D. (2003). Specialized nutrition support in critically ill patients. *Curr Opin Crit Care, 9*, 249–259.

48. Gurfinkel, V., et al. (2003). Hypertonic saline improves tissue oxygenation and reduces systematic and pulmonary inflammatory response caused by hemorrhagic shock. *J Trauma, 54*(6), 1137–1145.

49. Gutierrez, G., et al. (1992). Comparison of gastric intramucosal pH with measures of oxygen transport and consumption in critically ill patients. *Crit Care Med, 20*, 451–457.

50. Gys, T. (1988). The prognostic value of gastric intramural pH in surgical intensive care patients. *Crit Care Med, 16*, 1222–1224.

51. Hameed, S. M., Aird, W. C., & Cohn, S. M. (2003). Oxygen delivery. *Crit Care Med, 31*(12 Suppl.), 658–667.

52. Hochman, J. S. (2003). Cardiogenic shock complicating acute myocardial infarction. *Circulation, 107*, 2998–3002.

53. Hollenberg, S. M., et al. (2004). Practice parameters for hemodynamic support of sepsis in adult patients: 2004 update. *Crit Care Med, 32*(9), 1928–1948.

54. Ishida, T., et al. (2004). Right ventricular end-diastolic volume monitoring after cardiac surgery. *Ann Thorac Cardiovasc Surg, 10*(3), 167–170.

55. Ivatury, R. R., et al. (1995). Gastric mucosal pH and oxygen delivery and consumption indices in the assessment of adequacy of resuscitation after trauma. *J Trauma, 39*, 128–134.

56. Ivatury, R. R., et al. (1996). A prospective randomized study of endpoints of resuscitation after major trauma: global oxygen transport indices versus organ-specific gastric mucosal pH. *J Am Coll Surg, 183*, 145–154.

57. Jacobi, J., et al. (2002). Clinical practice guidelines for the sustained use of sedatives and analgesics in the critically ill adult. *Crit Care Med, 30*(1), 119–141.

58. Jesurum, J. (2001). Protocols for practice: SvO₂ monitoring. *Crit Care Nurse, 21*(1), 79–83.

59. Jin, X., et al. (2000). End-tidal carbon dioxide as a noninvasive indicator of cardiac index during circulatory shock. *Crit Care Med, 28*(7), 2415–2419.

60. Johnson, R. F., & Pebbles, R. S. (2004). Anaphylactic shock: pathophysiology, recognition, and treatment. *Semin Respir Crit Care Med, 25*(6), 695–703.

61. Kelley, D. (2005). Hypovolemic shock. *Crit Care Nurs Q, 28*(1), 2–19.

62. Kellum, J. A. (2002). Saline-induced hyperchloremic metabolic acidosis (editorial). *Crit Care Med, 30*(1), 259–261.

63. Kellum, J. A., & Pinskey, M. R. (2002). Use of vasopressor agents in critically ill patients. *Crit Care, 8*, 236–241.

64. Kern, J. W., & Shoemaker, W. C. (2002). A meta-analysis of hemodynamic optimization in high-risk patients. *Crit Care Med, 30*, 1686–1692.

65. Krassioukov, A., & Claydon, V. E. (2006). The clinical problems in cardiovascular control following spinal cord injury: an overview. *Prog Brain Res, 152*, 223–229.

66. Landry, D. W., & Oliver, J. A. (2001). The pathogenesis of vasodilatory shock. *N Engl J Med, 345*(8), 588–595.

67. Leeper, B. (2003). Monitoring right ventricular volumes: a paradigm shift. *AACN Clin Issues, 14*(2), 208–219.

68. Levine, R. L., Wayne, M. A., & Miller, C. C. (1997). End-tidal carbon dioxide and outcome of out of hospital cardiac arrest. *N Engl J Med, 337*, 301–306.

69. Light, T. D., et al. (2004). Real-time metabolic monitors, ischemia-reperfusion, titration endpoints, and ultra precise burn resuscitation. *J Burn Care Rehab, 25*, 33–44.

70. Magder, S., & Cernacek, P. (2003). Role of endothelins in septic, cardiogenic, and hemorrhagic shock. *Can J Physiol Pharmacol, 81*(6), 635–643.

71. Malbrain, M. (2004). Is it wise not to think about intraabdominal hypertension in the ICU. *Curr Opin Crit Care, 10*, 131–145.

72. Manikis, P. (1995). Correlation of serial blood lactate levels to organ failure and mortality after trauma. *Am J Emerg Med, 13*, 619–622.

73. Marr, A. B., et al. (2004). Preload optimization using "Starling curve" generation during shock resuscitation: can it be done? *Shock, 21*(4), 300–305.

74. Marik, P. E. (1993). Gastric intramucosal pH: a better predictor of multiorgan dysfunction syndrome and death than oxygen-derived variables in patients with sepsis. *Chest, 104*(1), 225–229.

75. Marik, P. (2001). Sublingual capnography: a clinical validation study. *Chest, 120*(3), 923–927.

76. Marik, P. E., & Bankov, A. (2003a). Sublingual capnometry versus traditional markers of tissue oxygenation in critically ill patients. *Crit Care Med, 31*(3), 818–822.

77. Marik, P. E. (2003b). The optimal endpoint of resuscitation in trauma patients (commentary). *Crit Care, 7*(1), 1862–1863.

78. Martin, M. J., et al. (2005). Use of serum bicarbonate measurement in place of arterial base deficit in the surgical intensive care unit. *Arch Surg, 140*, 745–751.

79. Maynard, N., et al. (1993). Assessment of splanchnic oxygenation by gastric tonometry in patients with acute circulatory failure. *JAMA, 270*, 1203–1210.

80. McKinley, B. A., et al. (2002). Normal versus supranormal oxygen delivery goals in shock resuscitation: the response is the same. *J Trauma, 53*(5), 825–832.

81. McNelis, J., et al. (2002). Predictive factors associated with development of abdominal compartment syndrome in the surgical intensive care unit. *Arch Surg, 137*(2), 133–136.

82. McNelis, J. (2001). Prolonged lactate clearance is associated with increased mortality in the surgical intensive care unit. *Am J Surg, 182*, 481–485.

83. Miami Trauma Clinical Trials Group (2005). Splanchnic hypoperfusion-directed therapies in trauma: a prospective, randomized control trial. *Am Surg, 71*, 252–260.

84. Miller, P. R., Meredith, J. W., & Chang, M. C. (1998). Randomized, prospective comparison of increased preload versus inotropes in the resuscitation of trauma patients: effects on cardiopulmonary function and visceral perfusion. *J Trauma, 44*(1), 107–113.

85. Moore, E. E. (2003). Blood substitutes: the future is now. *J Am Coll Surg, 196*(1), 1–16.

86. Moore, F. A., McKinley, B. A., & Moore, E. E. (2004). The next generation in shock resuscitation. *Lancet, 363*, 1988–1996.

87. Mullner, M., et al. (2005). Vasopressors for shock. *Cochrane Database Syst Rev, 2*: http://gateway.ut.ovid.com/gw1/ovidweb.cgi.

88. Oliveria, R. P. (2002). Clinical review; hypertonic saline resuscitation in sepsis. *Crit Care, 6*(5), 418–423.

89. O'Neil, M. (2002). Detection and measurement of sublingual CO₂. Sublingual Carbon Dioxide Reference Note #1. Nellcor Puritan Bennett.

90. Ott, K., Johnson, K., & Ahrens, T. (2001). New technologies in the assessment of hemodynamic parameters. *J Cardiovasc Nurs, 15*(2), 41–55.

91. Peterson, D. L., et al. (2004). Evaluation of initial base deficit as a prognosticator of outcome in the pediatric trauma population. *Am Surg, 70*(4), 326–328.

92. Pivots, H. P. (2000). Comparison between sublingual and gastric tonometry during hemorrhagic shock. *Chest, 118*(4), 1127–1132.

93. Rackow, E. C., et al. (2001). Sublingual capnometry and indexes of tissue perfusion in patients with circulatory failure. *Chest, 120* (5), 1633–1638.

94. Ramsey, J. D., & Tisdale, L. A. (1995). Use of ventricular stroke work index and ventricular function curves in assessing myocardial contractility. *Crit Care Nurse, 15*(1), 61–74.

95. Revel, M., Greaves, I., & Porter, K. (2003). Endpoints for fluid resuscitation in hemorrhagic shock. *J Trauma, 54*(5 Suppl.), 63–67.

96. Rhodes, A., & Bennett, D. E. (2004). Early goal directed therapy: an evidence based review. *Crit Care Med, 332*(11 Suppl.), 448–450.

97. Rivers, E., et al. (2001). Early goal-directed therapy in the treatment of severe sepsis and septic shock. *N Engl J Med, 345,* 1368–1377.

98. Rixen, D. (2001). Base deficit development and its prognostic significance in post-trauma critical illness: an analysis by the trauma registry of the Deutsche Gesellschaft für Unfallchirurgie. *Shock, 15,* 83–89.

99. Roberts, I., et al. (2005). Colloids versus crystalloids for fluid resuscitation in critically ill patients. *Cochrane Database Syst Rev, 2,* http://gateway.ut.ovid.com/gw1/ovidweb.cgi

100. Ruffolo, D. C., & Headley, J. M. (2003). Regional carbon dioxide monitoring. *AACN Clin Issues, 14*(2), 168–175.

101. Safcsak, K., & Nelson, L. D. (1999). Right heart volumetric monitoring; measuring preload in the critically injured patient. *AACN Clin Issues, 10*(1), 22–31.

102. Samuels, L. E., & Darze, E. S. (2003). Management of acute cardiogenic shock. *Cardiol Clin, 21*(1), 43–49.

103. Schulman, C. (2002). Endpoints of resuscitation: choosing the right parameters to monitor. *Dimens Crit Care Nurs, 21*(1), 2–14.

104. Seoudi, H. M., et al. (2003). The esophageal Doppler monitor in mechanically ventilated surgical patients: does it work? *J Trauma, 55*(4), 720–726.

105. Shoemaker, W. C., Appel, P. L., & Kram, H. B. (1988). Tissue oxygen debt as a determinant of lethal and non-lethal postoperative organ failure. *Crit Care Med, 16,* 1117–1120.

106. Shoemaker, W. C., et al. (1988). Prospective trail of supranormal values of survivors as therapeutic goals in high risk surgical patients. *Chest, 94,* 1176–1186.

107. Slone, S. D. (2004). Nutritional support of the critically ill and injured patient. *Crit Care Clin, 20,* 137–157.

108. Society of Trauma Nurses. (2003). Hemorrhagic shock. In *Advanced trauma course for nurses: provider manual.* Santa Fe: Society of Trauma Nurses, 21–34.

109. Squara, P. (2004). Matching total body oxygen consumption and delivery: a crucial objective? *Intensive Care Med, 30,* 2170–2179.

110. Stammers, A. H., et al. (2004). Utilization of rapid-infuser devices for massive blood loss. *Perfusion, 20,* 65–69.

111. Taylor, J. H., et al. (2005). Use of near-infrared spectroscopy in early determination of irreversible hemorrhage. *J Trauma, 58*(6), 1119–1125.

112. The SAFE Study Investigators. (2004). A comparison of albumin and saline for fluid resuscitation in the intensive care unit. *N Engl J Med, 350,* 2247–2256.

113. Tisherman, S. A., et al. (2004). Clinical practice guideline: endpoints of resuscitation. *J Trauma, 57,* 898–912.

114. Tremblay, L. N., Feliciano, D. V., & Rozycki, G. S. (2003). Are resuscitation and operation justified in injured patients with extreme base deficits. *Am J Surg, 186*(6), 597–600.

115. Trujillo, E. B., Robinson, M. K., & Jacobs, D. O. (2001). Feeding the critically ill patients: current concepts. *Crit Care Nurse, 21*(4), 60–69.

116. Turner, M. A. (2003). Doppler-based hemodynamic monitoring. *AACN Clin Issues, 14*(2), 220–231.

117. Vincent, J. L., & DeBacker, D. (2004). Oxygen transport-the oxygen delivery controversy. *Intensive Care Med, 30,* 1990–1996.

118. Vincent, J. L., & Gerlach, H. (2004). Fluid resuscitation in severe sepsis and septic shock: an evidence-based review. *Crit Care Med, 32*(11 Suppl.), S451–S454.

119. Weil, M. H., et al. (1999). Sublingual capnography: a new noninvasive measurement for the diagnosis and quantitation of severity of circulatory shock. *Crit Care Med, 27,* 1225–1229.

120. Waikar, S. S., & Chertow, G. M. (2000). Crystalloid versus colloids for resuscitation in shock. *Curr Opin Neph Hyper, 9,* 501–504.

121. Walker, J., & Criddle, L. M. (2003). Pathophysiology and management of abdominal compartment syndrome. *Am J Crit Care, 12*(4), 367–373.

122. Wilson, M., Davis, D. P., & Coimbra, R. (2003). Diagnosis and monitoring of hemorrhagic shock during the initial resuscitation of multiple trauma patients. *J Emerg Med, 24*(4), 413–422.

123. Zehtabchi, S., et al. (2005). Does ethanol explain the acidosis commonly seen in ethanol-intoxicated patients? *Clin Toxicol, 43*(3), 161–166.

CHAPTER 41

Optimizing Hemodynamics: Strategies for Fluid and Medication Titration in Shock

Deborah Tuggle

Hemodynamics is defined as the forces involved in circulating blood throughout the body. The primary purpose of blood circulation is to deliver oxygen, the most vital of cellular nutrients. Without optimal hemodynamics, cellular hypoxia, organ failure, and patient mortality inevitably follow. However, evidence-based guidelines for the management of hemodynamics are lacking. Confusion and uncertainty prevail in how to best titrate fluids and drug therapies to maximize organ perfusion.[60,63,77] As a result, critical care nurses often find themselves being guided by unscientific opinion, clinical tradition, or medical hearsay. This chapter is intended to assist nurses in understanding hemodynamic pathologies, the meaning of optimizing hemodynamics, and best practices in perfusion support. Physiologic concepts pertinent to this topic and employed in this chapter can be found in numerous textbooks and articles written for the bedside practitioner.*

HYPOPERFUSION STATES AND SYSTEMIC RESPONSES

Severe hypoperfusion is generally referred to as shock and characterized by tissue hypoxia and anoxia. Shock states can be categorized into threats to one of the three components of the cardiovascular system: the heart (pump), the blood (volume), or the vessels (resistance). Cardiogenic shock occurs when the heart is unable to pump enough blood to meet the body's demand for oxygen. The leading cause of cardiogenic shock is myocardial infarction (Box 41-1). Hypovolemic shock, the most prevalent form of hypoperfusion, occurs when the vascular system loses blood or fluid either externally or internally, leading to a fall in perfusion pressure (Box 41-2). Vasogenic shock (sometimes referred to as distributive shock) occurs when blood vessels dilate inappropriately; this condition may be accompanied by capillary leakage (Box 41-3). Septic shock is the predominant form of vasogenic shock seen in critical care.

Regardless of the origin of hypoperfusion, the body's response is patterned and nonspecific. The response to hypoperfusion is the same as the reaction to any number of other perceived threats. Whether real or imagined, physical or emotional, the body does not differentiate one crisis from another. Of all the systems that are activated in a crisis situation, the two most potent are the sympathetic nervous system (SNS) and the renin-angiotensin-aldosterone system (RAAS). SNS activation involves multiple and complex processes affecting the entire body (for purposes of this discussion, only the cardiovascular aspects will be covered). With SNS stimulation, catecholamines are released into the circulation from the adrenal medulla and at synaptic interfaces from systemic nerve endings. Release of epinephrine and norepinephrine leads to the following changes: increased heart rate (HR), increased cardiac contractility, and increased vascular tone (Figure 41-1). Vital organ vessels actually receive augmented flow via vasodilation, but the net effect is one of vasoconstriction and shunting of blood away from nonvital organs and toward vital organs (brain, heart, and skeletal muscle). Maintaining cerebral and cardiac perfusion is an obvious priority. However, the maintenance of skeletal muscle oxygenation appears inappropriate but is an important part of "fight or flight" to address crisis situations of all kinds.

The RAAS's primary purpose is to support blood pressure (BP) for efficient renal filtration and waste removal. With any fall in BP, the kidney secretes a tissue hormone called renin. Renin initiates a cascade of interactions that ultimately results in the release of aldosterone from the adrenal cortex and the production of angiotensin II from vessel linings (see Figure 41-1). Aldosterone induces the nephron to retain sodium and water, and angiotensin II causes vessels to constrict. In summary, hypoperfusion states activate the stress response mediated primarily by the SNS and RAAS. Together, these two systems elicit an upsurge in heart rate, contractility, vessel tone (afterload), and vascular volume (preload).

Although each of the hypoperfusion states varies in its pathology, the body's nonspecific response is more

---

*References 2, 11, 22, 35, 97, 103.

Box 41-1

Causes of Cardiogenic Shock

- Acute coronary syndromes
  - ST elevation myocardial infarction (STEMI)
  - Non-ST elevation myocardial infarction (non-STEMI)
- Reperfusion injury states (stunned myocardium)
- Exacerbated chronic heart failure
- Cardiomyopathy
- Infectious or inflammatory processes
- Traumatic chest contusion
- Cardiotoxic drug exposure
- Negative inotropic excess (beta-blockers, calcium channel blockers)
- Structural abnormalities (valvular dysfunction, septal disruptions)
- Obstructive pathologies (cardiac tamponade, pulmonary emboli, tension pneumothorax)

Box 41-2

Causes of Hypovolemic Shock

EXTERNAL LOSSES

- Decreased fluid intake
- Vomiting and diarrhea
- Diaphoresis
- Polyuria
- Hemorrhage
- Burns and wound exudate

INTERNAL LOSSES

- Interstitial shifting (third spacing)
- Bowel sequestration
- Internal hemorrhage
- Ascites

Box 41-3

Causes of Vasogenic Shock

- Sepsis
- Anaphylaxis
- Systemic inflammation of multiple causes (e.g., pancreatitis, fulminant hepatitis)
- Drug overdose
- Neurogenic insults (e.g., spinal cord injury, epidural drugs)

effective in some situations than in others. For example, hypovolemic shock is most appropriately managed by the body's stress reaction. Increasing HR and contractility improves cardiac output (CO), and therefore perfusion capability. Retaining sodium and water addresses the issue of hypovolemia, whereas vascular constriction creates a more balanced relationship between the volume and the vascular bed, improving perfusion pressure. Vasogenic shock, however, is not supported as efficiently by this response because of the inability of the vasculature to respond with increased tone. Nevertheless, fluid reabsorption and the HR and contractility augmentation are able to maintain perfusion to some extent in most forms of vasogenic shock.

In the case of cardiogenic shock, the body's response appears to be more life threatening than life supporting. First, there is no significant improvement in contractility because patients are already at maximum endogenous catecholamine levels. Patients in cardiogenic shock are generally incapable of contributing much more without external stimulation. In addition, forcing a failing heart to beat faster and to circulate greater venous volume against higher arterial resistance is counterproductive. This is why the fight-or-flight system is termed the "vicious cycle" in cases of pump failure (Figure 41-2).

When a patient becomes hypotensive and shows signs of hypoperfusion, it is vital to determine the underlying cause. Even though the body's response is nonspecific, successful therapeutic intervention must be targeted at the source of the problem. One way to approach hypoperfusion is to categorize it as involving the pump, volume, or vessels. To differentiate among these, ask, Is the patient having chest pain (pump)? Is there ST segment elevation (pump)? What was today's weight (volume)? Are neck veins distended or flat (volume)? Does the patient have a fever (vessel/sepsis)? Are there any medications or pathologies that could cause vasodilation (vessels)? The answers to these questions will help determine the source of shock so that targeted therapy can be initiated.

THE TRUTH ABOUT BLOOD PRESSURE

BP is commonly used to evaluate the adequacy of perfusion and overall cardiovascular function. However, shock is not a low BP, but hypoperfusion, and perfusion cannot be assessed by BP alone. Yet every day in critical care across the country, nurses receive orders to titrate powerful vasoactive and inotropic agents to arbitrary levels of BP. The level most commonly equated with adequate perfusion is a mean arterial pressure (MAP) of greater than 65 mm Hg (or a systolic pressure of greater than 90 mm Hg).[58] Unfortunately, this target BP has never been scientifically

Responder: Sympathetic nervous system

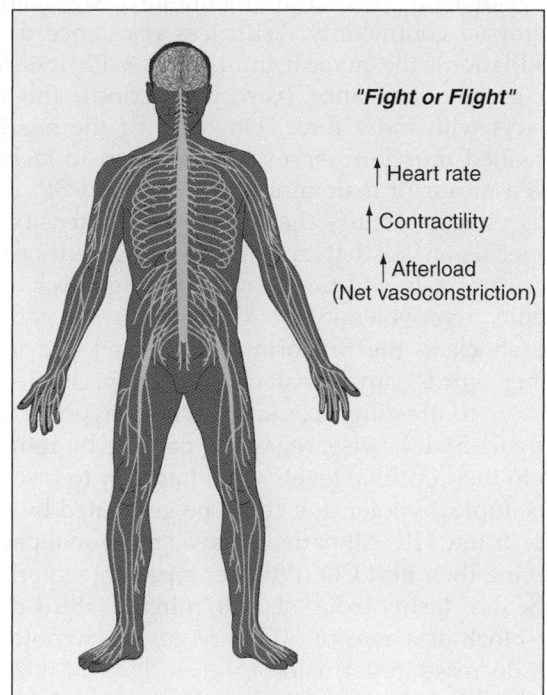

"Fight or Flight"

↑ Heart rate

↑ Contractility

↑ Afterload
(Net vasoconstriction)

Responder: Renin-angiotensin-aldosterone system

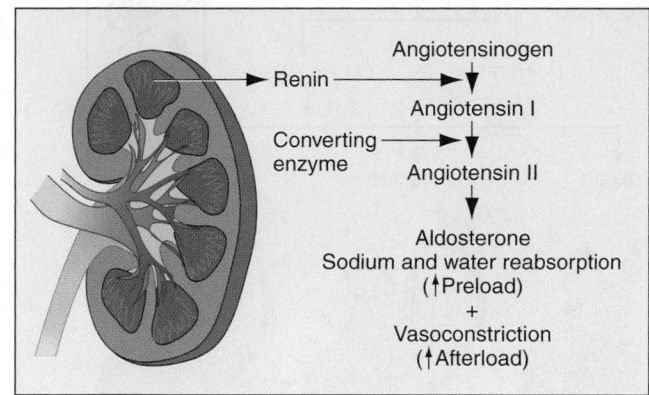

⬍FIGURE 41-1 Primary shock responders and their effects.

studied. It was merely proposed decades ago based on the fact that the kidneys cease to produce urine at pressures below 60 mm Hg and over time has been embraced as scientific fact.

BP measures are often unreliable. Patients with a low BP are not necessarily hypoperfusing, as evidenced by the many chronic cardiomyopathy patients with low BP who are warm, dry, alert, oriented, and producing adequate urine. There are critical care patients receiving high-dose vasopressor agents with a normal BP, but few signs indicating organ perfusion. At best, BP serves as a warning sign that hemodynamics may be threatened, with the true test being a review of body systems for signs of poor tissue oxygenation. Symptomatic hypotension is one of the recognized precursors to cardiac arrest and should be

Do the Responders Work?

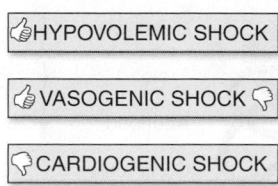

⬍FIGURE 41-2 The response to shock is the same regardless of the type. The stress responders help with hypovolemic shock, have minimal effect with vasogenic shock, and are harmful with cardiogenic shock.

aggressively managed as survival from arrest averages only 15% to 17%.[14]

Nurses need to better understand what BP actually assesses so they can troubleshoot hemodynamic compromise and provide interventions to address the source of the problem. BP is the product of CO and systemic vascular resistance (SVR). CO primarily creates systolic pressure and vascular resistance primarily determines diastolic pressure:

$$BP = CO \times SVR$$

CO is a product of HR and stroke volume (SV), the amount of blood ejected with each beat:

$$BP = CO \times SVR$$
$$HR \times SV$$

If SV is reduced to its determining parameters, the formula becomes

$$BP = CO \times SVR$$
$$HR \times SV$$

Preload
Afterload
Contractility

This formula is a function of preload, afterload, and contractility (Figure 41-3).

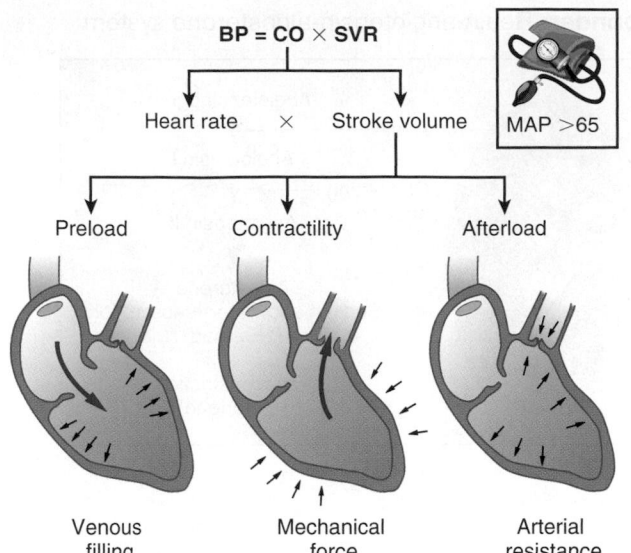

↕FIGURE 41-3 Blood pressure is a function of cardiac output and systemic vascular resistance. BP = Blood pressure, CO = cardiac output, SVR = systemic vascular resistance, MAP = mean arterial pressure.

Preload is the blood volume in the ventricle to be ejected. It is delivered to the heart by veins. Any manipulation in vascular volume or venous return affects preload. *Afterload* is the resistance to moving the preload. It is primarily determined by arterial vascular tone. Any manipulation in arterial caliber affects afterload. *Contractility* is the cardiac muscle's strength used to move preload against afterload. It is a complex and difficult parameter to measure as it is affected by both preload and afterload. Preload affects contractility via the Frank-Starling mechanism, with greater ventricular stretch resulting in greater cardiac contraction (Figure 41-4). This effect is limited, however, and

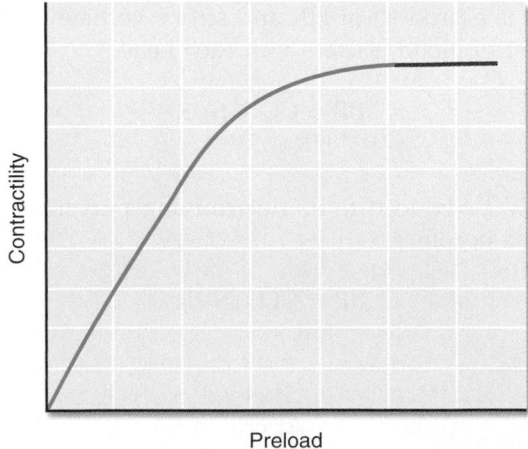

↕FIGURE 41-4 Frank-Starling mechanism. The greater the stretch, the greater the force of contraction, but only up to a point.

beyond a certain point, there is no increase in contractility even with preload augmentation. Afterload can also impact contractility. With less resistance to flow (vasodilation), the myocardium ejects with less force. With greater resistance (vasoconstriction), the heart contracts with more force. However, if the heart has diminished muscle reserves, it will resort to tachycardia as a means of maintaining SV, CO, and BP.

It is vital to identify the source of hypotension and hypoperfusion so that appropriate interventions can be performed. In addition to categorizing shock as cardiogenic, hypovolemic, or vasogenic, one can also relate shock to the BP formula reviewed previously. In other words, any imbalance in HR, preload, afterload, or contractility could provoke hypoperfusion (Figure 41-5). Likewise, regaining balance by returning them to their optimal levels would appear to resolve it. For example, hypotension could be generated by either a high or low HR. All patients have an optimal pace for achieving their best CO. Whether a patient experiences ventricular tachycardia at 160/min or third-degree heart block at a rate of 30, there can be hypotension and a decrease in perfusion.

Preload imbalance creates another potential threat to BP and tissue oxygenation. When preload decreases, patients can become hypovolemic, and in severe situations, deteriorate into hypovolemic shock. However, high preload can also cause hemodynamic compromise. As illustrated by the Frank-Starling curve in Figure 41-6, myocardium that is either understretched or overstretched can lose contractility, resulting in a decline in pump function. Preload excesses can be systemic, as in hypervolemia, or isolated to the heart chamber alone as in early pump failure. There is an optimal level of preload for best hemodynamic balance. High preload gives the heart more volume to pump, and low preload forces the heart to pump faster to maintain BP. High and low preload both burden the heart with additional work and a higher oxygen demand.

In an effort to reduce cardiac workload, clinicians may want to decrease preload. However, the reflex

TROUBLESHOOTING THE ETIOLOGY OF HYPOTENSION

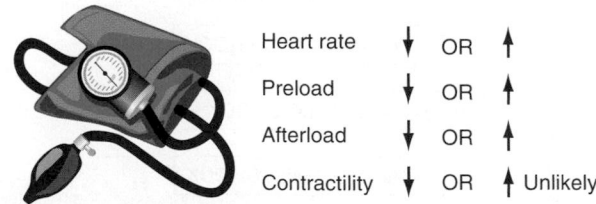

↕FIGURE 41-5 Hypotensive states should not be oversimplified because any of the parameters that can create blood pressure can be a factor in shock. In addition, both highs and lows can cause hemodynamic instability.

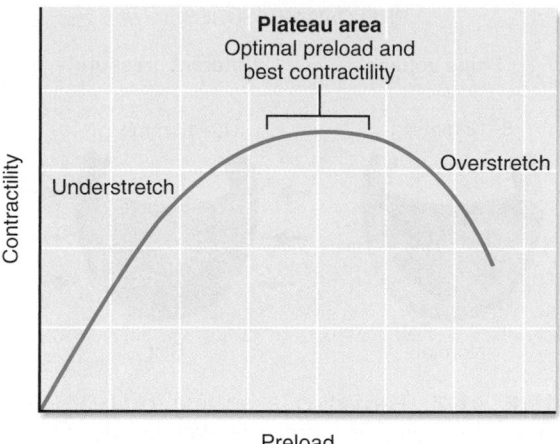

Plateau area
Optimal preload and
best contractility

Overstretch

Understretch

Contractility

Preload

✦**FIGURE 41-6** The law of optimal stretch. This curve illustrates the limits of the Frank-Starling mechanism. Both understretch and overstretch of the ventricle can lead to a fall in contractility and, therefore, a fall in blood pressure.

tachycardia and vasoconstriction stimulated by an underfilled vascular system can sabotage this strategy. Many consider diuretics, such as furosemide (Lasix), as BP-lowering drugs. In reality, a patient's BP response to furosemide depends on the location on the Frank-Starling curve. When patients are hypovolemic (understretched) or even euvolemic (optimally stretched), furosemide will generally lower BP. This is the reason it works well in treating hypertension. However, if patients are hypervolemic or in heart failure (overstretched), furosemide can reduce ventricular volume, optimize stretch, maximize contractility, and even elevate BP.

Afterload also has variable effects on BP. In states of vasodilation, BP is difficult to maintain, and perfusion declines. However, if arterial beds are constricted to improve BP, a critical point can be reached beyond which the heart can no longer overcome resistance and fails to maintain CO. This is most likely to occur in patients with depressed myocardial tissue and indicates the need for a vasodilator, such as nitroglycerin. Many perceive nitroglycerin and other vasodilators as medications that lower BP. Although they are appropriate for the treatment of hypertension, they also can be employed to reduce vascular tone and resistance to cardiac emptying. As with the other hemodynamic variables, there is an optimal level of afterload. Too high or too low afterload is detrimental to the maintenance of normal hemodynamics and effective tissue perfusion.

Contractility is low in all states of shock. In cardiogenic shock, contractility is diminished secondary to a direct myocardial insult. In hypovolemic shock, contractility is low as a consequence of poor stretch and inadequate stimulation of Frank-Starling mechanisms, all of which are reversed once preload is restored.

In vasogenic shock low contractility occurs as the result of vascular volume pooling in the periphery, and capillary leakage. In addition, vasogenic states lower afterload to levels that may inadequately stimulate the heart to respond with increased contractility. In the septic form of vasogenic shock, chemical mediators directly depress muscle function. Although rare, elevated contractility can also affect BP. Patients with hypertrophic cardiomyopathy have adequate muscle strength, but due to increased muscle mass, there is no room in the ventricle for preload, an antecedent to hypotension. In some cases, surgical myectomy is performed to debulk the muscle and create space for blood. Some centers perform catheter-based ablation procedures, infarcting the ventricular septum to enlarge the outflow tract and augment CO.[68] Although low contractility is the more common imbalance, there is an optimal level of contractility and both high and low levels are detrimental.

In summary, there are many factors that affect BP. Whether evaluating hypertensive or hypotensive patients, it is prudent to determine which parameter is out of balance and in which direction. Increased or decreased HR, preload, afterload, and contractility can all cause BP abnormalities, and identifying the problem is imperative to provide appropriate interventions.

IDENTIFYING AND INTERPRETING HEMODYNAMIC MEASURES

There are patients presenting in a state of hypoperfusion for which the cause and treatment are evident. However, in cases in which it is less discernible, or when the patient is unstable enough to warrant continual assessment, invasive hemodynamic monitoring is useful. This section is not intended to be a complete discussion of these devices, but instead a brief review of bedside measures used to direct therapy for hypoperfusion.[74] Criticism of the pulmonary artery catheter (PAC) has been prevalent in the literature almost since its inception because of the inability to prove a benefit in patient outcome through its use.* Some experts have proposed that this is more the fault of clinicians than the catheter.[50,55] For purposes of this discussion, it is assumed that the nurse understands proper techniques for deriving accurate hemodynamic measures. For more information, readers are referred to the American Association of Critical-Care Nurses Practice Alert "Pulmonary Artery Pressure Monitoring," at www.aacn.org, and to a free tutorial in hemodynamics at www.pacep.org.

---

*References 6, 10, 20, 41, 65, 73, 82, 85.

Arterial Blood Pressure

The most accurate measurement of BP is made via functional arterial lines.[84] These catheters are located directly inside the vessel and are able to eliminate a multitude of external variables affecting the accuracy of cuff readings, including disproportionate cuff size, misaligned cuff bladder, detaching cuff Velcro, low-quality stethoscopes, and overall poor technique. In addition, the vasoconstriction common to hypertension and hypotension hampers vessel vibrations and reduces Korotkoff sound transmission, making cuff pressures less dependable in abnormal pressure ranges. With the move from mercury to aneroid devices, cuff BP may be more questionable, even in normal pressure ranges.[80,101]

Arterial lines are the gold standard. If the catheter has been placed in an appropriate vessel, the transducer's stopcock properly leveled at the phlebostatic axis, and the system's dynamic response deemed adequate by square wave testing, the arterial line should be trusted. It is important to realize that arterial line pressures and cuff pressures are not expected to be the same and comparing the two is unnecessary.

Preload Measures

Preload can be assessed clinically by considering history, weight, intake and output, neck vein status, and other physical findings. It also can be appraised by a relatively new blood test called B-type natriuretic peptide (BNP). This chemical is secreted into the bloodstream by the ventricles when they are overly stretched. Serum levels greater than the normal upper limit of 100 pg/ml imply heart failure, but are felt to be reliable only in the absence of renal failure.[19,71] Preload can also be estimated invasively via central venous lines or the PAC. Central venous pressure (CVP) is used as a measure of right-ventricular preload and pulmonary artery wedge pressure (PAWP) as a measure of left-ventricular preload. However, there are concerns related to these measures, particularly PAWP due to its indirect nature and reliance on the state of the pulmonary vascular bed for proper evaluation of the left heart. Pressure changes may not reflect only volume changes but also ventricular compliance and pleural and intraabdominal pressure (Figure 41-7). In addition, obtaining accurate CVP and PAWP data is dependent on precise bedside monitoring techniques, making them prone to human error.

The normal preload ranges commonly quoted in critical care textbooks are a CVP of 2 to 6 mm Hg and a PAWP of 8 to 12 mm Hg. These ranges are based on studies of young, healthy, 70-kg resting males with normal heart function and do not apply to most critically ill patients. Adhering to the normal values listed in most textbooks for preload may result in inadequate fluid

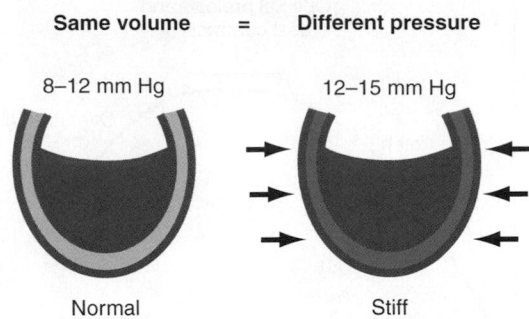

PRELOAD MEASURES

Same volume   =   Different pressure

8–12 mm Hg   12–15 mm Hg

Normal   Stiff

⇕FIGURE 41-7 Preload is a volume concept, yet it is traditionally measured as a pressure. Pressure does not equal volume; therefore, normal ranges for central venous pressure and pulmonary artery wedge pressure do not apply to the critically ill.

resuscitation, continued hypovolemia, and the use of a potentially dangerous drug when normal saline (NS) would have sufficed. Appropriate ranges for the critically ill are unclear due to a paucity of research and an abundance of patient variability. Some experts in hemodynamics have dismissed pressure-based measures of preload in favor of more sophisticated but not widely available technology. For example, the volumetric PAC can compute right ventricular end-diastolic volume, a superior measure of preload that's not available in many critical care units.[64]

Because they continue to be the most commonly used measure of preload, possible guidelines to address CVP and PAWP are offered here. First, it is important that treatment decisions not be made based on a single CVP or PAWP reading, but on data trends with comparisons to the clinical picture. Interpretation of readings must be individualized so that therapy can be directed to the unique needs of each patient. Secondary to the cardiac stiffening common in critical illness, CVP tends to reflect euvolemia in the typical critical care patient at higher than normal ranges. In the landmark study on early goal-directed therapy (EGDT) in severe sepsis by Rivers and associates,[86] a CVP range of 8 to 12 mm Hg was used. With mechanical ventilation, right ventricular compliance was deemed further diminished, and a CVP of 12 to 15 mm Hg was targeted. Using these CVP ranges for preload goals, a reduction in mortality of 34% was shown.[86]

Research has long shown that the majority of patients will develop pulmonary edema at PAWP levels of 18 mm Hg or more.[59,83] Therefore the most accepted guideline for PAWP has been to maintain levels lower than this point. Beyond that, there are few data to guide clinical practice. Due to reduced cardiac compliance observed in the critically ill, some have proposed a range of 12 to 15 mm Hg for the average critical care patient.[88] Young and previously healthy patients may do well at PAWP levels slightly less, and older clients with myocardial ischemia or infarction may require levels somewhat higher. The best method for determining optimal preload may be to evaluate the response to fluid administration. Whenever a patient has symptomatic hypotension of uncertain pathology, fluid administration should be the first consideration. If there is a favorable response to volume infusion, it should continue until the patient peaks and sustains the response. Measures of a favorable response to fluid therapy beyond actual filling pressures include increasing BP, CO, urinary output (UO), decreasing HR, and normalizing venous saturation (discussed later), along with an overall improvement in the patient's appearance and level of consciousness.

Afterload Measures

Afterload is measured by a mathematical equation and, as with preload, can be measured on both the right and left sides of the heart (Figure 41-8). Pulmonary vascular resistance (PVR) closely parallels pulmonary artery pressure (PAP), and is thus of limited interest in most clinical situations. SVR is useful when accurately computed and coupled with clinical assessment. Calculations of SVR higher than 1200 dynes imply vasoconstriction, and readings lower than 900 dynes imply vasodilation. Indexed ranges of SVR (resistance divided by body surface area to correct for patient size), though more discriminating, are not widely used.

Because SVR is computed rather than directly measured, it may be dismissed from consideration of the hemodynamic profile. However, clinical findings for the evaluation of afterload are limited to skin characteristics alone and tend to be subjective and unreliable. Hypovolemic and cardiogenic problems result in SNS- and RAAS-mediated vasoconstriction, causing patients to develop the classic cool and clammy appearance. Vasogenic shock, on the other hand, evokes vasodilation and the skin is generally flushed, even warm, early in the physiologic process. Though imperfect, afterload computations can be an important safety check when using vasopressor agents for the treatment of hypotension. Vasoconstriction can improve BP, but if excessive, can decrease CO and organ perfusion, which is contradictory to the intent of the treatment. Titrating vasopressors to BP without consideration of SVR can be particularly risky when the source of the BP is a radial arterial line, which may underestimate true BP when alpha constriction is prominent.[28]

Contractility Measures

Of all the variables affecting BP and hemodynamics, contractility is the most difficult to measure. As reviewed previously, contractility is affected by preload via the Frank-Starling curve. Although less

Afterload Measures

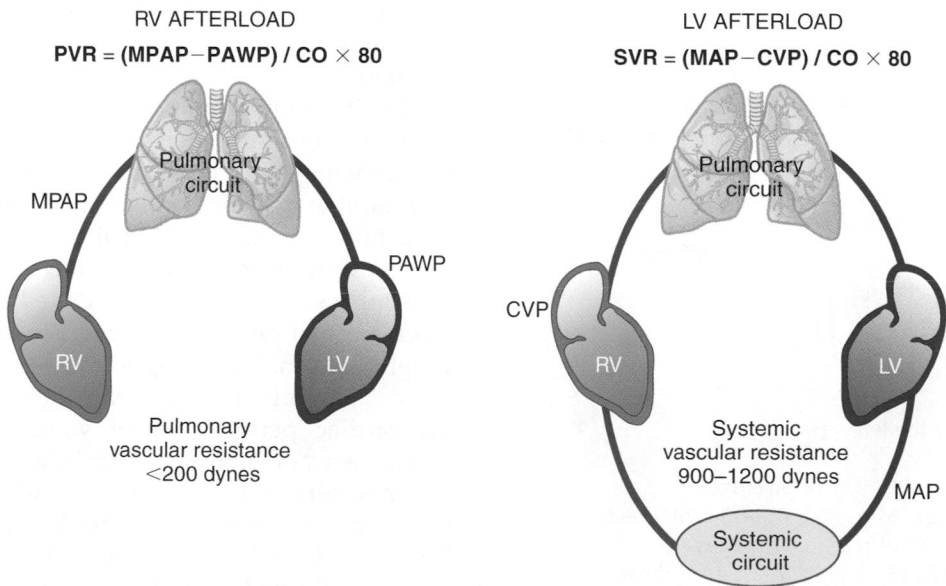

RV AFTERLOAD

$$PVR = (MPAP - PAWP) / CO \times 80$$

MPAP
Pulmonary circuit
PAWP
RV
LV
Pulmonary vascular resistance
<200 dynes

LV AFTERLOAD

$$SVR = (MAP - CVP) / CO \times 80$$

Pulmonary circuit
CVP
RV
LV
Systemic vascular resistance
900–1200 dynes
MAP
Systemic circuit

◆FIGURE 41-8 Afterload measures for the right and left ventricles. The number 80 in the formulas is a constant that converts resistance into a unit of measure known as dynes. RV = Right ventricle, PVR = pulmonary vascular resistance, MPAP = mean pulmonary artery pressure, CO = cardiac output, LV = left ventricle, SVR = systemic vascular resistance, MAP = mean arterial pressure, CVP = central venous pressure, PAWP = pulmonary artery wedge pressure.

emphasized, contractility is also influenced by afterload. When vessels constrict and afterload rises, normal hearts are stimulated to raise contractility to overcome resistance and maintain SV. Likewise, when vascular beds dilate and afterload declines, cardiac muscle is less stimulated and contractility also will decline. There are several measures used to evaluate contractility, but the most common is CO (Table 41-1). If a patient has a low CO, it may indicate actual myocardial depression (contractility). However, it may instead indicate inadequate myocardial stretch (low preload) excessive myocardial stretch (high preload), poor myocardial stimulation (low afterload), or excessive myocardial resistance (high afterload). Thus measures of contractility are meaningful reflections of actual muscle function and the need for inotropic support only when preload, afterload, and even HR are in their optimal ranges (Figure 41-9).

Measures other than CO are also equivocal. The right ventricle (RV) volumetric catheter measures

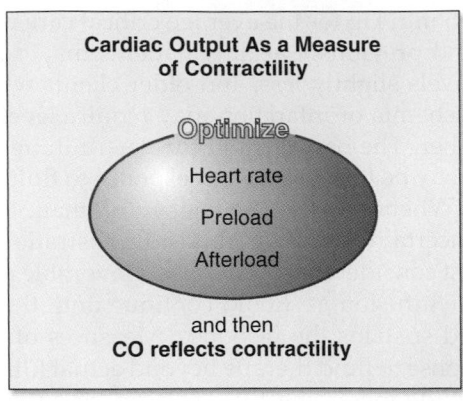

FIGURE 41-9 Cardiac output (CO) can only be considered a measure of contractility when the other factors affecting it are in the optimal range.

RV ejection fraction, probably the best gauge of contractility. But again, this catheter is not widely used because of possible increased cost and a lack of definitive research support. In some critical care units, stroke work index (SWI) is used to reflect cardiac strength, and as always, calculations are available to assess both right and left heart ventricular performance. Work relates to the mass moved and assesses cardiac strength by a formula that computes how many grams of blood the heart moves with every beat to each squared meter of the body. A rise in SWI means that the heart is moving more blood, not that it is necessarily working harder. The measure would be better termed "stroke productivity index" and should be viewed as a reflection of cardiac efficiency.

Despite being an imperfect measure of contractility, CO is still a useful criterion for assessing hemodynamics. Knowing how much blood the heart is pumping each minute does not explain the source of hypoperfusion, but only how critical the threat may be to the patient. Cardiac index (CI) is a measure of CO that corrects for body size, and is therefore helpful in setting a single normal range for patients of variable height and weight. Normal CI ranges are generally quoted as 2.5 to 3.5 L/min/m^2. However, this value is based on the cardiac performance of young, healthy, resting 70-kg men and may have no bearing on critically ill patients. Stroke volume index (SVI), a derivation of CI, is an even better parameter because it corrects for HR as well, typically averaging 40 to 50 ml/m^2/beat. Still, SVI doesn't pinpoint contractility, but includes preload and afterload. If a patient is deemed to have adequate vascular volume (preload) and relatively normal vascular tone (afterload), then SVI can be followed to guide inotropic therapy.

TABLE 41-1 Pulmonary Artery Catheter Measures Reflecting Contractility

CONTRACTILITY MEASURES	EXPECTED RANGES
Cardiac output	Different normal range for every body size Average 5–6 L/min
Cardiac index Controls for body size CO ÷ BSA	Average 2.5–3.5 L/min/m^2
Stroke volume index Controls for rate CI ÷ HR	Averages 40–50 ml/m^2/beat
Ejection fraction Special equipment; not readily available	Averages 50%-70%
Stroke work index A mathematical calculation; one for the left and right ventricle: LVSWI = (MAP–PAWP) × SVI × 1000 × 0.0136 RVSWI = (MPAP–CVP) × SVI × 1000 × 0.0136	Averages 40–80 g/m^2/beat Averages 7–12 g/m^2/beat

BSA = Body surface area, CI = cardiac index, CO = cardiac output, CVP = central venous pressure, HR = heart rate, LVSWI = left ventricular stroke work index, MAP = mean arterial pressure, MPAP = mean pulmonary artery pressure, PAWP = pulmonary artery wedge pressure, RVSWI = right ventricular stroke work index.

◆ Case Study 41-1, Part A

Hypertension

J.Q. is a 68-year-old man admitted to the cardiovascular surgery critical care unit following abdominal aortic aneurysm repair. He has multiple risk factors for cardiovascular disease including cigarette smoking, obesity, and hypertension. J.Q.'s history includes coronary artery and peripheral vascular disease, with coronary artery bypass surgery 3 years ago. His current problem started 18 months prior with the identification of an asymptomatic abdominal aortic aneurysm during a routine physical. The aneurysm was monitored for enlargement and when it reached 5 cm, surgical repair was scheduled after stenting was ruled out as a therapeutic option.

On arrival in critical care, J.Q. is lethargic but arousable. He is being mechanically ventilated and a warming blanket has been applied. He is in sinus rhythm with occasional premature ventricular contractions (PVCs), and lower extremity pulses are equal bilaterally. J.Q. has an arterial line, a pulmonary artery catheter, and a large abdominal dressing that is dry and intact. His vital signs on admission are:

Temp: 96° F
HR: 116 beats/min
RR: 12 beats/min
BP: 158/86 mm Hg

Decision point: To which parameter (HR, preload, afterload, or contractility) do you attribute J.Q.'s hypertension (158/86 mm Hg) on return from surgery?

J.Q.'s hemodynamic findings on arrival to critical care are as follows:

CVP: 9 mm Hg
PAWP: 17 mm Hg
PAP: 32/18 mm Hg
CO: 4.5 L/min
CI: 2.8 L/min
SVR: 1795 dynes

Decision point: What is your interpretation of each of these hemodynamic measures?

Approximately 2 hours after his arrival, J.Q. becomes cool and clammy, hypotensive, and tachycardic. At this time, the following profile is obtained:

Temp: 98.8° F
HR: 122 beats/min
RR: 16 beats/min
BP: 92/50 mm Hg
CVP: 5 mm Hg
PAWP: 9 mm Hg
PAP: 24/10 mm Hg
CO: 3.6 L/min
CI: 2.2 L/min
SVR: 1311 dynes

Decision point: To what do you attribute J.Q.'s hypotensive state?

BP = Blood pressure, CI = cardiac index, CO = cardiac output, CVP = central venous pressure, HR = heart rate, PAP = pulmonary artery pressure, PAWP = pulmonary artery wedge pressure, SVR = systemic vascular resistance, T = temperature, RR = respiratory rate.

Case continues on page 1127

Overall Cardiovascular Performance and Perfusion Indicators

Of all the information gleaned from hemodynamic monitoring, the most meaningful is venous oxygen saturation (SvO$_2$). This value is derived from the pulmonary artery via the distal port of the PAC and is used as a reflection of the balance between oxygen supply and demand. Normal ranges for SvO$_2$ are generally 70% to 80% and indicate stable oxygen balance. Neither a high nor a low SvO$_2$ is desirable. Both imply oxygen imbalance and serve as a warning to clinicians to evaluate the patient. When SvO$_2$ falls, it is secondary to either abatement of oxygen delivery or escalation of oxygen consumption. Likewise, when SvO$_2$ rises, it is related to either escalation of oxygen delivery or abatement of oxygen consumption. Oxygen delivery is determined by three factors: arterial oxygen saturation (SaO$_2$), the lung's ability to bring in oxygen; hemoglobin (Hgb), the blood's ability to carry oxygen; and CO, the heart's ability to transport oxygen. Oxygen consumption is determined by cellular extraction (Box 41-4).

To troubleshoot a rise or fall in SvO$_2$, the three oxygen delivery factors (SaO$_2$, Hgb, and CO) along with oxygen consumption must be considered. Unless there is an acute bleed, Hgb levels are fairly stable in most critically ill patients. Likewise, unless there is a sudden temperature spike, seizure activity, or acute agitation, most patients have high, but stable, oxygen consumption. Thus, SaO$_2$ and CO are the remaining factors most likely to alter SvO$_2$. SaO$_2$ can be continuously measured via pulse oximetry (SpO$_2$) and rapidly ruled in or out as the cause of a change in SvO$_2$. If SaO$_2$, Hgb, and oxygen consumption are deemed stable, then SvO$_2$ becomes a reflection of CO. Thus a fall in SvO$_2$ would be subsequent to a fall in CO. This may not appear to be a useful addition to the hemodynamic profile because it is already possible to *quantitatively* measure CO at the bedside. However, SvO$_2$ monitoring is capable of assessing CO *qualitatively*, addressing the more important question of whether blood oxygen supply is adequate to meet cellular oxygen demands.

Box 41-4

Clinical Conditions Associated With Changes in Venous Oxygen Saturation

CAUSES OF DECREASED VENOUS SATURATION
($Svo_2/Scvo_2$)

Decreased oxygen delivery
Decreased oxygen saturation
- Decrease in inspired oxygen
- Respiratory diseases (pneumonia, pulmonary edema, COPD, ARDS)
- Pulmonary emboli
- Any alveolar ventilation or perfusion mismatch

Decreased hemoglobin
- Hemorrhage
  - Anemia (decreased erythropoietin, as in renal failure; B_{12} deficiency; decreased iron intake)
  - Dysfunctional hemoglobin (sickle cell)

Decreased cardiac output
- Dysrhythmias
- Cardiogenic, hypovolemic or vasogenic shock
- Obstructive states (tamponade, tension pneumothorax, pulmonary emboli)
- Excessive levels of positive end-expiratory pressure

Increased oxygen consumption
- Increased activity (positioning, suctioning)
- Anxiety, pain, agitation, or restlessness
- High metabolic states (burns, trauma, fever, shivering)
- Hyperthermia

CAUSES OF INCREASED VENOUS SATURATION
($Svo_2/Scvo_2$)

Increased oxygen delivery
Increased Sao_2
- Supplemental oxygen therapy
- PEEP therapy
- Pulmonary disease resolution

Increased hemoglobin
- Blood transfusion
- Polycythemia (physiologic, as in COPD; pathologic)

Increased cardiac output
- Pacing therapy (HR)
- Fluid therapy (preload)
- Inotropic augmentation (contractility)
- Vasodilator therapy (afterload)

Decreased oxygen consumption
Decreased cellular need
- Hypothermia
- Neuromuscular blockade
- Analgesics, sedatives, anesthetic medications
- Antipyretics

Decreased cellular access
- Vasoconstriction
- Disseminated intravascular coagulation
- Microcirculatory inflammatory debris

Decreased cellular capability
- Cellular ischemia, injury, necrosis
- Cellular toxicity (cyanide, endotoxin, poisoning)

ARDS = Acute respiratory distress syndrome, CO = cardiac output, COPD = chronic obstructive pulmonary disease, HR = heart rate, PEEP = positive end-expiratory pressure, Sao_2 = arterial oxygen saturation, $Scvo_2$ = central venous oxygen saturation, Svo_2 = mixed venous oxygen saturation.

If low Svo_2 implies low CO, then it would seem reasonable to assume that a high Svo_2 implies high CO. However, a rise in Svo_2 is not often related to a rise in CO in the typical critical care patient. More likely, higher than normal Svo_2 readings are caused by an inability of cells to either access or extract oxygen. Limited cellular access to oxygen can be subsequent to excessive administration of vasopressors, disseminated intravascular coagulation, microcirculatory obstruction by inflammatory debris and other shock-related pathologies. Cellular extraction defects can result from extended periods of hypoperfusion followed by tissue hypoxia. Considering all the information possible via Svo_2 monitoring, many experts today view it as the gold standard for evaluating cardiovascular performance and determining global perfusion.[82] One advantage of using Svo_2 to guide therapy in shock is its reliability. The information it provides is not as dependent on proper technique as pressure transducer systems (CVP, PAP, PAWP), making it more efficacious and less prone to human error.

Another site for sampling venous oxygen saturation is in the vena cava. Measures can be taken intermittently or continuously using a specialized CVP catheter with oximetric capability.[87] Central venous oxygen saturation ($Scvo_2$) is generally about 10% higher than Svo_2 due to its location before the coronary sinus and the effect of venous admixture on Svo_2. Because of this, it is judicious to follow trends rather than individual values.[29] Although it is not a *mixed* venous specimen, $Scvo_2$-guided therapy has been found to reduce mortality in hypoperfused septic patients.[87] The primary advantages of this catheter are the ease of insertion and no need to traverse the heart to collect data. Newer catheters are being investigated that can be inserted peripherally, which would avoid the complications of subclavian artery cannulation, such as pneumothorax and central line infections.

Regardless how or where venous oxygen is measured, it reflects the final balance between oxygen delivery and uptake, which is the best appraisal of hemodynamic status. Bedside clinicians, however, tend to focus on BP or SpO_2. These values, though time-honored, can be deceiving, as illustrated in Box 41-5. In order to recognize hypoperfusion, $SvO_2/ScvO_2$, blood lactate, and base deficit are more meaningful. Some have proposed using SvO_2 venous oxygen saturation data as the cornerstone for directing therapy for all types of shock (Figure 41-10).[83]

Putting It Together: Differentiating Shock States

It is important to establish the type of shock so that therapy can be directed appropriately. Much of the hemodynamic information obtained in one of the shock states will trend in the same direction. For example, all three shock states decrease BP and SvO_2. These measures do not distinguish between the sources of shock, but serve as a warning that perfusion is threatened. Hypovolemic shock and cardiogenic shock can be differentiated by preload analysis. Hypovolemic shock has low filling pressures (CVP and/or PAWP), reflecting depleted vascular volume, whereas cardiogenic shock has high filling pressures, indicating poor ventricular emptying. Both have low CO secondary to either a lack of preload (hypovolemic) or a lack of contractility (cardiogenic). In addition,

both have SNS- and RAAS-mediated vasoconstriction and high SVR. Vasogenic shock has low filling pressures, but because of inappropriate vasodilation, the SVR is also low instead of high, as might be expected. In addition, CO may be elevated in vasogenic shock. In sepsis, the elevated CO is due to tachycardia, less resistance to flow (vasodilation), and shunting of blood from the microcirculation due to immune system cellular debris and disseminated intravascular coagulation. In today's era of mass beta-blocker use, however, this pathognomonic finding may be less common with hypotension accompanied by a normal CO (Table 41-2).

SHOCK-SPECIFIC THERAPY

Traditional approaches to shock therapy include unproven methodologies such as the titration of fluids and drugs to a target level of BP. Pressure does not guarantee perfusion, and BP has not been shown to be a valid measure of hemodynamic adequacy. Another strategy for managing hypotension, the Trendelenburg position, has been a ritual response to shock since it was first popularized in World War I. However, the evidence related to Trendelenburg position has linked it to a paradoxical fall in CO, compromised pulmonary function, increased intracranial pressure, and even retinal detachment.[54] The supine position with leg elevation has not been shown to be effective in hypotension either, but there are no data linking it to detrimental effects. Overall, there is insufficient research to guide practice in the treatment of shock. Successful reversal of cardiovascular collapse must focus on the cause and on improving cellular perfusion. A summary of the basic interventions for each of the three shock states is given in Box 41-6.

Hypovolemic Shock

The treatment for hypovolemic shock is to replace preload. The type of replacement fluid used depends on what is lost. If the patient is hypovolemic secondary to hemorrhage, blood transfusion will be the fluid of choice. The best Hgb level for the critically ill is controversial. For maximal oxygen-carrying capacity, a normal Hgb level seems desirable. However, research shows that transfused red blood cells lose deformability and may trigger an inflammatory response that actually diminishes oxygen perfusion.[42] To obtain the best cost-benefit ratio for patients, transfusions should be considered for Hgb levels less than 7 to 9 g/dl, figures that are much lower than the normal range.[23,42] For patients with cardiopulmonary compromise, a Hgb of 9 g/dl may be the safest target. In situations involving myocardial ischemia, anemia is poorly tolerated and should be treated to maintain levels of greater than 11 g/dl.[90]

Box 41-5

Unreliability of BP and Spo_2 in the Identification of Hypoperfusion

BP:	88/60
Spo_2:	88%
CI:	2.3 L/min/m²
SI:	31 ml/beat/m²
PAWP:	16 mm Hg
Svo_2:	67%

BP and Spo_2 indicate a possible problem, but Svo_2 shows oxygen balance.

BP:	112/64
Spo_2:	95%
CI:	2 L/min/m²
SI:	19 ml/beat/m²
PAWP:	19 mm Hg
Svo_2:	45%

Dobutamine indicated despite normal BP and Spo_2 due to dangerously low Svo_2.

BP = Blood pressure, CI = cardiac index, PAWP = pulmonary artery wedge pressure, SI = stroke index, Spo_2 = arterial oxygen saturation by pulse oximetry, Svo_2 = venous oxygen saturation. Modified from pacep.org.

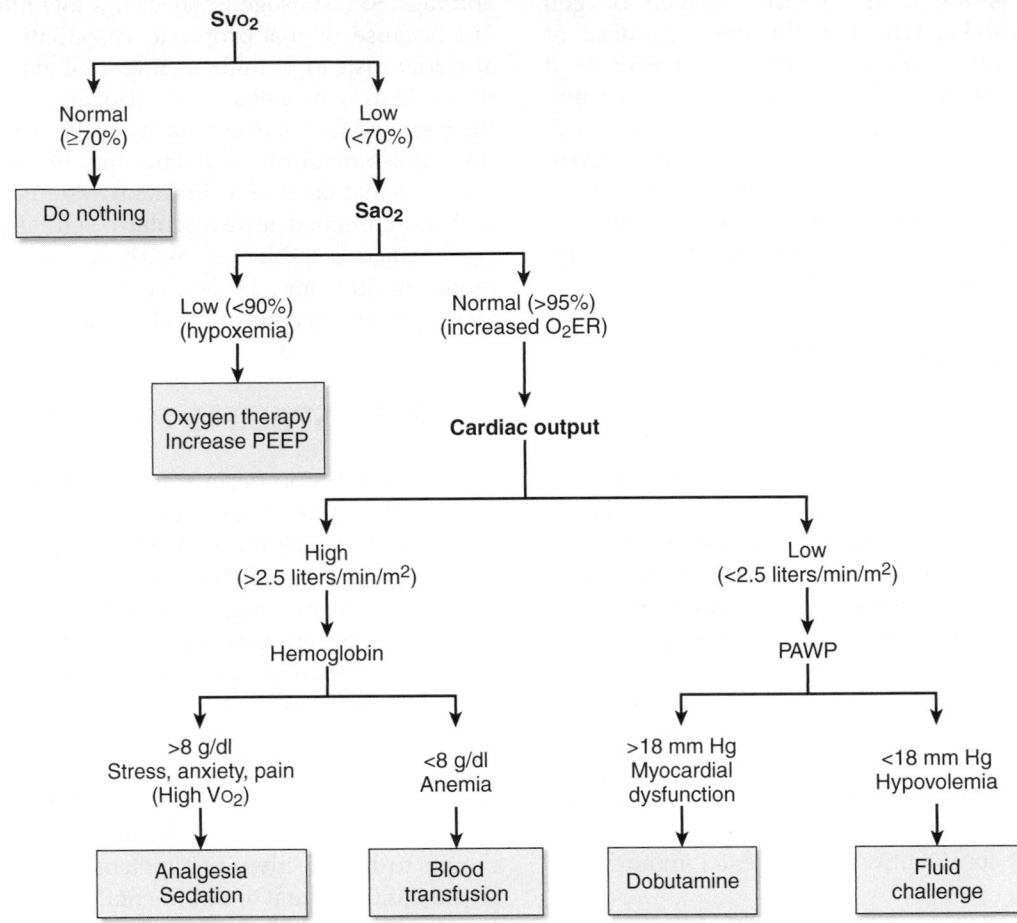

FIGURE 41-10 Diagnostic and therapeutic algorithm based on mixed venous oxygen saturation. Svo2 = Mixed venous oxygen saturation, Sao2 = arterial oxygen saturation, O2ER = oxygen extraction ratio, Vo2 = oxygen consumption, PAWP = pulmonary artery wedge pressure, PEEP = positive end-expiratory pressure.

TABLE 41-2 Hemodynamic Trends for Shock Differentiation

	HYPOVOLEMIC	LV CARDIOGENIC	RV CARDIOGENIC	VASOGENIC
Blood pressure	↓	↓	↓	↓
Cardiac index	↓	↓	↓	↑ ↔
Central venous pressure	↓	↑ ↔	↑	↓
Pulmonary artery wedge pressure	(↓)	(↑)	↑ ↔	↓
Systemic vascular resistance	↑	↑	↑	(↓)
Venous oxygen saturation	↓	↓	↓	↓

↑ = Increased, ↓ = decreased, ↔ = no change, ⬭ indicates most discriminating value for shock differentiation, LV = left ventricle, RV = right ventricle.

Box 41-6

Overview of Shock-Specific Strategies

HYPOVOLEMIC SHOCK

- Locate and resolve source of fluid loss
- Fluid resuscitation
    Normal saline or albumin or both to maintain
    PAWP 10–17 mm Hg
- Blood transfusion
    As needed to maintain Hgb 7–9 g/dl

VASOGENIC SHOCK

- Establish and address underlying cause
- Etiology-specific interventions (naloxone, airway support, antibiotics)
- Fluid resuscitation (as above)
- Vasopressors to maintain MAP greater than 65 mm Hg and SVR 900–1200 dynes
- For sepsis: early-goal directed therapy

CARDIOGENIC SHOCK

- Emergent revascularization (for myocardial infarctions)
- Inotropes
- To maintain cardiac index greater than 2.2 L/min/m^2
- Intraaortic balloon counterpulsation
- Vasodilators
    To reduce preload and afterload if warranted
- Vasopressors
    For cardiogenic shock accompanied by inflammation (SVR <900 dynes)
    For right ventricular cardiogenic shock
- Fluid therapy for preload augmentation
- Pacer therapy for bradycardia
- Pulmonary vasodilators if indicated

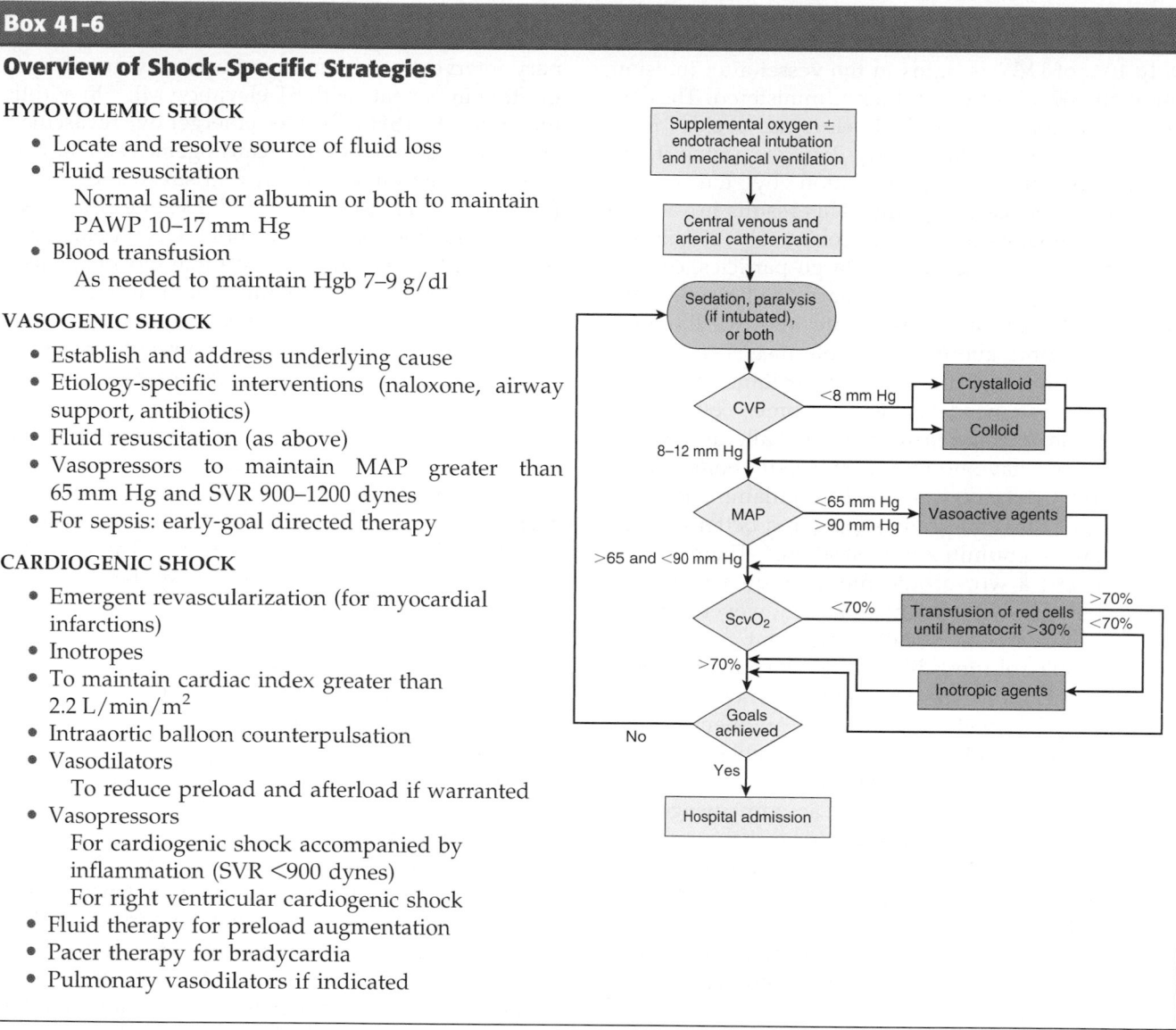

Hgb = Hemoglobin, MAP = mean arterial pressure, PAWP = pulmonary artery wedge pressure, SVR = systemic vascular resistance.

In hemorrhagic shock from trauma or abdominal aneurysm rupture, massive fluid resuscitation in the field and emergency department is now discouraged. Until hemostasis is achieved, augmenting vascular volume can encourage more bleeding due to higher intravascular pressure. "Permissive hypotension" is now recommended for the management of hemorrhagic shock.[30,37] Once bleeding has been controlled, fluid resuscitation can commence. It is not unusual in this extreme situation to employ vasopressor agents to maintain BP until vascular volume is restored. However, excessive use of these drugs may enhance hydrostatic forces inside the vessel and push the infusing fluid into the interstitium (third spacing). These patients are often thought to be refractory to therapy. More fluid is administered, but using high-dose vasopressors for BP control thwarts any actual improvement in vascular volume. As a result, perfusion may never be reestablished.

Intravenous fluid therapy is required to treat hypovolemia regardless of the cause. Research shows there is no difference in outcome using crystalloids or colloids, so NS, lactated Ringer's (LR), albumin, and Plasmanate are options for fluid resuscitation.[34,92,107] The challenge is not *what* to give, but how *much*. Measures for assessing adequate preload were discussed earlier; however, it is helpful to consider the dynamics of fluids and their effect on preload so that proper volumes can be anticipated. First, 5% dextrose and water (D$_5$W) is not used for preload restoration because it crosses all semipermeable membranes and distributes equally through all three fluid compartments (intracellular, interstitial, and intravascular). Only 10% of D_5W remains in the vessel after infusion, less than 100 ml for every liter administered. The electrolyte solutions—NS and LR—increase preload more efficiently with approximately 25% remaining in the vasculature due to manipulation by the cellular sodium and potassium pump. This results in vascular volume augmentation of approximately 250 ml per liter infused. Because of their large particles, colloids do not pass through the capillary wall readily, and thus 5% albumin and Plasmanate improve the intravascular volume about 100%. This means that 1 L of colloid will increase intravascular volume by 1 L. As a result of the need for less volume, colloids can replace preload losses faster than crystalloids, but they cost more and have no mortality benefit. Some studies have shown a trend toward less inflammation, less incidence of renal failure in sepsis, and better myocyte function with albumin administration.[34] There is also a trend toward a worse outcome in trauma with albumin, especially with brain injury. However, none of these findings are statistically significant.[34]

Hypertonic solutions like 3% or 5% sodium chloride and 25% (salt poor) albumin actually draw fluid from the cells and interstitial spaces to augment preload beyond what the solution itself could achieve. Because of this, hypertonic fluids may be of value in fluid resuscitation trauma patients with accompanying head injury.[79,104] In the past, fluids would be given to normalize preload at the risk of increasing intracranial pressure. With hypertonic solutions used in place of NS, mannitol administration may not be necessary. Hypertonic sodium chloride solutions must be used with caution, especially in situations of normal intracranial pressure. Rapid elevation of serum sodium levels can result in cerebral dehydration, cellular shrinkage, and even herniation. It is important to monitor serum sodium levels and administer isotonic solutions with hypertonic sodium chloride so that fluid movement from the intracellular to extracellular space is moderated.

Cardiogenic Shock

The heart is key to hemodynamic stability and tissue oxygenation. Ventricular dysfunction is common, and if refractory to treatment, lethal as well. The leading cause of cardiogenic shock is acute coronary syndrome (ACS) with myocardial infarction (MI), resulting in the loss of more than 40% of functional muscle.[47] Without adequate coronary flow, even powerful inotropes will be futile in improving hypotension. Therefore the most effective treatment of pump shock is coronary artery reperfusion.[45,46,94] A 1999 task force of the American College of Cardiology and the American Heart Association (ACC/AHA) gave a class I recommendation to the performance of primary percutaneous coronary intervention or emergent coronary artery bypass grafting in patients with ST elevation MI.[89] In addition, the SHOCK (SHould we emergently revascularize Occluded Coronaries in cardiogenic shocK?) trial showed an absolute difference in survival of 13.2% in favor of early revascularization.[31] Despite clearly established guidelines, 2002 data from the National Registry of Myocardial Infarction suggest that most patients did not receive reperfusion therapy.[5] In a recent European study, only 41.4% of ACS patients complicated by cardiogenic shock were shown to be urgently revascularized.[49] Thus mortality rates for cardiogenic shock remain at about 50% to 60%.[49]

Evidence from the SHOCK trial also uncovered a previously unrecognized systemic inflammatory response during cardiogenic shock involving complement activation, nitric oxide (NO) release, and the evolution of inflammatory cytokines.[33] These findings imply that cardiogenic shock may be more than reduced ventricular performance. An inappropriate vasodilatory reaction may complicate the clinical picture. It may be useful to monitor SVR to identify this phenomenon so treatment can be directed appropriately. SHOCK-2 (SHould we inhibit nitric Oxide synthase in patients with Cardiogenic shocK?) is being designed to test a novel NO inhibitor in a randomized trial of patients with persistent shock despite a patent infarct-related artery.[44]

In addition to correcting myocardial ischemia, electrolyte, acid-base, and medication imbalances that can depress muscle function should be addressed. Emergency surgical repair may be warranted in the event of structural complications such as tamponade, acute valvular regurgitation, or septal defects. If an underlying cause cannot be identified, or if the patient is acutely unstable during the diagnostic process, inotropic drugs are required. Data show an increased incidence of mortality when sympathomimetic agents are used for the treatment of acute decompensated heart failure.[33,67] To circumvent potential toxicity, many recommend the use of devices instead of drugs. Intraaortic balloon (IAB) counterpulsation is effective in the stabilization of the cardiogenic shock patient and recommended by the ACC/AHA.[7] In the European study, only 17.7% received IAB counterpulsation for ACS complicated by cardiogenic shock.[49]

Despite employment of revascularization and IAB counterpulsation, drug therapy for the support of patients in cardiogenic shock is generally necessary. Hypotension is addressed in this type of shock through contractility augmentation. Of all the available inotropic agents, dobutamine (Dobutrex) is probably the best tolerated by patients with heart disease.[33] Other inotropes may be more powerful and considered if the patient has profound hypotension and hypoperfusion. However, drugs such as norepinephrine (Levophed) or epinephrine cause vasoconstriction as well as contractility improvement. Vasoconstriction of veins and arteries increases preload and afterload, placing an even greater burden on an already failing ventricle. Although this strategy may improve the patient's BP, the increased ventricular workload does not improve long-term survival.

The long-term goal in managing cardiogenic shock is to decrease the heart's workload to allow for cardiac recovery. This is similar to the way respiratory failure is managed. The diaphragm, the body's air pump, is unloaded with a mechanical ventilator. Then, after a period of rest, work is reintroduced via the weaning process. The same approach applies to cardiac failure. The heart is unloaded with a mechanical device or drug therapy, and then work is reintroduced by gradually weaning the patient. The efficacy of IAB counterpulsation in managing cardiogenic hypotension illustrates the successful approach to this type of shock. The IAB pump mechanically reduces preload and afterload through rhythmic inflation and deflation of a balloon in the descending aorta. During diastole the balloon inflates, enhancing blood flow to the coronary circulation, reducing ischemia and improving contractility. During systole the balloon deflates, reducing afterload, the resistance to blood flow out of the ventricle. Both inflation and deflation help the ventricle to empty, which indirectly reduces preload. Vasodilators can medicinally achieve effects similar to the IAB pump through dilation of veins and arteries.

Vasodilators used to reduce preload and afterload in cardiogenic shock require careful titration. Administering nitroglycerin, for example, to a patient who is already hypotensive is challenging because of concerns that it will cause a further decline in BP:

$$CO \times SVR = BP$$
$$\leftrightarrow \quad \downarrow \quad \downarrow$$

In fact, this will occur if the patient is in hypovolemic or vasogenic shock. In cardiogenic shock, however, a modest drop in SVR would be more likely to improve CO with little or no change in BP:

$$CO \times SVR = BP$$
$$\uparrow \quad \downarrow \quad \leftrightarrow$$

Vasodilator therapy will not increase BP, but it will improve CO, preserve cardiac function (decreased workload), enhance tissue flow, and generally maintain baseline BP. Inotropes can be added to augment pressure, but vasopressors should be avoided in noninflammatory cardiogenic shock.

Thus far in this discussion of cardiogenic shock, the focus has been on failure of the left side of the heart. Right-sided failure is common with RV infarction, which occurs in 30% to 50% of patients with inferior or posterior wall MI. Hypotension is seen in at least 10% of these patients.[53,66,72] The diagnosis of RV infarction is confirmed by the presence of ST-segment elevations in right precordial leads or classic hemodynamic findings during right heart catheterization.[40] These findings include elevated right heart pressures accompanied by diminished pulmonary pressures and left heart filling.[74] Clinically, the nurse may note distended neck veins, but clear lungs in a patient with inferior wall MI, indicating primary RV failure rather than failure secondary to left ventricle (LV) dysfunction. Right-sided cardiac failure may go unnoticed when dominated by left-sided pathology. However, when the RV sustains significant damage, the LV will be underfilled, which can result in life-threatening hypoperfusion.

Because of its thin wall, failure of the pumping ability of the RV is generally complete, reducing the chamber to little more than a conduit for blood flow. Inotropic support is rarely helpful in improving RV contractility. As with an LV infarction, the single best strategy for RV infarction is emergent revascularization. Unlike the LV, however, the RV responds best to stretch and volume loading to maintain function. The goal is to augment preload to create enough pressure to drive blood through the lungs and into the LV. If the patient is bradycardic, a common finding due to right coronary artery pathology, pacing therapy or inotropes can be used to improve HR. RV cardiogenic shock leads to systemic congestion, not pulmonary congestion. However, if there is accompanying lung pathology, such as pneumonia or pulmonary hypertension, it will increase RV afterload and decrease forward flow to the left heart. Treatment of underlying lung diseases and reduction of PVR are important to reduce RV workload. Inhaled NO and epoprostenol (Flolan) infusions have been used in some centers for this purpose.[51] They are effective in dilating the pulmonary vasculature and reducing resistance to blood flow.

RV failure can also occur secondary to pulmonary pathology (cor pulmonale). Etiologies such as pulmonary emboli and tension pneumothorax require specific interventions such as fibrinolytics and pleural decompression, respectively. In chest trauma, the RV is the most vulnerable chamber because of its anterior location in the chest and propensity to contusion, which can seriously complicate fluid resuscitation efforts.

Vasogenic Shock

Vasogenic shock has several widely varied etiologies, all of which result in an inappropriate loss of vessel tone, hypotension, and hypoperfusion.[62] Some forms have a dual derangement, with vasodilation along with vessel leakage. Third spacing of vascular volume adds a hypovolemic component to the clinical picture, further complicating therapy. In either case, fluid resuscitation is appropriate and guidelines are similar to those discussed under hypovolemic shock. In addition to refilling the expanded and potentially depleted vascular space, perfusion pressure is restored by reversing dilation with vasopressive agents. Many vasogenic shock states are transient and respond to therapies other than hemodynamic medications. Drug overdose, for example, may respond to naloxone (Narcan), and spinal shock to the simple lapse of time and the body's assimilation of the loss of sympathetic innervation.

Sepsis is an etiology of vasogenic shock in which microorganisms in the bloodstream evoke widespread inflammation and trigger a cascade of cardiovascular insults, resulting in hemodynamic instability. In addition to vasodilation (vasogenic shock) and capillary leakage (hypovolemic shock), the toxins and mediators of sepsis can cause severe myocardial depression (cardiogenic shock). Thus it is said that septic patients suffer from all three forms of shock (Figure 41-11). In February 2004, the Surviving Sepsis Campaign was launched, releasing 45 therapeutic recommendations intended to reduce the mortality of sepsis by 25% over a 5-year period.[24] (A complete review can be found in Chapter 43; this section will review only the hemodynamic management of septic shock.)

Several landmark studies and papers have been written in the past decade addressing the cardiovascular support of septic patients.[23,48,86] In 2001, Rivers and colleagues published a breakthrough document describing a method termed EGDT.[86] In the past, goal-directed therapy had been tried, but there was little emphasis on intervening "early" and much focus on attaining "supranormal" levels of CO, all with inconclusive results.[59] However, Rivers' EGDT was found to decrease mortality by 34%, length of stay by 3.8 days, and cost of care by $12,000 per case. The premise of the study was early identification, even before hemodynamic findings of shock were apparent, and aggressive intervention to predetermined measures of perfusion. Occult hypoperfusion was uncovered by examining lactate levels. Patients with lactate levels greater than or equal to 4 mmol/L were treated the same as patients with hypotension and overt shock. Once identified, rapid restoration of normal cardiovascular function was sought primarily through fluid resuscitation at volumes approximately 50% higher than standard therapy or 5 L of crystalloid or more. Dobutamine, packed red blood cells, and vasopressors (dopamine [Intropin], norepinephrine, and vasopressin

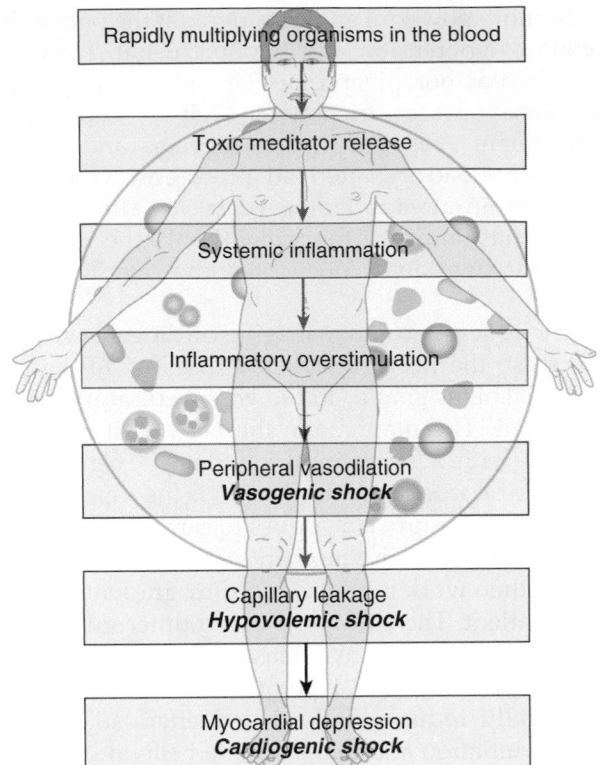

⬆FIGURE 41-11 Septic shock has a complicated pathophysiology. This diagram is only a reflection of the changes that lead to hemodynamic imbalance. As noted, the changes to the cardiovascular system give sepsis the characteristics of all three forms of shock.

[Pitressin]) also were used to maintain the following end points:

- UO greater than or equal to 5 ml/kg/min
- MAP greater than or equal to 65 mm Hg
- CVP 8 to 12 mm Hg (12–15 if on a mechanical ventilator)
- ScvO$_2$ greater than 70%

Consequent to its success, EGDT was embraced by the Surviving Sepsis Campaign and the Institute of Healthcare Improvement and was included in the Sepsis Resuscitation Bundle as a grade B recommendation (Box 41-7). The success of EGDT in sepsis has raised questions as to its application in other forms of cardiovascular collapse.

Another aspect of cardiovascular support in sepsis relates to the use of steroid therapy. Annane and coworkers found that septic patients requiring vasopressive agents frequently suffered from relative adrenal insufficiency.[3] High-dose steroid therapy has been ineffective; however, this recent study evaluated 7 days of replacement-dose steroid therapy only, and demonstrated earlier weaning of vasopressors and a significantly lower risk of death.[3]

Box 41-7

Sepsis Resuscitation Bundle

1. Serum lactate measured
2. Blood cultures obtained prior to antibiotic administration
3. From the time of presentation, broad-spectrum antibiotics administered within 3 hours for emergency department (ED) admissions and 1 hour for non-ED intensive care unit (ICU) admissions
4. In the event of hypotension and/or lactate greater than 4 mmol/L (36 mg/dl):
   - Deliver an initial minimum of 20 ml/kg of crystalloid (or colloid equivalent)
   - Apply vasopressors for hypotension not responding to initial fluid resuscitation to maintain mean arterial pressure (MAP) greater than 65 mm Hg
5. In the event of persistent hypotension despite fluid resuscitation (septic shock) and/or lactate greater than 4 mmol/L (36 mg/dl):
   - Achieve central venous pressure (CVP) of greater than 8 mm Hg
   - Achieve central venous oxygen saturation (Scvo$_2$) of greater than 70%

TITRATABLE MEDICATIONS USED IN MANAGING SHOCK

This section reviews three medication categories used in the treatment of hemodynamic compromise: cardiac inotropes, vasopressors, and vasodilators. Several of these drugs have more than one mechanism of action and are referred to as "inodilators" (combined inotropic and vasodilatory effects) or "inoconstrictors" (combined inotropic and vasoconstrictor effects). They are discussed under the heading that most describes their primary effect or clinical use. Because many of the agents act on the SNS, a brief review of adrenergic receptors is in order (Figure 41-12).

During the fight-or-flight response, catecholamines are released. Epinephrine and norepinephrine are secreted from the adrenal medulla into the circulation and norepinephrine is released from synaptic nerve endings on the heart and vasculature. The effect of catecholamines varies depending on the type of receptor that dominates within the target tissue. These receptors have been labeled as alpha adrenergic and beta adrenergic. The heart is driven by beta receptors, with the fight-or-flight response stimulating the receptors to increase HR and contractility for CO augmentation. The vasculature has both alpha and beta receptors, with vascular beta receptors, termed beta-2 receptors. Nonvital organ vessel beds primarily have alpha receptors,

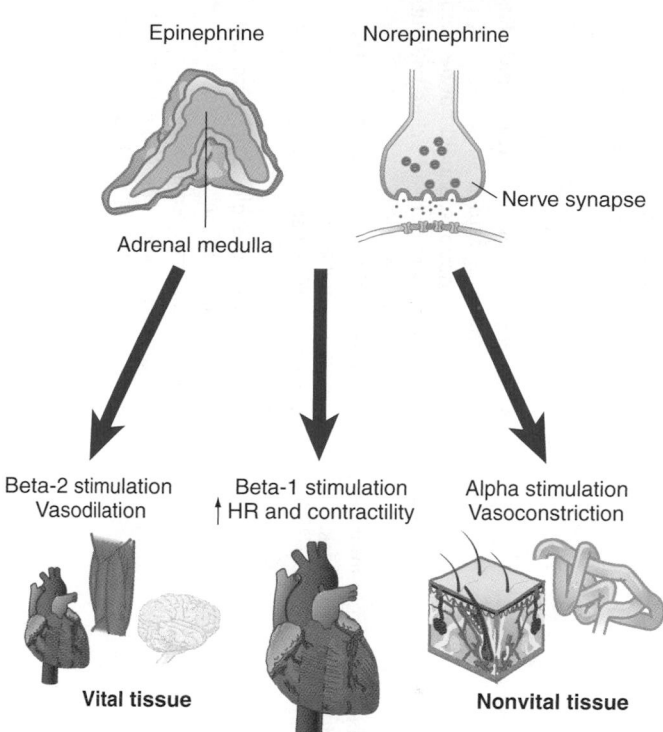

ADRENERGIC RECEPTORS
IN THE SYMPATHETIC NERVOUS SYSTEM

FIGURE 41-12 The stress response involves release of chemicals from both the adrenal gland and the sympathetic nervous system. These chemicals act at adrenergic receptor sites on many body structures, including in the heart and vasculature. HR = Heart rate.

whereas vital organ vessel beds primarily have beta-2 receptors. The vascular response to alpha stimulation is constriction, and the response to beta-2 stimulation is dilation. Thus during the stress response, when both receptors are stimulated, blood is shunted to vital organs (beta-2 vasodilation) and away from nonvital organs (alpha vasoconstriction).

In discussing the uses of titratable drugs for shock, it is a prerequisite to recognize that research is ill suited to guide clinical practice. There are no data definitively supporting the use of one cardiac inotrope or vasoactive agent over another.[60,77] In addition, because these drugs are generally titrated based on patient response, establishing dosage ranges is difficult. Titration implies infusing small increments until established goals or end points are reached. There is variation in what end points clinicians use. In addition, dosage ranges vary in the literature and may be reported in mg/min, mcg/min, mcg/kg/min, and units/min. Most of these drugs have very short half-lives—effects quickly subside when dosages are decreased or when the drug is stopped.

Text continues on p. 1122

ACTION, DOSING, AND SPECIAL CONSIDERATIONS FOR COMMONLY USED CARDIOTONIC AND VASOACTIVE DRUGS

MEDICATION	ACTION	DOSE	SPECIAL CONSIDERATIONS
Dobutamine (Dobutrex) *Inotrope*	Adrenergic stimulant. Beta-1 and beta-2 receptor effects. Used to improve contractility in cardiogenic shock. Effects on afterload fairly insignificant due to mild vasodilation limited to vital organ vessels (heart, brain, skeletal muscle).	**Continuous infusion only.** Titrate for desired effect. 2.5–10 mcg/kg/min on average. Occasionally 20–40 mcg/kg/min for desired effect. 5 mcg/kg/min has been shown to improve gastrointestinal tract perfusion in shock.	A first-line drug for pump failure including failure following cardiac surgery. As with any inotrope, should not be used for the treatment of heart failure without signs of hypoperfusion. Increases stroke volume, cardiac index, coronary artery perfusion. Decreases pulmonary artery wedge pressure (preload). Generally increases blood pressure, but may have little effect. May increase myocardial oxygen consumption, heart rate (especially with atrial fibrillation), and dysrhythmias, but less than other inotropes. May decrease blood pressure, especially with incomplete fluid resuscitation.
Dopamine (Intropin) *Inotrope (Vasopressor at higher dosages)*	Adrenergic stimulant. Used as first-line support of blood pressure in hypotension of uncertain etiology. Effects are dose dependent. *Low dose:* *dopaminergic receptor effects;* may increase urine output; may decrease central venous and pulmonary artery wedge pressure. *Moderate dose:* *beta-1 receptor effects;* increases stroke volume, cardiac index, and blood pressure; decreases pulmonary artery wedge pressure; may be best range for cardiogenic shock states. *High dose:* *alpha receptor effects;* increases systemic vascular resistance and blood pressure; may be best range for vasogenic shock states.	**Continuous infusion only.** Titrate for desired effect. *Low dose:* 2–5 mcg/kg/min *Moderate dose:* 5–10 mcg/kg/min *High dose:* 10–20 mcg/kg/min	Increases myocardial oxygen consumption, heart rate, and dysrhythmias. May decrease stroke volume, cardiac index, and organ perfusion (especially mesenteric perfusion) at high doses. Does not provide protection against renal failure and should be avoided, especially in the septic patient. In cardiogenic shock, vasoconstricting effects are undesirable and may increase preload and afterload, decrease cardiac output, aggravating pump dysfunction. May be administered concomitantly with low-dose vasodilators in support of patients with poor pump function. May be difficult to wean due to depletion of norepinephrine stores in synaptic nerve endings with long-term use. Consider switching to norepinephrine at doses greater than 20 mcg/kg/min.

MEDICATION	ACTION	DOSE	SPECIAL CONSIDERATIONS
Esmolol (Brevibloc) *Negative Inotrope*	Adrenergic blocker. Beta-1 effects. Slows heart rate primarily; decreases contractility and cardiac output. Used to decrease blood pressure. Used to slow supraventricular tachycardias and rapid ventricular rates in atrial fibrillation and atrial flutter.	Intravenous infusion. Titrate for desired effect. Immediate-control dosing: 80 mg bolus (approximately 1 mg/kg) over 30 seconds followed by 150 mcg/kg/min infusion if needed; may titrate up to 300 mcg/kg/min. Gradual-control dosing: loading dose: 0.25–0.5 mg/kg/min bolus IV over 1–2 minutes followed by a continuous infusion of 50–200 mcg/kg/min.	Should be avoided in situations of inadequate cardiac output. Hypotension is greatest during the first 30 minutes of infusion. Rapid, short-term control of ventricular rate. May cause cardiac failure, cardiogenic shock, bradycardic rhythms, heart block greater than first degree, myocardial ischemia, bronchospasm, and glycemic imbalances. Shortest half-life of all beta-blockers.
Epinephrine (Adrenalin) *Inotrope Vasopressor*	Adrenergic stimulant. Beta-1 and beta-2 receptor effects predominate at lower doses. Alpha receptor effects predominate at higher doses. Used to improve contractility associated with severe systolic dysfunction in cardiogenic shock. Used to improve vascular tone in vasogenic shock. May be best reserved for bolus therapy in cardiac arrest or anaphylaxis (beyond the scope of this table).	**Intravenous infusion only.** Titrate for desired effect. Beta-1 and beta-2 effects predominate at 0.01–0.05 mcg/kg/min. Beta-1 and alpha effects predominate at 0.05–2 mcg/kg/min. Pure alpha effects at dosages greater than 2 mcg/kg/min.	Powerful and indicated when other inotropes fail. Effects on heart rate may be beneficial with bradycardia. Reverses bronchoconstriction associated with anaphylactic reactions. Increases cardiac index, systemic vascular resistance, blood pressure. Extreme increases in myocardial oxygen consumption, heart rate, and dysrhythmias possible. May decrease stroke volume, cardiac index, and organ perfusion at excessive doses. May cause cardiac ischemia. Best reserved for patients without coronary artery disease. Has been shown to increase mesenteric ischemia, serum lactate, blood sugar.[28]
Labetalol (Normodyne) *Negative Inotrope*	*Vasodilator.* Adrenergic blocker. Alpha, beta-1, and beta-2 blockade; beta effects greater than alpha. Decreases heart rate, contractility, and systemic vascular resistance. Used to decrease blood pressure.	Titrate to effect. Intermittent boluses of 20–40 mg IV administered over 2 minutes, or as an infusion at 1–4 mg/min.	Longer-acting antihypertensive than esmolol. Helpful in the setting of acute aortic dissection to decrease blood pressure without reflexive increases in cardiac output and heart rate. May cause life-threatening hyperkalemia,

Table continues on page 1118

MEDICATION	ACTION	DOSE	SPECIAL CONSIDERATIONS
			especially in renal failure patients. Use cautiously; may cause profound hypotension. May cause cardiac failure, cardiogenic shock, bradycardic rhythms, heart block greater than first degree, myocardial ischemia, bronchospasm, and glycemic imbalances. Possible myocardial depression when used in conjunction with halothane, isoflurane, and cyclopropane anesthesia.
Milrinone (Primacor) *Inodilator*	Phosphodiesterase inhibitor (nonadrenergic) Increases systolic contractility and diastolic relaxation Dilates veins and arteries Long duration of action; dosage changes only every 4–8 hours	Relatively weak inotrope; inappropriate monotherapy for shock Increases stroke volume and cardiac index Decreases central venous pressure, pulmonary artery wedge pressure, and systemic vascular resistance Does not increase myocardial oxygen consumption Effective with beta blockade and overdose	May increase heart rate and dysrhythmias Less arrhythmogenic than catecholamines May decrease blood pressure, especially with hypovolemia Not titratable; long half-life May cause thrombocytopenia
		Optional bolus; maintenance 0.375–0.75 mcg/kg/min	
Nesiritide (Natrecor) *Vasodilator* *Natriuretic*	B-type natriuretic peptide (nonadrenergic). Dilates veins and arteries. Stimulates natriuresis and diuresis. Used to decrease preload and afterload in pump dysfunction.	**Continuous infusion only.** Optional bolus: 2 mcg/kg over 1 minute. Maintenance dose: 0.01 mcg/kg/min. Do not exceed recommended dosage.	Neurohormonal modulator. Decreases central venous pressure, pulmonary artery wedge pressure, and systemic vascular resistance. Increases stroke volume and cardiac index without increasing myocardial oxygen consumption. May decrease blood pressure and increase heart rate, especially with inadequate vascular volume. Discontinue infusion for 2 hours before drawing a BNP level. 30-day mortality *may* be higher than patients managed with other vasodilators and diuretic medications; further research required.

MEDICATION	ACTION	DOSE	SPECIAL CONSIDERATIONS
Nicardipine (Cardene)	*Vasodilator.* Calcium channel blocker (nonadrenergic). Blocks calcium channels primarily in the vasculature to decrease systemic vascular resistance. May have slight negative inotropic effects. Used to decrease blood pressure.	2.5 mg IV over 5 minutes (may repeat × 4), followed by an infusion at 2–4 mg/hr.	Provides stable control of blood pressure without the negative inotropic effects of other calcium channel blockers. May be used to treat angina. May also be used at a low dose (0.25 mcg/kg/min) to prevent spasm in radial artery grafts. Reduce dose in hepatic dysfunction.
Nitroglycerin (Tridil) *Vasodilator*	Nitric oxide releaser (nonadrenergic). Dilates primarily veins. Dilates arteries at higher dosages. Used to decrease preload and afterload in pump failure and cardiogenic shock (small amounts). Used to decrease blood pressure in hypertensive states.	**Continuous infusion only.** Titrate for desired effect. Ranges vary greatly; 0.1–100 mcg/kg/min or 5–200 mcg/min (higher doses have been reported). Venous dilation at rates less than 50 mcg/min (1 mcg/kg/min).	Increases stroke volume and cardiac index. Decreases central venous pressure, pulmonary artery wedge pressure, and systemic vascular resistance. Does not increase myocardial oxygen consumption. Effective coronary dilator. May decrease blood pressure and increase heart rate, especially with inadequate vascular volume or excessive dosage. Must be titrated slowly and in small increments for pump dysfunction, causing hypoperfusion. Less effective for the prevention of postoperative internal mammary artery vasospasm than diltiazem.
Nitroprusside (Nipride) *Vasodilator*	Nitric oxide releaser (nonadrenergic). Dilates veins and arteries; balanced effect. Used to decrease blood pressure in hypertensive states. May be used to decrease preload and afterload in pump failure and cardiogenic shock (small amounts).	**Continuous infusion only.** Titrate to desired effects. Initiate slowly, 0.1–8 mcg/kg/min.	Increases stroke volume and cardiac index. Decreases central venous pressure, pulmonary artery wedge pressure, and systemic vascular resistance. Does not increase myocardial oxygen consumption. Better afterload reducer than nitroglycerin. May undesirably decrease blood pressure and increase heart rate, especially with inadequate vascular volume or excessive dosage.

Table continues on page 1120

MEDICATION	ACTION	DOSE	SPECIAL CONSIDERATIONS
			Must be titrated slowly and in small increments for pump dysfunction, causing hypoperfusion. May cause coronary steal and cardiac ischemia. Inhibits hypoxic vasoconstriction and may reverse pulmonary autoregulation and decrease Pao_2 levels. Can cause methemoglobinemia, thiocyanate production, and cyanide toxicity, especially with high doses and/or prolonged therapy. Must not be used in patients with liver failure or renal failure (unless the patient is being dialyzed).
Norepinephrine (Levophed) *Vasopressor* *(Inotrope at lower dosages)*	Adrenergic stimulant. Alpha and beta-1 receptor effects. Used to improve contractility associated with severe systolic dysfunction in cardiogenic shock. Used to improve vascular tone in vasogenic shock, especially sepsis.	**Continuous infusion only.** Titrate to desired effects. Mean dosage range: 0.2 to 1.3 mcg/kg/min. Maximum dosage: 3.3 mcg/kg/min.	More potent than dopamine. Increases systemic vascular resistance and blood pressure. Increases stroke volume and cardiac index at low doses only. In cardiogenic shock, vasoconstricting effects may increase preload and afterload, decrease cardiac output, and aggravate pump dysfunction. Should be administered concomitantly with vasodilators in support of patients with poor pump function to counteract the negative effects of vasoconstriction on cardiac output. Increases myocardial oxygen consumption, heart rate, and dysrhythmias. May decrease stroke volume, cardiac index, and organ perfusion at excessive dosages (alpha effect). Associated with improved survival in patients with septic shock.

MEDICATION	ACTION	DOSE	SPECIAL CONSIDERATIONS
Phenylephrine (Neo-Synephrine) *Vasopressor*	Adrenergic stimulant. Alpha receptor effects only. Used to increase vascular tone and blood pressure in vasogenic forms of shock.	**Continuous infusion only.** Titrated to desired effect. Optional bolus dosing possible with severe hypotension: 2–5 mg. Infusion doses: average 40–60 mcg/min and can be as high as 180 mcg/min.	Increases systemic vascular resistance and blood pressure. Ideal in vasogenic shock states involving vasodilation only, such as spinal shock, spinal anesthesia, dilating drug overdose, and neurogenic shock. May decrease stroke volume, cardiac index, and organ perfusion at high doses. Generally does not increase heart rate. High doses can cause excessive vasoconstriction and a reflexive bradycardia.
Vasopressin (Pitressin) *Vasopressor*	Antidiuretic hormone (nonadrenergic). Stimulates V1 receptors. Used to increase vascular tone and blood pressure in vasogenic forms of shock when other vasopressors have failed. May be best reserved for bolus therapy in cardiac arrest (beyond the scope of this table).	**Intravenous infusion only.** Titrate only within specific parameters. Dosage safest at 0.01–0.04 unit/min. Do not exceed stated dosage ranges.	May decrease stroke volume, cardiac index, and perfusion to nonvital organs, especially the mesentery. Increases systemic vascular resistance and blood pressure. May be helpful in catecholamine-resistant shock and should be used primarily as salvage therapy. Should never be used as monotherapy for blood pressure control, but instead as a companion drug to catecholamines. May be most efficacious in treating the hypotension seen with sepsis and cardiopulmonary bypass due to hormone deficiency and a replacement effect. May be helpful in improving blood pressure in patients with massive blood loss until blood can be replaced. Incompletely studied except in cardiac arrest. Important to monitor for hyponatremia (water retention) and correct as needed. Use with caution; do not exceed dosage maximum.

BNP = B-type natriuretic peptide.

There is no absolute maximum dose for any of the commonly used agents (vasopressin is an exception and is discussed later). The titration of hemodynamic drugs is guided by animal studies and expert opinion, with few randomized studies or definitive data to standardize practice. Unfortunately, the use of BP as the goal for titration is common, and vasopressors are reliable in improving BP. Vasopressor overuse can mimic the effects of critical illness and organ failure, allowing their negative side effects to be attributed to the underlying disease instead of being recognized as a possible adverse drug event.

As with most medications, every drug used for shock has positive (therapeutic) and negative (nontherapeutic) effects. These are outlined in the Medication table on pp. 1116-1121. For example, inotropes increase contractility, SV, CI, and BP, and decrease preload, all considered positive effects when there is ventricular dysfunction. However, they can elicit a rise in HR, dysrhythmias, and myocardial oxygen consumption (Mvo_2), reduce preload and afterload, and increase SV and CI, similar to an inotrope, but without increasing Mvo_2. If used before adequate vascular volume replacement or in excessive dosage ranges, vasodilators can also increase HR and decrease BP. Lastly, vasopressors greatly enhance BP via arterial tone. Afterload augmentation is desirable in vasogenic shock, but can burden the heart in cardiogenic shock and lead to a fall in SV and CO. Vasopressors also increase HR and Mvo_2, which can further impair cardiac function. When used in excess, vasopressors can produce fluid extravasation and even perpetuate shock by decreasing blood flow and cellular perfusion. Without the needed evidence, the most critical guides for titration of cardiotonic and vasoactive drugs are an understanding of hemodynamics, an appreciation of cellular oxygenation, and a determination to use them to obtain the best cost-benefit ratio for the patient.

Inotropic Agents

Intravenous inotropes amplify the contractile force of the heart and are indicated for the support of heart failure causing hypoperfusion. All inotropes increase the influx of calcium into cardiac muscle cells to aid in myofibril shortening. One mechanism for augmenting calcium influx is to increase levels of cyclic adenosine monophosphate (cAMP), a molecule often referred to as the "second messenger," which regulates many cellular processes. Catecholamine drugs mimic SNS effects and increase contractility by increasing the production of cAMP. Pure beta-stimulating drugs include isoproterenol (Isuprel) and dobutamine. Dopamine, norepinephrine, and epinephrine are beta stimulating, but also have alpha effects and are generally thought of as "inoconstrictors." Another mechanism for increasing cAMP to improve calcium influx and contractility is by blocking its enzymatic degradation by phosphodiesterase. Phosphodiesterase inhibitors (PDIs) are noncatecholamine drugs used for inotropic support. Currently, there are only two drugs in this category in clinical practice: inamrinone and milrinone (Primacor). Inamrinone (amrinone was renamed due to confusion with amiodarone) is not widely used because of a strong propensity to induce thrombocytopenia. Milrinone, in addition to its inotropic effects, is a venous and arterial dilator. A new category of inotrope, termed calcium sensitizers, shows much promise in the support of the failing heart, but early studies have been disappointing. Like the PDI agents, these are also inodilators and include levosimendan. This drug increases troponin C's affinity for calcium to strengthen the heart and activates potassium channels to dilate venous, arterial, and coronary vasculature.[36]

Because of the importance of calcium in the efficacy of all these drugs, it may appear that a calcium infusion would work equally as well to support hypotension caused by myocardial depression. Calcium therapy does improve BP, but it is a short-term effect and caused primarily by vasoconstriction rather than contractility augmentation. Although transient improvement in CI is possible, calcium is more likely to decrease CI secondary to elevated afterload and the negative inotropic effects it can have on ischemic muscle. When used in combination, calcium has also been shown to attenuate the effects of dobutamine and even epinephrine.[15] Thus calcium administration is only appropriate when serum levels are deficient, when there is hyperkalemia requiring calcium stabilization, and in cases of calcium channel blocker overdose.

Dobutamine. Dobutamine is a common choice for cardiac dysfunction. Because it lacks vasoconstrictive effects, it is thought to cause less increase in the workload of the heart than most other inotropic agents. When compared with isoproterenol, a similar but older drug with pure beta-stimulating effects, it causes less of an increase in Mvo_2. Dobutamine has balanced beta-1 and beta-2 effects that improve not only contractility, but also coronary artery perfusion. Because it lacks vasopressor effects, some clinicians will consider initiating dobutamine only when systolic BP is greater than 80 mm Hg. Owing to its dromotropic effects, patients with atrial fibrillation should have their dysrhythmia converted or their rate slowed before starting dobutamine to prevent increases in ventricular response rate. Dosages for dobutamine usually range from 2.5 to 10 mcg/kg/min, but can range up to 20 mcg/kg/min. In rare circumstances, rates up to 40 mcg/kg/min have been required to reach the desired effect. Besides its use in cardiogenic shock, dobutamine is indicated in septic patients when CO measures indicate pump dysfunction.[86] Infusion of dobutamine at a rate of 5 mcg/kg/min also has been reported to improve gastrointestinal perfusion in patients with septic shock.[109]

In chronic heart failure, beta-1 receptors are less prevalent and less sensitive to stimulation (down-regulation) and the myocardium becomes beta-2 dependent. Therefore chronic heart failure patients with acute decompensation may respond better to dobutamine than other inotropes because of its beta-2 effect. There is much confusion surrounding the vasodilatory effects of dobutamine, with some considering it an inodilator. However, the vasodilatory effects of dobutamine are mild and limited primarily to vital tissue vessels (beta-2), a relatively small portion of the overall vascular bed. If vasodilation were a prominent effect, dobutamine would not be recommended in sepsis. Dobutamine may best be considered an inotrope that favors vital organ perfusion. Most of the afterload (SVR)-lowering effects of dobutamine can be attributed to improvements in CO, leading to a reflexive decline in sympathetic tone rather than direct vasodilation. Dobutamine's mild vasodilatory effects can decrease BP if volume resuscitation is not completed before initiation of the infusion. If dobutamine initiation results in a drop in BP, an evaluation of volume status should ensue, along with consideration of a fluid challenge. Like gravitational forces (orthostatic/postural hypotension) and increased intrathoracic pressures (ventilator-induced hypotension), mild vasodilation can detrimentally affect BP when there is even borderline hypovolemia.

Dopamine. Dopamine is a beta-1, alpha, and dopaminergic stimulant, depending on what dosage is being delivered (refer to the Medication table on pp. 1116-1121). Low-dose infusions have been used to improve renal and mesenteric perfusion. It was believed that dopaminergic levels of dopamine would help prevent renal failure and mesenteric ischemia. A meta-analysis done by Kellum and colleagues is considered a landmark paper virtually dispelling this belief.[57] Besides not helping with perfusion of nonvital organs, some studies have even indicated possible detrimental effects, especially in septic patients. The Surviving Sepsis Campaign does not support the use of dopamine in low doses for septic patients.[24] There is some evidence to suggest that a relatively new dopamine agonist, fenoldopam (Corlopam) (0.1 mcg/kg/min), may be helpful in improving renal and mesenteric perfusion in shock.[76]

Despite these challenges, dopamine is a versatile drug and can be used as an inotrope, an inoconstrictor, or a vasopressor, depending on the clinical situation. Myocardial depression responds best to ranges between 5 and 10 mcg/kg/min (contractility augmenting). Sepsis, involving both vasodilation and pump dysfunction,

might do best at levels from 10 to 20 mcg/kg/min (contractility and afterload augmenting). With primary vasodilatory states causing hypotension, levels at 20 mcg/kg/min or higher may be considered (afterload augmenting). Dopamine is more dysrhythmogenic than dobutamine. Although it may increase HR as one of its expected effects, tachycardia at low dosages warrants an assessment of fluid status. Hypovolemic states can exaggerate HR responses with virtually any inotropic agent.

Because of its varying and dosage-dependent effects, dopamine should be used cautiously. This is especially true with cardiogenic shock patients. Hypotension resulting from myocardial depression benefits most from inotropic levels of dopamine (5–10 mcg/kg/min). Beyond this range, or even before 10 mcg/kg/min in some patients, tachycardia and vasoconstriction (alpha effects) can occur, placing a further burden on the already failing heart. If orders are written to titrate dopamine to a target BP, it is possible that therapeutic levels of dopamine could be exceeded, rendering the therapy counterproductive. In situations such as this, it is important to consider alternative drugs, such as dobutamine.

Dopamine's effects on the cardiovascular system are both direct and indirect. The indirect effects come from its ability to trigger the release of norepinephrine at nerve endings. Thus when synaptic stores of norepinephrine are depleted, dopamine's effectiveness is attenuated. The time frame for depletion is variable, but is generally seen after about 48 hours of continual use and should be recognized as a characteristic of the drug and not a deterioration of the patient. This same norepinephrine depletion can cause difficulty during weaning of the drug. Some patients become dependent on small amounts to maintain normal cardiovascular function secondary to the lack of synaptic norepinephrine. Patients on as little as 0.5/mcg/kg/min have been known to decompensate into hypotension with drug termination. In these situations, it can be helpful to switch hemodynamic support to a low-dose norepinephrine infusion. This allows the synaptic granules to rebuild their stores of norepinephrine so that drug therapy can be successfully discontinued.

Epinephrine. Epinephrine is a beta-1, beta-2, and an alpha stimulant and the most potent inoconstrictor available. Like dopamine, its actions are dose dependent. At 0.01 to 0.05 mcg/kg/min it is mostly a beta-1 and beta-2 stimulant.[56] At 0.05 to 2 mcg/kg/min, it activates beta-1 and alpha receptors with more alpha effects as dosages increase. At dosages greater than 2 mcg/kg/min, epinephrine is strictly an alpha adrenergic. Appropriate uses for epinephrine include the reversal of laryngospasm and vasodilation in anaphylaxis, management of refractory bronchospastic asthma, and treatment of refractory bradycardia as well as a general cardiovascular stimulant in arrest states.[95] Although it has never been shown to be better than placebo for cardiac arrest, it continues to be the first choice despite recommendations for vasopressin.[39,106] Most of the data available on epinephrine use are from animal studies. It has been shown to elevate serum lactate concentrations, induce myocardial ischemia, lower mesenteric and renal circulation, and induce hyperglycemia and hypokalemia.[26,56,94] Epinephrine is highly dysrhythmogenic but generally safe for use in children and in heart transplant patients because of normal coronary circulation and the lack of ischemic substrate. Epinephrine administration triggers sensations of anxiety and fear in most patients, requiring frequent reassurance and appropriate sedation. Most experts agree that because of its potency and potential toxicity, epinephrine should be reserved for situations in which other agents have failed to improve hemodynamics.

Despite abundant precautions regarding epinephrine use, it remains a favorite in cardiovascular surgery settings. Postoperative hypotension is not uncommon following cardiac surgery, and its etiologies are varied (Chapter 14).[81] A thorough assessment is required to identify the source of hemodynamic compromise so therapy is properly directed. The most prevalent cause of any postoperative hypotension is hypovolemia, which is particularly common with surgeries requiring cardiopulmonary bypass (CPB). Hyperosmolar priming solutions for CPB pumps induce diuresis. Aortic cross-clamping can cause peripheral ischemia, resulting in intracellular fluid shift. The reperfusion process involved in coronary artery bypass operations also can induce a cardiogenic form of hypoperfusion. The myocardium may be severely depressed following cardiac surgery due to oxygen radical production and the resultant muscle "stunning" secondary to perioperative cardiac ischemia and infarction. Dysrhythmias also can negatively affect ventricular filling and pump function, particularly atrial fibrillation.

Postoperative vasoconstriction can contribute to poor CO and a fall in BP. Cardiac surgery patients can have massive narrowing of arterioles secondary to hypovolemia, hypothermia, the preoperative withdrawal of antihypertensive agents, and the overwhelming effects of SNS stimulation. If replacing vascular volume and warming the patient do not improve hemodynamics, modest vasodilatory support may be beneficial. Another cause of hypotension following CPB is an inflammatory response compounded by the vasodilatory effects of certain anesthetic agents. This vasogenic form of shock accounts for less than 10% of postoperative hypotension and may be the only type requiring the vasopressor support that epinephrine supplies.[4,81] A recent review of the literature published by Gillies and associates reported that the best-studied beta agonist and the one with the most favorable cost-benefit ratio is dobutamine.[38] Milrinone was found to enhance the likelihood of successful weaning from CPB support, magnify flow through arterial grafts, reduce mean pulmonary artery pressure, and improve right heart performance in pulmonary hypertension.[38]

Milrinone. Milrinone belongs to a unique class of inotropes known as bipyridines and has both inotropic and vasodilatory effects. Its ability to reduce preload and afterload allows it to stimulate contractility without increasing myocardial oxygen demands. Its mechanism of action is a result of the inhibition of phosphodiesterase. This enzyme induces the breakdown of cAMP, which in turn reduces calcium uptake. By inhibiting phosphodiesterase, cAMP is retained in greater concentrations and more calcium is available to enhance contractility. The fact that milrinone works outside the realm of the SNS affords certain advantages in the treatment of heart failure. With the widespread use of beta-blocking agents, beta stimulants may not be as effective secondary to diminished receptor availability. The ability of milrinone to improve contractility without accessing beta receptors is most advantageous in situations of beta-blocker overdose.[12]

Milrinone improves systolic function as well as diastolic relaxation, a plus for patients with lusitropic disturbances. It is also an effective pulmonary vasodilator and has been used to reduce the workload of the RV and reduce pulmonary hypertension in neonatal intensive care unit (ICU) settings.[8] Although it is less dysrhythmogenic than catecholamine drugs, an implantable cardioverter-defibrillator is recommended when it is used in home settings as a bridge to cardiac transplantation.[13]

Despite the benefits of milrinone, it remains a comparatively weak inotrope and is rarely effective with hypotensive cardiac failure when administered alone. Coupling milrinone with the more powerful beta stimulants, such as dobutamine, can have a synergistic effect by promoting inotropy on two levels. In addition, preload and afterload reduction can profoundly improve CO despite only modest improvements in BP. Milrinone is a far more potent vasodilator than dobutamine and cannot be expected to increase BP as much as it can improve hemodynamics and perfusion. The combination of inotropic and vasodilatory effects seen with milrinone drew interest in its use to "tune up" the myocardium of chronic heart failure patients in acute decompensation. The OPTIME study, however, did not support this strategy, showing no decrease in length of stay and an increase in adverse events (mostly dysrhythmias).[32] Thus the use of chronic IV inotropic therapy, either as a continuous or intermittent infusion, remains controversial.[21] There doesn't appear to be any significant difference in outcome between dobutamine and milrinone in the treatment of these patients, but milrinone does have a significantly higher cost.[108]

The pharmacokinetics of milrinone are different from other drugs used for hemodynamic support in hypoperfusion states. It is slower in reaching therapeutic levels and it has a long half-life, especially in patients with liver and renal insufficiency. Dosing involves an optional bolus of 50 mcg/kg over 10 minutes followed by a maintenance infusion of 0.375 to 0.75 mcg/kg/min. Because of its prolonged effect, dosage adjustments are generally made only every 4 to 8 hours.[12] Therefore milrinone is best used as a companion drug in the setting of cardiogenic hypotension with more potent and titratable inotropes as primary agents. Although far less problematic than its predecessor, inamrinone, milrinone can also propagate thrombocytopenia. Therefore platelet levels should be monitored and milrinone should be used cautiously with other platelet-lowering medications such as H_2 antagonists and heparin.

Vasopressor Agents

Vasopressor agents constrict vascular beds, increasing both preload and afterload. Vasoconstriction as a treatment for hypotension is best reserved for the reversal of a widespread loss of vascular tone as seen in vasogenic shock. However, because vasopressors are so reliable in raising BP, they are a common first choice in any hypotensive crisis. Recall that shock is not poor pressure but poor perfusion, and raising BP is not the same as resolving shock. Blood pressure is dependent on heart function and vascular tone (BP = CO × SVR). One can either augment CO or increase SVR to achieve a BP improvement. Increasing SVR is a reliable and relatively easy way to improve BP. Increasing CO is more challenging, more time consuming, and not as dependable. It is easy to understand why vasopressors are widely used in shock.

Vasopressors have several harmful effects. By increasing SVR they may create enough afterload to decrease CO and even induce pump failure. In addition, excessive vasoconstriction can intensify hydrostatic pressure and force fluid out of the vessels, creating a relative hypovolemia. Vasopressors can also divert blood flow from enough organ beds to further aggravate cellular hypoxia and perpetuate shock. In short, the misuse of vasopressor drugs can promote cardiogenic shock, hypovolemic shock, and even the multiple organ failure seen in vasogenic shock (sepsis). At best, vasopressors can dramatically improve perfusion pressure to the body. At worse, they can be as bad as the underlying hypoperfusion they were meant to correct.

Norepinephrine. Norepinephrine is a natural catecholamine with both beta-1- and alpha-stimulating effects. It is a powerful inoconstrictor, and like dopamine, the higher the dose the greater the vascular effects. Because of the wide variability in vasopressor use, average doses of norepinephrine are difficult to confirm. From clinical trials, mean dosages ranged from 0.2 to 1.3 mcg/kg/min with a maximum dosage of 3.3 mcg/kg/min.[69,94,105]

Norepinephrine has a colorful history. It was embraced historically as a wonder drug that could create BP in the sickest of patients, only to be later defiled as "leave 'em dead Levophed."[78] Today clinicians have a guarded yet positive view of this agent and its use is again widespread. Norepinephrine is recommended in the treatment of sepsis-induced hypoperfusion to reverse abnormal vasodilation and maintain perfusion pressure when fluid resuscitation is not enough. Septic patients with poor CO may require dobutamine along with norepinephrine to treat their cardiovascular collapse. This combination can be advantageous for many reasons. Data support the use of dobutamine for the improvement of mesenteric perfusion, a potential threat in septic patients.[109] In addition, its weak beta-2 vasodilation effects may temper some of the alpha vasoconstriction effects of norepinephrine to better support perfusion.

Norepinephrine also can be used to manage cardiogenic shock. It is a more potent beta stimulant than dobutamine or dopamine and possibly safer than epinephrine. However, when administered as monotherapy and titrated to BP in this type of shock, norepinephrine can be harmful because it can stress the LV with its vasoconstricting effects. Vasoconstriction increases both preload and afterload and could be detrimental unless there is evidence of vasodilation. Vasodilation may be present with severe pump failure due to inflammation, or in late-stage shock, as a result of acidosis. In cardiogenic shock, improvement in BP is seen with norepinephrine, but it is generally transient because vasoconstriction can decrease CO. To use this drug optimally in cardiogenic shock, it is best to couple it with a vasodilator such as nitroglycerin or nitroprusside to isolate the desired beta effects and reduce the undesired alpha response. It also can be used with milrinone. By stimulating inotropy through both beta stimulation and phosphodiesterase inhibition this combination may be especially beneficial to patients on beta-blockers and those with a diastolic component to their ventricular failure. Like nitroglycerin, milrinone can reduce preload and afterload but without as much concern about decreasing BP.

Phenylephrine. Phenylephrine (Neo-Synephrine) is a pure alpha stimulant and has no direct effect on the heart. Therefore it is used in hypotensive situations that do not require cardiac stimulation. Because phenylephrine does not affect beta receptors, less tachycardia and dysrhythmia is seen than with other vasoactive agents. It is used effectively following spinal or epidural blocks, which cause widespread vasodilation. Metaraminol and ephedrine have been used for this purpose in the past. Most of the recent literature regarding the use of phenylephrine discusses its use with spinal anesthesia for cesarean section.[18] Drug overdose and drug hypersensitivity causing vasodilation and hypotension also respond well to phenylephrine. For severe hypotension, a bolus of 2 to 5 mg can be attempted. Continuous infusion rates average 40 to 60 mcg/min, but can be as high as 100 to 180 mcg/min when rapid BP improvement is vital. Bradycardia is a side effect of any vasopressive agent, but most commonly with phenylephrine. Because of its lack of beta effects, phenylephrine's unopposed alpha constriction can stimulate a reflexive slowing of the heart by cardiopulmonary centers in the brain in an attempt to prevent excessive BP. This reflex reaction was employed for the treatment of supraventricular tachycardia before propranolol (Inderal) became available.[56]

Vasopressin. Vasopressin is an endogenous chemical known more commonly as antidiuretic hormone. It is produced by the hypothalamus and stored and secreted by the posterior pituitary gland in response to reduced plasma volume or increased serum sodium concentration. It promotes the retention of free water. Physiologically, the role of vasopressin is to regulate daily fluid balance. During hypotensive states, however, serum levels of vasopressin rise similarly to levels of epinephrine, cortisol, and other stress hormones. It is believed to be an influential vasoconstrictor mechanism in shock states. The pressor actions of vasopressin are complex and incompletely understood. It is distinctively different from other vascular constrictors, however, because it does not affect adrenergic receptors. Specialized arterial smooth muscle receptor sites for vasopressin are termed V1 receptors.[27]

Vasopressin has been shown to be effective, and perhaps superior to epinephrine, in the treatment of refractory ventricular fibrillation, pulseless ventricular tachycardia, and asystole.[96,106] Since it was added to advanced cardiac life support (ACLS) protocols it has been used in the critical care setting for the treatment of hypotension of any kind despite limited research for its use outside the setting of arrest. Three situations are associated with an inadequate endogenous elevation of vasopressin: massive hemorrhage, severe sepsis, and cardiopulmonary bypass.[27,75,99] The development of this relative vasopressin deficiency is poorly understood, but may be related to exhaustion of secretory stores following prolonged stimulation or impaired autonomic function with depressed baroreceptor-mediated release. Regardless, vasopressin use may be considered as salvage therapy in patients with

refractory shock despite adequate fluid resuscitation and high-dose conventional vasopressors.[9,17]

Vasopressin is not intended for use as an alternative to catecholamines in shock, but rather as a companion drug. It should never be ordered to be titrated to a target BP, but should be rigidly controlled to avoid dangerous outcomes, particularly that of mesenteric ischemia.[25] Adult rates for vasopressin infusion are 0.01 to 0.04 unit/min. As with all vasopressors, it may curtail stroke volume and impede cellular perfusion. Like epinephrine, vasopressin has been used mostly outside the cardiac arrest setting for the treatment of hypotension in postoperative cardiac surgery patients. It is important to thoroughly assess patients for the cause of shock before considering any vasopressor agent. Recall that in the cardiac surgery population, less than 10% are estimated to have vasodilatory hypotension warranting pressor support. Fluid, inotropic, and even vasodilator therapy may be more effective in long-term support. Another consideration with the use of vasopressin is the need for close serum sodium monitoring for the development of hyponatremia. Water retention is an innate characteristic of this drug (antidiuretic hormone) and can cause decreased levels of consciousness and seizures caused by cerebral swelling if sodium levels are not maintained.

Vasodilator Agents

As discussed, the body's response to hypotension is not helpful in the case of cardiogenic shock. The SNS and RAAS provide support in hypovolemic and vasogenic states, but they are detrimental in pump failure. Vasodilators can reverse the harmful cardiac effects of the stress response in patients with pump failure. Their efficacy is achieved through venous and arterial dilation and the resultant preload and afterload reduction. Reversing vascular constriction conserves cardiac energy and allows the heart to focus on contracting and moving blood instead of overcoming the obstacles placed on it by the body. Consider this analogy: A worker is instructed by his boss to move a mountain of heavy boxes onto a truck. He bends down, lifts a box, climbs onto the truck, and hoists it to the back. He repeats the process over and over until he is halfway through the task, but too weary to continue. Witnessing the worker's struggle, the boss provides him with an inclined plane, a lever and fulcrum, and a pulley and rope, instructing him on their use. The worker's load is so lightened, he is easily able to complete the remainder of the task. Vasodilators are the inclined plane, lever and fulcrum, and pulley and rope of cardiovascular support.

Vasodilators have been shown to be associated with significantly lower inhospital mortality from acute decompensated heart failure than inotropes.[1] To use vasodilators to treat cardiogenic shock, first stabilize the patient with inotropes. Vasodilators will then assist in lowering PAWP and the ventricular overstretch that compromises contractility beyond the original insult. They will also reduce SVR and the resistance to moving blood out to the body tissues. Preload and afterload reduction can actually improve CO and help reduce the need for inotropic support. In summary, vasodilators allow the heart to move blood more efficiently and with less oxygen consumption.

Nitroglycerin. William Murrel published the first article describing the therapeutic properties of nitroglycerin in the *Lancet* in 1879, and more than a century later it remains a staple in coronary critical care. Nitroglycerin induces the release of nitric oxide for the dilation of both veins and arteries. It is primarily a venodilator and preload reducer, especially at dosages less than 50 mcg/min (1 mcg/kg/min). It is used in treating acute coronary syndromes to balance oxygen supply and demand for the relief of ischemic pain and can be titrated up to 200 mcg/min. Because of its short duration of action, and a tendency for patients to become tolerant to it, higher doses have been reported. In cardiogenic shock secondary to myocardial infarction, nitroglycerin is often selected for vasodilation because of its effective dilation of coronary arteries. Following coronary bypass surgery with internal mammary artery grafting, however, diltiazem (Cardizem) provides better protection against vasospasm than does nitroglycerin.[98] In the setting of hypotension, nitroglycerin should be started at the lowest possible rate and titrated up according to patient tolerance. As with all vasodilators, it is critical that volume status be optimized before initiating the drug. If RV infarction is present, the preload-reducing characteristics of nitroglycerin may not be tolerated.

Nitroprusside. Although generally thought of as an antihypertensive agent, nitroprusside (Nipride) can be used in minute doses to reduce preload and afterload in pump failure. It rapidly and markedly improves cardiac function in patients with decompensated heart failure secondary to severe left ventricular systolic and aortic valve dysfunction, and thus provides a safe and effective bridge to aortic valve replacement or oral vasodilator therapy.[61] For patients awaiting heart transplantation, chronic intermittent nitroprusside infusions are more effective and safer than dobutamine in relieving symptoms and improving survival.[16] Whether chronic intermittent infusion of nitroprusside could represent a feasible medical strategy in an outpatient setting for patients with severe heart failure remains to be investigated. Some literature suggests an antiinflammatory role for nitroprusside in coronary artery bypass patients.[70]

◆ Case Study 41-1, Part B

Hypotension

J.Q. is given 500 ml of NS and 500 ml of albumin. His PAWP increases to 16, and his BP climbs to 138/78. Thirty minutes later, his BP again declines and another 500 ml of NS and 250 ml of albumin are administered.

Later on the day of his surgery, J.Q. again becomes hypotensive. His monitor shows sinus tachycardia with frequent PVCs and one nonsustained burst of ventricular tachycardia.

Temp:	98° F
HR:	124 beats/min
RR:	24 beats/min
BP:	88/68 mm Hg
CVP:	12 mm Hg
PAWP:	22 mm Hg
PAP:	44/24
CO:	3 L/min
CI:	1.8 L/min
SVR:	1680 dynes

Decision point: Is this too much fluid for a patient with heart disease?

Decision point: From the above clinical profile, what do you interpret to be the etiology of this hypotensive state?

ST segment depression and T wave inversion are noted by the nurse in bedside lead V3. A stat ECG, serum troponin, and BNP level are obtained. The ECG confirms ST depressions in V2-V6, and a normal troponin level rules out a non–ST-elevation MI. The BNP is elevated at 580 pg/ml, confirming ventricular dysfunction, and a diagnosis of anterior wall ischemia and failure is made.

Decision point: What therapy is recommended at this time?

BNP = B-type natriuretic peptide, BP = blood pressure, CI = cardiac index, CO = cardiac output, CVP = central venous pressure, ECG = electrocardiogram, HR = heart rate, PAP = pulmonary artery pressure, PAWP = pulmonary artery wedge pressure, SVR = systemic vascular resistance, T = temperature, RR = respiratory rate.

Case continues on page 1130

Nitroprusside is a balanced venous and arterial dilator that causes the release of nitric oxide, but through a different mechanism than nitroglycerin and without the problem of tolerance. Nitroprusside is a potent vasodilator and should be started at no more than 0.2 mcg/kg/min. It dilates the coronary arteries, but affects the smaller resistance vessels and can result in coronary steal in some patients. Chest pain, ST segment depressions, or ischemic ventricular ectopy should warrant a change to nitroglycerin. In pulmonary edema, not uncommon in cardiogenic states, nitroprusside has been known to reverse normal autoregulation in the lungs, causing arteriovenous shunting and a fall in partial pressure of arterial oxygen tension (Pa_{O_2}). For patients with borderline Pa_{O_2}, it is prudent to adjust oxygen and ventilator settings before initiating nitroprusside. Cyanide toxicity is a potential side effect of nitroprusside use, though unlikely at the small dosages used in this setting.

Nesiritide. Nesiritide (Natrecor) is not approved for the treatment of shock, but because of its use in the management of cardiac failure, it is reviewed here. Nesiritide is a BNP, an innate secretion of the ventricles that serves to counteract the effects of the SNS and RAAS. It is a vasodilator and a natriuretic that causes the excretion of large amounts of sodium in the urine to reduce vascular volume. Nesiritide has been promoted as a neurohormonal approach to the treatment of decompensated heart failure. It lowers preload and afterload and indirectly improves CO.[52] However, this drug is not truly titratable. It is initiated with an optional bolus of 2 mcg/kg, followed by a maintenance infusion of 0.01 mcg/kg/min. The primary side effect of nesiritide is hypotension, so dosages may need to be reduced in the setting of pump failure with hypoperfusion. Coupled with inotropic support, nesiritide has been shown to be at least as effective as standard vasodilator and diuretic therapy and with a higher survival to discharge than dobutamine or milrinone therapy.[1,93] Recently there have been questions regarding the safety of nesiritide and its effect on mortality beyond the hospital stay. A pooled analysis of seven nesiritide trials published by Sackner-Bernstein and colleagues reported a 30-day mortality of 5.3% in the nesiritide group compared with a 4.3% mortality in the group treated with other standard medications.[91] Many have been skeptical of this finding, and at this time, there is not enough information to definitively say that nesiritide treatment increases risk of death. One positive outcome from experiences with nesiritide is the revival of interest in vasodilators for the reduction of preload and afterload in the treatment of acutely decompensated heart failure.[100] Other intravenous vasodilators, such as nicardipine (Cardene) and enalaprilat (Vasotec), are available and effective preload and afterload reducers. However, because of negative inotropic effects and lengthy durations of action, they are better suited for the treatment of hypertension.

NURSING CARE OF THE SHOCK PATIENT

The complexities of caring for patients with hemodynamic compromise and oxygenation threats are challenging. Vigilant monitoring of all body organs

for cellular dysfunction due to hypoperfusion is crucial and may stimulate a reevaluation of therapy to improve oxygenation (Box 41-8). Critical care nurses make their greatest contribution by participating in multidisciplinary care focused on determining the best available therapies. The role of patient advocate includes making research-based recommendations accessible to all clinicians involved and developing protocols and daily goal sheets for improving care for future patients. The nurse needs to ensure that hypovolemic patients are adequately fluid resuscitated. If patients have cardiogenic shock secondary to myocardial infarction, implementation of the ACC/AHA guidelines[89] should be encouraged. The Research Utilization box on p. 1129 takes a closer look at this topic. With sepsis, EGDT should be considered for either

---

Box 41-8

Signs of Organ Dysfunction

CENTRAL NERVOUS SYSTEM DYSFUNCTION

Confusion
Psychosis
Deepening level of consciousness (LOC)

RESPIRATORY DYSFUNCTION

Tachypnea
Pa_{O_2} less than 70 mm Hg
Sa_{O_2} less than 90%
Pa_{O_2}: Fi_{O_2} ratio (P/F ratio) ≤ 300

GASTROINTESTINAL DYSFUNCTION

Excessive nasogastric drainage
Abdominal pain (ischemia)
Elevated liver enzymes
Jaundice
Decreased albumin

RENAL DYSFUNCTION

Oliguria
Elevated creatinine

HEMATOLOGIC DYSFUNCTION

Decreased platelets
Decreased activated partial thromboplastin time
Increased D-dimer
Acral cyanosis
Bleeding

METABOLIC DYSFUNCTION

Elevated lactate
Metabolic acidosis

Fi_{O_2} = Fraction of inspired oxygen, Pa_{O_2} = partial pressure of arterial oxygen tension, Sa_{O_2} = arterial oxygen saturation.

▲ RESEARCH UTILIZATION

Evaluating the Implementation of ACC/AHA and ESC Guidelines for the Treatment of Cardiogenic Shock Complicating Acute Coronary Syndrome

CLINICAL ISSUE

Research-based recommendations for the management of cardiogenic shock, secondary to acute coronary syndromes (ACS), have been established by the American College of Cardiology (ACC), the American Heart Association (AHA), and the European Society of Cardiology (ESC) since 1999. These guidelines recommend coronary angiography and revascularization as class I indications for patients who are within 36 hours of acute ST-elevation infarction or new left bundle branch block infarction who develop cardiogenic shock. They further suggest that patients be less than 75 years of age and that revascularization be performed within 18 hours of onset of cardiogenic shock. Use of intraaortic balloon (IAB) counterpulsation for hemodynamic support also is promoted. Clinical compliance with these recommendations has not been measured.

SUMMARY

This study sought to evaluate the implementation of ACC/AHA and ESC guidelines for the treatment of cardiogenic shock complicating ACS. The investigators reviewed the database known as the Euro Heart Survey of ACS. This was a prospective survey and included 10,136 ACS patients treated in Europe and the Mediterranean basin from September 2000 to May 2001. Cardiogenic shock occurred in 549 patients, or 5.4%. Of these, only 41.4% presenting with ST-elevation infarction and cardiogenic shock received early reperfusion therapy, 35.9% by primary percutaneous coronary intervention. In addition, IAB counterpulsation was used in only 17.7% of patients. Conclusions were that compliance with established guidelines was poor and that without improvement, mortality will remain extremely high, at more than 50%.

APPLICATION

Clinicians should be aware of the current recommendations for aggressive management of patients with cardiogenic shock as a complication of ACS and use revascularization and IAB counterpulsation when appropriate. Nurses should advocate for patients by encouraging physicians to follow the established guidelines. Nurse leaders can emphasize the importance of the guidelines during staff meetings, multidisciplinary committee meetings, and daily rounds. Advanced practice nurses can conduct studies to evaluate compliance in their institution and use the results to applaud staff or promote change. Nurse educators can incorporate these interventions into all cardiac-related programs, develop information sheets for distribution, and reinforce concepts during bedside consulting.

NEED FOR FURTHER STUDY

This review looked at a time frame after circulation of the new guidelines, but not in the recent past. Ongoing reviews of practice in this area are warranted. In addition, evidence-based approaches to championing change in the care of these patients would also be helpful.

Iakobishvili, Z., et al. (2005). Does current treatment of cardiogenic shock complicating the acute coronary syndromes comply with guidelines? *Am Heart J, 149*(1), 98–103.

---

hypotension or a lactate level of greater than 4 mmol/L. Bridging the gap from bench to bedside is vital in achieving the best patient outcome. The Multidisciplinary Plan of Care on pp. 1089-1093 outlines care of the patient with hemodynamic compromise.

While caring for hemodynamically unstable patients, it is easy to prioritize the manipulation of cardiovascular status and overlook less life-threatening needs. Skin breakdown is common in the shock patient and preventive care, including frequent turning and relief of pressure points, is important. Patients in shock require prophylaxis for deep vein thrombosis and pulmonary emboli. Anticoagulants may be contraindicated in certain trauma patients, and pneumatic compression devices are advised. Because most hypotensive patients require mechanical ventilation, peptic ulcer disease prophylaxis and head of bed elevation are also essential.

Maintaining the patient with hypotension in semi-Fowler's position at 30 to 45 degrees is challenging, but this strategy can significantly reduce the chances of ventilator-associated pneumonia (VAP). Oral care, though not definitively proven to reduce the incidence of VAP, is important for good hygiene and patient comfort. Central catheter placement and replacement should be managed with maximum barrier precautions and chlorhexidine site preparation to prevent infection. The specifics of prophylaxis for all of these issues can be found in Chapter 9.

Nutritional needs of the hypoperfusing patient are important to address. Enteral feeding is recognized as the preferred route. However, the gastrointestinal tract may not be adequately perfused during shock states, and a nutritional load could precipitate an oxygen imbalance and necrosis in addition to poor absorption of nutrients. The parenteral route for nutritional supplementation may be necessary. Glutamine is the primary nutrient for lymphocytes and enterocytes, assisting the body in fighting infection, regenerating tissue, and maintaining the normal gut barrier. Although it is a "nonessential" amino acid (the body synthesizes it from other protein building blocks), it is not manufactured adequately in critical illness. Supplementing glutamine may protect the gut from mucosal damage following shock and postischemia reperfusion. If available, parenteral glutamine is also an option, particularly for patients with trauma, burns, and possibly sepsis. Intensive insulin therapy for tight glycemic control is becoming a standard of practice for all critically ill patients and should be considered for this population as well.[43,102] For a review of current recommendations for nutritional support in critically ill adult patients, refer to Chapter 6.

◆ Case Study 41-1, Part C

Sources of Hypotension

The ischemic episode resolves with intervention and J.Q.'s BP, and overall hemodynamic status stabilizes. He remains sedated throughout the night and is maintained on dobutamine at 0.5 mcg/kg/min and nitroglycerin at 1.5 mcg/kg/min. Early on postoperative day (POD) 1, he remains sedated as part of an ischemia-reducing strategy, and a decision is made to postpone ventilator weaning until the following day. On POD2, J.Q. spikes a temp of 102.4° F. Urine and blood cultures are drawn, and a chest film is taken. No obvious source of infection is found, and empiric antibiotics are initiated. In the early morning hours of POD3, J.Q. becomes hypotensive once again.

Temp:	101.3° F (1 hr after acetaminophen)
HR:	128 beats/min
RR:	30 breaths/min
BP:	80/42 mm Hg
CVP:	8 mm Hg
PAWP:	14 mm Hg
PAP:	30/16 mm Hg
CO:	5.3 L/min
CI:	3.2 L/min
SVR:	709 dynes

Decision point: From this information, what is the source of J.Q.'s hypotension at this juncture?

Decision point: What therapy is indicated to treat this form of shock?

Fluid therapy is again initiated. J.Q.'s PAC is replaced with an oximetry catheter for Svo_2 monitoring. After 3 L of NS and 5 mcg/kg/min of dopamine, the following readings are obtained:

Temp:	100.8° F
HR:	124 beats/min
RR:	28 beats/min
BP:	92/48 mm Hg
CVP:	12 mm Hg
PAWP:	15 mm Hg
PAP:	40/24

CO:	4.7 L/min
CI:	2.8 L/min
SVR:	868 dynes
Svo_2:	60%
Lactate:	5.5 mmol/L

Decision point: What is your interpretation of these changes, and what interventions are appropriate?

Following the infusion of a total of 4 L of NS and 1 unit of packed red blood cells (PRBCs), and a change from dopamine to 2.5 mcg/kg/min of dobutamine, J.Q.'s vital signs have stabilized and his Svo_2 has climbed to 72%. He is then taken for an abdominal computed tomography (CT) scan in an effort to locate the source of infection. An abscess is identified at the graft site, and J.Q. returns to surgery for replacement of the graft.

On his fourth day in critical care, J.Q. remains ventilated and is now requiring a 70% Fio_2 and a PEEP of 14 mm Hg to maintain a saturation of 90%. He is obtunded, with a white blood cell count of 15,000 despite full antibiotic support. Despite aggressive fluid therapy, he is again hypotensive.

Decision point: What do these findings indicate?

J.Q.'s hospital course was long and protracted, but with continued adherence to the principles of EGDT and the Surviving Sepsis Campaign, he began to improve. He was gradually weaned from all vasoactive and inotropic agents (dobutamine and norepinephrine). Respiratory failure proved to be his biggest obstacle, and he required mechanical ventilation for a total of 18 days. After leaving critical care and going through rehabilitation therapy, he was discharged home on the 27th hospital day.

BP = Blood pressure, CI = cardiac index, CO = cardiac output, CVP = central venous pressure, Fio_2 = fraction of inspired oxygen, HR = heart rate, PAC = pulmonary artery catheter, PAP = pulmonary artery pressure, PAWP = pulmonary artery wedge pressure, PEEP = positive end-expiratory pressure, SVR = systemic vascular resistance, T = temperature, RR = respiratory rate, Svo_2 = venous oxygen saturation.

Throughout critical illness, it is important to maintain open lines of communication with the patient (when possible) and the family regarding treatment and prognosis. If the patient's chances of survival become unlikely, consideration should be given to limiting support. Critical care has traditionally been focused on curative therapy; however, this may not be consistent with the patient's or family's wishes. A realistic assessment of outcome must be made and shared. It is paramount to accept that a less aggressive approach to treatment or the withdrawal of life support may be in the best interest of the patient. Palliative care in critical care is becoming more prevalent and allowing patients to die with dignity more acceptable.

CONCLUSIONS

Managing patients with hemodynamic compromise is a challenging task with inadequate evidence-based guidelines for practice. Despite that, shock patients require our best scientific effort in reversing hypoperfusion and our most compassionate care when treatment becomes futile at the end of life.

REFERENCES

1. Abraham, W. T. (2005). In-hospital mortality in patients with acute decompensated heart failure requiring intravenous vasoactive medications: an analysis from the Acute Decompensated Heart Failure National Registry (ADHERE). *J Am Coll Cardiol*, 46(1), 65–67.
2. Ahrens, T. (1999). Hemodynamic monitoring. *Crit Care Nurs Clin North Am*, 11(1), 19–32.
3. Annane, D., et al. (2004). Corticosteroids for severe sepsis and septic shock: a systematic review and meta-analysis. *BMJ*, 329, 480–488.
4. Argenziano, M., et al. (1998). Management of vasodilatory shock after cardiac surgery: identification of predisposing factors and use of a novel pressor agent. *J Thorac Cardiovasc Surg*, 116(6), 973–980.
5. Babaev, A, et al. (2005). Trends in management and outcomes of patients with acute myocardial infarction complicated by cardiogenic shock. *JAMA*, 294(4), 448–454.
6. Barone, J. E., et al. (2001). Routine perioperative pulmonary artery catheterization has no effect on rate of complications in vascular surgery: a meta-analysis. *Am Surg*, 6, 674–679.
7. Barron, H. V., et al. (2001). The use of intra-aortic balloon counterpulsation in patients with cardiogenic shock complicating acute myocardial infarction: data from the National Registry of Myocardial Infarction 2. *Am Heart J*, 141(6), 933–939.
8. Baruch, L., et al. (2001). Pharmacodynamic effects of milrinone with and without a bolus loading infusion. *Am Heart J*, 141(2), 266–273.
9. Beale, R. J., et al. (2004). Vasopressor and inotropic support in septic shock: an evidence-based review. *Crit Care Med*, 32(11), S455–S464.
10. Bernard, G. R., et al. (2000). Pulmonary artery catheterization and clinical outcomes: National Heart, Lung, and Blood Institute and Food and Drug Administration Workshop Report. *JAMA, 283*, 2568–2572.
11. Bridges, E. J., et al. (2000). Monitoring pulmonary artery pressures: just the facts. *Crit Care Nurs*, 20(6), 59–80.
12. Bristow, M. R., et al. (2001). Inotropes and beta-blockers: is there a need for new guidelines? *J Card Fail*, 7(2 Suppl. 1), 8–12.
13. Brozena, S. C. (2004). A prospective study of continuous intravenous milrinone therapy for status IB patients awaiting heart transplant at home. *J Heart Lung Transplant*, 23(9), 1082–1086.
14. Buist, M., et al. (2004). Association between clinically abnormal observations and subsequent in-hospital mortality: a prospective study. *Resuscitation*, 62(2), 137–141.
15. Butterworth, J. F. (1993). Selecting an inotropic for the cardiac surgery patient. *J Cardiothorac Vasc Anesth*, 7(4 Suppl. 2), 26.
16. Capomolla, S., et al. (2001). Chronic infusion of dobutamine and nitroprusside in patients with end-stage heart failure awaiting heart transplantation: safety and clinical outcome. *Eur J Heart Fail*, 3(5), 601–610.
17. Chen, P. (2002). Vasopressin: new uses in critical care. *Am J Med Sci*, 324, 146–154.
18. Cooper, D. W., & Mowbray, P. (2004). Advantages of using a prophylactic phenylephrine infusion during spinal anaesthesia for caesarean section. *Int J Obstet Anesth*, 13(2), 124–125.
19. Cowie, M. R., et al. (2003). Clinical applications of B-type natriuretic peptide (BNP) testing. *Eur Heart J*, 24, 1710–1718.
20. Cruz, K., & Franklin, C. (2001). The pulmonary artery catheter: uses and controversies. *Crit Care Clin*, 17(2), 271–291.
21. Cuffe, M. S., et al. (2002). Short-term intravenous milrinone for acute exacerbation of chronic heart failure, a randomized controlled trial. *JAMA, 287*, 1541–1547.
22. Darovic, G. (2002). *Hemodynamic monitoring: invasive and noninvasive clinical application*. St. Louis: Saunders.
23. Dellinger, R. P. (2003). Cardiovascular management of septic shock. *Crit Care Med*, 31, 946–955.
24. Dellinger, R. P., et al. (2004). Surviving Sepsis Campaign guidelines for management of severe sepsis and septic shock. *Crit Care Med*, 32(3R), 858–873.
25. den Ouden, D. T., & Meinders, A. E. (2005). Vasopressin: physiology and clinical use in patients with vasodilatory shock: a review. *Neth J Med*, 63(1), 4–13.
26. Di Giantomasso, D., Bellomo, R., & May, C. N. (2005). The hemodynamic and metabolic effects of epinephrine in experimental hyperdynamic septic shock. *Intensive Care Med*, 31(3), 454–462.
27. Dinser, M., et al. (2001). The effects of vasopressin on systemic hemodynamics in catecholamine-resistant septic and postcardiotomy shock: a retrospective analysis. *Anesth Analg*, 93(1), 7–13.
28. Dorman, T., et al. (1998). Radial artery pressure monitoring underestimates central arterial pressure during vasopressor therapy in critically-ill surgical patients. *Crit Care Med*, 26(10), 1646–1649.
29. Dueck, M. H., et al. (2005). Trends but not individual values of central venous oxygen saturation agree with mixed venous oxygen saturation during varying hemodynamic conditions. *Anesthesiology*, 103(2), 249–257.
30. Dutton, R. P., MacKenzie, C. F., & Scalea, T. M. (2002). Hypotensive resuscitation during active hemorrhage: impact on in-hospital mortality. *J Trauma*, 52(6), 1141–1146.
31. Dzavik, V., et al. (2005). Outcome of patients aged greater than or equal to 75 years in the SHould we emergently revascularize Occluded Coronaries in cardiogenic shocK (SHOCK) trial: do elderly patients with acute myocardial infarction complicated by cardiogenic shock respond differently to emergent revascularization? *Am Heart J*, 149(6), 1128–1134.

32. Felker, G. M., et al. (2003). Heart failure etiology and response to milrinone in decompensated heart failure: results from the OPTIME-CHF study. *J Am Coll Cardiol*, *41*(6), 997–1003.

33. Felker, G. M., & O'Connor, C. M. (2001). Inotropic therapy for heart failure: an evidence-based approach. *Am Heart J*, *142*(3), 393–401.

34. Finfer, S. (2004). Lessons from the SAFE Study. Program and abstracts of the 24th International Symposium on Intensive Care and Emergency Medicine; March 30-April 2, 2004, Brussels, Belgium.

35. Fink, M. P. (2005). Non-invasive and invasive cardiovascular monitoring. In M. P. Fink (Ed.), *Textbook of critical care*. Philadelphia: Saunders.

36. Follath, F., et al. (2002). Efficacy and safety of intravenous levosimendan compared with dobutamine in severe low-output heart failure (the LIDO study): a randomised double-blind trial. *Lancet*, *360*(9328), 196–202.

37. Fowle, R., & Pepe, P. E. (2002). Fluid resuscitation of the patient with major trauma. *Curr Opin Anaesthesiol*, *15*, 173–178.

38. Gillies, M., et al. (2005). Bench-to-bedside review: inotropic drug therapy after adult cardiac surgery, a systematic literature review. *Crit Care*, *9*(3), 266–279.

39. Gottlieb, S. (2004). Vasopressin for cardiac arrest increases chances of survival. *BMJ*, *328*, 128.

40. Haji, S. A., & Movahed, A. (2000). Right ventricular infarction—diagnosis and treatment. *Clin Cardiol*, *23*, 473–482.

41. Harvy, S., et al. (2005). Assessment of the clinical effectiveness of pulmonary artery catheters in management of patients in intensive care (PAC-Man): a randomised controlled trial. *Lancet*, *366*(9484), 472–477.

42. Hebert, P. C., et al. (1999). A multicenter, randomized, controlled clinical trial of transfusion in critical care. *N Engl J Med*, *340*, 409–417.

43. Heyland, D. K., et al. (2003). Canadian clinical practice guidelines for nutrition support in mechanically ventilated, critically ill adult patients. *JPEN*, *27*, L355.

44. Hochman, J. S. (2003). Cardiogenic shock complicating acute myocardial infarction expanding the paradigm. *Circulation*, *107*, 2998.

45. Hochman, J. S., & Menon, V. (2002). Treatment of cardiogenic shock complicating acute myocardial infarction. *UpToDate*, *10.2*, 1–21.

46. Hochman, J. S., et al. (2001). One-year survival following early revascularization for cardiogenic shock. *JAMA*, *285*, 190–192.

47. Hollenberg, S. M. (2004). Recognition and treatment of cardiogenic shock. *Semin Respir Crit Care Med*, *25*(6), 661–671.

48. Hollenberg, S. M., et al. (2004). Practice parameters for hemodynamic support of sepsis in adult patients: 2004 update. *Crit Care Med*, *32*(9), 1928–1948.

49. Iakobishvili, Z., et al. (2005). Does current treatment of cardiogenic shock complicating the acute coronary syndromes comply with guidelines? *Am Heart J*, *149*(1), 98–103.

50. Iberti, T. J., et al. (1990). A multicenter study of physicians' knowledge of the pulmonary artery catheter. The pulmonary artery catheter study group. *JAMA*, *264*(22), 2928–2932.

51. Inglessis, I., et al. (2004). Hemodynamic effects of inhaled nitric oxide in right ventricular myocardial infarction and cardiogenic shock. *J Am Coll Cardiol*, *44*(4), 793–798.

52. Iyengar, S., et al. (2004). Nesiritide for the treatment of congestive heart failure. *Expert Opin Pharmacother*, *5*(4), 901–907.

53. Jacobs, A. K., et al. (2003). Cardiogenic shock caused by right ventricular infarction: a report from the SHOCK registry. *J Am Coll Cardiol*, *41*, 1273–1279.

54. Johnson, S., & Henderson, S. O. (2004). Myth: The Trendelenburg position improves circulation in cases of shock. *Can J Emerg Med*, *6*(1), 48–49.

55. Johnston, I. G., et al. (2004). Survey of intensive care nurses' knowledge relating to the pulmonary artery catheter. *Anaesth Intensive Care*, *32*(4), 564–568.

56. Kee, V. R. (2003). Hemodynamic pharmacology of intravenous vasopressors. *Crit Care Nurse*, *23*, 79–82.

57. Kellum, J. A., & Decker, J. M. (2001). Use of dopamine in acute renal failure: a meta-analysis. *Crit Care Med*, *29*(8), 1526–1531.

58. Kellum, J. A., & Pinsky, M. R. (2002). Use of vasopressor agents in critically ill patients. *Curr Opin Crit Care*, *8*, 236–241.

59. Kern, J. W., & Shoemaker, W. C. (2002). Early goal-directed therapy in shock. *Crit Care Med*, *30*(8), 1686–1692.

60. Khalaf, S., & DeBlieux, P. M. (2001). Managing shock: the role of vasoactive agents, part 1. *J Crit Illness*, www.findarticles.com.

61. Khot, U. N., et al. (2003). Nitroprusside in critically ill patients with left ventricular dysfunction and aortic stenosis. *N Engl J Med*, *348*(18), 1735–1736.

62. Landry, D. W., & Oliver, J. A. (2001). The pathogenesis of vasodilatory shock. *N Engl J Med*, *345*, 588–595.

63. Le Doux, D., et al. (2000). Effects of perfusion pressure on tissue perfusion in septic shock. *Crit Care Med*, *28*(8), 2729–2732.

64. Leeper, B. (2003). Monitoring right ventricular volumes: a paradigm shift. *AACN Clin Issues*, *14*(2), 208–219.

65. Levin, P. D., & Sprung, C. L. (2005). Another point of view: no swan song for the pulmonary artery catheter. *Crit Care Med*, *33*(5), 1123–1124.

66. Levin, T. (2002). Right ventricular myocardial infarction. *UpToDate*, *10.2*, 1–8.

67. Levine, B. S. (2000). Intermittent positive inotrope infusion in the management of end-stage, low-output heart failure. *J Cardiovasc Nurs*, *14*(4), 76–93.

68. Maron, B. J., & Kimmelstiel, C. (2004). Role of percutaneous septal ablation in hypertrophic obstructive cardiomyopathy. *Circulation*, *109*, 452–456.

69. Martin, G. S. (2003). Norepinephrine use in severe circulatory shock. *Online Medscape Critical Care*.

70. Massoudy, P., et al. (2000). Sodium nitroprusside in patients with compromised left ventricular function undergoing coronary bypass: reduction of cardiac proinflammatory substances. *J Thorac Cardiovasc Surg*, *119*(3), 566–574.

71. McKie, P. M., & Burnett, J. C. Jr. (2005). B-type natriuretic peptide as a biomarker beyond heart failure: speculations and opportunities. *Mayo Clin Proc*, *80*(8), 1029–1036.

72. Mehta, S. R., et al. (2001). Impact of right ventricular involvement on mortality and morbidity in patients with inferior myocardial infarction. *J Am Coll Cardiol*, *37*(1), 37–43.

73. Monnet, X., et al. (2004). The pulmonary artery catheter in critically ill patients. Does it change outcomes? *Minerva Anesthesiol*, *70*(4), 219–224.

74. Moore, K. (2002). Critical care hemodynamic parameters and pharmacologic interventions. *Crit Care Nurs Clin North Am*, *14*(1), 71–76.

75. Morales, D. L., et al. (2003). A double-blind randomized trial: prophylactic vasopressin reduces hypotension after cardiopulmonary bypass. *Ann Thorac Surg*, *75*(3), 926–930.

76. Morelli, A., et al. (2004). Effects of short-term fenoldopam infusion on gastric mucosal blood flow in septic shock. *Anesthesiology*, *101*(3), 576–582.

77. Mullner, M., et al. (2004). Vasopressors for shock. *Cochrane Database Syst Rev*, *3*, CD003709.

78. Nasraway, S. A. (2000). Norepinephrine: no more "leave 'em dead"? *Crit Care Med*, *28*(8), 3096–3097.

79. Nolan, J. (2001). Fluid resuscitation for the trauma patient. *Resuscitation*, *48*(1), 57–69.

80. O'Brien, E. (2003). Demise of the mercury sphygmomanometer and the dawning of a new era in blood pressure measurement. *Blood Press Monit*, *8*(1), 19–21.

81. Petersen, D. A. (2000). Managing hypotension after cardiac surgery: an algorithm for treatment. *Crit Care Nurse, 20*(2), 36–49.

82. Pinsky, M. R. (2003). Hemodynamic monitoring in the intensive care unit. *Clin Chest Med, 24*(4), 549–560.

83. Pinsky, M. R., & Vincent, J. L. (2005). Let us use the pulmonary artery catheter correctly and only when we need it. *Crit Care Med, 33*(5), 1119–1124.

84. Pittman, J. A., et al. (2004). Arterial and central venous pressure monitoring. *Int Anesthesiol Clin, 42*(1), 13–30.

85. Prentice, D., & Ahrens, T. (2001). Controversies in the use of the pulmonary artery catheter. *J Cardiovasc Nurs, 15*(2), 1–5.

86. Rivers, E. P., et al. (2001). Early goal-directed therapy in the treatment of severe sepsis and septic shock. *N Engl J Med, 345*(19), 1368–1377.

87. Rivers, E. P., et al. (2001). Central venous oxygen saturation monitoring in the critically ill patient. *Curr Opin Crit Care, 7*(3), 204–211.

88. Rosenthal, M. H. (1999). Intraoperative fluid management—what and how much? *Chest, 115*, 106S–112S.

89. Ryan, T. J., et al. (1999). 1999 update: ACC/AHA guidelines for the management of patients with acute myocardial infarction: a report of the American College of Cardiology/American Heart Association Task Force on Practice Guidelines (Committee on Management of Acute Myocardial Infarction). *J Am Coll Cardiol, 34*, 890–911.

90. Sabatine, M. S., et al. (2005). Association of hemoglobin levels with clinical outcomes in acute coronary syndromes. *Circulation, 111*(16), 2042–2049.

91. Sackner-Bernstein, J. D., et al. (2005). Short-term risk of death after treatment with nesiritide for decompensated heart failure: a pooled analysis of randomized controlled trials. *JAMA, 293*(15), 1900–1905.

92. SAFE Study Investigators. (2004). A comparison of albumin and saline for fluid resuscitation in the intensive care unit. *N Engl J Med, 350*, 2247–2256.

93. Sharma, M., & Teerlink, J. R. (2004). A rational approach for the treatment of acute heart failure: current strategies and future options. *Curr Opin Cardiol, 19*(3), 254–263.

94. Sharma, S., & Zevitz, M. E. (2005). Cardiogenic shock. www.emedicine.com/med/topic285.htm.

95. Smith, M. A. (2005). Use of vasopressors in the treatment of cardiac arrest. *Crit Care Nurse Clin North Am, 17*(1), 71–75.

96. Stiell, I., et al. (2001). Vasopressin versus epinephrine for inhospital cardiac arrest: a randomised controlled trial. *Lancet, 358*(9276), 105–109.

97. Summerhill, E. M., & Baram, M. (2005). Principles of pulmonary artery catheterization in the critically ill. *Lung, 183*(3), 209–219.

98. Tabel, Y., et al. (2004). Diltiazem provides higher internal mammary artery flow than nitroglycerin during coronary artery bypass grafting surgery. *Eur J Cardiothorac Surg, 25*(4), 553–559.

99. Talbot, M. P., et al. (2000). Vasopressin for refractory hypotension during cardiopulmonary bypass. *J Thorac Cardiovasc Surg, 120*(2), 401–402.

100. Tang, W. H., & Hobbs, R. E. (2005). Novel strategies for the management of acute decompensated heart failure. *Curr Cardiol Rev, 1*(1), 1–5.

101. Valler-Jones, T., & Wedgbury, K. (2005). Measuring blood pressure using the mercury sphygmomanometer. *Br J Nurs, 14*(3), 145–150.

102. Van den Berghe, G., et al. (2001). Intensive insulin therapy in the surgical intensive care unit. *N Engl J Med, 345*(19), 1359–1367.

103. Vender, J. S., & Franklin, M. (2004). Hemodynamic assessment of the critically ill patient. *Int Anesth Clin, 42*(1), 31–58.

104. Vialet, R., et al. (2003). Isovolume hypertonic solutes (sodium chloride or mannitol) in the treatment of refractory posttraumatic intracranial hypertension: 2 mL/kg 7.5% saline is more effective than 2 mL/kg 20% mannitol. *Crit Care Med, 31*(6), 1683–1687.

105. Vincent, J. L. (2001). Hemodynamic support in septic shock. *Intensive Care Med, 27*(1 Suppl.), S80–S92.

106. Wenzel, V., et al. (2004). A comparison of vasopressin and epinephrine for out-of-hospital cardiopulmonary resuscitation. *N Engl J Med, 350*, 105–113.

107. Wilkes, M. M., & Navickis, R. J. (2001). Patient survival after human albumin administration. A meta-analysis of randomized, controlled trials. *Ann Intern Med, 135*, 149–164.

108. Yamani, M. H., et al. (2001). Comparison of dobutamine-based and milrinone-based therapy for advanced decompensated congestive heart failure: Hemodynamic efficacy, clinical outcome, and economic impact. *Am Heart J, 142*(6), 998–1002.

109. Zhou, S. X., et al. (2002). Effects of norepinephrine, epinephrine, and norepinephrine-dobutamine on systemic and gastric mucosal oxygenation in septic shock. *Acta Pharmacol Sin, 23*(7), 654–658.

CHAPTER 42 Trauma

Christine Smith Schulman

The trauma patient population is one of the most diverse groups of patients seen in critical care, composed of people of all ages regardless of their socioeconomic status and preexisting health. The trauma victim often has multisystem injuries, and recovery may be long and fraught with complications. With today's sophisticated technology and coordinated trauma care systems, trauma patients stand an excellent chance of return to a productive life. For those who are critically injured, recovery is dependent on prompt, aggressive, and appropriate resuscitation in critical care.

Unique to the trauma patient is the etiology of critical illness: the transfer of kinetic energy to body tissues resulting in multisystem derangements. In addition to trauma-specific assessment, diagnostic testing, and interventions, these patients face similar physiologic challenges as do other critically ill patients: those with acute respiratory distress syndrome (ARDS), shock, neurologic compromise, gastrointestinal (GI) compromise, acute tubular necrosis (ATN), and infection, to name a few. Detailed information about the full spectrum of trauma care is covered in textbooks specific to the topic[119,127]; this chapter focuses on issues essential for any critical care nurse caring for injured patients.

EPIDEMIOLOGY

Trauma care has existed since ancient Egyptian and Greek civilizations described and treated a wide variety of wounds.[44] Trauma, or tissue injury resulting from the transfer of energy from the environment, affects people in the peak productive years of their lives. Trauma results from unintentional incidents (formerly referred to as "accidents") such as motor vehicle crashes (MVCs), falls, burns, and occasional firearm, recreational, and occupational mishaps. Intentional injury results from deliberate acts of violence such as assaults, child or elder abuse, shootings, and stabbings (the incidence and prevalence of trauma are described in Box 42-1). Alcohol use has a disturbingly high prevalence in trauma, especially MVCs. Influences of alcohol in

trauma are listed in Box 42-2, and the adverse effects of acute and chronic alcohol use are described in Box 42-3.

DEVELOPMENT OF THE TRAUMA SYSTEM

Military experience demonstrates optimal trauma care is provided when there is a coordinated, systematic approach to patient management utilizing the best available resources. The first attempt at a regional trauma system was the R. Adams Cowley Shock-Trauma Institute in Maryland in the early 1980s. This system was funded by the state legislature and provided for early triage of injured patients to the trauma center. The success of this first trauma center led to development of similar systems in the United States that now follow national standards developed by the American College of Surgeons Committee on Trauma (ACSCOT). Since then, ACSCOT has facilitated the development of numerous trauma systems in collaboration with National Highway Traffic Safety Administration (NHTSA) and the Division of Trauma and Emergency Medical Services (DTEMS). Patient morbidity and mortality have significantly improved nationally and internationally with the advent of trauma care systems.[39,93,123,145,146] Fundamental components of any trauma care system include regulations and policies, resource management, training programs, transportation, facilities, communication systems, public information and trauma prevention programs, designated medical directors, and formal evaluation programs. A network of trauma care facilities comprises any successful trauma care system. Trauma centers are categorized from Level I-IV depending on their level of resources;[57,120] characteristics of trauma centers are described in Table 42-1.

MECHANISMS OF INJURY

The term *mechanism of injury* refers to the underlying causes and physical forces resulting in physical injury. Knowledge of mechanism of injury provides for

Box 42-1

Incidence and Prevalence of Trauma

- Trauma is the fourth leading cause of death for all ages in the United States and the leading cause of death in people between ages 1 and 34.
- People between the ages of 17 and 24 have the highest trauma-related death rate.
- People older than the age of 85 have a greater likelihood of dying despite lower injury severity.
- Men are injured more frequently than women until the age of 70, after which time injuries to women are more common.
- Primary causes of unintentional injury are motor vehicle crashes (MVCs), falls and burns; MVCs involving cars, trucks, and motorcycles account for 48% of all trauma. Auto-pedestrian crashes and other modes of transportation such as snow vehicles, off-road vehicles, animal-drawn vehicles, and boats account for 9.7% of trauma.
- Falls account for 16.7% of trauma cases and for more than half of deaths occurring in the older adult; the peak incidence occurs after the age of 80.
- Intentional and unintentional injuries from firearms account for 5.4% of injuries and 19% of fatalities. The peak incidence of deaths related to firearms is between 12 and 20 years of age.
- Other intentional injuries from assaults, stabbing, and self-inflicted wounds account for 12% of all trauma cases.
- Alcohol is a factor in 40% of all traffic-related fatalities in which at least one driver or nonoccupant had a blood alcohol concentration (BAC) of 0.01 g/dl or higher.
- Alcohol is a major factor in intentional and interpersonal trauma, recreational trauma, and burns, and plays a large role in the incidence of traumatic brain injury.

Data from references 7, 15, 44, 105, 147, 151, 152, 165.

Box 42-2

Influences of Alcohol in Trauma

- Habitual drunken drivers have an increased risk of dying in an alcohol-related crash.
- There is no increase in complications in trauma patients who are acutely intoxicated at the time of injury, but there is a twofold increased risk of complications in patients with a history of chronic alcohol abuse.
- Intoxicated people are less likely to use seatbelts and are more likely to drive at high speeds.
- 69% of car occupants between 21 and 44 years of age killed in car crashes had blood alcohol concentration levels at or above 0.08 dg/d.
- More than 36% of all pedestrians older than 16 years of age killed in traffic crashes have elevated BAC.
- 47% of children killed in motor vehicle crashes are in crashes in which the driver had elevated BAC.
- The rate of alcohol involvement in fatal crashes is more than three times higher at night than during the day.
- 30% of all fatal crashes during the week are alcohol related, compared with 53% on weekends.
- Intoxicated drivers involved in fatal crashes are nine times more likely to have prior drinking and driving convictions than nonintoxicated drivers.
- Drinking drivers have higher hospitalization costs and longer lengths of stay independent of their age, gender, or injury severity.

Data from references 101, 112, 143, 147.

increased ease in injury identification and prediction of eventual patient outcomes.[199] In addition, it guides initial resuscitation and diagnostic activities and allows the critical care team to discover missed injuries and anticipate complications associated with specific injuries. Injuries are commonly diagnosed because a suspicious healthcare provider compared the physical findings with the patient's history, initiated further diagnostic workup, and identified a previously undiscovered injury.

Laws of Motion and Energy (Kinematics)

Trauma occurs when an acute exchange of mechanical, thermal, electrical, or chemical energy results in structural changes or physiologic imbalance.[128] Energy exchange is dependent on three basic principles of physics: an object in rest or motion will remain in that state until acted on by some outside force (Newton's first law of motion); energy is changed from one form to another, not created or destroyed; and the force of energy is a function of size and speed. Doubling the *size* of an object will result in a doubling of kinetic energy. Doubling the *speed* of an object results in a quadrupling of kinetic energy (kinetic energy: $KE = mass \times velocity^2$).[128] Force applied slowly and over a large surface area will result in less tissue destruction than force applied quickly over a small surface area.[199] Force puts

Box 42-3

Adverse Effects of Acute Alcohol Intoxication in the Injured Patient

- Vasodilation with exaggerated hypotension secondary to blood loss
- Hypovolemia from natriuresis and diuresis
- Impaired cardiovascular response to shock
- Metabolic acidosis secondary to alcohol substitutes (ethylene glycol, methanol, etc.)
- Excessive heat loss leading to hypothermia
- Pulmonary compromise secondary to aspiration
- Impaired response to hemorrhage

COMPLICATIONS OF CHRONIC ALCOHOL USE

- Electrolyte abnormalities (hyponatremia, hypokalemia, hypomagnesemia, hypophosphatemia, etc.)
- Nutritional deficiencies (hypoglycemia, hypovitaminosis, etc.)
- Loss of hepatic synthesis of coagulation factors
- Portal hypertension with refractory intraabdominal bleeding
- Cardiomyopathy and heart failure

From reference 113a.

TABLE 42-1 Characteristics of Trauma Centers

LEVEL	CHARACTERISTICS
Level I	• Typically located in larger cities, they are expected to admit at least 1200 trauma patients per year; at least 20% of these patients must be severely injured. • Responsible for teaching, research, and development of the regionalized trauma system. • Usually tertiary academic facilities with dedicated resources to support the personnel, education, equipment, and capacity to provide care for all phases of trauma care.
Level II	• Larger community hospitals that may or may not be academic centers. • Provide definitive trauma care to patients, but when resources are exceeded may need to transfer patient to highest level of care. • Does not have same expectations for education, research, and rehabilitation as Level I.
Level III	• Community hospital in a geographic area without Level I or Level II facilities. • Resuscitates and provides definitive surgical intervention. • Provides safe transfer to a higher level of care when the patient's needs exceed facility resources.
Level IV	• Usually smaller hospital in less-populated, rural areas. • Provides timely resuscitation and transfer of injured patients to higher level of care. • Establishes transfer agreements protocols with Level I and II centers.

Data from references 4, 32, 57, 120.

an object in motion; this motion will not change until a second force equal to or greater than the initiating force stops it. For example, a car will remain at a certain speed until acted on by an outside force, such as the application of brakes, another vehicle, or a tree. Rather than disappear, the kinetic energy of the moving car is absorbed by the other objects and body tissues of any passengers.

Tissue damage occurs as a result of acceleration, deceleration, shearing, or compressive forces. Acceleration is a change in the speed of a moving object[199] (e.g., a person standing by the side of the road is accelerated into motion when hit by an oncoming car). Conversely, deceleration is a decrease in the speed of a moving object[199] (e.g., a person riding a bicycle suddenly stops after hitting a parked car). Many injuries occur from a combination of acceleration and deceleration forces[128] (e.g., a person is thrown into motion after being hit by a car, and suddenly stopped by landing on the ground).

Shearing injuries result when structures move in opposite directions from each other, stretching and disrupting tissue planes and pulling organs away from their attachment points[199] (e.g., when the heart swings forward in the chest cavity while the aortic arch remains fixed to the thoracic spine). Finally, compressive forces overwhelm the ability of tissues to resist squeezing[199] (e.g., a person who falls from a height to land on the feet will sustain vertebral and long bone fractures along the axial plane, or when inflated lungs are squeezed during a sudden stop against a steering wheel, popping much like a closed paper bag).

Injuries can occur through either blunt or penetrating mechanisms, with the resultant injury dependent on the amount of energy delivered and the area of the body affected.[199] A thorough discussion of these mechanisms is beyond the scope of this chapter; however, an overview is provided here so that the critical care nurse can appreciate the forces responsible for the patient's injuries.

BLUNT TRAUMA

The combination of deceleration, acceleration, shearing, crushing, and compression result in blunt trauma. Blunt trauma is often more life threatening than penetrating trauma because distribution of destructive energy occurs across several body tissues. As a consequence, multiple injuries are common and identification of injuries can be difficult. MVCs, falls, assaults, explosions, and contact sports are associated with blunt force injuries.[128,199]

Motor Vehicle Crash

Different types of vehicle crashes produce predictable injury patterns. Types of MVCs include frontal impact collisions (with both "up-and-over" and "down-and-under" patient trajectories), lateral impact collisions, rear impact collisions, rotational collisions, and rollover crashes (Figure 42-1).[57] Having a high index of suspicion for specific injuries serves as a starting point to look for injuries varying from usual patterns.

Frontal impact collisions occur when a vehicle strikes an object ahead of it. The vehicle's occupants continue to move forward at the same speed as the vehicle until they hit the seatbelt, airbag, steering wheel, dashboard, or back of the front seat, depending on their position in the car. Two injury patterns are seen as a result of the unrestrained occupant's movement. The up-and-over pathway occurs as the head becomes the leading point of the body, striking the windshield or other supporting structures of the car. Once the head stops, the continued momentum of the torso pulls the body upward, forcing the chest and abdomen into the steering column or dashboard. The down-and-under pathway results as the occupant moves forward and down under the dashboard. The knee and femur are forced into the dash; the driver's chest and abdomen collide with the steering wheel (see Figure 42-1). As intrathoracic structures move forward, shearing acceleration forces result in tearing of organs from their vascular pedicles.[128]

Lateral impact collisions occur when the vehicle is struck at a 90-degree angle, changing the direction from a purely forward motion to a forward-lateral motion. Resultant injuries are due to compression and shearing as the occupants are hit on the side of impact or are thrown across the vehicle to hit the opposite side.[128]

Rear impact collisions cause the occupants to move forward at a faster speed than the vehicle's speed. If there is no head restraint, the head will fling backward and serious cervical spine injuries may result.[128]

Rotational collisions occur when an off-center part of the vehicle is struck by an object of lower speed, causing the vehicle to rotate around the point of impact. Occupants will continue movement in the original direction until they strike some object within the car. Shearing and compression injuries occur during rollover crashes as occupants are tossed in multiple directions in subsequent collisions as the car repeatedly rolls.[128] Injury patterns associated with specific collision types are illustrated in Figure 42-2.

Other Types of Collisions

Four collisions occur with any car crash, all of which have the potential to injure a passenger. They are often referred to as the "alphabet of collisions" and are described in Table 42-2.[128]

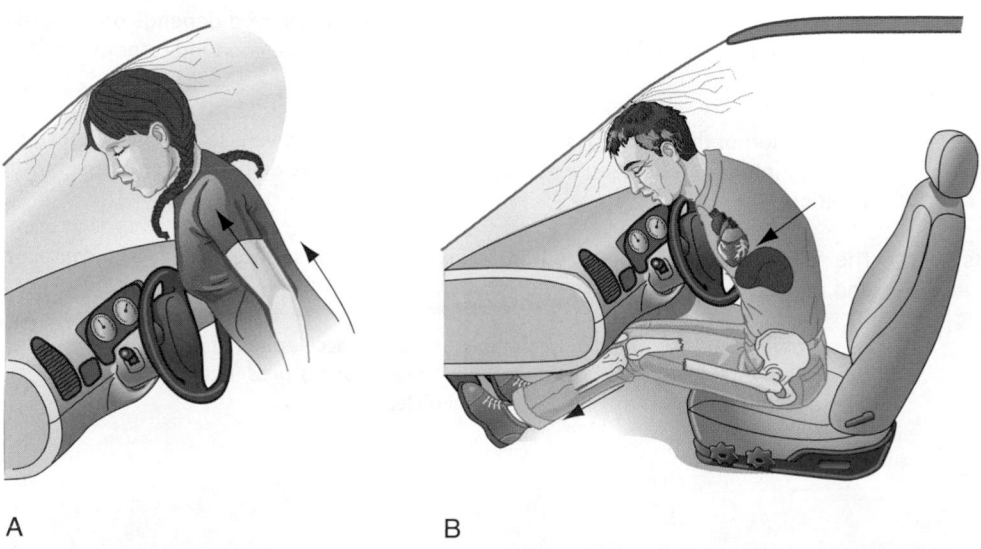

A   B

◆FIGURE 42-1 Up-and-over and down-and-under injury patterns. **A,** Up-and-over pathway. **B,** Down-and-under pathway.

Head-on collisions	Rear-end collisions
Up-and-over pathway Cervical spine compression and axial loading Skull fractures, brain injury Rib fractures, flail chest Pulmonary contusion and pneumothorax Myocardial contusion Liver, spleen, duodenum, and diaphragm lacerations Great vessel lacerations	Whiplash Rib fractures, flail chest Pneumothorax Pulmonary contusion
	Ejections Head injuries Cervical and thoracic spine compression fractures Pneumo/hemopneumothorax Liver, spleen, and pancreas lacerations Aortic tears Pelvic fractures, straddle fractures
Down-and-under pathway Cervical spine flexion Laryngeal trauma Carotid shearing Rib fractures, flail chest Pulmonary contusion and pneumothorax Myocardial contusion Aortic tears Pelvic and acetabular fractures Lower-extremity fractures	**Lateral collisions** Cervical ligamentous injuries Lateral rib fractures, flail chest Pneumothorax, pulmonary contusion Spleen or liver lacerations Pelvic, hip, and acetabular fractures Humerus and clavicle fractures

⬍FIGURE 42-2 Injury patterns resulting from different types of motor vehicle crashes.

TABLE 42-2 Types of Car Collisions

TYPE	DESCRIPTION
A: Auto collision	The collision of the vehicle into some object. The force involved depends on the distance required for the vehicle to stop. The extent of damage to the vehicle is a good indicator of the forces transmitted to the occupants.
B: Body collision	The collision of the occupant's body with the inside of the vehicle. Energy is transferred to the vehicle's interior and subsequently transmitted into tissue deformity, compression, stretching, and shearing.
C: Cavity contents collision	The collision of internal body contents against rigid body surfaces. Energy transmission damages tissues and organs as they collide with each other.
D: Debris collision	Loose objects in the car strike occupants as the car accelerates or decelerates. Coffee mugs, purses, briefcases, toolboxes, telephones, and even unrestrained passengers and animals become "debris" as they are thrown about the inside of the vehicle.

Data from reference 128.

Restraint-System Injuries. The primary protective mechanism of any motor vehicle is the structural design of its frame. Seatbelts, airbags, and infant restraint seats have decreased morbidity and mortality of trauma victims.* When restraints are properly applied, occupants slow at the same pace as their vehicles rather than being abruptly thrown against vehicle structures or ejected.[21,200] Even when worn correctly, a few injuries still result, requiring the healthcare team to consider associated injuries. Seatbelts have been shown to prevent deaths by 40%; however, there is an increased incidence of abdominal viscous injury.[200,203]

A properly applied seatbelt uses a three-point restraint system that crosses over the shoulder and the bony prominences of the pelvis, using these rigid body structures to hold the body securely in the seat. When the shoulder strap and the lap belt are used independently of each other, protective capabilities are significantly diminished and life-threatening injuries may result.[199] The classic Chance fracture occurs when a passenger violently flexes forward against a singular lap belt; the resulting low thoracic and lumbar spine fractures are associated with small bowel injuries. This association between lap belts, lower spine fractures, and small bowel lacerations is so strong that if a Chance fracture is diagnosed, a subsequent exploratory laparotomy is required to rule out intestinal injury.[128,204] This and similar injury patterns have led to the current requirements that all seatbelts in a vehicle have a three-point system.

---

*References 21, 48, 154, 156, 182, 200.

Since 1997, dual airbags have been federally required standard equipment in passenger vehicles in the United States. Despite the fact that airbag-related injuries still occur, NHTSA concluded that driver fatality has been reduced by 11% in all crashes and by 31% in purely frontal crashes, and overall injury is reduced by 60% when used together with three-point restraint systems.[148,149] Airbag injuries occur when occupants are out of position relative to the airbag compartment at the time of impact (e.g., with a person who is extremely short). They also occur if the occupant was bending over at the time of impact, had a pre-crash loss of consciousness, was asleep, if there was pre-crash braking, or if or an object was being held close to the face at the time of impact such as a coffee cup or cellular phone.[128] Airbags inflate and deflate in less than 50 microseconds via a contained explosion of nitrogen, carbon dioxide, and other gases. Airbags inflate only once and therefore offer no protection should there be an immediate second collision[128,148,149] (Box 42-4 lists injuries that occur from inappropriately worn seatbelts and airbag deployment).

Key Crash Information. Caregivers of the trauma patient should review the prehospital record to learn about the circumstances of the crash; many emergency medical services (EMS) systems now use digital cameras to photograph an accident scene. The images are downloaded for trauma team review for better appreciation of the amount of energy transfer involved. Important information to know about the crash is listed in Box 42-5.

Box 42-4

Injuries From Inappropriately Worn Seatbelts and Airbag Deployment

SEATBELTS

Lap Belt Only
- Fractured sternum, ribs, clavicles
- Blunt cardiac injury
- Torn thoracic aorta
- Mesenteric tears, bowel perforations, torn abdominal aorta
- Bladder rupture
- Chance fracture of lower thoracic or lumbar vertebrae

Shoulder Harness Only
- Cervical spine injuries
- Abrasions to neck, chest, and abdomen
- Carotid artery, laryngeal injuries

AIRBAGS
- Cervical spine injuries
- Bag slap injuries to face and neck
- Temporary hearing deficits
- Temporary hearing deficits
- Corneal abrasion, retinal detachment
- Upper extremity contusions
- Fracture/dislocations of thumb and wrist

Data from references 56, 128, 148, 149.

Key Questions Regarding Motor Vehicle Crashes

- What was the size and speed of the car?
- What did the car hit? A guardrail? An oncoming vehicle?
- What was the size and speed of the other vehicle?
- Where was the patient in the car? Driver? Front-seat passenger? Rear-seat passenger on the right or left?
- What was the amount of damage to the vehicle? How much intrusion was there into the passenger space?
- Where is the damage to the vehicle? Side of the car? Dashboard? Windshield? Steering wheel?
- What was the extrication time? A prolonged extrication time implies a delay of definitive treatment as well as extensive transfer of energy to the vehicle and its passengers.
- Was there death of an occupant in the car? What is the injury severity of others involved in the accident? The answers to these questions suggest the magnitude of energy transferred during the accident.
- Were restraint devices used, and were they used correctly?
- Did airbags deploy?

Data from references 56, 128, 199.

Auto-Pedestrian Accidents. When adults see an oncoming vehicle, they will turn and run and are subsequently hit on their side.[128] Different heights of the victim in relationship to the height of the vehicle also influence injury patterns; the taller the victim, the more likely the injuries will be in the lower extremities. Adults are initially struck by the bumper, resulting in fractures of the tibia and fibula. As they bend, their pelvis and upper femur are struck by the vehicle's hood, resulting in head, abdominal, and thoracic injuries as well as femur, pelvis, and spinal fractures. As they slide off of the hood, a third impact occurs in which the victim's head hits the ground, resulting in brain and cervical spine injuries.[128,148,149]

FALLS

Falls from more than three times the victim's height result in severe injury.[128] Circumstances of the fall allow anticipation of the amount of energy involved and likely injuries. Lower extremity fractures, dislocations, and abdominal shearing injuries are common in falls when the victim lands on the feet. In particular, bilateral calcaneal fractures are common if the person fell from a significant height and landed on a hard surface such as asphalt. Compressive forces are transmitted upward from the bottom of the foot to the tibia, femur, and spinal vertebrae, commonly referred to as the "Don Juan" syndrome. Should the victim land on his or her head, as commonly seen in diving injuries, serious head and cervical spine injuries result. In addition to how the victim landed, other influences on injury severity include the surface on which the person landed (a soft bush versus hard concrete), how far the victim fell, and whether anything was hit on the way down.[57,128]

BLAST INJURIES

Injuries sustained during explosion are the result of heat, chemicals, and concussive and acceleration-deceleration forces because victims are often thrown into the air.[128,199] Penetrating injuries can also occur as objects picked up by the blast become missiles. Knowledge of the circumstances of the explosion is necessary to discover all injuries, including thermal and chemical burns, blowout injuries of the lungs, and shearing injuries of abdominal organs. A complete discussion of blast injuries can be found in Chapter 44.

PENETRATING TRAUMA

Injuries resulting from penetration of foreign objects are considered penetrating trauma. Bullets, knives, and impalements from objects (branches and nails) cause penetrating wounds. Damage depends on the size of the penetrating object, its speed, and the elasticity and density of the affected tissues. In addition to the structural damage, serious infections are highly likely because penetrating objects introduce bacteria into wounds.[199]

Gunshot Wounds

The extent of damage created by firearms is influenced by the muzzle length, the size of the bullet, the distance of the victim from the weapon, and the amount of air friction on the missile. Low-velocity firearms (small handguns) create less damage than do high-velocity weapons (hunting rifles, large handguns). Shotguns are low-velocity weapons; they fire multiple lead pellets, each of which is considered a separate missile. The 9 to 200 small pellets in a shotgun shell create wounds that increase in size as the distance between the victim and weapon increases.[199]

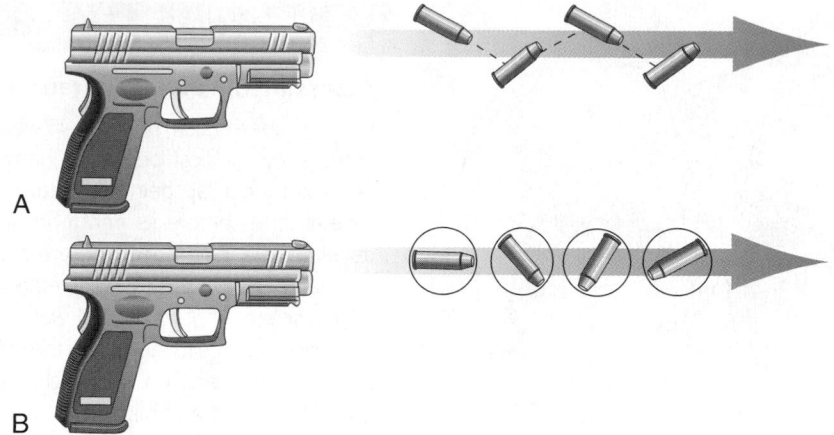

FIGURE 42-3 Wounding potential of a bullet. **A,** Yaw. **B,** Tumble.

A bullet will travel through and transfer energy to tissues, pushing tissues away from its path and creating a temporary tract that displaces tissues forward and laterally.[199] This process, known as cavitation, creates a temporary tract 20 to 25 times the diameter of the bullet that disappears once the bullet passes through the tissue.[128] The size of the cavity is directly proportional to the bullet's size and speed and produces injuries outside of the bullet's direct trajectory.[199] Muscle tissue expands to absorb energy with only a moderate amount of tissue damage; in contrast, liver, spleen, and especially bone do not expand to absorb the energy, and burst.[128,199]

Motion of the bullet as it travels through air and tissue contributes to tissue damage as well. Yawing occurs when the nose of the bullet wobbles back and forth as it moves forward after leaving the weapon's muzzle, creating a larger space than the diameter of the bullet. Yawing will cause a bullet to hit the body at an angle, rather than straight-on. Tumbling occurs when momentum carries the tail of the bullet forward in front of the nose, resulting in an end-over-end motion as it continues to move through air and then tissue. Fragmentation occurs when bullets break apart on impact to produce several smaller fragments, each causing damage to surrounding tissues.[128,199] The fragments lose speed as they travel through tissue, and there may not be enough remaining speed to create an exit wound.[61,190] Bullets yaw, tumble, and fragment as they pass through tissue, increasing the surface area damaged by the bullet. As a result, exit wounds are often larger than entrance wounds. Yaw and Tumble are illustrated in Figure 42-3, and cavitation is shown in Figure 42-4.

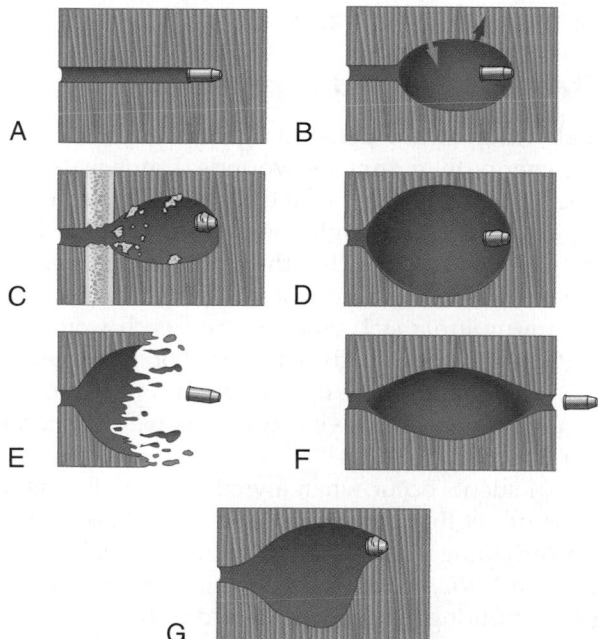

FIGURE 42-4 Wounds seen with cavitation and fragmentation. **A,** Low-velocity missile with small entrance and exit wounds and no cavitation. **B,** Higher-velocity missile with cavitation; tissue displaced in the direction of the arrows. **C,** High-velocity missile with cavitation of tissue and penetration of bone; bone fragments become secondary missiles. **D,** Extremely high-velocity missile with a small entry, resulting in significant cavitation; small exit wound. **E,** Extremely high-velocity missile with thin target; large exit wound with ragged edges. **F,** Relationship of missile velocity, size, and tissue thickness creates deep cavitation and small entrance and exit wounds. **G,** Cavity shape becomes irregular as bullet deforms and tumbles through tissue.

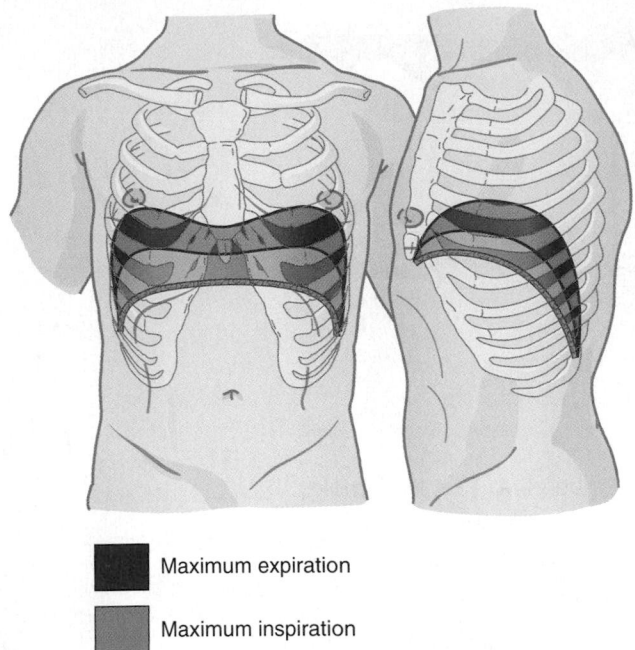

■ Maximum expiration

■ Maximum inspiration

♦FIGURE 42-5 Thoracic and abdominal areas that may be injured with a single stabbing incident.

Stab Wounds and Impalements

Stab wounds are penetrating injuries occurring at lower energy than gunshot wounds. Damage depends on the length and width of the stylette, affected tissues and vasculature, and angle the device enters the body. Damage is contained within the area of the wound. The concern with stab wounds, however, is that frequently there are multiple stab wounds, and each wound can extend into several body cavities. For example, any stab wound between the nipple line and the costochondral margin could involve thoracic as well as abdominal organs (Figure 42-5).[199]

Impalements occur when a victim forcefully collides with an object that penetrates tissue.[199] Impaled objects can be anything in the victim's path: a car door handle during an MVC, fence posts during a fall, arrows during bow hunting, or nails from hydraulic construction nail guns. Clothing fragments, organic materials, and bacteria often are introduced into these wounds, predisposing the patient to significant infection.[199]

APPLIED PATHOPHYSIOLOGY

The body's response to trauma is a global event; multiple processes are initiated at the moment of injury that respond to physiologic insult and promote healing. Compensatory, inflammatory, and hypermetabolic responses occur simultaneously while individual body structures react to injury and the hypoperfusion associated with shock. A comprehensive review of these

Case Study 42-1, Part A

Assessing the Patient's Trauma Circumstances

R.O., an obese (201 pounds) 17-year-old girl, was found by emergency medical personnel hanging upside down, suspended by her lap belt only, after her open-top jeep rolled several times before its front end hit a tree. She had been traveling at a high speed on an isolated rural highway; an estimated 60 minutes elapsed before medical personnel were at the scene. The windshield was shattered and there was extensive damage to the front of the vehicle. She denied having lost consciousness, but was slightly obtunded and only oriented to person and place. She had minor cuts and bruises about her face without significant facial bleeding or swelling. She complained of pain in her right lower extremity and midabdomen, denied difficulty breathing, and was able to move all four extremities. The following readings are obtained:

BP: 88/64 mm Hg
HR: 125 beats/min
RR: 28 breaths/min

Her skin was cool, pale and slightly diaphoretic, with weak radial pulses bilaterally; left pedal pulses were present but the right dorsalis pedis or posterior tibialis pulse was barely palpable. A rigid cervical collar was placed and she was extricated from the vehicle and immobilized on a backboard using full spinal precautions. High-flow oxygen via a nonrebreathing mask was applied. Two large-bore IVs with lactated Ringer's (LR) solution were started in each antecubital vein, a box splint was placed on her right lower leg, and she was covered in blankets, then transported to the closest emergency department at a Level II trauma center, 30 minutes away.

Decision point: What key pieces about this crash will assist the healthcare team in identifying injuries?

Decision point: What injuries are suspected in this patient?
Case continues on page 1178

responses is beyond the scope of this chapter, but the reader is referred to Chapters 6, 40, and 43 for additional information. This section provides an overview of the role of the physiologic responses to trauma, common physiologic sequelae that occur during the resuscitation phase, and pathophysiology of specific injuries.

PHYSIOLOGIC RESPONSES TO SHOCK

Shock

The most common type of shock following trauma is hypovolemic shock from overt hemorrhage;[192] significant third-space fluid losses also may occur from severe burns, large crush injuries, ischemic gut, and GI injuries. Intraperitoneal fluid accumulation can lead to abdominal hypertension and abdominal compartment syndrome, further compromising venous return to the heart and contributing to hypotension.[71] Hyperglycemia and administration of osmotic diuretics also deplete the vascular compartment.[192] Hemorrhagic shock not only results in life-threatening volume depletion, but also leads to inadequate oxygen-carrying capacity associated with red blood cell loss.[192]

Additional types of shock seen in trauma patients are obstructive shock, neurogenic shock, and cardiogenic shock. It is common for hypovolemic shock to occur simultaneously with these other causes of shock. Obstructive shock occurs when blood flow into or out of the heart is obstructed, commonly a result of tension pneumothorax, pericardial tamponade, and abdominal compartment syndrome. Neurogenic shock results when high-level cervical spine injuries transect or compress the sympathetic outflow tracts of the spinal cord, controlling peripheral vascular tone and heart rate (HR). It is not associated with injuries to the brain. Profound hypotension is caused by vasodilation and bradycardia, differentiating neurogenic shock from the other types. Cardiogenic shock occurs after a blunt force impact that bruises the heart. The right ventricle is most often affected because it swings forward in the thoracic cavity and hits the sternum during acceleration injuries. The contused and swollen myocardium is dyskinetic (has poor contractility), and decreased cardiac output results in cardiogenic shock.[8] (A complete discussion of the pathophysiology and hemodynamic consequences of shock can be found in Chapter 40.)

Following trauma, oxygen consumption will increase by 15% to 35% to compensate for impaired oxygen delivery.[43,181] Although tachycardia and tachypnea increase both oxygen delivery and oxygen consumption, this is particularly problematic in the hypovolemic trauma patient with cardiac or pulmonary injury. Oxygen consumption is significantly impaired because of failed oxidative metabolism within compromised cells; in late shock, oxygen use drops because cells cannot extract oxygen from hemoglobin (Hgb). Compensatory shunting of blood away from the vital organs exacerbates ischemia in distal tissue beds and contributes to the overall metabolic acidosis.[192]

Prolonged hypoperfusion and hypoxia stimulate multiple inflammatory pathways which, when continually stimulated, have devastating, multisystem consequences. Inflammatory mediators alter vascular and metabolic functions to such a degree that microvascular flow is impaired, metabolic functions become inadequate, and intracellular processes are disrupted. Anaerobic metabolism with profound lactic acidosis is the inevitable result; if they are not reversed, organ failure and death will occur.[104,192]

Systemic Inflammatory Response During Traumatic Shock

Under normal circumstances, a delicate balance exists between proinflammatory and antiinflammatory mediators, or cytokines. Following trauma, a complex inflammatory response is initiated that can overwhelm physiologic reserves. Appropriate and controlled release of inflammatory cytokines contains the insult, prevents bacterial invasion, and promotes healing. However, uncontrolled mediator release (e.g., severe trauma, under resuscitation, or sepsis) results in the systemic inflammatory response syndrome (SIRS). SIRS overwhelms an already compromised host because inflammatory mediators are continuously stimulated, adding to preexisting anaerobic metabolism and perpetuating secondary inflammatory responses. Cytokine release also initiates the immune and coagulation cascades, altering microvascular function, catecholamine release, neutrophil adhesion, chemotaxis, coagulation, and oxygen free radical and protease production.[104,192] Inflammatory mediators contribute to the cardiovascular manifestations of shock as well as end-organ dysfunction,[192] making prompt recognition and treatment of hypovolemia essential for the prevention of severe multisystem complications.

Hypermetabolic Response to Trauma

Following trauma, the body uses endogenous substrates, protein, and fat to support high physiologic demands. Glycogen stores are rapidly depleted because increased demands are coupled with poor intake (e.g., patients unable to ingest or digest food), quickly placing patients into catabolic states. Accelerated catabolic processes (e.g., proteolysis, gluconeogenesis, lipolysis, ketogenesis, and glycogenolysis) occur at a time when the patient needs maximal metabolic support to heal multiple injuries.[185] Basal metabolic rates increase immediately following injury because of increased catecholamine and other hormonal activity, a condition referred to as hypermetabolism. The hypermetabolic response supports survival, minimizes catabolism, and facilitates recovery by providing a constant supply of endogenous carbohydrates, proteins, and fats.[185] During hypermetabolism, the patient's resting energy expenditure may be elevated 120% to 155% above normal during the 10 days following injury (illustrated in Figure 42-6).[16,67,94,160] Sustained hypermetabolism results in significant loss of lean body mass and malnutrition, adversely affecting immune function and wound healing,

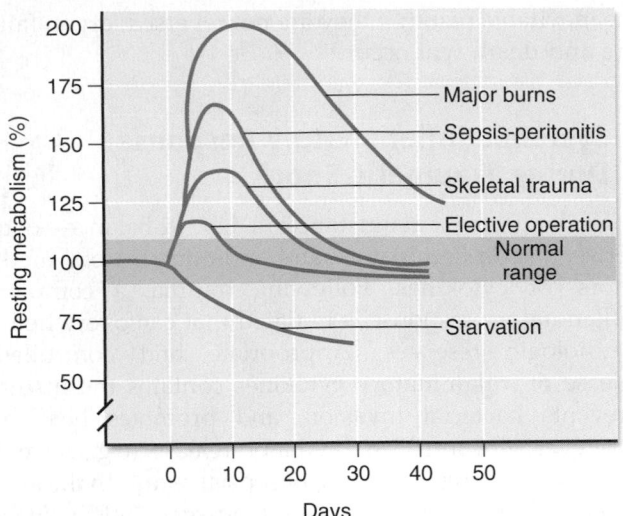

♦FIGURE 42-6   Stress-induced changes in resting metabolic expenditure.

and complicating recovery.[10] However, the ability to establish and maintain a hypermetabolic response to injury positively influences patient outcomes; patients unable to mount or maintain a stress response are likely to die from their injuries.[108,122]

Multiple factors influence the severity and duration of the hypermetabolic response, including the extent of injury, severity of complications, loss of protective barriers to infection, baseline nutritional status, age, and sex.[185] During the first 1 to 24 hours following injury, hypoxia, anoxia, hypovolemia, pain, and anxiety trigger the "ebb phase." Cardiac output, oxygen consumption, and temperature decrease, whereas catecholamines, glucagon, lactate, glucose, and free fatty acids (FFA) increase.[193] The nervous system and inflammatory cytokines (interleukin-1 and tumor necrosis factor) stimulate sustained glucagon, catecholamine, and cortisol release to increase the overall metabolic rate. In addition, catecholamines and cortisol promote lipolysis and the subsequent release of harmful FFAs. (As a side note, the hypermetabolic response does not occur in patients with spinal cord transection above the level of tissue damage.[193]) The "flow phase" begins when resuscitation is complete and injuries are treated, during which time the above-described responses resolve and physiologic parameters begin to normalize.[193] Figure 42-7 illustrates the complex metabolic changes occurring after injury.

Physiologic Sequelae During Trauma Resuscitation

Shock, inflammatory responses, and hypermetabolism following injury contribute to physiologic sequelae common in trauma. These clinical complications add to the physiologic stress in the already compromised patient and can be as difficult to manage as the original injuries themselves. The critical care team must be alert at all times for these complications.

Lethal Triad of Hypothermia, Acidosis, and Coagulopathy.   An altogether too common challenge in the critical care phase of trauma care is the lethal triad of hypothermia, acidosis, and coagulopathy. The triad presents early in the patient's course and is not only an indication of the interplay between the inflammatory and coagulation cascades, but is also considered an early sign of physiologic exhaustion.[54] As such, the triad is associated with more complications and high mortality.[40,77,135] A study by Farrar showed that hypothermic trauma patients who were acidotic despite adequate volume resuscitation were prone to coagulopathy.[62] The physiologic consequences associated with each factor have an additive effect, further impairing oxygen delivery and consumption. The physiologic consequence common to each of the three factors is inadequate oxygen delivery to the tissues (Figure 42-8).

Hypothermia.   The physiology of thermoregulation is discussed in detail in Chapter 7. The causes of hypothermia in trauma are multifactorial and somewhat unique. In normal circumstances, the baseline rate of thermogenesis adequately balances with ongoing heat losses to maintain normal body temperature. The environmental temperature range in which humans can maintain normal body temperature is between 25° and 30° C. Maintenance of normothermia in a cold environment requires additional oxygen as a substrate for heat production. Impaired oxygen delivery and consumption from hemorrhagic shock in a cool environment overwhelm thermoregulation and result in hypothermia.[87]

Trauma patients become hypothermic simply by being exposed to their environment, as described in Box 42-6. Hypothermia may also be a compensatory response to hemorrhagic shock.[113] During shock it is suggested that poor blood flow to the hypothalamus results in a lowering of the thermoregulatory set point, inhibiting shivering in hypotensive and hypoxic patients.[187]

Another possible explanation for hypothermia is that during refractory hemorrhagic shock, cells have extracted all available oxygen from hemoglobin. This results in inefficient cellular metabolism and lactic acid accumulation, and the stressed, hypoxic cells can neither use oxygen nor do cellular work to produce heat. Lactic acid accumulation in hypothermic, severely injured patients is common and is thought to support this theory.[176]

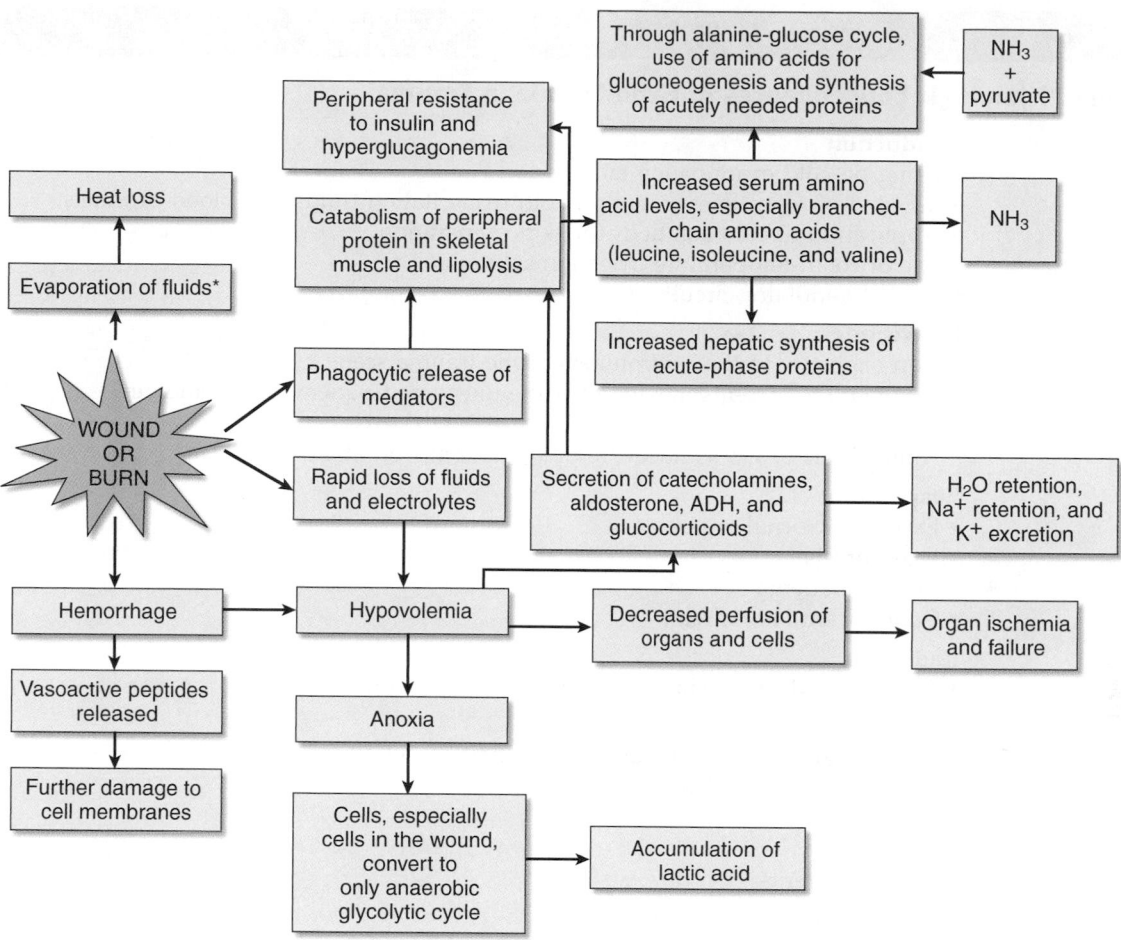

*Occurs mainly in patients with extensive burns

✦**FIGURE 42-7** Physiologic and metabolic changes immediately after an injury. ADH = Antidiuretic hormone, NH$_3$ = ammonia, Na$^+$ = sodium, K$^+$ = potassium.

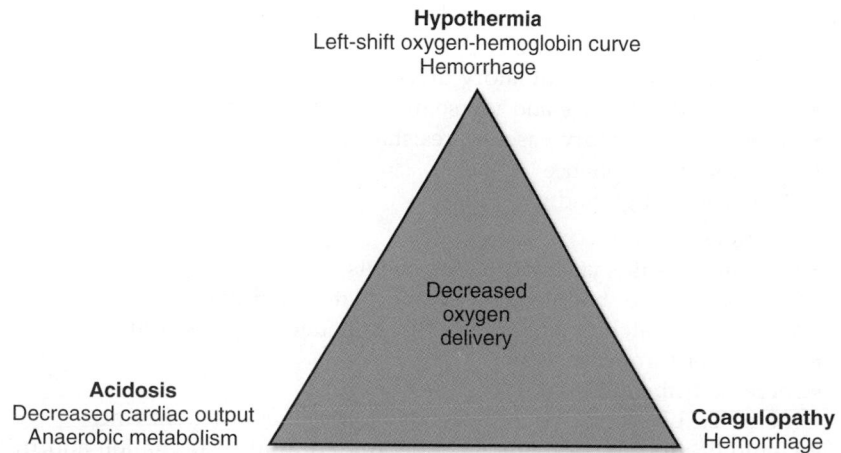

✦**FIGURE 42-8** Consequences of hypothermia, acidosis, and coagulopathy.

Box 42-6

Causes and Physiologic Consequences of Hypothermia in Trauma

Causes

Conduction
- Lying on cold examination tables
- Infusion of room-temperature or cold resuscitation fluids and blood products
- Application of cold solutions for skin preparation
- Use of room-temperature irrigation solutions
- Cooled ventilator circuit

Convection
- Skin exposure to the environment at the trauma scene
- Ambient air currents moving over the uncovered patient in the emergency department or radiology suite
- Ambient air drafts as uncovered patient is moved along hallways

Evaporation
- Exposed internal organs
- Diaphoresis
- Burned patients
- Cooled ventilator circuit

Radiation
- Patient's body temperature higher than room temperature

Medications
- Remove the ability to initiate heat-generating activities such as shivering, pulling on a warm blanket
- Alcohol
- Paralytics
- Sedative agents

Pathophysiologic consequences

Cardiovascular
- Initial increase in blood pressure due to release of catecholamines
- Subsequent decreases in blood pressure and cardiac output
- Increase in heart rate followed by bradycardia when body temperature falls below 32° C
- Increased myocardial workload from increased peripheral vascular resistance
- Increased CVP due to volume shunting from vasoconstriction
- T-wave inversion
- Prolonged PR, QRS, and QT intervals
- Atrial fibrillation
- J wave

Pulmonary
- Increased respiratory rate and drive, followed by a decrease in both when body temperature falls below 32° C
- Decreased hypoxic ventilatory drive
- Increased dead space and worsening $\dot{V}/\dot{Q}$ mismatch
- Increased pulmonary vascular resistance
- Worsening compliance
- Decreased cough and gag reflexes

Hematologic
- Decreased leukocyte and platelet counts
- Sequestration of both leukocytes and platelets in liver
- Change in platelet morphology, function, and response time
- Release of thromboplastin
- Increased fibrinolysis
- Increased bleeding due to reduced activity of clotting enzymes
- Hemodilution of coagulation factors due to fluid resuscitation and transfusions of blood products

---

Box 42-6—CONT'D

Metabolic
- Hyperglycemia due to insulin resistance
- Release of catecholamines
- Initial increase in metabolic rate followed by a decrease with profound hypothermia
- Left shift of oxygen-hemoglobin dissociation curve, resulting in decreased oxygen availability at the cellular level
- Combined respiratory and metabolic acidosis

Neurologic
- Confusion, anxiety, poor judgment, psychosis, short-term memory loss, and decreased level of consciousness
- Prolonged neurologic recovery time from anesthesia

Gastrointestinal
- Ileus
- Pancreatitis
- Oliguria
- Delayed hepatic lactate clearance
- Metabolic acidosis from poor renal buffering and excretion of organic acids
- Bacterial translocation from gut, predisposing patient to sepsis

Pharmacologic metabolism
- Increased drug half-life
- Decreased effects of medications on target organs
- Resistance to catecholamines

Modified from reference 175. Additional data from references 68, 75, 82, 84, 168, 169.
CVP = Central venous pressure, $\dot{V}/\dot{Q}$ = ventilation/perfusion.

Several studies show that mortality in trauma patients increases significantly when the core temperature falls below 34° C[102,114,137] and that serious hypothermic coagulopathies are present at slightly higher temperatures.[186,130,170,202] Hypothermia in trauma patients has multiple physiologic consequences (see Box 42-6).

Perhaps the most serious consequences of hypothermia in trauma are coagulopathy and cellular hypoxia. These two consequences worsen the situation in the patient who is already hemorrhaging from injuries and has inadequate oxygen delivery. Coagulopathy results in the loss of Hgb and its oxygen-carrying capacity. Cellular hypoxia results in a left shift of the oxygen-hemoglobin dissociation curve, representing an increase in hemoglobin's affinity for oxygen. The Hgb is well saturated, but oxygen is not released to the tissues.[84] The oxygen saturation as measured by pulse oximetry may be excellent, but this does not reflect the fact that the hemoglobin is not releasing oxygen at the cellular level where it is needed the most. Refer to Chapter 36 for a thorough understanding of the physiologic changes represented by the oxygen-hemoglobin dissociation curve.

Acidosis. Although respiratory acidosis may occur in trauma (e.g., hypoventilation from brain injury, spinal cord injury, or pulmonary injury), metabolic acidosis is of greater concern because it reflects the patient's degree of oxygen debt and resuscitation status. If the underlying cause of shock is not corrected, acidosis will worsen. Both respiratory and metabolic acidosis can be present trauma patients with airway compromise or pulmonary injury and hypovolemic shock. Acidosis with a pH of less than 7.20 can cause cardiac irritability, left ventricular failure, poor coronary perfusion, decreased catecholamine responsiveness, altered glucose metabolism, and cerebral swelling.[54,85] If unresolved, acidosis results in cellular death, disruption of cellular membranes, and release of intracellular toxins into the circulation. Cell death leads to organ death, multisystem organ dysfunction, and death.[85]

A *washout* phenomenon has been described in which the serum lactic acid (LA) level actually rises despite other resuscitation indicators within normal limits.

This is thought to be due to reestablishment of perfusion in previously ischemic tissue beds with mobilization of LA into the general circulation.[54] Metabolic acids, potassium (K^+), polymorphonuclear leukocytes, and other inflammatory mediators enter the circulation and may cause life-threatening hyperkalemia and cardiac dysrhythmias.[179] A full discussion of acidosis using serum LA levels and base deficit (BD) is found in Chapter 32.

Coagulopathy. Hemorrhage is the cause of death in a large percentage of trauma patients.[20,169] The presence of clotting abnormalities is an independent predictor of mortality, even in the presence of other risk factors such as injury severity.[116] Coagulopathic trauma patients, should they survive, are more likely to develop organ dysfunction and have longer critical care stays.[14,72] A life-threatening coagulopathy is present when the prothrombin time (PT) and activated partial thromboplastin time (aPTT) are more than two times that of laboratory control.[40,47]

Blood loss may be directly due to the injury itself, but several additional factors compound the problem. Cellular and humoral mediators cause a combination of consumption coagulopathy, excessive fibrinolysis, and activation of inflammatory pathways.[20] Tissue factor, a powerful anticoagulant, is released during massive tissue damage; the brain, mesenteric fat, and long bones are associated with profound clotting abnormalities from tissue factor release.[92,206] Hypothermia, as discussed earlier, causes inactivation of clotting enzymes, platelet sequestration and dysfunction, and increased fibrinolysis. Dilutional coagulopathy is seen when large volumes of crystalloids and red cells are infused without a balanced transfusion of coagulation factors. Consumptive coagulopathy occurs with consumption of clotting factors in excess of supply. Thrombocytopenia is common in patients receiving more than 1.5 times their blood volume in transfusions and exacerbated by consumption of platelets at injury sites.[47,54] Accelerated fibrinolysis destroys clots using plasmin, a proteolytic enzyme that breaks down many coagulation factors and plasma proteins.[111] Coagulopathies via the intrinsic pathways are exacerbated by severe acidosis.[54]

Abdominal Compartment Syndrome

A number of clinical conditions are associated with intraabdominal hypertension and abdominal compartment syndrome (ACS); in trauma patients, ACS is a clinical consequence of aggressive fluid resuscitation leading to profound tissue edema and accumulation of free fluid within the abdomen. It also can occur from intraabdominal hemorrhage and abdominal packing left in place after surgery.[136,157] ACS is yet another insult in the critically ill trauma patient who often has ongoing blood loss and severe multisystem injuries. In times past, these patients died a dramatic death in critical care because they could not be ventilated or perfused due to high abdominal pressure. With today's sophisticated ventilators and rapid infusers that allow immediate responses to the physiologic changes that occur after bedside decompression, these patients often can be saved. A full discussion of the clinical presentation and management of ACS is found in Chapter 29.

Rhabdomyolysis

Rhabdomyolysis is the release of injured skeletal muscle components into the circulation. There are many etiologies for rhabdomyolysis, but those most likely to be associated with trauma involve muscle compression seen with crush injury, vascular compromise of an extremity, soft-tissue infections, and electrical injuries. Improper operative positioning in the extended lithotomy and lateral decubitus positions, blunt extremity and torso trauma from beatings, and pneumatic antishock garments lead to muscle compression with development of rhabdomyolysis. Prolonged muscle ischemia results in anaerobic metabolism, a further decrease in adenosine triphosphate (ATP) production and subsequent release of anaerobic by-products and inflammatory mediators into the microvascular circulation. As sodium/potassium-ATPase activity is decreased, intracellular fluid and calcium (Ca^{++}) accumulate. Hyperphosphatemia follows and exacerbates the low Ca^{++} levels. Subsequent capillary permeability leads to interstitialization of fluids, hypovolemia, and decreased renal blood flow. An increased concentration of activated neutrophils develops once reperfusion has begun; these neutrophils further damage reperfused tissue by releasing proteolytic enzymes, generating free radicals, producing large amounts of metabolic acids and increasing microvascular resistance and vascular permeability. Tissue thromboplastin levels increase, leading to disseminated intravascular coagulation (DIC).[117]

The hallmark of rhabdomyolysis is the release of large amounts of myoglobin into the circulation, threatening kidney function.[117] Acute renal failure (ARF) occurs in 4% to 33% of patients with rhabdomyolysis, with a mortality rate of 3% to 50%.[183,197] ARF occurs from decreased renal perfusion, cast formation with renal tubular obstruction, and myoglobin toxicity. Myoglobin is a pigment protein in skeletal muscle that is filtered by the kidney. Increased levels of circulating myoglobin cause a dark tea-colored urine from myoglobinuria because the molecule is not reabsorbed in the renal tubules.[117]

PATHOPHYSIOLOGY OF SPECIFIC INJURIES

A thorough discussion of the pathophysiology of specific injuries is beyond the scope of this chapter. A brief overview of individual injuries is included here.

Brain and Spinal Cord Injury

Traumatic brain injury (TBI) and spinal cord injury are presented in detail in Chapters 22 and 24.

Facial Trauma

Injuries to the face are highly associated with severe brain and cervical spine injuries. The initial concern is for airway patency because profound swelling and significant bleeding are common; hemorrhagic shock can result because facial arteries do not constrict like arteries elsewhere in the body. The extent of injury is directly correlated with the velocity of the face at the time of impact. Penetrating wounds to the face are less common than those from lower-speed, blunt forces.

- Zygoma and orbital floor fractures involve the trigeminal nerve and affect eye movement. Severe comminuted zygomatic fractures cause acute enophthalmos because of severe loss of skeletal support. Entrapment of the facial nerves and muscle within the fracture lines restricts upper eye movement and causes facial paralysis and numbness. Occasionally the zygomatic arch can be displaced downward in such a way that it impedes opening of the mouth.[166]

- Mandibular fractures most frequently involve the body and condylar-subcondylar areas of the mandible. This results in malocclusion of the jaw. Although not directly life threatening, swelling from this and other facial injuries threatens airway patency.[166]

- LeFort maxillary fractures occur in three consistent patterns after significant blunt injury to the midface. Although not directly life threatening, patients often require tracheostomy for airway control until swelling resolves. LeFort I fractures separate the maxilla from the face, LeFort II fractures are a triangle-shaped separation of the nasomaxillary segment of the midface, and LeFort III fractures, also known as craniofacial dissociation, are characterized by a complete separation of the midface from the cranium. Fractures of the maxilla, zygomas, and nose are common. Distortion and movement of the midface suggest airway patency is threatened by severe swelling (Figure 42-9).[166]

Chest Trauma

Chest trauma is often associated with severe head and abdominal trauma, injuries with both blunt and penetrating etiologies. These injuries may occur as the result of blunt and penetrating trauma and often have extremely high mortality rates.

- Closed pneumothorax, hemothorax, and tension pneumothorax are due to accumulation of air or blood in pleural space, often from a lung laceration, a fractured rib, or a penetrating injury. These injuries may be unilateral or bilateral and, if

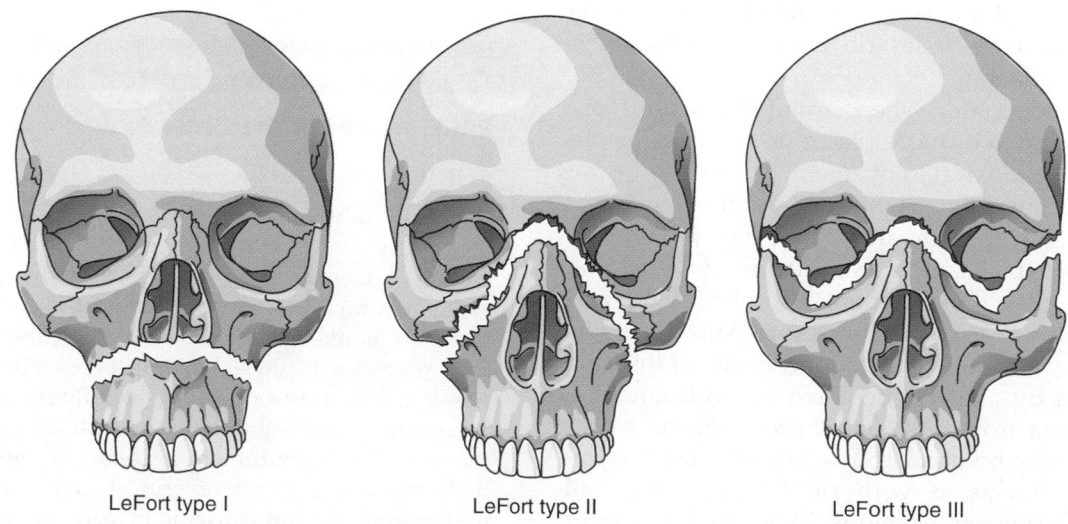

LeFort type I   LeFort type II   LeFort type III

⬍FIGURE 42-9 LeFort fractures. LeFort type I, transverse fracture of the maxillary process from the base of the maxilla and midface. LeFort type II, triangular fracture involving the entire maxilla and nasal bones. LeFort type III, craniofacial-midface disassociation.

unresolved, full respiratory and cardiovascular collapse result. Blood loss from hemothorax is not usually from pulmonary tissue but rather from injuries involving thoracic structures, including adhesions between pleura and the chest wall, the main pulmonary vessels, chest wall vessels, internal mammary arteries, and intercostal vessels.[50,164,180] Hemothorax of 1.5 to 4 L, or at least half of the patient's circulating blood volume, is considered a life-threatening injury because the chest has the capacity to hold most of the patient's circulating volume. It is usually associated with trauma to large systemic blood vessels or mediastinal structures; left-sided hemothorax frequently accompanies injuries to the thoracic aorta.[180]

- Tracheobronchial tears involve injuries at any bronchial level to within an inch of the carina. They are often fatal, with death occurring at the scene. For those who survived to hospital, continuity of the airway may have been maintained by surrounding fascia, or decompensation did not occur until after endotracheal intubation and positive pressure ventilation.[180]

- Rib fractures of the first and second ribs suggest high-energy impact and injury to underlying major vascular structures. Fractures of ribs three through nine are common with blunt trauma and are associated with lung injury; the lower ribs are frequently seen with abdominal injuries. Significant pain associated with these fractures impairs ventilation and secretion clearance, placing the patient at risk for both immediate and prolonged respiratory compromise.[180] A higher mortality is seen in the older adult, who may have only one or two fractures, when compared with younger patients with identical injury.[22] The Research Utilization box at right discusses rib fractures in the older adult population.

- Flail chest occurs when multiple fractures are present in two or more places on one side, resulting in paradoxical movement of the chest wall during respiration. Significant pulmonary contusion usually accompanies this injury. Hypoxia requiring mechanical ventilation is common because of altered dynamics of breathing and increased dead space from severe pain.[180]

- Pulmonary contusion is a direct bruise of the lung followed by alveolar hemorrhage, inflammation, and edema around the injury site. Pulmonary contusions may be unilateral or bilateral and are frequently associated with rib fractures and flail chest. Contusion develops 24 to 48 hours after injury and can cause life-threatening ventilation-perfusion mismatch and shunting. Aggressive fluid resuscitation may exacerbate the contusion because it contributes to pulmonary interstitial edema.[164,180]

- Cardiac tamponade occurs when bleeding into the pericardium or a small pericardial rupture follows high-speed blunt injury or penetrating trauma. The pericardium is a stiff, noncompliant sac; accumulation of more than 100 ml of air or blood into the pericardium produces cardiovascular collapse. The size of the pericardial leak and the opposing intrathoracic pressure determine the speed at which tamponade evolves; thus cardiogenic shock may not occur until well after the patient's admission to critical care.[180]

- Thoracic aorta injuries occur when the mobile aorta is torn at points of anatomic fixation with the thoracic spine. The most common sites for tears are at the aortic isthmus, distal to the left subclavian artery, at the ascending aorta where it leaves the pericardial sac, and where the aorta enters the diaphragm. Torn vascular intimal and medial layers bleed into the outer adventitial layer, creating a balloon, or pseudoaneurysm. If the expanding pseudoaneurysm is tamponaded by surrounding tissue, the patient may survive long enough to get to the operating room for definitive repair.[66] Injuries to the thoracic aorta are the leading cause of immediate death from MVC, auto-pedestrian collisions, and falls. Thirty-seven percent of those who survive to hospital die during initial resuscitation or while in surgery, 14% die postoperatively, and 19% of survivors develop paraplegia or sepsis.[66,141]

▲ RESEARCH UTILIZATION

Rib Fractures in the Older Adult Population

CLINICAL ISSUE

The older adult population is steadily increasing in the United States; the number of older adult trauma victims is increasing as well. Twenty-five percent of all trauma fatalities occur in older adults. The higher mortality is likely due to the fact that these patients have decreased physiologic reserves and compromised ability to respond to critical illness and injury. Seemingly minor injuries can have devastating consequences. Rib fractures are a common injury with a high mortality; therefore critical care nurses must understand the influence of this injury on the outcome of older adult trauma patients and plan care to minimize complications.

RESEARCH UTILIZATION—CONT'D

SUMMARY

This retrospective cohort study evaluated 277 patients older than the age of 65 who were admitted to a Level I trauma center over 10 years. The control group was 187 randomly selected patients with rib fractures between the ages of 18 and 64 years. The outcomes evaluated included number of pulmonary complications, number of ventilator days, length of intensive care unit and hospital stays, disposition, and mortality.

The two groups had similar mean abbreviated injury scores, injury severity scores, and number of rib fractures. However, the mean number of ventilator days, intensive care unit days, and length of stay were higher for older adult patients. Pneumonia and acute respiratory distress syndrome were more common in older adults than in the younger control group. Mortality in older adult patients with three or four rib fractures was 19%, with a pneumonia rate of 31%; mortality in older adult patients with more than six rib fractures was 31%, with a pneumonia rate of 51%. Older adults who received epidural analgesia had lower mortality than those who did not. The investigators concluded that mortality and thoracic morbidity of older adult patients is double that of younger patients with similar injuries. Furthermore, with each additional rib fracture, elder mortality increases by 19% and the risk of pneumonia increases by 27%.

APPLICATION

Close attention should be paid to the number of rib fractures in older patients when deciding where to admit the patient. To optimize outcomes, there should be a low threshold for admitting older adult trauma patients to critical care, particularly when comorbidities and additional injuries are present. Older adult patients with as few as three rib fractures should be hospitalized and receive adequate pain management and aggressive respiratory care.

NEED FOR FURTHER STUDY

Future studies are needed to determine the influence of pain management strategies for rib fractures in older adults on length of stay and patient outcome.

Bulger, E. M., et al. (2000). Rib fractures in the elderly. *J Trauma, 48* (6):1040–1046.

Blunt cardiac injuries (BCIs) include small symptomatic contusions, valvular tears, coronary artery dissection, or ventricular rupture. Rarely, BCIs are associated with "blowout" of the ventricular septum or flail injuries to mitral or tricuspid valves. Cardiac contusions are the most common result of BCIs. Dysrhythmias and dyskinesis of the right ventricle cause greatest concern.[66]

Abdominal Trauma

Knowledge of mechanism of injury is essential to determining site of injury. Abdominal injuries occur following both blunt and penetrating mechanisms, with the former being more common. Seldom is only one structure involved; furthermore, abdominal injuries are highly associated with multisystem trauma, particularly TBI and chest injuries. They carry high risk of exsanguination from blunt organ injury as well as transection of major mesenteric vessels. Late mortality from abdominal injuries is caused by infection from spilled abdominal contents into the peritoneum at the time of injury.[136]

- Diaphragmatic injury carries an extremely high morbidity and mortality and is associated with trauma to other chest structures. It is commonly the result of penetrating trauma; blunt injuries occur from sudden rises in intraabdominal pressure (at the time of impact) resulting in a "blowout" type of injury. It is more common on the left side because the liver "splints" the diaphragm on the right side. Diaphragmatic tears allow intestinal structures to enter the mediastinum, impeding respiration, contaminating the mediastinum, and causing severe pain. Late complications are the result of infection and inflammation of the mediastinum and include severe ARDS, pulmonary contusion, and infection.[136]
- Esophageal rupture is most commonly caused by penetrating trauma and usually involves the cervical esophagus; blunt esophageal injuries are extremely rare. Stomach contents escape into the mediastinum, causing severe life-threatening infection, abscess, empyema, fistulas, and ARDS. If definitive treatment is delayed, mortality is very high and is usually related to paraesophageal contamination and infection.[136]
- Splenic injury is the most common injury resulting from blunt trauma mechanism, although it is frequently affected with penetrating trauma of the left upper quadrant. Although the ribs protect from injury, they also may be the source of injury. Increasing injury severity is categorized by grades I through V: grade I implies a subcapsular, nonexpanding hematoma, grade V describes a completely shattered, hemorrhaging spleen. Isolated, low-grade splenic injury carries low mortality risk.[136] Conversely, high-grade injuries and those associated with multisystem injuries carry much higher risk of death. The initial threat to mortality is from uncontrolled hemorrhage.[60,136] Late mortality is a result of postsplenectomy sepsis, which can occur from 1 to 5 years after removal of the spleen; because

of the lifelong threat of infection for patients who have undergone splenectomy, the surgical team will make every effort to salvage, rather than remove, this organ.[60,136]

- Liver injury is a high risk following both blunt and penetrating injury because of its size and location in the right upper quadrant. Liver injuries carry high mortality rates when associated with other severe injuries. Increasing injury severity is described as grades I through VI: grade I describes a subcapsular, nonexpanding lesion involving a less than 10% surface area that may not require surgery. Grade V describes a large laceration involving at least 50% of a hepatic lobe with injuries to vascular structures around the liver. Grade VI describes complete hepatic avulsion.[136] Life-threatening blood loss is common when major vascular structures (e.g., the portal vein, hepatic artery, or hepatic vein) are involved, and significant coagulopathies develop when the injured liver cannot synthesize coagulation proteins necessary for hemostasis. Hypothermia and refractory acidosis are common challenges in resuscitating patients with high-grade liver injuries.[60] Later complications include ARDS, ATN, infection, hemobilia, hyperpyrexia, biliary fistula, arterial-portal venous fistula, difficulties with nutritional support due to altered liver metabolism, and liver failure.[60,136]

- Pancreatic injuries do not pose early threats to survival unless the splenic artery is involved. Although uncommon, most are caused by penetrating trauma; blunt injuries are the result of direct blows to the epigastric area.[100] Diagnosis of pancreatic injury is difficult and often delayed because of its proximity to other injured organs, particularly the spleen and the C-loop of the duodenum. As a consequence, prolonged spillage of highly caustic pancreatic enzymes contaminates the peritoneum, and subsequent pancreatitis is well established before injury is discovered. Major pancreatic complications such as pseudocyst, abscess, and sepsis are common.[100,136] The profound systemic inflammatory process associated with pancreatitis causes common complications of ARDS and left-sided pleural effusions.[100]

- Small-bowel injuries are common and caused by penetrating and blunt trauma although they are more common with penetrating mechanisms. There is an especially high incidence of duodenal injuries in high-speed MVCs when a patient wearing only a lap belt is thrown violently forward against the restraint and sustains an anterior lumbar spinal fracture (Chance fracture). Blood loss with small-bowel injuries is usually insignificant. However, shearing and penetrating injuries open the intestinal lumen, allowing spillage of intestinal contents into the peritoneum, peritonitis, and infection. Complications include hypovolemia secondary to third spacing and infection.[100,136]

- Large-bowel injuries are associated with extremely high mortality as a result of spillage of intestinal contents with high bacterial counts into peritoneum. The transverse colon is the most commonly injured because of its location, and is associated with lap-belt injuries. Blood loss is usually insignificant. Continued infection from ruptured bowel is managed by diverting colostomy.[136]

- Renal injuries are often associated with low posterior rib fractures and abdominal injuries. Technically in the retroperitoneum, avulsion of the kidney from its vascular pedicle and ureters is common in high-speed acceleration-deceleration crashes. The kidney is set in motion on its pedicle in relation to the more stable aorta; rotation around the pedicle tears the renal artery or vein and may cause renal artery thrombosis.[153] Renal contusion and fractures are seen with assaults and sports injuries. Penetrating injuries also are common. Ureteral trauma is usually caused by stretching when the kidney is compressed against the lower rib cage and upper lumbar spine.[79] Laceration of the ureter is also an iatrogenic event that occurs during surgery.[46] Although not usually a life-threatening injury in and of itself because most injuries are minor, mortality increases with injuries that extend deep into the renal cortex and medulla, and when ATN and renal failure develop as complications.[63]

Musculoskeletal Injuries

Most musculoskeletal injuries are not immediately life threatening, but many require prolonged recovery and result in serious disability. Injuries posing an immediate threat to life include those associated with significant blood loss and shock, such as traumatic amputations and massive pelvic fractures. Musculoskeletal injuries involve bone, muscles, tendons, ligaments, cartilage, nerves, blood vessels, and skin. The mechanism of injury is usually blunt trauma associated with MVCs, falls, assaults, and recreational injuries, but penetrating mechanisms seen with gunshot wounds (GSW) can result in significant bone and soft tissue injury. The direction and intensity of energy transferred to bones often influences the injury pattern (e.g., a patient landing on his feet after a fall from a significant height is likely to have fractures in both feet, calcanei, tibias, femurs, the pelvis, and the spine). Late complications and even death can result from infection that began when bacteria were introduced into open wounds accompanying fractures.[196]

An immediate limb-threatening complication is compartment syndrome, in which severe swelling and bleeding cause increased pressure and ischemic injury within a muscle compartment.[196] Burns and overly tight external splints also can cause compartment syndrome. The immediate inflammation following an extremity injury results in decreased distal blood flow and tissue hypoxia, release of inflammatory mediators, and permeability of capillary walls within the soft tissue. A vicious cycle of edema and ischemia is repeated and threatens limb viability.[159] Muscle ischemia occurs with intracompartmental pressures in excess of 30 to 40 mm Hg; irreversible muscle death occurs with pressures greater than 55 to 65 mm Hg.[159]

Another early complication occurring during resuscitation is fat embolism syndrome (FES). FES occurs in 3% to 4% of patients with long bone fractures and is thought to be caused by release of fat globules and inflammatory free fatty acids into the circulation. It can occur within 1 to 96 hours following injury, causing increased pulmonary capillary permeability, alveolar collapse, and hypoxia (Figure 42-10).[23,24]

- **Extremity injuries:** A fracture in which the skin integrity has not been broken is considered a closed fracture; any fracture associated with a wound is an open fracture. Fractures are classified based on the fracture line, whether the fracture line is oblique or comminuted, the anatomic location of the fracture, the type of displacement, and the position of displacement relative to bony fragments (Figure 42-11). Open wounds accompanying fractures increase the severity score of the fracture (Table 42-3). The incidence of significant infection increases for any fracture that does not receive irrigation and

debridement within 8 hours of injury. Bleeding associated with long bone fractures can be significant, with accumulations of blood from 500 ml (humerus fractures) to 3 L (femur fractures) in the surrounding soft tissues.[196]

- **Dislocation injuries:** Injuries to articulating joints are called dislocations. Joint movement is absent or limited and becomes unstable ("loose") when surrounding ligamentous structures are severely stretched or completely disrupted. Neurovascular structures are often injured, compromising sensation and perfusion of the distal extremity.[196] Subluxation injuries occur when only one portion of the articulating surface of a joint is disrupted. Neurovascular compromise often accompanies subluxation injuries, similar to dislocations.

- **Pelvic ring fractures:** Pelvic ring fractures are the third most common cause of death following MVCs, largely because of associated significant blood loss and injuries to neighboring organs. The pelvis has a large vascular network of collateral arterial and venous structures; disruption of the pelvic ring often involves laceration of multiple vascular structures and subsequent hemorrhage. Up to 6 L of blood can accumulate within the pelvis. The sciatic nerve, which innervates the pelvis and lower extremities, arises from the lumbosacral plexus and passes through the pelvis; injuries result in pelvic pain and decreased sensation in the lower extremities. Both the lower GI tract and genitourinary system have key structures that pass through the floor of the pelvis; fractures often perforate these structures, causing gross contamination and infection. FES (discussed later in this chapter) also contributes to mortality associated with pelvic fractures.[196]

- Two thirds of pelvic ring fractures are considered stable and non–life threatening, and are able to bear weight.[96] Although less common, unstable pelvic ring fractures are accompanied by hemorrhage, genitourinary trauma, sepsis, and chronic pain, and carry the potential for lifelong disability. Mortality from these injuries increases with open wounds and may be as high as 70% especially if puncture of the rectum or vagina has occurred.[205]

- A result of high-energy forces, the most common type of pelvic injury occurs when the anterior sacrum is crushed and the anterior pubic rami are displaced. This exerts pressure on the greater trochanter, disrupting the pubic rami into the anterior acetabulum. Even though these injuries are often considered stable, there may be significant soft tissue injury. An "open book" fracture occurs when a break of the symphysis pubis

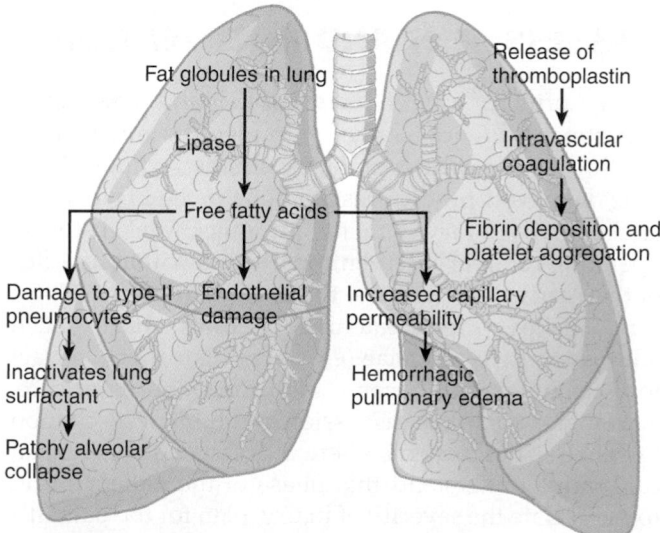

Fat globules in lung

Lipase

Free fatty acids

Release of thromboplastin

Intravascular coagulation

Fibrin deposition and platelet aggregation

Damage to type II pneumocytes

Endothelial damage

Increased capillary permeability

Inactivates lung surfactant

Hemorrhagic pulmonary edema

Patchy alveolar collapse

♦FIGURE 42-10 Pathophysiology of fat embolism syndrome.

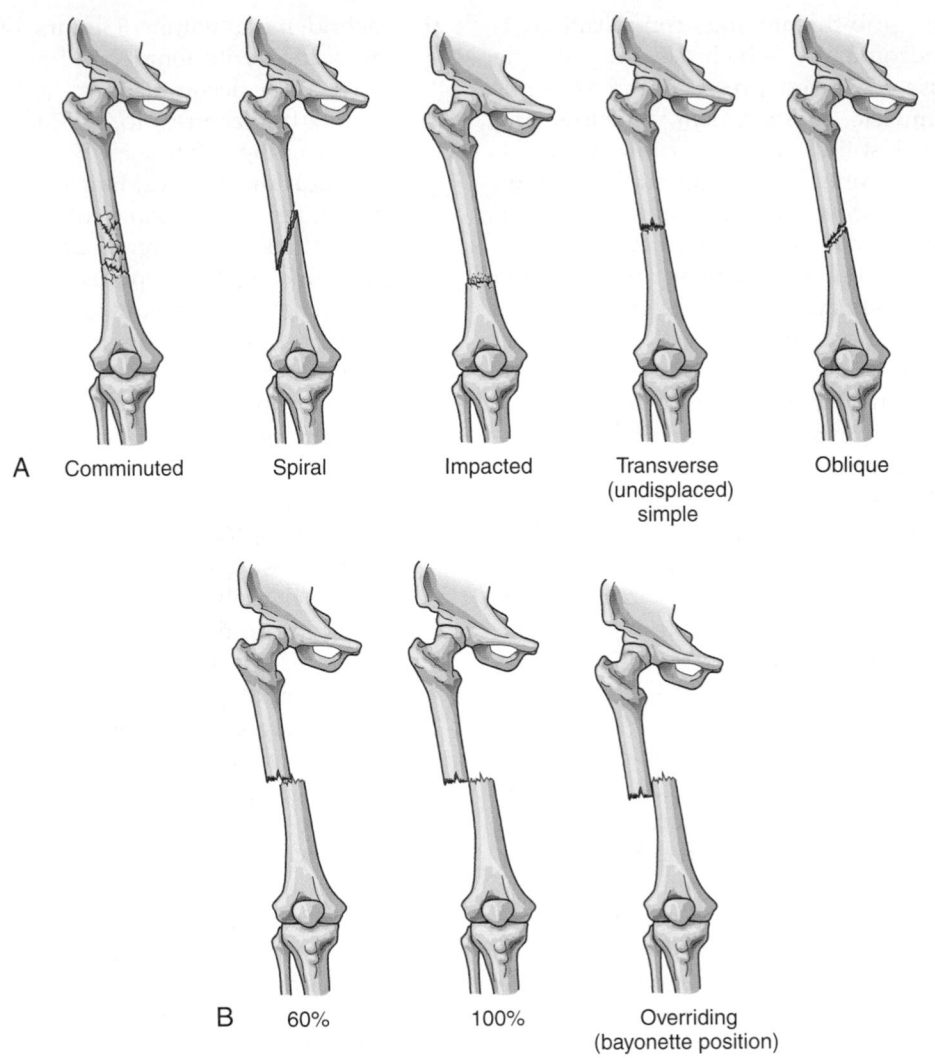

A Comminuted   Spiral   Impacted   Transverse   Oblique
                                        (undisplaced)
                                           simple

B   60%   100%   Overriding
                          (bayonette position)

♦FIGURE 42-11   A, Types of fractures. **B,** Degree of displacement.

occurs in conjunction with rupture of the anterior sacroiliac and sacrospinous ligaments.[196] Malgaigne fractures are unstable injuries involving both bone and soft tissue disruption and are the result of significant vertical shearing forces, such as those seen with falls and crush mechanisms. These fractures have the highest morbidity and mortality rates because of the high incidence of associated injuries to GI and genitourinary organs, as well as to vascular and neurologic structures.[96] Immediate complications of these injuries include hemorrhage, pain from muscle spasms and overriding bone ends, decreased venous and lymphatic return, increased swelling, neurovascular injury, and fat embolism. Long-term complications of pelvic fractures include chronic pain, decreased mobility, painful ambulation, and infection.[196]

ASSESSMENT AND INTERVENTION

The primary role of prehospital and emergency department (ED) personnel is to identify immediately life-threatening injuries and intervene accordingly. Multiple diagnostic procedures are done in the ED to locate and quantify injury; patients are quickly taken to the operating room or interventional suites within minutes of their arrival. By the time the patient arrives in critical care, major life-threatening injuries have been addressed; their sequelae (e.g., persistent shock, refractory coagulopathy) become the primary focus of care. Although a complete discussion of trauma resuscitation in the ED is not presented here, it is essential that critical care nurse understand this phase of the patient's care to appreciate the severity of injury, plan for the patient's admission, anticipate complications, and be aware of diagnostic procedures that may still need to be done.

TABLE 42-3 Classification of Fractures With Open Wounds

TYPE	DESCRIPTION
I	Wound less than 1 cm Moderately clean, minimal contamination Fracture—simple transverse or oblique with skin pierced by bone spike Minimal soft tissue damage
II	Wound greater than 1 cm Moderate contamination Fracture—moderate comminution/crush injury Moderate soft tissue damage (flaps or avulsions)
III	High degree of contamination Fracture—severe comminution and instability Extensive soft tissue damage involving muscle, skin, and neurovascular structures Traumatic amputation
III A	Soft tissue coverage of fracture is adequate Fracture—segmental or severely comminuted
III B	Extensive injury to or loss of soft tissue, periosteal stripping, and exposure of bone Massive contamination Fracture—severe comminution
III C	Any open fracture associated with arterial injury that must be repaired regardless of degree of soft-tissue injury

Modified from reference 183a.

The Emergency Nurses Association Trauma Nursing Core Curriculum and the American College of Surgeons Advanced Trauma Life Support course use primary and secondary surveys to guide systematic and organized assessment and treatment of injuries.[5,55] An "ABCD" mnemonic is used to prioritize care: "Airway-Breathing-Circulation-Disability." In critical care, nurses should perform a primary and secondary survey whenever a patient decompensates to identify problems and initiate further resuscitation.

PRIMARY SURVEY

The primary survey identifies life-threatening problems of the ABCDs, keeping in mind their trauma etiology (Box 42-7). Problems identified during the primary survey are treated before progressing to the secondary survey.[8,55]

Airway

Airway and breathing are top priorities for the trauma patient. Assessment and treatment of the airway are done while maintaining cervical spine immobilization. Inability to speak suggests a compromised airway. Common causes of airway obstruction include blood, vomitus, loose teeth, other foreign bodies, facial and mandibular fractures, and swelling of the tongue and facial soft tissues. The jaw thrust–chin lift maneuver is used to initially open the airway and inspect for obstruction. Nasal airways may be inserted in obtunded patients without evidence of facial trauma. Oral airways may be used in unconscious patients, but in most cases rapid-sequence intubation will be needed to secure a definitive airway. Occasionally, airway problems require surgical management (needle cricothyrotomy or emergent tracheostomy). Surgical airways are performed only in the prehospital or emergency setting for patients in extreme distress with high probability of significant anoxic insult. Performing either of these two procedures in an emergent situation can be challenging because of the presence of severe swelling and blood in the operative field.[8,55]

Breathing

Once the airway is secured, adequate oxygenation and ventilation must be assessed. Breathing is assessed by observing for spontaneous respirations, symmetry and depth of chest movement during respiration, respiratory rate (RR), pattern of breathing, use of accessory muscles, and auscultation of breath sounds. Skin color, thoracic bruises and wounds, chest wall tenderness, and the presence of neck vein distention or tracheal deviation also should be assessed. The patient with effective breathing should receive high-flow oxygen with a nonrebreather mask; the patient with ineffective or absent breathing should be supported with bag-valve-mask ventilation using an attached oxygen reservoir system until endotracheal intubation can be achieved. Life-threatening injuries that compromise breathing (e.g., tension pneumothorax, open pneumothorax, flail chest with pulmonary contusion, and hemothorax) require definitive intervention such as needle thoracostomy and chest tube placement.[8,55]

Circulation

Once the airway and breathing dynamics have been addressed, the circulatory system needs to be assessed. Cardiopulmonary resuscitation is indicated for the trauma patient without a palpable carotid pulse. Hemorrhage is the most common cause of shock in the trauma patient, although shock can also exist from

---

Box 42-7

Primary Survey for Trauma

Assessments	Interventions

A = Airway With Simultaneous Cervical Spine Stabilization or Immobilization

While maintaining spinal stabilization:

• Vocalization	• Position the patient
• Tongue obstruction	• Jaw thrust or chin lift
• Loose teeth or foreign objects	• Suction or remove foreign objects
• Bleeding	• Oro/nasopharyngeal airway
• Vomitus or other secretions	• Cervical spine stabilization
• Edema	• Endotracheal intubation
	• Needle or surgical cricothyrotomy

B = Breathing

• Spontaneous breathing	• Supplemental oxygen
• Chest rise and fall	• Bag-valve-mask ventilation
• Skin color	• Needle thoracentesis
• General rate and depth of respirations	• Chest tube
• Soft tissue and bony chest wall integrity	• Nonporous dressing taped on 3 sides
• Use of accessory and/or abdominal muscles	
• Bilateral breath sounds	
• Jugular veins and position of trachea	

C = Circulation

• Pulse general rate and quality	• Direct pressure over uncontrolled bleeding sites
• Skin cilor, temperature, degree of diaphoresis	• Two large-bore intravenous catheters with warmed lactated Ringer's solution or normal saline
• External bleeding	• Infuse fluid rapidly with blood tubing
	• Blood sample for typing
	• Pneumatic antishock garment
	• Pericardiocentesis
	• ED thoracotomy
	• Cardiopulmonary resuscitation and advanced life support measures
	• Blood administration
	• Surgery

D = Disability (neurologic status)

• Level of consciousness (AVPU)	• Perform further investigation
• Pupils (PERL)	• Hyperventilation, if indicated

From reference 58a.
AVPU = Alert, verbal, responsive to painful stimuli, responsive to verbal stimuli, PERRL = pupils equal, round, and reactive to light.

---

cardiac tamponade or blunt cardiac injury (cardiogenic shock), tension pneumothorax (obstructive shock), or spinal cord injury (neurogenic shock). The patient is assessed for tachycardia, hypotension, narrowed pulse pressure, poor peripheral pulses, cool and clammy skin, pallor, and any obvious signs of bleeding. An altered mental status, abnormally flattened neck veins or distended neck veins, and distant heart sounds also are signs of shock in the trauma patient. Uncontrolled external bleeding is managed by application of direct pressure to the bleeding site, elevation of a bleeding extremity, and application of pressure over proximal arterial pressure points; tourniquets should

be used only as a last resort when bleeding cannot be stopped and operative control is not immediately available.[55]

All trauma patients should receive two large-bore peripheral intravenous catheters; patients in shock should also receive at least one large single-lumen central venous catheter for rapid infusion of blood and resuscitation fluids. Fluids should be warmed to prevent hypothermia.[8,55,75,175] Uncrossmatched blood (O negative for females, O positive for males) may need to be given for the patient who is exsanguinating and cannot wait for typed and crossmatched blood products (refer to Chapter 36).[8,57] Pneumatic antishock garments are rarely used today but may be used for intraabdominal or pelvic hemorrhage.[55]

Emergency resuscitative thoracotomy (ERT) for cardiac arrest following trauma may be required if vital signs do not return. The role of ERT is controversial and hotly debated. In the face of spiraling healthcare costs, no trauma team is comfortable initiating a procedure that may save a previously healthy young patient's life, but result in a persistent vegetative state due to prolonged anoxia. While usually done in the ED, on occasion the procedure may be performed in critical care when a trauma patient decompensates despite ongoing resuscitation. In general, patients who have not yet suffered cardiac arrest despite severe cardiovascular collapse, patients demonstrating progressive bradycardia and persistent hypotension refractory to inotropic support and fluid resuscitation, and patients unresponsive to bilateral chest tube placement and needle pericardiocentesis may benefit from ERT.[11] Additional considerations for initiating ERT in the moribund patient include the location and mechanism of injury, signs of life at the scene and on ED admission, presence of cardiac electrical activity at thoracotomy, and systolic blood pressure (BP) response to aortic cross-clamping. Several policies restrict ERT to patients exhibiting electrical cardiac activity or who have sustained thoracic wounds.[11]

ERT has the best chance for successful outcome with penetrating trauma where pericardial tamponade was quickly relieved. It is of little benefit in blunt trauma patients. Successful resuscitation occurred in only 1% to 2% of patients following blunt trauma, regardless of whether vital signs were noted at presentation.[161] For patients with penetrating noncardiac injuries, 18% were resuscitated if they presented with hypotension and detectable vital signs and only 5% were salvaged if they presented without signs of life.[1,11,81,161] ERT is futile in blunt trauma patients requiring prehospital cardiopulmonary resuscitation (CPR) for more than 5 minutes and in penetrating trauma patients with more than 15 minutes of CPR.[81]

ERT allows for decompression of pericardial tamponade and control of bleeding from cardiac wounds via digital occlusion or hemostatic pledgets. Intrathoracic hemorrhage is controlled by direct pressure, application of clamps, and suture ligation. Control of massive air embolism and bronchopleural fistulae is achieved by placing a pulmonary hilar cross-clamp, vigorous cardiac massage, and aspiration of the aortic root and left ventricle for air. Should the heart chambers be empty from exsanguinating intraabdominal hemorrhage, the descending thoracic aorta is cross-clamped and blood flow redirected to the myocardial vessels and brain via manual cardiac massage. If a systolic pressure of 70 mm Hg is obtained, then the patient is rapidly transported to surgery for definitive management of the injuries.[11,81,161]

Disability

A brief neurologic assessment is performed once the airway, breathing, and circulation have been established and life-threatening injuries have been addressed. It is not practical to perform a thorough exam during aggressive resuscitation, nor is it likely to be accurate. A Glasgow Coma Scale (GCS) score and pupillary size and reaction are all that is needed during initial resuscitation. A head computed tomography (CT) exam is required for any patient with a GCS score of 12 or who experiences a decrease in their GCS of more than 2 points.[25] Pupillary size, symmetry, and reaction to light will help identify which side of the brain is injured. Alcohol and other drugs may affect the pupillary exam as well as the overall neurologic assessment.[8,57] Further neurologic assessment is deferred to the secondary survey. If the patient demonstrates any neurologic decompensation, short-term hyperventilation may be considered until the patient receives more definitive treatment during the secondary survey and in the operating room (OR).[25]

SECONDARY SURVEY

Once life-threatening injuries have been identified and treated, a thorough secondary survey is performed to identify and manage remaining injuries. A thorough head-to-toe assessment is performed, clothing must be removed, and hypothermia must be prevented by using warmers, warming blankets, and warmed IV fluids.[175] A full set of vital signs are obtained, including BP, HR, RR, and temperature (T); BP should be performed in both arms if the patient sustained trauma to the chest. Electrocardiogram monitoring, pulse oximetry, and end-tidal carbon dioxide (CO_2) monitoring are initiated.[55]

A Foley catheter is placed to monitor urine output unless contraindications are noted (e.g., blood at the meatus, blood in the scrotum, or suspicion of an anterior pelvic fracture). A gastric tube is placed to prevent aspiration of stomach contents; gastric tubes cannot be nasally placed in patients with severe facial fractures. Laboratory studies including blood typing, hematocrit (Hct), Hgb, coagulation studies, electrolytes, glucose, blood urea nitrogen (BUN), creatinine (Cr), blood alcohol, toxicology screen, arterial blood gas (ABG), BD, or serum LA should be sent; blood or urine should be sent for pregnancy tests for female patients of childbearing age.[55]

A full history of the incident is obtained, along with the patient's medical history, if known. Particular attention should be given to the patient's tetanus immunization history, allergies, and preexisting medical conditions. A full head-to-toe assessment, as described in Box 42-8, is performed. Assessment of

Box 42-8

Secondary Survey for Trauma

E = Expose Patient/Environmental Control (Remove Clothing and Keep Patient Warm)
- Remove clothing
- Blankets
- Warming lights

F = Full Set of Vital Signs: Five Interventions Facilitate Family Presence
- In addition to obtaining a complete set of vital signs
- Consider the five interventions:
  - Cardiac monitor
  - Pulse oximeter
  - Urinary catheter if not contraindicated
  - Gastric tube
  - Laboratory studies
- Facilitate family presence

G = Give Comfort Measures
- Verbal reassurance
- Touch
- Pain control

H = History
- Mechanism of injury, injuries sustained, vital signs, treatment (MIVT)
- Patient-generated information
- Past medical history

H = Head-to-Toe Assessment

Head and face	• Inspect for wounds, ecchymosis, deformities, drainage from nose and ears; check pupils. • Palpate for tenderness; note bony crepitus, deformity.
Neck	• Remove the anterior portion of the cervical collar to inspect and palpate the neck. Another team member must hold the patient's head while the collar is removed and replaced. • Inspect for wounds, ecchymosis, deformities, and distended neck veins. • Palpate for tenderness; note bony crepitus, deformity, subcutaneous emphysema, and tracheal position.
Chest	• Inspect for breathing rate and depth, wounds, deformities, ecchymosis, use of accessory muscles, paradoxical movement. • Auscultate breath and heart sounds. • Palpate for tenderness; note bony crepitus, subcutaneous emphysema, and deformity.
Abdomen and flanks	• Inspect for wounds, distention, ecchymosis, and scars. • Auscultate bowel sounds. • Palpate all four quadrants for tenderness, rigidity, guarding, masses, and femoral pulses.
Pelvis and perineum	• Inspect for wounds, deformities, ecchymosis, priapism, blood at the urinary meatus or in the perineal area. • Palpate the pelvis and anal sphincter tone.
Extremities	• Inspect for ecchymosis, movement, wounds, and deformities. • Palpate for pulses, skin temperature, sensations, tenderness, and deformities; note bony crepitus.

I = Inspect Posterior Surfaces

Posterior surface	• Maintain cervical spine stabilization and support injured extremities while the patient is log-rolled. • Inspect posterior surfaces for wounds, deformities, and ecchymosis. • Palpate posterior surfaces for tenderness and deformities. • Palpate anal sphincter tone (if not performed previously).

From reference 58b.

pain and sedation should also occur, which is often difficult in the confused or unresponsive patient. Of special note, providing analgesia in new trauma patients can be a challenge: although minimizing pain is important, the presence of pain helps identify injuries. During assessment, smaller doses of analgesics and sedatives may be given; full doses of these agents then can be given following identification of all injuries.[18]

Finally, additional diagnostic tests may be performed as part of the secondary survey to gather more information about injury location and severity. Cervical spine x-rays are done immediately on admission to the ED in patients involved in MVCs, auto-pedestrian collisions, and falls to identify atlanto-occipital dissociation, a lethal injury (suggesting additional resuscitation would be futile), and any other cervical injuries. The chest x-ray will identify lethal pulmonary injuries and correct placement of chest tubes and central venous catheters. A fast abdominal ultrasound for trauma (FAST) or diagnostic peritoneal lavage (DPL) assesses for bleeding in the hemodynamically unstable patient with likely abdominal injuries (Figure 42-14, p. 1166).[90] A flat plate of the pelvis is done should no life-threatening hemorrhage be located in the chest or abdomen.[8,55] Head CT scan is deferred until the patient is hemodynamically stable, and may be done en route to the critical care unit following surgery. Magnetic resonance imaging (MRI) scans to identify spinal cord injury must be delayed until the patient is completely hemodynamically stable; if the patient's neurologic exam suggests cord involvement, then a methylprednisolone infusion may be started prior to the MRI to control cord edema and secondary inflammation.[25] Extremity and facial films are taken once the patient is stable and considered safe to spend the several hours necessary in radiology to obtain all of the requested x-rays at one time.[178]

Early interventions for non–life-threatening injuries may be initiated during the secondary assessment. These basic interventions may include application of ice, splinting and elevation of fractures, administration of tetanus toxoid, and provision of emotional support and comfort. Repeated assessments of vital signs are important to determine resuscitation status and the need for additional interventions and diagnostic workup.[55] Following initial stabilization and identification of injuries, the patient may be admitted to critical care for continued resuscitation or taken to surgery or interventional suites for initial repair and hemorrhage control.

Definitive surgical repair is frequently not done on patients during their first trip to the operating room. "Damage control" surgery is the rapid termination of an operation following control of life-threatening hemorrhage and contamination.[171] These abbreviated operations are performed in patients with unresolved metabolic failure characterized by severe hypothermia, persistent acidosis, and coagulopathy refractory to surgical control. Time is of the essence because these patients are more likely to die from prolonged surgery and intraoperative metabolic failure than from the failure to finish definitive organ repairs.[28,137,138,142]

There are three stages of damage control.[65,171] During the first stage the operation is limited to control of hemorrhage and contamination. Conservative management of solid organ injuries may occur, along with resection without reanastomosis for major GI injuries and control of major vascular injuries in the trunk and extremities. Exploratory laparotomy, exploration of a hemorrhaging extremity, and packing of organs or spaces to control coagulopathy are also performed during the first stage.

The second stage occurs in the critical care unit, where priorities include vigorous rewarming, restoration of normal cardiovascular function, correction of clotting abnormalities, and supportive care for stunned lungs and kidneys. During the third and final stage of damage control, definitive surgical repair, identification of previously missed injuries, and incision closure occur. Trauma patients may return to surgery many times for follow-up to their initial operation. Each visit to the OR presents additional physiologic stresses from anesthesia and associated hypotension.[65,171]

Assessment and Intervention of Specific Injuries

Assessment and intervention of specific organ injuries involves multiple components, including the initial physical exam, laboratory results, and diagnostic procedures followed by surgical and nonsurgical interventions. A detailed discussion of every injury is beyond the scope of this text but is summarized in Table 42-4.

EARLY CRITICAL CARE RESUSCITATION

On arrival in critical care, the patient is settled and priorities for continued resuscitation established. A quick primary and secondary survey should be done on admission to establish a critical care baseline and allow comparison to what was seen in the ED. Clinical assessment of the patient's color, skin temperature, vital signs, urine output, wound and drain output, and bleeding should be frequently repeated. Assessment and care priorities during the initial hours of critical care are described in the Multidisciplinary Plan of Care on pp. 1167-1170.

TABLE 42-4 Assessment and Intervention of Specific Organ Injuries

ASSESSMENT	INTERVENTION
Brain Injury	Addressed in Chapter 22
Spinal Cord Injury	Addressed in Chapter 24

Facial Injury

Highly associated with brain and cervical spine injuries. Initial concern is for airway patency, requiring intubation and mechanical ventilation until swelling resolves and operative repair complete. Anticipate massive facial swelling; patient may be unrecognizable to family.

- Zygoma and orbital floor fractures: ecchymosis, tenderness along lower orbital rim, enophthalmos, and decrease in the height of the zygoma compared with the opposite side. Palpate for irregularities of the supraorbital and infraorbital ridges, depression of the zygomatic arch. Possible restriction in upper eye movement from entrapment of facial muscle in fracture line and associated damage to facial nerve. Assess visual acuity, pupillary response, full range of eye movement, and conjunctiva for hemorrhage or ruptured globe
- Mandibular fractures: assess for pain, subungual hematoma, offset of the bite, inability to open or close the jaw, pain with chewing.
- LeFort maxillary fractures: assess for facial asymmetry, swelling, and ability to breathe through the nose. Palpate for crepitus, tenderness, and irregularity along bony prominences. Gently manipulate the maxilla to assess for abnormal motion. Epistaxis and/or CSF may be present. Alterations of vision, smell, facial sensation should be assessed. Evaluate range of motion to determine cranial nerve involvement. Diplopia or dysconjugate gaze also may be present.

- Priorities of care are to protect the airway and stop hemorrhage. If injuries are not immediate threats to airway, breathing, and circulation, definitive operative repair is delayed.
- Photographs of the patient can help guide the surgeons during facial reconstruction.
- Tracheostomy is often required.
- Fractures are repaired using fixation devices, plates, and screws. Soft tissues are repaired with muscle, adipose, and vascular grafts.
- If the jaws are wired, wire cutters and suction should be kept at the bedside to clear the airway and mouth in the event of vomiting.
- Head of the bed should be elevated to help minimize swelling.
- Because the face so strongly influences self-image, provision of psychological support is essential to help patients tolerate the emotional sequelae to their injury.

Chest Injuries

A general inspection of the chest will help focus detailed assessment for specific injuries. Important to fully expose the chest to adequately assess for injuries. Observe and palpate all surfaces, looking for contusions, steering wheel marks, seatbelt marks, open wounds, bony asymmetry. Palpate for crepitus and unstable bone fragments. Assessment for upper abdominal bruising and wounds is necessary because organs extend to both compartments.

- Pneumothorax, hemothorax: respiratory distress or dyspnea, use of accessory respiratory muscles, loss of breath sounds on the affected side, increased tympany on the affected side for pneumothorax, but dullness to percussion with hemothorax. Patient may be anxious or confused. Cyanosis is a late sign of impaired oxygenation and ventilation. Subcutaneous emphysema over the chest wall may be palpated. Pain may be present from associated rib fractures. Decrease in oxygen saturation. ABGs reflect a fall in Pao_2 and a rise in $Paco_2$. A CXR is required to definitively determine whether blood or air occupies the pleural space. Signs and symptoms of hypovolemic shock with massive hemothorax (1.5–4 L of intrathoracic blood loss). Both can progress to tension pneumothorax unless treated.

- High-flow oxygen via nonrebreather mask or bag-valve-mask device. Airway support and intubation may be required.
- Emergent decompression accomplished with insertion of 14- to 16-gauge needle into pleural space at 2nd–4th intercostal space, midclavicular line will allow immediate escape of accumulated air.
- Chest tube placement at 4th or 5th intercostal space, midaxillary line with a 36 French tube will facilitate removal of air and blood from the pleural space.
- Additional chest tubes may be required if ventilation does not improve; bilateral chest tubes are quickly placed in severely compromised patients even before the specific side of injury is identified.
- Patient may require surgery if bleeding is excessive without signs of stopping (see Figure 42-12). Postinsertion CXR identifies placement of the tube and whether the lung(s) have reexpanded.
- Following placement, continually assess respiratory effort (if unintubated) or ventilator inspiratory pressures and exhaled tidal volumes (if intubated) for reaccumulation of pneumothorax, hemothorax, or tension pneumothorax.
- Medicate patient for pain during insertion and afterward because chest tubes are extremely uncomfortable.
- Dress chest tubes according to hospital policy and procedure. Document amount and characteristics of drainage.

ASSESSMENT	INTERVENTION
• Tension pneumothorax: same as for simple pneumothorax or hemothorax, but has progressed to the point of cardiopulmonary collapse. Early signs may be masked by shock and other injuries until significant tension pneumothorax has developed. Neck veins distended unless the patient is profoundly hypovolemic. Breath sounds decreased bilaterally, tracheal deviation, hypotension, tachycardia. CVP, PA, and PAWP will be elevated with dampened waveforms. If the patient is mechanically ventilated, high inspiratory pressure and low exhaled volume alarms will sound.	• Airway is obtained with endotracheal intubation with a standard ETT or tracheostomy. Double-lumen ETTs allow double lung ventilation: the uninjured lung is ventilated while ventilation to the affected lung is blocked. • Persistent pneumothorax, tension pneumothorax, and mediastinal air may require additional chest tube placements. • Care must be taken to not dislodge the ETT to prevent hypoxia, asphyxia, or reinjury of the bronchus. • Thoracotomy may be indicated if there is no air movement.
• Tracheal bronchial tears: dyspnea, hemoptysis, mediastinal subcutaneous emphysema, airway obstruction, difficulty with intubation, pneumothorax unresolved after chest tube insertion, tension pneumothorax. If chest tube present, persistent pleural air leak will be noted in the drainage collection unit; increases in amount of bloody drainage or size of air leak require immediate notification of the physician. CXR demonstrates early and significant atelectasis from blood and secretions obstructing the bronchus. Air embolism is manifested by sudden cardiovascular collapse without signs of bleeding and a change in level of consciousness.	• Diagnostic bronchoscopy will identify size and location of injury and determine needed repairs. Surgical repair is required for larger tears; small tears can be managed by stenting the bronchus with an ETT so that air movement is distal to the site of the tear. • Tension on postoperative incisions must be avoided; use gentle suctioning and manipulation of the head and neck. • If air embolus suspected, patient should be placed in Trendelenburg position to facilitate collection of air in the left ventricle; the nurse should prepare to assist with cardiocentesis or thoracotomy for control of the air leak.
• Rib fractures. • Simple, single fractures: pain aggravated by breathing and coughing, tenderness to palpation over fracture site • Complicated fractures with multiple fractures or underlying lung injury: severe chest wall pain, pneumothorax, hemothorax, atelectasis from decreased cough and accumulation of secretions. Associated injuries to liver and spleen with lower rib fractures. Upper rib fractures associated with clavicular fractures and neurovascular neck structures.	• Ensure that airway is patent and breathing is adequate; support as necessary as described above. All rib fractures require good pain control, which may include intercostal nerve blocks, intrapleural narcotic administration, patient-controlled analgesia, and epidural analgesia. A TENS unit also may be applied to decrease pain. Adequate analgesia is essential so that the patient tolerates the aggressive pulmonary care needed to prevent atelectasis and pneumonia. • Mechanical ventilation may be required if underlying pulmonary injuries are present.
• Flail chest: common triad of symptoms includes severe pain with respiration, accumulation of secretions, and ineffective ventilation from paradoxical (e.g., asymmetrical) chest wall movement during respiration). Respiratory distress, tachypnea, decreased oxygen saturation, hypoxia, respiratory acidosis, tachycardia, cyanosis, and crepitus.	• Flail chest injuries require definitive airway control, adequate analgesia, and oxygen. • Stabilization of the flail segment can be accomplished by placing the patient on the injured side, but is contraindicated if spinal injuries have not been ruled out. Internal "splinting" of the fractures is achieved using positive pressure ventilation. Internal fixation to stabilize the fracture is rarely required, but if necessary is accomplished by wiring bone fragments together or inserting metal plates. • Sedation and analgesia may be required in order to synchronize respiratory effort with the ventilator cycle and prevent unnecessary movement of the fractures. • Aggressive pulmonary care to include postural drainage, light percussion, and suctioning is necessary to prevent atelectasis and ventilator-associated pneumonia.
• Pulmonary contusion: during initial resuscitation, there may be respiratory distress, Pao_2 less than 60 mm Hg on room air, infiltrates on CXR, and bloody sputum. In critical care, CXRs show persistent patchy infiltrates and the sputum may have old blood, clots, or fresh blood. Wheezing may be evident, along with increased work of breathing. If the patient is mechanically ventilated, pulmonary compliance worsens, inspiratory and peak airway pressures increase, and Pao_2 falls despite appropriate ventilator changes.	• Oxygen therapy may be adequate initially, but early mechanical ventilation is required for adequate gas exchange. Severe contusions may require high-frequency ventilation or inverse I:E ventilation to minimize secondary inflammatory injury from barotrauma. • Aggressive fluid resuscitation necessary to achieve hemodynamic stability has been associated with severity of pulmonary contusion. Continued fluid administration should be carefully guided by monitoring of clinical and hemodynamic parameters in patients with persistent shock and pulmonary contusion.

Table continues on page 1162

ASSESSMENT	INTERVENTION
	• Meticulous pulmonary care is needed to clear the lungs of bloody secretions, clots, and pieces of dead tissue.
	• Continued monitoring of oxygen saturation, blood gases, capnography, and pulmonary compliance guides subsequent ventilator management.
• Cardiac tamponade: chest bruising and mechanism of injury suggest potential for immediate or delayed tamponade. Symptoms include distended neck veins, hypotension, narrowed pulse pressure, pulsus paradoxus, flattened hemodynamic waveforms, and rapidly falling cardiac output despite resuscitation.	• In the case of sudden or progressive decompensation, emergent needle pericardiocentesis may be required in the critical care unit (Figure 42-13). Following this, the patient will be taken to surgery for thoracotomy for identification and repair of the source of bleeding.
	• An emergency pericardiocentesis tray should be kept at the bedside for any patient at high risk for tamponade (e.g., high-force blunt injury to the sternum, penetrating trauma involving the myocardium, patients who had pericardotomy during their initial surgery).
• Thoracic aorta injuries: associated findings suggestive of these injuries include a pulse deficit in extremities, particularly the left arm; hypotension unexplained by other injuries, upper extremity hypertension compared with lower extremities, sternal pain, precordial or interscapular systolic murmur, hoarseness, dyspnea or respiratory distress, and lower extremity neuromuscular or sensory deficit. CXR demonstrates a widened mediastinum and requires confirmatory angiogram. Some institutions use a dynamic helical CT scan as the confirmatory test because it carries less risk than angiography. Following surgery or stenting, graft failure may present with increased bloody chest tube drainage, sudden hypotension, and high-pressure alarms on the ventilator. Monitor for postoperative complications such as paraplegia, bowel ischemia, and renal failure because these common complications are a result of aortic obstruction from the dissection or cross-clamping of the aorta during surgery.	• Rupture requires initial resuscitation of the ABC and treatment of other life-threatening injuries. Massive fluid and blood resuscitation is often required.
	• Dissecting injuries may require aggressive resuscitation, but if surgery is delayed, strict medical control of the blood pressure to keep MAP under 90 mm Hg is necessary because hypertension extends the dissection.
	• Surgery or stenting is required to treat the aneurysm, and cardiopulmonary bypass is often used.
	• Postoperative critical care management includes continued resuscitation and blood pressure control and monitoring for multisystem complications if the patient was in shock for an extended period. Invasive hemodynamic monitoring, frequent ABGs, lactic acid and/or base deficit, hematocrit, and coagulation tests should be drawn frequently to guide resuscitation.
• Blunt cardiac injury: a history of blunt trauma to the chest, presence of chest wall bruising, and fractures of the sternum and ribs raise the index of suspicion for BCI; 12-lead ECG shows abnormalities in only half of patients with BCI. There is no definitive test for BCI; elevations in cardiac enzymes, particularly the CK-MB and troponin may be present in some patients, although the literature does not strongly support serial monitoring of these enzymes. Continuous ECG monitoring and close clinical observation are necessary for symptomatic ventricular dysrhythmias and conduction defects. Echocardiogram or multigated angiography may detect cardiac wall movement abnormalities with low SV and EF. Chest pain may mimic angina and be difficult to differentiate from chest wall tenderness.	• Support of oxygenation and ventilation should be provided as indicated by the patient's condition.
	• Dysrhythmias are treated according to ACLS standards.
	• SV and EF may require treatment with dopamine, dobutamine, and digitalis.
	• Care must be taken to avoid overresuscitation with fluids because this may cause right ventricular dilation, which adversely affects contractility.

Abdominal Injury

Knowledge of mechanism of injury essential for identifying injuries. A common preventable cause of death is unidentified abdominal trauma. Associated with severe head and chest injuries.

Diagnosis of abdominal injury is made by combining physical signs and symptoms with FAST DPL in unstable patients (see Figure 42-14), and abdominal CT scan in hemodynamically stable patients.

• Diaphragmatic injury: respiratory distress, decreased breath sounds on the affected side, auscultation of bowel sounds in the chest, hemodynamic instability, difficulty in passing gastric tube, and chest pain. CXR may show stomach or loops	• Support of respiratory function and hemodynamics as indicated. Care must be taken for chest tube placement on affected side to avoid perforation of the abdominal organs and contamination of the chest with intestinal contents. Emergent surgical repair is

ASSESSMENT	INTERVENTION
of bowel in the chest field. Often complicated by severe ARDS, pulmonary contusion, and infection. Identification of right-sided rupture often delayed as liver covers the diaphragmatic tear.	usually required, although repair of right-sided tears may be deferred in patients with stable hemodynamic and respiratory status.
• Esophageal rupture: acute signs include respiratory distress, CXR infiltration, pain at the site of injury that may radiate to the neck, chest, shoulders, or abdomen, dysphagia, and intraperitoneal fluid or air. CXR changes and signs of sepsis (fever, elevated WBC) may be first indications of a small esophageal rupture; therefore a high index of suspicion for esophageal rupture is important if the mechanism of injury suggests a possibility of this injury.	• Support of hemodynamic and pulmonary function. Emergent surgical repair is indicated. Continued observation for and management of infection. Mechanical ventilation may be required if mediastinitis has resulted from a tear in the upper esophagus.
• Splenic injury: LUQ pain, Kehr's sign (referred shoulder pain), and pain around the injury site. Hemodynamic instability may be present if bleeding is not contained within the subcapsular space. Diagnostic tests include FAST scan and DPL (Figure 42-14, p. 1166) for unstable patients and abdominal CT scan for stable patients.	• Low-grade splenic injuries may not require surgery when close observation in critical care for at least 24 hours is an option. When surgery is needed, efforts to salvage the spleen by packing or resection are made to preserve long-term immunocompetence. In the case of life-threatening hemorrhage from multiple abdominal sources, the spleen will be removed as a quick fix to control a known source of bleeding while other abdominal sources are identified. Vaccinations for postsplenectomy sepsis are required after the patient transfers to acute care and before discharge from the hospital.
• Liver injury: abdominal pain, distention, bruising over RUQ, and hemodynamic instability from hemorrhagic shock. Lower right rib fractures may be present. Frequent hematocrit and coagulation tests are essential if nonoperative management is chosen and postoperatively if surgery was required.	• Every effort is made to not take the patient to surgery for liver injury alone because mortality risk increases simply by having surgery. A transfusion threshold of 4 to 6 units of PRBCs in 24 hours is often the decision criterion for surgery. Aggressive fluid, blood, and blood component resuscitation with warming measures is indicated pre- and postoperatively for hemodynamically unstable patients. During surgery, packing or resection may be required to control hemorrhage. Multiple trips to OR may be required before bleeding is stopped and packs are removed.
• Pancreas: not usually an immediately life-threatening issue unless splenic artery is involved. Symptoms may be delayed for 24–72 hours until leakage of pancreatic fluids and bile cause fever, elevated WBC, a continued need for fluid support, and abdominal pain. Continued postoperative assessment for development of pancreatitis is important for early management of sepsis.	• Surgical debridement, bleeding control, resection, and placement of drains to manage pancreatic fluids are required. Distal pancreatectomy or pancreatic duodenectomy may be needed for major injuries. Postoperative management includes pulmonary and hemodynamic support as indicated by the patient's condition.
• Small and large bowel injuries: knowledge of mechanism of injury an important guide in locating injury. Predominant finding is abdominal pain with signs of peritonitis, but this may be delayed if injury is subtle. FAST scan is not sensitive to bowel injuries, but DPL is very sensitive to the presence of WBC, bacteria, and intestinal contents suggestive of disruption of bowel integrity. Postoperative monitoring includes observation for sepsis, fistula formation, small bowel obstruction, suture line breakdown, bowel ischemia, and short-gut syndrome.	• Patients are taken to surgery for exploratory laparotomy if bowel injury is suspected for debridement, primary closure, and ligation of bleeding vessels. Resection is warranted if tears are multiple or are in proximity to each other, for massive destruction, and for significant mesenteric vascular injury, causing ischemia to distal bowel. Diverting colostomy or ileostomy may be required. Antibiotics are essential. Enteral feeding may be initiated if feeding tube can be placed well below the injury site.
• GU injuries: associated with complex or open pelvic fractures. Bleeding at the urinary meatus; genital bruising and swelling; flank, abdominal, and lumbar rib pain; flank mass. Palpation over the flanks or suprapubic region may indicate extravasation of blood or urine. Inability to void voluntarily or place an indwelling catheter suggests lower urinary tract injuries. Evaluation for vaginal tears should be deferred until bleeding from severe pelvic fractures has stopped because positioning of the legs may result in exsanguinating blood	• Medical management varies widely and is dependent on location of injury. Definitive reconstruction of injuries is deferred until after the patient is stable from other life-threatening injuries.
	• Catheterization should be avoided if blood is present at the urinary meatus. Only one catheterization attempt should be made in patients with suspected GU trauma; if unsuccessful, a urologist should be called. Catheters or stents may be also placed by a urologist. Suprapubic catheter may be required to

Table continues on page 1164

ASSESSMENT	INTERVENTION

loss. Gross hematuria correlates with lower urologic injury; microscopic hematuria suggests minor injury and may not require further diagnostic workup.

- Major renal injuries present with palpable flank mass, gross hematuria, hemorrhagic shock, bruising over lower ribs, abdominal tenderness, or microscopic hematuria.
- Radiographic studies include KUB x-ray, intravenous pyelogram, retrograde urethrogram, cystogram, ultrasound, renal angiography, and CT scan. Reabsorption of urine in patients with bladder rupture results in hyperkalemia, hypernatremia, uremia, and acidosis.

divert urine from the injury if a catheter cannot be placed. Infection must be prevented with antibiotic coverage for both Gram-positive and Gram-negative bacteria.

Orthopedic Injuries

- Fractures: signs and symptoms of fractures include pain, bruising, swelling, and changes in movement and distal sensation. Angulation, shortening, deformity, crepitus, muscle spasm, and open wounds and abrasions also may be present. Changes in color and decreases in peripheral pulses and capillary refill time indicate involvement of vascular structures. Hemorrhagic shock may accompany femur and pelvic fractures. Diagnostic studies include anterior and posterior plain x-rays. Inlet and outlet views are done for pelvic ring fractures.

- Long bone fractures require initial immobilization with splints, elevation, and application of ice packs to minimize swelling. Surgery for debridement and placement of external fixation devices is delayed until after the patient is hemodynamically stable.
- Pelvic fractures with severe hemorrhage may require PASG, external wrapping of sheets around the pelvis, or external fixation to control bleeding. Definitive control of hemorrhage is most often achieved via angiographic embolization.
- Antibiotics are indicated for any open wound or fracture requiring open fixation.
- Hemodynamic support, as indicated, for life-threatening hemorrhage associated with orthopedic injury.

- Traumatic amputations: signs of hemorrhagic shock are the hallmark presentation of amputations along with pain. Assess for wound infection. Postoperative assessment following reimplantation involves monitoring of color, temperature, swelling, bleeding, and sensation of the affected extremity.

- Fluid resuscitation as guided by physiologic and laboratory parameters. Efforts at reimplantation are considered in the context of "life-over-limb"; the patient's life should be salvaged even at the cost of sacrificing a limb. Care of the patient with a reimplanted limb includes pain control, elevation of the extremity, and a warm and humid room to promote vasodilation. Occasionally, medicinal leeches may be applied to remove venous congestion that is not drained by veins due to swelling.

- An early complication of orthopedic injuries that occurs even during resuscitation is compartment syndrome. Compartment syndrome presents as pain disproportionate to the injury and unrelieved by narcotics, numbness, and firmness to palpation. Early stages may present with rubor and bounding pulses, compensatory attempts to improve local blood flow. Coolness of the extremity, pallor, and decreased movement also may be noted. Late signs include loss of distal pulses and paralysis. When compartment syndrome is suspected or likely, slit and wick catheters connected to pressure monitoring systems may be placed within the muscle compartments to monitor pressures.

- Fasciotomy is indicated for intracompartmental pressures between 30–60 mm Hg. When patients are unconscious or unable to reliably describe pain and sensation, fasciotomy is usually recommended at lower compartmental pressures. Mannitol may relieve compartmental pressures by promoting osmotic diuresis. Fluid and blood resuscitation may be indicated following fasciotomy. Pain management and meticulous wound care are also essential.

- FES presents with sudden pulmonary and cardiovascular collapse. There is a transient appearance of petechiae about the trunk, face, mucous membranes, and conjunctiva. A rapid fever spike up to 40° C is a hallmark sign of FES. Lipuria (fat in the urine) and hematuria may be present. Thrombocytopenia as low as 50,000/mm^3 reflects platelet aggregation around fat globules. The diagnosis of FES cannot be made with laboratory tests or x-rays; it is a clinical diagnosis often made when there is no other explanation for the patient's sudden deterioration.

- Management involves hemodynamic and pulmonary support until FES resolves, and early fixation of fractures.

Data from references 5, 23, 24, 55, 90, 97, 103, 136, 153, 159, 164, 166, 178, 180, 196, 201, 204.
ABC = Airway, breathing, circulation, ABGs = arterial blood gases, ACLS = advanced cardiac life support, ARDS = acute respiratory distress syndrome, BCI = blunt cardiac injury, CK-MB = creatine kinase-myocardial bands, CSF = cerebrospinal fluid, CT = computed tomography, CVP = central venous pressure, CXR = chest x-ray, DPL = diagnostic peritoneal lavage, ECG = electrocardiogram, EF = ejection fraction, ETT = endotracheal tube, FES = fat embolus syndrome, GU = genitourinary, I:E = inspiratory: expiratory ratio, KUB = kidney, ureter, bladder, LUQ = left upper quadrant, MAP = mean arterial pressure, OR = operating room, PA = pulmonary artery, PaCO$_2$ = partial pressure arterial carbon dioxide, PaO$_2$ = partial pressure arterial oxygen tension, PASG = pneumatic antishock garment, PAWP = pulmonary artery wedge pressure, PRBCs = packed red blood cells, RUQ = right upper quadrant, SV = stroke volume, TENS = transcutaneous electrical nerve stimulation, WBC = white blood cell.

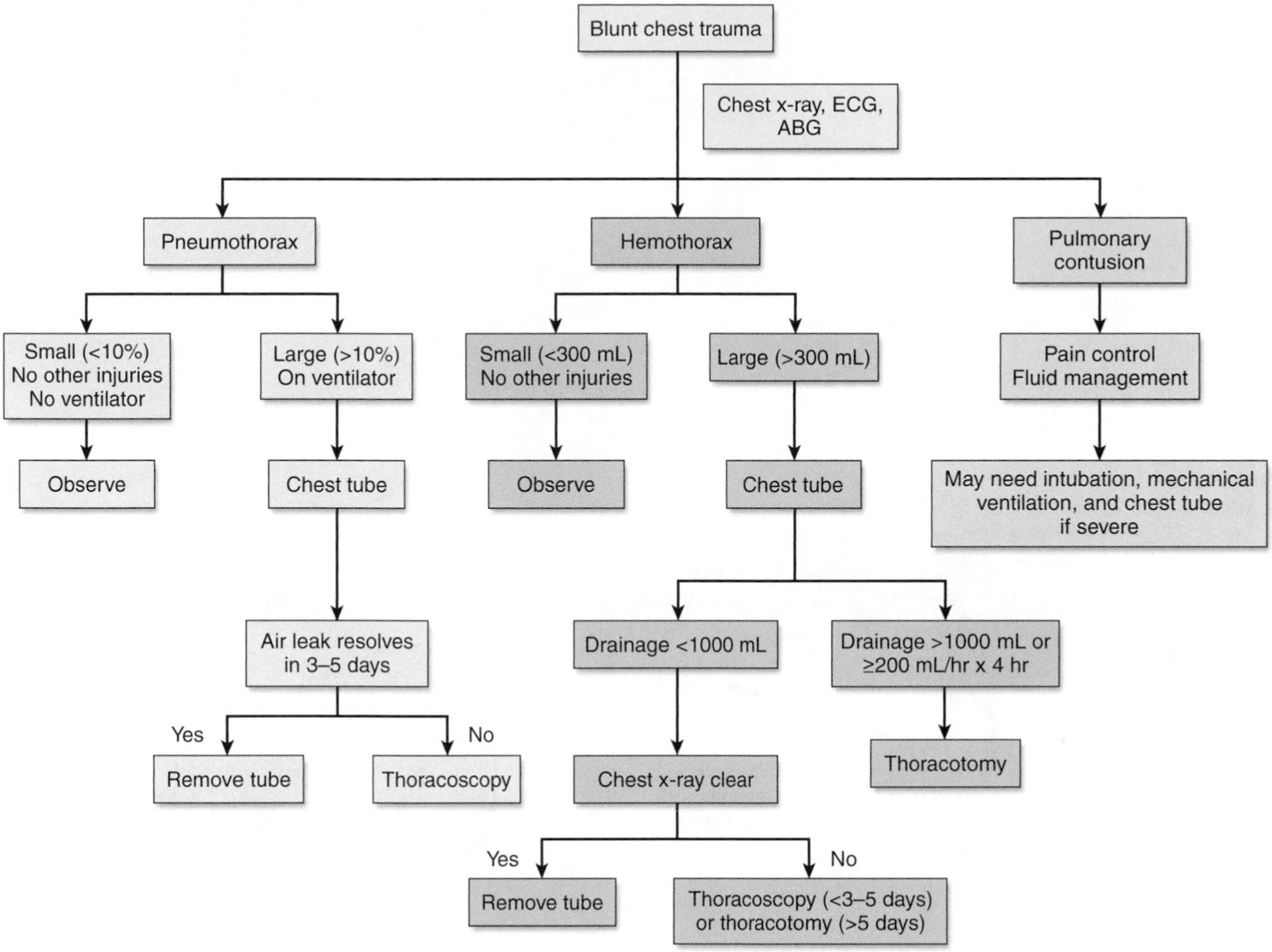

Blunt chest trauma
Chest x-ray, ECG, ABG
Pneumothorax
Hemothorax
Pulmonary contusion
Small (<10%) No other injuries No ventilator
Large (>10%) On ventilator
Small (<300 mL) No other injuries
Large (>300 mL)
Pain control Fluid management
Observe
Chest tube
Observe
Chest tube
May need intubation, mechanical ventilation, and chest tube if severe
Air leak resolves in 3–5 days
Yes
No
Remove tube
Thoracoscopy
Drainage <1000 mL
Drainage >1000 mL or ≥200 mL/hr x 4 hr
Thoracotomy
Chest x-ray clear
Yes
No
Remove tube
Thoracoscopy (<3–5 days) or thoracotomy (>5 days)

FIGURE 42-12 Blunt chest-trauma protocol. ECG = Electrocardiogram, ABG = arterial blood gas.

Neck veins distended
Brachial artery
Venous pressure elevated
Decreased arterial pressure and pulsus paradoxus
Brachial vein
45°
45°

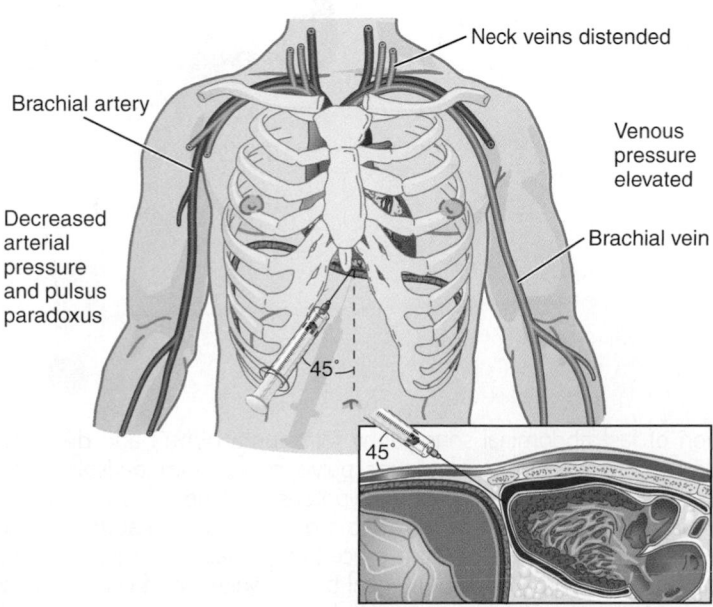

FIGURE 42-13 Needle pericardiocentesis for cardiac tamponade.

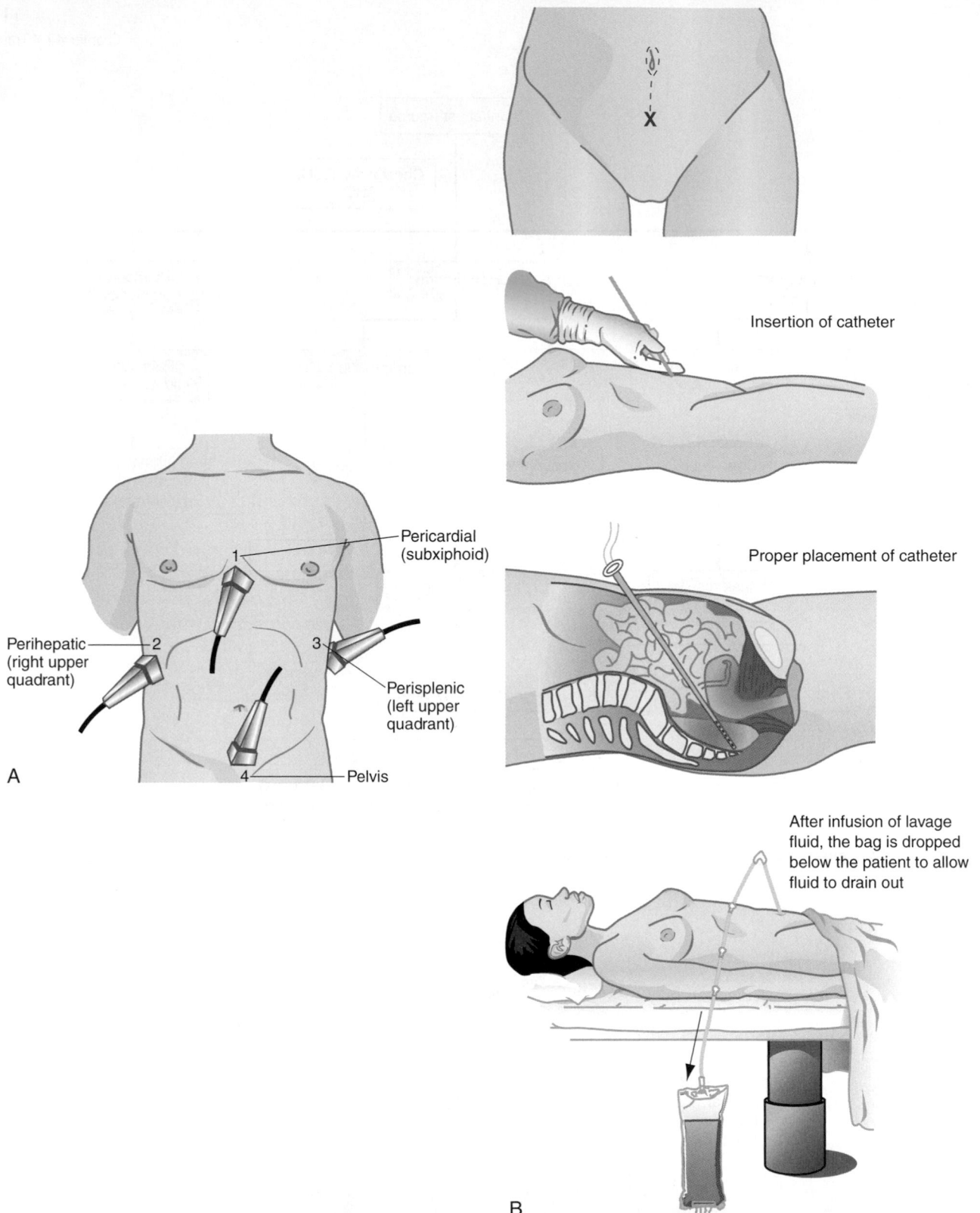

⬥FIGURE 42-14 Differentiation of fast abdominal sonography for trauma (FAST) and diagnostic peritoneal lavage (DPL) for abdominal trauma. **A,** A bedside FAST scan rapidly assesses the pelvis, pericardium, perisplenic, and perihepatic regions for fluid (blood) accumulation. Easily repeated in the event of sustained hypotension, it identifies location and volume of fluid but does not differentiate type of fluid. FAST is unreliable in patients with morbid obesity, multiple abdominal adhesions, ascites, or subcutaneous emphysema.[90,131,136,155] **B,** DPL is a simple, invasive procedure to diagnose intraabdominal hemorrhage or organ perforation. It is a very sensitive test for the presence of intraperitoneal blood, white blood cells, amylase, bacteria, fecal material, bile, and food particles, but it is not specific for the location or extent of damage. A small incision is made below the umbilicus, and warmed irrigating solution is infused using a peritoneal dialysis catheter. The solution is then allowed to drain via gravity, and a sample is sent to the lab for analysis. The stomach and bowel must be decompressed before the procedure to avoid inadvertent puncture of these organs.[27,90,136,139]

In figure A, labels read:
- Pericardial (subxiphoid) — 1
- Perihepatic (right upper quadrant) — 2
- Perisplenic (left upper quadrant) — 3
- Pelvis — 4

In figure B, labels read:
- Insertion of catheter
- Proper placement of catheter
- After infusion of lavage fluid, the bag is dropped below the patient to allow fluid to drain out

MULTIDISCIPLINARY PLAN OF CARE FOR ASSESSMENT AND CARE PRIORITIES DURING THE INITIAL HOURS OF CRITICAL CARE

PROBLEM	INTERVENTION	RATIONALE	EXPECTED OUTCOME	SPECIAL CONSIDERATIONS
Continued hemodynamic instability	• Continually assess for adequacy of resuscitation by evaluating multiple parameters to include HR, SBP, MAP, RR, temperature, and urine output. • Monitor hemodynamic parameters including CVP, PAWP, PA systolic and diastolic pressures, CO/CI, SVR, Svo_2, EDVI, SVI, Do_2I, Vo_2I, LVSWI, RVSWI. • Obtain baseline and repeated labs: ABG, lactic acid, base deficit, Hct, Hgb, platelets, INR, DIC screen, fibrinogen, electrolytes, and glucose. • Assist with placement of large central IV catheters for fluid and blood resuscitation. Place at least 2 large-bore peripheral IV catheters (if not already done). • Replace IVs started in the field as soon as possible. • Assist with placement of arterial catheter and PA catheter, if not already done. • Administer crystalloids, colloids, vasopressors, inotropes, blood and blood products as indicated by ongoing assessment and labwork. • Warm all fluids, blood, and blood products. • Assess for signs of ongoing bleeding: increased bloody output from drains, increasing abdominal circumference, increased bleeding from wounds. • Anticipate echocardiogram for sustained hypotension. • Repeat FAST or DPL. • Anticipate echocardiogram if hypotension sustained. • Assist with application of external fixator or wrapping of pelvis if source of bleeding is from a pelvic fracture. • Anticipate patient's return to OR or interventional suite to identify and control source of bleeding.	• Persistent hypoperfusion leads to multisystem organ failure. • Allows for rapid infusion of fluids and blood products. • Field IV starts are considered contaminated and should be restarted as soon as clinically appropriate to reduce the risk of IV-associated infection. • Prevents hypothermia, which causes coagulopathy and increases hemoglobin's affinity for oxygen. • Evaluates cardiac filling volumes and poor cardiac compliance as sources for hypotension. • Evaluates abdomen, pericardium, pelvis, perisplenic and subhepatic regions for accumulation of blood.	• Patient will have return of normal vital signs and other physiologic parameters. • Minimal or no organ dysfunction.	• Class I shock can persist even though vital signs and hemodynamic parameters have returned to normal. Therefore evaluation of multiple parameters is essential to determine the patient's resuscitation status. • Fluid resuscitation must be adequate before vasopressors are added. Overresuscitation of fluids can lead to pulmonary complications and abdominal compartment syndrome. • CT scans are contraindicated for acutely unstable patients suspected of abdominal bleeding.

Table continues on page 1168

PROBLEM	INTERVENTION	RATIONALE	EXPECTED OUTCOME	SPECIAL CONSIDERATIONS
Potential for pulmonary compromise	• Assess for compromised airway and plan for intubation as indicated by loss of consciousness, blood and secretions in airway, or inadequate respiratory effort. • Provide mechanical ventilation as indicated by ABGs and ventilator pressures. • Assess for development of ARDS (poor compliance, increased inspiratory pressures, refractory Pao_2 despite treatment, Pao_2/Fio_2 ratio less than 250. • Assist with placement of chest tubes for pneumothorax, hemothorax, tension pneumothorax. • Obtain chest x-ray to confirm endotracheal and chest tube placements.	• Hypoxia exacerbates any hypoperfusion and increases potential of multisystem organ failure and poor neurologic recovery. • ARDS occurs following inflammatory response to injury and is associated with resuscitation of large volumes of fluids. • Common causes of respiratory failure in trauma patients. Placement of multiple tubes is often needed.	• Adequate oxygenation and ventilation.	Bilateral needle thoracentesis is indicated for patients with known or suspected pulmonary injury who suddenly decompensate.
Potential for worsening injuries or missed injuries (refer to Chapters 22 and 24 for detailed information on traumatic brain injury and spinal cord injury).	• Repeat primary and secondary surveys on admission to critical care and whenever patient decompensates. • Perform neurologic exam every hour until the patient is awake; perform more frequently in patients with head injuries and ICP instability. • Maintain full spinal precautions with cervical collars and log-rolling until the spine is cleared of injuries. • Plan for full-spine x-rays (and MRI of cervical spine, if indicated), once patient is hemodynamically stable. • Obtain and/or repeat additional diagnostic tests, if not already done. • Cardiac enzymes, liver panel, alkaline phosphatase, amylase • Pregnancy and toxicology screens • 12-lead ECG for older adult patients, patients with preexisting cardiac disease, or with blunt cardiac injury • Portable x-rays of extremities	• Worsening or undetected injuries may be the source of continued hypoperfusion. • Subtle injuries requiring medical intervention are often discovered once life-threatening issues are under control • Head CT is performed once the patient is hemodynamically stable. Repeat CT may be indicated whenever a neurologic change occurs. • Sedation must be carefully administered and easily reversed so that neurologic exams are accurate. • Soft tissue (ligamentous) cervical spine injuries are often difficult to detect in unresponsive patients. • Assume injury is present by using cervical collars and log-rolling to maintain spinal alignment. • Establishes baseline data and determines whether patient is improving or getting worse. • Identifies injuries.	• All injuries will be identified and treated. • Prevents iatrogenic spinal cord damage until the patient is alert enough to cooperate with the exam.	

PROBLEM	INTERVENTION	RATIONALE	EXPECTED OUTCOME	SPECIAL CONSIDERATIONS
Pain and agitation (refer to Chapter 4).	• Provide analgesics and sedation as ordered.	• Pain and agitation increase oxygen consumption.	• Patients will report adequate pain control, if able; if unresponsive, physiologic manifestations of pain (tachycardia, hypotension, agitation) will be within normal limits. • Sedation will not interfere with reliable neurologic exam and allows patient to rest quietly in bed.	Evaluating for adequate pain control and anxiolysis is difficult in patients with neurologic injury. Do not assume that decreased LOC is due to oversedation or analgesics: evaluate any change in LOC with CT or good neurologic exam. Many patients have long-standing alcohol and drug abuse problems. If present, begin withdrawal prophylaxis protocols and obtain psychological consults as outlined by institutional policies.
Potential for psychosocial crisis and post-traumatic stress disorder	• Support family presence during resuscitation and invasive procedures. • Explain plan of care and critical care environment to patient and family. • Obtain early support from social worker and pastoral services. • Ask family to bring in pictures of loved one.	• Families cope better with crisis and/or patient death if able to be present during critical events. • Trauma patients often have prolonged recovery, requiring significant financial support to pay for large medical bills and long periods of unemployment. • Family dynamics and coping may decompensate under unexpected stress, such as trauma. • Many injuries are disfiguring, rendering the patient unrecognizable to family members. Pictures also help staff members identify the patient as a person with an active life and foster a relationship with patient and the family.	Patients and families will have effective coping and resolution of emotional stressors following trauma.	Early intervention provides the best chance of full psychosocial recovery.
Potential for complications and long-term care	• Participate in continued assessment of vital signs, hemodynamic measurements, neurologic assessments, laboratory tests, and other diagnostic procedures as indicated by clinical condition.	• Ongoing assessment identifies multisystem complications and problems before they become severe and/or irreversible.	• Complications will be identified and managed early. • There will be no long-term complications from underresuscitation.	Participation by multiple medical, nursing, and ancillary members of the healthcare team will be required for the critically ill trauma patient. Involvement is indicated by

Table continues on page 1170

PROBLEM	INTERVENTION	RATIONALE	EXPECTED OUTCOME	SPECIAL CONSIDERATIONS
			• Injuries will be identified and appropriately treated early in the hospitalization. • Discharge to home or rehabilitation facility.	specific injuries and may include, but is not limited to, consultation by specialists in neurology, neurosurgery, gerontology, orthopedic surgery, maxillofacial surgery, plastic surgery, vascular surgery, psychiatry, occupational therapy, physical therapy, nutritional support services, respiratory therapy.
	• Provide analgesia and sedation per protocol, including daily sedation holidays.	• Protocols for sedation and analgesia result in earlier weaning from mechanical ventilation.	• Patient is extubated as soon as possible when clinical condition allows. • No ventilator-associated pneumonia.	
	• Support nutritional needs within 3–4 days following injury; use enteral route if possible.	• Enteral nutrition supports overall gut immune function. Parenteral nutrition does not support the gut and is associated with increased complications such as infection.	• Daily nutritional requirements will be met with enteral nutrition until adequate oral intake is possible.	
	• Prevent DVT and PE using pharmacologic and mechanical interventions as indicated by injury pattern and clinical condition (refer to Chapter 9).	• DVT and PE are common and life-threatening complications in trauma patients.	• No DVT development. • Identified DVTs do not increase in size or mobilize to become PEs.	
	• Observe for infection. • Wound sites for drainage and redness • Fever • Elevated white blood cell counts • Purulent drainage in tubes and catheters • Sepsis or severe sepsis	• Infection in trauma patients is common due to wounds contaminated at the time of injury, perforating injury to abdominal organs, aspiration, surgical incisions, drains, catheters, tubes, invasive monitoring lines.	• Early identification and treatment of infections. • No infections.	
	• Promote early mobilization. Obtain early physical therapy and occupational therapy consults to develop patient-specific activity and rehabilitation plans.	• Minimizes pulmonary complications, supports skin integrity, enhances muscle function and growth, provides daytime activity so that patients can rest at night.	• No pressure ulcers. • Good muscle tone. • Return of range of motion. • Able to participate in ambulation as limited by injuries. • Patient is oriented and able to participate in rehabilitation.	

Data from references 2, 5, 8, 17, 18, 20, 25, 26, 31, 45, 50, 54, 55, 57, 58, 60, 70, 74, 100, 103, 109, 128, 144, 164, 166, 178, 180, 185, 192, 196, 203.
ABG = Arterial blood gas, ARDS = acute respiratory distress syndrome, CO/CI = cardiac output/cardiac index, CT = computed tomography, CVP = central venous pressure, DIC = disseminated intravascular coagulation, DO$_2$I = oxygen delivery index, DPL = diagnostic peritoneal lavage, DVT = deep venous thrombosis, ECG = electrocardiogram, EDVI = end diastolic volume index, FAST = fast abdominal sonography for trauma, FiO$_2$ = fraction of inspired oxygen, Hct = hematocrit, Hgb = hemoglobin, HR = heart rate, ICP = intracranial pressure, INR = international normalized ratio, LOC = level of consciousness, LVSWI = left ventricular stroke work index, MAP = mean arterial pressure, MRI = magnetic resonance imaging, OR = operating room, PA = pulmonary artery, PaO$_2$ = partial pressure arterial oxygen tension, PAWP = pulmonary artery wedge pressure, PE = pulmonary embolism, RR = respiratory rate, RVSWI = right ventricular stroke work index, SBP = systolic blood pressure, SVI = stroke volume index, SvO$_2$ = mixed venous oxygen saturation, SVR = systemic vascular resistance, VO$_2$I = oxygen consumption index.

Continued Resuscitation

Despite aggressive resuscitation in the ED and OR, during which time multiple liters of fluid and units of blood and blood components may have been given, the patient can still be in shock and require additional fluid resuscitation. Vasopressors may be added if the patient remains hypotensive despite adequate fluid resuscitation. Chapter 40 includes a detailed discussion of the use of crystalloids, colloids, and vasopressors for the resuscitation of hemorrhagic, neurogenic, and obstructive shock. Chapter 36 discusses the use of blood and blood components during the massive transfusion scenarios common in trauma. ABGs, LA, BD, Hct, and coagulation tests will help reveal the patient's metabolic state and to what extent that may be due to ongoing hemorrhage. These tests should be repeated frequently, at least as often as every hour, to stay current with the patient's resuscitation needs. The patient will probably return to the OR for surgical control of bleeding if persistent hypotension is believed to be caused by ongoing hemorrhage.

Using Hemodynamic Monitoring to Guide Resuscitation. Identifying optimal volume status and preload is difficult; a comprehensive review of hemodynamic monitoring in shock was addressed in Chapter 40 and will be discussed here only as it pertains to trauma. Traditional filling pressures such as central venous pressure (CVP) and pulmonary artery wedge pressure (PAWP) are measurements of *volume* under *pressure,* rather than specific volume measurements. Particularly in trauma, they are greatly influenced by many factors such as positive end-expiratory pressure (PEEP), pericardial tamponade, noncompliant myocardium, rigid chest or abdominal walls, ACS, and technical errors in measurement. A patient can be hypovolemic despite seemingly high filling pressures. Several studies suggest that these parameters are unreliable guides to determining volume status in trauma patients; using right ventricular end diastolic volume index (RVEDVI) better reflects preload in trauma patients.[33,49,132,195]

In one study, more than half of trauma patients demonstrated improved splanchnic perfusion when the RVEDVI was above $100 \, ml/m^2$.[33] In a different study, visceral perfusion occurred only after the RVEDVI was greater than $120 \, ml/m^2$, despite normal PAWP.[132] RVEDVI will not improve the cardiac index (CI) if pushed to more than $140 \, ml/m^2$ because the right ventricle is overstretched and loses contractile function.[49,195] RVEDVI is best used as a resuscitation target that tells the caregiver when additional volume will help improve the CI, and identifies the appropriate time to initiate inotropes.[33,49,171]

Caution must be used when interpreting RVEDVI values, and this parameter should not replace CVP or PAWP. These numbers are meaningful only if all are considered when determining the patient's volume status and cardiac function. When a patient requires additional fluid, the RVEDVI, CVP, PAWP, and CI should increase after a fluid bolus. However, if hypovolemia is not the source of the patient's hypotension, these numbers will not increase in concert with each other. For example, when fluid is infused into a noncompliant heart (seen with increased PEEP, myocardial edema, cardiac disease, and ACS), the stiff right ventricle does not stretch to accommodate the additional fluid. Increased hydrostatic forces push fluid into the pulmonary beds, and PAWP rises significantly, the RVEDVI may not change at all, and the CI decreases. In this scenario, the trauma patient's hypotension is not responsive to additional fluids and requires treatment with an inotrope to support cardiac output. Additional limitations of RVEDVI as a resuscitation parameter are addressed in Chapter 40.

Oxygen delivery index (Do_2I) and consumption index (Vo_2I) can supplement traditional pulmonary artery (PA) measurements and focus trauma resuscitation. Frequently, aberrations in all three components of oxygen delivery (cardiac output, hemoglobin saturation, and pulmonary function) can exist in the trauma patient. Analysis for the source of poor cardiac output, Hgb malfunction, and pulmonary dysfunction will identify the appropriate interventions to improve the Do_2I. Whereas normal Do_2I is $500 \, ml/min/m^2$, one study suggests that a Do_2I of $600 \, ml/min/m^2$ may improve outcomes.[125] Oxygen consumption levels can increase four to five times above normal in a critically injured trauma patient. Tachycardia, pain, agitation, shivering, posturing, and increased respiratory work will elevate oxygen demand beyond oxygen delivery. In late shock, oxygen use drops as cells are compromised and cannot extract oxygen from hemoglobin. Patients with abnormally high or low Vo_2I levels are not using oxygen at the cellular level and are in cellular shock.[144,173,192] Interventions to augment delivery and lower consumption in trauma patients to return the delivery-to-consumption ratio closer to the normal ratio of 4:1 are listed in Table 42-5.

PA catheters are not the mainstay of hemodynamic assessment in critically ill and injured patients that they once were because concerns over complication rates, measurement error, and variability in treatment called into question whether they positively affect morbidity and mortality.[37] Parameters measured with PA catheters do not measure cellular perfusion, the actual end point of resuscitation. Global and organ-specific parameters help clinicians assess end products of anaerobic metabolism. Global indexes (e.g., mixed venous oxygen saturation [Svo_2], LA, BD, and the difference between the $Paco_2$ and the mixed venous CO_2) reflect a mixing of oxygen debt from multiple

TABLE 42-5 Causes of and Interventions for Inadequate Oxygen Delivery and Consumption in Trauma Patients

INADEQUATE DELIVERY

CAUSES	INTERVENTIONS
Poor Cardiac Output	**Interventions**
• Hypovolemia	• Fluid resuscitation
• Blunt cardiac injury	• Blood product administration
• Pericardial tamponade	• Blood component transfusion
• Tension pneumothorax	• Inotropes for BCIs
• Cervical spine injury (neurogenic shock)	• Chest decompression
• Septic shock (late response)	• Vasopressors, once volume is adequate
• Liver shock (release of inflammatory mediators causing vasodilation)	• Pericardiocentesis
Hemoglobin Dysfunction	**Interventions**
• Hypothermia	• Rewarming
• Carbon monoxide poisoning (burns)	• Control of mechanical ventilation
• Decreased 2,3, DPG (from multiple blood transfusions)	• Limit blood product transfusions as soon as possible
• Alkalosis (cerebral hyperventilation)	• Give fresh PRBCs, if possible, to optimize 2,3 DPG function
	• High-flow oxygen
Pulmonary Dysfunction	**Interventions**
• Inadequate airway	• Airway control
• Pneumothorax, hemothorax, tension pneumothorax	• Oxygen administration
• Pulmonary contusion	• Mechanical ventilation
• Fat embolus syndrome	• Chest decompression
• Pulmonary embolus	• Bronchodilator therapy
• Bronchopleural fistula	• Antibiotics
• ARDS	• Suctioning
• Preexisting COPD	• Positioning
• Pneumonia	

INADEQUATE CONSUMPTION

CAUSES	INTERVENTIONS
Increased Consumption (Vo_2I >150 ml/min/m^2)	**Interventions**
• Tachycardia	• Support of ventilation
• Increased respiratory work	• Analgesics
• Brain injury	• Sedatives
• Pain	• Rewarming
• Agitation	• Paralysis
• Shivering	• Antipyretics, cultures, and antibiotics
• Posturing	• Anti-epileptic agents
• Seizures	• Coordinate nursing care to minimize oxygen needs
• Fever	• Tachycardia will improve if oxygen delivery is adequate
• Nursing care	
Decreased Oxygen Consumption (Vo_2I <100 ml/min/m^2)	**Interventions**
• Paralysis	• Evaluate and treat for refractory shock or sepsis
• Hypothermia	• Reverse induced paralysis if clinically indicated
• Deep sedation	• Rewarm
• Anesthesia	• Reverse anesthesia/deep sedation when clinically indicated
• Sepsis	
• Profound shock	

Data from references 144, 173, 192.
ARDS = Acute respiratory distress syndrome, BCIs = blunt cardiac injuries, COPD = chronic obstructive pulmonary disease, DPG = diphosphoglycerate, PRBCs = packed red blood cells, Vo_2I = oxygen consumption index.

vascular beds and quantify the patient's overall degree of hypoperfusion. They are influenced by a number of extraneous variables and are therefore more valuable as trended values than as isolated figures. Organ-specific parameters (e.g., gastric tonometry, sublingual capnometry, and near infrared spectroscopy) measure end-organ metabolic status because some organ beds remain underperfused despite global markers within normal limits.*

Ideally, the healthcare team should use multiple parameters and their interrelationships to guide resuscitation of the trauma patient. When considered together, traditional vital signs, hemodynamic targets, global end points, and organ-specific end points will identify the appropriate course of action. An important area for future research will be to determine whether goal-directed trauma resuscitation protocols improve patient outcome. A sample resuscitation protocol is illustrated in Figure 42-15.

Reversing the Lethal Triad of Hypothermia, Acidosis, and Coagulopathy

Hypothermia. Prompt reversal of hypothermia in trauma patients is a top priority because rewarming helps correct coagulation and returns the oxygen-hemoglobin dissociation curve to normal. Patients who are more rapidly rewarmed are more likely to survive resuscitation[77,78] Traditional active and passive methods for rewarming have been reserved for mildly hypothermic patients because they may take hours to rewarm a patient (see Box 42-6). Peripheral rewarming techniques warm the extremities and superficial body surfaces first, whereas core rewarming interventions use invasive techniques to warm the internal organs first. A thorough discussion of peripheral and core rewarming techniques is covered in Chapter 7. Continuous arteriovenous rewarming (CAVR), developed specifically for trauma patients, returns patients' body temperatures to 36° C within 39 to 180 minutes.[76,78] It is discussed in detail here.

CAVR uses a modification of the standard tubing used with the Sims Level 1 Rapid Infuser (Level 1, Inc., Rockland, Mass) (Figure 42-16). The tubing has a larger diameter to facilitate brisk blood flow, a T-connector side port for infusion of additional fluids and blood products, and a heparin-bonded interior surface to prevent blood from clotting without systemic anticoagulation. Blood is shunted from an 8.5 Fr femoral artery catheter through the warming chamber of the tubing and air filter. It is then returned to the patient's femoral, subclavian, or jugular vein through

a second 8.5 Fr catheter. CAVR requires a systolic blood pressure of at least 80 mm Hg to maintain a blood flow that will keep the system patent.[76] Less fluid and fewer blood products are required when compared with patients who receive standard rewarming measures such as warm blankets and IV fluids,[76] an important consideration when a patient has a life-threatening coagulopathy that in part is due to being cold. Nursing responsibilities during CAVR include frequent monitoring of temperature and hemodynamics along with checking to make sure that the system is patent. CAVR can be discontinued once the patient's temperature reaches 36° C, but the catheters should not be removed until the temperature remains stable for at least 2 hours and any coagulopathy has resolved. Because it is a self-driven circuit, it is not time intensive for the critical care nurse, making it a practical rewarming method during resuscitation.[78,174,175]

Acidosis. Trauma patients should undergo repeated ABG, LA, or BD testing to evaluate for severity and trend metabolic acidosis. A single value of either is not very informative, but repeated measurements over time better assess resuscitation progress. One study suggests that both parameters should be followed, if possible.[51] Practically speaking, if the LA or BD is worsening, then resuscitation activities need to be evaluated and revised. A full discussion about using LA and BD to guide resuscitation can be found in Chapter 40.

Treatment of metabolic acidosis includes reversal of the underlying source of shock; if the etiology of shock is controlled, the acidosis will be corrected. Multiple interventions should be initiated to improve oxygen delivery in trauma patients. The first is augmentation of preload using IV fluids to expand intravascular volume and red blood cell (RBC) transfusions to increase oxygen transport. Fluid resuscitation should be guided by several parameters, all of which are complementary (vital signs, urine output, PA pressures, CI, oxygen delivery and consumption, ABGs, LA and BD, Hct and Hgb). When the CI, Do_2I, and Vo_2I do not improve with additional fluids, vasoactive medications can be added to support cardiac output. Although vasopressor choice of varies among clinicians, epinephrine, dopamine (Intropin), and phenylephrine (Neo-Synephrine) commonly are used.[192] The patient should be warmed to facilitate oxygen off-loading of Hgb. Buffer therapy, such as sodium bicarbonate, is rarely justified because it does not treat the underlying cause of acidosis. Unfortunately, a paradoxical worsening of intracellular acidosis may occur as the bicarbonate binds with excess CO_2 associated with pulmonary compromise.[144] Shivering, anxiety, pain, and restlessness should be addressed to decrease oxygen demands in the face of impaired oxygen delivery.[173,192]

---

*References 6, 35, 36, 41, 80, 99, 124, 133, 173, 198.

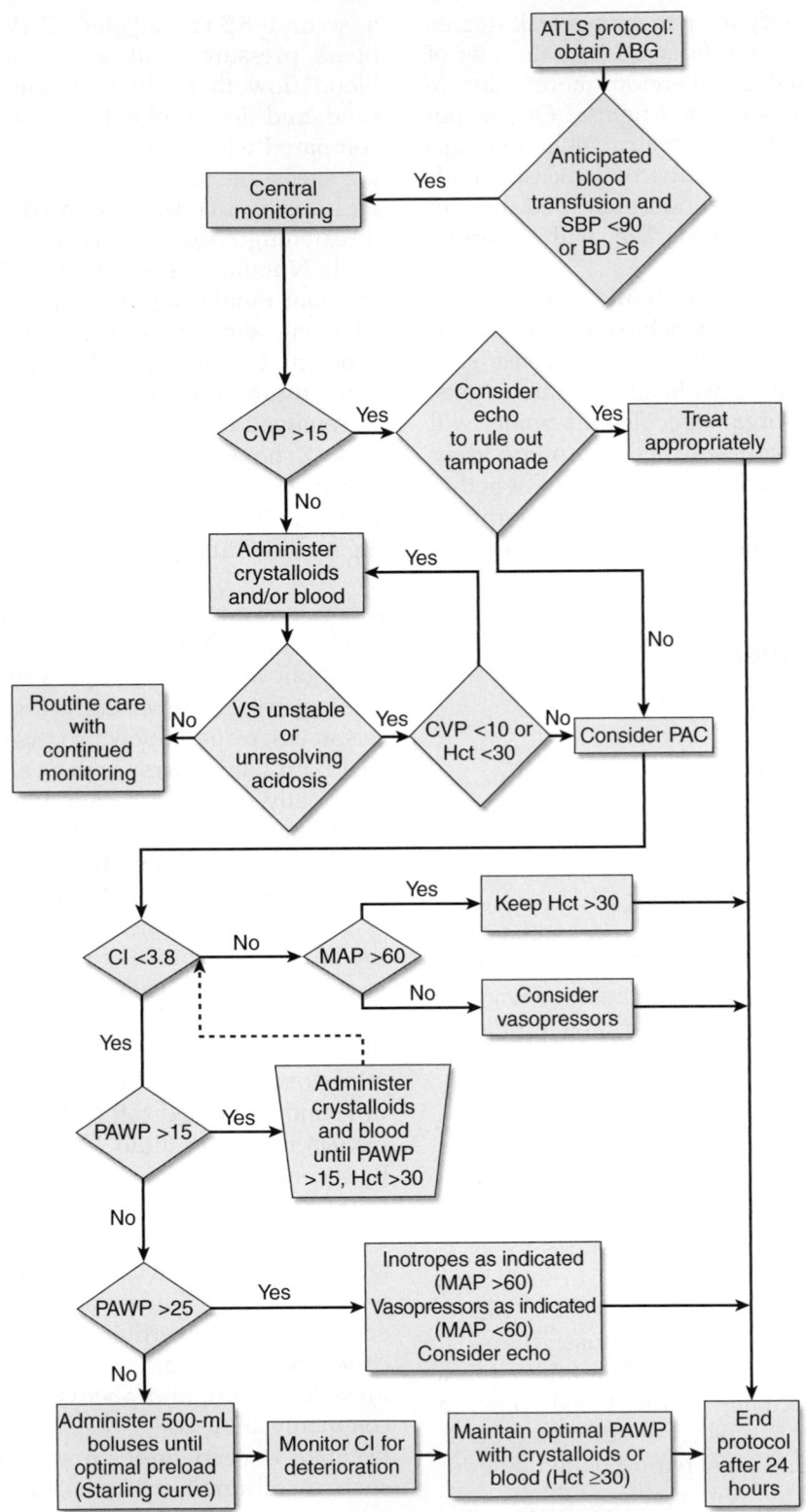

★FIGURE 42-15 Goal-directed resuscitation for trauma. ATLS = Advanced trauma life support, ABG = arterial blood gas, BD = base deficit, CI = cardiac index, CVP = central venous pressure, Hct = hematocrit, MAP = mean arterial pressure, PAC = pulmonary artery catheter, PAWP = pulmonary artery wedge pressure, SBP = systolic blood pressure, VS = vital signs.

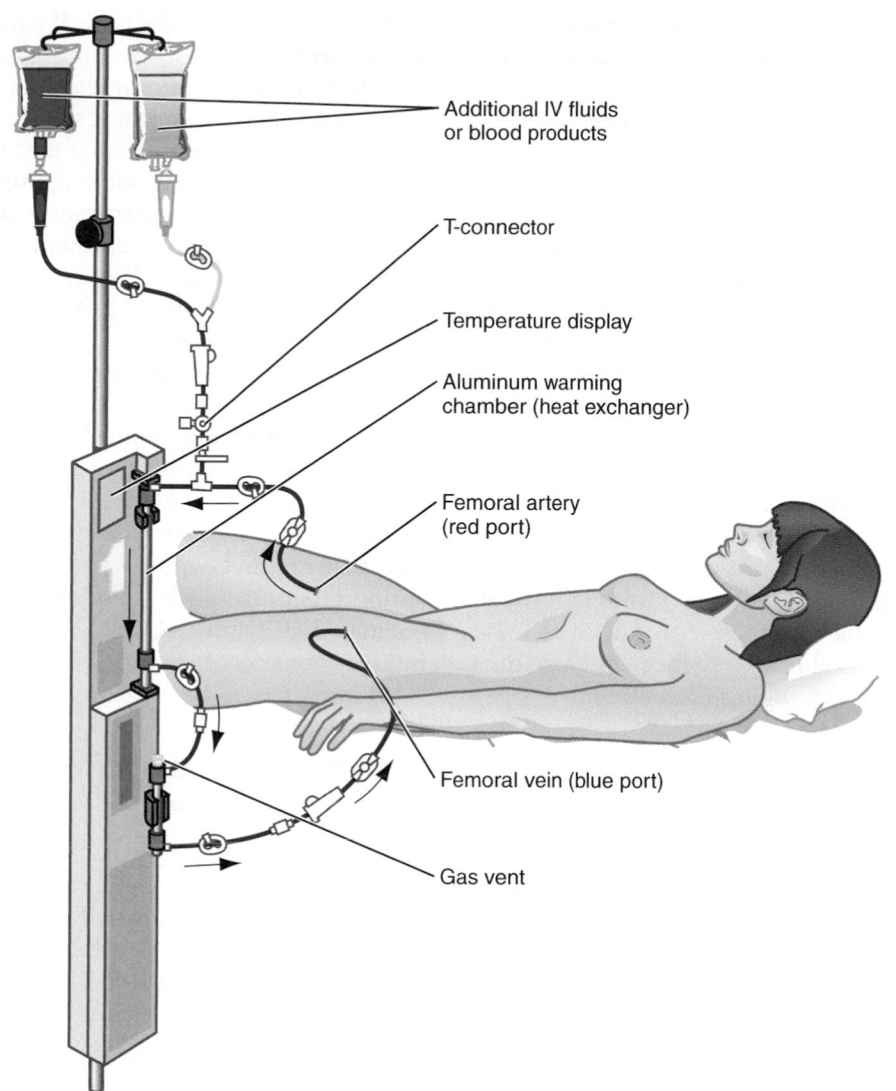

Additional IV fluids
or blood products

T-connector

Temperature display

Aluminum warming
chamber (heat exchanger)

Femoral artery
(red port)

Femoral vein (blue port)

Gas vent

⬥FIGURE 42-16 Continuous arteriovenous rewarming. Blood leaves the patient through a femoral artery catheter, passes through the aluminum warming chamber and gas vent before returning to the patient via a femoral (or jugular or subclavian) venous catheter. The circuit is powered by the patient's blood pressure.

Coagulation. The mainstay of coagulopathy monitoring is the clinical assessment of ongoing blood loss, either in the form of frank hemorrhage or diffuse oozing from cut surfaces, IV sites, surgical drains, or mucous membranes. The most beneficial lab studies with the fastest turnaround times include Hgb, platelet count, PT, aPTT, and fibrinogen.[54] These labs should be sent every 15 to 30 minutes for a patient with refractory hemorrhage. DIC screens, which include D-dimers and fibrinogen split products, provide useful information about the consumptive component of the coagulopathy but have long turnaround times that are often impractical during critical care resuscitation.[47]

Management of coagulopathy includes surgical control of hemorrhage, rewarming, reversal of

acidosis, and replacement coagulation factors. The current recommendation is to replace RBCs and coagulation factors based on actual lab values to conserve resources[47,144,192] At times, physicians may order blood products based on the clinical picture rather than wait for lab results and risk coagulopathy. When the laboratory cannot provide results quickly enough to keep up with excessive blood loss, platelets and plasma can be transfused while waiting for lab results. Plasma is indicated when the PT and aPTT are greater than 1.5 times laboratory control values and should not be used as a volume expander alone. Cryoprecipitate is indicated with fibrinogen levels less than 100 mg/dl. Platelets are infused when the platelet count is less than 50,000 in the presence of ongoing hemorrhage.[47,111] Complete discussions of blood replacement and management of coagulopathy can be found in Chapters 36 and 37.

Recombinant activated factor VIIa has been used to reverse traumatic coagulopathy. Historically used for treatment of patients with hemophilia and significant hepatic disease requiring surgery, a growing body of literature suggests it is successful in trauma patients.* Factor VIIa activates the extrinsic coagulation cascade by binding to exposed tissue factor at the site of injury. It is an attractive treatment alternative in trauma because it does not cause systemic hypercoagulability and bypasses the intrinsic coagulation system. It has a rapid onset and short half-life, with PT improvement within 5 minutes of IV administration; doses may be repeated one or two times until the rate of bleeding slows.[86,172]

New hemostatic dressings are used by the military to control hemorrhage following trauma. More research is needed before these products can be integrated into routine clinical practice, but preliminary results are very encouraging (Box 42-9).

Managing Abdominal Compartment Syndrome

Often the patient may be too unstable for the trip to the OR, and a decompressive laparotomy to relieve

---

*References 53, 88, 92, 98, 106, 118, 172.

ACS must be done in the critical care unit. The decision to perform a bedside decompression depends on a number of factors including the patient's age and underlying comorbidities, resources to support aggressive fluid resuscitation, confidence that the hypertension is caused by edema and not ongoing hemorrhage, and availability of surgical instruments and bedside cautery. Most clinical experts recommend that decompressive laparotomy is indicated only when significant cardiopulmonary compromise is present rather than as a response to a measurement.[69,95]

A high index of suspicion is critical for the early identification of ACS before it reaches a crisis point. Clinical examination alone does not consistently identify whether ACS is present. Intraaortic pressure (IAP) monitoring should be initiated in any patient with an inflammatory response causing capillary leak that requires volume resuscitation or vasopressor support because such patients are at risk for bowel edema, IAP, and ACS.[107,188] IAP monitoring and interventions for ACS are addressed in Chapter 39.

Identifying, Preventing, and Managing Rhabdomyolysis

Early identification of rhabdomyolysis is crucial and facilitated by having a high index of suspicion in patients with significant soft tissue crush or avulsion injuries. Patients with painful, swollen extremities following crush injuries should be monitored for rhabdomyolysis as well as compartment syndrome.[117] Dark

---

Box 42-9

Hemostatic Dressings

Dry fibrin sealant dressings	Dry, powdered human thrombin and fibrinogen compressed on a removable backing. Unlike fibrin glue used in the OR, this product requires no preparation, is stable at room temperature, and presents no infectious risk. When pushed into a wound, it coagulates on contact. The only limiting factor is that the product is dependent on adequate blood bank reserves because it is made from human blood.
Rapid deployment hemostat (RDH)	An acetylated poly-N-acetyl glucosamine dressing isolated from controlled aseptic, microalgal cultures. It is thought to work outside the coagulation cascade through red cell aggregate adhesion and vasoconstriction. FDA approval for its use in humans is pending.
Chitosan	A product made from shrimp shells, it is a biodegradable, nontoxic complex carbohydrate derivative of chitin. It is FDA approved and has been successfully used in military conflicts in the Middle East.
QuickClot	A granular zeolite that absorbs water and promotes clot formation. Because it contains no biological or botanical substances, it eliminates the danger of allergic reactions or disease transmission. A major drawback, however, is an exothermic reaction that produces heat when it absorbs fluids. The FDA has approved its use with external wounds.

Data from references 3, 89, 162, 194.
FDA = U.S. Food and Drug Administration, OR = operating room.

tea-colored urine that is dipstick positive for blood despite the absence of RBC on urinalysis suggests rhabdomyolysis is developing.[153] Serum creatine phosphokinase (CPK) levels are the quickest and least expensive screening test for rhabdomyolysis, but cardiac muscle must be ruled out as a source of the CPK elevation.[117] CPK levels are used instead of myoglobin levels because the results can be quickly obtained, are available in most institutions, and are relatively inexpensive.[183] A trigger for identifying and treating patients at risk for ARF secondary to rhabdomyolysis is a CPK level of 20,000 units/L.[117]

The primary goal of treating rhabdomyolysis is prevention of renal failure by early and aggressive resuscitation. This is accomplished by achieving hemodynamic stability without volume overload and maintaining urine output.[183] Large-volume resuscitation treats the hypovolemia and hypokalemia that contribute to rhabdomyolysis. Patients who receive large amounts of fluid before extrication have significantly better outcomes than those whose resuscitation was delayed.[9] Mannitol (Osmitrol) is given to diurese the patient and wash out tubular myoglobin, but can be used only when the patient is fully volume resuscitated and urine is being made. It also functions as a free radical scavenger and may therefore offer some renal protective effects.[207] Urine is alkalized with sodium bicarbonate to decrease cast formation and lessen myoglobin toxicity.[9] Large amounts of bicarbonate may be necessary to alkalize the urine to a pH of greater than 6.5.[117]

The source of inflammation and muscle necrosis causing the rhabdomyolysis may need to be removed. Crushed extremities may require early fasciotomy or amputation, forcing the trauma surgeon to sacrifice a limb in order to save the patient's life.[117]

Early signals of ARF include persistent hyperkalemia and acidosis despite volume resuscitation and bicarbonate administration. ARF from rhabdomyolysis is associated with poor outcomes in patients. Early initiation of continuous venovenous hemofiltration or daily hemodialysis to filter myoglobin and correct fluid overload and electrolyte abnormalities is recommended. These patients stand an excellent chance of full renal recovery if treated early and aggressively.[117]

A rhabdomyolysis treatment algorithm is provided in Figure 42-17. Additional research is needed to identify which specific interventions improve outcome.

Providing Analgesia and Sedation

Pain and anxiety contribute to morbidity and mortality in the critical care unit because they increase physiologic stress to an already compromised patient. Three general principles guide appropriate pain and sedation management of the trauma patient while in critical care. First, traumatic injuries are typically very painful, requiring aggressive analgesic therapy while avoiding hypotension. Analgesia should not be held for the painful patient with low blood pressure; rather, the blood pressure should be supported with IV fluids and, if necessary, vasopressors. This is frequently a challenge in the initial stages of critical care. Second, high injury severity often leads to lengthy stays in critical care and a prolonged need for sedation. Third, trauma patients often have a history of poly-substance abuse and are therefore at risk for potentially serious problems such as acute withdrawal syndromes and opioid and benzodiazepine tolerance.[115,184] A variety of opioid analgesics, anxiolytics, and antidelirium medications should be administered according to unit protocol. The critical care nurse plays a key role in ensuring that patients receive adequate pain control and sedation without physiologic compromise, as discussed in Chapter 4.

CRITICAL CARE MANAGEMENT OF COMPLICATIONS FOLLOWING TRAUMA

Following successful trauma resuscitation, multisystem sequelae and complications must be addressed (many of these considerations are addressed in other chapters in this book; those issues with especially unique considerations related to trauma are briefly discussed here).

Acute Respiratory Distress Syndrome

Originally known as "wet lung," "shock lung," and "Da Nang lung," ARDS was first recognized as a complication of hypotension associated with trauma. It is a secondary insult following injury, hypoperfusion, and resuscitation. Risk factors for ARDS associated with trauma include any type of shock, significant soft tissue destruction, direct pulmonary contusion, multiple orthopedic fractures, large-volume fluid resuscitation, multiple transfusions, aspiration, pneumonia, and major head injuries.[91,180,189] Critical care nurses must be alert for signs and symptoms of ARDS during resuscitation, in the days that follow initial resuscitation, and with any episode of sepsis. Clinical presentation and management of ARDS are discussed in detail in Chapter 19.

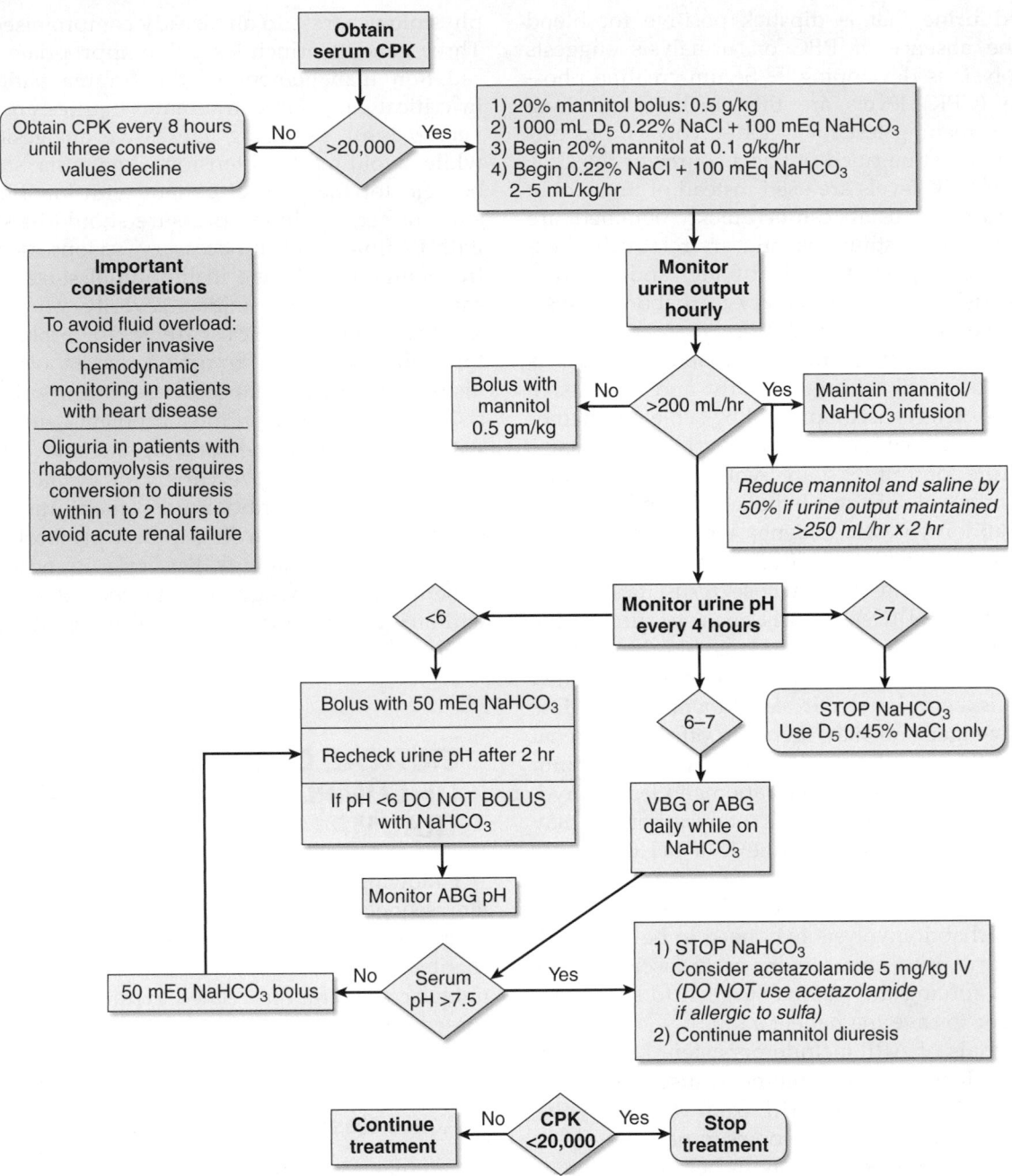

♦FIGURE 42-17 Treatment algorithm for patients with rhabdomyolysis. ABG = Arterial blood gas, CPK = creatine phosphokinase, NaHCO₃ = sodium bicarbonate, NaCl = sodium chloride, VBG = venous blood gas.

♦ Case Study 42-1, Part B

Determining Labs and Appropriate Diagnostic Tests

When R.O. arrived in the emergency department, primary and secondary surveys were performed. Her airway was patent, without foreign bodies or secretions in her mouth. Her breathing was rapid, with equal breath sounds bilaterally, although they were dim in both bases. Her skin remained cool and slightly diaphoretic, and vital signs (VS) remained unchanged despite the infusion of 2 L of warmed LR. She remained alert and oriented to person and place, with equal bilateral pupils. She denied neck pain and was able to move all extremities. Chest movement was symmetrical, with bruising over the left lower rib cage and pain on palpation and inspiration. Her abdomen was slightly distended and painful to light palpation over the midepigastrium and left upper quadrant. She complained of nausea without emesis. Her pelvis was stable on palpation. Her right lower leg was swollen with an obvious deformity of her tibia-fibula area and continued weak distal pulses and a pale foot after placement of the box splint.

Cervical-spine and chest x-rays were done concurrently with the head-to-toe assessment. A Foley catheter and nasogastric tube were placed. The patient was typed and crossed for 4 units of blood, and labs were sent. Despite morphine 4 mg IV for her abdominal pain, she complained of increasing belly pain. Her VS were now:

T: 34.2° C
BP: 78/50 mm Hg
HR: 135 beats/min
RR: 32 breaths/min

Her level of consciousness was diminishing. She was emergently intubated and received an additional liter of LR. After examination by the surgeon, she was quickly taken to the OR for an emergency exploratory laparotomy. In the OR, the following injuries were discovered: a grade V splenic laceration requiring splenectomy for hemorrhage control, avulsion of the duodenum from the base of her stomach with spillage of intestinal contents into the peritoneum, and a pancreatic contusion with laceration of the pancreatic duct. An additional very serious injury was also discovered: bilateral renal thrombosis, assumed to be caused by shearing injury during the multiple rollovers and constriction of the lap belt. Because the Level II facility did not have the resources to manage this unusual critical injury, the patient's abdomen was simply packed and covered and the surgeon arranged for her immediate transfer to the closest Level I trauma center.

In the OR at the Level I trauma center, one kidney was removed. Because the other had a hint of collateral circulation, vascular grafts were done in an effort to salvage the remaining organ. On arrival in critical care, the patient was hypotensive, hypothermic, and on a ventilator. After additional volume and PRBC resuscitation, her VS were:

T: 34.3° C
BP: 88/60 mm Hg
HR: 122 beats/min
RR: 14 breaths/min on pressure control of 25

Hemodynamics included the following:

CVP: 6 mm Hg
PAWP: 6 mm Hg
CI: 7.2 L/min

SVR:	345 dynes
Svo_2:	85%
Do_2I:	945 ml/min/m^2
Vo_2I:	135 ml/min/m^2
EDVI:	122
Hgb:	7.4
K$^+$:	3.8
Magnesium (Mg^{++}):	1.7
Ca^{++}:	0.9
Glucose:	155
Amylase:	203
LA:	4.5
BD:	4.8

Arterial blood gases revealed:

pH: 7.30
Pao$_2$: 125
Paco$_2$: 42
Bicarbonate (HCO$_3^-$): 14

The patient roused to verbal stimuli and was able to follow commands and move all four extremities. Morphine 4 mg IV was given every 30–60 minutes for pain. She was anuric. She received occasional PRBC transfusion when her Hct slowly dropped below 25. Electrolyte replacement and insulin protocols were put into place.

Decision point: What labs should be checked as part of the initial assessment in the emergency department?

Decision point: What is the most appropriate diagnostic test to assess for abdominal bleeding in this patient, and why?

Decision point: What are the likely explanations for her hemodynamic profile in the critical care unit?

Decision point: What are additional resuscitation and assessment priorities in the first hours following admission to critical care?

BD = Base deficit, BP = blood pressure, Ca^{++} = calcium, CI = cardiac index, CVP = central venous pressure, Do$_2$I = oxygen delivery index, EDVI = end diastolic volume index, HCO$_3^-$ = bicarbonate, Hct = hematocrit, Hgb = hemoglobin, HR = heart rate, K$^+$ = potassium, LA = lactic acid, LR = lactated Ringer's, Mg^{++} = magnesium, OR = operating room, Paco$_2$ = arterial carbon dioxide, PAWP = pulmonary artery wedge pressure, Pao$_2$ = arterial oxygen, PRBC = packed red blood cell, RR = respiratory rate, Svo$_2$ = mixed venous oxygen saturation, SVR = systemic vascular resistance, T = temperature, Vo$_2$I = oxygen consumption index, VS = vital signs.

Case continues on page 1183

Providing Nutritional Support

Nutritional therapy is a critical component of severely injured patients. Even in trauma patients who are young and well nourished, an unsupported hypermetabolic post-injury response will rapidly result in a starvation state. Immediate access to essential amino acids is required to facilitate healing and ward off infection. Early nutritional support has been shown to prevent development of sepsis and multiorgan dysfunction syndrome in trauma patients.[109,185] Special considerations for meeting the nutritional needs of

◆ NUTRITION

Nutritional Considerations for the Trauma Patient

Glycogen stores are rapidly depleted following trauma, forcing the body to use endogenous substrates, protein, and fat to support hypermetabolism following injury. The usual balance between anabolism and catabolism is disrupted, favoring protein catabolism. Profound catabolism, particularly in healthy, muscular patients, occurs when muscles are broken down to supply proteins for metabolic processes. An average loss of 6.4 kg of skeletal muscle can occur in blunt trauma patients within 21 days. Negative nitrogen balance following trauma is an indicator of the magnitude of injury rather than an indicator of how much protein is needed. Sacrifice of lean body mass results in poor wound healing, impaired immunologic function, inadequate pulmonary ventilation, cardiac insufficiency, and sustained elevations in oxygen consumption. The hypermetabolic phase peaks within 10 days following injury, and then gradually decreases.

Providing adequate nutritional support to trauma patients is a challenge for multiple reasons. Gastrointestinal (GI) function is impaired in most trauma patients because many have undergone extensive surgical interventions and have subnormal albumin and prealbumin concentrations secondary to the stress response. Furthermore, the GI tract is essentially useless for the first 42 to 48 hours because of repeated surgery, shock, and paralytic ileus. Direct injury to the GI tract and subsequent surgical repair can be a contraindication for the use of enteral nutrition unless a jejunostomy tube can be used for feeding. The patient with head and facial injuries may be unable to tolerate oral feedings because of altered level of consciousness, poor gag and swallow reflexes, or surgical fixation of the mandible.

A nutritional assessment within 24 hours after admission is indicated for trauma patients, particularly those at high risk for malnutrition and catabolism. High-risk patients are those who are young (e.g., males with significant muscle mass), have sustained brain and facial trauma, have multisystem injury, have GI injury, or have preexisting malnutrition (e.g., older adults). Indirect calorimetry is the best method to calculate energy expenditure and prevent overfeeding in trauma patients.

See guidelines for nutritional care on p. 1182

trauma patients are described in the Nutrition box above, and Chapter 6 provides a full discussion regarding nutritional and metabolic support of critically ill or injured patients.

Assessing and Treating Infection

A comprehensive review of trauma wound care is beyond the scope of this chapter and is not addressed here. However, because infection is a common complication and a major cause of morbidity and mortality in the injured patient, this chapter will provide a brief overview of the incidence of infection and of wound management following trauma. Infections can occur with any wound and as nosocomial events.[31] To prevent or control infection, the critical care nurse should assess the patient daily for signs of inflammation and infection, send multiple specimens for culture and sensitivity should the patient appear to be developing an infection, and perform wound care as ordered.

Traumatic wound infections can occur with any wound and have a variety of presentations. Knife wounds, for example, are relatively clean, whereas wounds from jagged instruments such as chain saws and farm equipment are associated with significant tissue destruction, wound hematomas, bacteria, and foreign bodies. Wounds that penetrate to the fascia require a high index of suspicion for necrotizing fasciitis, which carries an extremely high mortality. Gangrene is a deep infection seen with puncture wounds, leading to compartment syndrome, deep myonecrosis, and a "dishwater" appearance to wound drainage.[70]

Prevention of wound infections involves initial debridement and cleansing of the injury site, with removal of tissue until only viable, bleeding tissue remains. This may be done in the OR, but is frequently performed in the critical care unit for smaller, less severe wounds. Management of wound infections requires judicious use of antibiotics to minimize the development of resistance. Aggressive deep fascial debridement and amputation are required to arrest the progression of necrotizing fasciitis and gangrene; hyperbaric oxygen therapy also may be considered.[70]

Open fractures are at risk for infection because they contain skin fragments, devitalized bone, and foreign bodies such as the patient's clothing. Infection is prevented by thorough irrigation with antibiotic solutions and debridement as soon as possible after the injury; this may be done in the critical care unit if the patient is too hemodynamically unstable to go to the operating room for the procedure. The wound may be closed several days after the injury once it is clear that no infection is present. Repeated debridement and irrigation will be necessary so long as infection persists, including the removal of infected internal fixation hardware. Amputation is performed when irreparable vascular injury or osteomyelitis leaves little hope for a functional limb, or systemic compromise from infection threatens mortality.[196]

Intraabdominal infection usually begins with injury that disrupts the GI tract or biliary tree. Likelihood of infection is based on where the damage occurred: the risk is relatively small for stomach and duodenal injuries; however, there is significant risk if the lower intestinal tract, with high bacterial counts, is injured. Prevention of abdominal infection begins with prompt exploratory laparotomy; if intestinal contamination is found, reoperation and delayed closure may be necessary. Aggressive antibiotic therapy to cover both anaerobic and aerobic bacteria must be started immediately with frequent reevaluation of appropriateness of therapy.[70]

Nosocomial chest infections secondary to chest tube placement in the ED are quite common.[30] They may be a result of contamination from a penetrating injury, but they also may be caused by tube placement under less than ideal conditions. Ideally, strict sterile technique is followed during placement in controlled situations, but chaos during ED resuscitation frequently allows for breaks in sterility and inadequate skin preparation. Pulmonary infection and empyema create additional respiratory compromise in patients with decreased level of consciousness, disrupted chest wall integrity, thoracic or abdominal incisions, and paralysis.[31]

Empyema presents with fever, leukocytosis, and purulent chest tube drainage and is more likely in patients who had large amounts of bloody drainage or who have had their tube for more than 5 days. Empyemas are managed by antibiotics and placement of a second chest tube or catheter directly into the empyema cavity itself; this is occasionally done in CT scan to better guide placement of the tube. Daily chest x-rays monitor the response to therapy. Unresolved empyemas develop a thick "rind," requiring decortication of the pleural space, a surgical procedure that results in significant blood loss and postoperative pain.[70] The critical care nurse plays a key role in preventing empyema by performing daily chest tube dressings. Anchoring the tube to the chest wall will help prevent to-and-fro movements at the insertion site that drag bacteria into the wound.[180]

Central nervous system infections occur as meningitis, brain abscess, and empyema. They may be associated with open skull fractures and with facial fractures that involve the sinuses. As well, they are a potential complication of intracranial monitoring catheters. Sinusitis is associated with midface fractures and nasotracheal or nasogastric tubes because sinus drainage is obstructed by edema and injury.[31] This can be the underlying source of infection in a trauma patient when other obvious sources of fever have been ruled out.

Postsplenectomy sepsis is a life-threatening, fulminating infection in patients who underwent splenectomy for trauma; although it is more common in children, it is increasingly present in adults and is often fatal. The spleen has essential immunologic functions; when it is removed, patients become at risk for fulminant disseminated bacteremia.[70] The best preventive strategy is to salvage the spleen when possible. In the case of splenectomy, vaccination for *Pneumococcus*, *Meningococcus*, and *Haemophilus influenzae* must be done before discharge.[31]

Clostridium difficile enterocolitis is a colitis associated with antibiotics. The infection occurs in patients who were colonized by the microbe before their injury, which became opportunistic when normal gut flora were suppressed by IV antibiotics used to treat other infections. The best way to prevent *C. difficile* is with shorter courses of antibiotics. Severe cases, associated with toxic megacolon, may require surgical resection of the colon.[70]

Lastly, hospital-acquired infections are as common in this patient population as in other critically ill patients. Ventilator-associated pneumonia, aspiration-associated pneumonia, urinary tract infection, intravascular device infection, and GI microbial translocation all contribute to the overall morbidity and mortality of injured patients.

Preventing Deep Venous Thrombosis

A complete discussion of deep venous thrombosis (DVT) and pulmonary embolism (PE) pathology is found in Chapter 9, but warrants special attention here because of unique concerns found in the trauma population. After the coagulopathy during initial resuscitation has resolved, the trauma patient develops a hypercoagulable state in the post-injury recovery period. DVT, PE, and even death can occur, the latter of which is particularly frustrating because it often occurs when the patient is well on the way to recovery. The relationship between trauma and venous thrombosis is well known, with more than half of patients developing lower extremity thrombosis. Despite preventive interventions, approximately 5% of patients with specific injury patterns may go on to develop pulmonary embolus.[38,73,121,177]

The components of Virchow's triad (e.g., venous stasis, endothelial damage, and hypercoagulability) are well described in trauma. Immobility, often seen with head and spinal cord injury and lower extremity fractures, leads to venous stasis from loss of the leg muscle pump.[163] Direct vessel wall damage from penetrating injury, blunt energy forces, or stretch injury may directly damage endothelium and initiate the coagulation cascade. Thrombosis can occur near the sites of traumatic and iatrogenic injury (e.g., central venous catheter insertion site).[129] Trauma patients have low levels of antithrombin III, protein C, and protein S, leading to a procoagulant state, compounded by increased platelet adhesion and decreased fibrinolysis.[59,134,158] Risk factors for DVT and PE in trauma patients can be separated into three groups, listed in Table 42-6.

Because physical examination is not a reliable way to detect DVT, trauma centers perform routine surveillance screening in critical care patients using duplex ultrasound of lower extremity vessels.[167] Traditional interventions to prevent DVT are early ambulation, graded sequential compression devices, and low-dose anticoagulation. Depending on the patient's injuries, early ambulation may not be an option and anticoagulation is often contraindicated because of bleeding potential from injuries. Therefore sequential compression devices are recommended for patients with moderate risk of DVT. For high-risk patients who cannot be anticoagulated, a temporary or permanent inferior vena

---

TABLE 42-6 Risk Factors for Deep Venous Thrombosis and Pulmonary Embolus Specific to Trauma

At risk	Injury severity score >9
	Blood transfusion(s)
	Surgical procedure ≥2 hours
	Lower-extremity fracture
	Spinal cord injury
	Immobilization
	Excessive soft tissue trauma
	Shock states
At high risk	Femoral central venous catheter
	Glasgow Coma Scale score ≤8
	Spinal cord injury
	Pelvic fracture
	Femur/tibia fracture
	Venous injury
At very high risk	Spinal cord injury with paralysis
	Severe pelvic fracture
	Multiple long bone fractures (≥3)

Data from references 34, 74, 83, 126, 150, 167, 196.

Guidelines for Nutritional Support of Critically Ill Trauma Patients

Calculate total energy needs	25-30 kcal/kg (25 kcal/kg for older adults) as determined by indirect calorimetry. Amounts of protein, carbohydrate, and fat guided by laboratory values. Adjust body weight for amputees (decrease by 6% for below-knee amputations, 12% for above-knee amputations).
Monitor labs	• Chemistry (calcium, magnesium, liver function, phosphate) • Electrolytes, BUN, Cr • Serum triglycerides • CBC with differential • PT, aPTT • Albumin, prealbumin, and transferrin • Nitrogen balance
Follow these general guidelines	• Concentrations of serum proteins such as transferrin, prealbumin, somatomedin-C, fibronectin, and C-reactive protein are altered during the acute phase of trauma, reflecting the stressed state rather than nutritional status. • Patients with mild to moderate injury who are expected to tolerate oral feeding within 5–7 days may be supported with 5% dextrose in water, which provides 400–600 kcal/day. • Enteral nutrition is preferred for providing nutrition 3–4 days following injury. Feeding through a jejunostomy can begin when the patient is hemodynamically stable. Gastric feeding must wait until normal pyloric function has returned. • Specialized and immune-enhancing formulas containing branched-chain amino acids, arginine, glutamine, omega-3 fatty acids, and vitamins E and C may provide some benefit, but additional research is needed. • Parenteral nutrition is indicated if enteral feeding is expected to be delayed for 5 days or if the patient does not tolerate tube feedings. • Stool softeners, fluids, fiber, and bowel stimulants may be needed to regulate bowel movements. Metoclopramide (Reglan) may be effective in increasing gastric motility. • Physical therapy should be initiated early for activity that will promote muscle function and growth.

Data from references 16, 67, 94, 109, 110, 140, 185.
BUN = Blood urea nitrogen, CBC = complete blood cell count, Cr = creatinine, GI = gastrointestinal, PT = prothrombin time, aPTT = activated partial thromboplastin time.

cava filter may be appropriate. This has resulted in a decreased incidence of PE, although additional studies about their efficacy and long-term consequences are needed. Many guidelines exist about how to best prevent DVT and subsequent PE development.[74,150]

Providing Psychosocial Support

Crisis following trauma provides unique challenges to patients and their families because hospitalization may last for weeks, with many emergencies and complications during that time. Recovery may be prolonged and uncertain, subjecting families to long periods of anxiety and emotional stress. During the critical care phase of trauma care, patients may not be alert enough to manifest stress and require intervention. Families, however, may feel overwhelmed, out of control or angry, have difficulty breathing, shake, be unable to concentrate, and experience mood swings. Early psychosocial intervention by critical care nurses, social workers, and pastoral services is important to help patients and families struggling with an uncertain future.[42,64] Providing family support in critical care is addressed in Chapter 8.

Both the patient and the family are at risk for the development of post-traumatic stress disorder (PTSD) following a traumatic event. Symptoms can begin immediately after the event and persist for months, predisposing the person to long-term mental and emotional health problems. Those most likely to experience PTSD either experienced or witnessed an incident that resulted in death or injury. Patients with spinal cord injuries and facial injuries are also at high risk for PTSD.[2,12,13] Patients experience powerful flashbacks of the events, producing feelings of intense fear, helplessness, or horror that are so real they feel as if they are reliving the event. Victims are in a constant state of hyperarousal; extreme fear, grief, and anger cause continuous emotional distress. Relationships with family and friends often suffer as victims may be distant and unapproachable. Other symptoms include gastric upset, headaches, difficulty concentrating, insomnia, and irritability.[2]

PTSD is not always identified while the patient is in the critical care unit, but nurses should identify those at risk for the disorder and consult with appropriate services to provide early screening and interventions. Social workers, hospital chaplains, psychologists, and psychiatrists are skilled professionals who help patients and families deal with PTSD. Many patients respond well to counseling and other nonpharmacologic interventions, but occasionally benzodiazepines and serotonin reuptake inhibitors may be needed. Early interventions that restore a sense of control, reduce hyperarousal, and decrease feelings of guilt will facilitate full recovery.[2]

◆ Case Study 42-1, Part C

Follow-Up Care

R.O.'s K+, BUN, and Cr increased on day 4. Because she was hemodynamically stable, she was placed on daily hemodialysis. Of concern, however, her white blood cell count (WBC) elevated to 38,000, her temperature increased to 39.5° C, her HR increased, and her BP and SVR fell slightly. She was taken back to the OR for exploratory laparotomy, during which they found severe pancreatitis. Surgical drains were placed, and her abdominal wound was left open. Her reanastomosed kidney did not appear to have good perfusion.

Antibiotics were adjusted for greater sensitivity to organisms cultured from her peritoneum. Hyperalimentation for nutritional support was begun because her GI tract was not intact (2 weeks later a jejunostomy tube was placed and she tolerated enteral feedings well). Her pain was well regulated; she easily roused and communicated with nursing staff and her family. Physical therapy provided a plan for daily range of motion exercises and mobilization. DVT prophylaxis was initiated. Social services helped her family find lodging because they were from out of town and a prolonged hospitalization was anticipated.

She remained in the critical care unit for nearly 6 weeks, largely because of recurrent bouts of sepsis from pancreatitis. She progressed to being dialyzed every other day. At the beginning of week 7, she returned to the OR for examination of her pancreatitis and remaining kidney. Her pancreatitis was much improved, but her remaining kidney was necrotic and subsequently removed. Amazingly, within 48 hours of the nephrectomy, her BP and WBC stabilized, her color improved, her fever disappeared, and she was extubated without event. Clearly, the avascular kidney had caused a prolonged inflammatory response and sepsis-like picture that disappeared once it was removed.

She was weak and depressed, but willing to participate in physical therapy activities. She was tolerating tube feedings well, but despite seemingly adequate nutrition she had lost nearly 35 pounds during her hospitalization. Her pancreatitis was slowly resolving. Her pain was managed well with oxycodone. She was visited by friends and family, as well as the hospital's rehabilitation therapy dog every day. The patient was transferred to the acute care floor on week 8.

Decision point: What is the most appropriate intervention for DVT prophylaxis in this patient?

Decision point: Why was she losing weight despite tolerating her tube feedings well?

Decision point: What signs and symptoms would the patient exhibit if she were experiencing PTSD?

BP = Blood pressure, BUN = blood urea nitrogen, Cr = creatinine, DVT = deep venous thrombosis, GI = gastrointestinal, HR = heart rate, K+ = potassium, OR = operating room, PTSD = post-traumatic stress disorder, SVR = systemic vascular resistance, WBC = white blood cell.

CONCLUSIONS

Trauma is a multisystem phenomenon with immediate threat to life and long-term complications for the survivors of critical injury. The first hour after trauma, known as the "golden hour," sees the highest number of patient deaths[29,191]; for those who survive, the subsequent hours and days spent in critical care are no less important. An organized, systematic approach to managing these patients provides the best chance for meaningful outcome. The critical care nurse assesses and reassesses, monitors, infuses, assists, transports, applies pressure, explains, and comforts: a seemingly endless myriad of critical thinking and nursing activities. The nurse's attention to the clinical challenges addressed in this chapter, along with a high index of suspicion for decompensation at any time, are the patient's best chance for leaving the critical care unit in optimal condition to begin the long and difficult road of recovery.

REFERENCES

1. Ad hoc subcommittee on outcomes: working group. (2001). Practice management guidelines for emergency department thoracotomy. *J Am Coll Surg, 193*, 303–309.
2. Aguilera, D. (1998). *Crisis intervention: theory and methodology* (8th ed.). St. Louis: Mosby.
3. Alam, H. G., et al. (2004). Application of a zeolite hemostatic agent achieves 100% survival in a lethal model of complex groin injury. *J Trauma, 56*(5), 974–983.
4. American College of Surgeons Committee on Trauma. (1998). *Resources for optimal care of the injured patient.* Chicago: Author.
5. American College of Surgeons Committee on Trauma. (2004). *Advanced trauma life support course* (7th ed.). Chicago: American College of Surgeons.
6. Arbabi, S., et al. (1999). Near-infrared spectroscopy: continuous measurement of cytochrome oxidation during hemorrhagic shock. *Crit Care Med, 25*(1), 532–536.
7. Barillo, D. J., & Goode, R. (1996). Substance abuse in victims of fire. *BJ Burn Care Rehabil, 17*, 71–76.
8. Bell, R. M., & Krantz, B. E. (2000). Initial assessment. In K. L. Mattox, D. V. Feliciano & E. E. Moore (Eds.), *Trauma* (4th ed., pp. 153–169). New York: McGraw-Hill.
9. Better, O. S., & Stein, J. H. (1990). Early management of shock and prophylaxis of acute renal failure in traumatic rhabdomyolysis (comment). *N Engl J Med, 322*(12), 825–829.
10. Biesel, W. R. (1995). Herman award lecture, 1995: infection induced malnutrition from cholera to cytokines. *Am J Clin Nutr, 62*, 813–819.
11. Biffl, W. L., Moore, E. E., & Johnson, J. L. (2004). Emergency department thoracotomy. In K. L. Mattox, E. E. Moore & D. V. Feliciano (Eds.), *Trauma* (5th ed., pp. 239–254). New York: McGraw-Hill.
12. Binks, T. M., et al. (1997). Relationship between level of spinal cord injury and posttraumatic stress disorder symptoms. *Ann N Y Acad Sci, 821*, 430–432.
13. Bisson, J. I., Shepherd, J. P., & Manish, D. (1997). Psychological sequelae of facial trauma. *J Trauma, 43*, 496–500.

14. Blamback, M. (1985). Blood coagulation and fibrinolytic factors as well as their inhibitors in trauma. *Scand J Clin Lab Invest, 178* (Suppl.), 15–23.
15. Bombardier, C. H., & Thurber, C. A. (1998). Blood alcohol level and early cognitive status after traumatic brain injury. *Brain Inj, 12*, 725–734.
16. Boulanger, B. R., Nayman, R., & McLean, R. F. (1994). What are the clinical determinants of early energy expenditure in critically injured adults? *J Trauma, 37*, 969–974.
17. Bower, T. C. (1994). Maxillofacial and soft tissue injures. In V. D. Cardona, et al. (Eds.), *Trauma nursing: from resuscitation through rehabilitation* (2nd ed., pp. 587–615). Philadelphia: Saunders.
18. Bower, T. C., & Vanderheyden, V. A. (2002). Analgesia, sedation, and neuromuscular blockade in the trauma patient. In K. A. McQuillan, et al. (Eds.), *Trauma nursing: from resuscitation through rehabilitation* (pp. 324–365). Philadelphia: Saunders.
19. Brewer, R. D., Morris, P. D., & Cole, T. B. (1994). The risk of dying in alcohol-related automobile crashes among habitual drunk drivers. *N Engl J Med, 331*, 513–517.
20. Brohi, K., et al. (2003). Acute traumatic coagulopathy. *J Trauma, 54*(6), 1127–1130.
21. Bucklew, P. A., et al. (1992). Falls and ejections from pickup trucks. *J Trauma, 32*(4), 468–472.
22. Bulger, E. (2000). Rib fractures in the elderly. *J Trauma, 48*(6), 1040–1047.
23. Bulger, E. M., et al. (1997). Fat embolism syndrome. *Arch Surg, 132*, 435–439.
24. Bulger, E. M., Smith, D. G., & Maier, R. V. (1997). Fat embolus syndrome: a 10 year review. *Arch Surg, 132*, 435–439.
25. Bullock, M. R., Chesnut, R. M., & Clifton, G. L. (2000). Guidelines for the management of severe traumatic brain injury. In Brain Trauma Foundation and American Association of Neurological Surgeons (Ed.), *Management and prognosis of severe traumatic brain injury.* (pp. 7–165). New York: Brain Trauma Foundation.
26. Burch, J. M. (2000). Injury to the colon and rectum. In K. L. Mattox, D. V. Feliciano & E. E. Moore (Eds.), *Trauma* (4th ed., pp. 763–782). New York: McGraw-Hill.
27. Burch, J. M., Franciose, R. J., & Moore, E. E. (1999). Trauma. In S. I. Schwartz, et al (Eds.), *Principles of surgery* (7th ed., pp. 155–222). New York: McGraw-Hill.
28. Burch, J. M., et al. (1992). Abbreviated laparotomy and planned reoperation for critically injured patients. *Ann Surg, 215*, 476.
29. Cales, R. H., & Trunkey, D. D. (1985). Preventable trauma deaths. A review of trauma care systems development. *JAMA, 254*, 1059.
30. Caplan, E. S., et al. (1984). Empyema in the multiply traumatized patient. *J Trauma, 24*, 785.
31. Casper, P. B., & Manjari, J. (2002). Infection and infection control. In K. A. McQuillan, et al. (Eds.), *Trauma nursing: from resuscitation through rehabilitation* (pp. 223–259). Philadelphia: Saunders.
32. Champion, H. R., & Mabee, M. S. (1990). *An American crisis in trauma care reimbursement: an issue analysis monograph.* Washington, D.C.: The Washington Hospital Center.
33. Chang, M. C., et al. (1996). Preload assessment in trauma patients during large-volume shock resuscitation. *Arch Surg, 131*, 728–731.
34. Clagett, P. C., et al. (1998). Prevention of thromboembolism. *Chest, 111*, 531S–560S.
35. Cohn, S. M., Crookes, B. A., & Proctor, K. G. (2003). Near-infrared spectroscopy in resuscitation. *J Trauma, 54*(5 Suppl.), S199–S202.
36. Cohn, S. M., et al. (2001). Splanchnic perfusion evaluation during hemorrhage and resuscitation with gastric near-infrared spectroscopy. *J Trauma, 50*(4), 629–634.
37. Connors, A. F., et al. (1996). The effectiveness of right heart catheterization in the initial care of critically ill patients. *JAMA, 276*, 889–897.

38. Coon, W. W. (1977). Epidemiology of venous thromboembolism. *Ann Surg, 186*, 149.

39. Cooper, D. J., et al. (1998). Quality assessment of the management of road traffic fatalities at a level I trauma center compared to other hospitals in Victoria, Australia. *J Trauma, 45*(4), 772–779.

40. Cosgriff, N., et al. (1997). Predicting life-threatening coagulopathy in the massively transfused trauma patient: hypothermia and acidoses revisited. *J Trauma, 42*(5), 857–861.

41. Crookes, B. A., et al. (2005). Can near-infrared spectroscopy identify the severity of shock in trauma patients? *J Trauma, 58*(4), 806–813.

42. Cross, M. L., et al. (1996). Interaction between the trauma team and families: lack of timely communications. *Am J Emerg Med, 14*, 548–550.

43. Cuthbertson, D. P. (1942). Post-shock metabolic response. *Lancet, 1*, 433–436.

44. Davis, J. H., Pruit, J. H., & Pruitt Jr., B. A. (2000). History. In K. L. Mattox, D. V. Feliciano & E. E. Moore (Eds.), *Trauma* (4th ed., pp. 3–19). New York: McGraw-Hill.

45. Davis, J. W., et al. (1988). Base deficit as a guide to volume resuscitation. *J Trauma, 28*, 1464–1467.

46. De La Taille, A., Houdeletter, P., & Houlgatte, A. (1997). Ureteropelvic junction avulsion due to nonpenetrating abdominal trauma treated with caliceal ureterostomy. *J Urol, 157*, 1840–1844.

47. DeLoughery, T. G. (2004). Coagulation defects in trauma patients: etiology, recognition, and treatment. *Crit Care Clin, 20*(1), 13–24.

48. Denis, R., Allard, M., & Atlas, H. (1983). Changing trends with abdominal injury in seatbelt wearers. *J Trauma, 23*(11), 1007–1008.

49. Diebel, L. N., et al. (1992). End-diastolic volume: a better indicator of pre-load in the critically ill. *Arch Surg, 127*, 817–822.

50. Dunham, C. M., & Cowley, R. A. (1991). *Shock trauma/critical care manual*. Gaithersburg, Md: Aspen.

51. Durham, C. M., et al. (1991). Oxygen delivery and metabolic acidemia as quantitative predictors of mortality and the severity of the ischemic insult in hemorrhagic shock. *Crit Care Med, 19*, 231–243.

52. Dutton, R. P., Hess, J. R., & Scalea, T. M. (2003). Recombinant factor VIIa for control of hemorrhage: early experience in critically injured trauma patients. *J Clin Anesth, 15*(3), 184–188.

53. Dutton, R. P., et al. (2004). Factor VIIa for correction of traumatic coagulopathy. *J Trauma Nurs, 57*(4), 709–719.

54. Eddy, V. A., Morris, J. A., & Cullinane, D. C. (2000). Hypothermia, coagulopathy and acidosis. *Surg Clin North Am, 80*(3), 845–854.

55. Emergency Nurses Association. (2000). Initial assessment. In Emergency Nurses Association (Ed.), *Trauma nursing core course* (5th ed., pp. 39–64). Des Plaines, Ill: Emergency Nurses Association.

56. Emergency Nurses Association. (2000). Mechanism of injury. In Emergency Nurses Association (Ed.), *Trauma nursing core course* (5th ed., pp. 11–38). Des Plaines, Ill: Emergency Nurses Association.

57. Emergency Nurses Association. (2000). Stabilization, transfer, and transport. In Emergency Nurses Association (Ed.), *Trauma nursing core course* (5th ed.). Des Plaines, Ill: Emergency Nurses Association.

58. Emergency Nurses Association. (2001). *Presenting the option of family presence* (2nd ed.). Des Plaines, Ill: Emergency Nurses Association.

58a. Emergency Nurses Association (2000). Primary assessment. In Emergency Nurses Association (Ed.), *Trauma nursing core course* (5th ed., p. 313, Table 38). Des Plaines, Ill: Emergency Nurses Association.

58b. Emergency Nurses Association (2000). Secondary assessment. In Emergency Nurses Association (Ed.). *Trauma nursing core course*. (5th ed., p. 314, Table 39). Des Plaines, Ill: Emergency Nurses Association.

59. Engelman, D. T., et al. (1996). Hypercoagulability following multiple trauma. *World J Surg, 20*, 5.

60. Esposito, T. J., & Gamelli, R. L. (2000). Injury to the spleen. In K. L. Mattox, D. V. Feliciano, & E. E. Moore (Eds.), *Trauma* (4th ed., pp. 683–711). New York: McGraw-Hill.

61. Fackler, M. L. (1986). Wound ballistics. In D. D. Trunkey & F. R. Lewis (Eds.), *Current therapy of trauma* (pp. 94–101). Burlington, Ontario: B. C. Decker.

62. Farrar, A., et al. (1990). Hypothermia and acidosis worsen coagulopathies in the patient requiring massive transfusion. *Am J Surg, 160*, 515–518.

63. Farrar, J., Cottingham, C., & Rutter, M. M. (1994). Genitourinary injuries and renal management. In V. D. Cardona, et al. (Eds.), *Trauma nursing: from resuscitation to rehabilitation* (2nd ed., pp. 639–664). Philadelphia: Saunders.

64. Farrar, J. A. (2002). Psychosocial impact of trauma. In K. A. McQuillan, et al (Eds.), *Trauma nursing: from resuscitation through rehabilitation* (pp. 366–392). Philadelphia: Saunders.

65. Feliciano, D. V., Moore, E. E., & Mattox, K. L. (2000). Trauma damage control. In K. L. Mattox, D. V. Feliciano, & E. E. Moore (Eds.), *Trauma* (pp. 907–931). New York: McGraw-Hill.

66. Flynn, M. B., & Bonini, S. (1999). Blunt chest trauma: a case report. *Crit Care Nurse, 19*(5), 68–77.

67. Frankenfield, D. C., Omert, L. A., & Badelline, M. M. (1994). Correlation between measured energy expenditure and clinically obtained variables in trauma and sepsis patients. *JPEN, 18*, 398–403.

68. Fritsch, D. E. (1991). Hypothermia in the trauma patient. *AACN Clin Issues, 6*, 196–211.

69. Fritsch, D. E., & Steinmann, R. A. (2000). Managing trauma patients with abdominal compartment syndrome. *Crit Care Nurse, 20*, 48–58.

70. Fry, D. E. (2000). Prevention, diagnosis, and management of infection. In K. L. Mattox, D. V. Feliciano & E. E. Moore (Eds.), *Trauma* (4th ed., pp. 349–369). New York: McGraw-Hill.

71. Gallagher, J. J. (2006). Abdominal compression monitoring: ask the experts. *Crit Care Nurse, 26*(1), 67–70.

72. Gando, S., Tedo, L., & Kubota, M. (1992). Post-trauma coagulation and fibrinolysis. *Crit Care Med, 20*, 594–600.

73. Geerts, W. H., et al. (1994). A prospective study of venous thromboembolism after major trauma. *N Engl J Med, 331*, 1601.

74. Geerts, W. H., et al. (2004). Prevention of venous thromboembolism: the seventh ACCP conference on antithrombotic and thrombolytic therapy. *Chest, 126*(3), 338S–400S.

75. Gentilello, L. M. (1994). Practical approaches to hypothermia. *Adv Trauma Crit Care, 9*, 39–79.

76. Gentilello, L. M., et al. (1992). Continuous arteriovenous rewarming: rapid reversal of hypothermia in critically ill patients. *J Trauma, 32*, 316–327.

77. Gentilello, L. M., Jurkovich, G. J., & Stark, M. S. (1997). Is hypothermia in the victim of major trauma protective or harmful? A randomized prospective study. *Ann Surg, 226*, 642–647.

78. Gentilello, L. M., & Rifley, W. J. (1991). Continuous arteriovenous rewarming: report of a new technique for treating hypothermia. *J Trauma, 31*, 1151–1153.

79. Ghali, A. M. A., El Malik, E. M. A., & Ibrahim, A. I. A. (1999). Ureteric injuries: diagnosis, management, and outcome. *J Thromb Haemost, 46*, 150–158.

80. Gommersall, C. D., et al. (2000). Resuscitation of critically ill patients based on the results of gastric tonometry: a prospective, randomized controlled trial. *Crit Care Med, 28*(3), 607–614.

81. Grove, C. A., et al. (2002). Emergency thoracotomy: appropriate use in the resuscitation of trauma patients. *Am Surg, 68*(4), 313–317.

82. Gubler, K. D., et al. (1994). The effect of hypothermia on dilutional coagulopathy. *J Trauma, 36*, 847–851.

83. Gupta, R., et al. (1998). Pulmonary embolism prevention by clinical management guidelines in high risk trauma patients admitted to an ICU using duplex surveillance. *Crit Care Med, 26*, A48.

84. Guyton, A. C., & Hall, J. E. (2006). *Textbook of medical physiology.* (11th ed., pp. 911–922). Philadelphia: Elsevier.

85. Guyton, A. C., & Hall, J. E. (2006). *Textbook of medical physiology.* (pp. 383–401). Philadelphia: Elsevier.

86. Hedner, U. (2000). NovoSeven as a universal haemostatic agent. *Blood Coagul Fibrinolysis, 11*(1 Suppl.), S107–S111.

87. Hildebrand, F., et al. (2004). Pathophysiologic changes and effects of hypothermia on outcome in elective surgery and trauma patients. *Am J Surg, 187,* 363–371.

88. Holcomb, J. B. (2005). Use of recombinant factor VII to treat the acquired coagulopathy of trauma. *J Trauma, 58*(6), 1298–1303.

89. Holcomb, J. B., et al. (1998). Efficacy of a dry fibrin sealant dressing for hemorrhage control after ballistic injury. *Arch Surg, 133*(1), 32–35.

90. Hoyt, D. B., Coimbra, R., & Potenza, M. D. (2004). Management of acute trauma. In C. M. Townsend, et al (Eds.), *Sabiston textbook of surgery: the biological basis of modern surgical practice* (17th ed., pp. 483–532). Philadelphia: Elsevier.

91. Hudson, L. D., & Steinberg, K. P. (1999). Epidemiology of acute lung injury and ARDS. *Chest, 116*(1), 74S–82S.

92. Hulka, F., Mullins, R. J., & Frank, E. H. (1996). Blunt brain injury activates the coagulation process. *Arch Surg, 131,* 923–927.

93. Hulka, F., et al. (1997). Influence of a statewide trauma system on pediatric hospitalization and outcome. *J Trauma, 42*(3), 268–276.

94. Hwang, T., Shuang, S., & Chen, M. (1993). The use of indirect calorimetry in critically ill patients: the relationship of measured energy expenditure to injury severity score, septic severity score, and APACHE II score. *J Trauma, 34,* 247–251.

95. Ivatury, R. R., Sugerman, H. J., & Peitzman, A. B. (2001). Abdominal compartment syndrome: recognition and management. In J. L. Cameron (Ed.), *Advances in surgery* (vol. 35, pp. 1–19). St. Louis: Mosby.

96. James, C. (1998). Orthopedic and neurovascular trauma. In L. Newberry (Ed.), *Sheehy's emergency nursing: principles and practice* (4th ed.). St. Louis: Mosby.

97. James, M. D., & Gregis, R. M. (1998). Mannitol treatment for acute compartment syndrome. *Nephron, 79*(4), 492.

98. Jeroukhimov, K., et al. (2002). Early injection of high-dose recombinant factor VIIa decreases blood loss and prolongs time from injury to death in experimental liver injury. *J Trauma, 53*(6), 1053–1057.

99. Jin, S., et al. (1998). Decreases in organ blood flows associated with increases in sublingual Paco$_2$ during hemorrhagic shock. *J Appl Physiol, 85*(6), 1838–1843.

100. Jurkovich, G. J. (2000). Injuries to duodenum and pancreas. In K. L. Mattox, D. V. Feliciano & E. E. Moore (Eds.), *Trauma* (pp. 735–762). New York: McGraw-Hill.

101. Jurkovich, G. J., Frederick, P., & Rivara, F. J. (1993). The effect of acute alcohol intoxication and chronic alcohol abuse on outcome from trauma. *JAMA, 270,* 51–56.

102. Jurkovich, G. J., Greiser, W. B., & Luterman, A. (1987). Hypothermia: an ominous predictor of survival. *J Trauma, 27,* 1019–1022.

103. Kalb, R. L. (1999). Preventing the sequelae of compartment syndrome. *Hosp Pract, 34*(1), 105–107.

104. Kearney, M. L. (1996). Imbalance of oxygen supply and demand. In V. H. Secor (Ed.), *Multiple organ dysfunction and failure* (pp. 135–147). St. Louis: Mosby.

105. Kelly, M. P., et al. (1997). Substance abuse, traumatic brain injury, and neuropsychological outcome. *Brain Inj, 11,* 391–402.

106. Kenet, G., et al. (1999). Treatment of traumatic bleeding with recombinant factor VIIa. *Lancet, 354,* 1879.

107. Kirkpatrick, A. W., et al. (2000). Is clinical examination an accurate indicator of raised intra-abdominal pressure in critically injured patients? *Can J Surg, 43,* 207–211.

108. Kreymann, G., Grosser, S., & Buggish, P. (1993). Oxygen consumption and resting metabolic rate in sepsis, sepsis syndrome, and septic shock. *Crit Care Med, 21,* 1012–1019.

109. Kudsk, K. A., & Brown, R. O. (2000). Nutritional support. In K. L. Mattox, D. V. Feliciano & E. E. Moore (Eds.), *Trauma* (4th ed., pp. 1369–1405). New York: McGraw-Hill.

110. Kudsk, K. A., et al. (1992). Enteral vs. parenteral feeding: effects on septic morbidity following blunt and penetrating abdominal trauma. *Ann Surg, 215,* 503.

111. Lapointe, L. A., & von Rueden, K. T. (2002). Coagulopathies in trauma patients. *AACN Clin Issues, 13*(2), 192–203.

112. Li, G., Keyl, P. M., & Smith, G. S. (1997). Alcohol and injury severity: reappraisal of the continuing controversy. *J Trauma, 42,* 562–569.

113. Little, R. A., & Stoner, H. B. (1981). Body temperature after accidental injury. *Br J Surg, 68,* 221–227.

113a. Lucas, C. E., Ledgerwood, A. M., & Kline, R. A. (2000). Alcohol and drugs. In K. L. Mattox, D. V. Feliciano, & E. E. Moore (Eds.), *Trauma* (4th ed., p. 42). New York: McGraw-Hill.

114. Luna, G. K., et al. (1987). Incidence and effect of hypothermia in seriously injured patients. *J Trauma, 27,* 1019–1024.

115. Mackersie, R. C., Campbell, A. R., & Cammarano, W. B. (2000). Principles of critical care. In K. L. Mattox, E. E. Moore, & D. V. Feliciano (Eds.), *Trauma* (pp. 1231–1265). New York: McGraw-Hill.

116. MacLeod, J. B., et al. (2003). Early coagulopathy predicts mortality in trauma. *J Trauma, 55*(1), 39–44.

117. Malinoski, D. J., Slater, M. S., & Mullins, R. J. (2004). Crush injury and rhabdomyolysis. *Crit Care Clin, 20,* 191–192.

118. Martinowitz, U., et al. (2001). Treatment of traumatic bleeding with recombinant factor VIIa. *J Trauma, 51,* 431–439.

119. Mattox, K. L., Feliciano, D. V., & Moore, E. E. (2000). *Trauma* (4th ed.). New York: McGraw-Hill.

120. Maull, K. I., & Esposito, T. J. (2000). Trauma system design. In K. L. Mattox, D. V. Feliciano, & E. E. Moore (Eds.), *Trauma* (pp. 57–78). New York: McGraw-Hill.

121. McCartney, J. S. (1934). Pulmonary embolism following trauma. *Am J Pathol, 10,* 709.

122. McClave, S. A., & Snider, H. L. (1994). Understanding the metabolic response to critical illness: factors that cause patients to deviate from the expected pattern of hypermetabolism. *New Horiz, 2,* 139–146.

123. McConnell, K. J., et al. (2005). Mortality benefit of transfer to level I versus level II trauma centers for head-injured patients. *Health Serv Res, 40*(2), 435–457.

124. McKinley, B. A., et al. (2000). Tissue hemoglobin O$_2$ saturation during resuscitation of traumatic shock monitored using near infrared spectrometry. *J Trauma, 48*(4), 637–642.

125. McKinley, B. A., Valdivia, A., & Moore, F. A. (2003). Goal-oriented shock resuscitation for major torso trauma: what are we learning? *Curr Opin Crit Care, 9,* 292–299.

126. McMahon, D. J., et al. (1997). Efficacy of inferior vena cava filters in selected patients with very high risk for fatal pulmonary embolism. *Chest, 110,* 2S.

127. McQuillan, K. A., et al. (2002). *Trauma nursing: from resuscitation through rehabilitation* (3rd ed.). Philadelphia: Saunders.

128. McSwain, N. E. (2000). Kinematics of trauma. In K. L. Mattox, D. V. Feliciano, & E. E. Moore (Eds.), *Trauma* (pp. 127–152). New York: McGraw-Hill.

129. Meredith, J. W., et al. (1993). Femoral catheters and deep venous thrombosis: a prospective evaluation with venous duplex. *J Trauma, 35,* 187.

130. Michelson, A. D., McGregor, H., & Barnard, M. R. (1994). Reversible inhibition of human platelet activation by hypothermia in vivo and in vitro. *J Thromb Haemost, 71,* 633–640.

131. Miller, M. T., et al. (2003). Not so fast. *J Trauma, 52*(1), 52–60.

132. Miller, P. R., et al. (1999). Randomized, prospective comparison of increased preload versus inotropes in the resuscitation of trauma patients: effects on cardiopulmonary function and visceral perfusion. *J Trauma, 44*, 107–113.

133. Miller, P. R., et al. (1998). Threshold values of intramucosal pH and mucosal-arterial CO_2 gap during shock resuscitation. *J Trauma, 45*(5), 868–872.

134. Miller, R. S., et al. (1994). Antithrombin II and trauma patients: factors that determine low levels. *J Trauma, 37*, 442.

135. Mizushima, Y., Wanag, P., & Cioffi, W. G. (2000). Should normothermia be restored and maintained during resuscitation after trauma and hemorrhage? *J Trauma, 48*, 58–65.

136. Montonye, J. M. (2002). Abdominal injuries. In K. A. McQuillan, et al, (Eds.), *Trauma nursing: from rehabilitation through resuscitation* (3rd ed., pp. 591–619). Philadelphia: Saunders.

137. Moore, E. E. (1996). Staged laparotomy for the hypothermia, acidosis, and coagulopathy syndrome. *Am J Surg, 172*, 405.

138. Moore, E. E., et al, (1998). Staged physiologic restoration and damage control surgery. *World J Surg, 22*, 1184.

139. Moore, E. E., & Davis, J. H. (1987). Multiple injuries. In J. H. Davis, et al, (Eds.), *Clinical surgery* (pp. 2769–2823). St. Louis: Mosby.

140. Moore, F. A., et al. (1992). Early enteral feeding, compared with parenteral, reduces postoperative septic complications: the results of a meta-analysis. *Ann Surg, 216*, 172.

141. Morgan, P. B., & Buetcher, K. J. (2000). Blunt thoracic aortic injuries: initial evaluation and management. *South Med J, 93*(2), 173–175.

142. Morris, J. A., et al. (1993). The staged celiotomy for trauma: issues in unpacking and reconstruction. *Ann Surg, 217*, 576.

143. Mueller, B. A., Kenaston, T., & Grossman, D. (1998). Hospital charges to injured drinking drivers in Washington state: 1989–1993. *Accid Anal Prev, 30*, 597–605.

144. Mullins, R. J. (2000). Management of shock. In K. L. Mattox, D. V. Feliciano, & E. E. Moore (Eds.), *Trauma* (4th ed., pp. 195–232). New York: McGraw-Hill.

145. Mullins, R. J., et al. (2002). Survival of seriously injured patients first treated in rural hospitals. *J Trauma, 52*(6), 1019–1029.

146. Mullins, R. J., et al. (1996). Influence of a statewide trauma system on location of hospitalization and outcome in injured patients. *J Trauma, 40*(4), 536–545.

147. National Center for Statistics and Analysis. (2003). *Alcohol-related crashes and fatalities*: National Highway Traffic Safety Administration, Washington, DC.

148. National Highway Traffic Safety Administration. (1998). *Questions and answers regarding air gas, new occupant protection technology in 1998 vehicles, and supplemental questions and answers regarding air bags*. www.nhtsa.dot.gov.

149. National Highway Traffic Safety Administration. (1999). *Fourth report to congress effectiveness of occupant protection systems and their use*: National Highway Traffic Safety Administration, Washington, DC.

150. National Quality Forum. (2004 September). *National consensus standards for the prevention and care of deep vein thrombosis*. www.qualityforum.org/txDVTprojectsummaryFINAL.pdf.

151. National Safety Council. (1999). *Injury facts*. Chicago: National Safety Council.

152. National Trauma Data Bank Version 4. (2004). *American College of Surgeons*. www.facs.org/trauma/ntdbwhatis.html.

153. Nayduch, D. A. (2002). Genitourinary injuries and renal management. In K. A. McQuillan, et al (Eds.), *Trauma nursing: resuscitation through rehabilitation* (3rd ed., pp. 620–645). Philadelphia: Saunders.

154. Newman, R. J. (1986). A prospective evaluation of the protective effect of car seatbelts. *J Trauma, 26*(6), 561–564.

155. Ng, A. (2003). *Trauma ultrasonography: the FAST and beyond.* www.trauma.org.

156. O'Day, J., & Scott, R. (1984). Safety belt use: ejection and entrapment. *Health Educ Q, 11*(2), 141–146.

157. O'Keefe, G. E. (2003). Abdominal compartment syndrome. *Crit Care Alert, 11*(3), 29–32.

158. Owings, J. T., et al. (1996). Effect of critical injury on plasma antithrombin activity: low antithrombin levels are associated with thromboembolic complications. *J Trauma, 41*, 396.

159. Pellino, T. A., Polacek, L. A., & Preston, M. A. S. (1998). Complications of orthopaedic disorders and orthopaedic surgery. In A. B. Maher, S. W. Salmond, & T. A. Pellino (Eds.), *Orthopaedic nursing* (pp. 646–689). Philadelphia: Saunders.

160. Peterson, S. R., Holday, N. J., & Jeevanandam, M. (1994). Enhancement of protein synthesis efficiency in parenterally fed trauma victims by adjuvant recombinant human growth hormone. *J Trauma, 36*, 726–733.

161. Powell, D. W., et al. (2004). Is emergency department thoracotomy futile care? *J Am Coll Surg, 199*(2), 211–215.

162. Pusateri, A., et al. (2003). Effect of a chitosan-based hemostatic dressing on blood loss and survival in a model of severe venous hemorrhage and hepatic injury in swine. *J Trauma, 54*(1), 177–182.

163. Rhodes, M., & Cipolle, M. D. (1996). Deep venous thrombosis and pulmonary embolism. In K. Maull, A. Rodriguez, & C. E. Wiles (Eds.), *Complications in trauma and critical care* (p. 81). Philadelphia: Saunders.

164. Richardson, J. D., & Spain, D. A. (2000). Injury to the lung and pleura. In K. L. Mattox, D. V. Feliciano, & E. E. Moore (Eds.), *Trauma* (4th ed., pp. 523–543). New York: McGraw-Hill.

165. Rivara, F. J., Jurkovich, G. J., & Gurney, J. G. (1993). The magnitude of acute and chronic alcohol abuse in trauma patients. *Arch Surg, 128*, 907–912.

166. Robertson, B. C., & McQuillan, K. A. (2002). Maxillofacial trauma. In K. A. McQuillan, et al. (Eds.), *Trauma nursing: from resuscitation through rehabilitation* (3rd ed., pp. 463–483). Philadelphia: Saunders.

167. Rotondo, M. F., & Reilly, P. M. (2000). Bleeding and coagulation complications. In K. L. Mattox, D. V. Feliciano, & E. E. Moore (Eds.), *Trauma* (4th ed., pp. 1267–1285). New York: McGraw-Hill.

168. Rueler, J. B. (1978). Hypothermia: pathophysiology, clinical setting, and management. *Ann Intern Med, 89*, 519–527.

169. Sauaia, A., Moore, F. A., & Moore, E. E. (1995). Epidemiology of trauma deaths: a reassessment. *J Trauma, 38*, 185–193.

170. Schmied, H., Kurz, A., & Sessler, D. I. (1996). Mild hypothermia increases blood loss and transfusion requirements during total hip arthroplasty. *Lancet, 347*, 289–292.

171. Schreiber, M. A. (2004). Damage control surgery. *Crit Care Clin, 20*(1), 101–118.

172. Schreiber, M. A., et al. (2003). The effect of recombinant factor VIIa on non-coagulopathic pigs with grade V liver injuries. *J Am Coll Surg, 196*(5), 691–697.

173. Schulman, C. S. (2002). End points of resuscitation: choosing the right parameters to monitor. *DCCN, 21*(1), 2–12.

174. Schulman, C. S. (2005). Continuous arteriovenous rewarming. In D. J. Lynn-McHale & K. K. Carlson (Eds.), *AACN procedure manual for critical care* (5th ed., pp. 1004–1013). Philadelphia: Saunders.

175. Schulman, C. S., & Pierce, B. (1999). Continuous arteriovenous rewarming: a bedside technique. *Crit Care Nurse, 19*(6), 54–63.

176. Seekamp, A., et al. (1999). Adenosine-triphosphate in trauma-related and elective hypothermia. *J Trauma, 47*, 673–683.

177. Sevitt, S., & Gallagher, N. (1960). Venous thrombosis and pulmonary embolism: a clinico-pathologic study in injured and burned patients. *Br J Surg, 48*, 475.

178. Seyfer, A. E., & Hansen, J. E. (2000). Facial trauma. In K. L. Mattox, D. V. Feliciano, & E. E. Moore (Eds.), *Trauma* (4th ed., pp. 415–436). New York: McGraw-Hill.

179. Shackford, S. R., & Rich, N. H. (2000). Peripheral vascular injury. In K. L. Mattox, D. V. Feliciano, & E. E. Moore (Eds.), *Trauma* (4th ed., pp. 1011–1042). New York: McGraw-Hill.

180. Sherwood, S. F., & Hartsock, R. L. (2002). Thoracic injuries. In K. A. McQuillan, et al. (Eds.), *Trauma nursing: from resuscitation through rehabilitation* (3rd ed., pp. 543–590). Philadelphia: Saunders.

181. Siegel, J. H., et al. (1990). Early predictors of injury severity and death in blunt multiple trauma. *Arch Surg, 125*, 498–508.

182. Siegel, J. H., Mason-Gonzales, S., & Dischinger, P. (1993). Safety belt restraints and compartment intrusions in frontal and lateral motor vehicle crashes: mechanisms of injuries, complications, and acute care costs. *J Trauma, 5*(34), 736–759.

183. Slater, M. S., & Mullins, R. J. (1998). Rhabdomyolysis and myoglobinuric renal failure in trauma and surgical patients: a review. *J Am Coll Surg, 186*(6), 693–716.

183a. Snyder, P. (1998). In A. B. Maher, et al. (Eds.), *Orthopaedic nursing*. Philadelphia: Saunders.

184. Soderstrom, C., Dischinger, P., & Smith, G. (1992). Psychoactive substance dependence among trauma center patients. *JAMA, 267*, 2756.

185. Stanek, G. S., & Klein, C. J. (2002). Metabolic and nutritional management of the trauma patient. In K. A. McQuillan, et al. (Eds.), *Trauma nursing: from resuscitation through rehabilitation* (3rd ed., pp. 283–323). Philadelphia: Saunders.

186. Steinemann, S., Shackford, S. W., & Davis, J. S. (1990). Implications of admission hypothermia in trauma patients. *J Trauma, 30*, 200–202.

187. Stoner, H. B. (1969). Studies on the mechanisms of shock: the impairment of thermoregulation by trauma. *Br J Exp Pathol, 52*, 650–656.

188. Sugrue, M., et al. (2002). Clinical examination is an inaccurate predictor of intraabdominal pressure. *World J Surg, 26*, 1428–1431.

189. Sutchyta, M. R., et al. (1999). Epidemiology in ARDS. *Intensive Care Med, 25*(5), 538–539.

190. Swan, K. G., & Swan, R. C. (1980). *Gunshot wounds-pathophysiology and management*. Littleton, Mass: PSG Publishing.

191. Trunkey, D. D. (1983). Trauma. *Sci Am, 249*, 28.

192. Vary, T., McLean, B., & Von Rueden, K. T. (2002). Shock and multiple organ dysfunction syndrome. In K. A. McQuillan, et al. (Eds.), *Trauma nursing: from resuscitation through rehabilitation* (3rd ed., pp. 173–200). Philadelphia: Saunders.

193. Vitello, J. M. (1999). *Metabolic response to stress*. Paper presented at the 23rd Clinical Congress of the American Society for Parenteral and Enteral Nutrition: Nutrition support in stress and sepsis San Diego, Calif. Jan 31-Feb 3, 1999.

194. Vournakis, J. N., et al. (2003). The RDH bandage: hemostasis and survival in a lethal aortotomy hemorrhage mode. *J Surg Res, 113*(1), 1–5.

195. Wagner, J. G., & Leatherman, J. W. (1998). Right ventricular end-diastolic volume as a predictor of the hemodynamic response to a fluid challenge. *Chest, 113*(4), 1048–1054.

196. Walsh, C. R. (2002). Musculoskeletal injuries. In K. A. McQuillan, et al. (Eds.), *Trauma nursing: from resuscitation through rehabilitation* (3rd ed., pp. 646–689). Philadelphia: Saunders.

197. Ward, M. M. (1988). Factors predictive of acute renal failure in rhabdomyolysis. *Arch Intern Med, 148*(7), 1553–1557.

198. Weil, M. H., et al. (1999). Sublingual capnometry: a new noninvasive measurement for diagnosis and quantitation of severity of circulatory shock. *Crit Care Med, 27*(7), 1225–1229.

199. Wiegelt, J. A., & Klein, J. D. (2002). Mechanism of injury. In K. A. McQuillan, et al. (Eds.), *Trauma nursing: from resuscitation through rehabilitation* (3rd ed., pp. 148–168). Philadelphia: Saunders.

200. Wild, B. R., Kenwright, J., & Rastogi, S. (1985). Effects of seatbelts on injuries to front and rear seat passengers. *BMJ, 290* (6482), 1621–1623.

201. Willy, C., Gerngross, H., & Sterk, J. (1999). Measurement of intracompartmental pressure with use of a new electronic transducer-tipped catheter system. *J Bone Joint Surg, 81*(2), 158–168.

202. Winkler, M., Akca, O., & Birkenberg, B. (2000). Aggressive warming reduces blood loss during hip arthroplasty. *Anesth Analg, 91*, 978–984.

203. Wisner, D. H. (1996). Injury to the stomach and small bowel. In D. V. Feliciano, E. E. Moore, & K. L. Mattox (Eds.), *Trauma* (3rd ed., pp. 551–571). Stamford, Conn: Appleton & Lange.

204. Wisner, D. H. (2000). Stomach and small bowel. In K. L. Mattox, D. V. Feliciano, & E. E. Moore (Eds.), *Trauma* (4th ed., pp. 713–734). New York: McGraw-Hill.

205. Woods, R. K., et al. (1998). Open pelvic fractures and fecal diversion. *Arch Surg, 133*(3), 281–287.

206. Wright, M. M. (1999). Resuscitation of the multitrauma patient with head injury. *AACN Clin Issues, 10*, 32–45.

207. Zager, R. A. (1992). Combined mannitol and deferoxamine therapy for myohemoglobinuric renal injury and oxidant tubular stress: mechanistic and therapeutic implications. *J Clin Invest, 90*(3), 711–719.

CHAPTER 43

Systemic Inflammatory Response Syndrome and Multiple Organ Dysfunction Syndrome

Dennis J. Cheek, Sophia Chu Rodgers, and Christine Smith Schulman

Retrospective clinical studies found that patients do not die from their underlying disease or even a single complication, but rather from multiple organ dysfunction syndrome, or MODS.[8,19,32,72] Previously known as multiple system organ failure, MODS refers to a continuum of physiologic derangements. The term *dysfunction* identifies inadequate organ function, function not capable of maintaining homeostasis without intervention. The term *MODS* is used to describe the progressive dysfunction of two or more organ systems. Although sepsis and severe sepsis are the most common causes, MODS can also be initiated by any critical illness or traumatic injury that activates a massive systemic inflammatory response in acutely ill patients.[3,11] Other common triggers of MODS include major surgery, burns, shock, acute pancreatitis, acute renal failure, acute respiratory distress syndrome (ARDS), and necrotic tissue.[11] Despite the significant strides made in life support technology, pharmacology, and science as a whole, mortality for the MODS patient with two failing organ systems is 54% and rises to 100% when there are five failing organs.[11] In order to have a significant impact on this terminal syndrome, healthcare providers must be knowledgeable of the underlying pathophysiology. This chapter focuses on current definitions, developing theories of the underlying pathophysiology, early signs and symptoms, and current guidelines for evidence-based management of patients with sepsis and MODS.

DEFINITIONS AND PATIENT IDENTIFICATION

In 1992, an American College of Chest Physicians (ACCP) and Society of Critical Care Medicine Consensus Conference developed a set of definitions for use in patients with MODS.[18] The goal of the conference was to provide a standardized definition to assist the bedside clinician with early diagnosis of the syndrome and therefore early therapeutic intervention.[18] MODS is defined as the presence of altered organ function in an acutely ill patient such that homeostasis cannot be maintained without the intervention of healthcare providers.[18] Because the most common cause for MODS is sepsis and severe sepsis, the consensus guidelines have incorporated the definition for sepsis and its continuum. The definitions were updated in 2001 (Table 43-1).[56]

Systemic inflammatory response syndrome (SIRS) is present when at least two of the following criteria are present: temperature greater than 38° C or less than 36° C, heart rate (HR) greater than 90 beats per minute, respiratory rate (RR) greater than 20 breaths per minute or partial pressure of arterial carbon dioxide ($PaCO_2$) less than 32 mm Hg or need for mechanical ventilation secondary to respiratory failure, or white blood cell (WBC) count greater than 12,000 mm^3 or less than 4000 mm^3 or greater than 10% immature neutrophils.[18,56] Under normal conditions the inflammatory response is an essential and tightly regulated protective mechanism of local response to invasion of microorganism or local tissue damage. This local inflammatory response activates endothelial cells near the initial insult, releasing vasodilating mediators, such as nitric oxide (NO), histamine, and bradykinin, as well as influencing coagulation and fibrinolysis. This manifests clinically as capillary leak, microvascular thrombi, tissue hypoxia, impaired vascular tone, and free radical damage (Figure 43-1).[28,37,48] In SIRS, the inflammatory response becomes systemic, impacting the entire body. The body is overwhelmed by unregulated inflammation, impaired coagulation, fibrinolysis, and endothelial dysfunction. Clinically, this manifests as fever, peripheral edema, hypotension, tachycardia, impaired oxygenation, and elevated white blood cell count (see Figure 43-1).[18,28,56]

When patients have two of the four criteria in association with a known or suspected infection, they are considered to have sepsis.[18,56] Sepsis and its sequelae represent a continuum of clinical and pathophysiologic severity that affects prognosis. Severe sepsis is defined as the presence of a systolic blood pressure (BP) of less than 90 mm Hg or a reduction by 40 mm Hg or more from baseline in the absence of other causes for hypotension such as cardiogenic shock. Septic shock is defined as

TABLE 43-1 Definitions of Sepsis and Organ Failure

Infection,* documented or suspected, and some of the following†:

General variables

Fever (core temperature >38.3° C)

Hypothermia (core temperature <36° C)

Heart rate >90/min or >2 SD above the normal value for age

Tachypnea (>30 bpm)

Altered mental status

Significant edema or positive fluid balance (>20 ml/kg over 24 hr)

Hyperglycemia (plasma glucose >110 mg/dl or 7.7 mmol/L) in the absence of diabetes

Inflammatory variables

Leukocytosis (WBC count >12,000 µL)

Leukopenia (WBC count <4000 µL)

Normal WBC count with >10% immature forms (bands)

Plasma C–reactive protein >2 SD above the normal value

Plasma procalcitonin >2 SD above the normal value

Hemodynamic variables

Arterial hypotension† (SBP <90 mm Hg, MAP <70, or an SBP decrease >40 mm Hg in adults or <2 SD below normal for age)

Mixed venous oxygen saturation >70%†

Cardiac index >3.5 L/min/m²‡§)

Organ dysfunction variables

Arterial hypoxemia (Pao_2/Fio_2 <300)

Acute oliguria (urine output <0.5 ml/kg/hr or 45 mmol/L for at least 2 hr)

Creatinine increase ≥0.5 mg/dl

Coagulation abnormalities (INR >1.5 or aPTT >60 sec)

Ileus (absent bowel sounds)

Thrombocytopenia (platelet count <100,000 µL)

Hyperbilirubinemia (plasma total bilirubin >4 mg/dl or 70 mmol/L)

Tissue perfusion variables

Hyperlactatemia (>3 mmol/L)

Decreased capillary refill or mottling

From reference 56.

aPTT = Activated partial thromboplastin time, Fio_2 = fraction of inspired oxygen, INR = international normalized ratio, MAP = mean arterial blood pressure, Pao_2 = partial pressure of arterial oxygen, SBP = systolic blood pressure, SD = standard deviation, WBC = white blood cell.

*Infection is defined as a pathologic process induced by a microorganism.

†Values greater than 70% are normal in children (normally 75%–80%) and therefore should not be used as a sign of sepsis in newborns or children.

‡Values of 3.5 to 5.5 are normal in children and therefore should not be used as a sign of sepsis in newborns or children.

§Diagnostic criteria for sepsis in the pediatric population are signs and symptoms of inflammation plus infection with hyperthermia or hypothermia (rectal temperature >38.5° C or <35° C), tachycardia (may be absent in hypothermic patients), and at least one of the following indications of altered organ function: altered mental status, hypoxemia, elevated serum lactate level, or bounding pulses.

persistent hypotension despite fluid and vasopressor resuscitation.[12-13,18,56]

EPIDEMIOLOGY

MODS develops in about 15% of all patients admitted to critical care.[11] It accounts for 20% to 50% of patients admitted to critical care for multiple trauma and is responsible for 80% of all critical care deaths.[11,25] Unfortunately, this remains true even today, with mortality rates remaining at 70% to 80% for the past 25 years, despite numerous technologic advances in the healthcare arena.[11,25] The mortality of MODS increases with each organ system involved.[11] The estimated cost of MODS in critical care is $100,000, with a cost of $500,000 in survivors.[25,60] In order to continue tracking the true incidence and mortality of MODS, providers need to document it as a unique diagnosis as opposed to "respiratory failure" or "renal failure."[11,25,60]

PATHOPHYSIOLOGY OF MULTIPLE ORGAN DYSFUNCTION SYNDROME

MODS is a complex and unpredictable clinical syndrome. It is associated with multiple integrated responses. These major responses include increased inflammation, altered coagulation, and impaired fibrinolytic activity. There is also involvement of the endothelium, which becomes a central player in the development of SIRS and MODS.

Inflammation

As shown in Figure 43-1, when the body is exposed to bacteria, bacterial products, necrotic tissue, or other insult, an inflammatory cellular response is initiated. There is an increased production of inflammatory cytokines in the form of interleukin (IL)-1, IL-6, and tumor necrosis factor-alpha (TNF-α).[28] Although the early response of these cytokines plays a major role in the host's defense by attracting neutrophils to an infected site, it also contributes to the manifestations of the systemic inflammatory response.[28] The body attempts to maintain homeostasis by releasing antiinflammatory cytokines such as IL-4 and IL-10. Release of both the inflammatory and antiinflammatory mediators may lead to a state of primed inflammatory response (Figure 43-2).[28]

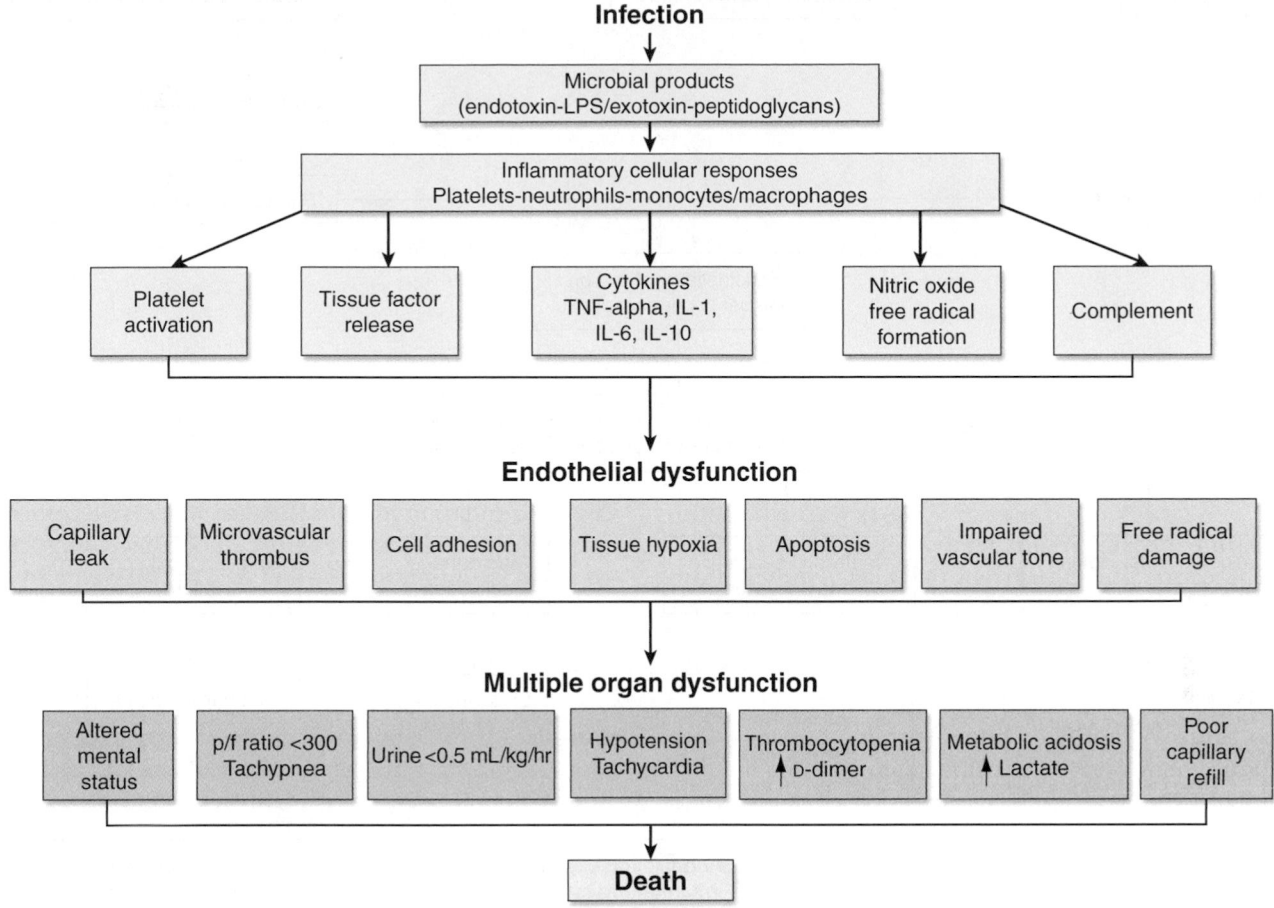

♣FIGURE 43-1 Endothelial dysfunction and multiple organ dysfunction. IL = Interleukin, P/F=partial pressure of arterial oxygen tension (Pao₂)/fraction of inspired oxygen (Fio₂), TNF = tumor necrosis factor.

Activation of Coagulation

Coagulation and inflammation are closely linked. It is believed that tissue factor is expressed by monocytes and endothelial cells following exposure to bacteria and it also stimulates the extrinsic coagulation cascade.[3,12,28,36] Through cross talk and feedback mechanisms, the intrinsic coagulation pathway also can be initiated.[3,4,12,28,36] Both pathways play an important role in coagulation. The intrinsic pathway is considered the initiator of coagulation and the extrinsic pathway is considered the amplifier. This accelerated coagulation process occurs at the capillary level of the various organs. When clots form at the microcirculatory level, distal cells become anoxic and consequently, if not dissolved, the organ becomes dysfunctional and eventually dies.[3,4,12,28,36] As a rule, coagulation reactions occur on activated cell surface membranes. This reaction is believed to be initiated by activated tissue factor. In the case of MODS, the coagulation cascade

may be activated by the inflammatory cytokine IL-6 acting on factor VIII.[13,28] Thrombin circulates in the form of prothrombin. The conversion of prothrombin to thrombin is mediated by factor Xa, which is activated by either factor VIIa of the extrinsic pathway or factor IXa of the intrinsic pathway. The result is that thrombin cleaves fibrinogen, forming fibrin, which then produces a clot.[3,4,12,28,36]

Impairment of Fibrinolysis

Normally clots are formed when bleeding occurs, but the vascular endothelium also has the ability to dissolve these clots using tissue plasminogen activator (tPA), which is released by endothelial cells. In severe sepsis, fibrinolytic activity is impaired due to increased production of plasminogen activator inhibitor-1 (PAI-1) and thrombin-activated fibrinolysis inhibitor (TAFI). These mediators suppress the activity of tPA, resulting in the

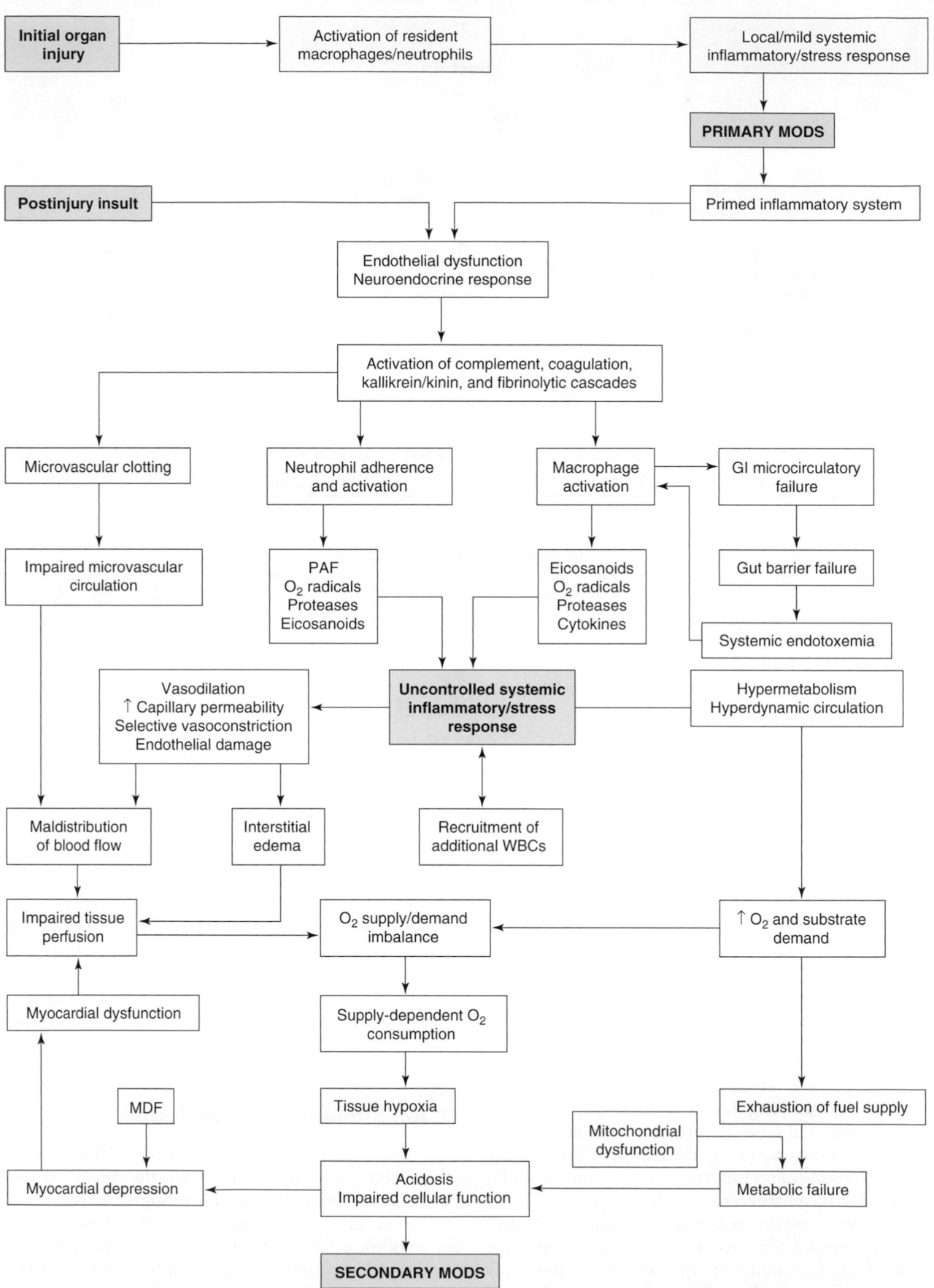

⬦FIGURE 43-2 Pathophysiology of multiple organ dysfunction syndrome.

loss of ability to dissolve clots. Consequently, an increase in the production of clot formation is compounded when the ability to lyse clots is impaired, resulting in diminished blood flow at the microcirculatory level and organ damage.[3,4,12,28,36]

Role of the Endothelium

For many years the endothelium was considered an inert layer, separating blood from underlying tissue. Over time we have learned that the endothelium is a highly active cell layer that has several functions including controlling vasomotor tone, trafficking nutrients, and maintaining blood fluidity.[21] The largest organ in the body, the endothelium plays a key role in the inflammatory, prothrombotic, and impaired fibrinolytic components of SIRS and MODS.* Progression of endothelial dysfunction results in maldistribution of blood flow secondary to increased microvascular permeability and formation of microthrombi (see Figure 43-1).[28] This is believed to be caused by either the production of inflammatory mediators and/or by the infecting organism or endotoxin.[3,4,76]

Normal endothelium has an anticoagulant property. Its outer membrane normally expresses various membrane-associated components with anticoagulant properties, among these a cell surface heparin-like molecule. In SIRS and MODS, proinflammatory mediators are released from monocytes and macrophages that cause injury to the endothelium (see Figure 43-1).[28] These mediators promote recruitment of neutrophils and accumulation of platelets to wall off infection but they can also continue to damage the endothelial layer. After injury, the endothelial cells may down-regulate the synthesis and expression of antithrombin molecules such as thrombomodulin, endothelial cell receptors for protein C, and tissue factor pathway inhibitor.[4,28,37]

Normally the endothelium produces a low level of adhesion molecules such as selectin. However, in severe sepsis and MODS, up-regulation of the adhesion molecules promotes interaction among the endothelium, white blood cells, and platelets. This interaction promotes accumulation of neutrophils and platelets that adhere to the endothelial wall and form further thrombi.[4,36]

In addition to the formation of clots, proinflammatory cytokines increase vascular permeability within 6 to 24 hours of the insult.[29] Physical disruption of the endothelium allows fluid and cells to move from the vascular compartment into the interstitial compartment, further adding to endothelial cell dysfunction, inflammation, and formation of edema. This is the mechanism responsible for the anasarca that critically ill patients develop.[4,18,28,36]

*References 3, 4, 21, 28, 33, 36, 37.

Vasomotor tone can also be affected. Normally the endothelium secretes substances such as NO and epoprostenol that promote a steady level of vasodilation. This becomes impaired when increased production of NO leads to abnormal and persistent vascular relaxation.[1,74] As MODS progresses, alterations in vasoregulation result in vasodilation, refractory hypotension, and impaired microcirculatory blood flow, which eventually lead to system-wide organ dysfunction (see Figure 43-2).[1,74]

MECHANISMS OF ORGAN DYSFUNCTION IN MODS

Cardiovascular System

Cardiovascular dysfunction is both the result and cause of hypoperfusion through several mechanisms. Changes in both systolic and diastolic ventricular function seen in SIRS and MODS result in decreased cardiac output (CO). Initially, ventricular function increases CO to maintain adequate BP in the presence of vasodilation because of the Frank-Starling mechanism.[12] However, older adult patients, and those with profound SIRS and preexisting heart disease, have an impaired ability to increase CO using contractility, resulting in hypoperfusion.[34] Myocardial contractility also may be depressed by the effects of hypoxia and acidosis of the myocardium or proinflammatory cytokines such as TNF, IL-1, or the myocardial depressant factor.[34]

In the regional circulation, vascular hyporesponsiveness induced by SIRS or MODS leads to considerable maldistribution of systemic blood flow among organ systems as well as hypotension. For example, organ dysfunction interferes with the normal ability to redistribute blood away from splanchnic organs (e.g., liver, gut) to essential organs (e.g., heart, brain) when oxygen delivery is depressed.[28,38] Blood volume pools in the distal organ beds rather than actively circulating to essential organs, creating a relative hypovolemia further contributing to poor CO and cardiovascular dysfunction.[28]

Microcirculatory blood flow may present as either "no flow" or intermittent flow.[29] Techniques including reflectance spectrophotometry and orthogonal polarization spectral imaging allow for in vivo visualization of the sublingual and gastric microvasculature. Compared with normal controls and critically ill patients without organ dysfunction, patients with severe organ dysfunction have an overall decrease in vessel density.[29] These changes may be due to extrinsic compression of the capillary by tissue edema and endothelial swelling, or plugging of the capillary lumen by leukocytes or red blood cells.[67] This capillary obstruction prevents blood flow to distal tissues, creating a significant derangement in metabolic autoregulation.

Metabolic autoregulation matches oxygen availability to changing tissue oxygen needs at the microvascular level. The initial release of inflammatory mediators causes appropriate vasodilation and increases microvascular permeability at the site of infection, a response intended to facilitate WBC movement through narrowed capillaries and into the interstitium to destroy bacteria. Among these mediators are the vasodilators epoprostenol and NO.[1,28,74] During septic shock, however, normal compensatory mechanisms become overwhelmed, and profound vasodilation and capillary permeability cause refractory hypoperfusion.[28] Subsequent blood flow stasis fails to deliver oxygen to the capillaries and cells, resulting in additional tissue ischemia and hypoperfusion (see Figure 43-2).[12,29]

In particular, NO has additional influences on cardiovascular failure accompanying septic shock.[74] It depresses the control mechanisms that match oxygen delivery to oxygen needs at all the central, regional, and microregional levels of the circulation. In addition, NO may trigger injury in the central nervous system in areas that regulate autonomic control such as heart rate and blood pressure via apoptosis or programmed cell death of the neurons located in the critical area of the central nervous system.[74] NO can react with superoxide radical anions to form peroxynitrite. This potent oxidizing agent not only induces lipid peroxidation, thus compromising cell wall integrity but also damages deoxyribonucleic acid (DNA). When DNA is damaged, the enzyme poly-ADP-ribosylpolymerase-1 is activated and uses nicotinamide adenine dinucleotide (NAD), an essential cofactor in a number of cellular reactions including the consumption of oxygen by the mitochondria, to repair DNA. During the repair process, NAD is consumed; without the availability of NAD, the cell's mitochondria cannot use oxygen.[12,19,27]

Another factor contributing to persistent cardiovascular dysfunction is impaired compensatory secretion of antidiuretic hormone (vasopressin). Vasopressin is a nonapeptide synthesized in the hypothalamus.[43,44,58,75] Vasopressin release is stimulated by hyperosmolality, hypotension, and hypovolemia as well as acidosis, pain, hypoxia, and hypercapnia.[43,44,58,75] Vasopressin acts on several different vasopressin receptors. Vasopressin-1 (V1) receptors stimulate vasoconstriction, V2 receptors regulate water balance, and V3 receptors stimulate adrenocorticotropin hormone (ACTH) release.[43,44,58,75] Normal vasopressin levels are 0.5 to 5.0 pg/ml in humans.[43,44,58,75] In one report, plasma vasopressin levels were much lower in 19 patients with septic shock

(3.1 pg/ml) than in 12 patients with cardiogenic shock who had similar systemic blood pressures (22.7 pg/ml).[39]

Yet another probable etiology of cardiovascular dysfunction in SIRS and MODS is relative adrenal insufficiency. In a double-blind, randomized study 300 patients underwent corticotropin stimulation testing; they were randomly assigned to receive either hydrocortisone and fludrocortisone or a matching placebo.[10] In this trial, those who met the criteria of relative adrenal insufficiency and received steroids had a lower incidence of death than those who received placebo. Vasopressors were also withdrawn earlier in the steroid group.[10]

Respiratory System

Pulmonary dysfunction results from and causes MODS. Pneumonia is the most common source for initiating the inflammatory process leading to pulmonary endothelial dysfunction and ARDS.[11,13,72]

Endothelial dysfunction in the pulmonary vasculature leads to disturbed capillary blood flow and increased microvascular permeability over a large surface area, resulting in interstitial and alveolar edema.[9,12,48] Neutrophil entrapment within the lungs' microcirculation initiates and/or amplifies this injury to the alveolar-capillary membrane.[27,29] Pulmonary edema is the clinical result, and is accompanied by ventilation-perfusion mismatch and arterial hypoxemia. This can develop into ARDS. Approximately 25% to 40% of ARDS cases originate from sepsis.[9,12,48]

Gastrointestinal System

The gastrointestinal (GI) tract is a particularly important target organ system for injury in organ dysfunction because it has the potential to provide a positive feedback loop in propagation of the injury.[25,27] This is even truer when the patient is intubated and unable to eat because bacteria may overgrow the upper GI tract and be aspirated into the lung, causing nosocomial pneumonia. Furthermore, the circulatory abnormalities seen during hypoperfusion may depress the gut's normal barrier function, allowing translocation of bacteria and endotoxin to enter the systemic circulation (possibly via the lymphatics), extending the inflammatory process.[12,28,48,53] Bacteria can be found in mesenteric lymph nodes as well as in the spleen and liver. Whether these findings are clinically important is not clear, although late infectious complications in SIRS/MODS are commonly caused by *Pseudomonas*, coagulase-negative staphylococcus, candida, and enterococcus, all common organisms found in the GI tract of critically ill patients.[38,53]

Hepatic System

By virtue of the liver's role in host defense and synthetic functions, liver dysfunction contributes to both the initiation and progression of SIRS and MODS. The reticuloendothelial system of the liver normally acts as the first line of defense in clearing bacteria and bacteria-derived products that entered the portal system from the gut. Liver dysfunction prevents the elimination of enteric-derived endotoxin and bacteria-derived products, precluding appropriate local cytokine response and permitting direct entry of these potentially injurious products into the systemic circulation.[12,28,38,48,53] The liver may also serve as a site for the release of acute-phase reactants (e.g., proinflammatory and antiinflammatory cytokines) during a hypoperfused state, leading to the development of centrilobular necrosis. If the liver is already at risk from other causes such as cirrhosis, hepatic failure will significantly affect formation and release of coagulation factors, also affecting any ongoing blood loss. Lastly, liver failure decreases albumin production. Hypoalbuminemia causes movement of intravascular fluids into interstitial compartments and peripheral and organ edema, further contributing to MODS.[28,38]

Renal System

The mechanisms by which endotoxemia and MODS might lead to acute renal failure are not clearly understood. Some of the etiology may be attributed to systemic hypoperfusion, direct renal vasoconstriction, release of cytokines such as tumor necrosis factor, and activation of neutrophils by endotoxin. Renal failure may also be a cause in the development of SIRS or MODS via the activation of endothelium located in the renal system, which induces the release of the vasoconstrictor, endothelin, and decreases production of the vasodilators NO and prostacyclin.[12,48]

Neurologic System

The pathogenesis of encephalopathy in MODS is poorly defined. Although a high incidence of brain microabscesses[48] was noted in one study, the significance of hematogenous infection as the principal mechanism of encephalopathy has been questioned.[28] It is also possible that with growing endothelial dysfunction, microvascular hypoperfusion will have an impact on the development of encephalopathy.[2,11,28] Continued hypoperfusion, seen with shock and cardiac arrest, leads to neurologic dysfunction and cerebral microvascular changes, causing cerebral edema, increased intracranial pressure, and herniation. Loss of cerebral autoregulation function causes continued cerebral and systemic hypotension, potentiating ischemic and inflammatory processes in the brain and throughout the body, that is, central nervous system infection and stroke can cause global hypoperfusion leading to inflammatory processes and MODS.[28]

Epidemiologic studies suggest that at least 25% of patients admitted to medical or surgical intensive care units have some degree of acquired paresis.[25,32,49,60] Most episodes present 7 or more days after the onset of critical illness. Affected patients manifest a sensorimotor polyneuropathy characterized clinically by limb muscle weakness and atrophy, reduced or absent deep tendon reflexes, loss of peripheral sensation to light touch and pinprick, and relative preservation of the cranial nerve function. Critical illness polyneuropathy is strongly associated with organ dysfunction and probably represents neurologic manifestations of the systemic inflammatory response.[28] A thorough review of critical illness polyneuropathy can be found in Chapter 25.

Hematologic System

Although disseminated intravascular coagulation (DIC) can occur in patients with organ dysfunction, the activation of the hemostatic system in patients with SIRS or MODS is not DIC. Increased D-dimers and decreased protein C levels are consistently seen in patients with organ dysfunction, but thrombocytopenia, prolonged activated partial thromboplastin time (aPTT) or prothrombin time (PT), or any combination is distinctly uncommon.[12,32] Therefore although the diagnosis of DIC is a clinicopathologic one, laboratory data suggest that the inflammatory and hemostatic changes of organ dysfunction are similar.[12,32] However, it is uncommon for the abnormal laboratory criteria seen with DIC, SIRS, or MODS to produce clinical bleeding.[3,9]

Decreases in protein C levels play an active role in the development of the hypercoagulable state in patients with severe sepsis, and are linked to the development of organ dysfunction and increased mortality.[12] A study of patients with cancer, chemotherapy-induced neutropenia (absolute neutrophil count [ANC] less than 1000/μL), severe sepsis, and septic shock demonstrated that protein C concentrations fall before the onset of fever or alterations in the leukocyte count. In fact, protein C levels decline 16 hours before severe sepsis is clinically diagnosed.[13] Protein C is a glycoprotein that is synthesized in the liver and circulates in the bloodstream. Activated protein C (APC) binds to the cell-surface-bound anticoagulant cofactor, protein S. The APC/protein S complex then lyses activated procoagulant cofactors such as factor VIII and factor V, reducing fibrin formation by preventing activation of procoagulant proteins such as factor X and prothrombin. Protein C deficiency is associated with an increased risk of thrombus formation. In addition to having anticoagulant properties, APC also appears to have profibrinolytic and antiinflammatory properties and preserves endothelial function.[12,48]

In one study, both tissue plasminogen activator and PAI-1 were high in survivors and nonsurvivors of sepsis, but survivors showed a progressive normalization of fibrinolytic parameters during the study period.[13] Low plasminogen levels and plasminogen/ alpha 2-antiplasmin ratios were found in both groups, with a trend toward normalization noted only in survivors. The differences reported were not apparent at the time of hospital admission. The investigators concluded that in the presence of fibrin formation, nonsurvivors maintained an imbalance in the fibrinolytic response determined by a higher PAI-1 plasma concentration.[13]

ASSESSMENT OF MULTIPLE ORGAN DYSFUNCTION SYNDROME

Much of our understanding of the progression of MODS comes from the work of Knaus and colleagues, using the Acute Physiology and Chronic Health Evaluation (APACHE) scoring systems at George Washington University.[49] Their work gave rise to a more consistent method for quantifying organ dysfunction and patient outcomes associated with MODS.[49] Organ dysfunction has been described using physiologic criteria that are based on clinical presentation and laboratory markers for the neurologic, pulmonary, hepatic, cardiovascular, renal, and hematologic systems.[48] These criteria, along with general clinical presentation of patients with MODS, are described later; a complete review of the pathophysiology and clinical presentation of individual organ dysfunction or failure is presented in organ-specific chapters elsewhere in this book.

A change in the level of consciousness is one of the most sensitive indicators of a failing neurologic system (Box 43-1). This change in mental status can be as subtle as an alteration in mental status to confusion or even deep coma. Most often, the critical care nurse will assess neurologic status using a specific scale such as the Glasgow Coma Scale (GCS).[49] The GCS is based on eye opening, verbal response, and motor response. The total possible score is 15; the lowest is a 3, indicating a patient in a total coma state. A patient with MODS will often have a GCS score of less than 6 in the absence of sedation.[49]

Manifestations of respiratory failure in MODS include a $PaCO_2$ of greater than 50 mm Hg, ventilator or continuous positive airway pressure dependence on the second day of organ dysfunction, and a partial pressure of arterial oxygen tension (PaO_2)/fraction of inspired oxygen (FiO_2) (P/F) ratio equal to, or less than, 300. The ACCP defines a P/F ratio of less than 200 as ARDS and P/F ratio of less than 300 as acute lung injury (ALI).[1,27] Clinical presentation also may include tachypnea, severe dyspnea, decreased oxygen saturation, cyanosis, respiratory acidosis, and refractory hypoxemia.[48]

Manifestations of hepatic failure include jaundice with bilirubin levels of greater than 6 mg/100 dl. Liver

---

Box 43-1

Commonly Used Markers of Acute Organ System Dysfunction

CARDIOVASCULAR

Tachycardia
Dysrhythmias
Hypotension
Elevated central venous and pulmonary artery pressures

RESPIRATORY

Tachypnea
Hypoxemia

RENAL

Oliguria
Anuria
Elevated creatinine levels

HEMATOLOGIC

Jaundice
Elevated levels of liver enzymes
Decreased concentration of albumin
Coagulopathy

HEPATIC

Thrombocytopenia
Coagulopathy
Decreased levels of protein C
Increased levels of D-dimers

NEUROLOGIC

Altered consciousness
Confusion
Psychosis

From reference 48.

enzymes are also elevated, including aspartate aminotransferase (AST) (formerly serum glutamic oxaloacetic transaminase [SGOT]), alanine aminotransferase (ALT) (formerly serum glutamic pyruvic transaminase [SGPT]), lactic dehydrogenase (LDH), and alkaline phosphatase. An increase in serum ammonia and decreases in serum albumin, prealbumin, and transferrin levels also may be present. A dysfunction in the regulation of the coagulation cascade is demonstrated by a PT 4 seconds greater than control. Any time a coagulopathy is noted in the absence of anticoagulant therapy, a full workup of liver function should be performed.[2,28,48] The clinical manifestation of hepatic dysfunction in MODS is hepatomegaly, jaundice, bleeding, and hepatic encephalopathy.[48]

Cardiovascular dysfunction associated with MODS presents in a number of ways. Early signs and symptoms of cardiovascular challenges include tachycardia, hypotension, pale mottled skin that is cool to the touch, and weak peripheral pulses.[48] Fulminant cardiac dysfunction in MODS is an ominous indication that compensatory requirements of hypoperfusion and shock are overwhelming.[2,28,48] When the cardiovascular system is unable to respond effectively to tissue demands and fluid resuscitation, the heart rate is usually below 60, mean arterial pressure (MAP) is less than 49 mm Hg, with increased central venous pressure

(CVP) and pulmonary arterial pressure. As systemic hypoperfusion continues, the microcirculation continues to deteriorate; decreased oxygen delivery as well as decreased consumption are evidenced by a serum pH less than 7.24 and a Pa_{CO_2} greater than 49 mm Hg.[28,48]

Criteria for renal dysfunction in MODS include urine output less than 479 ml/24 hr or less than 159 ml/8 hr, serum blood urea nitrogen (BUN) greater than 100 mg/dl, and/or serum creatinine greater than 3.5 mg/dl.[2,28,48] The cause of renal dysfunction in MODS may be due to renal hypoperfusion or possibly acute tubular necrosis. The clinical manifestation may be oliguria or anuria along with elevated BUN and serum creatinine.[48]

The last markers of organ dysfunction in MODS are abnormalities in hematologic function. Manifestations of hematologic failure include thrombocytopenia (platelets less than $20,000/mm^3$), prolonged PT (4 seconds greater than control), decreased protein C (normal level is 4 mcg/ml), leukopenia (less than $1000 cells/mm^3$), and an elevated D-dimer level (normal range is 0 to 0.4 mcg/ml).[4,13,48]

Quantification of organ function may be measured with one of several outcome prediction scores. The Logistic Organ Dysfunction Score (LODS) (Table 43-2), MODS score (Table 43-3), or the Sequential (formerly

TABLE 43-2 Logistic Organ Dysfunction Score System

VARIABLES	0	1	2	3	4
Glasgow Coma Scale	14–15	9–13	6–8	4–5	3
Pa_{O_2}/Fi_{O_2}	No ventilator	>250	150–249	50–149	<50
Heart rate	130–139	140–159	160	<30	
Blood urea nitrogen	<6	6–9.9	10–19.9	>20	
Creatinine	<1.2	1.2–1.6	>1.6		
Urine output (L/day)	0.75–9.99	0.5–0.74	<0.5		
White blood cell count	2.5–49.9	1.0–2.4 or >50	<1.0		
Bilirubin	<34.2	34.2–68.3	>68.3		
Platelets	≥50	<50			
Prothrombin time	≥25%	<25%			

From reference 54.
Fi_{O_2} = Fraction of inspired oxygen, Pa_{O_2} = partial pressure of arterial oxygen.

TABLE 43-3 Multiple Organ Dysfunction Syndrome Scoring System

ORGAN SYSTEM	0	1	2	3	4
Cardiovascular (heart rate, inotropes, lactate)	≤120	120–140	>140	Inotropes	Lactate >5
Respiratory, P_{O_2}/F_{IO_2}	>300	226–300	151–225	76–150	≤75
Renal (creatinine, mmol/L)	≤100	101–200	201–350	351–500	>500
Central nervous system (Glasgow Coma Scale score)	15	13–14	10–12	7–9	≤6
Hepatic (total bilirubin, mmol/L)	≤20	21–60	61–120	121–240	>240
Hematologic (platelet count × 10^3)	>120	81–120	51–80	21–50	≤20

Marshall, J.C., et al. (1995). Multiple organ dysfunction score: a reliable descriptor of a complex clinical outcome. *Crit Care Med, 23*(10), 1638–1652. Six domains of multiple organ dysfunction syndrome (MODS). The original cardiovascular component was defined by the heart rate times right atrial pressure. The modified cardiovascular component of MODS is defined as follows: 0, heart rate <120 beats per minute (bpm); 1, heart rate 120–140 bpm; 2, heart rate >140 bpm; 3, need for inotropes more than dopamine >3 mcg/kg/min; 4, serum lactate >5 mMol/L.

Sepsis-Related) Organ Failure Assessment (SOFA) (Table 43-4) are based on dysfunction of the respiratory, renal, hepatic, cardiovascular, hematologic, and neurologic systems and combine the severity of organ dysfunction from MODS into a single score. In 2002 Pettila and colleagues compared the predictive power for hospital mortality using the LODS, MODS, and SOFA tools along with the APACHE III and found that the discriminative power was strong among all the tools tested.[65] The study demonstrated that the greater the score and duration of organ dysfunction, the higher the mortality from MODS.[25,32,49,65]

The scoring systems were designed to describe the evolving morbidity and mortality and are employed primarily in clinical evaluation of interventions to treat MODS and sepsis.[25,32,49,65] In most of the scoring tools, the disease severity is evaluated using clinical presentation and laboratory data on the six specific organ systems.[25,32,49,65] In clinical practice, treatment is initiated as the scores increase, although there is no research defining at exactly what point on each scale interventions should start. The key for the critical care nurse is the early detection and treatment of dysfunctional organ systems to avoid subsequent organ failure. Mortality from MODS with failure of just two organ systems is 54%, and increases significantly to 100% when five or more systems have failed.[11]

INTERVENTIONS

Early detection or prevention of organ dysfunction is extremely important because there is no specific therapy for MODS once it occurs. In October 2003, 11 international critical care and infectious disease organizations collaborated to develop and publish management guidelines for the care of patients with sepsis and severe sepsis, known as the Surviving Sepsis Campaign (SSC).[31] This international effort focused on increasing the awareness and improving the outcomes of severe sepsis. Because sepsis is the most common etiology for MODS, many of the recommendations from the SSC may be applicable for any patient with multiple organ dysfunction. The majority of their recommendations are not supported by evidence but only by expert opinion. Furthermore, these are grouped by category and not by hierarchy.[31,35] The overall goal of the SSC is to prevent and respond to organ dysfunction before it becomes irreversible. A full review of individual organ system support is beyond the scope of this chapter, but is found elsewhere in this text. A schematic view of the interventions for a patient with MODS is shown in the Multidisciplinary Plan of Care on pp. 1200-1203. The following discussion focuses on the specific interventions prioritized by the SSC to avert MODS resulting from severe sepsis.

TABLE 43-4 Sequential Organ Failure Assessment Scoring System

ORGAN SYSTEM	Score				
	0	1	2	3	4
Respiratory Pao_2/Fio_2	>400	≤400	≤300	≤200	≤100
Renal creatinine, mmol/L	≤110	110–170	171–299	300–440	>440
Hepatic bilirubin, mmol/L	≤20	20–32	33–101	102–204	>204
Cardiovascular hypotension	No hypotension	Mean arterial pressure <70 mm Hg	Dopamine ≤5	Dopamine >5 or epinephrine ≤0.1 or norepinephrine ≤0.1	Dopamine >15 or epinephrine >0.1 or norepinephrine >0.1
Hematologic platelet count ($\times 10^{12}$/L)	>150	≤150	≤100	≤50	≤20
Neurologic Glasgow Coma Scale score	15	13–14	10–12	6–9	<6

From reference 78a.

Initial Resuscitation

Resuscitation of the patient with SIRS should begin as soon as the syndrome is recognized, without waiting until the patient is transferred to critical care; therefore, early therapy should be initiated in the emergency department. The basic principle of early goal-directed therapy (EGDT) is to redefine shock in terms of global tissue hypoxia. EGDT defines shock in terms of an imbalance between systemic oxygen delivery and demand and employs more sensitive measures to evaluate this imbalance.[70]

During the first 6 hours of EGDT, resuscitation goals should include all the following: CVP, 8 to 12 mm Hg (12 to 15 mm Hg if mechanically ventilated); MAP equal to or greater than 65 mm Hg, or systolic BP greater than 90 mm Hg; urinary output equal to or greater than 0.5 ml/kg/hr; and central venous oxygen saturation (Scvo2) equal to or greater than 70% or mixed venous oxygen saturation (Svo2) equal to or greater than 65%.

To achieve these goals, fluids may be administered at 1 to 2 L/hr.[22,24,34,73] Additional boluses of crystalloids (e.g., normal saline 500 to 100 mL) and colloids (e.g., albumin 300 to 500 ml) may be given and repeated until the desired resuscitation targets are achieved.[22,24,26] The choice of using colloids or crystalloids remains controversial. One issue that is not controversial is that crystalloid use requires about three times as much fluid as colloids to reach the same end point. Crystalloids have a larger distribution space and do not remain in the intravascular space, putting the patient at risk for significant edema. If the CVP or Svo2 targets cannot be reached, fluids, transfusion of packed red blood cells to a hematocrit (Hct) of 30%, and/or administration of dobutamine (Dobutrex) up to a maximum of 20 mcg/kg/min may be needed.[34] A discussion of the use of arginine vasopressin in patients with MODS appears in the Research Utilization box on p. 1204.

MULTIDISCIPLINARY PLAN OF CARE FOR MULTIPLE ORGAN DYSFUNCTION SYNDROME

PROBLEM	INTERVENTION	RATIONALE	EXPECTED OUTCOME	COMMENTS
Neurologic ischemia/ dysfunction	Perform neurologic assessment every hour, including assessment of changes in mentation or level of consciousness	Provides information regarding the status of cerebral blood flow and oxygenation	Patient will maintain adequate cerebral blood flow. Mental status will remain intact	
	Record and report any changes	Helps guide selection of appropriate interventions	Patient will return to pre-illness level of functioning	
Cardiovascular ischemia/ dysfunction	Monitor heart rate, rhythm, and blood pressure and other hemodynamic parameters as available	Monitors for early signs of microvasculature dysfunction, which lead to shock and hypotension	Maintenance of cardiovascular system function	
	Administer fluids and vasoactive agents as needed to maintain normovolemia and goal blood pressure Monitor and maintain acceptable Hct and Hgb			Dopamine and norepinephrine (with alpha, beta, and chronotropic properties) are agents of choice for MODS Dobutamine may be added as an adjuvant therapy to improve cardiac output but administered by itself may produce hypotension Arginine vasopressin may be added for refractory hypotension
Renal ischemia/ dysfunction	Monitor for urine output less than 0.5 ml/kg/hr, increase in urine specific gravity, elevation in serum BUN or Cr, abnormal serum electrolytes, low urine Na$^+$, K$^+$, protein and blood in urine, and metabolic acidosis	Assesses renal function		
	Administer fluids and diuretics as ordered to facilitate urine output		Patient will maintain urine output greater than 0.5 ml/kg/hr	
	Initiate CVVH or hemodialysis if acute renal failure develops		Patient's laboratory tests will confirm adequate renal function	

Table continues on page 1202

PROBLEM	INTERVENTION	RATIONALE	EXPECTED OUTCOME	COMMENTS
GI ischemia/ dysfunction	Perform daily weights	Identifies a possible complication of overtreatment; assesses GI function secondary to hypoperfusion	Patient's weight will not fluctuate more than 2 lb/day	
	Monitor signs and symptoms of fluid overload	Patients in MODS have profound metabolic demands		
	Monitor for presence of abdominal pain, distention, nausea, vomiting, anorexia, diarrhea, thirst; auscultate for bowel sounds		Patient will exhibit no abdominal discomforts	
	Initiate enteral or parenteral nutrition as soon as possible	Use of the gut supports immune function	Patient will tolerate ordered diet	
Peripheral vascular ischemia/ dysfunction	Monitor for presence of cool, pale, or cyanotic extremities; diminished or absent peripheral pulses; pain, tingling, or numbness in extremities; necrotic or gangrenous extremities; poor capillary refill	Indicates peripheral vascular ischemia	Parameters measuring metabolic function will be within normal limits	
	Report any changes in peripheral perfusion	Initiate prompt treatment as indicated by clinical findings Patient will exhibit no changes in peripheral perfusion	Patient will show no signs of peripheral ischemia	
	Initiate proper skin care measures	Maintain skin integrity and prevent pressure ulcers because they can develop quickly when immobility is combined with tissue ischemia Promote comfort and prevent vasoconstriction	Patient will remain free of skin breakdown	

PROBLEM	INTERVENTION	RATIONALE	EXPECTED OUTCOME	COMMENTS
Respiratory ischemia/ dysfunction	Monitor for altered respiratory rate and depth, dyspnea, use of accessory muscles, cyanosis, adventitious breath sounds, cough, abnormal chest x-ray	Development of respiratory failure may progress to ARDS and result in long critical care stays and poor outcome		
	Initiate oxygen and maintain Sao_2 ≥90%	Ensures adequate oxygenation	Patient's respiratory rate will not fluctuate from baseline	
	Monitor ABGs	Evaluates respiratory acidosis	Patient will remain adequately oxygenated as evidenced by an Sao_2 ≥90% Patient will maintain pH between 7.35 and 7.45	
	Auscultate and record breath sounds every 1–2 hr to determine presence of crackles, wheezes, and decreased or unequal breath sounds	Indicates impaired respirations	Patient will remain free of adventitious lung sounds	
	Assist patient to deep breathe	Opens up alveoli and improves gas exchange	Patient will turn, cough, and deep breathe on instruction from staff	
	Suction as needed	Removes secretions patient cannot remove independently	Patient will remain free of excess secretions	
	Maintain patent airway and prepare for possible intubation and mechanical ventilation	Ensures adequate oxygenation and ventilation	Patient will maintain adequate oxygenation and ventilation	
	Initiate protocol for prevention of ventilator-associated pneumonia	Secondary pneumonia can be a source of sepsis and potentiate MODS		

PROBLEM	INTERVENTION	RATIONALE	EXPECTED OUTCOME	COMMENTS
	Use good hand washing techniques Follow universal precautions Enforce infection control measures Wean mechanical ventilation as soon as possible Daily sedation holiday Monitor Hgb, Hct, WBC, PT, aPTT, fibrinogen, and platelets			
Hematologic dysfunction	Administer blood and blood components as necessary	Progressive coagulopathy may be indicative of endothelial dysfunction due to hypoperfusion	Hct, Hgb, WBC, and coagulation studies will remain within normal limits	Using low transfusion triggers will decrease potential for pulmonary complications
Potential for infection	Monitor temperature, WBC, drainage from wounds and drains	Any infection increases the risk of sepsis and potential for development of MODS	Presenting infections will be contained before MODS develops	
	Culture all suspected sources of infection and start antibiotics immediately	Early identification and treatment of infection are critical to avoid overwhelming sepsis	Secondary (nosocomial) infections will be prevented	

Data from references 30, 31, 40, 42, 65, 69, 77.
ABGs = Arterial blood gases, aPTT = activated partial thromboplastin time, ARDS = acute respiratory distress syndrome, BUN = blood urea nitrogen, Cr = creatinine, CVVH = continuous venovenous hemofiltration, GI = gastrointestinal, Hct = hematocrit, Hgb = hemoglobin, K^+ = potassium, MODS = multiple organ dysfunction syndrome, Na^+ = sodium, PT = prothrombin time, Sao_2 = saturation of arterial oxygen, WBC = white blood cell.

♦ RESEARCH UTILIZATION

Effects of Arginine Vasopressin Use in Patients With Multiple Organ Dysfunction Syndrome

CLINICAL ISSUE

In the critical care environment during initial resuscitation, adequate fluid resuscitation is employed as the first agent of choice for vasodilatory shock. If required, inotropes and vasopressors such as dopamine or norepinephrine may then be used to maintain blood pressure in vasodilatory shock. In some acute settings, the patient receiving dopamine or norepinephrine may still be hypotensive and require additional vasopressor support. The availability of another or alternate vasopressor in the treatment of vasodilatory shock of multiple organ dysfunction syndrome (MODS) is important.

SUMMARY

This retrospective study assessed the effects of arginine vasopressin (AVP) on hemodynamic, clinical, and laboratory variables and determined its adverse side effects in advanced vasodilatory shock in 316 patients. The result demonstrated that supplementary AVP infusion improved cardiocirculatory function in advanced vasodilatory shock, but an increase in liver enzymes and bilirubin, and a decrease in platelet count occurred during AVP therapy, particularly during simultaneous hemofiltration. In the treatment of vasodilatory shock, the first agent of choice is norepinephrine. Before the norepinephrine requirement exceeds a dose of 0.6 mcg/kg/min, the initiation of AVP infusion may improve outcome.

APPLICATION

The implementation of AVP infusion for those patients already receiving norepinephrine may improve the outcome of the patient in vasodilatory shock.

NEED FOR FURTHER STUDY

Additional large randomized clinical trials are required to determine the effectiveness of AVP in patients with MODS.

Luckner, G., et al. (2005). Arginine vasopressin in 316 patients with advanced vasodilatory shock. *Crit Care Med, 33*(11), 2659–2666.

♦ Case Study 43-1, Part A

Evidence-Based Care of the MODS Patient

L.M. is a 50-year-old Caucasian male who was brought to the emergency center by his wife with a 2-day history of hematemesis and melena. Three days earlier he was seen by his primary care physician with symptoms of anorexia, weakness, dizziness, and pain in bilateral lower extremities. He was given an acetaminophen 325 mg/oxycodone 5 mg (Percocet) prescription for presumptive peripheral neuropathy and sent home. His medical history was significant for alcohol abuse and hepatitis C diagnosed by liver biopsy. The patient stated he had abused alcohol in the past, but recently restarted because of being laid off from his job and admitted to drinking a bottle of wine and several beers daily. On initial assessment, his physical examination was as follows:

Physical Examination

- Vital signs
  - Temperature 36° C
  - HR 104 beats/min
  - RR 22 breaths/min
  - BP 88/57 mm Hg
- General
  - 71 kg, moderate distress
- Neurologic
  - Awake and oriented × 3, positive asterixis
- HEENT (head, ear, eye, nose, throat): scleral icterus

- Musculoskeletal: 2+ edema bilateral lower extremities, erythematous, warm and tender to palpation, especially both feet. Palpable pulses.
- Skin: spider angiomata, jaundice
- Abdomen: mildly distended, nontender, with normal active bowel sounds

Laboratory Values

- Sodium: 132 mEq/L
- Potassium: 3.9 mEq/L
- Chloride: 97 mEq/L
- CO_2: 17 mEq/L
- BUN: 54 mg/dl
- Creatinine: 1.8 mg/dl
- Glucose: 114 mg/dl
- WBC: 12.9 cells/mm^3
- Hgb: 9.9 g/dl
- Hct: 29.7%
- Platelets: 112,000/mm^3
- Neutrophils: 83%

Amylase, lipase, and liver function tests were normal except for a slight hyperbilirubinemia of 1.8. Ethanol (ETOH) was negative. His magnesium (Mg^{++}) was 1 mEq/L. He was admitted and transferred to the critical care unit with an initial diagnosis of a GI bleed.

Cultures were sent and empiric antibiotics started pending culture results. Fours hours later, more laboratory tests were obtained.

Laboratory Values

- pH: 7.33
- Pa_{CO_2}: 19.3 mm Hg
- Pa_{O_2}: 79.2 mm Hg
- HCO_3^-: 9.8 mEq/L
- Base excess: 14.6 on O_2 3 L/nasal cannula
- WBC: 2.9 cells/mm^3
- Hct: 26.2%
- Platelets: 93,000/mm^3
- Neutrophils: 33%
- Bands: 34%

Admitting orders included normal saline infusion at 125 ml/hr; pantoprazole (Protonix) infusion at 40 mg/hr; ETOH withdrawal prophylaxis including lorazepam (Ativan), thiamine, folate, and multiple vitamins; Mg^{++} replacement, ultrasound of abdomen, and repeat Hgb, Hct, and electrolytes every 4 hours. A GI consult was obtained and the gastroenterologist concluded that the bleeding may be secondary to gastritis, varices, or an ulceration.

Decision Point: Does L.M. show any signs of SIRS?

Decision Point: What are appropriate interventions and further diagnostic tests for the patient at this time?

Decision Point: What interventions should the critical care nurse anticipate in the event that the patient decompensates further?

Case continues on page 1207

Management of Infection

Source Identification. Early diagnosis, along with source identification and control are essential interventions for SIRS before it develops into severe sepsis. These activities should occur simultaneously with ongoing resuscitation, as indicated by the patient's clinical condition. Whenever possible, cultures of all potential infection sites should be obtained before antibiotics are given. To optimize identification of the causative organisms, at least two blood cultures should be obtained with one drawn from a vascular access and the other from venipuncture. If both cultures are positive, it suggests that the same organism is causing the severe sepsis. Moreover, if the culture from the vascular access is positive at a time earlier than the peripheral sample was drawn, it may offer support that the access is the source of the infection.[7–9] Other diagnostic studies (chest x-ray, ultrasound, computed tomography [CT] scan, lumbar puncture) should be performed promptly to determine the source of infection and the causative organism. However, the patient's safety and ongoing resuscitation should never be jeopardized for the sake of obtaining the cultures.[7–9]

Antibiotic Therapy. After appropriate cultures are obtained, broad-spectrum antibiotics should be started within the first hour of recognizing severe sepsis. Once the pathogen is identified, the drugs should be changed to organism-specific antibiotics to prevent superinfection and minimize development of resistant pathogens.[10–12] Forty-eight to 72 hours after starting antibiotics, the response to treatment should be reevaluated and changed as indicated. Antibiotics should be administered for 7 to 10 days and be guided by clinical response. Antibiotics should be discontinued if the clinical syndrome is due to a noninfectious source.[13–16]

Source Control. Patients should be examined for the source of infection and evaluated by an appropriate service for source control (e.g., interventionalist for abscess drainage or surgery consult for surgery). When a source of infection is identified, source control should be initiated as soon as possible after resuscitation. If an intravenous catheter is the likely source of infection, the device should be promptly removed after other access can be established. Benefit of the method of source control must outweigh the risk and the treatment used should be the one with the least physiologic upset.[11,31]

Additional Hemodynamic Support

Vasopressors. Vasopressors can be used if adequate fluid volume fails to restore blood pressure and organ perfusion (the Medication table in Chapter 41, pp. 1116-1121 provides comprehensive information about vasopressor agents). Either norepinephrine (Levophed) or dopamine (Intropin) through a central venous catheter can be used as first-choice vasopressors to correct septic shock.[30] Norepinephrine at 0.5 mcg to 30 mcg/min has been shown to be an excellent first choice for septic shock because it has less chronotropic effect, especially for patients who are already tachycardic.[30] A second vasopressor such as dopamine can be added if the first drug is at maximum dose.[30] Low-dose dopamine should not be used for renal protection as part of the treatment of severe sepsis.[30]

Several studies show that during early septic shock, vasopressin levels are elevated.[43,44,58] However, with continued shock, vasopressin concentration decreases to within a normal range in the majority of the patients within 24 to 48 hours. This is referred to as "relative vasopressin deficiency" because in the presence of hypotension, vasopressin should be elevated.

Vasopressin is a direct vasoconstrictor without inotropic or chronotropic effects and may result in decreased cardiac output and hepatosplanchnic flow. There are unique vasopressin receptor sites in the peripheral vasculature, explaining why this agent may be used when adrenergic agents have been ineffective. Vasopressin at a rate of 0.01 to 0.04 unit/min may be used to treat refractory shock despite adequate fluid resuscitation and high-dose conventional vasopressors. Doses of greater than 0.04 unit/min have been associated with myocardial ischemia, significant decreases in CO, and cardiac arrest.[36–38,44,58]

Inotropic Therapy. Dobutamine to augment myocardial contractility may be used in patients with low cardiac output despite adequate fluid resuscitation. Combined with vasopressor therapy, it can be used to increase BP and CO.[31] Infusion doses range from 2.5 to 20 mcg/kg/min. Increasing cardiac index to supranormal levels in order to achieve arbitrarily predefined targets is not recommended. Two large prospective clinical trials in critically ill patients failed to demonstrate benefit by increasing oxygen delivery to supranormal levels by using dobutamine.[30,40] (The Medication table in Chapter 41, pp. 1116-1121, provides comprehensive information about inotropic agents.)

Steroids. For patients with persistent septic shock despite adequate fluid resuscitation and vasopressors, intravenous corticosteroids are indicated.[31] One multicenter, randomized, controlled trial with patients in severe septic shock showed a high incidence of "relative" adrenal insufficiency as determined by a cortisol stimulation test.[78] To perform this test, three cortisol levels were drawn: a preadministration dose, following the administration of 250 mcg of ACTH, and 30 to 60 minutes after administration. Those patients whose serum cortisol levels were less than or equal to 9 mcg/dl, were classified as nonresponders and found to have a reduced mortality with the full course of steroid administration. With hypotensive patients, clinicians should not wait for ACTH results to administer corticosteroids.[10,17,26,31,78]

Hydrocortisone 200 to 300 mg/day is recommended for 7 days in three or four divided doses or by continuous infusion,[17,26,31] although there is much variability in practice. Some clinicians decrease steroid doses after resolution of septic shock, whereas others consider tapering doses at the end of therapy.[26] Oral fludrocortisone 50 mcg four times a day is often added to the steroid regimen to support mineralocorticoid function.[10] In the absence of shock, corticosteroids should not be administered for the treatment of sepsis. Doses of corticosteroids greater than 300 mg daily should not be used in severe sepsis or septic shock for the purpose of treating septic shock because high doses have been shown to be ineffective and even harmful.[17,26,31,78]

Recombinant Human Activated Protein C. For patients at high risk of death, recombinant human activated protein C (rhAPC) (drotrecogin alpha activated [Xigris]) is recommended (e.g., APACHE II greater than or equal to 25, sepsis-induced multiple organ failure, septic shock, or sepsis-induced ARDS) when there are no absolute contraindications related to bleeding risk or relative contraindications that outweigh its potential benefit.[12,31] This agent works by decreasing the inflammatory and procoagulant processes and increasing the profibrinolytic activity of severe sepsis.[12] Results from a landmark study demonstrated that the use of rhAPC improved overall mortality by 28%.[12] It is administered as a continuous infusion of 24 mcg/kg/hr for a total of 96 hours. Careful attention to indications and dosing requirements described on the packaging label is essential to avoid adverse consequences of this potent anticoagulant.[12,48]

Blood Product Administration. Red blood cell transfusion should be continued if hemoglobin (Hgb) remains below 7 g/dl. A level of 7 to 9 g/dl should be targeted as more conservative transfusion thresholds are associated with improved mortality in critically ill patients.[41] Red blood cell transfusion in septic patients improves oxygen delivery but not consumption.[57] Erythropoietin is not recommended as a specific treatment of anemia associated with severe sepsis but may be used for septic patients who may have other reasons for its administration, such as renal failure.[31]

Coagulopathy accompanying sepsis often requires administration of several blood products. Professional organizations have recommended fresh frozen plasma to treat coagulopathy associated with a documented deficiency of coagulation factors.[68,69] Routine use of fresh frozen plasma for volume resuscitation alone or to correct laboratory clotting abnormalities in the absence of bleeding or planned invasive procedure is not recommended.[68,69] Antithrombin administration is not recommended for the treatment of severe sepsis or septic shock.[80] In particular, high-dose antithrombin is associated with an increased risk of bleeding, especially when given with heparin.[80] Platelets should be administered to patients with severe sepsis, when counts are less than 5000/mm^3 regardless of apparent bleeding. Platelet transfusion may be considered when counts are 5000/mm^3 to 30,000/mm^3 and there is significant risk of bleeding. Platelet counts greater than 50,000/mm^3 are typically required for surgery or invasive procedures.[68,69]

◆ Case Study 43-1, Part B

Evidence-Based Care of the MODS Patient

L.M. developed acute respiratory failure and was emergently intubated by the intensivist. His pulmonary status continued to worsen, requiring maximal ventilatory support: Fio_2 100%, assist control rate of 34, inverse inspiratory/expiratory ratio (I: E) of 2:1, positive end-expiratory pressure (PEEP) of 14, with tidal volumes of 350 ml. He was sedated with fentanyl (Sublimaze) and propofol (Diprivan) infusions to tolerate the ventilator and for comfort; protocols for daily sedation holidays were initiated. A right subclavian $Scvo_2$ catheter and an arterial catheter were inserted with a $Scvo_2$ value of 55%. Because the patient remained hypotensive despite a CVP of 15, norepinephrine (Levophed) was started for worsening hypotension. Piperacillin sodium/tazobactam sodium (Zosyn) and gentamicin sulfate were empirically started. Delirium tremens (DTs) prophylaxis was continued (multivitamins, thiamine, folate, and magnesium 4 g).

Although some of his laboratory values appeared better at 0600 the next day, he was still critically ill. He was in septic shock and was developing MODS.

Physical Examination

- Neurologic
  - Sedated on fentanyl (Duragesic) 50 mcg/hr and propofol (Diprivan) 15 mcg/kg/hr
- Cardiovascular
  - BP 88/50 on norepinephrine, HR 132, sinus tachycardia with a few unifocal premature ventricular contractions (PVCs), Doppler-detected peripheral pulses, capillary refill >5 seconds, and cyanotic, mottled extremities. CVP of 16, $Scvo_2$ 55%.
- Respiratory
  - Bilateral interstitial infiltrates on the same ventilator settings. pH: 7.28, Pao_2: 66, $Paco_2$: 56, HCO_3^-: 16, oxygen saturation 94%.

- Renal
  - Urinary output 10 to 15 ml/hr of dark amber/brown, cloudy urine
- Extremities
  - Pitting edema, mottled, cold below the knees, hot around the thighs, Doppler-detected pulses, and small bilateral bullous skin lesions

Laboratory Values

- Sodium: 130 mEq /L
- Potassium: 3.6 mEq /L
- Chloride: 95 mEq /L
- CO_2: 20 mEq /L
- BUN: 52 mg/dl
- Creatinine: 2 mg/dl
- Glucose: 358 mg/dl
- WBC count: 1.2 cells /mm^3
- Hgb: 6.7 g/dl
- Hct: 18.8%
- Platelets: 45/mm^3
- Neutrophils: 11%
- Bands: 13%
- Prothrombin time/international normalized ratio (INR): 22.5/3.8%
- AST: 132 μ/L
- ALT: 63 μ/L
- Lactate: 12.4 mg/dl

Decision Point: How should his low $Scvo_2$ value be supported?

Decision Point: What other interventions are needed to provide multisystem support of this critically ill patient with MODS?

Case continues on page 1209

Mechanical Ventilation. High tidal volumes coupled with high plateau pressures should be avoided in ALI/ARDS because overventilation of affected alveoli potentiates the pulmonary inflammatory response.[1,42] Tidal volume should be targeted to 6 ml/kg of predicted body weight in conjunction with inspiratory plateau pressures of less than 30 cm H_2O.[31,42] Hypercapnia (allowing $Paco_2$ to increase above normal, called "permissive hypercapnia") can be tolerated in patients with ALI/ARDS who require minimized plateau pressures and tidal volumes for oxygenation without barotrauma.[42] The use of permissive hypercapnia is limited in patients with preexisting metabolic acidosis and is contraindicated in patients with increased intracranial pressure. In patients with preexisting metabolic acidosis, sodium bicarbonate infusion may be considered.[2,61] Chapter 19 has specific details and a discussion on management strategies.

Sedation, Analgesia, and Neuromuscular Blockade. Protocols should be used when sedation of critically ill mechanically ventilated patients is required. The protocol should include the use of a sedation goal as measured by a standardized subjective sedation scale.[31] Although either intermittent bolus or continuous drips may be used, the protocol should include a daily interruption or lightening of a continuous sedative infusion to determine whether sedative agents may be decreased.[50] This practice has been shown to decrease ventilator and critical care days and ventilator-associated pneumonia, thereby decreasing the risk of sepsis and MODS.[52]

Neuromuscular blockade agents should be discontinued as soon as possible. Train-of-four monitoring should be used to monitor the depth of block.[52] Chapter 4 discusses specific management strategies for sedation and neuromuscular blockade.

Glucose Monitoring. In a large single center trial of postoperative surgical patients, a significant improvement in survival was demonstrated when continuous insulin infusion was used to maintain glucose between 80 and 110 mg/dl.[77] Following initial stabilization of patients with severe sepsis, blood glucose should be maintained at a level of less than 150 mg/dl. With any protocol, glucose should be monitored frequently after initiation of insulin (every 30 to 60 minutes) and on a regular basis (every 4 hours) once the blood glucose concentration has been stabilized.[31,77] Glycemic control should also include a nutrition protocol with preferential use of the enteral route.[20,53] Chapter 34 provides comprehensive information on glycemic control.

Considerations for Nutrition. Patients with sepsis and MODS have increased energy requirements and numerous metabolic derangements. They are extremely hypermetabolic, as well. Total energy expenditure may be increased 15% to 100% above normal in hypermetabolic patients. Even though they appear quiet and sedated in a critical care bed, these patients are running a physiologic marathon. Typical findings of the septic patients include hyperglycemia, elevated free fatty acids, accelerated protein catabolism, and negative nitrogen balance.[20] The goal of nutrition support for septic patients is to provide enough calories, protein, and water to meet patients' metabolic demand and prevent catabolism.[20,31] Ultimately, adequate nutritional support improves resistance to the development of MODS.[20] The Nutrition box at right details the nutritional requirements for patients with MODS.

Renal Replacement. Intermittent hemodialysis and continuous venovenous hemofiltration (CVVH) result in equivalent outcomes in septic patients.[47] CVVH offers easier management in hemodynamically unstable patients. There is no current evidence to support the use of CVVH for the treatment of sepsis independent of renal replacement needs.[31,47] Chapter 33 provides more complete information about CVVH.

⬥ NUTRITION

Nutrition in Multiple Organ Dysfunction Syndrome

Calories
Indirect calorimetry is generally considered the standard for measuring energy expenditure through the measures of oxygen consumption, carbon dioxide production, and the ratio of carbon dioxide produced to oxygen consumed employing a metabolic cart. This method is relatively accurate in measuring calorie need of the mechanically ventilated critically ill patient, except for the patient with severe ARDS. Another reliable way to estimate calories needed for a patient with multiple organ dysfunction syndrome (MODS) is by employing the Harris-Benedict equation, which is an estimation of the patient's basal energy expenditure (BEE). Multiply the BEE by the patient's activity factor and stress factor.

Men: BEE (kcal/24 hr) = 66 + (13.7 × weight) + (5 × height in cm) − (6.7 × age in years)

Women: BEE (kcal/24 hr) = 655 + (9.6 × weight) + (5 × height in cm) − (4.7 × age in years)

Activity factor: confined to bed = 1.2 ; out of bed = 1.3.

Stress factor for sepsis = 1.8.

Protein
MODS creates a hypermetabolic state within the body. To provide adequate protein use the following formula: 1.8 to 3 g/kg of body weight.

Fluid
MODS generates increased fluid requirements. To provide adequate fluids use the following formula: 30 cm³/kg body weight/day. Glucose-containing intravenous solutions should be employed with caution because they can contribute to the hyperglycemia state.

Electrolytes
Electrolytes within normal limits are to be achieved and maintained.

Vitamins and Minerals
Provide supplementation as needed. Although it is controversial, critically ill patients have fewer complications when fed enteral formulas containing immunity-enhancing nutrients such as the amino acids arginine and glutamine, omega-6 and omega-3 fatty acids, vitamins E and C, and zinc.

Special Considerations
The patient with MODS is in a hypermetabolic state, which leads to hyperglycemia. By addressing the hypermetabolic and hyperglycemic states with nutrition support and glycemic control, mortality from MODS can be reduced.

Data from references 20, 52, 77.

Bicarbonate Therapy. Bicarbonate therapy for the purpose of improving hemodynamics or reducing vasopressor requirements is not recommended for treatment of hypoperfusion-induced lactic acidemia with pH greater than or equal to 7.15.[31,61] Administration of bicarbonate solely for metabolic acidosis masks the underlying cause—persistent hypoperfusion. Therefore effectiveness of resuscitation strategies should be evaluated and changed, if necessary, before the addition of a bicarbonate infusion.[61] The effect of bicarbonate administration on hemodynamics and vasopressor requirement at lower pH has not been studied.[61]

Deep Vein Thrombosis Prophylaxis. Severe sepsis patients should receive deep vein thrombosis (DVT) prophylaxis with low doses of either low-molecular-weight or unfractionated heparin. For septic patients with contraindications to heparin use, mechanical prophylactic devices or intermittent compression devices are recommended. For very high-risk patients such as those with severe sepsis or previous history of DVT, a combination of pharmacologic and mechanical therapy is recommended.[31,71] Chapter 9 covers specific management strategies for improving outcomes through prophylaxis.

Stress Ulcer Prophylaxis. Stress ulcer prophylaxis should be given to all patients with severe sepsis.[31] H_2 blockers are more effective than sucralfate and are the preferred agent.[23] Proton pump inhibitors have not been assessed in a direct comparison and therefore their relative efficacy is unknown. Chapter 9 covers specific management strategies for improving outcomes through prophylaxis.

Consideration for Limitation of Support. A final consideration must be given to limitation of support due to futility.[31] Advance care planning, including the communication of likely outcomes and realistic goals, should be discussed with patients and families. Decisions for less aggressive support or withdrawal of support may be in the patient's best interest.[19]

♦ Case Study 43-1, Part C

Evidence-Based Care of the MODS Patient

A surgery consult ruled out a diagnosis of necrotizing fasciitis, and a vascular consult concluded that the extremity cyanosis was caused by ischemia, probably from multiple emboli secondary to sepsis, and surgery was not indicated.

Around 0900 preliminary culture results demonstrated positive gram-negative rods in all four bottles of the blood cultures; urinalysis showed a few bacteria and WBC but was otherwise nonspecific. The bullous lesions were more pronounced. The gastroenterologist returned to see the patient and asked the wife if the patient had recently consumed raw oysters: she responded that 10 days previously they had been at a hot springs and they had eaten escargot and raw oysters. He explained that cirrhotic patients who consume raw oysters can develop a severe infection caused by *Vibrio vulnificus*, a gram-negative bacterium causing serious wound infections and bacteremia. The mortality for *V. vulnificus* is more than 50% for primary bacteremia and more than 90% in those who develop hypotension. Patients who survive the acute shock require prolonged hospitalization in critical care and suffer complications resulting from MODS.[15] An infectious disease consult was obtained for presumptive *V. vulnificus* infection; sodium/tazobactam sodium and gentamicin were discontinued and the patient was started on levofloxacin (Levaquin), ceftazidime (Fortaz), doxycycline (Vibramycin), and metronidazole (Flagyl).

At 1200, the patient's blood glucose dropped to 54 and the insulin drip was discontinued. One ampule of D_{50} was administered. His urine output decreased despite large continuous fluid infusions of 2 L/hr. At 1600, the bullous skin lesions worsened. At 1800, the patient was still hypotensive despite maximal adrenergic vasopressor support. At 2014, the patient's acidosis and oxygenation became worse: pH: 7.06, po_2: 54, $Paco_2$: 58 mm Hg, and HCO_3^-: 14.4. His lactic acid (LA) level was 12.8 mg/dl (normal is <2 mg/dl). A sodium bicarbonate drip was started for refractory metabolic acidosis. PEEP was increased to 18, but the cardiac output dropped, so the PEEP was decreased to 14. One hour later his blood gases were worse: pH: 6.99, po_2: 51, $Paco_2$: 51 mm Hg, HCO_3^-: 14.1 mEq/L, Sao_2: 64%. His $Scvo_2$ saturation was 36%. His peak pressure suddenly increased to 77, with a decrease in tidal volume and his oxygen saturation dropped to 35%.

Decision Point: What additional interventions might be initiated to further support this patient?

Decision Point: Which organ systems became dysfunctional in this patient and what is his likely prognosis based on the number of dysfunctional organ systems?

CONCLUSIONS

Patients with MODS do not die from their present disease or even a single complication, but rather from progressive and sequential organ dysfunction.[11] Goals for the bedside critical care nurse are the early identification and treatment of those patients whose organs are at risk for failure. The initial insult leads to microvascular hypoperfusion within each organ system. It is difficult to monitor, let alone identify, impending MODS. If unrecognized and untreated, hypoperfusion initiates systemic inflammatory responses, activates the coagulation cascade, impairs the fibrinolytic system, and causes endothelial dysfunction. This exacerbates hypoperfusion and results in further maldistribution of blood flow within individual organs, eventually leading to single organ failure and MODS. Despite the significant strides made in life-support technology, pharmacology, and science as a whole, the key to positive outcomes is early detection and treatment of every organ system at risk. The critical care nurse is in a strategic position to detect, identify, and facilitate treatment of those patients at risk for developing MODS.

REFERENCES

1. The Acute Respiratory Distress Syndrome Network. (2000). Ventilation with lower tidal volumes as compared with traditional tidal volumes for acute lung injury and the acute respiratory distress syndrome. *N Engl J Med, 342,* 1301–1308.

2. Ahrens, T., & Tuggle, D. (2004). Surviving severe sepsis: early recognition and treatment. *Crit Care Nurse* (supplement to October 2004) 2–15.

3. Aird, W. C. (2001). Vascular bed specific homeostasis and role of endothelium in sepsis pathogenesis. *Crit Care Med, 29*(7 suppl), 528–535.

4. Aird, W. C. (2003). The role of the endothelium in severe sepsis & MODS. *Blood, 101,* 3756–3777.

5. Ali, M. Z., & Goetz, M. B. (1997). A meta-analysis of the relative efficacy and toxicity of single daily dosing versus multiple daily dosing of aminoglycosides. *Clin Infect Dis, 24,* 796–809.

6. Amato, M. B., et al. (1998). Effect of a protective-ventilation strategy on mortality in the acute respiratory distress syndrome. *N Engl J Med, 338,* 347–354.

7. Amsden, G. W., Ballow, C. H., & Bertino, J. S. (2000). Pharmacokinetics and pharmacodynamics of anti-infective agents. In G. L. Mandell, J. E. Bennett, & R. Dolin (Eds.), *Principles and practice of infectious diseases* (5th ed.). Philadelphia: Churchill Livingstone.

8. Angus, D. C., et al. (2000). Caring for the critically ill patients: Current & projected work force requirement for care of the critically ill and patients with pulmonary disease: can we meet the requirement of an aging population? *JAMA, 284,* 2762–2770.

9. Angus, D. C., et al. (2001). Epidemiology of severe sepsis in the United States: Analysis of incidence outcome, and associated costs of care. *Crit Care Med, 29,* 1301–1310.

10. Annane, D., et al. (2002). Effects of treatment with low doses hydrocortisone and fludrocortisone on mortality in patients with septic shock. *JAMA, 288,* 862–887.

11. Awad, S. S. (2003). State-of-the-art therapy for severe sepsis and multisystem organ dysfunction. *Am J Surg, 186*(Suppl), 23S–30S.

12. Bernard, G. R., et al. (2001). Efficacy and safety of recombinant human activated protein C for severe sepsis. *N Engl J Med, 344,* 699–709.

13. Bernard, G. R. (2005). Acute respiratory distress syndrome: a historical perspective. *Am J Respir Crit Care Med, 172*(7), 798–806.

14. Bidani, A., et al. (1992). Permissive hypercapnia in acute respiratory failure. *JAMA, 272,* 957–962.

15. Bisharat, N., et al. (1999). Clinical, epidemiological, and microbiological features of *Vibrio vulnificus* biogroup 3 causing outbreaks of wound infection and bacteremia in Israel. *Lancet, 354,* 1421–1424.

16. Blot, F., et al. (1998). Earlier positivity of central venous versus peripheral blood cultures is highly predictive of catheter-related sepsis. *J Clin Microbiol, 36,* 105–109.

17. Bone, R. C., Fisher, C. J., & Clemmer, T. P. (1987). A controlled clinical trial of high-dose methylprednisolone in the treatment of severe sepsis and septic shock. *N Engl J Med, 317,* 653–658.

18. Bone, R. C., et al. (1992). Definitions for sepsis and organ failure and guidelines for the use of innovative therapies in sepsis. The ACCP/SCCM Consensus Conference Committee. *Chest, 101*(6), 1644–1655.

18a. Bota, D. P., et al. (2004). Body temperature alterations in the critically ill. *Intensive Care Med, 30,* 811–816.

19. Brealey, D., et al. (2002). Association between mitochondrial dysfunction & severity & outcome of septic shock. *Lancet, 360,* 219–223.

20. Cartwright, C. M. (2004). The metabolic response to stress: a case of complex nutrition support management. *Crit Care Nurs Clin North Am, 16,* 467–487.

21. Cheek, D. J., Smith, H., & Good, J. (2006). New respect for the humble endothelium. *Nursing 2006, 36*(3), 44–47.

22. Choi, P. T. L., et al. (1999). Crystalloids vs. colloids in fluid resuscitation: a systematic review. *Crit Care Med, 27,* 200–210.

23. Cook, D., et al. (1998). A comparison of sucralfate and ranitidine for the prevention of upper gastrointestinal bleeding in patients requiring mechanical ventilation. Canadian Critical Care Trials Group. *N Engl J Med, 338,* 791–797.

24. Cook, D., & Guyatt, G. (2001). Colloid use for fluid resuscitation: evidence and spin. *Ann Intern Med, 135,* 205–208.

25. Cook, R., et al. (2001). Multiple organ dysfunction: baseline and serial component scores. *Crit Care Med, 29*(11), 2046–2050.

26. Cronin, L., et al. (1995). Corticosteroid treatment for sepsis: a critical appraisal and meta-analysis of the literature. *Crit Care Med, 23,* 1430–1439.

27. Crouser, E. D., et al. (2002). Endotoxin induced mitochondrial damage correlates with impaired respiratory activity. *Crit Care Med, 30,* 276–284.

28. Cunneen, J., & Cartwright, M. (2004). The puzzle of sepsis: fitting the pieces of the inflammation response with treatment. *AACN Clin Issue, 15*(1), 18–44.

29. De Backer, D., et al. (2002). Microvascular blood flow is altered in patients with sepsis. *Am J Respir Crit Care Med, 166,* 98–104.

30. De Backer, D., et al. (2003). Effects of dopamine, norepinephrine, and epinephrine on the splanchnic circulation in septic shock: which is best? *Crit Care Med, 31,* 1659–1667.

31. Dellinger, R., et al. (2004). Surviving sepsis campaign guidelines for management of severe sepsis and septic shock. *Crit Care Med, 32,* 855–873.

32. Doig, C. J., et al. (2004). Study of clinical course of organ dysfunction in intensive care. *Crit Care Med, 32*(2), 384–390.

33. Futterman, L. G., & Lemberg, L. (2006). Coronary endothelium: a key to life expectancy. *Am J Crit Care, 15*(3), 315–320.

34. Gattinoni, L., et al. (1995). A trial of goal-oriented hemodynamic therapy in critically ill patients. *N Engl J Med, 333,* 1025–1032.

35. Girard, T. D., Opal, S. M., & Ely, E. W. (2005). Insights of severe sepsis in older patients: the epidemiology to evidence based management. *Clin Infect Dis, 40,* 719–727.

36. Gross, P. L., & Aird, W. C. (2000). The endothelium and thrombosis. *Semin Throm Hemost, 26,* 463–478.

37. Hack, C. E., & Zeerleder, S. (2001). The endothelium in sepsis: source of and a target for inflammation. *Crit Care Med, 29*(7 suppl), 521–527.

38. Hassoun, H. T., et al. (2001). Post injury multiple organ failure. The role of the gut. *Shock, 15,* 1–10.

39. Hatala, R., Dinh, T., & Cook, D. J. (1996). Once-daily aminoglycoside dosing in immunocompetent adults: A meta-analysis. *Ann Intern Med, 124,* 717–725.

40. Hayes, M. A., et al. (1994). Elevation of systemic oxygen delivery in the treatment of critically ill patients. *N Engl J Med, 330,* 1717–1722.

41. Hébert, P. C., et al. (1999). A multicenter, randomized, controlled clinical trial of transfusion in critical care. *N Engl J Med, 340,* 409–417.

42. Hickling, K. G., et al. (1994). Low mortality rate in adult respiratory distress syndrome using low-volume, pressure-limited ventilation with permissive hypercapnia: a prospective study. *Crit Care Med, 22,* 1568–1578.

43. Holmes, C. L., et al. (2001). Physiology of vasopressin relevant to management of septic shock. *Chest, 120,* 989–1002.

44. Holmes, C. L., et al. (2001). The effects of vasopressin on hemodynamics and renal function in severe septic shock: A case series. *Intensive Care Med, 27,* 1416–1421.

45. Hyatt, J. M., et al. (1995). The importance of pharmacokinetic/pharmacodynamic surrogate markers to outcomes. Focus on antibacterial agents. *Clin Pharmacokinet, 28,* 143–160.

46. Ibrahim, E. H., et al. (2000). The influence of inadequate antimicrobial treatment of bloodstream, infections on patient outcomes in the ICU setting. *Chest, 118,* 146–155.

47. Kellum, J., et al. (2002). Continuous versus intermittent renal replacement therapy: a meta analysis. *Intensive Care Med, 28,* 29–37.

48. Kleinpell, R. (2002). Advances in treating patients with severe sepsis. *Crit Care Nurse, 23*(3), 16–28.

49. Knaus, W. A., et al. (1991). The APACHE III prognostic system prediction of hospital mortality for critically ill hospitalized adults. *Chest, 100,* 1616–1640.

50. Kolleff, M. H., et al. (1998). The use of continuous IV sedation is associated with prolongation of mechanical ventilation. *Chest, 114,* 541–548.

51. Kreger, B. E., Craven, D. E., & McCabe, W. R. (1980). Gram negative bacteremia. IV. Re-evaluation of clinical features and treatment in 612 patients. *Am J Med, 68,* 344–355.

52. Kress, J. P. (2000). Daily interruptions of sedative infusions in critically ill patients undergoing mechanical ventilation. *N Engl J Med, 342,* 1471–1477.

53. Kudsk, K. A. (2001). Importance of enteral feeding in maintaining gut integrity. *Tech GI Endo, 3,* 2–8.

54. Le Gall, J. R., et al. (1996). The logistic organ dysfunction system. A new way to assess organ dysfunction in the intensive care unit. *JAMA, 276,* 802–810.

55. Leibovici, L., et al. (1998). The benefit of appropriate empirical antibiotic treatment in patients with bloodstream infection. *J Intern Med, 244,* 379–386.

56. Levy, M. M., et al. (2003). 2001 SCCM/ESICM/ACCP/ATS/SIS international sepsis definition conference. *Crit Care Med, 31*(4), 1250–1256.

57. Lorente, J. A., et al. (1993). Effects of blood transfusion on oxygen transport variables in severe sepsis. *Crit Care Med, 21,* 1312–1318.

58. Malay, M. B., et al. (1999). Low-dose vasopressin in the treatment of vasodilatory septic shock. *J Trauma, 47,* 699–705.

59. Marik, P. E., & Sibbald, W. J. (1993). Effect of stored-blood transfusion on oxygen delivery in patients with sepsis. *JAMA, 269,* 3024–3029.

60. Martin, G. S., et al. (2003). The epidemiology of sepsis in the United States from 1979 through 2000. *N Engl J Med, 348,* 1540–1546.

61. Mathieu, D., et al. (1991). Effects of bicarbonate therapy on hemodynamic and tissue oxygenation in patients with lactic acidosis: a prospective, controlled clinical study. *Crit Care Med, 19,* 1352–1356.

62. McCabe, W. R., & Jackson, G. G. (1962). Gram negative bacteremia. *Arch Intern Med, 110,* 92–100.

63. Mermel, L. A., & Maki, D. G. (1993). Detection of bacteremia in adults: consequences of culturing and inadequate volume of blood. *Ann Intern Med, 119,* 270–272.

64. Deleted in proofs.

65. Pettila, V., et al. (2002). Comparison of multiple organ dysfunction scores in the prediction of hospital mortality in the critically ill. *Crit Care Med, 30*(8), 1705–1711.

66. Phillips, J. K. (2003). Nursing management: shock and multiorgan dysfunction syndrome. In S. R. Dirksen, S. M. Lewis, & M. M. Heitkemper (Eds.), *Medical surgical nursing: assessment and management of clinical problems* (6th ed.). St. Louis: Mosby.

67. Piagnerelli, M., et al. (2003). Modification of red blood cell shape & glycoproteins membrane content in septic patients. *Adv Exp Med Biol, 510,* 109–114.

68. Practice guidelines for blood component therapy. (1996). A report by the American Society of Anesthesiologists Task Force on Blood Component Therapy. *Anesthesiology, 84,* 732–747.

69. Practice parameter for the use of fresh frozen plasma, cryoprecipitate, and platelets. (1994). Fresh-Frozen Plasma, Cryoprecipitate, and Platelets Administration Practice Guidelines Development Task Force of the College of American Pathologists. *JAMA, 271,* 777–781.

70. Rivers, E. P., et al. (2001). Early goal-directed therapy in the treatment of severe sepsis and septic shock. *N Engl J Med, 345,* 1368–1377.

71. Samama, M. M., et al. (1999). A comparison of enoxaparin with placebo for the prevention of venous thromboembolism in acutely ill medical patients. Prophylaxis in Medical Patients with Enoxaparin Study Group. *N Engl J Med, 341,* 793–800.

72. Sands, K., et al. (1997). Epidemiology of sepsis syndrome in 8 academic medical centers. *JAMA, 278,* 234–240.

73. Schierhout, G., & Roberts, I. (1998). Fluid resuscitation with colloid or crystalloid solutions in critically ill patients: a systematic review of randomized trials. *BMJ, 31,* 961–964.

74. Sharshar, T., et al. (2003). Apoptosis of neurons in cardiovascular autonomic centers triggered by inducible nitric oxide synthase after death from septic shock. *Lancet, 362,* 1799–1805.

75. Tsuneyoski, I., et al. (2002). Hemodynamic & metabolic effects of low dose vasopressin infusions in vasodilatory septic shock. *Crit Care Med, 29,* 487–493.

76. Vallet, B., & Weil, E. (2001). Endothelial cell dysfunction and coagulation. *Crit Care Med, 29*(7 suppl), 536–541.

77. Van den Berghe, G., et al. (2001). Intensive insulin therapy in the critically ill patients. *NEJM, 345,* 1359–1367.

78. The Veterans Administration Systemic Sepsis Cooperative Study Group. (1987). Effect on high-dose glucocorticoid therapy on mortality in patients with clinical signs of sepsis. *N Engl J Med, 317,* 659–665.

78a. Vincent, J. L., et al. (1996). The sepsis-related organ failure assessment (SOFA) score to describe organ dysfunction/failure. *Intensive Care Med, 22,* 707–710.

79. Vincent, J. L., et al. (2000). Effects of nitric oxide in septic shock. *Am J Respir Crit Care Med, 161,* 1781–1785.

80. Warren, B. L., et al. (2001). High dose antithrombin III in severe sepsis: a randomized controlled trial. *JAMA, 286,* 1869–1878.

81. Weinstein, M. P., et al. (1983). The clinical significance of positive blood cultures: a comprehensive analysis of 500 episodes of bacteria and fungemia in adults. I. Laboratory and epidemiology observations. *Rev Infect Dis, 5,* 35–53.

CHAPTER 44 Burns

Louis R. Stout

The treatment of burns has been a specialty concern recorded as far back as 1500 BC, with the Egyptians' application of salves, to the impregnated dressings used in ancient Greece (Box 44-1).[57] The focus has changed over time; however, some amazing similarities remain.[24,94] The care of the burn patient remains a highly specialized critical care field for all members of the healthcare team. The burn center concept has grown and changed over many decades with significant advances in the areas of technology, fluid resuscitation, synthetic skins or skin substitutes, and pharmacology. Outpatient and community programs have flourished, with emphasis on fire safety and burn prevention, the mandatory installation of smoke detectors and commercial fire suppression devices, and consumer product regulation for fire retardants. Prevention remains the key to this devastating injury. This progress has decreased the incidence and severity of burn injuries and thereby decreased mortality, decreased inpatient length of stay, and increased the percentage of procedures that can be completed as outpatient services. Specific interventions since the 1940s have increased the LD_{50} (the lethal dose for 50% of the population exposed) from 30% total body surface area (TBSA) burned to 80% TBSA burned.[76]

Although significantly reduced from the approximately 2 million per year in the late 1950s and early 1960s, more than 1.1 million burn injuries still occur annually throughout the United States; this prompts an estimated 700,000 emergency department (ED) visits, with 45,000 requiring hospitalization.[3,76] About half of these patients are admitted to the 125 specialized burn treatment centers across the nation.

More severe and complex burn patients benefit from treatment in a specialty unit.[5] In children, approximately 250,000 burn injuries result in 15,000 hospitalizations and 1100 deaths per year.[12] Despite dramatic advancements in technology and the increased availability of burn centers, there remains about a 6% mortality rate among patients admitted to burn centers. A significant number of these have suffered severe inhalation injuries.[3,76] As the population in the United States grew by 25% from 1971 to 1998, the deaths from fire and burns declined about 50%, resulting in a decline in the death rate by more than 60%.[3] The American Burn Association (ABA), in association with the American College of Surgeons, has established specific criteria for determining which patients should be transferred to a specialized burn center (Box 44-2). In some settings, the use of

---

Box 44-1

Timeline of Approaches to Burn Care and Major Interventions Associated With Decreases in Mortality

- **1500 BC:** Salve of resin and honey advocated by the Egyptians
- **600 BC:** Chinese use of tinctures and extracts from tea leaves
- **Ancient Greece:** Cleanse, apply animal fat and resin impregnated in bulky dressings
- **Roman Empire:** Cleanse, apply ashes and oil, herbs, then wrap
- **Middle Ages:** Wax plus herbs or boiling oil
- **16th and 17th centuries:** Use of frog and lizard skin as a "skin substitute"
- **1800s:** Heat or ice
- **Early 1900s:** Expose wound, apply tannic acid or variety of pigments to dry wound
  - Introduction of the use of skin substitutes from a variety of animals
- **1940s:** Penicillin
- **1950s:** Broad-spectrum antibiotics
  - Use of topical antibiotics using the exposure or the closed dressing method
  - Refinement of fluid therapy
- **1960s:** Rapid wound closure with surgery, skin, skin substitutes
  - Popularization of pigskin
  - The burn center concept
  - Topical therapy
  - Refinement of fluid therapy
- **1970s:** Aggressive nutrition
  - Aggressive excision

Data from references 24, 57, 94.

Box 44-2

Burn Center Referral Criteria

1. Partial-thickness burns greater than 10% total body surface area (TBSA).
2. Burns that involve the face, hands, feet, genitalia, perineum, or major joints.
3. Third-degree burns in any age-group.
4. Electric burns, including lightning injury.
5. Chemical burns.
6. Inhalation injury.
7. Burn injury in patients with preexisting medical disorders that could complicate management, prolong recovery, or affect mortality.
8. Any patient with burns and concomitant trauma (such as fractures) in which the burn injury poses the greatest risk of morbidity or mortality. In such cases, if the trauma poses the greater immediate risk, the patient may be initially stabilized in a trauma center before being transferred to a burn unit. Physician judgment is necessary in such situations and should be in concert with the regional medical control plan and triage protocols.
9. Burned children with any extent of burn if the hospital is without qualified personnel or equipment for the care of children.
10. Burn injury in patients who require special social, emotional, or long-term rehabilitative intervention.

Data from references 2, 5.

telemedicine may allow for the effective treatment of the burn-injured patient without movement to a regional burn center.[81]

Initial treatment must have the precedence of injuries that threaten life and limb. Although dramatic in presentation, the burn plan of care must wait to be defined until after primary organ system dysfunctions are effectively addressed.[2] The provider must appreciate that body systems may not respond as expected and must account for the effects of the burn injury; the balanced care plan must consider the patient holistically because the hypermetabolic burn response affects every facet of the body.

The consolidation of patients with burn injuries and primary diseases of the integument has shown to improve outcomes and decrease mortality, due in large part to specialty training and the necessary multidisciplinary approach involving nursing, physicians, respiratory therapy, rehabilitation services (physical and occupational therapy), operating room personnel, social work, nutritional services, infection control, behavioral

health or psychiatric services, and education.[2,90] Outside of specialized centers, burn care for most facilities is a low-volume, high-risk clinical area and is a perishable knowledge without repetitive exposure. The patient population requires appreciation of the subtlety of differences from other critical care cases.

◆ Case Study 44-1, Part A

Assessing a Patient With a Thermal Flash Injury

T.W. is a 34-year-old male who added accelerant to a barbecue pit, resulting in a thermal flash that caught his clothing on fire at approximately 6:00 PM. Emergency Medical Services (EMS) ambulance transports T.W. to the nearest emergency department, arriving at 6:45 PM. The emergency physician notes burns to the face with singed nasal and facial hairs, circumferential burns to bilateral upper extremities (BUE), the anterior torso, portions of the posterior torso, and scattered areas of the bilateral lower extremities (BLE). The burn size is estimated at 63% of total body surface area (TBSA). His preburn weight is 80 kg.

T.W. is a well-nourished, well-developed male in relative good health. He denies smoking or recreational drug use, but reports drinking 12 beers per week for the past 2 years. There is no history of significant past medical or surgical history. He is married with two small children. His family history indicates no significance of hypertension, diabetes, cardiac or renal disease, or cancer. Intravenous catheters are placed in bilateral antecubital fossae with lactated Ringer's infusions, and fentanyl (Duragesic) is given intravenously in 50- to 100-mcg increments as indicated for pain. An indwelling urinary catheter is inserted.

Decision point: Given the extent of his burns, would it be appropriate to transfer him to a burn center?

Case continues on page 1232

Overall, burns rank as the sixth leading cause of death related to unintentional injury.[48] The majority of burn deaths occur as a result of residential fires; structure fires (house fires) result in pediatric and geriatric casualties five to six times higher than all other age-groups because their mobility is greatly hindered and they have a decreased ability to protect their airway (i.e., hold breath, cover mouth and nose). This increases the incidence of inhalation injury and length of exposure to causative agents as they attempt to exit the structure; more than three quarters of the total deaths are related to inhalation of toxic substances.[74,76] Socioeconomic status (low-income housing, crowded living conditions), regional construction codes, and access to housing protective standards (absence of smoke detectors or effective commercial sprinkler systems) also influence death rates. As a direct reflection of income, minority children have three times the death rate in residential fires as white children.[76]

Patients at either extreme of age, the very young or very old, and pregnant females should be evaluated for potential abuse. Telltale signs are burn patterns inconsistent with the story received. Children should not have sock-like burn patterns or burns with clearly defined margins, because they should react aggressively as they move themselves away from the burning process, resulting in splash patterns.

APPLIED PHYSIOLOGY

The skin is the largest and heaviest organ of the body and has the following functions:

- Protection from injury and infection
- Tactile interaction with the environment (nerve endings and receptors process stimuli, such as heat, cold, pain)
- Fluid and electrolyte balance through water regulation (excretion and secretion)
- Temperature regulation through the controlled loss of heat
- Vitamin production
- Storage of fat
- Allows for motion and function
- Allows for personal and sexual identity

Loss of integrity of the skin disrupts the most basic protective mechanism of the body and makes the individual susceptible to a plethora of insults. Although the skin of the face tends to be the leanest, it is also some of the most vascular, contrasted by the significantly thicker soles of the feet and palms of the hand.

The skin is composed of two layers. The outer layer is the epidermis. It is thin, averaging from 0.07 to 0.12 mm (0.3 mm on the eyelids and 1.5 mm on the palms of the hands and soles of the feet[43]), and avascular. The cells of the epidermal layer receive their nourishment from the dermal layer; they continually slough and are replaced every 2 to 4 weeks. The dermis is the inner layer and is significantly thicker, from 1 to 4 mm.[43] It contains the vascular supply, which regulates body temperature through arterial and venous contraction and dilation. There are also sensory receptors, sebaceous glands, sweat glands, and hair follicles.[22,85] The subcutaneous tissue, or hypodermis, is a layer of loose connective tissue containing fat. This layer insulates the body for warmth. It also provides protective padding to the underlying muscles and organs through impact absorption and resistance against shearing forces (Figure 44-1; Box 44-3).

INITIAL ASSESSMENT

If the skin is exposed to a heat source beyond its protective abilities, a burn results. The severity of the injury depends on the length of exposure, the degree of the heat source, and the thickness of the integument in contact. The very young and the elderly tend to have thinner skin and are therefore more susceptible to burn exposure.[7,43,52,109]

Critical to the survival of the burn patient is the communication of events as accurately as possible throughout the chain of rescuers—from family, to pre-hospital care providers, to the emergency department (ED), to the receiving burn center. Key elements to be relayed are highlighted in Box 44-4.[89]

In burn patients who succumb to their wounds in the first 3 to 5 days of the injury, there is often a correlation with an underappreciation of threats to the primary assessment. As with all trauma patients, maintenance of cardiopulmonary function is the primary concern during initial assessment.[67]

The loss of the airway can occur rapidly if not secured early. Stridor or hoarseness is a good indicator of the probable need for intubation. Facial edema and/or airway edema quickly mounts as fluid resuscitation occurs, further complicating the intubation process or surgical airway if this becomes required (Figure 44-2). When the situation is questionable, the prudent healthcare provider should intubate early and sometimes prophylactically.

Most manufactured products contain materials that exude chemicals as they incinerate. This can result in the inhalation of many toxic compounds. High-flow oxygen (O_2) should be initiated immediately. Circumferential burns of the trunk may impair ventilation and must be closely monitored; decreased ventilatory compliance should be evaluated for potential escharotomies to the anterior thorax to decompress the restriction. Respiratory failure can ensue due to the smoke injury or to development of pneumonia or acute respiratory distress syndrome (ARDS).

Failure to adequately resuscitate a patient with fluid (under-resuscitation) can result from inaccurate calculation of fluid requirements or not being timely in responding to hemodynamic responses. Concurrently, over-resuscitation may result in life-threatening chronic complications. Missed nonthermal injuries can potentiate the under-resuscitation of the burn patient. If pulses are nonpalpable, Doppler examination should be used to determine circulatory deficit in a circumferentially burned extremity. It must be determined if the diminution of pulses is due to the burned tissue (eschar) or the result of hypovolemic or burn shock. Physical indicators of circulation deficit include decreased sensation, progressively severe deep tissue pain, diminished distal pulses, and slow capillary refill.

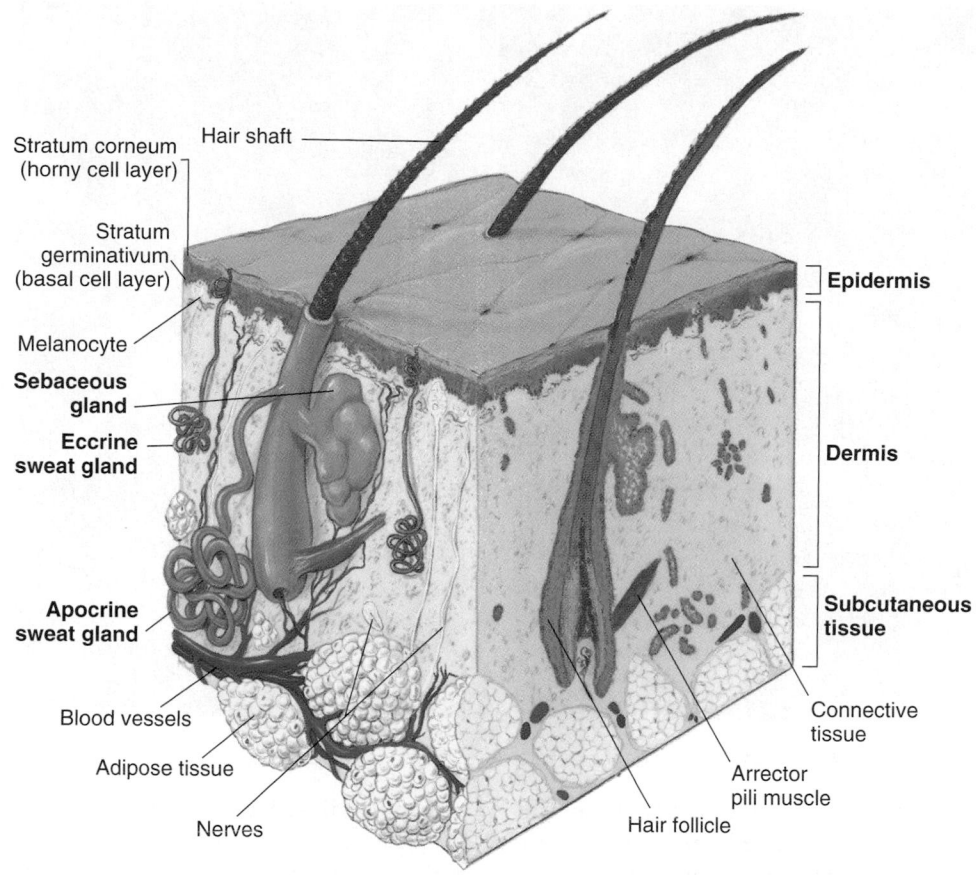

Stratum corneum
(horny cell layer)

Hair shaft

Stratum
germinativum
(basal cell layer)

Melanocyte

**Sebaceous
gland**

**Eccrine
sweat gland**

**Apocrine
sweat gland**

Blood vessels

Adipose tissue

Nerves

Epidermis

Dermis

**Subcutaneous
tissue**

Connective
tissue

Arrector
pili muscle

Hair follicle

⬍**FIGURE 44-1** Layers of the skin.[6]

Box 44-3

Functions of Skin

PRIMARY

- Protection from injury and infection
- Tactile interaction with the environment
- Fluid and electrolyte balance through water balance
- Temperature regulation

SECONDARY

- Storage of fat
- Allows for motion and function
- Allows for personal and sexual identity
- Vitamin production

Data from references 22, 43, 85.

Box 44-4

Key Communication Elements Between Providers

- Did the incident occur in an enclosed space? This increases the risk and suspicion of inhalation injury.
- Was there a blast or explosion? Assessment must include indications of concussive injury, such as hollow organ damage and fractures if the patient was thrown or fell.
- Is there indication of concomitant trauma?
- Was there loss of consciousness (LOC) at the scene? Was it witnessed? What was the length of time unconscious? What were the interventions and the patient's response?
- Is this an electrical injury?

Neurologic deficit is rarely related to the primary thermal burn injury but is indicative of concomitant trauma or subsequent injury, such as anoxic brain injury. Neurologic status should be routinely reassessed and intervention administered as indicated.

The maintenance of the patient's body temperature is a priority. Research indicates increased mortality in all trauma patients with uncontrolled exposure hypothermia.[33,104] The ambient temperature should be increased, up to or above body temperature. Warmed

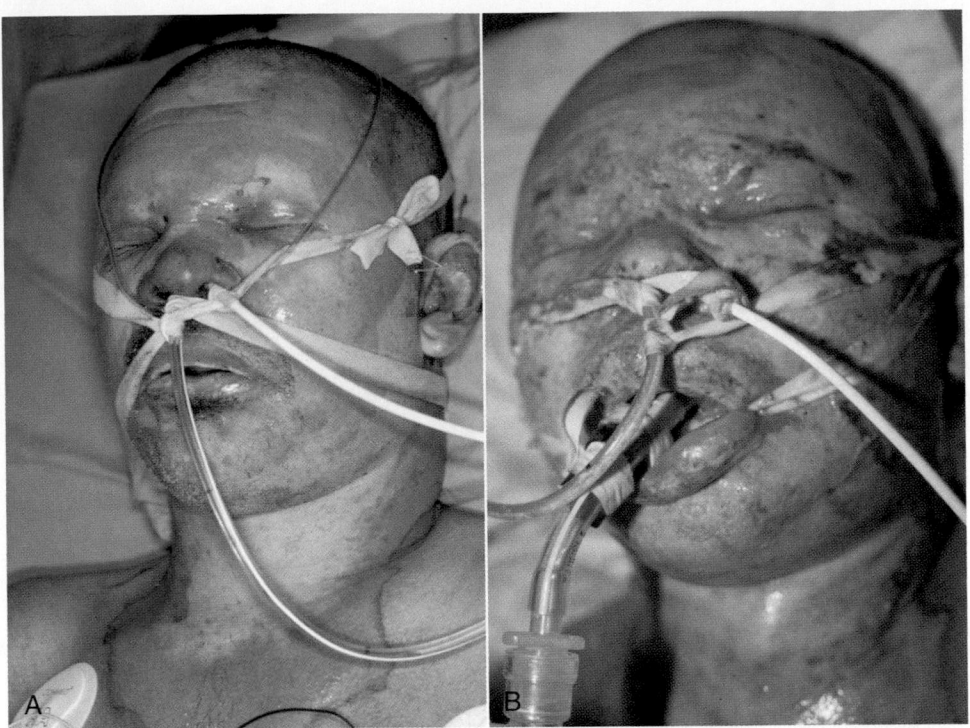

✦FIGURE 44-2 **A,** Facial edema before resuscitation. **B,** Facial edema after 24 hours.

intravenous fluids (37° to 40° C or 98° to 104° F) should be instilled; room temperature fluids are significantly lower than body temperature, causing increased metabolic demands. If the patient is to be transported to another facility or burn center less than 24 hours from the time of injury, wounds should be left intact and covered in clean, dry sheets and blankets (this is discussed in detail under Patient Transport).

The amount of edema formation in burn patients can be immense. Fluid requirements and titratable medications are always calculated from the preburn weight because this patient population's weight can increase by up to 15 kg with fluid resuscitation. The edema typically peaks at 12 to 24 hours and begins to mobilize after 3 to 5 days as the fluid shifts back from the interstitial space and returns to the vasculature.[67]

Mortality after the first 7 to 10 days is most often related to systemic infection. For this reason, burn centers are usually closed units, focusing on burn injuries and other injuries primarily affecting the integument, and the emphasis on infection control takes center stage.[111]

BURN STRESS RESPONSE

The body's response to the burn process is systemic and affects every organ system of the body. A burn of any significant size results in the massive release of inflammatory mediators both locally at the wound site and systemically.[111] Histamine, bradykinin,

prostaglandins, leukotrienes, and catecholamines have been proposed to explain the changes in capillary permeability and burn shock.[105] See Figure 35-1 in Chapter 35.

The general adaptation syndrome is one of initial peaked response (the alarm reaction) followed by a sustained response over time (the stage of resistance). The length of the response time is determined by the individual's ability to compensate, along with the healthcare team's ability to appropriately support the patient. The human body, without proper intervention, is limited in its ability to compensate and, in time, ceases to compensate and fails as it progresses through to the stage of exhaustion. The goal is to intervene and, through appropriate support, prevent the patient from ever arriving at the stage of exhaustion (Figure 44-15).

With any stressor, the autonomic nervous system (ANS) is stimulated in an attempt at self-preservation. The hormonal response to stress is the alarm reaction with the release of epinephrine, adrenocorticotropic hormone (ACTH), and antidiuretic hormone (ADH) primarily. This initiates a series of feedback mechanisms that allows the body to respond to the insult. The ANS has direct influence on the sympathetic nervous system and the anterior hypothalamus.

SYMPATHETIC NERVOUS SYSTEM

The sympathetic nervous system (SNS) is sensitive to baroreceptors found in the aortic arch and the carotid sinus. When stimulated, the SNS stimulates the adrenal medulla to release norepinephrine and epinephrine.

Epinephrine stimulates the beta-1 receptors to increase the heart rate (chronotropic) and increase myocardial contractility (inotropic), and the beta-2 receptors by increasing respiratory rate and vasodilatation of the coronary arteries, skeletal muscles, and brain. Other systemic responses include hepatic glycogenolysis increasing the body's circulating blood glucose, clotting, and inhibiting insulin secretion.

The release of norepinephrine occurs in higher concentrations during the stage of resistance. This leads to increased metabolic activity, the increased hydrolysis of fats, and the stimulation of alpha-1 receptors. The alpha-1 receptors directly affect peripheral vasoconstriction with manifestations in the skin of pallor and diaphoresis; the gastrointestinal tract with nausea, vomiting, anorexia; and the kidneys with decreased glomerular filtration rate (GFR), resulting in decreased urinary output (UOP).

The baroreceptors of the juxtaglomerular apparatus (JGA) of the kidneys are sensitive to the effects of norepinephrine when the renal blood flow is decreased. This, along with the osmoreceptor in the macula densa, stimulates the renin-angiotensin system. Increased renin combines with angiotensinogen from the liver to form angiotensin I. Angiotensin-converting enzyme (ACE) from the lungs converts angiotensin I to angiotensin II, a potent vasoconstrictor working primarily on the periphery and efferent arteriole.

The anterior hypothalamus is sensitive to the baroreceptors of the aortic arch and carotid sinus, the stretch receptors found primarily in the left atrium, as well as the osmoreceptors of the hypothalamus.

The release of corticotropic releasing factor (CRF) from the anterior hypothalamus stimulates the anterior pituitary to secrete adrenocorticotropic hormone (ACTH), which, like the renin-angiotensin system, has effects on the adrenal cortex. The adrenal cortex secretes cortisol, with systemic results. Among these are gluconeogenesis, subsequent increased blood glucose, broad antiinflammation, altered immune response with increased susceptibility to infection, protein catabolism, insulin antagonism, and polycythemia. These combined actions have a negative feedback mechanism on the anterior hypothalamus. Vasoactive substances (such as histamine, prostaglandins, and interleukins) are released systemically, initiating the systemic inflammatory response syndrome (SIRS). These mediators and cytokines (platelet-activating factor, tumor necrosis factor, serotonin, nitric oxide) decrease the flow of blood to the kidneys and gastrointestinal (GI) tract and deplete the intravascular volume. The release of platelet-activating factor (PAF) initiates neutrophil and white blood cell (WBC) activation and produces inflammation

of the tissues; PAF also contributes to the increased capillary permeability. Tumor necrosis factor (TNF) increases oxygen free radical formation, which leads to injury of the pulmonary system, kidneys, and GI tract. TNF further increases the production of cytokines, metabolic acidosis, and coagulopathy.[7]

Stimulation of the adrenal cortex with ACTH also increases the amount of circulating aldosterone. This directs the kidney to retain sodium (Na^+). Na^+ retention increases the serum osmolality. Via osmosis, water (H_2O) moves as the solute level increases with Na^+. As the kidney preserves Na^+, there is a consequent loss of potassium (K^+). This K^+ loss functions as a negative feedback loop, reducing the production of aldosterone.

The anterior hypothalamus also acts on the posterior pituitary's increased secretion of antidiuretic hormone (ADH). ADH directly stimulates the kidney to reabsorb H_2O, also increasing the circulating intravascular volume.

Use of Medications to Reduce Metabolic Demands

The use of medications to reduce the metabolic demands placed on the body during the burn healing process remains under review. Although it is more widely researched in the pediatric population and the elderly with preexisting comorbidities, the results in the adult burn population have not yet been significantly demonstrated in the literature. There has been some success with routine beta-blockade to limit the hypermetabolic response to circulating catecholamines with the use of an adjusted dose of propranolol to decrease the resting heart rate by 20% for up to 4 weeks.[20]

CAUSATIVE AGENTS

Sources of heat that cause burn injuries are divided into three main categories: thermal, chemical, and electrical. The first intervention is to stop the burning process while protecting the rescuer from harm.

Thermal Burns

Thermal burns are by far the most common burn injury encountered. They result from exposure to a flame source such as a house fire, explosion with ensuing fireball, or a scald burn from steam or hot object. Heated materials such as tar, asphalt, or plastic may cause a contact burn as they adhere to the skin; prolonged contact may also result in a chemical reaction at the cellular level. Removal from the heat source or application of cool water reduces the temperature of the object to stop the burning.

Electrical Burns

Electrical injuries are about 3% of the annual burn center admissions and result in almost 1000 deaths per year.[3] Exposure is most often from industrial sites and electricians or from contact with overhead powerlines. In the pediatric population, this type of injury often results from chewing on electrical cords and can cause significant damage to the oral commissure.

Electrical current flows along the path of least resistance; this flow is defined as Ohm's law:

$$\text{Amperage (Flow or intensity of current)} = \frac{\text{Voltage}}{\text{Resistance}}$$

The flow or intensity of current (I) is determined by a direct relationship of the amount of voltage (V), as it relates through an inverse relationship to the level of resistance (R), depicted as $I = V/R$.[27] The skin is not a good conductor of electrical current and is the most resistant organ of the body. Muscle tissue has the least resistance to electricity, and the largest mass of muscle is located along the bone; because bones do not conduct electricity, the current travels deeply; thus the injury pattern is often described by clinicians as "burning from the inside out." Electrical injuries can be the most difficult to fully appreciate because the cutaneous thermal damage does not reflect the potentially massive underlying tissue damage or predict outcome.

Along with length of exposure, the severity of electrical burns depends on several factors, including the type of current (alternating or direct), the voltage, the path of the current, the contact area(s), and the body's resistance. Electrical injuries are divided into low (less than 1000 volts), which most closely mimic thermal burns, and high voltage (1000 volts and greater). The higher the voltage, the more likely it is to overwhelm the body's limited resistance.[77] Electrical current can be either direct current (DC, continuous current flow in one direction) or alternating current (AC, periodic reversal in the current direction). Most homes and businesses are supplied with AC electricity. DC electricity is found in most electronics and many medical devices, where electricity is supplied by batteries or power supplies that convert AC from an electric socket to DC. The electrical current in the United States used in most dwellings is 60 Hz (the number of cycles completed in 1 second), 110-volt AC, whereas in Europe and Australia, 50 Hz AC is used. AC is more dangerous than DC; it may cause tetany, so that a person's grip on an electrical source tightens, which lengthens the exposure to the current.[27] DC tends to pass in one direction straight through the body.

AC transports as a sine wave at a frequency of 60 Hz. From a standpoint of cardiac susceptibility to fibrillation, it is the worst possible frequency. This is the standard electrical power in the United States. Direct current (DC) is the electrical power primarily in ships, mass transit vehicles, batteries, and welding equipment. It has poor penetration through intact skin. It does approximately one third of the tissue damage caused by AC.

The tissue damage occurs as the electrical current transforms to heat energy, measured in joules. The damage done by the joules (J) is a direct calculation of the current (I), multiplied by the resistance (R) and the length of contact or time (T), depicted as $J = I^2 \times R \times T$. The greatest heat is at the contact points.

Although there is a decreased incidence when compared with other traumatic events, lightning strikes are associated with an approximate 30% mortality and, of those who survive the event, almost 70% sustain serious long-term complications.[2] Lightning is an extremely high-voltage DC electrical discharge but differs in its effects on the body and clinical presentation because it more often travels over the body as opposed to through it. Immediate cardiac or respiratory arrest can occur from deep depolarization, but this mechanism of injury (flashover) often avoids much of the cardiac injury or muscular necrosis.[29]

Chemical Burns

Chemical burns occur after prolonged exposure to acids, alkalis, or organic compounds. Initial presentation may not be reflective of the extent of tissue damage that has occurred. There are more than 25,000 chemical compounds in both household and commercial products—from household cleaning products, to battery acid, to industrial solvents—that can cause burns.[37] The severity of the chemical injury is related to the agent, concentration, volume, extent of body surface involved, penetrability of the chemical, type of chemical, speed of action, and properties of the skin involved (Box 44-5). It is important to note that

---

Box 44-5

Severity of Chemical Injury

The severity of the chemical injury is related to the:
- Agent
- Concentration
- Volume
- Extent of body surface involved
- Penetrability of the chemical
- Type of chemical
- Speed of action
- Properties of the skin involved

Data from references 26, 37, 56, 83.

chemical exposure may account for only 3% of burns, but chemical injuries may account for approximately 30% of all burn deaths.[56]

Immediate Treatment. The immediate treatment of the chemical injury patient should occur in the prehospital or emergency department setting. Care must include appropriate precautions for all members of the health-care team. All clothing should be removed, including shoes and undergarments. Any apparel left in contact with the skin can harbor chemicals and continue to damage tissue; petroleum burns commonly occur with saturated clothing in a motor vehicle crash. Dry chemicals should be brushed from the skin. Do not attempt to neutralize the agent because this may generate heat and cause further injury. The patient should be subjected to prolonged water lavage, at least 30 minutes and as long as 2 to 3 hours. No element has been found superior to water in stopping the chemical burning process, but care must be shown to avoid the complicating effect of hypothermia. Hydrotherapy should be initiated immediately to decrease the concentration, and irrigation should continue until the pain is alleviated. The gentle flow of water is advised to avoid splashing the chemical into the eyes of the patient or healthcare provider or forcing the chemical deeper into the tissues. If required, irrigation of the eyes should continue until a staff ophthalmologist can evaluate.[26,83]

White phosphorus is used by the military in various munitions and to produce smoke; it is also used by industry in fertilizers, food additives, and cleaning compounds in the form of phosphoric acid and other chemicals, and in small amounts (in the past) in pesticides and fireworks. White phosphorus must be obscured from the ambient air by immersing immediately in water because contact with the atmosphere initiates a chemical reaction and burning.[1]

Hot tar burn is classified as a chemical burn, although it is in essence a contact burn. It is an insidious element because it cools on the outer layers while continuing to burn the skin. The molten material, hot bitumen, should be emergently cooled with cold water. Physical removal of the tar is not immediately necessary. It is best removed by emulsification with a petroleum-based product (such as mineral oil or white petroleum jelly); this breakdown may take as long as 24 hours.[3] The burn depth must be evaluated and is usually found to be quite deep.

Agents have been used for chemical warfare throughout history with the earliest reports of biological weapons in the sixth century BC.[99] Chemical weapons were used on large scales in World War I and have since become battlefield threats in military conflicts and as a tool of terrorism. Chemical agents are divided into the following types: blister agents/ vesicants (nitrogen mustard, lewisite), choking agents (chlorine, phosgene), and nerve agents (Sarin, VX).[2,39] Injury can be external as well as systemic. Definitive treatment should be referred to a burn center.[2]

Inhalation Injury

Of the patients admitted to burn centers, 15% to 30% have sustained inhalation injury; as an independent indicator, inhalation injury increases the risk of death by 20% more than the prediction by age and burn size alone.[15] A study of 1058 burn patients over a 5-year period at the U.S. Army Burn Center demonstrated that age and burn size–specific mortality was increased by 20% with the presence of inhalation injury, by 40% with pneumonia, and by 60% when both were present.[18,91] Inhalation injury is more common when the fire has occurred in an enclosed space, particularly in residential fires (Box 44-6), but prevention of pneumonia is key to reducing mortality.[30,80] A similar study of 1447 consecutive patients admitted to a civilian burn center also found a 20% incidence of inhalation injury but with a 31% mortality.[92]

Inhalation injury is divided anatomically into three types: injury above the glottis to the upper airways, injury below the glottis to the lower airways and pulmonary parenchyma, and/or systemic toxicity with the inhalation of carbon monoxide (CO) or cyanide.

Above the Glottis. In most instances, inhalation injuries suffered are limited to damage above the glottis, which includes the nasal cavity, nasopharynx, oropharynx, and larynx. These injuries are typically the result of thermal exposure as the victim inhales superheated air. The damage may produce upper airway

---

Box 44-6

Increased Suspicion of Inhalation Injury

- The burn injury occurred within an enclosed space, such as residential or vehicular fires.
- There were noxious fumes noted at the scene, especially in an industrial site.
- The patient has sustained significant facial burns.
- The patient is very old or very young—less able to adequately protect the airway.
- The patient has suffered a severe burn.
- Presence of carbonaceous sputum in the oropharynx.
- The patient relates a hoarse voice.
- Stridor is present or develops.

Data from references 15, 17, 18, 30.

obstruction, although the obstruction may develop late as the edema forms during fluid resuscitation; edema in burn resuscitation, to include the upper airway, generally peaks in the first 48 hours postburn. Hoarseness and stridor are primary signs of upper airway damage and airway obstruction. Obstruction can be complete and can occur rapidly in this population. Early intubation as a means to secure the airway is always prudent in these cases because the loss of anatomic landmarks potentiates the complication of this procedure. Cricothyroidotomy is rarely indicated and if necessary can be complicated by the diminution of landmarks.

Below the Glottis. Inhalation injury below the glottis is less common and usually limited to chemical exposure as opposed to thermal. Superheated air often causes laryngospasm, thereby closing the glottis and decreasing the incidence of thermal damage to the lungs. Water conducts heat approximately 30 times as efficiently as air; in an incident involving large amounts of steam the risk of injury is far greater because water has a heat-carrying capacity 4000 times greater than air.[67,98]

Products consumed in residential or commercial structure fires generate smoke containing noxious fumes and chemicals. The severity of damage from the chemical depends on the amount and type of volatile substance encountered, for example, smaller particles are more easily inhaled into the smaller bronchioles. Small children, older adults, or unconscious victims often remain within a burning structure for longer periods, sustaining greater damage.

Inhalation injuries below the glottis demonstrate such physiologic changes as impaired ciliary activity, erythema, edema, hyperemia, bronchospasm, bronchorrhea, or ulceration. This damage to the ventilatory tissue hinders the ability of oxygenation. The inflammation process is unpredictable based on the substance inhaled and its effects on the pulmonary tree; these patients should be observed for at least 24 hours. Intubation should be performed as needed.

Systemic Toxicity. The most commonly inhaled toxic substance is carbon monoxide (CO); this results from the incomplete combustion of carbon. CO binds with hemoglobin (Hgb) and thereby blocks the oxygen (O_2) from binding, creating an asphyxiation episode. CO has an approximately 200 times greater affinity for Hgb than O_2 and competes for the same binding sites; CO does not readily release itself from red blood cells (RBCs).[52] Inhalation of CO displaces oxygen and decreases the availability of oxygen for delivery to the tissues. The most vulnerable organs to the resultant hypoxemia are the nervous system and the heart; these organs require a continuous supply of O_2 to meet the persistent demand. Hypermetabolism from the burn injury compounds the demand by increasing the need for nutrients. The patient must be observed for decreasing levels of consciousness or dysrhythmia.

The patient who has inhaled CO presents with a cherry-red complexion because the hemoglobin is bound at the same site but not with O_2. The pulse oximetry reads a falsely elevated value because it is only a measure of bound hemoglobin and does not differentiate.[14] An arterial blood gas (ABG) with carboxyhemoglobin (COHgb) is the only evaluative method for determining the CO level in the blood. The signs of CO poisoning depend on the level of COHgb in the blood (Table 44-1). With increased COHgb levels in burn patients, there is an increased risk of aspiration, seizures, electrolyte abnormalities, or hypovolemic shock. An arterial blood gas remains unaffected by CO poisoning but is critical in determining the carboxyhemoglobin level.

TABLE 44-1 Effects of Carbon Monoxide Exposure

EXPOSURE	BLOOD CARBOXYHEMOGLOBIN	SIGNS AND SYMPTOMS
Mild	5%–15%	None significant; often found in smokers or those with exposure to heavy traffic (truckers, taxi drivers, etc.)
Moderate	16%–40%	Varying degrees of central nervous system effects: headache, confusion, nausea, impaired dexterity, visual changes, lethargy
Severe	41%–60%	Tachypnea, tachycardia, mental status changes (hallucinations, combativeness, delirium, coma), cardiovascular collapse, death (increased risk with COHgb >50%)
	>60%	Death within hours to minutes with rising levels

Data from references 88, 95.

When CO poisoning is suspected, the treatment is normobaric oxygen (NBO) therapy with 100% fraction of inspired oxygen (Fi_{O_2}) at a high flow until the COHgb is less than 15% to 20%.[2,101] If the COHgb is not known, 100% O_2 should be given until the level can be determined. The half-life of COHgb at room air is 250 minutes; at 100% Fi_{O_2} it is dramatically reduced to 45 minutes. The cardiovascular system must be monitored and supported against the detrimental effects of increased COHgb levels. Hyperbaric oxygen (HBO) therapy further reduces the COHgb half-life to between 15 and 23 minutes at 2.5 to 2.8 atmospheres of pressure. Although one of the primary indicators for HBO, its role remains controversial as studies comparing NBO and HBO have yielded conflicting results.[101]

Individual clinical course guides the decision to intubate. A patient presenting with mild symptoms should be observed in critical care. Many will elect for prophylactic intubation before completing a patient transport to a burn center. Upper airway edema due to inhalation injury can progress rapidly and lead to rapid death; there may be a delayed presentation as a result of hypovolemia. Maintenance of the elevation of the head of the bed reduces the risk of ventilator-associated pneumonia (VAP) and attempts to limit edema surrounding the airway.

ZONES OF BURN WOUNDS

Burn wounds are described in the percentage of TBSA affected as well as the depth, or zone, of the wound (Figure 44-3, Table 44-2). The area at the center of the injury that sustains the most damage is the *zone of coagulation*. The cells in this area are devitalized and necrotic, without the prospect of rejuvenation; they require surgical excision and grafting for recovery to occur. Circulation to this tissue is nonexistent.

The area peripheral to this (both adjacent and subjacent) is the *zone of stasis*. Subsequent to the burn injury and the resulting inflammatory process, the circulatory flow to this area is greatly compromised or "sluggish." With proper treatment during the burn resuscitation phase (approximately the first 48 to 72 hours after the time of injury), this area has the ability either to survive or, under less than ideal conditions, become necrotic and an extension of the zone of coagulation.

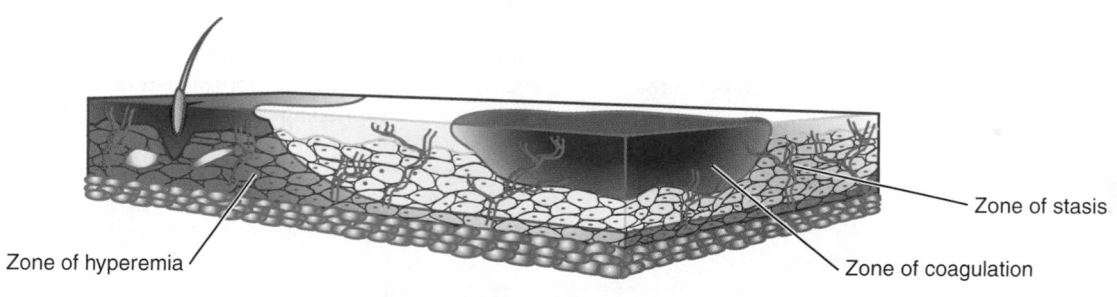

Zone of stasis

Zone of hyperemia

Zone of coagulation

♦FIGURE 44-3 Zones of burn wound.

TABLE 44-2 Zones of Burn Wound

	ZONE OF COAGULATION	ZONE OF STASIS	ZONE OF HYPEREMIA
Location	Focal point of burn injury	Adjacent and subjacent to zone of coagulation	Peripheral to zone of stasis
Appearance	White	Mottled red	Red
Circulation	None	Sluggish	Good
Recovery	None; requires surgical intervention	Questionable; dependent on ideal conditions and course of burn resuscitation	Should autorecover over next 10 days postinjury

Data from references 7, 109.

Surrounding the zone of stasis is the *zone of hyperemia*. In response to the burn injury, this area increases vascular flow through active and reactive hyperemia and the release of cytokines and other mediators into the systemic circulation. Vasodilation increases the flow of nutrients to the site of injury (active hyperemia) and removes metabolic waste products (reactive hyperemia). Reactive hyperemia is seen in patients in whom vascular compromise has been prolonged, and reperfusion is established with an escharotomy or fasciotomy.[111] There is good circulation, and this area will recover over the next 10 days postinjury.

DEPTH OF BURNS

There are many physical components to how the body reacts to contact with heat. Skin on some parts of the body is thinner than on others (backs of the hands, genitalia, face) and therefore more susceptible, as opposed to areas that are usually exposed to the environment or frequent use such as palms of the hands or soles of the feet. One's nutritional status and overall state of health help determine the amount of resistance. The very old and very young have less insulatory tissue (subcutaneous tissue) and sustain damage at a faster rate. Resistance in any age-group can be overcome based on the degree of heat and the duration of exposure (Table 44-3). Whereas the skin can tolerate varying degrees of thermal exposure, a fraction of a second of contact with an electrical source can cause severe damage.[27,66]

The extent of the burn wound is defined by the physical appearance. The depth of the injury determines the characteristics of the skin (Table 44-4). Burn wounds are classified by degrees (Figure 44-4).

TABLE 44-3 Temperature and Exposure

TEMPERATURE	LENGTH OF EXPOSURE	EXAMPLE
110° F (43° C)	Up to 6 hours	Hot tub
110° to 125° F (43° to 52° C)	Rate of destruction doubles with each degree rise in temperature	Water heater should be set to 124° to 130° (51° C to 54° C), and as low as 120° (49° C) for children or older adults Margarine and shortening melt between 120° and 130° F (49° C to 54° C)
118° F (48° C)	5 minutes to burn	
124° F (51° C)	3 minutes to burn	
126° F (52° C)	1 minute to burn	
130° F (54° C)	30 seconds to burn	Pure paraffin wax melts
133° F (56° C)	15 seconds to burn	
140° F (60° C)	5 seconds to burn	Wax paper, chocolate, construction adhesive, and beeswax melt
147° F (64° C)	2 seconds to burn	
150° F (66° C)		Film melts
155° F (68° C)	1 second to burn	
160° F (71° C)		Wood's metal (fusible metal) melts
160° to 180° F (71° C to 82° C)		Hot beverages

TEMPERATURE	LENGTH OF EXPOSURE	EXAMPLE
200° F (93° C)		Electric slow cooker
212° F (100° C)		Water boils
298° F (148° C)		Frying
392° F (200° C)		Baking
392° to 500° F (200° to 260° C)		Deep frying

Data from references 44 and 66.

TABLE 44-4 Depth of Burn Injury

	FIRST DEGREE	SECOND DEGREE		THIRD DEGREE
Cause	Sunlight exposure, very brief exposure to hot liquid, flash, flame, or chemical agent	Limited exposure to hot liquid, flash, flame, or chemical agent		Prolonged exposure to flame, hot object, or chemical agent. Contact with high-voltage electricity
Depth	Superficial	Superficial partial thickness	Deep partial thickness	Full thickness
Tissue	Involves only the epidermis	Epidermis, minimal dermis	Entire epidermis, more deeply into dermis	Dermis destroyed; extends to subcutaneous tissue
Characteristics	Skin intact and red	Mottled red color; blisters or weeping	Decreased moistness; skin pale in color; absent or prolonged blanching	Translucent, parchment-like or leathery appearance, charred; dry surface, thrombosed blood vessels; nonblanching
Pain	Painful, hypersensitive	Very painful, nerve endings exposed	Sensitive to pressure	Insensate; deep pressure only
Healing	Heals in 3–6 days	Usually heals in 10–14 days without surgery; minimal scarring	Some healing in 21–28 days, contractures; requires skin grafting	Requires grafting; self-generation destroyed

Data from references 7, 31, 111.

First-Degree Burns (Superficial)

First-degree burns, also referred to as superficial burns, involve mostly the epidermal layer and small amounts of the outer dermis (Figure 44-5). There is minimal epithelial damage; the skin remains intact and is reddened. The surface of the skin is dry and there are no blisters. It is painful and hypersensitive to tactile stimulation and normally treated with localized ointments or compresses. This type of burn heals in approximately 3 to 6 days without intervention and does not result in residual scarring. Care is palliative. Damaged tissue separates in conjunction with the normal replacement of the epidermal layer and reveals healthy tissue.

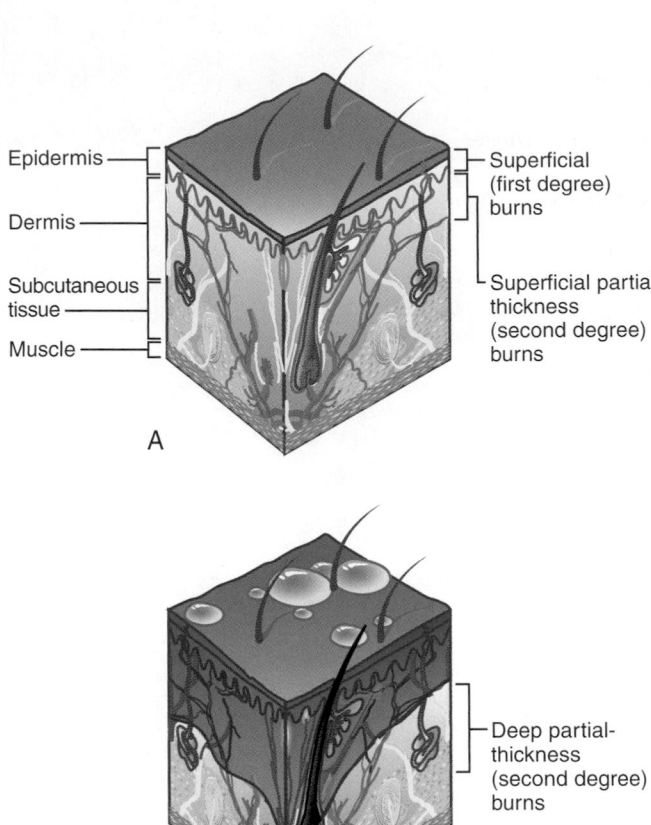

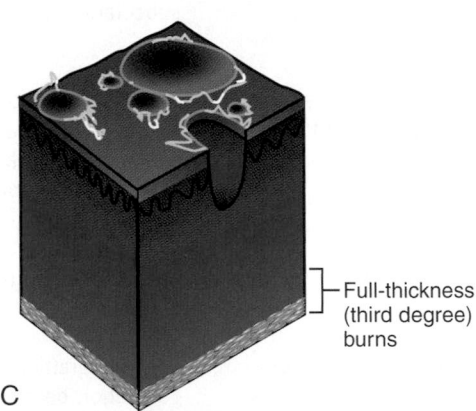

FIGURE 44-4 Layers of the skin and depth of burn wound. **A,** Superficial (first-degree) and superficial partial-thickness (second-degree) burn. **B,** Deep partial-thickness (second-degree) burn. **C,** Full-thickness (third-degree) burn.

Second-Degree Burns (Partial Thickness)

Second-degree burns involve the epidermis and extend into the dermal layer (Figure 44-6). Because the dermal layer is much thicker than the epidermis, second-degree burns are further classified as superficial partial thickness and deep partial thickness.

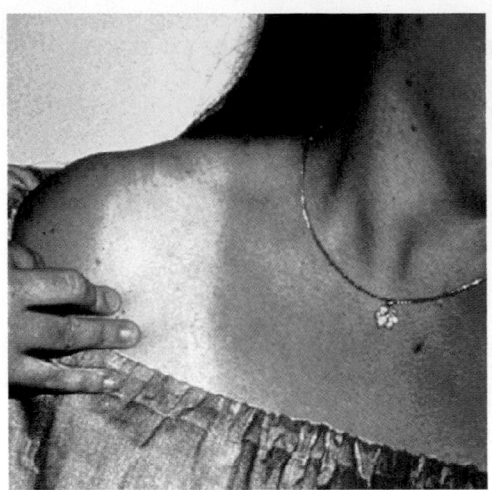

FIGURE 44-5 First-degree burn.

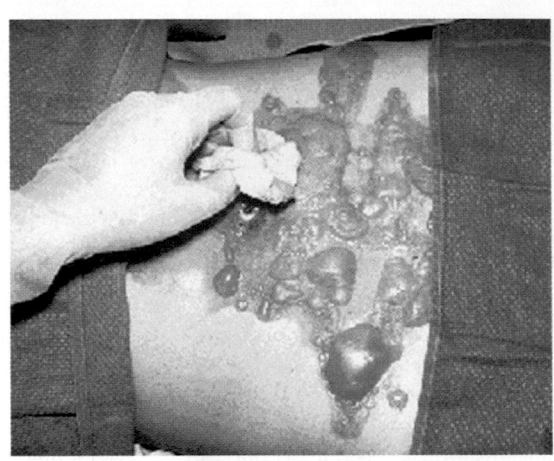

FIGURE 44-6 Second-degree burn.

Superficial partial-thickness burns involve the epidermis and parts of the dermis. The skin is typically mottled red. Blisters are formed, or the tissue is weeping serous fluid. These burns are very painful because the destruction of the epidermal layer has left nerve endings exposed. They usually heal spontaneously from preserved dermal appendages through epithelial migration in 10 to 14 days without surgical intervention and leave minimal scarring.[67] Often these burns can be covered with a synthetic dressing or skin substitute, and the patient can be treated on an outpatient basis; many synthetic dressings are available, and the products continually evolve. Selected synthetic dressings or skin substitutes are described in Table 44-5.

Deep partial-thickness burns involve the entire epidermal layer and extend more deeply into the dermis. There is decreased moistness as the glands become damaged and lose the ability to secrete. The skin is pale with absent or greatly prolonged blanching. There is some

TABLE 44-5 Skin Coverage

PRODUCT	MATERIAL	USE	ADVANTAGE	DISADVANTAGE
Biobrane	Mixture of highly purified peptides from porcine dermal collagen on semipermeable silicone membrane	Temporary wound covering for clean partial-thickness thermal burn wounds, donor sites, meshed autografts	Readily available Less expensive Long shelf-life without refrigeration	Higher infection rate, increased if not placed early on clean wound bed
Transcyte	Polymer membrane impregnated with newborn human fibroblast cells	Temporary wound covering of surgically excised full thickness and deep partial thickness; treatment of mid-dermal to indeterminate-depth burn wounds that typically require debridement and may be expected to heal without autografting	Transparent, allows direct visual monitoring of wound bed Stable coverage Readily available Some antiinfective effects	More expensive Transcyte must be stored frozen between −70° C and −20° C
Integra	Epidermal (Silastic) and dermal layer (animal collagen)	Coverage of surgically excised severe burn wounds, allows migration of fibroblasts and capillaries into material	Minimal contracture formation, less hypertrophic scarring Increased survivability of severe burns, improving functional and cosmetic outcomes Remove Silastic superficial layer and cover with very thin autograft after 2–3 weeks	Fragile framework
Homograft (allograft)	Cadaver skin (fresh or frozen/cryopreserved) Amniotic membrane (amnion) from human placenta	Temporary wound coverage	Placed at bedside or in operating room Cadaver skin vascularizes Best infection control, reduces bacterial colonization Amnion less expensive	Most expensive, limited availability Possibility of disease transmission (hepatitis or cytomegalovirus) Body will reject in about 2 weeks, antigenic Amnion does not vascularize
Xenograft (heterograft)	Skin from animals (usually pigskin–fresh, frozen, or freeze-dried)	Temporary coverage of clean wounds such as superficial partial thickness and donor sites	Readily available Adheres to clean superficial wounds allowing underlying wound to epithelialize Manufactured in multiple sizes Can be meshed or nonmeshed	Increased chance of infection Body will reject in 3–4 days, antigenic
Autograft	Autotransplanted from host donor site	Permanent coverage of excised burn wound	Permanent coverage Vascularizes Can be meshed or nonmeshed; meshing allows for increased coverage with less tissue Nonantigenic	Dependent on host's available donor sites, wound coverage may be greatly delayed Donor sites increase open body surface area and are painful Must be done in surgical suite

Data from references 11, 52, 85, 96, 111.

degree of healing in 21 to 28 days, but this depends on the burn size and location. Deep partial-thickness burns of significant size require surgical intervention. The technique of excision and grafting (E&G) is the definitive treatment to remove the necrotic tissue and accelerate the closure of the integument; this is described in detail under Surgical Excision and Grafting.

Third-Degree Burns (Full Thickness)

Third-degree burns are also called full-thickness burns because they involve all structures of the skin (Figure 44-7). In areas of full-thickness burns, the epidermal and dermal layers are destroyed. The skin is often translucent and has a parchment-like appearance; it may be charred. The cauterized skin is necrotic and forms an eschar that is leathery and without elasticity or turgor. The affected areas are painless because the sensory nerve endings have been destroyed (sensation to deep pressure will remain). Thrombosed blood vessels often are evident. This skin has lost the ability of autoregeneration and requires surgical grafting for repair.

Eschar tissue has acute as well as chronic concerns. Because of its loss of suppleness, the tissue beneath it is at increased risk for compartment syndrome. Circumferential burns to an extremity require continuous evaluation for potential escharotomy or fasciotomy because of fluid resuscitation and edema (these are discussed in detail separately later in this chapter under Compartment Syndrome, Escharotomy, and Fasciotomy). Eschar tissue is necrotic and increases the risk of infection the longer it remains.

Fourth-Degree Burns

The term fourth-degree burns is not a common term in the United States and is used to describe burns that are of such intensity as to extend completely through the dermal layer and subcutaneous tissue into deep structures, such as the underlying fat, fascia, muscle, tendon, or bone (Figure 44-8). Treatment requires elaborate debridement and, often, amputation.

After the initial assessment and life-threatening emergencies have been addressed, the burn wounds require initial classification, but final distinction between second- and third-degree burns can often be made only after the first 72 hours of treatment because the zones of the burn wound become delineated.

SEVERITY OF BURNS

Whereas the severity of the burn is based on multiple factors (Box 44-7), the depth (see Figure 44-3) and

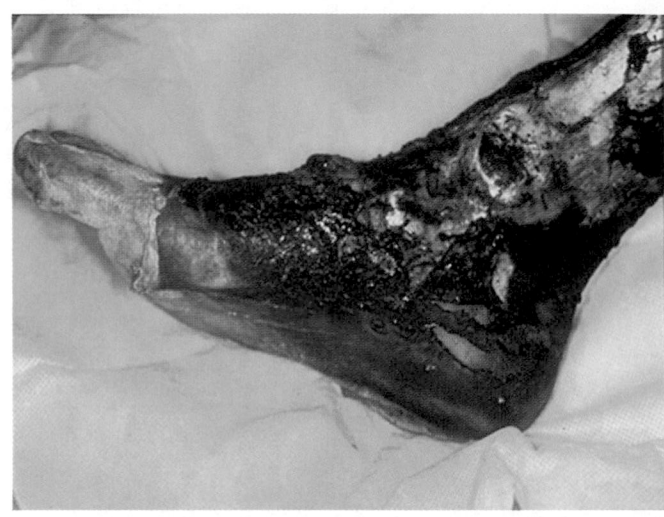

✦FIGURE 44-8 Fourth-degree burn.

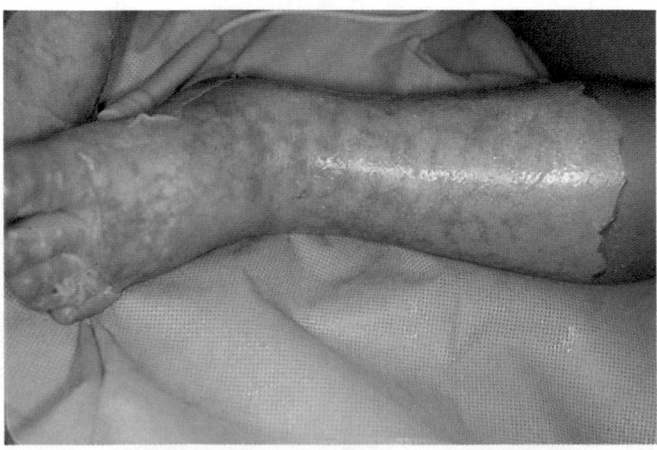

✦FIGURE 44-7 Third-degree burn.

Box 44-7

Factors Affecting Severity of Burn Injury

- *Presence of inhalation injury*—shown to independently increase mortality by 20% to 40%.
- *Age*—the very young and very old are more susceptible to the effects of the smallest of burns.
- *Physical and mental condition of the injured*—the outcome is highly dependent on the patient's ability or willingness to participate in the recovery process.
- *Location of the burn*—hands, feet, face, and genitalia require specific attention.
- *Source of the burn*—toxic or noxious fumes inhaled, electrical injury, and chemical exposure complicate the burn injury.

Data from references 5, 15, 76.

the extent of the TBSA affected are the key components in formulating the burn plan of care. Overestimation of TBSA burned is common.

There are several methods of estimating the burn size; the most common include the rule of palms, the rule of nines (Figure 44-9), and the use of the Lund and Browder chart (Figure 44-10). These are estimates only and are used for the initial calculation of fluid requirements and as a basis for the burn plan of care. The initial care algorithm includes admission to critical care or ward versus outpatient care; oral versus intravenous rehydration; number of projected surgical procedures; availability of host donor sites versus the use of allograft or synthetic material; and projected rehabilitation course or optimal functional outcome. There are several computer-based models to assist with the calculation of burn size and severity.

Each of the burn size calculation methods is to be inclusive of the second- and third-degree burns only. First-degree burns are not included because this tissue remains intact and thereby does not reflect a direct relationship to the increased caloric requirements and fluid resuscitation needs. This tissue also regenerates and does not require coverage with antimicrobial ointments, synthetic dressings or skins, or surgical correction. Functional outcome returns to the preinjury state.

Rule of Nines

The rule of nines (see Figure 44-9) is the most widely taught method of burn size calculation, dividing the body into multiples of nine: the head (to include the neck) counts for 9%, the anterior torso for 18%, the posterior torso for 18%, the upper extremities are 9% each,

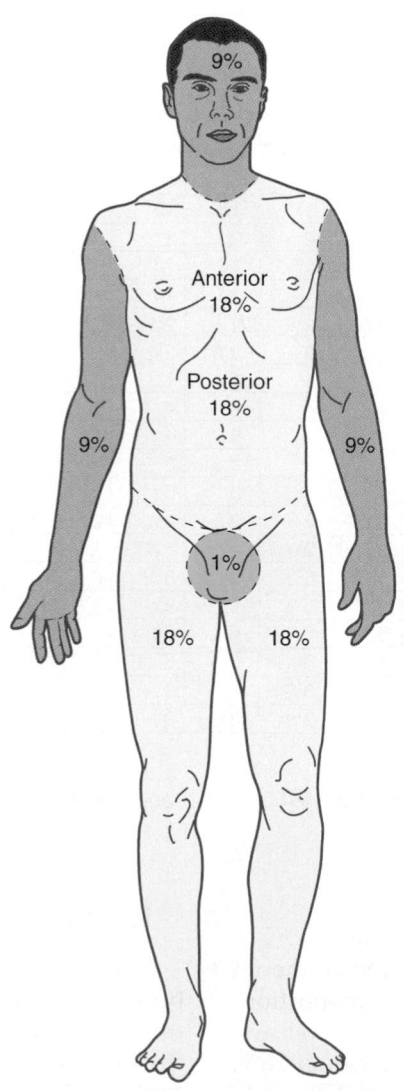

✦FIGURE 44-9 Burn surface area according to rule of nines (percentage for combined anterior and posterior surfaces).

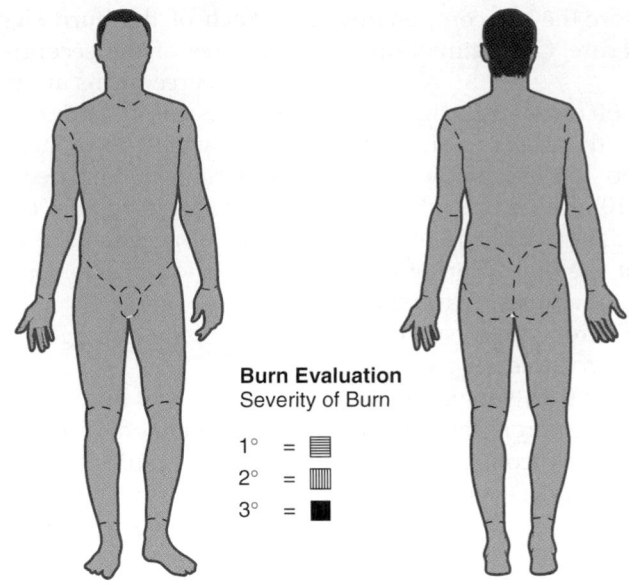

Burn Evaluation
Severity of Burn

1° = ▤
2° = ▥
3° = ■

Lund and Browder chart								
AREA	**AGE–YEARS**					% 2º	% 3º	% TOTAL
	0–1	1–4	5–9	10–15	ADULT			
Head	19	17	13	10	7			
Neck	2	2	2	2	2			
Ant. Trunk	13	17	13	13	13			
Post. Trunk	13	13	13	13	13			
R. Buttock	2½	2½	2½	2½	2½			
L. Buttock	2½	2½	2½	2½	2½			
Genitalia	1	1	1	1	1			
R.U. Arm	4	4	4	4	4			
L.U. Arm	4	4	4	4	4			
R.L. Arm	3	3	3	3	3			
L.L. Arm	3	3	3	3	3			
R. Hand	2½	2½	2½	2½	2½			
L. Hand	2½	2½	2½	2½	2½			
R. Thigh	5½	6½	8½	8½	9½			
L. Thigh	5½	6½	8½	8½	9½			
R. Leg	5	5	5½	6	7			
L. Leg	5	5	5½	6	7			
R. Foot	3½	3½	3½	3½	3½			
L. Foot	3½	3½	3½	3½	3½			
					Total			

⬍**FIGURE 44-10** Lund and Browder chart.

the lower extremities are 18% each, and the perineum counts for the remaining 1%. Children are proportionally different; therefore, the TBSA is divided as follows: the head is calculated as 18%, anterior torso as 16%, posterior torso as 16%, upper extremities are 10% each, lower extremities are 14% each, and the perineum counts for the remaining 1%.

Rule of Palms

The rule of palms is a technique best applied when burns are relatively small, not contiguous, or cover multiple areas of the body. Each "palm" size is 1% of the TBSA burned. The palm size is the patient's palmar surface, to include the fingers, not the healthcare provider's hand. The patient's palm size is visually estimated and then transposed over the burn injury.[2,111]

Lund and Browder Chart

The Lund and Browder chart (see Figure 44-10) gives a detailed breakdown of body surface areas and provides a means to account for variability of age from infants to adults. Further breaking down the parts of the body allows for a more accurate calculation of the burn size.[55]

Accurate determination of the depth and severity of the burn wound is essential for adequate fluid resuscitation and the avoidance of burn shock, proper wound care and agents, timely excision and grafting, and ultimately, the best functional and cosmetic outcome for the patient.

RESUSCITATION

Fluid Resuscitation in the First 24 Hours

A fluid resuscitation formula is a calculation used for the amount of fluid to be initially infused, accounting for the patient's preburn body weight and the percentage of TBSA burned. There are several formulas in use (Table 44-6), some of which have been blended to produce the ABA Consensus Formula[3]:

$$(2 - 4\,\text{ml Ringer's lactate}) \times (\text{Body weight in kg}) \times (\%\,\text{BSA burn})$$

TABLE 44-6 Burn Resuscitation Formulas

	FIRST 24 HOURS	SECOND 24 HOURS
American Burn Association consensus formula	Adult: (2–4 ml) × (kg body weight) × (% burned) Children: (3–4 ml) × (kg body weight) × (% burned)	Colloid-containing solution: (0.3–0.5 ml) × (kg) × (% burned) To maintain adequate urinary output (UOP): electrolyte-free fluid (adult), half normal saline (children)
Modified Brooke formula	LR: (2 ml) × (kg) × (% burned)	Colloid-containing solution: (0.3–0.5 ml) × (kg) × (% burned) To maintain adequate UOP: 5% dextrose in water
Brooke formula	LR: (1.5 ml) × (kg) × (% burned) Colloid: (0.5 ml) × (kg) × (% burned)	LR: (0.5–0.75 ml) × (kg) × (% burned) 5% dextrose in water (2000 ml)
Baxter (Parkland) formula	LR: (4 ml) × (kg) × (% burned)	Dextrose in water Potassium and colloid-containing fluid: (0.3–0.5 ml) × (kg) × (% burned)
Evans formula	0.9% normal saline: (1 ml) × (kg) × (% burned) Colloid solution: (1 ml) × (kg) × (% burned)	0.9% normal saline: (1 ml) × (kg) × (% burned) 5% dextrose in water (2 L)
Dextran (Demling) formula	Dextran 40 in saline: (2 ml) × (kg) per hour To maintain adequate UOP: LR	Fresh frozen plasma: (0.5 ml) × (kg) per hour for 18 hours To maintain adequate UOP: crystalloid
	First 24 Hours	
Infusion rate	From the time of the burn: half of the total fluid calculated is divided to be infused over the first 8 hours; the other half of the total fluid is divided to be infused over the next 16 hours	
Hypertonic (Monafo) formula	Hypertonic saline solution (250 mEq Na/L): to maintain adequate urinary output	
	First 16 Hours	
Modified hypertonic (Monafo) formula	First 8 hours to maintain adequate UOP: lactated Ringer's (LR) + 50 mEq NaHCO$_3^-$ (180 mEq Na/L) After 8 hours postburn: LR	

Data from references 2, 31, 105.

Lactated Ringer's solution (LR) is used for its tonicity and composition based on the burn patient's initial fluid requirements; when compared with normal saline (NS), its more nearly physiologic concentration of chloride ions makes LR the preferred solution (Table 44-7).[67] Prudent physicians agree that the best course of treatment is to initiate the infusion at the lowest rate calculated and titrate as indicated by hemodynamic response because it is easier to infuse more fluid than to remove it. (Sample resuscitations are shown in Table 44-8 and Box 44-8.) Dextrose solutions are not infused because they may cause osmotic diuresis, further complicating fluid resuscitation,[108] and because of early stress-induced glucose intolerance.[23]

Various factors can influence the burn patient's response (Box 44-9). Key parameters reflecting resuscitation efforts are urinary output, heart rate, blood pressure (particularly mean arterial pressure [MAP]), and

level of consciousness. Urinary output guidelines are given in Table 44-9.

Patients who tend to be "volume sensitive" to the fluid that is infused are those with preexisting cardiopulmonary disease or at either extreme of age, the very young or the very old. These groups should be very closely monitored and infusion rate changes made gradually.

The various fluid resuscitation formulas are an estimate only, and the amount of fluid should be titrated based on the patient's clinical presentation and response to treatments. The primary factors considered in the resuscitation are the patient's UOP and MAP. UOP in the adult thermal burn patient should be maintained between 30 and 50 ml/hr, or 0.5 ml/kg/hr (Table 44-9). The LR should be increased or decreased every other hour when the UOP is either less than 30 ml/hr or greater than 50 ml/hr for 2 consecutive

TABLE 44-7 Comparison of Commonly Used Fluid Components in Burns

	NORMAL SERUM RANGE	LACTATED RINGER'S (LR) SOLUTION	NORMAL SALINE (0.9% NaCl)	PLASMALYTE-A	DEXTROSE (5%) IN WATER (D_5W)	HETASTARCH 6% IN 0.9% NaCl (HESPAN)	ALBUMIN (5%)	ALBUMIN (25%)
Tonicity		Isotonic	Isotonic	Isotonic	Hypotonic	Hypertonic	Hypertonic	Hypertonic
		Crystalloid	Crystalloid	Crystalloid	Crystalloid	Colloid	Colloid	Colloid
Sodium (mEq/L)	136–145	130	154	140	–	154	130–160	130–160
Chloride (mEq/L)	96–106	109	154	98	–	154	130–160	130–160
Potassium (mEq/L)	3.5–5.0	4	–	5	–	–	<1	<1
Calcium (mEq/L)	8.5–10.8	3	–	–	–	–	–	–
Lactate (mEq/L)	0.5–1.5	28	–	–	–	–	–	–
Glucose (mg/dl)	80–110	–	–	23	50 g/L	–	–	–
Other	–	–	–	–	–	60 g/L starch	50 g/L albumin	250 g/L albumin
Osmolarity (mOsm/kg)	275–295	275	308	294	252	310	309	312
pH	7.35–7.45	6.5	5.0	7.4	4.0	5.5	6.4–7.4	6.4–7.4

Data from references 59–61.

TABLE 44-8 Example of Two Adult Burn Resuscitations	
38-YEAR-OLD FEMALE	**25-YEAR-OLD MALE**
Sustains 28% TBSA burn. Preburn weight is 60 kg.	Sustains 53% TBSA burn. Preburn weight is 85 kg.
(2 ml Ringer's Lactate) × (Body Weight in kg) × (% TBSA Burned) 2 (ml) × 60 (kg) × 28 (% TBSA)	2 (ml) × 85 (kg) × 53 (% TBSA)
Total Infusion of Ringer's Lactate Over First 24 Hours 3360 ml	9010 ml
Half of Total Amount Infused Over First 8 Hours *From the Time of the Burn* and Half Infused Over Next 16 Hours 1680 ml	4505 ml
Infusion Rate Over the First 8 Hours 210 ml/hr	563 ml/hr
Infusion Rate Over the Subsequent 16 Hours 105 ml/hr	282 ml/hr

Data from reference 2.

hours. Changes should be made more frequently only if the patient is hemodynamically unstable or symptomatic. MAP should be maintained at greater than 60 mm Hg to ensure adequate cerebral perfusion.[34]

One of the pitfalls of burn resuscitation is being less aggressive in decreasing the resuscitative fluid than in increasing it, resulting in complications from over-resuscitation; this can be as detrimental to the patient's outcome as under-resuscitation. Bolus therapy is to be avoided in this population because this potentiates loss of fluid into the interstitial space due to capillary leaking, increasing edema formation.

The resuscitative phase is usually considered the first 24 hours after a burn injury. The flux of mediators and closure of capillary leaks take place on a continuum, gradually occurring from 12 to 48 hours. The amount of fluid required to maintain UOP of 30 to 50 ml/hr should decrease progressively with resolution of the capillary leakage.[34]

Other factors to be considered in the resuscitation of the burn patient include clear mentation or level of consciousness, tachycardia (100-130 beats/min), gradual resolution of base deficit, and absence of hypotension (normotension does not necessarily indicate adequate

---

Box 44-8

Example of an Adult Burn Resuscitation

70-kg Male With 50% Total Body Surface Area (TBSA) Burn

Resuscitative fluid: Lactated Ringer's (LR) 2 ml × (Body weight in kg) × (% TBSA burned)
- 2 (ml) × 70 (kg) × 50 (% TBSA) = 7000 ml
- First 8 hours (from the time of the burn): 3500 ml/8 hr or 438 ml/hr
- Next 16 hours: 3500 ml/16 hr or 219 ml/hr

Albumin: (0.4 ml) × (Body weight in kg) × (% TBSA burned)
- 0.4 (ml) × 70 (kg) × 50 (% TBSA) = 1400 ml
- 1400 ml/24 hr = 58 ml/hr

D_5W: 1 (ml) × (Body weight in kg) × (% TBSA burned)
- 1 (ml) × 70 (kg) × 50 (% TBSA) = 3500 ml
- 3500 ml/24 hr = 146 ml/hr

Box 44-9

Patients Requiring More Intravenous Fluid Than the Resuscitation Formula Predicts

- Electrical injury
- Inhalation injury
- Patients with delayed resuscitation, either from delay in seeking healthcare or delay in the healthcare team's appreciating the complete fluid resuscitation needs
- Dehydration at time of injury, most commonly from alcohol or drug (e.g., methamphetamine) use or abuse
- Concomitant trauma

Data from references 2, 105.

TABLE 44-9 Goal Hourly Urinary Output

	URINARY OUTPUT
Adults	30–50 ml/hr (or 0.5 ml/kg/hr)
Electrical injury	75–100 ml/hr (or 2 ml/kg/hr)
Children (<30 kg)	1 ml/kg/hr

Data from reference 2.

resuscitation). The burn patient is hypermetabolic, with a heart rate in the adult of 100 to 130 beats per minute as a normal stress response to this insult (see Figure 35-1 and Figure 44-15). A heart rate greater than 140 beats per minute is considered significant tachycardia in this population; the patient must be evaluated for factors such as inadequate resuscitation, hypoxemia, proper analgesia, anxiolytics or sedatives, or stimulants. If patients are not demonstrating the appropriate hypermetabolic parameters, they must be evaluated for medications or drugs that may be suppressing this response (e.g., beta-blockers, calcium channel blockers, valium, illicit drugs, and so on).

Resuscitation should be projected at the 12-hour mark to predict the 24-hour total fluid resuscitation. Resuscitation in excess of 6 ml/kg/% TBSA burn has been associated with increased mortality, complications in hospital course, and decreased functional patient outcome.

Despite adequate crystalloid delivery, the resuscitation may be facilitated in the patient with persistent low UOP and MAP with colloid administration (albumin or fresh frozen plasma) after the capillary leak has closed. Typically infused between hours 24 and 48 postburn using the formula for 5% albumin of 0.3 to 0.5 ml/kg/% TBSA burned over 24 hours, infusion may begin at hour 12 to limit total crystalloid infusion. Alternatively, plasmapheresis may be indicated in a patient with ongoing fluid needs that exceed twice the estimated volume requirements. Early plasmapheresis (12 to 24 hours after injury) may decrease the incidence of complications from administration of excessive fluid; although unknown, plasmapheresis should theoretically remove inflammatory mediators that cause vasodilation and capillary leak.[34] Hypertonic solutions decrease the total fluid required for burn resuscitation, but the risk of hypernatremia is significant and the patient requires careful monitoring to avoid exceeding a serum sodium of 160 mEq/L.[23]

◆ Case Study 44-1, Part B

Fluid Resuscitation, Wound Care, Pain Control, and Infection Prevention

T.W. is transported and directly admitted to the burn intensive care unit, arriving 4 hours after the incident. Prior to his transport, T.W.'s fluid resuscitation was initiated using the ABA consensus formula for fluids during the first 24 hours after burn injury:

(2 ml LR) × (80 kg) × (48% TBSA burned) = 7680 ml to infuse over first 24 hours
½ over first 8 hours = 3840 ml or 480 ml/hr
½ over the next 16 hours = 3840 ml or 240 ml/hr

There is a high index of suspicion for inhalation injury, so he is placed on the Volumetric Diffusive Respiration (VDR-4), or high-frequency percussive ventilator. The pulses are immediately assessed, with a focus on the upper extremities secondary to the circumferential burns; pulses are present in all distal extremities but slightly diminished in the bilateral upper extremities.

Breath sounds are auscultated with coarse rhonchi. Heart sounds are normal, S_1S_2. Cardiac monitor demonstrates sinus tachycardia without ectopy. Initial vital signs are heart rate, 142 per minute; blood pressure, 108/64 mm Hg; respirations are assisted via the ventilator with a set rate of 10 breaths per minute; and the temperature via urinary catheter is 97° F (36.1° C).

A triple-lumen catheter and arterial line are placed in the left femoral vein and artery, respectively. Distal pulses on extremities with circumferential burns are palpable but weak and assessed every hour and more frequently in the upper extremities due to diminution. Carbonaceous sputum is observed in the oropharynx. Fiberoptic bronchoscopy is performed and reveals carbonaceous material in the bilateral upper airways with reddening throughout. Bilateral lower airways appear without injury. T.W. is placed on a continuous infusion of fentanyl at 200 mcg/hr and midazolam at 2 mg/hr for analgesic relief and sedation; additional dosing is given as indicated prior to interventions.

The Lund and Browder chart is completed, and a burn size of 48% total body surface area (TBSA) is calculated. The full-thickness burns account for 41% of the TBSA. These areas are insensate; the surface is dry, with thrombosed vessels observed, and the texture is leathery. The remaining partial-thickness burns are reddened, moist, and weeping serous fluid where the blisters have ruptured. The patient's weight is confirmed via a bed scale. Intravenous fluid continues as calculated. His urine output since placement of the urinary catheter has been 240 ml or an average of 60 ml/hr, above the goal of 30 to 50 ml/hr, but has been trending down, requiring close monitoring.

Admission labs are sent; chest roentgenogram is completed. Selected initial lab results are as follows:

Sodium:	143 mEq/L
Potassium	3.3 mEq/L
Chloride	106 mEq/L
Blood urea nitrogen (BUN):	18 mg/dl
Creatinine:	0.8 mg/dl
White blood cell count:	17,800 cells/mm^3
Hematocrit:	47.9%

Hematocrit reflects a hemoconcentrated value indicative of initial plasma loss and fluid shift, and demonstrates the need for continued fluid resuscitation. Radiology results are within normal limits without evidence of pneumothorax and confirming proper endotracheal (ET) tube placement.

The patient is taken to the shower room and all wounds are manually debrided. Silvadene cream (SVC) is applied to all partial- and full-thickness burns, bacitracin ophthalmic ointment around eyes, bacitracin ointment to the rest of the face, and Sulfamylon cream (SMC) to bilateral ears. The patient is placed on a pressure-relief mattress to decrease the incidence of decubitus, the head of the bed is elevated to 30 degrees, and bilateral upper extremities are placed in airplane slings to elevate the hands and abduct the axilla. The staff ophthalmologist arrives for examination of facial burns, which reveals no corneal abrasions. Lacrilube is ordered bilaterally every 2 hours for corneal protection.

The family arrives at the burn center and is met by the psychiatric clinical nurse specialist (CNS). A family meeting is held for a complete description of the wounds and the intensive care unit (ICU) environment. As they are prepared, family members are escorted into the ICU after demonstrating proper hand washing and donning personal protective equipment to protect the patient from additional exposure. Additional small doses of analgesia are administered as needed for signs of patient discomfort such as elevated heart rate and asynchrony with the ventilator.

Peripheral pulses in bilateral upper extremities (BUE) are no longer palpable at hour six but are biphasic via Doppler ultrasound. The forearms are showing increasing edema but remain supple. Intracompartmental (intramuscular) pressures (IMP) are measured at 26 mm Hg. T.W. is not hypotensive. Urinary output (UOP) for hours six and seven is 23 and 17 ml, respectively; intravenous rate is increased by 20% to 576 ml/hr. BUE pulses are no longer present per Doppler, and forearms are tight at hour nine, with IMP measured at 32 mm Hg. Escharotomies are performed to the medial and lateral aspects of both arms and the dorsum of the hands. Pulses are immediately palpable at the conclusion of this procedure. Wounds are closely observed for hemostasis.

A small-bore feeding tube is placed postpyloric and Osmolite HN, started at a trophic rate, is increased slowly every 8 hours as tolerated (goal is 105 ml/hr). Albumin 5% is added to fluid resuscitation between hours 24 and 48 at 48 ml/hr (0.3 ml/80kg/ 48% TBSA for 30% to 49% TBSA burn). The burn wound care plan is to cleanse the wounds with 4% chlorhexidine gluconate (CHG, Hibiclens) soap twice a day. Alternating solutions—mafenide acetate (Sulfamylon) in the morning and silver sulfadiazine (Silvadene) in the evening—are applied to all burn wounds except the face. Sulfamylon is always applied to the ears, bacitracin to the face, and bacitracin ophthalmic around the eyes. The exposed technique is used until excision and grafting (E&G) occurs. Passive range of motion is provided to all major joints frequently by nursing and rehabilitation personnel, with particular attention to the hands.

Decision point: During the patient's fluid resuscitation, what parameters need to be monitored to determine adequacy of resuscitation?

Decision point: What burn wound and skin care interventions are indicated in the first 24 hours after injury?

Decision point: What pulmonary complications is the patient most likely to experience in the first hours after injury? What are the signs and symptoms of these complications and how are the complications managed?

Case continues on page 1257

Pediatric Resuscitation

Pediatric patients have a greater TBSA in relation to their body mass index (BMI). This is a large factor in the fact that children require more fluid in relation to the size of their burn. In the child weighing less than 30 kg, the formula used for fluid resuscitation is (3 to 4 ml Ringer's lactate) × (body weight in kg) × (% TBSA burn).[2] This is the volume to be infused over the first 24 hours. As with adults, this is to be titrated to the patient's hemodynamic response to the fluids.

Pediatric patients have limited glycogen stores that, as with any traumatic scenario or stressful response, are rapidly depleted in the immediate postburn phase.

Therefore fluid resuscitation is supplemented with a maintenance dextrose-containing fluid, most often $D_5\frac{1}{2}NS$, particularly for children who weigh less than 20 kg. This fluid is infused at a constant rate and is not titrated.[9]

The pediatric burn patient responds as the adult does, with a hypermetabolic state and catecholamine response, but the hemodynamic parameters are variable and depend on the age. UOP in the child weighing less than 30 kg should be maintained at 1 ml/kg/hr. Pediatric patients have remarkable cardiopulmonary reserve and do not display clinical signs of hypovolemia until losing more than 25% of circulating volume, with low blood pressure and decreased UOP being late manifestations of shock and imminent cardiovascular decompensation.[9]

Difficult Resuscitation

The goal of education is to simplify approaches to medical care, but medicine is far from a simplistic skill. Burn resuscitation is no different, and the entire healthcare team continually strives to master the art of the science. Multiple complications may be encountered with any traumatic resuscitation. Over-resuscitation is not the answer and is found at the root of most complications occurring after the burn resuscitation phase. Appropriate consideration must be given to balance hypovolemia and the possible hypoperfusion of end organs with the comparably significant complications of interstitial fluid shift. Complications can include the following:

- Abdominal compartment syndrome—the need for decompressive celiotomy is associated with a high mortality
- Gastrointestinal dysfunction such as ileus, gastric ulcer, or superior mesenteric artery (SMA) syndrome leading to bowel necrosis
- Hypoperfusion of the zone of stasis and progression of wound depth
- Pneumothorax due to line placement
- Thoracic eschar syndrome and the inability to adequately ventilate or oxygenate the patient
- Extremity compartment syndrome
- Edema, specifically of the airway (leading to acute and rapid obstruction), but also cerebral or pulmonary
- Missed mechanical trauma
- Unplanned diuresis, further depleting the intravascular volume

Fluid Resuscitation in the Second 24 Hours (Hours 24 to 48)

The hypertonic properties of colloid infusion should decrease the overall crystalloid requirement and reduce the complication risk associated with overhydration. Colloids may be added as early as 12 hours postinjury but are avoided in the first 12 hours due to the diffuse capillary leakage, allowing colloids to move to the extravascular tissues. The infusion of colloids with capillary leakage increases the interstitial oncotic pressure and further the movement of fluid from the vasculature, potentiating the edema, increasing the risk of compartment syndrome, and furthering the hypovolemic process. As mentioned, plasmapheresis should also be considered when ongoing fluid needs exceed twice the estimated volume requirements.[34]

The modified Brooke formula for the adult burn patient includes the infusion of a colloid, albumin diluted to a 5% strength in normal saline (0.9% sodium chloride), during the second 24 hours (hours 24 to 48) from the time of the burn (Table 44-10; see also Table 44-6).[67]

Normal evaporative water loss is about 15 ml/m^2/hr, but loss from the burn wound is significant and may reach 300 ml/m^2/hr.[23] Evaporative loss continues until wound healing or skin closure occurs, either through synthetic dressing or surgical grafting.[23] In adults, 5% dextrose in water (D$_5$W) is added to replace the free water losses and the LR is titrated down. This is estimated at:

$$1 \text{ ml/kg/\% TBSA burn} = \text{ml/day}$$
or
$$(25 + \% \text{ burn}) \times (\text{Body surface area in m}^2) = \text{ml/hr}^{23}$$

This fluid can be titrated to assist with the correction of either hyponatremia or hypernatremia but runs the added risk of hyperglycemia. It is important to maintain glucose levels at 80 to 110 mg/dl; research has demonstrated the adverse effects of hyperglycemia on morbidity and wound healing.[100] Hypermetabolic requirements are excessive, and the treatment is aimed to provide caloric replacement through both glucose infusion and nutritional support.[23] Increased mortality, bacteremia, and decreased adherence of skin grafts have been associated in pediatric burn patients with poor glucose control.[35]

Fluid Resuscitation in the Third 24 Hours (Hours 48 to 72)

The albumin infusion should be stopped in the third 24 hours. The D$_5$W, or D$_5$ ½ NS in children, should continue to be infused and titrated as before to replace insensible water losses. Hyponatremia or hypernatremia is the most common electrolyte abnormality and is often addressed with the titration of 0.225% NS (¼ NS) or with the use of either NS or free-water gastric flushes.

TABLE 44-10 Colloid Solution in Burn Resuscitation

COLLOID	5% ALBUMIN IN NORMAL SALINE OVER SECOND 24 HOURS (HOURS 25–48)
30%–49% burn	0.3 ml/kg/% burn
50%–69% burn	0.4 ml/kg/% burn
70%–100% burn	0.5 ml/kg/% burn

Data from references 2, 105.

SPECIFIC BURN INJURY INTERVENTIONS

Electrical Injury

Electrical injury initially should be treated as polytrauma with a full evaluation. Concurrent injuries may be significant to include loss of consciousness, dysrhythmias, compartment syndrome, myoglobinuria, or fractures. Fractures, particularly spine and long bone, may occur from a subsequent fall or violent, tetanic skeletal muscle contraction; the cervical spine must be protected and compression fractures of vertebral bodies ruled out.[67,90] With the violent passing of high-voltage electricity, the hollow organs must also be evaluated for injury; prolonged contact may cause injury to the intestines or other visceral organs.

Causes of Cell Necrosis. Joule heating is the creation of heat by the movement of current through a resistor. Electroporation is the pulling of electrical dipoles, such as water molecules, by the electrical field into the cell membrane. This may generate pores whose diameter is sufficient to favor pore stabilization rather than closure. Permanent defects may result, leading to cell death. The electrical fields damage cell membrane proteins comprising voltage-gated ion channels, such as potassium channels. Muscle tissue that appears viable at first exploration is found, on subsequent operations, to have become necrotic. Reexploration should be planned approximately 48 hours after initial debridement. Often, repeated amputations are needed at levels that are more proximal.

Cardiac muscle has its intrinsic pacemaker cells; therefore it is very susceptible to the effects of electrical current passing through the body. Cardiac dysrhythmias, damage, and arrest are significant adverse effects of electrical injury. When exposed to current greater than 1000 volts, the patient should be observed for abnormalities even when asymptomatic—at a minimum, cardiac monitoring for 24 hours postinjury with serial examination of electrocardiograms and cardiac-specific enzymes. In cardiac arrest, the increased accessibility of automatic external defibrillators and decreased response time of emergency medical services have contributed to the increased survivability of electrical injury patients. With contact of less than 1000 volts, admission is required only when the patient is symptomatic or initial studies reveal abnormalities.

Due to Ohm's law, more than 40 volts is considered dangerous because of its ability to exceed the body's resistance (see equation on p. 1218).[23] Low-voltage AC injuries may cause immediate death as a result of ventricular fibrillation.[27] Later abnormalities are extremely rare. Local tissue damage is usually limited. Monitoring

for 24 hours, although frequently performed, is unnecessary if the electrocardiogram is normal on admission and there is no history of arrest or loss of consciousness. Secondary flash injuries can occur, causing thermal skin burns.

High-voltage AC and DC injuries are often devastating and more likely to produce transient ventricular asystole.[27] The death rate for those who arrive at the burn center alive is low, but there is a high amputation rate in this population, with long-term morbidity. Secondary to potential damage to the central and peripheral nervous systems, airway and breathing effectiveness must be continuously reassessed.

Contact points, commonly referred to as entry and exit points, are areas where the current density and tissue destruction are focal and greatest. These points are usually identified with full-thickness skin injuries. Arcing occurs when the current jumps or skips across adjacent parts of the body, such as the elbows or axilla. Skin resistance is reduced in sweaty areas.

Because electrical injuries tend to cause significantly more damage to structures other than the integument, the burn resuscitation formulas drastically underestimate the fluid requirements. The significant damage to structures other than cutaneous can lead to the breakdown of cellular tissue and the development of rhabdomyolysis. This disrupted tissue can become lodged in the filtration of the kidneys, leading to acute tubular necrosis (ATN) or myoglobinuric renal failure.[27] The urine must be continually observed for the development of pigmenturia (hemochromenuria or myoglobinuria) or darkening other than concentration. This should clear promptly with resuscitation fluid titrated to achieve UOP of 75 to 100 ml/hr or 2 ml/kg/hr to clear hemochromogens (see Table 44-9).

Sodium bicarbonate ($NaHCO_3^-$), added at 50 mEq/L of intravenous fluid, may be considered for judicious use to maintain slightly alkaline urine and may facilitate clearance of myoglobin by preventing its precipitation in the tubular cells.[67,90] If aggressive fluid resuscitation fails to increase UOP adequately and myoglobinuria is not resolving, in rare circumstances mannitol (Osmitrol) can be added with a bolus of 25 g and 12.5 g/L of intravenous fluid; caution must be used because its osmotic diuretic effect obscures the UOP as a reflection of the intravascular volume, and the placement of a pulmonary artery catheter should be considered for the invasive hemodynamic monitoring of preload (central venous pressure, pulmonary capillary wedge pressure).[67,90] When there is no pigmenturia or when the urine has cleared visually, the resuscitation fluid should be titrated to maintain UOP of 30 to 50 ml/hr, consistent with other burn patients.

Electrical injuries require early exploration for the extent of underlying necrotic tissue and excision.

Escharotomies and fasciotomies should be considered early because of potential deep tissue damage and the need to evaluate the muscle mass for compartment syndrome or necrosis. In wounds of limited extent with severe destruction, flap closure may be an attractive option. Contrary to this, the child with burns involving the commissure should be managed conservatively. The eschar needs to separate and reconstruction must be delayed because the amount of spontaneous healing is surprising, reducing the surgical intervention.[90]

Amputation is often the only solution to extensive myonecrosis. Nonstandard amputation flaps may be needed in order to preserve length and assist with prosthetic fitting. The devitalized lesion must be debrided to underlying healthy tissue.[23] Complications to electrical injuries are inherently different from other burn injuries, both acutely and in the long term. High-voltage injuries directly affect the central nervous system, resulting in neurologic impairment in approximately 50% of patients.[28,49] This can manifest on a wide spectrum from agitation, confusion, or visual disturbances to paralysis, aphasia, or coma.[27] The peripheral nervous system also may be affected with paresthesias manifesting often in the hands from contact with a power source; this may present immediately or be delayed, appearing as long as 2 years after the injury.[28] Patients must be evaluated for the absence of cataracts on admission; the formation of cataracts has been described from 4 weeks to 11 years after injury while showing no significant relationship to the voltage or contact points, although frequently associated with electrical injury to the head, neck, or upper chest.[28,77]

Chemical Burns

Chemical burns are divided into the following categories: acids, alkalis, and organic compounds. The concentration of the product and length of exposure are the key factors in the amount of damage sustained (see Box 44-5). Chemicals are found in alarming numbers throughout the country and range from the benign to the highly caustic in the home as well as the workplace. Acids tend to burn more rapidly (Figure 44-11), whereas alkalis penetrate deeply and cause severe tissue damage (Figure 44-12). Organic compounds not only cause cutaneous damage through contact but also can be absorbed systemically and damage the kidneys and liver. Whatever the chemical exposure, it is the disruption of a specific amino acid sequence or weak cellular bonds that leads to the denaturation of proteins.[83]

Acids are found in many household products, specifically bathroom cleaners (hydrochloric acid), rust removers (oxalic acid, hydrofluoric acid), swimming

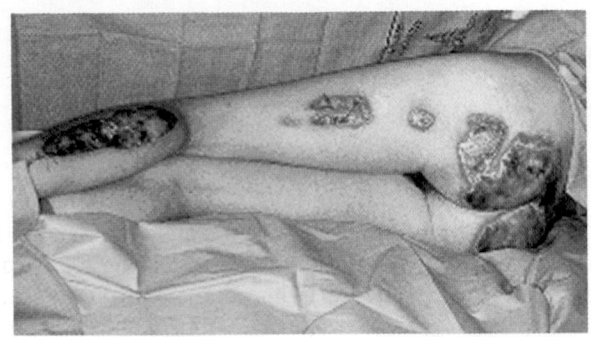

FIGURE 44-11 Acid burn.

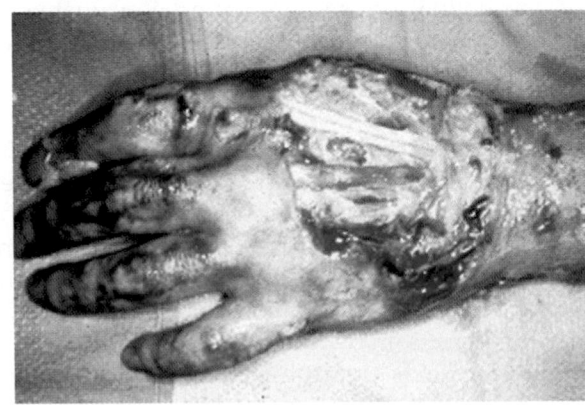

FIGURE 44-12 Alkali burn.

pool acidifiers (concentrated hydrochloric acid, muriatic acid), and industrial-strength drain cleaners (concentrated sulfuric acid, toilet bowl cleaners). Alkalis are most commonly found in oven and drain cleaners, industrial cleansers, fertilizers, and cement (pH of 12 when wet); they include hydroxides, potassium ammonium, lithium, and calcium. Organic compounds include petroleum and phenol products (deodorizers, sanitizers, and chemical disinfectants).[2,26,37]

The tissue damage done by acids tends to be of limited depth because the injury occurs through *coagulation necrosis* (the coagulation of protein causes the affected cells or tissue to convert into a dry, dull, homogeneous eosinophilic mass) and the precipitation of protein. This can form a tough, leathery eschar, which in turn forms a barrier and limits the deeper penetration of the acidic agent. Alkalis reduce the skin's resistance; they are less soluble in water, often take longer to clear, and should be flushed a minimum of 1 hour.[67] The damage can be deeper and more severe through liquefaction necrosis, saponification, and the denaturation of proteins (causing the gray to brown appearance of the tissue). Because they are a fat solvent, organic compounds damage the tissue by breaking down the cutaneous cell membranes; when these compounds are absorbed, extensive damage can occur to the liver and kidneys.[2,37,90] Phenol can cause extensive damage before being recognized by the patient because it acts as a local anesthetic.[26]

Another classification of chemicals, and perhaps more accurate, is by the damage that is done to proteins: oxidizing agents (sodium hypochlorite—Dakin's solution, Clorox), corrosives (phenols, white phosphorus), reducing agents (hydrochloric acid, nitric acid), desiccants (sulfuric acid, muriatic acid), vesicant (mustard gas, lewisite), or protoplasmic poison (hydrofluoric acid, acetic acid).[47,83]

Specific Chemical Burns and Potential Complications

Injury to the Eye. Two thirds of chemical injuries to the eyes involve an alkali compound. The eyes should be irrigated immediately and for a prolonged period with saline to limit damage. In the event of eyelid spasms, the lids should be forced open and facilitated with topical ocular anesthetics.[90] Irrigation may be accomplished in a multitude of fashions, to include the use of a Morgan lens or even a nasal cannula placed across the bridge of the nose (medial sulcus) with the patient supine and fluid flowing through the eyes and away from other orifices. Extreme caution must be observed with any method to avoid causing further ocular damage or transferring the chemical from one eye to the other. Irrigation should continue until the arrival of the staff ophthalmologist for a thorough examination.[2,102]

White Phosphorus. White phosphorus is found in varying professions, but the highest risk of exposure occurs in the military, where it is used in incendiary devices; agriculture, where it is contained in some fertilizers, insecticides, or rodenticides; and pyrotechnics, as a primary component of fireworks. White phosphorus can spontaneously ignite with exposure to the air, rapidly oxidizing and causing an exothermic reaction. It is identifiable with the production of a yellow flame, dense white smoke, and a garlic odor. The wound should be immediately immersed in water and the particles gently removed while remaining under water. Copper sulfate at 1% strength is then used to wash the wound, causing the remaining particles to become coated with copper phosphide; this combination fluoresces and can be removed in a darkened room or with a Wood's lamp.[37]

Treatment of white phosphorus exposure must follow the primary survey protocol. All clothing should be removed, the wounds irrigated with water, and the patient referred to the burn center. Re-ignition should be avoided. The material can be covered in saline- or water-soaked dressings. Topical antimicrobial agents can be used to block exposure to ambient air and delay the burning process. The patient needs to be monitored

and treated for hypocalcemia, hyperkalemia, and the increased risk of cardiac dysrhythmias.[37,69]

Anhydrous Ammonia. Anhydrous ammonia is a common fertilizer or industrial refrigerant. It is highly soluble in water, forming ammonium hydroxide. It is treated with lavage until the smell of ammonia is alleviated, early intubation if inhaled, topical antibiotics as indicated, and early excision. Extreme danger remains with the toxic cleanup of sites used in the production of methamphetamines because these are often found in poorly ventilated and clandestine locations. The fumes have been described as so toxic as to kill victims before they hit the floor.

Anhydrous ammonia is encountered as one of four main ingredients in the production of illicit methamphetamine. There were more than 6400 methamphetamine lab–related seizures by law enforcement in 2006 (down from almost 12,500 in 2005 and more than 17,000 in 2004 and 2003). Burn patients from explosions of these illegal labs may be coated by the chemicals used to produce the drug, including anhydrous ammonia.[62,84] These patients have an increased incidence of inhalation injury, requiring more ventilator days and a corresponding increased length of stay.[84] Almost complete destruction of the pulmonary mucosa has been observed secondary to the inhalation of ammonia gas.

Petroleum Exposure and Hydrocarbons. A motor vehicle crash with prolonged extrication time may leave the victim(s) in contact or saturated with petroleum products for extended periods. Petroleum products are highly lipid soluble; lingering integumentary exposure to petroleum products can result in the delipidation of the tissue. Partial- and full-thickness necrosis of the skin is common, although it may not be initially evident. The body may then absorb hydrocarbons, complicating subsequent therapy. The effects are usually evident 6 to 24 hours after exposure. Hydrocarbons are excreted through the pulmonary system; this process may produce chemical pneumonitis and bronchitis. Systemic toxicity may lead to organ failure, most commonly hepatic (hepatitis) or renal failure (glomerulonephritis), and cardiac instability.

Cutaneous absorption of lead containing petroleum has been described to manifest systemic lead poisoning; there should be a high index of suspicion, especially in the developing pediatric population, and serial levels should be drawn.[67,69]

Hydrofluoric Acid. Hydrofluoric acid is an occupational hazard in many industrial processes including producing semiconductors, cleaning air-conditioning equipment, refining petroleum, producing Teflon, and etching glass. Searching for a neutralizing agent is not useful with chemical exposure, but hydrofluoric acid is the exception. Although a weak acid, it is the most tissue-reactive inorganic acid because the fluoride ion binds to the tissue components. Fluoride activity continues to penetrate the tissue and ceases when combined with calcium or magnesium to produce an insoluble salt. Initially the wounds should be irrigated with copious water and calcium gluconate gel applied topically. A local injection of 10% calcium gluconate may be injected at 0.5 ml/cm^2 into the wound if pain does not subside. Hypocalcemia is the most serious side effect and must be treated as indicated.[40,67,69]

Circumferential Burns

If the burn completely envelops or nearly encompasses the extremity it can act as a tourniquet to the flow of blood and the lymphatic system because the eschar tissue has lost its elasticity. Referred to as eschar syndrome, this can result in necrosis to the distal tissue, neurologic compromise, or compartment syndrome. Inadequate perfusion may lead to the loss of distal extremities through amputation or extend the body surface area injury, such as the progression of hypoperfused tissue to necrotic tissue. Necrotic tissue has no benefit to the human body, and as a growth medium for bacteria or fungi, its presence exponentially increases the risks to the patient.

Any article of clothing or item that could be constricting to the patient (rings, watches, belt, clothing, or jewelry) should be immediately removed at the scene or in the ED. The extremities, especially the upper extremities, should be elevated to decrease the edema and assist with the long-term functional outcome of the patient. The head of the bed should be elevated to decrease edema, thereby reducing the risk of airway edema, the incidence of ventilator-associated pneumonia (VAP), and the risk of aspiration.

The distal pulses should be checked and neurovascular status (capillary refill, sensation, and color of the skin) evaluated at least hourly and documented. If the pulse is not palpable, an ultrasonic device should be used. The diminution or absence of a pulse is a late sign and indicates the need for an escharotomy (incision of the eschar).[7] Before the procedure, ensure that the patient is being adequately resuscitated and that this is not the result of hypovolemia. Escharotomy or fasciotomy may prevent the pressure occlusion of the microcirculation.[13]

Failure to identify adequate perfusion at any point in a timely manner may lead to reperfusion syndrome because circulation is restored to the affected extremity; the risk is greatest during the burn resuscitation phase but is possible throughout the disease process. Reperfusion syndrome is manifested by local as well as systemic responses; the level of inflammatory response is in direct relation to the extent of the region involved. Locally, tissue injury may be aggravated by limb swelling that follows reperfusion. The systemic response may result in organ failure and death. Irreversible muscle cell damage

starts after 3 hours of ischemia and is nearly complete after 6 hours.[13]

Active and passive range of motion (ROM) provides some assistance with the distal circulation. Patients should be encouraged to do all that they can actively, and given appropriate analgesia to assist with this. The entire healthcare team should conduct passive ROM as frequently as indicated, under the guidance of the rehabilitation staff as needed.

Escharotomy. Eschar syndrome is the restriction of blood flow to distal tissue due to the edema formation beneath an inelastic eschar. Eschar syndrome is diagnosed with a Doppler flowmeter verifying vascular compromise. In this event, the eschar tissue must be released with an escharotomy, creating an incision that penetrates the burned layers but does not exceed the underlying subcutaneous tissue.[64] Loss of blood should be minimal.[67]

Escharotomies are rarely indicated in the immediate postburn phase and should be completed only after consultation with a burn center. It must be ensured that the diminution or absence of a pulse is not secondary to insufficient fluid resuscitation. Indications for escharotomy increase as fluid is infused and the edematous process ensues (Box 44-10). Early escharotomies may be necessary in patients with deep circumferential limb or truncal burns (to maintain peripheral circulation or permit ventilation), high-voltage electrical injuries, or when resuscitation has been delayed.[2] A needle can be inserted subeschar or into the muscle compartment and attached to a hemodynamic monitor to measure pressure. Indications for escharotomy include a

---

Box 44-10

Indications and Rationale for Escharotomy

RATIONALE

- Full-thickness eschar
- Encircling a limb, or nearly so
- Burn wound edema
- Impaired venous return
- Impaired arterial inflow
- Ischemia, compartment syndrome
- Potential for muscle damage, nerve injury, or limb loss

INDICATIONS

- Progressive diminution of Doppler signal
- Loss of Doppler signal
- Cyanosis
- Neurologic dysfunction

Data from references 2, 64, 67, 111.

pressure in excess of 30 mm Hg, diminishing perfusion or temperature, or increased firmness.[63,67,111]

Escharotomy can be accomplished at the bedside with a scalpel or electrocautery device, ensuring appropriate analgesia. The patient should be placed supine and in the anatomically correct position to assist in identifying landmarks as the incisions are made; the body position shown in Figure 44-13 demonstrates the possible incision lines. Increased care should be employed with incisions crossing the joints because nerves and blood vessels tend to be most shallow at these locations and are in proximity to intended incision lines; for this reason, the ulnar nerve is of particular concern at the elbow and the radial nerve at the wrist. When possible, the incision is made from unburned tissue to an area of unburned tissue to adequately relieve the tourniquet-like effect of the eschar. This is not always possible in patients who have sustained massive burns in which the burn extends from the extremity to the torso. The incision depth is through the eschar to the subcutaneous layer and avoids viable tissue. Escharotomies are made on both the midlateral and midmedial line of each burned extremity. The incision lines are palpated to ensure that adequate pressure has been released and there are no bands that will continue to hinder vascular flow to the extremity. Document the restoration of pulses through palpation or use of the Doppler flowmeter. Subeschar or intramuscular compartment pressures can be remeasured to ensure adequacy of the procedure. Limbs are then elevated above the level of the heart to decrease edema.[2,63,64,111]

Circumferential burns of the trunk (anterior and posterior torso) may lead to the inability to adequately ventilate the patient through restriction of pulmonary excursion. Primary indicators for this are most often increased peak pressures, high-pressure alarming of the ventilator, impaired ventilation, decreased compliance, and impaired chest excursion on examination. This requires escharotomies of the tissue of the chest wall, in essence creating a flail segment of the tissue that allows for sufficient rise and fall of the chest; this is a lifesaving measure. Incisions are made along the anatomic clavicular line, along the anterior axillary lines, and across the upper abdomen along the costal margin. Incisions may be added to the sternum and extended across abdominal burns to decrease constriction (Figure 44-14).[2,64]

In burns involving the dorsum of the hand, in which the pulse in the palmar arch is not present but the radial and ulnar pulses have been verified, hand escharotomies to the dorsal surface may be indicated. In rare instances, escharotomies of the fingers also may be completed.[64] These should only be accomplished after direct consultation with a burn surgeon.

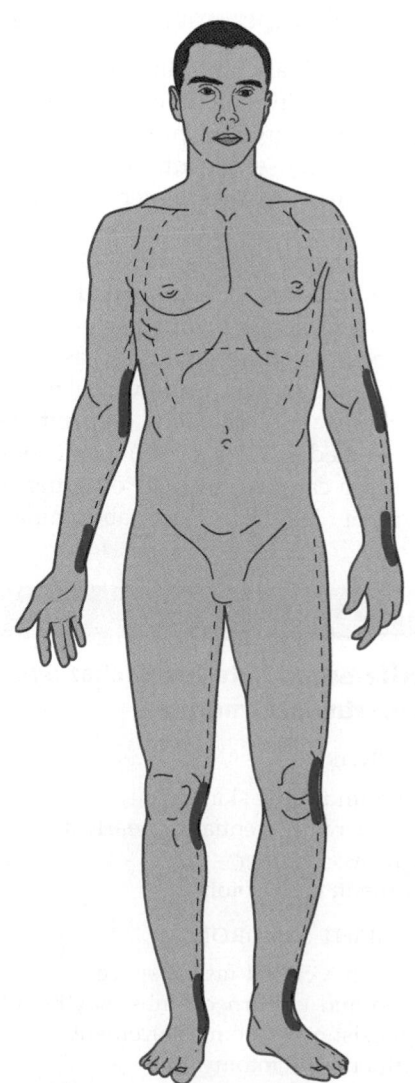

♦FIGURE 44-13 Escharotomy incision lines.

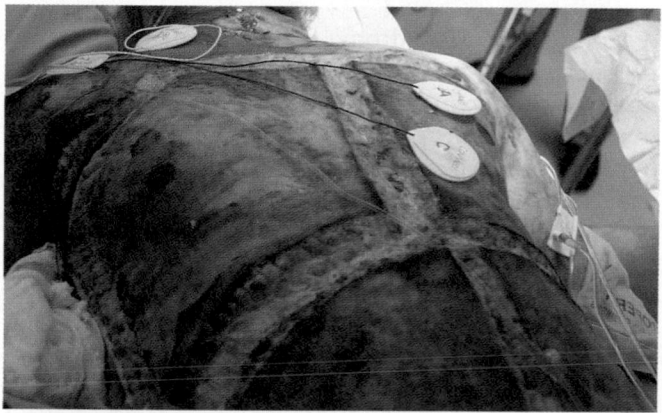

♦FIGURE 44-14 Chest escharotomies.

The inability to confirm reperfusion after any escharotomies requires a fasciotomy. Escharotomy incisions are ultimately repaired with the excision and grafting of the damaged tissue.

Fasciotomy. Although rarely indicated, fasciotomies may be required if escharotomies have already been accomplished and either the circulation fails to be restored to the distal extremity or the pulse is subsequently lost again with continued fluid resuscitation. Patients at risk include those with circumferential or near-circumferential limb burns, delayed or inadequate escharotomies, TBSA burn greater than 20%, high-voltage electrical injuries, and burn resuscitation in excess of 6 ml/kg/% TBSA burn. Burned and unburned limbs are at risk with over-resuscitation. Fasciotomies should be completed in the operating room secondary to the potential risks of this procedure because the incisions are made to the depth of the fascia[2,67] (see Figure 44-14). The incisions lines are the same anatomically as those for escharotomies. Hemostasis should be promoted and the wound closely monitored for bleeding secondary to the depth of the incision and potential exposure of large vessels. Hypothermia can result in coagulopathy and should be prevented to assist hemostasis.[2]

Fasciotomies are indicated when the compartment pressure exceeds 30 mm Hg and there are clinical indicators of compromised circulation. Surgical intervention releases the enclosing fascia along the entire length of the compartment. The wound may be covered with a biological dressing such as porcine heterograft and the extremity elevated to assist with the resolution of edema.[77] With early recognition and treatment, the result is generally good. Delay in treatment often results in nerve injury, muscle necrosis, loss of function, and possible amputation. Debridement should be reserved for 24 to 48 hours and the wounds left open and addressed with secondary closure or delayed grafting.[68]

Compartment Syndrome

Compartment syndrome is the result of increased pressure in a fascial compartment. In burns, this occurs most frequently with the increased leakage of fluid into the extravascular space and subsequent intravascular hypovolemia. Microvascular pressures during normal conditions usually maintain a near-equal balance between fluid filtration and lymph flow; studies in animals and humans demonstrate a large increase within 5 minutes of the burn injury in fluid filtration in burned tissue that exceeds lymph flow, causing rapid edema formation.[50] The compartments prone to developing elevated compartment pressures are those of the lower leg and the volar forearm.[103] With the tourniquet-like effect of eschar, the pressure continues to build as fluid

becomes trapped in the distal extremity, and edema forms. Pressure within a closed space impedes the blood supply and functioning of the tissue within that space. If not treated in a timely manner, this pressure can result in damage to the contents of the fascial compartment. Diminution or absence of pulses is a very late indicator of compartment syndrome; early signs include coolness to touch, delayed capillary refill, subjective numbness, and altered sensation.[63,77] Patients with high-voltage electrical injury remain at risk for the development of compartment syndrome for up to 48 hours postinjury.[77]

A patient may have both eschar and compartment syndrome simply due to the severity of injury and the required resuscitation (Box 44-11). This is generally a progressive presentation. Eschar syndrome usually precedes compartment syndrome. Delayed or inadequate escharotomy may result in the development of compartment syndrome. The entire healthcare team needs to be vigilant.

Abdominal Compartment Syndrome

Although abdominal compartment syndrome (ACS) is appreciated, the specific clinical conditions that define it are not agreed on; however, most clinicians agree the organ dysfunction caused by intra-abdominal hypertension (IAH) requiring surgical intervention with either decompressive celiotomy or laparotomy is considered to be ACS.[72] Most agree that intra-abdominal pressure (IAP) in excess of 25 mm Hg is defined IAH, impairing venous return and decreasing cardiac output; end organ damage has been described with IAP as low as 10 mm Hg.[67,72,73] ACS results in cardiovascular, pulmonary, renal, splanchnic, abdominal wall, and intracranial disturbances (detailed in Box 44-12) from elevated IAP regardless of the cause. Only 40% of patients with this severe form of increased intra-abdominal pressure

---

Box 44-11

Major Differences Between Eschar Syndrome and Compartment Syndrome

ESCHAR SYNDROME

- Edema under the skin
- Burn is circumferential or nearly so
- Diagnosis: Doppler
- Treatment: escharotomy

COMPARTMENT SYNDROME

- Edema in a closed fascial space
- Burned and unburned limbs may be affected
- Diagnosis: pressure measurement
- Treatment: fasciotomy

Data from references 50, 103.

Box 44-12

Diagnostic Points for Abdominal Compartment Syndrome

CARDIOVASCULAR

- Decreased cardiac output
- Decreased inferior and superior vena cava flow
- Increased systemic vascular resistance
- Decreased stroke volume and reflexive increased heart rate

PULMONARY

- Decreased compliance and increased peak inspiratory pressure
- Decreased total lung capacity, functional residual capacity, and residual volume
- Ventilation-perfusion ($\dot{V}/\dot{Q}$) mismatch displayed with hypoxia
- Hypoventilation with resultant hypercarbia

RENAL

- Inadequate renal perfusion caused by decreased cardiac output
- Corticomedullary shunting from renal vein compression and direct parenchymal pressure
- Increased renal vascular resistance
- Decreased renal blood flow
- Decreased glomerular filtration rate

CEREBRAL

- Increased intracranial pressure

survive.[20] The burn patients at greatest risk of ACS include the following:

- Those whose 12th-hour projected fluid resuscitation or actual 24-hour resuscitation is in excess of 6 ml/kg/% TBSA burn

- Those whose burns are >50% TBSA burned; Ivy and colleagues[45] established a 20% incidence in 10 patients with burns >20% TBSA
- Those who are being resuscitated for sepsis
- Those whose resuscitation exceeds 250 ml/kg; Hobson[41] described ACS in burn patients who received an average of 237 ml/kg over a 12-hour period. Oda and associates[70] found that most patients with severe burns required more than 300 ml/kg of resuscitation fluid for the first 24 hours after injury that led to ACS
- Those with reperfusion injury to the bowel, which has been described as a probable cause for ACS[36,46]

See Figures 35-1 and 44-15 for the neurohormonal response to stress.

Avoidance is the goal of ACS. Barring that, diagnosis is made with a urinary bladder pressure exceeding 30 to 35 mm Hg in the appropriate clinical setting. IAP can be conveniently measured via an indwelling urinary catheter and hemodynamic pressure monitor calibrated to atmospheric pressure. Per the recommendation of manufacturers of IAP kits, most facilities instill 50 ml of saline into the urinary bladder of the adult.[72] Caution should be used when instilling more fluid than this or instilling into smaller patients so as to avoid false readings. Abdominal computed tomography (CT) may reveal subtle findings such as round-belly sign, collapse of the vena cava, or bowel wall thickening with enhancement.[72]

The inability to sufficiently alleviate rising pressure and the life-threatening complications requires decompressive celiotomy. The opening of the abdominal compartment exposes the patient to untold risks and further complications. Percutaneous fluid drainage has had some recent success in burn patients as a procedure that can be completed at the bedside.[21,53,72]

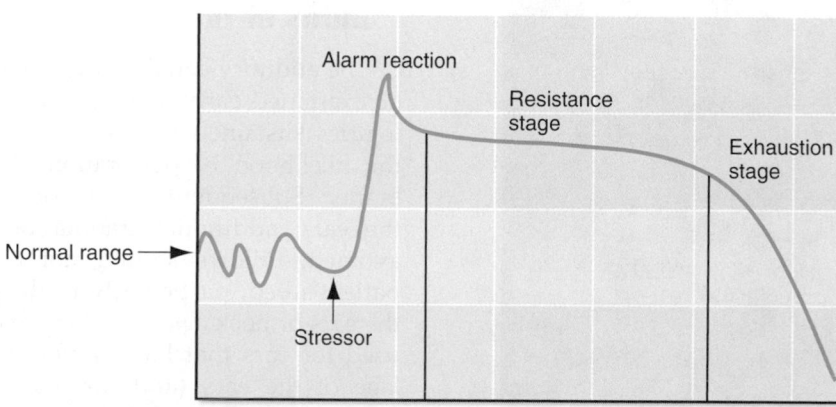

◆FIGURE 44-15 Neurohormonal response to stress.

SPECIFIC ANATOMIC BURNS

Extremity Burns

Any extremity sustaining significant burn wounds should be elevated to assist the vascular flow. Extremities may be placed on pillows or towels. Upper extremities should be placed on a properly padded airplane sling, especially if the burn extends to the axilla. This not only elevates the extremity, reduces edema, and promotes functional outcome, but also deters contraction of the axilla through abduction (Figure 44-16). Neurovascular checks, pulses, and sensation should be evaluated every hour or more, if indicated. Areas to check include the radial, ulnar, and palmar arch; digits in the upper extremities; and the dorsalis pedis and posterior tibialis in the lower extremities. Active and passive range of motion should be done frequently.

Facial Burns

Facial burns usually require hospitalization for sufficient observation and intervention. Extensive edema is common with any depth of facial burns, and airway compromise may develop late with a rapid onset. The head of the bed, whether the patient is intubated or spontaneously breathing, should be elevated to semi-Fowler's or high Fowler's position. The face should be cleansed with saline or water. On admission, hair should be shaved and cleansed where it is in proximity to any partial- or full-thickness burns because hair can harbor bacteria. Shaving of male patients manually debrides the uppermost layers of facial burn wounds and advances the healing process. All cephalically inserted

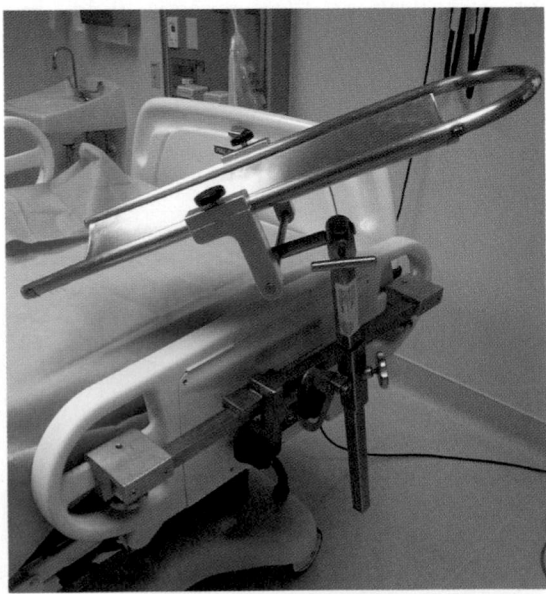

♦FIGURE 44-16 Airplane sling.

tubes (e.g., endotracheal or gastric) should be affixed with umbilical tape because the serous drainage from facial burns disrupts the adherence of any adhesive.[40]

The face is highly vascular, and healing often occurs spontaneously without surgical intervention. Intervention, when required, is usually delayed until late within the healing process and after other grafting has been completed. Common intervention consists of contraction release of the eyelids and of the oral commissure to allow mastication.

Burns of the Eyes

Fluorescein examination of the eyes with a Wood's lamp should occur early, before swelling hinders the ability to complete the procedure. This should be done for any patient with burns above the clavicles. Actual injury to the cornea or globe is uncommon because heat or smoke causes blepharospasm, although injury to the ocular adnexa is common with thermal exposure. Whenever available, ophthalmology should be consulted immediately for thorough evaluation. If corneal abrasion is present, ophthalmic antibiotic ointments should be initiated. Ophthalmic steroids are not indicated and should be avoided. The eyes should be protected with artificial tears, Lacri-Lube, or moisture chambers as appropriate. Chemical exposure of the eyes should be irrigated with copious amounts of saline until the staff ophthalmologist arrives. Increasing intraocular pressure (IOP) may compress the ocular vessels, compromising vascularity, potentially resulting in ischemia. Canthotomies may be indicated when the IOP exceeds 40 mm Hg and can be a vision-saving intervention. Any ocular defects should be evaluated daily because timely intervention is paramount. Lid releases and split-thickness skin grafts are indicated if the cornea is no longer protected; tarsorrhaphy may provide temporary corneal coverage but is dependent on the adequate availability of the lid margin.[2,67,78]

Burns of the Ears

The auditory canal and tympanic membrane should be examined early, before swelling occludes the view; injuries sustained with an explosion or blast increase the likelihood of perforation of the tympanic membrane.[2] Subsequent to the decreased vasculature of the ears, additional trauma or pressure should be avoided. Pillows should not be used on the burn patient's bed, particularly in the presence of burns to the ears or neck.[2] Sulfamylon cream (SMC) is routinely used for ears that have suffered any burns; the cartilage of the ears (and nose) is highly susceptible to chondritis, and the SMC's penetrating ability provides a necessary extra level of coverage.[85] Any infections to the ears are difficult to eradicate because the decreased vasculature of the area means that intravenous antibiotics do not arrive at the ears at high enough blood levels to be effective. Wound care should be done twice daily and SMC reapplied as needed to ear burns until healed.

Burns of the Hands and Feet

Secondary to the highly complex functionality, burns of any significance of the hands and feet should be referred to a burn center for evaluation. As early as possible in the burn treatment plan, burned hands and feet should be exercised actively, if possible, and passively for 5-minute intervals as often as possible. This should continue until debridement is initiated and then adapted in accordance with the interventions selected. Pulses should be verified frequently using a Doppler flowmeter if not palpable. Individual vascular flow checks of each digit are also highly recommended to monitor for alterations in perfusion. Full-thickness skin grafts are commonly used for the hands to optimize long-term functional outcome, leaving the surgical graft open for continual observation.[71] If a closed technique is used for burn wounds, dressings must be observed to avoid constriction. Reconstruction and rehabilitation of the hands and feet is a lengthy and complex process requiring coordinated efforts of the complete healthcare team and the continuous efforts of the patient.[63]

Burns of the Genitalia and Perineum

An indwelling urinary catheter should be inserted immediately to maintain urethral patency. A dorsal escharotomy of the penis is rarely needed. Scrotal swelling may be impressive but does not require specific treatment; elevation should be initiated as a comfort measure. A diverting colostomy is not necessary.[2] Maintaining cleanliness of the perineum in the face of burned or surgically grafted tissue can be a challenge for nursing personnel. Recent bowel management systems have assisted with this.

Other Burn Center Patients

Patients with wounds that primarily involve the integumentary system do better in a burn center as the unit is structured with the high levels of necessary resources to care for these patients. These patients include those with toxic epidermal necrolysis syndrome (TENS), staphylococcal scalded skin syndrome, and extensive cases of Stevens-Johnson syndrome. Other referrals include diseases that may result in the loss of large amounts of tissue such as bullous

pemphigoid, pemphigus vulgaris, or necrotizing fasciitis. Some areas of the country also routinely refer patients that suffer significant cold injuries to regional burn centers.[2]

APPROPRIATE DIAGNOSTIC EVALUATIONS

Knowledge of the mechanism of injury is critical to appropriately and efficiently order and prioritize interventions and diagnostic studies. Nonthermal injuries must be considered. Any burn patient who was involved in a violent incident or explosion, or in the event the history is unattainable, should receive the appropriate trauma workup, which may include CT, skeletal x-rays, and diagnostic peritoneal lavage (DPL).

Laboratory Testing

Initial assessment of the burn patient should include a trauma panel of laboratory studies with specific focus on chemistry panel (electrolytes, blood urea nitrogen [BUN], creatinine, lactate), hematology (hematocrit, coagulation studies), arterial blood gas with carboxyhemoglobin, urinalysis, and drug toxicology.

Radiologic Testing

Radiologic studies should be consistent with trauma guidelines. A baseline chest roentgenogram (CXR) allows for initial evaluation and subsequent comparison throughout hospitalization. Patients with electrical injuries should be evaluated because intense tetany can fracture long bones or spinous processes.

Fiberoptic Bronchoscopy

Bronchoscopy should be completed on every burn admission demonstrating a high suspicion of inhalation injury, primarily for the high correlation of inhalation injury to increased mortality. Direct visualization of the pulmonary tissue allows for evaluation of erythema, edema, ulceration, and enlarged vessels, as well as the primary removal of debris through lavage.

Other Diagnostic Interventions

Serial cardiac enzymes and electrocardiogram (ECG) should be completed on any electrical injury patient or on patients with a part history of cardiac disease. Diagnostic peritoneal lavage (DPL) should be completed following protocols for concomitant trauma or index of suspicion with concussive (blast) injuries.

PATIENT TRANSPORT

After initial treatment and stabilization, burn patients should be considered for transfer to a regional burn center for the expertise of a multidisciplinary team. The United States is divided into 10 regions; Canada is treated as a single region. Each region contains at least one tertiary burn center by geographic location, population base, and transport criteria. To be identified as a burn center, the facility must be capable of effectively delivering the specialized care required from acute care to rehabilitation, provide specialized training of personnel, and conduct burn research.[5]

If the patient is going to be transferred within 24 hours of the injury to a regional burn center or to a specialty facility with the ability to provide comparable definitive care, blisters should be left intact and topical agents need not be applied. Agents such as silver sulfadiazine (Silvadene) or mafenide acetate (Sulfamylon) interfere with the ability to maintain visualization of the burn wounds and with successful application of synthetic products (Biobrane or Transcyte) if it is determined that these products are indicated.

For transfer, the patient should be covered with clean, dry sheets. The movement of air over the wounds can be very painful because of the hypersensitivity of exposed nerve endings.[85] Wet dressings, although temporarily soothing to the patient, rapidly lower the patient's body temperature and increase the serious threat of hypothermia because dampened sheets increase the convective temperature loss of the patient's body heat. Dry sheets become moistened as the wounds weep serous fluid and should therefore be covered with blankets in accordance with local transport policies for either air or ground movement. Transport by rotary-wing aircraft is efficient, but decreased environmental control is an inherent problem.[82] Casualties of any significant burn size have lost the primary ability of the skin to regulate body temperature. Ice should never be applied to burn wounds. Analgesics must be considered early in the treatment plan and administered as appropriate.

Partial- and full-thickness burn injuries are contaminated open wounds, and tetanus vaccine should be prophylactically administered consistent with current guidelines. Documentation of administration or deferral is essential to ensuring proper delivery. Before transfer, the patient should remain NPO, insertion of a gastric tube should be considered for gastric decompression, and prophylactic intubation if indicated. For tar burns, after cooling has been ensured, removal is not necessary before transport.

The administration of antibiotics is not indicated in the early burn treatment plan. Antibiotics should be empirically initiated only if the patient demonstrates clinical signs and symptoms of infection. The antibiotic regimen should be modified at the earliest possible opportunity consistent with the organisms identified. The use of steroids is not indicated in the treatment of the burn casualty because of the negative effects these agents have on wound healing.[34]

Early and continued communication, verbal and written, with the regional burn center is paramount to successful transport.

Any temporary biologic or synthetic dressing should be applied within the first 24 hours of the injury to avoid high counts of bacterial colonization; products include allograft (cadaver skin), xenograft (pigskin), Transcyte, or Biobrane (see Table 44-5). These coverings decrease pain, decrease evaporative water losses, and reduce dressing changes.[111]

MONITORING

Hemodynamic Monitoring

Many parameters must be followed closely for early recognition of developing problems. Monitoring should be congruent with the availabilities of the facility in accordance with standards of care. Burn parameters are unique and require healthcare providers' familiarity with these differences. Intervention to physiologic changes will occur within different parameters from those of other trauma or critical care populations.

Despite all of the technologic advances, mean arterial pressure (MAP) remains the most reliable indicator of systemic tissue and organ perfusion. The MAP should be maintained above 60 mm Hg.[34] There is no evidence of effectiveness of a pulmonary artery (PA) catheter or monitoring of central venous pressure (CVP) in the burn resuscitation phase because these may inaccurately reflect the fluid volume status. The use of a PA catheter may lead to over-resuscitation and associated complications and should be restricted to cases of severe inhalation injury, massive fluid resuscitation, significant comorbidities, or requirement of diuretics or vasopressors.[23,34,67]

Arterial lines are not inherently necessary for hemodynamic monitoring in the burn population but are often inserted for the multiple and frequent lab draws for convenience and patient comfort. There may also be difficulty in locating a suitable location for a noninvasive cuff in the severely burned patient; Korotkoff sounds detected with a sphygmomanometer may be progressively moderated with edema, mimicking hypoperfusion. The arterial cannula may also lack complete accuracy with the circulation of increased catecholamine levels, which may trigger severe vasospasm.[67] It must be noted that arterial line insertion or repetitive arterial sticks risks further compromise to peripheral circulation.

Indwelling Urinary Catheter

One of the most critical monitoring devices in this patient population is the indwelling urinary catheter. Hourly monitoring, especially during the burn resuscitation phase, is paramount to the proper treatment of the patient (see Table 44-9). UOP is the most accurate reflection of tissue perfusion and should be followed closely well into the recovery phase. Significant end-organ damage can result from either insufficient fluid resuscitation or over-resuscitation; both are to be avoided.

The technology and availability of the digital urometer have vastly improved and help accurately calculate hourly UOP. Using technologies such as these, research is being done to develop automated programs ("closed loop") that may be able to adjust the intravenous fluid rate based on the hourly UOP and specific hemodynamic parameters.

MECHANICAL VENTILATION

Carboxyhemoglobin

The primary treatment is 100% oxygen. The half-life of carboxyhemoglobin (COHgb) at room air is 250 minutes; at 100% Fio_2 this is dramatically reduced to 45 minutes. Burn patients are at greater risk as the COHgb level rises. Truckers, smokers, or anyone who is routinely exposed to CO will be more tolerant of mild increases in COHgb. Everyone is at severe risk as COHgb exceeds 40% (see Table 44-1); this population needs to be intubated for airway protection and COHgb resolution.[15]

Interventions for Inhalation Injury

Despite advances in burn care, interventions for the patient with inhalation injury do little to alter the disease course.[15] Treatments are supportive, and it is prudent to intubate early, using the same criteria as any trauma patient but with perhaps a lower threshold. Edema can be limited with elevation of the head of the bed and use of aerosolized racemic epinephrine. Frequent tracheal suctioning may be all that is required to avoid atelectasis. Bronchoscopic lavage may be required in more severe cases with large amounts of inhaled particulates, thermally or chemically damaged pulmonary tissue, or obstruction from the physiologic response (protein, cellular debris, white blood cells) to the insult. High-frequency percussive ventilators such as the Volumetric Diffusive Respirator (VDR) have had significant success in the treatment of pulmonary injuries like inhalation injuries or pulmonary contusions by oxygenating at lower peak and mean airway pressures.[18,19] The avoidance of pneumonia is key to reducing mortality, and prevention is increased with high-frequency ventilation.[80] Respiratory compromise can progress in patients with inhalation injury and should be reevaluated frequently.[17]

Tracheostomy may be required in patients with significant production of secretions, endotracheal tube occlusion, or prolonged intubation (typically longer than 21 days) to avoid tissue erosion. The increased internal diameter will assist removal of debris and provide flexibility in weaning from the ventilator. Weaning in this population must be a concerted effort by the healthcare team and is a gradual process with reduction of support as function returns.

INTRAVENOUS FLUID

Lactated Ringer's is the most similar to the body's intravascular volume and is therefore the principal fluid used in the burn resuscitation. It is classified as an isotonic crystalloid volume expander (see Table 44-7). Albumin is also infused in an effort to maintain the intravascular volume. Care must be used when infusing to reduce the risk of the albumin moving into the interstitial space with capillary leakage and potentiating edema with increased interstitial oncotic pressure.

Dextrose 5% in water (D_5W) is infused to replace insensible water loss and to maintain glycogen stores in pediatrics or where enteral nutrition has not yet been initiated.[9] Use of 0.225% NS (¼ NS) intravenously or through enteral flush may be indicated to correct hypernatremia.

During maintenance therapy in some facilities, fresh frozen plasma is the colloid of choice when the albumin is less than 2 g/dl. Others use hypertonic lactated saline (HSL) with sodium at 250 mEq/L, adjusting the rate to maintain an adequate urine output[105] (see Table 44-6). Research studies with HSL have demonstrated a decrease in the total fluid requirements during burn resuscitation and avoidance of associated complications, but with reports as high as 40% to 50% of patients developing the potentially serious hypernatremia (serum Na^+ >160 mEq/L) and hyperosmolarity.[42,105]

The description written by Dr. Pruitt in 1981 remains true:

> The goal of burned patient fluid resuscitation is the maintenance of vital organ functions at the least immediate or delayed physiologic cost. The volume necessary to achieve this end is dependent on injury severity, age, physiologic status, and associated injuries, and the actual volume of fluids used for resuscitation should be modified according to the individual patient's response to the injury and therapy.[75]

Extensive literature compares the use of isotonic crystalloid, colloid, and a combined infusion of crystalloid and colloid without irrefutable conclusion. There remain benefits and drawbacks to all solutions, and the final fluid of choice must be infused judiciously and with suitable monitoring of hemodynamic parameters and electrolyte imbalance.[7,59,93,105]

ANALGESIA

Proper pain control remains one of the primary daily battles in burn care, from acute resuscitation through rehabilitation. Pain associated with burn wounds appears to respond equivalently to either morphine or fentanyl, with advantages and disadvantages for each. Patients respond differently to each, and consideration must be given to mechanism of delivery (intravenous, oral, or sublingual), time of onset, peak, duration of effect, and the intended intervention. Intramuscular or subcutaneous medications should generally be avoided in burn patients because of the systemic stress response and the decreased predictability of absorption; for this reason, only intravenous medications are recommended during resuscitation.

The intubated patient is a prime candidate for manually debriding the wounds while providing sufficient analgesia. Analgesics should typically be given in moderate amounts in 5- to 10-minute intervals during debridement. Additional care is required for the nonintubated patient because the patient may be overwhelmed by the analgesic effect as the painful stimulus of debridement is removed. Conscious sedation should be conducted at the earliest indication that analgesia is insufficient. Oral methadone is often added to the analgesic regimen as an adjunct to provide basal pain relief and thereby potentially reduce the total narcotic amount required for pain control. Propofol (Diprivan) is generally avoided but can be used with the caution of its fat emulsion content and the CO_2 production in its metabolism. Anesthesia services should be consulted in developing and maintaining an effective pain control regimen at all phases of the patient recovery. Nonpharmacologic interventions (imagery, relaxation techniques, music, distraction, etc.) should always be considered and employed when effective.[7]

Pediatric pain control is all the more necessary because children are not able to express their pain as adults do.[86] Children express their pain with behavior such as regression, anger, and tantrums, and the coping mechanisms learned may be necessary for years of recovery.[9] Acetaminophen is commonly used for basal pain control; additional medications are given for the management of procedural or episodes of severe pain.[110]

NUTRITIONAL SUPPORT

The induced stress response and hypermetabolic state increases the caloric needs of the burn patient dramatically in comparison to any other trauma scenario as discussed in the Research Utilization box on p. 1247. Metoclopramide (Reglan) or cisapride (Propulsid) often are administered to increase gastric motility; these may be supplemented with intermittent laxative or enema use[40] or an accepted bowel management system. Curling's ulcer (stress ulcer) is well described in the literature, and prophylaxis against gastric bleeding should be initiated and continued well into the recovery phase. Enteral feeds are the preferred method of delivery because burns do not disrupt the digestive tract directly.[4,40] The risks of parenteral nutrition on morbidity and mortality remain controversial, one of the most serious being catheter-related sepsis[8,32] or translocation of intestinal pathogens.

Practices vary by facility, but it is clear that nutritional support should be initiated at the earliest possible opportunity as indicated in the Nutrition box on p. 1248. A feeding tube should be placed postpyloric early and trophic feeds initiated, observing the patient for tolerance and increasing to the estimated caloric rate, which is calculated using the Harris-Benedict or equivalent formula (Table 44-11).[40] The instilled formula should include a significant fiber content and protein replacement. The interruption of feeds should be minimized. The goal is to maintain intestinal function throughout the burn recovery. Over-resuscitation can have deleterious effects on the bowel and hamper its proper function. If feeds are initiated through a nasogastric tube, it should be replaced with a nasoenteral feeding tube that is of smaller lumen and more pliable.[40]

Pediatric patients with burns greater than 30% TBSA require supplementation of their caloric needs; children with smaller injuries may be able to consume enough calories to sustain their metabolic needs because their wounds close more quickly.[9] Enteral feedings are preferred in pediatrics and may be tolerated as early as 2 hours postburn. Interruption of feedings for any significant period (i.e., operative procedure) should be considered based on the limited endogenous calorie stores.[60]

In a recent study of 103 adult patients with second- and third-degree burns of 10% to 80% TBSA, there was a 32.6% mortality for those patients who received less than 30 kcal/kg/24 hours enterally; in comparison, those who received 30 or more kcal/kg/24 hours had a 5.3% mortality ($p <0.01$). The caloric value of less than 30 kcal/kg/24 hours increased the frequency of pneumonia by 2 times and the frequency of sepsis by 1.8 times ($p <0.05$).[79]

necessary for patient transport by air and for surgical interventions.[17,40]

WOUND CARE

Although specific wound care protocols vary among burn centers and hospitals, all burns resulting in open wounds should be cleansed and dressed. Common cleansing techniques involve a comparable 4% chlorhexidine gluconate (CHG) solution (Hibiclens) and water or povidone-iodine (Betadine) and normal saline (NS). Frequency of wound care ranges from twice per day in the most severe burns to once a week with synthetic dressings in the outpatient setting.[65] Treatment regimen requires the clinician's knowledge of the benefits and limitations of the assorted agents and the use at varying stages of wounds. The development of topical antimicrobial agents in the 1960s and subsequent widespread clinical use has decreased invasive burn wound infections and ensuing fatal sepsis, with significant improvements in clinical outcome.[67,111] Early wound closure with definitive excision and grafting has proven the most beneficial clinical approach.[111]

For burn wound care, silver sulfadiazine cream (Silvadene/SVC), mafenide acetate cream (Sulfamylon/SMC), 0.5% silver nitrate, and bacitracin ointment remain the most commonly used agents.[85] Their employment may be similar to the following: patients who sustain less than 20% TBSA second-degree burns but require inpatient treatment should be cleansed twice a day and covered with silver sulfadiazine cream; burn wounds exceeding 20% TBSA or any third-degree burns should be treated with alternating agents of mafenide acetate cream in the morning and SVC in the evening (SMC penetrates eschar tissue and is described as uncomfortable by patients for 20 to 30 minutes; SVC is described as a more soothing cream in comparison and will be less distracting to the patient's rest[7,52,67]). Application every 12 hours will ensure continuous antimicrobial coverage. Either cream should be applied ⅛ inch thick and reapplied as necessary.[67]

Complete hydrotherapy, although approached differently in each facility, should be completed daily either in the patient's room or at a centralized location to completely remove previously applied agents, observe all wounds, and manually debride wounds. Procedure time should be limited to 20 minutes to avoid chilling and further increase of metabolic demand. Cross-contamination is the largest risk. There is concern that localized infection may be transposed to other burn wounds. For this reason, patient immersion in Hubbard tanks has become less common and portable shower trolleys with disposable covers are more widely used.[7,23]

◆ RESEARCH UTILIZATION

Hypermetabolic Response to Severe Burn Injury

CLINICAL ISSUE

The hypermetabolic response to severe burn injury causes a significant systemic stress response, which includes prolonged stimulation of the autonomic nervous system and subsequent alteration in immune response and increases in metabolic activity, hydrolysis of fats, and protein catabolism. It is hypothesized that aggressive burn wound intervention (early excision) and enteral feeding can markedly decrease the metabolic demands, reduce healing time, and positively influence outcome.

SUMMARY

This study enrolled 46 burned children into an analytic study, segregating according to time of burn to transfer to the burn facility for excision, grafting, and nutritional support. The subjects were excluded if they had previously undergone wound excision or received continuous nutritional support before transfer. The outcome variables measured were resting energy expenditure (REE), skeletal muscle protein kinetics, the quantitative cultures for degree of bacterial colonization, and burn sepsis incidence. It was found that the energy expenditure was not significantly reduced with the early, aggressive treatment (excision); however, early excision did markedly diminish muscle protein catabolism. The early treatment group also diminished the wound colonization and incidence of sepsis.

APPLICATION

Although early excision was not found to significantly reduce REE in this study, the benefits observed with protein catabolism, wound colonization, and sepsis indicate that this is a positive course of action in the treatment of severe burn patients. It is important for clinicians to be aware that this and similar studies may be limited in their scope and require implementation in a facility where this hospital course is supported.

NEED FOR FURTHER STUDY

Future studies are needed to increase the study size, replicate the results, and to study the effects in the adult burn population.

Hart, D. W., et al. (2003). Effects of early excision and aggressive enteral feeding on hypermetabolism, catabolism, and sepsis after severe burn. *J Trauma, 54*(4), 755–764.

Gastric Tube. Patients are at risk of gastric ileus development when deep burns cover more than 20% of the body surface area. A gastric tube reduces this risk and the risk of emesis or aspiration. It is also

◆ NUTRITION

Nutrition Considerations for the Critically Ill Burn Patient

CALORIES

The caloric requirement for any patient is dependent on the body size and metabolic requirements. Body size is calculated by the body surface area (BSA) using the Dubois equation, one of the simplified equations, or a nomogram. The basal metabolic rate (BMR) is the estimated baseline requirement (Fleisch equation) for any individual and is a factor of gender and age. The basal metabolic rate (BMR) (Table 44-11) is influenced by the body activity (activity factor) and stressors.

The key components considered for the activity factor are if confined to bed, ambulatory, or in a hyperthermic (fever) state. External stressors can be factored in the event of surgery, infection, burn injury (further divided by total body surface area burn size), ventilated, skin breakdown (decubitus), trauma, sepsis, and radiation therapy or chemotherapy.

Open wounds <20% TBSA: the body energy expenditure (Harris-Benedict formula), multiplied by the activity factor, and multiplied by the injury factor.

Open wounds ≥20% TBSA: the US Army Institute of Surgical Research (USAISR) equation is used for burns or other injuries with >20% TBSA open wounds to calculate estimated energy requirements (EER).

The hypermetabolic response and the subsequent increased caloric needs may remain elevated well beyond the acute phase and possibly after discharge from the hospital. Burn wound closure is the primary step to decreasing the caloric requirements of the patient.

PROTEIN

Protein needs also depend on the metabolic requirements and stressors of the body.

Open wounds <20% TBSA: 1.2–1.5 g/kg
Open wounds ≥20% TBSA: 1.5–2.5 g/kg proportional to burn size

NITROGEN

Nitrogen (N_2) is measured to evaluate whether the metabolic needs of the patient are being met.

+2 to +4 g N_2 indicates anabolism (desired)
−2 to +2 g N_2 indicates balance
<−2 g N_2 indicates catabolism

FLUID

The fluid requirements for the burn patient change as the patient proceeds through the phases of treatment and recovery. Closure of the burn wounds, either with synthetic skin products or definitively with surgical excision and grafting, is the key factor in reduction of fluid replacement needs. Lactated Ringer's (LR) most closely resembles the intravascular fluid and is the consensus fluid to meet the acute resuscitation needs of the burn patient. Dextrose 5% in water (D_5W) is also administered to provide for the glucose requirements of the patient and replacement of the insensible water lost through open wounds and respiration.

ELECTROLYTES

The intravascular electrolyte levels require close monitoring in the burn patient; all should be maintained within normal parameters. Electrolyte levels in burn patients are sensitive, and intervention should occur early because movement of electrolyte levels toward either extreme of normal limits may rapidly progress to critical values.

Sodium and chloride levels are treated primarily through titration of D_5W, ¼ normal saline (NS) (0.45% sodium chloride), or infusion of gastric flushes with either 0.9% NS (0.9% sodium chloride) or free H_2O.

Potassium and calcium should be replaced as indicated either intravenously or through the gastric system.

Maintenance of glucose levels as near to normal parameters as possible throughout hospitalization is consistent with decreased mortality levels.

VITAMINS AND MINERALS

Multivitamin and mineral supplements should be infused in the same manner as any trauma patient.

SPECIAL CONSIDERATIONS

Open wounds <20% TBSA: Fluid resuscitation and diet can be initiated enterally and switched to parenteral if complications develop or if the patient is unable to keep up with the required resuscitation. Intake should focus on high-protein, high-calorie supplements as needed for the healing process.

Open wounds ≥20% TBSA: Fluid resuscitation should be initiated intravenously and titrated to patient response. Nutritional supplements should be started as early as indicated and infused consistent with facility protocols; this may be via a gastric tube into the stomach or small-bore feeding tube—postpyloric infusion decreases the risk of aspiration. Burn injuries do not directly interfere with the function of the gut and should not prevent its utilization unless contraindicated. Total parenteral nutrition (TPN) is to be avoided.

TABLE 44-11 Nutritional Assessment Formulas

Desired body weight (DBW)	Male: 106 lb for first 5 feet, 6 lb for each additional inch Female: 100 lb for first 5 feet, 5 lb for each additional inch
	If %DBW is <125%, use actual weight for calculations If %DBW is >125%, calculate adjusted body weight (ABW): ABW = (actual wt − DBW) × (25%) + DBW
Body surface area (BSA)	$\dfrac{Ht\ (cm) \times Wt\ (kg)}{3600}$ or $\dfrac{Ht\ (in) \times Wt\ (lb)}{3131}$
	Dubois equation (1916): BSA (m^2) = (Wt in kg$^{0.425}$) × (Ht in cm$^{0.725}$) × 0.007184
Basal metabolic rate (BMR)	Fleisch equation (1951): Male: 54.337821 − (1.19961 × age) + (0.02548 × age^2) − (0.00018 × age^3) Female: 54.74942 − (1.54884 × age) + (0.03580 × age^2) − (0.00026 × age^3)
Harris-Benedict formula	Male: [(65.5) + (13.7) × (Wt in kg) + (5) × (Ht in cm) − (6.7 × age in yr)] × (AF) × (IF) Female: [(655.1) + (9.6) × (Wt in kg) + (1.8) × (Ht in cm) − (4.7 × age in yr)] × (AF) × (IF)
USAISR equation	EER = [BMR × (0.89142 + [0.01335 × TBSA])] × BSA × 24 × AF
	Protein requirement estimate: <20% TBSA: 1.2–1.5 g/kg ≥20% TBSA: 1.5–2.5 g/kg proportional to burn size
	Nitrogen (N$_2$) balance: +2 to +4 g N$_2$ indicates anabolism (desired) −2 to +2 g N$_2$ indicates balance <−2 g N$_2$ indicates catabolism
Waxman equation (N$_2$ loss estimate)	PBD 1–3: g N$_2$ = (0.3) × (BSA) × (%TBSA) PBD 4–16: g N$_2$ = (0.1) × (BSA) × (%TBSA) PBD >16: g N$_2$ = (0.1) × (BSA) × (actual %TBSA open)

Activity Factor		Injury Factor			
Confined to bed	1.2	Surgery	1.1–1.2	Burn Injury	
Ambulatory	1.3	Infection	1.2–1.6	<20%	1.2–1.4
Fever	1.13 for each° C >37° C	Trauma	1.4–1.8	20%–25%	1.6
		Sepsis	1.4–1.8	25%–30%	1.7
		Ventilator	1.3	30%–35%	1.8
		Skin breakdown	1.3–1.5	35%–40%	1.9
		Radiation therapy	1.6	40%–45%	2.0
		or chemotherapy		>45%	2.1

Data from references 16, 25, 38, 54, 58, 106.
AF = Activity factor, EER = estimated energy requirement, IF = injury factor, PBD = post-burn day, TBSA = total body surface [burned],
USAISR = U.S. Army Institute of Surgical Research.

Topical Antimicrobial Therapy

Silver Sulfadiazine. Silver sulfadiazine is a 1% suspension synthesized from silver nitrate and sodium sulfadiazine as a burn cream. It is painless with its topical application and does not cause staining of the tissue, primarily because of its limited solubility in water and thus limited penetration of eschar.[67,85] SVC is a broad-spectrum antimicrobial agent with bactericidal action against many gram-negative and gram-positive organisms,[85] primarily *Staphylococcus aureus, Escherichia coli, Klebsiella* sp., *Pseudomonas,* Enterobacteriaceae, proteus, and *Candida.* Care should be used in that this product is a sulfa derivative.

Adverse Effects. Subsequent to the application of Silvadene, the burn patient may demonstrate a transient leukopenia that cannot be associated with any other source. This often develops 2 to 3 days after the initiation of therapy.[23,85] There is a rare occurrence of acute hemolytic anemia in patients with glucose-6-phosphate dehydrogenase (G6PD) deficiency. Other rare complications associated with this medication are agranulocytosis, erythema multiforme, interstitial nephritis, and skin necrosis.

Mafenide Acetate. Mafenide acetate is a broad-spectrum antibacterial with bacteriostatic coverage against many gram-negative and gram-positive organisms similar to Silvadene.[85] It is nonstaining and indicated in the treatment of partial- and full-thickness burn wounds and their infections. Patients report a burning sensation with application thought to be associated with the medication's water solubility and rapid ability to penetrate eschar tissue.[67] Sulfamylon covers the following organisms: *Candida albicans*, Enterobacteriaceae, enterococci, *E. coli*, *Klebsiella* sp., *Citrobacter* sp., *Pseudomonas aeruginosa*, *Serratia* sp., *S. aureus*, and beta-hemolytic streptococci. This product is also a sulfa derivative.

Sulfamylon is also supplied in a powder form. Each packet contains 50 g of sterile mafenide acetate that is reconstituted in one liter of 0.9% sodium chloride irrigation or sterile water for irrigation, creating a 5% Sulfamylon solution (SMS). The 5% topical solution is most often used postexcision as a moistened dressing over meshed autograft tissue to provide antimicrobial coverage. It also can be used on burn wounds to promote the separation of eschar tissue.

Adverse Effects. Pain or discomfort may last 20 to 30 minutes after application.[67] Similar to Silvadene there is a rare occurrence of acute hemolytic anemia with disseminated intravascular coagulation in patients with G6PD deficiency. Other rare complications include metabolic acidosis, blood dyscrasias, pulmonary function impairment, or renal function impairment.

Silver Nitrate. Patients who demonstrate a hypersensitivity reaction to silver sulfadiazine or mafenide acetate, or general sensitivity to sulfa drugs, may be treated with 0.5% silver nitrate dressings.[67,85] This is maintained as a wet-to-wet dressing; the dressing must remain moistened at all times to prevent cytotoxic levels from forming if the silver nitrate becomes concentrated.[7,67] It is not effective in treating burn wound infection because it does not penetrate eschar, but it is the common treatment for patients with toxic epidermal necrolysis syndrome (TENS) because of its topical antimicrobial prophylaxis.[67]

Adverse Effects. Silver nitrate solution stains the tissue and all surfaces with which it comes into extended contact. Care must be exercised when using this solution on the patient and near healthcare members. It should never be applied near the eye because permanent scleral staining may occur. The patient's skin is typically stained for several months after its use is terminated until epidermal replacement occurs.

Methemoglobinemia is a rare but serious development with the use of silver nitrate.[85] Anticipate the transeschar leaching of sodium, potassium, chloride, and calcium and replace electrolytes as appropriate.[67]

Acticoat. The use of Acticoat has risen in recent years. It is a nonadherent burn wound dressing (urethane film) with nanocrystalline elemental silver impregnated into an absorbent middle layer. The silver has both bactericidal and fungicidal properties. Moisture, either from the wound exudate or from sterile water applied intermittently, sustains the release of silver. This dressing is intended for partial-thickness wounds and is used by some for TENS patients or donor site coverage. As with silver nitrate, the silver does not penetrate the eschar and is not effective against invasive burn wound infection. Unlike silver nitrate, it does not leach electrolytes because the silver does not precipitate from the dressing into the wound bed. The dressing should be observed daily and changed every 3 days or as needed.[67,85,97]

Primary Approaches to Wound Care

There are two primary approaches to wound care in burn centers: the exposure technique and the closed technique.

Exposure Technique. In the exposure technique, burn wounds are dressed with antimicrobial creams and left open with the thought that the wounds can be more routinely observed for potential complications. The wounds are more readily accessible for monitoring and intervention; there are no dressings present to impede range of motion or circulation. Agents are completely reapplied twice per day and intermittently as needed. Additional care must be observed with any proximity to the burn wounds secondary to the decreased barriers to the environment, such as increased diligence with infection control standards, control of ambient temperature and avoidance of air currents, and protection of pressure points. Bacterial growth is not enhanced as it is under dressings. This technique is used with severe burns in critical care units when the patient is mostly confined to the bed and there are sufficient partitions between the patients or separate rooms. It is also routinely used for wounds of the face, head, and hands.[23,85]

Closed Technique. The closed technique maintains all wounds covered with dressings that are opened only for cleansing, manual debridement or intervention, and reapplication of topical ointments. Topical agents are applied and then covered with gauze or nonadherent dressings. The closed technique is indicated when the patient leaves the unit for a procedure or gets out of bed for any reason. The closed technique is used on wards, when the patient is active or away from an isolated environment, or when the burn patient cannot be effectively separated from others. There is less risk of cross-contamination, decreased pain, and less heat loss with protection from the environment, and it reduces the need to reapply the creams throughout the day. There is the increased potential for bacterial growth beneath the dressings if they are not changed twice daily. The wound is less readily accessible and will take more time for dressing changes. The peripheral circulation must be checked intermittently for impairment.[23,85]

Neither approach has been found to have any significant difference in rates of infection. Any application can create an immersion syndrome and should be evaluated for potential maceration of underlying tissue. With any dressing that requires moistening, vigilance must be maintained to lightly dampen and avoid saturation. With either technique, all postexcision wounds are covered with appropriate dressings to increase adherence of grafts and decrease the risk of infection. Autograft is the ideal covering of excised tissue, but it may not be readily available[111] (see Table 44-5).

Bacitracin and bacitracin ophthalmic ointment should be applied to burn wounds of the face and around the eyes, respectively. SVC may be applied to severe facial burns but should be limited to inferior to the cheekbones to avoid contact with the eyes. Dressings can be cut into a facial mask and moistened with 5% SMS.

Surgical Excision and Grafting

Partial-thickness burns of less than 40% TBSA may be covered with synthetic products such as Biobrane or Transcyte (see Table 44-5) and allowed to heal spontaneously on an outpatient basis after brief observation. These products also may be used on patients with other dermatologic diseases processes, as with toxic epidermal necrolysis syndrome (TENS).

Full-thickness burns may be covered with allograft (tissue from another human donor or cadaver; also called homograft) or Integra until donor sites are available or until cultured cells can be produced. The conclusive intervention for wounds that are not expected to heal within 3 weeks postburn, deep partial-thickness burns of any significant size (>40% TBSA burned), and any full-thickness burns remains surgical excision and autograft. Awaiting spontaneous healing through conservative management usually entails painful dressing changes for prolonged periods, resulting in hypertrophic scarring and contractures that lead to poor functional and cosmetic outcome[110]; this practice is limited to older adult patients and in cases in which anesthesia and surgery are contraindicated.[111] Early surgical intervention is preferred after the resuscitation phase, when the patient is hemodynamically stabilized, with the goal to excise the majority of burned tissue in the first week postburn. This approach has decreased mortality

from the incidence of burn wound infection (subeschar sepsis).[67,111] Early wound closure decreases caloric and fluid replacement requirements, speeds the healing process, and decreases hospital length of stay.

Burn tissue is excised tangentially, removing the eschar to viable dermis or fat to the depth at which punctate bleeding is achieved (Figure 44-17).[67] The goal is to leave subcutaneous tissue intact whenever possible because of its cosmetic and protective properties. If vascularity is not encountered while excising through the dermal layers, the subcutaneous tissue must be removed to the level of fascia before the donor tissue is placed.[111] The wound bed must be meticulously cleansed before placement of the donor tissue, or the graft will be nonadherent.

Nonemergent surgical excision places significant demands on a body already under stress. The operative team must have identifiable end points before beginning the procedure; general practice guidelines vary among institutions, but some of the common points for ending surgical intervention include excision that produces blood loss equal to the patient's volume, 4 hours of operative time, worsening acidosis or base deficit in excess of -10 mmol/L, hypothermia unresponsive to increases in operative suite temperature, hypotension with repeated doses of vasopressors or initiation of continuous infusion, or excision of 20% to 40% TBSA.

Donor tissue of 0.008 to 0.012 inch thick is removed with a dermatome. The tissue may be "pie-crusted" and placed as a sheet graft on an area requiring thickness or cosmesis, such as the dorsum of the hands or the face. Tissue to cover more excised body surface area is meshed, typically expanded from 1½:1 to 4:1 and as wide as 9:1.[67] Mesh tissue is passed through a skin-meshing instrument that makes small incisions at regular intervals, allowing the tissue to cover a larger body surface area (Figure 44-18). Meshed tissue may be covered with cadaver skin, fresh or frozen, for additional protection while adherence and vascularization of the graft occur. Meshed tissue prevents the accumulation of material (e.g., blood, serum, purulent material) beneath the graft but decreases the cosmetic outcome and contributes to scar formation.[52] The

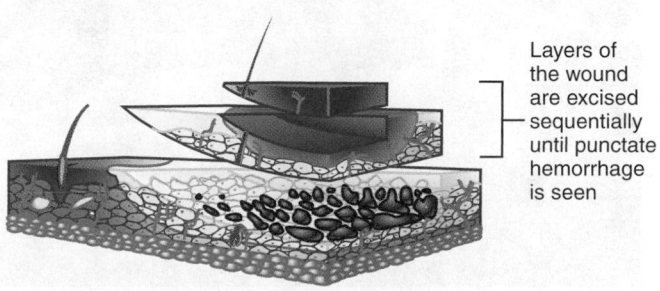

Layers of the wound are excised sequentially until punctate hemorrhage is seen

⬧FIGURE 44-17 Excision of burn wound.

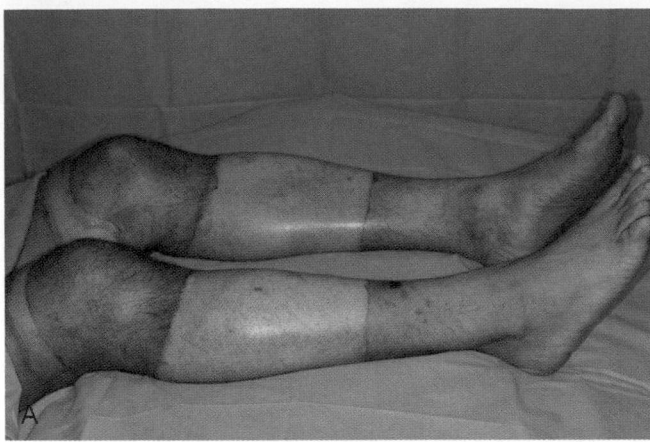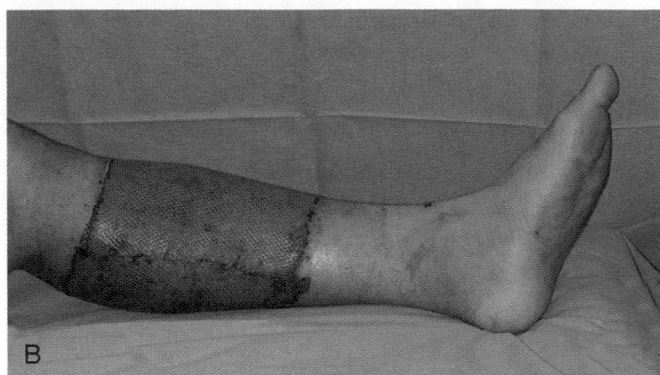

✦FIGURE 44-18   A, Leg burn wound before excision and grafting. **B,** Autograft mesh.

meshed openings are referred to as interstices and are observed daily after day 7 to determine when the skin is "closed." Once interstices have filled in, a topical moisturizing cream is applied to the graft sites.

Donor-site care varies widely from the use of xeroform gauze, to Scarlet Red, to coverage with Acticoat, among others.[85] Donor sites increase the open tissue by creating a partial-thickness wound for the patient and are extremely painful. Whatever the technique, the goal is for the rapid healing of the donor site with a minimization of scarring and to have the site ready for reharvesting at the earliest possible time if needed. The donor site should be elevated, if possible, when in contact with the bed surface. The goal is to decrease the moisture at the site. Heat lamps may be used to assist this process.[52]

In the massively burned patient, the current or future availability of donor sites to obtain autograft tissue can be extremely limited. A growing option is the coverage of burn wounds with cultured autologous keratinocytes—more facilities now provide the service. A cell sample is collected from the patient and sent to be grown into a tissue covering constructed of the patient's own cells. Time is still a limitation because a cell sample requires 3 or more weeks to be grown into an autograft that is only six or eight epidermal cells thick and very fragile.[67] A benefit is that if enough can be grown, the entire burn surface can be covered in one operative setting, a more attainable goal in the pediatric setting.[9] Skeletal traction can then be used after the application of cultured epidermal autograft to protect the tissue from even minimal shear forces (Figure 44-19).

Vacuum-Assisted Closure

The vacuum-assisted closure (VAC) device has provided dramatic changes in postoperative wound care. The VAC device increases adherence of the graft through controlled levels of negative pressure, and the sponge demonstrates a safe and effective method to protect the tissue from shearing forces; research has been associated with improved graft survival as measured by a reduction in number of repeated skin grafts.[87] Operative techniques range from small wound coverage to entire extremities. The VAC is also widely used in promoting granulation over exposed tendons before attempting to place an autograft.

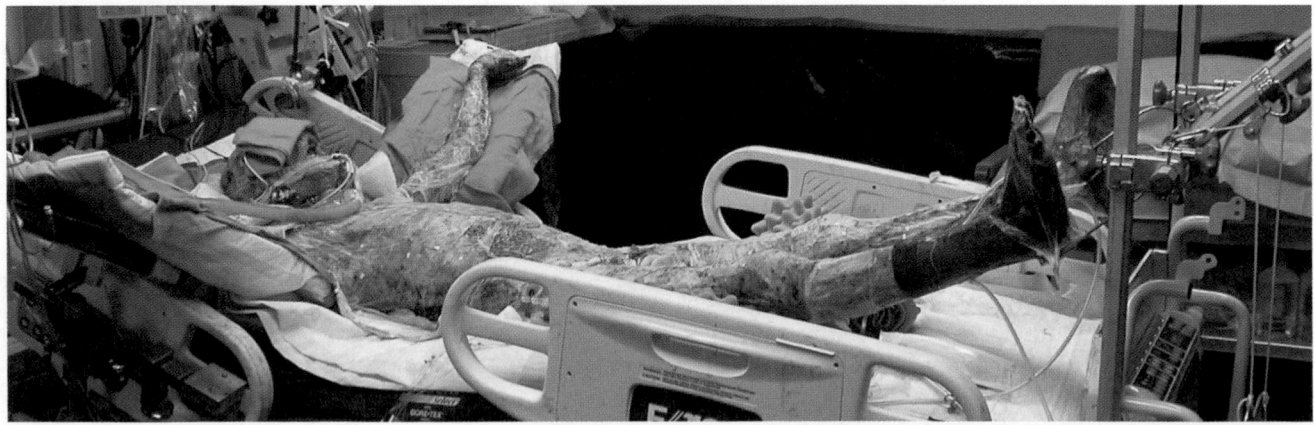

✦FIGURE 44-19 Patient with massive burn.

MULTIDISCIPLINARY PLAN OF CARE FOR THE BURN PATIENT

PROBLEM	INTERVENTION	RATIONALE	EXPECTED OUTCOME
Gas Exchange, Impaired	Assess carefully patients who present with: • Inhalation injury • Advanced age • Preexisting respiratory insufficiency	Early identification of patients allows for appropriate prophylactic intervention, especially in preparation for diagnostic testing or surgery.	Patients at risk for Impaired Gas Exchange are identified early.
	Elevate head of the bed to semi-Fowler's position at all times.	Decreased risk of pneumonia or ventilator-associated pneumonia, aspiration, and airway edema. Position to facilitate optimal breathing patterns.	Has no obvious congestion. Has normal respiratory pattern for the patient. Arterial blood gases (ABGs) within acceptable limits.
	Increase activity as tolerated.	To facilitate diaphragmatic excursion and support respiratory muscle function.	Maintain normal respiratory rate for the patient.
	Provide respiratory interventions as indicated, such as: • Cough and deep breathe • Incentive spirometry • Suction • Bronchodilators	Decreased risk of atelectasis or pneumonia and maintenance of airways for adequate oxygenation.	Absence of diminished breath sounds.
Airway Clearance, Ineffective	Assess ventilation and oxygenation as indicated, with careful consideration of patients who present with: • Inhalation injury • Extremes of age (very young or very old)	Patient with inhalation injury may obstruct airway rapidly, with increased risk during fluid resuscitation, or patients presenting with stridor or hoarseness.	Patients at risk for airway obstruction are identified and treated early.
Fluid Volume Deficit	Assess for signs/symptoms: • Inadequate urinary output • Tachycardia inconsistent with hypermetabolism • Decreased tissue perfusion • Decreased mentation	Burn patient will demonstrate plasma volume loss proportional to burn size and depth of wounds.	Burn wound progression and end-organ damage are minimized through proper fluid resuscitation.

Table continues on page 1254

PROBLEM	INTERVENTION	RATIONALE	EXPECTED OUTCOME
	Serial lab values with focus on: • Hematocrit/hemoglobin (Hct/Hgb) • Sodium • Chloride • Blood urea nitrogen (BUN) • Specific gravity	Adequate fluid resuscitation should be reflected with appropriate hemodilution and subsequent normalization throughout hospitalization.	Lab values within expected parameters.
Fluid Volume Excess	Assess for signs of compartment syndrome by: • Monitoring tissue for suppleness • Checking compartment pressure if firm to palpation • Decreasing fluid infusion if urine output above upper limits • Trending daily weights	Decreased tissue perfusion may result in burn wound progression, increased tissue loss, and decreased functional outcome.	Compartment pressures will remain within normal values to facilitate tissue perfusion.
Infection, Risk	Monitor for early indicators of infection: • Erythema • Foul-smelling wounds or drainage • Urinary sediment • Hyperthermia (>102.5° F) • Abnormal white blood cell (WBC) values	Early identification of patients allows for appropriate prophylactic intervention or treatment consistent with organism/source identified, especially in preparation for diagnostic testing or surgery.	Remain without infection or demonstrate recovery from infection.
	Appropriate healthcare interventions: • Good hand washing techniques • Visitors and healthcare workers with active infection avoid contact with patient • Minimize invasive procedures • Increased diligence with aseptic/sterile techniques with interventions • High-protein/high-carbohydrate foods/fluids	Prevention is the primary treatment in the patient who is already compromised.	

PROBLEM	INTERVENTION	RATIONALE	EXPECTED OUTCOME
	Protect wounds with appropriate antimicrobial coverage or skin coverage.	Disruption of integumentary barrier (impaired skin integrity) increases infection risk exponentially.	
Physical Mobility, Impaired	Increase mobility/activity as tolerated, passively and actively. Consult occupational or physical therapist as indicated.	Decrease the risk of skin breakdown with movement, maintain or increase muscle mass to reduce debilitation, and increase respiratory effort.	Maintain functional level at highest possible level.
	Reduce constriction and barriers to movement wherever indicated.	Allow for optimal circulation/tissue perfusion and assist passive and active ROM for best functional outcome.	
	Position in proper body alignment and reposition PRN.	Patient will move to position of comfort that may be contrary for best functional outcome.	
Imbalanced Nutrition: Less Than Body Requirements	Consult nutrition care early and throughout hospitalization for: • Calculation of requirements, accounting for hypermetabolic burn response and additional stressors • Appropriate patient education of dietary intake based on the healing process	Hypermetabolic response and surgical interventions greatly increase nutritional needs for a prolonged period. Caloric intake must be from appropriate sources (mixture of proteins, fats, etc.) for the individual while accounting for the phase of healing.	Patient receives appropriate dietary intake to meet nutritional needs orally whenever possible or with feeding tubes when necessary.
	Daily weight to allow for trends using same scale and with same equipment, linens, etc.	Trends in body weight are a reflection of intake and output over time.	
	When possible, accurate calculation of body fat.	Important to account for current weight while factoring changes in lean muscle mass of body fat percentage.	
Pain	Continuous analgesic relief when indicated, with appropriate dosing before expected painful intervention. Offer analgesics routinely.	Appropriate analgesia assists with patient's active participation and decreases the anxiety with expected and recurrent interventions.	Patient's pain is minimized to the lowest possible degree and interventions stopped when analgesia not controlled as evidenced by autonomic responses to acute pain.

Table continues on page 1256

PROBLEM	INTERVENTION	RATIONALE	EXPECTED OUTCOME
	Assess patient's level of pain before, during, and after any intervention either verbally or through monitoring of autonomic responses.	Patient's trust must be maintained with interventions. Success is increased with active and willing participation in the healing process.	Patient's response is minimized with: • Scale of 0 to 10 for pain severity • Increased blood pressure, pulse, respirations • Diaphoresis • Dilated pupils • Guarding • Facial mask of pain • Crying/moaning • Abdominal heaviness • Cutaneous irritation
	Maximize nonpharmacologic methods for reducing pain and promoting comfort: • Back rubs or comforting touch • Slow rhythmic breathing • Repositioning • Diversional activities such as music, TV, etc.		Patient develops techniques to potentiate analgesics when administered and for coping skills throughout hospital course and after discharge.
Disturbed Body Image	Address concerns with body image with the patient and family based on the ability of the participants. Involve external support systems whenever indicated such as: • Family (traditional or nontraditional) • Behavioral health team • Pastoral care • Burn survivor support groups	Recovery from burn wounds requires the active participation of the survivor and his or her support system. Acceptance is gradual and may take a prolonged period.	Patient continues to progress to acceptance of physical appearance and resultant functional limitations.

IDENTIFICATION OF TARGETED/ EXPECTED OUTCOMES

The physical and mental condition of the patient prior to the injury will greatly affect the outcome. Suicidal attempt through burning often results in the patient's demise because the patient refuses to participate in the recovery process or rehabilitation. The most optimal recovery of every burn patient requires the active participation of the entire healthcare team and, most important, the patient's belief in his or her survival and return to the highest level of function possible.

The three major risk factors for mortality with a burn injury have consistently been burn size, inhalation injury, and age. Although there has been little advance in reducing mortality in the presence of inhalation injury, the survivability of severe burns has increased. Age greatly contributes to a patient's ability to overcome the insult of a burn injury. The most accurate rule of thumb for predicting mortality after severe burn injury is still the Baux score (age + percent burn = mortality). This is variable because older adults have a significantly increased level of mortality in relation to the burn size based on their comorbidities and their reduced regenerative abilities.[20,107] The very young have higher regenerative ability but a less-developed stress response (see Figures 35-1 and 44-15). Many predictors have been studied, but the Baux score, the Edlich burn score, and the Zawacki score are highly correlated with patient outcome and length of stay using logistic regression techniques. On retrospective review, these scores more accurately predicted outcomes for burn patients with burns than did the Trauma Score–Injury Severity Score or the Glasgow Coma Scale score.[51] Indicators such as burn size, age, male sex, length of ICU stay, and the presence of mechanical ventilation have been linked to poorer outcome in another study; similarly, base deficit greater than −6 mmol/L during resuscitation has predicted far higher incidence of multiple organ dysfunction and death.[20]

The primary goal of burn care is to return the patient to the highest level of function possible. This requires every aspect of the burn healthcare team to be utilized, as shown in the Multidisciplinary Plan of Care on pp. 1253-1256. As the patient enters and leaves each phase, the focus of the burn care changes. Rehabilitative services must be actively engaged from admission to discharge to posthospitalization follow-up. Passive and active range of motion reduce edema, maintain motion, and should be initiated at the earliest possible time and continued routinely.[34] Extremities must be elevated to decrease edema and splinted or situated in a functional position. The hands require the most extensive care.

Case Study 44-1, Part C

Wound Care and Pain Management After Grafting

T.W. is taken to the operating room on postburn day 3 for a full excision and grafting (E&G). Estimates are that every burn patient will require one surgical procedure for every 10% TBSA burned. The donor sites are the areas of bilateral thighs not burned, and bilateral calves and are covered with xeroform gauze. The arms, right thigh, and posterior torso are covered with 3:1 autograft and wrapped with veil dressing and 5% Sulfamylon solution (SMS)–moistened gauze. The posterior torso is bolstered to protect from shearing forces. The dressings are moistened every 6 hours and whenever necessary to avoid tissue desiccation. To maximize donor tissue the anterior torso is excised and covered with Integra to close the wounds. The dorsum of the hands is covered with split-thickness sheet graft and left open; Integra is placed on the palms. The hands are splinted in a position of function. The sheet graft is observed hourly for the first 24 hours postop; blebs (subgraft fluid accumulation) are rolled to ensure graft take. After this, small hematomas are aspirated via tuberculin syringe. Donor sites are elevated on leg nets to expose to air. Heat lamps are applied at low setting to assist with drying.

T.W. is weaned from the ventilator postoperatively and extubated the morning of postburn day 4. Aggressive pulmonary toileting is initiated to reduce the risk of pneumonia. He is started on vancomycin for burn wound cellulitis; this is stopped after 5 days when resolved. T.W. is assisted to the bedside chair on postop day 4 (postburn day 7), and diet is advanced as tolerated. He is assisted to the standing table on postop day 8 (postburn day 11). Enteral feeds are changed to night feeds only when T.W. is tolerating 50% of his daily caloric needs orally and stopped when tolerating 75%. He is transitioned to oral doses of pain medication, receiving Percocet two tablets 30 to 60 minutes before any intervention. He begins ambulating on postop day 10 and is transferred to the ward. He receives Actiq 400 mcg transmucosally before rehabilitation exercises and slowly begins to increase his range of motion with recurrent intervention.

T.W. returns to the operating room on four more occasions for additional E&G procedures and to cover the Integra when donor sites are ready for reharvesting. His wounds are healing with minimal graft loss and without difficulty. On postburn day 53, T.W. is discharged to home with compression garments, returning daily to outpatient rehabilitation for continued strengthening and stretching of contracted tissue.

Decision point: What are the signs and symptoms of graft failure?

Decision point: What is the best way and when is the best time to initiate nutritional support for this patient?

Decision point: How should this patient's ongoing pain be managed?

Once the resuscitative and reparative phases are complete, rehabilitation becomes the primary focus. Proper caloric intake remains essential to continued burn wound healing, respiratory proficiency, and muscular rejuvenation. As hypermetabolism resolves, diet requires adjustment to meet the changing needs. This phase may last months for patients who have survived severe and debilitating burn injuries. The patient must be transitioned to function as an outpatient.

Rehabilitative services have made dramatic progress in keeping pace with the survival of the most severe burn wounds. Contractures and scar formation are largely preventable but are dependent on many factors. The patient assumes a position of comfort. Improper splinting or positioning even overnight can cause significant regression in the patient's care.[63] The patient must remain motivated and an active participant in the burn recovery plan. Rehabilitation may suffer numerous setbacks because additional surgical interventions or reconstructive procedures are required. Compression garments and facemasks must be checked for proper fit and wear frequently and may be required for 12 to 18 months. A common complaint of burn survivors is itching and the skin's sensitivity to the environment, particularly hot and cold. Recovering tissue needs to be protected from direct sunlight, and a mild nonirritating lotion may help keep skin lubricated.

CONCLUSIONS

Burn care is the ultimate expression of multidisciplinary care, and it was one of the first specialties to adopt a comprehensive multidisciplinary approach. Burn patients require the spectrum of intervention not only from specialized equipment but also all facets of the healthcare team, including nursing, burn surgeons, occupational and physical therapy, respiratory therapy, operating room staff, psychiatric and behavioral health services, dietary, social work services, and burn survivor groups.[34] The burn patient, the patient's family, and the entire healthcare team are invested physically as well as emotionally. A burn survival is not an acute event but a dynamic healing process that can last a lifetime.

REFERENCES

1. Agency for Toxic Substances and Disease Registry. (1997). *Tox-FAQ for white phosphorus.* Available at www.atsdr.cdc.gov/tfacts103.html.
2. American Burn Association. (2005). *Advanced burn life support course.* Chicago: Author.
3. American Burn Association. *Burn incidence and treatment in the US: 2000 fact sheet.* Available at http://ameriburn.org/pub/BurnIncidenceFactSheet.htm.
4. American Burn Association. (2001). Practice guidelines for burn care. *J Burn Care Rehabil,* Suppl, 1S–69S.
5. American College of Surgeons Committee on Trauma. (1999). Guidelines for the operation of burn units. In *Resources for optimal care of the injured patient.* Chicago: ACS.
6. Anatomical Chart Company. (2001). *Atlas of pathophysiology.* Springhouse, Pa, p. 361.
7. Appleby, T. (2004). Burns. In P. G. Morton, et al. (Eds.), *Critical care nursing: a holistic approach* (8th ed.). Philadelphia: Lippincott Williams & Wilkins.
8. Beghetto, M. G., et al. (2005). Parenteral nutrition as a risk factor for central venous catheter-related infection. *J Parenter Enteral Nutr, 29*(5), 367–373.
9. Benjamin, D., & Herndon, D. N. (2002). Special considerations of age: the pediatric burned patient. In D. N. Herndon (Ed.), *Total burn care* (2nd ed.). Philadelphia: Saunders.
10. Bickley, L. S., & Szilagyi, P. G. (2003). In L. S. Bickley, et al. (Eds.), *Bates' guide to physical examination and history taking* (8th ed.). Philadelphia: Lippincott Williams & Wilkins.
11. *Biobrane: temporary wound dressing.* Available at www.bertek.com/pdfs/biobrane.pdf.
12. Black, T. L., & Miller, J. P. (2005). Burns. In M. R. Dambro (Ed.), *Griffith's 5-minute clinical consult* (13th ed.). Philadelphia: Lippincott Williams & Wilkins.
13. Blaisdell, F. W. (2002). The pathophysiology of skeletal muscle ischemia and the reperfusion syndrome: a review. *Cardiovasc Surg, 10*(6), 620–630.
14. Bozeman, W. P., Myers, R. A., & Barish, R. A. (1997). Confirmation of the pulse oximetry gap in carbon monoxide poisoning. *Ann Emerg Med, 30,* 608.
15. Cancio, L. C., & Pruitt, B. A. (2002). Inhalation injury. In G. C. Tsokos & J. L. Atkins (Eds.), *Combat medicine: basic and clinical research in military, trauma, and emergency medicine.* Totowa, N.J.: Humana Press Inc.
16. Carlson, D. E., et al. (1991). Resting energy expenditure in patients with thermal injuries. *Surg Gynecol Obstet, 174,* 270–276.
17. Cheeseman, M. M, & Boozer, H. L. (2004). Burns and smoke inhalation. In C. K. Stone & R. Humphries (Eds.), *Current emergency diagnosis & treatment* (5th ed.). Norwalk, CT: Appleton & Lange.
18. Cioffi, W. G., & Rue, L. W. (1991). Diagnosis and treatment of inhalation injuries. *Crit Care Nurs Clin North Am, 3*(2), 191–198.
19. Cioffi, W. G., et al. (1991). Prophylactic use of high-frequency percussive ventilation in patients with inhalation injury. *Ann Surg, 213*(6), 575–580.
20. Cohen, R., & Moelleken, B. R. W. (2005). Disorders due to physical agents. In L. M. Tierney, M. A. Papadakis, & S. J. McPhee (Eds.), *Current medical diagnosis & treatment* (44th ed.). New York: McGraw-Hill.
21. Corcos, A. C., & Sherman, H. F. (2001). Percutaneous treatment of secondary abdominal compartment syndrome. *J Trauma, 51*(6), 1062–1064.
22. Davenport, J. (2005). Anatomy and physiology of the integumentary system. In P. G. Morton, et al. (Eds.), *Critical care nursing: a holistic approach* (8th ed.). Philadelphia: Lippincott Williams & Wilkins.
23. Demling, R. H. (2003). Burns & other thermal injuries. In L. W. Way (Ed.), *Current surgical diagnosis & treatment* (11th ed.). Norwalk, CT: Appleton and Lange.
24. Demling, R. H., DeSanti, L., & Orgill, D.P. *Evolution of burn wound care.* Available at www.burnsurgery.org/Betaweb/Modules/skinsubstitutes/sec2.htm.
25. Dickerson, R. N. (2002). Estimating energy and protein requirement of thermally injured patients: art or science? *Nutrition, 18,* 439–442.

26. Dimick, A. R., & Wagner, R. G. (1999). Burns. In G. R. Schwartz (Ed.), *Principles and practice of emergency medicine* (4th ed.). Baltimore: Williams & Wilkins.

27. Fish, R. M. (2004). Electrical injuries. In J. E. Tintinalli, G. D. Kelen, & J. S. Stapcznski (Eds.), *Emergency medicine: a comprehensive study guide* (6th ed.). New York: McGraw-Hill.

28. Fish, R. M. (2000). Electric injury: part II Specific injuries-changing concepts and taxonomy. *J Emerg Med*, *18*(1), 27–34.

29. Fish, R. M. (2004). Lightning injuries. In J. E. Tintinalli, G. D. Kele, & J. S. Stapcznski (Eds.), *Emergency medicine: a comprehensive study guide* (6th ed.). New York: McGraw-Hill.

30. Fitzpatrick, J. C., & Cioffi, W. G. (2002). Diagnosis and treatment of inhalation injury. In D. N. Herndon (Ed.), *Total burn care* (2nd ed.). Philadelphia: Saunders.

31. Flynn, M. B. (2002). Burn injuries. In K. A. McQuillan, et al. (Eds.), *Trauma nursing: from resuscitation through rehabilitation*. Philadelphia: Saunders.

32. Fuhrman, M. P. (1998). Management of complications of parenteral nutrition. In L. E. Matareseand & M. M. Gottschlich (Eds.), *Contemporary nutrition support practice: a clinical guide*. Philadelphia: Saunders.

33. Gentilello, L. M., et al. (1997). Is hypothermia in the victim of major trauma protective or harmful? A randomized, prospective study. *Ann Surg*, *226*(4), 439–447.

34. Gibran, N. S., & Hiembach, D. M. (2005). Management of the patient with thermal injuries. In D. W. Wilmoreet, et al. (Ed.), *ACS surgery: principles and practice*. New York: WebMD.

35. Gore, D. C., et al. (2001). Association of hyperglycemia with increased mortality after severe burn injury. *J Trauma*, *51*, 540–544.

36. Greenhalgh, D. G., & Warden, G. D. (1994). The importance of intra-abdominal pressure measurements in burned children. *J Trauma*, *36*, 685–690.

37. Harchelroad, Jr, F. P., & Rottinghaus, D. M. (2004). Chemical burns. In J. E. Tintinalliz, G. D. Kelen & J. S. Stapcznski (Eds.), *Emergency medicine: a comprehensive study guide* (6th ed.). New York: McGraw-Hill.

38. Hart, D. W., et al. (2002). Energy expenditure and caloric balance after burn: increased feeding leads to fat rather than lean mass accretion. *Ann Surg*, *235*(1), 152–161.

39. Helmenstine, A. M. *Chemical weapons and warfare agents*. Available at http://chemistry.about.com/cs/chemicalweapons/a/aa040303a.htm.

40. Hensell, D. O., & DeClement, F. (2001). Burns. In P. N. Lanken (Ed.), *The intensive care unit manual*. Philadelphia: Saunders.

41. Hobson, K. G., Young, K. M., & Ciraulo, A. (2002). Release of abdominal compartment syndrome improves survival in patients with burn injury. *J Trauma*, *53*(6), 1129–1133; discussion 1133–1134.

42. Huang, P. P., et al. (1995). Hypertonic sodium resuscitation is associated with renal failure and death. *Ann Surg*, *221*, 543–554.

43. Huether, S. E. (2002). Structure, functions, and disorders of the integument. In K. L. McCance & S. W. Huether (Eds.), *Pathophysiology: the biologic basis for disease in adults & children* (4th ed.). St. Louis: Mosby.

44. Hunt, J. L., & Purdue, G. F. (2002). Prevention of burn injuries. In D. N. Herndon (Ed.), *Total burn care* (2nd ed.). Philadelphia: Saunders.

45. Ivy, M. E., et al. (2000). Intra-abdominal hypertension and abdominal compartment syndrome in burn patients. *J Trauma*, *49*, 387–391.

46. Ivy, M. E., et al. (1999). Abdominal compartment syndrome in patients with burns. *J Burn Care Rehabil*, *20*, 351–353.

47. Jelenko, C. (1974). Chemicals that "burn." *J Trauma*, *14*, 65–72.

48. Kochanek, K. D., et al. (2004). Deaths: final data for 2002. *Natl Vital Stat Rep*, *53*(5), 1–116.

49. Koumbourlis, A. C. (2002). Electrical injuries. *Crit Care Med*, *30* (Suppl), S424.

50. Kramer, G. C., Lund, T., & Herndon, D. N. (2002). Pathophysiology of burn shock and burn edema. In D. N. Herndon (Ed.), *Total burn care* (2nd ed.). Philadelphia: Saunders.

51. Krob, M. J., D'Amico, F. J., & Ross, D. L. (1991). Do trauma scores accurately predict outcomes for patients with burns? *J Burn Care Rehabil*, *12*(6), 560–563.

52. LaBorde, P. J. (2004). Management of patients with burn injury. In S. C. Smeltzer & B. G. Bare (Eds.), *Brunner & Suddarth's textbook of medical-surgical nursing* (10th ed.). Philadelphia: Lippincott Williams & Wilkins.

53. Latenser, B. A., et al. (2002). A pilot study comparing percutaneous decompression with decompressive laparotomy for acute abdominal compartment syndrome in thermal injury. *J Burn Care Rehabil*, *23*(3), 190–195.

54. Lefton, J. (2003). Specialized nutrition support for the adult burn patients. *Support Line*, *25*(4), 19–25.

55. Lund, C., & Browder, N. (1944). The estimation of areas of burns. *Surg Gynecol Obstet*, *79*, 352–358.

56. Luterman, A., & Curreri, P. (1990). Chemical burn injury. In M. Jurkiewcz, T. Krizek, & S. Mathes (Eds.), *Plastic surgery: principles and practice*. St. Louis: Mosby.

57. Majno, G. (1973). *The healing hand Cambridge*. Cambridge, Mass: Harvard University Press.

58. Manelli, J. C., et al. (1998). A reference standard for plasma proteins is required for nutritional assessment of adult burn patients. *Burns*, *24*, 337–345.

59. Martin, G. S. (2005). *An update on intravenous fluids*. Available at: www.medscape.com/viewarticle/503138.

60. McDonald, W. S., Sharp, C. W., & Deitch, E. A. (1991). Immediate enteral feeding in burn patients is safe and effective. *Ann Surg*, *213*, 177–183.

61. The Merck Veterinary Manual. (2006). Crystalloids. In C. M. Kahn (Ed.). Available at www.merckvetmanual.com/mvm/index.jsp?cfile=htm/bc/160406.htm. Merck & Co, Inc.

62. Mitka, M. (2005). Meth lab fires put heat on burn centers. *JAMA*, *294*(16), 2009–2010.

63. Mlakar, J. M., & Dougherty, W. R. (2002). Reconstruction of the burned hand. In D. N. Herndon (Ed.), *Total burn care* (2nd ed.). Philadelphia: Saunders.

64. Mlcak, R. P., & Buffalo, M. C. (2002). Pre-hospital management, transportation, and emergency care. In D. N. Herndon (Ed.), *Total burn care* (2nd ed.). Philadelphia: Saunders.

65. Morgan, E. D., Bledsoe, S. C., & Barker, J. (2001). Ambulatory management of burns. *Amer Fam Phys*, *32*(9), 2015–2036.

66. Moritz, A. R., & Herriques Jr, F. C. (1947). Studies of thermal injuries: the relative importance of time and surface temperature in the causation of cutaneous burns. *Am J Pathol*, *23*, 695–720.

67. Mozingo, D. W., Cioffi, W. G., & Pruitt, Jr., B. A. (2003). Burns. In F. S. Bongard & D. Y. Sue (Eds.), *Current critical care diagnosis & treatment* (2nd ed.). New York: McGraw-Hill.

68. Muehlberger, T., Spies, M., & Vogt, P. M. (2002). Electrical injury: reconstructive problems. In D. N. Herndon (Ed.), *Total burn care* (2nd ed.). Philadelphia: Saunders.

69. Namias, N. (2003). Burn management. In R. S. Irwin & J. M. Rippe (Eds.), *Irwin and Rippe's intensive care medicine* (5th ed.). Philadelphia: Lippincott Williams & Wilkins.

70. Oda, J., et al. (2006). Resuscitation fluid volume and abdominal compartment syndrome in patients with major burns. *Burns*, *32* (2), 151–154.

71. Osborn, K. (2003). Nursing burn injuries. *Nurs Manage*, *34*(5), 49–56.

72. Paula, R. (2005). Compartment syndrome, abdominal. In J. Li, et al. (Eds.), *eMedicine*. Available online at www.emedicine.com/emerg/topic935.htm.

73. Peralta, R., & Hojman, H. (2001). Abdominal compartment syndrome. *Int Anesth Clin*, *39*(1), 75–94.

74. Price, D. P., Silverman, H., & Schwartz, G. R. (1999). Smoke inhalation. In G. R. Schwartz (Ed.), *Principles and practice of emergency medicine* (4th ed.). Baltimore: Williams & Wilkins.

75. Pruitt, B. A. (1981). Fluid resuscitation for the extensively burned patient. *J Trauma, 21,* S690–S692.

76. Pruitt, B. A., Goodwin, C. W., & Mason, Jr, A. D. (2002). Epidemiologic, demographic, and outcome characteristics of burn injury. In D. N. Herndon (Ed.), *Total burn care* (2nd ed.). New York: Saunders.

77. Purdue, G. F., & Hunt, J. L. (2002). Electrical injuries. In D. N. Herndon (Ed.), *Total burn care* (2nd ed.). New York: Saunders.

78. Remensnyder, J. P., & Donelan, M. B. (2002). Reconstruction of the head and neck. In D. N. Herndon (Ed.), *Total burn care* (2nd ed.). New York: Saunders.

79. Rimdeika, R. (2006). The effectiveness of caloric value of enteral nutrition in patients with major burns. *Burns, 32*(1), 83–86.

80. Rue, L. W., et al. (1993). Improved survival of burned patients with inhalation injury. *Arch Surg, 128,* 772–778.

81. Saffle, J. R. (2006). Telemedicine for acute burn treatment: the time has come. *J Telemed Telecare, 12*(1), 1–3.

82. Saffle, J. R., Edelman, L., & Morris, S. E. (2004). Regional air transport of burn patients: a case for telemedicine? *J Trauma, 57*(1), 57–64.

83. Sanford, A. P., & Herndon, D. N. (2002). Chemical burns. In D. N. Herndon (Ed.), *Total burn care* (2nd ed.). New York: Saunders.

84. Santos, A. P., et al. (2005). Methamphetamine laboratory explosions: a new and emerging burn injury. *J Burn Care Rehabil, 26* (3), 228–232.

85. Schallom, L. (2002). Burns. In L. D. Urden, K. M. Stacy, & M. E. Lough (Eds.), *Thelan's critical care nursing diagnosis and management* (4th ed.). St. Louis: Mosby.

86. Schecter, N., Allen, D. A., & Hanson, K. (1986). Status of pediatric pain control: a comparison of hospital analgesic usage in children and adults. *Pediatrics, 77,* 11–15.

87. Scherer, L. A., et al. (2002). The vacuum assisted closure device: a method of securing skin grafts and improving graft survival. *Arch Surg, 137*(8), 930–934.

88. Schwartz, G. R. (1999). The poisoned patient: overview. In G. R. Schwartz (Ed.), *Principles and practice of emergency medicine* (4th ed.). Baltimore: Williams & Wilkins.

89. Schwartz, L. R., & Balakrishnan, C. (2004). Thermal burns. In J. E. Tintinalli, G. D. Kelen, & J. S. Stapcznski (Eds.), *Emergency medicine: a comprehensive study guide* (6th ed.). New York: McGraw-Hill.

90. Sheridan, R. L. (2002). Burns. *Crit Care Med, 30*(11), S500–S514.

91. Shirani, K. Z., Pruitt, B. A., & Mason, A. D. (1987). The influence of inhalation injury and pneumonia on burn mortality. *Ann Surg, 205*(1), 82–87.

92. Smith, D. L., et al. (1994). Effect of inhalation injury, burn size, and age on mortality: a study of 1447 consecutive burn patients. *J Trauma, 37,* 655–659.

93. Sutcliffe, A. J. (April 8, 2001). *Fluid loading in the burn patient.* Available online at www.euroanesthesia.org/education/rc_gothenburg/13rc1.HTML.

94. Thomas, S., Barrow, R. E., & Herndon, D. N. (2002). History of the treatment of burns. In D. N. Herndon (Ed.), *Total burn care* (2nd ed.). New York: Saunders.

95. Traber, D. L., Herndon, D. N., & Soejima, K. (2002). The pathophysiology of inhalation injury. In D. N. Herndon (Ed.), *Total burn care* (2nd ed.). New York: Saunders.

96. Transcyte: Human fibroblast derived temporary skin substitute. Available at http://wound.smith-nephew.com/us/node.asp?NodeId=957.

97. Tredget, E. E., et al. (1998). A matched-pair, randomized study evaluating the efficacy and safety of Acticoat silver-coated dressing for the treatment of burn wounds. *J Burn Care Rehabil, 19,* 531.

98. University of Maryland Medical Center. (2004). *Inhalation injuries.* www.umm.edu/outdoor/inhalation_injuries.htm.

99. U.S. Army Office of the Surgeon General. History of chemical warfare and current threat. Available at www.nbc-Med.org/SiteContent/MedRef/OnlineRef/FieldManuals/medman/History.htm.

100. van den Berghe, G., et al. (2001). Intensive insulin therapy in the critically ill patients. *N Engl J Med, 345,* 1359.

101. Van Meter, K. W. (2004). Carbon monoxide poisoning. In J. E. Tintinalli, G. D. Kelen, & J. S. Stapcznski (Eds.), *Emergency medicine: a comprehensive study guide* (6th ed.). New York: McGraw-Hill.

102. Wagoner, M. D. (1997). Chemical injuries of the eye: current concepts in pathophysiology and therapy. *Surv Ophthalmol, 41,* 275–313.

103. Wallace, S., Goodman, S., & Smith, D. G. (2004). Compartment syndrome, lower extremity. In T. A. AmbroseII, et al. (Eds.), *eMedicine.* Available online at www.emedicine.com/orthoped/topic596.htm.

104. Wang, H. E., et al. (2005). Admission hypothermia and outcome after major trauma. *Crit Care Med, 33*(6), 1296–1301.

105. Warden, G. D. (2002). Fluid resuscitation and early management. In D. N. Herndon (Ed.), *Total burn care* (2nd ed.). New York: Saunders.

106. Waxman, K., et al. (1987). Protein loss across burn wounds. *J Trauma, 27*(2), 136–140.

107. Wibbenmeyer, L. A., et al. (2001). Predicting survival in an elderly burn patient population. *Burns, 27*(6), 583–590.

108. Wiebelhaus, P., & Hansen, S. L. (2001). Managing burn emergencies. *Nurs Manage, 32*(7), 29–36.

109. Williams, G. W. (2002). The pathophysiology of the burn wound. In D. N. Herndon (Ed.), *Total burn care* (2nd ed.). New York: Saunders.

110. Wolf, S. E., & Herndon, D. N. (1999). *Burn care.* Georgetown, Tex: Landes Bioscience.

111. Wolf, S. E., & Herndon, D. N. (2004). Burns and radiation injuries. In K. L. Mattox, D. V. Feliciano, & E. E. Moore (Eds.), *Trauma* (4th ed.). New York: McGraw-Hill.

CHAPTER 45

Mass-Casualty Competencies

Michael L. Schlicher*

Preparedness for mass-casualty incidents (MCIs) has taken on a new prominence in the United States since the terrorist events of September 11, 2001, and the massive destructive forces of Hurricanes Katrina and Rita in 2005. These events and other subsequent large-scale disasters have caused hospitals and providers around the world to shift their focus from preparing for the foreseeable to planning for the previously unforeseeable. Frequent training, simulations, and educational programs dealing with mass casualties have become necessary requirements to ensure preparedness for MCIs.[11] Critical care nurses are among those most essential in managing the consequences of any mass-casualty incident.

As hospitals and communities continue to develop mass-casualty response plans, critical care nurses must maintain prehospital readiness efforts and must precisely define the role of the advanced critical care clinician as a vital link in the entire mass-casualty process. The American Association of Critical-Care Nurses (AACN) fully recognizes the importance of critical care nurses in regard to the aftermath of any mass casualty and is dedicated to providing up-to-date, comprehensive education on mass casualties and terrorist attacks. The aim of this chapter is to provide an overview of mass-casualty preparedness for the critical care nurse to consider (Box 45-1).

By definition, MCIs are characterized by the destructive effects of natural or man-made forces producing a sudden influx of casualties large enough to disrupt a community's ability to properly allocate existing resources and provide adequate healthcare services.[3,26,27] Natural disasters (e.g., floods, earthquakes, hurricanes, and tornadoes) occur with striking regularity. More frightening, however, is the growing destructive character of man-made disasters (e.g., chemical explosions, nuclear meltdowns, and acts of terrorism). Terrorists in particular are now more willing and able to use weapons of mass destruction (WMD) against civilian targets. These deliberate attacks of aggression are likely to produce mass casualties that will stress and potentially overwhelm a community's medical infrastructure. MCIs have the horrific potential to cause vast numbers of human deaths and suffering, permanently transforming the character of an affected community.

Recent examples of MCIs include the following: Hurricanes Katrina and Rita of 2005; the 2005 Pakistani earthquake; the terrorist bombing of the London underground system in 2005; the devastating 2004 Indian Ocean tsunami; the destructive terrorist attacks of 2001 on the World Trade Towers in New York and the Pentagon in Washington, DC; the 1995 bombing of the Murrah Federal Building in Oklahoma City; and the 1995 sarin nerve agent attack in Tokyo. In all of these instances, critical care nurses were called upon to use critical thinking skills, provide advanced nursing care, alleviate suffering, allocate "limited" medical resources, and help bring order to an otherwise chaotic environment.

Inadvertently, these events also helped to reinforce the fact that overall hospital capacity, staffing, and critical care unit bed capacity are all major limiting factors associated with mass casualties and effective care.[17] For example, within a few hours of the Madrid bombing explosions in March 2004, 27 critically ill patients were admitted to the 2 closest hospitals, which had a maximum critical care capacity of 28 beds, most of which were already occupied.[13] After the 2002 terrorist bombing in Bali, victims were flown to the nearest Level 1 trauma center in Australia, with a capacity to care for a maximum of 12 ventilated patients. Air rescue arrived at the hospital with 20 critically ill patients, 15 of whom required mechanical ventilation.[23] Flooding caused by heavy rains in June 2001 crippled the Texas Medical Center in Houston and resulted in a sudden 75% loss of critical care bed capacity for a county consisting of more than 4 million residents.[22]

---

*The views expressed in this chapter are those of the author and do not reflect the official policy or position of the Department of the Army, the Department of Defense, or the U.S. Government.

Box 45-1

AACN Key Facts: Mass Casualties

KEY FACTS

- Bioterrorism and the potential result of mass casualties is a significant public health threat facing the United States. The nation's capacity to respond to this threat depends in part on the ability of healthcare professionals and public health officials to rapidly and effectively detect, manage, and communicate during an event resulting in mass casualties.
- Nurses represent the largest group of healthcare providers. Critical care nurses will be called upon to respond to mass-casualty situations. Education, training, and credentialing will be required in order to ensure nurses can skillfully care for victims of a terrorist attack.
- The value of preparedness and particularly bioterrorism education has recently been recognized. There is an urgent need to identify scientifically based resources for education and training of nurses and other healthcare professionals to be able to respond to a bioterrorism attack as well as radiation and chemical events. Awareness of the symptoms these agents produce, the routes of transmission, and the types of treatment required are important areas of knowledge that must be acquired.
- New federal legislation has been enacted to provide funding for training healthcare professionals to prepare for and respond to bioterrorism. The Public Health Security and Bioterrorism Response Act of 2002, signed into law during the Bush administration, authorized the spending of $4.3 billion to improve public health preparedness, enhance controls on deadly biological agents, and protect the nation's food, medication, and drinking water supplies.

From reference 3. Used with permission.

Case Study 45-1, Part A

The Mass-Casualty Incident

Seaside Community Hospital serves a population of about 3000 in a mid-size southeastern city. Seaside Community Hospital has an emergency department (ED) that sees about 20 patients daily, and has an 8-bed critical care unit and a 4-suite operating room. There is also a medical-surgical floor that contains 30 beds. Seaside is the only hospital this size that is available for 100 miles. The city is at risk for a number of environmental hazards as there is a chemical plant nearby where chlorine is produced. Because the city is located on the Atlantic coast, it is also at risk for hurricanes. As a critical care nurse of 15 years, J.S. arrives at work for a 12-hour shift along with three other nurses. It is a Friday evening at around 8:00 PM when she is notified that there has been a major explosion at the chemical plant and approximately 40 workers have been injured, several of whom are burned and others who are having a hard time breathing since chlorine was the agent involved. J.S. learns that patients will be arriving within the next 30 minutes.

Before hanging up the phone, J.S. questions who will be in charge of the MCI, if the rest of the hospital has been notified, and if any additional staff are being mobilized. As charge nurse, J.S. immediately surveys the unit and notifies the rest of her staff. Together, they quickly review the unit's MCI guidelines. J.S. understands that they will need as many open beds as possible, so she calls the charge nurse on the medical-surgical floor and requests that she send any additional staff to critical care to help transfer two of their patients who are not on ventilators as quickly as possible. Next, J.S. calls the pharmacy to request that additional pain medication be available since they are expecting several burn patients, and then she notifies respiratory support to have additional ventilators also available. Hospital administration was able to get three additional staff nurses to help out in critical care so the staff quickly orients the new nurses while making sure each room has additional burn supplies. While awaiting patients, J.S. reviews the following pages of the unit's MCI policy manual to make sure they are prepared and have not overlooked anything important.

Thirty-five minutes after initially being notified, J.S. learns that the ED has received five patients, all of whom have 50% total body surface area third-degree burns. The ED manager requests help from critical care. J.S. realizes that in order to maintain command and control of the unit she should not leave the unit at this time. Instead, she sends two critical care nurses who have worked in the ED before and has the additional staff nurses assume care of the current patients in the unit. J.S. explains to the nurses that they will each assume care of one patient in the ED and will follow that patient back to critical care when transfer is possible.

J.S. receives word that four of the burned patients are being transferred from the ED. She has one nurse for each patient. Knowing that the additional stress and long hours of an MCI can quickly lead to burnout, J.S. wonders if they will be able to maintain adequate manpower to handle the additional demands. The nurse manager and the hospital administrator on-call arrive on the unit.

Three nurses stayed to work double shifts. In addition to the nurses already scheduled to work, four more off-duty nurses came in to work double shifts, supporting unit staffing for another 16 hours. The nurse manager was present to handle phone calls, coordinate supply issues, and cover brief rest breaks for the nurses. Two attending physicians arrived to help the on-duty physician admit and stabilize the new patients; they were able to leave after 8 hours when the pace became manageable. Food from community restaurants was brought for staff and waiting family members. Other than the shortage of ventilators and burn dressings, supplies for providing patient care were not scarce because elective activities were canceled until the disaster needs were under control.

Decision point: In addition to the staff sent to help the critical care unit and ED, what are other sources of "reserve staff" that could help throughout the hospital as well as in the critical care area?

Decision point: What other community resources can be used during an MCI?

Decision point: What psychosocial stressors will be placed on the nurses who are working during this disaster?

Decision point: How might communications be supported, both to the general public and within the hospital?

Case continues on page 1269

Critical care bed capacity is not the only resource overwhelmed during an MCI. Damage to the physical and organizational structure of a healthcare institution may wipe out the entire patient care infrastructure. Victims of MCIs may include healthcare workers, limiting available critical care and other personnel. This was the case during the severe acute respiratory syndrome outbreak in Canada and Asia.[16] Viewed in the context of the everyday strain on currently available resources, the challenge to provide safe and adequate care becomes even greater.

Terrorist incidents are inherently more complex and add the emotional elements of anger and fear to an already complicated situation. Few critical care nurses have had much practical experience with mass-casualty emergencies. Therefore organization and preparation assume even greater importance for mass-casualty emergencies following terrorist acts.

The critical care component of many mass-casualty response plans is often incomplete. For example, many response plans fail to recognize the potential need to expand critical care beds and to add more staff. The fact is, until recently, mass-casualty training received very little attention.[21] Several studies have documented that the vast majority of hospitals are unprepared for a mass casualty secondary to a terrorist incident involving

WMD.[18,20] An analysis of the capacity of a 1200-bed hospital in the United States to handle patients in the setting of a toxic chemical exposure event revealed an ability to handle only 2 chemically contaminated patients at a time.[19] Equally important, routinely available critical care resources are almost always insufficient to respond to disasters that generate anything beyond a modest casualty stream.

AACN released a *Statement of Commitment to Mass Casualty and Bioterrorism Preparedness* recognizing that critical care nurses will be called on to respond to disaster/mass-casualty situations.[3] The statement includes the following: "Bioterrorism and the potential of mass casualties is a significant public health threat facing the United States. The nation's capacity to respond to this threat depends in part on the ability of the healthcare professionals and public health officials to rapidly and effectively detect, manage, and communicate during an event resulting in mass casualties. Critical care nurses maintain a diverse knowledge base, demonstrate astute assessment skills, and hold a strong commitment to public safety and service." These characteristics speak eloquently of the need for critical care nurses in any mass-casualty setting (Table 45-1). This topic is explored in the Research Utilization box on pp. 1264-1265.

TABLE 45-1 Disaster Type, Primary Casualty, and Expected Nursing Care*

DISASTER TYPE	PRIMARY CASUALTY	TYPE OF CRITICAL CARE NURSING REQUIRED
Armed conflict	Trauma/diseases	Burn/respiratory/trauma/surgical
Collapse of structures	Trauma/suffocation	Burn/respiratory/trauma/surgical
Earthquake	Trauma/burns	Respiratory/burn/surgical/trauma/medical

Table continues on page 1264

Table 45-1 Disaster Type, Primary Casualty, and Expected Nursing Care*—cont'd

DISASTER TYPE	PRIMARY CASUALTY	TYPE OF CRITICAL CARE NURSING REQUIRED
Fire	Burns/trauma	Burn/respiratory/trauma/surgical
Floods	Drowning/trauma/disease	Respiratory/medical/surgical/trauma
Industrial explosion	Blast injury/trauma/burns	Burn/respiratory/trauma/surgical
Landslide	Trauma/suffocation	Respiratory/trauma/surgical
Mass event	Trauma	Burn/respiratory/trauma/surgical
Terrorist attack	Blast injury/trauma/burns/diseases	Burn/respiratory/trauma/surgical
Tidal surge/hurricane	Drowning/trauma	Respiratory/medical/surgical/trauma
Transportation accident	Trauma/burns	Burn/respiratory/trauma/surgical
Volcanic eruption	Trauma/burns/respiratory	Burn/respiratory/trauma/surgical

Data from reference 8.
*Note that regardless of the type of disaster, all will require critical care nursing as a major component of care.

♦ RESEARCH UTILIZATION

Training of Hospital Staff to Respond to a Mass-Casualty Incident

CLINICAL ISSUES

Hospital disaster preparedness has taken on increased importance at local, state, and federal levels. Hospitals themselves are taking renewed interest in disaster preparedness, reexamining their disaster plans, and conducting disaster exercises. Preparing for a mass-casualty incident (MCI) is a daunting task, as unique issues must be considered with each type of event. For example, the systemic stress of a biothreat is entirely different from that of a chemical disaster or any other acute-onset disaster. These differences hold challenging implications for preparedness training.

Hospitals must play a key role in developing disaster preparedness plans, and they need to coordinate efforts with public health systems and appropriate governmental agencies. The Joint Commission (TJC) requires hospitals to test their emergency plan twice a year, including at least one community-wide drill. However, it is not known whether this type of training is effective.

The following key questions were addressed:
- What is the effectiveness of hospital disaster drills in training hospital staff to respond to an MCI?
- What is the effectiveness of computer simulations in training hospital staff to respond to an MCI?
- What is the effectiveness of tabletop or other exercises in training hospital staff to respond to an MCI?

- What methods or tools have been used to evaluate the effectiveness of hospital disaster drills, computer simulations, and tabletop exercises or other exercises in training hospital staff to respond to an MCI?

SUMMARY

Studies also varied in terms of targeted staff, learning objectives, identified outcomes, and evaluation methods. Because of the wide range of foci for the studies, it was difficult to draw definitive conclusions about the most effective approaches for training hospital staff to respond to an MCI.

APPLICATION

Some potentially valuable points could be identified in the literature:
- Internal and external communications were the key to an effective disaster response.
- A well-defined incident command center reduced confusion.
- Conference calls were an inefficient way to manage disaster response.
- Accurate phone numbers for key players were vital and regular updating was necessary.
- Disaster drills appeared to be an effective way to improve clinicians' knowledge of hospital disaster procedures.

- Computer simulation may be an economical method to educate key hospital decision makers and improve hospital disaster preparedness before implementation of a full-scale drill.
- A tabletop exercise can help to motivate hospital staff to learn more about disaster preparedness and can help to teach staff about aspects of disaster-related patient care in a way that simulates the practice setting.
- A regional exercise involving top government officials can help to increase awareness of the need for better disaster response planning.
- Video demonstrations may be an inexpensive, convenient way to educate a large number of staff about disaster procedures and equipment use in a short time.

NEED FOR FURTHER STUDY

The studies demonstrated that different types of training exercises may have different roles to play in educating hospital staff in disaster response. However, the evidence was insufficient to support firm conclusions about the effectiveness of specific training methods because of the marked heterogeneity of studies, weaknesses in study design, and the limited number of exercises that have been reported in the literature. Future disaster preparedness efforts would benefit from increased reporting of hospitals' experiences in disaster response training.

Hsu, E. B., et al. (April 2004). *Training of hospital staff to respond to a mass casualty incident.* Summary, Evidence Report/Technology Assessment: Number 95. AHRQ Publication Number 04-E015-1. Rockville, Md: Agency for Healthcare Research and Quality. Available at www.ahrq. gov.offcampus.lib.washington.edu/clinic/epcsums/hospmcisum.htm.

The potential roles of critical care nurses in an MCI may vary extensively because of diverse educational backgrounds, experiences, and practice settings within the community and healthcare system. These roles may include identifying when an MCI has occurred, responding to a call to go to the scene of an incident, working at a local hospital in the critical care unit, working in an emergency field hospital where victims are being treated, or relieving nurses who were initially involved in these activities.

Every critical care nurse should have sufficient knowledge and skills to recognize the potential for an MCI, identify when such an event may have occurred, know how to protect oneself, know how to provide immediate care for those individuals involved, recognize their own role and limitations, and know where to seek additional information and resources. Several studies have shown that nurses and other providers who plan, become better educated, and practice mass-casualty drills are more flexible and effective in providing improved patient outcomes.[7,14,26]

MASS-CASUALTY PREPARATION

The critical care nurse should begin mass-casualty preparation with a basic knowledge of specific disaster characteristics, the primary hazard or casualty expected, and the potential nursing care that might be required. Table 45-1 gives a quick overview of the overwhelming need for critical care nurses during any MCI. Knowing what patient types might be expected would help in overall planning, preparation, and organization.

TRIAGE AND DECONTAMINATION

The word *triage* is derived from the French verb *trier*, which literally means "to sort."[26] While the concept of triage is well known and recognized, the tangible act of triage is often difficult to demonstrate. The most commonly used system of triage involves sorting individual casualties into one of four categories according to the severity of injury and the need for immediate care: immediate, delayed, minimal, or expectant.

It should be apparent that there are no absolute criteria by which casualties are sorted into each individual category. Rather, the triage provider triages casualties based upon the available resources as well as the number of casualties anticipated.

In today's environment, patients are brought to the hospital and tremendous resources and manpower are applied to maximize survival. Conversely, during an MCI, the needs of the population as a whole must outweigh the needs of the individual. An MCI requires a change in mindset such that the greatest good is achieved for the greatest number of victims, rather than each individual casualty. Effective triage, therefore, requires advance preparation and planning, as well as education and training in basic mass-casualty principles.

Triage is performed most often by first responders (Figure 45-1). However, it also occurs within care settings (e.g., hospitals and alternative care sites), where individual victims may present for care independent of organized responses. Secondary triage may also be necessary within a facility (e.g., critical care unit) as demands on a system grow.[1]

Triaging during any MCI will not be an easy task. There are many associated challenges to be considered

CATEGORIZATION OF INJURY FOR TRIAGE

Group	Definition	Color	Examples of possible injuries
Immediate	Casualties who have life-threatening critical injuries that must be treated immediately	Red	• Upper-airway obstruction • Tension pneumothorax • Pelvic fracture
Delayed	Casualties who will require medical or surgical intervention but whose injuries are not life threatening	Yellow	• Fractures requiring operative reduction • Soft-tissue injury • Concussion
Minimal	Casualties who are not critically injured; injuries minor; self-care; little medical attention	Green	• Sprains • Minor burns • Post-traumatic stress disorder • Minor fractures
Expectant	Casualties who have suffered catastrophic injuries; not expected to survive	Black	• Cardiopulmonary arrest • Penetrating brain injury • Extensive body surface burns • Profound shock

⬍FIGURE 45-1 Common triage categories.

when triaging (e.g., staffing, resources, bed capacity). Triage in critical care might require movement of lower category patients to other floors in order to accommodate new higher-acuity patients.

During an MCI, most patients should arrive already decontaminated. The critical care nurse should, however, be aware of the potential for missed patients or those who are considered "walk-ins." Several decontamination solutions are available on the market, but for mass decontaminations, copious amounts of soap and water will be effective in most cases.

PERSONAL PROTECTIVE EQUIPMENT

The development and use of proven personal protective equipment (PPE) are essential to the health and safety of critical care nurses. PPE is equipment designed to protect providers from the risk of injury by creating a barrier against workplace hazards. It is of particular importance to terrorism preparedness and response to ensure worker health and safety. PPE has always played an important role in critical care

and must continue to be customized to mitigate the risks associated with chemical, biological, radiologic, nuclear, or other mass-trauma hazards. Of equal importance is training to ensure nurses can properly assess an environment's hazards and select the appropriate PPE.[25]

The type of PPE used varies with each situation. The types of PPE listed in Box 45-2 are general in nature. If an act of terrorism occurs, the type of PPE should already be determined within the unit's MCI plan of action. Box 45-2 provides additional information on the four levels of PPE. While these are general guidelines for typical equipment to be used in certain circumstances, other combinations of protective equipment may be more appropriate, depending upon specific site characteristics.[12,25]

COMMAND AND CONTROL

Command and control at the scene are essential components of any mass-casualty response.[10] A well-organized, well-planned approach to any mass-casualty

Box 45-2

Levels of Personal Protective Equipment

- **Level A protection** is required when the greatest potential for exposure to hazards exists and when the greatest level of skin, respiratory, and eye protection is required. Examples of Level A clothing and equipment include positive-pressure, full face-piece self-contained breathing apparatus (SCBA) or positive-pressure supplied air respirator with escape SCBA, totally encapsulated chemical- and vapor-protective suit, inner and outer chemical-resistant gloves, and disposable protective suit, gloves, and boots.

- **Level B protection** is required under circumstances requiring the highest level of respiratory protection, with a lower level of skin protection. Examples of Level B protection include positive-pressure, full face-piece self-contained breathing apparatus (SCBA) or positive-pressure supplied air respirator with escape SCBA, inner and outer chemical-resistant gloves, face shield, hooded chemical-resistant clothing, coveralls, and outer chemical-resistant boots.

- **Level C protection** is required when the concentration and type of airborne substances are known and the criterion for using air-purifying respirators is met. Typical Level C equipment includes full-face air-purifying respirators, inner and outer chemical-resistant gloves, hard hat, escape mask, and disposable chemical-resistant outer boots. The difference between Level C and Level B protection is the type of equipment used to protect the respiratory system, assuming the same type of chemical-resistant clothing is used. The main criterion for Level C is that atmospheric concentrations and other selection criteria permit wearing an air-purifying respirator.

- **Level D protection** is the minimum protection required. Level D protection may be sufficient when no contaminants are present or work operations preclude splashes, immersion, or the potential for unexpected inhalation or contact with hazardous levels of chemicals. Appropriate Level D protective equipment may include gloves, coveralls, safety glasses, face shield, and chemical-resistant, steel-toe boots or shoes.

planning for such events occurs at many levels, but often the preparedness of the local healthcare facility is overlooked in this planning process. A real mass-casualty event resulting from a weapon of mass destruction will stress the resources of any healthcare facility as it attempts to triage, decontaminate, and care for a potentially large number of victims while ensuring that the health of patients and employees already at the healthcare facility is not compromised.

This requires a well-designed, executable plan that ensures effective command and control; smooth coordination with local, state, and federal resources; secure communications; adequate staffing and supplies; and a system to track patients accurately. In addition, planning for the extra psychological care that staff and patients might need will be necessary. Public affairs support will be needed to handle the resultant media attention and possible public mass hysteria. Critical care physicians and nurse managers should establish command and control protocols clearly identifying who is in charge during an MCI, where the communication will come from, and who is responsible for maintaining it.

CRITICAL CARE UNIT PLANNING AND MANAGEMENT

The Incident Command System (ICS) is a generic command structure that has become ubiquitous in fire, police, emergency medical services (EMS), and military agencies. The ICS structure used within a hospital environment is commonly referred to as the Hospital Environment Incident Command System (HEICS). The HEICS employs a logical, scalable, managed structure incorporating defined responsibilities and clear reporting channels within each section of the hospital (Figure 45-2).

Once a hospital activates the overall HEICS, it is vital for the critical care sections to also activate their internal emergency disaster plan. In most instances, the charge nurse or nurse manager will be responsible for activating this plan. Three key areas that must be addressed are communication, coordination, and control. Communication provides the critical care staff with the information needed to perform their duties. Various forms of communication might be necessary (e.g., multichannel walkie-talkies, cell phones, communication boards). With effective communication in place, coordination can begin. This involves synchronizing activities toward desired goals of the overall disaster plan. Coordination occurs only through strong, effective leadership. Control is a manager's duty to ensure that staff perform in accordance with the

emergency is essential. Planning for mass casualties is standard practice for many healthcare facilities, but specific planning and training for possible terrorist events and potential weapons of mass destruction has only recently gathered much attention. Community-wide

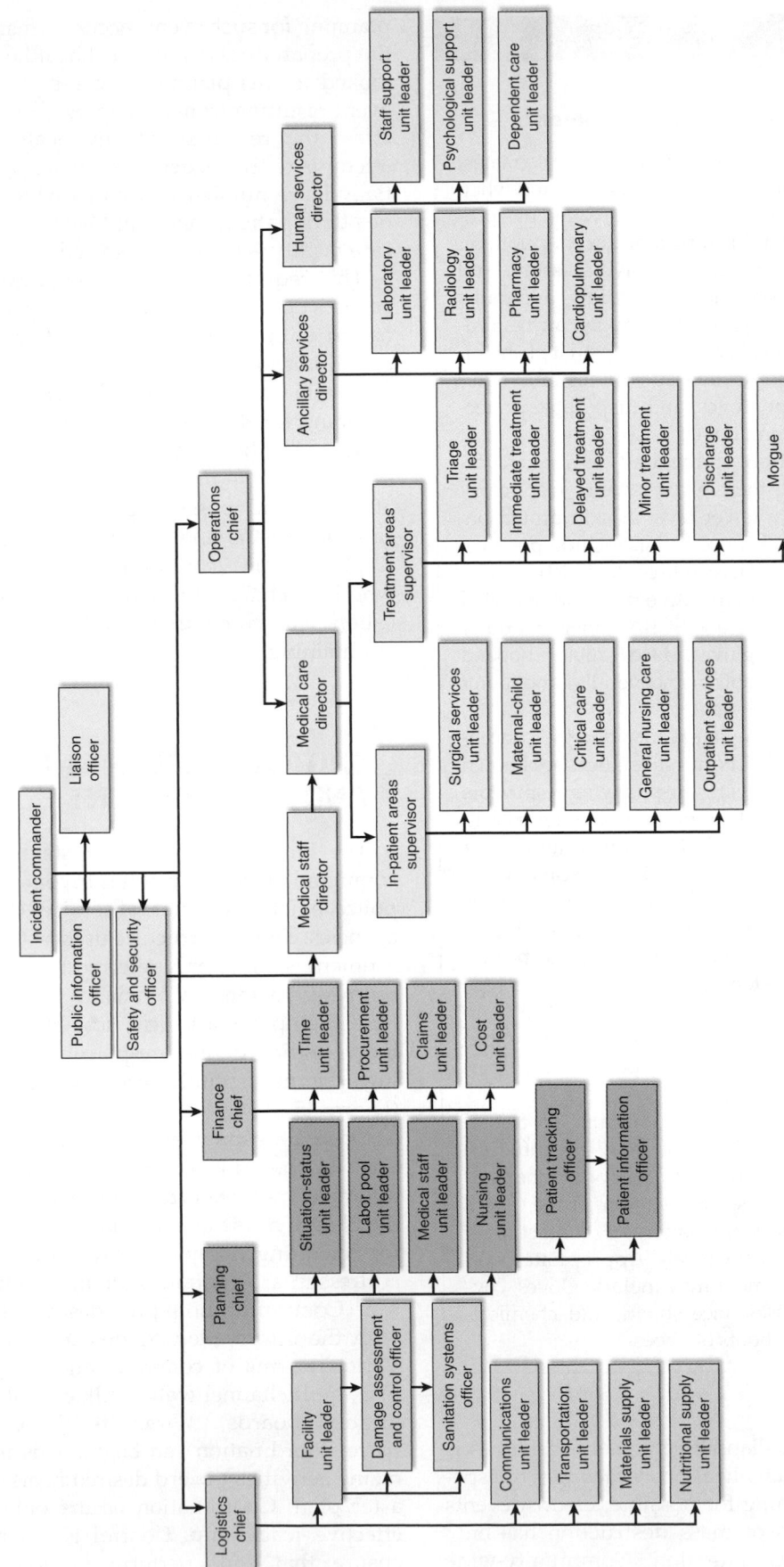

FIGURE 45-2 Example of a hospital environment incident command system.

Box 45-3

Special "Lessons Learned" Link

In response to the Hurricane Katrina disaster, the Department of Homeland Security has created a special Lessons Learned Information Sharing website, accessed through www.LLIS.dhs.gov, for members to gain relevant disaster recovery lessons learned, best practices, after-action reports, and other hurricane-related documents. LLIS.gov users also have the opportunity to submit comments, experiences, and observations from Katrina that will assist in the development of lessons learned. In addition, users can post questions, comments, and insights to a Katrina-specific message board at www.llis.dhs.gov/whats.cfm.

↕ Case Study 45-1, Part B

Triage and Patient Care Considerations

J.S. learns that four of the patients from the MCI will be admitted to critical care; three of the patients require mechanical ventilation. Presently, the unit is full, with eight mechanically ventilated patients. The respiratory therapist calls and explains that there are no more ventilators available. J.S. notifies the chief critical care resident and arranges transfer to the postanesthesia recovery unit (PACU) for four current, stable patients to make room for the burn casualties. These patients were ventilated by the PACU team using anesthesia ventilators; the critical care ventilators were quickly cleaned and made available for the new patients. The respiratory therapist supplied each room with backup manual ventilatory support. Air transport from the regional burn center was requested to transfer the burned patients as quickly as possible to that facility for maximal care, but they were unable to respond for several hours because of bad weather.

Decision point: What triage and patient care considerations should J.S. detail for her staff to help them prepare to receive multiple patients?

Case continues on page 1280

---

overall plan. Leadership is essential to control. In a disaster, flexibility is required, but staff should attempt to perform according to set standards and procedures whenever possible (Box 45-3).

Eventually the most critically ill patients will arrive to critical care, with the remainder of the patients admitted to other inpatient areas. Assessment of patient stability for transfer from critical care should be done and transfer accomplished as soon as possible. Following the Oklahoma City bombing, one hospital encountered difficulties in transferring patients to other areas of the hospital because of the overloaded or disrupted external communication system (e.g., inability to reach physicians for transfer orders) and internal communication system (e.g., difficulty in determining bed availability). In addition, transfer of patients was impeded by support personnel being quickly overwhelmed by the multiple tasks they were required to perform.[5] Critical care units should develop transfer protocols for mass-casualty events, should have alternative methods of communication available (e.g., walkie-talkies), and should ensure that a reliable "critical personnel" contact system has been established and tested. Other vital components of any MC plan should ensure that hospital police and security in conjunction with the public affairs department enact crowd and media control measures and provide psychosocial support for patients, families, and staff. The importance of critical incident stress management debriefings cannot be overstated.

CHEMICAL-BIOLOGICAL-RADIOLOGIC-NUCLEAR REVIEW

With terrorism posing a constant threat to countries and cities all over the world, the prospect of chemical, nuclear, or biological warfare has become a very real threat. The production of chemical and biological weapons has become easier, and the effects of these weapons can be deadly if found in the wrong hands. Chemical, biological, radiologic, and nuclear (CBRN) weapons can all result in mass illness or fatalities, with the severity of the effects dependent upon a number of factors such as type of agent used, concentration, and length of exposure time. To facilitate the rapid identification of any terrorist attack, critical care nurses should have basic clinical knowledge of the primary agents likely to be used, common signs and symptoms, and any potential treatment modalities. One specific emergency most critical care nurses are unprepared for is a radiologic or nuclear incident that may or may not be the result of an explosion. If nuclear detonation does involve an explosion, a daunting number of burn, flash, and blast injuries are likely to occur as a result of the fireball. Nuclear detonation also releases both immediate and delayed radiation effects adding to the injuries. It is also important to keep in mind that radiologic exposures can result from either deliberate or accidental release of radionuclides into the air, water, food supplies, or onto surfaces with which people come in contact.[25] Any attack has the definite potential to create a logistical, medical, and nursing nightmare; preparation and planning are the most important tools for improved survival rates.

One of the most significant differences between nuclear, chemical, and biological events will be the way in which medical consequences unfold over time. The Centers for Disease Control and Prevention's (CDC) *Strategic Plan for Preparedness and Response to Biological and Chemical Terrorism* notes that the medical casualties of chemical terrorism will be immediate and obvious.[12] Biological terrorism, on the other hand, may not have an immediate impact because of the delay between exposure and onset of illness. Nuclear terrorism will have both an immediate and a delayed impact. Because of these time differences, chemical and nuclear terrorism will have an identifiable incident scene while biological terrorism may not. Keep in mind that the casualties of chemical terrorism will be readily observable whereas the casualties of biological and radiologic terrorism may not even know that they are infected until many days after initial exposure. In any event, the primary consequence of a large-scale chemical, nuclear, or bioterrorist attack will be a catastrophically large number of medical casualties. What follows in this section is a highlighted clinical review of the more common agents that might be used during a terrorist attack.

Chemical Attack

A chemical weapon can employ any combination of chemical agents to cause illness and death. The contamination can be administered in a variety of ways, although the most likely is possibly contamination of air through agents used in gas, aerosol, or powder form. Depending on how the chemical agents are dispersed, exposure can occur through ingestion, breathing, absorption by the skin, and contact with the eyes. These weapons can be fast acting and extremely toxic, and effects of the agents can include breathing difficulties, eye irritation, skin abnormalities, nausea, respiratory problems, and chest or abdominal pain. Precise symptoms would depend on the agent used, and the severity of the symptoms can depend on the person's proximity to the contamination (Table 45-2).[12]

Other factors that can affect the effectiveness of these weapons include the direction of the wind (in the case of air contamination), the quantity used, the type of agent used, and the area exposed. The characteristics of likely agents would be those that:

- Survive in the environment for a long time
- Cause widespread disease and death

- Have highly toxic levels
- Result in conditions for which the onset of symptoms is fast or immediate
- Can stay active in the environment for a long time
- Require small doses for maximum effect

Types of chemical weapons

Nerve Agents. Nerve agents attack the body's nervous system, causing breathing difficulties, convulsions, paralysis, and death. Nerve agents can be inhaled or absorbed through the skin. Symptoms of nerve agent poisoning include runny nose, tightness of chest, dyspnea, excessive sweating, nausea, vomiting, dimness of vision, pinpointing of the pupils, convulsion, and death.[12]

Blister Agents. Blister agents attack the lungs, eyes, and skin. They blister both skin and mucous membranes.

Blood Agents. Blood agents interfere with the body's ability to absorb oxygen. The victim dies because the body tissues are starved of oxygen. Blood agents cause headaches, vertigo, and nausea before death.[12]

Choking Agents. Choking agents attack the lungs, causing them to fill with fluid. Choking agents are detected by their smell and their irritancy. The victim suffocates by drowning in his or her own body fluid. Choking agents cause coughing, choking, tightness of the chest, dyspnea, nausea, headache, and watering of the eyes (Table 45-3).[12]

Biological Attack

Potential agents of bioterrorism are classified into three categories: A, B, and C (Table 45-4). This section will highlight primarily the agents in category A, which are considered higher priority. High-priority agents include organisms that pose a risk to national security because they:

- Can be easily disseminated or transmitted from person to person
- Result in high mortality rates
- Might cause public panic and social disruption
- Require special action for public health preparedness

Bioterrorist weapons may employ a number of dangerous or deadly viruses and organisms. The primary goal of bioterrorist weapons is to cause widespread disease and death through contamination of water, food, or air.[25] Several of the agents can be used in aerosol form to contaminate the environment, or failing that, could be used to contaminate water supplies. Exposure can occur through breathing, skin contact, ingestion, and person-to-person contact.

TABLE 45-2   Common Chemical Weapons*

NAME	ODOR	RATE OF ACTION	INJURIES
CS	Pepper	Immediate	Irritation
Cyanogen chloride (CK)	Bitter almonds		Choking and dyspnea
Diphosgene (DP)	Freshly mowed hay, green corn	Immediate to 3 hr	Pulmonary capillary damage, edema, surfactant washout, hypoxia, respiratory failure
Hydrogen cyanide (AC)	Bitter almonds	Immediate	Toxic hypoxia
Lewisite (L)	Geraniums	Immediate	Poisoning/systemic failure
Mustard gas–distilled (MD)	Garlic	Hours to days	Blisters, injures blood vessels, destroys mucous membranes and tissue
Mustard gas–lewisite mix (HL)	Garlic	Immediate pain and blistering for 12 hr	Blisters, injures blood vessels, destroys tissues, poisons
Nitrogen mustard (HN)	Fishy or musty	12 hr or longer	Blisters, injures respiratory tract, destroys tissues
Phosgene (CG)	Freshly mowed hay, green corn	Immediate to 3 hr	Pulmonary capillary damage, edema, surfactant washout, hypoxia, respiratory failure
Phosgene oxime (CX)	Sharp, penetrating	Immediate	Irritates mucous membranes of eyes and nose
Sarin (GB)	Almost none	Immediate	Dyspnea/respiratory failure, cardiac compromise, death
Soman (GD)	Fruity, camphor odor	Immediate	Dyspnea/respiratory failure, cardiac compromise, death
VX	None	Immediate	Death

Modified from reference 24. Additional data from reference 12.
*NOTE: This chart is to be utilized as a rough guideline only. Odor, rate of action, and injuries can vary based on concentration and chemical purity.

Biological weapons can prove dangerous or fatal, and the extent of damage can depend on a number of factors, including the biological agent used, how it is dispersed, the quantity dispersed, whether it is infectious, and the area exposed. Symptoms can include skin lesions, eye problems, respiratory failure, internal organ failure, weight loss, fever, vomiting, and diarrhea.[12] The biological agents that would most likely be used are those that:

- Survive in the environment for a long time
- Cause widespread disease and death
- Have the ability to spread from person to person

- Result in conditions for which the onset of symptoms is fast or immediate
- Require small doses for maximum effect
- Are easy to deliver
- Are highly potent but not visible

By preparing for biological terrorism, critical care nurses will be better equipped to deal with both man-made biological terrorism and naturally occurring epidemics. This section summarizes some of the more common biological agents and highlights both clinical and epidemiologic clues helpful in recognizing possible bioterrorist events.

TABLE 45-3 Summary of Potential Chemical/Bioterrorism Syndromes

AGENTS	SIGNS	SYMPTOMS	CLINICAL DIAGNOSTIC TESTS	EXPOSURE ROUTE AND TREATMENT
Cyanides: Hydrogen cyanide (HCN) Cyanogen chloride	Moderate exposure: metabolic acidosis, venous blood oxygen level above normal, hypotension, "pink" skin color High exposure: above signs plus coma, convulsions, cessation of respiration and heartbeat	Moderate exposure: giddiness, palpitations, dizziness, nausea, vomiting, headache, eye irritation, increase in rate and depth of breathing (hyperventilation), drowsiness High exposure: immediate loss of consciousness, convulsions, and death within 1–15 min	Bitter almond odor associated with patient suggests cyanide poisoning Metabolic acidosis Cyanide (blood) or thiocyanate (blood or urine) levels Treat based on signs and symptoms; lab tests only for later confirmation	Inhalation, ingestion, and dermal absorption 100% oxygen by face mask; intubation with 100% Fio₂ if indicated Amyl nitrite via inhalation, 1 ampule (0.2 ml) every 5 min Sodium nitrite (300 mg IV over 5–10 min) and sodium thiosulfate (12.5 g IV) Additional sodium nitrite should be based on hemoglobin level and weight of patient
Nerve agents: Sarin (GB) Tabun (GA) Soman (GD) Cyclohexyl sarin (GF) VX Choking agents, other organophosphorus compounds including carbamates and pesticides	Pinpoint pupils (miosis) Bronchoconstriction Respiratory arrest Hypersalivation Increased secretions Diarrhea Decreased memory and concentration Loss of consciousness Seizures	Moderate exposure: diffuse muscle cramping, runny nose, difficulty breathing, eye pain, dimming of vision, sweating, muscle tremors High exposure: above plus sudden loss of consciousness, seizures, flaccid paralysis (late sign)	Red blood cell or serum cholinesterase (whole blood) Treat based on signs and symptoms; lab tests only for later confirmation	Inhalation and dermal absorption Atropine (2 mg) IV; repeat every 5 min, titrate until effective, average dose 6 to greater than 15 mg; use IM in the field before IV access (establish airway for oxygenation) Pralidoxime chloride (2-PAMCI) 600–1800 mg IM or 1 g IV over 20–30 min (maximum 2 g IM or IV per hr) Additional doses of atropine and 2-PAMCI depending on severity Diazepam (Valium) or lorazepam (Ativan) to prevent seizures if more than 4 mg atropine given Ventilatory support
Pulmonary/choking agents: Phosgene Chlorine Diphosgene	Pulmonary edema with some mucosal irritation (greater water solubility of agent = greater mucosal irritation) leading to ARDS or	Shortness of breath, chest tightness, wheezing laryngeal spasm, mucosal and dermal irritation and redness	No tests available but history may help identify source and exposure characteristics	Inhalation Management of secretions; oxygen therapy; consider high-dose steroids to prevent pulmonary edema (demonstrated benefit only for oxides of nitrogen)

AGENTS	SIGNS	SYMPTOMS	CLINICAL DIAGNOSTIC TESTS	EXPOSURE ROUTE AND TREATMENT
Chloropicrin Oxides of nitrogen Sulfur dioxide Ricin (castor bean oil extract)	noncardiogenic pulmonary edema Pulmonary infiltrate injury; circulatory collapse and shock, tracheobronchitis, pulmonary edema, necrotizing pneumonia	Ingestion: nausea, diarrhea, vomiting, fever, abdominal pain Inhalation: chest tightness, coughing, weakness, nausea, fever	(majority of incidents generating exposures to humans involve trucking, with labels on vehicle) ELISA from commercial laboratories	Treat pulmonary edema with PEEP to maintain Pao$_2$ above 60 mm Hg Supportive care For ingestion: consider charcoal lavage
T-2 mycotoxins: *Fusarium,* *Myrothecium,* *Trichoderma,* *Verticimonosporium,* *Stachybotrys*	Mucosal erythema and hemorrhage (intestinal necrosis) Red skin, blistering Increased salivation Pulmonary edema Seizures and coma Liver/renal dysfunction	Dermal and mucosal irritation; blistering, necrosis Blurred vision, eye irritation, tearing Nausea, vomiting, and diarrhea Ataxia, coughing, and dyspnea	ELISA from commercial laboratories Gas chromatography/mass spectroscopy in specialized laboratories	Inhalation and dermal contact No antidote Supportive care For ingestion: charcoal lavage Consider high-dose steroids
Vesicants/blister agents: Sulfur mustard Lewisite Nitrogen mustard Mustard lewisite Phosgene-oxime	Skin erythema and blistering; watery, swollen eyes; upper airway sloughing with pulmonary edema; metabolic failure; neutropenia and sepsis (especially sulfur mustard, late in course)	Burning, itching, or red skin Mucosal irritation (prominent tearing, burning and redness of eyes) Shortness of breath, nausea, and vomiting	Often smell of garlic, horseradish, or mustard Oily droplets on skin from ambient sources Urine thiodiglycol tissue biopsy	Inhalation and dermal absorption Mustards: no antidote For lewisite and lewisite/mustard mixtures: British antilewisite (BAL or dimercaprol) IM (rarely available) Thermal burn therapy; supportive care (respiratory support and eye care)

Modified from reference 24. Additional data from reference 12.
ARDS = Acute respiratory distress syndrome, ELISA = enzyme-linked immunosorbent assay, Fio$_2$ = fraction of inspired oxygen, Pao$_2$ = partial pressure of arterial oxygen, PEEP = positive end-expiratory pressure.

TABLE 45-4 Summary of Category A Bioterrorism Syndromes

DISEASE	SIGNS AND SYMPTOMS	INCUBATION TIME	DIAGNOSIS	POSTEXPOSURE PROPHYLAXIS FOR ADULTS	TREATMENT FOR ADULTS
Anthrax *Bacillus anthracis* A. Inhalation B. Cutaneous	Flu-like symptoms (fever, fatigue, muscle aches, dyspnea, nonproductive cough, headache), chest pain; possible 1–2 day improvement, then rapid respiratory failure and shock Meningitis may develop Intense itching followed by painless papular lesions, then vesicular lesions, developing into eschar surrounded by edema	1–6 days (up to 6 weeks) 1–12 days	Chest x-ray evidence of widening mediastinum; obtain sputum and blood culture Sensitivity and specificity of nasal swabs unknown; do not rely on for diagnosis Peripheral blood smear may demonstrate gram-positive bacilli on unspun smear with sepsis	Prophylaxis for 60 days: ciprofloxacin (Ciloxan) 500 mg PO every 12 hr or doxycycline (Vibramycin) 100 mg PO every 12 hr Alternative (if strain susceptible and above contraindicated): amoxicillin (Augmentin) 500 mg PO every 8 hr In vitro studies suggest that levofloxacin (Levaquin) 500 mg PO every 24 hr, gatifloxacin (Tequin) 400 mg PO every 24 hr, or moxifloxacin (Avelox) 400 mg PO every 24 hr could be substituted	Inhalation anthrax: Combined IV/PO therapy for 60 days; ciprofloxacin 500 mg every 12 hr or doxycycline 100 mg every 12 hr, AND 1 or 2 additional drugs: vancomycin (Vancocin), rifampin (Rifadin), imipenem (Primaxin), clindamycin (Cleocin), chloramphenicol (Chloromycetin), clarithromycin (Biaxin) If susceptible, penicillin or ampicillin for cutaneous anthrax
Botulism *Clostridium botulinum* toxin	Afebrile, excess mucus in throat, dysphagia, dry mouth and throat, dizziness, then difficulty moving eyes, mild pupillary dilation and nystagmus, intermittent ptosis, indistinct speech, unsteady gait, extreme symmetric descending weakness, flaccid paralysis; generally normal mental status	Inhalation: 12–80 hr Foodborne: 12–72 hr (2–8 days)	Laboratory tests available from CDC or public health dept; obtain serum, stool, gastric aspirate; suspect foods before administering antitoxin Differential diagnosis includes polio, Guillain-Barré, myasthenia, tick paralysis, cerebrovascular accident, meningococcal meningitis	Pentavalent toxoid (types A, B, C, D, and E) 0.5 ml subcutaneous may be available as investigational product from the United States Army Medical Research Institute for Infectious Diseases	Botulism antitoxins from public health authorities Supportive care and ventilatory support Avoid clindamycin and aminoglycosides

DISEASE	SIGNS AND SYMPTOMS	INCUBATION TIME	DIAGNOSIS	POSTEXPOSURE PROPHYLAXIS FOR ADULTS	TREATMENT FOR ADULTS
Gastrointestinal *Clostridium perfringens*	Abdominal pain, nausea and vomiting, severe diarrhea, gastrointestinal bleeding, and fever	1–7 days	Culture blood and stool	Recommendations same for pregnant women and immunocompromised persons	Ciprofloxacin 500 mg PO every 12 hr or doxycycline 100 mg PO every 12 hr Recommendations same for pregnant women and immunocompromised persons
Pneumonic plague *Yersinia pestis*	High fever, cough, hemoptysis, chest pain, nausea and vomiting, headache Advanced disease: purpuric skin lesions, copious watery or purulent sputum production; respiratory failure in 1–6 days	2–3 days (2–6 days)	Presumptive diagnosis may be made by Gram, Wayson, or Wright stain of lymph node aspirates, sputum, or cerebrospinal fluid with gram-negative bacilli with bipolar (safety pin) staining	Doxycycline 100 mg PO daily every 12 hr or ciprofloxacin 500 mg PO every 12 hr	Streptomycin 1 g IM every 12 hr or gentamicin 2 mg/kg; then 1–1.7 mg/kg IV every 8 hr Alternatives: doxycycline 200 mg PO load, then 100 PO mg every 12 hr; or ciprofloxacin 400 mg IV every 12 hr
Smallpox Variola virus	Prodromal period: malaise, fever, rigors, vomiting, headache, backache After 2–4 days, skin lesions appear and progress uniformly from macules to papules to vesicles and pustules, mostly on face, neck, palms, soles, and subsequently progress to trunk	12–14 days (7–17 days)	Swab culture of vesicular fluid or scab, send to BL-4 laboratory All lesions similar in appearance and develop synchronously as opposed to chickenpox Electron microscopy can differentiate variola virus from varicella	Early vaccine critical (in less than 4 days) Call CDC for vaccinia	Supportive care Previous vaccination against smallpox does not confer lifelong immunity Potential role for cidofovir

Modified from reference 25. Additional data from reference 12.

Anthrax. Anthrax is an acute infectious disease caused by spore-forming bacteria. For centuries, anthrax has caused disease in animals and, uncommonly, serious illness in humans throughout the world. Research on anthrax as a biological weapon began more than 80 years ago. Today, at least 17 nations are believed to have offensive biological weapons programs; it is uncertain how many are working with anthrax. Anthrax spores are very tenacious. They can live in soil and survive there at least 40 years; when animals feed, sometimes they ingest these spores.[12,25]

Symptoms.

- *Dermal infection:* Symptoms usually appear within 1 to 7 days, but can take 14 days or as long as 60 days after exposure.
- *Respiratory:* Initial symptoms may resemble a common cold including fever, malaise, fatigue, and sometimes a dry cough. Following this there is often a period of improvement that lasts from a few hours to 2 to 3 days. Afterward, decompensation occurs, resulting in severe dyspnea, sweating, and cyanosis. The patient usually goes into shock and dies 24 to 36 hours after the severe symptoms begin.
- *Dermal (skin):* Approximately 95% of infections occur when bacteria enter a cut or abrasion on the skin. It begins as a raised, itchy bump that looks like an insect bite. Within 1 to 2 days it changes into a painless blister, usually ⅓ to 1 inch in diameter with a black center. Adjacent lymph glands may swell.
- *Intestinal:* Intestinal contamination may follow eating contaminated meat and is characterized by acute inflammation of the intestinal tract. Initial signs include nausea, loss of appetite, vomiting, and fever followed by abdominal pain, vomiting of blood, and severe diarrhea.

NOTE: These types are all from the same spore. It is the point of entry into the body that determines the form the disease takes and, ultimately, the likelihood of recovery. Anthrax is NOT contagious, i.e., person-to-person. On the skin, it needs a place of entry such as a cut; otherwise, it might not even be dangerous. To breathe it, however, could be fatal. Humans can become infected with anthrax by handling products from infected animals, by eating undercooked meat from infected animals, or by inhaling anthrax spores.

Mortality. Untreated, anthrax in all forms can lead to blood poisoning and death. A lethal dose of inhaled anthrax is considered to be 10,000 spores, but depending upon a person's immune system and state of health, that level might be as high as 50,000 anthrax spores. To put this size in perspective, 1 gram of anthrax culture contains 1 trillion spores, theoretically enough for 100 million fatal doses. When inhaled, anthrax is usually fatal. When spread though open skin, death is rare when appropriate antimicrobial therapy is prescribed. It is fatal in 20% of untreated cases. Intestinal spread is associated with a fatality rate of 25% to 60%. Incineration of corpses is essential to prevent further contamination.

How does it spread? There currently are no warning systems to detect an aerosol cloud of anthrax spores—the attack would most likely not be discovered until patients arrived in hospitals.

Diagnosis. Anthrax is diagnosed by isolating the bacteria from the blood, skin lesions, or respiratory secretions or by measuring specific antibodies in the blood. Nasal swabbing is one of the most common methods. Necessary diagnostic samples include blood cultures or stool cultures if gastrointestinal disease is suspected.

Treatment. To be effective, treatment must be done early. This is especially true when anthrax spores have been inhaled. Antibiotics (e.g., amoxicillin [Augmentin], ciprofloxacin [Ciloxan], erythromycin, gentamicin) treat skin and intestinal infections successfully, but respiratory anthrax is very hard to treat and nearly always fatal. Most natural strains of anthrax are sensitive to penicillin, but some strains resist this antibiotic, so it is not a sure treatment. Respiratory support may be required.

Vaccine. While the vaccine is 93% effective, the current supply is reserved for military personnel. Regardless of how it is stored, the anthrax vaccine's shelf life is guaranteed a maximum of 3 years from date of manufacture, but may last as long as 6 years.

Botulism. *Clostridium botulinum* is a group of bacteria commonly found in soil. Proliferating in low-oxygen environments, the bacteria form spores that allow them to survive dormant until the right conditions develop for growth. There are seven types of botulism, but only three make humans sick. The three main kinds of botulism are the following: foodborne botulism, caused by eating foods that contain botulism; wound botulism, caused by toxin produced from a wound infected with *Clostridium botulinum;* and infant botulism, caused by eating spores of the bacteria, which then grow in the intestines and release toxin. Though rare, all forms can be fatal and are considered medical emergencies. On average, 100 cases are reported in the United States yearly. Terrorists have already attempted to use botulinum toxin as a bioweapon. Aerosols were dispersed at multiple sites in downtown Tokyo, Japan, and at U.S. military installations in Japan on at least three occasions between 1990 and 1995. These attacks failed because of faulty microbiological technique, deficient aerosol-generating equipment, or internal sabotage.[12]

Symptoms. Symptoms include double or blurred vision, drooping eyelids, slurred speech, difficulty swallowing, dry mouth, and muscle weakness. Infants with botulism appear lethargic, feed poorly, are constipated, and have a weak cry and poor muscle tone. These are all symptoms of the muscle paralysis caused by the bacterial toxin. If untreated, symptoms may cause paralysis of arms, legs, trunk, and respiratory muscles. In foodborne botulism, symptoms generally begin 18 to 36 hours after eating the contaminated food but can occur as early as 6 hours to as late as 10 days.

Mortality. Botulism can result in death attributable to respiratory failure. In the last 50 years, the number of patients who die from botulism has decreased from 50% to 8%.[12] Patients who survive this poisoning may be tired and experience shortness of breath for years. Long-term therapy may be needed.

How does it spread? Botulism spreads through ingestion, inhalation, or absorption through eyes or breaks in the skin and can cause profound intoxication and death. Aerosol-released botulinum toxin could incapacitate or kill 10% of persons within 0.3 mile downwind.[12]

Diagnosis. Because botulism mimics other diseases, blood, stool, or gastric secretions should be collected and transported to the local state health department lab or the CDC to confirm a diagnosis. Respiratory failure and paralysis may require mechanical ventilation for weeks plus intensive medical care. After several weeks, paralysis slowly improves. If diagnosed early, foodborne and wound botulism can be treated with an antitoxin, preventing symptoms from worsening. Antitoxin is not routinely given to infants. Instead, induced vomiting or enemas are used. Wounds should be treated, usually surgically, to remove the source of the toxin-producing bacteria.

Treatment. Table 45-4 outlines specific treatments for the patient impacted by botulism.

Vaccine. Along with state health departments, the CDC maintains intensive surveillance for botulism in the United States. Every case of foodborne botulism is treated as a public health emergency. If antitoxin is needed, it can be quickly delivered to a physician anywhere in the country. Skin testing for hypersensitivity should be performed before equine antitoxin is given.

Clostridium. *Clostridium perfringens* is a common anaerobic bacillus that produces at least 12 toxins. Spores survive cooking and then germinate and multiply from storage at ambient temperature, slow cooling, or inadequate rewarming. *C. perfringens* lives in soil and the gastrointestinal tract of healthy persons and animals. The primary threat is to the respiratory tract. This would result in pulmonary disease vastly different from the naturally occurring diseases associated with *C. perfringens*. The toxin may also be combined with other toxins to produce a variety of symptoms.[12]

Symptoms. Incubation is short, about 6 hours, and produces respiratory distress syndrome and respiratory failure. Absorbed toxin can lead to intravascular hemolysis, thrombocytopenia, and liver damage. Early symptoms beginning within minutes of exposure include burning skin pain, redness, tenderness, blistering, and progression to skin death, with leathery blackening and sloughing of large areas of skin. Upper respiratory tract exposure may result in nasal itching, pain, sneezing, epistaxis, and runny nose. Pulmonary/ tracheobronchial toxicity produces difficulty breathing, wheezing, and coughing. Mouth and throat exposure causes pain and blood-tinged saliva and sputum. Loss of appetite, nausea, vomiting, and watery or bloody diarrhea occur with gastrointestinal toxicity. Eye pain, tearing, redness, foreign body sensation, and blurred vision may follow ocular exposure.

Skin symptoms occur in minutes to hours and eye symptoms in minutes. Systemic toxicity can occur via any route of exposure, and results in weakness, prostration, dizziness, ataxia, and loss of coordination. Irregular heartbeat, hypothermia, and hypotension follow in fatal cases. The most common symptoms are vomiting, diarrhea, skin involvement with burning pain, redness and pruritus, rash or blisters, bleeding, and difficulty breathing. A late effect of systemic absorption is pancytopenia, predisposing to bleeding and sepsis.

Mortality. Prognosis is poor. Death may occur within minutes, hours, or days of exposure.

How does it spread? Gas gangrene results from wound contamination with soil containing spores of *C. perfringens*. Clostridial food poisoning follows eating foods contaminated with soil or feces and then stored under conditions that allow the organism to reproduce. This toxin is not communicable person to person.

Diagnosis. *Clostridium perfringens* exposure should be suspected if an aerosol attack occurs in the form of "yellow rain" with droplets of variously pigmented oily fluids contaminating clothes and the environment. Confirmation requires testing of blood, tissue, and environmental samples.

Treatment. There are no specific antitoxins or antidotes available. Medical management is symptom based and consists of mechanical ventilation, management of adequate cardiac output, skin and wound care, and supportive care. Patients may require a tracheotomy.

Vaccine. There is no vaccine available. There is also no preexposure or postexposure prevention.

Plague. Plague is an infectious bacterial disease affecting both animals and humans. In the United States, the last urban plague epidemic occurred in Los Angeles in 1924 to 1925. Since then, human plague in the United States has occurred mostly as scattered cases in rural areas. Globally, the World Health Organization reports 1000 to 3000 cases of plague every year. Since reports of mass production and aerosol dissemination of plague exist, the ready availability of this bacterium in microbe banks around the world, the high fatality rate in untreated cases, and the potential for secondary spread make an attack using plague a serious biological concern.[12]

Symptoms. Within 1 to 6 days after exposure, the first signs of illness are demonstrated—fever, headache, and weakness, which can lead to shock and death within 2 to 4 days. It takes three major forms depending on what part of the body the disease primarily affects. With septic plague, signs and symptoms include fever, shaking, chills, extreme exhaustion, abdominal pain, and shock and bleeding into skin and other organs. Complications of septicemia include septic shock, blood clotting disorder, coma, and meningitis. In pneumonic plague, signs and symptoms include high fever, shaking chills, coughing up blood, and difficulty breathing because of severe pneumonia. Rapid shock and death follow if not treated early. Bubonic plague is manifested by enlarged, tender lymph nodes, usually in the groin, armpits, or cervical areas, and the most readily identifiable symptoms of plague—fever, chills, and extreme exhaustion.

Mortality. Mortality is 50% to 90% in untreated cases and 15% of treated cases. The mortality of untreated pneumonic plague approaches 100%.[12]

How does it spread? It can move from animal to animal and from animal to human by the bites of infected fleas or by handling an infected animal. It can also be transmitted by aerosolization of droplets following a cough by an infected person or animal. However, person-to-person transmission is not common and has not been seen in the United States since 1924. Wild rodents (e.g., ground squirrels, prairie dogs, wood rats, mice in the western United States) can be infected with plague. Human outbreaks are usually associated with infected rats and rat fleas.

Diagnosis. As soon as a diagnosis is made, the patient should be hospitalized and medically isolated, and local and state health departments should be notified. To verify the diagnosis, lab work will include serum for capsular antigen testing, blood cultures, and culture of sputum or tracheal aspirates.

Treatment. Antibiotic drug therapy should begin as quickly as possible, within 24 hours of the first symptoms. Streptomycin, tetracycline (Sumycin), and chloramphenicol (Chloromycetin) are highly effective if begun early. Chloramphenicol is specifically indicated in treating plague meningitis. Critical care resuscitative support such as mechanical ventilation and fluid management may also be required.

Vaccine. Primary preventive measures are reducing the threat of infection in humans in high-risk areas through environmental management, public health education, preventive drug therapy, and vaccines.

Smallpox. Smallpox poses a serious bioterrorist threat because it has a high fatality rate, spreads easily in any climate and season, is highly infectious by aerosol, is environmentally stable, and can retain infectivity for long periods. Additionally, the majority of the U.S. population has no immunity, little vaccine is readily available, and no effective treatment exists for the disease. Those who do not die from the disease usually experience severe scarring. An aerosol release of smallpox virus disseminates readily given its considerable stability in aerosol form, with epidemiologic evidence suggesting the infectious dose is very small. As few as 50 to 100 cases would likely generate widespread concern or panic and a need to invoke large-scale, perhaps national emergency control measures.[12,25]

Symptoms. After a 7- to 17-day incubation period, symptoms begin acutely with high fever, headache, chills, malaise, muscle pain, vomiting, and abdominal and back pain. During the initial phase, 15% of patients become delirious in 2 to 3 days and lesions appear that quickly change into pus-filled blisters, especially on the extremities and face. Patients are most infectious 3 to 6 days after the onset of fever. Virus is shed from the scabs and respiratory secretions.

Mortality. Two types of smallpox are generally recognized. Variola major, the most severe form, has a fatality rate of 30% in unvaccinated individuals and 3% in those previously vaccinated. Variola minor, a milder form of smallpox, is lethal in only 1% of unvaccinated individuals.[12]

How does it spread? Smallpox spreads directly from person to person, primarily by spray expelled from the back of the mouth of an infected person or by aerosol. Contaminated clothing or bed linen can also spread the virus. Special precautions need to be taken to ensure that all bedding and clothing of patients are autoclaved.

Disinfectants (e.g., hypochlorite, quaternary ammonia) should be used for washing contaminated surfaces.

Diagnosis. Smallpox is usually diagnosed after looking at blister scrapings under an electron microscope. Sometimes a modified silver stain is used; however, these tests cannot distinguish between smallpox, monkeypox, and cowpox. Smallpox is differentiated from chickenpox by the centrifugal distribution of its rash and the presence of lesions at the same stage of development everywhere on the body.

Treatment. Strict quarantine with respiratory isolation for 17 days should be applied to all people in direct contact. Negative airflow should be used. People exposed to either weaponized smallpox or clinical cases must be vaccinated immediately. Vaccination within a few days will lessen severity or prevent illness altogether. Vaccinia immune globulin (VIG) is given to patients who cannot take the vaccine; examples include persons with impaired immune systems or HIV infection, pregnant women, persons with a history or evidence of eczema, or persons who have current household, sexual, or other close physical contact with person(s) possessing one of these conditions. Specifics on treatment can be found in Table 45-4.

Vaccine. Vaccination ceased in this country in 1972. Anyone vaccinated before that time no longer has immunity. Vaccination with a verified clinical "take" (vesicle with scar formation) within the past 3 years is considered immune to smallpox. Smallpox vaccine (a weakened form of the virus) is administered by injection, resulting in a permanent scar. A blister usually appears 5 to 7 days after inoculation that scabs over and heals over the next 1 to 2 weeks. Reactions include low-grade fever and enlarged lymph nodes. VIG can be obtained from the CDC and is administered intramuscularly at a dose of 0.6 ml/kg.

Special transport requirements for biological agents. Specimen packaging and transport must be coordinated with local and state health departments and the FBI. A chain of custody document should accompany the specimen from the moment of collection. For specific instructions, contact the *Bioterrorism Emergency Number at the CDC Emergency Response Office, (770) 488-7100.* Advance planning may include identification of appropriate packaging materials and transport media in collaboration with the clinical laboratory at individual facilities.

Nuclear and Radiologic Attacks

The threat of a nuclear terrorist attack seems to be looming more strongly than ever during recent years.

There are several types of danger involved in a nuclear attack (e.g., shockwave injury, fire, radiation fallout contamination). As with any disaster, advance planning may help protect against many of these dangers.[12]

If a healthcare institution survives a nuclear or radiologic attack, the critical care units would undoubtedly be called upon to function as an extension of a burn center since total body surface burns and internal injuries would be anticipated.

Blasts and shockwaves. The location of the attack will play a large part in determining whether or not survival is possible. Shelter or no shelter, living in an area close to the attack could result in death simply from the blast. Atmospheric air pressure surrounding a detonation causes a shockwave that moves at alarming speeds and with great force. The intensity of the wave often results in perforated eardrums of victims, so keep in mind that patients may not hear anything for several hours after the blast. A victim who looks directly at the blast can also experience temporary blindness, retinal burning, or permanent eye damage. Concussive forces often result in internal injuries (e.g., pulmonary contusion, cardiac contusion, and, in some cases, cardiac-pulmonary arrest).

Fire risk. The effect of the blast combined with the pulse of the nuclear weapon cause ignition of combustible materials, so fire is a high risk, particularly in areas very close to the detonation. The critical care team should plan for a large number of burn patients during any nuclear attack and ensure that adequate supplies and medications are available. In addition, several patients may arrive to critical care with smoke inhalation injuries and may require mechanical ventilation.

Radiation. The initial radiation following the nuclear blast can prove particularly hazardous, especially to those in close proximity. Radiation forms during the first minute following detonation. There are three main types of radiation: alpha, beta, and gamma. Alpha radiation is normally stopped by the outer layer of the skin; however, high quantities of ingestion or inhalation can result in internal damage. Beta radiation can cause skin burns if contaminated particles make contact with the skin and can be quite penetrative. Gamma radiation is the most dangerous of the three, causing extensive internal and external damage, destroying organs, skin, bones, and blood. In large doses, gamma radiation causes serious illness and death.

Fallout. The fallout, or the widespread distribution of nuclear contamination, occurs as earth matter from the center crater is transformed into hot gas and dust and rises up in the form of a fireball. As the fireball rises, radioactive materials from the detonated weapon attach themselves to dust and dirt particles. Eventually, the fire cools into a cloud formation, where the wind carries it and spreads it into different areas. Radioactive particles fall out of the air and scatter to anything on ground level. The fallout from the first 24 hours following detonation is the most dangerous as the particles are still highly radioactive. Fallout can continue for months to years;[12] however, within a couple of weeks, fallout radiation levels will be a tiny fraction of the levels at the time of detonation.

Health effects. There are many short-term and long-term effects that come with exposure to nuclear warfare. The effects can be spread far and wide, and can continue to affect us and our families for generations. The obvious risk from exposure to nuclear warfare is immediate death from the blast, from the explosion, from flying debris, from fire, and from vaporization caused by gamma rays.

Despite initial survival, negative health effects from nuclear exposure are many. In addition to burns, rashes, and smoke inhalation, other consequences include vomiting, diarrhea, fatigue, fainting, dehydration, hair loss, loss of appetite, and bleeding from the nose, mouth, rectum, or gums. The severity of these effects will depend upon the level of exposure. Some people may experience both immediate and delayed effects, which can ultimately end in death. Some effects will be obvious immediately following exposure. However, other ill effects may not reveal themselves for many years. Even a small dose of radiation could cause enough damage to put an exposed person at increased risk of developing diseases such as cancer.[12,25]

In most cases, patients in critical care will also be battling the effects of acute radiation syndrome. There are four stages of this syndrome:

- Prodromal stage: The classic symptoms of this stage are nausea, vomiting, and possibly diarrhea (depending on dose) that occur from minutes to days following exposure. The symptoms may last (episodically) for minutes up to several days.
- Latent stage: The patient looks and feels generally healthy for a few hours or even up to a few weeks.
- Manifest illness stage: The symptoms depend on the specific syndrome and last from hours up to several months.
- Recovery or death: Most patients who do not recover will die within several months of exposure. The recovery process lasts from several weeks up to 2 years (Table 45-5).

Educational Competencies for Registered Nurses Related to Mass-Casualty Incidents

The International Coalition for Mass Casualty Education (INCMCE) is an organization that aims to facilitate the systematic development of sustainable and scalable educational policies related to mass-casualty events as they impact nursing practice.[15] The INCMCE has developed core MCI competencies for all nurses. Critical care nurses should work toward development of these competencies as the foundation for any MCI preparation program (Box 45-4).

◆ Case Study 45-1, Part C

Preparation for a Future Incident

By the end of the disaster, the entire staff was exhausted. Within 36 hours all care was back to normal routine in critical care, and all four of the MCI patients were transferred to the regional burn center for definitive care. Each person was stressed beyond the call of duty, but each person appreciated the time spent earlier planning, preparing, and practicing for similar disasters. As a result, a stressful situation was turned into a positive outcome for a majority of those involved.

In the following debriefing, many staff had suggestions about how to do things differently should another disaster occur. J.S. documented all of these suggestions for review by the hospital's emergency preparedness committee for consideration.

Decision point: What suggestions might the staff nurses make to be better prepared for a future disaster of similar or greater magnitude?

Decision point: How might the special demands of an MCI change the way a hospital delivers patient care?

CONCLUSIONS

Today's complex disasters, especially those involving terrorism and weapons of mass destruction (chemical, biological, or nuclear), have the potential to unleash great destruction and chaos. Critical care nurses must be ready for any MCI in any environment. Many MCIs will result in a severe environment—an extended practice arena for most critical care nurses.[9] As significant partners in preparedness, critical care nurses must add disaster-specific knowledge and patient management to their current set of unique skills. Preparation, education, and training for any type of MCI will ensure that critical care nurses maintain the highest standard of care available during a mass-casualty emergency.

TABLE 45-5 Acute Radiation Syndrome

SYNDROME	DOSE	PRODROMAL STAGE	LATENT STAGE	MANIFEST ILLNESS STAGE	RECOVERY
Bone marrow	0.7–10 Gy (70–1000 rad) Mild symptoms may occur as low as 0.3 Gy or 30 rad	Anorexia, nausea, and vomiting Occurs 1 hr to 2 days after exposure Lasts for minutes to days	Stem cells in bone marrow are dying, though patient may appear and feel well Lasts 1–6 weeks	Drop in all blood cell counts for several weeks Anorexia, fever, malaise Primary cause of death is infection and hemorrhage Survival decreases with increasing doses Most deaths occur within a few weeks	In most cases, bone marrow cells will begin to repopulate marrow Should be full recovery for large percentage of individuals from a few weeks up to 2 years after exposure Death may occur in some individuals at 1.2 Gy (120 rad)
Cardiovascular and central nervous system	Greater than 50 Gy (5000 rad) Some symptoms may occur as low as 20 Gy or 2000 rad	Extreme nervousness, confusion, severe nausea, vomiting, and watery diarrhea; loss of consciousness; burning sensations of skin Occurs within minutes of exposure Lasts for minutes to hours	Patient may return to partial functionality May last for hours but often is less	Return of watery diarrhea, convulsions, coma Begins 5–6 hr after exposure Death within 3 days of exposure	No recovery
Gastrointestinal	10–100 Gy (1000–10,000 rad) Some symptoms may occur as low as 6 Gy or 600 rad	Anorexia, severe nausea, vomiting, cramps, and diarrhea Occurs within a few hours after exposure Lasts about 2 days	Stem cells in bone marrow and cells lining GI tract are dying, though patient may appear and feel well Lasts less than 1 week	Malaise, anorexia, severe diarrhea, fever, dehydration, electrolyte imbalance Death is due to infection, dehydration, and electrolyte imbalance Death occurs within 2 weeks of exposure	

Data from reference 12; www.bt.cdc.gov/radiation/pdf/arsphysicianfactsheet.pdf.

Box 45-4

Core Competencies for Mass-Casualty Preparedness

CRITICAL THINKING

- Use an ethical and nationally approved framework to support decision making and prioritizing needed in disaster situations.
- Use clinical judgment and decision-making skills in assessing the potential for appropriate, timely individual care during a mass-casualty incident (MCI).
- Use clinical judgment and decision-making skills in assessing the potential for appropriate, individual ongoing care after a mass-casualty incident.
- Describe at the predisaster, emergency, and postdisaster phases the essential nursing care for:
  - Individuals
  - Families
  - Special groups (e.g., children, older adults)
  - Communities
- Describe accepted triage principles specific to MCIs.

ASSESSMENT

- Assess the safety issues for self, the response team, and victims in any given response situation in collaboration with the incident response team.
- Identify possible indicators of a mass exposure (e.g., clustering of individuals with the same symptoms).
- Describe general signs and symptoms of exposure to selected chemical, biological, radiologic, nuclear, and explosive agents (CBRNE).
- Demonstrate the ability to access up-to-date information regarding selected nuclear, biological, chemical, explosive, and incendiary agents.
- Describe the essential elements included in an MCI scene assessment.
- Identify special groups of patients that are uniquely vulnerable during an MCI (e.g., the very young, aged, immunosuppressed).
- Conduct a focused health history to assess potential exposure to CBRNE agents.
- Perform an age-appropriate health assessment, including:
  - Airway and respiratory assessment
  - Cardiovascular assessment, including vital signs and monitoring for signs of shock
  - Integumentary assessment, particularly a wound, burn, and rash assessment
  - Pain assessment
  - Injury assessment from head to toe
  - Gastrointestinal assessment, including specimen collection
  - Basic neurologic assessment

- Musculoskeletal assessment
- Mental status, spiritual, and emotional assessment
- Assess the immediate psychological response of the individual, family, or community following an MCI.
- Assess the long-term psychological response of the individual, family, or community following an MCI.
- Identify resources available to address the psychological impact (e.g., critical incident stress debriefing [CISD] teams, counselors, psychiatric/mental health nurse practitioners [P/MHNPs]).
- Describe the psychological impact on responders and healthcare providers.

TECHNICAL SKILLS

- Demonstrate safe administration of medications, particularly vasoactive and analgesic agents, via oral, subcutaneous, intramuscular, and intravenous administration routes.
- Demonstrate the safe administration of immunizations, including smallpox vaccination.
- Demonstrate knowledge of appropriate nursing interventions for adverse effects from medications administered.
- Demonstrate basic therapeutic interventions, including:
  - Basic first aid skills
  - Oxygen administration and ventilation techniques
  - Urinary catheter insertion
  - Nasogastric tube insertion
  - Lavage technique (e.g., eye and wound)
  - Initial wound care
- Assess the need for and initiate the appropriate CBRNE isolation and decontamination procedures available, ensuring that all parties understand the need.
- Demonstrate knowledge and skill related to personal protection and safety, including the use of personal protective equipment (PPE) for:
  - Level B protection
  - Level C protection
  - Respiratory protection
- Implement fluid/nutrition therapy, taking into account the nature of injuries or agents of exposure and monitoring hydration and fluid balance accordingly.
- Assess and prepare the injured for transport, if required, including provisions for care and monitoring during transport.
- Demonstrate the ability to maintain patient safety during transport through splinting, immobilization, monitoring, and therapeutic interventions.

Box 45-4

Core Competencies for Mass-Casualty Preparedness—Cont'd

- Demonstrate use of emergency communication equipment and information management techniques required in an MCI response.

COMMUNICATION

- Describe the local chain of command and management system for emergency response during an MCI.
- Identify your role, if possible, within the emergency management system.
- Locate and describe the emergency response plan for one's place of employment and its role in community, state, and regional plans.
- Identify one's own role in the emergency response plan for the place of employment.
- Discuss security and confidentiality during an MCI.
- Demonstrate appropriate emergency documentation of assessments, interventions, nursing actions, and outcomes during and after an MCI.
- Identify appropriate resources for referring requests from patients, media, or others for information regarding MCIs.
- Describe principles of risk communication to groups and individuals affected by exposure during an MCI.
- Identify reactions to fear, panic, and stress that victims, families, and responders may exhibit during a disaster situation.
- Describe appropriate coping strategies to manage self and others.

HEALTH PROMOTION, RISK REDUCTION, AND DISEASE PREVENTION

- Identify possible threats and their potential impact on the general public, emergency medical system, and the healthcare community.
- Describe community health issues related to MCI events, specifically limiting exposure to selected agents; contamination of water, air, and food supplies; and shelter and protection of displaced persons.

HEALTHCARE SYSTEMS AND POLICY

- Define and distinguish the terms *disaster* and *MCI* in relation to other major incidents or emergency situations.
- Define relevant terminology, including:
  - CBRNE
  - Weapons of mass destruction
  - Triage

- Chain of command and management system for emergency response
- PPE
- Scene assessment
- Comprehensive emergency management
- Describe the four phases of emergency management: preparedness, response, recovery, and mitigation.
- Describe the local emergency response system for disasters.
- Describe the interaction between local, state, and federal emergency response systems.
- Describe the legal authority of public health agencies to take action to protect the community from threats, including isolation, quarantine, and required reporting and documentation.
- Discuss principles related to an MCI site as a crime scene (e.g., maintaining integrity of evidence, chain of custody).
- Recognize the impact MCIs may have on access to resources and identify how to access additional resources (e.g., pharmaceuticals, medical supplies).

ILLNESS AND DISEASE MANAGEMENT

- Discuss the differences/similarities between an intentional biological attack and that of a natural disease outbreak.
- Describe, using an interdisciplinary approach, the short-term and long-term effects of physical and psychological symptoms related to disease and treatment secondary to MCIs.

INFORMATION AND HEALTHCARE TECHNOLOGIES

- Describe use of emergency communication equipment that you will be required to use in an MCI response.
- Discuss the principles of containment and decontamination.
- Describe procedures for decontamination of self, others, and equipment for selected CBRNE agents.
- Describe how nursing skills may have to be adapted while wearing PPE.

ETHICS

- Identify and discuss ethical issues related to MCI events:
  - Rights and responsibilities of healthcare providers in MCIs (e.g., refusing to go to work or report for duty, refusal of vaccines)
  - Need to protect the public versus an individual's right for autonomy (e.g., right to leave the scene after contamination)
  - Right of the individual to refuse care, informed consent

Continued

Box 45-4

Core Competencies for Mass-Casualty Preparedness—Cont'd

- Allocation of limited resources
- Confidentiality of information related to individuals and national security
- Use of public health authority to restrict individual activities, require reporting from health professionals, and collaborate with law enforcement
- Describe the ethical, legal, psychological, and cultural considerations when dealing with the dying or the handling and storage of human remains in a mass-casualty incident.
- Identify and discuss legal and regulatory issues related to:
  - Abandonment of patients
  - Response to an MCI and one's position of employment
  - Various roles and responsibilities assumed by volunteer efforts

HUMAN DIVERSITY

- Discuss the cultural, spiritual, and social issues that may affect an individual's response to an MCI.
- Discuss the diversity of emotional, psychosocial, and sociocultural responses to terrorism or the threat of terrorism on oneself and others.

PROFESSIONAL ROLE DEVELOPMENT

- Describe these nursing roles in MCIs:
  - Researcher
  - Investigator/epidemiologist
  - EMT or first responder

- Direct care provider, generalist nurse
- Direct care provider, advanced practice nurse
- Director/coordinator of care in hospital/nurse administrator or emergency department nurse manager
- On-site coordinator of care/incident commander
- On-site director of care management
- Information provider or educator, particularly the role of the generalist nurse
- Mental health counselor
- Member of planning response team
- Member of community assessment team
- Manager or coordinator of shelter
- Member of decontamination team
- Triage officer
- Identify the most appropriate or most likely health-care role for oneself during an MCI.
- Identify the limits to one's own knowledge/skills/abilities/authority related to MCIs.
- Describe essential equipment for responding to an MCI (e.g., stethoscope, registered nurse license to deter imposters, packaged snack, change of clothing, bottles of water).
- Recognize the importance of maintaining one's expertise and knowledge in this area of practice and of participating in regular emergency response drills.
- Participate in regular emergency response drills in the community or place of employment.

REFERENCES

1. Altered standards of care in mass casualty events: bioterrorism and other public health emergencies. (April 2005). *AHRQ Publication No. 05–0043*. Rockville, Md: Agency for Healthcare Research and Quality. www.ahrq.gov/research/altstand.
2. Altered standards of care in mass casualty events. Prepared by Health Systems Research Inc. under contract 290-04-0010. (April 2005). *AHRQ Publication No. 05–0043*. Rockville, Md: Agency for Healthcare Research and Quality.
3. American Association of Critical-Care Nurses. *Statement of commitment on mass casualty and bioterrorism preparedness*. www.aacn.org/AACN/pubpolcy.nsf/vwdoc.
4. American College of Critical Care Medicine, Society of Critical Care Medicine. (2000). Consensus report for regionalization of services for critically ill or injured. *Crit Care Med, 28,* 236–239.
5. Anteau, C., & Williams, L. (1997). The Oklahoma bombing: lessons learned. *Crit Care Nurs Clin North Am, 9*(2), 231–235.
6. Barbera, J., & Macintyre, A. (2003). *Jane's mass casualty handbook: hospital emergency preparedness and response.* Surrey, U.K.: Jane's Information Group, Ltd.
7. Bradley, R. (2000). Health care facility preparation for weapons of mass destruction. *Prehosp Emerg Care, 4*(3), 261–269.
8. Bridges, E. J. (2003). Military and disaster nursing. *Crit Care Nurs Clin North Am, 15*(2), 12–14.
9. Briggs, S., & Cox, E. (2004). Disaster nursing: new frontiers for critical care. *Crit Care Nurse, 24*(3), 16–22.
10. Burkle, F. M. (2002). Mass casualty management of a large-scale bioterrorist event: an epidemiological approach that shapes triage decisions. *Emerg Med Clin North Am, 20,* 409–436.
11. Carter, G. (2001). New Jersey Hospital Association Testimony—Senate Law and Public Safety Committee. New Jersey's Disaster Preparedness Hearing. Clifton City Hall, Clifton, NJ.
12. Centers for Disease Control and Prevention (CDC). (2005).www.bt.cdc.gov.

13. de Ceballos, J. P. G., et al. (2005). The terrorist bomb explosions in Madrid, Spain—an analysis of the logistics, injuries sustained and clinical management of casualties treated at the closest hospital. *Critical Care, 9*, 104–111.

14. Inglesby, T., et al. (2000). Preventing the use of biological weapons: improving response should prevention fail. *Clin Infect Dis, 30*(6), 926–929.

15. International Coalition for Mass Casualty Education. (2004). www.INCMCE.org.

16. Johannigman, J. (2005). Disaster preparedness: it's all about me. *Crit Care Med, 33*(1, suppl), S22–S28.

17. Lingard, L., et al. (2004). The rules of the game: interprofessional collaboration on the intensive care unit team. *Crit Care, 8*, R403–R408.

18. Macintyre, A., et al. (2000). Weapons of mass destruction events with contaminated casualties: effective planning for health care facilities. *JAMA, 283*, 242–249.

19. Murray, V., & Goodfellow, F. (2002). Mass casualty chemical incidents—towards guidance for public health management. *Public Health, 116*, 2–16.

20. O'Connell, K., et al. (2002). Issues in preparedness for biological terrorism: a perspective for critical care nursing. *AACN Clin Issues, 13*(3), 452–469.

21. Pesik, N. (1999). Do U.S. emergency medicine programs provide adequate training for bioterrorism? *Ann Emerg Med, 34*, 173–176.

22. Romans, J. (2002). Tropical storm Allison: the Houston flood of June 9th, 2001. *Internet J Rescue Disaster Med, 6*(1).

23. Southwick, G., et al. (2002). Australian doctors in Bali: the initial medical response to the Bali bombing. *Med J, 177*, 624–626.

24. U.S. Army Medical Research Institute of Chemical Defense—USAMRIID 2005. Available at http://https://ccc.apgea.w.army.mil.

25. U.S. Army Medical Research Institute of Infectious Diseases—USAMRIID. 2005. www.usamriid.army.mil/education/instruct.htm.

26. Veenema, T. G. (Ed.). (2003). *Disaster nursing and emergency preparedness for chemical, biologic, and radiological terrorism and other hazards*. New York: Springer Publishing.

27. Wheeler, D., & Poss, W. (2003). Mass casualty management in a changing world. *Pediatric Ann, 32*(2), 98–105.

CHAPTER 46

Caring for the Patient in the Immediate Postoperative Period

Denise O'Brien and Sharon Dickinson

The immediate postanesthesia period is a time when patients are vulnerable and dependent secondary to the residual effects of anesthesia and the surgical procedure. Nursing care during this time focuses on assessment, anticipation, and prevention of adverse outcomes and complications, especially those related to the respiratory and cardiovascular systems. From the arrival of the patient into the postanesthesia care unit (PACU) or critical care until the patient is ready for discharge or transfer to the next level of care, the patient requires intensive and observant monitoring by nurses oriented and educated to address the special needs of this population.

Patients who have undergone major surgical procedures, with comorbidities, or who have suffered perioperative complications may require observation and monitoring in critical care. Practices vary among institutions regarding the disposition of the immediate postanesthesia patient; some institutions initiate direct operating room (OR) to critical care transfers; others require an initial transfer from the operating room to the PACU and then to critical care when the patient stabilizes. Wherever recovery from anesthesia occurs, the patient should receive the same standard of nursing care. Understanding anesthesia agents and techniques, anticipating common postanesthesia complications and emergencies, and knowledge of and adherence to the American Society of PeriAnesthesia Nurses (ASPAN) *Standards of Perianesthesia Nursing* will assist the critical care nurse to provide quality patient care regardless of the practice setting.[8]

PATIENTS AT RISK FOR POSTOPERATIVE COMPLICATIONS

Patients undergoing operative procedures with anesthesia may be at increased risk for intraoperative and postoperative complications because of preexisting medical conditions or medications. For elective surgical procedures, these comorbidities require preoperative evaluation and potential intervention to optimize the patient's physical condition for surgery.

First introduced by Saklad in 1941, the American Society of Anesthesiologists (ASA) physical status classification scale identifies patient risk for anesthetic morbidity and mortality based on history and physical examination.[60] The classification system offers the anesthesia provider information regarding the patient's status concisely and simply. The ASA physical status classification predicts risk based on the patient's coexisting medical conditions and not based on the surgical procedure (Table 46-1).

Patients are evaluated before surgery to identify risk for anesthesia and postoperative complications. Factors known to increase the patient's risk for intraoperative and postoperative complications include history of pulmonary disease (e.g., chronic obstructive pulmonary disease [COPD], smoking, reactive airway disease),

TABLE 46-1	ASA Physical Status Classification
ASA PHYSICAL STATUS	**CLASSIFICATION**
ASA or PS 1	A normal healthy patient
ASA or PS 2	Patient with mild systemic disease
ASA or PS 3	Patient with severe systemic disease
ASA or PS 4	Patient with severe systemic disease that is a constant threat to life
ASA or PS 5	Patient critically ill who will die within 24 hours with or without operative procedure
ASA or PS 6	Declared brain dead patient whose organs are being removed for donor purposes
E	Emergency, added to any of the above

ASA = American Society of Anesthesiologists, PS = physical status, E = emergency.

obesity, cardiovascular disease (e.g., coronary artery disease, hypertension, peripheral vascular disease), diabetes, extremes of age, poor nutritional status, operative procedures over 3 hours long, significant blood loss, renal or hepatic disease, and use of herbal and vitamin supplements.* These preexisting conditions can lead to increased length of hospitalization, impaired wound healing, surgical site infection, prolonged postoperative mechanical ventilation, and an overall increase in morbidity and mortality.[21,30,72]

---

*References 9, 13, 21, 23, 30, 32, 59, 62, 72.

◆ Case Study 46-1, Part A

Assessing Risk Factors of a Patient With Abdominal Aortic Aneurysm

T.R. is a 54-year-old male, ASA physical status classification 3, recently diagnosed with a 6-cm abdominal aortic aneurysm (AAA). His medical history is significant for an MI, cardiac stent placement, diabetes mellitus type 2, hypercholesterolemia, and gastroesophageal reflux disease. His social history is significant for cigarette smoking (1 ppd × 40 years) and occasional alcohol use (3 to 4 beers/week). He has no recent history of weight loss and has adequate subcutaneous fat stores. It is anticipated that he will resume eating in 2–3 days.

Home medications include the following:

Atorvastatin (Lipitor) 80 mg every day
Aspirin 81 mg every day
Nifedipine (Procardia XL) 30 mg every day
Furosemide (Lasix) 40 mg PO three times a day
Potassium (K-Dur) 20 mEq PO tid
Nitroglycerin sublingual PRN
Metoprolol (Lopressor) 25 mg twice a day
Glipizide (Glucotrol) 10 mg every day
Garlic tablets (2) every day (he stopped taking 3 weeks ago following his preoperative visits to his surgeon and anesthesia care provider)

He takes no other herbal or vitamin supplements.

Allergies: No known drug allergies; no known food or environmental allergies/sensitivities. One hour before his surgical procedure, T.R. is given cefazolin (Kefzol) 1 g IV for antibiotic prophylaxis. General anesthesia was planned based on his history, physical assessment, and surgical needs. His anesthesia was induced with propofol. Anesthesia with endotracheal intubation was maintained with isoflurane, nitrous oxide, opiates, and neuromuscular blockade throughout the 4-hour procedure.

Decision point: What are T.R.'s risk factors for his surgery and anesthesia?

Case continues on page 1300

OVERVIEW OF ANESTHESIA AND THE ANESTHETIC AGENTS

Prior to administering any anesthesia, the anesthesia care provider evaluates the patient and develops a plan based on the patient's physical status, operative procedure, and surgeon preference. Anesthesia can consist of general or regional techniques or a combination of both techniques.

GENERAL ANESTHESIA

General anesthesia is defined as "a reversible state of unconsciousness, produced by anesthetic agents, with absence of pain sensation over the entire body and a greater or lesser degree of muscular relaxation. The drugs producing this state can be administered by inhalation, intravenously, intramuscularly, or rectally."[15] Therefore general anesthesia produces amnesia, analgesia, blunting of autonomic nervous system reflexes, and some degree of muscle relaxation.[63]

Inhalation agents, introduced in the mid-1800s, are administered as vapors or gases that diffuse across air spaces and are carried by the blood to the brain to produce anesthesia. The inhalation agents first introduced included ether and nitrous oxide.[39] Ether was used until the 1960s and was replaced by halothane, the first halogenated inhalation agent.[65] Halothane was nonflammable and sweet smelling. Today, newer inhalation agents that are less toxic and less soluble have replaced halothane. Nitrous oxide, although still in use after 150 years, is not a complete anesthetic agent. It is used primarily as a carrier agent for the other gases and to diminish awareness under anesthesia.

Although inhalation agents are defined as gases, nitrous oxide is technically the only gas; the other agents are vapors of volatile (i.e., evaporate) liquids.[65] Speed of action and administration via the lungs are unique features of the inhalation agents. Establishing a partial pressure or concentration in the central nervous system produces the anesthetic state. This partial pressure is initially created in the lungs and equilibrates with the brain and spinal cord. The inhalation agents affect ventilation and perfusion. Recovery, like induction, depends on the agent's solubility and the patient's ventilation and cardiac output (CO). The inhalation agents all produce respiratory depression, vasodilation, and some degree of myocardial depression. In general, minimal metabolism of the agents occurs in the body, and elimination is primarily through the lungs. The Medication table on p. 1291 lists medications used as inhalation agents for general anesthesia.

MEDICATIONS USED AS INHALATION AGENTS FOR GENERAL ANESTHESIA

AGENT	METABOLISM/ ELIMINATION	ADVANTAGES	DISADVANTAGES
Nitrous oxide (N_2O) "gas" (1844)	Elimination via exhalation	Carrier agent Amnesia Analgesia	Fills air-containing spaces (avoid in ear, brain, bowel procedures) May increase risk of postoperative nausea and vomiting
Halothane (1956)	Primary—exhalation	Sweet-smelling, nonirritating to airway	Risk of immune-mediated hepatitis ("halothane hepatitis") Malignant hyperthermia triggering agent
Isoflurane (Forane) (1970)	Primary—exhalation	Inexpensive Nontoxic Coronary artery vasodilator	Malignant hyperthermia triggering agent
Sevoflurane (Ultane) (1984)	Primary—exhalation	Minimal odor, pungency; potent bronchodilator	Expensive May precipitate emergency agitation/ delirium, pediatrics more than adults Malignant hyperthermia-triggering agent
Desflurane (Suprane) (1990)	Least soluble, rapid elimination—exhalation	Very rapid emergence	Airway irritant Requires specialized vaporizer Expensive Malignant hyperthermia-triggering agent

Data from references 14 and 48.

Postoperatively, patients who have received the inhalation anesthetic agents require monitoring of respiratory rate and rhythm, oxygen saturation monitoring, supplemental oxygen if desaturation occurs, and stimulation and encouragement to ventilate (deep breathe). Depending on the surgical procedure and hemodynamic status, elevation of the head of bed may help the patient's oxygenation and ventilation. The newer volatile agents are rapidly eliminated from the lungs in the spontaneously breathing patient. Patients with airway obstructions or inadequate ventilatory efforts may require additional supportive care.

INTRAVENOUS AGENTS

Intravenous agents used to provide anesthesia include hypnotics/nonhypnotics, barbiturates, benzodiazepines, and analgesics. Combining intravenous agents to produce analgesia, amnesia, and muscle relaxation is called *balanced anesthesia,* or "anesthesia that uses a combination of drugs, each in an amount sufficient to produce its major or desired effect to the optimum degree and keep its undesirable or unnecessary effects to a minimum."[15]

The hypnotic agents in use today include sodium thiopental (Pentothal) and methohexital (Brevital). These barbiturates are induction agents that produce hypnosis and loss of consciousness. Nonhypnotic agents used for induction are propofol (Diprivan) and etomidate (Amidate). The benzodiazepines (diazepam [Valium], midazolam [Versed], and lorazepam [Ativan]) are agents used for anxiolysis and to produce amnesia before induction and intraoperatively. Analgesics are used to blunt cardiovascular stimulation during induction and intraoperatively, and for pain relief. The Medication table on pp. 1292-1293 lists medications commonly used for intravenous anesthesia techniques and in combination with inhalation anesthetic agents to produce general anesthesia. More comprehensive sedation and analgesia information is addressed in Chapter 4.

While not specifically anesthetic agents, antacids, gastrokinetic agents, and histamine blockers are routinely administered as part of the anesthesia plan. Antacid prophylaxis may be administered to patients at increased risk for aspiration because of a history of hiatal hernia, gastroesophageal reflux disease, and gastroparesis.[3] More information on the use of these agents is found in the Medication table on pp. 1292-1293.

MEDICATIONS USED FOR INTRAVENOUS ANESTHESIA

MEDICATION	ACTION	DOSE RANGE	SPECIAL CONSIDERATIONS
Induction Agents—Promote Unconsciousness			
Propofol (Diprivan)	Non-barbiturate hypnotic agent for induction/general anesthesia	2–2.5 mg/kg Elderly, debilitated: 1–1.5 mg/kg Maintenance: 0.1–0.2 mg/kg/min	Anti-emetic properties; pain at injection site; systemic vasodilator
Etomidate (Amidate)	Non-barbiturate hypnotic agent; induction/maintenance of general anesthesia; useful for hemodynamically unstable patients	0.2–0.6 mg/kg over 30–60 sec Maintenance: 5–20 mcg/kg/min	Pain at injection site; blocks normal stress-induced increase in adrenal cortisol production for 4–8 hr; myoclonus
Thiopental (Pentothal)	Barbiturate; induction of general anesthesia	3–5 mg/kg Maintenance: 25–100 mg as needed	May see emergence delirium, prolonged somnolence, hiccups
Methohexital (Brevital)	Barbiturate; induction of general anesthesia, cardioversion, electroconvulsive shock therapy	50–120 mg initially, 20–40 mg every 4–7 min IV	Myoclonus, hiccups, seizures
Sedatives/Amnesic Agents (Provide Amnesia and Anxiolysis)			
Midazolam (Versed)	Benzodiazepine; anxiolysis, sedation	Preoperative sedation: 0.02–0.04 mg/kg, repeat every 5 min; titrate to effect Sedation for procedures: 0.05–0.2 mg/kg	Dose needs to be individualized: reduce dose in hepatic dysfunction, elderly, COPD, CHF, concomitant CNS depressants
Diazepam (Valium)	Benzodiazepine; anxiolysis, sedation	2–10 mg	Paradoxical excitement/rage may be seen; phlebitis, pain with injection
Lorazepam (Ativan)	Benzodiazepine; anxiolysis, sedation	Preoperative sedation: 0.04–0.05 mg/kg IV, maximum 2 mg; induction agent 0.1–0.25 mg/kg IV	Given slowly and diluted
Analgesics (to Blunt Response to Surgical Stimulus and for Pain)			
Morphine	Opioid analgesic; preanesthetic medication, adjunct to general or regional anesthesia	2.5–20 mg	Hypotension, nausea, vomiting, respiratory depression
Fentanyl (Sublimaze)	Synthetic opioid analgesic; preoperative medication, adjunct to general or regional anesthesia	Preoperative sedation: 25–100 mcg Adjunct to general anesthesia (GA): 2–50 mcg/kg IV	Rapid infusion may lead to chest wall rigidity: hypotension, nausea/vomiting, respiratory depression
Remifentanil (Ultiva)	Synthetic opioid analgesic; induction (in combination with other agents)/maintenance of general anesthesia	Induction or sedation: 1 mcg/kg IV; continuous infusion: 0.5–1 mcg/kg/min	Risk of respiratory depression/muscle rigidity; ultra-short-acting—potent

MEDICATION	ACTION	DOSE RANGE	SPECIAL CONSIDERATIONS
Hydromorphone (Dilaudid)	Opioid analgesic; blunt surgical stimulus	1–4 mg IV titrated doses	Respiratory depression; less nausea/vomiting than morphine/fentanyl
Meperidine (Demerol)	Synthetic opioid analgesic; postoperative shivering	50–150 mg	Not recommended for analgesia; may precipitate serotonin syndrome*; active metabolite: normeperidine—not reversible with naloxone

Data from references 14, 48.
CHF = Congestive heart failure, CNS = central nervous system, COPD = chronic obstructive pulmonary disease, IV = intravenous.
*Serotonin syndrome can be triggered by a drug or combination of drugs (e.g., selective serotonin reuptake inhibitors [SSRIs], tricyclic antidepressants [TCAs], monoamine oxidase inhibitors [MAOIs], and other serotonergic drugs) that increase CNS serotonin receptor stimulation. Signs and symptoms include cognitive changes (disorientation, confusion), altered behavioral status (agitation, restlessness), autonomic nervous system instability (fever, shivering, diaphoresis, tachycardia, diarrhea), and neuromuscular changes (tremors, hyperreflexia, myoclonus, ataxia). The addition of a second serotonergic drug may trigger these symptoms.[24]

NEUROMUSCULAR BLOCKING AGENTS

Neuromuscular blocking agents (NMBAs) include depolarizing agents (agents that mimic acetylcholine) and nondepolarizing agents (agents that interfere or block the action of acetylcholine).[65] The only depolarizing agent used in the United States is succinylcholine (Anectine), a rapid-acting skeletal muscle relaxant used for intubation and rapid-sequence induction of anesthesia. It has an onset of approximately 30 to 60 seconds and duration of 3 to 5 minutes. Adverse effects of succinylcholine include myalgias, hyperkalemia, increased intracranial pressure, and increased intraocular pressure). It is also known to be a triggering agent for malignant hyperthermia. Patients with histories of pseudocholinesterase deficiency, either hereditary or from disease processes (e.g., febrile disorders, hepatic disease, use of echothiophate eye drops), will have prolonged neuromuscular blocks, often requiring endotracheal intubation and mechanical ventilation.[65] Drugs such as the anticholinesterases do not antagonize.[20]

Nondepolarizing agents are either spontaneously reversible or reversible with pharmacologic intervention. Pharmacologic reversal includes an anticholinesterase (e.g., neostigmine [Prostigmin]) and anticholinergic (e.g., glycopyrrolate to counteract the muscarinic effects of the anticholinesterase agent). Muscarinic effects include bradycardia, salivation, miosis, and hyperperistalsis.[16]

The nondepolarizing agents are not known to trigger malignant hyperthermia crisis. Metabolism and elimination of the NMBAs vary with the agents. Atracurium (Tracrium) and cisatracurium (Nimbex) are eliminated through Hofmann degradation; warming may speed reversal of these agents. Hofmann degradation, or elimination, is a spontaneous, nonbiologic process in plasma at normal pH and temperature and does not depend on circulating esterases.[16,61] Pancuronium (Pavulon) is primarily excreted by the kidneys and mivacurium (Mivacron) through pseudocholinesterase; vecuronium (generic) has primarily renal but some hepatic elimination.

REGIONAL ANESTHESIA

Regional anesthesia is "the production of insensibility of a part by interrupting the sensory nerve conductivity from that region of the body. It may be produced by field block, the creation of walls of anesthesia encircling the operative field by means of injections of a local anesthetic; or nerve block, injection of the anesthetic agent close to the nerves whose conductivity is to be cut off. These are also called blocks, blockages, block a., and conduction a."[15]

Local Anesthetics

Local anesthetics are used to produce the anesthesia or analgesia when using regional techniques, as indicated in the Medication table on p. 1294. The agents are either esters or amides. Ester local anesthetics include cocaine (used topically), procaine (Novocain) (used topically, by infiltration, or nerve block applications), chloroprocaine (Nesacaine) (low risk of systemic toxicity), and tetracaine (longest duration). These agents are not as widely used as the amide local anesthetics. Esters are less stable than amides and may cause rare allergic reactions.[37]

MEDICATIONS COMMONLY USED AS LOCAL ANESTHETICS

AGENT	USE	SPECIAL CONSIDERATIONS
Amides		
Lidocaine	Topical, infiltration, field block, spinal, epidural, caudal (also used as an antidysrhythmic)	Most versatile; rapid onset, intense analgesia Class Ib antidysrhythmic agent
Bupivacaine	Infiltration, nerve block, spinal, epidural	Most widely used
Ropivacaine	Spinal, epidural (labor)	Less cardiotoxic, less potent than bupivacaine
Levobupivacaine	Infiltration, spinal, epidural	Similar to bupivacaine
Mepivacaine	Infiltration, nerve block	Derivative of lidocaine, slower metabolism, ineffective topically
Dibucaine	Topical agent	
Etidocaine	Epidural, nerve block	Rare use; less sensory nerve blockade, similar to bupivacaine in cardiotoxic properties
Esters		
Cocaine	Topical	CNS depression/stimulation; tachydysrhythmias
Chloroprocaine	Nerve block, epidural	
Tetracaine	Spinal, topical	Long duration of action

Data from references 37, 48, 52.
CNS = Central nervous system.

Amide local anesthetics include lidocaine (Xylocaine), bupivacaine (Marcaine), mepivacaine (Carbocaine), levobupivacaine (Chirocaine), ropivacaine (Naropin), dibucaine (Nupercainal), and etidocaine. Allergic reactions are extremely rare with amide local anesthetic agents.

Systemic toxicity may occur following an inappropriately high dose or accidental intravascular injection.[37] Early signs involve the central nervous system including circumoral numbness, dizziness, slurred speech, tinnitus, confusion, and restlessness. Cardiovascular signs may be bradycardia, with subsequent conduction block, multifocal ectopic beats, reentrant dysrhythmias, tachycardia, and ventricular fibrillation. Treatment is supportive and may include oxygen supplementation, fluids, anticonvulsants, and vasoconstrictor and inotropic medications. Dysrhythmias may be treated with amiodarone (Cordarone). Recent evidence suggests lipid emulsion infusions and clonidine (Catapres) may be useful in these toxic reactions.[37]

Central Neuraxial Blocks. Spinal anesthesia, also referred to as intrathecal, subarachnoid, or SA block, produces sensory, motor, and sympathetic block of the nerve roots. Injection of the local anesthesia agents into the cerebrospinal fluid at the level of L3-4 or L4-5 provides variable duration of lower abdominal and lower extremity anesthesia. Loss of sympathetic tone can result in significant hypotension, usually responsive to ephedrine intravenously. Other complications include bladder atony, high spinal block, hematoma formation, post–dural puncture headache, and low back pain.[50,53] Infrequently, neurologic injury can occur from local anesthetic toxicity or inadvertent intravascular injection.

Epidural anesthesia (injection of local anesthesia into the epidural space) provides sensory and motor blockade, and less sympathetic block than spinal anesthesia. Epidural approaches may be used as the sole anesthetic or in combination with spinal anesthesia or general anesthesia techniques. Lumbar and thoracic approaches are used depending on the level of anesthesia or analgesia required for the operative procedure (Figure 46-1). The epidural catheter may remain in place after the surgery for postoperative pain

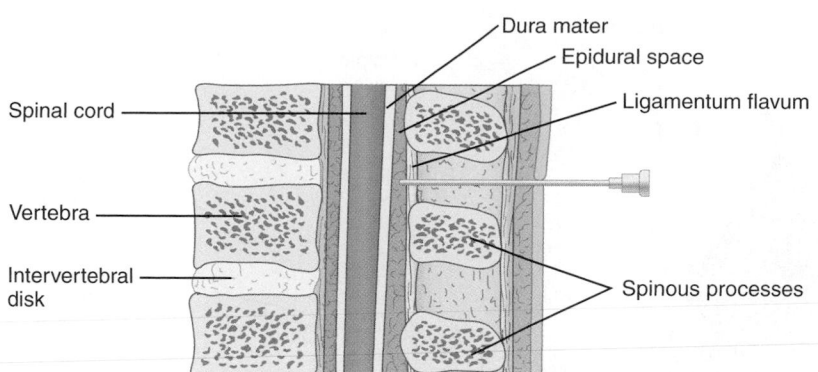

⬍FIGURE 46-1 Anatomy for epidural placement.

management or removed following the operative procedure. An epidural catheter may also be placed preoperatively for postoperative analgesia and attached to a pump after surgery for continued postoperative pain management. Potential complications include epidural hematoma formation, catheter migration or break, intravascular injection, post–dural puncture headache, and local anesthetic systemic toxicity.[50]

Local anesthesia injected through the lower back into the caudal space leading to sacral and perineal sensory block is called "caudal anesthesia." It is rarely used in adults and has a failure rate of 3% to 5%.[11]

Peripheral Nerve Blocks. Peripheral nerve blocks are used for anesthesia and postoperative analgesia. Blocks may be appropriate as adjuncts to general anesthesia or used as the sole anesthetic. Benefits include decreased pain and use of postoperative opioids, and subsequently less nausea, vomiting, and sedation.[18] Patients who have had these blocks may be seen in critical care either postoperatively after procedures during which the blocks were used, or as the result of complications resulting from block placement or local anesthetic side effects.

Cervical Plexus. Cervical plexus blocks provide anesthesia for surgical procedures in the distribution of C2 to C4, including lymph node dissections, plastic repairs, and carotid endarterectomy (Figure 46-2).[74] Patients remain awake; neurologic status should be monitored continuously. Tracheostomy and thyroidectomy can be performed using a bilateral cervical plexus block. Complications include intravascular injection producing blockade of the phrenic and superior laryngeal nerves, and spread of local anesthetic solution into the epidural and subarachnoid spaces.

Brachial Plexus. An interscalene brachial plexus block is commonly used to provide anesthesia and analgesia for shoulder and upper arm surgery (Figure 46-3).[18,74]

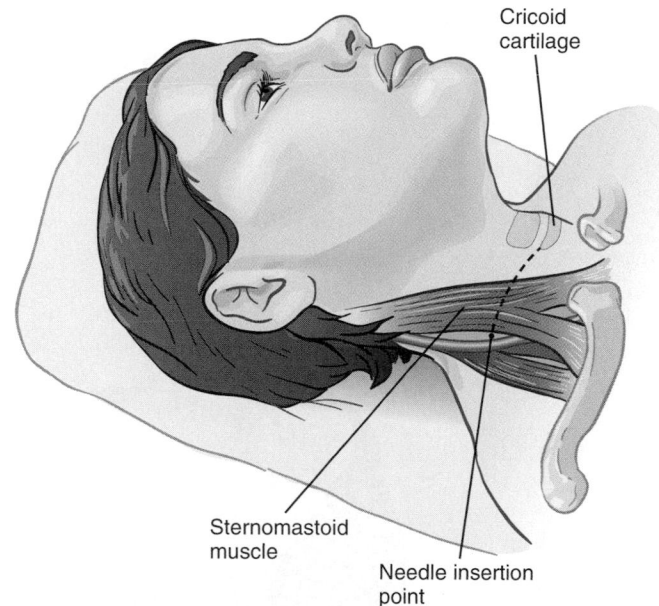

⬍FIGURE 46-2 Superficial cervical plexus block.

Complications include ipsilateral phrenic nerve block with diaphragmatic paralysis and, rarely, severe hypotension and bradycardia (i.e., Bezold-Jarisch reflex).[74]

Supraclavicular blocks are indicated for operations on the elbow, forearm, and hand (Figure 46-4). Pneumothorax is a potential complication of this block, and onset of symptoms is usually delayed for up to 24 hours. Other complications include frequent phrenic nerve block (40% to 60%), Horner syndrome, and neuropathy.[74] Horner syndrome, caused by paralysis of the cervical sympathetic nerve trunk, is characterized by contraction of the pupil, partial ptosis of the eyelid, enophthalmos, and sometimes loss of sweating on the ipsilateral side of the block.[67] The phrenic block or cervical sympathetic block is self-limited. The patient needs reassurance the effects are temporary and will resolve in time.

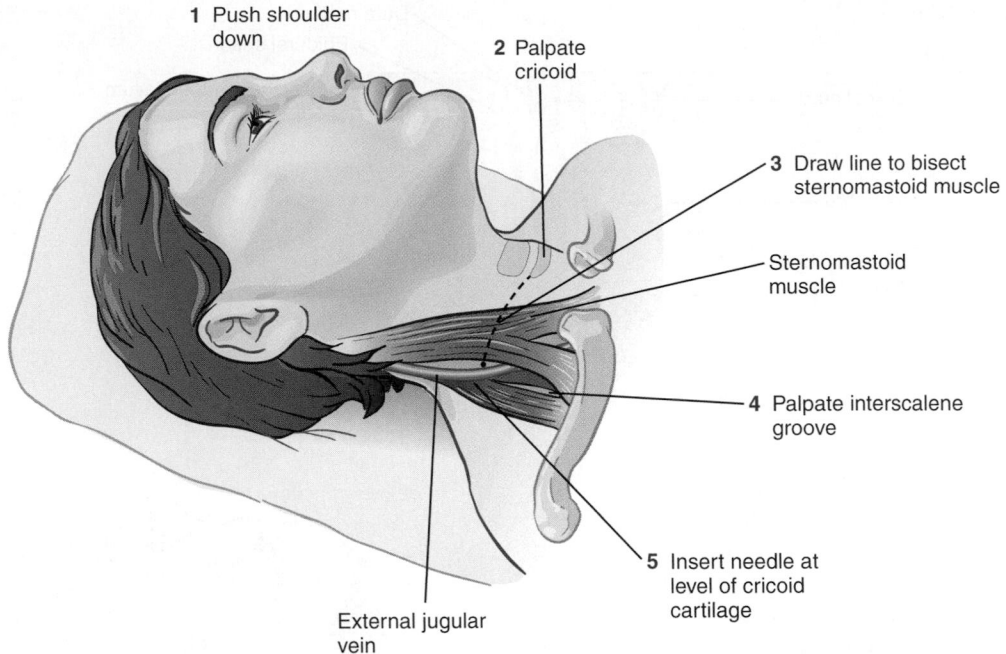

1 Push shoulder down

2 Palpate cricoid

3 Draw line to bisect sternomastoid muscle

Sternomastoid muscle

4 Palpate interscalene groove

5 Insert needle at level of cricoid cartilage

External jugular vein

FIGURE 46-3 Interscalene approach to brachial plexus block.

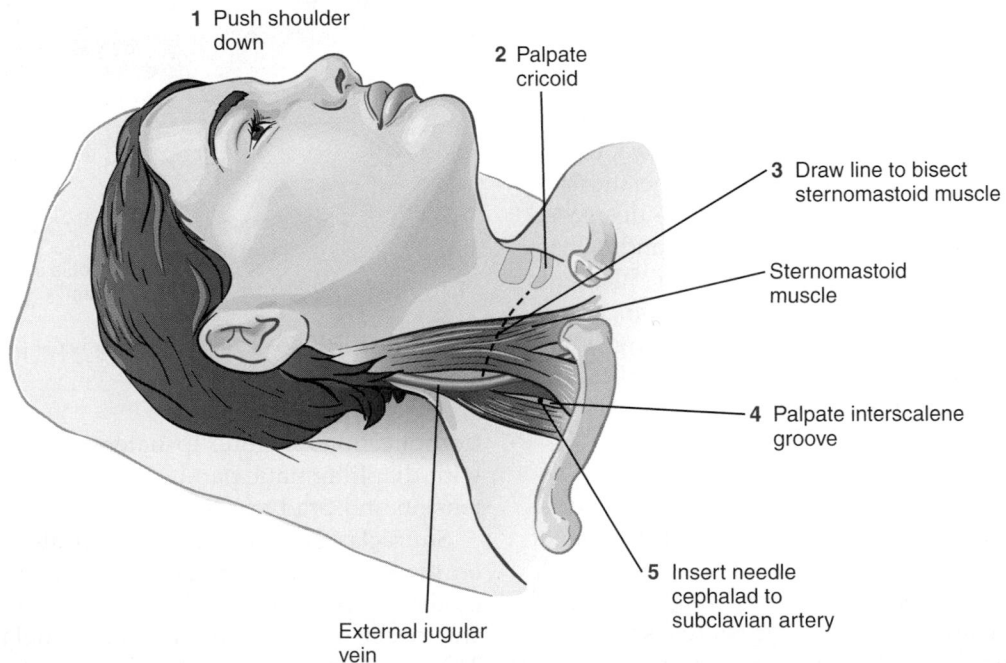

1 Push shoulder down

2 Palpate cricoid

3 Draw line to bisect sternomastoid muscle

Sternomastoid muscle

4 Palpate interscalene groove

5 Insert needle cephalad to subclavian artery

External jugular vein

FIGURE 46-4 Supraclavicular approach to brachial plexus block.

The infraclavicular block provides anesthesia to the arm and hand. The approach to the plexus is blind, thus increasing the risk of intravascular injection.[74] Other complications include pneumothorax, infection, and hematoma.[74]

Forearm, hand, and elbow surgery may be performed with an axillary block (Figure 46-5).[18,74] This technique may be used for vascular access procedures. Significant complications include nerve injury and systemic toxicity from intravascular injection. Hematoma

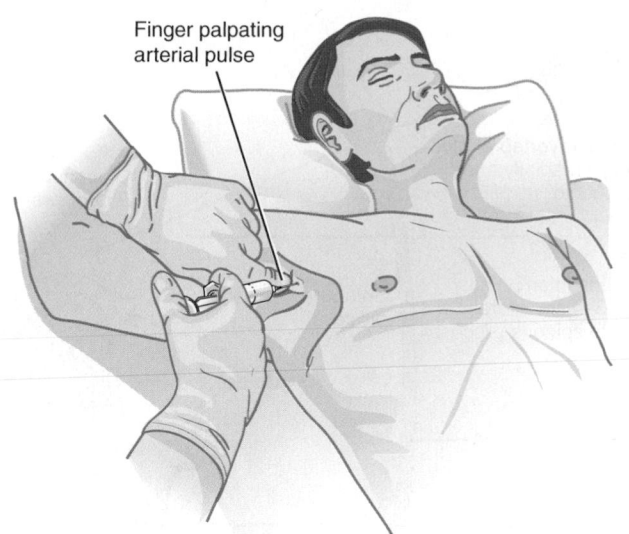

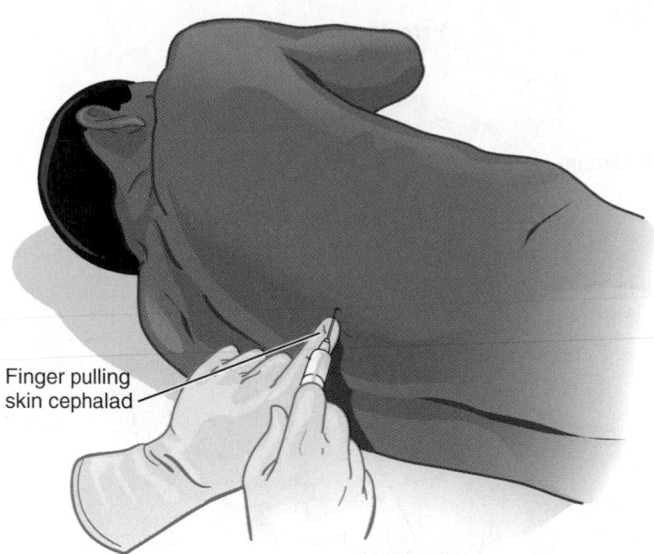

⬍FIGURE 46-5 Approach and needle insertion position for axillary block.

⬍FIGURE 46-6 Approach and needle insertion position for intercostal nerve block.

and infection are rare complications. Unlike the risk with the other brachial plexus approaches, central neural blockade and pneumothorax are not complications of the axillary approach.[74]

Intercostal Nerve Block and Interpleural Catheter Placement. Patients with contraindications to neuraxial blockade may have intercostal nerve blocks or interpleural catheters placed (Figures 46-6 and 46-7). When combined with celiac plexus blocks and light general anesthesia, they may also be used for intra-abdominal

procedures.[74] Pneumothorax is the most common complication of the intercostal nerve block.[74]

Celiac Plexus Block. The celiac plexus block can be combined with intercostal block to provide anesthesia for intra-abdominal surgery (Figure 46-8).[74] Reduction of stress and endocrine responses to operative procedures is possible with this block because of autonomic nervous system blockade. Complications that may occur include hypotension; spinal, epidural, or intravascular injection; pneumothorax; puncture of the kidney, ureter, or intestine; and retroperitoneal hematoma.[74]

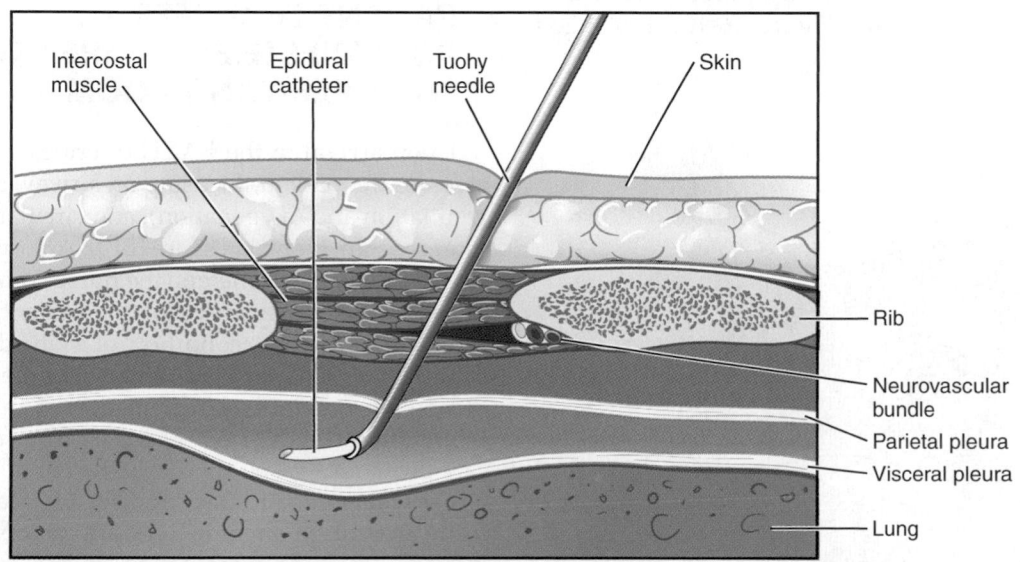

⬍FIGURE 46-7 Placement of epidural catheter for interpleural block.

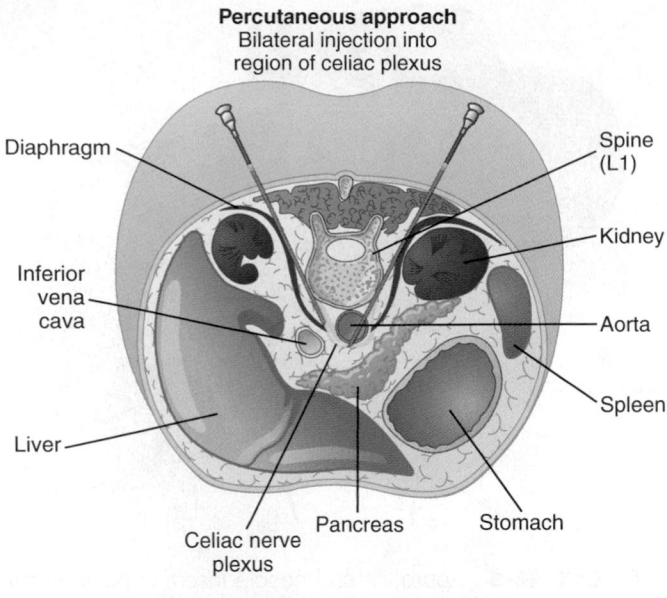

FIGURE 46-8 Celiac plexus block.

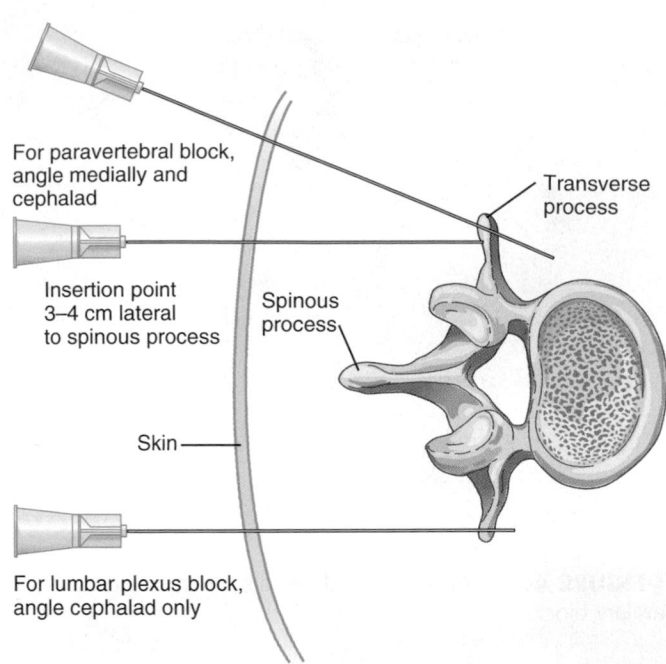

FIGURE 46-10 Needle insertion points for lumbar plexus blocks.

Paraverterbral Block. The paravertebral block may be used to provide anesthesia and analgesia for thoracic, abdominal, pelvic, and upper leg surgery (Figure 46-9). Local anesthetic injection in the epidural or subarachnoid space is possible because of the proximity of the central neuraxis during placement.[74] There is a risk of intravascular injection through the lumbar vessels, vena cava, or aorta. Although this block has multiple uses and advantages over thoracic epidural anesthesia and is less difficult to place, it is not widely used at this time.[18]

Lumbar Plexus. Three main terminal nerves (femoral, lateral femoral cutaneous, and obturator) can be reliably anesthetized for knee and hip procedures with a block of the lumbar plexus (Figure 46-10). Prolonged

postoperative analgesia can be achieved using continuous catheter techniques.[18] Single-injection blocks may regress over 10 to 18 hours after the local anesthetic injection, reducing the benefits of blocks for postoperative pain management. Potential risks include epidural, subarachnoid, or intravascular injection and peripheral nerve damage.[74]

PATIENT TRANSFER TO POSTANESTHESIA CARE FROM THE OPERATING ROOM

Upon arrival to the PACU or critical care, the nurse assesses the patient, focusing on airway, breathing (i.e., ventilation and oxygenation), and circulation (i.e., heart rate/rhythm, blood pressure [BP]). After the initial evaluation of these parameters, the nurse completes a quick "head-to-toe" assessment of the patient, determining intravenous access; condition of skin, dressings, and drains; and comfort status. Following the initial assessment of the patient and management of any acute issues, the nurse receives a verbal report from the anesthesia care provider.

Components of the transfer of care summary from anesthesia include relevant preoperative status (history, physical examination, mental/emotional status); anesthesia/sedation technique and agents used;

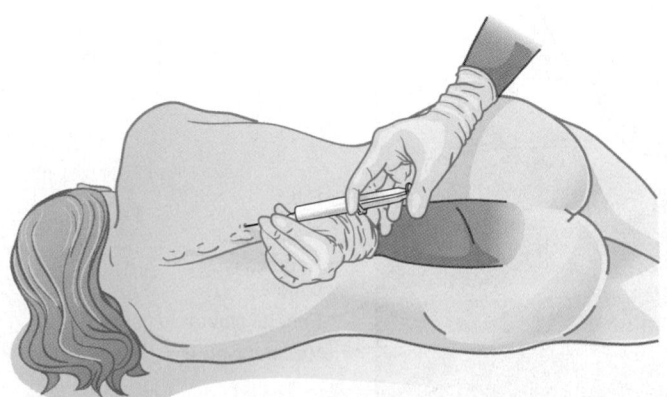

FIGURE 46-9 Approach and needle insertion position for thoracic paravertebral block.

reversal agents given; procedure(s) performed; length of anesthesia/sedation and operative procedure; analgesics and review of postoperative pain management plan; medications administered; estimated fluid/blood loss and replacement; and complications during anesthesia and operative course, treatment, and response (Table 46-2).[8]

Following report, the nurse indicates verbal acceptance of transfer of care and responsibility for the patient from the anesthesia care provider. If questions remain related to the patient's safety or physical status, the nurse should not accept the transfer. The plan of care for the immediate postanesthesia period includes pain and comfort management, fluid management, establishment of hemodynamic stability, and management of potential complications (e.g., postoperative nausea, vomiting, or postanesthetic shivering).

The American Association of Critical-Care Nurses (AACN) produces *Standards for Critical Care Nursing* with recommendations for monitoring, staffing, and patient care. The ASPAN establishes *Standards of Perianesthesia Nursing Practice* for all postanesthesia patients. These standards include assessment, monitoring, and staffing guidelines for this postanesthesia patient population. Regardless of the location of the postanesthesia care, whether in critical care or the PACU, the same standards for recovery and stabilization apply (AACN/ASPAN/ASA Joint Statement on ICU Overflow).[8] Full details can be found in the ASPAN *Standards of Perianesthesia Nursing Practice.*[8]

Although one normally thinks of operative complications occurring in the OR, they often occur wherever the patient is during the postoperative period. For example, decreased stimulation, delayed drug absorption, or slow drug elimination may contribute to residual sedation or cardiopulmonary depression. Currently, there are insufficient data to examine the effects of post-procedural monitoring on patient outcomes in the postoperative period. However, it is widely accepted that continuous observation and monitoring of the patient during this critical period can decrease the likelihood of adverse events. Therefore patients should be observed in an appropriately staffed and equipped area (i.e., PACU or critical care) until they are near their baseline level of consciousness and are no longer at risk for cardiopulmonary compromise.

TABLE 46-2 Transfer of Care Summary

PREOPERATIVE	OPERATIVE	POSTOPERATIVE
History—including chronic medical conditions	Procedure performed and complications	Procedure performed and complications
Allergies	Allergies Pertinent history and medications	Level of consciousness
Physical exam (focus on cardiovascular, respiratory, endocrine, skin assessment)	Airway management (e.g., ease of intubation or difficult airway management)	Vital signs
Mental/emotional status	Anesthetics given Length of anesthesia	Airway and ventilation status
Medications—pertinent (status of medications: taken, held)	Reversal agents used	IV access points, fluid rates, blood products, intake/output
Fasting status	Other medications given (including antiemetics, anxiolytics/sedatives, analgesics)	Analgesics given
Pain assessment and management plan	Estimated blood loss, urinary output, other losses/output	Pain management plan
	Fluids and blood products given	Other medications given
	Pain management plan	Medications/allergies

Assessing and Managing a Postoperative Patient With Abdominal Aortic Aneurysm

T.R. had an uneventful intra-operative AAA repair, during which he received 1 unit of packed red blood cells, 1 L of colloid, and 3 L of crystalloid for an estimated blood loss of 1100 ml. He was extubated in the OR and transported to critical care for postanesthesia recovery. He had a lumbar epidural catheter (L2) placed preoperatively for pain management, which was utilized on arrival to critical care. Vitals signs are the following: BP 165/70 mm Hg, heart rate 65 beats/min, respiratory rate 24 breaths/min; SpO_2 97% on 3 L of oxygen via nasal cannula. His temperature is 36.4° C. He is pink, with an oxygen saturation of 97%. The pulmonary artery catheter readings are as follows: pulmonary artery pressure 42/17 mm Hg, PAWP 17 mm Hg, CVP 13 mm Hg, mixed venous oxygen saturation, 69%. His extremities are warm and well perfused, with a capillary refill time of 2 seconds. He has a nasogastric tube in place, draining yellow fluid. A urine catheter is draining clear straw-colored urine. Abdominal dressing is dry and intact. Bilateral pedal pulses palpable. Head of bed is elevated 30 degrees. T.R.'s breath sounds are clear in all lung fields. He is awake and alert, responding to verbal commands, moving all 4 extremities, not agitated, and resting peacefully. He moves all extremities on command; he denies numbness in lower extremities. Self-reported pain score 4 (0–10 scale); he states he is nauseated. T.R.'s initial electrolytes are sodium 140 mEq/L, potassium 3.7 mEq/L, chloride 110 mEq/L, HCO_3^- 23 mEq/L, creatinine 1.2 mg/dl, magnesium 1.6 mEq/L, ionized calcium 4 mg/dl, and glucose 155 mg/dl. The epidural solution is a combination of bupivacaine 0.0625% and hydromorphone 10 mcg/ml at the following settings: continuous rate of 6, demand of 3, lock out of 15 minutes.

Decision point: What is your interpretation of his postoperative status and what interventions are needed?

Most patients recover from anesthesia or surgery without incident. However, there is a group of patients who have preexisting comorbid states that put them at a higher risk for life-threatening complication status. The staff needs to anticipate these complications and react with immediate and thoughtful intervention.

As is the case with much of critical care, initial postanesthesia care should be managed in terms of the ABCs: airway (patency), breathing (respiratory status, breath sounds, oxygen therapy, and oxygen saturation), and circulation (BP, pulse, cardiac rhythm, fluid and electrolyte balance including urine output, and hemodynamic readings from central venous catheters and pulmonary artery catheters [PACs]). After the ABCs are stabilized, ongoing assessment and management should include, but not be limited to, monitoring neurologic status including level of consciousness, mentation, and sensorimotor functioning; thermoregulation, promoting normothermia; pain management as well as physical and emotional comfort; and procedural/surgical specific care.

Respiratory Complications

Respiratory complications are perhaps the most common and dangerous in the immediate postoperative patient. PACU and critical care staff should anticipate and closely monitor the development of respiratory compromise. The signs and symptoms of respiratory compromise include tachypnea, dyspnea, increased work of breathing, shallow respirations, and decreased oxygen saturation. Other, nonrespiratory signs of respiratory distress include agitation and an altered level of consciousness.

Respiratory complications can be divided into upper airway dysfunction and alterations in pulmonary mechanics or breathing.[43] Upper airway dysfunction can be subtle in the postoperative patient. Initially, there may only be some dyspnea that can be easily overlooked. However, even though the work of breathing has increased, observant staff will notice a decrease in breath sounds and air movement. This is followed by a decrease in oxygen saturation. The most common cause of upper airway obstruction is a loss of muscle tone often with the tongue falling posteriorly. This can be treated with a jaw thrust that pulls the tongue anteriorly (Figure 46-11) or with placement of an oral airway. Occasionally the loss of muscle tone can result from oversedation. In this instance, it can be effectively treated with pharmacologic reversal agents. Laryngospasm is another cause of upper airway obstruction that generally requires intubation. Lastly, upper airway obstruction can occur as the result of external trauma or by airway damage, or edema as the result of the operative procedure itself.

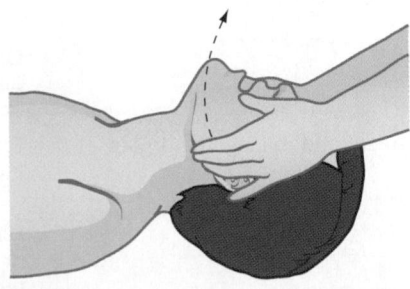

◆**FIGURE 46-11** Jaw-thrust airway maneuver.

In this situation, intubation or tracheostomy may be necessary.

Postoperative patients are also at risk for developing alterations in breathing or lower respiratory tract dysfunction. This most commonly results from atelectasis. Effects of pain (especially from chest or abdominal incisions) and sedation can increase the incidence of atelectasis. Rales or crackles can often be auscultated in dependent portions of the lungs of patients with atelectasis. Atelectasis can be treated with adequate pain control to encourage coughing and deep breathing.[75] Pneumothorax can develop, compressing the lung, and may be a complication of chest or neck surgery, or central line placement. Occasionally patients with preexisting significant COPD can rupture a bleb while being ventilated, causing a pneumothorax. With a pneumothorax, reduced breath sounds will be auscultated on the affected side. Accumulation of more air in the pleural space may lead to further collapse of the affected lung and displacement of the trachea and mediastinal structures to the opposite side. In general, a pneumothorax of less than 20% is asymptomatic and will not require chest tube placement. In patients who are symptomatic, a chest tube may be needed.

Lower respiratory tract dysfunction in postoperative patients can result from pulmonary edema. Operative patients often accumulate interstitial fluid, requiring additional fluids throughout the procedure to maintain preload and CO. These additional fluids may lead to hypervolemia; occasionally, this fluid accumulates in the lungs, resulting in pulmonary edema. The stress of surgery can also lead to cardiac dysfunction, further exacerbating pulmonary edema. Treatment of pulmonary edema involves fluid restriction or diuretics. An additional sign of fluid overload may be a falling hematocrit (Hct) as the excess intravascular fluid dilutes the red blood cells. However, extreme caution should be used in assuming that a falling Hct is a sign of fluid overload. It may be a sign of blood loss and the need for additional fluids.

Cardiovascular Complications

Postoperative patients frequently develop cardiovascular complications. The primary manifestation of cardiovascular dysfunction is poor perfusion. Signs and symptoms of this include tachycardia, hypotension, and poor peripheral perfusion as demonstrated by cool, pale extremities and poor capillary refill (greater than 3 seconds). However, poor peripheral perfusion can be misleading in patients with preexisting peripheral vascular disease.

Diminished CO could be due either to primary cardiac dysfunction or to insufficient preload causing secondary cardiac dysfunction. Differentiation between these two states can best be made by examining the central venous pressure (CVP) or the pulmonary artery wedge pressure (PAWP). In cardiac disease, these pressures are often elevated, whereas if insufficient preload is the problem, CVP and PAWP will be low. Insufficient preload is common in the postoperative patient.

Insufficient preload in the postoperative patient can result from bleeding at the operative site, occult bleeding in the gastrointestinal tract (e.g., stress gastritis or peptic ulcer disease), or bleeding from other organs. If bleeding is suspected, the Hct should be checked and vital signs monitored closely. Large amounts of blood can escape the vascular space without obvious outward signs. The abdominal cavity, pleural space, or thighs may sequester large blood volumes following injury or operative procedures with inadequate hemostasis. When bleeding is present, red blood cells should be replaced, along with attempts made to correct low platelet counts and abnormal blood coagulation as measured by the prothrombin time (PT) and partial thromboplastin time (PTT), if necessary. A more common cause of insufficient cardiac preload is the movement of fluid into the interstitial space that often occurs during surgery. Frequently, patients just out of the OR will continue to require large amounts of crystalloid solution to maintain their CVP and CO. Lastly, some surgeries include treatment of infectious sites, such as abscesses. This can lead to endotoxemia, sepsis, and interstitial fluid movement in the immediate postoperative period. Additional fluids will be required.

Cardiac causes of poor CO are also quite common in the postoperative patient. The stress of a major surgery, stimulating a neuroendocrine response, can worsen preexisting coronary artery disease, leading to myocardial infarction (MI). Unlike a nonoperative patient, postoperative patients are often sedated or given analgesics. Therefore patients may not complain of chest pain even in the presence of a significant MI. Another cause of cardiac dysfunction, as the result of the interstitial fluid shifts, is pulmonary edema.

Stressful stimuli (e.g., surgical incisions, organ manipulation) can elicit an adrenergic response precipitating transient increases in heart rate and BP.[57] This stress of surgery can lead to cardiac dysfunction and exacerbate pulmonary edema. Patients with histories of coronary artery disease frequently are taking beta-blocker medications. Beta blockade does not reduce the neuroendocrine response. This suggests that the beta blockade is not responsible for improved cardiovascular outcomes.[77] Several advantages can be gained from use of beta blockers, including decreased analgesic requirements, faster recovery from anesthesia, and improved hemodynamic stability.[77]

Hypertension in postoperative patients is usually the result of a preexisting condition, aggravated by withholding the patient's medications before or during surgery.[27] Although postoperative patients often require large amounts of crystalloid, too much fluid may also lead to hypertension, especially in patients with a history of renal disease or after operations that involve the urinary tract. Hypertension can also be an early sign of pain or fluid overload.

Postoperative patients are often immobilized for prolonged periods of time both in the OR and in critical care, leading to deep vein thrombosis (DVT). DVT prophylaxis (see Chapter 9) has received a great deal of attention recently; there are several therapeutic maneuvers to prevent this often life-threatening complication. Previously, restrictive stockings were thought to be sufficient to prevent DVTs. However, sequential compression devices (SCDs) and foot-pump devices have been found more effective.[33] SCDs encircle the lower extremities and are sequentially inflated and deflated to compress the legs and move venous blood to the heart. Although SCDs are somewhat effective for the legs, DVTs can form in other large veins. Thus anticoagulation with subcutaneous heparin, including low molecular weight (LMW) heparin, is more effective. LMW heparin is much more expensive than heparin and not generally considered a first-line agent. Warfarin (Coumadin) can take several days to fully anticoagulate a patient and is not used in the immediate postoperative period. Although anticoagulation is often the preferred method of DVT prophylaxis for hospitalized patients, great care should be used because of the risk of bleeding at the operative site. Thus many postoperative patients receive SCDs.

Central Nervous System Complications

Unless patients are intentionally sedated postoperatively, emergence from anesthesia should occur rapidly and predictably. Return to baseline neurologic status is expected in the immediate postanesthesia period. Level of consciousness, response to commands, and ability to move extremities purposefully are assessed and documented. Orientation to person, place, and time begins as the patient awakens. Muscle strength is evaluated through hand grasps, ability to raise head, and plantar extension. Any deviation from baseline status is noted and reported.

Patients undergoing procedures with potential neurologic injury or following trauma require close observation and assessment. Complete neurologic status is examined. The Glasgow Coma Scale is commonly used to quickly and consistently monitor neurologic status.

Infrequently, either patients will awaken abruptly, agitated and unresponsive to commands, or emergence will be delayed. Emergence delirium or excitement is characterized by restlessness, disorientation, crying, moaning, and inappropriate behavior.[54] Initial assessment includes oxygenation and ventilation status to rule out hypoxemia or pain as a cause of the excitement. Other causes include preexisting agitation or anxiety, drugs, incomplete reversal of neuromuscular blocking agents, withdrawal from alcohol or drugs, full bladder, acid-base disturbances, and electrolyte abnormalities. If pain is determined to be the cause of agitation, it is difficult to determine when to administer additional analgesia. Obviously, allowing the agitated patient to return to a full level of consciousness before analgesic administration might result in a great deal of needless pain. However, one should not jump to this conclusion without careful consideration of other causes of agitation. Premature analgesic administration may delay the treatment of these causes.

Delayed emergence from anesthesia may be due to prolonged drug effects, metabolic problems, or neurologic injury.[54] Drug effects may include overdosage, inadequate reversal, or altered metabolism or elimination of drugs. Electrolyte imbalances may result in decreased awareness or an altered level of consciousness. Neurologic injury may be the result of tissue damage or an anoxic event. The response is that the patient fails to respond as expected during emergence from anesthesia. Maintenance of adequate ventilation, oxygen saturation, and CO is essential while potential causes are evaluated. A thorough review of the anesthesia course is initiated, metabolic disturbances are corrected, and, if no other cause is identified, a complete neurologic examination is performed.

Electrolytes

Assessment of the serum electrolyte values and potential interventions are a vital component in caring for a critically ill patient in the postoperative period. Electrolyte concentrations influence metabolic activities as well as fluid movement within and between body compartments. Abnormal electrolyte values may be the result of fluid shifts, acid-base imbalances, or renal or endocrine dysfunction. Monitoring of the patient's electrolyte status, specifically potassium, calcium, and magnesium, in the immediate postoperative period can prevent hemodynamic instability and cardiac dysfunction.

The most common electrolyte disturbances seen in the postoperative period include hypokalemia from fluid resuscitation or nasogastric losses; hyperkalemia from tissue catabolism or acidosis; hypocalcemia from alkalosis, administration of citrated blood, or hemodilution; and hypomagnesemia from gastrointestinal or urinary losses. Hypomagnesemia has been associated with a higher mortality and worse clinical outcomes in the critical care setting (see Chapter 32).[69]

Nutrition

Nutrition (see Chapter 6) is important for the rapid and complete recovery of the postoperative patient. Good nutrition improves wound healing, decreases the time patients require mechanical ventilation, results in fewer infectious complications, and reduces length of stay.[55] A nutritional assessment should be made soon after the patient is admitted to critical care (Figure 46-12).

The first consideration is to determine if the patient is already malnourished. Many critically ill postoperative patients have had prolonged illnesses before surgery that can result in malnutrition. The nutritional assessment should include pertinent historical data such as weight loss or decreased caloric intake. On physical exam, malnourished patients may have a decrease in weight and a loss of subcutaneous fat in the triceps or buttocks. If a patient is malnourished, nutritional management should be considered as soon as the patient is stabilized.[58] The gastrointestinal tract is the preferred choice because it has far fewer complications (e.g., infection) than intravenous or parenteral nutrition. Most critically ill patients cannot take sufficient calories orally, and a feeding tube must be used.[55] Tube feedings are usually begun continuously at small volumes and then increased as tolerated by the patient. It should be remembered that even very small amounts of tube feedings (5 to 10 ml/hour) have beneficial effects on the gut.[44] Patients usually cannot tolerate the large glucose loads initially, because they may precipitate hyperglycemia. Recent studies have shown a markedly improved survival for critical care patients who receive tight glucose level control.[12,73]

Thermoregulation

Thermoregulation during the perioperative period ranges from the hypothermic to the hyperthermic state. Normothermia is defined as a core temperature between 36° and 38° C. Temperature is assessed when the patient arrives in the PACU or critical care and periodically throughout the patient's recovery and postoperative care.

Hypothermia is defined as a core temperature below 36° C. Patients who are hypothermic should have temperatures assessed every 30 minutes until normothermia is achieved.[6] Hypothermia normally results in an increased catecholamine level, causing tachycardia, peripheral vasoconstriction, and hypertension. However, anesthetic agents blunt the peripheral vasoconstriction, resulting in little change in BP in the postoperative patient. Hypothermia can produce patient discomfort, untoward cardiac events, adrenergic stimulation, impaired platelet function, altered drug metabolism, and impaired wound healing with increased risk of infection.[6] Active warming measures include application of a forced-air warming system, passive

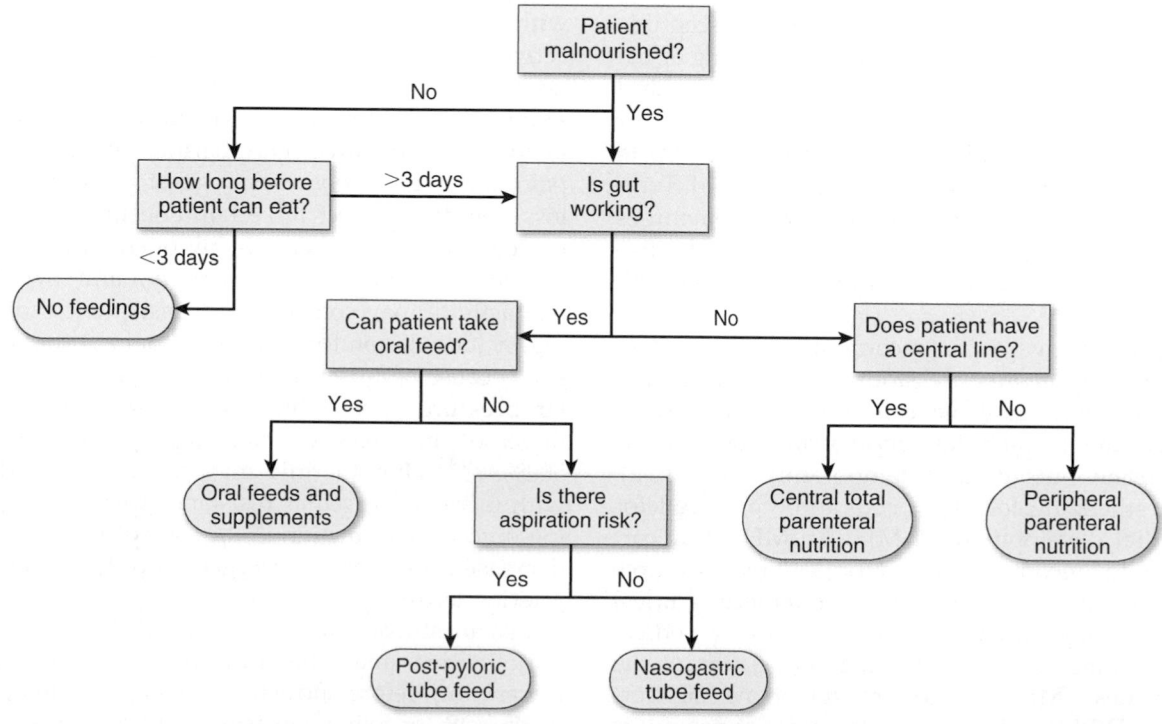

⇕FIGURE 46-12 Postoperative nutrition algorithm.

insulation (with warm blankets, socks, head coverings, circulating water mattress/pads), increased room temperature, warmed intravenous solutions, and humidified and warmed supplemental oxygen.[6]

Hyperthermia, at the other end of the temperature spectrum, is rare in the postanesthesia population. Core temperatures above 38° C may be due to sepsis, preexisting infectious processes, drug fever, trauma, blood transfusions, or, rarely, malignant hyperthermia. Hyperthermic patients may also have tachycardia with increased CO, increased respiratory rates, and peripheral vasodilation with a widening of the pulse pressure—all designed to remove heat from the body. Five syndromes of drug-induced hyperthermia have been described. The syndromes include malignant hyperthermia, neuroleptic malignant syndrome, anticholinergic poisoning, sympathomimetic poisoning, and serotonin syndrome.[28] Treatment includes medications (anti-infectives, antipyretics) and cooling measures (cool cloths, cooling blankets).

Malignant hyperthermia (MH), known as the disease of anesthesia, is a rare, life-threatening pharmacogenetic disorder triggered by volatile anesthetic agents (halothane, isoflurane, sevoflurane, desflurane) and succinylcholine in genetically susceptible patients. It is a state of hypermetabolism and skeletal muscle rigidity. The incidence ranges from 1:10,000 to 1:50,000 patients.[45] It occurs more frequently in children, but has been reported in older adults. Development of MH during the perioperative period frequently led to death (over 70%) before the introduction of dantrolene (Dantrium) in 1979.[2] When triggering agents are given to susceptible individuals, the initial response may be doubling or tripling of the end-tidal carbon dioxide concentration and unexplained tachycardia (Box 46-1). This can occur within 30 minutes of induction of anesthesia or up to 24 hours after the triggering agent is administered. Temperature elevation is a late indicator and is sometimes absent. Prompt recognition and treatment with dantrolene can reduce morbidity and mortality to less than 5% to 10%.[2,45]

Treatment begins with recognition. Once recognized, triggering agents are stopped, 100% oxygen is administered, and dantrolene is administered. Additional treatment includes monitoring of cardiac rhythm, urine output, and temperature (Box 46-2). Every anesthetizing location needs to be prepared for the potential development of MH. An MH kit or cart stocked with recommended supplies and resource materials (posters, pocket cards, reference guides) should be readily available to the nursing and medical staff. The Malignant Hyperthermia Association of the United States (MHAUS) offers telephone support (1-800-MHHYPER) 24 hours daily to assist providers managing an MH crisis.

Box 46-1

Signs of Malignant Hyperthermia

EARLY

- Doubling or tripling of end-tidal CO_2
- Hypoxemia
- Metabolic acidosis
- Muscle rigidity
- Skin flushing
- Tachycardia
- Tachypnea
- Ventricular dysrhythmias

LATE*

- Elevated creatinine phosphokinase
- Hyperkalemia
- Hyperthermia†
- Mixed metabolic and respiratory acidosis
- Myoglobinuria
- Skin mottling
- Sweating

Data from references 2, 28, 45.

*These signs may not be present with early recognition and treatment.

†Correlates with severity of malignant hyperthermia.

Postanesthesia Shivering

Postanesthesia patients frequently experience shivering.[1] Shivering is more common in young adults, with longer anesthesia or surgery times, and if no active perioperative rewarming was used.[1] There is no definitive explanation for why postanesthesia shivering occurs. Most common causes are thought to include perioperative hypothermia and postoperative pain, although hypotheses suggest perioperative heat loss, the direct effect of certain anesthetics, hypercapnia or respiratory alkalosis, pyrogens, hypoxia, early recovery of spinal reflex activity, and sympathetic overactivity may contribute.[1] Consequences of shivering include discomfort, increased pain at the operative site because of muscle contractions, increased intraocular pressure after ophthalmological surgery, and an increase in oxygen consumption by 200% to 500%.[1,10,42] Hypothermia may cause vasoconstriction, with increased vascular resistance further compromising myocardial function in the patient with preexisting decreased myocardial oxygen supply secondary to arteriosclerosis.[35]

Postanesthetic shivering caused by perioperative hypothermia may be prevented by skin surface rewarming before induction, raising the temperature in the OR, or using rewarming intravenous solutions and active warming during the surgical procedure.

Box 46-2

Treatment of a Malignant Hyperthermia Crisis

- Call for help.
- Stop triggering agents.
- Evaluate need for invasive monitoring, mechanical ventilation.
- Hyperventilate with 100% oxygen (increase minute ventilation to decrease end-tidal carbon dioxide concentration).
- Prepare and administer dantrolene (2.5 mg/kg initial dose, up to 10 mg/kg recommended but may be exceeded).
- Begin cooling measures for hyperthermia—iced solutions; ice packs to axilla/groin, neck; iced nasogastric lavage; cool water mist and fans. Stop cooling at 38.5° C.
- Treat dysrhythmias—do not use calcium channel blockers; may use lidocaine.
- Obtain blood gases, electrolytes, creatine kinase (CK) level, coagulation studies, blood and urine for myoglobin level.
- Treat hyperkalemia with bicarbonate, IV glucose, and insulin.
- Maintain urine output at 2 ml/kg/hr with mannitol, furosemide, fluids.
- Observe in intensive care unit for 36 hours minimum.
- Postacute episode: continue dantrolene at 1 mg/kg IV every 4–6 hours for 24–36 hours.
- Counsel patient and family; refer patient and family to Malignant Hyperthermia Association of the United States.

Data from references 2, 28, 45.

Shivering may also exist in the absence of hypothermia (cutaneous vasodilation or nonthermoregulatory shivering); its cause is not known.[1] Treatment may include medications such as low doses of meperidine (Demerol), tramadol (Ultram), and, in some cases, clonidine.

Acute Postoperative Pain and Comfort Management

Evidence exists that postoperative pain remains suboptimally treated.[66] Pain may cause changes in immune system function, decreased healing, diminished ability to function, needless suffering, and chronic pain. Pain and comfort guidelines have been published for the assessment and management of acute postoperative pain.[4,7] The reader is directed to the guidelines at www.aspan.org/painandcomfort.htm and to Chapter 4 of this text for an in-depth discussion

of pain assessment and management in the critical care setting.

Acute postoperative pain needs to be assessed and reassessed frequently and managed aggressively. Continuous catheter techniques (epidural, other peripheral nerve blocks) can be used in the critical care setting to provide adequate pain management. Protocols for monitoring and observation of the catheter sites and devices guide critical care nurses' care of the patient in pain. Algorithms or procedures for troubleshooting inadequate pain relief and nonfunctioning catheters are essential for each institution.

Patient comfort needs are also assessed with pain management needs. Comfort includes more than the assessment and management of pain. According to Kolcaba, comfort includes four contexts: physical, psychospiritual, environmental, and sociocultural.[34] Meeting the postanesthesia patient's comfort needs is important to the patient's overall recovery. Survey tools and questionnaires are available to assess the patient's comfort needs.[34]

Postoperative Nausea and Vomiting

Nausea and vomiting occurs in 25% to 30% of postoperative patients—an incidence unchanged over the past 40 years.[24,70] Risk factors for postoperative nausea and vomiting (PONV) are female gender, nonsmoker, history of motion sickness, history of previous PONV, and operative procedure longer than 180 minutes. Certain anesthetic agents (nitrous oxide) and commonly used drugs (opioids, anticholinesterases) are known to increase the risk of PONV, while other agents (propofol) may help minimize the incidence. Adequate hydration, pain management, anti-emetic prophylaxis, and avoidance of triggering agents and other stimuli may minimize PONV.[24,71]

Treatment includes medications that are serotonin, dopamine, acetylcholine, and histamine antagonists (see the Medication table on p. 163 in Chapter 9). Nonpharmacologic treatment is also recommended (e.g., peppermint oil, isopropyl alcohol inhalation, oxygen, and fluid hydration). Studies have shown that the effectiveness of these nonpharmacologic therapies varies, and further research is necessary.*

Other Complications: Risks Associated With the Use of Herbal or Vitamin Supplements

Patients using herbal and vitamin supplements may increase their risk of adverse events, such as bleeding

---

*References 17, 26, 38, 40, 48, 49, 51, 68, 76.

and drug interactions, during the perioperative period.[29] Patients may fail to disclose usage of supplements, and healthcare professionals may be less aware of the risks associated with the use of these supplements. The supplements may interfere with platelet adhesion, increase sedation, cause hypoglycemia, increase or decrease anticoagulant effects of warfarin, alter cardiac glycoside levels, or potentiate the effects of anesthetics.[29,30,36]

Patients must be asked before operative or interventional procedures about their use of herbal and vitamin supplements. General recommendations suggest stopping the supplements 2 weeks before operative and interventional procedures, and when the patient will receive anesthetics or sedating medications for noninvasive procedures.[30] Table 46-3 summarizes the common herbal and vitamin supplements and potential risks associated with their use by patients undergoing anesthesia and operative or interventional procedures.

THE SURGICAL CARE IMPROVEMENT PROJECT

The Surgical Care Improvement Project (SCIP) evolved from the Surgical Infection Prevention (SIP) project implemented by the Centers for Medicare and Medicaid Services and the Centers for Disease Control and Prevention in 2002. The SIP project focused on the prevention of surgical-site infections with goals related to appropriate prophylactic antibiotic use, perioperative glycemic control, maintenance of normothermia, and operative site hair removal. The SIP project objective was "to decrease the morbidity and mortality associated with postoperative infection in the Medicare patient population."[64] In July 2004, the Joint Commission on Accreditation of Healthcare Organizations (JCAHO), now known as The Joint Commission, began including goals related to appropriate prophylactic antibiotic use for surgical-site infection prevention as core measures (Box 46-3).[31]

TABLE 46-3 Herbal and Vitamin Supplements

HERBAL OR VITAMIN PRODUCT	USE	EFFECTS	POTENTIAL DRUG INTERACTIONS
Echinacea	Immune stimulant	Immunosuppression, poor wound healing, and infection with prolonged use (longer than 8 weeks)	
Garlic	Hypertension, hyperlipidemia, antibacterial	Causes hypoglycemia	Antidiabetic agents
		Inhibits platelet aggregation	Aspirin, NSAIDs may enhance antiplatelet activity
Ginkgo	Dementia, memory loss, antioxidant, peripheral vascular disease	Bleeding Increases anticoagulant effects	NSAIDs, aspirin, warfarin
Ginger	Antinauseant, antispasmodic	May prolong bleeding time	Warfarin, antiplatelet agents
Ginseng	Stress, learning and memory, diuretic	Causes hypoglycemia	Antidiabetic agents
		Interferes with BP control	Antihypertensives
		Potentiates or increases effects	Corticosteroids
		Elevates levels	Digoxin
		Decreases effects	Diuretics, warfarin

HERBAL OR VITAMIN PRODUCT	USE	EFFECTS	POTENTIAL DRUG INTERACTIONS
St. John's wort	Depression, anxiety, menopausal symptoms	Excessive sedation; delayed emergence	Anesthetics
		Serotonin syndrome	Antidepressants, dextromethorphan
		Decreases sleep time	Barbiturates
		Increases sedative effect	Benzodiazepines
		Reduces levels	Cyclosporine, digoxin
		Decreases anticoagulant effects	Warfarin
Valerian	Insomnia, sleep disorders, migraine	Excessive sedation; delayed emergence Prolongs sleep time Excessive sedation	Anesthetics, barbiturates, benzodiazepines
Vitamin E	Antioxidant, skin conditions	Increased risk of death at doses larger than 400 units/day; bleeding—interferes with platelet adhesion	

Data from reference 29.
BP = Blood pressure, NSAIDs = nonsteroidal antiinflammatory drugs.

Box 46-3

Surgical Infection Prevention Goals

QUALITY INDICATORS: NATIONAL SURGICAL INFECTION PREVENTION PROJECT

Quality Indicator #1
Proportion of patients who receive antibiotics within 1 hour before surgical incision

Quality Indicator #2
Proportion of patients who receive prophylactic antibiotics consistent with current recommendations

Quality Indicator #3
Proportion of patients whose prophylactic antibiotics were discontinued within 24 hours of surgery end time

Data from reference 45.

The SCIP was established in 2004 with a goal "to reduce preventable surgical morbidity and mortality by 25% by 2010."[46] Four preventable complication modules are included: surgical infection prevention, cardiovascular complication prevention, venous thromboembolism prevention, and respiratory complication prevention. Performance measures include the continuance of the SIP goals, use of perioperative beta-blocker therapy, prevention of venous thromboembolism using deep vein thrombosis prophylaxis, and application of evidence-based measures to prevent ventilator-associated pneumonia.

MULTIDISCIPLINARY PLAN OF CARE

Most patients do very well after surgery. However, there are many potential complications that a nurse must assess in order to begin therapy before the complications result in morbidity or mortality. An initial plan of care for the postoperative patient, outlined in the Multidisciplinary Plan of Care on pp. 1308-1309, is similar to that for any hospitalized patient and begins with the ABCs: airway, breathing, and circulation.

Because many patients receive general anesthesia via an endotracheal tube, they are at risk for developing swelling and airway obstruction. Other common causes of airway obstruction include the decreased tone of the genioglossal muscle from the relaxant effects of anesthesia and analgesia. Nurses need to assess the respiratory rate, auscultate breath sounds, and monitor oxygen saturation by pulse oximetry (SpO_2) regularly. Early intervention of an obstructed

MULTIDISCIPLINARY PLAN OF CARE FOR POSTOPERATIVE PATIENTS

PROBLEM	INTERVENTION	RATIONALE	EXPECTED OUTCOME
Risk for respiratory obstruction/ compromise	Monitor respiratory status and oxygenation: • Respiratory rate between 14 and 25 • Auscultate breath sounds on admission and every hour until stable • Supplemental oxygen to keep SpO_2 greater than 92% • Provide patient stimulation • Forward displacement of jaw to relieve pharyngeal obstruction • HOB elevated at least 30 degrees • Encourage coughing and deep breathing	Early identification of respiratory compromise allows for appropriate prophylactic intervention Decreased tone of genioglossal muscle, leaving airway unable to protect itself from complications or laryngospasm Decreased risk for aspiration Prevents atelectasis and accumulation of secretions	Patients at risk for respiratory compromise/ obstruction will be identified early.
Risk for cardiovascular compromise	Monitor vital signs, hemodynamic parameters: • BP, MAP, HR • PAP, PAWP, CVP, SvO_2, CO, CI, SVR • Urine output • CBC • Electrolyte panel • PT/PTT/INR • Abdominal girth (if appropriate) • Change in LOC • GI bleeding	Hypertension places these patients at risk for bleeding from graft site Hypotension places major organs at risk for further ischemia and graft failure Adequate hydration Hypertension increases SVR, which increases workload of heart and places patient at risk for myocardial infarction	Early changes in vital signs and hemodynamic parameters will be identified.
	Monitor ECG and lab values • 12-lead ECG • Potassium level at 4.5 mEq/L • Magnesium level at 3 mEq/L • Ionized calcium 1.2 mmol/L • Troponin • CK	Tachycardia decreases diastolic filling time; thus coronary blood flow is compromised Magnesium deficiency has been associated with hypokalemia, hypocalcemia, tetany, dysrhythmia, and free radical release	Routine monitoring will promote electrolyte replacement.
Risk for ischemia, inadequate organ perfusion	Monitor presence/absence of peripheral pulses; ankle/arm index; signs and symptoms of lower extremity ischemia: • Pain • Pallor • Paralysis • Pulselessness • Paresthesias Monitor motor function and sensation in lower extremities, capillary refill, color, pain Auscultate bowel sounds	Cross-clamping during surgical procedure impairs blood flow distally	Early changes in perfusion will be identified and corrected.
Risk for complications	Thermoregulation Monitor temperature, maintain	Postanesthesia period is the time when the patient is vulnerable to	Complications will be minimized or avoided;

PROBLEM	INTERVENTION	RATIONALE	EXPECTED OUTCOME
	normothermia; apply warming/cooling devices as appropriate Observe for signs/symptoms of malignant hyperthermia Identify triggers for postanesthetic shivering; treat with warming/medications	residual effects of anesthesia and surgical procedure	when identified, they will be treated appropriately.
	CNS Monitor LOC, Glasgow Coma Scale, motor strength/movement *PONV* Monitor signs and symptoms of nausea/vomiting; check patency of nasogastric tube; maintain HOB greater than 30 degrees or side lying; treat complaints of nausea/vomiting with anti-emetics, fluids *Pain & comfort* Monitor patient self-report of pain intensity; if patient unable to respond, use behavioral observation scale; medicate to reduce pain response; nonpharmacologic therapies: positioning, environmental changes		

BP = Blood pressure, CBC = complete blood cell count, CI = cardiac index, CK = creatine kinase, CNS = central nervous system, CO = cardiac output, CVP = central venous pressure, ECG = electrocardiogram, GI = gastrointestinal, HOB = head of bed, HR = heart rate, INR = international normalized ratio, LOC = level of consciousness, MAP = mean arterial pressure, PONV = post-operative nausea and vomiting, PAP = pulmonary artery pressure, PAWP = pulmonary artery wedge pressure, PT = prothrombin time, PTT = partial thromboplastin time, SpO_2 = oxygen saturation by pulse oximetry, Svo_2 = mixed venous oxygen saturation, SVR = systemic vascular resistance.

airway can prove to be life-saving. Other measures to protect the airway include elevating the head of the bed to 30 degrees to decrease the risk of postoperative aspiration with vomiting. To aid in breathing and to prevent atelectasis and pneumonia, nurses should encourage their patients to cough and deep breathe.

Circulatory or cardiovascular complications are also quite common after surgery. Surgery can result in bleeding during and after the operation. Fluid shifts associated with general anesthesia complicate cardiovascular function. Lastly, major cardiovascular events (e.g., myocardial infarction and stroke) are seen more frequently in the perioperative period. Monitoring of circulation can be as simple as recording the pulse and BP and observing the peripheral perfusion by skin color and temperature. In the event of a suspected complication, more invasive cardiovascular monitoring with central venous and invasive arterial access may be necessary. Thus the skilled postoperative nurse should be familiar with monitoring the CVP, pulmonary artery pressure (PAP), PAWP, systemic venous oxygenation, cardiac index, and systemic vascular resistance. Other important indications of

cardiovascular stability include the urine output, serum electrolytes, and a complete blood count. Hypotension can arise from bleeding either at the operative site or in the gastrointestinal tract. Bleeding can be exacerbated by abnormal blood clotting as measured by the PT and PTT. Hypertension can arise from the pain associated with surgery or overzealous fluid administration. Hypertension increases the afterload on the heart, which increases the risk of myocardial infarction.

Although hypotension can lead to generalized ischemia, ischemia of single organs or limbs can also be observed in the postoperative period. Ischemia can be manifested by pain, pallor, paralysis, pulselessness, or paresthesia of the affected organ or limb. These complications are more likely to arise following operations that require cross-clamping of the blood supply to an organ or limb during the operative procedure. They can also occur when patients lie in one position or on a limb for a prolonged time while under anesthesia. Pain must be monitored as well as pulses, capillary refill, motor function, and sensation to ensure prompt identification of ischemia.

The patient's temperature must also be monitored for hypothermia. Postoperative patients are at risk for hypothermia because of the vasodilation and heat loss that occurs during anesthesia and the heat lost from body cavities during major open cases of the abdomen and chest. Nurses should warm the patient to prevent complications and shivering. Although much less common, hyperthermia can occur in association with infection or a drug reaction or malignant hyperthermia. Complications will be avoided if malignant hyperthermia is promptly recognized and treated.

Postoperative nurses must also monitor the patient's return to consciousness. The Glasgow Coma Scale is a valuable reproducible tool that is commonly used. In addition, motor strength and sensation should also be monitored since limb deficits are quite common.

PONV continues to be a common complication of surgery and can lead to increased recovery time, expanded nursing care, and increased total healthcare costs.[22] Persistent vomiting may result in electrolyte abnormalities and dehydration, as well as put tension on suture lines and increase the risk of pulmonary aspiration. The nurse should seek the most effective method to prevent and treat PONV.

Pain and comfort measures begin with assessment of pain and comfort, using the patient's self-report of pain and comfort when possible. Acute severe pain may lead to hypertension, tachycardia, or agitation. Therapeutic interventions include pharmacologic and nonpharmacologic approaches.

Good preoperative skin assessment and evaluation of preoperative risk factors are important first steps in preventing postoperative pressure ulcer development. As indicated in the Research Utilization box at right, attention must be paid to all patients undergoing operative procedures and especially to those who are female, who have low ASA or New York Heart Association (NYHA) status (poor physical status), or who are nutritionally depleted or have poor food intake. Awareness of the patients at greater risk should increase vigilance.[41]

CONCLUSIONS

The immediate postoperative period is challenging for the patient and the nurse. The patient is vulnerable to pain and discomfort, hemodynamic alterations, respiratory compromise, and other complications. Nurses must remain vigilant and aware of the risks associated with anesthesia and surgical intervention. Critical and comprehensive monitoring along with an understanding of anesthesia agents and adjuncts, postoperative care, and complications will provide a sound basis for caring for patients in the immediate postoperative period.

◆ RESEARCH UTILIZATION

Risk Factors for Developing Pressure Ulcers in Adult Surgical Patients

CLINICAL ISSUE

Pressure ulcers increase length of stay and morbidity in hospitalized patients. Identification of patients at high risk for developing pressure ulcers is especially important in the perioperative population where lengthy operative procedures and immobilization increase patient risk.

SUMMARY

This study was a prospective, comparative study of 286 adult patients undergoing surgery. Data were collected preoperatively, daily for 7 days postoperatively, and once a week for up to 12 weeks. Perioperative data were also collected. The Risk Assessment Pressure Sore (RAPS) scale was used to identify patients at risk for pressure sore development. The scale measures general physical condition, activity, mobility, sensory perception, friction and shear, body temperature, serum albumin level, and moisture, food, and fluid intake. Scores range from 10 to 39; the lower the score, the greater the risk of pressure ulcer development. The RAPS scale has been validated for reliability. Forty-one (14.3%) patients developed a total of 57 pressure ulcers: 9 (15.8%) developed more than 1 pressure ulcer. Twenty-nine (22.5%) of the women developed pressure ulcers; 12 (7.6%) of the men developed pressure ulcers ($P < 0.001$). The most common locations for the pressure ulcers were the sacrum (29.8%), heels (19.3%), and ischial tuberosities (14%). Patients who had epidural/spinal analgesia tended to have greater risk than patients undergoing general anesthesia. Risk factors identified in multiple stepwise logistic regression analysis were female gender, American Society of Anesthesiologists (ASA) or New York Heart Association (NYHA) status, and food intake.

APPLICATION

Preoperative skin assessment and evaluation of preoperative risk factors are important first steps in preventing postoperative pressure ulcer development. Attention must be paid to all patients undergoing operative procedures, and especially those who are female, who have low ASA or NYHA status (poor physical status), or who are nutritionally depleted or with poor food intake. Awareness of the patients at greater risk should increase vigilance.

NEED FOR FURTHER STUDY

Future studies are needed to further investigate the relationship of having surgery to risk factors for pressure ulcer development.

Lindgren, M., et al. (2005). Pressure ulcer risk factors in patients undergoing surgery. *J Adv Nurs, 50*(6), 605–612.

REFERENCES

1. Alfonsi, P. (2001). Postanaesthetic shivering: epidemiology, pathophysiology, and approaches to prevention and management. *Drugs, 61*(15), 2193–2205.

2. Ali, S. Z., Taguchi, A., & Rosenberg, H. (2003). Malignant hyperthermia. *Best Pract Res Clin Anaesthesiol, 17*(4), 519–533.

3. American Society of Anesthesiologists. (1999). *Practice guidelines for preoperative fasting and the use of pharmacologic agents to reduce the risk of pulmonary aspiration: application to healthy patients undergoing elective procedures.* A Report by the American Society of Anesthesiologists. www.asahq.org/publicationsAndServices/NPO.pdf.

4. American Society of Anesthesiologists. (2003). *Practice guidelines for acute pain management in the perioperative setting.* www.asahq.org/publicationsAndServices/pain.pdf.

5. Anderson, L. (2001). Abdominal aortic aneurysms. *J Cardiovasc Nurs, 15*(4), 1–14.

6. ASPAN. (2002). *Clinical guideline for the prevention of unplanned perioperative hypothermia.* www.aspan.org/PDFfiles/HYPOTHERMIA_GUIDELINE10-02.pdf.

7. ASPAN. (2003). *ASPAN pain and comfort clinical guideline.* www.aspan.org/PDFfiles/pain&comfort.pdf.

8. ASPAN. (2004). *Standards of perianesthesia nursing.* Cherry Hill, NJ: American Society of PeriAnesthesia Nurses.

9. Barkhordarian, S., & Dardik, A. (2004). Preoperative assessment and management to prevent complications during high-risk vascular surgery. *Crit Care Med, 32*(4 suppl), S174–S185.

10. Bay, J., Nunn, J. F., & Prys-Roberts, C. (1968). Factors influencing arterial P_{O_2} during recovery from anaesthesia. *Br J Anaesth, 40,* 398–407.

11. Brown, D. L. (2005). Spinal, epidural, and caudal anesthesia. In R. D. Miller (Ed.), *Miller's anesthesia* (6th ed). Philadelphia: Saunders.

12. Butler, S. O., Btaiche, I. F., & Alaniz, C. (2005). Relationship between hyperglycemia and infection in critically ill patients. *Pharmacotherapy, 25*(7), 963–976.

13. den Herder, C., et al. (2004). Risks of general anaesthesia in people with obstructive sleep apnea. *BMJ, 329,* 955–959.

14. Donnelly, A. J., et al. (2005). *Anesthesiology & critical care drug handbook* (6th ed.). Hudson, Ohio: Lexi-Comp.

15. *Dorland's illustrated medical dictionary* (29th ed.). Philadelphia: Saunders.

16. Drain, C. B. (2003). Muscle relaxants. In C. B. Drain (Ed.), *Perianesthesia nursing: a critical care approach* (4th ed.). Philadelphia: Saunders.

17. Ernst, E., & Pittler, M. H. (2000). Efficacy of ginger for nausea and vomiting: a systematic review of randomized clinical trials. *Br J Anaesth, 84,* 367–371.

18. Evans, H., et al. (2004). Peripheral nerve blocks and continuous catheter techniques. *Anesthesiol Clin North Am, 23,* 141–162.

19. Feitelson-Winkler, M., et al. (1989). Use of retinol-binding protein and pre-albumin as indicators of response to nutritional therapy. *J Am Diet Assoc, 89,* 684–687.

20. Fisher, D. M. (1997). Muscle relaxants. In D. E. Longnecker & F. L. Murphy (Eds.), *Dripps/Eckenhoff/VanDam introduction to anesthesia* (9th ed.). Philadelphia: Saunders.

21. Fleischmann, K. E., et al. (2003). Association between cardiac and noncardiac complications in patients undergoing noncardiac surgery: outcomes and effects on length of stay. *Am J Med, 115,* 515–520.

22. Gan, T. J., et al. (2003). Consensus guidelines for managing postoperative nausea and vomiting. *Anesth Analg, 97*(1), 62–71.

23. Glister, B. C., & Vigersky, R. A. (2003). Perioperative management of type 1 diabetes mellitus. *Endocrinol Metab Clin North Am, 32,* 411–436.

24. Golembiewski, J. (2002). Safety concerns with meperidine. *J Peri-Anesth Nurs, 17*(2), 123–125.

25. Golembiewski, J. A., & O'Brien, D. (2002). A systematic approach to the management of postoperative nausea and vomiting. *J Perianesth Nurs, 17*(6), 364–376.

26. Greif, R., et al. (1999). Supplemental oxygen reduces the incidence of postoperative nausea and vomiting. *Anesthesiology, 91,* 1246–1252.

27. Halaszynski, T. M., Juda, R., & Silverman, D. G. (2004). Optimizing postoperative outcomes with efficient preoperative assessment and management. *Crit Care Med, 32*(4 suppl), S76–S86.

28. Halloran, L. L., & Bernard, D. W. (2004). Management of drug-induced hyperthermia. *Curr Opin Pediatr, 16,* 211–215.

29. Heyneman, C. A. (2003). Preoperative considerations: which herbal products should be discontinued before surgery? *Crit Care Nurse, 23*(2), 116–124.

30. Hodges, P. J., & Kam, P. C. A. (2002). The peri-operative implications of herbal medicines. *Anaesthesia, 57,* 889–899.

31. Joint Commission on Accreditation of Healthcare Organizations. (2005). www.jcaho.org/pms/core+measures/aligned_manual.htm.

32. Kaafarani, H. M. A., et al. (2004). Thirty-day and one-year predictors of death in noncardiac major surgical procedures. *Am J Surg, 188,* 495–499.

33. Kaboli, P., Henderson, M. C., & White, R. H. (2003). DVT prophylaxis and anticoagulation in the surgical patient. *Med Clin North Am, 87,* 77–110.

34. Kolcaba, K. (2001). *Comfort theory and practice.* New York: Springer.

35. Kranke, P., et al. (2002). Treatment of postoperative shivering. *Anesth Analg, 94,* 453–460.

36. Kuhn, M. A. (2002). Herbal remedies: drug-herb interactions. *Crit Care Nurse, 22*(2), 22–35.

37. Lagan, G., & McClure, H. A. (2004). Review of local anaesthetic agents. *Curr Anaesthesia Cri Care, 15,* 247–254.

38. Langevin, R. B., & Brown, M. M. (1997). A simple, innocuous, and inexpensive treatment for postoperative nausea and vomiting. *Anesth Analg, 84*(suppl), 16.

39. Larson, M. D. (2005). History of anesthetic practice. In R. D. Miller (Ed.), *Miller's anesthesia* (6th ed, pp. 3–53). Philadelphia: Saunders.

40. Lee, A., & Done, M. L. (1999). The use of nonpharmacologic techniques to prevent postoperative nausea and vomiting: a meta-analysis. *Anesth Analg, 88,* 1362–1369.

41. Lindgren, M., et al. (2005). Pressure ulcer risk factors in patients undergoing surgery. *J Adv Nurs, 50*(6), 605–612.

42. Macintyre, P. E., Pavlin, E. G., & Dwersteg, J. F. (1987). Effect of meperidine on oxygen consumption, carbon dioxide production, and respiratory gas exchange in postanesthesia shivering. *Anesth Analg, 66,* 751–755.

43. Mandel, M. B. (2005). *Respiratory complications.* www.pitt.edu/~mandel/resp.htm.

44. Marik, P. E., & Zaloga, G. P. (2001). Early enteral nutrition in acutely ill patients: a systematic review. *Crit Care Med, 29*(12), 2264–2270.

45. McCarthy, E. J. (2004). Malignant hyperthermia: pathophysiology, clinical presentation, and treatment. *AACN Clin Issues, 15* (2), 231–237.

46. Medqic. (2005). *Surgical care improvement project: a national quality partnership.* www.medqic.org/scip/.

47. Merritt, B. A., Okyere, C. P., & Jasinski, D. M. (2002). Isopropyl alcohol inhalation: alternative treatment of postoperative nausea and vomiting. *Nurs Res, 51,* 125–128.

48. Micromedex Healthcare Series, Thomson Micromedex, Greenwood Village, Colo (2007).

49. Ming, J. L., Kuo, B. I. T., Lin, J. G., et al. (2002). The efficacy of acupressure to prevent nausea and vomiting in post-operative patients. *J Adv Nurs, 39,* 343–351.

50. Molnar, R., & Pian-Smith, M. C. M. (2002). Spinal, epidural, and caudal anesthesia. In W. E. Hurford (Ed.), *Clinical anesthesia procedures of the Massachusetts General Hospital* (6th ed.). Philadelphia: Lippincott Williams & Wilkins.

51. Monti, S., & Pokorny, M. (2000). Preop fluid bolus reduces risk of postop nausea and vomiting: A pilot study. *Internet J Adv Nurs Practice*, p. 4. www.ispub.com/ostia/index.php?xmlFilePath_journals/ijanp/front.xml.

52. Moore, C. H. (2003a). Local anesthetics. In C. B. Drain (Ed.), *Perianesthesia nursing: a critical care approach* (4th ed, pp. 339–345). Philadelphia: Saunders.

53. Moore, C. H. (2003b). Regional anesthesia. In C. B. Drain (Ed.), *Perianesthesia nursing: a critical care approach* (4th ed, pp. 346–353). Philadelphia: Saunders.

54. O'Brien, D. (2003). Care of the perianesthesia patient. In C. B. Drain (Ed.), *Perianesthesia nursing: a critical care approach* (4th ed., pp. 393–408). Philadelphia: Saunders.

55. O'Leary-Kelly, C., et al. (2005). Nutritional adequacy in patients receiving mechanical ventilation who are fed enterally. *Am J Crit Care*, 14(3), 222–231.

56. Pinnock, C. A., Fischer, H. B. J., & Jones, R. P. (1996). *Peripheral nerve blockade*. London: Churchill Livingstone.

57. Reves, J. G., & Flezzani, P. (1985). Perioperative use of esmolol. *Am J Cardiol*, 56(11), 57F–62F.

58. Roberts, S. R., Kennerly, D. A., Keane, D., et al. (2003). Nutrition support in the intensive care unit: adequacy, timeliness and outcomes. *Crit Care Nurse*, 23(6), 49–57.

59. Rock, P., & Passannante, A. (2004). Preoperative assessment: pulmonary. *Anesthesiol Clin North Am*, 22, 77–91.

60. Saklad, M. (1941). Grading of patients for surgical procedures. *Anesthesiology*, 2(3), 281–284.

61. Shafer, S. L., & Schwinn, D. A. (2005). Basic principles of pharmacology related to anesthesia. In R. D. Miller (Ed.), *Miller's anesthesia* (6th ed., pp 67–194). Philadelphia: Saunders.

62. Smetana, G. W. (2002). Preoperative pulmonary assessment of the older adult. *Clin Geriatr Med*, 19, 35–55.

63. Stanski, D. R., & Shafer, S. L. (2005). Measuring depth of anesthesia. In R. D. Miller (Ed.), *Miller's anesthesia* (6th ed., pp. 1227–1264). Philadelphia: Saunders.

64. Stimler, C. (2003). *Overview of national SIP Medicare QI collaborative*. http://providers.ipro.org/shared/sip/040703/stimler_qi.pdf.

65. Stoelting, R. K., & Hillier, S. C. (2006). Inhaled anesthetics. *Handbook of pharmacology & physiology in anesthetic practice.* (2nd ed., pp. 45–79). Philadelphia: Lippincott Williams & Wilkins.

66. Strassels, S. A., McNicol, E., & Suleman, R. (2005). Postoperative pain management: a practical review, part 1. *Am J Health Syst Pharm*, 62, 1904–1916.

67. *Taber's cyclopedic medical dictionary* (20th ed.). Philadelphia: F.A. Davis.

68. Tate, S. (1997). Peppermint oil: a treatment for postoperative nausea. *J Adv Nurs*, 26, 543–549.

69. Tong, G. M., & Rude, R. K. (2005). Magnesium deficiency in critical illness. *J Intensive Care Med*, 20, 3–17.

70. Tramer, M. R. (2001). A rational approach to the control of postoperative nausea and vomiting: evidence from systematic reviews. Part 1. Efficacy and harm of antiemetic interventions, and methodological issues. *Acta Anaesthesiol Scand*, 45, 4–13.

71. Tramer, M. R. (2004). Strategies for postoperative nausea and vomiting. *Best Pract Res Clin Anaesthesiol*, 18(4), 693–701.

72. Trayner, E., & Celli, B. R. (2001). Postoperative medical complications: postoperative pulmonary complications. *Med Clin North Am*, 85(5), 1129–1139.

73. Van den Berghe, et al. (2003). Outcome benefit of intensive insulin therapy in the critically ill: insulin dose versus glycemic control. *Crit Care Med*, 31, 359–366.

74. Wedel, D. J., & Horlocker, T. T. (2005). Nerve blocks. In R. D. Miller (Ed.), *Miller's anesthesia* (6th ed., pp. 1685–1718). Philadelphia: Saunders.

75. Westerdahl, E., et al. (2005). Deep-breathing exercises reduce atelectasis and improve pulmonary function after coronary artery bypass surgery. *Chest*, 128(5), 3482–3488.

76. Zarate, E., et al. (2001). The use of transcutaneous acupoint electrical stimulation for preventing nausea and vomiting after laparoscopic surgery. *Anesth Analg*, 92, 629–635.

77. Zaugg, M., et al. (1999). Beneficial effects from beta-adrenergic blockade in elderly patients undergoing noncardiac surgery. *Anesthesiology*, 91(6), 1674–1686.

CHAPTER 47 Caring for the Critically Ill Pregnant Patient

Julene B. Kruithof

Caring for the critically ill obstetric patient presents the critical care team with unique management challenges. In the past, the specialties of obstetrics and critical care have been widely separated; the usual normalcy of pregnancy and the severe illness-orientation of critical care seem diametrically opposed. However, current trends including higher maternal age and pregnancy in women with preexisting diseases have led to an increase in the number of pregnant women cared for in critical care. Studies have documented that increasing maternal age is associated with specific adverse pregnancy outcomes.[19] Current public health priorities include the goal of reducing maternal mortality to 3.3 maternal deaths per 100,000 live births or less, although the current rate is close to 12 maternal deaths per 100,000 live births.[70] Race-specific pregnancy-related mortality trends demonstrate that African-American women are more than four times as likely to die from pregnancy-related causes as are Caucasian women.[70] These concerns underscore the need for critical care nurses who, in addition to their critical care knowledge and skills, also understand the unique needs of the critically ill obstetric patient.

There are three management priorities for the critically ill pregnant woman, including optimizing maternal physiologic functioning, enhancing fetal growth and development, and supporting the maternal and family experience. Understanding the unique body of knowledge surrounding critical care obstetrics will help to achieve the positive outcomes for both the woman and the child. Common obstetric terms are highlighted in Box 47-1, and a broad overview of fetal development is provided in Figure 47-1.

PREGNANCY AND CRITICAL ILLNESS

Obstetric patients requiring critical care fall into two groups. The first group includes women with preexisting disease who become pregnant and require advanced care and management. Examples of preexisting diseases that might compromise a woman's condition and necessitate admission to critical care include diabetes, heart valve disease, corrected or uncorrected congenital heart disease, asthma, spinal cord injury, or neuromuscular disease (e.g., multiple sclerosis). The second group includes women who experience critical illness or injury during an otherwise normal pregnancy. Examples of critical illnesses or injury that may arise during or as a result of pregnancy include thromboembolic disease,

---

Box 47-1

Common Obstetric Terms

- Acceleration: visually apparent abrupt increase in fetal heart rate above the baseline
- Deceleration: visually apparent decrease in fetal heart rate
- Effacement: shortening and thinning of the cervix during the first stage of labor
- First trimester: weeks 1 through 13 of pregnancy
- Gravida: woman who is pregnant
- Multipara: woman who has completed two or more pregnancies to the stage of fetal viability
- Nullipara: woman who has not completed a pregnancy with a fetus who has reached the stage of viability
- Preterm: pregnancy that has reached 20 weeks of gestation but before completion of 37 weeks of gestation
- Primigravida: woman who is pregnant for the first time
- Second trimester: weeks 14 through 26 of pregnancy
- Term: describes a pregnancy from the beginning of the 38th week of gestation to the end of the 42nd week of gestation
- Third trimester: weeks 27 through 40 of pregnancy
- Tocolytic therapy: administration of medications that inhibit uterine contractions
- Viability: capacity to live outside the uterus, currently about 22 to 24 weeks of gestation, or weight of fetus greater than 500 g

Data from reference 54.

First Trimester

Primitive heart starts to beat

Many internal organs form and begin to function

Facial features and limbs become apparent

Nervous system develops the ability to respond

Spontaneous breathing movements begin

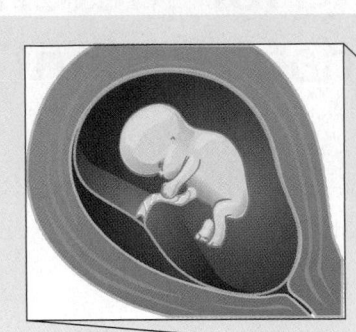
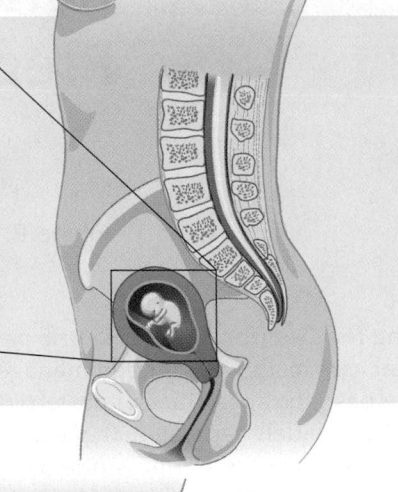

Fetus in 9th week of development

Second Trimester

Muscles begin to develop

Spontaneous movements can be observed

Details form, such as eyelids, nails, genitalia, sweat glands, and hair

Internal organs mature

Bones strengthen and harden

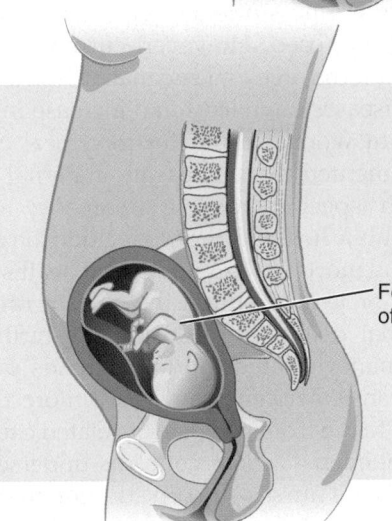

Fetus in 18th week of development

Third Trimester

Organs continue to mature

Fat layers begin to form

Brain grows rapidly

Lungs mature

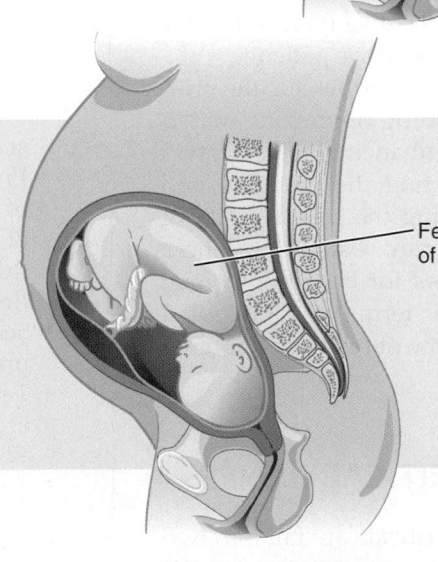

Fetus in 32nd week of development

⬥FIGURE 47-1 Stages of fetal development.

myocardial infarction, peripartum cardiomyopathy, anaphylactoid syndrome, pneumonia, trauma, or hypertensive disease. Any of these conditions may necessitate critical care for the pregnant or recently delivered woman. Critical care nurses must be prepared to deal with the unique management concerns during pregnancy.

NORMAL PHYSIOLOGIC CHANGES IN PREGNANCY

Physiologic changes occur during pregnancy impacting nearly every organ system. These changes alter baseline assessment and laboratory data findings, potentially confounding diagnosis and management. Physiologic changes occur in pregnancy to maintain the pregnancy and allow for fetal growth and development. Hormonal increases in progesterone, estrogen, and human placental lactogen account for many of these changes. Nearly every body system is affected. Some adaptations are so profound that they would be considered pathologic if occurring outside of pregnancy. The physiologic changes begin as early as the first week of gestation and continue up to 6 weeks or more following delivery. Changes associated with critical illness or injury are highlighted in the following text.

Reproductive System

Reproductive organs undergo dramatic changes during pregnancy. The capacity of the uterus grows from 10 ml to between 4.5 and 5 liters. As the uterus grows out of the pelvis, abdominal contents are displaced and diaphragmatic elevation occurs. The uterine vascular bed expands dramatically, and uterine blood flow increases from 50 ml/minute at 10 weeks to 500 ml/minute at 40 weeks.[11,33]

Cardiovascular System

During pregnancy, the cardiovascular system undergoes dramatic changes in blood volume and cardiac output (CO). Total blood volume increases approximately 30% to 40%, approximately 1 to 1.5 liters over normal volume. This increase in volume maximizes between weeks 26 and 34 of gestation. Red blood cell volume increases approximately 20%, plasma volume increases 45% to 50%, and total body water increases by approximately 6 to 8 L.[65] Together these changes produce a dilutional anemia and a decrease in colloid oncotic pressure. Expected hemoglobin (Hgb) and hematocrit levels in pregnancy are approximately 10 to 14 g/dl and 32% to 44%, respectively.[50,72] Pregnancy is considered a

hypercoagulable state with increases in the levels of factors I, II, VII, VIII, IX, and X.[81] In addition to the increased levels of clotting factors, fibrinolytic activity is decreased, further promoting coagulability.[27] Hemodynamic status in normal pregnancy is discussed in the Research Utilization box below.

In addition to the volume changes, structural changes in the cardiovascular system occur as well. The heart is displaced upward and to the left because of the elevation of the diaphragm. Left axis deviation can occur as a result of the mechanical displacement, but there are no other characteristic electrocardiographic changes. Hypertrophy of the cardiac muscle can occur to meet

---

◆ RESEARCH UTILIZATION

Assessment of Cardiovascular Hemodynamics in Normal Pregnancy

CLINICAL ISSUE

Factors affecting cardiac output during normal pregnancy are controversial and multifactorial. Understanding hemodynamic changes during pregnancy is essential to optimization of maternal-fetal outcomes.

SUMMARY

This study examined cardiac performance in 35 healthy pregnant women from early second trimester until 6 to 12 weeks postpartum. The study demonstrated an expected increase in cardiac output of 46% to 51%, with approximately half of the increase occurring by 28 weeks of gestation. Data from this study demonstrated that the peak occurred in the early to mid third trimester and was maintained or had only very slight increases after that until term. This study also concluded that the initial mild increase in cardiac output early in pregnancy can be attributed to an increase in heart rate, but the progressive increase seen in the latter half of pregnancy is due to an increase in stroke volume.

APPLICATION

It is important for clinicians to understand the mechanisms behind the cardiac output increases during pregnancy, so that expected increases in heart rate and stroke volume can be monitored and supported.

NEED FOR FURTHER STUDY

Further studies are needed to continue to clarify the exact timing and mechanisms of cardiac output changes during pregnancy.

Desai, D. K., Moodley, J., & Naidoo, D. P. (2004). Echocardiographic assessment of cardiovascular hemodynamics in normal pregnancy. *Obstet Gynecol, 104*(1).

TABLE 47-1 Positional Cardiac Output Changes in Third-Trimester Pregnancy

MATERNAL POSITION	CARDIAC OUTPUT (L/min)
Knee-chest	6.9 ± 2.1
Right lateral	6.8 ± 1.3
Left lateral	6.6 ± 1.4
Sitting	6.2 ± 2
Supine	6 ± 1.4
Standing	5.4 ± 2

Data from reference 17.

the volume demands. During physical assessment, changes in heart sounds may be noted such as S_1 split in 90% of women and S_3 development in 90% of the population.[60] These are considered normal physiologic changes in pregnancy. Approximately 50% of women develop a systolic murmur during pregnancy.[60] These murmurs, which typically resolve following delivery, are considered pathologic only if it is a loud systolic, grade II/IV, or diastolic murmur.[60]

Pregnancy also brings many blood pressure (BP) variations. Typically, BP decreases slightly during the first trimester, reaches a low point during the second trimester, and then returns to normal. Supine positioning can cause vena cava compression by the gravid uterus,

decreasing venous return and CO, potentially causing postural hypotension. To meet the physiologic demands of pregnancy, CO undergoes dramatic changes. Normal CO during pregnancy is considered to be 6 to 7 L/minute, generally a 30% to 50% increase from prepregnancy values.[22] Changes in CO begin in the first trimester and peak during the second trimester. Increases in blood volume and progesterone-induced decreases in vascular resistance contribute to the increase in CO. Increases in heart rate during the second trimester help to support this increase in CO as well. Unique to pregnancy are the positional CO changes that occur (Table 47-1).[17] Normal hemodynamic values in pregnancy are referenced in Table 47-2.[16,65]

Pulmonary System

As pregnancy progresses, diaphragmatic elevation occurs, shortening lung length by approximately 4 cm. However, hormonal changes allow anteroposterior and circumferential enlargement of approximately 5 to 7 cm, compensating for the shorter thoracic cavity.[44] Tidal volume increases approximately 40%, to a normal of 500 to 600 ml, and the respiratory rate increases slightly. Respiratory reserve volume and functional residual capacity both decrease by approximately 5% to 15%. Together, these changes enhance minute ventilation to 9 to 13 L/minute. All together, pulmonary physiologic changes allow the mother to have increased minute ventilation by approximately 50% at term.[31] This normal hyperventilation causes changes in arterial blood gas values during pregnancy. Hyperventilation causes the maternal partial pressure of arterial carbon dioxide

TABLE 47-2 Hemodynamic Changes Associated With Term Pregnancy

PARAMETER	NORMAL VALUE	CHANGE
Mean arterial pressure	90 ± 6 mm Hg	No significant pressure change
Central venous pressure	4–8 ± 2 mm Hg	No significant change
Pulmonary artery wedge pressure	4–7 ± 2–3 mm Hg	No significant change
Heart rate	75–95 beats/min	Increase 10–20 beats/min
Cardiac output	6.2 ± 1 L/min	Increase 30%–50%
Systemic vascular resistance	1210 ± 266 dynes/sec/cm^{-5}	Decrease 20%
Pulmonary vascular resistance	78 ± 22 dynes/sec/cm^{-5}	Decrease 34%
Left ventricular stroke work index	43–48 ± 6–9 gm/m^2	No significant change

Data from references 4, 16, 17, 47, 59.

(Paco$_2$) level to drop between 28 and 32 mm Hg. A mild respiratory alkalosis results, compensated by an increase in renal excretion of bicarbonate.

Maternal oxygen demands increase 15% to 25% during pregnancy, primarily to meet fetal oxygen demands. To meet these requirements, normal maternal partial pressure of arterial oxygen tension (Pao$_2$) is 101 to 108 mm Hg,[44,65] and arterial oxygen saturation should be maintained at greater than 95%. To facilitate oxygen exchange from the mother to the fetus, the maternal oxyhemoglobin dissociation curve shifts slightly to the right.

Gastrointestinal System

The maternal gastrointestinal (GI) system undergoes changes in both structure and function, attributable to hormonal changes as well as interference from the growing uterus. GI motility decreases, intestinal secretion slows, and water absorption increases, placing the woman at risk for constipation and aspiration. In addition, the gravid uterus causes displacement and potential incompetence of the gastroesophageal junction, further enhancing aspiration risk. Vascular congestion occurs in many mucosal tissues, including gums, nose, pharynx, larynx, trachea, bronchi, urethra, and bladder, because of the influence of progesterone.[54] This hyperemia can lead to bleeding gums and impaired gallbladder emptying as well as decreased gallbladder activity, leading to gallstones and cholecystitis.

Renal System

Structural renal changes include slight enlargement of the kidneys, dilation of pelvic and ureteral structures, displacement of the bladder forward and upward, and impairment of blood and lymph drainage. Functional renal changes are primarily caused by changes in renal blood flow. Renal blood flow increases 25% to 50%, up to 1250 to 1500 ml/minute. Glomerular filtration increases about 50%, up to 140 to 170 ml/minute, and renal blood flow increases 35%, to approximately 700 to 900 ml/minute.[22,44,60] However, because glomerular filtration increases more than blood flow, renal clearance is enhanced, lowering the plasma concentration of many substances, including maternal creatinine and blood urea nitrogen (BUN). Since even these waste products are excreted more effectively, serum levels in pregnant women are reduced. The normal upper limit for serum creatinine level in pregnancy is 0.8 mg/dl;[91] BUN levels are 8.2 mg/dl.[22,60] Although glomerular filtration is enhanced, the maternal tubular capability to reabsorb glucose and protein does not change; therefore both glycosuria and proteinuria are common in pregnancy. These findings may be normal, but require further investigation as they may be indicators of serious pathology.

MONITORING OF THE CRITICALLY ILL OBSTETRIC PATIENT

Monitoring of both mother and fetus is essential to provide the healthcare team with information regarding the status and tolerance of therapies and activities. Gestational age plays a significant role in the decision-making process of determining appropriate monitoring strategies. The current range for fetal viability is between 22 and 24 weeks of gestation, with fetal weight greater than 500 grams[54] (0.5 kg). In light of these parameters, management efforts should be focused primarily on maternal outcomes before 23 to 26 weeks of gestation. Once fetal viability has been reached, however, it is critical to evaluate both maternal and fetal response to interventions and physiologic status. Currently, many authorities concur that until approximately 32 to 34 weeks of gestation, the fetus is generally supported better in utero rather than outside of the uterus.[21] At times, situations may be encountered where fetal viability, fetal outcome, and maternal stability are uncertain. Each clinical decision must be weighed while considering maternal and fetal risk and benefit.

Maternal Monitoring

Monitoring of the pregnant woman is similar to monitoring other critically ill patients. The American College of Obstetricians and Gynecologists (ACOG) has defined specific indications for hemodynamic monitoring in pregnancy (Box 47-2).[7] These indications, along with standard indications for monitoring,

---

Box 47-2

Indications for Hemodynamic Monitoring in Pregnant Patients

- Adult respiratory distress syndrome
- Cardiovascular decompensation during intrapartum or intraoperative periods
- Chronic disease during labor or intraoperatively (New York Association Classification III or IV cardiac disease)
- Massive hemorrhage or volume replacement needs
- Pulmonary edema, oliguria, or heart failure refractory to treatment or of unknown etiology
- Severe pregnancy-induced hypertension with persistent oliguria or pulmonary edema
- Shock of unknown etiology
- Sepsis with oliguria or refractory hypotension

Data from reference 7.

provide practitioners excellent guidelines for physiologic monitoring of the critically ill obstetric patient.

Monitoring of laboratory and radiologic studies is also an important aspect of caring for the critically ill obstetric patient. Practitioners should keep in mind the normal dilutional anemia of pregnancy, arterial blood gas changes, and BUN and creatinine level changes as well as the normal presence of mild glycosuria and proteinuria. Careful attention should be paid to therapeutic levels of medications. Larger than normal doses of medications may be required because of enhanced renal clearance during pregnancy. Each abnormal laboratory result should be evaluated to determine if the change is due to normal physiologic changes in pregnancy or potential pathology. Radiologic studies also provide important insights into maternal treatment. However, each radiologic study may provide radiation exposure to the growing fetus, posing a risk to fetal development. Proper shielding helps to reduce the risk to the fetus; each radiologic study should be considered with a risk/benefit ratio before performing it. In general, exposure to radiation is not typically of great concern until a threshold of 5 to 15 rad (cGy) has been exceeded (Table 47-3).[25,34,43,84]

Fetal Monitoring

Fetal monitoring provides caregivers with important information regarding overall fetal and maternal status. Adequate uterine blood flow and oxygen content, sufficient placental size and function, and a normal umbilical cord are necessary for effective transfer of oxygen and carbon dioxide between the mother and the fetus.[78] The uteroplacental bed is a passive, low-resistance system without autoregulation, having few, if any, compensatory mechanisms. Therefore changes in uteroplacental perfusion can significantly affect fetal oxygenation and well-being. The uteroplacental system receives approximately 10% to 17%[60,65] of maternal CO; however, it is considered to be a peripheral, nonessential organ during physiologic stress, preferentially shunting perfusion away from the fetus and back into maternal circulation. Monitoring of fetal heart rate patterns is undertaken to determine fetal well-being. Collaboration with obstetric experts in fetal monitoring will provide critical care practitioners with information about the mother's ability to provide optimal fetal perfusion.

There is a lack of agreement on definitions and interpretations surrounding fetal monitoring. However, in general, reassuring fetal heart patterns indicate that the fetus is receiving adequate oxygenation to meet demands. Reassuring characteristics include a baseline fetal heart rate between 110 and 160 beats/min, moderate baseline variability, and periodic accelerations with

TABLE 47-3 Radiation Dose from Radiologic Studies	
RADIOLOGIC STUDY	**ESTIMATED FETAL DOSE*** $(1 \times 10^{-5}$ Gy$)$
Chest x-ray	8
Skull x-ray	4
Cervical spine x-ray	2
Thoracic spine x-ray	402
Lumbar spine x-ray	275
Abdominal x-ray	185
IV/retrograde pyelography	585
Upper GI x-ray	330
Lower GI x-ray	465
Pelvimetry	750
Hip x-ray	100
Lower extremity x-ray	1

Data from references 25, 34, 43, 83.
*Gy = Gray, IV = intravenous, GI = gastrointestinal.

fetal movement. Variability refers to irregular fluctuations in the baseline fetal heart rate.[83] Accelerations and decelerations refer to visually apparent abrupt increases or decreases in the fetal heart rate above the baseline rate.[83] Fetal heart rate patterns that may indicate a less than optimal fetal environment include changes in the baseline heart rate, either bradycardia or tachycardia; late, variable, or prolonged decelerations; and absent or minimal variability.[78] It is essential that an obstetric practitioner trained in fetal monitoring interpret all fetal monitor tracings in the critical care environment.

MULTIDISCIPLINARY PLAN OF CARE

Alterations in the plan of care are required when caring for pregnant, critically ill patients. The primary change is the collaboration required between critical care and obstetric practitioners. To maximize maternal outcomes, it is essential that all disciplines be actively involved. Each brings its own expertise in patient management, and, together, optimal outcomes for both mother and fetus can be achieved. This collaboration is highlighted in the Multidisciplinary Plan of Care below and on pp. 1320 and 1321.

Environment of Safety

Central to the care of the critically ill obstetric patient is ensuring an optimal environment for safe care of the mother and fetus. Conscious decision making should occur during the admission process, beginning with placement decisions addressing whether the woman is best cared for in critical care, labor and delivery, or an antepartal unit. Decisions should be based upon optimal care for the woman, and resources then mobilized to meet those needs. If the woman is placed in the labor and delivery or antepartal unit, critical care support should be mobilized, including physiologic monitoring if required. Although there are no specific criteria or guidelines,

MULTIDISCIPLINARY PLAN OF CARE FOR CRITICALLY ILL PREGNANT PATIENTS

PROBLEM	INTERVENTION	RATIONALE	EXPECTED OUTCOMES
Potential for decreased CO	Monitor HR, BP, and hemodynamic parameters Maintain natural hypervolemic state and fluid balance with administration of fluids/diuretics as appropriate Maintain optimal volume status for patient Administer inotropic medications as appropriate (Chapter 41) Monitor and correct acid-base and electrolyte imbalances Monitor ECG for dysrhythmias Keep gravid uterus off IVC Optimize maternal position Maintain CO at 6–7 L/min Monitor for signs of fluid overload (crackles, edema) Monitor overall maternal circulatory status (capillary refill, extremity warmth, color, urine output) Assess adequacy of uteroplacental perfusion Consider impact of preexisting or pregnancy-induced cardiovascular disease states on woman's ability to support adequate CO	Optimize maternal cardiac output to support maternal stability and optimal fetal oxygenation and outcomes	HR, BP, and hemodynamic parameters in expected range CO maintained at 6–7 L/min Adequate uteroplacental perfusion
Adjustment to maternal role	Establish a trust relationship with patient and family unit Access obstetric resources to supplement care Encourage infant visitation and bonding Encourage parent(s) to hold and cuddle infant Use pictures, recordings of fetal heartbeat, or maternal voice Support maternal decision to breast-feed Facilitate a minimum of 8 feeds per day Enhance flow of milk using a hospital-grade breast pump Collaborate with obstetric and pharmacy resources to determine storage or disposal of breast milk	Critical illness can interfere with the normal maternal role adjustments that occur during postpartum period	Support of maternal and infant attachment, promotion of breast-feeding choice

Table continues on page 1320

PROBLEM	INTERVENTION	RATIONALE	EXPECTED OUTCOMES
Potential fetal intolerance of decreased uteroplacental perfusion	Consider impact of gestational age Collaborate with obstetric resources for analysis of electronic fetal monitoring Collaborate with obstetric resources for monitoring of uterine status/contraction pattern Consider impact of uterine status on fetal perfusion Recognize normal fetal HR range of 110–160 beats/min Recognize presence of accelerations as reassuring sign Recognize presence of variability as reassuring sign Recognize presence of decelerations as potential sign of fetal distress Anticipate need for maternal interventions if signs of fetal distress persist Consider FDA drug category of maternal medications and potential fetal impact Use vasopressors (Chapter 41) with caution to avoid additional decrease in uteroplacental perfusion Anticipate need for immediate delivery with acute, severe maternal or fetal decompensation Access resources if fetal demise occurs	Signs of fetal distress may require the critical care nurse to consider how maternal status can be optimized to facilitate oxygen delivery to the fetus	Reassuring fetal HR, presence of accelerations, absence of decelerations
Risk for deep vein thrombosis/pulmonary embolism	Monitor peripheral pulses, edema, capillary refill, color and temperature of extremities Monitor for pain in extremities Administer anticoagulation as ordered Encourage position change, leg and ankle exercises to reduce venous stasis Provide pain relief and comfort measures Monitor laboratory values Monitor for occult or overt bleeding if on anticoagulation therapy	Assist to control/reduce already elevated maternal risk for development of deep vein thrombosis/pulmonary embolism	Absence of deep vein thrombosis
Impaired gas exchange leading to maternal or fetal hypoxia	Monitor overall pulmonary status: respiratory rate, rhythm, effort of respirations and breath sounds Monitor pulse oximetry and arterial blood gases Maintain mild maternal respiratory alkalosis Maintain oxygen saturation greater than 95% Reduce aspiration risk (stomach decompression, head of bed elevation) Position for maximal ventilation potential Remove secretions by encouraging coughing or by suctioning Monitor effects of position changes on pulmonary status	Optimize maternal oxygenation to support and promote optimal maternal and fetal outcomes	Adequate gas exchange and ventilation Absence of aspiration Maintenance of normal mild respiratory alkalosis

PROBLEM	INTERVENTION	RATIONALE	EXPECTED OUTCOMES
	Monitor for symptoms of respiratory failure Provide mechanical ventilatory support if necessary Adjust mechanical ventilatory settings to accommodate physiologic normal values during pregnancy Keep emergency airway and resuscitative equipment readily available Anticipate site alteration for chest tube placement or cricothyrotomy Consider impact of natural dilutional anemia on maternal oxygen delivery		
Potential for postpartum complications	Consult with obstetric resources Monitor urinary elimination including frequency, odor, volume, and color as appropriate Monitor wound(s) for signs of infection Monitor temperature Monitor for nausea and vomiting and medicate as appropriate Monitor lochial flow characteristics, amount and presence of clots Monitor for excessive blood loss Provide pain relief Monitor fundal height and firmness; provide fundal massage as appropriate Provide perineal hygiene to prevent infection	Early and continuous monitoring for complications can reduce their presence and impact on overall recovery	Absence of postpartum complications
Anxiety related to change in health status, serious nature of illness, potential or perceived threat to well-being of self or fetus	Establish trust relationship with patient and family unit Use a calm, reassuring approach Explain all procedures and sensations Provide pain management Encourage verbalization of feelings, perceptions, and fears Seek to understand patient's perception of situation Identify changes in level of anxiety Observe for verbal and non-verbal signs of anxiety Support appropriate use of defense mechanisms Control stimuli as appropriate Encourage use of relaxation techniques Encourage family involvement as appropriate Acknowledge spiritual/cultural background Administer medication as appropriate Appraise effectiveness of non-pharmacologic and pharmacologic interventions Consider MSW/chaplain referral	Assisting patient/family unit to identify and control anxiety may aid in overall recovery and adjustment process	Control of anxiety response Use of coping strategies Optimal sleep/rest pattern Verbalization of feelings and concerns

BP = Blood pressure, CO = cardiac output, ECG = electrocardiogram, FDA = U.S. Food and Drug Administration, HR = heart rate, IVC = inferior vena cava, MSW = medical social worker.

once mechanical ventilation is required, many institutions prefer placement in critical care. If care will be provided in critical care, obstetric and neonatal resources should be ensured. Rapid availability of fetal monitoring and delivery equipment, neonatal warmer, and infant resuscitation equipment is vital. Safe labor and delivery can take place in critical care with appropriate obstetric and neonatal resources. Regardless of patient location, collaboration and open communication among practitioners provide the optimal benefit to the patient.

Psychosocial Care

Pregnancy has an inherent set of maternal psychosocial tasks, and fathers have specific psychological tasks to accomplish as well. One of the confounding factors of critical care obstetrics is that the usual normalcy and joyful expectation typically associated with pregnancy and delivery is marred. Encountering critical illness or injury during pregnancy challenges the coping mechanisms of any individual and the family unit. In addition, stress may occur because of a real or perceived threat to life or functional outcome of both mother and baby. In the event of fetal demise, collaboration with individuals who have received advanced training in fetal demise can provide essential support to the maternal family unit through that experience. Critical situations may bring a variety of values (personal, cultural, social, spiritual, or ethical) into conflict. All members of the healthcare team should discuss management options and proceed with collaborative decision making with patient or family members.

Maintenance of Cardiac Output

Ensuring adequate blood volume and correct positioning of the critically ill obstetric patient is essential to optimize CO. The normal hypervolemic state of pregnancy should be maintained; however, blood loss can be easily underestimated with subsequent inadequate fluid replacement. Supine positioning should be avoided to prevent the associated vena caval compression and reduction in venous return. Either right or left side-lying position is acceptable, or at least a 30-degree tilt from the supine position. In initial traumatic injury, the entire backboard can be tilted to alleviate impairment of venous return. If tilting or side-lying positioning is not able to be accomplished, manual displacement of the uterus can provide the same outcome.

Airway and Oxygenation Support

General pulmonary care considerations in the management of critically ill obstetric patients include continuous assessment as well as maintenance of maternal oxygenation, protection of airway, and provision of ventilatory support. Assessment of maternal status may be confounded by the normal hyperventilation and dyspnea associated with pregnancy. High-flow oxygen should be administered through use of a face mask since nasal passages tend to be hyperemic and mouth breathing is common during pregnancy. The goal is to maintain the physiologic maternal PaO_2 level of 101 to 104 mm Hg.[65]

If advanced adjuncts are required, airway management in a pregnant patient should be rapidly accomplished with an oral endotracheal tube to help meet oxygen needs and reduce risk of aspiration. Noninvasive mechanical ventilation should be avoided or used with caution because of the aspiration risk.[35]

◆ Case Study 47-1, Part A

Stabilizing a Pregnant Patient With Premature Contractions

B.F. is a 36-year-old female, pregnant with her first child. She has had adequate prenatal care and is currently at 34 weeks of gestation. She has no significant medical history, and an essentially normal pregnancy to date. During her past two prenatal visits, her BP readings were 146/88 and 154/90 mm Hg. She was instructed to decrease her activity level and return for weekly BP reviews. During the evening before her next prenatal visit, she begins to experience nausea, headache, and some contractions. During a telephone consultation, the obstetrician instructed her to proceed to the hospital's antepartal unit for evaluation.

On admission to the antepartal unit, B.F.'s vital signs include a temperature of 36.9° C, heart rate 124 beats/min, respiratory rate 25 breaths/min, BP 188/122 mm Hg, and pulse oximetry 94%. Laboratory studies demonstrate a white blood cell count 11,500/mm³, Hgb level 10.2 g/dl, platelet count 250,000/mm³, BUN 9 mg/dl, and creatinine 0.8 mg/dl. Urinalysis results include moderate glycosuria and significant proteinuria. Physical examination is essentially unremarkable with the exception of moderate peripheral edema, oliguria, and the presence of a faint systolic murmur. B.F. is having irregular, mild contractions. Vaginal examination reveals cervical dilation of 1 cm with no cervical effacement. Fetal heart rate monitoring demonstrates a reassuring pattern, with fetal heart rate baseline of 130s, normal variability, and periodic accelerations.

Decision point: What immediate interventions should be initiated?

Case continues on page 1334

Ventilatory support should mimic physiologic changes in respiratory rate, depth, and minute ventilation mentioned previously. Gastric decompression with an orogastric or small nasogastric tube should be accomplished to prevent gastric reflux and aspiration. If emergency cricothyrotomy or tracheotomy is needed, it should be performed above the usual site because of the upward displacement of thoracic structures. In addition, the entry point for chest tube insertion may need to be reassessed because of the increase in anteroposterior diameter of the chest and decrease in length.

Infection Control

Pregnancy poses several infection risks to maternal well-being. The risk of pulmonary infection from aspiration is a significant concern. Incompetence of the gastroesophageal mechanism and delays in gastric emptying enhance the aspiration risk. Obstetric patients are generally treated as "full stomach" patients, requiring longer nothing by mouth times before procedures. Ventilator-associated pneumonia (VAP) risks are also higher in the obstetric population; careful attention should be paid to standard VAP prevention techniques, including oral care and elevation of the head of the bed. Chapter 9 provides more details on the prevention of VAP. The potential for urinary stasis also increases the risk for urinary tract infections during pregnancy.[72] Diagnosis of infection can be confounded by a normal leukocytosis,[72] with a normal white blood cell range of 11,000 to 16,000 per mm^3.

Pharmacologic Concerns

Use of medications in critically ill obstetric patients requires thoughtful consideration of the likelihood of obtaining therapeutic results and of the risk/benefit ratio for both mother and fetus. The Medication table below and on p. 1324 summarizes medications used in pregnancy in the critical care unit. The U.S. Food and Drug Administration (FDA) has developed categories for drug use in pregnancy, shown in the Medication table on p. 1324, that are useful in guiding decision making.[10,58] Since renal clearance during pregnancy is enhanced, careful attention to therapeutic levels must be observed. In addition, certain medications may have teratogenic effects on the developing fetus. Many vasoactive medications commonly used in the critical care setting (e.g., epinephrine, dopamine) may have negative effects on uteroplacental perfusion. Use requires consideration of the risk/benefit ratio, keeping in mind that adequate maternal perfusion is required, in spite of vasoconstriction, for fetal perfusion to occur. The Medication table on p. 1324 lists FDA ratings for drug use in pregnancy. The table on pp. 1325-1326 lists the pregnancy drug categories for medications commonly used in critical care.

MEDICATIONS USED IN PREGNANCY IN THE CRITICAL CARE UNIT

MEDICATION	ACTIONS	DOSAGE	SPECIAL CONSIDERATIONS
Magnesium	Blocks neuromuscular transmission; decreases amount of acetylcholine released at motor plate	IV: Bolus of 4–6 g, then infusion rate of 1–2 g/hr to maintain serum level of 4–7 mEq/L	Monitor maternal vital signs, deep tendon reflexes, duration and frequency of contractions; monitor fetal HR
Terbutaline (Brethine)	Relaxes uterine muscle; inhibits uterine contractions	IV: 2.5–10 mcg/min Can be slowly increased every 15–20 min up to 17.5–30 mcg/min	Monitor maternal vital signs, duration and frequency of contractions; monitor fetal HR
Ritodrine (Yutopar)	Relaxes uterine muscle; inhibits uterine contractions	IV: 50–350 mcg/min PO: Initial, 10 mg 30 min before IV is discontinued, then 10 mg every 2 hr for 24 hr Maintenance: PO: 10–20 mg every 4–6 hr until term (or until 37th week of gestation) or as medical judgment dictates Max daily oral dose is 120 mg	Monitor maternal vital signs, duration and frequency of contractions; monitor fetal HR

Table continues on page 1324

MEDICATION	ACTIONS	DOSAGE	SPECIAL CONSIDERATIONS
Oxytocin (Pitocin)	Contracts uterine smooth muscle; used to control postpartum bleeding	IV: 10–40 units in 1000 ml at rate sufficient to control uterine atony IM: 10 units (total dose) following delivery	Monitor maternal vital signs, duration and frequency of contractions; notify MD/NP if contractions last longer than 1 min or occur more frequently than every 2 min; monitor fetal HR
Indomethacin (Indocin)	Inhibits prostaglandin production, resulting in inhibition of preterm labor	Rectal suppository: 50–100 mg loading dose, followed by 2.5 mg every 6–8 hr orally	
Glucocorticoids Betamethasone (Celestone)	Increases fetal maturation: reduces perinatal mortality, ARDS, and intraventricular hemorrhage	IM: Two 1-mg doses given 24 hr apart	Monitor maternal vital signs, monitor for infection
Dexamethasone (Decadron)	Increases fetal maturation: reduces perinatal mortality, ARDS, and intraventricular hemorrhage	IM: Four 6-mg doses given 12 hr apart	Monitor maternal vital signs, monitor for infection

ARDS = Acute respiratory distress syndrome, HR = heart rate, NP = nurse practitioner.

FDA DRUG USE-IN-PREGNANCY RATINGS

CATEGORY	DESCRIPTION
A	Adequate, well-controlled studies in pregnant women have not shown an increased risk of fetal abnormalities.
B	Animal studies have revealed no evidence of harm to fetus; however, there are no adequate and well-controlled studies in pregnant women. **or** Animal studies have shown an adverse effect, but adequate and well-controlled studies in pregnant women have failed to demonstrate risk to fetus.
C	Animal studies have shown an adverse effect and there are no adequate and well-controlled studies in pregnant women. **or** No animal studies have been conducted and there are no adequate and well-controlled studies in pregnant women.
D	Studies, adequate well-controlled or observational, in pregnant women have demonstrated risk to fetus. However, benefits of therapy may outweigh potential risk.
X	Studies, adequate well-controlled or observational, in animals or pregnant women have demonstrated positive evidence of fetal abnormalities. Use of product is contraindicated in women who are or may become pregnant.

Data from reference 58.

FDA PREGNANCY DRUG CATEGORIES OF CRITICAL CARE DRUGS

MEDICATION	FDA PREGNANCY DRUG CATEGORY	MEDICATION	FDA PREGNANCY DRUG CATEGORY
Abciximab (ReoPro)	C	Enoxaparin (Lovenox)	B
ACE inhibitors	C in 1st trimester, D in 2nd and 3rd trimesters	Epinephrine	C
Acetaminophen (Tylenol)	B	Epoprostenol (Flolan)	B
Adenosine (Adenocard)	C	Eptifibatide (Integrilin)	B
Albuterol (Proventil)	C	Etomidate (Amidate)	C
Aminoglycosides	C	Famotidine (Pepcid)	B
Amiodarone (Cordarone)	D	Fentanyl	C
Amphotericin B	B	Furosemide (Lasix)	C
Ampicillin	B	Heparin	C
Aspirin	C if less than 150 mg/day, D if more	Ibuprofen (Motrin)	B, D in 3rd trimester
Atenolol (Tenormin)	D	Insulin	B
Atropine	C	Ketorolac (Toradol)	C
Atorvastatin (Lipitor)	X	Labetalol (Normodyne)	C
Aztreonam (Azactam)	B	Lidocaine	B
Barbiturates	D	Lorazepam (Ativan)	D
Bumetanide (Bumex)	C	Magnesium	B
Calcium channel blockers	C	Metformin (Glucophage)	B
Cephalosporins	B	Metoprolol (Toprol)	C
Clopidogrel (Plavix)	B	Midazolam (Versed)	D
Codeine	C	Milrinone (Primacor)	C
Diazepam (Valium)	D	Morphine	C
Digoxin (Lanoxin)	C	Nesiritide (Natrecor)	C
Diltiazem (Cardizem)	C	Nitroglycerin	B
Dobutamine (Dobutrex)	B	Nitroprusside (Nipride)	C
Dopamine (Inocor)	C	Norepinephrine (Levophed)	C
Drotrecogin alpha (Xigris)	C	Pancuronium (Pavulon)	C

Table continues on page 1326

MEDICATION	FDA PREGNANCY DRUG CATEGORY	MEDICATION	FDA PREGNANCY DRUG CATEGORY
Penicillin	B	Propofol (Diprivan)	B
Pentobarbital	D	Propranolol (Inderal)	C
Phenobarbital (Luminal)	D	Pneumococcal vaccine	C
Phenylephrine (Neo-Synephrine)	C	Reteplase (Retavase)	C
Phenytoin (Dilantin)	D	Vasopressin (Pitressin)	C
Potassium chloride	C	Vecuronium (Norcuron)	C
Procainamide (Pronestyl)	C	Warfarin (Coumadin)	D

Data from references 10, 58.

Nutritional Considerations/ Glycemic Control

Maternal metabolic rate increases approximately 15% to 20% during pregnancy.[54] Nutritional support provided during critical illness or injury must meet these increased demands, as outlined in the Nutrition box below. Total daily caloric intake should be based on ideal body weight. Glucose maintenance during pregnancy can present significant challenges during critical illness or injury as well. Secretion of human placental lactogen (also known as known human chorionic somatomammotropin), progesterone, and cortisol antagonize insulin, sparing glucose for the developing fetus.[12,54] These hormones also cause maternal breakdown of lipids and fatty acids, promoting maternal hyperglycemia. Many pregnant women are able to enhance insulin production and therefore maintain normal blood glucose levels;[38] however, gestational diabetes can develop. Diabetes during pregnancy, either preexisting or gestational, causes both maternal and fetal complications and increases morbidity. Major tenets of diabetic care in pregnancy

---

♦ NUTRITION

Caloric Requirements During Pregnancy

Nutrition is one of many variables, including family dynamics, education, motivation, income, and health, that influence the outcome of pregnancy. Consideration must be given to the increased nutritional needs that critical illness or injury presents in addition to those required because of pregnancy. Maternal weight gain is normal and expected during pregnancy, and maternal and fetal risks are incurred when weight gain is too much or too little. In general, pregnancy is a time to replace empty-calorie foods with nutrient-dense foods. The Institute of Medicine[45] has established ideal ranges of weight gain based on prepregnancy body mass index (BMI):

- Women with prepregnancy BMI of less than 19.8 should gain between 12.5 and 18 kg.
- Women with prepregnancy BMI of 19.8 to 26 should gain between 11.5 and 16 kg.
- Women with prepregnancy BMI of 26 to 29 should gain between 7 and 11.5 kg.

- Women with prepregnancy BMI of greater than 29 should gain at least 7 kg; however, caution should be taken to limit additional weight gain.

Prepregnancy: Women considering pregnancy should obtain the ideal body weight and ingest a minimum of 400 mcg of folic acid daily to decrease the risk of neural tube defects.

First trimester: During this time there should be minimal changes in the recommended nutritional goals from prepregnancy goals. Starting in the first trimester and throughout a normal pregnancy, women should ingest at least 1.5 to 2 L of fluid daily.

Second and third trimesters: During this time the fetus uses and deposits energy stores; therefore caloric needs increase approximately 300 calories per day over prepregnancy requirements. In addition, vitamin and mineral needs increase, specifically in the need for iron, zinc, iodine, magnesium, folic acid, thiamine, riboflavin, and niacin as well as vitamins E, C, B_6, and B_{12}.[62] These increased requirements should be met with diet and multivitamin supplementation.

are similar to conventional diabetic therapy: blood glucose level monitoring, diet, exercise, and patient education. Glycemic targets endorsed by the ACOG include a fasting value less than 96 mg/dl and 2-hour postprandial values less than 120 mg/dl.[5] Glycemic control should be reassessed frequently throughout pregnancy and in the postpartum period. Aggressive management of diabetic ketoacidosis (DKA) during pregnancy is required to prevent maternal dehydration, acidosis, organ dysfunction, and electrolyte imbalances.[12] Recent analysis reports perinatal mortality rates between 9% and 35% with even a single episode of DKA during pregnancy.[12]

Prevention of Deep Venous Thrombosis

Prevention of venous thrombosis (DVT) and subsequent pulmonary embolism requires aggressive measures. The risk of DVT is 5 times higher in pregnant women as compared with nonpregnant women[81] and is responsible for 17% of all maternal deaths.[27] Untreated DVT may result in pulmonary embolism (PE) in up to 24% of pregnant patients.[89] The three major underlying factors in venous thrombosis—hypercoagulability, venous stasis, and vascular damage—all occur in pregnancy. Venous stasis occurs by the end of the first trimester and continues throughout the pregnancy.[36] Vena cava compression can cause endothelial damage; most cases of DVT in pregnancy are ileofemoral rather than calf vein thrombosis.[27] Diagnosis of DVT in the pregnant patient is as difficult as in the nonpregnant patient, since most do not exhibit classic signs and symptoms. DVT in pregnancy can be associated with lower abdominal pain that can confound the diagnosis. While most diagnostic tests are identical to those for nonpregnant patients, D-dimer testing is not reliable in pregnancy.[28,80]

Management of thromboembolism is generally completed with unfractionated heparin or low molecular weight heparins. Warfarin (Coumadin) is rated as a category D drug and is not recommended for use in the first trimester because of its known teratogenic risks.[10] Standard management adjuncts (e.g., anti-embolic devices, bedrest, and analgesia) should be included. Patients who are anticoagulated require a carefully planned delivery to avoid potentially negative outcomes. Postpartum patients should continue treatment for between 6 weeks and 6 months after delivery to reduce the risk of PE.[27]

Labor and Delivery Considerations

Additional stress is incurred during labor and delivery—the process of moving the fetus, placenta, and membranes out of the uterus and through the birth canal. Normal labor is considered to occur when the pregnancy is at or near term, there are no complications, and the process is completed within 24 hours. Critical care nurses caring for antepartum patients should monitor for signs of labor. These may include urinary frequency because of lightening (descending of the fetal presenting part into the pelvis), increase in vaginal mucus ("bloody show"), backaches, contractions, nausea, or rupture of membranes. Normal labor includes a regular progression of uterine contractions, effacement (thinning) and dilation of the cervix, and progress in the descent of the presenting part of the fetus through the birth canal.[55] The presence and strength of contractions can be assessed through fundal palpation. During a contraction, a fundus that feels like the tip of the nose is considered to be a contraction of mild strength. Moderate strength contractions feel like touching a finger to the chin, and during strong contractions, the fundus feels like touching a finger to the forehead.[69]

The normal labor and delivery process occurs in four stages (Table 47-4 and Figure 47-2). Throughout each of these stages, dramatic physiologic changes occur. These changes are due in part to the pain and anxiety associated with labor, but are also due to physiologic alterations. The most dramatic changes are seen in the cardiovascular system. Each contraction produces an

TABLE 47-4	Stages of Labor
LABOR STAGE	**DEFINITION/CHARACTERISTICS**
First stage	Onset of regular uterine contractions through full dilation of cervix. Typically lasts between 1 and 20 hours.
Latent phase of first stage	Progression of effacement and little descent of fetus. Typically ends at between 3 and 5 cm of dilation.
Active phase of first stage	Rapid dilation of cervix and increased rate of fetal descent.
Transition	Fetal head crowning occurs.
Second stage	From full cervical dilation through fetal delivery. Typically lasts 20 to 50 minutes.
Third stage	Birth of fetus through placental delivery. Typically lasts 3 minutes to 1 hour.
Fourth stage	First 2 hours after placental delivery. Immediate recovery phase and until initial homeostasis is achieved.

Data from references 22, 55.

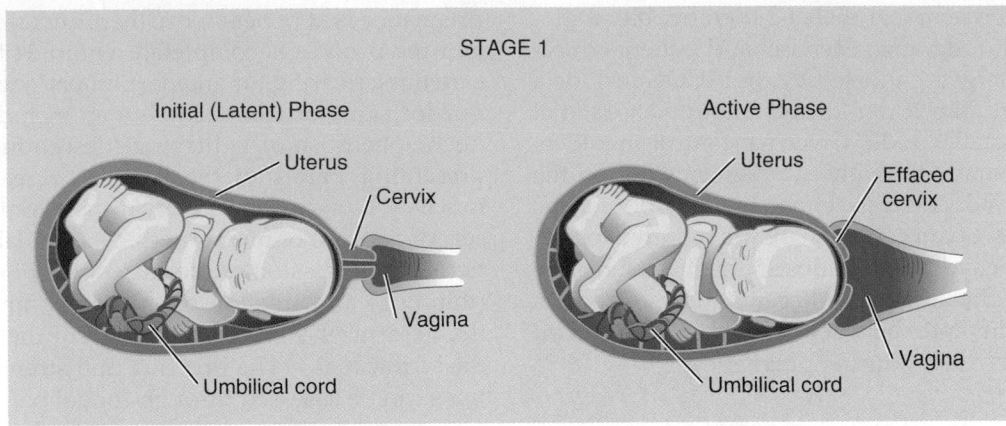

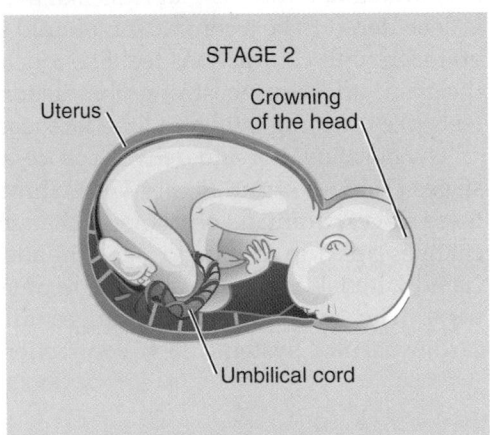

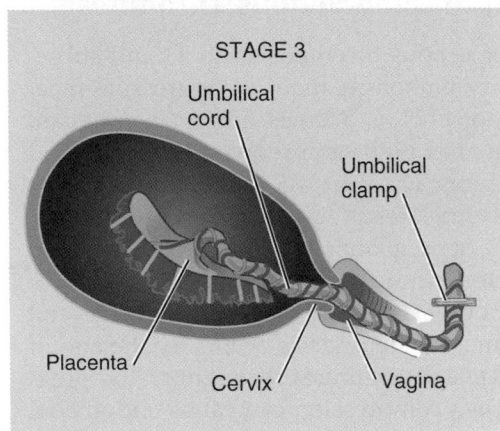

⬍**FIGURE 47-2** Stages of labor.

autotransfusion of approximately 300 to 500 ml; delivery produces a final maternal autotransfusion of approximately 1000 ml.[44] Because of these autotransfusions, CO changes dramatically during each phase of labor and in the immediate postpartum period. These changes are summarized in Table 47-5.[15,82] Blood loss also occurs

TABLE 47-5 Cardiac Output Changes in Labor and Delivery

LABOR STAGE	CHANGE IN CARDIAC OUTPUT
Early first stage of labor	Increased approximately 15%
Last first stage of labor	Increased approximately 30%–35%
Second stage of labor	Increased approximately 45%
First 5 minutes postpartum	Increased approximately 50%–65%
First hour postpartum	Increased 40%–50%

Data from references 64, 81.

during delivery and is generally estimated to be approximately 600 ml from a vaginal birth and 1000 ml from a cesarean birth.[60,76] Since these dramatic changes typically occur over a short length of time, mothers must be monitored carefully to assess tolerance and watch for potential decompensation. Critical care and obstetric collaboration are essential during the labor and delivery process, and the necessary equipment must be available (Box 47-3). Obstetric emergencies during the labor process include the development of non-reassuring fetal heart rate patterns, inadequate uterine relaxation, vaginal bleeding, or umbilical cord prolapse.[55]

Preterm labor is defined as cervical change and uterine contractions occurring between 20 weeks and 37 weeks of pregnancy. Preterm labor is multifactorial in nature and can lead to preterm birth, defined as any birth occurring before the end of 37 weeks of pregnancy.[29] Management of preterm labor includes prevention with prenatal care, lifestyle modifications to avoid activities presumed to initiate preterm labor, and restriction of physical activity. Tocolytic therapy—the administration of pharmaceutical agents, including ritodrine (Yutopar), terbutaline (Brethine), magnesium sulfate, or indomethacin (Indocin),[29] that suppress uterine activity—is a mainstay of therapy. Tocolytic therapy

Box 47-3

Suggested Supplies for Childbirth

- Birthing table
- Case cart with instruments, sutures, bulb syringe
- Infant crib with overhead radiant heat source
- Overhead lights
- Mirror
- Emergency equipment for both maternal and infant resuscitation
- Items for scrubbing (e.g., brushes)
- Sterile gowns and gloves, masks and goggles
- Sterile towels and drapes
- Anesthetic solutions and supplies
- Sterile basin
- Supplies for cleansing the perineum (solution, sponges, diluent)
- Infant identification materials
- Infant receiving blankets
- Material for prophylactic infant eye care and vitamin K administration
- Additional items for cesarean section may be required, such as indwelling Foley catheter, wedge for uterine displacement, surgical instruments required for procedure

Modified from reference 69.

can provide a window of opportunity for administration of glucocorticoids (e.g., betamethasone [Celestone] or dexamethasone [Decadron]), which can stimulate fetal lung maturity and reduce infant complications.

Labor induction is the chemical or mechanical initiation of uterine contractions before the natural onset of spontaneous labor. Labor induction is usually accomplished when the maternal and fetal risks of labor and birth are less than the risk of continuing the pregnancy.[68] The most common methods for labor induction include cervical ripening with prostaglandin agents or mechanical induction through artificial rupture of the membranes along with administration of oxytocin (Pitocin) to stimulate uterine contractions.

Pain Management

Pain management, outside of labor pain management, in critically ill obstetric patients is essentially similar to that for other critically ill patients. Consideration must be given to maternal and fetal tolerance of medications administered. Many narcotics decrease maternal BP, which can, in turn, reduce uteroplacental perfusion and subsequently cause non-reassuring fetal status.

Unique to the critically ill obstetric patient's pain management plan is pain management during labor. The ACOG Committee on Obstetric Practice states that pain management should be provided whenever medically indicated and that maternal request is a sufficient medical indication for pain relief during labor.[2] Labor pain management is best managed with collaborative expertise from obstetric and anesthesia colleagues. This is frequently accomplished with epidural analgesia, allowing the woman to maintain alertness and participation in the labor process with the fewest negative effects for the fetus. Epidural placement can cause vasodilation, commonly managed with a preplacement fluid bolus. Careful consideration of the woman's ability to tolerate the fluid bolus must be undertaken before administration.

POSTDELIVERY CARE

Management of the postdelivery patient requires collaboration between critical care and obstetric practitioners. Highlights of postpartum care are presented here in three broad categories: prevention of hemorrhage, support of breast-feeding, and support of maternal-infant bonding.

Prevention of Hemorrhage

Monitoring of lochial flow is essential. Immediate postdelivery lochial flow is generally to be considered normal if it is less than or equal to one pad per hour. Clots, quarter-sized or less, can be expected, but greater flow or larger clots warrant further investigation. Lochial flow is generally bright red for the first day (ruborous) and progresses to a more normal serosanguineous color after 2 to 3 days. Patients experiencing more than normal bleeding postdelivery should be assessed to determine the source of bleeding and for potential signs of shock. Appropriate lab studies (e.g., complete blood cell acount, type and crossmatch, coagulation studies) should be obtained and venous access ensured for volume resuscitation.

Postpartum hemorrhage may be due to coagulopathy. If coagulopathy is suspected, assess for the underlying cause, provide appropriate fluid and blood replacement therapy, and, if necessary, initiate pharmacologic support with vasopressors and uterotonic agents, such as oxytocin.[56] Surgical intervention may be required. Another major cause of postpartum bleeding is a nondelivered placenta. If the placenta has not yet been delivered, tocolytic therapy is typically implemented while the obstetric team is preparing to manually remove the placenta. Supportive therapy with fluid and blood replacement therapy as well as vasopressor support is also continued. If bleeding is not controlled following removal, surgical intervention may be required. Most major hemorrhages occur within the first hour postpartum.[11] Assessment of fundal height and character is done to ensure uterine firmness and recession. The top of the fundus is described as the number of finger breadths below the umbilicus, and the fundus should be firm, not boggy or mushy. If the fundus is not firm, uterine massage may be performed to stimulate uterine contractions and regression. Concerns about fundal height and character or the presence of continued bleeding require immediate consultation with obstetric colleagues. Cervical or vaginal lacerations should be ruled out and repaired if possible. If bleeding continues, uterine atony may be the cause and surgical intervention may be required. Ongoing supportive therapy and monitoring of maternal physiologic status is essential.[56]

Support of Breast-Feeding

Many mothers wish to breast-feed their newborn infants; this request should be honored and supported unless absolutely impossible. Consideration must be given to maternal medications and their safety for the infant. Consultation with obstetric and pharmacy colleagues is recommended to determine whether the mother's milk can be stored for later infant consumption or whether it should be discarded. If it is to be stored for later consumption, strict attention should be paid to institution policies for handling and storage of breast milk. General guidelines include storage in a separate refrigerator, with freezing of milk if storage is predicted to be longer than 3 days. Pumping with a hospital-grade electric pump should be initiated as soon as possible. General guidelines for pumping are to pump simultaneously for a minimum of 15 minutes on each breast every 2 to 4 hours. Assisting the mother to don a nursing support bra should be accomplished as soon as is feasible. Consultation with lactation or obstetric colleagues can enhance success for all involved.

Support of Maternal-Infant Bonding

Maternal-infant bonding is essential during the immediate postpartum period, and of special significance is the ability of the mother to hold her newborn infant. Although severe physiologic instability of either the infant or the mother may prohibit visitation, great strides should be taken to facilitate visitation if at all possible. Other mechanisms, such as pictures and recordings of infant or maternal voices, should be employed to enhance bonding as much as possible. Infant visitation in critical care should be accomplished whenever possible, and collaboration with neonatal or nursery staff can facilitate this experience. There is not an increased risk of infection to either the mother or the infant during visitation.

CARDIAC DISEASE IN PREGNANCY

General Considerations

Cardiac disease accounts for 15% of pregnancy-related mortality[13] and may be the result of preexisting conditions or may develop during pregnancy. Pre-pregnancy counseling is highly recommended for women with known cardiac disease to provide insight into the maternal and fetal risks associated with pregnancy[1] (Table 47-6) as well as open the discussion into appropriate timing of pregnancy. Some preexisting or congenital cardiac diseases may require intervention before conception to maximize maternal and fetal outcomes. Fetal risks include congenital heart disease, prematurity, intrauterine growth restriction (IUGR), and intrauterine fetal demise (IUFD).

General principles of antenatal management address four areas: coagulation, heart rate, volume status, and antibiotic prophylaxis. Anticoagulation is frequently recommended because of the normal hypercoagulable state of pregnancy. As mentioned previously, anticoagulation with heparin is recommended because of the teratogenic effects of oral agents.[10] Heart rate must be carefully monitored, and although mild tachycardia is expected, caution must be taken to avoid significant

TABLE 47-6 Maternal Mortality Risks		
GROUP 1 MORTALITY <1%	**GROUP 2 MORTALITY** 5%–15%	**GROUP 3 MORTALITY** 25%–50%
• Atrial septal defect • Ventricular septal defect • Patent ductus arteriosus • Pulmonic tricuspid disease • Corrected tetralogy of Fallot • Bioprosthetic valve • Mitral stenosis, NYHA Classes I and II • Marfan syndrome with normal aorta	• Mitral stenosis with atrial fibrillation • Artificial valve • Mitral stenosis, NYHA Classes III and IV • Aortic stenosis • Coarctation of aorta, uncomplicated • Uncorrected tetralogy of Fallot • Previous myocardial infarction	• Pulmonary hypertension • Coarctation of aorta, complicated • Marfan syndrome with aortic involvement

Data from reference 14.
NYHA = New York Heart Association.

tachycardia, which could compromise CO. Management is generally accomplished with beta blockade. Careful attention must be paid to maternal volume status to maintain as optimal euvolemia as possible. Pulmonary edema may be easily induced because of the natural decrease in colloid osmotic pressure. Antibiotic prophylaxis may be used to prevent endocarditis.

Problematic during pregnancy is that physiologic changes of pregnancy (e.g., murmur development, shortness of breath) may be accepted as routine when they actually are due to pathology. Cardiac monitoring is recommended through all stages of labor. Management of the pregnant woman with cardiac disease mandates collaboration between obstetric and cardiology colleagues to carefully monitor progress throughout pregnancy, as well as plan for delivery. Method and timing of delivery are decided primarily by obstetric needs, but must consider the woman's ability to tolerate the stress and cardiac demands of labor. Frequently, induction is planned to provide maximal resources during the labor and delivery process. Induction may be targeted to occur after cervical ripening has already begun to ease the cardiac workload. In addition, shortening the second or pushing stage of labor may be accomplished through use of vacuum- or forceps-assisted delivery techniques to alleviate prolonged cardiac stress. Patients who have received antenatal anticoagulation are generally changed to intravenous anticoagulation in the inpatient setting to allow careful titration of therapy. Pain management is crucial, as pain and anxiety can lead to tachycardia and potentially negative impacts on cardiac function. As a general rule, most patients tolerate epidural anesthesia better than general anesthesia, although attention must be paid to the risk of vasodilation. Intravenous fluid resuscitation should be immediately available. Aggressive control of bleeding should be accomplished in order to lessen fluid volume shifts in the immediate postpartum period.[47]

Pregnancy in Women With Preexisting Valvular Heart Disease

The significant physiologic changes during pregnancy can pose problems for patients with preexisting valvular heart disease. Pregnant women tolerate valve incompetence better than stenosis because of the decreased systemic vascular resistance (SVR) that helps to reduce the effects of regurgitation.[30] Generally, women with New York Heart Association (NYHA) Class I or II disease have a favorable prognosis in pregnancy, while those with Class III or IV have a difficult time tolerating the physiologic requirements. Approximately 62% of women can expect to have a worsening of their NYHA classification during pregnancy, 38% will develop heart failure, and up to 23% will experience adverse fetal outcomes.[40]

Mitral Valve Stenosis. The severity of mitral stenosis directly correlates with the frequency of adverse maternal cardiac, fetal, or neonatal events.[47] Decompensation in patients with mitral stenosis is generally associated with two primary causes: volume overload, causing pulmonary congestion and edema; and tachycardia, decreasing left ventricular filling time and CO as well as promoting pulmonary congestion. The risk for onset of atrial fibrillation and thromboembolism poses additional dangers to the mother. Management follows the general considerations in the antenatal period; percutaneous balloon mitral valvotomy may be recommended.[47] During labor and the immediate postpartum period, careful monitoring of cardiac and pulmonary status is required because of the fluid shifts that occur and resultant required CO changes. Patients with relatively fixed cardiac outputs because of the presence of mitral stenosis may rapidly decompensate during this time and develop acute pulmonary edema. Invasive hemodynamic monitoring may be employed. Recommended pulmonary artery wedge pressure before delivery is 14 mm Hg or less, to proactively accept the typical increase of up to 16 mm Hg in the immediate postpartum period.[15]

Aortic Stenosis. Management of mild to moderate aortic stenosis is typically conservative with the following general considerations. Depending on the severity of the lesion, stroke volume may be relatively fixed by the obstructed valve, causing heart rate to be the primary determinant of CO.[47] Careful attention must be paid to volume status, since hypovolemia can cause rapid decompensation. Decreases in preload from causes such as vasodilation from epidural anesthesia, diuresis, or postpartum hemorrhage can cause reflex tachycardia, which worsens the effects of aortic stenosis. Shortening of the second stage of labor is recommended because of the dramatic CO demands during this phase.[47]

Prosthetic Heart Valves. The natural hypercoagulable state of pregnancy provides additional challenges when attempting to maintain adequate anticoagulation for patients with mechanical heart valves. Biological valves require lower levels of anticoagulation.[47]

Pregnancy in Women With Congenital Heart Disease

Women with congenital heart disease must face two realities during pregnancy: the risk of cardiac decompensation and the potential for transmission of the congenital defect to the fetus. Proactive correction of maternal congenital defects may be advised. In general, women with corrected lesions tolerate pregnancy and the associated cardiac demands well. In addition to the general considerations and management during pregnancy, patients with congenital disease should be monitored with echocardiography and evaluated for the development of pulmonary hypertension. The development of pulmonary hypertension has a negative and rather dramatic impact on both maternal and fetal prognosis.[47] However, favorable outcomes using an epoprostenol (Flolan) infusion during pregnancy have been reported.[80] Epoprostenol, a naturally occurring prostaglandin manufactured in the vasculature, promotes pulmonary vasodilation, thereby reducing pulmonary vascular resistance. Several congenital defects are highlighted in the following paragraphs.

- **Left to right shunts.** Defects causing a left to right shunt (e.g., atrial septal defects, ventricular septal defects) are commonly well tolerated during pregnancy because of the natural hypervolemia. Logically, the size of the defect impacts the ability of the woman to meet the increased cardiac demands. Most typical complications are dysrhythmias, heart failure, and thromboembolism; proactive management should be employed to maximize outcome.
- **Marfan syndrome.** The prognosis of a pregnant woman with Marfan syndrome is primarily based upon aortic root diameter, with a significant increase in aortic dissection and mortality when the aortic root exceeds 4 to 4.5 cm.[46,73,75] Hypertension and aortic wall stress should be avoided and are typically managed with beta blockade.
- **Cyanotic lesions.** Cyanotic congenital heart diseases such as tetralogy of Fallot, transposition of the great arteries, tricuspid atresia, and others are frequently significant enough to require repair during the childhood years. Women with corrected cyanotic lesions often tolerate pregnancy well, although careful observation for and management of dysrhythmias, heart failure, thromboembolism, and pulmonary hypertension are essential.

Cardiac Disease Arising During Pregnancy

Peripartum Cardiomyopathy. Peripartum cardiomyopathy is defined as symptoms of heart failure that become apparent in the last month of pregnancy or within 5 months postpartum in patients who have no preexisting heart disease and no other obvious etiology for heart failure.[23] Etiology is unknown, although multiple hypotheses, including viral myocarditis, immune-mediated injury, selenium deficiency, cardiac stress of pregnancy, and myocarditis, have been proposed.[63] Symptoms and management of peripartum cardiomyopathy are similar to those seen with classic heart failure. Management is typically accomplished with preload optimization, afterload reduction, and inotropic support. Unique to pregnancy is the inability to provide afterload reduction

with angiotensin-converting enzyme (ACE) inhibitors. Administration of ACE inhibitors during the second and third trimesters of the antenatal period is associated with fetal renal dysfunction.[42] Alternatives including hydralazine (Apresoline) or nitroglycerin are considered safe. Controversy continues regarding the risk of peripartum cardiomyopathy in subsequent pregnancies; follow-up with echocardiography is recommended. Fortunately, research has demonstrated that contractile reserve during dobutamine stress echocardiography correlated with subsequent recovery of left ventricular function, indicating that for some women the diagnosis of peripartum cardiomyopathy is benign.[26]

Ischemic Heart Disease. The incidence of myocardial infarction during pregnancy is increasing and is more common in patients with hypertension, diabetes, and advanced maternal age.[49] Mortality ranges from 35% to 45% and partially depends on the timing of the myocardial event, with higher mortality if delivery and myocardial events are within 2 weeks of each other.[14,47] Diagnosis and management of acute ischemic heart disease during pregnancy is similar to conventional management, with general and pharmacologic considerations for pregnancy taken into consideration. Both thrombolytic use and primary coronary intervention in the pregnant patient have been reported[74,77,88] with positive outcomes.

Shock. Shock requires aggressive management of both the underlying cause and the current clinical status. Management must consider the enhanced physiologic cellular oxygen requirements during pregnancy. Therapies used are similar to conventional therapy, and practitioners must focus on maternal stabilization in order to provide an optimal uterine environment for the fetus. Special consideration should be given to fetal well-being when vasoconstrictors are employed, since uteroplacental insufficiency may result. Abruptio placentae, uterine rupture, placenta previa, and postpartum hemorrhage are examples of causes of hemorrhagic shock unique to pregnancy.[11] As discussed previously, postpartum hemorrhage may be caused by uterine atony, genital tract lacerations, hematoma formation, retained placenta, or uterine prolapse.[11] Unique causes of septic shock in the pregnant patient include chorioamnionitis, septic abortion, and postpartum pyelonephritis.[52]

Cardiac Arrest. Should cardiac arrest occur during pregnancy, the primary goal is to resuscitate the mother rapidly, thereby minimizing negative fetal effects. With a viable fetus, survival and outcome of the infant are directly proportional to the interval of time between maternal death and delivery. Fetal outcomes are usually enhanced if delivery is accomplished as soon as possible, and preferably within 5 minutes of cardiac arrest.[57] If perimortem cesarean section is to be performed, cardiopulmonary resuscitation should be continued during the procedure, performed by the most skilled available provider, and not be delayed for consent reasons. Neonatal services should be available to support the infant.[57] Perimortem cesarean section may improve CO and actually play a role in maternal survival as well. If the fetus has not yet reached the age of viability, there is little evidence as to whether perimortem cesarean section is beneficial.[57]

American Heart Association recommendations[9] for basic life support include minor changes from standard procedures for the pregnant patient. Ensuring venous return is essential and can easily be accomplished through lateral displacement of the uterus. Manual uterine displacement or placement of a wedge under the woman's hip will reduce vena caval compression and facilitate venous return. Risk for complications from cardiopulmonary resuscitation, including fractured ribs or sternum, hemothorax, hemopericardium, and internal organ damage, is greater during pregnancy.

There are no specific alterations of advanced life support guidelines for resuscitation during pregnancy. Electrical interventions (i.e., defibrillation, cardioversion, pacing) are acceptable during pregnancy. Defibrillation should occur at the same energy levels as in nonpregnant women.[57] Early aggressive airway support followed by oral intubation should be performed to address the increased oxygen demands, greater aspiration risk, and risk for mucosal bleeding. Advanced life support[9] pharmacologic interventions should be undertaken as usual. Vasoconstriction associated with epinephrine and vasopressin (Pitressin) administration may decrease placental perfusion; the maternal benefits likely outweigh the risk of administration. Sodium bicarbonate administration is controversial; most authorities recommend correction of maternal circulation and hypoxia to combat fetal acidosis rather than pharmacologic intervention.[57]

Hypertensive Disease

Hypertensive disease occurs in approximately 12% to 22% of pregnancies and is responsible for approximately 17% of maternal deaths.[3] Maternal compromise can be seen in the cardiovascular, pulmonary, renal, neurologic, and hepatic systems.[32,37,67] Fetal consequences include uteroplacental insufficiency, placental abruption, prematurity, IUGR, and IUFD.[90]

Classification. There are four classifications of hypertension during pregnancy, all with a systolic BP greater than or equal to 140 mm Hg and a diastolic pressure greater than 90 mm Hg.[85] Chronic hypertension is defined as hypertension present before conception or occurring before 20 weeks of gestation. Gestational hypertension is described as hypertension without proteinuria occurring after 20 weeks of gestation. The presence of proteinuria greater than 300 mg in 24 hours advances the diagnosis to preeclampsia;[85] the additional presence of seizures advances the diagnosis to eclampsia.[64,67] Specific criteria substratify hypertensive disease into mild and severe forms, based upon systolic and diastolic readings. The division point between mild and severe forms is based upon a systolic BP cut-off point of 160 mm Hg and a diastolic BP cut-off point of 105 to 110 mm Hg.[85]

Pathology. The pathology of preeclampsia is thought to be primarily related to vasospasms in the arterial system that result in endothelial damage, platelet aggregation, and decreased vascular volume. These arteriolar vasospasms result from abnormal sensitivity to vasoconstrictor substances such as angiotensin II, prostacyclin, and thromboxane A_2.[32,87] These generalized cyclic vasospasms lead to tissue ischemia and eventually end-organ dysfunction.[32] In addition, the damage done by vasospasm may lead to a decrease in circulating plasma volume, which is typically seen in proportion to the severity of disease.[24]

Management. Hypertensive disease in pregnancy should be managed to maximize maternal and fetal outcomes. Optimization of maternal fluid status is an essential component of preeclampsia management. This is typically accomplished with infusions of normal saline or lactated Ringer's solution at 100 to 125 ml/hour with boluses as required.[24] Monitoring the efficacy of replacement therapy is confounded because oliguria may not reflect actual volume depletion and because preeclamptic patients have been shown to have a poor central venous pressure (CVP) to pulmonary artery wedge pressure (PAWP) correlation.[24] Not all patients require fluid; preeclamptic patients can present with low, normal, or elevated PAWP readings.[24]

The goal of therapy is to maintain systolic pressure between 130 and 160 mm Hg and diastolic pressure between 80 and 110 mm Hg.[24] ACOG recommends methyldopa (Aldomet) or labetalol (Normodyne) as first-line therapy for severe hypertension.[6] Calcium channel blockers can be used, but are considered second-line agents.[90] Diuretic use poses concerns about altering the normal hypervolemic state of pregnancy, thereby decreasing perfusion to the placenta and potentially causing fetal compromise. ACE inhibitors are contraindicated during the second and third trimesters because of increases in fetal or neonatal morbidity and mortality.[85] Intravenous vasodilators such as hydralazine (Apresoline) or intravenous beta blockers such as labetalol are commonly employed for acute management of hypertensive crisis in the hospital setting. More potent vasodilators such as sodium nitroprusside (Nipride) are rarely used because of concerns about fetal toxicity. Most often, use during pregnancy is restricted to situations in which other agents have failed and delivery is imminent. ACOG relates that there is no clear benefit or enhancement in prenatal outcome that warrants treatment of women with uncomplicated mild hypertension.[3]

In addition to BP control, continuous assessment and management of both mother and fetus should be a collaborative effort between obstetric and critical care practitioners. Ongoing assessment of cardiovascular, pulmonary, renal, and neurologic systems provides early indications of potential maternal complications secondary to hypertension. Ongoing monitoring of fetal well-being is required, and accomplished through fetal monitoring, biophysical profile assessment, and fetal lung maturity testing through amniocentesis.

Management strategies include bedrest, seizure prevention, and delivery. Bedrest reduces the oxygen demand of the mother, allowing for fetal oxygenation. Seizure prevention and management are essential components of therapy.

Magnesium sulfate is the mainline therapy in the obstetric population rather than anticonvulsant therapies because of the vasospastic nature of the disease. Magnesium decreases neuromuscular irritability, decreases cardiac conduction, and decreases central nervous system irritability. Magnesium infusions of 1 to 2 g per hour are given following a loading bolus dose of 4 to 6 g in order to achieve serum magnesium levels of 4 to 7 mEq/L. Ongoing assessment during magnesium therapy includes monitoring of blood pressure, heart rate, respiratory rate, urine output, and deep tendon reflexes. Early signs of magnesium toxicity include nausea, feelings of warmth, flushing, muscle weakness, slurred speech, and a decrease in reflexes.[71] Outright seizure activity is controlled by administration of a 4- to 6-g intravenous magnesium sulfate bolus over 5 to 10 minutes.[86] Anticonvulsants such as phenytoin (Dilantin) may be indicated if magnesium is ineffective or cannot be tolerated, such as in a patient with impaired renal function. The ultimate management strategy is delivery of the fetus.

Complications. Complications of hypertensive disease include hemolysis, elevated liver enzymes, low platelets (HELLP) syndrome, and disseminated intravascular coagulation (DIC). HELLP syndrome is a cluster of symptoms reflecting the negative impact of arteriolar vasospasms. Vasospasm causes red blood cell hemolysis. Liver dysfunction causes elevated liver enzymes and platelet consumption, evidenced as thrombocytopenia. Although associated with hypertensive

---

◆ **Case Study 47-1, Part B**

Monitoring, Assessing, and Managing a Compromised Pregnant Patient

B.F. is placed in a side-lying position and given two 1000-ml normal saline fluid boluses. Magnesium therapy via bolus and infusion is initiated, as well as labetalol and betamethasone administration. Oxygen is provided at 4 L/min per nasal cannula. Over the next several hours, B.F.'s condition begins to deteriorate. Heart rate is now 128 beats/min, respiratory rate 32 breaths/min, BP 198/120 mm Hg, and pulse oximetry 91%. B.F. remains oliguric despite the fluid boluses. Contractions have eased, but fetal heart rate monitoring reveals a baseline rate of 110s with a loss of variability. The decision is made to transfer B.F. to consult critical care for further evaluation and management.

Decision point: What physiologic and technical monitoring does the critical care nurse need to institute to monitor this pregnant patient and her fetus?

Decision point: Which hemodynamic findings would suggest that this mother is compromised?

Decision point: What interventions are needed to support her cardiovascular and pulmonary status?

Decision point: What findings would suggest that the fetus is compromised? What does the critical care nurse need to do to support the fetus and anticipate emergent delivery or C-section?

Decision point: How should this pregnant patient's pain be managed in a way that is safe for the fetus?

Case continues on page 1337

disease in approximately 4% to 12% of patients, approximately 10% to 20% of pregnant patients with HELLP syndrome will not have elevated BP.[24,51] Patients are critically ill and may require invasive monitoring and aggressive supportive management. Complications of HELLP include abruptio placentae, liver hematoma, DIC, pulmonary edema, liver rupture, and acute renal failure.[24] Preeclampsia-eclampsia, along with abruptio placentae, dead fetus syndrome, septic abortion, and amniotic fluid embolus, are all obstetric-related causes of DIC. Management is similar to conventional management, with the additional caveats of treating the obstetric-specific cause, if applicable.

PULMONARY DYSFUNCTION IN PREGNANCY

Oxygen requirements are elevated during pregnancy, and since fetal oxygenation is directly dependent on maternal oxygen supply, compromise of maternal respiratory function places both mother and fetus at risk for harm. Maternal hypoxia can be caused by various conditions, including, but not limited to, pneumonia, asthma, trauma, acute respiratory distress syndrome (ARDS), and PE.

Mechanical Ventilation

Mechanical ventilation settings should mimic physiologic tachypnea, increased tidal volume, enhanced minute ventilation, and decreased functional residual volumes of pregnancy. In addition, the physiologic $Paco_2$ of 30 to 32 mm Hg should be maintained. Sedation and analgesia to enhance tolerance of therapy are similar to conventional therapy. Fetal impact of sedative and analgesic agents administered must be considered; obstetric colleagues should be aware of medications used when analyzing fetal well-being. Neuromuscular blocking agents may be required during pregnancy for facilitation of mechanical ventilation. Care providers must recognize that only skeletal muscle is affected; therefore the uterine smooth muscle can still contract. In addition, neuromuscular blocking agents cross the placental barrier and paralyze the fetus as well. If delivery occurs, neonatal resuscitation will be required for fetal support.

Asthma

The prevalence of asthma during pregnancy is currently between 3.7% and 8.4%.[41,48] Adverse outcomes associated with asthma include preterm labor, low birth weight infants, preeclampsia, hyperemesis gravidarum, gestational diabetes, labor complications, IUGR, and IUFD.[31] Approximately one third of women will see improvement in their asthma symptoms, one third will see no change, and one third will see their symptoms worsen during pregnancy. If asthma exacerbation occurs, it will most likely take place during the second and third trimesters.[41]

Management recommendations are similar to conventional therapies, including avoidance of triggers, monitoring of peak flow, and routine use of medications. Peak flow rate does not change during pregnancy,[35] so it serves as a reliable indicator of maternal pulmonary function. A change in peak flow rates to the "yellow" zone, indicating a decrease to 50% to 80% of the patient's norm, requires physician notification for a symptom and management plan review. A decrease in peak flow rates into the "red" zone, or less than 50% of the patient's norm, requires immediate attention and physician notification for aggressive intervention.[31] Pharmacologic front-line therapies such as inhaled bronchodilators (beta agonists) and cromolyn sodium (Crolom) are considered safe during pregnancy.[31] Inhaled corticosteroids are preferred over oral corticosteroids for safety reasons.[41] In the postpartum period, breast-feeding while

receiving asthma medications is considered both beneficial to the mother and safe for the infant.[31]

Acute Respiratory Distress Syndrome

ARDS can result from a variety of conditions. Causes rather unique to pregnancy include tocolytic administration leading to pulmonary edema, preeclampsia, eclampsia, placental abruption, postpartum hemorrhage, amniotic fluid embolism/anaphylactoid syndrome, septic abortion, and IUFD. However, regardless of whether the cause of ARDS is unique to pregnancy or seen in the general population, management is similar to conventional therapy with the addition of the pregnancy-specific pulmonary management considerations mentioned previously. Target tidal volume of 6 ml/kg of predicted body weight, inspiratory plateau pressures of less than 30 cm of water, supplemental oxygenation, and appropriate positive end-expiratory pressure settings are all recommended therapies during pregnancy.[21] Caution must be used to avoid significant hypercarbia, because of the normal respiratory alkalosis of pregnancy.[21] Rotational and prone therapies can be accomplished during the antenatal period.

Pulmonary Embolism

PE has recently surpassed infection, hemorrhage, and preeclampsia-eclampsia as a leading cause of maternal mortality[81] and is linked to the incidence of venous thromboembolism. The immediate postpartum period is a high-risk period for PE and will be fatal in almost 15% of patients.[81] Presentation and diagnosis of PE are similar to those in nonpregnant patients, although practitioners must have a high index of suspicion. Management is accomplished with standard supportive care and anticoagulation. Heparin and low molecular weight heparins do not cross the placenta, but higher doses than normal may be required to maintain therapeutic anticoagulation.[81] Thrombolytic therapy is relatively contraindicated during pregnancy, although case reports have demonstrated low maternal mortality. Vena cava filters can be used safely during pregnancy.[81]

Amniotic Fluid Embolism/Anaphylactoid Syndrome of Pregnancy

Amniotic fluid embolism (AFE) is a highly catastrophic condition that occurs during labor and delivery or the immediate postpartum period because of the presumed exposure of amniotic fluid to the maternal circulation. It is believed that the event is triggered by the release of vasoactive substances into the maternal circulation. Reported, but inconsistently supported, risk factors include turbulent labor, trauma, multiparity, oxytocin use, increased maternal age, increased gestational age, male fetus, and cesarean sections.[61] Pulmonary artery spasm occurs, with resultant severe and sudden hypoxemia, pulmonary hypertension, and heart failure, causing shock out of proportion to blood loss. Total cardiovascular collapse, seizures, and DIC may rapidly follow. Diagnosis is essentially clinical, made on the basis of clinical presentation of a woman presenting with profound shock, cardiovascular collapse, and severe respiratory distress while in labor or shortly after delivery.[61] Management requires aggressive airway management, oxygenation, cardiovascular support with fluids and inotropic therapy, rapid delivery, and correction of coagulopathies. Fortunately, incidence is reported in ranges from 1 in 8000 to 1 in 83,000 deliveries.[61] Mortality rates reported in 1995 for AFE were 61%;[18] however, improved care has dropped mortality rates to 30% or less.[33]

ACUTE FATTY LIVER OF PREGNANCY

Acute fatty liver of pregnancy (AFLP) occurs rarely, with incidence estimates varying between 1 in 6659 and 1 in 13,000 births.[39] AFLP most likely occurs because of an enzyme deficiency that increases levels of long-chain fatty acids, causing hepatic overload and hepatotoxicity. Women present with abdominal pain, fatigue, nausea, or vomiting. Unfortunately, these symptoms can be easily overlooked; therefore sometimes jaundice, altered mentation, hepatic encephalopathy, or hypoglycemia are the initial presenting symptoms. As the disease progresses, renal failure, acidosis, and coagulopathies ensue. Frequently, AFLP is associated with hypertensive diseases or HELLP syndrome. Diagnosis is confirmed by liver biopsy. Management includes delivery, which stops the overload of long-chain fatty acids, and appropriate supportive therapies.[39]

TRAUMA IN PREGNANCY

The primary cause of trauma in pregnancy is motor vehicle crashes; however, other types of injuries, such as falls, assaults, and burns, also occur. The presence of blunt trauma, especially injuries involving the face, head, abdomen, or breasts, should raise the suspicion of domestic violence.[4,53] The first trimester accounts for approximately 10% of injuries during pregnancy, the second trimester 40%, and the remaining 50% in the third trimester.[79] Proper maternal seatbelt use, with the belt positioned under the pregnant abdomen and the shoulder harness between the breasts, should be encouraged as typically only 46% of pregnant trauma patients are restrained.[59] Life-threatening trauma is

associated with a 40% to 50% risk of fetal loss; however, fetal loss frequently also follows relatively minor trauma.[59] Mechanisms of injury are similar in the pregnant and nonpregnant populations. Management of trauma during pregnancy is similar to conventional management (Chapter 42), with few alterations. Assessment findings may be altered by the normal physiologic changes of pregnancy.

General Pregnancy Considerations

First Trimester. Before fetal viability, resuscitative efforts must be focused on establishing maternal stability. Providing optimal maternal status is the best management plan for the fetus. Fortunately, the fetus is well protected from external trauma since the uterus remains a pelvic organ until after the twelfth week of gestation. Spontaneous abortion can occur, however, so careful monitoring of vaginal bleeding or discharge is required.

Second Trimester. As the fetus and uterine environment grow, maternal abdominal organs are displaced, a consideration during physical assessment. Women who experience even minor traumatic injury beyond 22 to 24 weeks of gestation should undergo observation and fetal monitoring for between 4 and 48 hours to assess fetal well-being and observe for latent injuries or premature labor. Once the fetus has reached the stage of viability, all therapeutic interventions must be weighed in terms of risk/benefit ratio for both mother and fetus. Emergent delivery may be required.

Third Trimester. The risk of falls increases as the fetus grows and changes the woman's gait and center of gravity. Throughout the early weeks of gestation, the fetus is well cushioned by the uterus, amniotic fluid, and the maternal abdominal wall. As the antenatal period continues, risk for traumatic fetal injury increases. Fetal skull injury and intracranial hemorrhage may occur as the fetus begins to settle into the pelvis in preparation for birth. Fetal death is most commonly the result of a fetal skull fracture, or secondary to placental abruption or preterm birth.[20]

Cardiovascular Considerations

Practitioners should keep in mind that the volume expansion in pregnant women provides a physiologic reserve for blood loss, so blood loss and hypoperfusion may occur before typical symptoms would be seen.[11,20] Upper extremity or central access should be obtained for fluid resuscitation, as venous return may be impeded if infusing volume through lower extremity sites. Generally, 3 ml of volume resuscitation should occur for each milliliter of blood lost, with careful monitoring to prevent volume overload and pulmonary edema (Chapter 41). Hgb levels should be monitored carefully, since blood loss can significantly impact maternal and fetal oxygenation. Venous return must be maximized either through lateral displacement of the uterus or by tilting the woman at least 30 degrees to one side. In extreme circumstances, pneumatic antishock garments may be applied without inflation of the abdominal compartment.[59]

Abdominal and Pelvic Considerations

Presence of the gravid uterus and subsequent displacement of abdominal organs pose challenges for healthcare providers following maternal abdominal trauma. Traditional assessment and pain locations may be altered, confounding diagnosis. Classic peritoneal signs such as tenderness, rigidity, and rebound tenderness are unreliable. Diagnostic peritoneal lavage, if required, is typically accomplished with open technique through a supra-umbilical site. The pelvic vasculature and all pelvic organs are engorged. This requires caution when performing vaginal or rectal assessments and caution when placing urinary catheters, and increases the risk of retroperitoneal hemorrhage.

Reproductive System Considerations

A comprehensive maternal and fetal assessment should be performed as soon as possible. Information gathered should include gestational age, the number of fetuses, obstetric history, obstetrician, Rh factor, and any prenatal complications to date. Obstetric physical assessment should determine fetal presentation, status of amniotic membrane, and the presence of fetal parts or umbilical cord in the vagina. Monitoring of fundal height; uterine size, position, and tone; and also fetal heart rate should be performed. Ultrasound assessment will provide insight into fetal position and placental location and condition. Amniocentesis may be performed to assess for the presence of red blood cells in amniotic fluid and to analyze fetal lung maturity through use of the lecithin/sphingomyelin (L/S) ratio and presence of phosphatidylglycerol. Tocolytic therapy to stop contractions may be required.

Neurologic System Considerations

Whether spinal cord injury (SCI) is acute or chronic, there are several considerations during the labor and delivery process. Generally speaking, vaginal delivery is possible for most SCI patients. Women with injuries above the T6 level are more prone to autonomic dysreflexia, and may require assisted vaginal delivery or a cesarean section.[8,66] Provision of epidural analgesia early in labor may help avoid the autonomic dysreflexia associated with uterine contractions. Women with injuries above T10 are unable to feel uterine contractions because of spinal cord insertion of the uterine sensory nerves at the T11 to L1 level. Uterine palpation and associated symptoms such as shortness of breath or abdominal spasms must be relied upon to determine the onset of labor.

Multisystem Considerations

Final multisystem considerations should occur after initial stabilization of the mother. Toxicology results should be carefully reviewed with consideration given to the fetal effects of substances ingested. Necessary radiology studies should be performed, with appropriate shielding to reduce fetal radiation exposure. Administration of tetanus toxoid is safe since it does not cross the placenta. Rh-negative mothers must receive immune globulin (RhoGAM) if there is a possibility that they have been exposed to Rh-positive blood. This can occur through administration of Rh-positive blood in an emergency situation, or if the placental integrity of an Rh-positive fetus has been violated. The Kleihauer-Betke test is used to detect the presence of fetal blood in the maternal bloodstream, and if positive, it indicates the need for RhoGAM administration. Guidelines for administration are 300 mcg initially and an additional 300 mcg for every 30 ml of estimated fetomaternal transfusion.[59]

◆ Case Study 47-1, Part C

Multidisciplinary Care After Emergency Cesarean Section

Following cesarean section, B.F.'s vital signs include a temperature of 36.6° C, heart rate 110 beats/min, respiratory rate 14 breaths/min, BP 156/98 mm Hg, and pulse oximetry 99%. Hemodynamic data reveal cardiac output 6.2 L/min, pulmonary artery pressure (PAP) 36/24 mm Hg, PAWP 20 mm Hg, SVR 1800 dynes/sec/cm^{-5}, and CVP 8 mm Hg. B.F. recovers from the general anesthetic without complications and is able to wean from mechanical ventilatory support within 12 hours. Diuresis continues, and within 24 hours hemodynamics improve and the pulmonary artery catheter is removed. Critical care and obstetric collaboration provide B.F. and her daughter with frequent visits and condition updates. Lactation is consulted to assist with facilitation of B.F.'s request to breast-feed. B.F. is transferred to the postpartum unit on day 2 and is discharged home with her daughter on day 5.

Decision point: What are three complications associated with pregnancy that the critical care nurse should anticipate? What are significant findings and interventions for each problem?

CONCLUSIONS

Caring for the critically ill obstetric patient presents unique challenges to critical care practitioners. Optimizing care for mother and fetus requires interdisciplinary collaboration and a conscious awareness of the impact of interventions and medications on both mother and fetus. Maternal assessment and management must be undertaken with constant consideration of pregnancy physiologic alterations. Immediate access to obstetric colleagues is essential. The multidisciplinary team should continually focus on the maternal-fetal relationship, with the goal of optimizing maternal status so as to provide an optimal in utero environment for the fetus. Obstetric patients may require critical care services during pregnancy because of preexisting disease or critical illness or injury that arises during pregnancy. Each interaction brings unique challenges, but is also an opportunity to optimize the maternal-family experience.

REFERENCES

1. American College of Obstetricians and Gynecologists. (1992). *Cardiac disease in pregnancy*. Technical Bulletin 168.
2. American College of Obstetricians and Gynecologists. (2004). Committee Opinion 295: *Pain relief during labor*.
3. American College of Obstetricians and Gynecologists. (2002). *Diagnosis and management of preeclampsia and eclampsia*. ACOG Practice Bulletin 33.
4. American College of Obstetricians and Gynecologists. (1999). *Domestic violence*. Educational Bulletin 257, December.
5. American College of Obstetricians and Gynecologists. (2001). *Gestational diabetes*. ACOG Practice Bulletin 30, Washington, DC.
6. American College of Obstetricians and Gynecologists. (2001). *Hypertension in pregnancy*. ACOG Practice Bulletin 29, Washington, DC.
7. American College of Obstetricians and Gynecologists. (1988). *Invasive hemodynamic monitoring in obstetrics and gynecology*. Technical Bulletin 121.
8. American College of Obstetricians and Gynecologists. (2002). *Obstetric management of patients with spinal cord injuries*. Committee Opinion 275.
9. American Heart Association. (2002). *Textbook of advanced cardiac life support*. Dallas, Tex: American Heart Association.
10. Briggs, G., Freeman, R., & Yaffe, S. (2005). *Drugs in pregnancy and lactation* (7th ed.). Baltimore: Williams & Wilkins.
11. Burton, R., & Belfort, M. A. (2004). Etiology and management of hemorrhage. In G. Dildy, et al. (Eds.), *Critical care obstetrics* (4th ed.). Malden, Mass: Blackwell Publishing.
12. Carroll, M. A., & Yeomans, E. R. (2005). Diabetic ketoacidosis in pregnancy. *Crit Care Med, 33*(10), S347–S353.
13. Chang, J., et al. (2003). Pregnancy-related mortality surveillance—United States, 1991–1999. *MMWR, 52*(SS02), 1–8.
14. Clark, S. (1987). Structural cardiac disease in pregnancy. In S. L. Clark, D. B. Cotton, & P. Pehlan (Eds.), *Critical care obstetrics*. Oradell, NJ: Medical Economics Books.
15. Clark, S., et al. (1985). Labor and delivery in the presence of mitral stenosis: central hemodynamic observations. *Am J Obstet Gynecol, 152*, 984–988.
16. Clark, S., et al. (1989). Central hemodynamic assessment of normal term pregnancy. *Am J Obstet Gynecol, 161*, 1439–1442.
17. Clark, S., et al. (1991). Position change and central hemodynamic profile during normal third-trimester pregnancy and post partum. *Am J Obstet Gynecol, 164*, 883–887.
18. Clark, S., et al. (1995). Amniotic fluid embolism analysis of the National Registry. *Am J Obstet Gynecol, 172*, 1158–1167.
19. Cleary-Goldman, J., et al. (2005). Impact of maternal age on obstetric outcome. *Am J Obstet Gynecol, 105*(5).
20. Colburn, V. (1999). Trauma in pregnancy. *J Perinat Neonat Nurs, 3*, 21–32.
21. Cole, D. E., et al. (2005). Acute respiratory distress syndrome in pregnancy. *Crit Care Med, 33*(10), S269–S278.
22. Cunningham, F. G., et al. (2005). *Williams obstetrics* (22nd ed.). Norwalk, Conn: Appleton & Lange.
23. Demakis, J. G., et al. (1971). Natural course of peripartum cardiomyopathy. *Circulation, 44*, 1053–1062.
24. Dildy, G. (2004). Complications of pre-eclampsia. In G. Dildy, et al. (Eds.), *Critical care obstetrics* (4th ed.). Malden, Mass: Blackwell Publishing.
25. DiSaia, P. J. (2003). Radiation therapy in gynecology. In J. R. Scott, et al. (Eds.), *Danforth's obstetrics and gynecology* (9th ed.). Philadelphia: Lippincott.
26. Dorbala, S., et al. (2005). Risk stratification of women with peripartum cardiomyopathy at initial presentation: a dobutamine stress echocardiography study. *J Am Soc Echocardiography, 18*(1), 45–48.
27. Doyle, N., & Monga, M. (2004). Thromboembolic disease in pregnancy. *Obstet Gynecol Clin North Am, 31*, 319–344.
28. Francalanci, I., et al. (1995). D-dimer concentrations during normal pregnancy, as measured by ELISA. *Thromb Res, 78*, 399–405.
29. Freda, M. C. (2000). Preterm labor and birth. In D. L. Lowdermilk, S. E. Perry, & I. M. Bobak (Eds.), *Maternity and women's health care* (7th ed.). St. Louis: Mosby.
30. Fujitani, S., & Baldisseri, M. R. (2005). Hemodynamic assessment in a pregnant and peripartum patient. *Crit Care Med, 33*(10), S354–S361.
31. Gardner, M., & Doyle, N. (2004). Asthma in pregnancy. *Obstet Gynecol Clin North Am, 31*, 385–413.
32. Gilbert, E., & Harmon, J. (2003). *Manual of high risk pregnancy and delivery* (3rd ed.). St. Louis: Mosby.
33. Gilbert, W., & Danielson, B. (1999). Amniotic fluid embolism: decreased mortality in a population-based study. *Obstet Gynecol, 93*, 973–977.
34. Goodsitt, M. M., & Christodoulou, E. G. (2004). Image safety during pregnancy. In M. D. Pearlman, J. E. Tintinalli, & P. Dyne (Eds.), *Obstetric and gynecologic emergencies*. New York: McGraw-Hill.
35. Graves, C. R. (2002). Acute pulmonary complications during pregnancy. *Clin Obstet Gynecol, 45*(2), 369–376.
36. Greer, I. A. (1999). Thrombosis in pregnancy: maternal and fetal issues. *Lancet, 353*, 1258–1265.
37. Gregg, A. (2004). Hypertension in pregnancy. *Obstet Gynecol Clin North Am, 31*, 223–241.
38. Griffith, J., & Conway, D. (2004). Care of diabetes in pregnancy. *Obstet Gynecol Clin North Am, 31*, 243–256.
39. Guntupalli, S. R., & Steingrub, J. (2005). Hepatic disease and pregnancy: an overview of diagnosis and management. *Crit Care Med, 33*(10), S332–S339.
40. Hameed, A., et al. (2001). The effect of valvular heart disease on maternal and fetal outcome of pregnancy. *J Am Coll Cardiol, 37*(3), 893–899.
41. Hanania, N. A., & Belfort, M. A. (2005). Acute asthma in pregnancy. *Crit Care Med, 33*(10), S319–S324.
42. Hanssens, M., et al. (1991). Fetal and neonatal effects of treatment with angiotensin-converting enzyme inhibitors in pregnancy. *Obstet Gynecol, 78*, 128–135.
43. Harrison, B. P., & Crytal, C. S. (2003). Imaging modalities in obstetrics and gynecology. *Emerg Med Clin North Am, 21*, 711–735.

44. Harvey, M. G. (1991). Physiologic changes of pregnancy. In C. J. Harvey (Ed.), *Critical care obstetrical nursing*. Gaithersburg, Md: Aspen.

45. Institute of Medicine. (1992). *Nutrition during pregnancy and lactation: an implementation guide*. Washington, DC: National Academy Press.

46. Jelsema, R., & Cotton, D. (1999). Cardiac disease. In D. K. James, et al. (Eds.), *High risk pregnancy: management options* (2nd ed.). Philadelphia: Saunders.

47. Klein, L., & Galan, H. (2004). Cardiac disease in pregnancy. *Obstet Gynecol Clin North Am, 31*, 429–459.

48. Kwon, H., Belanger, K., & Bracken, M. (2003). Asthma prevalence during pregnancy in the United States: estimates from national health surveys. *Ann Epidemiol, 13*, 317–324.

49. Ladner, H., Danielsen, B., & Gilbert, W. (2005). Acute myocardial infarction in pregnancy and the puerperium: a population based study. *Obstet Gynecol, 105*, 480–484.

50. Lange, S., & Jenner, M. (2004). Myocardial infarction in the obstetric patient. *Crit Care Nurs Clin North Am, 16*, 211–219.

51. Leicht, T. G., & Harvey, C. J. (1999). Hypertensive disorders in pregnancy. In L. K. Mandeville & N. H. Troiano (Eds.), *High-risk intrapartum nursing*. Philadelphia: Lippincott.

52. Leonardi, M. R., & Gonik, B. (2004). Septic shock. In G. Dildy, et al. (Eds.), *Critical care obstetrics* (4th ed.). Malden, Mass: Blackwell Publishing.

53. Lipsky, S., et al. (2003). Impact of police reported intimate partner violence during pregnancy on birth outcomes. *Obstet Gynecol, 102*(3), 557–564.

54. Lowdermilk, D. L. (2000). Anatomy and physiology of pregnancy. In D. L. Lowdermilk, S. E. Perry, & I. M. Bobak (Eds.), *Maternity and women's health care* (7th ed.). St. Louis: Mosby.

55. Lowdermilk, D. L. (2000). Labor and birth processes. D. L. Lowdermilk, S. E. Perry, & I. M. Bobak (Eds.), *Maternity and women's health care* (7th ed.). St. Louis: Mosby.

56. Lowdermilk, D. L. (2000). Postpartum complications. In D. L. Lowdermilk, S. E. Perry, & I. M. Bobak (Eds.), *Maternity and women's health care* (7th ed.). St. Louis: Mosby.

57. Mallampalli, A., & Guy, E. (2005). Cardiac arrest in pregnancy and somatic support after brain death. *Crit Care Med, 33*(10), S325–S331.

58. Mattox, K. L., & Goetzl, L. (2005). Trauma in pregnancy. *Crit Care Med, 33*(10), S385–S389.

59. Meadows, M. (May-June 2001). Pregnancy and the drug dilemma. *FDA Consumer Magazine, 35*(3).

60. Monga, M., & Creasy, R. (2004). Maternal cardiovascular and renal adaptation to pregnancy. In R. Creasy, R. Resnik, & J. Iams (Eds.), *Maternal-fetal medicine* (5th ed.). Philadelphia: Saunders.

61. Moore, J., & Baldisseri, M. R. (2005). Amniotic fluid embolism. *Crit Care Med, 33*(10), S279–S285.

62. Moore, J. C. (2000). Maternal and fetal nutrition. In D. L. Lowdermilk, S. E. Perry, & I. M. Bobak (Eds.), *Maternity and women's health care* (7th ed.). St. Louis: Mosby.

63. Murali, S., & Baldisseri, M. R. (2005). Peripartum cardiomyopathy. *Crit Care Med, 33*(10), S340–S346.

64. National High Blood Pressure in Pregnancy Education Program Working Group. (2000). *Working group report on high blood pressure in pregnancy*. NHBPEP Publication.

65. Norwitz, E. R., et al. (2004). Pregnancy-induced physiologic alterations. In G. Dildy, et al. (Eds.), *Critical care obstetrics* (4th ed.). Malden, Mass: Blackwell Publishing.

66. Pereira, L. (2003). Obstetric management of the patient with spinal cord injuries. *Obstet Gynecol Survey, 58*(10), 678–686.

67. Peters, R. M., & Flack, J. M. (2004). Hypertensive disorders of pregnancy. *JOGN, 33*(2), 209–214.

68. Piotrowski, K. A. (2000). Labor and birth complications. In D. L. Lowdermilk, S. E. Perry, & I. M. Bobak (Eds.), *Maternity and women's health care* (7th ed.). St. Louis: Mosby.

69. Piotrowski, K. A. (2000). Nursing care during labor. In D. L. Lowdermilk, S. E. Perry, & I. M. Bobak (Eds.), *Maternity and women's health care* (7th ed.). St. Louis: Mosby.

70. Poole, J., & Long, J. (2004). Maternal mortality—a review of current trends. *Crit Care Nurs Clin North Am, 16*, 227–230.

71. Poole, J. (2000). Hypertensive disorders in pregnancy. In D. L. Lowdermilk, S. E. Perry, & I. M. Bobak (Eds.), *Maternity and women's health care* (7th ed.). St. Louis: Mosby.

72. Poole, J. (2004). Multiorgan dysfunction in the perinatal patient. *Crit Care Nurs Clin North Am, 16*, 193–204.

73. Pyeritz, R. E. (1981). Maternal and fetal complications of pregnancy in the Marfan syndrome. *Am J Med, 71*, 784–790.

74. Roth, A., & Elkayam, U. (1996). Acute myocardial infarction associated with pregnancy. *Ann Intern Med, 125*, 751–762.

75. Rutherford, J. D., & Hands, M. (2002). Preexisting heart disease. In P. S. Douglas (Ed.), *Cardiovascular health and disease in women* (2nd ed.). Philadelphia: Saunders.

76. Sacks, D. A. (2004). Blood component replacement therapy. In G. Dildy, et al. (Eds.), *Critical care obstetrics* (4th ed.). Malden, Mass: Blackwell Publishing.

77. Schumacher, B., Belfort, M. A., & Card, R. J. (1997). Successful treatment of acute myocardial infarction during pregnancy with tissue plasminogen activator. *Am J Obstet Gynecol, 176*, 716–719.

78. Simpson, K. (2004). Fetal assessment in the adult intensive care unit. *Crit Care Nurs Clin North Am, 16*, 233–242.

79. Stallard, T. C., & Burns, B. (2003). Emergency delivery and perimortem C-section. *Emerg Med Clin North Am, 21*, 679–693.

80. Stewart, R., et al. (2001). Pregnancy and primary pulmonary hypertension: successful outcome with epoprostenol therapy. *Chest, 119*, 973–975.

81. Stone, S. E., & Morris, T. A. (2005). Pulmonary embolism during and after pregnancy. *Crit Care Med, 33*(10), S294–S300.

82. Troiano, N. H. (1999). Cardiac diseases in pregnancy. In L. K. Mandeville & N. H. Troiano (Eds.), *High-risk intrapartum nursing*. Philadelphia: Lippincott.

83. Tucker, S. M. (2000). Fetal assessment. In D. L. Lowdermilk, S. E. Perry, & I. M. Bobak (Eds.), *Maternity and women's health care* (7th ed.). St. Louis: Mosby.

84. VanHook, J. W. (2002). Trauma in pregnancy. *Clin Obstet Gynecol, 45*(2), 414–424.

85. Vidaeff, A. C., Carroll, M. A., & Ramin, S. M. (2005). Acute hypertensive emergencies in pregnancy. *Crit Care Med, 33*(10), S307–S312.

86. Villar, M., & Sibai, B. (1988). Eclampsia. *Obstet Gynecol Clin North Am, 15*(2), 355–377.

87. Walsh, S. (1985). Preeclampsia: an imbalance in placental prostacyclin and thromboxane production. *Am J Obstet Gynecol, 152*, 335–340.

88. Webber, M. D., Halligan, R. E., & Schumacher, J. A. (1997). Acute infarction, intracoronary thrombolysis, and primary PTCA in pregnancy. *Cathet Cardiovasc Diagn, 42*, 38–43.

89. Whitty, J. E., & Dombrowski, M. P. (2002). Respiratory diseases in pregnancy. In S. G. Gabbe, J. K. Niebyl, & J. L. Simpson (Eds.), *Obstetric normal and problem pregnancies* (4th ed.). Philadelphia: Churchill Livingstone.

90. Yankowitz, J. (2004). Pharmacologic treatment of hypertensive disorders during pregnancy. *J Perinatal Neonatal Nurs, 18*, 230–240.

91. Yeomans, E. R., & Gilstrap, L. C. (2005). Physiologic changes in pregnancy and their impact on critical care. *Crit Care Med, 33*(10), S256–S258.

CHAPTER 48

Caring for the Pediatric Patient in an Adult Critical Care Unit

Mary Frances D. Pate

A fundamental position is that society has a special obligation to address the needs of children because they must depend on others for the protection of their health and safety and have no political voice of their own.[59]

This chapter is designed to be a resource for those nurses who care predominantly for critically ill adults. The saying goes that "children are not little adults." While skilled in caring for adult patients, these same critical care nurses are often acutely aware of this fact, especially if only a small number of pediatric patients are admitted to their units, decreasing the opportunity to care for children on a regular basis. Maintaining pediatric skills and competencies becomes an ongoing challenge.

All critically ill children should be admitted to designated pediatric critical care beds.[7] An American Hospital Association survey found that pediatric intensive care units (PICUs) were found in only 9% of the counties in the United States, with the majority located in urban areas.[62,77,83] While the reasons for admission to a PICU vary, guidelines for the development of admission and discharge criteria have been published by the American Academy of Pediatrics (AAP) in collaboration with the Society of Critical Care Medicine (SCCM), so that available beds can be optimized and care appropriate to a child's condition can be provided (Box 48-1).[79]

LEVELS OF PICU CARE

Guidelines and levels of care for PICUs were developed and represent the elements necessary to provide the highest quality of care possible.[79,86] Level 1 PICUs provide multidisciplinary care for a wide range of complex, progressive, rapidly changing medical, surgical, and traumatic disorders for children (excluding premature newborns).[86] Level 2 PICUs care for patients who are less complex, with some units providing care for children with moderate illness severity. Level 2 PICUs may also provide stabilization to children requiring transfer to another center.[86] The same standards of quality of care must be applied regardless of level.

MODELS OF CO-RESIDENCE

In the United States, some hospitals without PICUs provide co-residence of adult and pediatric patients. These co-residential units can provide mechanical ventilation and monitoring of vascular and intracranial pressure.[102] Fewer of these types of patient care settings offer nitric oxide, hemodialysis, or hemofiltration for children.[102] Two models regarding the co-residence of children and adults have been described in the literature.[31]

Service Line Model

One model is to place children and adults in the same critical care unit along service lines.[31] An example of this would be having a cardiac or trauma critical care unit where the staff cares for patients along the age continuum.

Geographic Model

The second model of co-residence is that of intermingled adult and pediatric patients in general medical-surgical units.[31] Some primarily adult critical care units where children are cared for have designated pediatric areas within the unit. These areas may be decorated for the pediatric population and stocked with pediatric equipment and supplies. Other co-residential units may instead intermingle pediatric patients with adult patients while having pediatric-focused carts that can be rolled to the bedsides of children who are admitted to critical care. These carts can be stocked with pediatric equipment and pediatric reference materials.[80]

REGIONALIZATION OF CARE

In 2000 the AAP and SCCM concluded the evidence supporting regionalized care for critically ill children was strong. Additional studies support the view that regionalization of PICU services in large, tertiary centers

---

Box 48-1

Common Reasons for Pediatric Intensive Care Unit Admissions

- Respiratory disease processes
- Injuries (leading cause of death in children and young adults)
  Motor vehicle injuries
  Pedestrian injuries
  Bicycle injuries
  Firearms injuries
  Nonaccidental trauma
  Burns
- Near-drowning/drowning
- Congenital heart defect repair
- Infectious processes/sepsis
- Diabetic ketoacidosis
- Ingestions
- Shock

---

leads to improved health outcomes when compared to small units with limited tertiary pediatric services.[93,106] One study in New York State found significant variations in the care and mortality rates noted in the eight regions of the state in non-PICU hospitals.[61] Sanchez, Lucas, and Feustel compared the outcomes of adolescent trauma patients admitted to an adult surgical critical care unit versus a PICU.[90] The adolescents admitted to the PICU were less likely to be intubated and to have pulmonary artery catheters placed, had fewer ventilator days, and had a decreased length of stay compared to those admitted to the adult unit.

Pediatric Intensivist Coverage

An association has been shown between improved patient outcomes and 24-hour coverage by intensivists in the PICU.[50] For units without pediatric intensivists, telemedicine has been implemented and allows for remote PICU management in rural or other locations that lack staffing depth.[64,65] The use of telemedicine to provide pediatric critical care consultation in trauma patients in a rural adult critical care area has been studied; the clinical outcomes showed that mortality rates and length of stays were comparable to 33 national PICUs.[65]

Tiered Care

Another solution for providing optimal pediatric critical care is organizing critical care resources in a tiered manner, following the example of trauma

centers. Utilizing such a model would channel children in need of more intensive or complex services to the needed resources.[45]

Localized Community Care

Though there is much support for regionalization of pediatric services, the importance of pediatric patients remaining in local communities has been shown to be important to healthcare providers and families; some healthcare insurance plans mandate care at certain facilities.[80] It is also possible that some lengthy, risky, and expensive patient and family transports can be avoided when care is provided locally.[66] Some nontertiary hospitals are set up with the intent of transferring the more critically ill children to the regional PICUs and caring for the less acutely ill patient in their own facility. However, some of the more ill may remain in the community hospital because of family preferences, while those not acutely ill may be transferred to regional tertiary center PICUs, again because of family preference.[66] The development of clear transfer guidelines can assist healthcare providers in the decision-making process of whether or not to transfer pediatric patients to tertiary care centers.[59]

STANDARDIZING CARE FOR CHILDREN

It is essential that institutions caring for children require pediatric-specific competency validation for all disciplines involved with the population. Pediatric-specific policies, procedures, standards, and protocols can be developed or pediatric-specific information can be integrated into existing adult documents (Box 48-2). Pediatric procedure books and pediatric-specific standards have been developed by the American Association of Critical-Care Nurses (AACN) and SCCM, and can be used to guide practice.

Ensuring that all areas are child-ready can be challenging to implement across an entire institution or health system that cares for mostly adult patients. The AAP and SCCM co-developed *Guidelines and Levels of Care for Pediatric Intensive Care Units,*[7] updated in 2004.[8] The guidelines are helpful to PICUs in determining the scope of care to pediatric patients, organizational and administrative structures, hospital facilities and services, personnel needs, drugs and equipment needs, quality monitoring, and educational needs.[7,86] While these guidelines were not written for units without distinct, separate[86] PICUs, they may be helpful for those facilities with small inpatient pediatric populations.[86] A Multidisciplinary Plan of Care focused on pediatric care considerations is provided on pp. 1342-1347.

Box 48-2

Admission of the Child to the Adult Critical Care Unit

- Obtain report from emergency department/transport team/acute care floor/other.
- Contact
  1. Pediatric respiratory therapist for supplemental oxygen/ventilatory support
  2. Pediatric pharmacist so that medications; maintenance intravenous fluids; vasoactive, analgesic, and anxiolytic drips will be set up and ready to start upon arrival to unit
  3. Child life therapy/pediatric-specific social worker/chaplain to assist with family support
  4. Physician upon patient admission
- Bed space setup
  1. Adequate number of infusion pumps including syringe pumps with the ability to administer small fluid volumes down to 0.5 ml/hr
  2. Pressure tubing for transduced lines
  3. Isolation room/equipment if appropriate
  4. Emesis basin

5. Chart with pediatric-focused documentation
6. Weight-specific resuscitation medications sheet
7. Set cardiorespiratory monitor to correct mode (i.e., adult/pediatric/neonatal)
- Age/size-specific equipment (as needed)
  1. Electrocardiogram leads
  2. Gown
  3. Diapers
  4. Crib/bed (if scale in bed, zero with linens)
  5. Chest tubes
  6. Foley catheter
  7. Blood pressure cuff
  8. Intravenous catheters
  9. Pulse oximetry probes
  10. Central venous line tray
  11. Pediatric laboratory tubes
  12. Resuscitation bag and mask
  13. Suction catheters/bulb syringes/oral suction
  14. Cervical spine collar (if prehospital collar improperly fitted)

MULTIDISCIPLINARY PLAN OF CARE FOR PEDIATRIC CARE CONSIDERATIONS

FOCUS	INTERVENTION	RATIONALE
Respiratory Considerations		
Smaller upper and lower airways	In the trauma patient, open the airway using the jaw-thrust maneuver. Repositioning often may be the only intervention needed to maintain a patent airway.	Foreign matter such as blood, mucus, and vomit and also teeth easily obstruct small airways. Small amounts of edema can obstruct the airway, markedly increasing airway resistance.
Tongue is larger relative to oropharynx	Oropharyngeal airways can be used in the unresponsive child.	In the trauma patient, open the airway using the jaw-thrust maneuver. Repositioning often may be the only intervention needed to maintain a patent airway.
Cartilage of the larynx is softer	Place child in "sniffing" position with chin-lift maneuver. Use jaw-thrust in the trauma patient.	Hyperextension or hyperflexion of the neck can compress and obstruct the airway.
Larger head/body ratio	Place a small towel roll under the child's shoulders to maintain the "sniffing" position.	Neck may be in flexion when the child is immobilized on a backboard.
Infants are obligate nose breathers for the first several months of life	Suction nares frequently. Nasopharyngeal airway may be placed.	Obstructed nasal passages can produce significant respiratory distress in the infant.
Larynx is positioned more anteriorly and cephalad	Use cricoid pressure to compress the esophagus against the spine during bag-mask ventilation to help prevent gastric insufflation and aspiration. This maneuver also assists	There is an increased risk of aspiration. Direct visualization of the vocal cords is more difficult during intubation.

FOCUS	INTERVENTION	RATIONALE
	with visualization of the vocal cords during intubation attempts.	
Shorter tracheal length	Pay meticulous attention to initial endotracheal tube position (centimeter mark at the gum). Perform recurrent reassessment of tube placement with postintubation chest x-ray films. Maintain head in midline position and prevent extension or flexion of the neck.	There is an increased chance of mainstem intubation. Changes in head position will cause movement in the endotracheal tube. Flexion of the neck displaces the tube farther into the trachea, and extension of the neck moves the tube farther out of the trachea.
Cricoid cartilage is the narrowest portion of the airway	In the in-hospital setting a cuffed endotracheal tube is as safe as an uncuffed tube for children beyond the newborn period. Cuff pressures should be less than 20 cm H_2O.	Cricoid ring provides a natural seal for the endotracheal tube. Cuffed tubes with high pressure may cause airway damage in younger children.
Cartilaginous ribs of the infant and small child are twice as compliant as those of an adult	Closely observe the child with continuous monitoring of heart rate, respiratory rate and effort, and pulse oximetry. Deliver highest possible concentration of oxygen to infants and children in respiratory distress. Provide nonthreatening environment and avoid noxious stimuli. Allow alert child to maintain own position of comfort to optimize respiratory effort. Allow parents to remain with child if their presence is comforting to the child.	Retractions are more common and reduce the infant's or small child's ability to maintain functional residual capacity or generate adequate tidal volume.
Intercostal muscles are poorly developed	If possible, maintain patient in upright position to support diaphragmatic function. Avoid abdominal distention by inserting a nasogastric or orogastric tube to decompress the stomach.	Generation of tidal volume depends on diaphragmatic function. Anything impeding diaphragm movement can lead to respiratory failure.
The child's respiratory system has less compensatory reserve than the adult's respiratory system	Closely observe the child with continuous monitoring of heart rate, respiratory rate and effort, and pulse oximetry. Deliver highest possible concentration of oxygen in a nonthreatening manner. Consider blood gas analysis.	The younger child may develop respiratory distress and failure more rapidly than an adult.
Infants with respiratory distress often grunt during exhalation	Provide high concentration of supplemental oxygen and consider ventilatory support.	Grunting is a result of premature glottic closure during exhalation. Infants grunt to increase airway pressure, lung volume, and functional residual capacity.
Infants and small children have less elastic and collagen tissue in their lungs	Maintain high index of suspicion for pneumothorax, pneumomediastinum, and pulmonary edema. Obtain chest x-ray films as necessary.	Liquid or air can enter an infant's pulmonary interstitium more easily than in the older child or adult, making the infant more susceptible to air leaks and edema.
Infants and small children have thin chest walls	Frequently reassess bilateral breath sounds with side-by-side comparison of difference in pitch and intensity. Breath sounds should be auscultated over the anterior and posterior chest wall and in the axillary areas using a pediatric stethoscope. Obtain chest x-ray films as necessary.	Breath sounds are easily transmitted across the chest wall and over the abdomen.

Table continues on page 1344

FOCUS	INTERVENTION	RATIONALE
The ventilated child	Noninvasive ventilation may be an option for some pediatric patients (e.g., cystic fibrosis, musculoskeletal disease). When conventional ventilation is used, tidal volume may escape around an uncuffed ETT, so the lowest effective tidal volume should be used. Suction catheters should not touch mucosa or the carina, so the end of the catheter should not extend more than 0.5 cm past the end of the ETT. Suctioning and instillation of normal saline should not be performed on a routine basis, but individualized according to patient assessment. Suction settings should be set between 80 and 120 cm H_2O.	Lower tidal volumes, low suction settings, individualized suctioning, and premeasured suction depths prevent barotrauma.

Circulatory Considerations

FOCUS	INTERVENTION	RATIONALE
Myocardium is less compliant and has less contractile tissue compared with that of an adult	Provide continuous ECG monitoring with attention to trends in heart rate. Tachycardia is the earliest clinical manifestation in compensated shock, but it also may be a result of anxiety, pain, fever, or increased activity. If other signs of compensated shock are present (delayed capillary refill time, cool extremities, duskiness or mottling of the skin, diminished peripheral pulses, narrowing pulse pressure, tachypnea), rapid intravenous access is established and fluid resuscitation is initiated.	Stroke volume is not easily adjusted; therefore children increase their heart rate in response to falling cardiac output.
Infants and children have a smaller overall blood volume	Carefully estimate blood loss, including blood drawn for laboratory analysis. Serial hemoglobin and hematocrit analysis should be obtained as necessary.	Although the child's circulating blood volume is greater per kilogram of body weight compared with an adult (child 80 ml/kg vs. adult 70 ml/kg), the circulating volume is significantly less. Smaller amounts of blood loss can cause volume depletion.
Most dysrhythmias are clinically insignificant in the pediatric patient and do not require treatment	Provide continuous ECG monitoring. Establish and maintain patent airway.	Bradycardia and SVT are the two most common significant dysrhythmias in children.
Bradycardia is the most common terminal cardiac rhythm in children, whereas ventricular tachycardia or fibrillation is the usual terminal rhythm in the adult	Provide adequate oxygenation and ventilation. Establish intravenous access. If severe cardiorespiratory compromise (as evidenced by poor perfusion, respiratory distress, or hypotension) is present, follow the PALS guidelines for bradycardia or tachycardia with poor perfusion.[11]	Bradycardia is often a result of hypoxia and is not well tolerated in children because it significantly reduces cardiac output. SVT usually is well tolerated in infants and children, but can lead to cardiovascular collapse.
A greater percentage of total body weight is water in infants and children	Calculate maintenance fluids based on each child's weight in kilograms and clinical condition.	Infants and young children will lose larger amounts of water through evaporation than will the adult.

FOCUS	INTERVENTION	RATIONALE
There is a larger surface area/volume ratio	Record all sources of fluid intake and fluid loss to calculate fluid balance and adjust fluid therapy accordingly.	Children have greater potential for dehydration. Maintenance fluid requirements per kilogram of body weight are higher in children.
Infants and children have smaller, more difficult to cannulate veins	Establish a protocol that addresses obtaining intravenous and intraosseous access in critically ill or injured children utilizing PALS guidelines.	Rapid establishment of intravenous access is more difficult in infants and children.
Neurologic Considerations		
The head of the infant and young child is larger and heavier in proportion to the rest of the body	Anticipate head injury in the traumatically injured child. Suggest use of stress preventive measures, such as seat belts, car seats, and helmets, to patients and family members.	If an infant or child falls or is thrown a significant distance, the initial impact more often will be to the head, which predisposes the child to head injury.
The skull is thinner during infancy and childhood	Same as above.	The thin skull provides less protection for the brain. Head trauma can result in severe brain injury in children.
Cranial sutures do not fuse until approximately age 16 to 18 months	Measure occipital frontal circumference with neurologic examinations in the child up to age 16–18 months at risk for increasing intracranial pressure.	If intracranial volume increases during this time, head circumference may increase. The ability to expand may better accommodate gradual increases in intracranial volume than in an adult. Increased intracranial pressure may still develop, especially with acute increase in intracranial volume.
Anterior and posterior fontanelles are open in infants	Assess fontanelles for size and tension in the infant age 16–18 months or younger.	The anterior fontanelle is the junction of the coronal-sagittal and frontal bones and does not close until age 16–18 months. The posterior fontanelle is the junction of the parietal and occipital bones and closes at approximately age 2 months. The fontanelles will be tense or bulging in the event of increased intracranial pressure and will be sunken if the infant is dehydrated.
Spinal cord injuries are less common in the pediatric trauma patient than in the adult trauma patient	Children with head and/or neck injuries should be presumed to have a spinal cord injury until proven otherwise. Stabilize and immobilize the cervical spine with a hard cervical collar, long spine board, and a commercial immobilization device or foam blocks, rolled towel, and tape. Remember, the child's prominent occiput places the neck in flexion when lying flat on a spine board. Place padding under the child's torso to elevate it approximately 2 cm, bringing the head into neutral position.	The child's spine, especially the cervical spine, is more elastic and mobile. When a child sustains a spinal cord injury, it is often present without radiographic abnormality, described as spinal cord injury without radiographic abnormality

Table continues on page 1346

FOCUS	INTERVENTION	RATIONALE
Musculoskeletal Considerations		
Children's bones are more flexible because of incomplete bone calcification	Suspect injury to internal structures underlying fractures and areas subjected to significant forces as evidenced by contusions, swelling, and tenderness. Obtain surgical consultation as necessary. Monitor for signs of internal hemorrhage: decreasing level of consciousness, poor peripheral perfusion, decreased urinary output, tachycardia, tachypnea, and narrowing pulse pressure. Obtain hemoglobin and hematocrit analysis as necessary.	Significant force generally is necessary to break children's bones. Underlying injury may be present without fracture.
There is increased elasticity and compliance of the chest wall because the ribs and sternum are more cartilaginous in infants and young children	Suspect pneumothoraces and/or hemothoraces in the child who has significant chest trauma with or without rib fractures. Monitor respiratory effort and oxygen saturation. Obtain chest x-ray films as necessary. Be prepared for needle thoracostomy or chest tube insertion in the event of a tension pneumothorax.	There is a low incidence of rib or sternal fractures in children. Increased chest wall compliance allows traumatic forces to be transmitted to underlying thoracic structures. Pneumothorax is the most common result of thoracic trauma in children and may be more likely to progress to a tension pneumothorax because of the increased mobility of the mediastinal structures.
Abdominal muscles are less developed in children	Obtain surgical consultation as necessary. Monitor for signs of shock secondary to internal hemorrhage. Obtain serial abdominal girth measurements. Follow serial hemoglobin and hematocrit analysis.	Children are at an increased risk of sustaining abdominal injuries. The spleen and the liver are the most commonly injured abdominal organs in children.[36]
Pseudosubluxation of C2 on C3	Maintain cervical spine immobilization and suspect spinal cord injury in any child with head and neck injuries. Perform thorough serial neurologic examination. Do not rule out cervical spine injury on the basis of negative radiographic studies only. Obtain neurosurgical consultation.	Seen in up to 40% of children age <7 years and in ≤20% of children age <16 years. This is a normal variation caused by increased ligamentous laxity.[48]
Metabolic and Thermoregulatory Considerations		
Infants and young children have a larger body surface area/body mass ratio, and less insulating subcutaneous tissue and fat stores	Monitor temperature frequently. Cover children with warm blankets or place them under warming lights if they cannot be covered. Use warmed intravenous fluids or blood for volume resuscitation. Warm and humidify supplemental oxygen if possible. Place warming pads (such as K pads) or chemically activated warming devices (such as portable warmers) under children. Follow manufacturer's directions for the use of these devices.	A great deal of heat is lost to the environment through radiation and evaporation, especially from the child's proportionally large head. Infants and children can become hypothermic very easily. Hypothermia can cause metabolic acidosis, hypoglycemia, coagulopathies, central nervous system depression, respiratory depression, and myocardial irritability, making resuscitation more difficult.
Infants younger than 3 months old cannot produce heat by shivering and must burn their limited fat stores for thermogenesis	Same as above. Consider placing small infants in isolettes with overbed warmers. Attach skin probe for continuous skin temperature monitoring to avoid overheating and thermal injury.	There is an increased risk of hypothermia in the small infant. The burning of fat increases oxygen consumption, which can lead to hypoxia.

FOCUS	INTERVENTION	RATIONALE
Infants and young children have less glycogen stores than adults	Monitor glucose level frequently during and after resuscitation. Administer glucose as ordered.	The ill or injured child is at increased risk for developing hypoglycemia.
Children have higher metabolic rates than adults	Provide supplemental oxygen to all seriously ill or injured children. Consult with physician and dietitian to provide early, adequate nutritional support to the compromised child.	Higher metabolic rates increase oxygen consumption. The child's nutritional needs are higher per kilogram of body weight than in an adult.
Pain Management Considerations		
Children may receive too little pain medication or none at all	Maintain awareness of misconceptions regarding pain in children and advocate, assess, and provide for evidence-based pain management.	Children express pain in a variety of ways. Younger children may not say that they are in pain because they feel the pain is punishment for misbehavior, or they may fear an injection. Older children may not admit pain in front of peers. Just because children are asleep does not mean that they are not experiencing pain.

Additional data from references 11, 52–54, 58, 73, 75, 81, 87, 96, 102, 107.
Adapted with permission from Rupp, L. A. & Day, M. W. (2003). Children are different: Pediatric differences and the impact on trauma. In Moloney-Harmon, P. A. & Czerwinski, S. J. (2003). *Nursing care of the pediatric trauma patient*. St. Louis: Saunders.
ECG = Electrocardiogram, ETT = endotracheal tube, PALS = pediatric advanced life support, SVT = supraventricular tachycardia.

Standardized Equipment

It is important that all areas of the hospital where children will be seen have child-appropriate equipment and services available (e.g., surgery, postanesthesia care unit, radiology, emergency department) and the resources to provide pediatric resuscitation. Pediatric equipment should be standardized across institutions[18] to include resuscitation equipment and intravenous pumps that can deliver volumes less than 1 ml/hour.[80] The Medication table on p. 1348 summarizes medications for treatment of pediatric dysrhythmias and on p. 1349 summarizes medications used in non-dysrhythmic emergencies. Having child-safe hospital beds available to accommodate infants, toddlers, and preschoolers is imperative (Figure 48-1). Dietary and nutrition services will need to be versed in pediatric diets and nutrition, as discussed in the Nutrition box on p. 1349. Blood banks should have the ability to have blood products available in aliquots for the small amounts that pediatric patients require. Hospital laboratories will need to obtain equipment for running the small volumes of blood required for pediatric laboratory samples. Pediatric-sized tubes for blood draws should be available in all areas where children are served, since minor blood losses can have a significant impact on a child. Pharmacy must ensure that

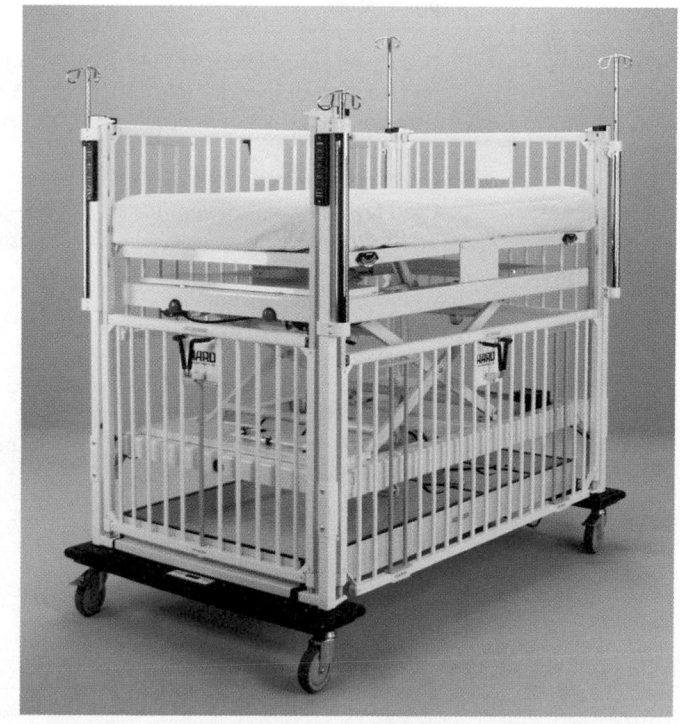

✦FIGURE 48-1   Pediatric crib.

MEDICATIONS FOR PEDIATRIC DYSRHYTHMIAS

MEDICATION	ACTIONS	DOSAGE	SPECIAL CONSIDERATIONS
Adenosine (Adenocard)	Slows impulse formation in the SA node; slows conduction in the AV node Used for treatment of supraventricular tachycardias	Initial dose: 0.1 mg/kg IV/IO (maximum dose 6 mg); if ineffective, may repeat in 1–2 min at 0.2 mg/kg IV/IO (maximum dose 12 mg)	Give FAST IV push, followed by normal saline flush. May cause temporary heart block or asystole
Amiodarone (Cordarone)	Decreases SA node function; slows conduction in the AV node Used for treatment of ventricular dysrhythmias	For pulseless rhythms: 5 mg/kg IV/IO (maximum bolus dose 300 mg); repeat as needed up to maximum daily dose 15 mg/kg IV/IO (2.2 g in adolescent)	Monitor QT interval Give over 20–60 min
Atropine	Competes with acetylcholine for binding sites; blocks muscarinic receptors Used for treatment of symptomatic bradycardic arrhythmias	0.02 mg/kg IV/IO; may repeat once after 5 min (minimum dose 0.1 mg in children with maximum single dose of 0.5 mg; maximum single dose 1 mg in adolescents); maximum total child dose 1 mg; maximum adolescent dose 2 mg. 0.04 to 0.06 mg/kg ETT*	
Epinephrine (1:10,000 preparation; 0.1 mg/ml or 1:1000 preparation; 1 mg/ml)	Stimulates alpha receptors to cause vasoconstriction and beta receptors to cause increased heart rate and contractility Used in the treatment of pulseless dysrhythmias and symptomatic bradycardia	0.01 mg/kg IV/IO 1:10,000; maximum dose 1 mg. 0.1 mg/kg ETT* 1:1000	Repeat every 3–5 min as needed Monitor blood pressure and ECG continuously
Lidocaine	Decreases automaticity in the myocardium during diastole Used for treatment of ventricular dysrhythmias	1 mg/kg IV/IO; 2–3 mg via ETT* Infusion: 20–50 mcg/kg/min	Follow bolus with continuous infusion
Magnesium sulfate	Used for treatment of ventricular dysrhythmias Used in treatment of cardiac arrest when hypomagnesemia is suspected or if the dysrhythmia is torsades de pointes	25–50 mg/kg IV/IO Maximum dose: 2 g	Usually administered over 10–20 min; may be given more quickly as determined by the patient's rhythm Monitor BP and ECG continuously
Procainamide (Pronestyl)	Decreases myocardial excitability, conduction velocity, depresses contractility Used to treat atrial and ventricular dysrhythmias	15 mg/kg IV/IO	Give initial bolus slowly over 30–60 min; follow with continuous infusion Monitor QT interval

Data from references 11, 13, 14.
*Flush with 5 ml of normal saline and follow with 5 ventilations.
ECG = Electrocardiogram, IO = intraosseous, ETT = endotracheal tube.

MEDICATIONS USED IN PEDIATRIC EMERGENCY SITUATIONS

MEDICATION	ACTIONS	DOSAGE	SPECIAL CONSIDERATIONS
Calcium chloride 10%	Used in the management of hyperkalemia, hypocalcemia, or calcium channel blocker toxicity	20 mg/kg IV/IO; may be repeated in 10 min if needed	IV/IO SLOW push during cardiac arrest if hypocalcemia known or suspected. Otherwise, infuse over 30–60 min. Monitor BP and ECG continuously
Glucose	Used in the treatment of hypoglycemic emergencies	0.5–1 g/kg IV/IO Different glucose preparations are available. $D_{25}W$: usual dose is 2–4 ml/kg $D_{10}W$: usual dose is 5–10 ml/kg	Maximum recommended concentration for bolus administration is $D_{25}W$ ($D_{50}W$ can be mixed 1:1 with sterile water
Naloxone (Narcan)	Displaces opiates on opiate receptors in the central nervous system. Used to treat opiate-induced sedation and respiratory depression	Total reversal: 0.1 mg/kg IV/IO/IM/ subcutaneously every 2 min as needed up to 2 mg. Reversal titrated to effect: 1 to 5 mcg/kg IV/IO/IM/ subcutaneously.	Dose may need to be repeated as half-life of opioid being reversed may be longer than that of naloxone
Sodium bicarbonate	Provides bicarbonate ions used to treat metabolic acidosis and severe hyperkalemia	1 mEq/kg IV/IO	Give SLOWLY. Do not give more than 8 mEq daily for children ≤2 years of age Monitor pH and ECG

Data from references 11, 13, 14.
ET = Endotracheal tube, IO = intraosseous.

medications can be delivered in the smaller doses needed for the pediatric population and that the staff is educated to prepare and dispense medications for children.[4,35]

Standardizing Emergency Equipment

Resuscitating an infant or child is different in that medication dosages are based on the child's weight and the point when resuscitation is initiated. In addition, cardiac compression rate and depth as well as the number of resuscitation breaths are not the same as those for an adult. Administering weight-based resuscitation medications may be made easier through the use of precalculated emergency medication sheets. There are software programs available that allow these emergency sheets to be prepared upon the child's admission to critical care and placed at the bedside for quick retrieval in case of deterioration in patient status. If the precalculated sheets are not available, a Broselow/Luten pediatric resuscitation tape can be used as a guide (Figure 48-2). The child is measured with the tape, and at each increment on the tape, the endotracheal tube size, precalculated medication for weight, and joules for defibrillation are noted. Products such as a Broselow/Hinkle resuscitation cart can be used in conjunction with the tape measurement

♦ NUTRITION

Nutritional Assessment of the Critically Ill Child

Compared to adults, children are much more vulnerable to malnutrition in the critical care unit because of increased basal energy requirements and limited nutritional reserves. Without adequate nutritional support, children develop protein-calorie malnutrition within 5 to 7 days. Once the resuscitation phase of critical care has resolved, nutritional support should be initiated to promote wound healing, immune function, and overall recovery.[73] See the table on p. 1350 for a list of conditions that leave patients more vulnerable to malnutrition.

As with adults, the enteral route is preferred in order to promote normal physiologic function of the gut. Total parenteral nutrition (TPN) can be used if the enteral feedings are poorly tolerated because of diarrhea or large residuals. Careful selection of the appropriate TPN or enteral formula is essential to avoid excess protein intake and complications such as electrolyte imbalance, hyperglycemia, hypoglycemia, and fat and carbohydrate imbalances.[73] For those patients able to take in oral nutrition, providing favorite foods with high nutritional value will increase the child's interest in eating.

Conditions That May Predispose Patients to Malnutrition

MEDICAL CONDITION	ASSOCIATED CLINICAL MANIFESTATIONS

Cardiac disease
  Congenital heart disease
  Congestive heart failure
	Fatigue, dyspnea, diaphoresis, cyanosis, decreased oral intake, vomiting, gastric distention, anorexia, early satiety, and inability to coordinate suck, swallow, and respiration

Pulmonary disease
  Respiratory syncytial virus
  Bronchopulmonary dysplasia
  Pneumonia
  Cystic fibrosis
	Fatigue, dyspnea, diaphoresis, cyanosis, decreased oral intake, vomiting, gastric distention

Liver disease	Anorexia, vomiting, gastric distention, malabsorption
Renal disease	Vomiting, loss of appetite, anorexia, poor growth, reflux, uremia
Inborn errors of metabolism	Inability to metabolize various substrates, severe dietary restrictions, anorexia
Oncology	Anorexia, nausea, vomiting, increased energy demands, poor growth
HIV/AIDS	Anorexia, nausea, vomiting, diarrhea, malabsorption, failure to thrive, increased energy demands, medication side effects

Trauma
  Multiple fractures
  Burns
	Increased energy demands, inability to take oral diet, nutrient losses from wounds

Gastrointestinal disorders
  Short-bowel syndrome
  Inflammatory bowel syndrome
  Gastroesophageal reflux
  Gastric surgery
	Impaired absorption of nutrients, altered gastric motility, delayed gastric emptying

Developmental disabilities	Poor suck and swallow, impaired motor and oral skills

Data from reference 23.
AIDS = Acquired immunodeficiency syndrome, HIV = human immunodeficiency virus.

(Figure 48-3). The drawers on the code cart are color-coded to match the resuscitation tape and are stocked with equipment accordingly. Some units use the Brose-low/Hinkle carts and precalculated medication sheets together. Staff members place colored dots that correspond with the color on the corresponding cart drawer on the precalculated medication sheets, so the proper drawer can be retrieved in a rapid manner. Other units print precalculated emergency medication sheets on colored paper that corresponds with the correct code cart drawer so that time will not be lost in crisis situations.

Standardizing Documentation Across the Institution

Pediatric-specific documentation in areas caring for children will also be needed and may be able to be integrated into preexisting adult-focused documentation. An admission database that addresses the pediatric patient's development is essential. This document should include the child's regular routine, food preferences, and comfort items. When normal routines are altered, the child can feel loss of control and have decreased coping skills.[70]

CHILD AND FAMILY-CENTERED CARE

Highlighting the child's usual routine can also be accomplished by completing an "All About Me" poster that highlights the child's preferences and lists the names of his or her loved ones (Figure 48-4). Participating in poster completion can provide a needed distraction for families, especially at the time of admission to

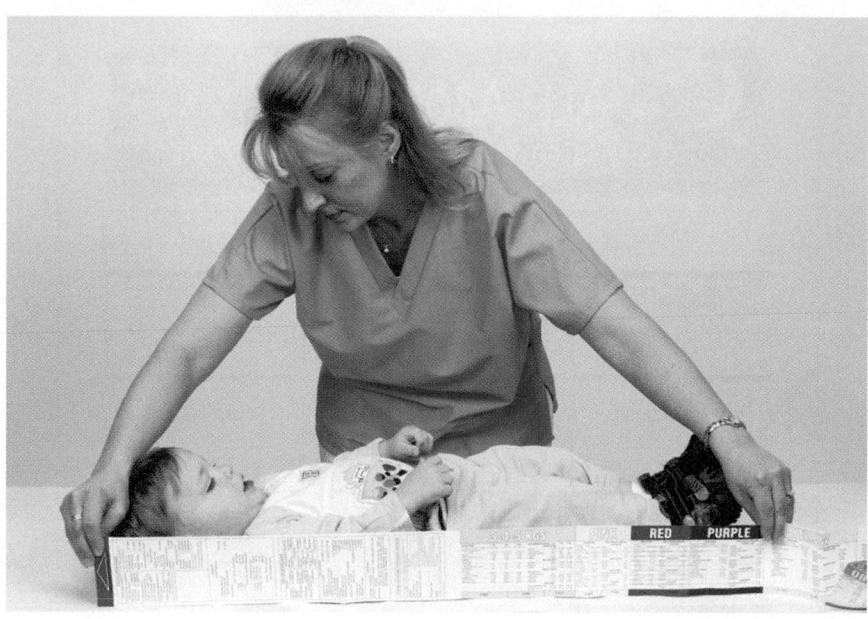

✦FIGURE 48-2 Broselow/Luten tape. (Courtesy Armstrong Medical Ind.)

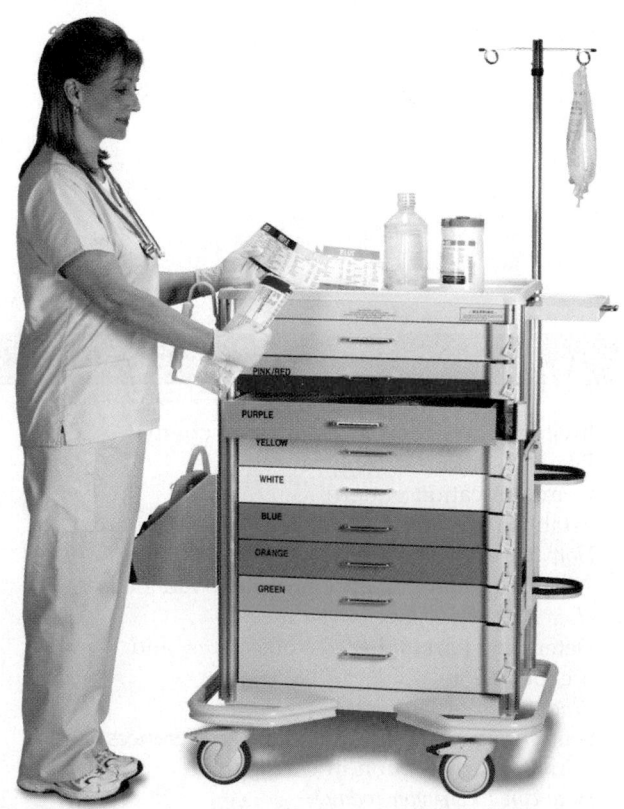

✦FIGURE 48-3 Broselow/Hinkle cart. (Courtesy Armstrong Medical Ind.)

critical care. Pictures of the child and family are sometimes added to the posters, to allow healthcare providers to see "what the child was like" before the illness/injury.

It has been said that no one knows the child better than loved ones. Members of the family can serve as interpreters of the child's behaviors and symptoms. The Nursing Mutual Participation Model of Care emphasizes the family's role in caring for the child and stresses the importance of a strong partnership with the healthcare team (Box 48-3).[36–38]

Decreasing Family Stressors

The experience of having a child admitted to critical care is stressful for family members. Spending time orienting loved ones to the unit can decrease stressors. This orientation can include the purpose of monitoring equipment, the types of alarms and their significance, and reasons why staff may respond at a different pace to certain alarms.[25] Ensuring that alarm limits are set so they are not continually, needlessly sounding can help to decrease family stress.[25]

Other areas of stress that families may encounter during the time in critical care include changes in the child's behavior, emotions, and appearance; unfamiliar sights and sounds; and procedures that are frightening to the child, especially ones in which needles and tubes

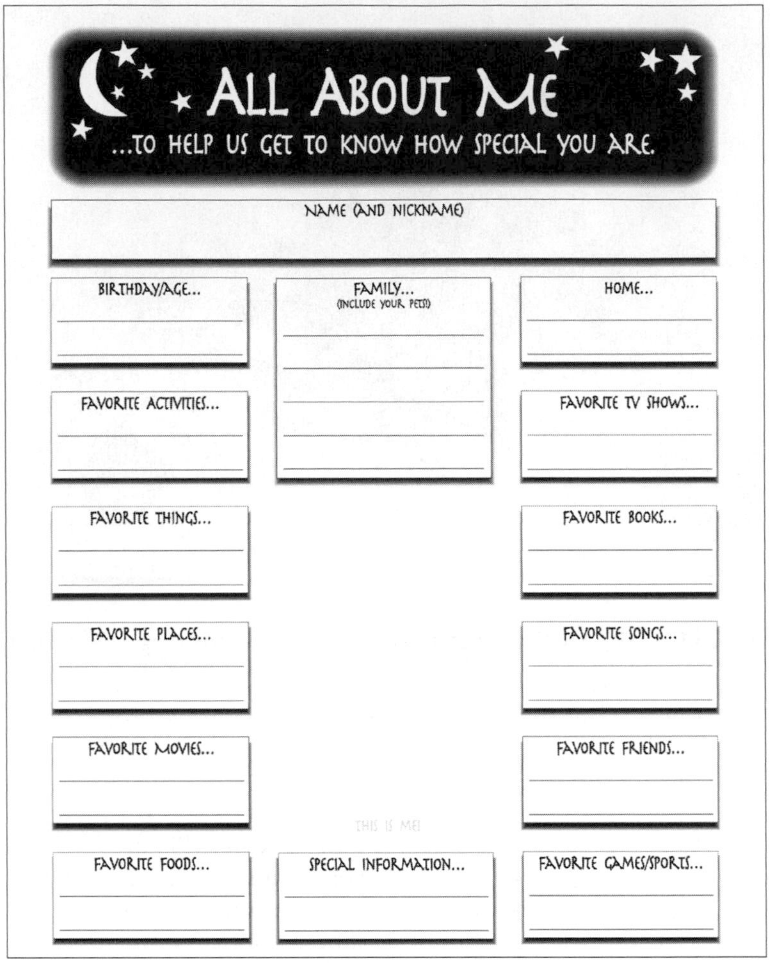

⬥FIGURE 48-4 "All About Me" poster.

Box 48-3

Nursing Mutual Participation Model of Care

ADMISSION

- Extend our care to include parents
- Acknowledge their importance

DAILY BEDSIDE CONTACT

- Enabling strategies that provide parents with system savvy
  Information—teach and clarify
  Anticipatory guidance—illness trajectory
  Provide instrumental resources
- Facilitate transition to "parent-to-a-critically ill child"
  Enhance parent-child unique connectedness
  Role model interactions

Invite participation in nurturing activity
Provide options during procedures
- Communication pattern
  Establish a caring relationship with the parent
  How are you doing today?
  Assist parental perception of the child's illness
  How does she/he look to you today?
  Determine parental goals, objectives, and expectations
  What troubles you most?
  Seek informed suggestions and preferences, and invite participation in care
  How can I help you today?

are placed in the child.[24–26] The behavior of the critical care staff and "too many people talking" have also been shown to increase family stress.[24–26] Of the stressors identified by families, parental role change is the hardest with which to cope.[24,25]

Family Presence

A sound scientific basis for restricting visitors in critical care units does not exist.[95] Families who have children admitted to critical care have identified being with their child as their priority need.[95] In carrying out the family-centered care philosophy of AACN that promotes care that is driven by the needs of patients and their families, this need can be met through open visitation policies for all critical care patients, not only for the children. Parents should be given the option of staying to support their child even when procedures are performed, since the majority of parents want to stay.[24,25] Berwick and Kotagal[22] write that strict visiting in critical care is "neither caring, compassionate, nor necessary." Open visitation has been found to have a beneficial effect for 88% of families and decreased anxiety in 65% of families.[93] These types of open policies also engender trust in families, creating a better working relationship between hospital staff and family members.[22] Adult critical care patients rated visiting as a nonstressful experience because visitors offered reassurance, comfort, and calming effects.[49] So there is no need to have different visiting policies for the children and adults sharing the same intensive care unit. The AACN *Practice Alert: Family Presence During CPR and Invasive Procedures*[9] addresses the importance of families in the critical care environment. The practice alert states that "family members of all patients undergoing cardiopulmonary resuscitation (CPR) and invasive procedures should be given the option of being present at the bedside." The Emergency Nurses Association[44] and the American College of Chest Physicians also support this philosophy of care.[7] Family-centered care (Chapter 8) is a philosophy, and not just one intervention,[95] such as open visitation or family presence. Referring to family and friends as "visitors" gives them a decreased significance,[95] when it is the healthcare providers who are the visitors to the patient and family situation.

Siblings and Childhood Friends

Siblings and friends should also be allowed to visit with the pediatric patient. Before visiting, these special visitors should be screened for exposure to contagious illnesses such as chickenpox, measles, or mumps so that these illnesses are not spread to any patients or families.

Allowing siblings and young friends to visit decreases the chance that their imaginations will have them envision a reality of the hospitalized child's illness or injury that is far worse. Child life therapists (CLTs) can be an important support to siblings and friends, especially if they feel, in some real or imagined way, responsible for the illness/injury. These special visitors will need preparation before visiting the bedside to have questions answered,[95] and after visiting the critically ill child, a debriefing may be needed by younger loved ones. CLTs are specifically educated to assist with this process.

QUALITY MONITORING

A program of performance improvement must be in place at the outset of the initiation of pediatric care to assess and improve the critical care systems and processes.[46] Taking time to assess indicators such as pain management, accidental breakdown of extubations, and nosocomial infections is important for maintaining quality care. The Research Utilization box below and on p. 1354

◆ RESEARCH UTILIZATION

Unplanned Extubations

CLINICAL ISSUE

Unplanned extubations can contribute to increased patient morbidity and mortality, but may be preventable. Past research has identified the use of restraints, sedation and anxiolytic policies, and various endotracheal tube securing methods as possible interventions to reduce this occurrence. Research has shown nursing care to be related to quality patient outcomes, but the relationship between unplanned extubations and nurse experience and staffing has not been reported.

SUMMARY

At a university-affiliated children's hospital, unplanned extubations were assessed over a 4-year period. During this time, 55 of 1004 intubated patients (5.5%) had an unplanned extubation. Factors associated with unplanned extubations included the documentation of patient agitation and a nurse-to-patient ratio of 1:2 relative to a nurse-to-patient ratio of 1:1. Years of PICU nursing experience, use of patient restraints, and the method of sedation delivery (continuous infusion vs. intermittent bolus) were not associated with unplanned extubations.

Box continues on p. 1354

APPLICATION

Pediatric patients are more likely to experience an unplanned extubation when being cared for by a nurse assigned to two patients. To provide safe patient care, healthcare policymakers and hospital administrators should consider the nurse-to-patient ratio and its potential association with adverse events in hospitalized children.

NEED FOR FURTHER STUDY

Future studies of care processes and medical errors should be continued to identify factors that can improve the overall quality of care.

Marcin, J. P., et al. (2005). Nurse staffing and unplanned extubation in the pediatric intensive care unit. *Pediatr Crit Care Med, 6,* 254–257.

explores unplanned extubations. Participation in national PICU databases allows caregivers to compare their outcomes to similar institutions. Regular multidisciplinary pediatric mortality and morbidity conferences can also provide a time for the multidisciplinary team to review pediatric cases and make improvements when necessary.

THE CHILD'S RESPONSE TO CRITICAL CARE

A child's response to surgery and hospitalization will reflect experience, age, and family support. Children tend to regress to a previous developmental level when stressed. In general, care should be directed toward developmental age rather than chronologic age (Box 48-4).[69] Children who are admitted to critical care are exposed to a multitude of environmental stimuli that can be overwhelming. With the addition of a severe illness and the invasive procedures endured, the child has the potential to have lasting effects. Some children have been able to recall their intensive care experience in great detail, while others have been amnesic of the event.[33] One study found that, for the youngest pediatric patients, the number of invasive procedures endured and the severity of the illness had the longest effects postdischarge.[84] These findings underscore the potential need for long-term support that can be provided by advanced-practice nurses, clinical psychologists, child life and music therapists, social workers, discharge planners, and case managers specializing in pediatric care.

Box 48-4

Age-Specific Variations for Working With Hospitalized Children

INFANT

- Give family choice to be involved in procedures.
- Use analgesics as needed.
- Keep family in infant's line of vision.
- If family members cannot remain with infant, place familiar object near infant.
- Have consistent caregivers and limit stranger contact.
- Comfort child during and after procedures.
- Keep harmful objects out of reach.
- Keep frightening objects out of view.
- Use nonintrusive procedures when possible (e.g., oral medications, axillary temperatures).

TODDLER

Use same approaches as for infant with these additions:
- Explain what child will see, hear, taste, smell, and feel.
- Emphasize when cooperation is needed (e.g., lie still).
- Let child know that it is okay to cry, scream, yell to express discomfort/fear.

- Ignore temper tantrums.
- Use distraction techniques.
- Use simple terms familiar to child, using one direction at a time.
- Show small replicas of equipment and allow child to hold.
- Use play to demonstrate procedures, but not child's favorite toy; child's imagination may believe that the toy can feel procedure.
- Prepare child immediately before procedures.
- Tell child when procedures are complete.
- Allow choices and child's participation whenever possible.

PRESCHOOL-AGE CHILD

- Encourage family presence as a comforter, not to restrain child.
- Provide analgesia as needed.
- Use simple terms to explain procedures.
- Demonstrate equipment and allow child to play with equipment or miniature.
- Allow child to use play to demonstrate procedures to clarify misconceptions.

Box 48-4—CONT'D

- Allow child to point out on doll exact location of procedure to decrease fantasy of multiple body parts being involved.
- Allow child to wear underpants and realize that procedures involving genitals are anxiety producing.
- Explain all unfamiliar things.
- Involve child in care, but avoid delays in procedures.
- Praise child continually.
- Use concrete words (e.g., rolling bed versus stretcher; child may believe bed can "stretch" child).
- Allow child to verbalize.
- Provide information regarding procedures shortly before actual procedure.
- Explain the reason procedure is being performed and allow child to say why a procedure is done (e.g., children may imagine they are being punished).
- Keep equipment out of sight.
- Use nonintrusive procedures when possible (e.g., oral medications, axillary temperatures).
- Apply a bandage; children may fantasize "leakage" of "insides."
- Involve child in care whenever possible, avoiding excessive delays.

SCHOOL-AGE CHILD

- Explain procedures using correct terminology.
- Explain procedures by using simple diagrams.
- Explain function of equipment in concrete terms and allow to hold and model use.
- Allow time before and after procedure for questions and discussion.
- Prepare in advance of procedure.

- Gain child's cooperation, explaining what is expected of child.
- Suggest ways of maintaining control (e.g., taking a deep breath, counting).
- Allow child to assist with simple tasks and include in decision making when feasible (e.g., time of day to perform, preferred site).
- Encourage active participation (e.g., opening packages).
- Provide privacy during procedures.

ADOLESCENT

- Explain procedure including why it is beneficial/ necessary, and long-term consequences.
- Encourage questioning regarding fears, risks, options, and alternatives.
- Provide privacy.
- Discuss how procedure may affect appearance and how to minimize.
- Realize that immediate effects are more significant than long-term benefits.
- Involve in decision making and planning (e.g., clothing to wear).
- Impose as few restrictions as possible, allowing patient to maintain control.
- Suggest ways of maintaining control and accept aggression as method of coping.
- Realize adolescents may have difficulty accepting new authority figures and may resist complying with procedures.
- Allow adolescents to talk with other adolescents who have had same experience.

Data from reference 3.

CONSIDERATIONS IN PEDIATRIC CARE

Pediatric Assessment

Blood Pressure. The age and size of the child should be considered when obtaining vital signs (Table 48-1). Blood pressure measurement is most accurate when the cuff's bladder encompasses 80% to 100% of the arm's circumference and has a bladder width of approximately 40% of the circumference of the child's upper arm.[17] When attempting to obtain a diastolic blood pressure in children, the disappearance of sound may not occur until zero. Some institutions and healthcare providers may choose to only document a systolic value. If a change occurs in the sounds at a point during auscultation of the blood pressure, this value can also be noted, such as 90/50/0.[17]

Pulse. During auscultation of an apical pulse, the healthcare provider should listen at the fourth intercostal space medial to the left midclavicular line in children under 7 years of age. After age 7, the apical impulse is located at the fifth intercostal space at the left midclavicular line. The healthcare provider should make sure that the stethoscope used during the assessment is the appropriate size for infants and children.

Temperature. Historically, healthcare providers have assumed that rectal temperatures are 1° C higher and that axillary temperatures are 1° C lower than oral temperatures. Studies have demonstrated that the difference is much smaller.[55,56] The temperature measurement site and instrument should be based on the child's physiologic stability and age, not "one size fits all." For consistency, the same method and instrument should be used

TABLE 48-1 Pediatric Vital Signs

AGE	HEART RATE (beats/min)	RESPIRATIONS (breaths/min)	SYSTOLIC BLOOD PRESSURE (mm Hg)
Infant	100–160	30–60	87–105
Toddler	80–110	24–40	95–105
Preschooler	70–110	22–34	80–110
School-age	65–110	18–30	97–112
Adolescent	60–90	12–16	112–128
Normal Hemodynamic Values in Children			
Central venous pressure	4–8 mm Hg		
Systolic pulmonary artery pressure	20–30 mm Hg		
Diastolic pulmonary artery pressure	<10 mm Hg		
Mean pulmonary artery pressure	<20 mm Hg		
Pulmonary artery wedge pressure	4–12 mm Hg		

Data from references 52, 53, 54, 72, 73.

to trend the individual patient's temperature over time.[68] The axillary route for temperature assessment may be the safest for neonates and small infants, whereas the tympanic and rectal routes may be best for children with poor perfusion.[68] It must be noted that the rectal route should not be "the norm," but that the temperature route and instrument should be individualized according to the child's needs.

Respiratory Rate. The respiratory rate should be assessed when the child is at rest. Any condition that increases oxygen needs can cause increased respiration (e.g., fever, fear, respiratory distress). Children with a sustained respiratory rate greater than 60 breaths per minute should be assessed for hypoxemia.[17]

Fluid Balance in Children

Placing an intravenous (IV) catheter into the small vein of a child, when one is not used to it, can be a daunting task. No one wants a child to endure repeated attempts at locating a vessel, but skill at pediatric IV placement is difficult to maintain without consistent opportunities for practice. Repeated attempts may be a catalyst for negative physiologic consequences in the child (e.g., oxygen desaturations, bradycardia). Many hospitals limit the number of times an

individual healthcare provider may attempt IV placement to 2 to 3 times. IV catheter selection is individualized for each child for gauge and length. Following catheter insertion, an infusion pump is used for fluid and IV medication administration. Some children require very low volumes, so infusion pumps that can deliver increments of 0.1 ml should be available.[20]

In the event an IV line cannot be inserted, intraosseous infusions may be used to gain vascular access in children. This is an effective, safe, and accessible route for fluid resuscitation, blood sampling, blood product transfusion, and vasoactive infusions (Figure 48-5).[11] Although rare, complications include subcutaneous infiltration and leakage from the puncture site after needle removal. Extended intraosseous infusions and infusion of hypertonic fluids have been associated with infections.[73]

Small changes in fluid and electrolyte balance may cause complications in a child. Those under the age of 2 years are more dependent on adequate intake than adults, because of the greater proportion of daily fluid losses. Problems such as fever, increases in metabolic rate, vomiting, and diarrhea that occur can increase fluid losses. Conversely, children can experience fluid excesses from chronic renal disease and rapidly flowing IVs.[17] Maintenance fluids for a child can be calculated based on kilograms of body weight (Table 48-2).

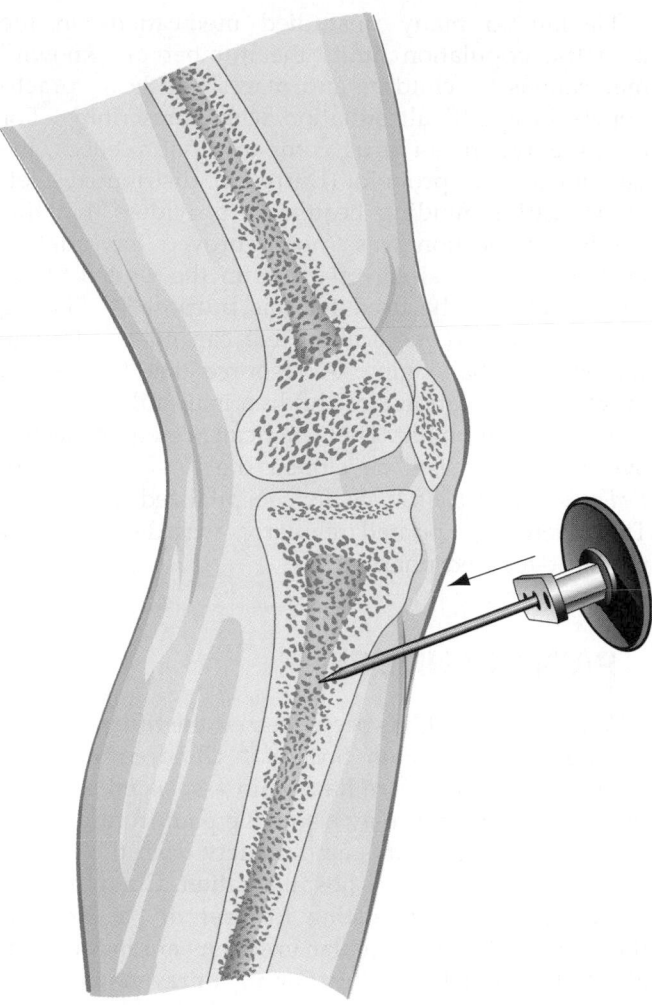

↕FIGURE 48-5 Intraosseous needle.

TABLE 48-2 Calculation of Maintenance Fluids (Per 24 Hours) in Children

WEIGHT (kg)	KILOGRAM BODY WEIGHT FORMULA
0–10	100–120 ml/kg
11–20	1000 ml for first 10 kg and 50 ml/kg for each kilogram over 10 kg
21–30	1500 ml for first 20 kg and 25 ml/kg for each kilogram over 20 kg

Data from reference 73.

To monitor small losses and gains, strict fluid intake and output as well as daily weights (taken at the same time of day with the same scale) are documented so that trends can be assessed. Urine output for infants and incontinent children can be measured by using a gram scale, since 1 g of weight equals 1 ml of urine volume. A rapid weight gain over a 24-hour period is most likely due to the accumulation of fluid.[17]

Additional volume losses can occur when blood is drawn for laboratory specimens. Pediatric tubes should be used, obtaining the smallest sample possible. Closed blood drawing systems can be used so the blood loss is only the sample needed, and there are no "discards" or wasted blood (Figure 48-6). Each time blood is drawn, the amount should be documented so that cumulative totals of blood loss are easily retrievable.

Medication Administration in Children

The administration of medication in the pediatric population may be challenging to those not used to the small doses and weight-based calculations. Because of the weight variability for each age of child, having standard doses for pediatrics is not possible. Because of variations in child weight, body surface area, and organ maturity, the ability to metabolize and excrete medications can be affected.[4] Pediatric medications are weight-based, so it is critical that an accurate weight in kilograms is obtained upon patient admission and that the weight is documented in a standard area of the patient's chart. According to the United States Pharmacopoeia Medication Reporting Program, incorrect administration of intravenous fluids was the most common pediatric medication error noted.[35] The number of pediatric medication errors has been reported to be as high as 1 in 6.4 orders (Box 48-5).[5,67] In response to the high numbers of errors, in 2003 the AAP developed a policy statement related to the prevention of medication errors in the pediatric inpatient setting as a commitment to preventing such errors.

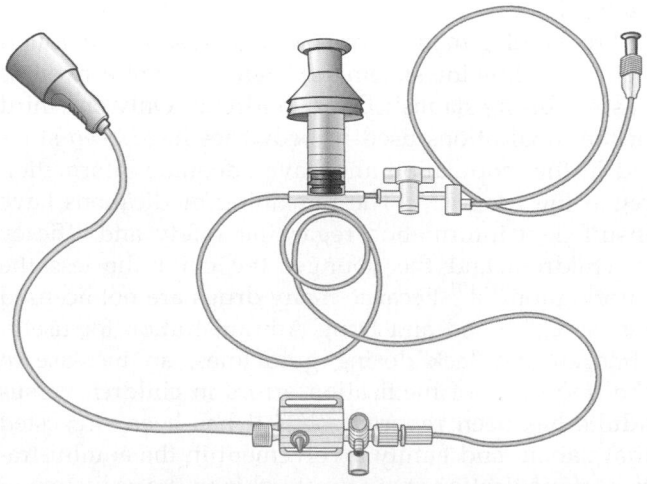

↕FIGURE 48-6 Vamp drawing.

Prevention of Pediatric Medication Errors

1. Provide adequate numbers of nurses and pharmacists that are educated to prepare, dispense, and administer medications to children.
2. Establish and maintain a functional pediatric formulary.
3. Standardize the following throughout the institution:
   - Pediatric infusion pumps
   - Weight scales
   - Measurement systems, e.g., all kilograms or all pounds
   - Pediatric medication physician order sheets
4. Confirm that child's weight is correct, and dose does not exceed adult dose.
5. Avoid use of a terminal zero to minimize 10-fold dosing errors (e.g., use 4 rather than 4.0).
6. Use a zero to the left of a dose less than 1 to avoid dosing errors (e.g., use 0.25 rather than .25).
7. Double-check calculations.
8. Verify unusually large or small volumes or dosages.
9. Listen when the patient or caregiver questions whether a medication should be administered.

Data from references 4, 35.

It has been shown that the presence of a critical care pharmacists, as part of the critical care multidisciplinary team, can enhance patient outcomes related to fluid management, adverse drug events, medication administration errors, and ventilator-associated pneumonias.[60] Institutions caring for children will want to ensure that they have a pharmacist who specializes in the administration of fluids and medications in the pediatric population.

Frequently, medication package inserts are found with the following statement: "Safety and effectiveness has not been established for children." Only one third of the medications used in pediatrics have been studied in this population and have adequate information regarding usage.[34,85] The remaining medications have insufficient information regarding safety and efficacy in children, and the younger the child the less the information.[85,101] Because many drugs are not licensed by the U.S. Food and Drug Administration for use in children and lack dosing guidelines, an increase in the frequency of medication errors in children versus adults has been reported.[5,35,40] It has been suggested that patient and family involvement in the administration of medications may be of value in the reduction of errors.[1]

Having so many unstudied medications in the pediatric population limits the number of "known" medications for children and places healthcare practitioners in a difficult situation when prescribing. For example, one major drug company, AstraZeneca, the manufacturer of propofol (Diprivan), distributed a letter in 2001 reminding healthcare providers that this specific medication was "not approved for sedation in pediatric critical care patients in the United States and should not be used for this purpose."[16] Having pediatric-focused medication text can make administration less challenging. A resource that focuses on injectable medications for children is useful in the critical care environment. The American Society of Health-System Pharmacists developed the *Teddy Bear Book: Pediatric Injectable Drugs* for hospitalized children.[14] This reference, updated regularly, was developed by pediatric-focused pharmacists.

PAIN IN CHILDREN

Pain assessment has been deemed the fifth vital sign by the American Pain Society.[32] Children who are admitted to critical care have pain associated with the illness or injury, but may also have pain from medical and nursing procedures, and anxiety from the experience of the critical care hospitalization. Children may deny that they are hurting for fear of "a shot" as the remedy.[51] Intramuscular injections are inappropriate if the child has a functioning intravenous line.[51] During IV placement and needle sticks for blood drawing, the use of local anesthetic creams is desirable.[91] Consultation with a multidisciplinary Pediatric Pain Service can assist the pediatric healthcare provider with pain management in children with complex pain issues; however, there are estimated to be only a dozen such teams in the United States.[100] The AAP has developed guidelines that can be used to ensure the safe administration and monitoring of patients receiving sedation and analgesia in the pediatric population (Box 48-6).[5,7]

A pain assessment should occur upon admission to the hospital, and on an ongoing basis according to institution policies. "Attempting to assess and measure another person's pain is like trying to speak a foreign language that you don't understand."[63] Assessment of the child in pain can be a challenging task especially if the child is preverbal or has developmental delays, and nurses have consistently rated children's pain levels lower than the children themselves have rated their pain.[28] Children respond to pain behaviorally and physiologically,[27] and there are pain assessment tools that can be helpful in measuring both types of responses (Boxes 48-7, 48-8, and 48-9 and Table 48-3). Children who are older than 7 years of age can use a

Box 48-6

Overview of Pediatric Sedation Guidelines

1. The child must undergo a documented presedation medical evaluation, including a focused airway examination.
2. There should be an appropriate interval of fasting before sedation.
3. Children should not receive sedative or anxiolytic medications without supervision by skilled medical personnel (i.e., medication should not be administered at home or by a technician without medical supervision from a practitioner who, by virtue of training, education, certification, or applicable licensure, law, or regulation, is qualified to supervise the delivery of medical care). The individual may be a physician, nurse, dentist, or other appropriately trained health professional.
4. Sedative and anxiolytic medications should be administered only by or in the presence of individuals skilled in airway management and cardiopulmonary resuscitation.
5. Age- and size-appropriate equipment and appropriate medications to sustain life should be checked before sedation and be immediately available.
6. All patients sedated for a procedure must be continuously monitored with pulse oximetry.
7. An individual must be specifically assigned to monitor the patient's cardiorespiratory status during and after the procedure; for deeply sedated patients, that individual should have no other responsibilities and should record vital signs at least every 5 minutes.
8. Specific discharge criteria must be used.
9. The *Guidelines for Monitoring and Management of Pediatric Patients During and After Sedation for Diagnostic and Therapeutic Procedures* apply regardless of the settings in which sedatives are administered or the specific training or profession of the practitioners involved.
10. At least one individual must be present who is trained in, and capable of, providing pediatric basic life support, and who is skilled in airway management and cardiopulmonary resuscitation; training in pediatric advanced life support is strongly encouraged.
11. Children who receive sedative medication with a long half-life may require extended observation.

Data from references 4, 5.

Box 48-7

Behavioral Indicators of Pain

INFANT

- Facial expression: brows lowered and drawn together, broadened nasal root, eyes tightly closed and angular, squarish mouth with a taut tongue
- Irritability
- Restlessness
- Continuous crying/whimpering
- Crying when stimulus applied
- Intense crying
- Knees drawn to chest
- Clenched fists
- Refusal to eat
- Hyper-alertness
- Restless sleep, inability to sleep
- Hypersensitivity to touch
- Muscle tension

TODDLER

- Says he or she "hurts" or has an "owie"
- Intense or continuous crying
- Aggressive behavior
- Rubbing, pulling, guarding, touching affected body part

- Inability to be comforted
- Regressive behavior
- Resistance to being helped
- Irritability/restlessness
- Nightmares, inability to sleep
- Decreased activity tolerance
- Lowered frustration tolerance
- Change from usual play behavior
- Seeking of comfort objects (e.g., blanket)
- Seeking of comfort from family

PRESCHOOL-AGE CHILD

Similar to toddler with the following additions:
- Denies pain in the presence of other behavioral cues and physical injury
- Repetitive verbalizations such as "it hurts, it hurts, it hurts"
- Refusal to allow touching of affected body part by others

SCHOOL-AGE CHILD

- Denial of pain in the presence of behavioral cues
- Resistance of movement

Box continues on p. 1360

Box 48-7—CONT'D

- Grimacing
- Nightmares
- Low frustration tolerance
- Guarding
- Emotional withdrawal
- Irritability/restlessness/thrashing

TEENAGER

- Muscle tension
- Guarding
- Change in activity level
- Nightmares
- Change in eating pattern
- Irritability/restlessness/thrashing
- Increased sleeping in the absence of pain control measures

- Low frustration tolerance
- Grimacing
- Nonverbal/neurologic damage
- Facial grimacing/flushing
- Increased muscle tension
- Hypersensitivity to the environment/touch
- Grinding of teeth
- Seizure activity
- Clenched fists
- Inability to be comforted
- Continuous crying
- Extremity spasms
- Vomiting
- Inability to tolerate lying in the same position

Data from references 2, 27, 57.

numerical 0 to 10 rating scale. Sedation scales can be used in conjunction with pain assessment scales. One such scale is the Modified Motor Activity Assessment scale (Table 48-4).[40,76]

As with adults, nonpharmacologic strategies for pain relief (distraction, touch, sucking) can be utilized, but the comfort that they provide may cease when the intervention stops,[94] so adequate pharmacologic sedation/analgesia must still be employed.[51] Dosing guidelines for these agents are listed in the Medication table on p. 1363. When it comes time to wean the patient from sedation/analgesia, weaning protocols that allow these

---

Box 48-8

Physiologic Responses to Pain in Children

- Increased pulse rate, blood pressure, respiratory rate
- Increased depth of respirations
- Flushing or pallor
- Diaphoresis
- Dilated pupils
- Decreased oxygen consumption/saturation
- Muscle tension
- Nausea and/or decreased gastric motility

Additionally, infants may have the following:

- Apnea
- Color changes
- Seizures
- Stooping
- Hiccupping

Data from reference 27.

medications to be reduced slowly can decrease the physical signs and symptoms of withdrawal (Box 48-10). These symptoms may be affected by the child's age, underlying illness, and cognitive state.[99]

Diarrhea; vomiting; problems with feeding, sucking, and swallowing; high-pitched crying; and irritability may be signs of withdrawal in neonates and infants, but may be attributed to reasons other than withdrawal.[97]

Neuromuscular Blockade

Chemical relaxation with neuromuscular blocking agents is used in the pediatric population for reasons such as rapid-sequence intubation, ventilatory control, and the prevention of increased arterial blood pressure from isometric muscle contraction.[105] Some care providers continue to mistakenly believe that these agents have analgesic and anxiolytic properties[76] and fail to provide adequate pain relief and sedation for the children receiving them. Train-of-four testing with a peripheral nerve stimulator, and drug holidays can be used to assess the appropriate level of chemical relaxation for the patient's condition and to prevent the complication of prolonged weakness following neuromuscular blockade. In children who are chemically paralyzed or who have no blink response, eyes should be kept protected and moist by creating a moisture chamber. This can be achieved by instilling normal saline drops every 2 hours, covering the eyes with plastic wrap, and changing the wrap daily or more frequently to prevent infection.[82] Earplugs can be used to eliminate the noise in critical care. These should be removed any time patients will be touched so they can be apprised of what will be occurring. The nurse should reassure the patient

Box 48-9

FACES Pain Rating Scale*

ORIGINAL INSTRUCTIONS:

Explain to the person that each face is for a person who feels happy because he has no pain (hurt) or sad because he has some or a lot of pain.

- **Face 0** is very happy because he doesn't hurt at all.

- **Face 1** hurts just a little bit.

- **Face 2** hurts a little more.

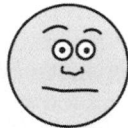

- **Face 3** hurts even more.

- **Face 4** hurts a whole lot.

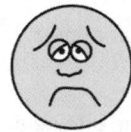

- **Face 5** hurts as much as you can imagine, although you don't have to be crying to feel this bad.

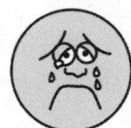

Ask the person to choose the face that best describes how he is feeling.

Data from references 2, 108.
*This rating scale is recommended for persons age 3 years and older.

that the inability to move is only temporary. To reduce stress, using the word "relaxation" versus "paralyzed" may be helpful when discussing neuromuscular blockade with the child and family.

INTENTIONAL INJURIES IN THE PEDIATRIC PATIENT

Reports of child abuse in the United States are increasing, and those children who are admitted to PICUs have the highest rates of mortality. These children most often present with severe head injury, and the victims tend to be younger in age.[110] Clinicians should also be aware that inconsistencies in the child's patient history might also be indicative of Munchausen syndrome by proxy, the fabrication of a child's illness.[100] A summary of factors to assess in children with suspected intentional injuries is given in Box 48-11.

Role of the Nurse

Healthcare providers are mandated by law to report suspected abuse to child protective services and law enforcement personnel. It is not their role to identify the perpetrator or prove that abuse occurred.[39] The focus should be on care of the patient and family in a professional, nonjudgmental manner. Unit visitation policies should be followed in the usual manner unless the child is taken into protective custody or there is a reason to believe the child is in danger. Documentation should be focused on detailed objective data that include history of the injury with timelines, actual behaviors of child and family, and physical findings that may include radiographs, photographs and body diagrams.[39,89]

In the event of death from an intentional injury, the child may still be considered for organ donation. It is imperative that there is collaboration between law enforcement, medical examiners, coroners, the critical care team, and the transplant surgeon to ensure that evidence is preserved and there is meticulous documentation of the transplant procedure.[110] Flawed criminal investigations or prosecutions related to organ donation have not been reported.[48]

Regardless of the patient's outcome, dealing with intentional injuries to a child can be difficult. Participation in unit-level debriefing sessions, increased peer-to-peer support, and individual self-care measures can be helpful in coping with this patient situation.

PARENTAL PERMISSION AND CHILD ASSENT

In the United States parents have legal authority in matters of concern for their minor children, and limits to parental authority occur only when the child's interests are clearly severely threatened by parental action.[15] Some states recognize "mature minors" as those who can understand proposed treatments and the potential consequences.[15] While state statutes vary,

TABLE 48-3 FLACC Scale for Assessing Postoperative Pain in Children Ages 2 to 7

	SCORING*		
CATEGORIES	0	1	2
Face	No particular expression or smile	Occasional grimace or frown, withdrawn, uninterested	Frequent to constant quivering chin, clenched jaw
Legs	Normal position or relaxed	Uneasy, restless, tense	Kicking, or legs drawn up
Activity	Lying quietly, normal position, moves easily	Squirming, shifting back and forth, tense	Arched, rigid, or jerking
Cry	No cry (awake or asleep)	Moans or whimpers; occasional complaint	Crying steadily, screams or sobs, frequent complaints
Consolability	Content, relaxed	Reassured by occasional touching, hugging, or being talked to, distractible	Difficult to console or comfort

Data from references 70, 71.
*Each of the 5 categories—(F) Face; (L) Legs; (A) Activity; (C) Cry; (C) Consolability—is scored from 0 to 2, which results in a total score between 0 and 10.

TABLE 48-4 Modified Motor Activity Assessment Scale

SCORE	DESCRIPTION	DEFINITION
−3	Unresponsive	Minimal or no response to noxious* stimulus; does not communicate or follow commands
−2	Responsive only to noxious stimuli	Opens eyes or raises eyebrows or turns head toward stimulus or moves limbs with noxious stimulus
−1	Responsive to touch or name	Opens eyes or raises eyebrows or turns head toward stimulus or moves limbs with touch or when name is spoken; drifts off after stimulation; follows simple commands
0	Calm and cooperative	No external stimulus is required to elicit movement; calm, awakens easily, and follows commands
+1	Restless and cooperative	No external stimulus is required to elicit movement; picking at tubes but consolable
+2	Agitated	No external stimulus is required to elicit movement; attempting to sit or move limbs to get up and inconsolable despite frequent attempts; requires physical restraint, biting ETT
+3	Dangerously agitated, uncooperative	No external stimulus is required to elicit movement; patient unsafe—attempting to pull at ETT/catheters; desaturating; thrashing side-to-side; climbing over rail; striking at staff

Data from references 41, 76.
*Suctioning or 5 seconds of nail bed pressure.
ETT = Endotracheal tube.

emancipated minors are generally recognized as adolescents younger than 18 years of age who are one of the following: in the military, married, an unmarried mother, or not living at home and self-supporting.[15] Those living in states with mature minor statutes, or who are emancipated, are generally allowed to make personal healthcare decisions. The traditional view is that children are not competent to make medical decisions;[109] while refusal of treatment is allowed by competent adults, children are not afforded the same rights in the United States.[77] One may argue that children are not always rational; however, "rationality

SUGGESTED GUIDELINES FOR DOSING OF SEDATIVE AND ANALGESIC AGENTS

AGENT	DOSE*	COMMENTS
Fentanyl (Duragesic)	2–4 mcg/kg/hr	Neonates may be more sensitive to chest wall rigidity and respiratory depression than adults.
Morphine	10–30 mcg/kg/hr	Chest wall rigidity and hypotension may occur with rapid administration.
Midazolam (Versed)	0.05–0.15 mg/kg/hr	Contains benzyl alcohol 1%, which may cause fatal gasping syndrome in neonates.
Lorazepam (Ativan)	0.025–0.05 mg/kg/hr	Contains benzyl alcohol 2% and propylene glycol, which may cause adverse effects in neonates.
Ketamine (Ketalar)	1–2 mg/kg/hr	Use with caution in those at risk for increased intracranial pressure. Laryngospasm and apnea may occur.
Pentobarbital (Nembutal)	1–2 mg/kg/hr	Is an alkaline solution so may cause tissue necrosis with extravasation.

Modified from reference 99 with additional data from references 13 and 14.
*These infusion rates represent suggestions for starting doses. The infusion should be supplemented with as-needed bolus doses to provide the desired level of baseline sedation/analgesia. In patients requiring frequent bolus doses, the infusion rate should be increased by 10% to 20%. If patients require no bolus doses and are excessively sedated, the infusion rate should be decreased by 10% to 20%.

Box 48-10

Sedative/Analgesic Weaning for Administration Longer Than Approximately 5 Days

1. A weaning schedule should be developed for children who have received sedative/analgesic infusions or frequent dosing for greater than approximately 5 days.
2. Medication dosing should be changed from continuous infusions to around-the-clock intermittent IV/oral administration.
3. Intravenous medications the patient is receiving should be converted to equianalgesic oral dosing as soon as possible before discharge.
4. During medication weaning, the baseline original daily dose should be reduced 10% to 20% every 1 to 2 days. For example, a dose of 60 mg would be reduced by 6 to 12 mg every 1 to 2 days. In patients receiving high doses of medication, it may be necessary to decrease the rate by smaller increments every 12 hours to reduce withdrawal symptoms.

Data from references 97, 99.

Box 48-11

Assessment of Intentional Injuries

- Unbelievable/inconsistent patient history
- Delay in seeking medical assistance
- New adult partner in household
- Prior history of abuse/suspected abuse
- Multiple injuries in various stages of healing
- Absence of primary caretaker at onset of illness
- Unexplained neurologic deterioration, shock, cardiac arrest

---

Children may be more capable of making health-related decisions than first thought, and it is reasonable to ask for a child's consent to treatment while giving parents the opportunity to give informed permission.[109] The AAP concluded that, "patients should participate in decision-making commensurate with their development . . . parents and physicians should not exclude children and adolescents . . . without persuasive reasons."[6]

The wishes of those children who refuse consent in order to gain a better understanding or refuse because of fear should be respected, and coercion to treat should be avoided.[6,92] When there is persistent objection, medical interventions performed for the child's "own good" are disrespectful to the child. Any time this occurs, an apology to the child should occur.[19] For healthcare providers who were not treated with this type of

might not be a necessary criterion for a minor to make his or her own medical decision, given that medical decisions by adults need not be rational."[6,109] Children may only be deemed competent when they make the decision that the doctor wants them to make.[42]

decision-making respect as children, it may not be easy for them to respect children in this manner.[19] It may also be hard for parents to view the child as a decision maker when that role may not be supported in the child's home environment.[19] A collaborative model of decision making that involves the child, the family, and healthcare providers is optimal.[34]

Unfortunately, there are times when the child's best interest can get buried in controversies, family tensions, and medical technology.[15] The pediatric critical care nurse is in a prime position to ensure that the child is the focus of all decisions and not the individual personalities involved.

TRANSITIONS FOR THE CHILD AND FAMILY IN CRITICAL CARE

Out of the PICU

As the child's health improves, the child and family must be prepared for transfer out of the critical care unit or for discharge home. Transitioning to a general care unit after a critical care admission may be a source of anxiety for the child and family.[103] Utilization of a transfer protocol for pediatric patients from the critical care unit has been shown to decrease family stress while increasing family satisfaction with the transfer process (Figure 48-7).[103] Bent et al. found that parents felt unprepared to care for their child after discharge home from a critical care admission and that the time following discharge was extremely stressful and uncertain.[21]

Palliative Care

Forty to sixty percent of all deaths in the PICU occur following a decision to limit life-sustaining therapies.[29,30] Therefore a commitment and a plan to provide palliative care to children and families are needed in institutions that have made the decision to provide care at the end of life for this population. It is also important to provide multidisciplinary healthcare provider debriefing sessions, bereavement rounds to allow for the open discussion of end-of-life issues, and verbalization of healthcare provider stress and emotions.[30,47]

PEDIATRIC RESUSCITATION PRIORITIES

Unlike adults, children exhibit subtle changes that must be identified early to prevent decompensation (Table 48-5). In children, respiratory failure is the primary cause of an arrest, with cardiac arrest being secondary, most often from hypoxemia and acidosis. Basic life support sequences are dependent on the age of the victim.

TABLE 48-5 Warning Signs of Potential Decompensation

SYSTEM	ASSESSMENT FINDINGS
Respiratory	Child self-positions Requires interventions (head positioning, suctioning, adjunct airways) Tachypnea* Bradycardia* Hypoxemia Hypercarbia Change in responsiveness Decreased chest movement with respiration Labored breathing, retractions, nasal flaring, grunting, head bobbing, wheezing, stridor Decreased or absent air exchange upon auscultation
Cardiovascular	Heart rate is absent, irregular, bradycardic, or tachycardic* Blood pressure decreases (sign of late decompensation: 10-mm decrease is significant) Pallor, cyanosis, mottled skin Cool extremities Diminished or absent peripheral pulses Capillary refill >2 seconds despite warm ambient temperature Worried appearance Decreased urine output
Neurologic	Irritable Lethargic Obtunded or comatose Decreased or absent reaction to pain Decreased muscle tone Decreased or absent pupillary response Unequal pupils

Data from references 11, 52–54, 72–74, 96, 107.
*All vital signs must be evaluated according to individual patient's age, baseline values, and clinical condition.

When children do have cardiac arrest, the American Heart Association algorithms should be followed for fast, slow, and absent rhythms (Figures 48-8, 48-9, and 48-10, respectively).[11-13] These protocols are included in the Multidisciplinary Plan of Care on pp. 1342-1347.

COMPETENT PEDIATRIC INTENSIVE CARE NURSING

Studies by Tilford et al.[98] and Ruttimann et al.[88] showed improved patient outcomes were related to higher

Instructions:
Answer every question by completely filling in the correct circle. If you are unsure about how to answer a question, please give the best answer you can. *There are no right or wrong answers.*

This survey is **voluntary.** Your answers will be kept **in strict confidence.**

Thinking about your child's transfer from the PICU to the general pediatric floor, how would you rate each of the following:

	Poor	Fair	Good	Very Good	Excellent	Not Applicable
1. Helpfulness of nursing staff in preparing you for transfer of your child to the general pediatric floor.	①	②	③	④	⑤	⑥
2. Clear and complete explanation provided by nursing staff about:						
a. Time of day for your child's transfer.	①	②	③	④	⑤	⑥
b. Your child's medical condition leading to transfer.	①	②	③	④	⑤	⑥
c. Increased number of patients each floor nurse cares for.	①	②	③	④	⑤	⑥
d. Frequency of the floor nurse checking on your child.	①	②	③	④	⑤	⑥
e. Your role in providing care to your child on the pediatric floor.	①	②	③	④	⑤	⑥
3. Amount of notice you were given before the transfer.	①	②	③	④	⑤	⑥
4. Promptness and efficiency of the transfer process.	①	②	③	④	⑤	⑥
5. Introduction by the floor nurse to your child on arrival.	①	②	③	④	⑤	⑥
6. Helpfulness of nursing staff in giving you a tour of the floor.	①	②	③	④	⑤	⑥
7. Information shared between units about your child's needs.	①	②	③	④	⑤	⑥
8. Overall quality of the transfer process from ICU to the floor.	①	②	③	④	⑤	⑥

9. How much notice were you given before your child was transferred?

None	Less than 1 hour	1 to 2 hours	2 to 4 hours	More than 4 hours
①	②	③	④	⑤

10. Time of day transfer occurred:

Morning (6 AM to 12 noon)	Afternoon (12 noon to 6 PM)	Evening (6 PM to 12 midnight)	Night (12 midnight to 6 AM)
①	②	③	④

11. Length of time in ICU:

1 day	2 to 3 days	4 to 5 days	More than 5 days
①	②	③	④

We welcome any addtional comments you may have:

_____
_____
_____
_____

Thank You! Your opinions are important to us.

▲FIGURE 48-7 Transfer guidelines survey form.

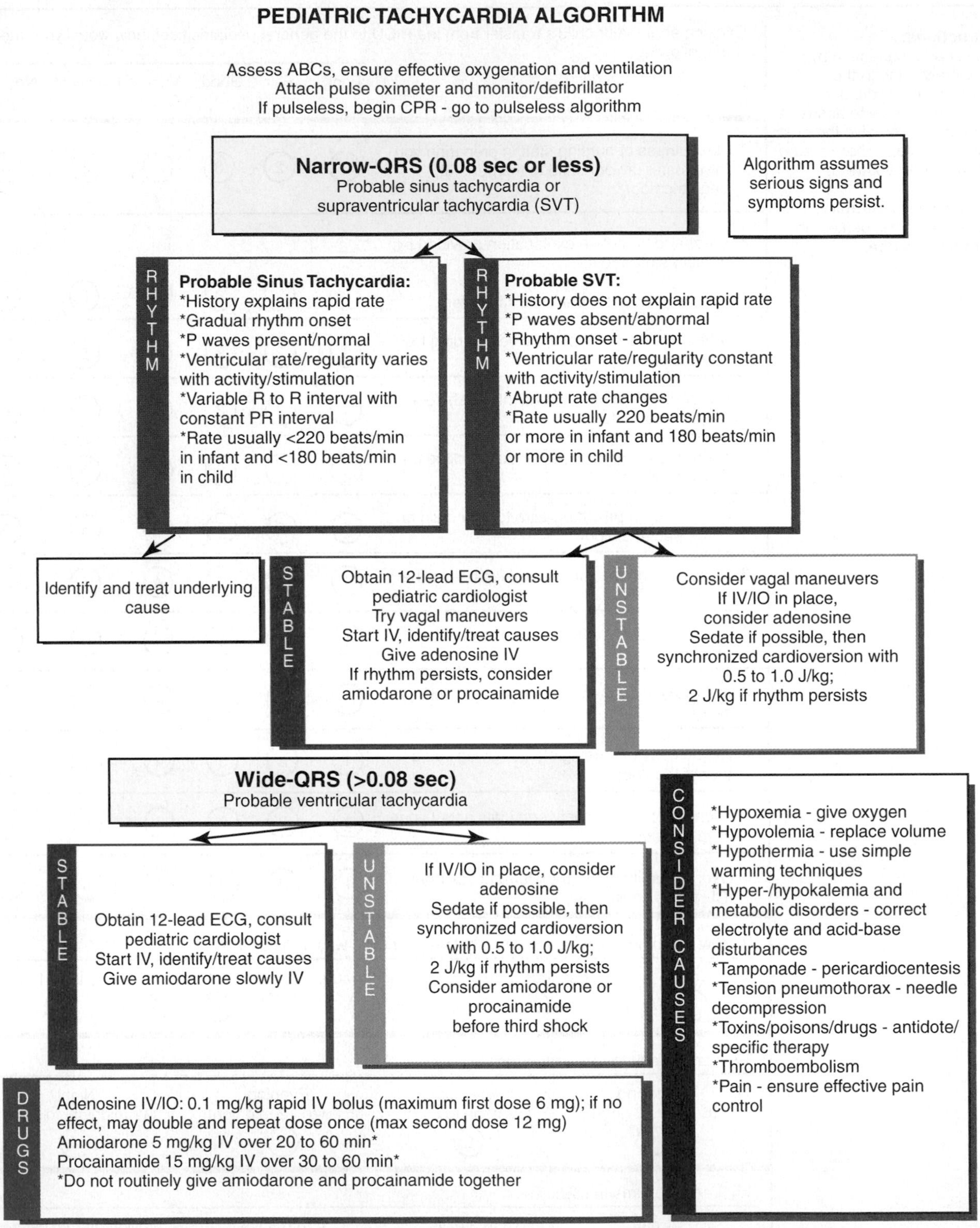

PEDIATRIC TACHYCARDIA ALGORITHM

Assess ABCs, ensure effective oxygenation and ventilation
Attach pulse oximeter and monitor/defibrillator
If pulseless, begin CPR - go to pulseless algorithm

Narrow-QRS (0.08 sec or less)
Probable sinus tachycardia or
supraventricular tachycardia (SVT)

Algorithm assumes serious signs and symptoms persist.

RHYTHM

Probable Sinus Tachycardia:
*History explains rapid rate
*Gradual rhythm onset
*P waves present/normal
*Ventricular rate/regularity varies
with activity/stimulation
*Variable R to R interval with
constant PR interval
*Rate usually <220 beats/min
in infant and <180 beats/min
in child

RHYTHM

Probable SVT:
*History does not explain rapid rate
*P waves absent/abnormal
*Rhythm onset - abrupt
*Ventricular rate/regularity constant
with activity/stimulation
*Abrupt rate changes
*Rate usually 220 beats/min
or more in infant and 180 beats/min
or more in child

Identify and treat underlying cause

STABLE

Obtain 12-lead ECG, consult
pediatric cardiologist
Try vagal maneuvers
Start IV, identify/treat causes
Give adenosine IV
If rhythm persists, consider
amiodarone or procainamide

UNSTABLE

Consider vagal maneuvers
If IV/IO in place,
consider adenosine
Sedate if possible, then
synchronized cardioversion with
0.5 to 1.0 J/kg;
2 J/kg if rhythm persists

Wide-QRS (>0.08 sec)
Probable ventricular tachycardia

STABLE

Obtain 12-lead ECG, consult
pediatric cardiologist
Start IV, identify/treat causes
Give amiodarone slowly IV

UNSTABLE

If IV/IO in place, consider
adenosine
Sedate if possible, then
synchronized cardioversion
with 0.5 to 1.0 J/kg;
2 J/kg if rhythm persists
Consider amiodarone or
procainamide
before third shock

CONSIDER CAUSES

*Hypoxemia - give oxygen
*Hypovolemia - replace volume
*Hypothermia - use simple
warming techniques
*Hyper-/hypokalemia and
metabolic disorders - correct
electrolyte and acid-base
disturbances
*Tamponade - pericardiocentesis
*Tension pneumothorax - needle
decompression
*Toxins/poisons/drugs - antidote/
specific therapy
*Thromboembolism
*Pain - ensure effective pain
control

DRUGS

Adenosine IV/IO: 0.1 mg/kg rapid IV bolus (maximum first dose 6 mg); if no
effect, may double and repeat dose once (max second dose 12 mg)
Amiodarone 5 mg/kg IV over 20 to 60 min*
Procainamide 15 mg/kg IV over 30 to 60 min*
*Do not routinely give amiodarone and procainamide together

◆FIGURE 48-8 Algorithm for pediatric tachycardia with poor perfusion.

volumes of pediatric critical care admissions. Remaining competent in an area with little chance to utilize skills is challenging, and orienting an entire adult critical care unit's staff to pediatric patients and maintaining ongoing competencies may be time and cost prohibitive. Unit leaders can identify a multidisciplinary cadre of healthcare providers who have an interest in caring for the pediatric population, versus those drafted into the situation.

SYMPTOMATIC BRADYCARDIA ALGORITHM

Perform an initial assessment
Assess ABCs, ensure effective
oxygenation and ventilation
Attach pulse oximeter and monitor/defibrillator
If pulseless, begin CPR - go to pulseless algorithm

Serious signs and symptoms persist?

YES

NO

Observe
Support ABCs, give O$_2$ if needed
Consider cardiology consult

Heart rate <60/min and poor perfusion present despite oxygenation and ventilation?

YES

NO

Start chest compressions

Start IV
Give epinephrine

Give atropine
(if increased vagal tone
or primary AV block)

Consider causes

Consider pacing

DRUGS

Epinephrine IV/IO: 0.01 mg/kg (1:10,000)
every 3 to 5 min
Epinephrine ET: 0.1 mg/kg (1:1000), max 10 mg

Atropine IV/IO: 0.02 mg/kg (minimum dose 0.1 mg)
Max single dose 0.5 mg for child, 1.0 mg for adolescent

CONSIDER CONTRIBUTING CAUSES

*Hypoxemia - give oxygen
*Hypovolemia - replace volume
*Hypothermia - use simple warming techniques
*Hyper-/hypokalemia and metabolic disorders - correct
electrolyte and acid-base disturbances
*Head injury - provide oxygenation and ventilation
*Heart block - consider atropine, chronotropic drugs
early pacing; consult pediatric cardiologist
*Heart transplant (special situation) - may require pacing
or large doses of sympathomimetics
*Tamponade - pericardiocentesis
*Tension pneumothorax - needle decompression
*Toxins/poisons/drugs - antidote/specific therapy
*Thromboembolism
*Increased vagal tone, AV block - give atropine

⬦FIGURE 48-9 Algorithm for pediatric bradycardia.

Children and families, especially those who are hospital savvy, are highly skilled at recognizing those who truly enjoy the care of pediatric patients.

Initial Pediatric Orientation

For the identified cadre of nurses, attendance and competency at a pediatric advanced life support (PALS) class is essential. These classes are just a starting point, with the focus being pediatric emergency care only, and do not a pediatric critical care nurse make. Preparing to care for children in the adult critical care unit takes initial educational preparation that may include the following: a pediatric-focused internship, didactic lectures by experts/consultants, PALS classes, simulated admissions and emergencies, and bedside pediatric clinical competency validation by a preceptor at a regional tertiary PICU.[80]

Ongoing Competencies

To provide ongoing pediatric clinical focus after the initial orientation, the following are recommended: reassessment of pediatric skills and bedside competencies,

CARDIAC ARREST ALGORITHM

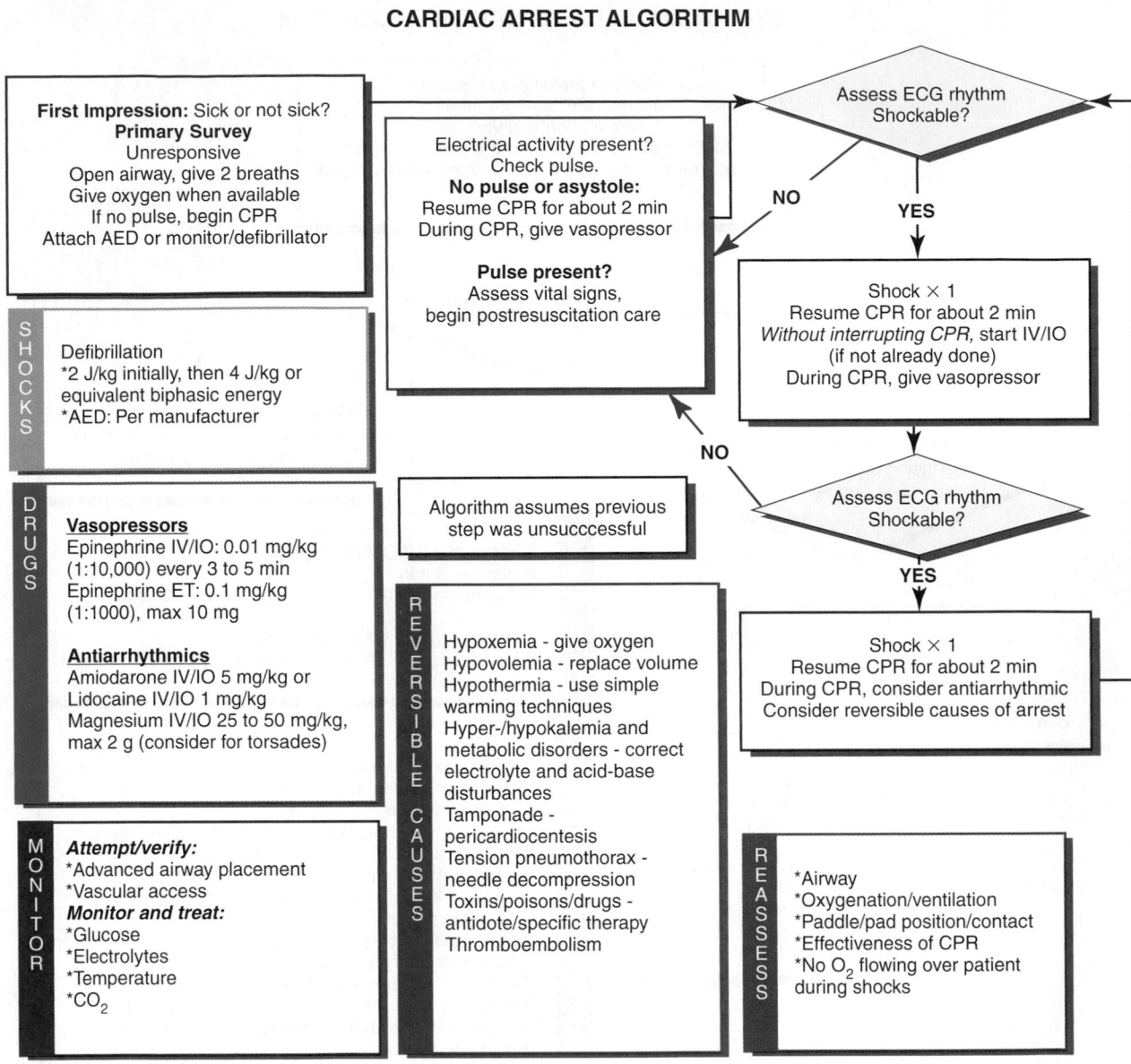

First Impression: Sick or not sick?
Primary Survey
Unresponsive
Open airway, give 2 breaths
Give oxygen when available
If no pulse, begin CPR
Attach AED or monitor/defibrillator

Electrical activity present?
Check pulse.
No pulse or asystole:
Resume CPR for about 2 min
During CPR, give vasopressor

Pulse present?
Assess vital signs,
begin postresuscitation care

Assess ECG rhythm Shockable?

NO   YES

S H O C K S
Defibrillation
*2 J/kg initially, then 4 J/kg or
equivalent biphasic energy
*AED: Per manufacturer

Shock × 1
Resume CPR for about 2 min
Without interrupting CPR, start IV/IO
(if not already done)
During CPR, give vasopressor

D R U G S
Vasopressors
Epinephrine IV/IO: 0.01 mg/kg
(1:10,000) every 3 to 5 min
Epinephrine ET: 0.1 mg/kg
(1:1000), max 10 mg

Antiarrhythmics
Amiodarone IV/IO 5 mg/kg or
Lidocaine IV/IO 1 mg/kg
Magnesium IV/IO 25 to 50 mg/kg,
max 2 g (consider for torsades)

Algorithm assumes previous
step was unsucccessful

NO

Assess ECG rhythm Shockable?

YES

Shock × 1
Resume CPR for about 2 min
During CPR, consider antiarrhythmic
Consider reversible causes of arrest

M O N I T O R
Attempt/verify:
*Advanced airway placement
*Vascular access
Monitor and treat:
*Glucose
*Electrolytes
*Temperature
*CO_2

R E V E R S I B L E   C A U S E S
Hypoxemia - give oxygen
Hypovolemia - replace volume
Hypothermia - use simple
warming techniques
Hyper-/hypokalemia and
metabolic disorders - correct
electrolyte and acid-base
disturbances
Tamponade -
pericardiocentesis
Tension pneumothorax -
needle decompression
Toxins/poisons/drugs -
antidote/specific therapy
Thromboembolism

R E A S S E S S
*Airway
*Oxygenation/ventilation
*Paddle/pad position/contact
*Effectiveness of CPR
*No O_2 flowing over patient
during shocks

♦FIGURE 48-10 Algorithm for pediatric asystole and pulseless arrest.

attendance at pediatric educational sessions, and the opportunity to provide care for pediatric patients on a regular basis. If there are not ample pediatric admissions, a repeat precepted bedside experience at a tertiary PICU should be considered. For units with low pediatric admissions, skill labs and simulation labs with products such as SimBaby and MegaCode Kid (Figure 48-11) and mock resuscitations can also provide pediatric content reinforcement. However, simulation can never take the place of actual, hands-on pediatric patient care.

Daily bedside multidisciplinary pediatric team rounds can also provide an opportunity for learning and have been shown to improve communication and collaboration among the participants[104] and decrease patient length of stay.[43] Family members should be given a chance to participate in rounds. With families present at rounds, the importance of family involvement in the care process is reinforced. Pediatric pocket reference guides that can be utilized on a moment's notice—such as the *AACN Pediatric Reference Card,* the *PALS Pocket Reference* by the American Heart Association, and the *Harriet Lane Handbook*—all are quick fingertip resources, some with software available for personal digital assistants.

Pediatric advanced-practice nurses can promote evidence-based practice in the critical care environment. These clinical experts can provide mentoring and reinforce pediatric best practices with the bedside nurse.

Nurses working with children, meeting the designated requirements, should strongly consider taking the certification exam to become a pediatric critical care

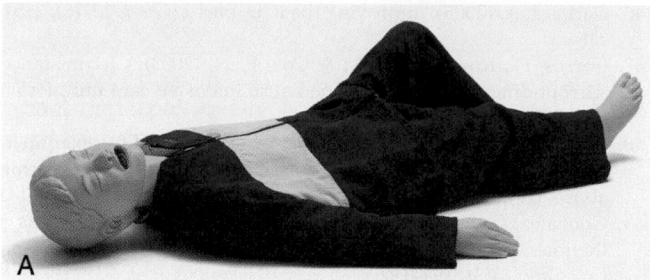
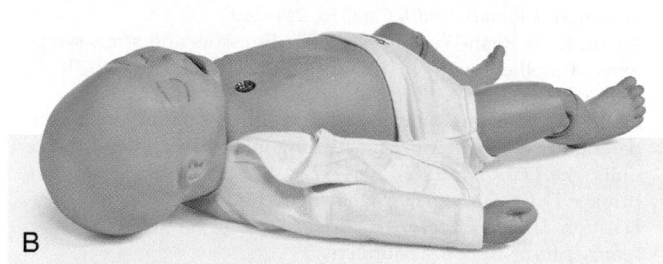

✦FIGURE 48-11   A, MegaCode Kid, and **B,** SimBaby.

registered nurse. Certification offers employers and patients validation that nurses possess the specialty knowledge, skills, and experience to effectively and safely deliver care. Fewer medical errors, increased job satisfaction, and increased self-confidence have been linked to certification.[10]

To remain current in the care of pediatric patients, AACN and the SCCM provide pediatric-focused resources in the form of current books, journal articles, web pages, and live educational sessions. SCCM offers the Pediatric Critical Care web site as a resource at http://pedsccm.wustl.edu. Joining the PICU listserv provides an opportunity for networking with others in the specialty.

CONCLUSIONS

Caring for children in an adult critical care unit can be an exciting challenge. With appropriate orientation, competency maintenance, and performance improvement monitoring, the multidisciplinary team can provide quality care to children and their families.

REFERENCES

1. Agency for Healthcare Research and Quality. (2000). *Patient fact sheet: 20 tips to help prevent medical errors in children.* Rockville, Md: Agency for Healthcare Research and Quality. Publication No. 00-P038.
2. Algren, C. (2005). Family-centered care of the child during illness and hospitalization. In M. J. Hockenberry (Ed.), *Wong's essentials of pediatric nursing* (7th ed.). St. Louis: Elsevier Mosby.
3. Algren, C., & Arnow, D. (2005). Pediatric variations of nursing interventions. In M. J. Hockenberry (Ed.), *Wong's essentials of pediatric nursing* (7th ed.). St. Louis: Elsevier Mosby.
4. American Academy of Pediatrics, Committee on Drugs. (2002). Guidelines for monitoring and management of pediatric patient during and after sedation for diagnostic and therapeutic procedures: addendum. *Pediatrics, 110*(4), 836–838.
5. American Academy of Pediatric Committee on Drugs and Committee on Hospital Care. (2003). Prevention of medication errors in the pediatric inpatient setting. *Pediatrics, 112*(2), 431–435.
6. American Academy of Pediatrics Committee on Bioethics. (1995). Informed consent, parental permission, and assent in pediatric practice. *Pediatrics, 95*(2), 314–317.

7. American Academy of Pediatrics, Committee on Drugs. (1992). Guidelines for monitoring and management of pediatric patient during and after sedation for diagnostic and therapeutic procedures. *Pediatrics, 89,* 1110–1115.
8. American Academy of Pediatrics Committee on Hospitals. (1993). Guidelines and levels of care for pediatric intensive care units. *Pediatrics, 92*(1), 166–175.
9. American Association of Critical-Care Nurses. (2004). *Practice alert: family presence during CPR and invasive procedures.* Aliso Viejo, Calif: AACN.
10. American Association of Critical-Care Nurses & AACN Certification Corp. (2002). Safeguarding the patient and the profession: the value of critical care nurse certification. *Am J Crit Care, 2003, 12,* 154–164.
11. American Heart Association. (2005). 2005 American Heart Association guidelines for cardiopulmonary resuscitation and emergency cardiovascular care. *Circulation, 112*(24 suppl I).
12. American Heart Association in Collaboration with the International Liaison Committee on Resuscitation. (2000). Guidelines for cardiopulmonary resuscitation and emergency cardiovascular care: an international consensus on science, *Circulation, 102*(suppl 1), 291–342.
13. American Heart Association & American Academy of Pediatrics. (2002). *PALS provider manual.* Dallas: American Heart Association.
14. American Society of Health-System Pharmacists. (2004). *Teddy bear book: pediatric injectable drugs* (7th ed.). Bethesda, Md: American Society of Health-System Pharmacists.
15. Ariff, J. L., & Groh, D. H. (2001). In the best interest of the child: ethical issues. In M. A. Q. Curley & P. A. Moloney-Harmon (Eds.), *Critical care nursing of infants and children* (2nd ed.). Philadelphia: Saunders.
16. AstraZeneca. (March 26, 2001). *Letter.* Wilmington, Del.
17. Ball, J. W., & Bindler, R. C. (2005). Pediatric and newborn assessment. In J. W. Ball & R. C. Bindler (Eds.), *Child health nursing: partnering with children and families.* Upper Saddle River, NJ: Pearson Prentice Hall.
18. Barnes-McDowell, B. M. (1998). Ask the experts: pediatric patients in adult ICUs. *Crit Care Nurse, 18*(3), 1–2.
19. Bartholome, W. G. (1995). Informed consent, parental permission, and assent in pediatric practice (Letter to the editor). *Pediatrics, 95* (5), 981–982.
20. Beauman, S. S. (2001). Didactic components of a comprehensive pediatric competency program. *J Infusion Nurs, 24*(6), 367–374.
21. Bent, K. N., Keeling, A., & Rouston, J. (1996). Home from the PICU: are parents ready? *Matern Child Nurs, 21,* 80–84.
22. Berwick, D. M., & Kotagal, M. (2004). Restricted visiting hours in the ICU: time to change. *JAMA, 292*(6), 736–737.
23. Bettler, J., & Roberts, K. A. (2000). Nutrition assessment of the critically ill child. *AACN Clin Issues, 11*(4), 498–506.

24. Board, R. (2004). Father stress during a child's critical care hospitalization. *J Pediatr Health Care, 18,* 244–249.

25. Board, R., & Ryan-Wenger, N. (2003). Stressors and stress symptoms of mothers with children in the PICU. *J Pediatr Nurs, 18*(3), 195–202.

26. Board, R., & Ryan-Wenger, N. (2000). State of the science on parental stress and family functioning in pediatric intensive care units. *Am J Crit Care, 9*(2), 106–122.

27. Brinker, D. (2003). Pain management in children. In P. A. Moloney-Harmon & S. J. Czerwinski (Eds.), *Nursing care of the pediatric trauma patient.* St Louis: Saunders.

28. Broome, M. E., & Huth, M. M. (2002). Nursing management of the child in pain. In N. L. Schechter, C. Berde & M. Yaster (Eds.), *Pain in infants, children, and adolescents* (2nd ed.). Philadelphia: Lippincott Williams & Wilkins.

29. Burns, J. P., et al. (2000). End of life care in the pediatric intensive care unit after foregoing of life-sustaining treatment. *Crit Care Med, 28*(8), 3060–3066.

30. Burns, J. P., & Rushton, C. H. (2004). End-of-life care in the pediatric intensive care unit: research review and recommendations. *Crit Care Clin, 20,* 467–485.

31. Campbell, J. (2001). Unique solutions in pediatric critical care. *Pediatr Nurs, 27*(5), 483–491.

32. Campbell, J. (1995). *Pain: the fifth vital sign: advocacy and policy.* American Pain Society. Accessed 08/10/05 at www.ampainsoc.org/advocacy/fifth.htm.

33. Carnavale, F. A. (1997). The experience of critically ill children: narratives of unmaking. *Intensive Crit Care Nurs, 13,* 49–52.

34. Cote, C., et al. (1996). Is the "therapeutic orphan" about to be adopted? *Pediatrics, 98,* 118–123.

35. Crowley, E., Williams, R., & Cousins, D. (2001). Medications errors in children: a descriptive summary of medication error reports submitted to the United States Pharmacopeia. *Curr Ther Res, 26,* 627–640.

36. Curley, M. A. Q. (1988). Effects of the nursing mutual participation model of care and parental stress in the pediatric intensive care unit, *Heart Lung, 17,* 682–688.

37. Curley, M. A. Q., & Wallace, J. (1992). Effects of the nursing mutual participation model of care on parental stress in the pediatric intensive care unit—a replication. *J Pediatr Nurs, 7,* 377–385.

38. Curley, M. A. Q., & Meyer, E. C. (2001). Caring practices: the impact of the critical care experience on the family. In M. A. Q. Curley & P. A. Moloney-Harmon (Eds.), *Critical care nursing of infants and children* (2nd ed.). Philadelphia: WB Saunders.

39. Czerwinski, S. J., & Moloney-Harmon, P. A. (2003). Intentional injuries. In P. A. Moloney-Harmon & S. J. Czerwinski (Eds.), *Nursing care of the pediatric trauma patient.* St Louis: Saunders.

40. D'Antonio, Y. C., & Cohen, M. R. (1999). Pediatric medication errors. In M. R. Cohen (Ed.), *Medication errors.* Washington, DC: American Pharmaceutical Association.

41. Devlin, J. W., et al. (1999). Motor activity assessment scale: a valid and reliable sedation scale for use with mechanically ventilated patient in an adult surgical intensive care unit. *Crit Care Med, 27,* 1271–1275.

42. Dixon-Woods, M., Young, B., & Henry, D. (1999). Partnerships with children. *BMJ, 319,* 778–780.

43. Dutton, R. P., Cooper, C., Jones, A., et al. (2003). Daily multidisciplinary rounds shorten length of stay for trauma patients. *J Trauma, 55*(5), 913–919.

44. Emergency Nurses Association. (2000). Pediatric trauma. In B. Bennett-Jacobs (Ed.). *Trauma nursing core course provider manual,* Park Ridge, Ill: Emergency Nurses Association.

45. Ewart, G. W., et al. (2004). The critical care medicine crisis: a call for federal action. *Chest, 125,* 1518–1521.

46. Garland, A. (2005). Improving the ICU: part 1. *Chest, 127*(6), 2151–2164.

47. Garros, D., Rosychuk, R. J., & Cox, P. N. (2003). Circumstances surrounding end of life in a pediatric intensive care unit. *Pediatrics, 112*(5), e371–e379.

48. Goldstein, B., Shafer, T., & Greer, D. (1997). Medical examiner/coroner denial for organ donation in brain dead victims of child abuse: controversies and solutions. *Clin Intensive Care, 8,* 136–141.

49. Gonzalez, C. E., et al. (2004). Visiting preferences of patients in the intensive care unit and in a complex care medical unit. *Am J Crit Care, 13*(3), 194–197.

50. Goh, A. Y., Lum, L. C., & Abdel-Latif, M. E. (2001). Impact of 24-hour critical care physician staffing on case-mix adjusted mortality in pediatric intensive care. *Lancet, 357,* 445–446.

51. Gregg, T. L. (1998). Pediatric pain management in an adult critical care unit. *Crit Care Nurs Q, 21*(2), 42–58.

52. Hazinski, M. F. (1992). *Children are different. Nursing care of the critically ill child.* St. Louis: Mosby.

53. Hazinski, M. F. (1997). Anatomic and physiologic differences between children and adults. In D. Levin & F. Morriss (Eds.), *Essentials of pediatric intensive care* (2nd ed). New York: Churchill Livingstone.

54. Hazinski, M. F. (1999). *Children are different. Manual of pediatric critical care.* St. Louis: Mosby.

55. Holtzclaw, B. J. (1998). New trends in thermometry for the patient in the ICU. *Crit Care Nurs Q, 21,* 1.

56. Holtzclaw, B. J. (1993). Monitoring body temperature. *AACN Clin Issues Nurs, 4,* 49.

57. Johnston, C. C., & Strata, M. E. (1986). *Pain management in children.* Milwaukee, Wis: MaxiShare Corp.

58. Inaba, A. S., & Seward, P. N. (1991). An approach to pediatric trauma unique anatomic and pathophysiologic aspects of the pediatric patient. *Emerg Med Clin North Am, 9,* 523–548.

59. Institute of Medicine, Committee on Pediatric Emergency Medical Services. (1993). In J. S. Durch & K. N. Lohr (Eds.), *Emergency medical services for children.* Washington, DC: National Academies Press.

60. Kane, S. L., Weber, R. J., & Dasta, J. F. (2003). The impact of critical care pharmacists on enhancing patient outcomes. *Intensive Care Med, 29,* 691–698.

61. Kanter, R. K. (2002). Regional variation in child mortality at hospitals lacking a pediatric intensive care unit. *Crit Care Med, 30*(1), 94–99.

62. Kelley, M. A., et al. (2004). The critical care crisis in the United States. *Chest, 125,* 1514–1517.

63. Kuttner, L. (1996). *A child in pain: how to help, what to do.* Vancouver, BC: Hartley & Marks.

64. Marcin, J. P., et al. (2004). The use of telemedicine to provide pediatric critical care consultations to pediatric trauma patients admitted to a remote trauma intensive care unit: a preliminary report. *Pediatr Crit Care Med, 5*(3), 251–256.

65. Marcin, J. P., et al. (2004). Use of telemedicine to provide pediatric critical care inpatient consultations to underserved rural Northern California. *J Pediatr, 144,* 375–380.

66. Marcin, J. P., et al. (2005). Nurse staffing and unplanned extubation in the pediatric intensive care unit. *Pediatr Crit Care Med, 6,* 254–257.

67. Marino, B. L., et al. (2000). Prevalence of errors in a pediatric hospital medication system: implications for error proofing. *Outcomes Manag Nurs Pract, 4,* 129–135.

68. Martin, S. A., & Kline, A. M. (2004). Can there be a standard for temperature measurement in the pediatric intensive care unit? *AACN Clin Issues, 15*(2), 254–266.

69. Mason, K. J. (1998). Neuromuscular scoliosis: a case of the pediatric patient in the adult ICU. *Crit Care Nurs Q, 21*(2), 64–81.

70. Merkel, S. I., et al. (1997). The FLACC: a behavioral scale for scoring postoperative pain in young children. *Pediatr Nurs*, 23(3), 293–298.

71. Merkel, S. I., et al. (2003). FLACC behavioral pain assessment scale: a comparison with the child's self-report. *Pediatr Nurs*, 29(13), 195–199.

72. Moloney-Harmon, P. A., & Rosenthal, C. H. (1992). Nursing care modification for the child in the adult ICU. In S. Stillwell (Ed.), *Mosby's critical care nursing reference*. St. Louis: Mosby.

73. Moloney-Harmon, P. A. (2002). Pediatric trauma. In K. McQuillan, K. Von Rueden, & R. Hartstock, et al. (Eds.), *Trauma nursing: from resuscitation to rehabilitation* (3rd ed., pp. 747–771). Philadelphia: Saunders.

74. Moloney-Harmon, P. A. (2005). The critically ill pediatric patient. In P. Gonce Morton, et al. (Eds.), *Critical care nursing: a holistic approach* (8th ed.). Philadelphia: Lippincott Williams & Wilkins.

75. Mullen, J., & Pate, M. F. D. (2006). Caring for critically ill children and their families. In M. Slota (Ed.), *AACN core curriculum for pediatric critical care nursing* (2nd ed.). Aliso Viejo, Calif: AACN.

76. Oakes, L. (2001). Caring practices: providing comfort. In M. A. Q. Curley & P. A. Moloney-Harmon (Eds.), *Critical care nursing of infants and children* (2nd ed.). Philadelphia: Saunders.

77. Odetola, F. O., et al. (2005). A national survey of pediatric critical care resources in the United States. *Pediatrics*, 115(4), e382–e386.

78. Omnibus Reconciliation Act of 1990. Title IV, Section 4206. Congressional Record. Oct 26, 1990, h12456-h12457.

79. Pediatric Section Task Force on Admission and Discharge Criteria. (1999). Society of Critical Care Medicine In Conjunction with the American College of Critical Care Medicine and the Committee on Hospital Care of the American Academy of Pediatrics. *Crit Care Med*, 27(4), 843–845.

80. Paladichuk, A. (1998). Children in the adult ICU: interview with Mary Fran Hazinski. *Crit Care Nurse*, 18(6), 82–87.

81. Pate, M. F., & Zapata, T. (2002). How deeply should I go when I suction an endotracheal (ETT) or tracheostomy tube (TT)? *Crit Care Nurse*, 22, 130–131.

82. Quigley, S. M., & Whitney, D. E. (2001). Skin integrity. In M. A. Q. Curley & P. A. Moloney-Harmon (Eds.), *Critical care nursing of infants and children* (2nd ed.). Philadelphia: Saunders.

83. Randolph, A. G., et al. (2004). Growth of pediatric intensive care units in the United States from 1995 to 2001. *J Pediatr*, 144, 792–798.

84. Rennick, J. E., et al. (2002). Children's psychological responses after critical illness and exposure to invasive technology. *J Dev Behav Pediatr*, 23(3), 133–144.

85. Roberts, R., et al. (2003). Pediatric drug labeling: improving the safety and efficacy of pediatric therapies. *JAMA*, 290(7), 905–911.

86. Rosenberg, D. I., & Moss, M. M. (2004). American College of Critical Care Medicine of the Society of Critical Care Medicine. Guidelines and levels of care for pediatric intensive care units. *Crit Care Med*, 32(10), 2117–2127.

87. Rupp, L. A., & Day, M. W. (2003). Children are different: pediatric differences and the impact on trauma. In P. A. Moloney-Harmon & S. J. Czerwinski (Eds.), *Nursing care of the pediatric trauma patient*. St. Louis: Saunders.

88. Ruttimann, U. E., Patel, K. M., & Pollack, M. M. (2002). Relevance of diagnostic diversity and patient volumes for quality and length of stay in pediatric intensive care units. *Pediatr Crit Care Med*, 1, 133–139.

89. Salassi-Scotter, M., Jardine, J. M., & Lawson, L. (1994). Child maltreatment. In D. P. Henderson & D. Brownstein (Eds.), *Pediatric emergency nursing manual*. New York: Springer Publishing.

90. Sanchez, J. L., Lucas, J., & Feustel, P. (2001). Outcome of adolescent trauma admitted to an adult surgical intensive care unit versus a pediatric intensive care unit. *J Trauma*, 51(3), 478–480.

91. Schechter, N. L., et al. (1997). The ouchless place: No pain, children's gain. *Pediatrics*, 99(6), 890–894.

92. Shield, J. P. H., & Baum, J. D. (1994). Children's consent to treatment: listen to the children—they will have to live with the decision. *Br Med J*, 308, 1182–1183.

93. Simon, S. K., et al. (1997). Current practices regarding visitation policies in critical care units. *Am J Crit Care*, 6, 210–217.

94. Slonim, A. D., & Ognibene, F. P. (1998). Sedation for pediatric procedures, using ketamine and midazolam, in a primarily adult intensive care unit: a retrospective evaluation. *Crit Care Med*, 26(11), 1900–1904.

95. Slota, M., et al. (2003). Perspectives on family-centered, flexible visitation in the intensive care unit setting. *Crit Care Med*, 31(5), S362–S366.

96. Smith, M. F., & Lyons, A. (2001). In M. A. Q. Curley & P. A. Moloney-Harmon (Eds.), *Critical care nursing of infants and children* (2nd ed.). Philadelphia: WB Saunders.

97. Tejedor-Sojo, J. (2002). Analgesia and sedation. In V. L. Gunn & C. Nechyba (Eds.), *The Harriet Lane handbook: a manual for pediatric house officers*. Philadelphia: Mosby.

98. Tilford, J. M., et al. (2000). Volume-outcome relationships in pediatric intensive care units. *Pediatrics*, 106, 289–294.

99. Tobias, J. D. (2002). Pain management for the critically ill child in the pediatric intensive care unit. In N. L. Schechter, C. Berde, & M. Yaster (Eds.), *Pain in infants, children, and adolescents* (2nd ed.). Philadelphia: Lippincott Williams & Wilkins.

100. Turner, H. N. (2005). Complex pain consultations in the pediatric intensive care unit. *AACN Clin Issues*, 16(3), 388–395.

101. U.S. Food and Drug Administration. (2001). *Pediatric exclusivity provision: status report to congress*. Rockville, Md: Food and Drug Administration.

102. Vanore, M. L. (2000). Care of the pediatric patient with brain injury in an adult intensive care unit. *Crit Care Nurs Q*, 23(3), 38–48.

103. Van Waning, N. R., Kleiber, C., & Freyenberger, B. (2005). Development and implementation of a protocol for transfers out of the pediatric intensive care unit. *Crit Care Nurse*, 25(3), 50–55.

104. Vazirani, S., Hays, R. D., Shapiro, M. F., et al. (2005). Effect of a multidisciplinary intervention on communication and collaboration among physicians and nurses. *Am J Crit Care*, 14(1), 71–77.

105. Vernon-Levett, P. (2001). Skin integrity. In M. A. Q. Curley & P. A. Moloney-Harmon (Eds.), *Critical care nursing of infants and children* (2nd ed.). Philadelphia: Saunders.

106. Watson, R. S. (2002). Location, location, location: regionalization and outcome in pediatric critical care. *Curr Opin Crit Care*, 8, 344–348.

107. Winkelstein, M. (2005). The child with respiratory dysfunction. In M. J. Hockenberry (Ed.), *Wong's essentials of pediatric nursing* (7th ed.). St. Louis: Elsevier Mosby.

108. Wong, D., & Baker, C. (1988). Pain in children: comparison of assessment scales. *Pediatr Nurs*, 14(1), 9–17.

109. Zawistowski, C. A., & Frader, J. E. (2003). Ethical problems in pediatric critical care: consent. *Crit Care Med*, 31(5), S407–S410.

110. Zenel, J., & Goldstein, B. (2002). Child abuse in the pediatric intensive care unit. *Crit Care Med*, 30(11), S515–S523.

CHAPTER 49

Caring for the Critically Ill Elderly Patient

Laura M. Criddle

THE AGING POPULATION

Demographics

Americans are living longer than ever before. Older adults constitute the fastest-growing segment of the U.S. population. The number of Americans age 65 and over is expected to increase from a current level of 30 million to 54 million by the year 2020,[91] accounting for almost 13% of the total population.[74] This represents a threefold increase in the number of persons in this age-group since 1900. Between 1900 and 1990, the number of older Americans increased by 2.6 million, or 8%, while the under-65 population grew by only 6%.[80] Moreover, the population of elderly persons in the United States is expected to double in the next 30 years, reaching 70 million by 2030.[70] By the year 2050, it is estimated that worldwide the number of people over the age of 65 will total 2.5 billion, comprising 20% of the earth's population.[25]

There is a lack of uniformity regarding the specific age that qualifies a patient to be considered "geriatric," and various sources set the lower cutoff for "elderly" anywhere between the ages of 50 and 75.[21,26,33,85,97] Nevertheless, 65 years, the age of Medicare eligibility, is the age most commonly selected to define the "older" adult in the United States. Because an individual may live to be well over 100 years, the "elderly" category encompasses a very large group, many of whom may be much closer to age 100 than they are to 50.[115]

If mortality rates remain constant, those who were age 65 in 2000 can expect to live an average of 18 additional years, compared to 65-year-olds in 1900, who had a remaining life expectancy of only 12 years. However, life expectancy at age 65 is almost 2 years less for African Americans than for Caucasians.[70] The most rapidly growing segment of the elderly population is the over-85 age-group. Their number is projected to increase sixfold, to nearly 20 million, by 2050.[87] In fact, approximately one third of Americans now live beyond 85 years, and at least 10% of persons over age 90 can expect to live until 99 years.[2]

This increase in life expectancy during the twentieth century has been a remarkable achievement. However, senescence (growing old) is accompanied by increased risk for many diseases and disorders. Although older Americans enjoy generally good heath, many elderly adults have physical disabilities;[80] a significant proportion of seniors suffer from chronic health conditions. Fortunately, despite the presence of chronic disease, the rate of disability among older people has actually declined in recent years.[70] Besides enjoying better health than previous generations of seniors, the current cohort of older Americans is more highly educated than any previous generation. In 1998 about 11% of older women and 20% of older men were college graduates. This trend toward better educated seniors will continue.[70]

FACTORS THAT INFLUENCE AGING

Age-Related Changes

Regardless of chronologic age, senescence is a highly individual process; no two people age at the same rate or in the same way. Some aging processes are universal. Over time, the number of normally functioning cells in the body is reduced, oxygen consumption is decreased, and response to physiologic stressors is blunted.[80] However, a significant interaction between genetic, environmental, physiologic, psychological, and social aspects of life exists. There are major differences between individuals' physiologic reserves and their disease exposure, severity, and its functional impact. This difference between chronologic and physiologic aging is reflected in the adage, *"It's not the years but the mileage."*

As age advances, the incidence of disease increases; cardiovascular and neoplastic diseases become the most common causes of death.[23] Although physiologic decline and disease processes influence each other, the body's normal aging process does not produce significant dysfunction or impairment in the absence of disease.[23,80] Therefore it is important to distinguish age-related changes from those associated with chronic conditions or acute illness in order to avoid prematurely attributing findings to advanced age, when they are actually caused by a disease state.[80]

Social and Environmental Factors

Some changes commonly associated with aging are a result of long-term exposure to a variety of environmental and social conditions (Box 49-1). Over the course of a lifetime, socioeconomic status, lifestyle, and personal health habits leave their mark on everyone.

Cumulative Health History

Long life span is associated with an increased prevalence of chronic and acute illnesses. Many conditions take years or even decades to manifest, and their number accumulates over time. The cumulative effects of life are borne by all; no one reaches old age without a medical history, often a very extensive one.

Comorbidities

Other disorders found in association with senescence are not universal, but are instead the result of comorbidities common to the elderly population. A comorbid condition is defined as any additional disease state that will significantly affect the patient's response to the present illness or injury. Box 49-2 lists comorbidities common

---

Box 49-2

Comorbidities Common to the Geriatric Patient

- Arthritis
- Hypertension
- Cardiovascular disease
- Neoplasms
- Chronic pulmonary disease
- Obesity
- Dementia
- Renal insufficiency
- Hepatic disease
- Stroke
- Hyperlipidemia
- Type 2 diabetes

Data from references 10, 12, 13, 15, 47, 48, 57.

---

among geriatric patients. Each of the environmental, social, and comorbidity factors previously described is strongly influenced by genetics, particularly a family history of certain disorders (e.g., coronary artery disease, stroke, dementia, and cancer).

THE GERIATRIC CRITICAL CARE PATIENT

Demographics

The characteristic processes of tissue and organ changes associated with aging—in conjunction with the prevalence of chronic conditions—contribute to the high number of geriatric patients treated in critical care.[23] Even though senior citizens currently constitute approximately one eighth of the U.S. population, they consume more than one fourth of all critical care and trauma resources.[87] Inpatient admission rates have dropped for all other age-groups, yet the admission rate for those over age 65 has increased 23% during the past 3 decades. In 1970 only 20% of hospital beds and one third of hospital days were used by the elderly. By 2000 these numbers had climbed to 40% of admissions and 50% of all hospital days.[43] Driven by demographics and increased life expectancy, the total number of older patients treated in critical care can be expected to rise dramatically over the next quarter century.[23]

Currently, half of all patients admitted to critical care in the United States are older than 65 years.[57] In fact, 20% of Americans will die in critical care.[112] The leading causes of death among older patients are heart disease, malignancies, stroke, influenza, and chronic obstructive pulmonary disease. However, with advancing age, the need for critical care management of chronic disease

---

Box 49-1

Environmental and Social Factors Associated With Aging

ENVIRONMENTAL EXPOSURES

- Inhalants—tobacco smoke, wood fires, asbestos, coal dust
- Toxins—heavy metals, radon
- Ultraviolet light

POVERTY

- Lack of adequate primary care, including immunizations
- Reduced access to care
- Self-care knowledge and skills deficits
- Undertreatment of acute and chronic conditions

LIFESTYLE

- Absence of an effective social support system
- Chronic stress
- Deficient personal hygiene practices
- Inadequate sleep
- Poor nutritional status, including obesity
- Repetitive-use injuries
- Sedentary behaviors
- Substance abuse—alcohol, tobacco, prescription and recreational drugs

Data from references 23, 31, 35, 69.

exacerbations also results in frequent critical care admissions.[80] Practitioners caring for critically ill seniors are routinely faced with difficult decisions regarding aggressive treatment, outcome optimization, and rationing of resources. In order to understand the basis for such decisions, healthcare providers must appreciate the normal changes associated with aging and their implications for care.[115]

Critical care nurses need to be cognizant of the differences in outcomes and complications experienced by critically ill elders.[115] Senescence has a profound impact on individual physiologic performance. In every body system, the elderly patient's physiologic reserves are limited and function can deteriorate rapidly, even with expert medical and nursing attention. Their declining physiologic status can force seniors to use "reserves" just to maintain homeostasis. Therefore when reserves are required to meet the increased demands of acute illness or surgical stress, but are no longer present, organ system failure ensues.[101]

Traumatic Injury

In addition to experiencing frequent acute illnesses and exacerbations of chronic conditions, the elderly are overrepresented in the number of trauma patients admitted to surgical critical care units. Trauma—once considered predominantly a disease of the young—has long been the leading cause of death in the United States for individuals between the ages of 1 and 44 years. However, of the 11 million people over the age of 65 hospitalized annually in the United States, more than 8% have a first-listed diagnosis of injury or poisoning. More than 900,000 seniors require hospitalization for trauma each year, and half of these patients have one or more fractures.[25]

Although the incidence of major traumatic injury remains lower in the geriatric population than in any other age-group, both longevity gains and increasingly active lifestyles have contributed to rising injury rates.[64,91] Trauma is the number 4 cause of mortality in those over the age of 55 and the seventh leading cause of death in persons 75 years and older.[74] In some areas of the United States, the number of elderly women hospitalized for injury now exceeds that of young men.[16,42] Following major injury, seniors experience an in-hospital mortality two to six times greater than younger adults with equivalent injuries. Although older persons comprise only 12.5% of the population, almost one third of the deaths from injury occur in the 65-plus age-group.*

In the elderly patient, poor outcomes following traumatic injury are related to both the normal changes of aging and the prevalence of preexisting comorbid

conditions. As a result of reduced physiologic reserves and chronic disease, injured geriatric patients are hospitalized for trauma at a rate twice that of the general population.[91] On average, trauma care expenditures for geriatric patients are two and a half times those of younger individuals. These higher costs are attributed to greater frequency and duration of critical care admissions, an increased incidence of complications, and overall longer hospital stays.[25]

There are significant differences between older and younger patients related both to injury patterns and to the frequency and type of complications experienced following trauma. Despite a typically less severe mechanism of injury, older adults experience a greater number of post-injury complications than do their younger counterparts. Preexisting medical conditions, particularly cardiovascular disease, have a profound effect on patients' ability to manage the stresses of injury.

Mechanisms of Injury. Falls are the leading trauma mechanism among persons over the age of 65 years.[49] Many factors associated with aging contribute to the high incidence of falls in this population. In the over-75 age-group, falls are also the leading cause of death from trauma.[25] Dementia, decreased visual acuity, obesity, neurologic and musculoskeletal impairments, gait and balance disturbances, and medication use can all be contributory factors. The majority of falls (84%) occur at home, and approximately 13% are attributed to some acute medical condition.[25]

By the year 2020, the number of drivers in the United States greater than age 65 will total 33 million.[25] Although the number of miles driven annually decreases in individuals over the age of 55, seniors have a total motor vehicle crash rate second only to that of 16- to 25-year-olds. However, the elderly (particularly those 75 years or older) suffer a post-collision fatality rate greater than any other age-group. In contrast to younger individuals, seniors are more likely to crash during daylight hours, in good weather, and close to home. Older adults are also more prone to collisions involving intersections, traffic sign violations, right-of-way decisions, and another vehicle. However, compared with younger cohorts, the older adult is less likely to have ingested alcohol. Age-related declines in cognitive function, decreased auditory acuity, changes in direct and peripheral vision, impaired coordination, and increased reaction time all contribute to crashes in elderly motorists.[25,49,78]

Automobile versus pedestrian incidents are a major source of musculoskeletal and head injury in older patients and are the third most common cause of traumatic mortality in those over the age of 65 years. In fact, seniors have the highest pedestrian mortality rate of any age-group.[25,49] In addition to slowed ambulation, many seniors suffer from kyphosis, which

---

*References 5, 8, 32, 40, 41, 64, 91, 95.

produces a stooped posture, making it difficult to raise the head to see oncoming traffic. Increased reaction time, vision and hearing losses, limited neck rotation, medication use, substance abuse, and poor judgment also contribute to geriatric pedestrian injury.[25,78]

Critical Care Outcomes Following Injury. The elderly are predisposed to serious post-trauma sequelae and suffer an increased incidence of multiple organ system dysfunction, wound healing problems, sepsis, and other infections.[25] These differences between geriatric and younger patients suggest the need for prompt diagnosis and aggressive treatment of the older population. However, there is still considerable debate regarding whether routine critical care admission, invasive hemodynamic monitoring, and hemodynamic "optimization" really lead to improved survival following geriatric trauma. Outcomes in the critically injured elderly are often affected by the presence of complications, some of which have significant effects on an individual's long-term status. Functional recovery in the subset of elderly trauma patients with major brain injury or extensive burns is notoriously poor, with mortality and disability rates more than twice those of younger patients.[91,96]

Even minor trauma may result in a substantial loss of preinjury function.[74] Nevertheless, most injured seniors without significant neurologic insults will return home and as many as 85% eventually resume independent function.[47] This suggests that an initial aggressive approach to geriatric trauma patient management should be pursued. However, more attention must be paid to long-term outcomes (e.g., quality of life and functional ability), and not just survival to hospital discharge. Without these long-term predictors, we may fail to treat those older adults who would survive, and instead pursue futile interventions in other critically injured seniors.[115]

Minimizing Potential Critical Care Problems

The goals of patient management in critical care are to maintain optimum cellular oxygen delivery, provide adequate substrate for tissue healing, and control pain. As a result of the physiologic changes and coexisting organ dysfunction common to the geriatric population, some of our usual patient care strategies may need to be adjusted.[87]

CARDIOVASCULAR SYSTEM

Cardiovascular decline has been one of the most studied aspects of aging, yet the functional implications of these changes are difficult to separate from normal age-related alterations in body composition, metabolic rate, and general state of fitness, all of which affect cardiac performance.[109] In the healthy elderly, exercise capacity is commonly restricted by noncardiac functions that limit exercise ability (e.g., neurologic, pulmonary, or musculoskeletal disorders).[23]

Age-Related Changes

Decreased Beta-Adrenergic Receptors. Aging is associated with changes in the sympathetic and parasympathetic nervous systems. Receptors present on the senescent myocardium become less sensitive, producing an impaired response to beta-adrenergic stimulation that attenuates maximal heart rate (HR). This is particularly important during exercise or other physiologic stressors such as major injury or critical illness. From a pharmacologic standpoint, HR responses to drugs (e.g., beta-blockers, digoxin, and parasympatholytic agents) are less in the elderly population.[4]

Decreased Exercise Tolerance and Cardiac Reserve. In the older patient at rest, cardiac output (CO), stroke volume (SV), and ejection fraction are not substantially changed.[23] These functions are maintained despite the increase in afterload imposed by stiffening of the outflow tract. However, senescence is associated with a decline in exercise performance.[102] Patients 65 years and older have decreased pump function as a result of progressive fibrosis of the myocardium. Thickening of the left ventricular wall, along with stiffening of the aortic and mitral valves, makes it more difficult for the aging heart to maintain adequate contractile strength.[48]

Healthy older persons have no major age-associated decline in CO during exercise, but maximal HR, maximal aerobic capacity, peak exercise CO, and peak ejection fraction slowly decline with advancing years. Notably, the mechanism by which CO is maintained during exercise differs between elderly and younger persons. In young adults, output is sustained by increasing HR. In contrast, the aging heart becomes less responsive to beta-adrenergic stimulation and instead maintains CO by recruitment of reserves to increase ventricular filling and SV.[109]

Increased Dysrhythmias. With aging, much of the heart's autonomic tissue is replaced by connective tissue and fat. These progressive changes cause conduction abnormalities throughout the intranodal tracts and bundle of His, contributing to a high incidence of sick sinus syndrome, atrial dysrhythmias, and bundle branch blocks. About 50% of elderly persons have abnormalities on their resting electrocardiograms (ECGs), most commonly PR or QT interval prolongation, intraventricular conduction abnormalities, reduced QRS voltage, and a leftward shift of the QRS axis. Elderly men have ECG abnormalities more frequently than do equivalent-age women.[80]

The most prominent dysrhythmia in older adults is premature ventricular contractions. Other symptoms of increasing myocardial irritability include sinus node dysfunction (e.g., atrial fibrillation, atrial flutter, paroxysmal supraventricular tachycardia) and atrioventricular conduction defects. Because the majority of dysrhythmic patients are asymptomatic, the routine use of antidysrhythmics is not recommended. The side effects and toxicities related to antidysrhythmic use frequently pose a greater risk to the elderly than does the dysrhythmia itself. On the other hand, pharmacologic therapy is warranted in symptomatic patients. Those with malignant ventricular dysrhythmias (e.g., ventricular fibrillation or sustained ventricular tachycardia) should be considered for automated implantable cardiac defibrillator placement.[23]

Orthostatic Hypotension. Abrupt reductions in blood pressure (BP)—caused by alterations in peripheral resistance, CO, or blood volume—are sensed by the baroreceptors. Baroreceptor stimulation results in increased impulse frequency in the medullary vasomotor center. This produces a rise in HR as well as vasoconstriction of the peripheral vasculature. Both of these effects are designed to restore BP. However, baroreceptor function is blunted with aging, predisposing elderly patients to episodes of orthostatic hypotension that can be further exacerbated by certain common medications. The prevalence of orthostatic hypotension is greater in institutionalized older adults who take anti-hypertensive medications.[23] In addition, many geriatric patients can readily become hypotensive as a result of vagal stimulation. In this population, a Valsalva maneuver can easily cause a drop in BP and even produce syncope.

Heart Rate Changes. With advancing age, the heart maintains a rate not substantially changed from that of younger adults. However, the maximal HR achieved during exercise is attenuated. Fortunately, this decreased HR response is accompanied by an increase in both left ventricular end-diastolic volume and SV, which serve to maintain CO during exercise. If the HR response becomes restricted—from diseased myocardium or beta-blockade—an elderly person's capacity to respond to exercise or stress will be severely limited.[23] Conversely, tachycardias are also poorly tolerated in the elderly. When left ventricular filling time is shortened by a tachydysrhythmia, cardiac performance is significantly decreased.[109]

Decreased Diastolic Filling. Despite an age-related reduction in early diastolic filling, preload is maintained

because left atrial contraction becomes more vigorous, thereby increasing late diastolic filling of the left ventricle (LV). In a poorly compliant LV, left atrial contraction can contribute up to 50% of LV filling. As a result of this vigorous atrial contraction, it is not uncommon to note a compensatory S_4 heart sound. Loss of atrial "kick," the atrial contribution to preload, will substantially impair cardiac function. Consequently, in older adults, the onset of atrial fibrillation can cause a marked reduction in CO.[80] Because ventricular filling and relaxation are energy-dependent processes, even mild hypoxemia can prolong relaxation, increase diastolic pressures, and aggravate pulmonary congestion, subsequently leading to diastolic dysfunction. In patients over the age of 80 years, diastolic dysfunction is responsible for up to 50% of heart failure cases.[87]

Vascular Changes. Senescence induces gradual thickening of the intimal vascular layer, primarily the result of an increase in the number of smooth muscle cells and the amount of connective tissue.[23] Arteriosclerosis (thickening and loss of elasticity in the arterial walls) and atherosclerosis (lipid deposition and thickening of the intimal cell layers within the arteries) cause the arteries to become progressively less distensible. The narrowing vascular diameter then alters the vessels' pressure-volume relationship. These changes are clinically significant because even small alterations in intravascular diameter are accompanied by a disproportionate increase in systolic BP.[23] Atherosclerotic disease not only elevates BP but also is associated with a concomitant reduction in blood flow to vital organs, and a decrease in physiologic reserve.

The vascular changes of aging are not limited to the small vessels. Calcification and fibrosis cause progressive stiffening of the cardiac valves, the great vessels, and the heart's outflow tract, resulting in increased resistance to ventricular emptying, a modest increase in pulmonary artery pressure, and compensatory ventricular hypertrophy.[23] The progressive aortic calcification associated with aging, along with osteoporosis of the thoracic vertebrae, can result in more calcium visible in the aorta than in the spine on the chest radiographs of some elderly patients. Because of these vascular changes, peripheral pulses, particularly in the feet, may be diminished or absent in seniors.[48,91]

Blood Pressure Changes. The vascular changes of senescence produce a gradual but linear rise in systolic BP. Diastolic pressure is less affected by time and generally remains the same or may even drop as the patient ages.[23]

Decreased Left Ventricular Compliance. With advancing years, there is progressive loss of myocytes—in both the left and right ventricles—and an increase in myocardial collagen content (type I). Although the muscle fibers that line the endocardium atrophy with age, the left ventricular wall thickens, producing left ventricular hypertrophy (LVH). This LVH is primarily the result of myocyte hypertrophy related to an increase in myocyte cell volume. LVH causes a moderate reduction in left ventricular cavity size and a compensatory rise in systolic BP. These changes all combine to increase myocardial stiffness, limit diastolic filling, and produce an overall decline in ventricular compliance. Therefore the LV must develop a higher filling pressure for a given increase in ventricular volume. The functional consequence of this is heightened myocardial oxygen consumption, which puts patients at risk for the development of myocardial ischemia.[23]

Decreased Number of Pacemaker Cells. Another change associated with cardiac senescence is a progressive reduction in the number of pacemaker cells in the sinus node. By the age of 75 years, older individuals have only 10% of the number of pacemaker cells they had at age 20.[80] This explains the frequency of sinus dysrhythmias in the elderly and partially accounts for seniors' reduced compensatory response to stressors.

Common Problems and Management Strategies

Coronary Artery Disease. The incidence of cardiovascular disorders—coronary artery disease, acute coronary syndrome, and myocardial infarction—all increase markedly with age. Cardiac disease is also the most common comorbid condition in the elderly, with 83% of all cardiovascular deaths occurring in patients over the age of 65. Although the functional impact of this disease significantly affects geriatric morbidity and mortality, its presentation is frequently atypical and nonspecific.[109]

Chest pain is still the leading symptom of myocardial infarction (MI) in all age-groups, yet the elderly often present a very different clinical picture than younger persons with acute MI. Individuals with altered cardiac pain perception (e.g., the elderly and persons with long-standing diabetes mellitus) regularly present with anginal-equivalent syndromes rather than classic ischemic chest pain. In older patients, typical anginal-equivalent symptoms include weakness, shortness of breath, syncope, acute confusion, and stroke.[87] The most frequently encountered anginal-equivalent chief complaint is dyspnea, usually resulting from pulmonary edema. Unexplained sinus tachycardia, cardiogenic asthma, and new-onset lower extremity edema have also been reported as anginal-equivalents in the elderly.[10] Among the very old, an acute MI may present

with neurologic symptoms (e.g., acute mental status changes, new-onset weakness, and stroke).[10] In the Framingham Heart Study, persons ages 75 to 84 years were found to have an asymptomatic MI incidence of greater than 40%.[87]

Myocardial ischemia treatment strategies for patients between the ages of 65 and 75 years are similar to those used in the younger population. Limited data are available regarding the treatment of patients 75 to 84 years of age. In the very old, those over 85 years, diagnosis and therapy must be highly individualized.[109] The high incidence of atypical MI symptoms means that older patients often arrive at the hospital later than their younger counterparts. Unfortunately, this eliminates the possibility of fibrinolytic therapy if the 6-hour window of opportunity has expired. In addition, comorbid conditions (e.g., hypertension, dysrhythmias, or previous stroke) frequently contraindicate fibrinolysis in the elderly.[109]

In older patients undergoing surgery, the use of preoperative beta-adrenergic blockade has been shown to reduce the incidence of postoperative cardiac morbidity and mortality in patients at increased cardiac risk. In fact, published guidelines on perioperative cardiac risk management now include the use of beta blockers.[79]

Seniors are more prone to the development of cardiogenic shock after acute MI than are younger adults,[63] but augmentation of CO and SV in response to dobutamine is less in older patients because of decreased beta-receptor sensitivity. With the stiffening of the outflow tract that accompanies aging, afterload reduction is a particularly useful management strategy in older patients with cardiac dysfunction.[109]

Shock. Normal cardiovascular changes in the elderly affect how the body responds to shock states. Left ventricular wall thickening, myocardial irritability, calcification and fibrosis of the heart valves, loss of myocardial compliance, and decreased SV combine to limit the body's response to stress and increased oxygen demands. These age-related cardiac changes make it considerably more difficult for the geriatric patient to respond to hypovolemic, distributive, or cardiogenic shock states.

Because of the prevalence of hypertension in the elderly, BP may appear normal despite significant reduction from baseline. This loss of elasticity and vasomotor tone decreases the body's ability to adapt to changing oxygen needs. In individuals with a history of hypertension, hypotensive episodes may be difficult to detect. Common medications (e.g., digoxin [Lanoxin] and beta blockers) will blunt compensatory reactions to shock by inhibiting the normal tachycardic response.[5] As a result of the geriatric patient's dependence on preload, even minor hypovolemia can produce significant compromises in cardiac function.[4] The senescent myocardium is less sensitive to both endogenous and exogenous catecholamines, restricting its ability to mount a normal, compensatory tachycardic response to hypovolemia.[109]

Fluid administration in hypovolemic and distributive shock states must be judiciously monitored to provide adequate volume replacement while preventing overload. Nonetheless, under-resuscitation must be strictly avoided because CO in the aging heart is highly dependent on adequate preload. Hypovolemia will worsen diastolic dysfunction, decrease renal and coronary perfusion, and impair tissue oxygen delivery, leading to myocardial ischemia and wound-healing failures.[49] In the injured elderly, shock represents the primary cause of death.[74] Therefore an aggressive approach to resuscitation of the older patient in traumatic shock has been recommended, and pulmonary artery catheters are frequently used to guide fluid resuscitation.[49,74] Once the geriatric patient has been fluid resuscitated, the need for high doses of vasopressors to achieve adequate BP must be weighed against the increased myocardial workload these agents produce.

Because seniors are poorly able to raise CO to meet oxygen demands, consider early transfusion rather than the infusion of large volumes of crystalloids or colloids to the patient in hypovolemic shock. Many elders are at increased risk for bleeding because of the use of warfarin (Coumadin), aspirin, ibuprofen (Advil), and other anticlotting agents. Administration of packed red blood cells promotes oxygen-carrying capacity without fluid overload. The practice of limiting transfusion volume, even in the severely injured elderly, is currently unjustified.[19] Whenever possible, all blood products should be warmed before transfusion. Vasopressors should be used cautiously and only after adequate volume has been restored. When large-volume resuscitation is necessary (e.g., sepsis, hemorrhage), subsequent fluid mobilization may take up to four times as long as it does in younger patients.[87]

Cardiac Arrest. Complications resulting from cardiopulmonary resuscitation increase with age. Even when chest compressions are performed correctly, rib fractures can result. Less frequent complications include sternal fractures, pneumothorax, hemothorax, pulmonary contusions, lacerations of the liver and spleen, and separation of the ribs from the sternum.[45] Each of these conditions is poorly tolerated in the geriatric patient.[60]

RESPIRATORY SYSTEM

As the result of both chest wall and lung changes, a gradual decline in respiratory function accompanies aging. The normal respiratory rate in older adults is 20 to 22 breaths per minute. Typically, these modifications occur progressively as age advances; they should not alter an elderly person's ability to breathe effortlessly.[23] Nonetheless, factors such as frequent exposure to environmental pollutants (particularly cigarette smoke) and recurrent pulmonary infections will accelerate age-related changes, making it difficult to distinguish expected alterations in pulmonary function from disease states.[23] Even when the patient presents with a nonrespiratory condition, careful assessment and management of respiratory status are essential. For example, elderly postsurgical patients have up to a 40% incidence of respiratory complications, depending on the site of surgery.[5]

Age-Related Changes

Decreased Lung Compliance. Physiologic changes in the senescent lungs lead to diminished elastic recoil as a result of an increase in the ratio of elastin to collagen in the interlobular septa and pleura.[23] This loss of lung elasticity reduces pulmonary compliance, which leads to small airway collapse, uneven alveolar ventilation, and air trapping. Collapse of the small airways during forced expiration affects dynamic lung volumes and limits flow rates. These anatomic changes are reflected by an increase in residual volume and a decline in forced expiratory volume.[23]

Ventilation/Perfusion Imbalance. Age-associated changes in the morphology of the alveolar parenchyma are related to a reduction in the alveolar surface area available for gas exchange.[94] This produces an increase in the amount of physiologic dead space and leads to a ventilation/perfusion mismatch, which in turn causes a decline in the partial pressure of arterial oxygen tension (Pa_{O_2}).[94] The expected reduction in Pa_{O_2} accompanying aging may be roughly estimated using the following equation:[39]

$$100 \text{ mm Hg} - 0.3 \times \text{the number of years of age over 25}$$

Age alone does not affect ventilation. The partial pressure of carbon dioxide (Pa_{CO_2}) in healthy elders remains unchanged despite the increase in dead space.[94] However, because many older patients suffer from pulmonary disorders that reduce carbon dioxide elimination (e.g., chronic obstructive pulmonary disease), elevated Pa_{CO_2} levels are not an uncommon finding in the geriatric population.[94]

Thoracic Changes. With advancing age, the chest wall and vertebrae (thoracic skeleton) undergo progressive osteoporotic changes and vertebral collapse, producing kyphosis. Contractures of the intercostal muscles and calcification of the costal cartilage result in a decline in rib mobility and reduced chest wall compliance. The functional effect of these transformations is a decrease in thoracic wall excursion.[23] Progressive loss of strength in the respiratory muscles is accompanied by a decline in maximum inspiratory and expiratory force by as much as 50%.[87]

Decreased Efficacy of Ventilatory Exchange. Starting at about 40 years of age, there is a gradual and linear decrease in the efficacy of ventilatory exchange. Changes include a reduction in the number of functional alveoli and pulmonary capillaries, an increase in atelectasis and fibrosis, and enlargement of the alveolar ducts.[48] Capillary blood volume and surface area also decline with advancing age.[23] In addition to remodeling of the small airways, anatomic alterations occur in the large airways as well. The cartilage of the trachea and bronchi becomes stiffer and less compliant. Bronchial enlargement then displaces inhaled air away from the alveoli that line the alveolar ducts, limiting the area available for gas exchange.[23] These modifications combine to diminish diffusion capacity, which is a function of both surface area and capillary blood volume.[23] A summary of age-associated changes in respiratory parameters is given in Table 49-1.

Decreased Ventilatory Response to Hypoxia and Hypercarbia. The control of ventilation is also affected by senescence. Geriatric patients have a diminished response to hypoxia and hypercarbia because chemoreceptor sensitivity is decreased.[48] Therefore ventilatory responses to hypoxemia and hypercapnia fall by 50% and 40%, respectively. The exact mechanism of this decline has not been well defined, but it may be the result of reduced chemoreceptor function either at the peripheral or at the central nervous system level.[13] Importantly, respiratory center sensitivity to narcotics increases with advancing age.[48]

Increased Susceptibility to Atelectasis and Infection. A number of age-related changes diminish the geriatric patient's respiratory defense mechanisms and increase susceptibility to atelectasis and pulmonary infections. Because of atrophy of the epithelial lining, mucociliary clearance is reduced and it becomes progressively more difficult to clear bacteria from the bronchi. Even the mucus itself changes. The submucosal glands decrease mucus production, causing dryness and thickening of secretions.[23] Impaired mucociliary clearance and thickened secretions promote chronic gram-negative colonization of the upper airways, predisposing patients to pneumonia. Elderly individuals with impaired cough and swallowing mechanisms are at heightened risk for pneumonia secondary to

TABLE 49-1 Age-Associated Changes in Respiratory Parameters for the Critically Ill Elderly Patient

PARAMETER	CHANGE
Chest wall compliance	Decreased
Forced vital capacity	Decreased
Forced expiratory volume	Decreased
Functional residual capacity	Mildly increased
Maximum expiratory force	Decreased
Maximum inspiratory force	Decreased
P_{AO_2}	No change
Pa_{O_2}	Decreased
P_{CO_2}	No change
Residual volume	Increased
Total lung capacity	No change
Vital capacity	Decreased

aspiration.[58] In addition, older adults experience alterations in the ability of the respiratory system to protect against pathogens. As an accompaniment of normal aging, cough strength decreases and there is a progressive reduction in T-cell function and decreased IgA production, which unite to increase susceptibility to viral and bacterial infections.[94]

Common Problems and Management Strategies

Acute Lung Injury and Acute Respiratory Distress Syndrome. The incidence of acute lung injury and acute respiratory distress syndrome (ALI/ARDS) increases with age.[115] However, most ALI/ARDS trials in the United States have reported relatively younger average patient ages. In the geriatric population, the combination of decreased chest wall elasticity, increased chest wall rigidity, impaired respiratory defense mechanisms, and weaker respiratory muscles all promote the need for respiratory interventions. Mechanical ventilation and prolonged ventilatory support are both associated with increased morbidity and mortality in older adults.[94] These differences between elderly and younger ALI/ARDS patients have not been thoroughly addressed in clinical trials. Ely and colleagues[24] evaluated the important questions of how age affects survival from ALI, and whether there is delayed physiologic recovery in seniors, and found that a patient age of 70 years or older was a strong predictor of in-hospital death.[24]

Pneumonia. The incidence of pneumonia is almost six times greater in those over age 75 than it is in persons under 60.[72] Elderly nursing home patients in particular have a substantially higher mortality rate than other individuals with community-associated pneumonia.[72] A diminished cough reflex, fewer cilia, a decline in surfactant production, a decrease in immune system effectiveness, and an increased frequency of oropharyngeal colonization with gram-negative organisms all place the geriatric patient at risk for the development of pneumonia.[61]

Most pneumonias in older adults result from microaspiration. Seniors, particularly those with impaired airway protection or a gastrointestinal condition that predisposes them to reflux, can aspirate large volumes of bacteria.[72] The high incidence of pneumonia among elderly inhabitants of long-term care facilities is largely related to the prevalence of dysphagia.[72] Pneumonia is also strongly associated with nutritional status because of the relationship between protein adequacy and immune system function. One landmark study found that only 16% of geriatric patients with pneumonia were considered well nourished, while 47% had a kwashiorkor-like malnutrition.[82]

In general, pneumonia symptoms in seniors are less prominent than in adults under 65 years old. The elderly are prone to atypical pneumonia presentations characterized by subacute illness and nonrespiratory symptoms (e.g., headache and diarrhea). Cough, the most common finding in about 80% of all pneumonia patients,[72] is less prominent in the elderly, especially nursing home residents and those with serious comorbidities. Other atypical pneumonia symptoms include falling, failure to thrive, altered functional capacity, and deterioration of existing illnesses. Delirium and acute confusion frequently signal pneumonia in older adults.[72] Individuals over the age of 80 years are less likely to present with pleuritic chest pain, headache, or myalgias than are younger patients, but are more likely to exhibit altered mental status. The absence of clear-cut respiratory symptoms, the lack of fever, and the presence of pleuritic chest pain are all related to an increased risk of death from pneumonia.[72]

Chest Trauma. As a result of progressive osteoporosis and reduced chest wall compliance, older trauma patients are more likely to have rib fractures—or even a flail segment—than are young adults. Rib fractures and chest wall contusions are intensely painful and lead to splinting and hypoventilation. This is especially detrimental to the geriatric patient with little respiratory reserve. Incentive spirometry, early mobilization, and keeping the head of the bed elevated at least 30 degrees are all well-established methods of reducing post–chest trauma respiratory complications.[49]

Prompt and adequate pain relief is essential for promoting pulmonary health in the elderly patient with thoracic compromise. Inadequate pain control increases the work of breathing, elevates oxygen demand, and can easily progress to respiratory failure in seniors. Epidural catheters are particularly effective for controlling rib fracture and thoracotomy pain without heavy sedation, while simultaneously decreasing the incidence of pulmonary complications. For geriatric patients, an epidural infusion of opioids combined with a local anesthetic agent is an excellent method of pain control, providing excellent analgesia with minimum sedation.[48] To be most effective, epidural analgesia should be initiated early in the course of care. Unfortunately, because of degenerative changes, the elderly spinal canal may not be easy to cannulate.

Mechanical Ventilation. Obtaining and maintaining a definitive airway is essential in the older patient with respiratory failure. Because even mild hypoxia can initiate a downward spiral in seniors, it is best to err on the side of early ventilatory support. Evaluation of the need for preintubation removal of dental appliances in the mechanically ventilated geriatric patient is essential. Although many retrospective and a few prospective studies have reported that age is an independent predictor of outcome following mechanical ventilation, other research counters this finding.[28] Persons older than 70 years are especially susceptible to long-term ventilator dependence.[55] Elderly chronic obstructive pulmonary disease patients in respiratory failure have poor outcomes. However, these outcomes appear to be more related to the disease process itself than to the patient's age per se.[93]

Successful weaning from mechanical ventilation does not appear to be directly correlated with age, but age-related changes clearly impact the respiratory fitness of a particular patient and contribute to weaning failure.[94] Few studies have specifically addressed the role of monitoring weaning parameters or other common ventilatory issues (e.g., timing of tracheostomy in the elderly population).[27] The benefits of several new and heavily promoted devices for the prevention of ventilator-associated pneumonias (e.g., subglottic suction or silver-coated endotracheal tubes) have not been well established in the elderly population.

NEUROLOGIC SYSTEM

The nervous system regulates cognitive, behavioral, motor, sensory, and homeostatic functions throughout the body. Age-related physiologic changes to the nervous system are complex and far-reaching. Sensory perception declines steadily with normal aging; the incidence of neurologic disorders increases with every decade of life.[105]

Age-Related Changes

Brain Atrophy. Between the ages of 40 and 70 years, a 10% reduction in brain size occurs as a result of the progressive, scattered loss of approximately 20% of cerebral cortex neurons.[91] As brain weight decreases, cerebral blood flow is concomitantly reduced. Neuronal loss is accelerated by Alzheimer's disease and alcoholism.[106] As the brain loses neurons, the number of neuroglial cells increases. Neuronal loss is associated with slowed impulse conduction through nerves, along nerve fibers, and across synapses.[106] This diminishes the body's ability to deal with multiple stimuli, respond to information, and recover from stressors.

Cognitive Decline. Intellectual functioning normally peaks at age 20 to 30 years and then plateaus until the mid-80s, at which time function starts to decline.[23] Cognitive dysfunction in the elderly postsurgical patient has been shown to persist for up to 3 months in a significant percentage of elderly patients.[87] Cognitive decline is accompanied by a modest loss of short-term memory and reduced sensory and perceptual acuity.[65,106] Sleep disturbances include longer time to fall asleep, less time spent in rapid eye movement sleep, and alterations in sleep patterns such as daytime sleeping.[35] Additional neurologic changes include impaired judgment, poor memory, and a reduced ability to process new information.[105]

Vascular Disease. The development of age-associated atherosclerotic disease is not limited to the heart. Vessels in the brain are similarly affected, and the incidence of stroke jumps markedly with age. In addition to ischemic strokes, seniors are also at increased risk for hemorrhagic stroke. There is a rising incidence of intracranial aneurysms associated with advancing age and the female gender. Although not as strongly suggestive as genetics and heredity, risk factors acquired over a lifetime are the most important etiologies of intracranial aneurysms and subarachnoid hemorrhage (SAH). Hypertension, smoking, traumatic brain injury, and sepsis are among the acquired factors that contribute to the intracranial aneurysm formation and subsequent SAH in elderly individuals.[76]

Peripheral Nerve and Metabolic Changes. An age-related decline in peripheral nerve function—associated with thickening of the leptomeninges in the spinal cord—reduces the body's ability to maintain homeostasis efficiently.[80] In addition, the elderly blood-brain barrier becomes more permeable, leading to increased sensitivity to many medications.[105]

Sensory Decline

Hearing. Elderly persons lose auditory acuity for a variety of reasons. Normal senescence is accompanied by anatomic and functional changes in the auditory and vestibular apparatus, causing decreased sensitivity to sound and altered frequency discrimination. Changes include loss of auditory neurons, angiosclerosis of the ear, and degeneration of neural receptors in the cochlea, eighth cranial nerve, and the central nervous system. These alterations produce both loss of hearing (from high to low frequencies) and difficulty hearing, especially in the presence of background noise or when speech is rapid or involves consonants. Presbycusis, a sensorineural hearing loss, is the most common cause of hearing loss in older adults. This condition is characterized by a gradual, progressive, bilateral, symmetrical high-frequency, perceptive hearing loss associated with poor speech discrimination.[65] In addition, cerumen production increases with age, and impaction may cause conductive hearing loss. Older patients should be evaluated for cerumen impaction and have it removed as necessary. Hearing loss leads to social isolation, but elderly patients may not have adequate resources to obtain auditory aids.[23,74,80]

Vision. With aging, many transformations occur in the eye and the central visual pathways. Anatomic changes include decreased rod and cone function and pigment accumulation. The ciliary muscles atrophy and the iris loses its ability to accommodate rapidly to light and dark.[65] The elderly lens yellows, increases in size, and becomes less flexible. Pupils decrease in size and become less responsive to light as a result of pupil sphincter hardening. Intraocular pressure in the senescent eye rises, and there is a drop in tear production associated with eye dryness and irritation.[65]

These anatomic changes limit visual acuity, depth perception, peripheral vision, tolerance to glare, and speed of eye movements. Impaired light/dark adaptation and other age-related effects heighten an older person's need for ambient light and reduce the geriatric patient's ability to differentiate blues, greens, and violets.[65] Elevated intraocular pressure and lens inflexibility combine to increase the prevalence of glaucoma in seniors. In addition, the high incidence of macular degeneration, retinal tears, cataracts, and diabetic retinopathy in the elderly all contribute to visual impairment.[65]

Strategies for working with seniors with visual impairment include use of materials with large print, selection of contrasting colors for printed material, assurance of adequate glare-free lighting, and facing the patient directly when speaking. Touch and visual cues can also be used to facilitate communication.[23,74,80]

Smell and Taste. There is a reduction in the number of olfactory and gustatory nerve fibers accompanying normal aging. This limits one's ability to perceive and discriminate both pleasant and noxious odors and flavors. Decreased taste perception is associated with a declining food intake in the elderly. In addition to smell and taste, hunger and thirst are affected by age—both at the end-organ level and in the hypothalamus. Seniors develop an increased threshold for certain flavors such as salt. The satiety center in the hypothalamus can become hypersensitive, leading to anorexia, while the hypothalamically mediated thirst response to hyperosmolarity is reduced, making the elderly less sensitive to their need for water.[80]

Touch and Balance. Two-point discrimination and both tactile and vibratory sensation all diminish with aging. Proprioception, balance, and postural control likewise decline. Elderly persons experience changes in coordination, an altered "righting" reflex, and difficulty with balance. Together these transformations—in conjunction with distorted depth perception and musculoskeletal deterioration—make the older individual less able to respond to environmental changes and more susceptible to falls, particularly in unfamiliar surroundings (e.g., critical care).[105]

Pain. The sensory changes of aging can reduce an elder's ability to perceive, respond to, or express pain, yet pain is one of the most pervasive and undertreated problems of senescence.[111] Pain in the elderly, both acute and chronic, is associated with depression, decreased socialization, poor nutrition, sleep disturbances, impaired mobility, and increased healthcare costs.[111] Pain assessment in seniors can be challenging, particularly in those who are cognitively impaired. Pain is frequently expressed nonverbally as facial grimacing, guarding, or restlessness. Other common geriatric pain manifestations are psychobehavioral and include withdrawal, irritability, anxiety, crying, or fearfulness.[6]

Age-associated respiratory, neurologic, and gastrointestinal changes complicate pain management in the elderly. Seniors who are opiate naïve, and those with neuromuscular or pulmonary disease, are very sensitive to the side effects of narcotic analgesics[48] (i.e., respiratory depression, altered mental status, weakness, and constipation). See Chapter 4 for in-depth information on pain management techniques.

Common Problems and Management Strategies

Stroke and Transient Ischemic Attack. Stroke is one of the leading health problems in the United States today, with 600,000 new or recurrent cerebral ischemic events occurring annually.[75] Three important factors characterize stroke in the elderly. First, the incidence of stroke is highest in this age group. Seventy-five percent of all "brain attacks" occur in persons age 65 years and older.[1] In fact, age is the single most important risk factor for stroke and reversible ischemic neurologic deficits.[60] Second, the risk factors contributing to stroke continue to increase with age; stroke is now the third most common cause of death among Americans.[89] As a consequence of population aging, the stroke death rate in the United States has been increasing despite advances in care.[75] African Americans have a 38% higher adjusted incidence of ischemic stroke than do Caucasians and suffer greater stroke mortality.[75]

The third reason stroke is a major public health problem in older individuals is that the ongoing burden of this disease is huge. In the United States, stroke has become the principal cause of long-term disability, primarily in the elderly population.[75] There are approximately 4.5 million stroke survivors alive today, most of them over the age of 65. The economic toll of stroke is estimated at $43 billion each year in the United States.[29]

Stroke is a broad category of neurologic deficits with many etiologies. There are several vascular mechanisms that lead to stroke, including large-artery atherosclerosis with occlusion, distal embolization, aneurysm rupture, and small penetrating arterial disease with lacunar infarction. The incidence of each of these conditions increases with advancing age. Approximately 85% of all strokes are ischemic, and almost 60% are attributable to atherothrombotic disease. The location of this disease can be anywhere in the vasculature from the carotid arteries to the small vessels of the brain. Although the smaller vessels are the most common site, extracranial arterial occlusion from carotid atherosclerosis accounts for about 20% of all strokes in geriatric patients.[75] Cardiac dysrhythmias, primarily atrial fibrillation, may be either the cause or the consequence of a stroke.[60]

Dysphagia. Each year, approximately 500,000 Americans are affected by dysphagia resulting from neurologic disorders.[72] Many elderly individuals with ischemic or degenerative diseases of the central nervous system—Alzheimer's disease, amyotrophic lateral sclerosis, Parkinson's disease, multiple sclerosis, and stroke—will develop dysphagia. Dysphagia generally occurs early in the course of the disease; its severity does not necessarily correlate with the overall severity of the neurologic condition. Aspiration pneumonia is a major cause of death in these patients.[72] Considering the prevalence of cerebrovascular and degenerative neurologic diseases in nursing home dwellers, it is not surprising that dysphagia has been reported to occur in 50% to 75% of this population.[58] This fact explains the extremely high incidence of pneumonia among residents of long-term care facilities.[58]

Head Trauma. Atrophic changes in the aging brain increase the amount of intracranial dead space. As a result, the distance between the skull and the brain surface increases and the bridging veins between the brain and dura mater are stretched, making them prone to tear and bleed. These anatomic transformations place older patients at a significantly increased risk for acute, chronic, and subacute subdural hematoma formation following even minor traumatic injury.[25] Unfortunately, significant cerebral atrophy can mask signs of an expanding hematoma in the elderly; there may be substantial intracranial hemorrhage before definitive neurologic symptoms are present.[18] Subtle changes in level of consciousness, an early indicator of intracranial hemorrhage, may be difficult to detect, particularly in persons with dementia.[54] In the geriatric trauma patient, computed tomographic brain scans should be used liberally to assess any patient with a potential head injury.[47]

Spinal Cord Injury. Although seniors may sustain a variety of spinal cord injuries, one type of cord trauma is more prevalent in the geriatric age-group than in other populations.[30] Central cord syndrome, an incomplete injury, is uncommon in younger individuals and usually occurs in older trauma patients with preexisting cervical spinal stenosis or spondylosis. The elderly most often develop central cord syndrome following a forward fall. This mechanism causes cervical hyperextension. Neurologic dysfunction is secondary to ischemia in the central portion of the spinal cord, particularly near the distribution of the anterior spinal artery. Patients with central cord syndrome generally retain lower extremity motor and sensory function with deficits noted in the upper extremities.[25,90]

As is true in younger persons, the spine of the geriatric trauma patient must be stabilized with a rigid cervical collar, rigid backboard, and a head immobilization device until the patient is clinically or radiographically cleared.[25] However, because of kyphosis, elderly individuals are frequently difficult to stabilize effectively.[49] Adequate padding to reduce discomfort and removal of all immobilization devices as soon as possible to minimize skin breakdown and other complications of immobility should be encouraged.[5] Magnetic resonance imaging scans may be required to evaluate compression of the spinal cord and detect injury to the stabilizing ligaments.

Dementia and Delirium. The person with dementia has a preexisting or baseline cognitive impairment (e.g., Alzheimer's disease). Although rarely the admitting diagnosis for a critically ill patient, dementia is a common comorbidity in the hospitalized elderly. In fact, the dementia rate in older Americans doubles with every 5-year increase in age—from 1.5% in those ages 65 to 70, to nearly 25% in people over the age of 85.[87] Because dementia is part of a patient's baseline status, interventions focus on symptom management and not on cure.

In contrast, the patient with delirium has a transient organic mental syndrome characterized by a cognition disorder, global attention deficits, a reduced level of consciousness, abnormal psychomotor activity patterns, and disturbed sleep-wake cycles. Delirium adversely affects mental processing, perception, thinking, memory, and, frequently, behavior.[105] Despite its behavioral manifestations, the root cause of delirium is not psychiatric. Any condition that affects brain function can potentially lead to delirium.[57,67]

Up to one half of persons over the age of 65 admitted to critical care will develop some kind of delirium during their hospitalization.[57] Risk factors for delirium include advanced age, preexisting cognitive impairment, poor functional status, hemodynamic or respiratory instability, ethanol abuse, sensory overload, metabolic imbalances, pain, anxiety, alterations in the sleep-wake cycle, malnutrition, bladder catheterization, sleep deprivation, polypharmacy, and the use of physical restraints. Delirium may also be the first manifestation of a previously unrecognized disease. However, the number one risk factor for delirium is baseline dementia.[5,57,115]

Regrettably, in the critically ill older adult, the behavioral disturbances of delirium are all too often dismissed as critical care psychosis and the patient is treated with sedatives and antipsychotic medications. In older individuals, the likelihood of medication-induced delirium is high. Analgesics can alter cognitive function, especially when used in combination with many other substances. Nevertheless, withholding medications—particularly undertreating pain—can also cause delirium.[57]

Appropriate assessment and intervention are essential for a positive outcome in the patient with delirium. In the acutely agitated or aggressive patient with hyperactive delirium, medicines such as haloperidol (Haldol) can sedate and rest the patient.[51] The primary treatment goal, however, involves identifying and removing the underlying causes of delirium. For mild agitation, interventions include decreasing environmental stimuli (lights and noise) and clustering care. Friends or volunteers can help reorient, mobilize, and feed the patient. Clocks, calendars, family photos, glasses, and hearing aids are also means of assisting orientation.[57,115] The hypoactive form of delirium is the most common type of delirium in the elderly; it is difficult to recognize and is associated with poor outcomes. This condition is manifested by a quiet state of withdrawal, apathy, and decreased arousal.[67]

Evidence-Based Care of the Critically Ill Elderly Patient

R.S., a 92-year-old retired accountant, cannot recall what happened, but his neighbor found him lying unconscious on the kitchen floor. On hospital arrival, R.S.'s respirations are regular and unlabored, his oxygen saturation is normal, he denies chest pain, and there are no obvious signs of a head injury. R.S.'s chief complaint is severe pain in his obviously deformed right upper arm. R.S. states that he has had mild diarrhea for the past 2 days. A brief neurologic exam reveals no gross focal or cognitive deficits. R.S. is in sinus rhythm at a rate of 47 beats/min, with frequent premature ventricular beats and a BP of 96/45 mm Hg.

When R.S. reaches critical care, he is alert and cooperative but in a lot of pain from his upper arm injury. R.S. has a history of atrial fibrillation, treated with digoxin and warfarin. R.S. has also been taking metoprolol (Lopressor) since his myocardial infarction 3 years ago. In addition, R.S. suffers from gout and osteoarthritis of the knees. A 12-lead ECG is obtained. It indicates an old anterolateral wall infarction, but no acute changes are noted. Basic laboratory studies, including a troponin level, are all within normal limits.

A 2-L infusion of normal saline brings R.S.'s BP up to 127/52 mm Hg and his HR is now 86 beats/min. The physician orders a computed tomographic scan of R.S.'s head and plain radiographs of his right arm and cervical spine. During the imaging procedure, while still strapped to a long backboard, R.S. begins to vomit. He is turned onto his left side and his secretions are suctioned. However, since the vomiting event, R.S. has had a persistent cough. R.S. receives 5 mg of IV morphine sulfate and obtains some relief from his humeral fracture pain. Thirty minutes later, his nurse notes that R.S.'s room air saturation level has dropped to 87%. He is started on 3 L of oxygen by nasal prongs.

Decision point: What are likely etiologies of R.S.'s initial episode of loss of consciousness?

Decision point: What impact will routine beta-blocker use have on R.S.'s physiologic response to his injury and hospitalization?

Decision point: What factors might be responsible for R.S.'s dwindling oxygen saturation?

Case continues on page 1391

MUSCULOSKELETAL SYSTEM

Normal senescence is accompanied by a number of important changes to the musculoskeletal system. An overall decrease in muscle mass, strength, and agility leads to alterations in gait (wide-based, shorter steps) and posture (flexed forward).[80] These alterations, in combination with loss of bone mass, put older persons at risk for musculoskeletal injury, particularly those with sedentary lifestyles.

Age-Related Changes

Muscular Changes. As the body ages, there is a concomitant decline in the total amount of body water and an increase in the percentage of body fat.[48] Changes in growth hormone metabolism have been implicated in muscle mass decline, as have alterations in androgen secretion.[87] Not only is muscle mass diminished, but the remaining myocytes lose functional capacity because of a reduction in myosin adenosine triphosphate (ATP) activity in the cells.[80] This diminishes the muscle cells' ability to extract and utilize oxygen, which increases fatigue. These changes serve to reduce overall muscle strength.[5]

Skeletal Changes

Osteoporosis. The high incidence of osteoporosis in the geriatric population leads to a rate of fractures greater than in any other age-group. Osteoporosis occurs as a result of decreased osteoblastic activity, which reduces production of new bone cells.[80] The resultant loss of mass is associated with bone fragility and predisposes the older adult to bony fractures following even minor trauma. Much attention has been given to osteoporosis in women, but both elderly men and women have brittle skeletons.[25] With decreased bone density there is a loss of total body height, attributable in large part to a decrease in the height of the vertebral bodies. Other degenerative changes to the cervical spine include narrowing of the cervical canal secondary to osteophytes (bony spurs).[107]

Osteoarthritis. Osteoarthritis, previously known as degenerative joint disease, is the most common form of arthritis. This condition, a common accompaniment of senescence, causes chronic joint pain. Osteoarthritis is a leading cause of disability in the United States.[14] Nearly 70 million Americans, or one of every three adults, suffer from chronic joint symptoms.[14] However, the risk of developing osteoarthritis increases substantially with age, becoming especially prevalent in individuals over 60 years old.[14] Elderly women are disproportionately affected by osteoarthritis, but this condition also affects many older men.[12]

Osteoarthritis is a disease of both weight-bearing and non–weight-bearing joints. Damage is caused by mechanical stresses that injure areas of articular cartilage and subchondral bone. Biochemical changes in the joint surface, the synovium, and synovial fluid play a role in osteoarthritis etiology as well. Symptoms include joint pain, morning stiffness lasting less than 30 minutes, and loss of function.[12]

Connective Tissue Changes. The amount of connective tissue and collagen continues to increase with age. This is most prominently manifested by a nose and ears that continue to grow in size. These transformations are largely cosmetic and have few functional implications. Other changes, such as deterioration and drying of the joints and cartilage, have clinical ramifications, producing joint pain and stiffness.[80]

Common Problems and Management Strategies

Fractures. Although it is unclear whether the incidence of fractures is a surrogate for preexisting fragility in the elderly or the actual cause of decline, several studies of isolated fractures in older individuals have documented serious outcomes subsequent to even "minor" injuries. Following isolated hip fracture, Irwin[46] noted a 60-day mortality of 9.7%; one third of Rose and Maffulli's hip fracture patients were not alive 1 year post-injury.[86] Even an isolated distal radius fracture in an geriatric patient is associated with a significantly decreased life span. Rozenthal and colleagues found that the cumulative estimated survival at 7 years in their cohort of 325 older radial fracture patients was only 57% compared to the expected value of 71% for the U.S. population.[88]

The rate of hip fractures increases with advancing years. The most common mechanism of injury in geriatric patients is falling. However, evidence suggests that some individuals have such osteoporotic hips that a spontaneous fracture actually precedes the fall.[25] Cervical spine fractures in seniors tend to involve more than one level, commonly occur at C1-C2, and are frequently unstable.[47] As with hip fractures, the leading cause of pelvic fractures in the elderly is falls. Following pelvic fracture, older patients suffer mortality rates three to five times greater than their under-55-year-old counterparts. Bone healing time is prolonged in the geriatric patient. Patient interventions (e.g., physical therapy, range-of-motion exercises, occupational therapy) focus on facilitating mobility and restoring function, while simultaneously preventing complications of immobility (e.g., thromboembolic disease and pressure ulcers).[5]

INTEGUMENTARY SYSTEM

Assessment of the elderly person's skin (i.e., presence of peripheral vascular disease, edema, deformities, lesions, discoloration, wounds, scars, medical devices) can provide a large amount of information about the patient's medical history, surgical history, and current health status. Because of decreased skin elasticity, the common practice of using skin turgor as a measure of hydration status may be inaccurate in the elderly.[56]

Age-Related Changes

Decreased Protective Functions. Aging is associated with decreased effectiveness of several of the skin's protective functions. Subcutaneous fat is lost, particularly the fatty pads that protect bony prominences. Both the dermis and the epidermis thin, making delicate, aging skin susceptible to tears.[74] Changes also occur in the structure of interstitial tissues, which predispose to soft tissue injury.[87] Loss of skin moisture, decreased elasticity, diminished tensile strength, and reduced turgor all lead to wrinkling and skin laxity.[23] Both dryness and pruritus are common dermal complaints in older individuals and may lead to scratching.[80] The number of nerve cells in the skin also declines with advancing age, making the elderly less aware of dermal injury or ischemia. These senescent changes are accompanied by a reduction in the number melanocytes, which heightens seniors' need for sun protection.[80]

Delayed Wound Healing. All aspects of wound healing appear to be influenced by senescence. Responses in both the inflammatory and the proliferative wound healing phases are decreased. Angiogenesis, epithelialization, and wound remodeling are all delayed. Fibroblast proliferation and collagen synthesis also diminish with aging.[98] Furthermore, the high frequency of routine aspirin or ibuprofen use in the older population, combined with capillary fragility, contributes to wound bleeding tendencies and ecchymosis. Once the body's protective layers are breached, external barriers to bacterial invasion are removed, promoting wound infection. This is aggravated by the immune system alterations that accompany aging, which limit the older adult's ability to mount an adequate response to infection.[5,49] Nutritional deficits, particularly vitamins A and C and trace minerals (e.g., zinc), adversely affect the enzyme systems necessary for wound healing.[87]

Common Problems and Management Strategies

Pressure Ulcers. In the geriatric patient, atrophic changes in the skin and a limited capacity to heal contribute to the high incidence of pressure ulcer formation.[35] Skin breakdown in the elderly can be initiated by a variety of factors including sensory or motor loss, bed rest, reduced vasomotor tone, hypovolemia, poor nutrition, and age-related changes in skin composition.[98] Pressure ulcers may develop virtually anywhere on a patient's body, but are most common over the bony prominences of the sacrum, heels, ischium, elbows, occiput, and pinna.[98] Importantly, rigid backboards must be used only as extrication and stabilization devices. Older individuals should be removed from spine boards as soon as possible. Pressure ulcers can form rapidly in immobilized seniors; tissue ischemia has been reported to occur within 20 to 30 minutes of rigid immobilization.[25,44]

The elderly require exceptional skin care, and skin integrity must be monitored frequently for signs of impairment. Strategies to prevent skin damage in the critically ill older adult include gentle handling of the patient, avoidance of shearing forces, padding of bony prominences with additional layers, and frequent repositioning.[25] Use of a nonalcoholic, nondrying cleanser to keep the skin clean may be helpful. Skin moisturizers and protective lotions should be applied liberally, and bony prominence contact with beds and chairs should be minimized. For geriatric patients at high risk—and those with signs of skin disruption—the use of special air or rotating beds might be considered. The number of products and treatment options currently available for pressure ulcer care is staggering.[35] Consultation with a wound and ostomy nurse for help with selecting the most appropriate interventions is often beneficial.

Burns. Elderly individuals are at increased risk for thermal injuries because many of the physical and cognitive changes of normal aging render seniors poorly equipped to respond to fires and smoke. Impaired thermal perception, diminished manual dexterity, slowed reaction time, limited vision, hearing loss, an attenuated sense of smell, and possible cognitive impairment all render the older person vulnerable to burns. Alcohol abuse, cigarette smoking, poverty, sedating medications, and altered sleep patterns also contribute to injury.[5,56]

Once burned, elderly patients are more adversely affected than are younger individuals with similar injuries.[56] Despite advances in burn care, postburn mortality in the geriatric population remains extremely high. For example, between the ages of 3 and young adulthood, the 50% mortality for a burn (the level at which half of all patients would die) is 80% of body surface area (BSA). After age 70, the 50% mortality drops dramatically to between 20% and 30% BSA.[5] All together, burns claim the lives of approximately 1200 to 1500 persons over the age of 65 each year in the United States.[25]

Variables influencing outcome following thermal injuries in the elderly include previous heath status, burn severity (i.e., location, depth, and extent), adequacy of resuscitation, and any post-injury complications.

Providing appropriate fluid resuscitation to the geriatric burn patient is especially challenging. Preexisting comorbid conditions—particularly cardiovascular or pulmonary disease—make fluid resuscitation problematic. Post-resuscitation, older burn patients are prone to pneumonia and sepsis, particularly those with inhalation injuries.[56] Burn wound care presents special challenges in the elderly, and complications of healing occur frequently in this population. Following even minor burns, wounds generally exhibit poor or delayed healing. Delayed healing, or failure to heal, affects not only partial-thickness wounds but also skin graft beds and split-thickness donor sites as well.[56]

URINARY SYSTEM

With increasing age, a substantial number of anatomic and physiologic changes occur that directly impact the urinary system. In addition, alterations to other systems (e.g., a decreased sense of thirst and changes in cardiovascular status) have an indirect effect on renal function.

Age-Related Changes

Voiding Pattern Changes. Several normal transformations of aging impact voiding in the elderly, including reduced bladder muscle tone, diminished bladder capacity, and a heightened sense of urgency.[35] In the aging bladder, increased collagen content limits distensibility and impairs emptying. In females, decreased circulating levels of estrogen and decreased tissue estrogen responsiveness cause urethral sphincter changes that predispose to urinary incontinence. In older males, prostate enlargement may impede urinary flow, impairing bladder emptying.[35] Together, these factors lead to urinary incontinence in approximately 10% to 15% of seniors living in the community and 50% of hospitalized elders.[35]

Nephron Loss. The total number of glomeruli decreases by 30% to 40% by the eighth decade of life.[80] Nephron loss is accompanied by a drop in the number of renal tubular cells. Glomerular sclerosis produces a gradual reduction in blood flow to the glomerular capillary tufts and the small vessel walls, resulting in atrophy of the afferent and efferent arterioles.[80] Sclerotic changes begin in the cortical regions of the kidneys and then progress toward the medullary portion. These processes eventually cause renal blood flow to decline by approximately 50%.[87] To compensate, the remaining functional nephrons hypertrophy. Nevertheless, by the age of 65 years, there is an overall reduction in renal mass of 20% to 40%. Over time, this nephron loss causes the geriatric patient's renal reserve to dwindle.[23] However, because of large renal reserves, the body's ability to maintain adequate fluid and acid-base homeostasis is not appreciably altered until the number of functioning nephrons falls below 10% to 20%.[99]

Decreased Glomerular Filtration Rate.
Glomerular filtration rate (GFR) declines with advancing age as a result of both nephron loss and reduced renal blood flow.[23] Total renal blood flow begins to drop after the fourth decade of life because of hyaline arteriosclerosis. By age 80, arteriolar hyalinization has reduced renal mass by about 20%.[23] With an ever-decreasing number of nephrons left to do the work of the kidney, there is a yearly decline in GFR of about 1 ml per minute that begins at around the age of 40.[38]

Altered Renal Clearance.
Serum creatinine levels do not undergo significant changes in older patients because of the normal decrease in lean body mass, which reduces overall creatinine production. Therefore a normal serum creatinine level does not necessarily mean normal kidneys; creatinine levels tend to overestimate renal function in the geriatric population. In the senescent kidney, the declining GFR is reflected by a slight drop in creatinine clearance (approximately 0.75 ml per minute per year in healthy older males). However, creatinine clearance remains a better indicator of renal function than does serum creatinine level.[116] The following formula can be used to estimate creatinine clearance in healthy older persons although it may be influenced by critical illness or medications that affect renal function.[91]

$$\text{Creatinine clearance} = \frac{(140 - \text{Age in years}) \times (\text{Weight in kilograms})}{72 \times (\text{Serum creatinine in mg/dl})}$$

Decreased Ability to Concentrate or Dilute Urine.
As renal tubular function declines with age, the kidneys' ability to conserve sodium and excrete hydrogen ions is diminished. This reduces the older adult's capacity to maintain fluid and acid-base balance. Seniors are prone to develop volume depletion (prerenal conditions) because the senescent kidney does not compensate for nonrenal sodium and water losses with the typical mechanisms of enhanced renal sodium retention, increased urinary concentration, and heightened thirst.[116] These changes occur secondary to renin-angiotensin system attenuation and decreased end-organ responsiveness to antidiuretic hormone (ADH).[116]

Dehydration in older individuals can be missed because of their limited ability to concentrate urine. In the aged, urine specific gravity will remain relatively low despite significant volume loss.[38] This finding makes urine specific gravity an unreliable indicator of volume status in elderly persons. As age increases, urine production over a 24-hour period becomes more constant (loss of diurnal variation). This reduces the kidneys' ability to conserve fluid volume on demand.[116] Conversely, volume overload can occur because of both a drop in GFR and functional impairment of the diluting segment of the nephron. This phenomenon is exacerbated in critically ill patients by the elevation in levels of ADH seen postoperatively and during other periods of physiologic stress.[100]

Common Problems and Management Strategies

Altered Drug Excretion.
Changes in renal status have important implications for the type and dosage of drugs used in the elderly. Although drugs are managed by the kidneys in a variety of ways, most alterations in renal drug processing correspond with the decline in GFR. Therefore creatinine clearance is a good marker of clearance for most agents processed by the kidneys; dosages can be adjusted accordingly.[116] Two classes of drugs commonly consumed by older individuals are nonsteroidal antiinflammatory agents and angiotensin-converting enzyme inhibitors. Both of these drugs have adverse effects on renal regulatory mechanisms.[38] Other nephrotoxic substances frequently prescribed to critically ill patients include iodinated contrast media and diuretics. Aminoglycosides (e.g., vancomycin and gentamicin) require careful monitoring of serum levels to avoid toxicity in the geriatric patient.[51,92]

Acute Renal Failure.
The incidence of chronic renal failure increases with age because of anatomic and physiologic changes to the kidneys associated with age and comorbidities. In the critically ill older adult, diminished baseline renal function, polypharmacy, and an elevated risk for nephrotoxicity combine to increase the incidence of acute renal failure (ARF) as well. However, geriatric patients may also exhibit atypical signs of uremia. Unexplained exacerbations of well-controlled heart failure and unexplained mental status or personality changes may be evidence of failing renal function.[38]

ARF in critically ill elders is often found in conjunction with sepsis. This disease combination carries a mortality rate of 65% to 80%.[115] Overall, outcomes for persons with ARF are not improving.[71] The likely explanation for this finding is we are now treating older and more difficult ARF cases. In a classic review of 1347 patients treated between 1956 and 1988, Rodgers and colleagues[84] demonstrated that the ARF population had become progressively older and sicker. Examining patients who had both sepsis and ARF, they compared two cohorts—one from the 1960s, the other from the 1980s. Over the 20-year period, average age rose from 51 to 63 years, the number of patients requiring mechanical ventilation climbed from 2% to 41%, and survival fell from 49% to 37%. Given this demographic shift in the ARF population, it is not surprising that outcome does not appear to be improving despite significant advances in healthcare in general.[115] See Chapter 33 for details on ARF and its treatment.

Urinary Tract Infections. Urinary tract infections (UTIs) are among the most common infections in older adults in the community, in long-term care facilities, and in critical care. With age, there is an increasing incidence of asymptomatic bacteriuria. UTIs in geriatric patients are usually asymptomatic. In older adults, the prevalence of asymptomatic bacteriuria (significant bacterial counts in the urine, without other symptoms) ranges from 15% to 30% in men and from 25% to 50% in women. Those living in long-term care facilities have the highest incidence of both asymptomatic bacteriuria and UTIs.[37]

UTIs are a major source of bacteremia and sepsis in the older adult, causing significant morbidity and mortality.[37,81] A discussion of the problem of sepsis in the elderly patient appears in the Research Utilization box below. Among the elderly, UTIs are responsible for 30% to 50% of all community-acquired bacteremias.[87] The presence of an indwelling urinary catheter dramatically increases the incidence of bacteriuria, pyuria, and symptomatic UTIs. Early discontinuation of indwelling catheters is recommended.[81]

GASTROINTESTINAL SYSTEM

Although gastrointestinal (GI) complaints are common in old age, in general GI function is well preserved in the healthy older adult. Importantly, some of the age-associated changes that affect GI function—such as loss of abdominal muscle strength, reduced appetite, and decreased fluid intake—actually take place in other body systems.[31]

Age-Related Changes

Supragastric Changes. With senescence, fibrosis and atrophy of the salivary glands decrease salivation, resulting in dry mouth.[104] There is a concomitant atrophy and loss of taste buds, dulling the sense of taste, particularly altering the ability to distinguish sweet and salty foods. Bitter and sour tastes remain largely unchanged. In addition, esophageal emptying slows, increasing risk for esophageal spasm.[104]

Gastric Changes. Gastric acid secretion does not decrease as a result of normal aging, but there is a rising incidence of gastritis and GI bleeding, commonly caused by *Helicobacter pylori*. Delayed gastric emptying has been demonstrated in some studies of elderly subjects. Aspiration, secondary to unrecognized gastric atony, is not uncommon.[104]

Bowel Changes. Small-bowel motility and the absorption of most nutrients are unchanged with age. Only calcium absorption falls significantly; this is primarily

---

♦ RESEARCH UTILIZATION

Care of the Septic Elderly Patient

CLINICAL ISSUE

The incidence of severe sepsis skyrockets with aging. Care of the septic geriatric patient remains a major challenge in critical care.

SUMMARY

This research examined the epidemiology of severe sepsis. Although sepsis can occur throughout the life span, it is overwhelmingly a disease of older adults. The incidence of sepsis in children is only 0.2 per 1000, but this number increases more than 100-fold with age, soaring to 26.2 per 1000 in persons older than 85 years. Not only incidence but also mortality increases with aging. Only 10% of septic children will die, yet for 38.4% of those over the age of 85, sepsis will be their final diagnosis.

APPLICATION

Bacteremias can be seeded from any infected location, but the most common sites in geriatric patients are the pulmonary and urinary tracts. The focus is on critical care nurses, and other healthcare professionals, to reduce mortality by taking all possible measures to prevent sepsis in the vulnerable elderly population.

NEED FOR FURTHER STUDY

Much research remains to be done to determine optimum treatment of the septic geriatric patient (see Chapter 43). Simultaneously, the impact of nursing interventions (e.g., urinary catheter care, head-of-bed positioning, oral care, suctioning, weaning protocols) on sepsis prevention and treatment in older adults must also be better described.[3]

Angus, D. C., et al. (2001). Epidemiology of severe sepsis in the United States: analysis of incidence, outcome, and associated costs of care. *Crit Care Med, 29,* 1303–1310.

attributed to a decrease in renal production of 1,25-hydroxycholecalciferol and reduced intestinal calcium binding.[104] Iron and many drugs are absorbed more slowly or less effectively in older adults as a result of atrophy of the mucosal lining. In addition, the senescent gut stabilizes and absorbs cholesterol less efficiently. Decreased muscle tone in the bowel delays bowel emptying, putting seniors at risk for constipation, diverticular disease, and bacterial translocation (see Chapter 29). The etiology of constipation in the elderly is multifactorial; sedentary lifestyle, poor diet, dehydration, anorectal and colonic pathology, systemic illness, and medications can all contribute to abnormal bowel function.[104] A history of multiple abdominal surgeries, tumors, or adhesions increases the incidence of bowel obstruction in geriatric patients.

Hepatobiliary Changes. In association with advancing age, there is a reduction in the number of hepatocytes and overall liver size. However, there is a compensatory increase in cell size, cell sensitivity, and proliferation of the bile ducts.[104] Hepatic blood flow decreases by approximately 1% per year so that blood flow has dropped to almost half by age 85.[15,87] The most common hepatobiliary disorder in the elderly population is gallstones and gallstone-related complications. The prevalence of gallstones rises steadily with age, varying somewhat with the cohort studied. However, biliary stones have been documented in up to 80% of nursing home residents over the age of 90 years. Biliary tract disease is the most common indication for abdominal surgery in older adults.[87]

Although standard liver function tests remain unchanged in healthy seniors, metabolism of, and sensitivity to, certain substances is altered.[31] Metabolism of drugs requiring microsomal oxidation (phase I reactions) before conjugation (phase II reactions) slows, whereas substances requiring only conjugation will continue to be cleared at a normal rate. Drugs such as warfarin, which acts directly on the liver cells, will produce therapeutic effects at lower doses in the elderly because of increased hepatocyte sensitivity.[87] There is also a drop in the liver's first-pass extraction of some pharmacologic agents, including propranolol (Inderal) and verapamil (Calan), which reduces hepatic clearance of these substances.[80,114]

Common Problems and Management Strategies

Malnutrition. Malnutrition, a decrease in nutrient reserves, occurs in approximately 9% to 15% of community-dwelling elders, 12% to 50% of older patients in acute care hospitals, and 25% to 60% of seniors living in long-term care facilities.[31,87] There are countless reasons for malnutrition in the elderly, only some of which involve the GI system. A variety of social, cognitive, functional, and physiologic factors contribute to poor nutritional status in the geriatric population. These include limited financial or physical ability to obtain and prepare food, poor dentition, depression, alcohol abuse, anorexia, drug-nutrient interactions, and the loss of a spouse. Additionally, chronic medical conditions—such as congestive heart failure, diabetes, lung disease, and renal failure—make it difficult to keep ill seniors adequately fed and hydrated.[15] Gastroesophageal reflux disease, chronic diarrhea, and many medications also interfere with appetite or nutrient metabolism among this population.[31,87] Moreover, malabsorption secondary to bacterial overgrowth is found in a large percentage of older adults with nutritional deficits unexplained by dietary factors.[87] Measuring nutritional status in the geriatric patient can be difficult; criteria for the interpretation of biochemical markers in this age-group have not been well established. Unfortunately, standard anthropomorphic measurements do not take into account the body composition and structural alterations that accompany senescence.

Several simple measurements have been used to predict outcome related to nutritional deficits in critically ill elders, but they should be applied with caution. The simplest of these measures is body mass index (weight in kilograms divided by the height in meters, squared).[31] A body mass index less than $22 \, kg/m^2$ signals undernutrition. A body mass index less than $20 \, kg/m^2$ is considered an indicator of malnutrition and has been shown to predict mortality in community-dwelling older adults.[31]

Malnutrition places the elderly at heightened risk for morbidity and mortality. Protein-energy malnutrition, together with immobility, leads to deconditioning, and deconditioning involves changes to all major organ systems.[31] The incidence of poor wound healing, pneumonia, prolonged ventilatory support, and postoperative complications is increased in patients with nutritional deficits.[31] In fact, impaired nutritional status, present at the time of admission to critical care, has been shown to predict 6-month mortality in older individuals who require ventilatory support.[20] Despite reduced metabolic demands, normal GI changes associated with aging predispose the elderly to nutritional deficits by reducing the absorption of lipids, proteins, and carbohydrates. Serum albumin level is a strong predictor of outcome in critically ill geriatric patients. Low serum albumin levels (less than 3.3 mg/dl) in the elderly correlate with increased length of stay and an increased rate of all-cause mortality. In surgical patients, a low albumin level strongly correlates with postoperative outcomes, regardless of whether it is related to poor nutritional status or to an unidentified chronic illness.[87] However, because the half-life of albumin is 20 days, it does not detect early protein malnutrition. Prealbumin has a half-life of only 1 to 2 days. This makes it an excellent marker for recent-onset malnutrition and is more appropriate for assessment of the geriatric patient in a critical care setting.[31] A decrease in the hypothalamically mediated thirst response to hyperosmolarity makes the elderly less sensitive to their need for water.[80,87] Seniors with limited cardiac or renal function poorly tolerate high sodium loads, and individuals taking diuretics or digoxin frequently require potassium supplementation. Enhanced intake of calcium is instrumental in both the prevention and treatment of osteoporosis in the at-risk elderly population.[17] Routine micronutrient supplementation should be provided because deficiencies are common among geriatric patients. Enteral vitamins and trace mineral supplementation have been shown to improve immunologic responses and to decrease infections.[87] Steps should be taken to avoid long periods of "nothing by mouth" in the geriatric patient. When feasible, enteral nutrition is the preferred route.[31] Enteral nutrition (either oral or through a feeding tube) is considerably safer and less expensive than parenteral nutrition. The Nutrition box below summarizes geriatric nutritional needs.

Moreover, enteral nutrition helps the GI tract maintain its physiologic processes and may protect against bacterial translocation from the gut to the bloodstream via the mesenteric lymph nodes.[31] In elderly patients who are adequately nourished, postoperative parenteral nutrition has actually been associated with increased complications and, therefore, should be used only in seniors with severe nutritional deficits in whom the enteral route is unavailable.[68]

♦ NUTRITION

Nutritional Concerns in the Elderly Patient

CALORIC REQUIREMENTS

Both undernutrition and obesity are common findings in older adults.

- Evaluate caloric needs based on body mass index (BMI):
  - BMI $<20 \text{ kg/m}^2$ is consistent with malnutrition
  - BMI $20-22 \text{ kg/m}^2$ indicates undernutrition
  - BMI $23-24 \text{ kg/m}^2$ is normal
  - BMI $25-30 \text{ kg/m}^2$ is considered overweight
  - BMI $>30 \text{ kg/m}^2$ is obese

PROTEIN REQUIREMENTS

An elderly patient's protein needs must be individualized on the basis of preexisting previous nutritional status and current medical condition.

- Monitor serum prealbumin levels. Reference values depend on patient age, gender, sample population, and test method. Norms will also vary by lab.
- Low prealbumin levels indicate:[87]
  - Undernutrition
  - Severe or chronic illness
  - Hyperthyroidism
  - Liver disease
  - Serious infection
  - Certain digestive disorders
- Higher levels of prealbumin are common in patients with:
  - High-dose corticosteroid therapy
  - Hyperadrenalism
  - High-dose nonsteroidal antiinflammatory medication use
  - Hodgkin's disease

CARBOHYDRATE REQUIREMENTS

- Older adults' carbohydrate needs must be adjusted in accordance with their protein-calorie requirements.
- Carbohydrates should compromise 40%–60% of total calories.
- Consider hidden sources of carbohydrates (5% dextrose in IVs, dextrose in dialysate).
- Maintain glucose level at or below 110 mg/dl.

FAT REQUIREMENTS

- Limit fat intake to 1.5 g/kg of body weight.
- Fats should compromise 20%–40% of total calories.
- Fats should provide 4% of total fat calories to prevent essential fatty acid deficiency.

ELECTROLYTES

- Seniors with limited cardiac or renal function poorly tolerate high sodium loads.
- Individuals taking diuretics or digoxin frequently require potassium supplementation.
- Calcium supplementation can both prevent and treat osteoporosis.[17]

SPECIAL CONSIDERATIONS

- Gastric feeding is the preferred route for nutrition.[31]
- Routine micronutrient supplementation should be provided.[87]
- Avoid long periods of "nothing by mouth" in the geriatric patient.

Evidence-Based Care of the Critically Ill Elderly Patient

R.S. has now received a third liter of normal saline and states he needs to urinate. R.S. is unable to sit up and cannot void in a supine position, so an indwelling catheter is placed. Because of benign prostatic hypertrophy, catheter insertion is very difficult and results in urethral bleeding. The urine retrieved is cloudy and foul-smelling. The operating room notifies R.S.'s nurse that they are ready to perform R.S.'s humeral repair. As his nurse prepares him for surgery, she notes that R.S. is moderately agitated, cannot remember why he is in the hospital, and is trying to climb out of bed to look for his wife. R.S.'s skin is dry and flushed; his temperature is 37.9° C.

Just 3 hours after hospital arrival, and only 4 hours after waking up in his own home feeling fine, R.S. is on his way to surgery. He leaves critical care still in pain, with a serious orthopedic injury, occasional-to-frequent premature ventricular beats, a large skin tear, a small urethral tear, and early symptoms of fluid overload, aspiration pneumonia, delirium, and a sacral pressure ulcer.

Decision point: What musculoskeletal changes of aging predispose this patient to fractures?

Decision point: What additional possible reason for R.S.'s hypotension, flushed skin, and altered level of consciousness is suggested by his cloudy, foul-smelling urine; flushed skin; and moderate temperature elevation?

Case continues on page 1395

It is important to start early enteral supplementation in the undernourished or malnourished geriatric patient. Limited data suggest that enteral protein supplementation preoperatively can reduce negative outcomes in malnourished patients.[7] In critically ill older adults with declining renal function, protein needs may require adjustment. However, basal protein requirements may be slightly higher rather than lower. Other interventions to prevent or reverse malnutrition or feeding problems in the critically ill elderly patient include the following: provide small, frequent meals to avoid discomfort and increase intake; encourage fluids and fiber to improve bowel function; and obtain early nutritional consultation.[31]

ENDOCRINE/METABOLIC SYSTEM

The metabolic and endocrine changes associated with senescence are wide ranging, affecting every system in the body. Metabolic responses, in particular, influence the geriatric patient's ability to cope with the stresses of critical illness.

Age-Related Changes

Metabolic Needs. Caloric requirements are lower in older adults. Both basal metabolic rate and daily energy expenditure decrease over time. At age 80, resting energy expenditure is approximately 15% lower than at age 40.[87] Maximum oxygen consumption and maximum energy expenditure are also reduced. These decreases are primarily the result of a decline in physical activity and a loss of lean muscle mass. In the presence of acute illness or injury, resting energy expenditure and oxygen consumption normally rise to support the additional cardiopulmonary work, tissue repair, and immunologic responses that accompany healing. In seniors, however, the magnitude of this increase is smaller and the hypermetabolic state is less pronounced.[31]

In the face of stress, the older patient's metabolic response is characterized by increased requirements for energy and protein. However, the increase in catabolism—from illness, injury, infection, or surgery—is frequently not matched by an equal rise in energy intake. This condition is further exacerbated in patients with a preexisting poor nutritional status. Endogenous protein stores are depleted just to meet basic metabolic demands. Serum albumin is consumed and hepatic function declines, further impairing protein synthesis. Decreased muscle mass causes a reduction in muscle strength, particularly detrimental in the respiratory muscles. Cells with high turnover (e.g., skin, red and white blood cells, GI organs) fail first, leading to loss of barrier function, delayed wound healing, increased susceptibility to infection, and further impairment of nutrient absorption.[31]

Changes in Insulin Sensitivity. Aging is associated with a decline in glucose tolerance because of decreased peripheral receptor insulin sensitivity.[103] Elderly individuals have a fasting blood glucose level that is normal to slightly elevated under optimal circumstances. An increase in blood glucose level to 200 mg/dl occurs in approximately half of all people over the age of 70 years.[80] In times of acute illness, insulin responsiveness declines even further.[103] This fact explains why hyperglycemia is common in critically ill patients, even those without preexisting diabetes.[110]

Other Hormonal Changes. Secretion of many hormones decreases with aging. Elderly individuals experience a drop in the production of growth hormone, thyroid hormone, aldosterone, adrenal androgens, testosterone, and estrogen.[80,108]

Older adults have an increased incidence of thyroid nodularity, thyroid fibrosis, and other thyroid disorders, particularly hypothyroidism. A reduction in thyroid function is manifested by a decrease in triiodothyronine (T_3) levels with a concomitant elevation in levels of thyroid-stimulating hormone. Adrenal androgen levels also decline, limiting patients' immune system responsiveness to stress.[80] Significant changes in sex hormone levels occur with aging but seldom play an important role in critical illness.[113]

Common Problems and Management Strategies

Hyperglycemia. In a study examining age-related differences in metabolic responses to trauma, hyperglycemia was more pronounced in the elderly (over the age of 60 years) than in younger patients, despite similar carbohydrate intake.[34] Glycemic control becomes difficult in the geriatric patient because the usual insulin resistance to stress is exacerbated by the declining glucose tolerance associated with normal aging. In recent years, the importance of limiting insulin resistance has been demonstrated by a marked improvement in the outcome of critically ill patients who were placed on insulin protocols to maintain strict glycemic control. In a landmark study, both morbidity and mortality were decreased by more than 40% in the group in which glucose levels were tightly managed compared to control subjects.[110] Careful glucose regulation is particularly important in the elderly patient. Closely monitored blood glucose levels and the administration of exogenous insulin according to a protocol designed to maintain blood glucose level within a strict range are recommended.

Hypoadrenalism. Adrenal insufficiency is a rare disorder with an overall incidence of less than 0.01% in the general population (see Chapter 35). However, up to 28% of seriously ill patients have been found to have occult or unrecognized hypoadrenalism. Notably, the incidence among patients over the age of 55 years is two and a half times greater than that of younger individuals.[83] Adrenal insufficiency is a potentially life-threatening condition that results from marked stimulation of the neurohumoral hypothalamic-pituitary-adrenal axis, causing signs of sodium and volume depletion. In the setting of critical illness, patients with insufficient cortisol release, who fail to mount an appropriate neurohumoral stress response, can develop vasopressor-dependent refractory hypotension.[115]

Severe hypoadrenalism is characterized by a high CO and a markedly reduced systemic vascular resistance, a clinical picture that mimics and is often misinterpreted as sepsis.[83] Adrenal insufficiency is diagnosed by measuring a baseline serum cortisol level (normal is more than 20 mcg/dl) and response to the adrenocorticotropic hormone (ACTH) stimulation test.[59] Treatment involves a high index of suspicion for adrenal insufficiency and the immediate administration of steroids (hydrocortisone) to elderly patients at risk in order to alleviate potential adrenal crisis.

THERMOREGULATION

Thermoregulatory responses are decreased in older persons (see Chapter 7). Cognitive and functional decline, certain medications, social factors, loss of muscle mass, skin thinning, and systemic conditions (e.g., thyroid disease, diabetes, and malnutrition) all reduce tolerance to temperature extremes. Therefore abnormalities of body temperature are both more common and more prolonged in seniors.[87] Not surprisingly, the majority of both cold-related and heat-related deaths occur in elderly people.[52]

Age-Related Changes

Hypothalamic Decline. The hypothalamus is the body's thermoregulatory control center. With advancing age, declining hypothalamic function and a decreased basal metabolic rate combine to produce an overall reduction in the older patient's capacity to maintain thermal balance.[108]

Aging is also associated with a normal reduction in the threshold for peripheral vasoconstriction and shivering, reducing the body's ability to generate and conserve heat.[50] Because of sweat gland atrophy, the ability to sweat decreases with normal aging, thus reducing the body's ability to regulate heat when exposed to high ambient temperatures or exertion.[98]

Lower Baseline Temperature. Hypothalamic, metabolic, and body fat changes combine to cause older adults to experience a reduction in baseline body temperature. Normal temperature drops to 35.5° to 36.1° C.[53] Axillary temperature measurements tend to be poor indicators of core temperature in the geriatric population because skin temperature may be several degrees cooler than core temperature as a result of decreased peripheral circulation. Tympanic or oral temperature measurements are generally considered acceptable in the critically ill elder, but bladder or pulmonary artery thermometers provide a more accurate assessment of core thermal status.[50]

Attenuated Febrile Response and Immunosenescence.
In addition to a reduced ability to self-warm, geriatric patients have a blunted febrile reaction to infection as a result of immunosenescence. A significantly smaller percentage of older individuals generate a febrile response to stress than do their younger counterparts, and this febrile response is often attenuated.[87] With aging, there is a progressive decrease in T-cell function, defects in B-cell function, an increase in the number of autoantibodies and monoclonal immunoglobulins, and increased tumorigenesis.[87] Neutrophil counts do not drop, but the ability of the bone marrow to increase white blood cell production in response to infection is impaired. When combined with the stresses of critical illness, injury, or surgery, these cellular changes make it more likely that the geriatric patient will contract an infectious disease and will then be less able to eradicate it.[36]

Common Problems and Management Strategies

Hypothermia. There are far more cold-related deaths than heat-related deaths in the United States, Europe, and almost all countries outside the tropics. The majority of deaths are due to common illnesses that are exacerbated by cold rather than the direct result of severe hypothermia. Coronary and cerebral thrombosis constitute about 50% of cold-related deaths; respiratory diseases account for almost half of the rest.[52]

Hypothermia has profound effects on all components of the coagulation system. When exposed to cold stress, the body's first adjustment is to limit blood flow to the skin in order to conserve body heat. This vasoconstriction shifts blood from the skin to the core, which increases central blood volume and results in hypertension.[22] To compensate, sodium and water are shunted from the vessels into the interstitial space and are eventually excreted ("cold diuresis"). Left behind as the plasma volume drops are red cells, white cells, platelets, and fibrinogen. This increase in blood viscosity and concentration of thrombogenic factors promotes clotting.[52] Besides increased clotting, the high incidence of morbid cardiac events among hypothermic geriatric patients is likely attributable to the increased level of circulating norepinephrine required to produce vasoconstriction and maintain shivering. With more severe degrees of hypothermia, conduction abnormalities and myocardial irritability are common. Dysrhythmias in the hypothermic older adult are usually resistant to medications, countershock, and electrical pacing.[22]

The elderly individual may arrive at the hospital in a hypothermic state. However, iatrogenically induced hypothermia also puts seniors at risk. Intraoperative hypothermia in the geriatric patient with cardiac risk

factors is an independent predictor of postoperative cardiac events.[50] In the postoperative period, ventricular tachycardia, hypertension, angina, and hypoxemia have been demonstrated to occur more frequently in mildly hypothermic elderly patients than in normothermic individuals. Because the elderly are at an increased risk for hypothermia, every effort should be made to prevent heat losses. Use of forced-air heating blankets, warmed intravenous solutions, heated ventilator circuits, and higher room temperatures when patients are uncovered are all appropriate interventions.[5]

Hyperthermia. During a 3-week period in the summer of 2003, a heat wave rolled through France, leaving 14,800 persons dead in its wake. The majority of victims were over the age of 75 years. Although this is the most severe incident of heat-related deaths in recorded history, hyperthermia kills hundreds of seniors each year.[9]

Like cold-related deaths, most heat-related deaths in the elderly are due to the indirect effects of temperature rather than to high temperature per se.[52] However, when persons are exposed to air close to or above body temperature for long periods, a substantial number of heat-related deaths will be due to simple hyperthermia. Hyperthermia elevates temperature to a point where body proteins denature. In addition to reduced sweating mechanisms, many cognitive, social, and functional changes predispose older adults to heat-related illnesses. A wide range of drugs, particularly psychiatric medications and those with anticholinergic or narcotic actions, further impair sweating and other responses to heat.[52]

Coronary and cerebral thromboses account for many heat-related deaths because the salt and water losses from sweating produce hemoconcentration. Other heat-related deaths result from a range of factors that are poorly understood, but which probably include cardiac strain from trying to provide additional blood flow to the skin to increase heat loss. In the frankly hyperthermic patient (above 40° C), immediate and aggressive cooling can be life-saving. However, measures that induce shivering, which causes vasoconstriction and adds excess stress to the elderly heart, should be avoided.[52]

DRUG METABOLISM

Compared to younger adults, the elderly typically take more drugs, have more underlying organ dysfunction, are more susceptible to malnutrition, are more likely to have diminished or exaggerated responses to medications, and experience more interindividual variations in drug disposition.[11] The majority of older patients admitted to critical care are already taking a number of medications. Each drug is associated with an adverse risk profile that only worsens when combined with systemic disease and additional medications. This fact underscores the importance of obtaining a thorough medication and health history from the patient, family, or caregiver.[57]

Age-Related Changes

Altered Body Habitus. Several age-associated changes alter drug distribution in the elderly. With senescence, the portion of lean body mass decreases, the percent of body water drops, and the relative amount of adipose tissue increases. These alterations result in greater distribution of lipophilic drugs into the fat, producing a longer half-life for agents such as anesthetics, barbiturates, and benzodiazepines.[11]

Changes in Drug Processing, Absorption, Metabolism, and Excretion. Although the total amount of drug absorbed is basically unchanged, elderly patients experience a decline in the rate of drug absorption. Decreased serum albumin levels alter drug availability in substances that are protein-bound, enhancing the amount of bioactive agents. Both liver and kidney function decline with advancing age, which reduces clearance of many substances. The net effect of these senescent changes is an increase in the incidence of drug toxicity related to accumulation of metabolites.[11]

Common Problems and Management Strategies

Adverse Drug Reactions. Age-related changes in pharmacologic responses place the elderly at increased risk for adverse drug reactions. In fact, when the number of drugs per day exceeds 5, the incidence of adverse reactions doubles.[77] The hepatic and renal impairment that occurs with aging can quickly lead to elevated drug concentrations, even in fully compliant patients on standard therapeutic dosing regimens. Agents with a high potential for adverse reactions in older adults include anticoagulants, antidysrhythmics, calcium-channel blockers, digoxin, diuretics, narcotics, and theophylline.[77] Cardioactive substances in particular are problematic for the geriatric patient. These agents have an inherently narrow therapeutic range, which is further reduced in the elderly by an age-related decline in intrinsic heart rate (HR) and slowing of conduction through the atrioventricular node.[77]

The first step in reducing adverse medication reactions in the elderly involves obtaining a complete medication history (drug reconciliation) on each patient at the time of admission. This history must include prescription medications, over-the-counter agents, recreational drugs, and nutritional supplements as well as herbal, homeopathic, naturopathic, and folk medications.[57] Other strategies for reducing adverse medication reactions in seniors include weaning drugs as appropriate, increasing doses cautiously, monitoring closely for untoward effects, dosing according to renal function, and consulting with a pharmacist regarding age-appropriate dosages.[11]

PSYCHOSOCIAL AND FUNCTIONAL FACTORS

Regardless of initial circumstances, when a potentially life-threatening medical condition, injury, or complex surgical procedure has occurred, older persons suddenly find themselves in a strange and scary environment where they experience pain, anxiety, loss of familiar surroundings, loss of independence, and sleep deprivation.[57]

Age-Related Changes

As part of the normal aging process, the elderly experience a number of changes in social interaction. Friends, siblings, spouses, and other family members are often dead or dying. Many geriatric patients have lost their life partner as the result of either death or severe cognitive impairment. Even while managing their own healthcare needs, older adults frequently serve as caregivers for a spouse, parent, sibling, neighbor, child, or even great-grandchild. A huge number of elderly persons are cared for by those who are senior citizens themselves. The individual caring for a 94-year-old patient is likely to be the 92-year-old spouse or a 70-year-old child. Despite the decremental losses associated with aging, most elders perceive their lives as satisfying. Older adults exhibit a strong need to remain independent, maintain and develop meaningful relationships, and have a purpose in life.

Common Problems and Management Strategies

Functional Decline. Up to half of all geriatric patients admitted to hospitals experience a significant decline in function, or loss of the ability to perform activities of daily living. Specific factors associated with loss of function in the elderly include preexisting chronic illness, delirium, immobility, malnutrition, depression, and uncontrolled pain.[77] Sleep disturbances also accelerate functional decline. Approximately 5 million older Americans have serious sleep disorders. Sleep problems are only exaggerated by the stresses of critical care.[77]

Another condition that can cause severe functional decline in elderly persons is alcoholism. When the geriatric patient experiences hallucinations, tremors, or seizures, the possibility of alcohol withdrawal must be considered. The onset of alcohol withdrawal usually occurs in the first 48 to 72 hours of admission. Patients with a known history of alcohol abuse can be treated to prevent or attenuate the effects of delirium tremens. However, unrecognized abuse can lead to life-threatening alcohol withdrawal with consequences that can negatively affect the patient's critical care course and create long-term morbidity.[57]

End-of-Life Concerns. A tremendous amount of healthcare resources—and a large percentage of Medicare expenditures—are being consumed by geriatric patients in the last weeks of life.[112] In general, age alone does not predict a poor outcome for the critically ill elder.[87] However, a central problem complicating end-of-life decision making is the difficulty predicting outcomes in critically ill older adults. Yet the combination of multiple coinciding medical problems and rapidly changing clinical status makes predicting remaining life span a very difficult task.[112] Attempts have been made to generate models of projected mortality in critically ill seniors. Factors entered into these formulas include such variables as age, gender, HR, independent activities of daily living, dependent activities of daily living, number of critical care interventions, and the number of organ system failures.[73] Despite some predictive success in certain facilities, no system of geriatric critical care mortality determination has yet been widely validated or adopted.[73]

One of the greatest potential critical care problems in the elderly is the decision to withhold or withdraw support. This decision is a complex one that may reflect the personal biases of healthcare providers, patients, and family members.[112] Aggressive treatment of the critically ill geriatric patient may be contrary to the individual's own expressed wishes. Unfortunately, only about 15% to 20% of patients have an advance directive at the time of hospital admission.[112] When they exist, advance directives are often inadequate, except in cases of the most obvious treatment decisions, because they are too vague, using phrases such as "terminal illness" and "little chance of recovery."[112] Even when a patient's wishes are clear, many physicians are wary of ignoring the requests of a living surrogate, especially if it is a spouse or other close family member.[112]

Research regarding older adults' end-of-life preferences often seems confusing or contradictory. Despite the fact that 90% of Americans polled said that they would prefer to die at home, about 80% continue to go to some sort of healthcare facility to die. Sixty percent will die in an acute care hospital, and 20% will die in critical care.[112] In one study, most seniors who survived

to critical care discharge stated that they would be willing to undergo similar treatment again.[66] However, in another study published the same year, 56% of older patients claimed they were "very unwilling" or would "rather die" than enter a nursing home.[62]

MULTIDISCIPLINARY PLAN OF CARE

Meeting the needs of the critically ill geriatric patient requires careful assessment, individualized planning, teamwork, and frequent reevaluation, as shown in the Multidisciplinary Plan of Care on pp. 1396-1397. Areas of special concern in this population include: comorbidities, delirium, diminished physiologic reserves, hypothermia, pain, polypharmacy, potential for skin breakdown, and sensory deficits.

◆ Case Study 49-1, Part C

Evidence-Based Care of the Critically Ill Elderly Patient

Except for intraoperative blood loss greater than anticipated, the open reduction and internal fixation of R.S.'s right humerus is uneventful. However, his pulmonary status declined, and R.S. was unable to be weaned from mechanical ventilation after surgery. Despite a forced-air warming blanket and a warmed, humidified ventilator circuit, R.S.'s bladder temperature remains approximately 35.6° C. Postoperatively, there is substantial bloody oozing from R.S.'s surgical site and he is persistently hypotensive. R.S.'s pulmonary status continues to deteriorate and he is now requiring a fraction of inspired oxygen (Fio_2) of 80% to maintain an oxygen saturation of 90%. R.S.'s airways are suctioned frequently for copious, tan endotracheal secretions. Urine output for the last 3 hours has totaled only 67 ml.

Decision point: What are the probable effects of hypothermia on this patient?

Over the course of the night shift, R.S. progresses to sepsis and acute renal failure, and begins to have short bursts of ventricular tachycardia. By morning R.S. is unresponsive to noxious stimuli, requires 100% Fio_2, and is receiving phenylephrine (Neo-Synephrine), dobutamine (Dobutrex), amiodarone (Cordarone), and furosemide (Lasix) drips, as well as three different antibiotics. R.S.'s nurse and attending physician requested a family conference to determine R.S.'s wishes regarding life-sustaining care. With the help of a neighbor, the critical care social worker is able to learn that R.S. and his wife are estranged from their only living child and R.S. has no advance directive. R.S.'s wife, suffering from Alzheimer's disease, is unable to grasp her husband's dismal prognosis.

Decision point: What do you do in this situation?

MULTIDISCIPLINARY PLAN OF CARE FOR THE CRITICALLY ILL ELDERLY PATIENT

PROBLEM	INTERVENTION	RATIONALE	EXPECTED OUTCOME
Comorbidities	Assess the patient for chronic disease conditions that can significantly impact the admitting diagnosis, including: 　Chronic obstructive pulmonary disease 　Hyperlipidemia 　Cardiovascular disease 　Hypertension 　Type 2 diabetes 　Renal insufficiency	A comorbid condition is any additional disease state that significantly affects the patient's response to the present illness or injury.	Comorbid conditions will be identified and managed to minimize their impact on the critically ill patient.
Delirium	Identify and remove underlying causes of delirium Treat acutely agitated or aggressive patients with antipsychotic agents to provide rest and promote safety (see Chapter 50) Decrease environmental stimuli by limiting visual, auditory, and tactile stimulation Engage family members, friends, or volunteers to help reorient, mobilize, and feed the patient Use clocks, calendars, family photos, glasses, and hearing aids to assist orientation	Delirium in critical care is associated with higher morbidity and mortality. In older individuals, the likelihood of medication-induced delirium is high. Appropriate assessment and intervention are essential for a positive outcome in the patient with delirium.	Efforts will be made to identify the source of delirium and reduce its impact on the critically ill patient.
Diminished physiologic reserves	Minimize the stressors placed on each body system: 　Pulmonary 　Cardiovascular 　Renal 　Neurologic 　Gastrointestinal 　Musculoskeletal 　Integumentary 　Immune	In every body system, the elderly patient's physiologic reserves are limited and function can deteriorate rapidly. A declining physiologic status forces seniors to use "reserves" just to maintain homeostasis. When reserves are required to meet the increased demands of critical illness or surgical stress, but are no longer present, organ system failure ensues.	
Hypothermia	Aggressively prevent heat loss Use forced-air heating blankets, warmed intravenous solutions, heated ventilator circuits; keep room temperatures high when patients are uncovered	Hypothermia is associated with adverse cardiac events in the geriatric patient. Even mild hypothermia (core temperature decreased by 1° C) can cause significant alterations in normal immune responses.	Patients will be normothermic throughout their critical care stay.
Pain	Determine whether the patient had any chronic pain conditions before hospitalization Assess for the presence of acute pain related to the patient's disease, injury, or surgical	Many older adults suffer from some form of chronic pain (e.g., back pain, arthritis). When hospitalized, elders experience acute-on-chronic pain.	The geriatric patient will have his or her pain needs met without oversedation. With pain adequately controlled, elderly patients will be able to

PROBLEM	INTERVENTION	RATIONALE	EXPECTED OUTCOME
	intervention Tailor pharmacologic and nonpharmacologic pain relief mechanisms to the individual elder Closely monitor the patient's response to analgesics to prevent toxicity	The opiate-naïve geriatric patient is very sensitive to the side effects of narcotic analgesics, including oversedation, nausea, and constipation.	participate in their care and resume mobility as early as possible.
Polypharmacy	Reconcile the patient's complete drug list at the time of admission and critical care discharge Minimize the number of drugs to which the elderly patient is exposed Monitor renal and hepatic function as recommended Reduce drug doses as indicated, particularly for agents with a high potential for adverse reactions in older adults Obtain a pharmacology consult for the management of patients receiving multiple drugs	Age-related changes in pharmacologic responses place the elderly at increased risk for adverse drug reactions. The hepatic and renal impairment that occurs with aging can quickly lead to elevated drug concentrations, even in fully compliant patients on standard therapeutic dosing regimens.	The geriatric patient will be free from adverse drug reactions and toxicities.
Potential for skin breakdown	Handle the patient gently Avoid shearing forces Pad bony prominences with additional layers Reposition the patient frequently Use a nondrying cleanser to keep the skin clean Apply skin moisturizers and protective lotions liberally Consider the use of special air or rotating beds Consult a wound and ostomy nurse Remove elderly patients from spine boards as soon as possible	Pressure ulcers may develop virtually anywhere on the geriatric patient's body, but are most common over the bony prominences of the sacrum, heels, ischium, elbows, and pinna. Pressure ulcers can form rapidly in immobilized seniors.	Elderly patients at risk for skin disruption will be identified at the time of admission.
Sensory deficits	Use patient teaching materials with large type fonts Select contrasting colors for printed material Ensure adequate, glare-free lighting Face the patient directly when speaking Use touch and visual cues to facilitate communication Assist patients with glasses and hearing aids	Anatomic changes of senescence limit visual acuity, depth perception, peripheral vision, tolerance to glare, and speed of eye movements. Impaired light/dark adaptation heightens the older person's need for ambient light. Normal aging is accompanied by anatomic and functional changes in the auditory and vestibular apparatus that cause decreased sensitivity to sound and altered frequency discrimination.	While in critical care, elderly patients will be assisted to see and hear at their preadmission level of function.

From reference 91.

CONCLUSIONS

Demographic shifts, longevity gains, and advances in healthcare in the last 50 years have dramatically increased the number of older persons in U.S. critical care. The proportion of critically ill patients who are elderly is projected to continue to increase well into the middle of the twenty-first century. Senescence affects every system in the body, but in the geriatric patient, normal age-related transformations can be difficult to distinguish from alterations caused by illness, environmental, social, functional, and comorbid conditions. These changes interact to threaten seniors' ability to survive and recover from critical illness or injury.

REFERENCES

1. American Heart Association. (2000). *2001 Heart and stroke statistical update*. Dallas, Tex: American Heart Association.
2. Anderson, R. N. (2000). A method for constructing complete annual U.S. life tables. *Vital Health Statistics Series, 2*(129), 1–28.
3. Angus, D. C., et al. (2001). Epidemiology of severe sepsis in the United States: analysis of incidence, outcome, and associated costs of care. *Crit Care Med, 29*(7), 1303–1310.
4. Asuncion, M., & Kaushik, V. (2000). Management of shock. In T. Yohikawa & D. Norman (Eds.), *Acute emergencies and critical care of the geriatric patient*. New York: Marcel Dekker.
5. Atwell, S. (2002). Trauma in the elderly. In K. McQuillan et al. (Eds.), *Trauma nursing: from resuscitation through rehabilitation* (3rd ed.). Philadelphia: Saunders.
6. Baird, M., Keen, J., & Swearingen, P. (2005). *Manual of critical care nursing* (5th ed.). St. Louis: Elsevier.
7. Beattie, A., Prach, A., & Pennington, C. (2000). A randomized controlled trial of the use of enteral nutritional supplements postoperatively in malnourished surgical patients. *Gut, 46*, 813–818.
8. Bergeron, E., et al. (2003). Elderly trauma patients with rib fractures are at greater risk of death and pneumonia. *J Trauma Injury Infect Crit Care, 54*(3), 478–485.
9. Bouchama, A. (2004). The 2003 European heat wave. *Intensive Care Med, 30*(1), 1–3.
10. Brady, W., et al. (2005). Acute coronary syndromes: pathophysiology and diagnosis. In M. Fink et al. (Eds.), *Textbook of critical care* (5th ed.). Philadelphia: Elsevier.
11. Brundage, R., & Mann, H. (2005). General principles of pharmacokinetics and pharmacodynamics. In M. Fink et al. (Eds.), *Textbook of critical care* (5th ed.). Philadelphia: Elsevier.
12. Burks, K. (2005). Osteoarthritis in older adults: current treatments. *J Gerontol Nurs, 31*(5), 11–19.
13. Campbell, E. (2000). Physiologic changes in respiratory function. In R. A. Rosenthal, M. Zenilman, & M. Katlic (Eds.), *Principles and practice of geriatric surgery*. New York: Springer-Verlag.
14. Centers for Disease Control and Prevention. (2002). Prevalence of self-reported arthritis or chronic joint symptoms among adults—United States, 2001. *JAMA, 288*(24), 3103–3104.
15. Chambers, J. (2001). Gastrointestinal alterations. In M. Sole, M. Lamborn, & J. Hartshorn (Eds.), *Introduction to critical care nursing* (3rd ed.). Philadelphia: WB Saunders.
16. Clark, D. E., & Chu, M. K. (2002). Increasing importance of the elderly in a trauma system. *Am J Emerg Med, 20*(2), 108–111.
17. Committee on Nutrition Services for Medicare Beneficiaries. (2000). *The role of nutrition in maintaining health in the nation's elderly*. Washington, DC: National Academy Press.
18. Criddle, L. M. (2005). Head trauma. In L. Newberry & L. M. Criddle (Eds.), *Sheehy's manual of emergency care* (6th ed.). St. Louis: Elsevier.
19. Criddle, L. M., Eldredge, D. H., & Walker, J. (2005). Variables predicting trauma patient survival following massive transfusion. *J Emerg Nurs, 31*(3), 236–242.
20. Dardaine, V., et al. (2001). Outcome of older patients requiring ventilatory support in intensive care: impact of nutritional status. *J Am Geriatr Soc, 49*(5), 564–570.
21. Demetriades, D., et al. (2001). Old age as a criterion for trauma team activation. *J Trauma, 51*(4), 754–756.
22. Denke, N. (2005). Environmental emergencies. In L. Newberry & L. M. Criddle (Eds.), *Sheehy's manual of emergency care* (6th ed.). St. Louis: Elsevier.
23. Draude, B. (2004). Gerontologic alterations. In L. Urden, K. Stacy, & M. Lough (Eds.), *Priorities in critical care nursing* (4th ed.). St. Louis: Elsevier.
24. Ely, E. W., et al. (2002). Recovery rate and prognosis in older persons who develop acute lung injury and the acute respiratory distress syndrome. *Ann Intern Med, 136*(1), 25–36.
25. Emergency Nurses Association. (2000). *Trauma nursing core course*. Des Plaines, Ill: Emergency Nurses Association.
26. Empana, J. P., Dargent-Molina, P., & Breart, G. (2004). Effect of hip fracture on mortality in elderly women: the EPIDOS prospective study. *J Am Geriatr Soc, 52*(5), 685–690.
27. Epstein, C. D., El-Mokadem, N., & Peerless, J. R. (2002). Weaning older patients from long-term mechanical ventilation: a pilot study. *Am J Crit Care, 11*(4), 369–377.
28. Epstein, C. D., et al. (2002). Oxygen transport and organ dysfunction in the older trauma patient. *Heart Lung, 31*(5), 315–326.
29. Farrell, C. (2004). Poststroke depression in elderly patients. *Dimens Crit Care Nurs, 23*(6), 264–269.
30. Fazio, J. (2005). Spinal cord and neck trauma. In L. Newberry & L. M. Criddle (Eds.), *Sheehy's manual of emergency care* (6th ed.). St. Louis: Elsevier.
31. Fick, D., & Schumacher, L. (2001). Nutrition. In T. Fulmer, M. Foreman, & M. Walker (Eds.), *Critical care nursing of the elderly*. New York: Springer.
32. Finelli, F. C. J., et al. (1989). A case control study for major trauma in geriatric patients. *J Trauma Injury Infect Crit Care, 29*(5), 541–548.
33. Forsen, L., et al. (1999). Survival after hip fracture: short- and long-term excess mortality according to age and gender. *Osteoporos Int, 10*(1), 73–78.
34. Frankenfield, D., et al. (2000). Age-related differences in the metabolic response to injury. *J Trauma, 48*(1), 49–56.
35. Fulmer, T., & Foreman, M. (2001). Common geriatric problems. In T. Fulmer, M. Foreman, & M. Walker (Eds.), *Critical care nursing of the elderly*. New York: Springer.
36. Ginaldi, L., & Sternberg, H. (2003). The immune system. In P. Timiras (Ed.), *Physiological basis of aging and geriatrics* (3rd ed.). Boca Raton, Fla: CRC Press.
37. Goldrick, B. A. (2005). Infection in the older adult: long-term care poses particular risk. *Am J Nurs, 105*(6), 33–34.
38. Goshorn, J. (2001). Acute renal failure. In M. Sole, M. Lamborn, & J. Hartshorn (Eds.), *Introduction to critical care nursing* (3rd ed.). Philadelphia: Saunders.
39. Gross, R., & Dellinger, R. (2005). Arterial blood gas interpretation. In M. Fink et al. (Eds.), *Textbook of critical care* (5th ed.). Philadelphia: Elsevier.
40. Grossman, M. D., et al. (2002). When is an elder old? Effect of preexisting conditions on mortality in geriatric trauma. *J Trauma Injury Infect Crit Care, 52*(2), 242–246.
41. Gubler, K. D., et al. (1997). Long-term survival of elderly trauma patients. *Arch Surg, 132*(9), 1010–1014.

42. Hall, M. J., & Owings, M. F. (2000). Hospitalizations for injury: United States, 1996. *Advance Data, 318,* 1–9.

43. Hall, M. J., & Owings, M. F. (2002). 2000 National hospital discharge survey. *Adv Data Vital Health Statis, 329*(1).

44. Hauswald, M., & McNally, T. (2000). Confusing extrication with immobilization: the inappropriate use of hard spine boards for interhospital transfers. *Air Med J, 19*(4), 126–127.

45. Hirshon, J. (2004). Basic cardiopulmonary resuscitation in adults. In J. Tintinalli, G. Kelen, & J. Stapczynski (Eds.), *Emergency medicine: a comprehensive study guide* (6th ed.). New York: McGraw-Hill.

46. Irwin, Z. N., et al. (2004). Variations in injury patterns, treatment, and outcome for spinal fracture and paralysis in adult versus geriatric patients. *Spine, 29*(7), 796–802.

47. Jacobs, D. G. (2003). Special considerations in geriatric injury. *Curr Opin Crit Care, 9*(6), 535–539.

48. Johnson, C., Ashley, S., & Steen, S. (2000). Emergency anesthesia. In T. Yohikawa & D. Norman (Eds.), *Acute emergencies and critical care of the geriatric patient.* New York: Marcel Dekker.

49. Johnson, K., & Johnson, S. (2001). Trauma care. In T. Fulmer, M. Foreman, & M. Walker (Eds.), *Critical care nursing of the elderly.* New York: Springer.

50. Joaquin, A. (2000). Hypothermia and hyperthermia. In T. Yohikawa & D. Norman (Eds.), *Acute emergencies and critical care of the geriatric patient.* New York: Marcel Dekker.

51. Karch, A. (2003). *2003 Lippincott's nursing drug guide.* Philadelphia: Lippincott Williams & Wilkins.

52. Keating, W. R., & Donaldson, G. C. (2004). The impact of global warming on health and mortality. *South Med J, 97*(11), 1093–1099.

53. Keen, J., & Swearingen, P. (Eds.). (1997). *Mosby's critical care nursing consultant.* St. Louis: Mosby.

54. Klein, D. (2001). Trauma. In M. Sole, M. Lamborn, & J. Hartshorn (Eds.), *Introduction to critical care nursing* (3rd ed.). Philadelphia: Saunders.

55. Kleinhenz, M. E., & Lewis, C. Y. (2000). Chronic ventilator dependence in elderly patients. *Clin Geriatr Med, 16*(4), 735–756.

56. LaBorde, P., & Willis, J. (2001). Burns. In M. Sole, M. Lamborn, & J. Hartshorn (Eds.), *Introduction to critical care nursing* (3rd ed.). Philadelphia: Saunders.

57. Litton, K. A. (2003). Delirium in the critical care patient: what the professional staff needs to know. *Crit Care Nurs Quart, 26*(3), 208–213.

58. Marik, P. E. (2001). Aspiration pneumonitis and aspiration pneumonia. *N Engl J Med, 344*(9), 665–671.

59. Marik, P. E., & Zaloga, G. (2005). Adrenocortical insufficiency. In J. Hall, G. Schmidt, & L. Wood (Eds.), *Principles of critical care.* New York: McGraw-Hill.

60. Martin, M. (2001). Code management. In M. Sole, M. Lamborn, & J. Hartshorn (Eds.), *Introduction to critical care nursing* (3rd ed.). Philadelphia: Saunders.

61. Martinis, M., & Timiras, P. (2003). The pulmonary respiration, hematopoiesis and erythrocytes. In P. Timiras (Ed.), *Physiological basis of aging and geriatrics* (3rd ed.). Boca Raton, Fla: CRC Press.

62. Mattimore, T., Wenger, N., & Desbiens, N. (1997). Surrogate and physician understanding of patients' preferences for living permanently in a nursing home. *J Am Geriatr Soc, 45,* 818–824.

63. McKinley, M., & Robinson, C. (2001). Shock. In M. Sole, M. Lamborn, & J. Hartshorn (Eds.), *Introduction to critical care nursing* (3rd ed.). Philadelphia: Saunders.

64. McMahon, D. J., Shapiro, M. B., & Kauder, D. R. (2000). The injured elderly in the trauma intensive care unit. *Surg Clin North Am, 80*(3), 1005–1019.

65. Meisami, E., Brown, C., & Emerle, H. (2003). Sensory systems: normal aging, disorders, and treatments of vision and hearing in humans. In P. Timiras (Ed.), *Physiological basis of aging and geriatrics* (3rd ed, pp. 141–165). Boca Raton, Fla: CRC Press.

66. Mick, D. J., & Ackerman, M. H. (1997). Neutralizing ageism in critical care via outcomes research. *AACN Clin Issues, 8*(4), 597–608.

67. Milisen, K., et al. (2001). Delirium. In T. Fulmer, M. Foreman, & M. Walker (Eds.), *Critical care nursing of the elderly.* New York: Springer.

68. Morrison, R., Carney, M., & Manfredi, P. (2000). Pain management. In R. Rosenthal, M. Zenilman, & M. Katlic (Eds.), *Principles and practice of geriatric surgery.* New York: Springer-Verlag.

69. Murray, M., et al. (2002). *Critical care medicine: perioperative management* (2nd ed.). Philadelphia: Lippincott Williams & Wilkins.

70. National Center for Health Statistics. (2000). *Older Americans 2000: key indicators of well-being.* Washington, DC: Federal Interagency Forum on Aging Related Statistics.

71. Neild, G. H. (2001). Multi-organ renal failure in the elderly. *Int Urol Nephrol, 32*(4), 559–565.

72. Niederman, M. (2005). Community-acquired pneumonia. In M. Fink, et al. (Eds.), *Textbook of critical care* (5th ed.). Philadelphia: Elsevier.

73. Nierman, D. M. S., et al. (2001). Outcome prediction model for very elderly critically ill patients. *Crit Care Med, 29*(10), 1853–1859.

74. Novak, A. (2005). Geriatric trauma. In L. Newberry & L. M. Criddle (Eds.), *Sheehy's manual of emergency care* (6th ed.). St. Louis: Elsevier.

75. Pasternak, R. C., et al. (2004). Atherosclerotic Vascular Disease Conference: Writing Group I: epidemiology. *Circulation, 109*(21), 2605–2612.

76. Pfohman, M., & Criddle, L. M. (2001). Epidemiology of intracranial aneurysm and subarachnoid hemorrhage. *J Neurosci Nurs, 33*(1), 39–41.

77. Prevost, S. (2001). Individual and family response to the critical care experience. In M. Sole, M. Lamborn, & J. Hartshorn (Eds.), *Introduction to critical care nursing* (3rd ed.). Philadelphia: Saunders.

78. Pudelek, B. (2002). Geriatric trauma: special needs for a special population. *AACN Clin Issues, 13*(1), 61–72.

79. Redelmeier, D., Scales, D., & Kopp, A. (2005). Beta blockers for elective surgery in elderly patients: population based, retrospective cohort study. *Br Med J, 331*(7522), 22.

80. Resnick, B. (2005). The critically ill older patient. In P. Morton et al. (Eds.), *Critical care nursing: a holistic approach* (8th ed.). Philadelphia: Lippincott Williams & Wilkins.

81. Richards, C. L. (2004). Urinary tract infections in the frail elderly: issues for diagnosis, treatment and prevention. *Int Urol Nephrol, 36*(3), 457–463.

82. Riquelme, R., et al. (1997). Community-acquired pneumonia in the elderly. Clinical and nutritional aspects. *Am J Respir Crit Care Med, 156*(6), 1908–1914.

83. Rivers, E. P., et al. (2001). Adrenal insufficiency in high-risk surgical ICU patients. *Chest, 119*(3), 889–896.

84. Rodgers, H., et al. (1990). Acute renal failure: a study of elderly patients. *Age Ageing, 19*(1), 36–42.

85. Rogers, F. B., et al. (2001). A population-based study of geriatric trauma in a rural state. *J Trauma, 50*(4), 604–609.

86. Rose, S., & Maffulli, N. (1999). Hip fractures. An epidemiological review. *Bull Hosp J Dis Orthop Inst, 58*(4), 197–201.

87. Rosenthal, R. A., & Kavic, S. M. (2004). Assessment and management of the geriatric patient. *Crit Care Med, 32*(4 suppl).

88. Rozenthal, T. D., et al. (2002). Survival among elderly patients after fractures of the distal radius. *J Hand Surg Am, 27*(6), 948–952.

89. Rozzini, R., et al. (2004). Stroke units and acute care for elders model of care. *J Am Geriatr Soc, 52*(9), 1587–1588.

90. Russo-McCourt, T. (2002). Spinal cord injuries. In K. McQuillan, et al. (Eds.), *Trauma nursing: from resuscitation through rehabilitation* (3rd ed.). Philadelphia: Saunders.

91. Schwab, C. W., Shapiro, M. B., & Kauder, D. R. (2000). Geriatric trauma: patterns, care, and outcomes. In K. Mattox, D. Feliciano, & E. Moore (Eds.), *Trauma* (4th ed.). New York: McGraw-Hill.

92. Semla, T. (2001). Pharmacologic therapy. In T. Fulmer, M. Foreman, & M. Walker (Eds.), *Critical care nursing of the elderly*. New York: Springer.

93. Sevransky, J. E., & Haponik, E. F. (2003). Respiratory failure in elderly patients. *Clin Geriatr Med, 19*(1), 205–224.

94. Sue, D. (2000). Acute respiratory failure. In T. Yohikawa & D. Norman (Eds.), *Acute emergencies and critical care of the geriatric patient*. New York: Marcel Dekker.

95. Susman, M., et al. (2002). Traumatic brain injury in the elderly: increased mortality and worse functional outcome at discharge despite lower injury severity. *J Trauma Injury Infect Crit Care, 53*(2), 219–223.

96. Susman, M., et al. (2002). Traumatic brain injury in the elderly: increased mortality and worse functional outcome at discharge despite lower injury severity [see comment]. *J Trauma, 53*(2), 219–223.

97. Taheri, P. A., et al. (1997). Physician resource utilization after geriatric trauma. *J Trauma, 43*(4), 565–568.

98. Timiras, M. (2003). The skin. In P. Timiras (Ed.), *Physiological basis of aging and geriatrics* (3rd ed.). Boca Raton, Fla: CRC Press.

99. Timiras, M., & Leary, J. (2003). The kidney, the lower urinary tract, body fluids and the prostate. In P. Timiras (Ed.), *Physiological basis of aging and geriatrics* (3rd ed.). Boca Raton, Fla: CRC Press.

100. Timiras, P. (2003). The adrenal and pituitary. In P. Timiras (Ed.), *Physiological basis of aging and geriatrics* (3rd ed.). Boca Raton, Fla: CRC Press.

101. Timiras, P. (2003). Aging as a stage of life, common terms related to aging, methods used to study aging. In P. Timiras (Ed.), *Physiological basis of aging and geriatrics* (3rd ed.). Boca Raton, Fla: CRC Press.

102. Timiras, P. (2003). Cardiovascular alterations with aging: atherosclerosis and coronary heart disease. In P. Timiras (Ed.), *Physiological basis of aging and geriatrics* (3rd ed.). Boca Raton, Fla: CRC Press.

103. Timiras, P. (2003). The endocrine pancreas, diffuse endocrine glands and chemical mediators. In P. Timiras (Ed.), *Physiological basis of aging and geriatrics* (3rd ed.). Boca Raton, Fla: CRC Press.

104. Timiras, P. (2003). The gastrointestinal tract and liver. In P. Timiras (Ed.), *Physiological basis of aging and geriatrics* (3rd ed.). Boca Raton, Fla: CRC Press.

105. Timiras, P. (2003). The nervous system: functional changes. In P. Timiras (Ed.), *Physiological basis of aging and geriatrics* (3rd ed.). Boca Raton, Fla: CRC Press.

106. Timiras, P. (2003). The nervous system: structural and biochemical changes. In P. Timiras (Ed.), *Physiological basis of aging and geriatrics* (3rd ed.). Boca Raton, Fla: CRC Press.

107. Timiras, P. (2003). The skeleton, joints, and skeletal and cardiac muscles. In P. Timiras (Ed.), *Physiological basis of aging and geriatrics* (3rd ed.). Boca Raton, Fla: CRC Press.

108. Timiras, P. (2003). The thyroid, parathyroid, and pineal glands. In P. Timiras (Ed.), *Physiological basis of aging and geriatrics* (3rd ed.). Boca Raton, Fla: CRC Press.

109. Tresch, D., & Poornima, I. (2000). Cardiac emergencies. In T. Yohikawa & D. Norman (Eds.), *Acute emergencies and critical care of the geriatric patient*. New York: Marcel Dekker.

110. van den Berghe, G., et al. (2001). Intensive insulin therapy in the critically ill patients. *N Engl J Med, 345*(19), 1359–1367.

111. Wallace, M., & Flaherty, E. (2001). Pain. In T. Fulmer, M. Foreman, & M. Walker (Eds.), *Critical care nursing of the elderly*. New York: Springer.

112. Ward, N., & Levy, M. (2005). End-of-life issues in the intensive care unit. In M. Fink, et al. (Eds.), *Textbook of critical care* (5th ed.). Philadelphia: Elsevier.

113. Wise, P. (2003). The female reproductive system. In P. Timiras (Ed.), *Physiological basis of aging and geriatrics* (3rd ed.). Boca Raton, Fla: CRC Press.

114. Wong, F., & Rho, J. (2000). Drug dosing and life-threatening drug reactions in the critically ill patient. In T. Yohikawa & D. Norman (Eds.), *Acute emergencies and critical care of the geriatric patient*. New York: Marcel Dekker.

115. Wood, K. A., & Ely, E. W. (2003). What does it mean to be critically ill and elderly? *Curr Opin Crit Care, 9*(4), 316–320.

116. Yamaguchi, D. (2000). Acute renal failure. In T. Yohikawa & D. Norman (Eds.), *Acute emergencies and critical care of the geriatric patient*. New York: Marcel Dekker.

CHAPTER 50 Caring for the Critically Ill Patient With a Neuropsychiatric Disorder

Kathleen M. Baldwin

The prevalence of patients with neuropsychiatric disorders in acute care settings is high. Estimates range from 20% to 35%.[59] Deinstitutionalization, a laudable human rights movement begun in the early 1960s, has placed an increasing number of patients with severe and chronic neuropsychiatric disorders into the community and onto the streets.[57] Nurses working in critical care can expect to encounter these patients in their practice. Attitudes of nurses toward patients with neuropsychiatric disorders in a critical care setting are mixed.[5] Perceptions about the purposes of critical care and the appropriateness of caring for patients with neuropsychiatric disorders may be based on unquestioned assumptions, prejudice, and social stigma.

Most neuropsychiatric disorders seen in critical care are comorbid conditions. These disorders may be long-standing and play a major role in development of an acute illness or injury, but are usually not responsible for the critical care admission. Neuropsychiatric disorders may develop following the critical care admission and complicate recovery. Dealing with a critically ill patient is challenging enough. Neuropsychiatric symptoms and their treatment can complicate the management of multisystem conditions and lead to emergency situations. The symptoms and treatment of medical conditions may exacerbate neuropsychiatric disorders.

This chapter differs from others in many respects. Whereas other chapters in this book are devoted to single disorders (e.g., acute renal failure), this chapter encompasses many and varied disorders. In the first half of this chapter, six common disorders are classified and described. In the second half a multidisciplinary plan of care is provided for treatment of patients who are anxious, confused, elated, hostile, manipulative, suicidal, suspicious, or withdrawn.

DEFINITIONS

Neuropsychiatric illnesses are disorders of the brain. Although these disorders may be associated with gross structural changes (cortical atrophy, enlarged ventricular spaces) of that complex and highly plastic organ, most of the structural changes in neuroanatomy are at cellular and molecular levels. For example, widespread loss of cholinergic neurons is characteristic of Alzheimer's-type dementia, whereas schizophrenia and delusional disorders are caused by an increase in the number and sensitivity of dopaminergic and serotonergic receptors. In short, neuropsychiatric disorders represent flaws in brain chemistry.

Neurochemicals (acetylcholine, dopamine, gamma-aminobutyric acid [GABA], noradrenaline, and serotonin) increase or decrease communication between and among nerve cells. Because the brain's purpose is to transmit electrochemical impulses, these chemicals (known as neurotransmitters) must be present in the right amount. For convenience, neuropsychiatric disorders may be classified as excesses or deficiencies of specific chemicals (Table 50-1). Similar to hormone modulation for hyperadrenalism, hypothyroidism, or diabetes, treatment is frequently lifelong and focuses on eliminating surplus chemicals or replacing those chemicals that are in short supply.

Genetic predisposition for a particular mix of brain chemicals does not necessarily cause a neuropsychiatric disorder. Although brain chemistry is an important factor in the development of neuropsychiatric disorders, environmental triggers usually prompt the onset of symptoms. These triggers may include psychosocial stressors (e.g., surviving physical, emotional, or sexual trauma; living in relentless poverty; or experiencing profound loss, such as the death of a loved one or a disabling disease). Other triggers include autoimmune responses, biologic or industrial toxins, viral infections, chronic illnesses, medical emergencies, malnutrition, and crisis events (e.g., the 9/11 terrorist attacks or Hurricane Katrina). Genetics plus environment yields changes in brain chemistry that cause neuropsychiatric disorders.

Neuropsychiatric disorders are defined by behavior. The *Diagnostic Statistical Manual of Mental Disorders, Fourth Edition, Text Revision (DSM-IV-TR)*[2] is the primary diagnostic compendium used by all mental health professionals. The *DSM-IV-TR* lists defining criteria for hundreds of neuropsychiatric, personality, and substance

TABLE 50-1 Neuropsychiatric Disorders as Excesses or Deficiencies of Specific Neurotransmitters

NEUROPSYCHIATRIC DISORDERS	LEVELS	SPECIFIC NEUROTRANSMITTER
Schizophrenia and other psychoses*	Excess Deficiency	D2, NE, serotonin 5-HTP GABA
Bipolar disorder—mania*	Excess Deficiency	Epinephrine, NE, serotonin 5-HTP GABA
Anxiety-related disorders*	Excess Deficiency	D2, epinephrine, NE, serotonin 5-HTP GABA
Dementia—Alzheimer's type	Deficiency	Acetylcholine (parasympathomimetic)
Depression	Deficiency	D2, epinephrine, NE, serotonin 5-HTP
Delirium	Variable	Synergistic effect

D2 = Dopamine, GABA = gamma-aminobutyric acid, NE = norepinephrine.
*CNS excitement in each of these disorders is a product of both excess neurostimulation (e.g., serotonin 5-HTP) and deficient neuroinhibition (e.g., GABA). GABA is a CNS inhibitor; it causes subcortical depression.

abuse disorders. These defining criteria include specific symptom manifestations such as apathy, irritability, delusions, hallucinations, euphoria, loosely associated thoughts, strange or extreme emotional reactions, impoverished or garrulous speech, poor interpersonal relationships, disturbed sleep, short attention span, impulsivity, and low self-esteem. For a definitive diagnosis, symptoms must be present for a while (usually 2 weeks to 3 months). Behavior is the clinician's clue to chemical substrates causing a neuropsychiatric disorder; therefore, behavior becomes a target for determining effectiveness of treatment. Selection and adjustment of pharmacologic and nonpharmacologic interventions is determined by the effect on patient behavior.

AT-RISK PATIENTS

Patients with a history of psychiatric hospitalization, diagnosis, and treatment are at risk; however, many high-risk individuals do not possess this history. Patients who have known genetic susceptibility, a generational trend, recent loss, or other environment triggers also are at risk. Risk factors associated with specific neuropsychiatric disorders are detailed later in this chapter.

◆ Case Study 50-1, Part A

Seeking the Cause of Abnormal Behavior

Seventy-year-old J.C., a resident of an assisted living facility, was admitted to critical care at 1600 yesterday for treatment following a motor vehicle crash. J.C. has a fractured right wrist, a fractured sternum, a severe right ankle sprain, multiple contusions, and abrasions. Her admission orders included:

- Continue usual medications
- Give meperidine (Demerol) via patient controlled analgesia (PCA) as needed for pain
- Administer promethazine (Phenergan) 25 mg IVP every 4 hours PRN for nausea

The night nurse reports that J.C. received promethazine three times during the night and the meperidine PCA was discontinued at 0200. Apparently, J.C. became hyperactive around midnight; she was verbally abusive and angry. Following this episode of hyperactivity, she became somnolent and difficult to arouse. In referencing the medication administration record, you note that J.C. used her PCA pump frequently until 0200. On entering J.C.'s room, you see she is awake, restless, and agitated. She has attempted to climb out of bed, and her right leg is entangled in the side rail. When you attempt to readjust J.C.'s right leg and move her up in bed, she curses at you and claws at your forearms and face.

Decision point: Based on above information, what might account for J.C.'s restlessness and agitation?

Decision point: What additional assessment data do you need to plan J.C.'s care?

Decision point: What are J.C.'s most urgent nursing care needs?

Case continues on page 1411

TYPES OF NEUROPSYCHIATRIC DISORDERS

Although the official classification system for neuropsychiatric disorders is the *DSM-IV-TR*, neuropsychiatric disorders may be classified in various ways. This chapter divides disorders into two general groups with respect to specific neurochemical concentrations and their effects. Delirium, dementia, and depression represent neurochemical deficiencies or synergistic effects, whereas schizophrenia, mania, and anxiety represent excesses of central nervous system (CNS) activity.

The Three Ds: Delirium, Dementia, and Depression

This section addresses three conditions that are often confused with one another and are frequently misdiagnosed (e.g., delirium diagnosed as dementia) or underdiagnosed (e.g., depression). From a neurochemical standpoint, these disorders are characterized by deficiencies or synergistic effects of acetylcholine, dopamine, norepinephrine, and serotonin. Patients with delirium, dementia, and depression may exhibit highly variable and unpredictable behaviors.[5]

Delirium. Delirium is an acute confusional syndrome resulting in dramatic yet reversible behavioral changes. It is a potentially life-threatening medical emergency.[3] Delirium is often misdiagnosed and inappropriately treated as Alzheimer's-type dementia despite its sudden onset and transient course. To complicate matters further, manifestations of delirium are under-recognized, particularly in patients with concomitant dementia.[16]

Delirium increases morbidity and mortality, complicates and prolongs patient hospitalizations, and increases the cost of care.[47] The 3-month mortality rate from a diagnosis of delirium in the acutely delirious patient is 34%.[14] Delirium can occur at any age but is more common in older adults. Delirium is estimated to occur in 5% to 80% of hospitalized patients ages 65 and older, 6% to 30% of the general hospital population,[14] and 7% to 52% of patients following surgery.[4,16,21,29,50]

Causes of delirium vary and may include disease exacerbations, metabolic disorders, fluid and electrolyte imbalances, and alcohol or medication intoxication or withdrawal. Infections, sepsis, hypoxia, fractures, pain, nutritional deficiencies, sleep deprivation, immobility, sensory deficits, intracranial insults, urinary retention, and fecal impaction also cause delirium.[4,14,21,26,58] Underlying medical conditions predisposing patients to delirium include hypertensive encephalopathy, seizure, sequelae of head trauma, and focal lesions of the right parietal lobe.[2]

Among older adults, delirium commonly results from polypharmacy, medication interactions, and medication toxicity, particularly from sedative hypnotics, diuretics, and anticholinergics. Many medications have anticholinergic properties that severely alter mental status. The effects of anticholinergic medications are additive if a patient is taking more than one. Box 50-1 shows common medications with anticholinergic properties. Correctly diagnosing and treating the underlying cause are the most important caveats for managing delirium.[14]

There are three categories of delirium: hyperactive (the most common), hypoactive, and mixed.[21] Patients with hyperactive delirium are restless and agitated, patients with hypoactive delirium may present in stupor and be barely responsive, and those with mixed delirium exhibit hyperactive as well as hypoactive symptoms. Because symptoms vary depending on type, the diagnosis and treatment of delirium become more challenging. Any acute change in cognition,

---

Box 50-1

Medications That Can Cause Delirium

Amantadine (Symmetrel)
Amitriptyline (Elavil)
Atenolol (Tenormin)
Atropine (Atropine)
Benztropine (Cogentin)
Chlorpheniramine maleate (Chlor-Trimeton)
Chlorpromazine (Thorazine)
Cimetidine (Tagamet)
Digoxin (Lanoxin)
Diphenhydramine (Benadryl)
Disopyramide (Norpace)
Doxepine hydrochloride (Doxepin)
Furosemide (Lasix)
Homatropine (Isopto)
Hydroxyzine (Vistaril)
Imipramine pamoate (Tofranil)
Lithium (Eskalith, Lithobid)
Meperidine (Demerol)
Methyldopa (Aldomet)
Metoprolol (Lopressor, Toprol)
Nifedipine (Adalat, Procardia)
Prazosin (Minipress)
Prednisolone (Prednisone)
Procainamide (Procanbid)
Prochlorperazine maleate (Compazine)
Promethazine (Phenergan)
Propranolol (Inderal)
Quinidine (Quinate)
Ranitidine (Zantac)
Scopolamine (Scopolamine)
Theophylline (Theo-Dur)
Thioridazine (Mellaril)
Trihexyphenidyl (Artane)
Verapamil (Calan)

Data from references 9, 10, 14.

---

consciousness, or both should be considered delirium until proven otherwise. Table 50-2 compares and contrasts delirium, dementia, and depression. Delirium is distinguished by a disturbance of consciousness that develops quickly and fluctuates over the course of the day.[2]

Prevention of delirium should be the major goal of care although there is no established, effective protocol. Interventions to prevent or treat delirium can be subdivided into four areas: physiologic, environmental, patient safety, and pharmacologic. Physiologic intervention begins with identification of patients at risk for delirium and proceeds to early diagnosis and treatment of underlying causes. Early identification and correction of dehydration and electrolyte imbalance,

TABLE 50-2 Delirium, Dementia, and Depression Differentiation

PARAMETER	DELIRIUM	DEMENTIA	DEPRESSION
Onset	Rapid, acute, often occurs at night	Slow, insidious	Rapid, related to specific events
Distinguishing feature	Fluctuating levels of consciousness with decreased attention	Memory impairment	Sadness, loss of interest
Duration	Hours or days, less than 1 month	Years	Variable, can be persistent or episodic
Course	Short, fluctuation worse at night	Long-term, progressive course	Variable, related to causative factors
Prognosis	Potentially reversible	Irreversible, progressive	Potentially reversible
Triggers	Multiple physical and psychological factors	Vary with the cause of dementia	Personal loss, stress, medication toxicity
Acuity	Medical emergency	Chronic, progressive disease	Episodic disease
Awareness	Reduced	Clear	Clear, but selective
Alertness	Fluctuates, can be abnormally high or low	Usually normal	Normal
Attention	Impaired, fluctuating	Generally normal	Minimal impairment, but distracted
Activity	Increased or decreased	Decreased in later stages	Lethargic or agitated
Memory	Impaired recent and immediate memory	Impaired recent and remote memory	Forgetfulness
Thinking	Disorganized, distorted, fragmented, can be slow or accelerated	Impaired abstract thinking, word finding, and judgment	Inability to concentrate
Speech	Incoherent and rambling	Inappropriate or incorrect, but may be close to correct	Apathetic. Often responds "Don't know"
Mood/affect	Labile, with rapid swings	Fluctuating, depressed, apathetic, uninterested	Consistent, from extreme sadness to anxiety or irritability
Sleep-wake cycle	Disturbed, cycles reversed	Fragmented, awakens often at night	Insomnia or hypersomnia
Delusions	Yes	Yes	Yes
Hallucinations	Yes	Yes	Not usually
Disabilities	Acute, new deficits	Slow onset and may conceal them	Recognizes deficits

recognition of concomitant dementia, adequate oxygenation, and correction of nutritional deficits are key aspects of physiologic intervention.

Environmental interventions for delirium include early mobilization, adequate and uninterrupted sleep, and noise control, which are difficult to regulate in critical care. Using glasses and hearing aids to compensate for sensory deficits, keeping familiar objects in the patient's room, varying light intensity to distinguish night and day, and providing a television or radio for stimulation may forestall or prevent delirium. Safety interventions include integrating reality orientation into casual conversations with the patient, preventing hospital-acquired infections, allowing the patient to participate in care, using bed alarms and wander guards, placing the patient in a room close to the nurses' station, providing clocks and calendars in the patient's room, and minimizing the number of room changes and transfers.

Pharmacologic interventions for delirium include using neuroleptics or benzodiazepines to manage symptoms, completing a medication evaluation to determine if the additive effects of medicines are causing the delirium, and managing the patient's pain. Risperidone (Risperdal) is rapidly replacing haloperidol as the medication of choice for patients with delirium.[26] Haloperidol (Haldol) is notorious for producing brutal parkinson-like extrapyramidal reactions; however, at only slightly higher than normal doses, risperidone yields similar neuromotor effects, which include tremors, slurred speech, restlessness, and muscle rigidity.

Dementia. Dementia is the eighth leading cause of death in the United States.[4] It has an insidiously gradual onset with progressive cognitive decline. Unlike other chronic illnesses, dementia does not remit, and brain insult results in global loss of intellectual functioning.[52] Alzheimer's disease is the most common type of dementia, and it accounts for 53% to 65% of all dementias.[4,14] It is followed by vascular dementia, accounting for 15% to 23% of dementias.[14] The remaining 14% to 20% of dementias are caused by other pathologic processes, including diffuse Lewy body disease, Pick's disease, Huntington's disease, Creutzfeldt-Jakob disease, Parkinson's disease, substance-induced dementia, human immunodeficiency virus (HIV) dementia, normal-pressure hydrocephalus, vitamin deficiencies, and endocrine abnormalities.[4,14]

Dementia occurs most commonly in older adults; incidence increases with age. About 1% of individuals younger than age 65 have dementia, in contrast to 10% to 22% of individuals ages 65 to 85, and 40% to 50% of individuals older than age 85.[14,29] The incidence of Alzheimer's disease and vascular dementia increases with age, so the number of people affected by both processes will rise as the population of older adults mushrooms in the decades ahead.

Alzheimer's disease results in a slow, unrelenting deterioration of mental and self-care capacities that change a patient's personality. The disease usually lasts 8 to 10 years, always culminating in death. Because of its slow course, early identification of Alzheimer's disease may be missed. Memory impairment can be masked in the early stages by social skills and memory aids.[52] Senile plaques and neurofibrillary tangles develop throughout the brain. As these plaques and tangles increase, patients experience difficulty with memory, decision making, communication, and ability to care for themselves.[14] Although the precise cause of Alzheimer's disease is unknown, current theories include loss of neurotransmitter stimulation, genetic mutations, loss of the protein that binds with beta amyloid, and influx of excess calcium into the brain.

Diagnosis of dementia is made by identifying an impairment in two or more of the following brain functions: language, memory, personality, cognition, and visuospatial perception.[3] Box 50-2 contains several evidence-based assessment tools useful in confirming a diagnosis of dementia. The Confusion Assessment Method; Folstein Mini-Mental State Exam; The Clox: An Executive Clock-Drawing Test; and the Geriatric Depression Scale could all be used in the critically ill patient because they take little time to complete and do not deplete the patient's reserves.

Treatment for dementia depends on the cause. If the cause can be corrected, appropriate measures should be taken. Otherwise, the treatment is supportive and includes pharmacologic and nonpharmacologic approaches. Significant dementia research is being conducted, particularly in Alzheimer's disease. A new class of memory-enhancing medications has been developed that can slow the decline of intellectual function, but rarely raise cognitive ability. Known as cholinesterase inhibitors, these medications increase acetylcholine levels and include donepezil (Aricept), rivastigmine (Exelon), and galantamine (Reminyl). Memantine (Namenda) is a medication approved by the U.S. Food and Drug Administration (FDA) in October 2003 for treatment of moderate to severe Alzheimer's disease. When used in conjunction with donepezil or other cholinesterase inhibitors, memantine appears to work by regulating the activity of glutamate, a brain chemical that plays a specialized role in learning and memory functions.[38]

Atypical second-generation antipsychotic medications—olanzapine (Zyprexa), aripiprazole (Abilify), risperidone (Risperdal), and quetiapine (Seroquel)—have been used to treat behavioral symptoms in dementia; however, the FDA recently issued a warning that they are associated with increased mortality. Other medications used for the treatment of dementia include

Box 50-2

Evidence-Based Assessment Tools

Process	Tool
Delirium	Confusion Assessment Method
	Neecham Confusion Scale
	The Memorial Delirium Assessment Scale
Dementia	Folstein Mini Mental State Exam
	Cognitive Capacity Screening Exam
	The Clox: An Executive Clock-Drawing Test
	Activities of Daily Living Exam
	Instrumental Activities of Daily Living Exam
	Neuropsychiatric Inventory
	Behavioral Pathology in Alzheimer's Disease Scale
	Cohen-Mansfield Agitation Inventory
	Agitated Behavior Dementia Scale
Depression	Center for Epidemiological Studies Depression Scale
	Geriatric Depression Scale
	Beck Depression Inventory
	Hamilton Rating Scale for Depression
	Zung Depression Scale
	Hopkins Symptom Checklist
	Montgomery Asberg Depression Rating Scale
	Inventory for Depressive Symptoms

vitamins, ginkgo biloba, antiinflammatory agents, statins, estrogen, antidepressants, and mood stabilizers.[60]

The goals of nonpharmacologic treatment are to maintain functional capacity, independence, and quality of life. Nonpharmacologic treatment measures include reducing stress, providing cues to prompt memory, using sensory enhancements, adjusting daily routines to focus on the person, encouraging socialization to prevent sensory deprivation and isolation, and offering structured activities to alleviate agitation and boredom.[52] Most patients require continual care and institutionalization in the latter stages of dementia. The burden to caregivers who keep patients with dementia at home is significant; therefore decisions about when and where to discharge the patient should be started early.

Depression. Depression is a common psychiatric disorder. According to an Institute of Medicine report, unipolar depression will be the leading cause of global disability within the next decade.[30] An estimated 8.3% of adolescents, 5.3% of adults, and 6% of elders have been diagnosed with major depression in the United States.[45] Depression is underdiagnosed and undertreated, particularly among older adults, and is seen in 20% to 30% of patients with dementia.[26]

Although the incidence of depression is similar across all races and ethnic groups,[17] there are gender differences—more women than men are affected worldwide. Depression frequently accompanies acute and chronic illness with prevalence rates as high as 70%.[29] Treatment and lost productivity due to depression cost billions of dollars annually. The cause of depression is thought to be dysregulation of the neurotransmitters serotonin, norepinephrine, epinephrine, and dopamine.[17] The underlying medical conditions predisposing people to depression (and carrying the greatest risk for suicide) include chronic, incurable, and painful conditions (e.g., malignancy, spinal cord injury, peptic ulcer disease, Huntington's disease, acquired immunodeficiency syndrome [AIDS], and end-stage renal disease).[2]

Depression slows all bodily processes, including elimination; therefore, clinically depressed patients must be observed for signs of constipation and urinary retention. Depression also slows cognition, leading mental health professionals to use the term *pseudodementia*[29] when referring to depressive symptoms (e.g., poor attention span and memory loss). Diagnosis of depression begins with a comprehensive assessment. Presenting symptoms include insomnia or hypersomnia; tiredness; lack of energy; overeating or undereating; difficulty concentrating and making decisions; lack of interest in personal appearance; sexual dysfunction; avoidance of interpersonal interactions; delusions; hallucinations; vague somatic complaints; feelings of sadness, despair, misery, self-loathing, and guilt; and suicidal ideation.[1] Several evidence-based depression assessment scales are identified in Box 50-2. Physiologic processes that mimic depression (e.g., vitamin deficiencies, hypothyroidism) must be ruled out as causes.

Treatment of depression is aimed at eliminating symptoms, reducing recurrence, and increasing quality of life.[14] Both pharmacologic and nonpharmacologic therapies are used to treat depression. Major nonpharmacologic therapies for depression are psychotherapy and electroconvulsive therapy. Other therapies include phototherapy, increased physical exercise to raise serotonin levels, transcranial magnetic stimulation, vagus nerve stimulation, and herbal remedies (St. John's wort).[17] The four classes of antidepressant medications are selective serotonin reuptake inhibitors (SSRIs), tricyclic antidepressants (TCAs), monoamine oxidase inhibitors (MAOIs), and atypical antidepressants. Agents in these classes are summarized in the Medication table on pp. 1407-1410. All antidepressants interact with other medications. The most frequently used and safest

MEDICATIONS USED IN THE TREATMENT OF NEUROPSYCHIATRIC DISORDERS

MEDICATION	ACTIONS	DOSAGE	SPECIAL CONSIDERATIONS
Antianxiety			
Buspirone hydrochloride (BuSpar)	Binds to serotonin, dopamine at presynaptic neurotransmitter receptors in the CNS	5 mg 2 or 3 times daily PO or 7.5 mg 2 times/day PO. May increase in 5-mg increments/day at intervals of 2–4 days. Maintenance: 15–30 mg/day in 2 or 3 divided doses. Maximum dose 60 mg/day	Can cause hypotension, sedation, nausea, and dry mouth. Interacts with CNS depressants, alcohol, and other antidepressants. Can cause moderate to severe renal or hepatic impairment. May increase serum transaminase levels. May displace digoxin from serum binding, increasing the risk for drug toxicity.
Benzodiazepines	Enhance action of inhibitory neurotransmitters in the brain	Alprazolam (Xanax): 0.25–0.5 mg PO tid, may titrate every 3–4 days to a max dose of 4 mg/day in divided doses Clonazepam (Clonapam; Klonopin): 1.5 mg PO daily, may titrate, do not exceed maintenance dosage of 0.2 mg/kg/day Lorazepam (Ativan): PO: 2–6 mg/day in 2 or 3 divided doses. Max dose is 10 mg/day	Observe for paradoxical reaction. Can cause respiratory depression. Can transiently elevate serum transaminases and alkaline phosphatase. Can reach toxic levels if there is renal impairment. Abrupt withdrawal may result in pronounced restlessness, irritability, insomnia.
Antidepressants			
SSRIs	Inhibit reuptake of serotonin by CNS neurons	Paroxetine hydrochloride (Paxil): 10–50 mg PO daily Sertraline hydrochloride (Zoloft): 50-200 mg PO daily. Fluoxetine (Prozac): 10–80 mg PO daily Escitalopram (Lexapro): 10–20 mg PO daily	Can cause hypotension, sedation, nausea, and dry mouth. Interacts with CNS depressants, alcohol, and other antidepressants. Patients with hepatic or renal impairment need a lower dose. May cause hyponatremia. May cause swings in glucose levels.
TCAs	Inhibit reuptake of norepinephrine and serotonin from the synaptic gap	Amitriptyline (Elavil, Amitril): 75–300 mg PO in 1–3 divided doses daily Amoxapine (Asendin): 50-100 mg PO tid Clomipramine (Anafranil): 75–300 mg PO daily	Can cause sedation, orthostasis, dry mouth, urinary retention, and constipation. Can interact with cimetidine, oral contraceptives, clonidine, guanethidine, alcohol, and other CNS depressants.
Atypical	Balance neurotransmitters in the brain. May inhibit reuptake of either dopamine, serotonin or norepinephrine depending on the drug	Duloxetine (Cymbalta): 20–30 mg PO bid Bupropion (Wellbutrin): 100 mg PO bid or tid Max total daily dose is 450 mg Venlafaxine (Effexor): 37.5–75 mg PO daily tid; max total daily dose is 225 mg	Can increase blood pressure and heart rate. Can cause dizziness, nausea, vomiting, dry mouth, somnolence, and sweating. Use cautiously in patients with renal and hepatic impairment. Can increase suicidal ideation. Bupropion is contraindicated in patients with seizure disorders. Bupropion is also the active

Table continues on page 1408

MEDICATION	ACTIONS	DOSAGE	SPECIAL CONSIDERATIONS
			ingredient in Zyban, a smoking cessation drug. Do not give concomitantly with bupropion.

Mood Stabilizers

MEDICATION	ACTIONS	DOSAGE	SPECIAL CONSIDERATIONS

Lithium (Lithobid)	Accelerates catecholamine destruction, inhibits neurotransmitter release, and decreases the sensitivity of postsynaptic receptors	Loading dose:
		  Total of 1800 mg PO over 24 hours in either 600-mg tablets tid or 900-mg sustained-release tablets bid
		Maintenance dose:
		  300-mg tablets PO tid or qid
			NSAIDs, diuretics, and ACE inhibitors increase lithium levels. Theophylline, caffeine, sodium, and acetazolamide decrease lithium levels. Methyldopa, carbamazepine, calcium channel antagonists, antipsychotics, and SSRIs increase the chance for lithium toxicity. Monitor serum lithium levels; toxicity can occur even when lithium levels are within therapeutic range. Watch for extrapyramidal reactions. Monitor renal function.

Carbamazepine (Tegretol)	Decreases sodium, calcium ion influx into neuronal membranes, reducing post-tetanic potentiation at synapse	Initially 100 mg PO 2 times/day. May increase by 100 mg 2 times/day up to 400–800 mg/day Maximum dose 1200 mg/day	Toxic reactions appears as blood dyscrasias. Can cause respiratory depression and heart block. Do not abruptly withdraw medication after long-term use. Carbamazepine induces its own metabolism; may take 3–5 weeks to achieve fixed therapeutic dose.
Valproic acid (Depakene)	Directly increases concentration of the inhibitory neurotransmitter gamma-aminobutyric acid	Manic episodes: initially 750 mg/day PO in divided doses; loading regimens of 20–30 mg/kg/day have been used to rapidly achieve therapeutic levels	Observe for hepatotoxicity, especially in first 6 mo of therapy. Can cause liver failure, pancreatitis, and bone marrow depression. Therapeutic serum level is 50-100 mcg/ml. Toxic reactions appear as blood dyscrasias. Do not discontinue therapy abruptly.

Antipsychotics

MEDICATION	ACTIONS	DOSAGE	SPECIAL CONSIDERATIONS
Haloperidol (Haldol)	Blocks postsynaptic dopamine receptors, interrupts nerve impulse movement, increases turnover of dopamine in the brain	Psychotic disorder: initially, 0.5–5 mg PO 2 or 3 times daily Dosage gradually adjusted as needed Older adults 0.5–2 mg 2 or 3 times/day Typical dose range is 1–15 mg daily	Observe patient for parkinson-like extrapyramidal reaction: tremors, slurred speech, restlessness, and muscle rigidity. Can cause neuroleptic malignant syndrome, agranulocytosis, laryngospasm, and respiratory depression.
Chlorpromazine (Thorazine)	Blocks dopamine neurotransmission at	IM/IV: initially 25 mg; may repeat in 1–4 hr. May gradually increase to	Extrapyramidal symptoms appear to be dose related and are divided

MEDICATION	ACTIONS	DOSAGE	SPECIAL CONSIDERATIONS
	postsynaptic dopamine receptor sites. Possesses strong anticholinergic, sedative, antiemetic effects	400 mg every 4–6 hr, maximum 300–800 mg/day. IV—incompatible with many other medications PO: 30–800 mg/day in 3–4 divided doses	into 3 categories: Akathisia Parkinsonian symptoms Acute dystonias Can cause sudden, unexplained death. ECG changes can occur—prolonged QT and PR intervals, blunted T waves, and ST depression. Can cause neuroleptic malignant syndrome.
Fluphenazine decanoate (Prolixin)	Antagonizes dopamine neurotransmission at synapses by blocking postsynaptic dopaminergic receptors in the brain	IM: 2.5–10 mg/day in divided doses at 6- to 8-hr intervals PO: 2.5–10 mg/day in divided doses at 6- to 8-hr intervals	Extrapyramidal symptoms appear to be dose related and are divided into three categories: Akathisia Parkinsonian symptoms Acute dystonias May cause impaired thermoregulation, agranulocytosis, hypotension.

Second-Generation Antipsychotics

MEDICATION	ACTIONS	DOSAGE	SPECIAL CONSIDERATIONS
Aripiprazole (Abilify)	Provides partial agonist activity at dopamine and serotonin receptors and antagonist activity at serotonin receptors	10–15 mg once daily. May increase up to 30 mg/day	Extrapyramidal symptoms, NMS rarely occur. Monitor diabetic patients for loss of glucose control. May cause orthostasis.
Olanzapine (Zyprexa)	Antagonizes dopamine, serotonin, muscarinic, histamine, alpha$_1$-adrenergic receptors. Produces anticholinergic, histaminic, CNS depressant effects	PO: 5–15 mg/day; may titrate to desired effect. Maximum 20 mg/day IM: 2.5–10 mg; may repeat in 2 hr after first dose and 4 hr after second dose. Maximum 30 mg/day	NMS and extrapyramidal symptoms can occur. May enhance hypotensive effects of antihypertensive medications. Monitor diabetic patients for loss of glucose control. Monitor LFTs, particularly in patients with liver disease. Can cause orthostasis.
Quetiapine (Seroquel)	Interacts with neurotransmitter receptors, including dopamine, serotonin, histamine, alpha$_1$-adrenergic receptors	Maintenance dose: 300–800 mg per day PO	Overdosage produces heart block, decreased BP, hypokalemia, tachycardia. Monitor diabetic patients for loss of glucose control. Can lower the seizure threshold.
Risperidone (Risperdal)	Dopamine, serotonin receptor antagonism	Psychotic disorder: initially, 0.5–1 mg PO bid; reduce in older adults to 0.25–2 mg/day PO in 1 or 2 divided doses. Range 2–8 mg/day Mania: initially, 2–3 mg PO as a single daily dose. May increase at 24-hr intervals of 1 mg/day. Range 2–6 mg/day	Observe patient for signs of neuroleptic malignant syndrome and tardive dyskinesia. Can elevate LFTs. Monitor diabetic patients for loss of glucose control. Can prolong the QTc interval and cause tachycardia.

Table continues on page 1410

MEDICATION	ACTIONS	DOSAGE	SPECIAL CONSIDERATIONS
Ziprasidone (Geodon)	Antagonizes dopamine, serotonin, histamine, alpha$_1$-adrenergic receptors; inhibits reuptake of serotonin, norepinephrine	Initially 20 mg 2 times/day PO with food; titrate at intervals of no less than 2 days. Maximum dose: 80 mg PO bid	Prolongation of QT/QTc interval as seen on ECG. May produce torsades de pointes. Do not administer to patients with known cardiac disease. Monitor diabetic patients for loss of glucose control.

Cholinesterase Inhibitors—Anti-Alzheimer's Dementia Agents

MEDICATION	ACTIONS	DOSAGE	SPECIAL CONSIDERATIONS
Donepezil hydrochloride (Aricept)	Enhances cholinergic function by increasing the concentration of acetylcholine through inhibition of the hydrolysis of acetylcholine by the enzyme acetylcholinesterase	Alzheimer's disease: 5–10 mg/day as a single dose	Overdosage may result in cholinergic crisis. Use cautiously in patients with cardiac disease, GI bleeding, and pulmonary disease. Monitor for GI bleeding, especially if the patient is on an NSAID.
Rivastigmine tartrate (Exelon)	Increases the concentration of acetylcholine through reversible inhibition of its hydrolysis by cholinesterase	Alzheimer's disease: initially, 1.5 mg twice a day. Increase dosage after a minimum of 1–2 wk. Maximum 6 mg twice a day	Overdosage may result in cholinergic crisis. May exacerbate muscle reactions to paralytics. Monitor diabetic patients for loss of glucose control.
Galantamine (Reminyl)	Elevates acetylcholine concentrations in cerebral cortex by slowing degeneration of acetylcholine released by still-intact cholinergic neurons	Alzheimer's disease: initially, 4 mg twice a day (8 mg/day). If tolerated after a minimum of 4 wk, may increase dosage. Range is 16–24 mg/day in two divided doses. Max total daily dose is 32 mg	Overdosage may result in cholinergic crisis. Not recommended in patients with severe renal or hepatic dysfunction. May cause orthostasis.
Memantine hydrochloride (Namenda)	Decreases the effects of glutamate, the principal excitatory neurotransmitter in the brain	Alzheimer's disease: initially, 5 mg once/day, with target dose of 20 mg/day. Increase in 5-mg increments to 10 mg/day, 15 mg/day, 20 mg/day. Total dosage should be given in 2 doses. Recommended dose increases are in 1-wk increments	Use cautiously in moderate to severe renal impairment. Can cause hypertension and cardiac failure. Monitor diabetic patients for loss of glucose control. Can cause hallucinations, ataxia, aggression, and agitation.

Data from references 20, 21, 31.
ACE = Angiotensin-converting enzyme, BP = blood pressure, CNS = central nervous system, ECG = electrocardiogram, GI = gastrointestinal, LFTs = liver function tests, NMS = neuroleptic malignant syndrome, NSAIDs = nonsteroidal antiinflammatory drugs, SSRIs = selective serotonin reuptake inhibitors, TCAs = tricyclic antidepressants.

are the SSRIs, including escitalopram (Lexapro), paroxetine (Paxil), and sertraline (Zoloft) and the atypical agents, including venlafaxine (Effexor XR), duloxetine (Cymbalta), and bupropion (Wellbutrin).

Serotonin syndrome, a rare but potentially lethal condition, can occur when two or more medications that enhance serotonin transmission are given together. Serotonin syndrome occurs when mixing any of the following medications: SSRIs, MAOIs, TCAs, dextromethorphan, meperidine, and lithium. Symptoms include autonomic instability, hyperreflexia, shivering, diaphoresis, hypertension, tremors, mental status changes, and ataxia.[1,17,48] Immediate recognition and intervention are needed to prevent the potentially fatal complications of rhabdomyolysis, multiple organ dysfunction syndrome, and disseminated intravascular coagulation. The offending medication should be discontinued and the physician notified.

◆ **Case Study 50-1, Part B**

A Review of Background Information and Medical Records

After situating J.C. comfortably in bed, you sit by her bedside and begin to review her chart. According to the chart, she presented as "a pleasant, slightly confused elderly woman in moderate pain" when admitted late yesterday afternoon with multiple injuries from a motor vehicle accident. J.C.'s daughter accompanied her mother to critical care. J.C.'s daughter told the admitting nurse that her mother "moved to an assisted living facility 6 months ago and is able to care for herself in her own apartment." The daughter also confided that J.C. has suffered a gradual cognitive decline over the past 2 years and was recently diagnosed with early Alzheimer's disease.

When you look up from J.C.'s chart, you notice that J.C. still thrashes about in bed, but she seems comforted by your quiet presence. Continuing your review of the chart, you note that hypertension, degenerative joint disease, and hypothyroidism

are listed in the past medical history. Her medications prior to admission included:

- Donepezil 10 mg daily
- Levothyroxine (Synthroid) 0.05 mg daily
- Celecoxib (Celebrex) 200 mg daily
- Nifedipine (Procardia) 20 mg twice daily
- Furosemide (Lasix) 20 mg daily

Decision point: What type of delirium is J.C. experiencing?

Decision point: What diagnoses does J.C. have that put her at risk for delirium?

Decision point: What medications is J.C. taking that might predispose her to delirium?

Decision point: What are two major treatment goals for delirium?

Schizophrenia, Mania, and Anxiety

This section discusses commonalities and differences among psychotic, mood, and anxiety-related disorders. From a neurochemical standpoint, these disorders are characterized by excesses of dopamine, norepinephrine, and serotonin. Patients with schizophrenia, mania, or acute anxiety exhibit excitation and hypersensitivity to internal and external stimuli.[39] In short, their CNS is supercharged.

Schizophrenia. The schizophrenias are a group of psychotic disorders characterized by disturbed or loosely associated thoughts, misperceived or falsified interpretations of reality, altered sense perceptions, apathy, ambivalence, lack of emotional responsiveness, and impaired interpersonal and vocational functioning. To think of schizophrenia as a single disorder is akin to thinking of heart disease as one malady, rather than several clearly distinguishable conditions (myocardial infarction, heart failure, cardiomyopathy). Types of schizophrenia include catatonic, disorganized, paranoid, residual, or undifferentiated. Each of these disorders manifests differently.

Schizophrenia exists in all cultures and socioeconomic groups. Approximately 1% of the population worldwide will develop this severe and disabling condition over the course of a lifetime.[30] Schizophrenia is responsible for longer hospitalizations, higher costs to individuals and governments, more chaos in families, and more public fear (usually unfounded) than any other neuropsychiatric disorder. Schizophrenia is a condition in which thoughts are fragmented and emotions are compartmentalized. Causes of schizophrenia are

complex. Schizophrenia most likely results from a combination of biologic, psychologic, and environmental influences on a person vulnerable to the illness. Abnormal levels of dopamine, norepinephrine, serotonin, and GABA have been implicated.[6,23]

Schizophrenia usually develops in stages. Premorbid behavior includes aloof indifference to others. People who will later become schizophrenic have difficulty forming and maintaining relationships. As they become more socially withdrawn, their lifestyle grows more eccentric. They begin to neglect personal hygiene, communicate in peculiar ways, and fail to perform in mature adult roles. Tasks that constitute the normal transition from adolescence to adulthood, such as establishing occupational capacities, are the very things that tend to pose the greatest difficulties for schizophrenic patients. Poor prognosis is associated with an earlier onset of symptoms, failure to complete college or high school, inability to hold a job, and lack of familial support. Even when prognostic indicators are in the person's favor, a severely distorted, internal representation of the illness makes sustained compliance with treatment unlikely. People with schizophrenia may not agree that they are ill (or ill enough) to warrant costly treatment.[11]

Schizophrenia is a chronic illness that follows predictable patterns with respect to chronicity. In acute exacerbations or relapses, positive symptoms predominate. Far from positive in the sense of being desired or desirable, positive symptoms of schizophrenia include intense reactions, such as full-blown delusions and hallucinations. Delusions are false ideas unmediated by logic; hallucinations are sensory experiences, usually auditory, without basis in reality. Delusions and hallucinations are stress-related reactions that respond favorably to hospitalization and medication.[36] After stabilization, the person with schizophrenia experiences remission of positive symptoms; however, negative symptoms of schizophrenia remain. Negative symptoms refer to lack of motivation, apathy, thought blocking, and dulled emotions—the insidious, often unrecognized silent suffering of schizophrenic patients. If antipsychotic medications are held during a critical care stay, some break-through of psychotic symptoms, including anxiety, confusion, suspicion, and withdrawal may be expected. These symptoms can be managed using interventions discussed in the Multidisciplinary Plan of Care section starting on p. 1413.

Treatment modalities for schizophrenia and other psychotic disorders may include psychotherapy and social skills training. These therapies are successful, however, only when used in conjunction with antipsychotic medications (neuroleptics). Older medications, including chlorpromazine (Thorazine), fluphenazine (Prolixin), and haloperidol, were effective for curbing positive symptoms, but they possessed troublesome anticholinergic properties and neuromotor side effects. The newer medications, including olanzapine, ziprasidone (Geodon), and aripiprazole, treat positive and negative symptoms and produce fewer neuromotor effects; however, they are known to cause obesity, glucose metabolism errors, and electrocardiogram changes, specifically prolongation of the QT interval.[54] Close and careful monitoring of neuroleptic therapy prevents the most serious adverse reactions (e.g., neuroleptic malignant syndrome, tardive dyskinesia, and seizure). Antipsychotic medications achieve their therapeutic benefit by exerting alpha-adrenergic blockade on the CNS. Sedation and orthostatic hypotension are common side effects. Because these medications are also beta-agonists, tachycardia leading to fatal dysrhythmias may occur with moderate to high doses.[19]

Psychosis is a generic term referring to schizophrenia and the schizophrenic-like behaviors of people with other medical conditions, including neoplasms, stroke, meningitis, Huntington's disease, hypoadrenalism, hypoxia, and hypoglycemia.[2] Fluid and electrolyte imbalances and adverse medication reactions may produce similar symptoms. For instance, a rarely reported sequela of procainamide (Pronestyl) use is medication-induced psychosis. Procainamide is used to treat atrial and ventricular dysrhythmias in physiologically compromised patients. If a patient reports experiencing an adverse reaction to procaine in the dentist's office, critical care nurses should be alert to the possibility of procainamide-induced psychosis. To avoid mistaking the schizophrenic-like symptoms for critical care psychosis, listening to family and client cues is helpful.

Critical care psychosis is a type of delirium caused by sensory overload, sleep deprivation, or pain; it reportedly occurs after 48 hours. Medication-induced psychosis usually occurs sooner.[24]

Mania. Mania is associated with bipolar illness. The person with bipolar illness experiences a range of moods from incapacitating depression to acute mania. During mania, clients describe their experience as an intense feeling of well-being, extreme cheerfulness, or oneness with the universe. The median age of onset is 19 years.[8] Although depression is more prevalent in women than men, bipolar illness occurs equally between genders.

As the height of bipolar mood swing, mania begins with euphoria, progresses through expansive exultation, and sometimes ends in frenzy. Symptoms of mania are categorized by severity. Hypomanic symptoms are not sufficiently severe to impair social or occupational functioning, and they do not warrant hospitalization. In acute mania, the person's overjoyous mood seems out of proportion to the circumstances. With boundless enthusiasm, energy, and self-confidence, the person with acute mania knows no strangers. Friendly and talkative, manic patients often claim to be on a quixotic quest and frequently grow irritable when others fail to appreciate the great quest they are undertaking. Manic patients can be belligerent, intrusive, and quick to anger. With the belief that they possess great wealth, power, and prestige, they may squander their life savings or accumulate excessive credit card debt. Hospitalization is required for acute mania. Delirious mania is the gravest form of mania, characterized by intense manic symptoms, self-neglect, clouding of consciousness, and psychotic features. According to the kindling theory,[39] one severely manic episode tends to yield another. Increased neuroreceptor sensitivity is responsible for this kindling effect.

Like schizophrenia, the causes of mania are complex; strong hereditary influence has been reinforced by study of the human genome.[8] Physiologic reasons for mania include brain lesions, medication side effects, and electrolyte imbalances, particularly increases in intracellular sodium and calcium. Biochemical abnormalities of dopamine, norepinephrine, serotonin, and GABA are implicated.[6]

Treatment for mania is primarily pharmacologic. In the high pitch of acute mania, patients require antipsychotic medications to rein in their expansive mood. Mood stabilizers are used to keep the mood on an even keel. Lithium is an effective medication for stabilizing mood; it is a mineral salt with a therapeutic blood level of 0.8 to 1.3 mEq/L. As a salt, lithium binds freely with sodium receptors. This competition for receptor sites can deplete sodium and cause lithium toxicity (levels equal to or greater than 2 mEq/L). The physiologic signs and symptoms of lithium toxicity are the signs and symptoms of hyponatremia, familiar to critical care nurses (Chapter 32). Consequently, other medications that increase the elimination of sodium, including diuretics and angiotensin-converting enzyme inhibitors, should be avoided or used with extreme caution when the patient is taking lithium.[8] Selected anticonvulsants, such as carbamazepine (Tegretol) and valproic acid (Depakene), are also useful as mood stabilizers; each has its own side effect profile, including blood disorders and hepatotoxicity, respectively.

Anxiety. Anxiety is both a symptom and a class of neuropsychiatric disorders. Levels of anxiety range from mild to moderate to severe. Panic is the most extreme form of anxiety. A person with mild to moderate anxiety usually feels energized or tense, exhibits discriminating attention, and solves problems with speed. Conversely, a person with severe to panic-level anxiety often feels threatened, distorts reality, and experiences excessive autonomic stimulation, poor motor coordination, diminished hearing and pain sensation, scattered perception, and inattentiveness.

Anxiety is pathologic if the response is greatly disproportional to the threat, continues after the danger abates, impairs everyday functioning, or leads to somatic consequences (e.g., colitis or dermatitis).[25] Specific types of anxiety disorders include phobia, obsessive-compulsive disorder, conversion reaction, post-traumatic stress disorder (PTSD), and hypochondria. As their name suggests, panic attacks are episodic. Their onset is sudden, and patients frequently present in the hospital emergency department with a pervasive feeling of terror, fear of impending doom, and intense physical discomfort. The previous traumas experienced by PTSD patients may predispose them to flashbacks, nightmares, and confusion in critical care.

Treatment modalities for anxiety disorders include cognitive and behavioral therapies as well as medications. The medications used depend on the cause or source of the anxiety. Sometimes antidepressants are recommended[18]; because antidepressants are psychostimulants, their use seems paradoxical; however, their use is justified if the anxiety is symptomatic of an underlying, chronic depression. Anxiolytic (or antianxiety) medications are most often used to treat acute anxiety and incorporate use of the benzodiazepines, including alprazolam (Xanax), clonazepam (Klonopin), and lorazepam (Ativan), along with buspirone (BuSpar) and beta-blockers.[41] Buspirone is less potentially addictive than the benzodiazepines; it achieves similar CNS depression without compromising patient alertness or arousal. By slowing heart rate, beta-blockers relieve the autonomic manifestations that patients associate with anxiety. Any of these medications must be monitored judiciously, particularly in a critical care setting. Interactions with alcohol and other medications are common and can prove catastrophic.

◆ Case Study 50-2

Drug Overdose

By mid-morning, J.C., your 70-year-old patient with mixed delirium appears calmer and quieter. You prepare to receive the next admission. At 1035, a 52-year-old male, K.E., is admitted to critical care following treatment in the emergency department (ED) for drug overdose. He is feverish and shaky, and his pupils are dilated. K.E. claims to see his recently deceased mother standing by the window. He angrily argues with her and pleads with you and "other people" in the room to let him die. According to the ED record, K.E. has suffered from depression for many years. After several sleepless nights, K.E. swallowed 25 of his 50-mg nortriptyline (Pamelor) tablets around 0500 today. Nortriptyline is a tricyclic antidepressant (TCA). Treatments in the ED included gastric lavage, central venous catheter, and arterial line insertion. K.E. is admitted for observation of probable TCA toxicity.

Decision point: What anticholinergic effects would you expect to see in K.E.?

Decision point: What cardiac effects would you expect to see in K.E.?

Decision point: What central nervous system effects would you expect to see in K.E.?

Decision point: What medications would you anticipate for TCA overdose?

Decision point: What nursing interventions should you implement for K.E.?

Decision point: What is K.E.'s prognosis?

Medications used in the treatment of the neuropsychiatric disorders are multiple and varied. See the Medication table on pp. 1407-1410 for specific information.

MULTIDISCIPLINARY PLAN OF CARE

It is difficult to develop a multidisciplinary care plan that addresses all critically ill patients with a neuropsychiatric disorder. Some relevant treatment approaches have been discussed. In this section, behavior-specific strategies for dealing with diverse patients are covered. Table 50-3 lists eight kinds of behaviors frequently seen among patients with neuropsychiatric disorders: anxious, confused, elated, hostile, manipulative, suicidal, suspicious, and withdrawn. These behaviors are identifiable and distinguishable through patient actions and statements. Verbal and nonverbal indicators of these behaviors are fairly easy to detect even in complicated clinical situations and critical care areas. To respond appropriately, critical care nurses do not need to know the nuances of every *DSM-IV-TR* diagnosis,[46] but need to master the ability to identify and distinguish these

TABLE 50-3 The Eight Most Frequently Seen Behaviors in Neuropsychiatry

BEHAVIORS	EXAMPLES OF NEUROPSYCHIATRIC, PERSONALITY, AND SUBSTANCE ABUSE DISORDERS
Anxious	Undifferentiated schizophrenia Alcohol withdrawal
Confused	Psychosis due to a medical condition Delirium, dementia
Elated	Bipolar illness—mania Acute psychosis
Hostile	Medication-induced psychosis Delirium, dementia
Manipulative	Bipolar illness—mania Antisocial personality
Suicidal	Depression Alcohol intoxication
Suspicious	Paranoid schizophrenia Cocaine intoxication
Withdrawn	Catatonic schizophrenia Depression

eight behaviors when clients, visitors, or co-workers manifest them.

Patients with neuropsychiatric disorders have overt behaviors. The expert psychiatric nurse can recognize each behavior and knows how to respond quickly, safely, and accurately. Symptom identification is familiar to critical care nurses. Becoming familiar with the behaviors associated with different psychiatric disorders will facilitate prompt recognition and, therefore, appropriate intervention for each disorder.

The Anxious Patient

In *The Meaning of Anxiety*, Rollo May distinguishes between fear and anxiety.[37] According to May, fear is a threat to the periphery of an individual's experience, but anxiety is a threat to the foundation and center of human existence. The anxious patient exhibits a number of autonomic symptoms that include pupillary dilation, palpitations, sweating, trembling, shortness of breath, dry mouth, throat constriction, choking, chest pain, nausea, dizziness, crying, fear of losing control, numbness, tingling, and chills.

Even under the best of circumstances, critically ill patients can feel afraid and anxious. Gently approaching the scared patient and demonstrating acceptance of nervously heightened activity or increasingly bizarre behavior are important. Patients who are intubated or delusional cannot express their feelings easily. Giving voice to anxious feelings, particularly if the patient cannot, may be helpful. If a delusional patient becomes more delusional and irrational, the nurse should not appeal to reason, defend her actions, or request detailed explanations. Instead, responding to the process would be appropriate. The nurse should stop what she is doing and say, "I think you are getting more anxious." Then she should sit quietly with the patient. If possible, she should not leave the patient's bedside; leaving or walking to another part of the room may increase the patient's anxiety. Anxious patients may use rituals or avoidance behaviors to manage their anxiety. The nurse should not interfere with ritualistic behaviors unless they pose a legitimate and imminent threat, such as compulsively drinking fluids[44] or repeatedly dialing 911. Patients with PTSD (e.g., combat or rape trauma) may startle easily, so they should be warned about sudden, loud noises or unexpected activity.

Because anxiety can be contagious, the nurse should create as calm an emotional climate as possible. A patient who is anxious may fear losing control. For the patient to whom losing control is a major concern, the nurse should gently explain that a response team and other resources are in place to assist in managing out-of-control behavior. Explaining a plan in matter-of-fact terms may reassure the anxious patient. To avoid sounding like a threat, which heightens rather than allays anxiety, this verbal intervention requires the finesse that comes with experience. The nurse can enlist the help of a psychiatric liaison nurse or clinical nurse specialist as needed.

The Confused Patient

The unfamiliar setting of critical care may be disorienting to a patient, especially if that patient is hypoxemic, ketoacidotic, or otherwise at risk for delirium. A confused patient may be mute or mumble incoherently, appear clueless when asked simple questions, fail to respond or respond slowly when given a command, reply to unseen voices, see people who aren't present, or behave in odd and eccentric ways.

When dealing with a critically ill patient who is visibly confused, the nurse should offer explanations that are short and simple. The patient's environment should be structured and the schedule kept as predictable as possible. If a change is necessary, he should be prepared for it early. Consistency is crucial. No more than one caregiver should be assigned per shift. The nurse should set few limits, offer frequent reminders, and be lenient.[15,43] She should use tangible and familiar objects to orient and reorient the patient. The nurse should introduce herself, casually integrating the date, time, and location into the conversation, but cease reality orientation if the patient reaches a tolerance threshold or becomes agitated. A list can be posted to remind the patient's family and other nurses of the patient's routine activities and care. The nurse should accept regressive or infantile behavior from such patients. If a confused patient exposes himself or openly masturbates, the nurse should realize that he is expressing primitive impulses, much as a young child does. She should cover the patient and offer privacy.

The nurse should acknowledge hallucinations as *real* for the patient and convey understanding for how the patient is affected by them. For instance, once she has determined that a patient is hearing voices (about which it is okay, even prudent, to ask), the nurse might say, "I don't hear the voices, but I can see how upset you are by them." With a patient who is actively hallucinating, the nurse should avoid abrupt handling, accidental touching, hugging, or other gestures that could be misinterpreted.[3,15] She should reassure confused patients they will not be harmed by frighteningly unfamiliar objects, such as an oxygen compressor, nasal cannula, or rebreather mask. Even common objects such as a hairbrush, cup of lukewarm tea, or "razor-sharp" apple slice may appear strange and scary. The nurse should not assume that a confused patient is in full control of his language and behavior. Conversely, she should not act as if he has no control over his behavior. Exhorting the confused patient to exercise whatever degree of control he can muster at the moment is a reasonable expectation.

The Elated Patient

Although elation is most frequently associated with major mood disorders, other causes include primary endocrine dysfunction (e.g., thyrotoxicosis),[51] steroid use, and psychostimulant intoxication, such as amphetamine or cocaine abuse.[9] Medical treatment is the paramount concern, but dealing with an elated patient means staying alert to behavioral cues. An elated patient will display a persistently elevated and expansive mood, inflated self-esteem, incessant talkativeness, insomnia, hypersexual impulses, excessive movement, and racing thoughts. Intrusiveness, distractibility, irritability, and agitation are commonly observed.

When addressing the critically ill patient who is elated, the nurse can use mild persuasion and cajolery. Despite his constant motion and flightiness, an elated patient doesn't respond agreeably to being hurried.[28,39]

Too many people and too much activity can easily agitate an elated patient. It is important to limit his choices and reduce environmental stimuli, which are ubiquitous in critical care. As the main source of stimulation in the patient's environment, the nurse should speak and move slowly. She should avoid calling the elated patient by his nickname or speaking sharply. If elation reaches a feverish and frenzied pitch, the nurse can encourage hygiene, nutrition, and rest. She should also monitor fluid and electrolyte imbalances and provide replacement therapy, especially if the client is taking lithium.

The Hostile Patient

Aggression and hostility are more commonplace in nonpsychiatric settings than they once were. Because patients are sicker and healthcare resources are inadequate, patients as well as their families experience frustration without an appropriate outlet for its expression. People diagnosed with the subtype of schizophrenia known as paranoid may become easily agitated and combative, but contrary to the popular stereotype, people with schizophrenia are no more likely than members of the general population to exhibit violent behavior.[15] Other risk factors for aggressive or hostile behavior include a diagnosis of delirium or dementia, alcohol intoxication or misuse of other medications, youthfulness, overt threats against others, angry outbursts, and direct provocation within the treatment milieu. The number one risk factor for hostile behavior is a history of violence.[20,34] Shouting, shoving, and brandishing a weapon are the most salient clues.

When dealing with a hostile and potentially violent patient, visitor, or co-worker, the nurse must be alert, evaluate the situation, and solicit help. She should listen to the aggressive person, let him vent frustration or anger, and not argue or demand better behavior. She should strive to psychologically disarm a hostile person while communicating an expectation of self-control. For instance, the nurse might calmly say, "I can see that you're worried. Tell me what's bothering you in a way that doesn't hurt you or anyone else." Saying no too quickly and insisting that others do things our way are the biggest mistakes nurses make.[20,44] The nurse should avoid taking verbal or physical attacks personally, lower her voice, and adopt a nonconfrontational posture. Standing at a right angle to the hostile person and keeping hands visible are ways to minimize the patient's perception of a threat. Demonstrating the universal "no weapons" gesture and avoiding a locked stare with the patient send the same message.

The nurse can ensure safety of other patients and staff by assisting the hostile person to a safe place. She should use seclusion or restraint only as a last resort and always in the least restrictive way possible. A nurse should never approach a hostile person from behind, never block his access to an exit, and never attempt to subdue a patient or visitor who has a weapon. For example, suppose an agitated critical care visitor grabs a large pair of scissors from the nurses station and displays them menacingly. The nurse would move a safe distance away, motion others to do the same, and firmly instruct, "Put the scissors down."

The Manipulative Patient

When a critically ill patient cannot express his wishes clearly or is unable to read cues about acceptable behavior, he may try to manipulate nurses and other healthcare professionals. Manipulative behavior may be difficult to detect. People who frequently resort to manipulation may appear sincere and quite charming at first. They present themselves as victims; their stories are convincing. The target of manipulative behavior feels used and angry. Nurses may experience tremendous guilt for being angry at a patient, and they may need to debrief with a colleague or supervisor about the incident.

To deal effectively with manipulative patients, critical care nurses should establish and enforce limits firmly, consistently, and without exception. (NOTE: This approach to limit setting departs dramatically from the tactic taken with a confused patient.) Avoid giving ultimatums and making deals; limit responses to the present situation. The nurse should not offer choices when there are none, and should not argue facts. She should identify her feelings in order to avoid being drawn into defending her position.[4,55] She should respond to suggestive talk and sexually inappropriate behavior in a no-nonsense manner. The manipulative patient will be disappointed when he doesn't get his way, so the nurse must be prepared for sweet seduction to morph into rage when the patient is thwarted. She can acknowledge that the manipulative patient has been deprived of something important. She should explain that the patient's manipulative behavior may cause others to reject him. The patient should be held to standards. His self-esteem can be built with praise for socially appropriate accomplishments.

The Suicidal Patient

Although Thomas Szasz, professor emeritus of psychiatry at Syracuse University, asserts that suicide is the most autonomous human act, the majority of healthcare providers and bioethicists argue *against* the right of a suicidal person to kill himself.[53] Suicide intervention is mandated in order to preserve the person's autonomy for the future. Despite the link to major depression, a suicidal impulse, plan, or attempt is not a neuropsychiatric diagnosis.

Suicidal patients are not merely acting out or staking a dramatic bid for attention. A suicidal gesture is an intentional act of self-harm, which seems to contradict the value of human life that nurses hold sacrosanct. Suicidal patients present a great challenge to nurses, particularly those who work in intensive care. Critical care nurses experience mixed emotions about treating patients who have attempted suicide and wish to die. Critical care nurses may question the appropriateness of caring for suicidal patients in critical care, and they often feel inadequately prepared to manage suicidal patients.[5,10] Nurses without a background in psychiatric care often fear that if patients are suicidal, then talking about suicide will precipitate suicidal behavior. On the contrary, patients may experience relief that someone is willing to listen to their concerns, rather than leaving them to feel alone and isolated in a conspiracy of silence. If a nurse does not have the time or feels uncertain of how to deal with a suicidal patient, she can solicit help from the psychiatric consultation team or from a clinical nurse specialist.

Suicidal patients may have a history of physical, verbal, or sexual abuse. They may have survived the suicide or sudden death of a close friend or family member. Besides bereavement, other risk factors include loss of job, onset or progression of a chronic or disabling illness, threat of incarceration, and social isolation. Suicidal patients may voice veiled intent or speak openly about suicide; they may give away personal belongings, make funeral arrangements, write a will, and withdraw from loved ones. Suicidal patients typically exhibit a deadly triad of depression, hostility, and impulsivity.[56]

When dealing with a critically ill patient who is suicidal, the critical care nurse must maintain close surveillance and activate suicide precautions. She should recognize a sudden burst of energy, improved appetite and sleep, or an unexpected lift in mood as a cue that the depressed patient has mobilized the wherewithal to devise a plan and act on it. She should take all suicide threats seriously and determine the lethality of the threat. Even indirect statements such as "I don't see much hope for the future" should alert the nurse to inquire directly about suicide plans. Although most suicidal patients are not psychotic, the nurse should ask the actively hallucinating patient to describe auditory imperative or command hallucinations (e.g., "What are the voices telling you to do?"). Potentially harmful devices and instruments of mutilation should be retrieved. The patient should be observed for opportunities to hoard and overdose on antidepressant or other medications.

A suicidal patient may speak in ironic terms (e.g., "I don't like it *here*"), which nurses tend to interpret literally. Rather than clarify lived ironies or delve deeply into their meaning, the nurse should encourage the patient to talk (e.g., "Tell me more"). Evidence of the patient's ambivalence should be observed. Glimmers of hopefulness, happy memories, or expressions of moral uncertainty (e.g., "I can't leave my kids alone") provide occasions for the nurse to intervene. Without inflicting guilt or shame, the nurse can secure a verbal or written nonsuicide agreement and contract with the suicidal patient to tell someone if he cannot resist his suicidal thoughts. The nurse can provide genuine reassurance and life support if an attempt is made. She should be sensitive to the fact that a failed suicide is construed by the suicidal patient as an example of his ineptitude—another failure in a life characterized by a long succession of perceived failures.[27,56]

The Suspicious Patient

Even mentally healthy patients who voluntarily enter the hospital acknowledge that events and activities done on their behalf seem to be done *to* them rather than *for* them. If the patient is psychotically suspicious, this perception is multiplied exponentially. Although the structured environment and treatment patterns of critical care may actually help to bridge the gap between external and internal stimuli that fuel perceptual distortions of a suspicious patient,[42] critical care nurses must proceed with caution. A suspicious patient generally isn't reassured by touch. He may misinterpret it as an assault or a sexual advance. If you must touch him to administer care, explain why and limit your contact to only what is necessary.

Most suspicious patients are uncomfortable in open spaces. They may think that someone is coming up behind them. They should not be positioned in bed with their backs toward the door. If a suspicious patient must sit up, the chair should be arranged so that the patient's back is against the wall. Extremes of light or darkness may be another source of stress. Suspicious patients exhibit hypervigilance; they frequently dart their eyes around the room, turn their heads from side to side, and hide their personal belongings. They have a low tolerance for ambiguity,[7] become impatient with routine questions, and may make insulting or derogatory remarks meant to offend or repel others.

The critical care nurse should try to maintain a physical and emotional distance from the suspicious patient. She should be honest and direct, make promises clear and abide by them, speak in brief declarative sentences, and avoid making critical statements. The nurse should avoid secretive gestures, whispering, or figures of speech. Even common medical abbreviations may be ominously misconstrued with an unintended message (e.g., "PRN" may be interpreted as "Persecute Robert Now!").

Gaining and preserving trust are goals with a suspicious patient. The patient's delusion should never be challenged or denied. The nurse who either validates or denies a patient's delusion will become part of the perceived conspiracy against the suspicious patient. Instead, the nurse should look for and respond to the underlying concern. For example, if the suspicious patient says, "You're out to kill me; I have to leave," the nurse should not argue, defend herself, or openly disagree with the delusion. To convey empathic understanding, she might say, "Being in a strange hospital and not knowing what's going on must be very frightening." She should focus on what is real in the patient's immediate situation and anticipate the patient's refusal to accept food or prescribed treatment. Foods and medicine can be offered whole or in "tamper-proof" containers. For instance, a whole pear, rather than fruit cocktail, can be requested for the patient's dinner tray, and the patient can be allowed to tear open individually wrapped, unit-dose oral medications.[12]

The Withdrawn Patient

Admission to critical care is an overwhelming experience for patients and their families. It may be so overwhelming that critically ill patients may shut down emotionally to preserve their sanity over the short term. For clinically depressed or catatonic patients, the social and emotional withdrawal will be more pronounced and can interfere with medical treatment. Symptoms of withdrawal include little or no eye contact, a blank facial expression, slowed responses, barely discernible speech, blunted or dulled affect, sluggish or no movement, urinary retention, constipation, and poor personal hygiene. Grooming may underscore separation from others. For example, a bushy mustache or unkempt beard covers the patient's mouth, and oily hair worn in long bangs conceals the patient's eyes.

When dealing with a severely withdrawn patient, the critical care nurse must urge the patient to express feelings of anger, fear, or guilt. Clinical depression is not the same as sadness; in fact, the critically ill patient who presents tearfully and feels sad is exhibiting a normal response to a stressful situation. A clinically depressed or catatonic patient experiences an emotional vacuum or void. The nurse should provide simple diversion and distracting conversation without obligating the withdrawn patient to participate and can enlist the patient's help with basic care.

Malignant catatonia and clinical depression often look alike. Both conditions exacerbate the critically ill patient's medical compromise and hamper recuperation.[32,35,49] The stuporously withdrawn patient must be protected from the effects of self-neglect. The nurse should assist with feeding, perform passive range-of-motion exercises, administer medications that prevent thrombus formation, aid with elimination, and promote restful sleep. The severely withdrawn patient should be approached slowly and cautiously. Although the withdrawn patient seems totally unresponsive and motionless, he may react suddenly and forcefully when startled.

CONCLUSIONS

Underlying, unrecognized baseline neuropsychiatric disorders complicate the care of critically ill patients with serious medical illnesses or traumatic injuries. This chapter provides an overview of selected neuropsychiatric disorders and eight behaviors frequently seen in patients experiencing them. Nursing interventions to treat patients exhibiting these eight behaviors also are provided. The nursing care goal should be early recognition of neuropsychiatric disorders and rapidly instituted, appropriate treatment interventions to decrease or prevent morbidity and mortality. Referral to a mental health professional for diagnosis and treatment recommendations will facilitate patient-centered care for the critically ill patient with a neuropsychiatric disorder.

REFERENCES

1. Adams, M. P., Josephson, D. L., & Holland, L. N. (2005). *Pharmacology for nurses: a pathophysiologic approach.* Upper Saddle River, NJ: Pearson Prentice Hall.
2. American Psychiatric Association. (2000). *Diagnostic and statistical manual of mental disorders* (4th ed., Text Revision). Washington, DC: American Psychiatric Association.
3. Arnold, E. (2005). Sorting out the 3 Ds: delirium, dementia, depression. *Holistic Nurs Pract, 19,* 99–104.
4. Arnold, E., & Hallinan, K. (2000). Mind over matter: helping a mentally ill patient in an acute care setting. *Nursing, 30,* 50–54.
5. Bailey, S. R. (1998). An exploration of critical care nurses' and doctors' attitudes towards psychiatric patients. *Aust J Adv Nurs, 15,* 8–14.
6. Benes, F. M. (2004). The development of "mis-wired" limbic lobe circuitry in schizophrenia and bipolar disorder. *Psychiatr Times, 21,* 48–49.
7. Bentall, R. P., & Swarbrick, R. (2003). The best laid schemas of paranoid patients: autonomy, sociotropy and need for closure. *Psychol Psychother Theory Res Pract, 76*(part 2), 163–171.
8. Borovicka, M. C., & Love, R. C. (2005). Mood disorders II: bipolar disorders. In M. A. Koda-Kimble, et al. (Eds.) *Applied therapeutics: the clinical use of drugs* (8th ed., p. 80-1 to 80-18). Philadelphia: Lippincott Williams & Wilkins.
9. Ciraulo, D. A., et al. (2005). Nefazodone treatment of cocaine dependence with comordid depressive symptoms. *Addiction, 100*(suppl 1), 23–31.
10. Clinical research update: attempted suicide clients given poorer care in ICU. (1998). *Aust Nurs J, 5,* 34.
11. Dearing, K. S. (2004). Getting it together: how nurse patient relationships influence treatment compliance for patients with schizophrenia. *Arch Psychiatr Nurs, 18,* 155–163.
12. Detective work needed to solve paranoia in older adults. (2004). *Senior Care Manage, 7,* 11.
13. Edmands, M. S. (1995). "Murder!" she said: a case of iatrogenic delirium. *Issues Ment Health Nurs, 16,* 109–116.
14. Edwards, N. (2003). Differentiating the three D's: delirium, dementia, and depression. *Medsurg Nurs, 12,* 347–357.
15. Favro, D. (1993). Management of the schizophrenic patient on a medical-surgical unit. *Medsurg Nurs, 2,* 139–142.
16. Fick, D., & Foreman, M. (2000). Consequences of not recognizing delirium superimposed on dementia in hospitalized elderly individuals. *J Gerontol Nurs, 26,* 30–40.
17. Finley, P. R., Laird, L. K., & Benefield, W. H. (2005). Mood disorders 1: major depressive disorders. In M. A. Koda-Kimble, et al. (Eds.), *Applied therapeutics: the clinical use of drugs* (8th ed., p. 79-1 to 79-32). Philadelphia: Lippincott Williams & Wilkins.
18. Flynn, C. A., & Chenn, Y. C. C. (2003). Antidepressants for generalized anxiety disorder. *Am Fam Phys, 68,* 1757–1758.
19. Glassman, A. H. (2005). Schizophrenia, antipsychotic drugs, and cardiovascular disease. *J Clin Psychiatry, 66*(suppl 6), 5–10.
20. Haddad, A. (2005). Ethics in action: where do you draw the line between protecting yourself and caring for a potentially violent patient? *RN, 68,* 30.
21. Hanley, C. (2004). Delirium in the acute care setting. *Medsurg Nurs, 13,* 217–225.
22. Harrigan, R. A., & Brady, W. J. (1999). ECG abnormalities in tricyclic antidepressant ingestion. *Am J Emerg Med, 17,* 387–393.
23. Harrison, P. J. (1999). The neuropathology of schizophrenia: a critical review of the data and their interpretation. *Brain, 122*(part 4), 593–624.
24. Harrongton, L. (1993). Procainamide-induced psychosis. *Crit Care Nurs, 13,* 70–72.
25. Henningsen, P., et al. (2005). Somatization revisited: diagnosis and perceived causes of common mental disorders. *J Nerv Ment Dis, 193,* 85–92.
26. Henry, M. (2002). Descending into delirium: confusion, isolation, forgetfulness, lethargy: as one case study shows, older people with dementia and depression are especially vulnerable to the vagaries of delirium. *Am J Nurs, 102,* 49–56.
27. Horgan, D. (2002). Practical management of the suicidal patient. *Aust Fam Phys, 31,* 819–822.
28. Hummelvoli, J. K., & Severinsson, E. (2002). Nursing staffs' perceptions of persons suffering from mania in acute psychiatric care. *J Adv Nurs, 38,* 416–424.
29. Insel, K. C., & Badger, T. A. (2002). Deciphering the 4 D's: cognitive decline, delirium, depression, and dementia—a review. *J Adv Nurs, 38,* 360–368.
30. Institute of Medicine. (2005). *Nervous system disorders in developing countries.* Washington, DC: IOM Board on Global Health.
31. Keis, N. A. (1992). Cardiotoxic side effects associated with tricyclic antidepressants overdose. *AACN Clin Issues Crit Care, 3,* 226–232.
32. Krch-Cole, E., & Barnes, S. (1997). Malignant catatonia: a medically compromised psychiatric patient. *Nurs Spectrum, 10,* 10–11.
33. Levy, D. B. (1999). Managing the TCA overdose. *Emergency, 21,* 20–24, 27–29.
34. MacKay, I., Paterson, B., & Cassells, C. (2005). Constant or special observations of inpatients presenting risk of aggression or violence: nurses' perceptions of the rules of engagement. *J Psychiatr Ment Health Nurs, 12,* 464–471.
35. Madan, R. (2003). Catatonia in late-life: the importance of recognizing an uncommon syndrome. *Clin Geriatr, 11,* 26–28.
36. Marland, G. R. (1999). Atypical neuroleptics: autonomy and compliance? *J Adv Nurs, 29,* 615–622.
37. May, R. (1979). *The meaning of anxiety.* New York: Pocket Books (classic).

38. McShane, R. H. (2004). Memantine plus donepezil improves physical and mental health in people with Alzheimer's disease. *Evid Based Ment Health*, 7, 76.

39. Murphy, K. (2005). The separate reality of bipolar disorder and schizophrenia. *Nursing Made Incredibly Easy*, 3, 6–19.

40. Nelson, L., & Hoffman, R. S. (1994). What to do when drug poisoning causes tachycardia: standard guidelines may not yield successful resuscitation. *J Crit Ill*, 9, 831–842.

41. Nutt, D. J. (2005). Overview of diagnosis and drug treatments of anxiety disorders. *CNS Spectrums*, 10, 49–56.

42. Paranoia (2004). *Harv Ment Health Lett*, 21, 1–3.

43. Parker, B. A. (1992). When your medical-surgical patient is also mentally ill. *Nursing*, 22, 66–68.

44. Porth, C. M., & Erickson, M. (1992). Physiology of thirst and drinking: implication for nursing practice. *Heart Lung*, 21, 273–284.

45. *Prevalence and incidence of depression.* Available at:www.wrong-diagnosis.com/d/depression/prevalence_printer.htm.

46. Regan-Kubinski, M. J. (1995). Patient management consultation: learning the language of the DSM-IV. *Medsurg Nurs*, 4, 317–319.

47. Samuels, S. C., & Evers, M. M. (2002). Delirium pragmatic guidance for managing a common, confounding, and sometimes lethal conditions. *Geriatrics*, 57, 33–38.

48. Sato, A., et al. (2004). Life-threatening serotonin syndrome in a patient with chronic heart failure and CYP2D6*1/*5. *Mayo Clin Proc*, 79, 1444–1448.

49. Sheps, D. S., & Rozanski, A. (2005). From feeling blue to clinical depression: exploring the pathogenicity of depressive symptoms and their management in cardiac practice. *Psychosom Med*, 67 (suppl 1), S2–S5, S74-S76.

50. Sherman, F. T. (2002). Delirium: more than stroke; it befuddles both clinicians and seniors. *Geriatrics*, 57, 5–6.

51. Siconolfi, L. A. (1994). The forgotten system: endocrine dysfunction during multiple system organ dysfunction. *Crit Care Nurs Q*, 16, 16–26.

52. Smith, M., & Bockwalter, K. (2005). Behaviors associated with dementia. *Am J Nurs*, 105, 40–52.

53. Szasz, T. (2002). Fatal freedom: the ethics and politics of suicide. Syracuse, NY: Syracuse University Press.

54. Taylor, D. M. (2002). Prolongation of QTc interval and antipsychotics. *Am J Psychiatry*, 159, 1062–1064.

55. Trimpey, M., & Davidson, S. (1998). Nursing care of personality disorders in the medical surgical setting. *Nurs Clin North Am*, 33, 173–186.

56. Valente, S. (2002). Overcoming barriers to suicide risk management. *J Psychosoc Nurs Ment Health Serv*, 40, 22–23.

57. Walker, C. (1998). Homeless people and mental health: a nursing concern. *Am J Nurs*, 98, 26–32.

58. Webb, J. M., Carlton, E. F., & Geehan, D. M. (2000). Delirium in the intensive care unit: are we helping the patient? *Crit Care Nurs Q*, 22, 47–60.

59. Wintz, C. J. B. (1998). Nursing management of psychotropic drug reactions. *Nurs Clin North Am*, 33, 217–231.

60. Xiong, G., & Doraiswamy, M. (2005). Combination therapy for Alzheimer's disease: what is evidence-based and what is not? *Geriatrics*, 60, 22–26.

CHAPTER 51

Caring for the Bariatric Patient

Sandra L. Schutz

Obesity is the Latin word for "to overeat," and today in the United States there is an epidemic of overweight and obesity.[169] In 2000, 64.5% of the adult population met the criteria for being either overweight or obese.[66] Of those, 31% met the criteria for being obese.[84] When comparing the data from 1976 to 1980 with data from 1999 to 2000, a 40% increase in the incidence of over-weight individuals is seen. The prevalence of obese individuals has risen 110% using the same data for comparison.[169]

The adverse impact of obesity on health is over-whelming. Obesity affects at least nine organ systems in the human body.[105] It is estimated that 300,000 deaths per year in the United States are attributable to obesity,[5,82,92] making excess weight from poor diet and inactivity the second leading preventable cause of death today.[123] Compared with individuals of normal weight, individuals who are obese have a 50% to 100% increased risk of premature death from all causes.[178] Obesity also increases the risk of death in the hospitalized patient.[117] In addition to the risk of premature death, being over-weight and obese will result in many debilitating conditions that negatively impact physical, behavioral, and emotional health. The cost of obesity-related illnesses is staggering. It is estimated to consume nearly 5% of the total healthcare costs—$117 billion in the United States, of which $61 billion is related directly to the medical costs and $56 billion to indirect costs associated with diseases attributable to obesity.[178] These diseases include type 2 diabetes, coronary artery disease (CAD), and hypertension.[194]

The escalating epidemic of overweight and obese individuals and their requirement for obesity-related medical care has given rise to a new field in medicine known as bariatric medicine, which is devoted solely to obesity. *Bariatric* is derived from the Greek word *baro* meaning "weight" and *iatrics* meaning "treatment." The bariatric healthcare provider specializes in the causes, prevention, and treatment of obesity and obesity-related conditions.

A recent study by Nasraway et al. found 26.7% of critically ill surgical critical care admissions were obese or extremely obese.[130] The study also found commonalities in these obese patients, such as they were younger, were more likely to be female, and had sustained a significantly higher critical care and hospital mortality rate when compared to all other patients admitted with a prolonged length of stay. In obese patients with a prolonged length of stay, the odds of death increased greater than 700%.[129]

DEFINING AND CLASSIFYING OBESITY

The terms *overweight* and *obese* have meant different things to different people in the past. People who were considered overweight were defined by simply being over one's ideal body weight, a term that was defined by the insurance industry. Obesity has also been defined as a chronic disease associated with an abnormally high percentage of body weight without precise categorization of the degree or amount of fat.[111] Because direct measurement of body fat is difficult, obesity was defined as excess body weight. In 1991 the World Health Organization and the National Institutes of Health defined being over-weight or obese based on body mass index (BMI).[133] This criterion allows a more exact method of quantifying and defining the degree of obesity. BMI is determined by dividing the weight in kilograms by the height in meters squared. A person's BMI is a mathematical expression of his or her weight, adjusted for height (Box 51-1).

A healthy BMI range is 18.5 to 24.9 kg/m^2. Over-weight is defined as a BMI from 25 to 29.9 kg/m^2, and obesity is defined as a BMI of at least 30 kg/m^2. Obesity is further classified into three classes or subsets. Class I obesity is a BMI of 30 to 34.9 kg/m^2. Class II obesity is defined as a BMI of 35 to 39.9 kg/m^2 and the person is 40% greater in weight than ideal body weight.[129] A BMI of 40 kg/m^2 or more defines class III and is considered extreme obesity. This class is also labeled as morbid obesity. Other definitions of extreme obesity include patients who are at least 100% over their ideal body weight.[48,89] Super obese individuals are defined as having a BMI of 50 to 59.9 kg/m^2 or being 225% over ideal body weight.[48,89,111,116] The super-super obese have a BMI of 60 kg/m^2 or more.[89]

Box 51-1

Calculating BMI

The steps for calculating BMI are as follows:
1. Multiply weight in pounds by 703.
2. Divide that answer by height in inches.
3. Divide that answer again by height in inches

Data from reference 186.

THE PHYSIOLOGIC EFFECTS OF OBESITY

Obesity is a chronic, complex metabolic and behavioral disorder in which there is an imbalance of energy ingested in calories over the energy expended. It represents a condition of excess body fat relative to lean body mass.[24] This results when the body consumes more energy than it uses, leaving the body with an excess of energy. When this excess energy is not used, fat cells enlarge or increase in number.[22] The exact etiology of obesity is unknown but is believed to be a complex interaction of genetic, physiologic, environmental, and psychological factors that determine how energy is stored and used, and how fat is mobilized. A number of molecular mechanisms have been identified that lead to obesity or its negative consequences.

The fat cell in adipose tissue, the adipocyte, is considered a type of endocrine cell, with adipose tissue considered an endocrine organ.[22] The major function of the adipocyte is to store triglycerides for use as future energy.[96] The hyperplasia and hypertrophy of fat cells are the pathologic mechanisms of obesity. Adipose cells secrete the peptide leptin.[22] The role of leptin is to regulate fat stores by signaling the brain when there is depletion or accumulation of fat stores relative to total body adipose mass.[193] Central resistance to leptin has been suggested to be a prominent feature of obesity.[111] The obese appear to be resistant to the hypothalamic effects of leptin, maintaining excess body weight by interruption or inactivation of the neural triggers designed to reduce appetite and increase energy expenditure.[193] Leptin has also been linked to the increased sympathetic activity[81] and the increased inflammatory state found in obesity.[111] Leptin and its receptors share structural and functional similarities to the family of proinflammatory interleukin-6 (IL-6) cytokines.[88] IL-6 cytokines stimulate the release of tumor necrosis factor-alpha, which increases inflammation. Obese individuals have elevated leptin levels, but whether this is a result of obesity or a cause of obesity remains unclear.[50]

Insulin resistance also plays a role in the negative consequences of obesity. Insulin and catecholamines are hormones that influence the rate of lipolysis.[96] Insulin inhibits lipolysis of stored triglycerides in the adipocyte, whereas catecholamines stimulate lipolysis. In the absence of insulin, fat storage is reversed and lipolysis proceeds. Lipolysis causes the release of fatty acids and glycerol, which in turn promote conversion of the fatty acids into phospholipids and cholesterol in the liver. In turn, the elevated levels of free fatty acids will block insulin-induced uptake of glucose in muscle tissues, further worsening insulin resistance.[19] The high lipid concentration leads to the development of atherosclerosis.[78] Resistance to the action of insulin may also lead to overeating and weight gain.[164] Resistin, an adipocyte-secreted factor, has been thought to be associated with the insulin resistance causative factor of obesity. Recent studies have not proven that to be true, making the role of resistin and insulin resistance unclear.[36,109] Resistin also has not been shown to be a causative factor of obesity as previously reported.[109]

Other gastrointestinal hormones have been identified as possibly having a role in obesity. Ghrelin, produced in the stomach and duodenum,[45,98] is a hormone that stimulates appetite, as well as releases growth hormone.[165] Ghrelin levels are known to increase just before a meal, during acute fasting, and in food-restricted eating disorder patients (e.g., anorexia).[8,43] Plasma ghrelin levels fall shortly after standard meal consumption, and are abnormally lower in patients who have undergone gastric bypass surgery when compared to patients who are obese with no alteration in their digestive system.[44,51]

Many studies have evaluated the contributions of genetics and environmental control as combined culprits of obesity. Although results vary from study to study, approximately 30% to 40% of the variance in BMI can be attributed to genetics and 60% to 70% to environment.[152] Though there is no single genetic cause of obesity, the following two factors are genetically associated: the risk of developing obesity based on a family history of obesity and the age at onset of obesity. It has been suggested that biological relatives exhibit similarities in maintenance of weight and the degree of effectiveness of diet and physical activity on weight.[178] The presence of one or more biologically obese parents raises the risk of offspring obesity significantly. Individuals who are obese in childhood with obese parents show a stronger pattern of childhood to adult obesity.[108] Genes also play a role in the regulation of body weight through multiple processes in the brain and gastrointestinal tract that normally influence appetite. A person's eating patterns are affected by satiety centers in the hypothalamus and pituitary glands that react to high fat stores and hunger.

Three metabolic factors have been reported to be predictive of weight gain: a low level of habitual physical activity; a low resting metabolic rate for a given

◆ Case Study 51-1, Part A

Defining Obesity

J.W. is a sedentary 48-year-old Caucasian male who was admitted to the hospital for laparoscopic gastric bypass surgery. He is 6 feet 4 inches tall and weighs 214.55 kg (472 pounds). He has a long history of obesity, weighing 200 pounds by the age of 12 and 300 pounds by age 18. He reports that there is a long history of overweight individuals in his family, including maternal grandparents, his mother, and three of his four siblings. His obesity has been refractory to diet and exercise.

Decision point: What is J.W.'s BMI?

Decision point: Is J.W. considered extremely obese, super obese, or super-super obese?

Decision point: Another way of defining obesity is by class of obesity. What class of obesity is J.W.?

Decision point: What risk factors does J.W. have for the development of obesity?

Case continues on page 1435

body mass and body composition; and a high respiratory quotient in the fasting state in which the tendency is to oxidize more carbohydrates than lipids. A fourth metabolic factor may be high insulin sensitivity.[179] In addition, dietary patterns of modern society have been shown to promote weight gain and obesity, such as a high-fat diet and eating rapidly. These dietary patterns are often accompanied by more sedentary lifestyles. Of all the factors, low energy expenditure appears to be the fundamental determinant in obesity today.[179] Medical causes of obesity include drug-induced obesity, trauma, and neuroendocrine abnormalities.

COMPLICATIONS OF OBESITY

Health risks associated with obesity are the most prevalent and costly medical problems seen in this country.[84] Obesity increases the risk of or causes about 30 serious medical conditions, and it is associated with decreased quality of life and increased early death (Table 51-1 and Box 51-2). Complications occur either

TABLE 51-1 Physiologic Consequences of Obesity

SYSTEM	PATHOPHYSIOLOGY	CLINICAL MANIFESTATIONS
Pulmonary	Decreased residual lung volume from abdominal pressure on the diaphragm Pulmonary shunting following alveoli collapse Decreased compliance Increased carbon dioxide production Increased chest wall thickness Increased intrathoracic pressure	Decreased functional residual capacity Atelectasis Hypercarbia Hypoxemia Sleep apnea
Cardiovascular	Hypertension Increased blood volume (increased preload and afterload) Hyperkinetic circulation	Hypertension Elevated central venous pressure, pulmonary artery pressure, pulmonary artery wedge pressure, systemic vascular resistance, cardiac output Tachycardia
Renal	Increased renal blood flow Increased renin and aldosterone levels	Increased clearance of renally excreted drugs Fluid and electrolyte abnormalities
Hematologic	Increased blood viscosity Decreased fibrinolysis Increased plasminogen activator inhibitor Antithrombin III deficiency	Elevated fibrinogen levels Venous stasis leading to venous thrombosis Pulmonary embolism

Table continues on page 1423

SYSTEM	PATHOPHYSIOLOGY	CLINICAL MANIFESTATIONS
Gastrointestinal	Increased intra-abdominal pressure	Increased incidence of hiatal hernia
Metabolic/endocrine	Increased insulin and pancreatic polypeptides production Insulin resistance	Hyperglycemia
Immunologic	Endothelial inflammation Changes in cellular immunity Impaired neutrophil function	Increased tumor necrosis factor-alpha Increased interleukin-6 Increased risk for infection

Data from references 113, 150.

Box 51-2

Obesity-Related Medical Complications and Comorbidities

PULMONARY

Obstructive sleep apnea
Obesity-related hypoventilation syndrome
Gastroesophageal reflux–induced asthma or aspiration
Pulmonary hypertension
Pickwickian syndrome

CARDIOVASCULAR

Hypertension
Atherosclerotic coronary artery disease
Cardiomyopathy
Congestive heart failure
Dyslipidemia
Stroke
Pulmonary embolism
Varicose veins
Venous thromboembolic disease
Cor pulmonale

NEUROVASCULAR

Intracranial hypertension
Pseudotumor cerebri

HEMATOLOGIC

Hypercoagulability

DERMATOLOGIC

Hirsutism
Cellulitis
Venous and stasis ulcers
Acne
Intertrigo
Striae distensae (stretch marks)
Acanthosis nigricans/skin tags
Lymphedema
Stasis pigmentation of legs

PSYCHOLOGICAL

Depression
Poor self-image
Poor quality of life
Body image disturbance

GI/ABDOMINAL

Gallbladder disease (usually associated with cyclic weight loss and gain)
Gastroesophageal reflux disease
Recurrent ventral hernias
Nonalcoholic fatty liver disease

ENDOCRINE

Type 2 diabetes
Metabolic syndrome
Gout
Impaired glucose tolerance
Insulin resistance
Hyperlipidemia
Hypercholesterolemia

GU/REPRODUCTIVE

Recurrent urinary tract infections
Stress urinary incontinence
Irregular menstruation
Infertility
Polycystic ovarian syndrome
Obstetric complications
Fetal abnormalities

MUSCULOSKELETAL

Degenerative osteoarthritis of the knees, hips, feet
Intervertebral disk herniation
Restrictive mobility
Chronic low back pain

OTHER

Cancer (breast, endometrium, colon, and prostate)
Accident prone
Social stigmatization

because of the weight or mass of the extra adipose tissue or because of the increased secretion of free fatty acids and many peptides from the enlarged fat cells.[22] Evidence of comorbid consequences can be found in individuals with a BMI of 30 kg/m² or greater who have been obese for more than 1 year.[128] Of significance is the increased distribution of intra-abdominal fat and its link to an increased number of complications. The proportion of intra-abdominal fat continues to increase solely as a process of aging.[13] At the cellular level, upper body abdominal and visceral fat is more metabolically active and has a greater alpha-adrenergic lipolytic sensitivity than femoral and gluteal fat in the "pear"-shaped body.[168,177] Visceral fat increases production of interleukin-6 and tumor necrosis factor-alpha, which are significant in the development of insulin resistance.[168] The rates of insulin resistance, hypertension, diabetes, unfavorable lipid profiles, stroke, and CAD are all higher in persons with upper body fat patterns when compared to those with lower body fat distributions.[167,177] Box 51-3 lists cardiovascular risk factors associated with visceral obesity.

Metabolic Complications

Metabolic abnormalities are worse in the obese than in the normal weight individual.[112] Among the more

---

Box 51-3

Cardiovascular Risk Factors Associated With Visceral Obesity

- Blood pressure greater than 135/85 mm Hg
- Insulin resistance or hyperinsulinemia
- Low high-density lipoprotein cholesterol concentrations
- High triglyceride concentrations
- Increased apolipoprotein B concentrations
- Small, dense low-density lipoprotein cholesterol particles
- Increased fibrinogen concentrations
- Increased plasminogen activator inhibitor levels
- Increased C-reactive protein levels
- Increased tumor necrosis factor-alpha levels
- Increased interleukin-6 levels
- Microalbuminuria
- Increased blood viscosity
- Increased systolic and pulse pressures
- Increased left ventricular hypertrophy
- Premature atherosclerosis (coronary heart disease and stroke)
- Nonalcoholic fatty liver

Data from reference 168.

---

serious consequences is type 2 diabetes. BMI, abdominal fat distribution with a greater intra-abdominal fat accumulation (visceral obesity), and weight gain are critical factors in the development of type 2 diabetes. It is estimated that between 70% and 90% of individuals with type 2 diabetes are obese.[6,112] Data from the National Health and Nutrition Examination Survey III found that those patients with type 2 diabetes had a BMI of 27 kg/m² or greater, and the risk of diabetes increased linearly with BMI.[131] For a BMI of 30 kg/m² or greater, the risk rises to a sixtyfold to eightyfold increase for diabetes.[190] Elevated lipid levels are common in the obese. High triglyceride levels, low high-density lipoprotein (HDL) cholesterol levels, and increased low-density lipoprotein (LDL) levels are associated with increased abdominal fat (Table 51-2).[176]

Metabolic syndrome, also known as syndrome X, is a specific body phenotype of abdominal obesity associated with a group of metabolic disorders believed to be risk factors for CAD.[84] The syndrome is associated with a waist circumference greater than 40 inches in men and greater than 35 inches in women and is characterized by hypertension, high triglyceride levels, low HDL cholesterol levels, and impaired glucose tolerance.[84] Abdominal fat distribution also places the patient at increased risk of CAD. Although once thought to be due to the hypertension, dyslipidemia, and impaired glucose intolerance/diabetes found in syndrome X, it has recently been found that obesity and overweight are independent risk factors for CAD.[87,120]

Pulmonary Complications

Obesity can cause changes in respiratory mechanics, respiratory muscle strength, endurance, pulmonary gas exchange, control of breathing, and exercise intolerance.[112] The principal effect of obesity is to decrease the residual lung volume from abdominal pressure on the diaphragm. Men are more likely to be subject to changes in ventilatory capacity, possibly from the distribution of fat into a visceral fat pattern.[22] This is due in part to the elevation of the diaphragm from abdominal fat and the decreased ability of the diaphragm to flatten in inspiration, which reduces functional residual capacity to one third of normal.[146] This loss of volume leads to collapse of alveoli in the bases of the lung, resulting in pulmonary shunting,[146] which increases exponentially as body mass increases.[147] Fat deposited around the ribs, diaphragm, and in the abdomen impairs the ability of the lung to be inflated or compliant. The net effect is to increase the work of breathing.[146] The work of breathing is further increased when the obese individual moves from the sitting to a supine position, and from an increased carbon dioxide (CO_2) production that may exacerbate the respiratory load.[150] The overweight and

TABLE 51-2 Classification of Overweight by Body Mass Index, Waist Circumference, and Associated Risk

CLASSIFICATION	BODY MASS INDEX*	OBESITY CLASS	Disease Risk (for type 2 diabetes, hypertension, cardiovascular disease) Relative to Normal Weight-to-Waist Circumference	
			MEN ≤102 cm (≤40 in) WOMEN ≤88 cm (≤35 in)	MEN ≥102 cm (≥40 in)* WOMEN ≥88 cm (≥35 in)
Underweight	<18.5†	NA	NA	NA
Normal	18.5–24.9	NA	NA	NA
Overweight	25–29.9	NA	Increases	High
Obesity	30–34.9	I	High	Very high
	35–39.9	II	Very high	Very high
Extreme obesity	≥40	III	Extremely high	Extremely high

Data from reference 105.
*Calculated as weight in kilograms divided by height in meters squared: weight (kg) ÷ height (m^2). Conversion factor: (weight in pounds) ÷ (height in inches)^2 × 703.
†Measure waist circumference at the level of the iliac crest. An increased waist circumference may indicate increased disease risk even at a normal weight.

obese experience increased episodes of chronic bronchitis,[154] and these individuals are at increased risk of atelectasis, severe hypoxemia, pulmonary embolism, aspiration pneumonia, and acute ventilatory failure in critical illness.[97]

Obese individuals are also at high risk of sleep apnea from partial or complete upper airway obstruction, which may cause severe consequences and lead to episodes of apnea or hypopnea.[84] Sleep apnea is considerably more common in obese men than in women.[22] However, the degree of obesity is a greater predictor of sleep apnea when compared to age or gender.[46] Individuals with sleep apnea have an increased snoring index with an increased maximal nocturnal sound intensity.[22] The intensity of the snoring is related to the increasing inspiratory narrowing, which increases the work of breathing.[62,140] Loud snoring often accompanies respiratory-mediated arousal in sleep apnea.[140,187] Nocturnal oxygen saturations are also significantly reduced.[22] This may accompany such minor problems as daytime somnolence and morning headache. Ultimately, this may lead to systemic hypertension, a worsening of current hypertension, and eventually pulmonary hypertension.[84] At extremes of weight, obesity-hypoventilation syndrome, also called "pickwickian syndrome," may occur.

Arterial hypercapnia (partial pressure of arterial carbon dioxide [Paco$_2$] greater than 45 mm Hg) while awake is found in some patients with a BMI of greater than 30 kg/m^2. This hypercapnia is seen in the absence of any other known causes of hypoventilation.[139] Clinically, patients may present with symptoms such as excessive daytime sleepiness, fatigue, mood disorders, or morning or nocturnal headaches, which are similar to the symptoms seen in obstructive sleep apnea–hypopnea syndrome.[104,172] Instead, what is seen in patients with obesity-hypoventilation syndrome is daytime hypercapnia and hypoxemia associated with pulmonary hypertension and right-sided heart failure (cor pulmonale).[95] A study done on obese hospitalized patients with a BMI of 35 kg/m^2 or greater found that 31% had daytime hypercapnia unexplained by any other disorder.[137] Although weight alone did not predict which patients were at risk of hypoventilation, almost half of the patients with a BMI of 50 kg/m^2 or greater had chronic daytime hypoventilation.[139]

There is no exact known cause of the syndrome, although it has been suggested that it results from a complex interaction of impaired respiratory mechanics, abnormal central ventilatory control, possible sleep disordered breathing, neurohormonal abnormalities, increased neck circumference, and fat deposits in the pharyngeal area.[22,97,158] It has also been suggested that hypoventilation syndrome in the obese is under-recognized and undertreated[137] and is associated with a significant increase in mortality.[140] An arterial blood gas will confirm the presence of daytime hypercapnia and compensated respiratory acidosis and hypoxemia.[140]

Treatment may be necessary with nighttime continuous positive airway pressure and noninvasive mechanical ventilation.[140]

Hypoventilation associated with obesity is discussed in the Research Utilization box below.

Cardiovascular Complications

The cardiovascular complications of obesity reflect the increased energy requirements associated with moving an expanded body mass as well as perfusing excess tissue to meet metabolic demands.[111] Severe obesity is characterized by an increased cardiac output and an increased total circulating blood volume. Stroke volume increases without an increase in cardiac rate.[49] The increased cardiac output results in increased mean oxygen consumption, and the consumption increases linearly with increasing body weight.[49] Increased oxygen consumption in the presence of increased risk of cardiovascular disease and poor ventilation places the patient at an increased risk of cardiovascular event.

Hypertension is common in the overweight individual. Excess weight gain is a major cause of essential hypertension, and the resulting abnormal kidney function appears to be a cause as well as a consequence of obesity hypertension.[80] Increased sodium reabsorption results from a number of factors. It is believed to be one of the causes of obesity-induced hypertension, as well as a contributing factor to the increased circulating volume. In addition, a diet high in fat will cause increased sodium reabsorption.[59] Obesity is also associated with activation of the renin-angiotensin system from elevated aldosterone levels, increased sympathetic nervous system activity, and hyperinsulinemia, all contributing to increased sodium reabsorption.[80,111] Adipose tissue binds the aldosterone-angiotensin converting enzyme.[111] In addition to the increased pressures in the kidney, there is an inappropriately small natriuretic response.[80] The volume expansion creates hyperdynamic circulation, increasing glomerular wall stress and provoking glomerulosclerosis, proteinuria, microalbuminuria, and loss of nephron function in the kidney.[59] These changes occur before microscopic structural changes are seen.[59] Renal tubule flow rates are reduced, which also leads to increased sodium reabsorption. Other causes of hypertension are related to the chronic inflammatory state associated with obesity.[59] With prolonged obesity, there is increasing

---

◆ RESEARCH UTILIZATION

Hypoventilation (Hypercapnia) Associated with Obesity

CLINICAL ISSUE

As the population of severely obese hospitalized patients increases, the impact of the complications of severe obesity will affect the course of their hospitalization and the costs of healthcare. Hypoventilation syndrome is a common complication of obesity and yet may not be diagnosed before admission. This syndrome, if unrecognized, places the patient at a higher risk of morbidity and mortality. The study examined a cohort of hospitalized adults to determine the frequency, effects, and outcome of hypoventilation (hypercapnia) associated with obesity.

SUMMARY

Over a 6-month period, 4332 admissions were screened for the presence of severe obesity, defined as a body mass index of equal to or greater than $35 \, kg/m^2$. Of the admissions, 277 patients (6%) were found to be severely obese. Of these, 150 were enrolled in the study. Hypoventilation was present in 31% of subjects who did not have other reasons for hypercapnia. Decreased objective attention/concentration and increased subjective sleepiness were present in patients with obesity-associated hypoventilation compared with severely obese hospitalized patients without hypoventilation. There were higher rates of intensive care, long-term care at discharge, and mechanical ventilation among subjects with obesity-associated hypoventilation. At 18 months after discharge, mortality was 23% in the obesity-associated hypoventilation group compared to 9% in the obesity without hypoventilation group.

APPLICATION

In caring for obese patients, it is essential that the nurse be aware that patients may not be diagnosed as having hypoventilation syndrome but may in fact have it. This syndrome will impact responsiveness to sedation and pain medications and impact recovery from anesthesia, and in general places the patient at risk of significant hypoxemia that is preventable.

NEED FOR FURTHER STUDY

Based on the above findings, utilization of oximetry monitoring in the routine care of the obese patient and use of arterial blood gas measurements in those patients recognized as having decreased attention/concentration and increased daytime sleepiness may identify those patients not suspected as having hypoventilation syndrome and reduce the risks associated with the syndrome.

Nowbar, S., et al. (2004). Obesity-associated hypoventilation in hospitalized patients: prevalence, effects and outcome. *Am J Med, 116* (1), 1–7.

urinary protein excretion and gradual, worsening nephron dysfunction. This results in exacerbation of the hypertension, making obesity-related hypertension a risk factor for end-stage renal disease.[82] These changes also contribute to the excess volume load seen in obesity.[111]

Overweight and hypertension also have a secondary impact on cardiac function, in particular the left ventricular structure and function. Hypertension produces concentric hypertrophy of the heart, with thickening of the left ventricle. Although this change is seen in the obese, eccentric dilatation is also seen, with greater preload and stroke work required for normal function.[94] Increased cardiac work results from increased weight, both of the body and of the heart. The increased cardiac work associated with overweight may produce cardiomyopathy and heart failure in the absence of diabetes, hypertension, or atherosclerosis.[22] Increasing severity and duration of obesity influence the degree of these changes.[94] The higher levels of proinflammatory cytokines (tumor necrosis factor-alpha and IL-6) found in adipose tissue further decrease cardiac function.[76,180,182,197] The obese also have elevated levels of

C-reactive protein, which is a predictor of heart failure[94] and cardiomyopathy.[22,111] These changes predispose them to the increased risk of cardiac dysrhythmias and sudden death.[111] Figure 51-1 illustrates the role of increased body fat mass in the pathophysiology of hypertension and congestive heart failure.

The dyslipidemia seen in obese individuals also places them at greater risk of cardiovascular disease.[22] The abdominal adipose tissue distribution pattern in particular is associated with increased risk of CAD, as it is related to hypertension, dyslipidemia, and diabetes.[94] In those individuals who experience an acute myocardial infarction, obese individuals are at higher risk of recurrent events when compared to non-obese individuals and when adjusted for other clinical risk factors.[157]

There are electrocardiogram (ECG) and rhythm changes associated with the severely obese. There is a leftward shift in the axes of the P wave, QRS complex, and T waves attributed to the horizontal orientation of the heart in the mediastinum, which results from the restricted upward diaphragmatic expansion because of the obese abdomen as well as left ventricular hypertrophy.[7] The voltage of the QRS complex in standard leads is lower,

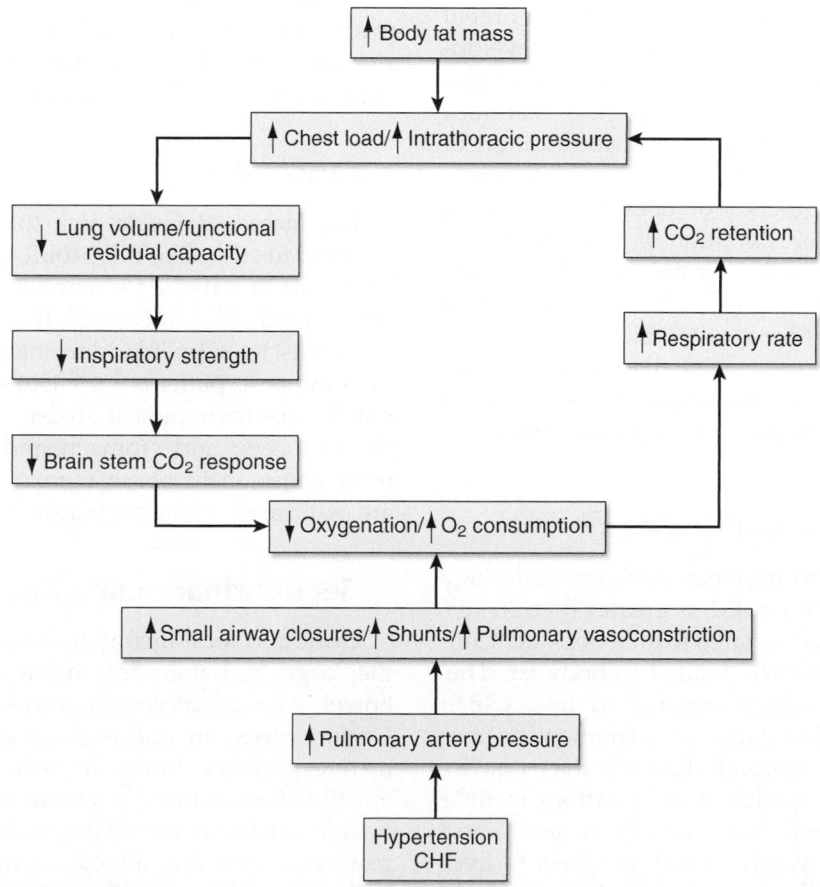

♦FIGURE 51-1 Role of increased body fat mass in the pathophysiology of hypertension and congestive heart failure. CHF = Congestive heart failure, CO_2 = carbon dioxide, O_2 = oxygen.

which correlates with excessive chest wall adipose tissue and epicardial fat.[7] The loss of voltage is believed to contribute to under-diagnosis of left ventricular hypertrophy by ECG criteria.[7] Obesity increases the risk of atrial fibrillation by 50%.[178]

Renal Complications

Renal function is also altered as a consequence of progressive renal injury. The obese patient's kidney shares functional abnormalities similar to the diabetic kidney, which increases the risk of susceptibility to insult and damage.[34] This in part is due to the presence of chronic hypertension and the impact of high pressures on the kidney, as well as the presence of insulin resistance and hyperglycemia from the metabolic syndrome of obesity.[9] The obese patient will have high renal plasma flow, increased glomerular filtration, and enhanced albumin excretion rates.[34,151] The presence of high pressure and high flow stretches the glomerular capillary wall and causes injury to the endothelial and epithelial cells.[34] This damage is thought to be the basis of the decline of glomerular filtration and development of glomerulosclerosis.[82,196] The glomerulopathy presents as nephrotic syndrome, with or without evidence of renal failure.[34] As body weight increases, the risk of developing kidney disease also increases.[69,183] Estimation of glomerular filtration rate (GFR) using the standard equations of Cockcroft-Gault (CG) or Modification of Diet in Renal Disease (MDRD) does not provide a reliable estimate in the presence of obesity.[181] Verhave et al. found marked overestimation of GFR by the CG equation and underestimation by means of the MDRD formulation.[181] Uncorrected, absolute GFR provides a more accurate picture of renal function.[34] With visceral or central obesity, compression of the kidneys occurs from adipose tissue and increased intra-abdominal pressures, leading to increased intrarenal pressures.[80]

Gastrointestinal Complications

Cholelithiasis is the primary hepatobiliary pathology associated with those whose BMI is greater than 30 kg/m^2. The risk of gallstones is related to total body fat. Cholesterol production is linearly related to body fat. This increased cholesterol is then secreted in bile, which increases the likelihood of gallstone formation.[22] Other complications include nonalcoholic fatty liver disease or nonalcoholic steatohepatitis. Manifestations include hepatomegaly, abnormal liver functions tests, and abnormal liver histology, which may progress to liver fibrosis or cirrhosis.[84] Obesity is regarded as an important contributing factor to gastroesophageal reflux symptoms.[138] The obese patient is at 1.5-fold to 2-fold more risk of the symptoms of gastroesophageal reflux disease (GERD) than normal-weight individuals.[60]

Mobility Complications

There is a 2.5 times greater functional limitation in the obese than in the nonobese.[185] They are frequently dependent on canes and wheelchairs and are at risk of ruptured or compressed vertebral disks.[148] Osteoarthritis, primarily in the knees and ankles, is significantly increased in overweight individuals.[22] Mostly it is from the trauma on those joints from the excess weight;[64] however, osteoarthritis in non–weight-bearing joints suggests that being overweight may alter cartilage and bone metabolism.[22] Excess body weight is also a risk factor in rheumatoid arthritis and gout.

Gynecologic Complications

Obese women experience irregular menses, amenorrhea, and infertility.[77] Anovulation is seen in women with a BMI greater than 30 kg/m^2.[77] The incidence of polycystic ovarian disease and hirsutism is increased.[22] Pregnancy is associated with increased risk of maternal death and fetal demise, and a tenfold increased risk of pregnancy-induced high blood pressure (BP).[178] The risk of birth defects, particularly neural tube defects such as spina bifida, is also increased.[178]

Cancer Risk

The increased levels of insulin seen in obesity are believed to stimulate cell proliferation and decrease cell death, making tissue vulnerable to uncontrolled abnormal growth.[106] Cancers of the esophagus, pancreas, renal cells, liver, gallbladder, colon, and rectum are common in obese patients.[84,112] Obese women are more at risk for postmenopausal breast, endometrium, and cervical cancers; and stomach and prostate cancers are more common in obese men.[112] Cancers in the obese are associated with a higher death rate.[112]

Genitourinary Complications

Urine and fecal incontinence are common because of the large abdomen impinging on the bladder and bowel, causing increased intra-abdominal pressure.[12] Urinary stress incontinence is seen in obese women; men experience lower urinary tract symptoms and erectile dysfunction.[127] Often, obese individuals are unable to adequately cleanse following toileting, which results in odors and infections. Infertility is common in both sexes. Women with a BMI greater than 30 kg/m^2 are at increased risk of urinary tract infections, particularly during pregnancy and postpartum.[3]

Dermatologic Complications

Dermatologic changes also occur. Stretch marks, or striae, are common in the obese and are from pressure on the skin. Acanthosis nigricans, with deepening pigmentation in the folds of the neck, knuckles, and extensor surfaces, occurs in many overweight individuals and is associated with metabolic syndrome.[22] Intertrigo (cutaneous inflammation that results from the friction of opposing skin surfaces rubbing together) commonly occurs in the groin, axillae, and inframammary folds, but can also be found in the antecubital fossae; umbilical, perineal, or interdigital areas; neck creases; and the folds of the eyelids.[90] Moisture trapped in deep skinfolds where air circulation is limited facilitates its development. The moisture can become a source of a secondary bacterial or fungal infection that causes odor or drainage.[90] The skins folds are also at risk of breakdown and ulceration from pressure[35] and cutaneous infections.[63] Lower extremity edema, lymphedema, stasis dermatitis, and leg ulcers are common.[53,72] Lymphedema in turn may lead to or exacerbate lower extremity cellulitis,[53,63,72] which usually develops in areas of skin breakdown, but can develop in normal healthy skin.[72] The injury can range from acute erythema with or without blisters to an open wound with extensive necrosis and exudate.[72]

Cerebrovascular Effects

Though the pathophysiologic source is unknown, it is believed that patients who are obese and have undergone a recent weight gain are at risk of pseudotumor cerebri (PTC).[71] The syndrome consists of increased intracranial pressure in the absence of a space-occupying or vascular lesion without enlargement of the cerebral ventricles; no causative reason has been identified.[10] The incidence in the general population is 0.9/100,000. However, in women ages 20 to 44 years who are 20% over their ideal body weight, the incidence increases to 19.3/100,000.[71] The link with obesity is speculated to be from the effect of central obesity causing an increase in the intra-abdominal filling pressure, increasing cardiac filling pressure, which limits venous return from the brain and causes increased intracranial pressure.[175] The clinical manifestations include headaches, asymmetric papilledema, and brief episodes of partial or complete vision loss, pulsatile tinnitus, blurred vision, diplopia, depression, and anxiety.[71] In one study, there was a resolution of the headache and increased intracranial pressure at 38 ± 8 months postoperatively following surgical treatment for obesity.[174]

Hematologic Effects

Hypercoagulability and the resulting development of thromboembolic lesions occurs at a higher rate because of increased viscosity, increased levels of fibrinogen and plasminogen activator inhibitor I, decreased levels of antithrombin III, and decreased fibrinolysis.[111,168] Human adipose tissue, in particular visceral adipose tissue, also releases thrombin-activatable fibrinolysis inhibitor (TAFI).[111,168] Increased levels of TAFI are seen with increasing BMI and insulin resistance, and are believed to be related to the hypofibrinolysis.[86] The result is recurrent or persistent thrombosis that is believed to contribute to premature atherosclerosis (Figure 51-2).[111]

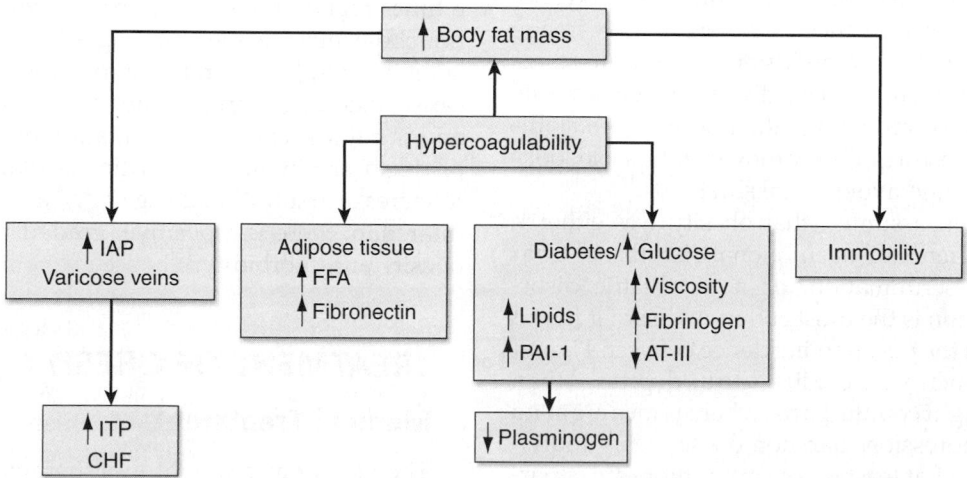

✦FIGURE 51-2 Contribution of increased body fat mass to thrombogenesis in obesity. AT-III = Antithrombin-III, CHF = congestive heart failure, FFA = free fatty acids, IAP = intra-abdominal pressure, ITP = intrathoracic pressure, PAI-1 = plasminogen activator inhibitor-1.

Immunologic Effects

The chronic inflammatory state found in obesity also has an effect on immunity.[111] Neutrophils have impaired chemotaxis and activation and are unable to migrate normally to sites of inflammation.[41,111] This loss of function places the obese individual at a higher risk of infection and may be the mechanism for the increased rates of cancer.[41] Cell-mediated immunity seems to correlate with the degree of injury and thus impacts the obese patient undergoing an open surgical procedure.[111] Infection risk is increased because of the hypovascularized adipose layer, which is a rich medium for bacterial growth.[111]

Psychosocial Impacts

There is significant prejudice and discrimination against individuals who are overweight or obese. They experience significant public condemnation with constant pressure to achieve the valued "thin" standard of beauty.[22] These biases have persisted even with the increased population of obese individuals. Healthcare providers are also among those who misunderstand, ridicule, and reject the obese.[155] There is a strong anti-fat bias in the media, schools, businesses, and in everyday conversation.[163] The view is that obese individuals are responsible for their excess weight and that their weight can and should be controlled.[155] Being teased about weight or receiving negative comments about size is common.[155] Society places a strong importance on thinness as a symbol of beauty, with the "perfect" body weight becoming increasingly lower in women.[192] In men, the leaner, muscular male who is well proportioned and has the classic "six-pack abs" is the social norm.[107]

Body image dissatisfaction with physical appearance is very common in the obese, especially with childhood obesity.[162,163] Interestingly, as they lose weight, body image improves,[162] although in some instances there are residual body image problems.[163] This dissatisfaction prompts these individuals to camouflage their bodies with clothing, change their posture or body movements, avoid looking at themselves, and avoid social situations.[162]

It has also been assumed that obesity was either a cause or a consequence of an emotional disturbance from prejudice and discrimination, or a psychiatric disorder.[14,124] Depression is the most common disorder found in the obese, with the reported incidence between 4% and 80%.[17] Obese women are more likely to be depressed than their average-weight counterparts, whereas men are at no greater risk of depression than non-obese men.[14] Individuals with a BMI of at least 40 kg/m^2 or more are at particular risk of significant depression, though the relationship between extreme obesity and depression is not well understood.[14] It has been suggested that more

extremely obese individuals experience a greater prejudice and discrimination than those who are less obese, which places the extremely obese at greater risk of depression.[14] Another theory is that the poor quality of life in the extremely obese because of limitations in daily functions is related to BMI and symptoms of depression.[14] In the extremely obese, there are no differences in depression seen between men and women.[141] The risk of depression in extremely obese women was nearly four times greater than in normal-weight women, and the risk in extremely obese men was nearly eight times greater than in normal-weight men.[141] Extremely obese individuals with a binge-eating disorder were also at higher risk of a mood disorder.[184] Suicidal ideation and actual attempts were found more frequently in obese women.[33]

Socioeconomic effects have been determined to be related to obesity. Young obese women are less likely to be married, have completed fewer years of education, and have lower household incomes than normal-weight individuals.[75,192] Males are also less likely to be married, but there appears to be no impact of weight on education.[75,192] Increased or excess weight may impact being employed, especially in women.[159] Many obese individuals report a decreased quality of life because of decreased vitality, social and occupational impairment, and bodily pain.[155] Other factors impacting quality of life include pathologic hunger, sexual impairment, excessive perspiration, urinary incontinence, and inability to clean oneself.[103] Obese individuals experience embarrassment dealing with public chairs, hallways, and aisles that are too small to accommodate them.[70] Regular-sized assistive devices, such as walkers and wheelchairs, in medical settings are unusable.[67]

The risk of death is significantly increased by excess weight—12 times higher in men ages 25 to 34 years and 6 times higher in men ages 35 to 44 years, compared to nonobese men of the same age-groups.[56] In the non-smoking adult, the relative risk of death from any cause increases abruptly above a BMI of 30 kg/m^2, and is not associated with a history of disease. The risk of death attributable to cardiovascular disease begins to increase at a BMI of 25 kg/m^2,[31] and postmyocardial infarction, there is a positive, graded relation between obesity and morbidity.[156]

TREATMENT OF OBESITY

Medical Treatment

The goal of any weight loss therapy is to produce a negative energy balance without side effects,[144] while at the same time reduce the disability and morbidity and improve the quality of life of the individual.[51]

TABLE 51-3 Choices of Treatment by Body Mass Index and Comorbidities

TREATMENT CHOICES FOR DIFFERENT BMIs	25–26.9	27–29.9	30–34.9	35–39.9	≥40
Diet, physical exercise, and behavioral therapy	With comorbidities	With comorbidities	Use regardless of comorbidities	Use regardless of comorbidities	Use regardless of comorbidities
Drug therapy		With comorbidities	Use regardless of comorbidities	Use regardless of comorbidities	Use regardless of comorbidities
Bariatric surgery				With comorbidities	Use regardless of comorbidities

Data from reference 125.

Small, incremental weight losses over time are preferred.[153] There are multiple strategies designed to promote weight loss, including dietary therapy, physical activity, behavioral modification therapy, pharmacotherapy, combination therapy, and bariatric or weight loss surgery. The choice of treatment approach is guided by BMI and the presence or absence of comorbidities (Table 51-3). Diet, physical activity, and behavioral therapy are suggested for all levels of obesity, with drug therapy and surgical therapy added in the more obese.[125]

Treatment of overweight and obesity consists of two principal processes: assessment to determine the degree of obesity and the absolute degree of risk or presence of comorbid conditions; and management, which involves weight loss, maintenance of the lower weight, and implementation of measures to control other risk factors.[51] An area of controversy in all forms of weight loss therapy is determining the appropriate, sufficient, healthy, or optimal weight goals for the severely obese.[128] The National Institutes of Health and the National Heart, Lung and Blood Institute obesity guidelines recommend losing 10% of body weight within 6 months and making lifestyle changes, such as diet, exercise, and behavioral modifications.[122] These recommendations are indicated for the adult population, but there are questions as to whether these recommendations are safe for elderly adults.[122]

Diets, combined with behavioral therapy and exercise, are the hallmark of conservative approaches to weight loss therapy. Dietary treatment of obesity is simply to reduce energy intake.[173] The desired outcomes of dietary changes are to lose body fat, while sparing muscle protein, normalizing blood lipid levels, stabilizing blood glucose level, and reducing hypertension.[173] A low calorie diet is usually 500 to 1000 calories below daily energy needs and will produce a weight loss of 1 to 2 pounds (0.5 to 1 kg) per week. In patients who are extremely obese and in whom the medical risks of remaining obese are great, a very low calorie diet may be used. This diet consists of less than 800 calories per day, supplying the minimal amount of energy and enough essential nutrients to avoid negative consequences.[173] Unfortunately, no dietary approach alone has achieved long-term success in treating extreme obesity.[47,48] This is due to counter-regulatory mechanisms that cause an increase in appetite and a decrease in energy expenditure in the presence of a decrease in caloric intake as a preventive measure against starvation.[110]

The goals of behavioral therapy are directed at modifying eating habits, increasing physical activity, and increasing patient insight by promoting better health and weight management.[144] Weight loss therapy should include a behavioral assessment to gather information about weight loss history, previous weight loss attempts, environmental circumstances and social support, and any comorbid psychiatric disturbances that may complicate the course of treatment.[125] Though this can be a successful strategy, studies have shown that the weight loss is not sustained. One study showed that one third of patients who lost weight using behavioral therapy maintained the loss for only 52 weeks before they began gaining again.[68] Nonoperative methods for treating extreme obesity have been ineffective in achieving medically significant long-term weight loss in severely obese adults.[48] In fact, it has been shown that the majority of patients regain the majority, if not all, of their weight loss over the next 5 years.[149]

Weight loss medications usually are reserved for patients who have failed more standard behavioral interventions of diet and exercise[93] or for individuals whose BMI is 27 kg/m^2 or greater with obesity-related comorbidities.[100,125] Pharmacologic therapies include agents that influence eating behaviors, food intake, nutrient absorption, and energy expenditure. Drug treatment is considered effective when used as an adjunct to diet- and exercise-based behavioral therapies. The addition of pharmacologic therapy typically increases the amount of weight loss by 4% to 6% over 1 to 2 years.[143] The three drugs that have been approved specifically for the treatment of obesity are phentermine (Ionamin), sibutramine (Meridia), and orlistat (Xenical). Studies for each drug suggest that the action is to cause the weight-regulatory systems to adjust the weight and energy setpoints downward rather than actually causing weight loss.[93] For each agent and each patient, there appears to be a maximum weight loss achievable.[93] National Institutes of Health guidelines recommend that if a chosen medication does not produce a 2-kilogram weight loss in the first month of treatment, the dose should be adjusted or the medication discontinued.[134] Phentermine is a noradrenergic agent approved for short-term use (up to 3 months). It acts by inhibiting the reuptake of norepinephrine and dopamine in the hypothalamus, resulting in appetite suppression.[100,122] Sibutramine inhibits norepinephrine, dopamine, and serotonin reuptake. Though ineffective as an antidepressant, it reduces body weight by reducing appetite and increasing satiety.[100] Orlistat binds to ingested fat and is an inhibitor of pancreatic and gastrointestinal lipases; it prevents absorption of approximately 30% of dietary fat.[100,136] Both sibutramine and orlistat have been approved for long-term use. Weight regain within 12 months usually occurs after discontinuing either drug.[23]

Many of the agents have undesirable side effects caused by their therapeutic mechanism of action. These undesirable effects include the euphoric and addictive effects of amphetamines, the hypertensive and dysrhythmogenic effects of adrenergic agents, and the steatorrhea associated with orlistat. These and other side effects often limit the use of these drugs.[93] All of the drugs approved for use produce weight loss, but the loss is less and for a shorter period of time than would be considered ideal.[93] Other agents with off-label indications for weight loss include bupropion (Wellbutrin), metformin (Glucophage), topiramate (Topamax), and zonisamide (Zonegran), as shown in the Medication table below.

Future drug therapy for obesity is directed at a number of mechanisms regulating the balance of energy intake and use. With knowledge emerging about the regulation of energy by the hypothalamus, new agents can be developed targeting the neuropeptides and their receptors. In addition to development of agents to change the relationship of leptin to the neural receptors, agents that suppress the appetite-stimulating

MEDICATIONS USED IN THE TREATMENT OF OBESITY

MEDICATION	TYPICAL DOSING	CLASSIFICATION	COMMON ADVERSE EFFECTS
Approved by FDA specifically for weight loss indication*			
Phentermine (Adipex-P)[†]	15–37.5 mg/day	Adrenergic agent	Tachycardia, hypertension
Sibutramine (Meridia)[†,‡]	10–15 mg/day	Serotonergic/adrenergic	Hypertension, tachycardia
Orlistat (Xenical)	120 mg three times daily	Lipase inhibitor	Malabsorption, steatorrhea
Approved by FDA for other indications[§]			
Bupropion (Wellbutrin)[†]	150–300 mg/day[¶]	Depression	Anticholinergic, agitation
Metformin (Glucophage)	500–1000 mg/day[¶]	Type 2 diabetes	Hepatic oxidative injury
Topiramate (Topamax)	50–100 mg/day[¶]	Seizure disorder	Cognitive impairment
Zonisamide (Zonegran)	400–600 mg/day[¶]	Seizure disorder	Cognitive impairment

Data from reference 93.
*Phentermine is approved by the FDA for short-term use, and sibutramine and orlistat are each approved without time limitation. Use in clinical practice varies widely.
[†]Use of phentermine, sibutramine, or bupropion in patients taking monoamine oxidase inhibitors (MAOIs) is strongly contraindicated because of the risk of severe cardiovascular events.
[‡]Use of sibutramine in patients taking selective serotonin reuptake inhibitors (SSRIs) is relatively contraindicated because of the risk of serotonin syndrome.
[§]These agents typically are approved for life-long use for their specific indication.
[¶]Typical dosing for use as a weight loss agent. Effective doses for primary indication may be higher.

hormone ghrelin may impact weight loss and long-term regulation of weight and appetite.[100] In animal studies it was found that those animals that were given ghrelin had increased food intake and energy consumption, which suggests a role for the development of a ghrelin antagonist in the treatment of obesity.[51]

An increased understanding of other neurohormones secreted in the gastrointestinal tract may also provide direction for new drug development. The peptide YY$_{3-36}$, also known as PYY, is normally secreted after eating in proportion to the calories ingested. PYY decreases food intake by slowing gastric motility and induces a sense of fullness.[100] Obese individuals exhibit a blunted postprandial PYY response when compared to lean subjects.[100] Development of a PYY agonist potentially can impact weight loss.

Surgical Treatment

The concept of bariatric surgery was first introduced in 1954 after surgeons first observed that patients who had undergone gastric resection for gastric cancer or peptic ulcers experienced weight loss. Today, three types of bariatric procedures are done: malabsorptive procedures that involve the anatomy and function of the gastrointestinal tract and limit the digestion and absorption of food; restrictive procedures that reduce the gastric capacity and limit the intake of food and calories; and combination procedures (Box 51-4). Bariatric surgery is not considered a cosmetic procedure and does not involve the removal of adipose tissue by suction or excision.

The number of patients undergoing bariatric surgery has grown tremendously, from approximately 16,000 in 1992 to an estimated 103,000 in 2003.[170] Surgery is believed to be the most effective treatment of obesity in terms of the degree of weight loss and duration of the weight loss.[51]

Box 51-4

Bariatric Surgical Procedures Categorized by Technique

RESTRICTIVE

Adjustable gastric banding (AGB)
Vertical banded gastroplasty (VBG)
Laparoscopic gastric banding (Lap-Band)

MALABSORPTIVE

Biliopancreatic diversion (BPD) with or without duodenal switch

COMBINATION

Roux-en-Y gastric bypass (RYGB)

The 1991 National Institutes of Health multidisciplinary conference defining management options for the problem of obesity concurred that surgical intervention was the only method proven to have a significant long-term impact on the disease of extreme obesity.[132] The goal of surgical treatment for obesity is to enhance satiety or reduce hunger signals to create undernutrition.[32] Further goals include decreasing the rate of eating or limiting the absorption of nutrients that contribute to weight.[111] In simpler terms, the treatment goal for bariatric surgery is to decrease the quantity of consumed food, reduce caloric intake, and help ensure that the patient practices behavioral modification by slowly eating small amounts of well-chewed foods.

PATIENT SELECTION FOR BARIATRIC SURGERY

Generally, surgery for weight loss is reserved for people who are severely overweight, who have health problems as a result of the obesity, and who have failed the nonsurgical treatments of dieting, exercise, psychotherapy, and drug treatment. According to guidelines developed by the National Heart, Lung and Blood Institute and by the North American Association for the Study of Obesity, surgery for obesity may be considered in an individual if the BMI is 40 kg/m^2 or the BMI is 35 to 39.9 kg/m^2 with significant documented comorbidity.[132] Those comorbidities include diabetes, hypertension, hyperlipidemia, sleep apnea syndrome, obesity-hypoventilation syndrome, PTC, degenerative joint dysfunction, disk disease, GERD, severe venous stasis disease, and abdominal wall hernia.[111] Reversal of comorbidities is significant with weight loss. All treatable causes of obesity must be eliminated or treated before consideration for surgery.[171]

In addition to these requirements, there are several other important aspects that should be considered in the evaluation of patients. These considerations include the patient as a pivotal factor in the success of the procedure. The long-term outcomes of anti-obesity surgery, both positive and negative, are independent of the technical operative procedure and more dependent on the patient.[128] Typically, the majority of patients who seek bariatric surgical intervention are self-referred, determined to achieve change, and committed to making personal lifelong sacrifices to achieve their goals. However, other patients may have certain eating and lifestyle issues that may not be conducive to a good outcome following bariatric surgery. Anti-obesity surgery can be considered behavioral surgery without a curative intent.[128] Box 51-5 lists the patient factors that influence postoperative complication rates and outcomes.

Evaluation of the expected health benefits and acceptable risks of bariatric surgery for each individual patient

Box 51-5

Factors That Influence Postoperative Complication Rates and Outcomes in Severely Obese Subjects

POSITIVE

> Employed
> Married
> Age younger than 40
> Social support
> Realistic expectations
> Appointment keeping
> Diet compliance
> Preoperative weight loss
> Female sex
> Quitting smoking
> Knowledge of eating rules
> Higher education
> Well-informed

NEGATIVE

> Minnesota Multiphasic Personality Inventory
> psychopathology
> Previous psychiatric admission
> Negative life events
> Alcohol, drug use
> African-American ethnicity
> Codependent
> Childhood abuse
> Denial of disease
> Secondary gain

Data from reference 128.

must be done. Of importance for patients to consider are the risks they may encounter without any intervention, and the risks of being treated by medical methods versus the risks and benefits of surgery in terms of net morbidity, prolongation of life, and improvements in quality of life.[128] It is recommended that the patient be evaluated by a multidisciplinary team including a surgeon, medical physician, behavioral health practitioner, and nutritionist. In addition, a comprehensive screening of existing living conditions, life stresses, family relationships, childhood experiences, and present-day coping responses is required. As with medical treatment of obesity, the best results for bariatric surgery are achieved with a fully informed patient who has realistic expectations and is prepared to engage in healthy eating behaviors and regular physical activity. A patient who expects to achieve a total or near-total weight loss from anti-obesity surgery alone, without making any changes in eating or lifestyle, will be very dissatisfied with the outcome of the surgery.[51] Patients should be aware that

bariatric surgery will not make them thin but rather will return them to a more healthy range and reduce their short- and long-term risks for morbidity and mortality.[171] Additionally, the patient is evaluated for the ability to carry out postoperative care and potential dietary and eating restrictions. General dietary guidelines are outlined in the Nutrition box below. Patients must be able to comply fully with the restrictions or limitations on eating and must fully accept the consequences of the procedure.

A further goal of an extensive preoperative evaluation is to identify risk factors that may modify the perioperative course.[1] The number of comorbidities, particularly those that are cardiac related, must be considered. Patients are placed in low (1 or no risk factors), intermediate (2 to 3 risk factors), or high (more than 3 risk factors) stratified groups. Clinical management and preoperative noninvasive testing are then guided by the level of risk.[1]

♦ NUTRITION

General Dietary Guidelines After Gastric Surgery

> Meals may be liquid for the first 2 weeks; at week 2, meals should consist of small quantities of food and be pureed, or soft, or cut easily with a fork; at week 6, textured foods can be introduced that are easily chewed to a pureed consistency before swallowing.
> Meals need to last 20 minutes or more to avoid bolus eating and to allow satiety to occur.
> High-protein foods should be eaten preferentially at meals.
> Sixty grams of protein is recommended per day to avoid protein malnutrition.
> Liquids should be ingested well before meals or at least 30 to 60 minutes afterward.
> Foods that are dry (roast beef, turkey), sticky (peanut butter), gummy (fresh bread), or stringy (celery, fibrous fruit and vegetables) should be avoided.
> Daily vitamin/mineral supplementation is recommended.
> Chew food thoroughly.
> Stop eating when fullness is felt.
> If vomiting occurs:
> - Identify the reason(s).
> - Wait 4 hours before drinking.
> - Advance the diet only if tolerated.
> - If not tolerated, nothing by mouth until the next day.
> Limited amounts or no alcohol is recommended.

Patients may be rejected based on overt untreated psychiatric illness including depression, severe situational stress, active substance abuse (alcohol and illegal drug use), insufficient motivation or understanding to comply with postoperative guidelines, demonstrated noncompliance with previous medical care, or lack of adequate environmental support.[11,73] Active peptic ulcer disease is also a contraindication.[21] Patients with conditions that are not likely to improve with weight loss or who have an illness that will reduce life expectancy, such as cancer, are a contraindication to bariatric surgery.[171]

◆ Case Study 51-1, Part B

Obesity-Related Traits and Complications

J.W. presents with the following medical conditions: sleep apnea treated with nocturnal CPAP; hypercholesterolemia; hypertriglyceridemia; hypertension treated with beta blockers; degenerative joint disease in his feet and knees that requires use of a cane or walker for ambulation; significant back pain on standing or walking; chronic lower extremity edema with past episodes of cellulitis; gastroesophageal reflux disease with a small hiatal hernia; and uncontrolled type 2 diabetes with oral agents and insulin. His hemoglobin A_{1C} level is 8.2%. He has left ventricular hypertrophy. His blood gases are normal on room air. He has been told that he has a "fatty" liver, but his liver enzymes are normal. He had asthma in childhood, but has not had an attack in 10 years. He is dyspneic with moderate activity. His obesity has been refractory to diet and exercise, having tried Jenny Craig, LA Weight Loss, Weight Watchers, Atkins, OPTIFAST, and hypnosis. He has tried to exercise, but has been unable to sustain his efforts for any period of time. He did lose 50 pounds on orlistat but stopped the drug because of unsatisfactory and embarrassing side effects. Within 6 months of stopping the drug, he has regained the 50 pounds plus 20 more. He is unmarried, lives alone, and did complete high school. He is unemployed as a result of his limited mobility. He does not date and has not had a significant relationship. He is very anxious to have a gastric bypass, believing this is his only chance at survival.

Decision point: What obesity-related complications does J.W. have?

Decision point: What common psychosocial obesity-related traits does he have?

Decision point: What treatments has he tried to lose weight?

Decision point: What criteria does J.W. meet for qualification for bariatric surgery?

Case continues on page 1445

BARIATRIC SURGICAL PROCEDURES

The first widely used procedure for bariatric surgery occurred over 40 years ago. This procedure, the jejunoileal intestinal bypass, produced weight loss by causing malabsorption. Following this procedure, the patient could eat large amounts of food, but food would be poorly digested or passed along the digestive tract too quickly for the body to absorb calories. The problems associated with the early intestinal bypass procedures were significant and life threatening. Severe metabolic side effects resulted from the nonfunctional portion of the intestinal tract that remained, which allowed bacterial overgrowth and their byproducts to be absorbed into the portal venous system, causing liver failure. Other side effects included severe diarrhea with severe electrolyte losses of magnesium and potassium, protein malnutrition, and kidney stones.[52,136]

Of the three types of procedures done today, the most common is the restrictive procedure. Purely restrictive procedures only limit food intake and do not interfere with the normal digestive process. With the restrictive technique, a small pouch is created out of the top of the stomach, allowing food to enter from the esophagus. The narrowed outlet at the lower end of the pouch serves to delay the emptying of food from the pouch into the larger part of the stomach, causing the patient to experience a feeling of fullness.[99] Restrictive procedures are typically easier to perform and are generally safer than the malabsorptive technique, but patients often lose less weight compared to those who have a malabsorptive procedure.[99] One of the most common risks of the restrictive technique is nausea and vomiting, which can occur when the patient consumes too much or the narrow passage into the larger part of the stomach becomes obstructed.

Vertical banded gastroplasty (VBG) is a restrictive procedure that accounts for 15% of all weight reduction procedures in the United States each year (Figure 51-3).[111] A polypropylene band is placed around the lesser curvature, and four to six vertical rows of staples are aimed at the angle of His (near the gastroesophageal junction), creating a small pouch of 10 to 45 ml along the lesser curvature and a narrow passage, usually 10 to 11 mm in diameter, from the pouch into the larger remainder of the stomach.[111,171] Postoperatively, patients may not tolerate solid foods, which may lead to vomiting. Other problems occurring with VBG procedures are staple-line failure and development of maladaptive eating patterns that lead to weight gain. Early weight loss is reported to be at 60%,[1] with a subsequent weight gain reported at 3 to 5 years.[21] In a study of patients done at the Mayo Clinic, only 20% lost and maintained the loss of at least half of their excess body weight, and another 19% of

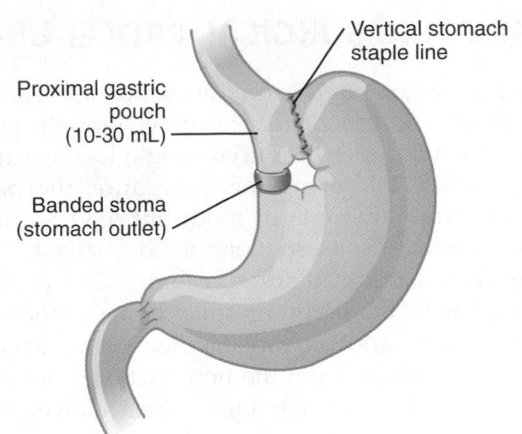

FIGURE 51-3 Vertical banded gastroplasty.

the patients required a second procedure to convert to a different type of weight loss surgery because of inadequate weight loss following VBG.[11]

An alternative procedure is the placement of a constricting inflatable ring completely around the cardia of the stomach (Figure 51-4). This creates an hourglass effect that limits the size of the stomach by creating a small distal pouch with a large remnant of stomach below.[12,48] The size of the gastric pouch is then regulated by a small reservoir placed in the subcutaneous tissues of the abdominal wall, allowing the size of the gastric opening to be expanded or reduced.[111] The absence of a staple line and the concomitant risk of staple-line disruption are the advantages of this technique.[51] Approximately 89% of patients undergoing this procedure experience side effects including nausea, vomiting, heartburn, abdominal pain, and band slippage.[51] Sarker et al.[160] reported a mean excess weight loss of 53.3% at a 3-year follow-up in patients undergoing laparoscopic gastric banding. Other studies have suggested that the

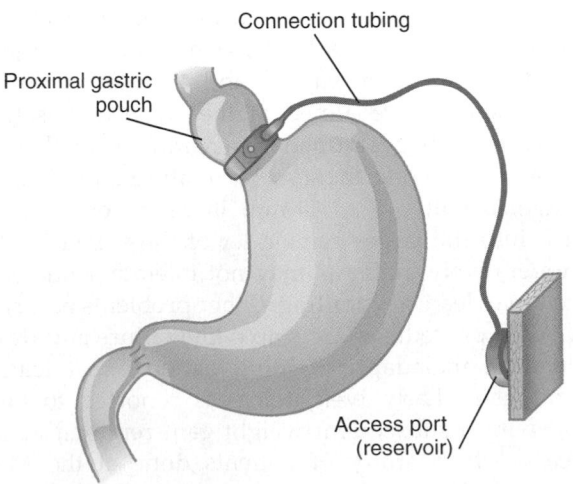

FIGURE 51-4 Adjustable gastric banding.

2- to 3-year effective weight loss is between 55% and 60%.[65] One study reported that there is an approximately 35% conversion to another type of anti-obesity surgery because of insufficient weight loss.[188]

Restrictive procedures may fail to reduce weight because they only limit the intake of solid food. Liquid and semisolid, high-calorie foods can pass through the restricted outlet and do not produce a sense of satiety.[51] This enables some patients to maintain or regain the excessive weight, particularly in the extremely obese sweet-eaters.[47]

The Roux-en-Y gastric bypass procedure is a combination restrictive-malabsorptive technique (Figure 51-5). The procedure creates a small stomach reservoir separated from the rest of the stomach. This pouch is anastomosed to a segment of the proximal jejunum, called a Roux limb, bypassing the remaining stomach and duodenum.[171] The gastric pouch is usually 15 to 30 ml with the Roux limb (which serves as the attachment segment) being 75 to 150 cm in length. The amount of food intake at any one time is restricted, and food exposure to normal digestive enzymes is limited, which creates malabsorption. The longer the Roux limb, the greater the malabsorption and the greater the weight loss.

Combination restrictive and malabsorptive procedures typically produce more weight loss when compared to the restrictive technique alone. The success of the procedure is found in the negative conditioning that results from the uncomfortable symptoms of dumping syndrome that occur with a high-carbohydrate liquid meal.[51] In fact, patients who have combination restrictive and malabsorptive bariatric procedures generally lose two thirds of their excess weight within 2 years.[134] The long-term data for weight loss show that this procedure is the optimal choice for clinically severe obesity.[1]

Biliopancreatic diversion with or without duodenal switch is another procedure that combines the restrictive and malabsorptive approaches (Figure 51-6). In the biliopancreatic diversion without a duodenal switch, the distal two thirds of the stomach is removed and the 200- to 300-cm remnant is connected to the ileum, bypassing the duodenum and jejunum. A common channel is created that allows bile and pancreatic enzymes to mix and be delivered about 50 cm above the ileocecal valve, allowing bile and pancreatic digestive juices to mix with undigested food.[136] This procedure limits the exposure of food to digestive enzymes, allowing significant weight loss to occur because of malabsorption.[136] Significant loss of essential nutrients, electrolytes, and vitamins occurs with this procedure. The more common diversion surgery done is the biliopancreatic diversion with a duodenal switch. This procedure consists of a sleeve gastrectomy that removes the greater curvature of the stomach and creates a tube from the stomach fundus that preserves

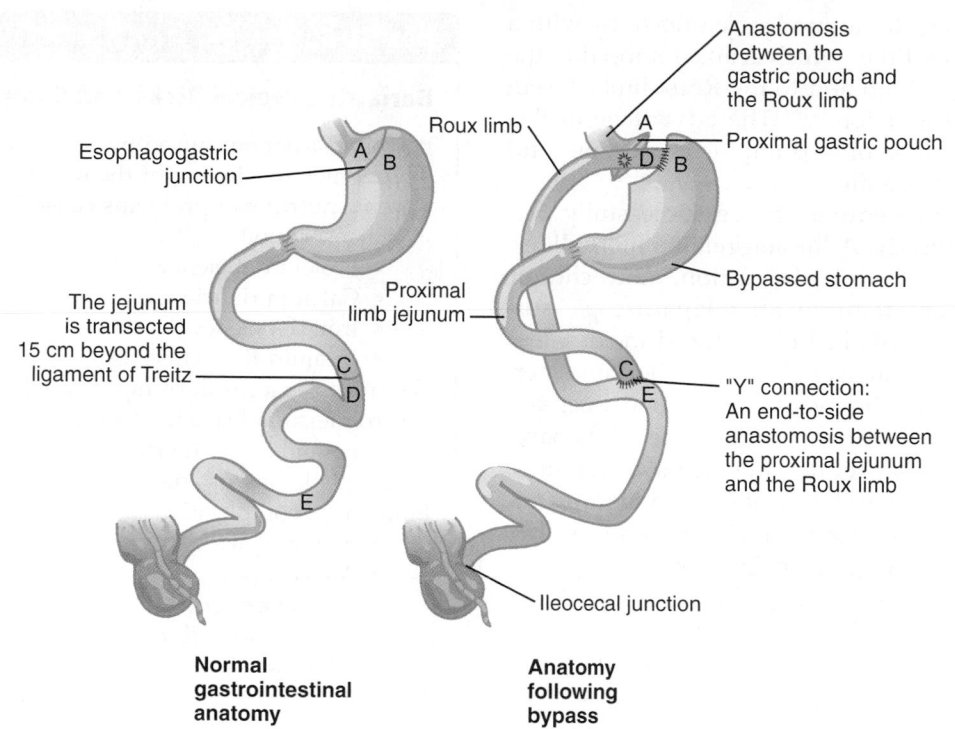

Esophagogastric junction

Roux limb

Anastomosis between the gastric pouch and the Roux limb

Proximal gastric pouch

The jejunum is transected 15 cm beyond the ligament of Treitz

Proximal limb jejunum

Bypassed stomach

"Y" connection: An end-to-side anastomosis between the proximal jejunum and the Roux limb

Ileocecal junction

Normal gastrointestinal anatomy

Anatomy following bypass

✦**FIGURE 51-5** Comparison of normal gastrointestinal anatomy to Roux-en-Y gastric bypass anatomy. *A-E* show how the anatomy is reconstructed for the bypass.

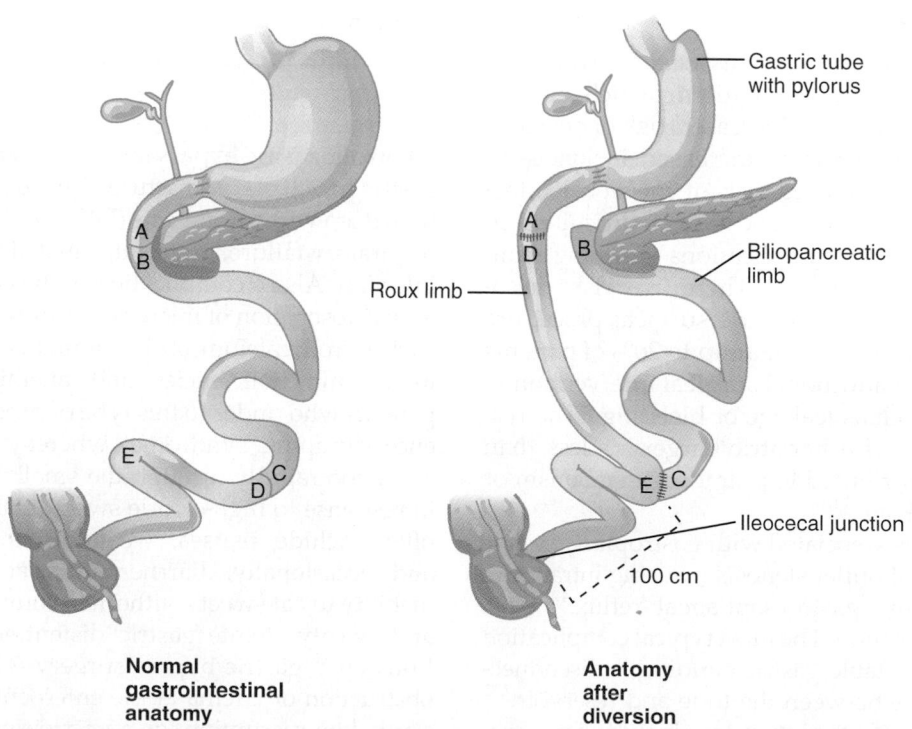

Gastric tube with pylorus

Roux limb

Biliopancreatic limb

Ileocecal junction

100 cm

Normal gastrointestinal anatomy

Anatomy after diversion

✦**FIGURE 51-6** Normal gastrointestinal anatomy to biliopancreatic diversion with duodenal switch anatomy. *A-E* show how the anatomy is reconstructed for the diversion.

the pylorus. This creates a duodenojejunostomy with a 200- to 250-cm Roux limb, which is anastomosed to the long biliopancreatic limb and to the Roux limb 100 cm from the ileocecal junction.[12,48] The advantage of this procedure is that it avoids dumping syndrome and reduces the loss of vitamins and iron.[136]

Many bariatric procedures can be successfully performed laparoscopically. Adhesion-related morbidities, such as infertility, bowel obstruction, and chronic abdominal pain, are reduced after laparoscopic surgery. Additional benefits include reduced incidence of wound infections, seromas, dehiscence, incisional hernia, and thromboembolic events; less blood loss; and less need for postoperative critical care.[142] Laparoscopic procedures also reduce the stress response of the body when compared to open abdominal cases, which is believed to reduce the incidence and severity of stress-response–related complications.[42]

The decision to undergo weight loss surgery is complex, intensely personal, and of great magnitude. Despite the surge in popularity, bariatric surgery is not for every obese patient. It is considered a major procedure, accompanied by significant and indefinite lifestyle changes, risks, and side effects. Consideration regarding the best type of bariatric procedure for each individual patient is essential.

Surgical Risks and Complications of Bariatric Surgery

There are inherent problems associated with performing surgery on an obese patient, which include respiratory insufficiency (i.e., increased risk of developing postoperative pneumonia), increased incidence of venous thrombosis, increased risk of incisional infections, increased wound complications, difficulties in proper positioning, and complications resulting from preexisting comorbidities.[41,111] There are risks associated with every type of bariatric surgical procedure (Box 51-6). Evidence suggests that up to 20% of patients require some type of additional surgical intervention to correct problems such as leakage or bleeding.[2] The risk of death associated with bariatric surgery is less than 1% and is usually attributed to pulmonary embolism or gastrointestinal leakage.[115]

The complications associated with gastroplasty procedures include stomal outlet stenosis (causing intractable vomiting) and severe gastroesophageal reflux.[47] Both require surgical correction. The most typical complication associated with adjustable gastric banding is disconnection at the portal site between the tube and reservoir.[135] Other complications of gastric banding include band erosion, erosive esophagitis, upward herniation of the stomach into the band, and band migration.[47] Complications

---

Box 51-6

Bariatric Surgical Risks and Complications

Bowel obstruction caused by scar tissue in the abdomen or kinking of the bowel

Chronic nutritional problems caused by malabsorption:
- Protein deficiency
- Calcium deficiency
- Iron deficiency
- Vitamin B_{12} deficiency

Gallstones as a result of rapid weight loss

Gastrointestinal leakage of stomach contents into the abdominal cavity (peritonitis) from a dehiscence of the staple line or anastomosis

Pulmonary complications:
- Pneumonia
- Atelectasis
- Pulmonary emboli
- Respiratory failure

Stomal stenosis

Ulcer at the margin where the new stomach pouch is connected up to the small bowel

Wound-related complications:
- Infection
- Dehiscence
- Hernia at the surgical incision
- Abscess formation in the abdomen
- Stricture where the stomach pouch is connected to the bowel

Death

---

following gastric bypass include leak at the anastomosis, gastric pouch outlet stricture, jejunojejunostomy obstruction, deep vein thrombosis (DVT), pulmonary embolism, respiratory failure, gastrointestinal bleeding, and wound infection. Also a complication of the gastric bypass is the loss of absorption of micronutrients from the duodenum, such as iron, calcium, and vitamin B_{12}.[37,47] This will result in vitamin deficiencies and anemia.[111] In addition, patients who undergo this type of procedure may experience dumping syndrome, whereby stomach contents move too rapidly through the small intestine, occurring in response to high-calorie sweet intake.[47,166] Symptoms often include nausea, weakness, sweating, faintness, and, occasionally, diarrhea after eating, as well as the inability to eat sweets without becoming extremely weak and sweaty. Acute gastric distention may occur after Roux-en-Y gastric bypass surgery. This may be due to obstruction or edema at the enteroenterostomy, causing staple-line disruption, or a gastrojejunostomy leak. The patient will complain of a bloated feeling and may complain of the hiccups.[30]

The clinical signs of anastomosis leaks may be subtle and the complication often not recognized until signs of severe sepsis are evident. A persistent fever; increased white blood cell count; left shoulder, pelvic, or back pain; anxiety; restlessness; hiccups; unexplained tachycardia of 120 beats/min or greater; and tachypnea are signs and symptoms of sepsis.[113,171] Abdominal pain is variable, depending on the size of the patient, with some very large patients having little to no abdominal pain.[113] In patients who do have pain, increasing pain can be an indicator.[12] Other potential indicators include bile drainage from the wound and unexplained oliguria.[111] When a dehiscence occurs, a possible leak of the anastomosis or staple line should be considered.[113] This complication is not seen as often because of the significant increase in laparoscopic procedures currently being performed. An anastomotic leak will precipitate the development of peritonitis, which predisposes the patient to multisystem organ failure and death.[27,171]

Pulmonary embolism represents a devastating complication of bariatric surgery. Risk is highest in the presence of presurgical comorbidities of a BMI greater than 60 kg/m^2, truncal obesity, venous stasis disease, and sleep apnea/obesity-hypoventilation syndrome in combination.[161] Perioperatively, with laparoscopic procedures, risk is increased because of positioning in reverse Trendelenburg position for long periods and pneumoperitoneum impediment of venous return, though the incidence of such events is similar when evaluating the whole hospitalization.[4]

Inadequate weight loss is experienced by many patients undergoing bariatric surgery. This may result from the unrealistic goal of expecting to be normal ideal weight, which is rarely possible.[114] Patients will remain overweight even with the weight loss from surgery.[184] The expected final weight loss is one third of the initial total body weight, but many patients will gradually regain lost weight 2 to 3 years following surgery (Table 51-4).[114] This may bring the patient back for technical repair of the prior procedure or for another procedure. A higher rate of major postoperative complications is seen in obese patients undergoing revisional bariatric surgical procedures. Early complication rates range from 15% to 50%, with mortality approaching

TABLE 51-4 Negative and Positive Predictors of Weight Loss Outcome After Gastric Bypass or Gastric Restrictive Surgery

	NEGATIVE PREDICTORS	POSITIVE PREDICTORS
Psychiatric/ psychological factors	Severe psychological problems Generalized anxiety Acute depression Psychosocial crisis Suicidal ideation Binge-eating disorder or redevelopment of binge eating Increased extrapunitiveness Personality disorder	Higher levels of psychological stress Increased phobia scores High self-esteem Marital dissatisfaction Realization (preoperatively) that overeating was cause of obesity
Eating pattern/ behavioral factors	High-calorie liquid or soft food consumption Drinking carbonated beverages Sweet-eating behavior Non–sweet-eating behavior Lack of exercise Eating poorly balanced meals or grazing and snacking	Eating in response to a sense of accomplishment Eating in response to pleasant feelings Moderate alcohol consumption Low food contacts Drinking water Eating three balanced meals and two snacks daily Regular exercise Sleeping 7 hours per night Taking multivitamins, iron, and calcium
Demographic/biological factors	Older age Increased body mass index Poor physical ability African-American ethnicity Diabetes mellitus	Younger age Body mass index less than 50 Higher initial weight

Data from reference 155.

10%.[21] The incidence of gastrointestinal leaks after revision procedures is 5 to 10 times higher than that from primary procedures.[111]

Rhabdomyolysis has been reported as a complication from unrelieved muscle pressure during bariatric surgery. This reported risk increases with massively obese patients who undergo prolonged surgical procedures.[38] In a series of six cases reported by Bostanjian et al.,[20] all of the patients presented with an area of buttock skin breakdown initially. Five of the six patients were male, with a median BMI of 67 kg/m^2, and an operation time of 5.7 hours. Three of the six patients developed renal failure and died.[20] In a series of patients undergoing laparoscopic procedures, Mognol reported 22.7% of 66 consecutive patients experienced rhabdomyolysis.[126] All patients with elevated serum creatine phosphokinase levels had BMIs greater than 60 kg/m^2. No patients experienced renal failure and no deaths were reported.[126] In addition to gluteal involvement, rhabdomyolysis can also affect the lower limbs and lumbar regions.[150] Though patients may lack symptoms, a common presentation of rhabdomyolysis is numbness and muscular pain.[150] Rhabdomyolysis should be suspected if the patient's urine is brown in color, suggesting the presence of myoglobinuria.[150] The urine should be tested to confirm the presence of hemoglobin and, if positive, treatment immediately started.

Long-term complications of bariatric surgery vary widely and depend on the procedure performed.[121] Protein-calorie malnutrition can be seen in any procedure, but is seen particularly in the biliopancreatic diversion procedure.[4] Complications of malabsorptive procedures may include iron deficiency anemia from decreased absorption and decreased activity of gastric intrinsic factor; vitamin B$_{12}$ depletion, leading to neurologic complications; and calcium deficiency, leading to bone demineralization.[4,30] Vitamin D deficiency is a significant complication of weight reduction surgery. Preoperatively, many obese patients may exhibit higher parathyroid hormone levels and lower vitamin D levels.[121] Incisional hernias, intestinal obstructions, and anastomotic ulceration have also been reported long term.[4] In the restrictive procedure of gastric banding, though the complications are fewer, vitamin B$_{12}$ deficiency, severe thiamine deficiency, nutrient-related neuropathy, and bone density loss have been reported.[121] Wernicke's encephalopathy can occur from severe thiamine (vitamin B$_1$) deficiency. Cases have been reported to occur as soon as 2 weeks postoperatively and as long as 13 years after surgery.[3,121] Acute post-gastric reduction surgery neuropathy is a unique neuropathy seen following bariatric surgery and consists of progressive vomiting, weakness, and hyporeflexia[121] Impairment of vision, hearing, attention, and memory may occur, accompanied by pain, numbness, and incontinence.[121]

MANAGEMENT OF THE CRITICALLY ILL OBESE PATIENT

Caring for the critical ill obese patient presents many unique and complex challenges. These postoperative patients are at greater risk of respiratory events, such as unanticipated hypoxia, hypoventilation, or upper airway obstruction, than nonobese patients.[117] Once an event occurs, this patient population requires longer ventilator support, is more difficult to extubate, and requires more supplemental oxygen during the course of their hospital stay.[61] This is especially evident in obese patients who have undergone abdominal and thoracic surgery.

Atelectasis is common, may be the result of pain with respiratory effort and immobility,[1] and may be associated with fever and tachycardia during the first 24 hours postoperatively.[111] Though laparoscopic techniques have limited the incidence of atelectasis, early ambulation, adequate pain control, and use of incentive spirometry are encouraged.[1] Patients also may benefit from supplemental oxygen for the first 3 postoperative days.[171] Continuous positive airway pressure (CPAP) may be required in some patients.[111] During the postoperative period, sudden respiratory decompensation may be an indication of a pulmonary embolism.[111]

Airway management is daunting in severely obese patients, as they may desaturate more quickly than nonobese patients.[15] Oxygenation is more difficult because of decreased lung and chest wall compliance, increased airway resistance, and a reduced functional capacity requiring higher-than-normal ventilatory pressures.[26,97] Respiratory assessment is critical and may require displacement of all skinfolds over the area of auscultation to adequately hear breath sounds.[79] The patient may also have to breathe as deeply as possible to hear air movement.

In the supine position, the patient experiences increased work of breathing and may benefit from a more upright position to improve pulmonary function.[26] The pulmonary changes seen are amplified by being sedated, paralyzed, and supine, which worsens arterial oxygenation.[145] Tidal volumes increase and respiratory rates decrease when obese patients are placed in a 45-degree reverse Trendelenburg position.[29] This was not found to be as true at 0- or 90-degree positions. Pulse oximetry can be unreliable because of increased finger tissue thickness and poorly transmitted light waves that are needed for determination of oxygen saturation.[26] Preoxygenation in a more upright posture (at 25 degrees) provides greater oxygen storage in larger lung volumes.[55] To achieve higher ventilatory pressures when bag-valve-mask ventilation is required, the addition of a positive end-expiratory device may be needed or the pop-off valve may need to be occluded.[26] Early ambulation within 2 hours of surgery and minimal time spent in the supine position while in bed are emphasized to decrease the risk of serious complications.[150]

Because of the increased incidence of sleep apnea in the obese population, monitoring of respiratory function with pain medications and during hours of rest is critical. The most common treatment for obstructive sleep apnea is nasal CPAP, which provides one continuous level of pressure in both inspiration and expiration.[58] Another device used to treat obstructive sleep apnea is noninvasive positive pressure ventilation, which allows bi-level pressure differences for inspiration and expiration and a lower mean airway pressure and is more comfortable in patients who require high levels of pressure to keep the airways open.[58] If the patient has sleep apnea and uses continuous CPAP at home, it should be instituted during the hospital stay as well.[150]

Endotracheal intubation remains the choice for controlling the airway of the obese patient in respiratory failure or requiring airway protection or support.[26] The relatively short, wide necks and additional oropharyngeal tissue make even elective intubation difficult.[150] Other potential factors that may make intubation difficult include limited neck mobility, limited mouth opening, and the presence of an underbite or receding chin.[26] Obese patients require much greater elevation of their head, neck, and shoulders to produce the same anatomic alignment necessary for laryngoscopy and intubation. The "ramped" position may be used by elevating the upper body and head until horizontal alignment between the ear and the sternal notch is achieved.[39] Elevation of the bed to 30 to 45 degrees may also be useful in oral intubation.[26] It has been reported anecdotally that absent or reduced cricoid pressure could improve glottal opening visualization.[85] Fiberoptic bronchoscopy may be needed for intubation. The laryngeal mask airway or the intubating laryngeal mask airway may also be useful in airway management.[26,40] At the time of intubation, equipment for emergent airway management, including surgical instrumentation, should be readily available.[179]

The critically ill obese patient requiring mechanical ventilation will require an adjustment of tidal volume based on ideal body weight rather than actual weight. Use of the patient's actual weight will result in high airway pressures and alveolar overdistention.[179] Further manipulation of tidal volume should be guided by inflation pressures and arterial blood gases.[26,111] Although the prone position has been shown to improve pulmonary function,[147] it may be impossible in the obese; however, the benefits of rotational therapy are well-known.[118] The use of positive end-expiratory pressure is recommended to prevent end-expiratory closure and atelectasis, particularly in dorsal lung regions.[179] The use of end-tidal CO_2 monitoring is not suggested because

of the widened alveolar-arterial gradients present in most obese patients.[61] Once intubated, resting of the respiratory muscles becomes important to lessen respiratory muscle fatigue and replenish energy stores.[28] Patients can be rested with pressure support ventilation, either alone or with a backup rate;[35] however, the workload must be offset with an appropriate pressure support level to lower spontaneous breathing rates to less than or equal to 20 breaths per minute and to attain a tidal volume of 6 to 10 ml/kg.

Ventilator weaning is best accomplished with the head of the bed at 45 degrees.[29] Failure to wean places the patient at risk for ventilator-associated pneumonia or may be an indication of anastomotic leak.[111] Nasraway[129] recommends that evaluation of the patient's ability to wean be conducted at 7 days. The decision is based on assessment of potential for successful weaning. If anticipated by day 14, maintaining the endotracheal tube in place is acceptable. If weaning is not predicted, then early tracheostomy should be considered,[129] which may be difficult. An open tracheostomy wound in an obese patient is often extensive because of the necessary dissection of the trachea within the larger neck. Care should be directed at preventing infection and excessive movement of the tube within the trachea and protecting the skin surrounding the area.[129] The use of percutaneous dilatational tracheostomy, once thought to be difficult in the obese because of the difficulty of identification of neck anatomy, has been found to be a safe and effective alternative to an open tracheostomy.[83] Consideration of the size of tracheostomy tubes required must also take place because regular-sized tubes may be inadequate for the size of the patient's neck.

The risk of pneumonia and aspiration is increased in the critically ill obese patient because of increased intraabdominal pressure from the large abdominal size, panniculus, hiatal hernias, lower gastric pH, and higher gastric fluid volumes in the fasting state.[26] Combined with a lack of mobility, altered white cell function, and an inability to breathe deeply, the patient should be monitored for evidence of decreasing or abnormal breath sounds. Prophylactic use of histamine antagonists in the nonsurgical obese patient is recommended.[178]

Use of continuous sedative and analgesic infusions requires special consideration. Midazolam (Versed) accumulates in adipose tissue and may result in need for increased dosing, which may produce prolonged sedative effect from a delayed elimination half-life.[111,150] Benzodiazepines should be dosed on absolute body weight.[150] If used for a long period, fentanyl may result in prolonged ventilation because of chest wall rigidity, which may prevent extubation.[111] Dosing of fentanyl is suggested to be based on ideal body weight.[150] Propofol (Diprivan) is a lipophilic sedative hypnotic and will accumulate in adipose tissue, which may delay awakening after discontinuation.[35] Dosing of propofol should be based on absolute body weight.[150]

Many other pharmacologic agents are also altered in obese patients because of the higher GFR with normal renal function,[34,119,151] which increases the clearance of drugs that are both filtered and secreted by the kidney. There is still no one description of the influence of body size on both clearance and volume distribution of various medications for the obese. A number of variables have been used to relate body weight and medications in the obese, including body weight, lean body weight, ideal body weight, body surface area, BMI, fat-free mass, percent ideal body weight, adjusted body weight, and predicted normal body weight.[63] Obese patients show increased volume distribution and clearance for vancomycin (Vancocin) and aminoglycosides, which correlates better with total body weight than with ideal body weight.[63] With the variable nature of the pharmacokinetics of the extremely obese, careful monitoring of clinical end points, signs of toxicity, clinical response, and serum drug levels is critical.[179] With known renal dysfunction, the dosing of renal-excreted drugs should be based on measured, rather than calculated, creatinine clearance.[119] Subcutaneous and cutaneous routes of administration will be less effective because of poor perfusion of the adipose tissue; therefore intravenous or enteral is the preferred route of administration of medications.[35]

Analgesia is crucial in the postoperative obese patient. Good pain control will allow the patient greater mobility and decrease pulmonary and skin complications. A variety of methods can be used depending on patient acuity and on the type of operative procedure. For open procedures, epidural analgesia may be preferred. The use of a pain pump with low-dose local anesthetic delivered continuously into the fascial layer may also provide pain control.[1] Patient-controlled analgesia is also an effective method of pain control. Ketorolac (Toradol) may be needed to address postoperative and degenerative joint disease pain in the absence of renal dysfunction. Acetaminophen/hydrocodone (Lortab) elixir may be used when the patient is able to take oral fluids.[1]

As a result of the many cardiac changes associated with obesity, fluid volume loading may not be tolerated as well as in a non-obese patient, even in the asymptomatic patient.[179] Heart failure and pulmonary edema can be exacerbated and physical assessment for signs of heart failure may be limited. Breath and heart sounds are difficult to hear; it may be difficult to move the patient into an upright position. In the patient at risk for heart failure because of known left ventricular dysfunction, hemodynamic monitoring may be needed to guide fluid balance and effective cardiac pump function.[119] While volume loading may not be tolerated,

maintenance of a higher preload may be necessary. A loss of the higher volume and a drop in BP to a level less than the patient's norm may result in a renal insult.

Although the need for central venous and pulmonary artery monitoring may be required more frequently and for a longer time, placing central venous lines is problematic because of the short neck anatomy, loss of landmarks, and increased distance from the skin to the central vessels.[25] This may result in a higher incidence of catheter malpositions and local puncture complications in the obese.[150,179] Femoral venous placement may also be limited as a result of severe intertrigo.[179] Once placed, the risk of catheter-related bacterial infection is increased by threefold over non-obese patients.[25] A recent study found the determination of cardiac index with the use of bioimpedance technology in the obese patient population provided an alternative to invasive monitoring. A correlation was found between cardiac index values determined by bioimpedance and thermodilution in severely injured obese patients with a BMI of 30 kg/m^2 or greater.[25] By using a noninvasive method to obtain cardiac parameters, some of the difficulties in caring for obese patients may be alleviated.[25]

Peripheral venous access may be equally difficult in the obese. If able to be placed, peripheral catheters are often subjected to extreme stress with patient movement, especially when getting in and out of bed. Utilization of hand-held venous ultrasound may be helpful, and early placement of a peripherally inserted central catheter (PICC) is recommended.[179] A PICC is also valuable in that it can be used for measuring and trending central venous pressures.[18]

Systolic and diastolic BP measurements using noninvasive techniques can also be difficult in the obese, as they require the correct-sized cuff. Too small a cuff results in an erroneously high pressure. The largest-sized cuffs for sphygmomanometer and for automatic systems are often too small for the super obese patient.[129] The use of thigh cuffs for arm pressures may be limited by the fat distribution of the upper arm, reducing the arm surface available to wrap the cuff. A trend of the pressures can be used with consideration for consistent sampling.[129] Radial artery pressures can also be used and should be measured 13 cm below the elbow with auscultation or palpation of the radial pulse.[189] The same technique can be used with an oscillometric automated pressure device with the measurement device directly over the radial artery. Placement of an indwelling arterial catheter may be required for continuous arterial pressure monitoring.[129]

Cardiac rhythm may be altered because of infiltration of the conduction system by fat and fibrosis of the bundle branches, producing dysrhythmias that may be silent in nature but place the patient at risk of a fatal cardiac event.[16] Continuous cardiac monitoring with review of stored cardiac rhythm events in the bedside monitor is essential.

Skin breakdown, pressure sores, and delayed wound healing are often found because of decreased vascularity of the adipose tissue.[191] The inability to turn or reposition themselves in bed or to assist care providers to do so is a precursor to pressure-related injuries.[191] For the patient in bed for a prolonged time, pressure point protection is critical and positional changes of the arms and legs are helpful when patients cannot be turned.[191] Moisture and incontinence are also risk factors for skin breakdown. Folds of the breasts, back, abdomen, and perineum must be inspected for existing infections, such as yeast or bacterial infections. Thorough and meticulous skin care, especially in the perineal area, must be a nursing priority. The use of powders in the skinfolds is discouraged as the particles in the powder along with the weight of the fold may lead to skin breakdown; however, the use of gauze or soft cloths in the folds to keep them dry is helpful.[12,79]

Nutrition cannot be overlooked. A common misconception is that the individual who is obese is well nourished. Though there are excess body fat stores, obese patients have increased resting energy expenditure secondary to increased BMI with central adipose tissue being more metabolically active.[150] The patient will likely develop energy malnutrition in response to metabolic stress[111] and will mobilize more protein and less fat when stressed.[91] This is due to a block in lipolysis and fat oxidation shifting to a carbohydrate source of fuel for glyconeogenesis.[91] Unfortunately, energy expenditure equations are unreliable in the critically ill obese.[178] If indirect calorimetry is unavailable as a means to measure energy expenditure, it is recommended that patients receive 20 to 30 kcal/kg/day based on their obesity-adjusted weight (obesity-adjusted weight = ideal body weight (IBW) + [actual weight − IBW] × 0.25),[179] where IBW is ideal body weight. Hypocaloric formulas have been suggested as an option to provide protein while avoiding muscle wasting.[57] Protein recommendations are 1.5 to 2 g/kg IBW per day.[57,179] The goal of nutrition in the obese is nitrogen equilibrium.[57] Enteral nutrition is preferred if possible.[179] Most calories should be given as carbohydrate and fat to prevent essential fatty acid deficiency.[111] Nutrition is of equal importance in the patient who has undergone weight loss from bariatric surgery. Protein-caloric malnutrition and vitamin and mineral deficiencies are common complications.[113] Folate and iron deficiencies are also seen, particularly in the patient having a malabsorptive-type procedure.[113]

Hyperglycemia from stress was found to be similar in the obese patient to that of other critically ill patients.[74] The response to this metabolic stress is likely to develop energy malnutrition despite fat stores.[111] Close monitoring of blood glucose level postoperatively is important even in the nondiabetic patient. Elevated untreated glucose levels place the patient at further risk of infection. Insulin is less metabolically effective in the severely ill surgical patient.[111] In the diabetic patient, subcutaneous insulin may need to be replaced by an insulin infusion or dosages adjusted as a result of the delayed action of insulin caused by the lack of blood supply to adipose tissue.[179] Therefore these patients require close monitoring.

The obese patient, and in particular the postoperative patient, is at risk of DVT and pulmonary embolism. This is in part due to the baseline-limited mobility, venous stasis, pulmonary hypertension, and impaired coagulation. Obese patients who had limited mobility preoperatively are at greater risk.[113] The surgical procedure also increases the risk, especially if the patient was supine during the procedure for more than 30 minutes.[111] DVT is manifested by the sudden onset of lower extremity edema, usually unilateral.[113] A consensus statement on DVT prophylaxis for the bariatric surgery patient is unavailable.[111] Prevention is the best management approach. The use of sequential compression devices intraoperatively and postoperatively concomitant with early ambulation is an excellent preventive measure. Anticoagulation, at the physician's discretion, may be necessary until the patient is fully ambulatory.[195] Pulmonary embolism is the most severe postoperative complication and is attributed to one to two out of three deaths in the bariatric surgical patient.[111] The sudden onset of profound hypoxia and hypotension should also be considered as signs of pulmonary embolism.[113]

Early ambulation in this patient population is essential. Assisting this patient will require adequate help, including the assistance of physical and occupational therapists. The use of double overhead trapezes is also helpful. Knowledge of how the patient gets out of bed at home is helpful,[79] and attempts should be made to allow as much of the patient's normal movement routine as possible. Many obese patients may use assistive or support devices such as canes or walkers and may need them when ambulating in the hospital. Utilizing a bariatric bed that can be placed into a full sitting position may allow the patient to stand from the sitting position. Caution should be taken when moving an obese patient to limit as much as possible the friction of skin moving on skin, which can cause skin breakdown and lead to ulceration.[191] Dionne[54] offers a technique for assisting in moving the patient that provides for the safety of both the patient and the nurse (Box 51-7).

The severely obese surgical patient does not manifest complications in the same manner as the nonobese postoperative patient.[113] This is compounded by the obese patient's limited physiologic reserves.[113] An example is the obese postsurgical patient with peritonitis. This

---

Box 51-7

Moving the Obese Patient Safely

The technique assumes the patient is able to participate in a non-exertional manner with the transfer. Preparation includes ensuring maximal inflation of an overlay mattress, if used; padding of the leading edge of the bed to avoid trauma; placing the bed height to the lowest position; and placing a friction-reducing material (e.g., a Gore-Tex sheet, silicone-based transfer sheet, or transfer mattress) between the patient and the mattress. Flat spin the patient with the transfer sheet to a perpendicular supine position. Deflate all air-filled or driven devices. Pre-position the patient's thigh to a level position with the knee joint aligning the hip joint. A foot stool may be needed to achieve this alignment. The foot stool will be used only to position the patient to a sitting position. This pre-positioning will prevent sliding of the patient toward the floor. Once positioned, the patient can be assisted to a sitting position while maintaining contact with the patient's knee. Should the patient begin to slide, the patient can be lowered to a supine posture to stop the slide. In those patients who cannot participate in their transfer, mechanical devices that can support the patient's weight should be used.

When moving the patient to a wheelchair capable of supporting the patient's weight, Dionne recommends positioning the bed against the wall with the brake locked to prevent bed movement.[54] Utilize two transfer sheets under the bed. The second sheet will provide a "backup" should the first sheet become dislodged with the additional movement from the bed to the chair. Adjust the bed height 1 inch higher than the wheelchair. This will use gravity in the transfer to the chair. Before moving the patient, place a lift sheet in the chair. This will aid in using a lift to move the patient back to the bed should the patient tire and be unable to safely return to bed. The wheelchair should be positioned so that the front nearest corner of the wheelchair is next to the bed, and as close to the patient's thigh as possible. Once the chair is placed, it should be locked. Position the patient as in moving him or her to a sitting position. The team member closest to the patient's knee that is nearest the wheelchair will block the anterolateral aspect of the patient's knee. This allows for better control. The patient is instructed to lean forward and move toward the wheelchair in an inch-by-inch scoot. The head-forward position allows un-weighting of the patient's gluteal region. Slow movement allows the patient and the team time to correct positions, to adjust placement of lines and tubing, and to ensure safety. Once on the side of the bed, the patient can begin shifting the hips to the direction of the wheelchair. Support the patient to a standing position and movement to the wheelchair.

---

patient will not generate a fever, may not have abdominal pain or tenderness or an elevated white blood cell count.[113] In addition, diagnostic studies may be limited in some obese patients as a result of their size. Being knowledgeable of possible complications and having a strong sense of suspicion when patients are not progressing as expected are essential in the care of the obese patient (Box 51-8).[113]

UNIQUE CARE REQUIREMENTS

While caring for obese patients can be a challenge because of their multiple physiologic and medical needs, there are also challenges in having equipment and supplies that can accommodate or assist an extremely obese or super obese individual. Items placed around or on an obese patient should be sufficiently large for the patient. Equipment used in the care of the bariatric patient should be appropriate for the individual's weight, height, and girth. Examples of such items include patient gowns, abdominal binders, compression stockings, BP cuffs, nonskid socks, scales that can weigh above 350 pounds or 159 kilograms, wheelchairs, commodes, and standard room

---

Box 51-8

Factors Associated With Admission to Critical Care in the Immediate Postoperative Period

- Male gender
- Age greater than 50 years
- Body mass index greater than 60 kg/m²
- Comorbid conditions (cardiovascular disease, diabetes mellitus, pulmonary disease, venous stasis)
- Obstructive sleep apnea syndrome
- Syndrome X
- Intraoperative or postoperative surgical complications

Data from references 113, 150.

---

chairs. Many of these patients will require larger beds, as well as lifts and transfer devices that can support larger patients. Gait belts will need to be at least 60 inches in size. Standard hospital beds may not be wide enough to allow for movement or turning. The mattress may not support the patient's weight. Floor-mounted toilets are necessary to support an obese patient. Longer intravenous access devices and the ability to visualize vessels with a hand-held vascular ultrasound device may be needed for intravenous access. Regular-sized tracheostomy tubes may be inadequate for the size of the patient's neck.

Both the patient and the multidisciplinary team will benefit from proper-sized items and necessary equipment. It is important to be sensitive to the patient's special requirement and not place the patient in embarrassing situations, such as a chair that is too small or cannot support the patient's weight. Of equal importance is to ensure the safety of both the patient and the nurse. These issues are addressed in the Multidisciplinary Plan of Care on pp. 1446-1448.

◆ Case Study 51-1, Part C

Surgery and Its Complications

J.W. undergoes laparoscopic gastric bypass surgery that is uneventful. Postoperative day 1 he complains of soreness, with his abdomen soft and only slightly tender. He is reluctant to get up and walk, but does walk a few steps with encouragement. He is using his incentive spirometer and has faint bibasilar rales. Vital signs are stable with his peak temperature 38.1° C, BP 103–136/50–70 mm Hg, heart rate 70–100 beats/min, respiratory rate 16–22 breaths/min; he is 95% oxygenated on 2 liters of oxygen by nasal cannula. His Gastrografin swallow study is negative, and he is started on water 30 ml every 30 minutes as tolerated. He is reluctant to drink for fear of causing a leak. He is using a patient-controlled analgesia device. On day 2 he complains of increasing abdominal pain and is unable to void following removal of his urinary catheter. He is straight-cathed with return of 150 ml of urine that is darkly colored. He is encouraged to drink, but continues to do so very cautiously and limitedly. He begins walking up to 50 feet and is in the chair for 90 minutes. Vital signs day 2 include peak temperature of 38.6° C, BP 90–120/45–65 mm Hg, heart rate 90–110 beats/min, respirations 18–24 breaths/min with oxygen saturation 94% on 3 liters by nasal cannula. On day 3 the indwelling urine catheter is reinserted because of his inability to void. Urine remains dark and concentrated and he continues to not drink fluids. A bolus of 1 liter of normal saline is started for a BP of 88/50 mm Hg, and then IV fluids are increased to 200 ml/hour. J.W.'s other vital signs are within his normal limits with his heart rate now 110–120 beats/min. His creatinine level was noted to be 1.9 mg/dl. On day 4 he becomes confused and disoriented. He is complaining of nausea without emesis. Because of decreasing oxygen saturation levels, his oxygen was increased to 6 liters via face mask. His pain is unchanged. His BP continues to fall despite fluid boluses of 1 liter times 4 with his heart rate greater than 120 beats/min for the preceding 4 hours and continued low urine output. He begins to leak bile from his lower right abdominal incision. He is taken back to the operating room and discovered to have an anastomosis leak. Following his small bowel resection and reanastomosis, he is transferred to critical care and intubated on a ventilator, requiring dopamine (Intropin) and fluid boluses to maintain his mean BP above 60 mm Hg. He is receiving pro-pofol (Diprivan) and fentanyl IV continuously for sedation and pain control and is started on total parenteral nutrition. During day 5 postoperatively he continues to require frequent fluid boluses and vasopressors. Arterial blood gases show pH 7.45, $Paco_2$ 30 mm Hg, partial pressure of arterial oxygen tension (Pao_2) 72 mm Hg, bicarbonate 20 mEq/L with a base excess of −3.3 on an Fio_2 of 0.50. Vital signs include a BP of 80–130/40–60 mm Hg with heart rate in the 90s. Systemic inflammatory response syndrome is diagnosed. On day 6, with continued need for vasopressors, a pulmonary artery catheter is placed with right atrial pressure 16 mm Hg, pulmonary artery pressure 42/22 mm Hg, pulmonary artery wedge pressure 22 mm Hg, cardiac output 10.8 L/min, cardiac index 5 L/min/m^2, and systemic vascular resistance 304 dynes/sec/cm^{-5}. Subsequent blood gases indicate a decrease in tidal volume to 700 and addition of positive end-expiratory pressure of 5 cm; ABGs were pH 7.44, $Paco_2$ 37 mm Hg, Pao_2 104 mm Hg, bicarbonate 22 mEq/L with a base excess of −1.7 on an Fio_2 of 0.50. The patient subsequently went into full sepsis and remained ventilated for the next 18 days. Pressors were weaned on postoperative day 6 and restarted on day 9. On day 10 he developed pulmonary edema following a fluid bolus. During his critical care stay, he developed extensive skin breakdown under his pannus, chest folds, and groin with yeast overgrowth.

Decision point: What signs and symptoms of a leak did J.W. have?

Decision point: Why did he not complain of increasing abdominal pain?

Decision point: What other complications of surgery does this patient face postoperatively?

Decision point: Given this patient's return to surgery, what special needs would he have had postoperatively?

Decision point: What preventable complication did he develop?

Decision point: What possible further complications might be anticipated related to his need for continued mechanical ventilation support?

MULTIDISCIPLINARY PLAN OF CARE FOR THE BARIATRIC PATIENT

PROBLEM	INTERVENTION	RATIONALE	EXPECTED OUTCOME
Potential for pneumonia	Instruct patient to cough and deep breathe Use of incentive spirometry Early ambulation	Compliance of respiratory system is 35% lower in bariatric patient related to lung or chest wall compliance, and chest wall expansion is impaired because of abdominal mass	No pulmonary infection
Potential for ineffective breathing and ventilation	Position head of bed at least 30 degrees Properly secure endotracheal tube to prevent displacement Use CPAP or BiPAP during sleep hours if indicated or used at home before hospitalization	Increased abdominal mass increases workload of breathing when patient is flat Bariatric patient can be difficult to re-intubate because of increased neck size Bariatric patient often has obstructive sleep apnea	Normal breathing and ventilation
Potential for nontherapeutic medication effects	Consult pharmacist	Distribution is affected by obesity: lipophilic drugs are typically dosed on patient's TBW; hydrophilic drugs are normally dosed on patient's IBW or DW Clearance is affected by obesity and may require shorter or longer dosing frequency	Medication dosing and frequency regimen will be based on pharmacist recommendations
Potential for skin breakdown	Perform full body skin assessment daily Assess tubes, lines, and drains to ensure that they are not trapped in skin folds Use padding on any surface area where excess skin is likely to make contact (e.g., bedside rails, wheelchair arms) Separate skin folds with dry linens or pads Use extra precaution when turning a patient with pendulous breasts or abdomen Use specialty bed to accommodate bariatric patient Institute treatment with antifungal powders to areas that are moist or show evidence of existing infection	Prone to early skin breakdown because of increased body size/weight	No skin breakdown
Potential for postoperative malnutrition	Consult dietitian	Provision of adequate energy to preserve functional lean body mass is of utmost importance when feeding morbidly obese patient; bariatric patients should be fed expeditiously as critical illness produces significant	Adequate nutrition

PROBLEM	INTERVENTION	RATIONALE	EXPECTED OUTCOME
		catabolism and starvation places patient at risk of increased loss of lean body mass	
Depression	Consult psychiatrist or psychiatric clinical nurse specialist Administer antidepressant medication as ordered	Depression is common in the bariatric patient; treat the obese patient as you would any other patient; it is essential to remember that obesity is a disease and not a character flaw	No signs of clinical depression
Immobility or restricted mobility from degenerative joint disease or prolonged bed rest	Consult PT/OT for assistance and care planning on moving the patient in and out of bed	Moving the patient will be a team effort The goal is to assist the patient with minimal embarrassment and minimal injury to the patient and caregivers	The patient will be able to move with minimal assistance and without injury in and out of bed
	Identify the patient's normal method of getting in and out of bed	This allows the patient participation in the care planning process as well as utilizes the normal routine for getting in and out of bed if possible	This allows the patient a greater sense of participation in care and control of movements
	Use devices that allow movement, limiting skin friction	Limiting skin friction will limit the injury to the patient as well as make the patient easier to move	There will be no skin breakdown from friction or pressure
	Obtain proper size bed, allowing the patient to be turned from side to side	Use of a bariatric bed sized for the patient, considering side to side and weight, will allow the patient to be turned, and turn more easily	
	Utilize double overhead trapezes	In those capable patients this allows greater leverage ability with their excess tissue; it also allows them greater ability to move themselves, relieving pressure points	
	Obtain a rotational therapy bed if unable to oxygenate or be mechanically ventilated	This will allow the patient to be turned and allow greater ventilation of the full lung surface	
	Obtain mobility devices used at home or sized to the bariatric patient	Obtaining walkers, canes, commodes, and wheelchairs that are properly sized will allow greater mobility	
Potential for postoperative bariatric surgery complications	Identify those complications common to the type of procedure and have knowledge of their presentation postoperatively	Bariatric patients do not present in the same fashion as nonobese patients may present	Early identification of the unique signs and symptoms of this population may prevent long-term complications

Table continues on page 1448

PROBLEM	INTERVENTION	RATIONALE	EXPECTED OUTCOME
Potential for excessive stress response and hyperglycemia	Monitor the patient's blood glucose level closely	Obese patients may have an excessive response to stress, placing them at risk for hyperglycemia, or may have preexisting type 2 diabetes or metabolic syndrome with insulin resistance	Blood glucose level will be maintained as close to normal as possible
	If hyperglycemia is found, administer appropriate therapy, realizing subcutaneous administration of insulin may not be effective	Blood flow to the subcutaneous tissues in the obese patient may also be limited, which limits the action of administered insulin	
	If the patient normally uses insulin at home for glycemic control, additional insulin may be required during critical illness because of excessive glycolysis or ineffective insulin response	Elevated undetected blood glucose levels may enhance susceptibility to infection or poor wound healing	

BiPAP= Bi-level positive airway pressure, CPAP = continuous positive airway pressure, DW = dosing weight, IBW = ideal body weight, OT = occupational therapy, PT = physical therapy, TBW = total body weight.

CONCLUSIONS

The obese patient in acute and critical care presents unique challenges. The presence of excess tissue changes the normal physiology and places the patient at risk for many comorbid diseases and conditions. Knowledge of the pathologic conditions associated with obesity, the unique presentation of certain complications, and the risks found in the obese will allow both acute and critical care nurses to meet and anticipate the needs of the bariatric patient population in a sensitive and caring manner. Acute and critical care nurses should be familiar with the special needs of this patient population, including monitoring and managing the airway, maintaining hemodynamic stability, managing pain, providing complex nutritional support, caring for the postoperative surgical and medical patient, ensuring safe mobilization, and providing education and emotional support. Acute and critical care nurses have a pivotal role in helping this special patient population achieve optimal health outcomes.

REFERENCES

1. Abir, F., & Bell, R. (2004). Assessment and management of the obese patient. Crit Care Med, 32(4 suppl), S87–S91.
2. Albrecht, R. J., & Pories, W. J. (1999). Surgical intervention for the severely obese. Best Pract Res Clin Endocrinol Metab, 13(1), 149.
3. Al-Fahad, T., et al. (2006). Very early onset of Wernicke's encephalopathy after gastric bypass. Obesity Surg, 16(5), 671–672.
4. Ali, M. R., et al. (2005). Bariatric surgical outcomes. Surg Clin North Am, 85(4), 835–852.
5. Allison, D. B., et al. (1999). Annual deaths attributable to obesity in the United States. J Am Med Assoc, 282(16), 1530–1538.
6. Allison, D. B., & Saunders, S. E. (2000). Obesity in North America: an overview. Med Clin North Am, 84(2), 305–333.
7. Alpert, M. A., et al. (2001). Effect of weight loss on the ECG of normotensive morbidly obese patients. Chest, 119(2), 507–510.
8. Ariyasu, H., et al. (2001). Stomach is a major source of circulating ghrelin, and feeding state determines plasma ghrelin-like immunoreactivity levels in humans. J Clin Endocrinol Metabolism, 86(10), 4753–4758.
9. Bagby, S. P. (2004). Obesity-initiated metabolic syndrome and the kidney: a recipe for chronic kidney disease? J Am Soc Nephrol, 15(11), 2775–2791.
10. Ball, A. K., & Clarke, C. E. (2006). Idiopathic intracranial hypertension. Lancet Neurol, 5(5), 433–442.
11. Balsiger, B. M., et al. (2000). Ten and more years after vertical banded gastroplasty as primary operation for morbid obesity. J Gastrointestinal Surg, 4(6), 598–605.
12. Barth, M. M., & Jenson, C. E. (2006). Postoperative nursing care of gastric bypass patients. Am J Crit Care, 15(4), 378–388.
13. Baumgartner, R. N., Heymsfield, S. B., & Roche, A. F. (1995). Human body composition and the epidemiology of chronic disease. Obesity Res, 3(1), 73–95.
14. Berkowitz, R. I., & Fabricatore, A. N. (2005). Obesity, psychiatric status, and psychiatric medications. Psychiatric Clin North Am, 28(1), 39–54.
15. Berthoud, M. C., Peacock, J. E., & Reilly, C. S. (1991). Effectiveness of preoxygenation in morbidly obese patients. Br J Anesthesia, 67, 464–466.

16. Bharati, S., & Lev, M. (1995). Cardiac conduction system involvement in sudden death of obese young people. *Am Heart J, 129*(2), 273–281.

17. Black, D. W., Goldstein, R. B., & Mason, E. E. (1992). Prevalence of mental disorder in 88 morbidly obese bariatric clinic patients. *Am J Psychiatry, 149*(2), 227–234.

18. Black, I. H., Blosser, S. A., & Murray, W. B. (2000). Central venous pressure measurements: peripherally inserted catheters versus centrally inserted catheters. *Crit Care Med, 28*(12), 3833–3836.

19. Boden, G. (1999). Free fatty acids, insulin resistance and type 2 diabetes mellitus. *Proc Assoc Am Physicians, 111*(3), 241–248.

20. Bostanjian, D., et al. (2003). Rhabdomyolysis of gluteal muscles leading to renal failure: a potentially fatal complication of surgery in the morbidly obese. *Obesity Surg, 13*(2), 302–305.

21. Brolin, R. E. (2001). Gastric bypass. *Surg Clin North Am, 81*(5), 1077–1095.

22. Bray, G. A. (2004). Medical consequences of obesity. *J Clin Endocrinol Metabolism, 89*(6), 2583–2589.

23. Bray, G. A. (2005). Drug treatment of obesity. *Psychiatric Clin North Am, 28*(1), 193–217.

24. Bray, G. A., & Greenway, F. L. (1999). Current and potential drugs for treatment of obesity. *Endocrine Rev, 20*(6), 805–875.

25. Brown, C. V. R., et al. (2005). The effect of obesity on bioimpedance cardiac index. *Am J Surg, 189*(5), 547–550.

26. Brunette, D. D. (2004). Resuscitation of the morbidly obese patient. *Am J Emergency Med, 22*(1), 40–47.

27. Buckwalter, J. A., & Herbst, C. A. (1988). Leaks occurring after gastric bariatric operations. *Surgery, 103*(2), 156–160.

28. Burns, S. M. (2005). Ventilatory management—volume and pressure modes. In D. J. L. Wiegand & K. K. Carlson (Eds.), *AACN procedure manual for critical care* (5th ed.). St. Louis: Saunders.

29. Burns, S. M., et al. (1994). Effect of body position on spontaneous respiratory rate and tidal volume in patients with obesity, abdominal distension and ascites. *Am J Crit Care, 3*(2), 102–106.

30. Byrne, T. K. (2001). Complications of surgery for obesity. *Surg Clin North Am, 81*(5), 1181–1193.

31. Calle, E. E., et al. (1999). Body-mass index and mortality in a prospective cohort of U.S. adults. *N Engl J Med, 341*(15), 1097–1105.

32. Cannizzo, F., & Kral, J. G. (1998). Obesity surgery: a model of programmed under nutrition. *Curr Opin Clin Nutrition Metabolic Care, 1*(4), 363–368.

33. Carpenter, K. M., et al. (2000). Relationships between obesity and DSM-IV major depressive disorder, suicide ideation, and suicide attempts: results from a general population study. *Am J Public Health, 90*(2), 251–257.

34. Chagnac, A., et al. (2003). The effects of weight loss on renal function in patients with severe obesity. *J Am Soc Nephrol, 14*(6), 1480–1486.

35. Charlebois, D., & Wilmoth, D. (2004). Critical care of patients with obesity. *Crit Care Nurse, 24*(4), 19–27.

36. Chu, M. C., et al. (2006). Insulin resistance in postmenopausal women with metabolic syndrome and the measurements of adiponectin, leptin, resistin, and ghrelin. *Am J Obstet Gynecol, 194*(1), 100–104.

37. Collene, A. L., & Hertzler, S. (2003). Metabolic outcomes of gastric bypass. *Nutrition Clin Pract, 18*(2), 136.

38. Collier, B., Goreja, M. A., & Duke, B. E., III (2003). Postoperative rhabdomyolysis with bariatric surgery. *Obesity Surg, 13*(6), 941–943.

39. Collins, J. S., et al. (2004). Laryngoscopy and morbid obesity: a comparison of the "sniff" and "ramped" positions. *Obesity Surg, 14*(9), 1171–1175.

40. Combes, X., et al. (2005). Intubating laryngeal mask airway in morbidly obese and lean patients. *Anesthesiology, 102*(6), 1106–1109.

41. Cottam, D. R., et al. (2003). Dysfunctional immune-privilege in morbid obesity: implications and effect of gastric bypass surgery. *Obesity Surg, 13*(1), 49–57.

42. Cottam, D.R, Mattar, S. G., & Schauer, P. R. (2003). Laparoscopic era of operations for morbid obesity. *Arch Surg, 138*(4), 367–375.

43. Cummings, D. E., et al. (2001). A preprandial rise in plasma ghrelin levels suggests a role in meal initiation in humans. *Diabetes, 50*(8), 1714–1719.

44. Cummings, D. E., & Shannon, M. H. (2003). Ghrelin and gastric bypass: is there a hormonal contribution to surgical weight loss? *J Clin Endocrinol Metabolism, 88*(7), 2999–3002.

45. Date, Y., et al. (2000). Ghrelin, a novel growth hormone-releasing acylated peptide, is synthesized in the distinct endocrine cell type in the gastrointestinal tracts of rats and humans. *Endocrinology, 141*(11), 4255–4261.

46. Dealberto, M. J., et al. (1994). Factors related to sleep apnea syndrome in sleep clinic patients. *Chest, 105*(6), 1753–1758.

47. DeMaria, E. J., et al. (2001). High failure rate after laparoscopic adjustable silicone gastric banding for treatment of morbid obesity. *Ann Surg, 233*(6), 809–818.

48. DeMaria, E. J., & Jamal, M. K. (2005). Surgical options for obesity. *Gastroenterol Clin North Am, 34*(1), 127–142.

49. de Divitiis, O., et al. (1981). Obesity and cardiac function. *Circulation, 64*(3), 477–482.

50. Denke, M. A. (2002). Anorexia nervosa, bulimia nervosa and obesity. In M. Feldman, et al. (Eds.), *Sleisenger & Fordtran's gastrointestinal and liver disease* (7th ed.). St. Louis: Saunders.

51. DeWald, T., et al. (2006). Pharmacological and surgical treatments for obesity. *Am Heart J, 151*(3), 604–624.

52. DeWind, L. T., & Payne, J. H. (1976). Intestinal bypass for morbid obesity. Long term results. *J Am Med Assoc, 236*(20), 2298–2301.

53. Dimant, J. (2005). Bariatric programs in nursing homes. *Clin Geriatric Med, 21*(4), 767–792.

54. Dionne, M. (2005). Watch your back. *Rehab Management, 18*(6), 30, 32–33, 50.

55. Dixon, B. J., et al. (2005). Pre-oxygenation is more effective in the 25° head-up position than in the supine position in severely obese patients. *Anesthesiology, 102*(6), 1110–1115.

56. Drenick, E. J., et al. (1980). Excessive mortality and causes of death in morbidly obese men. *J Am Med Assoc, 243*, 443–445.

57. Ecklund, M. M. (2004). Meeting the nutritional needs of the bariatric patient in acute care. *Crit Care Nurs Clin North Am, 16*(4), 495–499.

58. Ecklund, M. M., & Kurlak, S. A. (2004). Caring for the bariatric patient with obstructive sleep apnea. *Crit Care Nurs Clin North Am, 16*(3), 311–317.

59. El-Atat, F., et al. (2003). Obesity and hypertension. *Endocrinol Metabolism Clin North Am, 32*(4), 823–854.

60. El-Serag, H. B. (2005). Obesity and disease of the esophagus and colon. *Gastroenterol Clin North Am, 34*(1), 63–82.

61. El-Solh, A. A. (2004). Clinical approach to the critically ill, morbidly obese patient. *Am J Crit Care Med, 169*(5), 557–561.

62. Fajdiga, I. (2005). Snoring imaging: could Bernoulli explain it all? *Chest, 128*(2), 896–901.

63. Falagas, M. E., & Kompoti, M. (2006). Obesity and infection. *Lancet Infectious Dis, 6*(7), 438–446.

64. Felson, D. T. (2004). An update on the pathogenesis and epidemiology of osteoarthritis. *Radiol Clin North Am, 42*(1), 1–9.

65. Fielding, G. A., & Ren, C. J. (2005). Laparoscopic adjustable gastric band. *Surg Clin North Am, 85*(1), 129–140.

66. Flegal, K. M., et al. (2002). Prevalence and trends in obesity among US adults. *J Am Med Assoc, 288*(14), 1723–1727.

67. Fontaine, K. R., et al. (2002). Quantitative prediction of body diameter in severely obese individuals. *Ergonomics, 45*(1), 49–60.

68. Foreyt, J. P., & Goodrick, G. K. (1993). Evidence for success of behavior modification in weight loss and control. *Arch Internal Med, 119*(7), 698–701.

69. Fox, C. S., et al. (2004). Predictors of new-onset kidney disease in a community-based population. *J Am Med Assoc, 291*(7), 844–850.

70. Fox, K. M., et al. (2000). Understanding the bariatric surgical patient: a demographic lifestyle and psychological profile. *Obesity Surg, 10*(5), 477–481.

71. Friedman, D. I. (2004). Pseudotumor cerebri. *Neurologic Clin North Am, 22*(1), 99–131.

72. Gallagher, S. (2005). *The challenges of caring for the obese patient.* Edgemont, Pa: Matrix Medical Communications.

73. Gertler, R., & Ramsey-Stewart, G. (1986). Pre-operative psychiatric assessment of patients presenting for gastric bariatric surgery (surgical control of morbid obesity). *Australian New Zealand J Surg, 56*(2), 157–161.

74. Gniuli, D., et al. (2001). Glucose disposal in morbidly obese patients in the early post-operative period. *Obesity Surg, 11*(6), 686–692.

75. Gortmaker, S. L., et al. (1993). Social and economic consequences of overweight in adolescences and young adulthood. *N Engl J Med, 329*(14), 1036–1037.

76. Gottdiener, J. S. (2000). Predictors of congestive heart failure in the elderly: the cardiovascular health study. *J Am Coll Cardiol, 35*(6), 1628–1637.

77. Grodstein, F., Goldman, M. B., & Cramer, D. W. (1994). Body mass index and ovulatory infertility. *Epidemiology, 5*(2), 247–250.

78. Guyton, A. C., & Hall, J. E. (1996). *Textbook of medical physiology.* Philadelphia: Saunders.

79. Hahler, B. (2002). Morbid obesity: a nursing care challenge. *Med Surg Nurs, 11*(2), 85–90.

80. Hall, J. E. (2000). Pathophysiology of obesity hypertension. *Curr Hypertension Rep, 2*(2), 139–147.

81. Hall, J. E., Hildebrandt, D. A., & Kuo, J. (2001). Obesity hypertension: role of leptin and sympathetic nervous system. *Am J Hypertension, 14*(6), 103S–115S.

82. Hall, J. E., et al. (2004). Is obesity a major cause of chronic kidney disease? *Adv Renal Replacement Therapy, 11*(1), 41–54.

83. Heyrosa, M. G., et al. (2006). Percutaneous tracheostomy: a safe procedure in the morbidly obese. *J Am Coll Surgeons, 202*(4), 618–622.

84. Hill, J. O., Catenacci, V., & Wyatt, H. R. (2005). Obesity: overview of the epidemic. *Psychiatric Clin North Am, 28*(1), 1–23.

85. Ho, A. M., et al. (2001). Airway difficulties caused by improperly applied cricoid pressure. *J Emergency Med, 20*(1), 29–31.

86. Hori, Y., et al. (2002). Insulin resistance is associated with increased circulating level of thrombin-activatable fibrinolysis inhibitor in Type 2 diabetic patients. *J Clin Endocrinol Metabolism, 87*(2), 660–665.

87. Hubert, H. B. (1983). Obesity as an independent risk factor for cardiovascular disease: a 26 year follow-up of participants in the Framingham Heart Study. *Circulation, 67*(5), 968–977.

88. Hukshorn, C. J. (2004). Leptin and the proinflammatory state associated with human obesity. *J Clin Endocrinol Metabolism, 89*(4), 1773–1778.

89. Inge, T. H., et al. (2005). A critical appraisal of evidence supporting a bariatric surgical approach to weight management for adolescents. *J Pediatrics, 147*(1), 10–19.

90. Janniger, C. K., et al. (2005). Intertrigo and common secondary skin infections. *Am Family Physician, 72*(5), 833–838.

91. Jeevanandam, M., Young, D. H., & Schiller, W. R. (1991). Obesity and the metabolic response to severe multiple trauma in man. *J Clin Investigation, 87*(1), 262–269.

92. Johnson, D. A. (2005). Obesity. *Gastroenterol Clin North Am, 34*(1), xi–xiii.

93. Kaplan, L. E. (2005). Pharmacological therapies for obesity. *Gastroenterol Clin North Am, 34*(1), 91–104.

94. Kenchaiah, S., Gaziano, M. J., & Vasan, R. S. (2004). Impact of obesity on the risk of heart failure and survival after the onset of heart failure. *Med Clin North Am, 88*(5), 1273–1294.

95. Kessler, R., et al. (1996). Pulmonary hypertension in the obstructive sleep apnea syndrome: prevalence, causes, and therapeutic consequences. *Eur Respir J, 9*, 787–794.

96. Klein, S., & Romijn, J. A. (2003). Obesity. In P. R. Larsen, et al. (Eds.), *Williams' textbook of endocrinology* (10th ed.). St. Louis: Saunders.

97. Koenig, S. M. (2001). Pulmonary complications of obesity. *Am J Med Sci, 321*(4), 249–279.

98. Kojima, M., & Kangawa, K. (2005). Ghrelin: structure and function. *Physiol Rev, 85*(2), 495–522.

99. Kolanoski, J. (1997). Surgical treatment for morbid obesity. *Br Med Bulletin, 53*(2), 433–444.

100. Korner, J., & Aronne, L. J. (2004). Pharmacological approaches to weight reductions: therapeutic targets. *J Clin Endocrinol Metabolism, 89*(6), 2616–2621.

101. Kral, J. G. (2001). Selection of patients for anti-obesity surgery. *Int J Obesity, 25*(suppl 1), S107–S112.

102. Kral, J. G. (2001). Morbidity of severe obesity. *Surg Clin North Am, 81*(5), 1039–1061.

103. Kral, J. G., Sjostrom, L. V., & Sullivan, M. B. (1992). Assessment of quality of life before and after surgery for severe obesity. *Am J Clin Nutrition, 55*(2), 611S–614S.

104. Kryger, M. H. (1992). Management of obstructive apnea. *Clin Chest Med, 13*, 481–492.

105. Kushner, R. F., & Roth, J. L. (2005). Medical evaluation of the obese individual. *Psychiatric Clin North Am, 28*(1), 89–103.

106. Kuchta, K. F. (2005). Pathophysiologic changes of obesity. *Anesthesiol Clin North Am, 23*(3), 421–429.

107. Labre, M. P. (2005). The male body ideal: perspectives of readers and non-readers of fitness magazines. *J Men's Health Gender, 2*(2), 223–229.

108. Lake, J. K., Power, C., & Cole, T. J. (1997). Child to adult body mass index in the 1958 British birth cohort: associations with parental obesity. *Arch Diseases Childhood, 77*(5), 376–381.

109. Lee, J. H., et al. (2003). Circulating resistin levels are not associated with obesity or insulin resistance in humans and are not regulated by fasting or leptin administration: cross-sectional and interventional studies in normal, insulin-resistant, and diabetic subjects. *J Clin Endocrinol Metabolism, 88*(10), 4848–4856.

110. Leibel, R. L. (2002). The role of leptin in the control of body weight. *Nutrition Rev, 60*(10, pt 2), S15–S19.

111. Levi, D., et al. (2003). Critical care of the obese and bariatric surgical patient. *Crit Care Clin, 19*(1), 11–32.

112. Li, Z., Bowerman, S., & Heber, D. (2005). Health ramifications of the obesity epidemic. *Surg Clin North Am, 85*(4), 681–701.

113. Livingston, E. H. (2005). Complications of bariatric surgery. *Surg Clin North Am, 85*(4), 853–868.

114. Livingston, E. H., et al. (2001). Biexponential model for predicting weight loss after gastric surgery for obesity. *J Surg Res, 101*(2), 216–224.

115. Maggard, M. A., et al. (2005). Meta-Analysis: surgical treatment of obesity. *Ann Internal Med, 142*(7), 547–559.

116. Manson, J. E., et al. (1995). Body weight and mortality among women. *N Engl J Med, 333*(11), 677–685.

117. Marik, P. E. (2006). The paradoxical effect of obesity on outcome in critically ill patients. *Crit Care Med, 34*(4), 1251–1253.

118. Marik, P. E., & Fink, M. P. (2002). One good turn deserves another! *Crit Care Med, 30*(9), 2146–2148.

119. Marik, P. E., & Varon, J. (1998). The obese patient in ICU. *Chest, 113*(2), 492–498.

120. Mason, E. E., et al. (1987). Super obesity and gastric reduction procedures. *Gastroenterol Clin North Am, 16*(3), 495–502.

121. Mason, M. E., Jalagani, H., & Vinik, A. I. (2005). Metabolic complications of bariatric surgery: diagnosis and management issues. *Gastroenterol Clin North Am, 34*(1), 25–33.

122. Mathys, M. (2005). Pharmacologic agents in the treatment of obesity. *Clin Geriatric Med, 21*(4), 735–746.

123. McGinnis, J. M., & Foege, W. H. (1993). Actual causes of death in the United States. *J Am Med Assoc, 270*(18), 2207–2212.

124. Mills, J. K. (1995). A note on the interpersonal sensitivity and psychotic symptomatology in obese adult outpatients with a history of childhood obesity. *J Psychol, 129*(3), 345–348.

125. Mitchell, J. E., & Myers, T. C. (2005). Behavioral assessment and treatment overview. *Psychiatr Clin North Am, 28*(1), 105–116.

126. Mognol, P., et al. (2004). Rhabdomyolysis after laparoscopic bariatric surgery. *Obesity Surg, 14*(1), 91–94.

127. Mydlo, J. H. (2004). The impact of obesity in urology. *Urologic Clin North Am, 31*(2), 275–287.

128. Naslund, E., & Kral, J. G. (2005). Patient selection and the physiology of gastrointestinal antiobesity operations. *Surg Clin North Am, 85*(4), 725–740.

129. Nasraway, S. A., Hudson-Jinks, T. M., & Kelleher, R. M. (2002). Multidisciplinary care of the obese patient with chronic critical illness after surgery. *Crit Care Clin, 18*(3), 643–657.

130. Nasraway, S. A., et al. (2006). Morbid obesity is an independent determinant of death among surgical critically ill patients. *Crit Care Med, 34*(4), 964–970.

131. National Task Force on Prevention and Treatment of Obesity. (2000). Overweight, obesity and health risk. *Arch Intern Med, 160*(7), 898–904.

132. National Institutes of Health Conference. (March 25–27, 1991). *Gastrointestinal surgery for severe obesity: consensus development conference panel.* Bethesda, Md: NIH.

133. National Institutes of Health Consensus Development Panel. (1991). Gastrointestinal surgery for severe obesity. *Ann Internal Med, 115*(12), 956–961.

134. National Institutes of Health. Publication 98–4083. Retrieved 04/14/05 from www.nhlbi.nig.gov/guidelines/obesity/sum-evid.htm.

135. Nehoda, H., et al. (2001). Results and complications after adjustable gastric banding in a series of 250 patients. *Am J Surg, 181*(1), 12–15.

136. Neligan, P. J., & Williams, N. (2005). Nonsurgical and surgical treatment of obesity. *Anesthesiol Clin North Am, 23*(3), 501–523.

137. Nowbar, S., et al. (2004). Obesity associated hypoventilation in hospitalized patients: prevalence, impact, and outcome. *Arch Internal Med, 116*(1), 1–7.

138. O'Brien, P. E., & Dixon, J. B. (2002). The extent of the problem of obesity. *Am J Surg, 184*(6B), 4S–8S.

139. Olson, A. L., & Zwillich, C. (2005). The obesity hypoventilation syndrome. *Am J Med, 118*(9), 948–956.

140. Olson, E. J., Park, J. G., & Morgenthaler, T. I. (2005). Obstructive sleep apnea-hypopnea syndrome. *Primary Care Clin Office Practice, 32*(2), 329–359.

141. Onyike, C. U., et al. (2003). Is obesity associated with major depressions? Results from the third national health and nutrition examination survey. *Am J Epidemiol, 158*(12), 1139–1147.

142. Oria, H., & Moorehead, M. (1998). Bariatric analysis and reporting outcome system (BAROS). *Obesity Surg, 8*, 487–497.

143. Padwal, R., Li, S. K., & Lau, D. C. (2003). Long-term pharmacotherapy for overweight and obesity: a systematic review and meta-analysis of randomized controlled trials. *Int J Obesity Related Metabolic Disorders, 27*(12), 1437–1446.

144. Patel, M. R., et al. (2005). Clinical trial issues in weight-loss therapy. *Am Heart J, 151*(3), 633–642.

145. Pelosi, P., et al. (1996). Prone positioning improves pulmonary function in obese patients during general anesthesia. *Anesthesia Analgesia, 83*(3), 578–583.

146. Pelosi, P., et al. (1996). Total respiratory system, lung, and chest wall mechanics in sedated-paralyzed postoperative morbidly obese patients. *Chest, 109*(1), 144–151.

147. Pelosi, P., et al. (1998). The effects of body mass on lung volumes, respiratory mechanics and gas exchange during general anesthesia. *Anesthesia Analgesia, 87*(3), 654–660.

148. Pender, J. R., & Pories, W. J. (2005). Surgical treatment of obesity. *Psychiatric Clin North Am, 28*(1), 219–234.

149. Perri, M. G., & Fuller, P. R. (1995). Success and failure in the treatment of obesity: where do we go from here? *Medicine Exercise Nutrition Health, 4*, 255–272.

150. Pieracci, F. M., Barie, P. S., & Pomp, A. (2006). Critical care of the bariatric patient. *Crit Care Med, 34*(6), 1796–1804.

151. Pinto-Sietsma, S. J., et al. (2003). A central body fat distribution is related to renal function impairment, even in lean subjects. *Am J Kidney Diseases, 41*(4), 733–741.

152. Pi-Sunyer, X. F. (2002). The obesity epidemic: pathophysiology and consequences of obesity. *Obesity Res, 10*, 97S–104S.

153. Plodkowski, R. A., & St. Jeor, S. T. (2003). Medical nutrition therapy for the treatment of obesity. *Endocrinol Metabolism Clin North Am, 32*(4), 935–965.

154. Poulain, M., et al. (2006). The effect of obesity on chronic respiratory diseases: pathophysiology and therapeutic strategies. *Canad Med Assoc J, 174*(9), 1293–1299.

155. Puzziferri, N. (2005). Psychologic issues in bariatric surgery—the surgeon's perspective. *Surg Clin North Am, 85*(4), 741–755.

156. Rana, J. S., et al. (2003). Obesity and the risk of death after acute myocardial infarction. *Am Heart J, 147*(5), 841–846.

157. Rea, T. D., et al. (2001). Body mass index and the risk of recurrent coronary events following acute myocardial infarction. *Am J Cardiol, 88*(5), 467–472.

158. Rochester, D. (1998). Obesity and pulmonary function. In M. A. Alpert & J. K. Alexander (Eds.), *The heart and lung in obesity* (pp. 109–131). Armonk, NY: Futura Publishing.

159. Roe, D. A., & Eickwort, K. R. (1976). Relationship between obesity and associated health factors with unemployment among low income women. *J Am Med Women's Assoc, 31*(5), 193–194.

160. Sarker, S., et al. (2006). Three-year follow-up weight loss results for patients undergoing laparoscopic adjustable gastric banding at a major university medical center: does the weight loss persist? *Am J Surg, 191*(3), 372–376.

161. Sapala, J. A., et al. (2003). Fatal pulmonary embolism after bariatric operations for morbid obesity: a 24 year retrospective analysis. *Obesity Surg, 13*(6), 819–825.

162. Sarwer, D. B., Thompson, J. K., & Cash, T. F. (2005). Body image and obesity in adulthood. *Psychiatric Clin North Am, 28*(1), 69–87.

163. Schwartz, M. B., & Brownell, K. D. (2004). Obesity and body image. *Body Image: Int J Res, 1*(1), 43–56.

164. Schwartz, M. W., & Niswender, K. D. (2004). Adiposity signaling and biological defense against weight gain: absence of protection or central hormone resistance? *J Clin Endocrinol Metabolism, 89*(12), 5889–5897.

165. Schwartz, M. W., et al. (2000). Central nervous system control of food intake. *Nature, 404*(6778), 661–671.

166. Schauer, P., et al. (2000). Outcomes after laparoscopic roux-en-y gastric bypass for morbid obesity. *Ann Surg, 232*(4), 515–529.

167. Sjorstrom, C. D., Lissner, L., & Sjostrom, L. (1997). Relationships between changes in body composition and changes in cardiovascular risk factors: the SOS Intervention Study. *Obesity Res, 5*(6), 519–530.

168. Sowers, J. R., & Frohlich, E. D. (2004). Insulin and insulin resistance: impact on blood pressure and cardiovascular disease. *Med Clin North Am, 88*(1), 63–82.

169. Stein, C. J., & Colditz, G. A. (2004). The epidemic of obesity. *J Clin Endocrinol Metabolism*, *89*(6), 2522–2525.

170. Steinbrook, R. (2004). Surgery for severe obesity. *N Engl J Med*, *350*(11), 1075.

171. Stocker, D. J. (2003). Management of the bariatric surgery patient. *Endocrinol Metabolism Clin North Am*, *32*(2), 437–457.

172. Strumpf, D. A., Millman, R. P., & Hill, N. S. (1990). The management of chronic hypoventilation. *Chest*, *98*, 474–480.

173. Stumbo, P., Hemingway, D., & Haynes, W. G. (2005). Dietary and medical therapy of obesity. *Surg Clin North Am*, *85*(1), 703–723.

174. Sugerman, H. J., et al. (1995). Effects of surgically induced weight loss on idiopathic intracranial hypertension in morbid obesity. *Neurology*, *45*(9), 1655–1659.

175. Sugerman, H. J., et al. (1997). Increased intra-abdominal pressure and cardiac filling pressure in obesity-associated pseudotumor cerebri. *Neurology*, *49*(2), 507–511.

176. Terry, R. B., et al. (1989). Regional adiposity patterns in relation to lipids, lipoprotein cholesterol, and lipoprotein subfraction mass in men. *J Clin Endocrinol Metabolism*, *68*(1), 191–199.

177. Tung, A. (2005). The biology and genetics of obesity and obstructive sleep apnea. *Anesthesiol Clin North Am*, *23*(3), 445–461.

178. United States Department of Health and Human Services. *The Surgeon General's call to action to prevent and decrease overweight and obesity*. (Jan 1, 2005). Accessed 06/01/06 at www.surgeongeneral.gov/topics/obesity/calltoaction/toc.htm.

179. Varon, J., & Marik, P. (2001). Management of the obese critically ill patient. *Crit Care Clin*, *17*(1), 187–200.

180. Vasan, R. S., et al. (2003). Inflammatory markers and risk of heart failure in elderly subjects without prior myocardial infarction: the Framingham Heart Study. *Circulation*, *107*(11), 1486–1491.

181. Verhave, J. C., et al. (2005). Estimation of renal function in subjects with normal serum creatinine levels: influence of age and body mass index. *Am J Kidney Diseases*, *46*(2), 233–241.

182. Visser, M., et al. (1999). Elevated C-reactive protein levels in overweight and obese adults. *J Am Med Assoc*, *282*(22), 2131–2135.

183. Vupputuri, S., & Sandler, D. P. (2003). Lifestyle risk factors and chronic kidney disease. *Ann Epidemiol*, *13*(10), 712–720.

184. Wadden, T. A., et al. (2001). Psychosocial aspects of obesity and obesity surgery. *Surg Clin North Am*, *81*(5), 1001–1024.

185. Weil, E. (2002). Obesity among adults with disabling conditions. *J Am Med Assoc*, *288*(10), 1265–1268.

186. Well Connected. Weight control and diet. www.wellconnected.com.

187. Westbrook, P. R., et al. (2005). Description and validation of apnea risk evaluation system: a novel method to diagnose sleep apnea-hypopnea in the home. *Chest*, *128*(4), 2166–2175.

188. Westling, A., Ohvall, M., & Gustavsson, S. (2003). Roux-en-Y gastric bypass after previous unsuccessful gastric restrictive surgery. *J Gastrointestinal Surg*, *6*(2), 206–211.

189. Whalen, D. A., & Kelleher, R. M. (1998). Cardiovascular patient assessment. In M. R. Kinney, et al. (Eds.), *AACN's clinical reference for critical care nursing* (4th ed.). St. Louis: Mosby.

190. Willett, W. C., Dietz, W. H., & Colditz, G. A. (1999). Guidelines for healthy weight. *N Engl J Med*, *341*(6), 427–434.

191. Wilson, J. A., & Clark, J. J. (2003). Obesity: impediment to wound healing. *Crit Care Nurs Quart*, *26*(2), 119–132.

192. Wing, R. R., & Klem, M. L. (2001). Obesity. In J. L. Jacobson & A. M. Jacobson (Eds.), *Psychiatric secrets* (2nd ed.). Philadelphia: Hanley & Belfus.

193. Wisse, B. E. (2004). The inflammatory syndrome: the role of adipose tissue cytokines in the metabolic disorders linked to obesity. *J Am Soc Nephrol*, *15*(11), 2792–2800.

194. Wolf, A. M. (1998). What is the economic case for treating obesity? *Obesity Res*, *6*(suppl 1), 2S–7S.

195. Wu, E. C., & Barba, C. A. (2000). Current practices in the prophylaxis of venous thromboembolism in bariatric surgery. *Obesity Surg*, *10*(7), 7–13.

196. Yoshida, Y., Fago, A., & Ishikawa, I. (1989). Glomerular hemodynamic changes vs. hypertrophy in experimental glomerular sclerosis. *Kidney Int*, *35*(2), 654–660.

197. Yudkin, J. S., et al. (1999). C-reactive protein in healthy subjects: associations with obesity, insulin resistance and endothelial dysfunction: a potential role for cytokines originating from adipose tissue? *Arteriosclerosis Thrombosis Vascular Biol*, *19*(4), 972–978.

CHAPTER 52

Oncologic Emergencies

Roberta Kaplow

A diagnosis of cancer produces a number of physical and psychologic responses for patients and their significant others. Additionally, serious conditions caused by treatment modalities as well as the effects of disease itself may complicate the patient's therapy. Although many patients have complication-free treatment following diagnosis, others experience treatment-associated complications. Some complications of treatment for cancer are life threatening and require admission to critical care.

Six oncologic emergencies, identified by the Oncology Nursing Society, including hypercalcemia of malignancy (HCM), acute tumor lysis syndrome (ATLS), syndrome of inappropriate antidiuretic hormone (SIADH) secretion, spinal cord compression (SCC), superior vena cava syndrome (SVCS), and cardiac tamponade, are discussed in this chapter. Three additional emergencies, including sepsis, increased intracranial pressure, and disseminated intravascular coagulation, are discussed elsewhere in this text.

Development of these oncologic emergencies may be subtle or rapid in onset. Given their life-threatening nature, prompt recognition and management are required for patient survival.[24]

HYPERCALCEMIA OF MALIGNANCY

HCM is demonstrated by an elevated serum calcium and defined as a total serum calcium level greater than 10.5 mg/dl corrected for low albumin levels.[24,32] It is considered a paraneoplastic syndrome, a clinical condition associated with cancer not directly related to the physical effects of the tumor or associated metastasis.[3]

Hypercalcemia occurs in 10% to 20% of patients with cancer,[15] but may affect as many as 30% of patients during the disease trajectory.[52] Up to 40% of patients with either breast or lung cancer or multiple myeloma may be affected by HCM.[37]

Patients at Risk

Cancer of the breast, lung (squamous cell), head and neck, kidney, esophagus, gastrointestinal tract, and cervix as well as lymphomas, leukemia, multiple myeloma, and melanomas are the most frequently reported malignancies associated with the development of HCM.[24,32,38] HCM also has been seen with other cancers (e.g., renal, prostate).[52]

Additional risk factors for the development of HCM include dehydration, excessive intake of calcium and vitamin D, decreased parathyroid hormone levels, immobility, Paget's disease, vitamin A intoxication, hyperparathyroidism, and thiazide diuretic or lithium use.[9,15,24,38] Other therapies (e.g., estrogen, antiestrogen agents, all-transretinoic acid) also have been associated with the development of transient HCM.[24]

Pathophysiology

HCM is an outcome of an aberration in calcium control[52] and most often results from bone metastasis, causing osteoclastic bone resorption and release of calcium. This causes an imbalance between bone formation and resorption, resulting in additional calcium in the blood.[3] HCM also can result from the tumor's releasing substances with parathyroid hormone–like action or from inadequate calcium clearance by the kidney.[50]

There are two types of HCM: osteolytic and humoral. Osteolytic hypercalcemia is caused by direct bone destruction by a tumor or metastasis. It arises when tumor growth in the bone results in calcium release into the blood. Humoral hypercalcemia, accounting for up to 80% of reported cases, results from circulating factors secreted by cancer cells (e.g., parathyroid hormone–related protein [PTHrP], growth factors, interleukin-1, tumor necrosis factors, and interleukin-6), that cause calcium to be pumped out of the cells and into the bloodstream.[50]

Physical Assessment Findings

Clinical manifestations of HCM vary depending on effects of calcium on the different body systems, rate of the rise of calcium levels, patient's stage of disease and overall condition, renal function, and severity of the HCM (Table 52-1). Mild, moderate, and severe HCMs

TABLE 52-1 Physical Assessment Findings of Hypercalcemia of Malignancy

SYSTEM	FINDINGS
Cardiovascular	Hypertension, electrocardiogram changes (slowed conduction, prolonged PR interval, widened QRS complex, shortened QT interval, shortened or absent ST segments, widened T waves), dysrhythmias, bradycardia, bundle branch block, incomplete or complete atrioventricular block, increased myocardial contractility, myocardial irritability, increased sensitivity to effects of digitalis glycosides, vascular calcification, asystole, cardiac arrest
Gastrointestinal	Anorexia, nausea, vomiting, increased gastric acid production, constipation, abdominal pain, ileus, abdominal distention, anorexia, dry mouth or throat, pancreatitis, peptic ulcer disease
Muscular	Fatigue, muscle weakness, hyporeflexia, muscle weakness, bone pain, ataxia, pathologic fractures
Neurologic	Restlessness, apathy, fatigue, depression, moodiness, irritability, confusion, somnolence, delirium, obtundation, visual disturbances, headache, lethargy, psychosis, diminished deep tendon reflexes, symptoms of personality change, impaired concentration and memory, stupor, corneal calcification, disorientation, incoherent speech, hallucinations, delusions, coma
Renal	Nocturia, polyuria, polydipsia, renal tubular acidosis, oliguric renal failure, azotemia, loss of urinary concentrating ability, decreased glomerular filtration rate, calcium phosphate crystals in renal tubules, renal failure, nephrogenic diabetes insipidus, dehydration
Skeleton	Osteopenia, osteoporosis, soft-tissue calcification, arthritis, pathologic fractures
Other	Pruritus, keratitis, conjunctivitis

Data from references 3, 9, 15, 29, 37, 38, 52, 53.

are defined as a corrected calcium level of less than 12 mg/dl, 12 to 15 mg/dl, and greater than 15 mg/dl, respectively. Onset of symptoms may be insidious or rapid.[24,52] Patients with mild HCM can be asymptomatic; diagnosis may be made serendipitously when routine blood work is obtained. The history and physical assessment of a patient with any degree of HCM should focus on the clinical manifestations, risk factors, causative agents, and a family history of hypercalcemia-associated conditions (e.g., kidney stones).[9]

Laboratory Findings

Laboratory findings associated with HCM include abnormalities in serum creatinine, calcium, electrolytes, magnesium, and phosphorus.[52] Patients also may have an elevated alkaline phosphatase.[15]

Diagnostic Evaluation

The diagnosis of HCM is based on serum calcium levels as compared with serum albumin levels. Patients with normal serum calcium levels and hypoalbuminemia may be considered to have HCM.[24] Calcium levels should be corrected based on albumin levels because 40% of calcium is bound to albumin. Two formulas are proposed[53]:

Corrected calcium (mg/dl) = measured calcium (mg/dl) + 0.8 (4 − measured albumin [g/dl])

Or

Corrected calcium (mg/dl) = measured calcium (mg/dl) − measured albumin (g/dl) + 4

Multidisciplinary Plan of Care

The management of HCM can be challenging and is based on the severity of symptoms, the patient's quality of life, and the options for cancer treatment.[24,52] The primary therapy of HCM is treatment of the underlying malignancy, the only effective long-term measure, which can entail chemotherapy, radiation therapy, hormonal therapy, surgical resection, or any combination of these.[32] Irrespective of severity, management should include treatment of any underlying nondisease-related causes. This may include withholding any medications contributing to the condition. The Multidisciplinary Plan of Care on p. 1455 discusses care of the patient with HCM.

Patients with mild HCM (corrected calcium level less than 12 mg/dl) may only require monitoring. Because some underlying tumors respond faster than others to cancer therapies, it is suggested that if the tumor will likely have a slower response to treatment, interventions to manage symptoms and stabilize the

MULTIDISCIPLINARY PLAN OF CARE FOR THE PATIENT WITH HYPERCALCEMIA OF MALIGNANCY

PROBLEM	INTERVENTION	RATIONALE	EXPECTED OUTCOME
Deficient fluid volume	Fluid replacement with isotonic (0.9%) saline. Fluid challenges of 250 ml over 15 minutes may be administered until therapeutic end points are reached. Avoid loop diuretics until fluid volume status is corrected.	Patients with moderate to severe HCM may require 5–10 L to restore euvolemia. Hydration reduces calcium and promotes urinary sodium and calcium excretion. Dehydration will be exacerbated, resulting in a decrease in calcium excretion.	Patient's extracellular fluid volume status will be restored.
Increased osteoclast activity	Administration of bisphosphonates	Bisphosphonates inhibit action of osteoclasts, which results in a decrease in calcium levels.	Patient's serum calcium level will be normalized.
Immobility	Encourage mobility. Collaborate with physical therapist specific to weight bearing.	Activity stresses the ends of long bones, which will result in osteoblast (cells that make bone) activity.	Mobility will be enhanced. Patient will not develop additional HCM related to immobility.
Mental status changes	Collaborate regarding strategies to manage delirium or other mental status changes.	Some patients develop clinically significant and distressing mental status changes related to HCM.	Patient's mental status changes will be controlled and resolved with supportive therapies and treatment of the underlying cause.
Potential impaired hemodynamic status	Monitor cardiac and hemodynamic status. Monitor for dysrhythmias and ECG changes.	Patients who received cardiotoxic cancer treatment are at risk for fluid volume overload.	Normal hemodynamic status will be attained and maintained. Dysrhythmias and ECG changes will be detected and treated early.

Data from references 15, 24, 32, 52.
ECG = Electrocardiogram, HCM = hypercalcemia of malignancy.

patient's metabolic status should be initiated.[38] Patients with moderate to severe HCM require aggressive, immediate treatment to prevent further complications.

Rehydration. If patients are able to tolerate oral fluids, they should be instructed to drink 1 to 2 liters of fluid per day.[52] Patients with moderate to severe HCM may require 5 to 10 liters of fluid resuscitation to restore extracellular fluid balance. Aggressive intravenous administration of isotonic saline may be required, depending on severity of symptoms and amount of volume repletion required.[32] Patients usually show an improvement within 24 hours of initiation of volume repletion. Therapeutic end points include a sustained improvement in vital signs, hemodynamic status, mental status, and urinary output. Administration of loop diuretics, which inhibits calcium reabsorption and enhances urinary calcium excretion, should be avoided

until volume status has been restored, because further dehydration and a decrease in urinary calcium excretion may result.[52] A loop diuretic in moderate doses, once the patient has been rehydrated, may be necessary to control volume overload.[38]

Antiresorptive Therapy. In addition to rehydration, patients with HCM require administration of antiresorptive therapy with intravenous bisphosphonates. Although the precise mechanism of action of the bisphosphonates on bone cells and bone resorption is not completely understood, it involves inhibition of the function of osteoclasts (cells that break down bone and are responsible for bone resorption) in a variety of ways, for example, by producing a direct toxic effect on the resorbing osteoclasts, by promoting programmed cell death, or by inhibiting the differentiation of the osteoclasts into mature osteoclasts.[44] Antiresorptive therapy should be started when rehydration has been established.[45] The most frequently used bisphosphonates are pamidronate (Aredia) and zoledronic acid (Zometa).

Corticosteroid Therapy. Patients with HCM caused by steroid-responsive tumors may benefit from corticosteroid therapy. Such tumors include lymphomas and myeloma. Glucocorticoids work by enhancing calcium excretion in the urine and inhibiting calcium reabsorption in the gastrointestinal tract.[38]

Renal Replacement Therapies. If HCM results in renal failure (due to hypoperfusion from hypovolemia), dialysis therapy may be used. Peritoneal dialysis, hemodialysis, and ultrafiltration are effective methods of removing calcium. Patients receiving any of these therapies require careful monitoring of phosphorus levels. As phosphorus is lost, hypophosphatemia may develop and aggravate a hypercalcemic condition.[38]

Symptom Management. Management of hypercalcemia also may entail symptom management and increasing mobility, as clinically indicated. Collaboration with physical therapists may be indicated if patients have been immobile for long periods.[52]

Treatment of HCM will likely palliate many of the distressing symptoms associated with the condition. Although polyuria, polydipsia, central nervous system, and some of the gastrointestinal symptoms may be relieved, other symptoms such as anorexia, malaise, and fatigue may not subside as readily.[38]

Psychosocial Support. Patients with HCM may develop distressing mental status changes, depending on level of severity. Such changes include agitation, delirium, and confusion. Oral or intravenous neuroleptic agents like haloperidol (Haldol) with or without benzodiazepines may be indicated. The mental status of some patients will not resolve for several days or a week after normalization of serum calcium levels. While patients are experiencing mental status changes, care must be given to prevent patient injury.[38]

ACUTE TUMOR LYSIS SYNDROME

ATLS is an oncologic emergency that can develop from cancer itself or from treatment for cancer. It results from the release of intracellular components of destroyed cancer cells into the bloodstream[1] and calls for prompt treatment to prevent renal failure, multiple organ dysfunction syndrome, or death.[8]

The incidence of ATLS in all cancer patients is not known.[12] Patients with leukemia and lymphoma are reported to have a 5% to 25% incidence rate.[17]

Patients at Risk

Patients with cancer and various preexisting conditions are at risk for developing ATLS. These conditions include renal dysfunction, elevated serum creatinine levels, decreased glomerular filtration rate , anuria, oliguria, volume depletion, hyperuricemia, and elevated lactic dehydrogenase (LDH) levels. The latter has a correlation with high tumor burden if the levels exceed 1500 units/L. Patients receiving supplementation of potassium or phosphorus, enteral feedings, or parenteral nutrition also are at risk.[1,5,8,12,17,22]

Antineoplastic therapy administration places the patient at risk for ATLS. Some of the treatments implicated in its development include chemotherapy, biologic response modifiers, radiation therapy (less often), and corticosteroids; these appear in Box 52-1.

ATLS occurs most frequently in patients with hematopoietic malignancies (i.e., leukemia and lymphoma), and in patients with bulky tumors made of rapidly proliferating cells. Tumors in which ATLS has been reported include Burkitt's lymphoma, acute lymphoblastic leukemia, acute lymphoblastic lymphoma, advanced

---

Box 52-1

Antineoplastic Therapies Associated With the Development of Acute Tumor Lysis Syndrome

Chemotherapy
- amsacrine
- ara-C
- cisplatin (Platinol)
- cladribine (Leustatin)
- cytarabine (Cytosar-U)
- doxorubicin (Adriamycin)
- etoposide (Toposar)
- fludarabine (Fludara)
- intrathecal methotrexate (Folex)
- mitoxantrone (Novantrone)
- paclitaxel (Taxol)

Radiation therapy (less often)
Immunotherapy/biologic response modifiers
- alemtuzumab (Campath)
- gemtuzumab (Mylotarg)
- imatinib mesylate (Gleevec)
- interferons
- interleukins
- rituximab (Rituxan)
- tumor necrosis factor

Corticosteroids
Hormonal therapy
- tamoxifen (Nolvadex)

Data from references 1, 8.

non-Hodgkin's lymphoma, chronic leukemias, and rarely, solid tumors (e.g., small cell lung cancer [SCLC]). The solid tumors implicated in the development of ATLS include those that "respond to chemotherapy" (e.g., SCLC, metastatic medulloblastoma, breast cancer, germ cell tumors, ovarian cancer, soft tissue sarcoma, thymoma, vulvar cancer, metastatic seminoma, rhabdomyosarcoma, and metastatic melanoma).[1,8,17,43]

Pathophysiology

ATLS may occur when a large number of cancer cells are killed (or lysed) either spontaneously or via antineoplastic therapy. Normal intracellular components are potassium, phosphorus, and nucleic acids. When cancer cells are killed, these intracellular ions leave the cell and enter the bloodstream. The result is hyperkalemia along with hyperphosphatemia with secondary hypocalcemia as calcium and phosphorus bind. Nucleic acids are converted in the liver to uric acid. When cells are destroyed, hyperuricemia results. In some patients, especially those with baseline renal insufficiency, the acute increase in the electrolytes may exceed the kidneys' elimination abilities. This results in life-threatening levels (i.e., potassium level greater than 6.5 mEq/L).[1]

Physical Assessment Findings

The signs and symptoms that a patient with ATLS manifests reflect the electrolyte imbalances and their respective effects on the body. These clinical manifestations are summarized in Table 52-2.

Laboratory Findings

Laboratory data indicative of ATLS are related to the pathophysiologic changes that occur when antineoplastic therapy kills cancer cells. Patients exhibit

TABLE 52-2 Clinical Manifestations of Acute Tumor Lysis Syndrome

	HYPERKALEMIA	HYPERPHOSPHATEMIA	HYPOCALCEMIA	HYPERURICEMIA
Cardiac	Tachycardia, bradycardia, pulseless electrical activity, ventricular tachycardia, ventricular fibrillation, asystole, peaked T waves, flattened P waves, widened QRS, sudden death	Hypertension, edema	Hypotension, prolonged QT interval, inverted T wave, ventricular dysrhythmias, heart block, cardiac arrest/ sudden death	Edema, hypertension (if severe), endocarditis (if severe)
Gastrointestinal	Diarrhea, increased bowel sounds, nausea, vomiting		Diarrhea	Nausea, vomiting, diarrhea, anorexia
Neurologic	Tingling, paresthesias, twitching, paralysis, lethargy, syncope		Muscle twitching, tetany, paresthesias, depression, hallucinations, confusion, syncope, seizures, mental status changes, anxiety, carpopedal spasms, positive Chvostek's sign, positive Trousseau's sign	
Renal		Oliguria, anuria, renal insufficiency/failure, azotemia, exacerbation of preexisting renal compromise		Compromised renal function, renal failure (if severe), oliguria, anuria, azotemia, flank pain, hematuria, colic (rare), metabolic acidosis, acute uric acid nephropathy
Other	Muscle cramps, muscle weakness	Muscle cramps	Muscle cramps, bronchospasm, laryngospasm	Gout, pruritus, fatigue, malaise, weakness

hyperuricemia, hyperkalemia, hyperphosphatemia, and hypocalcemia.[12] They also manifest an elevated LDH, decreased creatinine clearance, elevated blood urea nitrogen (BUN), elevated serum creatinine, decreased pH, and elevated bicarbonate levels. Urinalysis reveals uric acid crystals and hematuria.[1]

- Approximately 6 to 12 hours after antineoplastic therapy, hyperkalemia is the first electrolyte abnormality to manifest.
- Hyperphosphatemia and resultant hypocalcemia usually develop 24 to 48 hours after onset of treatment.
- Hyperuricemia usually occurs 24 to 48 hours after initiation of antineoplastic therapies and can result in renal failure if uric acid levels are not controlled. Patients usually present with clinically significant findings when uric acid levels are greater than 10 mg/dl.[8,12,30]

Multidisciplinary Plan of Care

The primary goals of treatment of ATLS are prevention and prompt management to correct any metabolic or electrolyte derangements that do occur despite preventive strategies. The Multidisciplinary Plan of Care below outlines care of the patient with ATLS.

Prevention of ATLS is essential for all patients at risk. This can be accomplished with a number of interventions. Collaboration among members of the multidisciplinary team is vital. Healthcare providers can identify patients at risk, including those with tumors with rapidly proliferating cells, those who will be receiving any of the treatment modalities that have been implicated in the development of this complication, and those with preexisting conditions that place a patient at risk.[8,22,48] Any factors further compromising preexisting renal dysfunction should be eliminated, including nephrotoxic agents (e.g., aminoglycosides, amphotericin B, nonsteroidal antiinflammatory agents). Treatments that can cause electrolyte imbalances should similarly be discontinued.

A key preventive strategy is vigorous hydration 24 to 48 hours before initiating antineoplastic treatment.[48] Once hydration has been initiated, further preventive strategies can continue with forced diuresis. This can be accomplished with either a loop or osmotic diuretic (furosemide [Lasix] or mannitol [Osmitrol], respectively). The furosemide dose is 1 to 2 mg/kg IV every 6 to 8 hours; the dose of mannitol is 0.5 g/kg IV every

MULTIDISCIPLINARY PLAN OF CARE FOR THE PATIENT WITH ACUTE TUMOR LYSIS SYNDROME

PROBLEM	INTERVENTION	RATIONALE	EXPECTED OUTCOME
Potential electrolyte or metabolic imbalances	Initiate preventive measures: hydration with isotonic fluids (3 L/24 hr) Forced diuresis Alkalization of urine with sodium bicarbonate 50–100 mEq/L	Prevents hyperuricemia. Volume depletion is a risk factor for ATLS. Prevents conversion of nucleic acids to uric acid.	Maintain specific gravity <1.010. Urinary output of at least 3 L/24 hr Urinary pH ≥7
	Monitor intake and output	To assess hydration status and for signs of renal failure.	
	Administer allopurinol		
	Monitor lab values after initiating antineoplastic therapy		
Hyperuricemia	Administer allopurinol PO or IV or rasburicase. Alkalize urine using sodium bicarbonate. Avoid drugs that block reabsorption of uric acid by renal tubules (e.g., aspirin, thiazide diuretics).	Prevents and treats hyperuricemia. Treats hyperuricemia. Promotes uric acid solubility.	Serum uric acid level will be normalized.

Data from references 8, 43, 48.
ATLS = Acute tumor lysis syndrome.

6 to 8 hours if urine output is not maintained with fluids and furosemide. A urine output of at least 150 ml/hour should be maintained.[8,48] A specific gravity less than 1.010 is a good indicator of dilute urine.

Urinary alkalization is accomplished with the administration of sodium bicarbonate. Alkalization is started 24 to 48 hours before administration of antineoplastic therapy. This helps prevent precipitation and promotes excretion of uric acid. Concerns of alkalization are the increased possibility of calcium phosphate precipitation in the renal tubules and enhanced hypocalcemia secondary to elevated pH.[28] Urinary alkalization should be stopped with urine pH levels greater than 7.5 or when normal uric acid levels have been attained. Administration of acetazolamide (Diamox) 250 to 500 mg/day may be considered if bicarbonate does not adequately alkalize the urine. Acetazolamide works by decreasing bicarbonate reabsorption.

Allopurinol (Zyloprim), a xanthine oxidase inhibitor is administered to decrease uric acid levels. Xanthine oxidase is the enzyme needed to help convert nucleic acids to uric acid. Patients should receive a loading dose of 600 to 900 mg and be placed on a maintenance dose of 100 to 300 mg daily or twice a day.[28] If patients are unable to tolerate oral allopurinol, an intravenous form is available. Rasburicase (Elitek), a recombinant form of the enzyme urate oxidase, also may be used to treat hyperuricemia.[43] Rasburicase is contraindicated for use in patients with glucose-6-phosphate dehydrogenase deficiency because there is a risk for hemolytic anemia. The main side effect of this agent is hypersensitivity reaction.[5]

Following the initiation of antineoplastic therapy, laboratory data must be monitored to help ensure early detection of any metabolic derangements. A level of 6 mEq/L of potassium, phosphorus level greater than 10 mg/dl, uric acid level greater than 10 mg/dl, or BUN and creatinine levels twice the patient's baseline are all considered clinically significant.[8]

Hyperkalemia can be treated with one or more of the interventions described in the Multidisciplinary Plan of Care on p. 1458. The clinician should minimize potassium administration. Medications such as heparin, potassium-sparing diuretics, and angiotensin-converting enzyme inhibitors can increase potassium levels.[8,48] Enteral and parenteral nutrition and dietary and oral supplementation of potassium should be eliminated.[48] Renal replacement therapies are rarely required for the acute management of hyperkalemia associated with ATLS. It is estimated that approximately 20% of patients will require dialysis to manage ATLS.[43]

Administration of oral or intravenous allopurinol helps prevent the development of hyperuricemia. Rasburicase may be indicated if the patient is unable to take or tolerate allopurinol. Rasburicase metabolizes uric acid into a soluble form and can be used to treat severe hyperuricemia.[8,43]

SYNDROME OF INAPPROPRIATE ANTIDIURETIC HORMONE SECRETION

SIADH is a condition related to water intoxication. It is characterized by inappropriate production and secretion of antidiuretic hormone (ADH) (also known as arginine vasopressin), causing increased tubular water reabsorption with subsequent water retention, hyponatremia, decreased serum osmolality, and increased urine osmolality.[19,32,51] The discernible secretion of ADH occurs despite adequate circulating fluid volume and urinary sodium excretion.[3,51]

SIADH occurs in 1% to 14% of patients.[32] Patients with SCLC have an incidence up to 10%.[8]

Patients at Risk

SCLC is the most common cancer associated with the development of SIADH. Others include non–small cell lung cancer (NSCLC); carcinoid tumors; breast and brain tumors; squamous cell carcinoma of the head and neck, prostate, esophagus, pancreas, and colon; thymoma; uterine; bladder; neuroblastoma; ovarian; duodenal; mesothelioma; Hodgkin's disease; non-Hodgkin's lymphoma; and leukemia. It also can be caused by metastasis to the central nervous system.[19,24,32]

Administration of certain chemotherapeutic agents also places patients at risk for the development of SIADH. The agents include vincristine (Oncovin), vinblastine (Velban), cyclophosphamide (Cytoxan), ifosfamide (Ifex), cisplatin (Platinol), and melphalan (Alkeran). Each of these agents can cause elevated arginine vasopressin[23,24,57] and hyponatremia.

Several non–cancer-related etiologic factors for SIADH have been identified. Medications such as opioids, antidepressants, nonsteroidal antiinflammatory drugs , thiazide diuretics, barbiturates, and anesthetic agents have been implicated. Nonmalignant causes consist of central nervous system disorders (i.e., infections, brain abscesses, brain herniation, hemorrhage, head trauma) and pulmonary disorders including infection, pneumonia, tuberculosis, and lung abscess. Pain, stress, and nicotine also are associated with SIADH.[19,57]

Pathophysiology

SIADH may result from an underlying tumor secreting a protein similar to ADH. This protein is not reactive to normal body feedback mechanisms. SIADH also may be caused by chemotherapy provoking the posterior pituitary to secrete ADH. Both of these mechanisms cause inappropriate and disproportionate secretion of ADH. When ADH is secreted, there is stimulation of water absorption in the distal tubules and collecting ducts. This results in decreased urinary excretion, concentration of urine, dilution of plasma, decreased serum osmolality, and dilutional serum hyponatremia.[32]

Physical Assessment Findings

Patients present with a variety of symptoms, often related to their dilutional hyponatremia, hypocalcemia, or hypokalemia. Signs and symptoms of SIADH are listed in Table 52-3.

Laboratory Findings

Laboratory data consistent with a diagnosis of SIADH include a urinary sodium greater than 40 mEq/L, elevated urinary osmolality greater than 1000 mOsm/L, serum hypo-osmolality, and serum hyponatremia.[32]

Multidisciplinary Plan of Care

Ongoing assessment of the patient's neuromuscular, cardiac, gastrointestinal, and renal status is important in order to detect subtle changes in a patient's clinical status. Assessment of fluid and electrolyte status and for side effects of cancer treatment is equally essential. Collaboration among the physician, pharmacist, and nurse to manage anxiety and depression may help optimize patient outcomes because many medications used to treat these disorders lead to development of SIADH

TABLE 52-3 Signs and Symptoms of Syndrome of Inappropriate Antidiuretic Hormone

BODY SYSTEM	ASSOCIATED SYMPTOMS
Cardiac	Hypotension or normal blood pressure and heart rate, fluid retention
Central nervous system	Headache, lethargy, changes in behavior, ataxia, fatigue, malaise, mental status changes, irritability, disorientation, tremors, somnolence, hallucinations, confusion, hyporeflexia, weakness, myoclonus, agitation, obtundation, coma, unexplained seizures
Gastrointestinal	Anorexia, abdominal cramping, nausea, vomiting, diarrhea
Musculoskeletal	Muscle cramps, weakness
Renal	Thirst, incontinence, weight gain without edema, oliguria
Respiratory	Inability to mobilize secretions

Data from references 3, 19, 24, 32.

and may require modification.[19] The Multidisciplinary Plan of Care below summarizes care of the patient with SIADH.

When feasible, treatment of the underlying cause of SIADH should be implemented. Treatment modalities may include chemotherapy, radiation therapy, corticosteroids, or a combination of these.[32]

MULTIDISCIPLINARY PLAN OF CARE FOR THE PATIENT WITH SYNDROME OF INAPPROPRIATE ANTIDIURETIC HORMONE

PROBLEM	INTERVENTION	RATIONALE	EXPECTED OUTCOME
Water excess/ hyponatremia	Strict intake and output		Patient's fluid and electrolyte status will normalize
	Fluid restriction of 800–1000 ml/day Administer demeclocycline 600–1200 mg/day If severe hyponatremia, administer 3% sodium chloride	To decrease dilutional hyponatremia	
	Consider loop diuretic administration	To increase water excretion	

The cornerstone of management is fluid restriction of 800 to 1000 ml/day until there is improvement in hyponatremia.[19,32] In addition to fluid restriction, administration of demeclocycline (Declomycin) 600 to 1200 mg/day is recommended if the former is not effective. Demeclocycline, an oral antibiotic, causes nephrogenic diabetes insipidus by decreasing tubular response to ADH. Side effects of demeclocycline include nausea, photosensitivity, and azotemia.[19,32,57]

If patients have acute hyponatremia and severe neurologic symptoms, 3% sodium chloride should be administered IV at a rate of 300 to 500 ml over 4 to 6 hours. This infusion should continue until the serum sodium is 125 mg/dl.[14] Serum sodium should be corrected at a rate no faster than 1 to 2 mEq/hr to prevent complication of therapy (e.g., pulmonary edema, hypernatremia, mental status changes, seizures).[19] Diuretics may also need to be administered to prevent fluid overload.

SIADH resolves quickly (usually less than 3 weeks) when treatment of the underlying cause has been started. Symptoms frequently return if there is tumor progression.[3,19] Patients do not require long-term management of SIADH but should be educated about possible symptoms during and following cancer treatment.

SPINAL CORD COMPRESSION

SCC is compression of the thecal sac by a tumor in the epidural space. The tumor applies pressure on the spinal cord, affecting its vascular supply. The decreased blood flow to the spinal cord can lead to infarction or vertebral collapse. The compression can be located in the spinal cord or at the level of the cauda equina.[20,42]

The incidence of SCC depends on the tumor's starting point. In one study, the reported probability of developing SCC ranged from 0.2% to 7.9%.[36] Other data suggest that 5% to 30% of patients with cancer can develop SCC.[15,34,39-41] There is an incidence of 10%, 70%, and 20% in the cervical, thoracic, and lumbosacral spine, respectively. SCC is seen on adjoining levels in 10% to 38% of cases.[15]

Patients at Risk

SCC often results from metastatic tumors. The most frequently reported tumors with metastases to the skeleton are lung, breast, and prostate. Others include lymphoma, melanoma, gastrointestinal cancers, seminoma, neuroblastoma, sarcoma, myeloma, and renal cell carcinoma. Patients with primary cancers of the spinal cord (i.e., ependymoma, astrocytoma, hemangioblastomas, oligodendrogliomas, mixed gliomas) also are at risk.[21,23,24,32,57]

Pathophysiology

SCC is usually caused by tumors that metastasize to the spine. SCC is classified as either intramedullary (within the spinal cord), intradural (within the dura mater), extramedullary (outside the spinal cord), or extradural (outside the dura mater).[32] The extradural is the most common type.[20,57] Cancer can spread to specific areas on the spine. Specifically, lung, breast, or prostate cancer usually (70% of the time) metastasizes to the thoracic area. Gastrointestinal and prostate tumors may metastasize to the lumbosacral spine. When a tumor spreads to the spinal cord, it breaks up the vertebral body, causing it to collapse. The spinal cord compresses as tumor or particles of bone are pushed into the epidural space.[20]

Most tumors spread to the spinal cord as an embolic process through the paravertebral and extradural venous plexus to bone marrow. This causes the vertebral body to collapse and an epidural mass to form.[20] Growth of a tumor in the epidural space may also result from adenopathy of the prevertebral lymph nodes. Central nervous system cancer can also spread to the cerebrospinal fluid. This results in spread to the subarachnoid space, brain, and spinal cord.[20] As the cancer spreads, blood flow to affected tissues is impaired, edema of the tissues and nerves, and neural distortion, ischemia, and tissue death result.[57]

Assessment Findings

Patients with SCC may present in a variety of ways, depending on the location and extent and etiology of the compression, blood supply involvement, and the speed at which the compression has developed. Effects can be sensory, motor, autonomic, or any combination of these.[20,24] Clinical manifestations are listed in Table 52-4.

Patients most frequently report back or neck pain.[15,21,32] Pain may be localized at the site at of the tumor. The pain is constant, dull, or aching. Pain may also be radicular (aggravated by movement or constant and may be alleviated by sitting) or medullary. The pain may intensify when lying supine.[21,32] The patient may experience pain for 3 months before developing sensory deficits, and usually intensifies with time. The pain may develop slowly over months before other neurologic symptoms or quickly, over hours before complete, irreversible damage to the spinal cord.[15] Patients also may report pain upon coughing or sneezing, a sudden change in pain that has been present, or pain that waxes and wanes. Patients may further report unilateral or bilateral radiating leg pain.[54] Vertebral invasion by tumor, or periosseous and osseous nerve stimulation can account for localized pain and tenderness.[24]

TABLE 52-4 Clinical Manifestations of Spinal Cord Compression

MOTOR SYMPTOMS	AUTONOMIC SYMPTOMS	SENSORY SYMPTOMS
Ataxia	Bladder distention	Decrease in strength
Easy fatigue	Changes in bowel and bladder	Decreased light touch, joint, position sense,
Gait disturbance	function	and proprioception
Hyporeflexia	Constipation	Lhermitte's sign
Hypotonicity	Decreased anal tone	Loss of deep pressure sensation
Leg pain	Hesitancy	Loss of thermal sense
Loss of coordination	Impotence	Loss of vibration sensation
Motor weakness, usually in lower	Lack of ability to bear down	Numbness
extremities	Lack of urge to defecate	Paresthesia
Neck or back pain	Obstipation	Sensory loss to level of compression
Paralysis	Sphincter disturbances	Severe pain
	Urinary incontinence	
	Urinary overflow	
	Urinary retention	

Data from references 21, 24, 34, 57.

Sensory changes usually begin distally and rise to the level of the compression.[21] Patient reports of weakness usually occur over some time following pain.[15] Patients with compression of the cervical spine have quadriplegia. Patients with compression of the thoracic spine have paraplegia. When a patient has compression of the cauda equina, sensory loss is bilateral. Patients usually experience sensory and motor symptoms prior to autonomic dysfunction.

The most vital data to assist in the diagnosis of SCC are the patient history and clinical evaluation. Patient history is key to evaluating spinal lesions.[2] A comprehensive initial history, physical, and neurologic assessment, and evaluation of pain, sensory, motor, and autonomic functions are essential. Ongoing assessments, including pain assessments, intake and output, and vital signs every 1 to 2 hours, are indicated to monitor for changes.[32]

It is essential that a patient with reported back or neck pain be thoroughly evaluated. This is because the strongest prognostic indicator of a patient with SCC is neurologic status prior to starting treatment. A patient's ability to ambulate at diagnosis will significantly predict ability to ambulate following treatment. Prompt recognition and immediate intervention are essential to avert irreversible neurologic function.[21]

The patient's history should include determination of characteristics of the symptoms (intensity, quality, onset, and duration), presence of sensory, motor, and autonomic symptoms. A thorough examination of the neurologic and musculoskeletal systems is imperative in any patient who is at risk for development of SCC and who is symptomatic, even if pain is the only presenting symptom. The patient should be asked to perform a straight-leg raise. If the patient is experiencing radicular pain, it will increase with this movement. Sharp pain on dorsiflexion suggests nerve root compression.[21]

Evaluation of pain, temperature, touch, vibration, and position should be conducted. The area of sensory loss can determine the level of the compression. Positive sensation is usually one or two levels below the site of the compression.[16,21] The patient will usually report tenderness to percussion at the site of the compressed vertebrae.[15]

Sensory changes will progress if interventions are not initiated. Paresthesia will advance to sensory loss. Patients may report a tingling sensation in the arms or trunk that occurs with neck flexion. This known as Lhermitte's sign.[54]

Motor changes progress without intervention. Initial weakness may advance to problems with coordination and finally, motor loss. Weakness usually begins in the feet and moves proximally.[54]

Patients should be evaluated for gait disturbances, muscle strength, involuntary movements, and coordination. Reflexes also should be assessed. Tendon reflexes are increased below the level of the compression, absent at the level of the compression, and normal above the level of the compression.[21] A patient who displays a positive Babinski's sign likely has motor involvement.

Any reported autonomic dysfunction requires further evaluation, especially if the patient is at risk for developing SCC. Autonomic dysfunction is a poor prognostic indicator.[24]

Respiratory distress may occur if the compression is at the cervical level. Assessment for impaired oxygenation and ventilation is pivotal, especially in patients with tumor involvement at the C4 level or above. These patients require airway protection with intubation.[32]

Any findings on physical examination may help in the diagnosis of SCC. It should be noted, however, that lack of signs and symptoms does not rule the diagnosis. A patient at risk for SCC who reports sudden onset of back pain and leg weakness should be evaluated.[54]

Radiology Findings

Spinal radiograph is the initial diagnostic study for SCC. It may be normal or reveal fracture, damage, or erosion to vertebrae or reveal a lesion in up to 85% of the vertebrae. It might detect epidural metastasis in the majority of cases.* Radiograph will not discern early SCC, because 50% of bone must be destroyed for compression to be viewed.[21]

Magnetic resonance imaging (MRI) is the most definitive tool to determine the exact location of the compression, evaluate extent of disease, and determine the presence of tumors of the vertebrae.[15] It also visualizes soft tissue, the spinal cord, and cauda equina. The entire spine should be visualized because metastasis can occur in multiple sites. Either MRI or computed

---

*References 15, 21, 24, 32, 54, 55.

tomography (CT) scan may identify the location and extent of trauma to the spinal cord as well as assess for bone destruction. A myelogram may be done; however, MRI is preferable because it is noninvasive, does not require contrast injection, and can image the entire spine.[21,55]

CT with contrast will detect paraspinal masses and early lesions but does not image the entire spine.[21] CT scan may be used to confirm SCC and to fully determine the level and extent of the lesion.[24] Positron emission tomography can substantiate data received from MRI or CT.[21] A bone scan may reveal the extent of bone involvement and spinal level 20% of the time and detect abnormalities that are not detected on radiograph.[21,24,35]

Multidisciplinary Plan of Care

Spinal cord compression is an oncologic emergency requiring immediate intervention to prevent permanent disability.[15,21,32,40,54] Options for management include surgery, steroids, radiation therapy, and chemotherapy.[24,39] Goals of therapy are to provide pain relief, restore neurologic function, treat the underlying malignancy, and prevent permanent disability.[21,24,32] Treatment depends on the type of underlying tumor, location, and characteristics.[21] The Multidisciplinary Plan of Care below and on p. 1464 outlines the care of patients with SCC.

MULTIDISCIPLINARY PLAN OF CARE FOR THE PATIENT WITH SPINAL CORD COMPRESSION SYNDROME

PROBLEM	INTERVENTION	RATIONALE	EXPECTED OUTCOME
Immobility	Rehabilitation with PT and OT when stable/indicated.	Helps patient cope with disability and recover from injury. Patients may benefit from rehabilitation	
	Bed rest and logroll	To stabilize patient's condition	
	Antiembolic precautions	To prevent complications and further damage	
Potential for side effects of treatment	Monitor for GI bleeding, hyperglycemia, psychosis, myopathy	Side effects of steroids	Side effects of therapy will be prevented or recognized and treated early
	Taper steroids, as tolerated	Prevent adrenal insufficiency	
	Monitor for fatigue, skin changes (erythema, pigmentation, desquamation)	Side effects of radiation therapy	

Table continues on page 1464

PROBLEM	INTERVENTION	RATIONALE	EXPECTED OUTCOME
	Observe for signs and symptoms of stroke, for hematoma, DVT, pulmonary embolism, wound dehiscence	Potential complications of surgical intervention	
Pain	Administer steroids	Decreases swelling and edema	Comfort will be promoted
	Radiation therapy	Treatment of underlying cause of compression	
	Thorough pain assessment		
	Assess for musculoskeletal and neurologic changes	Early detection and intervention can prevent further damage	
	Administer opioids		
	Attempt nonpharmacologic interventions	First line of therapy for pain/discomfort	
Bowel and bladder dysfunction	Assess bowel and bladder function Intermittent bladder catheterization Bladder retraining Implement bowel regimen Refer for sexual counseling	Nerves that control bowel and bladder function have been altered or are dysfunctional Patients may have sexual dysfunction related to SCC	Autonomic functioning will be optimized
Inadequate coping and potential for depression	Assess patient/family modes of coping in past Psych consult if indicated	Patients with SCC may develop depression or impaired coping related to SCC	Patient coping will be optimized
Potential for further dysfunction	Thorough neurologic assessment and reassessments Check for sensory, motor, and autonomic function Monitor vital signs and I/O	Symptoms must be recognized early to prevent permanent disability	Signs and symptoms will be recognized and treated promptly
Potential for respiratory compromise	Assess for impaired oxygenation and ventilation Intubate, as indicated	Respiratory distress may occur if compression is at the cervical level. Airway protection may be required	Patient will maintain optimal oxygenation and ventilation

Data from references 21, 32, 34.
DVT = Deep vein thrombosis, GI = gastrointestinal, I/O = intake and output, OT = occupational therapy, PT = physical therapy, SCC = spinal cord compression.

Surgery. Surgery should be the first line of therapy in patients with spinal instability, bony compression, or paraplegia on initial presentation.[34] Surgical decompression may be used to alleviate pain and stabilize the spine, which can be accomplished by resection of a vertebral body with spinal immobilization.[24,34] Surgery usually is considered when the underlying tumor does not respond to radiation therapy or if the area has already been treated with that therapy.[21] Surgery also is indicated in patients whose neurologic status continues to deteriorate despite radiation therapy. Excision and fusion as well as complete or partial removal of the tumor may be required.[15,32]

Radiation Therapy. Radiation therapy is the definitive treatment for SCC. A total of 3000 to 4000 cGy is administered in fractionated doses.[24,57] The radiated area usually includes the affected vertebrae, and extends one or two vertebral bodies above and below the compression.[21] Radiation therapy should be the first line of therapy in ambulatory patients and for patients who are asymptomatic with epidural SCC.[34] Radiation therapy is used to minimize the size of the tumor, to decompress the spinal cord, and for pain relief. Approximately 85% of patients report pain relief with radiation therapy; approximately 50% of patients are stabilized.[32]

Corticosteroid Therapy. Steroids are commonly used initially in managing SCC until treatment of the underlying cause (with radiation therapy or surgery) can be implemented.[15,21] They are used to decrease edema, inflammation, and pain.[24,32] Patients are given a loading dose of dexamethasone (Decadron) with subsequent tapering.[21] Significant side effects can occur with high-dose steroids and these should be closely monitored. For patients who are not paretic and ambulatory, high-dose steroids and radiation therapy are recommended.[34] Use of high-dose steroids has resulted in a decreased incidence and severity of permanent neurologic damage.[54]

Chemotherapy. Patients with lymphoma, SCLC, or germ cell tumors may benefit from chemotherapy as a treatment of the underlying malignancy of SCC. Chemotherapy may be used in patients who are not candidates for radiation therapy or surgery. Patients with breast or prostate cancer may benefit from hormonal therapy.[23,24]

SUPERIOR VENA CAVA SYNDROME

SVCS is a manifestation of cancer of the bronchus. It is depicted by swelling of the neck and venous distention over the chest. It results from obstruction of the superior vena cava (SVC). The obstruction may be above or below the azygos vein from an intravascular clot, tumor in the right main upper lobe bronchus, or large amounts of lymphadenopathy of the mediastinum. The last is usually due to right paratracheal or precarinal lymph node areas.[24,27,46,61]

Occlusion of the SVC occurs frequently because of its location, its thin walls, and its being surrounded by structures that don't compress. Because blood flow in the SVC is under low pressure, when regional lymph nodes or the aorta enlarge, the SVC constricts and blood flow becomes sluggish, often resulting in occlusion.[24]

Meta analyses revealed an incidence of 2.4% to 1.1% of lung cancer patients.[46] An incidence rate of 10% of patients with a right-sided malignant metastatic mass has been reported.[34]

Patients at Risk

More than 90% of the cases of SVCS are a result of malignancy. Of these, 80% are caused by adenocarcinoma or squamous cell carcinoma of the lung and non-Hodgkin's lymphoma.[3,32,58] A small number of cases of SVCS are due to metastasis from breast or testicular cancer. T-cell leukemia causes mediastinal adenopathy and enlargement of the thymus, which can compress the SVC. Rare cases of SVCS are attributed to Kaposi's sarcoma, esophageal cancer, thymoma, mesothelioma, and Hodgkin's disease. Some patients without cancer are at risk, such as those with tuberculosis, indwelling central venous catheters, pacemaker wires, Silastic catheters, dialysis catheters, histoplasmosis, aneurysm of the aortic arch, or constrictive pericarditis.[24,32]

Pathophysiology

Of those patients with lung cancer, SVCS is usually due to direct extension or lymph node metastasis.[3,34] The obstruction impairs blood flow from the SVC to the right atrium and venous drainage above the upper thorax is impaired. This results in a decreased venous return to the heart.[32]

Assessment Findings

The signs and symptoms of SVCS vary and depend on the degree, severity, and location of the obstruction (above or below the azygos vein). The more rapid the development of the obstruction, the more severe the symptoms will be because of the body's inability to compensate.[24] As shown in Table 52-5, symptoms tend to be more severe when they are below the azygos vein.[46]

Radiology Findings

Both CT and MRI are useful to determine the extent of the underlying tumor. A contrast-enhanced spiral CT or multislice CT can identify the site of the obstruction and the presence of associated thrombus. A venogram, which is usually done before stenting, can be used to determine if the obstruction of the SVC is a result of stenosis or obstruction, and the extent of a thrombus.[46]

Chest CT can also help determine location of mediastinal lymph nodes.[23] A Doppler ultrasound can detect obstruction of the SVC if the patient cannot tolerate a CT.[4,24]

Multidisciplinary Plan of Care

Treatment of SVCS is aimed at symptom management and treatment of the underlying cause, as shown

TABLE 52-5 Clinical Manifestations of Superior Vena Cava Syndrome

BODY SYSTEM	ASSOCIATED SYMPTOMS
Cardiac	Edema of face, arm, and upper chest; congestion of collateral veins of neck and anterior chest wall; erythema of eyelids; dilated veins in upper torso, shoulders, and arms; jugular venous distention; tachycardia; chest pain; hypotension
Central nervous system	Headache, dizziness (especially if bending forward), confusion, anxiety, mental status changes, drowsiness, blurred vision, syncope
Respiratory	Dyspnea, shortness of breath, hoarseness, cyanosis, cough, dysphagia, stridor, epistaxis
Other	Tightness of neck (Stokes' sign), periorbital edema.

Data from references 3, 23, 24, 32.

in the Multidisciplinary Plan of Care below and on p. 1467. Customarily, treatment has consisted of steroids and either chemotherapy or radiation therapy. Steroids are generally indicated in patients receiving radiation therapy because of the potential for radiation-induced edema. It is further suggested that high-dose steroids should be used for a limited amount of time.[46]

Treatment of the underlying malignancy has been reported to relieve SVCS in varying percentages, depending on disease and treatment modality. Chemotherapy and radiation therapy are the two common treatments of choice.[27,32] A meta-analysis revealed 77% of patients with SCLC who received chemotherapy, radiation therapy, or both, had relief. In patients with NSCLC, 60% had relief following chemotherapy, radiation therapy, or both. A short-lived increase in signs and symptoms and increase in dyspnea within the first 3 days were observed in patients receiving chemotherapy. Data further indicated reaccumulation in 17% to 19%, respectively, in these patients.[46] It has been suggested that radiation therapy and chemotherapy should be withheld until the cause of the obstruction has been determined. If the patient's signs and symptoms are minimal, treatment may not be needed.[27,61]

MULTIDISCIPLINARY PLAN OF CARE FOR THE PATIENT WITH SUPERIOR VENA CAVA SYNDROME

PROBLEM	INTERVENTION	RATIONALE	EXPECTED OUTCOME
Obstruction of SVC	Treat underlying cause	Treatment of underlying cause is essential to reduce obstruction and for survival	Obstruction will be alleviated
	Ongoing assessment and maintenance of patent airway	Airway compromise or tracheal obstruction is possible	
	Administer diuretics and steroids if indicated Consider treatment strategies Maintain head of bed elevated 45–90 degrees	Reduce airway edema	
	Maintain Spo$_2$ higher than 95% with oxygen Keep suction equipment available at bedside	May provide temporary relief	
Potential for bleeding from thrombolytic therapy, anticoagulation, perforation, or hematoma from endovascular procedures	Monitor CBC and coagulation profiles Maintain bleeding precautions Monitor blood pressure with arterial line. Avoid blood pressure cuff in upper extremity	To identify complications of treatment High risk for thrombocytopenia Inflation of blood pressure cuff may result in more venous congestion in the affected area	Bleeding will be prevented or recognized and treated promptly

PROBLEM	INTERVENTION	RATIONALE	EXPECTED OUTCOME
Potential for infection from antineoplastic therapy, steroids, or endovascular procedures	Monitor WBC count Consider prophylactic antibiotics	To identify complications of treatment To treat potential infection	Infection will be prevented or recognized and treated promptly
	Reverse isolation, if neutropenic	To prevent infection	
Potential for dehydration, electrolyte imbalance, hypotension from diuretic therapy	Maintain fluid and electrolyte balance and adequate cardiac output Monitor vital signs Strict intake/output	To identify progression of symptoms	Dehydration will be prevented or recognized and treated promptly
Potential for skin breakdown	Meticulous skin care Elevate extremities Keep skin clean, dry, especially in skinfolds Protect areas from trauma	Patients are at risk for skin breakdown from edema, radiation therapy, or both	Skin will remain intact
Anxiety	Administer sedatives that do not act on central nervous system Provide oxygen therapy, if indicated Provide quiet environment Provide emotional support and reassurance	Patients typically present with anxiety due to respiratory distress, poor prognosis, or body image changes	Anxiety will be alleviated

Data from references 24, 32.
CBC = Complete blood cell count, Spo₂ = oxygen saturation by pulse oximetry, SVC = superior vena cava, SVCS = superior vena cava syndrome, WBC = white blood cell.

Radiation Therapy. If the patient develops respiratory distress, immediate radiation therapy is indicated. Almost 50% of patients have reported relief with radiation therapy.[59]

Chemotherapy. Chemotherapy is indicated for chemosensitive tumor etiologies (e.g., SCLC, lymphoma).[23,24,58] Patients have reported relief of symptoms in 7 to 10 days and complete resolution of symptoms within 2 weeks.[24]

Diuretic Therapy. Data support use of diuretic therapy in patients with SVCS. The likely indication is edema of the airway.[32,46] Use of diuretics may reduce preload by decreasing venous return. This will decrease pressure on the SVC, resulting in symptom relief. Diuretics should be avoided in patients who have a pericardial effusion, cardiac tamponade, or are at risk for dehydration. Furosemide is the diuretic administered most often, with dosages ranging from 20 to 80 mg orally. This can be repeated in 6 to 8 hours, as needed.[24]

Endovascular techniques (i.e., thrombolysis, angioplasty, stenting) can be done in conjunction with antineoplastic therapies.[24] Thrombolysis should be initiated if the cause of the obstruction is a thrombus. Administration of thrombolytics should be started within a few days of onset to be effective. The best results are seen in patients who receive treatment within 2 days. Tissue plasminogen activator, streptokinase, or urokinase may be used.[24] Anticoagulation in conjunction with thrombolysis prevents further thrombus formation.[32] Percutaneous placement of expandable metallic stents into the SVC reopens the SVC. This has resulted in return of normal blood flow and resolution of signs and symptoms in most patients. Immediate relief of signs and symptoms has been reported.[58] Research reveals stent insertion relieved the obstruction 90% to 95% of the time.[10,34,46] Concerns about stent placement revolve around their being time consuming and costly. Recurrence of SVC may occur, requiring retesting. A small, but clinically significant, incidence of complications is reported with stents, especially when thrombolytics are used.[46] Balloon angioplasty may be indicated to enlarge the vessel lumen for proper stent placement.[34]

Continuous monitoring and maintenance of a patent airway is essential for a patient with SVCS. Although rare, it is possible for the patient to develop airway compromise or tracheal obstruction.[24] Airway management strategies are described in the Multidisciplinary Plan of Care box for SVCS on pp. 1466-1467.

Corticosteroid Therapy. Glucocorticoids are indicated to decrease edema that is surrounding the tumor.[58] The dosage of methylprednisolone is 125 to 250 mg IV as a loading dose, then 0.5 to 1 mg/kg/dose every 6 hours for 5 days or 5 to 60 mg orally (two to four times daily) of prednisone. Dosage should be tapered over a 2-week period as symptoms resolve.[24]

CARDIAC TAMPONADE

Cardiac tamponade is compression of the heart as a result of accumulation of fluid in the pericardial sac.[25] The fluid in the pericardial sac can cause enough pressure to prevent the atria and ventricles from filling completely during diastole. This results in a decrease in cardiac output (CO), stroke volume (SV), and hypotension. The body attempts to compensate with tachycardia.[25] Eventually, the compensatory mechanisms fail. Cardiac tamponade occurs when the pericardial effusion results in hemodynamic instability with compensatory mechanisms no longer being effective.[31]

Because many of the signs and symptoms of cardiac tamponade are often subtle, the diagnosis is often overlooked. Malignancies are the most common cause of cardiac tamponade, occurring in up to 21% of patients with cancer.[6]

Patients at Risk

Pericardial effusions, which can ultimately result in tamponade, may arise from direct expansion of a tumor or from metastasis through the lymphatic vessels of the mediastinum.[28] Primary malignancies of the pericardium or myocardium, although rare, can put the patient at risk for development of a pericardial effusion. These include mesothelioma and sarcomas. Patients with benign tumors of the pericardium or mediastinum, such as teratomas, fibromas, or angiomas also maybe at risk because these tumors may cause fluid to collect in the pericardium.[18,28] Chemotherapeutic agents including daunorubicin (Cerubidine), doxorubicin (Adriamycin), paclitaxel (Taxol), and docetaxel (Taxotere) have been implicated.[18,31]

Cancers that metastasize to the heart put the patient at risk for developing cardiac tamponade. These cancers include lung, breast, esophageal, Hodgkin's and non-Hodgkin's lymphomas, leukemia, melanoma, liver, gastric, thymic, sarcomas, and pancreatic cancers.[11,18]

Cardiac tamponade can develop following surgery, radiation therapy, or chemotherapy, or from constriction of the pericardium by tumor.[31,33] Patients who have received mediastinal radiation therapy (more than 4000 cGy) are at risk because of development of postradiation pericarditis.[18,31]

Several non-cancer causes of cardiac tamponade include renal failure, myocardial infarction, viral or bacterial infection, transvenous pacemaker insertion and other invasive cardiac procedures, pericarditis, chest trauma, immune disorders, hypoalbuminemia, hypothyroidism, aneurysm, improper central venous catheter insertion, complications from angioplasty, and any other cause of injury or inflammation to the pericardium.[18,25,49]

Pathophysiology

The pericardial sac consists of the visceral and parietal layers. There is normally up to 50 ml of plasma-like fluid between them. The fluid lubricates the heart as it contracts.[25] When more than the normal amount of fluid is in the pericardial sac, a pericardial effusion has developed.

As cancer invades the pericardium, the cancer or the pericardium itself can produce excess fluid in response to the malignant process. Pericardial fluid can accumulate when lymphatic and venous flow is blocked by tumor, thereby preventing fluid reabsorption. Tumors can bleed, causing accumulation that results in cardiac tamponade.[18]

As fluid accumulates in the pericardial sac, the pericardium has the ability to stretch.[18,56] The pericardial sac can accommodate an approximate 1- to 2-L increase in fluid if the fluid accumulation occurs slowly; the hemodynamic effects occur gradually because the body has a chance to compensate. If fluid accumulates rapidly, the pericardium is unable to stretch quickly enough to accommodate the excess fluid, and hemodynamic compromise ensues.[26] As little as 200 ml of fluid accumulating over a short time can result in hemodynamic compromise. As fluid collects, the heart chambers become progressively smaller. The compression hinders blood flow from the right to left side, thus impairing ventricular filling with resultant decrease in SV and CO.[25]

Right ventricular filling is dependent on a gradient between central venous pressure and right ventricular diastolic pressure. The increased intrapericardial pressure that occurs with fluid accumulation in the pericardial sac affects this gradient and the right ventricle is unable to fill adequately. A decrease in right ventricular preload and compression leads to a decrease in the amount of blood leaving that chamber. This reduces the amount of blood flowing to and from the left heart. As pressure in the pericardium increases, intrapericardial pressures increase, equalizing right and left ventricular end-diastolic pressures.[13,31]

The right atrium and ventricle may initially compensate by causing tachycardia in an effort to increase or maintain stroke volume. Eventually the compensatory mechanisms fail and patients become symptomatic or develop cardiovascular collapse.[13,28,31]

Assessment Findings

Early signs and symptoms of cardiac tamponade may be unremarkable and undetected.[26] The presentation of cardiac tamponade depends on a number of factors, including how quickly the fluid collects in the pericardium and the underlying cause. The onset of symptoms may be impressive if the fluid accumulates quickly.

Patients most frequently present with progressive shortness of breath, chest pain, and cough. Other symptoms are summarized in Table 52-6. Three classic symptoms of cardiac tamponade, known as Beck's triad, include hypotension, distended neck veins, and distant heart sounds. This triad of symptoms is rarely seen clinically.[28]

Although not unique to cardiac tamponade, a pulsus paradoxus is a sign of this condition. This is a decrease in systolic blood pressure of greater than or equal to 10 mm Hg on inspiration. It may be noted when more pulse beats are palpated on expiration than inspiration or when a palpable pulse is lost on inspiration.[26] It is possible for patients with cardiac tamponade with severe hypotension or other cardiac conditions (e.g., atrial septal defect, severe aortic stenosis, left ventricular dysfunction) not to have a pulsus paradoxus.

A frequent finding on physical examination is a pericardial friction rub. This is best auscultated at the left lower sternal border or the apex when the patient is sitting forward.[60]

Early signs and symptoms of cardiac tamponade include dyspnea and retrosternal chest pain that increases when the patient is in a supine position and is relieved when leaning forward. This is caused by compression on the heart. Patients also manifest dysphagia, hoarseness, or hiccoughs from mechanical compression on nerves of the esophagus, bronchi, or trachea; dizziness; light-headedness or agitation due to hypoxia; and weakness, fatigue, or malaise related to decreased CO. Gastrointestinal complaints include anorexia, nausea, or vomiting from visceral congestion and venous stasis.[18]

Late signs and symptoms include retrosternal chest pain, progressive dyspnea, and orthopnea related to

TABLE 52-6 Signs and Symptoms of Cardiac Tamponade	
SYSTEM	**SIGNS AND SYMPTOMS**
Cardiovascular	Tachycardia, jugular venous distention, pulsus paradoxus, pericardial friction rub (uncommon), hypotension, cyanosis, narrowing pulse pressure (decreased systolic blood pressure, increased diastolic blood pressure), increased SVR, increased ventricular diastolic pressure, increased pulmonary venous pressure, distant or absent apical pulse, elevated CVP, palpitations, nonspecific chest pain that is relieved when leaning forward and worsens with deep inspiration, diaphoresis, edema, dysrhythmias (PACs, PVCs), decreased stroke volume, decreased cardiac output, muffled heart sounds, sharp stabbing chest pain that radiates to shoulder, back, or abdomen
Gastrointestinal	Hepatic enlargement/congestion, ascites, dysphagia, anorexia, hepatojugular reflux (elevation in jugular venous pressure by $\geq$1 cm), abdominal distention
Neurologic	Mental status changes, dizziness, drowsiness, restlessness, loss of consciousness, light-headedness, fainting, anxiety
Respiratory	Shortness of breath, dyspnea on exertion that progresses to air hunger, tachypnea, crackles at bases, hoarseness, cough, orthopnea
Other	Pallor, fatigue, weakness, malaise, low-grade fever, chills

Data from references 13, 18, 26, 31, 56, 60.
CVP = Central venous pressure, PACs = premature atrial contractions, PVCs = premature ventricular contractions, SVR = systemic vascular resistance.

decreased CO and hypoxia; peripheral edema from venous congestion; and confusion, restlessness, and apprehension due to hypoxia and decreased cerebral perfusion.[18]

Several tests assist in the diagnosis of cardiac tamponade. These include chest radiograph, CT scan, MRI, pulmonary artery catheterization, echocardiogram, and electrocardiogram (ECG).[28]

Radiology Findings

A chest film of a patient with cardiac tamponade may reveal cardiac enlargement from the increased fluid in the pericardial sac and mediastinal widening or hilar adenopathy.[18] However, if the fluid accumulates rapidly, radiographic findings may be normal. If the fluid accumulates slowly, the pericardial sac may hold 1 to 2 L of fluid. In these cases, the radiograph reveals a "water bottle" heart.[18,28] At least 250 ml of pericardial fluid must have collected for it to be visible on x-ray.[26]

CT may be used in conjunction with clinical findings to help diagnose and manage cardiac tamponade.[47] It reveals a pericardial effusion and differentiates this diagnosis from superior vena cava syndrome.

MRI may be used in conjunction with clinical findings to help manage cardiac tamponade.[47] MRI has partial value in the diagnosis of cardiac tamponade. It shows large pericardial effusions and provides an estimate of the extent of an effusion Both CT and MRI may be less readily available and are usually not needed unless Doppler echocardiography is not available.[56]

Diagnostic Evaluation

Electrocardiogram. Findings on ECG are usually nonspecific. Electrical alternans, a change in the axis from beat to beat, is caused by excessive heart movement in the increased pericardial fluid.[18,28,49] Tachycardia, premature contractions, change in shape and amplitude of P waves, ST segment elevation or depression, and low-voltage QRS complexes also are noted.[18,26,31]

Echocardiogram. Echocardiogram is the quickest and most accurate method to diagnose cardiac tamponade.[18,26] With an echocardiogram, ultrasonic waves produced with a probe create a picture of the heart and portray cardiac functioning. It reveals fluid in the pericardial sac and compression of the heart chambers. Echocardiograms also provide an estimate of ejection fraction, can detect a pericardial mass, and further assess hemodynamic sequela of cardiac tamponade.[31,33]

Pulmonary Artery Catheterization. Evaluation of pulmonary artery pressures reveals equalization of right- and left-sided heart pressures, decreased CO and elevated systemic vascular resistance (SVR), central venous pressure, left atrial pressure, pulmonary artery pressures, and pulmonary artery wedge pressure. Pulmonary artery catheterization is an invasive procedure and is associated with several risks; therefore catheterization is not routinely used as a diagnostic tool.[31]

Multidisciplinary Plan of Care

Overall management of cardiac tamponade centers on relieving pressure on the heart and enhancing cardiac function.[26,31] Other goals include fluid removal, prevention of reaccumulation of fluid, and minimizing complications.[31] The Multidisciplinary Plan of Care below and on p. 1471 summarizes management of the patient with cardiac tamponade.

Initial management strategies of the patient with cardiac tamponade should be intended to stabilize the

MULTIDISCIPLINARY PLAN OF CARE FOR THE PATIENT WITH CARDIAC TAMPONADE

PROBLEM	INTERVENTION	RATIONALE	EXPECTED OUTCOME
Hemodynamic compromise	Administer oxygen to keep SpO_2 ≥92% Monitor ECG for dysrhythmias, monitor for hypotension and electrical alternans	Decreases tissue demands, helps reduce myocardial workload, respiratory distress, and anxiety.	Patient will attain and maintain systolic blood pressure greater than 90 mm Hg. Filling pressures will be optimized.
	Administer IV fluids (0.9% NS or LR) or blood/blood products	Increases filling pressures, cardiac output.	
	Prepare to administer inotropes	Improves myocardial contractility and enhances preload.	
	Avoid sudden changes in preload and increases in SVR	These changes can lead to rapid clinical deterioration.	

PROBLEM	INTERVENTION	RATIONALE	EXPECTED OUTCOME
	Avoid beta blockers and diuretics	Beta-receptor antagonist. Decreases circulating volume, ventricular filling	
	Consider use of vasodilators Maintain patient on bed rest in semi-Fowler's position	May decrease cardiac workload.	
Pain and anxiety	Administer mild anxiolytics	Cardiac tamponade is an emergency that can cause pain and anxiety.	Patient's pain and anxiety will be relieved.
	Administer pain medication with caution	Opioids can contribute to hypotension.	
	Provide emotional support as needed Position changes, as tolerated	Admission to critical care can be anxiety provoking.	
Deficient knowledge	Teach patient/family S/S to report if at risk for development of cardiac tamponade Provide explanation of anticipated interventions and associated sensations Allow patient to verbalize concerns	Early intervention is essential to minimize complications and improve patient outcomes	Patient and family will be informed about signs and symptoms to report and of anticipated procedures
Potential for fluid reaccumulation	Ongoing assessment of systems Investigate signs and symptoms of reaccumulation immediately Intervene as indicated and described	Patients have reaccumulation of fluid following treatment	

Data from references 13, 18, 26, 31.
ECG = Electrocardiogram, LR = lactated Ringer's, NS = normal saline, Spo$_2$ = oxygen saturation by pulse oximetry, S/S = signs and symptoms, SVR = systemic vascular resistance.

patient. Patients may require maintenance of a patent airway and volume resuscitation to enhance right-sided preload and stroke volume.[28] Maintaining adequate filling pressures and enhancing myocardial contractility and cardiac output are essential in managing the patient.[13] Positive pressure ventilation should be avoided, if possible, because it further decreases cardiac output.[31,56]

Agents that decrease SVR or those that rapidly decrease preload (e.g., vasodilators) should be avoided because these patients are sensitive to changes in intrathoracic pressure and SVR.[13]

Treatment depends on cause and severity of the tamponade.[26] Patients with severe hemodynamic compromise require decompression with pericardiocentesis. Patients who are more stable may respond to supportive measures.[13]

Pericardiocentesis. Percutaneous pericardiocentesis entails insertion of a catheter into the pericardial space to drain the fluid. The catheter can be left in place for up to 24 hours to drain additional accumulation of fluid.[18,26]

In patients with significant hemodynamic compromise, removal of a small amount of pericardial fluid (50 to 100 ml) may improve the patient's condition. If possible, the catheter should be allowed to remain in place to drain fluid.[28] When less than 50 ml per day drains, the catheter can be removed.[56]

Complications associated with pericardiocentesis include dysrhythmias, pneumothorax, laceration of the coronary arteries, laceration of the lung, puncture of the right atrium or ventricle, trauma to abdominal organs (e.g., liver), infection, introduction of air into the heart, and hypotension.[31] The likelihood of these complications occurring is decreased when the procedure is done under direct visualization or when there is a large effusion.[31,56]

Echocardiogram-Guided Pericardiocentesis.

Echo-guided pericardiocentesis is considered the procedure of choice to remove pericardial fluid. The direction of the needle and depth of needle advancement are confirmed with echocardiography.[60] The needle tip is visualized with imaging and the optimal point of penetration of the pericardium can be determined.[56]

Pericardial Window.

Pericardial window procedures usually are performed on patients who do not respond to other treatments. This procedure entails removing a section of the pericardium, creating an opening in the pericardium to drain fluid from the pericardial sac if cardiac tamponade is recurrent.[26] Complications of this procedure include infection, atelectasis, pleural effusion, pneumothorax, pain, and dysrhythmias.[31,32] Because the procedure is not tolerated well in critically ill patients, stabilization of the patient's condition should be done first.

Balloon Pericardiotomy.

A pericardiocentesis provides temporary relief of signs and symptoms until the underlying malignancy is treated. Balloon pericardiotomy is another option to prevent fluid accumulation.[7,31,32,33] This procedure involves the insertion of a catheter with a balloon tip into the pericardial sac. The catheter tears the pericardium and creates a window for drainage of fluid. The chance of fluid reaccumulation is minimized because the balloon decreases the space. Once the balloon is inserted, there is an opening in the pericardium that facilitates internal drainage and fluid reabsorption. When the balloon is in place, it is dilated to form a pericardial window, which allows fluid to drain.[7,31]

Sclerotherapy.

Sclerotherapy may be indicated for patients with recurrent cardiac tamponade. It entails insertion of a catheter into the pericardial sac with subsequent administration of a sclerosing agent. The effusion is resolved because of an inflammatory response from the agent, connecting the visceral and parietal layers of the pericardium.[18,26]

Common sclerosing agents include bleomycin (Blenoxane), doxycycline (Vibramycin), cisplatin, fluorouracil (5FU), minocycline (Minocin), nitrogen mustard, thiotepa (Thioplex), and radioisotopes.[7,31,32] Side effects of sclerotherapy include pain, nausea, fever, and dysrhythmias.[31]

Pericardiectomy.

A pericardiectomy is the excision of part or all of the pericardium that involves a thoracotomy or median sternotomy. The pericardium is resected to enhance drainage of fluid into the pleural space.[31] A pericardiectomy is indicated for patients with pericarditis or those with cancer with constriction caused by radiation therapy.[7,31] This surgical procedure can be used in patients with recurrent malignant cardiac tamponade.[18] Complications include laceration of the myocardium, bleeding, scarring, and infection.[31]

Poststabilization.

On stabilization, treatment of the underlying malignancy should begin. Depending on the patient's disease and condition, management may include radiation therapy or chemotherapy.[18]

MEDICATIONS USED IN ONCOLOGIC EMERGENCIES

MEDICATION	ACTIONS	DOSAGE	SPECIAL CONSIDERATIONS
Hypercalcemia of Malignancy			
Bisphosphonates	The precise mechanism of action of the bisphosphonates on bone cells and bone resorption is not completely understood. It involves inhibition of the function of osteoclasts in a variety of ways (e.g., by producing a direct toxic effect on the resorbing osteoclasts, by promoting programmed cell death, or by inhibiting the differentiation of the osteoclasts into mature osteoclasts). Inhibits calcium reabsorption and enhances urinary calcium excretion.	Pamidronate (Aredia): serum calcium 12–13.5 mg/dl: 60–90 mg IV over 4 hr Serum calcium higher than 13.5 mg/dl: 90 mg IV over 4 hr Zoledronic acid (Zometa): if serum calcium equal to or greater than 12 mg/dl, 4 mg IV over at least 15 min	Should be started when rehydration has been established. Dose may be repeated if needed after 7 days.

MEDICATION	ACTIONS	DOSAGE	SPECIAL CONSIDERATIONS
Loop diuretics: Furosemide (Lasix)	Increases elimination of fluid and calcium by the kidney. Inhibits calcium reabsorption by the kidneys and protects against volume overload.	Up to 100 mg IV every 1–4 hr may be given	If administered as continuous IV infusion, should be given at rate ≤4 mg/minute.
Corticosteroids	Enhances calcium excretion in the urine and inhibits calcium reabsorption in the gastrointestinal tract. Part of treatment of underlying malignancy.	Variable; depends on protocol to treat underlying malignancy	Should be avoided until volume status has been restored. Carefully monitor magnesium and potassium values.
Tumor Lysis Syndrome			
Sodium bicarbonate	Alkalizes urine to prevent uric acid crystal formation.	50–100 mEq added to each L of hydration. Can be started 1–2 days prior to starting chemotherapy	Maintain urine pH greater than 7.5
Allopurinol (Zyloprim)	Xanthine oxidase inhibitor. Decreases uric acid formation.	PO: 100 mg daily IV: 200–400 mg/m^2. Maximum of 600 mg/day	
Rasburicase (Elitek)	Recombinant urate-oxidase enzyme.	0.15–0.20 mg/kg IV over 30 min daily for 5 days	Can cause severe hemolysis in patients with glucose-6-phosphate dehydrogenase deficiency. Can cause severe anaphylactic reactions. Has been associated with methemoglobinemia.
SIADH			
Demeclocycline (Declomycin)	Causes nephrogenic diabetes insipidus.	600–1200 mg daily PO in three or four divided doses, then decrease dose to 600–900 mg/day in divided doses	
Spinal Cord Compression			
Corticosteroids: Dexamethasone (Decadron)	Decreases inflammatory response to underlying tumor and edema surrounding the tumor that may damage the spinal cord.	Loading dose: 4–100 mg IV, followed by 16–96 mg/day in divided doses	Taper over several days.
Superior Vena Cava Syndrome			
Diuretics: Furosemide (Lasix)	Decreases right-sided preload (venous return), which will decrease pressure on the SVC.	20–80 mg PO; may repeat in 6–8 hr	
Corticosteroids: Methylprednisolone (Solu-Medrol)	Decreases inflammatory response to underlying tumor and edema surrounding the tumor.	Loading dose: 125–250 mg IV Maintenance dose: 0.5–1 mg/kg IV every 6 hr for up to 5 days	

SIADH = Syndrome of inappropriate antidiuretic hormone, SVC = superior vena cava.

CONCLUSIONS

Patients undergoing treatment for cancer require ongoing support. This need is intensified when patients develop a potentially life-threatening complication of the disease or its treatments. When these emergencies occur, the multidisciplinary team plays a pivotal role in helping the patient and family cope. Focused monitoring and prompt intervention of preventive and management approaches are essential to promote quality of life and reduce morbidity and mortality. The knowledge of the critical care nurse regarding these oncologic emergencies is essential for attaining these quality patient outcomes. A summary of the common medications used for each of the oncologic emergencies appears in the Medication table on pp. 1472-1473.

REFERENCES

1. Altman, A. (2001). Acute tumor lysis syndrome. *Semin Oncol, 28* (2, Suppl 5), 3–8.
2. Arch, D., Sass, P., & Abul-Khoudou, H. (2001). Recognizing spinal cord emergencies. *Am Fam Phys, 64*(4), 631–638.
3. Beckles, M. A., et al. (2003). Initial evaluation of the patient with lung cancer: symptoms, signs, laboratory tests, and paraneoplastic syndromes. *Chest, 123*(1), 97S–104S.
4. Benenstein, R., et al. (2003). Doppler diagnosis of acute occlusion of the superior vena cava. *Echocardiography, 20*(1), 97–98.
5. Brant, J. M. (2002). Rasburicase: an innovative new treatment for hyperuricemia associated with tumor lysis syndrome. *Clin J Oncol Nurs, 6*(1), 12–16, 25–26.
6. Bullock, B. L. (2000). Altered cardiac function. In B. L. Bullock & R. L. Henze (Eds.), *Focus on pathophysiology.* Philadelphia: Lippincott Williams, & Wilkins.
7. Camp-Sorrell, D. (2001). Cardiac tamponade. In R. A. Gates & R. M. Finks (Eds.), *Oncology nursing secrets.* Philadelphia: Hanley & Belfus.
8. Cantril, C. A., & Haylock, P. J. (2004). Tumor lysis syndrome. Prevention and early detection are crucial in caring for patients with cancer. *Am J Nurs, 104*(4), 49–52.
9. Carroll, M. F., & Schade, D. S. (2003). A practical approach to hypercalcemia. *Am Fam Phys, 67*(9), 1959–1966.
10. Chatziioannon, A., et al. (2003). Stent therapy for malignant superior vena cava syndrome. Should be first line or simple adjunct to radiotherapy. *Eur J Radiol, 47*(3), 247–250.
11. Cheng, M., et al. (2005). Cardiac tamponade as a manifestation of advanced thymic carcinoma. *Heart Lung, 34*(2), 136–141.
12. Cope, D. (2004). Tumor lysis syndrome. *Clin J Oncol Nurs, 6*(1), 415–416.
13. Cousineau, A., & Savitsky, E. (2005). Cardiac tamponade presenting as an apparent life-threatening event. *Pediatr Emerg Care, 21* (2), 104–108.
14. Crook, N. (2002). Vasopressin V receptor antagonists. *J Clin Pathol, 53,* 883.
15. Crossno, R. J. (2004). Dying in the emergency department: what emergency physicians should know about palliative medicine. *Top Emerg Med, 26*(1), 19–28.
16. DeMichele, A., & Glick, J. (2001). Cancer-related emergencies. In R. Lenhard, R. Osteen & T. Gansler (Eds.), *Clinical oncology.* Atlanta: American Cancer Society.
17. Doane, L. (2002). Overview of tumor lysis syndrome. *Semin Oncol Nurs, 18*(3), 2–5.
18. Flounders, J. A. (2003a). Cardiac emergencies: pericardial effusion and cardiac tamponade. *Oncol Nurs Forum, 30*(2), E48–E53.
19. Flounders, J. A. (2003b). Syndrome of inappropriate antidiuretic hormone. *Oncol Nurs Forum, 30*(3), E63–E68.
20. Flounders, J. A. (2003c). Oncology emergencies modules: spinal cord compression. *Oncol Nurs Forum, 30*(1), E17–E21.
21. Flounders, J. A., & Ott, B. B. (2003). Oncology emergency modules: spinal cord compression. *Oncol Nurs Forum, 30*(1), E17–E23.
22. Gobel, B. H. (2002). Management of tumor lysis syndrome: prevention and treatment. *Semin Oncol Nurs, 18*(3), 12–16.
23. Gucalp, R., & Dutcher, J. (2001). Oncologic emergencies. In E. Braunwald, et al. (Eds.), *Harrison's principles of internal medicine* (15th ed.). New York: McGraw-Hill.
24. Gullatte, M. M., Kaplow, R., & Heidrich, D. (2005). Oncology. In K. K. Kuebler, et al. (Eds.), *Palliative practices. An interdisciplinary approach.* St. Louis: Mosby.
25. Hawley, J., & Dreher, H. M. (2002). Cardiac tamponade: the pressure's on. *Nursing, 32*(4), 32cc1–32cc4.
26. Hawley, J., Dreher, H. M., & Vasso, M. (2003). Under pressure: treating cardiac tamponade. *Nurs Manage, 34*(2), 44D, F, H.
27. Hemann, R. (2001). Superior vena cava syndrome. *Clin Excell Nurse Pract, 5*(2), 85–87.
28. Hemphill, R. R., & Ismach, R. B. (2001). Oncologic emergencies: diagnosis, triage, and management. *Emerg Med Rep, 22*(15), 1–11.
29. Inzucchi, S. E. (2004). Understanding hypercalcemia. Its metabolic basis, signs, and symptoms. *Postgrad Med, 115*(4), 69–76.
30. Kaplow, R. (2002). Pathophysiology, signs and symptoms of acute tumor lysis syndrome. *Semin Oncol Nurs, 18*(3), 6–11.
31. Kaplow, R. (2005). Cardiac tamponade. In C. H. Yarbro, M. H. Frogge, & M. Goodman (Eds.), *Cancer nursing principles and practice* (6th ed.). Boston: Jones and Bartlett.
32. Kaplow, R., & Reid, M. (2006). Oncologic emergencies. In H. M. Schell & K. A. Puntillo (Eds.), *Critical care nursing secrets.* Philadelphia: Hanley & Belfus.
33. Keefe, D. L. (2000). Cardiovascular emergencies in the cancer patient. *Semin Oncol, 27*(3), 244–255.
34. Kvale, P. A., Simoff, M., & Prakash, V. B. (2003). Palliative care. *Chest, 123*(1), Suppl, 284S–311S.
35. Levack, P., et al. (2002). Don't wait for a sensory level—listen to the symptoms: a prospective audit of the delays in the diagnosis of malignant cord compression. *Clin Oncol, 14*(6), 472–480.
36. Lublaw, D. A., Laperriere, N. J., & Mackillop, W. J. (2003). A population-based study of malignant spinal cord compression in Ontario. *Clin Oncol, 13*(4), 211–217.
37. National Coalition for Cancer Survivorship. Hypercalcemia. Available at http://cancer.nccs.drtango.com.
38. National Cancer Institute. Hypercalcemia. Available at: http://cancerweb.ncl.ac.uk/cancernet.
39. Osowski, M. (2002). Spinal cord compression. An obstructive oncologic emergency. *Top Adv Pract Nurs, 2*(4), 7p.
40. Pease, N. J., Harris, R. J., & Finlay, I. G. (2004). Development and audit of a care pathway for the management of patients with suspected malignant spinal cord compression. *Physiotherapy, 90*(1), 27–34.
41. Purdue, C. (2004). Clinical diagnosis and treatment of malignant spinal cord compression. *Nurs Times, 100*(38), 38–41.
42. Quinn, J., & DeAngelis, L. (2000). Neurologic emergencies in the cancer patient. *Semin Oncol, 27,* 311–321.
43. Ribeiro, R. C., & Pui, C. (2003). Recombinant urate oxidase for prevention of hyperuricemia and tumor lysis syndrome in lymphoid malignancies. *Clin Lymphoma, 3*(4), 225–232.
44. Rogers, M. J. (2003). New insights into the molecular mechanisms of action of bisphosphonates. *Curr Pharm Des, 9,* 2643–2658.

45. Ross, J. R., et al. (2004). A systematic review of the role of bisphosphonates in metastatic cancer. *Health Technol Assess, 8*(4), 1–176.

46. Rowell, N. P., & Gleeson, F. V. (2005). Steroids, radiotherapy, chemotherapy, and stents for superior vena caval obstruction in carcinoma of the bronchus. *Cochrane Database Syst Rev*, (4): CD001316.

47. Sagrista, S. J. (2003). Clinical decision making based on cardiac diagnostic imaging techniques (I). Diagnosis and therapeutic management of patients with cardiac tamponade and constrictive pericarditis. *Rev Esp Cardiol, 56*(2), 195–205.

48. Sallan, S. (2001). Management of acute tumor lysis syndrome. *Semin Oncol, 28*(2, Suppl 5), 9–12.

49. Shatzer, M., & Castor, A. (2004). Drug challenge (eye on diagnostics). *Nursing, 34*(3), 73–74.

50. Sherwood, L. (2004). *Human physiology from cells to systems.* Belmont, CA: Brooks/Cole.

51. Shirland, L. (2001). SIADH: a case review. *Neonat Netw, 20*(1), 25–32.

52. Shuey, K. M., Brant, J. M. (2004). Hypercalcemia of malignancy: Part II. *Clin J Oncol Nurs, 8*(3), 321–323.

53. Solimando, D. A. (2001). Overview of hypercalcemia of malignancy. *Am J Health Syst Pharm, 58*, S4–S7.

54. *Spinal cord compression: a palliative care emergency.* Available at: www.palliative.org.

55. *Spinal cord trauma.* Available at:www.nlm.nih.gov/medlineplus/ency.

56. Spodick, D. H. (2003). Current concepts: acute cardiac tamponade. *N Engl J Med, 349*(7), 684–690.

57. Tan, S. (2002). Recognition and treatment of oncologic emergencies. *J Infus Nurs, 25*(3), 182–188.

58. Thirlwell, C., & Brock, C. S. (2003). Emergencies in oncology. *Clin Med, 3*(4), 306–310.

59. Vachani, C. (2006). Superior vena cava syndrome. Available at: www.oncolink.com/resources/article.cfm?c=16&s=46&ss=205&id=893.

60. Valley, V. T. (2003). Pericarditis and cardiac tamponade. Available at:www.emedicine.com/EMERG/topic412.htm.

61. Wudel, L. J., & Nesbitt, J. C. (2001). Superior vena cava syndrome. *Curr Treat Options Oncol, 2*(1), 77–91.

CHAPTER 53 Chemical Dependency

Sandra L. Schutz

The chemically addicted patient presents unique patient care challenges in the critical care setting. Alcoholism and drug dependence are believed to be associated with 25% to 50% of all general hospital admissions.[78] The addicted patient can be admitted to critical care for a number of reasons. Admission may be due to an illness or injury that is the direct result of the patient's addiction, or the patient may have an illness complicated by the addiction. Regardless of the reason for admission to critical care, addicted patients are at risk of withdrawal from addicted substances during their stay.

In each of the above circumstances, the nurse is faced with the challenge of identifying and understanding the physiologic effects of the addictive substance or substances. Withdrawal may be evident as a single physiologic event, or may complicate a particular illness or injury. The nurse must also have knowledge of the presenting signs and symptoms of withdrawal from a particular substance and the appropriate management of the withdrawal state. At the same time, the nurse must anticipate and attempt to prevent complications from withdrawal. Last, the nurse must have an understanding of the physiologic, behavioral, or psychoactive states of withdrawal, and of pharmacologic agents that may impact withdrawal directly or indirectly.

PATIENT ASSESSMENT

A thorough assessment of the patient's substance use is vital in the identification and management of withdrawal syndromes. It may be difficult for the nurse to make inquiries of patients or their families regarding possible or known addictive substance use. Often, patients are reluctant to report the extent of their substance use. This reluctance may be out of shame or fear of social or legal consequences. There also may be denial that the use of a given substance is problematic, minimizing reporting. The best way for the nurse to obtain the information needed is to be supportive and to inform the patient and family or support system of the importance of accurate information both for predicting possible withdrawal and for treating withdrawal. Asking how much or how often is effective for most low to moderate substance users, while these questions may result in underreporting in the heavy user. Exploring whether the heavy user has experienced poor control over the substance or experienced deleterious social or behavioral consequences may be more effective.[78]

A complete list of substances used and the amount and the manner in which they are used is essential. The frequency and duration of use is also useful. Additionally, the time of last use of the substance is helpful in establishing a correlation between the signs and symptoms seen or the anticipated signs and symptoms of withdrawal. Of particular importance is the assessment of poly substance abuse, as the combination of certain substances, such as alcohol and benzodiazepines, can complicate withdrawal. It is common for one substance to be used in exchange for another or for multiple substances to be used simultaneously.[78] Also helpful is knowledge of the severity of prior withdrawal episodes and if there have been any periods of sobriety in the past.

Once substance use information is known, it can be used to assist in the anticipation of withdrawal, including the possible timing of the onset and course of withdrawal, and to allow for earlier medical, nursing, and psychosocial management of the patient (Box 53-1).

ALCOHOL ADDICTION

In 2004, 121 million Americans ages 12 or older were current drinkers of alcohol and 55 million (22.8%) had participated in binge drinking—defined as five or more drinks on at least one occasion in the 30 days before the National Survey on Drug Use and Health.[77] It is believed that approximately one third of drinkers of alcohol are women.[20] The prevalence of alcohol abuse and dependence in the inpatient and outpatient settings is between 15% and 40%.[59] Every fifth patient admitted to a general hospital abuses alcohol.[53] Excessive alcohol consumption is the third leading cause of preventable death in the United States after cigarette smoking and obesity.[59] Alcohol or its withdrawal will impact the hospital course and the nursing care of the patient either directly or indirectly.

Box 53-1

Assessment of Chemically Addicted Patients

- Complete list of substances used
- Amount used
- Manner of use
- Frequency of use
- Duration of use
- Date and time of last use of each substance
- Withdrawal history
- Periods of sobriety

Pathophysiology of Alcohol Addiction

An understanding of the chemical effects of alcohol on the brain and the subsequent tolerance of the brain to repeated doses of alcohol is essential to understanding the clinical syndrome seen in acute alcohol withdrawal. The primary effect of alcohol on the brain is as a neural depressant, resulting in decreased overall brain excitability.[1] This effect results from the enhancement of the inhibitory neurotransmitter gamma-aminobutyric acid (GABA). GABA receptors involve motor control, visual acuity, and regulation of anxiety. The effects of alcohol on the brain are also attributable to the release of opioid peptides and dopamine (the major excitatory neurotransmitter), the inhibition of glutamate receptors, and the interaction of serotonin systems.[24] The combined neurologic changes cause a decrease in overall brain excitability. This results in sedative-hypnotic effects (e.g., sedation, muscle relaxation, and a raised seizure threshold). The resulting signs of these neural changes include the classic signs and symptoms of alcohol intoxication, including ataxia, slurred speech, mood lability, decreased concentration and memory, poor judgment, facial flushing, enlarged pupils, and nystagmus.[33] The relative deficiency of GABA is believed to be the predisposing factor for seizure activity seen with alcohol withdrawal.[45] The brain compensates for the chronic exposure to alcohol by upregulating the excitatory neurotransmitters.[1]

Alcohol also inhibits the sensitivity of the brain to the autonomic adrenergic systems.[45] With chronic alcohol use, there is an upregulation that in withdrawal results in a rebound overactivity of the brain and peripheral noradrenergic systems.[45] The symptoms of tachycardia, hypertension, tremor, diaphoresis, and anxiety are in part due to this increased sympathetic autonomic activity in the brain.[45]

Tolerance is a state of adaptation in which repeated exposure to a substance over time induces changes that result in diminution of one or more of the drug's effects.[79] The brain develops tolerance to alcohol over time with repeated exposure. Tolerance to alcohol is manifested as a reduced sensitivity to the effects of alcohol.[89] Over time, an individual will see fewer effects with greater amounts of alcohol until the threshold is reached where effects are then seen and felt. As use progresses, tolerance becomes dependence. *Dependence* is that physiologic state in which the adaptation to a specific substance, such as alcohol, is characterized by a state of withdrawal in the absence of the substance.[78] At some point the body becomes accustomed to a certain level of alcohol on a regular basis. When taken in amounts less than the accustomed levels, withdrawal will occur even in the presence of alcohol.

Withdrawal will manifest itself as the exact opposite presentation of alcohol, resulting in a hyperexcitable neurologic state.[60] Hyperexcitability is also seen in the peripheral noradrenergic systems secondary to the activity in the brain. The resulting symptoms of withdrawal are from the sudden stimulation of excitability receptors previously inhibited by alcohol. Withdrawal can occur at any time the level of alcohol drops below the level to which the brain has become adapted. This activity manifests in the physical symptoms of tachycardia, hypertension, tremor, diaphoresis, and anxiety.[45] The extreme anxiety associated with alcohol withdrawal is due in part to increased corticotropin-releasing factor (CRF) in the brain, which can rise to approximately 500% of baseline levels within 12 hours after the cessation of alcohol ingestion.[7] CRF is a neuropeptide that induces behavioral and physiologic changes similar to those seen in the stress response. In addition to anxiety, the patient in withdrawal may also experience depressive-like symptoms.[7]

Acute Alcohol Withdrawal Syndrome

Acute alcohol withdrawal is a physiologic condition of hyperexcitability of the brain that, if left undertreated or untreated, can be fatal. Symptoms have been suggested to relate proportionately to the amount of alcohol intake and the duration of the patient's recent drinking pattern.[1] This is generally true except in the patient who has had a long-term steady alcohol intake with no prior withdrawals (e.g., long-term older adult drinker).[84] These patients may show limited or minimal signs of withdrawal. The minimal withdrawal patient is contrasted with the patient who has undergone a number of previous withdrawal episodes or is a binge drinker. This latter patient will potentially experience a more difficult withdrawal.

A thorough assessment, if possible, of the patient's normal alcoholic intake is essential. The assessment should include the amount consumed per episode, the type of alcoholic beverage, the duration of drinking per episode, and the age at which drinking started. Knowledge of the drinking pattern, constant or binge, is very helpful. An assessment of the time of the last drink, prior withdrawal episodes, and time sober between relapses as well as determination of seizure activity in withdrawal is valuable. A history of previous withdrawals involving delirium tremens (DTs) is also important. Patients who have experienced DTs or seizures previously in withdrawal are at greater risk of recurrence of the same states.[1,45] If the patient is unable to provide this information, the family can be a helpful resource or can validate the patient's statements. All of this information is helpful in planning for management and serves as a best predictor of the possible severity of the withdrawal course.

Alcohol withdrawal progresses in stages of increasing severity, with the symptoms very slight or mild in the beginning to extreme in the later stages. A common misconception is that the patient with evidence of alcohol in the bloodstream cannot be in withdrawal. Symptoms of withdrawal can be present with a measurable blood alcohol level provided the alcohol level is below the patient's customary level.[45] In general, the symptoms of alcohol withdrawal relate proportionately to the amount of alcohol consumed and the duration of the patient's recent drinking routine.[1]

The onset of withdrawal symptoms can vary. Some authors report the onset of minor symptoms can begin within 4 hours after stopping or suddenly decreasing the amount of alcohol intake[33] and others report 6 to 12 hours after the last drink[1,24,42] and as late as 24 hours after the last drink.[45] Minor or mild symptoms include insomnia, mild to moderate anxiety, and mild tremulousness. Visible tremors are usually preceded by tremors that can be felt under the skin (e.g., in the finger tips or upper arm). Other symptoms include gastrointestinal upset, headache, diaphoresis, tachycardia, and hypertension. If minor symptoms go untreated, a more severe withdrawal state can be seen at 24 to 72 hours after the last drink.[1,45] Symptoms include marked restlessness, agitation, moderate visible tremulousness, constant eye movement, marked diaphoresis, nausea, vomiting, diarrhea, and marked tachycardia. Systolic blood pressures can be greater than 160 mm Hg. Patients may be disoriented and appear confused, but reorientation is possible.[2] Patients may experience perceptual distortions of a visual, auditory, or tactile nature, such as lights being too bright, sounds being too loud, or being startled.[45] Overall symptoms are reported to peak at 36 to 48 hours and subside in approximately 5 days.[33]

Generalized tonic-clonic seizures can occur at anytime 8 to 24 hours after the last drink. Seizures may also occur before the blood alcohol level returns to zero.[45] Seizure activity may be limited to a single seizure or may occur in a burst of several seizures over a period of 1 to 6 hours.[45] A small percentage of patients experiencing seizures in withdrawal, fewer than 3%, can go on to develop status epilepticus.[45] The risk of seizures increases in patients who have had previous seizures in withdrawal or in patients who have undergone repeated withdrawal episodes. The risk of seizure activity is further increased in patients who are undergoing withdrawal concurrently from alcohol and benzodiazepines or other sedative-hypnotic drugs.[45]

Patients who have stopped drinking 72 to 120 hours prior and received no or limited treatment are at risk of alcohol withdrawal delirium, also known as delerium tremens (DTs).[24] This can progress into a severe, life-threatening condition accompanied by an autonomic storm.[45] DTs affect about 5% of patients who have been drinking fairly heavily for a decade or more.[24] Symptoms of DTs include frequent frank visual or auditory hallucinations, extreme agitation and severe disorientation, drenching sweats, hyperthermia, hypertension, incontinence, and tachycardia. There may be severe psychomotor activity and severe disruption of the normal sleep-wake cycle, marked by the absence of clear sleep for several days.[45] The duration of this stage of withdrawal is variable, but peaks at 5 days.[1]

Risk factors for developing alcohol withdrawal delirium include concurrent acute medical illness (e.g., pneumonia, daily heavy alcohol use or an extended period of binge drinking, previous delirium tremens or withdrawal seizures, older age, abnormal liver function, and evidence of severe withdrawal symptoms on presentation).[1] Mayo-Smith reports that individuals who have a high alcohol level at the time of presentation (greater than 300 mg/dl) or who present after having a withdrawal seizure appear to be at higher risk for severe withdrawal or DTs.[45] The risk of death in this stage is 1% to 5%, with an increased risk in the presence of delayed diagnosis, inadequate treatment, and concurrent medical pathology such as underlying cardiac disease.[44] Causes of death associated with DTs include head trauma, cardiovascular complications, infections, aspiration pneumonia, and fluid and electrolyte abnormalities.[2]

The onset of withdrawal symptoms may be delayed by treatment with benzodiazepines given for other reasons (e.g., sedation during mechanical ventilation). This may mask the signs and symptoms of withdrawal. If benzodiazepines are given for sedation in small doses, withdrawal from alcohol will continue. If they are given in large doses or continually, alcohol withdrawal may stop; no symptoms will be seen. Since benzodiazepines act on their own receptor sites coupled to the GABA receptor sites, they have the same effect as alcohol in the brain; secondary withdrawal from benzodiazepines will begin after discontinuation. This can occur especially if the discontinuation of the benzodiazepine is done abruptly, without dose tapering.

♦ Case Study 53-1, Part A

Alcohol

M.M. is a 76-year-old male. On the day before his admission, the patient experienced multiple bouts of emesis, possibly as many as 12. He reported having had 7 beers, none of which he could keep down. When the vomiting became almost continuous, he called 911 and was brought to the emergency department. He states that he takes pantoprazole (Protonix) daily and ranitidine (Zantac) PRN, but it is unclear if he is compliant with these medications. He normally drinks 18–20 beers and up to a fifth of vodka per day. The last drink he was able to keep down was 24 hours before his admission. This is his fifth admission in 2 years for alcohol withdrawal, and he has been noted to have severe DTs in the past. He has had withdrawal seizures in past admissions and has a distant history of alcoholic-related pancreatitis. His labs in the emergency department (ED) were white blood cells (WBC) 7.5%, hemoglobin (Hgb) 13.1 g/dl, hematocrit (Hct) 38%, sodium 142 mEq/L, potassium 3.6 mEq/L, chloride 97 mEq/L, total carbon dioxide (CO_2) 30 mEq/L, blood urea nitrogen (BUN) 25 mg/dl, creatinine 1.2 mg/dl, glucose 206 mg/dl, total bilirubin 1.6 mg/dl, liver enzymes within normal limits.

Decision point: What predictors exist from admission about the possible severity of his withdrawal?

Decision point: Would you anticipate seizure activity with this withdrawal?

Case continues on page 1484

The withdrawal from benzodiazepines will appear identical to alcohol withdrawal and will require treatment in the same symptomatic approach as is done in alcohol withdrawal; the overall goal is tapering the amount of drug to facilitate slow withdrawal.

Management of Acute Alcohol Withdrawal

Early identification of the symptoms of withdrawal or the potential for withdrawal is crucial in management of the critically ill patient withdrawing from alcohol. The purpose of early identification and anticipation is to allow rapid intervention and to prevent progression to more extreme states and increased risk of death. Assessment of the patient should also include identification of any coexisting psychiatric or medical conditions, including alcohol-related medical complications that might impact or mimic withdrawal (Table 53-1).[1,31] Lastly, an assessment of any other substance taken in addition to alcohol, such as benzodiazepines, is important.

Three goals of treatment have been identified by the American Society of Addiction Medicine (ASAM)

TABLE 53-1 Alcohol-Related Complications

SYSTEM/REALM OF PROBLEM	COMPLICATIONS
Nervous system	Intoxication Withdrawal Cognitive impairment Cerebellar degeneration/atrophy Peripheral neuropathy Hepatic encephalopathy Wernicke-Korsakoff syndrome Amblyopia Central pontine myelinolysis
Cardiovascular system	Supraventricular dysrhythmias Chronic nonischemic cardiomyopathy Systolic and diastolic hypertension
Liver	Fatty liver Alcoholic hepatitis Cirrhosis Hepatoma
Hematopoietic	Anemia Loss of white cell production, thrombocytopenia Loss of platelet function Loss of humoral and cell-mediated immunity Macrocytosis
Gastrointestinal tract	
Esophagus	Chronic inflammation Malignancies Mallory-Weiss tears Esophageal varices
Stomach	Gastritis Peptic ulcer disease
Pancreas	Acute pancreatitis Chronic pancreatitis
Nutritional	Vitamin deficiencies of folate, thiamine, pyridoxine, niacin, and riboflavin Electrolyte deficiencies of magnesium, zinc, calcium, phosphate Protein deficiency
Metabolic	Hypoglycemia Hyperlipidemia Hyperuricemia Alcoholic ketoacidosis Gout

Table continues on page 1480

Table 53-1 Alcohol-Related Complications—cont'd

SYSTEM/REALM OF PROBLEM	COMPLICATIONS
Other medical problems	Cancers: mouth, oropharynx, esophagus Pneumonia Tuberculosis Pseudo-Cushing's syndrome Testicular atrophy Amenorrhea Osteopenia
Psychiatric	Depression Anxiety Suicide
Behavioral and psychosocial	Injuries Violence Crime Child/partner abuse Tobacco, other drug abuse Unemployment Legal problems

Data from references 24 and 59.

(Box 53-2). Treatment of alcohol withdrawal is directed at reducing the physiologic effects and managing the resulting symptoms sufficiently to allow minimal withdrawal to continue until completed without adverse effects from the withdrawal state or from withdrawal medications (Box 53-3).[31]

The challenge experienced in the management of the critically ill patient is differentiating symptoms of alcohol withdrawal from those of other causes (e.g.,

---

Box 53-2

American Society of Addiction Medicine Goals of Alcohol Withdrawal Treatment

1. To provide a safe withdrawal from the drug(s) of dependence and enable the patient to become drug-free
2. To provide a withdrawal that is humane and thus protects the patient's dignity
3. To prepare the patient for ongoing treatment of his or her dependence on alcohol or other drugs

Data from reference 31.

Box 53-3

Alcohol Withdrawal Pharmacologic Treatment Regimens

MONITORING

- Monitor the patient every 4 to 8 hours using the CIWA-Ar (see Box 53-4) until the score has been below 8 to 10 for 24 hours.
- Repeat the CIWA-Ar 1 hour after every dose to assess the need for further medications.

SYMPTOM-TRIGGERED MEDICATION REGIMENS

Administer **one** of the following medications every hour when the CIWA-Ar is greater than 8 to 10:
- chlordiazepoxide (Librium) 50–100 mg
- diazepam (Valium) 10–20 mg
- oxazepam (Serax) 30–60 mg
- lorazepam (Ativan) 2–4 mg

(Other benzodiazepines may be used at equivalent substitutions.)

STRUCTURED MEDICATION REGIMENS

To prevent mild to moderate withdrawal, **one** of the structured regimens can be used:
- chlordiazepoxide 50 mg every 6 hours for four doses, then 25 mg every 6 hours for eight doses
- diazepam 10 mg every 6 hours for four doses, then 5 mg every 6 hours for eight doses

- lorazepam 2 mg every 6 hours for four doses, then 1 mg every 6 hours for eight doses

(Other benzodiazepines may be used at equivalent substitutions.)

It is very important that patients receiving medication on a predetermined schedule be monitored closely and that additional medication be provided should the doses given prove inadequate.

AGITATION

For the patient who displays increasing agitation or hallucinations that have not responded to oral benzodiazepines alone, one of the following medications can be used:
- haloperidol 2 to 5 mg IM alone or in combination with 2 to 4 mg of lorazepam
- Intravenous diazepam given slowly every 5 minutes until the patient is lightly sedated; begin with 5 mg for two doses, and if needed increase to 10 mg for two doses, then 20 mg every 5 minutes

Given the risk of respiratory depression, the patient on this regimen should be closely monitored, with equipment for respiratory support immediately available.

(Other phenothiazines and benzodiazepines may be substituted at equivalent substitutions.)

CIWA-Ar: Clinical Institute Withdrawal Assessment Scale for Alcohol, Revised.

metabolic disturbances, hypoxia, or dementia). Alcohol withdrawal in many critical care patients may not be identified as withdrawal until the patient has progressed well into severe withdrawal. If treatment is delayed until more severe symptoms appear, management of the patient may be very difficult and frustrating. Another impacting factor is that patients who have undergone repeated withdrawal episodes in the past appear to have a worsening of withdrawal with each subsequent detoxification. This is thought to be related to the phenomenon of "kindling." Long-term changes in the brain occur with repeated detoxifications. This is postulated to increase obsessive thoughts or alcohol craving during and after withdrawal and to worsen withdrawal with repeated withdrawals.[1]

Administration of benzodiazepines, either long-acting or short-acting, remains the standard treatment of alcohol withdrawal.[47] Benzodiazepines enhance the effect of GABA sedation in the same manner as alcohol. A specific benzodiazepine receptor site has been identified on the GABA receptor complex.[45] The common approach to alcohol withdrawal is to base the dose and the frequency of benzodiazepine administration on the severity of alcohol withdrawal symptoms. Defining the severity of withdrawal from nurse to nurse can result in an erratic course of withdrawal. To avoid this, the use of a scoring tool, such as the Clinical Institute Withdrawal Assessment for Alcohol instrument, is suggested. Commonly referred to as the CIWA, the tool is very effective in quantifying severity of withdrawal (Box 53-4). A score of 9 or less indicates mild withdrawal, a score of 10 to 18 indicates moderate withdrawal, and a score greater than 18 suggests severe withdrawal.[45] Pharmacologic management is begun at CIWA scores between 8 and 10.

The choice of benzodiazepine is based on a number of factors including duration of action, rapidity of onset, and cost.[47] Chlordiazepoxide (Librium) is commonly used in the patient able to take oral fluids who is under 60 years of age or free of liver disease.[1,84] Chlordiazepoxide is limited to oral administration only because of the erratic absorption with intramuscular injections. The onset of action may be slower than in other benzodiazepines such as diazepam (Valium), lorazepam (Ativan), or oxazepam (Serax). In those patients unable to take oral agents, or in whom there is evidence of liver disease or who are older than age 60, lorazepam or oxazepam is the more commonly used short-acting benzodiazepine.[1] It requires more frequent dosing to maintain a constant effect on the brain. If needed, intramuscular injections of lorazepam can be considered in the treatment of withdrawal because the absorption is predictable.[1] Lorazepam is used frequently for the patient unable to take oral medications who requires intravenous administration. Lorazepam infusions have been used in severe withdrawal. A recommended infusion starting point is at 1 mg/hour and then titrated to effect.[42] An alternative continuous benzodiazepine infusion is midazolam (Versed); dosing begins with a 2- to 4-mg intravenous loading dose followed by a continuous infusion of 2 mg/hour titrated to effect.[42] The benzodiazepine, long- or short-acting, should be administered until the symptoms of withdrawal are minimal but not totally abated. If all symptoms are abated, then withdrawal may stop and rebound with the withdrawal of benzodiazepines. In patients with moderate to severe withdrawal symptoms and at risk of withdrawal seizures, administration of the benzodiazepine should continue for approximately 24 to 48 hours and then gradually taper until the risk of withdrawal seizure activity has passed.[45] Research has shown that longer-acting agents may be more effective in preventing withdrawal seizures and can contribute to a smoother withdrawal with fewer rebound symptoms.[47]

Using the CIWA score to guide treatment, it is essential that patient assessments and reassessments be done frequently. The assessment score will provide a guide to the amount of drug administered. Following administration, a reassessment of the CIWA score will provide knowledge of the drug and dosage effectiveness. If the CIWA score remains unchanged or is continuing to increase, then repeating the dose or adding an adjunctive agent is appropriate. If the CIWA score is lower at the time of reassessment, the dosing was adequate to reduce the severity of withdrawal. The frequency of assessments will vary by patient. In the patient who is actively withdrawing, assessments every 30 minutes to 1 hour may be required until withdrawal is controlled at a lesser level. It is suggested that monitoring of the patient be at least every 4 to 8 hours until the CIWA score is below 8 to 10 for 24 hours.[45]

The dosing of benzodiazepines can be problematic because it is often done on an irregular frequency. Often one or several nursing shifts will medicate heavily and subsequent shifts will decrease the dosage. The decreased dosage may occur either because of the belief that the patient has been medicated too heavily and is presumably overmedicated or as a result of workload dosing intervals becoming prolonged. In either case, the risk of the patient experiencing rebound withdrawal is high. Any time the level of benzodiazepine is less than the brain receptors require for calming, the patient will return to the withdrawal state. They may return to the same level they were at the time initial therapy was instituted or to a more severe level of withdrawal. This phenomenon frequently occurs with benzodiazepine infusions that are frequently decreased and then increased based on the perceived level of sedation. In either case, once the symptoms of withdrawal have been minimized, the level of the infusion or dosing should remain constant or slowly tapered until all symptoms of withdrawal cease.

Box 53-4

Clinical Institute Withdrawal Assessment Scale for Alcohol, Revised (CIWA-Ar)

Total score is a simple sum of each item score (maximum score is 67).

NAUSEA AND VOMITING

0   No nausea or vomiting
1
2
3
4   Intermittent nausea with dry heaves
5
6
7   Constant nausea, frequent dry heaves and vomiting

PAROXYSMAL SWEATS

0   No sweats visible
1   Barely perceptible sweating, palms moist
2
3
4   Beads of sweat obvious on forehead
5
6
7   Drenching sweats

ANXIETY

0   No anxiety, at ease
1
2
3
4   Moderately anxious, guarded
5
6
7   Acute panic state, consistent with severe delirium or acute schizophrenia

AGITATION

0   Normal activity
1   Somewhat more than normal activity
2
3
4   Moderately fidgety and restless
5
6
7   Paces back and forth during most of the interview or constantly thrashes about

TREMOR

0   No tremor
1   No visible tremor, but can be felt at finger tips
2
3
4   Moderate when patient's hands extended
5
6
7   Severe, even with arms not extended

HEADACHE

0   Not present
1   Very mild
2   Mild
3   Moderate
4   Moderately severe
5   Severe
6   Very severe
7   Extremely severe

AUDITORY DISTURBANCES

0   Not present
1   Very mild harshness or ability to frighten
2   Mild harshness or ability to frighten
3   Moderate harshness or ability to frighten
4   Moderately severe hallucinations
5   Severe hallucinations
6   Very severe visual hallucinations
7   Continuous visual hallucinations

TACTILE DISTURBANCES

0   None
1   Very mild paresthesias
2   Mild paresthesias
3   Moderate paresthesias
4   Moderately severe hallucinations
5   Severe hallucinations
6   Extremely severe hallucinations
7   Continuous hallucinations

ORIENTATION AND CLOUDING OF SENSORIUM

0   Oriented and can do serial additions
1   Cannot do serial additions
2   Disoriented for date by no more than 2 calendar days
3   Disoriented for date by more than 2 calendar days
4   Disoriented for place or patient

From Addiction Research Foundation, Toronto, Ontario, Canada.

Adjunctive therapies provide supportive treatment. The pharmacologic management of alcohol withdrawal, in addition to benzodiazepines, includes sympatholytics, anticonvulsants, and antipsychotics.[31] Haloperidol (Haldol) may be required for the treatment of extreme, increasing agitation in the absence of any other withdrawal symptoms or in the patient experiencing increasing agitation despite adequate benzodiazepine therapy. It is also recommended for treatment of hallucinations, although it can lower the seizure threshold.[1] Beta blockers may be required for the treatment of hypertension or tachycardia not responding to adequate withdrawal management. Beta blockers should be considered in patients who have underlying coronary artery disease and may not tolerate the increased cardiovascular demands placed on the heart by withdrawal. Nicotine patches may lessen the anxiety of not smoking in those patients who smoke.

Carbamazepine (Tegretol) may be used for the prophylactic treatment of seizures in those patients at risk. When attempting to get a patient out of bed or ambulating, caution should be taken in the patient receiving carbamazepine because it may cause ataxia. Valproate (Depakote) can also be used for the prevention of withdrawal seizures. Though there is little scientific evidence that either of these agents can fully prevent seizures, anecdotal evidence supports their use because of their secondary effect of potentially reducing the symptoms of withdrawal.[84] Phenytoin (Dilantin) does not treat withdrawal seizures, but can be considered in a patient with an underlying seizure disorder.[1]

All patients in alcohol withdrawal should be treated with thiamine as soon as their potential or actual withdrawal is recognized. Chronic alcohol use may lead to malnutrition and result in a thiamine deficiency. This deficiency, if untreated, places the patient at risk of Wernicke's syndrome or Wernicke-Korsakoff syndrome, which potentially results in permanent neurologic damage (Box 53-5).[11,34,45] Thiamine 100 mg should be given IM, preferably before administration of oral or intravenous glucose.[34] Administration of intravenous glucose may deplete already deficient B vitamins.[34,45] Patients who exhibit the classic triad of mental disturbances, paralysis of eye movements, and ataxia indicative of Wernicke's disease require immediate treatment on admission to prevent permanent memory deficits.[45] Immediate treatment with parenteral administration of thiamine 50 mg IV and 50 mg IM should be given to the symptomatic patient.[45] Correction of fluid deficits and electrolyte imbalances, which are common in the alcoholic, must also occur.

The treatment of a patient who is in acute alcohol withdrawal delirium can be very difficult as the patient may become refractory to benzodiazepine therapy or benzodiazepine therapy may place the patient at severe risk of respiratory complications or prolonged sedation. The ASAM has published guidelines for treatment of DTs in alcohol withdrawal, recommending benzodiazepine choice be guided by the following considerations: agents with rapid onset control agitation more quickly, for example, oral or intravenous diazepam has a more rapid onset than other agents;

agents with long durations of action (e.g., diazepam) provide a smooth treatment course with less breakthrough symptoms; agents with shorter duration of activity (e.g., lorazepam) may have lower risk when there is concern about prolonged sedation, such as in patients who are elderly or who have substantial liver disease or other serious concomitant medical illness (Box 53-6).[31] If a patient demonstrates agitation that is not controlled with extremely large doses of benzodiazepines, use of pentobarbital or propofol (Diprivan) can be considered.[46] Currently, there are few cases reported in the literature documenting the effects of propofol in the treatment of DTs in patients refractory to benzodiazepines.[1,79] All cases reported are in patients who have airway protection with endotracheal intubation and mechanical ventilation. No studies on the routine use of propofol in alcohol withdrawal without delirium have been reported.

Box 53-5

Wernicke-Korsakoff's Syndrome

WERNICKE'S SYNDROME

Evolves over days to weeks
Clinical features:
1. Abnormal eye movements, which begin as nystagmus and progress to partial or complete ophthalmoplegia, usually with pupillary sparing
2. Ataxia of gait and stance, often accompanied by lower-limb intention tremor and dysarthria
3. Altered mentation, the earliest signs of which are inattentiveness, mental slowing, and impaired memory
4. Wernicke's aphasia is characterized by an inability to comprehend spoken or written word

Can progress to extreme lethargy, coma, and death

KORSAKOFF'S AMNESTIC SYNDROME

Emerges as the acute confusional delirium of Wernicke's syndrome subsides
Clinical features:
1. Profound isolated loss of memory for recent events
2. Placid lack of insight, leading to total disorientation
3. Absurd conversation or absurd answers to questions (confabulation)

Data from references 24 and 60.

Box 53-6

Benzodiazepine Choice Guidelines for Treatment of Delirium Tremens

Benzodiazepine choice should be guided by the following considerations:

1. Agents with **rapid onset** control agitation more quickly; for example, oral or intravenous diazepam has a more rapid onset than other agents.
2. Agents with **long duration** of action (e.g., diazepam) provide a smooth treatment course with less breakthrough symptoms.
3. Agents with **shorter duration** of activity (e.g., lorazepam) may have lower risk when there is concern about prolonged sedation, such as in older adult patients who have substantial liver disease or other serious concomitant medical illness.

Data from reference 32.

◆ Case Study 53-1, Part B

Alcohol

In the ED M.M.'s vital signs were blood pressure 167/101 mm Hg, heart rate 130 beats/min, respiratory rate 24 breaths/min, oxygen saturation 92% on room air. He was severely tremulous in the ED and profoundly diaphoretic but denies visual or auditory disturbances. He states he is feeling a little anxious. He is oriented to person, time, and place. He is a smoker, smoking 1.5 to 2 packs of cigarettes per day. He was started on IV fluids and given a total of 4 mg of IV lorazepam in the ED. He was then transferred to the medical-surgical nursing floor with an admitting diagnosis of alcohol dependence and withdrawal.

Decision point: From the information provided, you would estimate his CIWA score in the ED at what value?

Decision point: At what level of CIWA points is it suggested that benzodiazepine therapy should begin?

Decision point: From the information provided, what would you estimate as his CIWA score now?

Decision point: Does the CIWA score suggest that further benzodiazepine therapy should be administered?

Decision point: What would be the goal for this patient's therapy?

Decision point: What other therapies should be anticipated in this patient?

Case continues on page 1486

Alcohol withdrawal is also complicated by the co-addiction to benzodiazepines. It is crucial for the nurse to assess not only for an addiction to alcohol but also for the possible use of and addiction to benzodiazepines (e.g., alprazolam [Xanax]). Concurrent withdrawal from alcohol and benzodiazepines places the patient at severe risk of withdrawal seizures and a prolonged, difficult withdrawal. Initially, the patient is treated as an alcohol withdrawal patient using benzodiazepines and requires careful tapering with scheduled dosing following completion of the alcohol withdrawal.[84] Abrupt discontinuation of the benzodiazepines should not be done and will result in return of withdrawal symptoms or precipitation of seizure activity. This phenomenon may also be seen in a patient who is being administered long-term sedation for other reasons. If the sedation is not tapered, withdrawal may be precipitated.

Medical Sequelae of Alcohol Exposure

A patient may be admitted for a medical condition that is the direct result of excessive or prolonged alcohol intake and not be in withdrawal or admitted because of withdrawal. Knowledge of the many comorbid conditions associated with excessive alcohol intake may be helpful in anticipation of possible withdrawal or may help explain conditions that can be exacerbated or complicated by continued alcohol exposure (see Table 53-1). This may lead the nurse to question possible or anticipate pending withdrawal in the patient with no withdrawal symptoms on admission.

An increase in infections can be anticipated or expected in the alcoholic patient. White blood cell production is decreased in the alcoholic patient because of bone marrow suppression. This results in a decrease in white blood cells as well as a loss of white cell immune function.[60] Alcoholic patients are at high risk for infectious diseases such as pneumonia and tuberculosis. Additionally, it is estimated that 80% to 90% of alcoholics are regular and heavy smokers.[33,34] This dual addiction places the patient at further risk. A study done by Spies et al.[72] demonstrated that when combined with smoking, an alcohol addiction increased the postoperative risk of infectious complications, with pneumonias often being the basis for admission to the critical care unit. The organism *Streptococcus pneumoniae,* including drug-resistant strains, is common in the alcoholic patient.[43]

In addition to pneumonias, the respiratory system is further impacted during the withdrawal phase. The alcoholic patient who is sedated or obtunded is at risk for aspiration pneumonia. This is particularly true in the older adult patient, in part because of greater impairment of swallowing and respiratory clearance mechanisms.[28] Chronic alcoholism also presents an even higher risk factor for development of acute lung injury or acute respiratory distress syndrome (ARDS) as a consequence of aspiration as well as pneumonia and trauma.[30] The risk further increases in the chronic alcoholic patient who develops septic shock.[54]

Alcohol abuse is the leading cause of liver disease in the United States.[60] Though men generally drink alcohol in larger amounts than women, alcohol-dependent women have greater physical impairment once they begin drinking heavily.[9] Women develop alcohol-related liver disease, heart disease, and brain disorders earlier in their drinking careers than men.[9] Alcoholic liver disease includes three main features that may occur independently or be related: fatty liver, acute alcoholic hepatitis, and cirrhosis.[16,85] Patients with more advanced cirrhosis may present asymptomatic but may have associated symptoms of jaundice, ascites, and coagulopathy. Cirrhosis may lead to active bleeding from esophageal varices or Mallory-Weiss tears of the esophagus.[59]

Secondary consequences of alcoholic liver disease include thrombocytopenia, anemia, increased bleeding times, and increased mean corpuscular volume. Portal hypertension leads to ascites and esophageal varices development with subsequent gastrointestinal bleeding. It has been reported that 70% of patients with chronic pancreatitis abuse alcohol.[21] Although pancreatitis does occur in patients who abstain from alcohol, a pathologic link has been suggested to exist between alcohol drinking and chronic and acute pancreatitis. It appears that alcohol is not a direct cause of acute pancreatitis, but it lowers the threshold for initiation of acute pancreatitis from other sources.[44]

The alcoholic patient's nutritional status may be compromised. Alcoholic patients often receive the majority of their calories from alcohol and may be malnourished on admission. The ingestion of alcohol results in lower serum levels of vitamins, decreased storage of ingested vitamins, and a decreased ability to convert vitamins to their metabolically active forms.[42] Vitamin B complex is often absent in patients who consume large amounts of alcohol. Thiamine deficiency is associated with Wernicke's encephalopathy, which is an acute and chronic disorder of the central nervous system (see Box 53-5). Wernicke's encephalopathy limits a patient's ability to follow verbal directions, impacting patient safety. Thiamine deficiency may also be associated with alcoholic polyneuropathy. This relative deficiency forms the basis for administration of thiamine intramuscularly on admission. Niacin and vitamin B_6 may also be depleted and result in neurologic, hematologic, and dermatologic disorders. Mineral stores may also be impacted by chronic alcohol ingestion.

In addition to the secondary effects of alcoholic liver disease, decreased production of platelets may result from the direct toxic effects of alcohol on the bone marrow. A further insult to the bone marrow may occur from a deficiency of vitamin B_{12} and folate, a common deficiency in the alcoholic patient.[65] The resulting thrombocytopenia may place the patient at risk of bleeding or may answer the question as to why the patient is bleeding or presents with extensive bruising.[65,84]

Electrolyte disorders can also be anticipated in the chronic alcoholic intake patient. Hypocalcemia may be due to hypoalbuminemia but also can result from vitamin D deficiency, deficient calcium intake, and excessive renal losses and malabsorption of calcium as well as from hypomagnesemia. Alcoholic patients presenting with acute pancreatitis will demonstrate low calcium levels.[42]

Neurologic changes can result from chronic alcohol abuse and result in cerebral atrophy and signs of dementia as early as age 40.[24] Acute Wernicke's disease patients can present clinically with confusion and delirium; they are often drowsy or semistuporous, have an ataxic gait, and use incomprehensible dysarthric speech. They may have partial or complete external ophthalmoplegia and nystagmus. The alcoholic patient may also be hypothermic and hypotensive, experience diffuse inability to feel pain, or have a lessened sensation to pain. They may have a loss of short-term memory. The loss of memory may be associated with a lack of insight and total disorientation. The patient may have no ability to carry on a conversation or may provide incongruous answers to questions.[24] These neurologic changes can lead to difficulty managing the patient's safety. This is particularly significant related to patient fall prevention. The patient may not understand verbal or written instructions to call the nurse for needs such as toileting, and when up independently may be unable to walk without falling.

There are also cardiac consequences of chronic long-term alcohol consumption. Dilated nonischemic cardiomyopathy represents the most common cardiovascular complication of alcohol abuse.[47,58,59] It has been estimated that up to 40% of cases of idiopathic cardiomyopathy are alcohol related; up to 30% of alcohol-dependent patients demonstrate evidence of cardiac dysfunction.[82] Alcohol and its direct metabolite acetaldehyde are cardiotoxins both acutely and chronically.[73] The alcoholic patient may present in heart failure. The onset of failure may be gradual but also may be acute. The patient may or may not have atrial or ventricular dysrhythmias with failure.[47] Cardiac dysrhythmias in the absence of cardiomyopathy or failure are also common in this patient population and include atrial fibrillation and supraventricular tachycardias.[60]

◆ Case Study 53-1, Part C

Alcohol

After 4 hours on the medical-surgical floor, M.M.'s CIWA score remains less than 8. While he is in telemetry his CIWA scores continue to range between 16 and 20 when he is awake. He is given Ativan 2–4 mg every 1 to 2 hours. He becomes somnolent and difficult to arouse after 24 hours. He is noted to have coarse rhonchi that do not clear with coughing and is febrile to 102.4° F (39.1° C); he is diagnosed with aspiration pneumonia. His vital signs become unstable, with his blood pressure dropping to 70 mm Hg palp, heart rate 156 beats/min, respiratory rate 30 breaths/min, and oxygen saturation 76% on room air. He is transferred to critical care on 100% oxygen via non-rebreather mask.

Decision point: What is the basis for his somnolence after 24 hours?

Decision point: Aspiration pneumonia places the patient at what additional risks?

Decision point: What other potential complications could be anticipated?

Alcohol Dependence in the Older Adult

Alcohol dependence and withdrawal in the older adult present a unique set of physiologic circumstances. The estimates of the number of alcohol-affected older adults range from 3% to 25%, depending on the population sampled.[68] Hybels and Blazer[26] report a greater incidence of drinking in older men than older women. As the body ages, a number of changes that naturally occur will impact older adults' tolerance of alcohol. Smaller amounts may produce more harmful effects and may contribute to worsening of medical and mental conditions found in older adults.[68]

There are a number of factors contributing to an increased negative impact of alcohol in this population. As the body ages, there is a decrease in lean body mass and total body water with an increase in total body fat. A decrease in total body volume distribution results; therefore the amount of alcohol present in the bloodstream increases even when there is no increase in alcohol consumption.[70,81] Older alcoholic patients have decreased gastric concentrations of alcohol dehydrogenase, an enzyme that partially metabolizes alcohol during absorption. With fewer enzymes available, the amount of alcohol metabolized is reduced, leading to greater absorption of alcohol. Overall, the higher blood alcohol levels result in greater negative physiologic consequences.[81]

Other factors impacting the older patient include the loss of liver function that occurs after the age of 60 years. For every 1 year over 60, there is a loss of 1%

of hepatic blood flow.[66] This has an impact on maintaining a higher blood alcohol level and also influences the metabolism of benzodiazepines given for withdrawal. Therefore short-acting benzodiazepines (e.g., lorazepam) are essential in the management of withdrawal in the aged population.

Attention must also be placed on renal function in the elderly. As the kidney ages, renal blood flow can drop as much as 50%.[66] Renal tubular function also declines with aging; the kidney loses its ability to conserve sodium and excrete hydrogen ion. Dehydration becomes a problem because the kidney does not compensate for nonrenal losses of sodium and water. Older adults also experience a marked decline in the subjective feeling of thirst.[66] Renal insufficiency may exist before withdrawal. If an older patient becomes dehydrated from a lack of oral or intravenous fluids when in withdrawal, there is an increased risk of renal compromise and the risk of acute renal failure increases. Monitoring intake and output and measuring levels of electrolytes are essential during the sedation period of withdrawal treatment.

Assessment of withdrawal symptoms is complicated by the normal cognitive changes that occur with aging as well as by alcoholic-related dementia. Mental status changes can also occur from too rapid rehydration or changes in electrolytes, particularly sodium. Patients can be undertreated or overtreated because of a misinterpretation of confusion symptoms. Confusion occurring in the absence of any other signs or symptoms of alcohol withdrawal is generally related to another mental status or cognitive change.

The central nervous system in an older individual may have an impact on the course of withdrawal. Whereas elevated vital signs are typically seen in patients withdrawing from alcohol, this elevation may be less obvious in the older patient, in particular the patient prescribed beta blockers.[13] Cognitive function also declines with age. Some older patients may have underlying dementia that becomes evident with the stress of withdrawal. Organic brain syndrome may also be present at the time of withdrawal, making the diagnosis of withdrawal confusing and difficult. Sensory perception and vision decline with aging. There is a decreased sensitivity to sound and altered frequency discrimination. Tactile sensation, vibratory sensation, and ability to maintain balance decline. These changes coupled with a change in environment may result in more significant confusion and depression and place the older withdrawal patient at a greater risk of falling.[66]

Many older adults who drink also smoke.[81] As the patient experiences nicotine withdrawal, he may be agitated from an inability to smoke. Again, this agitation may be misinterpreted as alcohol withdrawal. Nicotine patches are essential in this population to prevent nicotine craving.

DRUG ADDICTION

Based on the 2004 National Household Survey on Drug Abuse (NHSDA), 19.1 million people ages 12 years or older used illicit drugs in the month before the survey.[77] Hopper and Shafi[24a] proposed that drug dependence should be seen as a chronic medical illness. Marijuana was the most commonly used substance in 2004.[77] It is estimated that 2.7 million people in the United States have used heroin at some point; 1 million are actually addicted to heroin.[6] An equal number are estimated to misuse pain relievers each year.[68] Though the prevalence of reported use of drugs was higher among men (8.7%) than women (5.5%), the risks for health consequences of drug use are more serious for women.[65] It has been suggested that from 0.4% to 27% of pregnant women, depending on the population sampled, are substance abusers.[5] The discussion in this section will be limited to those withdrawal states in which there are physiologic consequences that may be manifested during or complicate a critical illness.

Pathophysiology of Drug Addiction

A diagnosis of substance abuse requires the recurrent use of a substance over 12 months with subsequent adverse consequences or placement of an individual in a high-risk situation.[68] Drug addiction is considered a chronic, relapsing illness typified by compulsive drug-seeking behaviors and substance use.[68] The basis for this repeated use is both physiologic and psychological. Activation of the pleasure responses of the brain is the neurologic basis for habitual drug use. The changes in the brain occur within the mesolimbic dopaminergic system. Different substances will affect this system differently. Some substances increase the dopamine activity in the upper centers of the brain.[7,64] Other drugs will mimic the effects of neurotransmitters and still others will block the reuptake of neurotransmitters such as dopamine. Stimulation of the neurologic system involved in pleasure, in combination with external stimuli or internal moods, thoughts, or behaviors, generates a positive or rewarding response. Repeated and frequent substance use induces adaptations in the brain associated with the acute rewarding effects of the drug. This response will result and be sought by using the same substance again.[38]

Getting "high" is a common reference to the pleasure experienced from using drugs and provides insight into the lure of drug addiction. Samet[67] describes the high phenomenon in relationship to the high of heroin: "Heroin's initial effect is an intense euphoria described as a 'rush' or 'kick' compared to the intensity and pleasure with an orgasm, lasting from 45 seconds to several minutes. The initial effects may be perceived as a turning in

the stomach with tingling and warmth. The intense euphoria is followed by an intoxicated pleasant feeling referred to as "nodding," with decreased respiration and peristalsis. This brings about sedation, mental clouding, decreased visual acuity, heavy feeling in the extremities, light sleep with vivid dreams, and a reduction in anxiety."[67] This reward/response lasts until tolerance to the substance develops, at which time more substance is required to achieve the same high.

Any act that increases the activity of the reward centers of the brain will lead to more activity that will achieve stimulation of the same craving pathway. This stimulation leads to drug-seeking behaviors.[64] Repeated use of the substance will result in tolerance, dependence, dysphoria, and sensitization.[38,58] With habituated use, diminishing physiologic responses to the abused substance result, leading to greater and more frequent use. Repeated exposure also may lead to upregulation of metabolism of the substances, changing the onset of effects, the duration of effects, and half-life elimination as tolerance and dependence develop (Table 53-2).[64]

The action of opioids is primarily at the mu receptors, resulting in diminished sensation of pain. Repeated exposure to opioids causes molecular adaptations that result in upregulation of the receptors and a lessening of the effect of the previous repeated dose. As the cells adapt to continued suppression, the firing rates reset themselves, causing greater pain.[24] To achieve the same level of diminished pain effect, the patient will require more of the substance or drug used. When the drug is abruptly stopped, the pain receptors fire at an abnormally high level, leading to the intense pain sensation. The pain then leads to use of more drug, thus continuing the cycle of abuse.

The physical and neurologic adaptations combine to result in the withdrawal syndrome that is felt when administration of the drug of abuse is abruptly stopped. These two factors lead to intense craving following cessation of drug self-administration. This drug craving leads in turn to drug-seeking behaviors and ultimately continued use to diminish the pain experienced and to achieve the rewards associated with the drug.

Acute Drug Withdrawal Syndrome

Identification of all substances taken and the manner taken is essential in management of the patient in drug withdrawal. Urine drug testing aids in the identification of specific substances used as well as providing an approximate time reference for when substances were used last (Table 53-3). Once all substances are known, several things must be taken into account. First, the onset of withdrawal is dependent on a number of factors. The half-life of the substance is the greatest predictor. This will in part be determined by the manner in which the

TABLE 53-2 Pharmacologic Properties of Common Drugs of Abuse

DRUG	TIME TO ONSET	ELIMINATION HALF-LIFE	METABOLISM	EFFECTS
Heroin			Other opioids are metabolized to morphine Morphine undergoes N-demethylation, 6-glucuronidation, and 3-glucuronidation conjugation with sulfate or glucuronide for excretion	Specific opioid receptors; mu is most important
Injected	7–8 min	1–2 hr		
Intranasal	10–15 min	1–2 hr		
Smoked	10–15 min	1–2 hr		
Morphine	30 min	2–4 hr		
Hydrocodone	30 min	3.8 hr		
Methadone	Peaks at 4 hr	15–40 hr; average 24 hr; average 10 hr in pregnancy	Reduction to hydroxyl form: aromatic hydroxylation of one aromatic ring	
Cocaine			Hydrolysis of benzoate and methyl esters	Blocks dopamine reuptake in nucleus accumbens
Injected	Immediate	20–30 min		
Smoked	Immediate	20–30 min		
Intranasal	Less than 10 min	60–90 min		
Ingested	Less than 10 min	60–90 min		
Marijuana (smoked)	Immediate	7 days	Extensively metabolized to long-acting forms	Cannabinoid receptors, decreases GABAergic inhibition at ventral tegmental area, thereby increasing dopamine release at nucleus accumbens
Nicotine			Metabolized to cotinine, nicotine N^1-oxide, 3-hydroxycotinine, and conjugated derivatives	Nicotinic cholinoceptor, a ligand-gated ion channel in the locus coeruleus, ventral tegmental area, and in nucleus accumbens; also has peripheral autonomic effects
Smoked	Immediate	Hours		
Transdermal	Immediate	Hours		

drug is taken. Not all drugs are taken intravenously or orally. Examples of other administration methods include heroin injected under the skin, a practice known as skin popping; this method is often used when vascular access cannot be obtained. A popular practice is to destroy the protective covering on slow-release formulations of oxycodone (e.g., OxyContin) by crushing or chewing the pills; the powder is then consumed by oral ingestion, by injection, or by snorting. It is believed that this will yield effects similar to those seen with heroin.[68] Brewing teas or other liquid forms using the raw material, such as the opium poppy, is an alternative method for ingesting drugs.

Withdrawal symptoms will begin as the substance effects wear off. The duration of action of many abused opiates varies widely. Heroin has a half-life of 30

TABLE 53-3 Urine Testing for Abused Drugs

DRUG	COMPOUND DETECTED	URINE DETECTION TIME
Heroin	Morphine 6-acetylmorphine	1–3 days
Codeine	Codeine Morphine	1–3 days
Methadone	Methadone	2–4 days
Cocaine	Benzoylecgonine	1–3 days
Amphetamine	Amphetamine	2–4 days
Methamphetamine	Methamphetamine Amphetamine	2–4 days
Marijuana	Tetrahydrocannabinol (THC)	1–3 days for casual use; up to 30 days for chronic use
Phencyclidine	Phencyclidine	2–7 days for casual use; up to 30 days for chronic use
Benzodiazepines	Oxazepam Diazepam Other benzodiazepines	Up to 30 days
Barbiturates	Amobarbital Secobarbital Other barbiturates	2–4 days for short acting; up to 30 days for long acting

minutes with a duration of action of 4 to 5 hours.[88] Withdrawal from heroin will begin approximately 4 to 8 hours after the last dose, with peak effects of withdrawal occurring within 36 to 72 hours and subsequently subsiding over the next 5 to 7 days.[69] Methadone has a prolonged elimination half-life of 35 hours; onset of withdrawal from methadone may be seen in 36 to 72 hours, peaking in 96 to 144 hours and lasting 14 to 21 days.[4]

The second important element in consideration of the care of a patient who has a current opioid use history is attempting to foresee the degree of withdrawal.

A predictor of the degree of withdrawal from opiates is found in the amount of drug taken and the duration of use. Though this information is valuable, it is important to realize that low to moderate users will report use, whereas the heavy user may underreport use.[79] Despite the potential for underreporting, it is still useful to try to estimate the amount of drug used, as this will impact the likelihood and severity of withdrawal.[89]

Not all patients who report substance abuse or are suspected of substance abuse are at risk for drug withdrawal syndromes. Illicit drugs such as stimulants, cocaine, hallucinogens, amphetamines, and cannabis (marijuana) do not have associated physiologic withdrawal syndromes but may be taken at toxic levels. The outcome from stopping any of the above substances is psychological in nature, primarily manifested by intense drug craving.

Opiate drugs—such as heroin, acetaminophen with hydrocodone (Vicodin), oxycodone (OxyContin), and acetaminophen with oxycodone (Percocet)—all have an associated physiologic withdrawal syndrome when the drug is stopped abruptly. Opiates produce an intensive withdrawal that is subjectively severe, but the withdrawal by itself is usually not life threatening.[25] Opiate withdrawal when combined with alcohol, barbiturates, or benzodiazepines is life threatening and requires the treatment of opiate withdrawal be secondary to the withdrawal from alcohol, barbiturates, or benzodiazepines. Opioid withdrawal can be fatal in the presence of underlying conditions that place the patient at risk, such as cardiovascular disease or severe dehydration from vomiting or diarrhea. Opioid withdrawal in pregnancy can result in fetal death from premature onset of labor[25] and will be discussed separately.

The central nervous system effects of opioids include analgesia, sleepiness, mood changes, and impaired mentation. Abrupt cessation of the drug will result in an overactivity of those receptor sites that have been suppressed from the constant drug use. The signs and symptoms of acute opiate withdrawal syndrome include a heightened sense of intense pain, particularly in the joints and muscles, gastrointestinal distress such as diarrhea and vomiting, fever, insomnia, and marked anxiety and agitation and dysphoria (Box 53-7).[61] Other signs include the following: heart rate greater than 10 beats/min over baseline or more than 90 beats/min if there is no history of tachycardia and the baseline is unknown; systolic blood pressure 10 mm Hg or more above baseline or more than 160/90 mm Hg in patients without hypertension; dilated pupils; gooseflesh; diaphoresis; rhinorrhea; lacrimation; insomnia; labile mood swings; and drug-seeking behavior.[61,79]

Box 53-7

Clinical Manifestations of Opioid Withdrawal

Early symptoms
- Myalgia
- Nausea
- Rhinorrhea
- Lacrimation
- Increased production of phlegm
- Yawning

Intermediate symptoms
- Sweats
- Fever
- Chills
- Piloerection ("cold turkey")

- Insomnia or restless sleep
- Muscle spasms, often in the lower limbs ("kicking")
- Bone pain (often in thighs)

Late symptoms
- Vomiting
- Diarrhea
- Hypertension
- Tachycardia
- Hyperventilation

At any stage
- Dilated pupils
- Anxiety
- Irritability

◆ Case Study 53-2, Part A

Opiates

B.S. is a 36-year-old male who is admitted to critical care from the ED at 1600 following a motor vehicle crash in which he sustained a fractured arm, fractured leg, and pneumothorax. A chest tube has been placed, and his arm and leg placed in immobilizers. He is scheduled for surgery later in the day. He is in excruciating pain on admission, profoundly diaphoretic, and begging for more pain medication. He states his pain is 10 out of 10 despite 40 mg of morphine in the ED. He is noted to be tremulous with his arms at his side. Vital signs are blood pressure 172/110 mm Hg, heart rate 143 beats/min, and respiratory rate 26 breaths/min with an oxygen saturation of 92% on 4 liters of oxygen per nasal prongs. He is nauseated with dry heaving, his pupils are slightly dilated, and he is profoundly diaphoretic. He is complaining that he is anxious and feeling panicked. He appears acutely ill. He reports drinking alcohol daily for many years, up to 10 drinks per day, predominantly gin and bourbon with some beer. He does get tremulous and very nauseated when he does not have regular alcohol. His last drink was 5 hours earlier. He also reports using opiates in the form of acetaminophen with hydrocodone and acetaminophen with oxycodone, obtained primarily from friends and the Internet, with his daily use approximately 10 to 20 pills per day for the past 3 years. These are taken primarily orally. His last pill was this morning at 0600. He also reports use of oxycodone when he can get it, and this is chewed. He

also uses cocaine on a daily basis but is unable to quantify the amount. He further uses citalopram (Celexa), which he takes with alcohol to enhance the effects of both substances. He has also used amphetamines and diazepam on an intermittent basis. He has not previously withdrawn from alcohol, but does experience opiate withdrawal if he does not take some opiate every 4 hours. His labs in the ED were WBC 14.6%, Hgb 12.4 g/dl, Hct 35.7%, sodium 141 mEq/L, potassium 3.8 mEq/L, chloride 104 mEq/L, total CO_2 28 mEq/L, BUN 9 mg/dl, creatinine 1.1 mg/dl, glucose 102 mg/dl, with a urine toxicology screen positive for cocaine and opiates. His blood alcohol level (BAL) is 0.28 mg/dl; he is a nonsmoker. He is started on morphine via patient-controlled analgesia.

Decision point: What potential withdrawal states may impact his critical care stay?

Decision point: Which withdrawal state can be fatal if untreated—alcohol or opiate?

Decision point: What substances will not result in withdrawal states?

Decision point: Would you anticipate seizure activity with this withdrawal?

Decision point: What are the potential signs of alcohol withdrawal present on the initial assessment?

Case continues on page 1492

Management of Acute Opiate Withdrawal

Essential to the management of the patient undergoing opiate withdrawal is the understanding that patients will have a heightened pain response coupled with a severely decreased pain tolerance.[25] Patients who have associated psychoactive disorders may experience more severe pain than patients without these disorders.[25] Healthcare providers' misconceptions and value judgments about injection drug use affect their ability to assess and adequately treat pain.[25] Any patient complaining of severe pain not relieved by conventional means should be assessed for signs and symptoms of withdrawal.

There are several approaches that can be taken in the management of acute opiate withdrawal. Virtually any opioid can be administered to relieve acute withdrawal symptoms. Though short-acting opiates can be controlled in their delivery, they require frequent monitoring and dose adjustment. Patients are likely to experience further withdrawal symptoms near the end of the dosing period. While the use of short-acting opiates may work well in the critical care setting, adjustment would be needed upon transfer to another level of care where there is less frequent patient interaction.[89] With the continued use of narcotics, such as morphine, the patient should be observed for persistent signs and symptoms of withdrawal or signs of overmedication or excess sedation with each dose. These signs and symptoms can be used to guide further dosing.

Another common approach is an opiate taper using a long-acting opiate. Desan and Powsner suggest providing 10 mg of methadone initially, followed by additional doses of 5 to 10 mg given for objective signs of withdrawal over the next 24 hours.[13] Though it has been suggested that 10 to 30 mg of methadone in 24 hours is adequate for most street users, consideration must be given to patients who have been or are on methadone maintenance, where typical doses of 80 to 120 mg are seen.[13,80] Patients who are receiving antiretroviral drugs also require high doses because of the lower serum methadone concentrations.[13] Other known drug interactions with methadone include rifampin and phenytoin, which can lower the methadone concentration and effectiveness.[75,81] If the patient has been in a methadone program and used additional substances, it is critical that patient-reported doses are verified with the methadone program to confirm the correct dose used on a daily basis and the time of the last dose, allowing continuation of that amount.[80] Management should include receiving additional short- to intermediate-acting opioids in addition to the usual dose of methadone.[80] It is not advisable to increase the usual dose of methadone. If methadone is to be discontinued within or after a hospital stay, it can be tapered over a 21-day period.[80]

Buprenorphine (Suboxone) can also be used for detoxification from opioids. Buprenorphine is a partial agonist at the mu receptor and, when administered, displaces all opioids on the receptor.[31] If buprenorphine is given to a patient with active opiate on the mu receptor at the time of administration, active abrupt withdrawal can be precipitated.[31] Thus the patient must be into full withdrawal before administration. If the withdrawal has not peaked in intensity, administration of the drug will worsen the patient's physical and subjective experience, resulting in abrupt onset of withdrawal. Buprenorphine is administered sublingually and effects last 8 to 10 hours. Test dosing is recommended, as it allows for determination of improvement in symptoms or worsening of symptoms. Recommended test dosing of buprenorphine is 2/0.5 mg sublingual with institution of an 8/2 mg dose two to three times daily if the test dose does not worsen symptoms. If the test dose worsens symptoms, then further dosing of buprenorphine should be delayed 4 to 6 hours until the patient is further into withdrawal.[83] Buprenorphine is also an antagonist of the kappa opioid receptor, which may produce a positive mood and feelings of well-being and prevent the depression that is common in opiate withdrawal.[31]

Adjunctive medications are also helpful in management of opiate withdrawal and do not require waiting until the patient is in full withdrawal. These medications may include acetaminophen or nonsteroidal anti-inflammatory drugs, benzodiazepines, antidiarrheals, or antispasmodics. Clonidine (Catapres) may be useful in lessening the adrenergic hyperactivity of opiate withdrawal as well as the perceived restlessness and anxiety that occur with withdrawal. Swift suggests on day 1 of withdrawal, 0.1 mg of clonidine be given every 8 hours with the dose gradually increasing on days 2 through 4.[78] Typical doses are 0.6 to 1.2 mg by day 4, with this dose continuing until day 7, after which it is reduced by 0.2 to 0.3 mg per day until discontinued.[78] Adjunctive therapy is useful between doses of pain medications, with drugs such as muscle relaxants and anti-nausea agents used to treat the symptoms of withdrawal. Benzodiazepines are not recommended for use as muscle relaxants.[84]

The patient on maintenance buprenorphine presents a unique and difficult management problem for the nurse. The agent is used for the prevention of opiate relapse use and usually taken daily. Buprenorphine blocks the effect of narcotic medications and leaves the patient with no pain relief at all. Use of non–opiate-based agents (e.g., ketorolac [Toradol]) is suggested initially and for up to 48 hours.[84] If narcotic medications are used, the nurse can anticipate exceedingly large doses to be required for up to 48 hours, after which more normal dosing will be required.[84]

Management of Acute Opiate Withdrawal in the Pregnant Woman. Management of the pregnant woman who is using opiates during pregnancy is directed toward preventing the onset of early labor and subsequent delivery of the fetus. The accepted treatment in this population is the use of methadone until the completion of the pregnancy.[4,62,84] Treatment with low-dose methadone should begin immediately if the patient is able to take oral medications. Methadone is given in small amounts, such as 10- and 20-mg doses, until evidence of withdrawal no longer exists or there is evidence of excessive drug effect (e.g., somnolence, slurred speech, and other signs and symptoms of excessive drug use). Methadone peaks in action within 4 hours, and repeated dosing should take this into account to prevent overdosing due to too-frequent administration.[83] It may take several days to stabilize the pregnant patient; most pregnant patients will stabilize at between 30 and 150 mg daily.[84] Once a maintenance dose is achieved, it can be given on a daily basis or in divided doses. Splitting the dose to morning and evening is the preferred method of daily dosing.[87] The dose should be continued throughout the pregnancy to delivery. Methadone requirements may increase during the third trimester of the pregnancy because of increased plasma volumes, reduced protein binding, increased tissue binding, and increased metabolism of the mother. A stable methadone dose reduces variability in the mother's opioid levels, which reduces stress on the baby.[89] Without treatment to prevent withdrawal and the associated severe muscle cramping, labor will be induced and the fetus delivered at any point in the pregnancy. In addition to labor, withdrawal may precipitate spontaneous fetal loss or intrauterine fetal demise.[84]

▲ Case Study 53-2, Part B

Opiates

B.S. is determined to be in alcohol withdrawal and is reasonably sedated between doses of benzodiazepines. When he is awake he continues to complain of extreme pain that is not relieved by the pain medicine he is receiving. He is switched from morphine to hydromorphone (Dilaudid) but continues to complain of muscle cramping and severe back pain. He is rapidly labeled as a drug seeker by the staff.

Decision point: Is the label "drug seeker" appropriate?

Decision point: What nursing actions can be taken to help this patient?

Medical Sequelae of Drug Exposure

There are many detrimental medical complications of drug use. Knowledge of the consequences of drug abuse may provide insight into the possibility of drug abuse or possible withdrawal. The most challenging are the chronic infectious diseases (e.g., viral hepatitis B, hepatitis C, human T-lymphotropic virus, and human immunodeficiency virus) that are most commonly associated with intravenous drug use.[70] Skin infections and acute bacterial endocarditis are common bacterial infections in the drug-addicted patient. The

pathogen most frequently cited is *Staphylococcus aureus*.[69] Other cardiac complications include cardiomyopathy, perivalvular abscess, and abnormalities of the conduction system, including prolonged QT intervals, ST-T wave changes, and cor pulmonale.[69] Pulmonary hypertension can result from impurities in the injected drug (e.g., talc, which causes talc granulomatosis). Acute pulmonary edema, bronchospasm, septic pulmonary emboli, and infectious or chemical mediastinitis are other pulmonary complications.[69]

Neurologic complications can result from infectious or noninfectious sources. They include seizures, usually noninfectious in nature and resulting from respiratory depression and hypoxia and cerebral infarction.[69] Meningitis, mycotic aneurysm, and abscesses are infectious complications related to intravenous drug injections.[69]

Psychiatric Disorders and Addiction

The experience of many nurses is that the addicted patient is a difficult patient. This is in part because of their difficult behavior. Alcoholics are often viewed as patients without self-control, who are to blame for their situation. Drug abusers are frequently labeled as drug seeking and manipulative in their behavior in an effort to get more drug or special favors, such as smoking. Often these patients are regarded as socially deviant, a burden to society, manipulative, and not intelligent enough to make good choices or decisions.[25] What is often unknown is that a large percentage of the addicted patient population has some co-occurring psychiatric disorder impacting their behavior. Many addicted patients suffer from anxiety or affective personality disorder and the behaviors exhibited are not all related to drug seeking or withdrawal from a desired substance, but may result from the psychiatric disorder itself.

It is estimated that 27% of the general population have diagnosable substance abuse or dependence.[33] The National Institute of Mental Health Epidemiologic Catchment Area study estimated that 45% of individuals addicted to alcohol and 72% of individuals with drug addiction had at least one co-occurring psychiatric disorder.[63] The National Comorbidity study found approximately 78% of alcohol-dependent men and 86% of alcohol-dependent women met the criteria for a psychiatric disorder in addition to their drug addiction.[36] Kennedy reports the presence of substance abusers in specific psychoactive disorder populations: 50% of schizophrenia patients, 84% of antisocial personality patients, 24% of anxiety disorder patients, 32% of affective personality disorder patients, and 56% of bipolar disorder patients are substance abusers.[32] Individuals with the combined diagnoses of substance abuse and a psychiatric disorder are identified as dual-diagnosis patients.

Depression may significantly increase the use of alcohol. The risk for alcohol dependence was 4.8 times higher among depressed women and 3.1 times higher among depressed men when compared with the general population.[36] At the same time, depression may result from alcohol abuse.[33] Women who are alcohol dependent have a higher incidence of anxiety disorders, mood disorders, phobias, and posttraumatic stress disorder compared to men who drink.[9] In comparison, alcoholic men were more likely to have antisocial personality disorder.[23] Findings were similar in drug-addicted patients.

An appreciation of the behavior patterns specific disorders have on patient behavior may help the nurse better understand and deal with the behaviors seen in the addicted patient. It is believed that some individuals with psychoactive disorders may be self-medicating psychiatric symptoms with the substances abused.[56] Alcohol may relieve anxiety or decrease manic symptoms, whereas stimulants may reverse depression. Psychiatric symptoms may also be induced by chronic substance abuse. Patients may experience acute psychosis from stimulants or hallucinogenic substances. It may be difficult while the patient is in critical care to differentiate if these symptoms are from the abuse or are the result of underlying psychoactive disease.[33] Anxiety disorders and affective disorders are common in opioid-dependent patients.[79]

Patients with personality disorders such as schizoid, paranoid, or schizotypal are often described as odd or eccentric. They are uncomfortable in interpersonal situations, emotionally distant, difficult to engage, and isolative.[86] The patient may present initially as hostile or in conflict with others when placed in a very stressful situation or forced into contact with others. Patients with antisocial, borderline, histrionic, or narcissistic personality disorders are described as dramatic or erratic and are characterized as labile, unpredictable, unlikable, and impulsive. Coexisting mood disturbances, such as depression, anger, and anxiety, are frequent findings in such patients.[19] Furthermore, the patient can be very demanding, manipulative, emotionally unstable, and interpersonally inappropriate. Antisocial patients exhibit a disregard for the rights of others, and are deceitful and impulsive.[86] Healthcare providers often experience strong negative emotional reactions to antisocial patients.[86] Organic brain disorders, such as Wernicke's encephalopathy (which is seen with repeated alcohol use), may also result in personality changes that are difficult to handle. This patient may have difficulty with short-term memory and be unable to understand instructions.

Management of the difficult patient is not easy but may be guided by several useful approaches. Treatment of both illnesses, addictive and psychoactive, is critical in dual-diagnosis patients. To achieve this outcome, the assessment of the psychiatric disorder is of great importance. Asking if a patient has seen a mental health professional and subsequently been treated for a mental health disorder is useful. If the patient was previously prescribed antidepressants or other pharmacologic psychoactive treatment, resumption of these medications as soon as possible is advised. Such medications may lessen their symptoms or behaviors considerably.

If the use of pharmacologic agents is not possible or the use of prior medications is unable to be identified, responding to the patient in a specific manner may be helpful in controlling behavior. Setting limits in a calm, non-hostile, and nonjudgmental manner and reinforcing the limits in the same manner can be helpful. Avoid frustration as the care provider by expecting the patient to have difficulty in following rules consistently. Consistency among providers also can be useful in reinforcing limits. Outline behaviors that are and are not acceptable. Attempt to not react to outbursts.[40,56] Many of these patients may have unreasonable requests. Spickerman[71] recommends rather than saying no outright, use what is called the toddler principle of saying, "I won't give you that, but I would love to give you this." Offering an acceptable alternative is often helpful. If the patient requests the same thing from multiple staff members, having a consistent reason for saying no is essential. Avoid arguing with the patient.[71]

Also important in the management of the difficult patient is the treatment of the identified substances from which the patient is withdrawing. Appropriate withdrawal treatment will eliminate the possible effect of the abused substance on the patient's behavior. Often symptoms of the personality disorder are worsened or increase in severity as a result of withdrawal and will abate with treatment of withdrawal.[19] Evaluation of the other causes of behavior is also warranted. Elevated ammonia levels or severely decreased sodium levels in the alcoholic patient may be causes of erratic behavior. The presence of hallucinogenic substances may also alter behavior. Hyperthyroidism can be a source of sudden behavior changes as can early dementia.[87]

ILLICIT DRUG ABUSE AND TOXIC OVERDOSE

There may be circumstances in which a patient is admitted to critical care for treatment of a substance that has no withdrawal state, but the substance imposes additional risks to the patient's care. There are three circumstances in which this may occur. The patient is admitted because the substance is toxic or at overdose levels; because of the consequences of the substance alone or in combination with other substances; or because of the impact of the substance on another physiologic process. In addition, patients may experience consequences from the manufacturing of the drug, as some illicit substances are manufactured without control of purity or specified chemicals. Illicit drugs are estimated to be responsible for 5% of critical care admissions, with neurologic complications especially significant from drug abuse.[10] It is estimated that 10% of strokes are related to drug abuse.[10] Diagnosis of intoxication may be at best difficult and requires knowledge of some of the more common substances associated with intoxication (Box 53-8).[52] The Medication table on pp. 1495-1496 offers further information on this topic. Knowledge of patient management related to toxic substance levels or overdose will assist the nurse in the care of a patient suffering from a toxic exposure. Discussion will be limited to stimulant drugs and psychoactive drugs known as club drugs. Additionally discussed will be the toxicity of cyclic antidepressants because of the life-threatening consequences of this class of drugs at toxic levels.

Stimulant drugs in large doses represent a class of drugs that can be very harmful to the body because of severe increased physiologic activity. The two most commonly used stimulants are cocaine and those in the amphetamine group (Table 53-4). Neither of these drugs has a withdrawal syndrome other than intense craving, but both stimulants when taken in large amounts pose an extreme risk to the patient. Amphetamines and amphetamine-like drugs are stimulants that have increased dramatically in use in the United States in the past decade.[53] Amphetamines as a chemical substance can be found in many prescription and nonprescription drugs for use as appetite suppressants, and drugs used to treat hyperactivity disorders. Examples of such medications include methylphenidate (Ritalin), dextroamphetamine (Dexedrine), and amphetamine

---

Box 53-8

Drugs That Affect Temperature, Heart Rate, and Pupil Size

Hypothermia	Hyperthermia	Tachycardia	Bradycardia	Miosis	Mydriasis
Alcohols	Amphetamines	Amphetamines	Antidysrhythmics	Barbiturates	Amphetamines
Barbiturates	Anticholinergics	Anticholinergics	Beta blockers	Carbamates	Anticholinergics
Cyclic antidepressants	Antihistamines	Antihistamines	Calcium channel blockers	Clonidine	Antihistamines
Hypoglycemic agents	Cocaine	Caffeine	Carbamates	Ethanol	Cocaine
Opioids	Cyclic antidepressants	Carbon monoxide	Clonidine	Isopropyl alcohol	Cyclic antidepressants
Phenothiazines	Drug withdrawal	Clonidine	Cyclic antidepressants	Organophosphates	Dopamine
Colchicine	LSD	Cocaine	Digoxin	Opioids (meperidine may cause mydriasis)	Opiate withdrawal
Akee fruit poisoning	Monoamine oxidase inhibitors	Cyanide	Lithium	PCP	Glutethimide
Lithium	Phencyclidine (PCP)	Cyclic antidepressants	Metoclopramide	Phenothiazines	LSD
	Psychotropic (neuroleptic malignant syndrome)	Drug withdrawal	Opioids	Physostigmine	Monoamine oxidase inhibitors
	Phenothiazines	Ephedrine	Organophosphates	Pilocarpine	PCP
	Butyrophenones	Hydrogen sulfide	Phenylpropanolamine		
	Clozapine/ olanzapine	Phencyclidine (PCP)	Physostigmine		
	Risperidone	Phenothiazines	Propoxyphene		
	Salicylates	Pseudoephedrine	Quinidine		
	Serotoninergic antidepressants	Theophylline			
	Serotonin syndrome	Thyroid hormones			

COMMON TOXIDROMES

TOXIDROME	FEATURES	DRUGS/TOXINS	DRUG TREATMENT
Anticholinergic "Hot as a hare, dry as a bone, red as a beet, mad as a hatter"	Blurred vision Coma Seizures Dry skin Fever Flushing Hypertension Ileus Mydriasis Myoclonus Psychosis Tachycardia Urinary retention	Antihistamines Atropine Baclofen Benztropine Phenothiazines Propantheline Scopolamine Tricyclic antidepressants	Physostigmine (for life-threatening events; do not use in cyclic antidepressant overdose because of potential of worsening of conduction disturbances)
Alpha-adrenergic	Bradycardia Hypertension Mydriasis	Phenylephrine Phenylpropanolamine	Treat hypertension with phentolamine or nitroprusside, beta blockers, but not as sole treatment alone
Beta-adrenergic	Hypotension Tachycardia Tremor	Albuterol Caffeine Terbutaline Theophylline	Beta blockade (caution in asthmatics) Potassium replacement
Beta- and alpha-adrenergic	Diaphoresis Dry mucous membranes Hypertension Mydriasis Tachycardia	Amphetamines Cocaine Ephedrine Phencyclidine Pseudoephedrine	Benzodiazepines Beta blockers
Cholinergic "SLUDGE"	Bradycardia Bronchorrhea Diaphoresis Diarrhea Emesis GI cramps Lacrimation Miosis Salivation Urination Wheezing	Carbamate Organophosphates Physostigmine Pilocarpine	Atropine Pralidoxime for organophosphates
Epileptogenic	Hyperreflexia Hyperthermia May mimic stimulant patterns Tremors	Anticholinergics Camphor Chlorinated hydrocarbons Cocaine Isoniazid Lidocaine Lindane Nicotine Phencyclidine Strychnine Xanthines	Antiseizure medications Pyridoxine for isoniazid Extracorporeal removal of drug (lindane, camphor, xanthines) Physostigmine for anticholinergic agents Avoid phenytoin for theophylline-induced seizures

Table continues on page 1496

TOXIDROME	FEATURES	DRUGS/TOXINS	DRUG TREATMENT
Extrapyramidal	Choreoathetosis Hyperreflexia Opisthotonos Rigidity/tremor Trismus	Haloperidol Olanzapine Phenothiazines Risperidone	Benztropine Diphenhydramine
Hallucinogenic	Hallucinations Psychosis Panic Fever Mydriasis Hyperthermia Synesthesia	Amphetamines Cannabinoids Cocaine Lysergic acid diethylamide Phencyclidine (may present with miosis)	Benzodiazepines
Narcotic	Altered mental status Slow, shallow breaths Miosis Brachycardia Hypotension Hypothermia Decreased bowel sounds	Dextromethorphan Opiates Pentazocine Propoxyphene	Naloxone Urinary alkalinization for phenobarbital
Sedative/hypnotic	Apnea Confusion Slurred speech Stupor and coma		Flumazenil
Serotonin	Diaphoresis Diarrhea Fever Flushing Hyperreflexia Irritability Myoclonus Tremor Trismus	Clomipramine Fluoxetine Meperidine Paroxetine Sertraline Trazodone	Benzodiazepines Withdrawal of drug Cyproheptadine
Solvent	Confusion Depersonalization Derealization Headache Incoordination Lethargy Restlessness	Acetone Chlorinated hydrocarbons Hydrocarbons Naphthalene Toluene Trichloroethane	Avoid catecholamines Withdrawal of toxin
Uncoupling of oxidative phosphorylation	Hyperthermia Metabolic acidosis Tachycardia	2,4-Dichlorophenol Aluminum phosphide Dinitrophenol Glyphosphate Pentachlorophenol Phosphorus Salicylates Zinc phosphide	Sodium bicarbonate for metabolic acidosis Patient cooling Avoid atropine and salicylates Hemodialysis in refractory acidosis

TABLE 53-4 Commonly Abused Amphetamines and Their Derivatives

STREET NAME	COMMON NAME	SPECIAL FEATURES
Speed, uppers	Amphetamine and dexamphetamine Methamphetamine hydrochloride	
Crank, speed	Mixed isomers	
Ice, crank, crystal	D-Isomer	Smokable
	Propylhexedrine	
Khat	Cathionine, catha edulis plant	
Serenity, tranquility, peace	Designer amphetamines	
	4-Methyl-2,5-dimethoxyamphetamine (DOM, STP)	Hallucinations
Golden eagle, LSD-25, tile, MOA	4-Bromo-2,5-dimethoxyamphetamine (DOM, STP)	Hallucinations
	Para-methoxyamphetamine (PMA)	Hallucinations
Love drug, love pill	3,4-Methylenedioxyamphetamine (MDA)	Hallucinations
Adam, ecstasy	3,4-Methylenedioxymethamphetamine (MDMA)	Euphoria
Eve	3,4-Methylenedioxyethamphetamine (MDEA)	Euphoria
Cat	Methcathinone	Euphoria Hallucinations

dextroamphetamine (Adderall), all used to treat hyperactivity disorders. Pemoline (Cylert) is used primarily for the sleep disorder narcolepsy and attention-deficit disorder. Diethylpropion (Tenuate) and phentermine (Teramine) are used for weight loss.[53] Designer forms of methamphetamine are known on the street as crank, speed, go, and ecstasy. The street forms of the drug are easily manufactured for illicit use as tablets, capsules, powders, and gelatin or impregnated into pieces of paper that can be smoked.[10] "Ice" and "crystal" are the pure hydrochloride salt forms of methamphetamine and are used for smoking, inhaling, or injection.[10] The physiologic effects of amphetamine include central nervous system stimulation, peripheral release of catecholamines, inhibition of reuptake of catecholamines, or inhibition of monoamine oxidase. Monoamine oxidase in turn inactivates dopamine, serotonin, norepinephrine, and epinephrine.[77] Amphetamine substances also have hallucinogenic properties primarily from the stimulation of the dopamine and serotonin receptors.[10] The duration of clinical effect is 24 hours.[10]

An overdose of amphetamines causes confusion, tremor, anxiety, agitation, and irritability. Other symptoms include pupil constriction, tachydysrhythmias, myocardial ischemia, hypertension, hyperreflexia, hyperthermia, rhabdomyolysis, renal failure, coagulopathy, and seizures.[53] Also seen are diaphoresis, pallor, nystagmus, blurred vision, and intraretinal hemorrhages. Muscles may be rigid, muscle spasms may be present, and patients may grind their teeth. Nausea, vomiting, and diarrhea may occur.[10] Methamphetamine is associated with the sensation of ants or bugs crawling under the skin, causing patients to pick at themselves and engage in self-mutilation.[10]

Mortality from an overdose of methamphetamine primarily occurs in two different timeframes. Early deaths occur secondary to cardiac dysrhythmias, seizures, and depression of the central nervous system, whereas late deaths, 24 to 48 hours, result from complications of malignant hyperthermia, such as rhabdomyolysis, renal failure, disseminated intravascular coagulation, metabolic acidosis, and ultimately circulatory collapse.[10] Death may also occur from fulminant liver failure.[53]

Management of a toxic level of amphetamine is directed at supportive therapies to lessen the physiologic effects of the drug. Severe hypertension requires intravenous vasodilation.[10,53] The use of beta blockers to treat tachydysrhythmias is controversial. Esmolol (Brevibloc) or propranolol (Inderal) has been suggested by some authors,[53] while others[10] recommend beta blockers be avoided because possible unopposed alpha effects may result in coronary and peripheral arterial vasoconstriction. It has further been suggested that intravenous diltiazem (Cardizem) may be safe.[10] Benzodiazepines and haloperidol can be used for seizure activity and agitation.[10,53] Cooling measures may be required for core temperatures greater than 40° C.[53]

The effects of cocaine are similar to those of methamphetamines. The most toxic effects from excessive cocaine occur because of the excessive central nervous system stimulation and inhibition of the neural uptake of catecholamines. Onset of action depends on the route of administration, the dose, and the patient's tolerance (Table 53-5). The most rapid onset is with smoking or intravenous injection, with symptom production within 1 to 2 minutes. Onset of action with oral use is delayed, with onset of symptoms at 20 to 30 minutes. The half-life of cocaine is up to 60 minutes but is detectable in the urine for 24 to 36 hours after use. Cocaine is often mixed with other abused substances, including heroin ("speedball"), phencyclidine, and alcohol. In the presence of ethanol, cocaine undergoes a change in the liver, making the drug last longer and become more toxic.[53] The toxic cocaine patient is euphoric, anxious, agitated, psychotic, and delirious, and may seize. Vasospasm may lead to chest pain, myocardial ischemia or myocardial infarction, or cardiac dysrhythmias, resulting in sudden death. Cerebral infarcts may also result from vasospasm. Other cardiovascular complications include heart failure, tachycardia, pulmonary hypertension, pulmonary edema, endocarditis, and aortic dissection. Respiratory complications include status asthmaticus, upper airway obstruction with stridor, barotraumas, and alveolar hemorrhage. Severity of the respiratory complications can vary from mild to severe, requiring endotracheal intubation and mechanical ventilation. The patient may have severe muscle rigidity leading to rhabdomyolysis, with hyperthermia and altered mental status.[53]

The seizures, hyperthermia, and agitation require immediate treatment after securing the airway and circulation. Hyperthermia requires cooling, and agitation requires benzodiazepines to lessen the further sympathetic insult. Intubation and mechanical ventilation may be required. Activated charcoal may be administered to lessen further absorption of the drug when taken orally. Chest pain may be treated with nitrates and calcium channel blockers. Beta blockers should be avoided because of blockage of beta$_2$-mediated vasodilation and unopposed beta alpha-adrenergic stimulation.[53]

Club drugs are psychoactive drugs frequently used to intensify social experiences. They are frequently used at dance parties, raves, and night clubs. The most prominent club drugs are 3,4-methylenedioxymethamphetamine (MDMA), also known as ecstasy; gamma-hydroxybutyrate (GHB); flunitrazepam (Rohypnol); and ketamine (Ketalar) (Table 53-6).[17] These drugs are often described as "entactogens," providing the individual taking them with a sense of physical closeness, empathy, and euphoria.[17]

MDMA increases the release of serotonin, dopamine, and norepinephrine from presynaptic neurons and prevents their metabolism by inhibiting monoamine oxidase.[17] Hyperthermia and serotonin syndrome are the most dangerous potential outcomes. In addition to hyperthermia, manifestations of serotonin syndrome include rigidity, myoclonus, and autonomic instability that can result in rhabdomyolysis and acute renal failure, hepatic failure, ARDS, and coagulopathy.[17] Other adverse effects occur from the sympathetic overload and include tachycardia, mydriasis, diaphoresis, tremor, hypertension, dysrhythmias, parkinsonism, medial deviation of the eyes, and urinary retention.[17] There is a direct rise in the release of antidiuretic hormone. The patient may experience confusion, delirium, paranoia, headache, anorexia, depression, insomnia, irritability, and nystagmus. Symptoms may last a few weeks.[17]

TABLE 53-5 Cocaine Pharmacology by Route of Administration

ROUTE	FORMULA	ONSET OF ACTION	PEAK EFFECT	DURATION
Inhalation	"Crack"	8 sec	2–5 min	10–20 min
Intranasal	Cocaine HCl	2–5 min	5–10 min	30 min
Intravenous	Cocaine HCl	Seconds	2–5 min	10–20 min
Oral	Cocaine HCl	10 min	30–60 min	60 min

TABLE 53-6 List of Common Street Names for Club Drugs

CHEMICAL COMPOUND/DRUG NAME	CLUB DRUG STREET NAME
BD (1,4-butanediol, chemical precursor of GHB)	Revitalize plus Serenity Thunder nectar Weight belt cleaner
Flunitrazepam (Rohypnol)	Circles Forget-me pill La rocha Mexican valium R2 Roche Roofies Rope Rophies
GBL (gamma-butyrolactone, chemical precursor of GHB)	Blue nitro Gamma G GH revitalizer
GHB (gamma-hydroxybutyrate)	Bodily harm G Gib Grievous Liquid ecstasy Nitro Scoop Soap
Ketamine (Ketalar)	Cat Jet K Keets Kit-kat Special K Super acid Super K Valiums Vitamin K
MDMA (3,4-methylenedioxymethamphetamine)	Adam Beans Clarity E Ecstasy Hug drug Lover's speed M Rolls X XTC

GHB is a derivative of the inhibitory neurotransmitter gamma-aminobutyric acid; when taken orally produces euphoria, progressing with higher doses to dizziness, hypersalivation, hypotonia, and amnesia.[18] Overdose may result in Cheyne-Stokes respirations, seizures, coma, and death.[17] Coma may be interrupted by agitation, with the appearance similar to a drowning swimmer fighting for air.[14,15] Bradycardia and hypothermia may occur in approximately one third of patients and appears correlated with the level of consciousness.[15] Chronic use of GHB may produce dependence and a withdrawal syndrome that includes anxiety, insomnia, tremor, and, in severe cases, treatment-resistant psychoses.[15]

Flunitrazepam (Rohypnol) is a potent benzodiazepine with very rapid onset. The potency is approximately 10 times that of diazepam with the same effects as other benzodiazepines. At high doses, the drug produces anterograde amnesia, lack of muscular control, and loss of consciousness. Effects occur about 30 minutes after ingestion, peak within 2 hours, and may last up to 8 to 12 hours.[17] Chronic use can produce dependence, with a withdrawal syndrome that includes headache, tension, anxiety, restlessness, muscle pain, photosensitivity, numbness and tingling of the extremities, and increased seizure potential.[48]

Ketamine is a phencyclidine derivative used as an anesthetic agent that produces anesthesia without respiratory depression.[17,76] Onset of drug action is rapid, with duration 30 to 45 minutes. The drug produces sensations of floating outside of the body, visual and auditory hallucinations, and a dreamlike state from the loss of ability to perceive gravity.[27,76] The dreams and hallucinations can persist for up to 24 hours and may progress to a state of delirium.[76]

As a result of the illicit manufactured sources of club drugs and their relative impurities, club drugs must be considered as unknown substances to some degree.[17] The greatest concern with this type of toxic drug exposure is airway support, in particular when these drugs are combined or taken with alcohol.[17] Gastric decontamination with activated charcoal may be useful if done within 60 minutes of drug ingestion.[17] Hypertension and tachycardia generally will resolve with the management of anxiety or agitation. Severe hypertension can be treated with labetalol or nitroprusside.[17] Benzodiazepines can be used for agitation. Flumazenil can be used for reversal of Rohypnol. Hyperthermia can be treated with standard methods of cooling. The use of dantrolene (Dantrium) is not recommended.[87]

Cyclic antidepressants, when taken at higher-than-normal levels, can be very toxic. The Medication table on p. 1500 provides expanded information on tricyclic and tetracyclic antidepressants. Toxic levels of cyclic antidepressants affect the central nervous and cardiovascular

CYCLIC ANTIDEPRESSANTS

TYPE OF ANTIDEPRESSANT	GENERIC NAME	TRADE NAME
Tricyclic	Amitriptyline	Elavil
	Amoxapine	Asendin
	Clomipramine	Anafranil
	Desipramine	Norpramin
	Doxepin	Sinequan
	Imipramine	Tofranil
	Nortriptyline	Pamelor
	Protriptyline	Vivactil
	Trimipramine	Surmontil
Tetracyclic	Maprotiline	Ludiomil

systems, with the potential to cause abrupt and unpredictable deterioration of the patient. Doses greater than 2 grams can be lethal.[26] Toxicity primarily results from the anticholinergic effects, inhibition of neural uptake of norepinephrine or serotonin, peripheral alpha-adrenergic blockade, and cardiac cell membrane depressant effect.[51] Patients present with signs and symptoms of an anticholinergic syndrome, including mydriasis, ileus, urinary retention, fever, flushing, sinus tachycardia, central nervous system depression ranging from lethargy to coma, and seizures.[39] Patients have orthostatic hypotension because of alpha-adrenergic receptor blockade. Prolongation of the QRS complex results from blockage of sodium channels in the His-Purkinje system and ventricular myocardium.[39] QRS prolongation of greater than 0.10 second predicts seizures, and a QRS longer than 0.16 second is associated with heart block and ventricular dysrhythmias.[3,8,22] Cardiac complications account for 2% to 3% of deaths from cyclic antidepressants[26] and usually occur within the first 24 hours of admission.[51]

Treatment involves serum alkalinization with intravenous sodium bicarbonate (1 to 2 mEq/kg) when there is widening of the QRS. This will decrease the fraction of free drug in the blood.[51] Sodium bicarbonate is continued until the QRS narrows to 0.10 sec or until the pH increases to 7.55.[84] Hypotension is treated with crystalloids and vasopressor support.[84] Gastric decontamination can be considered up to 12 hours after ingestion, with activated charcoal the preferred method.[26,51] Emesis should be avoided, as should the use of ipecac.[26] Cardiac dysrhythmias should be treated after correction of hypoxia, hypotension, and acidosis. Sodium bicarbonate is indicated before initiation of antidysrhythmic drugs.[26] Ventricular tachycardia should be treated with intravenous lidocaine or countershock.[50] Phenytoin should not be used in the treatment of ventricular tachycardia or seizures, as it increases the frequency and duration of ventricular tachycardia.[84] Treatment of seizures is done with administration of intravenous lorazepam or diazepam. Refractory seizures have been treated with phenobarbital or propofol.[84]

MULTIDISCIPLINARY PLAN OF CARE

Caring for critically ill patients who are also experiencing withdrawal from addictive substances is challenging. A multidisciplinary approach is necessary; special problems in patient care are addressed in the Multidisciplinary Plan of Care below and on pp. 1501-1504.

MULTIDISCIPLINARY PLAN OF CARE FOR ADDRESSING SPECIAL PROBLEMS AMONG ADDICTED PATIENTS

PROBLEM	INTERVENTION	RATIONALE	EXPECTED OUTCOME
Patient fear of judgment by the staff if addictive behavior is disclosed or denial of an addictive behavior	Develop a trusting, nonjudgmental relationship with the patient or family/support system	This creates a system of trust that the care provider is concerned for the patient's welfare and is not judgmental; allows for anticipation of problems that will affect the course of hospitalization or care as well as prevent any unexpected physiologic states that may place the patient at risk of death.	A relationship will be developed that allows the patient or family/support system to provide open and honest information that permits care planning for the duration of the patient's stay.

PROBLEM	INTERVENTION	RATIONALE	EXPECTED OUTCOME
Risk of developing withdrawal in patient with no presenting signs of withdrawal on admission for non-withdrawal hospitalization	Careful assessment of risk factors for withdrawal: • Complete list of **all** substances used • History of use including duration of use, frequency of use, age of first use, date of last use, and amount of last use • If alcohol is used, the type of alcohol • If illicit substances are used, where obtained • If prescription drugs are used, reason for initial use • Sobriety duration • Prior withdrawal events • Severity of prior withdrawals • If alcohol or benzodiazepines are used: seizure with prior withdrawal • With alcohol, type of drinker: constant or binge • Prior delirium tremens episodes	Assessment of use of substances that place the patient at risk of withdrawal allows identification of the substance or substances early and anticipation of the possibility of withdrawal during the course of hospitalization.	Substances will be identified early and withdrawal treated early in the stay before the development of negative outcomes that impact the hospital stay, the clinical condition, or the patient's life.
	Monitor the patient for signs and symptoms of substance withdrawal: • From identified substances • From unidentified substances when the physiologic condition does not correlate with the expected clinical presentation or standard therapies have not been effective	If substance use has been identified, then monitoring of the signs and symptoms allows initiation of treatment early. If substance use has not been identified, monitoring the signs and symptoms of possible withdrawal allows the nurse to identify those signs and symptoms that do not correlate with the expected clinical presentation and anticipate the need for treatment.	Substances will be identified early and withdrawal treated early in the stay before the development of negative outcomes that impact the hospital stay, the clinical condition, or the patient's life.
	Assess the patient for comorbid conditions that may indicate the presence of substance use, such as the presence of alcoholic liver disease in the alcohol user, infected wounds in the IV drug user, pain not controlled by conventional pain medications and appropriate dosing, the presence of unexplained confusion, or extreme anxiety	Knowledge of those conditions that may be the result of substance use may provide the nurse the basis for suspicion or anticipation of withdrawal.	If the patient has comorbid conditions, the nurse will evaluate the patient for the possible impact of the patient's continued substance use on the clinical condition or reason for admission.
The pregnant patient admitted to critical	A complete assessment of the pregnant patient who is	This will allow the RN to immediately institute	The pregnant patient will not go into labor

Table continues on page 1502

PROBLEM	INTERVENTION	RATIONALE	EXPECTED OUTCOME
care who goes into withdrawal is at risk of spontaneous delivery, fetal demise, or spontaneous fetal loss	admitted to critical care for any possible substance abuse with related withdrawal syndromes	withdrawal therapies and prevent fetal harm. It will also allow for the involvement of the obstetric nurse in the care planning process.	during the course of stay in critical care/hospital and the fetus will not be delivered early.
	Treat with appropriate withdrawal medication: • Alcohol–benzodiazepines • Opiates–methadone	This will prevent early delivery or loss of the fetus.	
	Monitor and assess the patient frequently for: • Continued signs of withdrawal in the presence of treatment • Vital signs to ensure the patient is not experiencing any untoward side effects of the withdrawal therapy • Oxygen saturations done with each vital sign • Patient is weighed daily • Frequent urinalysis for protein	If withdrawal continues despite treatment, then more withdrawal medication must be given. Monitoring for untoward side effects of the therapy allows for assurance that the patient does not experience hypoxemia or respiratory suppression as a result of treatment, ensuring the fetus continues to be well oxygenated. Monitoring of blood pressure, weight, and frequent urinalysis for excreted protein allows for early detection of preeclampsia.	The mother and fetus will experience no untoward side effects of withdrawal therapy.
The patient who goes into alcohol withdrawal is at risk of progressing into a higher or more dangerous state of withdrawal, placing the patient at risk of seizure activity or death	Signs and symptoms of alcohol withdrawal are identified and monitored Severity of withdrawal is based on a clinical tool such as the CIWA scale	Identification of the signs and symptoms of alcohol withdrawal allows for earlier therapy with limitation of progression of the withdrawal state, allowing withdrawal to progress until completed.	The patient will have therapy instituted early, and the severity of withdrawal will not progress.
	Alcohol withdrawal therapy is instituted early: • Therapy is based on the severity of withdrawal • Dosing is based on appropriate intervals • Appropriate therapy is based on age and presence of liver compromise	With early onset of treatment, the patient will have a smoother withdrawal without progression to worsening withdrawal or becoming oversedated.	The patient will receive sufficient therapy based on symptoms that allows withdrawal to complete without complications.
	A chemical dependency counselor/social worker sees the patient	This will allow for development of a discharge plan at the time alcohol abuse is determined and provide the patient a plan	The patient will be discharged to long- term rehabilitation.

PROBLEM	INTERVENTION	RATIONALE	EXPECTED OUTCOME
		for follow-up long-term alcohol rehabilitation.	
The patient in alcohol withdrawal or alcohol and benzodiazepine withdrawal is at risk of complications resulting from the withdrawal or from the therapy for the treatment of withdrawal	Preventive measures are taken to reduce the risk of complications: • Thiamine 100 mg is administered on admission • Patient is placed in upright position of 30–45 degrees when heavily sedated • Intake and output are monitored when patient is heavily sedated or is unable to drink fluids on own • Airway protection measures are instituted such as thickened liquids, eating only in the upright position when unable to fully protect airway • Fall risk is assessed and fall prevention protocols instituted • Seizure precautions instituted if identified as seizure risk	Interventions to prevent complications are critical in this population.	The patient will not have any complications as a result of withdrawal or treatment of withdrawal.
	Patient is assessed regularly for complications of withdrawal: • Aspiration pneumonia • Hypoxia • Hypoventilation • ARDS • Dehydration • Overhydration • Urinary retention • Electrolyte imbalance • Vitamin insufficiency • Neurologic complications, such as Wernicke's syndrome • Seizure activity • Liver failure • Renal insufficiency/failure	Monitoring and assessment of the patient allow for early identification of complications and institution of appropriate therapies.	If patient does experience complications, they will be identified and treated early.
The patient who goes into benzodiazepine withdrawal is at risk of progressing into a higher or more dangerous state of withdrawal, placing the patient at risk of	Preventive measures are taken to reduce the risk of complications: • Patient is placed in upright position of 30–45 degrees when heavily sedated • Intake and output are monitored when patient is	Interventions to prevent complications are critical in this population.	

Table continues on page 1504

PROBLEM	INTERVENTION	RATIONALE	EXPECTED OUTCOME
seizure activity or death	heavily sedated or is unable to drink fluids on own • Airway protection measures are instituted such as thickened liquids, eating only in the upright position when unable to fully protect airway • Fall risk is assessed and fall prevention protocols instituted • Seizure precautions instituted if identified as seizure risk • Liver function is monitored frequently		
	Patient is assessed regularly for complications of withdrawal: • Aspiration pneumonia • Hypoxia • Hypoventilation • ARDS • Dehydration • Overhydration • Urinary retention • Electrolyte imbalance • Vitamin insufficiency • Neurologic complications, such as Wernicke's syndrome • Seizure activity • Liver failure • Renal insufficiency/failure	Monitoring and assessment of the patient allow for early identification of complications and institution of appropriate therapies.	
	A chemical dependency counselor/social worker sees the patient	This will allow for development of a discharge plan at the time alcohol abuse is determined and provide the patient a plan for follow-up long-term alcohol rehabilitation.	The patient will be discharged to long-term rehabilitation.

ARDS = Acute respiratory distress syndrome, CIWA = Clinical Institute Withdrawal Assessment.

CONCLUSIONS

Caring for the chemically addicted patient requires the nurse both to understand the physiologic effects of the substance or substances used and to identify the signs and symptoms of withdrawal. The nurse must be able to recognize withdrawal and provide appropriate therapy, allowing the completion of withdrawal without negative outcomes to the patient's well-being. A critical component in caring for the chemically addicted patient is a full assessment of the substances used. This assessment will allow for anticipation of the onset of withdrawal or the possibility of potential withdrawal as well as guide the course of withdrawal therapy. The chemically addicted patient may also present with difficult behavior. An understanding of addiction and the possibility of psychoactive co-pathology will allow for better behavior management of the patient. The goal of withdrawal management is to provide a safe withdrawal without harm to the patient, and the nurse at the bedside is instrumental in this care.

REFERENCES

1. Bayard, M., McIntyre, J., Hill, K. R., et al. (2004). Alcohol withdrawal syndrome. *Am Family Physician, 69*(6), 1443–1450.

2. Blondell, R. D. (2005). Ambulatory detoxification of patients with alcohol dependence. *Am Family Physician, 71*(3), 495–502.

3. Boehnert, M. T., & Lovejoy, F. H. (1985). Value of QRS duration versus the serum drug level in predicting seizures and ventricular arrhythmias after an acute overdose of tricyclic antidepressants. *N Engl J Med, 313*(8), 474–479.

4. Bogenschutz, M. P., & Geppert, C. M. A. (2003). Pharmacologic treatments for women with addictions. *Obstet Gynecol Clin, 30*(3), 523–544.

5. Bolnick, J. M., & Rayburn, W. F. (2003). Substance use disorders in women: special considerations during pregnancy. *Obstet Gynecol Clin, 30*(3), 545–555vii.

6. Borg, L., & Kreek, M. J. (2003). The pharmacology of opioids. In A. W. Graham, et al. (Eds.), *Principles of addiction medicine* (3rd ed.). Chevy Chase, Md: American Society of Addiction Medicine.

7. Bruijnzeel, A. W., Repetto, M., & Gold, M. S. (2004). Neurobiological mechanisms in addictive and psychiatric disorders. *Psychiatr Clin North Am, 27*(4), 661–674.

8. Buckley, N. A., O'Connell, D. L., Whyte, I. M., et al. (1996). Interrater agreement in the measurement of QRS interval in tricyclic antidepressant overdose: implications for monitoring and research. *Ann Emerg Med, 28*(5), 515–519.

9. Chander, G., & McCaul, M. E. (2003). Co-occurring psychiatric disorders in women with addictions. *Obstet Gynecol Clin, 30*(3), 469–481.

10. Colucciello, S. A., & Tomaszewski, C. (2002). Substance abuse. In J. A. Marx, et al. (Eds.), *Rosen's emergency medicine: concepts and clinical practice* (5th ed.). St. Louis: Mosby.

11. Coomes, T. R., & Smith, S. W. (1997). Successful use of propofol in refractory delirium tremens. *Ann Emerg Med, 30*(6), 825–828.

12. Counihan, T. J. (2001). Focal brain disease. In T. E. Andreoli, et al. (Eds.) *Cecil essentials of medicine* (5th ed.). Philadelphia: Saunders.

13. Desan, P. H., & Powsner, S. (2004). Assessment and management of patients with psychiatric disorders. *Crit Care Med, 32*(4), S166–S173.

14. Dyer, J. E. (1991). Gamma-hydroxybutyrate: a health-food product producing coma and seizure like activity. *Am J Med, 9*(4), 321–324.

15. Dyer, J. E., Roth, B., & Hyma, B. A. (2001). Gamma-hydroxybutyrate withdrawal syndrome. *Ann Emerg Med, 37*(2), 147–153.

16. Fallon, M. B., et al. (2001). Acute and chronic hepatitis. In T. E. Andreoli, et al. (Eds.), *Cecil essentials of medicine* (5th ed.). Philadelphia: Saunders.

17. Gahlinger, P. M. (2004). Club drugs: MDMA, gamma-hydroxybutyrate (GHB), rohypnol, and ketamine. *Am Family Physician, 69*(11), 2619–2626.

18. Garrison, G., & Mueller, P. (1998). Clinical features and outcomes after unintentional gamma hydroxybutyrate (GHB) overdose. *J Clin Toxicol, 36*(5), 503–504.

19. Giese, A. A. (2001). Personality and personality disorders. In Jacobson (Ed.), *Psychiatric secrets* (2nd ed.). Philadelphia: Hanley & Belfus.

20. Greenfield, S. F., Manwani, S. G., & Nargiso, J. E. (2003). Epidemiology of substance use disorders in women. *Obstet Gynecol Clin, 30*(3), 413–446.

21. Hanck, C., & Whitcomb, D. C. (2004). Alcoholic pancreatitis. *Gastroenterol Clin, 33*(4), 751–765.

22. Harrigan, R. A., & Brady, W. J. (1999). ECG abnormalities in tricyclic antidepressant ingestion. *Am J Emerg Med, 17*(4), 387–393.

23. Hesselbrock, M. N., Meyer, R. E., & Keener, J. J. (1985). Psychopathology in hospitalized alcoholics. *Arch Gen Psychiatry, 42*(11), 1050–1055.

24. Holcomb, T. E., & Clothier, J. L. (2001). Alcohol and substance abuse. In T. E. Andreoli, et al. (Eds.), *Cecil essentials of medicine* (5th ed.). Philadelphia: Saunders.

24a. Hopper, J. A., & Shafi, T. (2002). Management of the hospitalized injection drug user. *Infect Dis Clin North Am, 16*: 571–87.

25. Huber, M. G., & Taylor, G. J. (2000). Psychologic disorders, street drugs and drug abuse. In G. J. Taylor (Ed.), *Primary care management of heart disease*. St. Louis: Mosby.

26. Hybels, C. F., & Blazer, D. G. (2003). Epidemiology of late-life mental disorders. *Clin Geriatr Med, 19*(4), 663–696.

27. Jansen, K. L. (1993). Non-medical use of ketamine. *Brit Med J, 306*(6878), 601–602.

28. John, A. D., & Sieber, F. E. (2004). Age associated issues: geriatrics. *Anesthesiol Clin North Am, 22*(1), 45–58.

29. Jones, H. E. (2004). Practical considerations for the clinical use of buprenorphine. *Science Practice Perspect, 2*(2), 4–16.

30. Kantrow, S., & deBoisblanc, B. P. (2004). Mysteries of the drunken lung. *Crit Care Med, 32*(3), 833–884.

31. Kasser, C., et al. A. Detoxification: principles and protocols. American Society of Addiction Medicine. www.asam.org/publ/detoxifications.htm.

32. Kennedy, J. A. (2001a). Psychoactive substance disorders. In J. L. Jacobson & A. M. Jacobson (Eds.), *Psychiatric secrets* (2nd ed.). Philadelphia: Hanley & Belfus.

33. Kennedy, J. A. (2001b). Alcohol use disorders. In J. L. Jacobson & A. M. Jacobson (Eds.), *Psychiatric secrets* (2nd ed.). Philadelphia: Hanley & Belfus.

34. Kennedy, J. A. (2001c). Opioid use disorders. In J. L. Jacobson & A. M. Jacobson (Eds.), *Psychiatric secrets* (2nd ed.). Philadelphia: Hanley & Belfus.

35. Kessler, R. C., et al. (1996). The epidemiology of co-occurring addictive and mental disorders: implications for prevention and service utilization. *Am J Orthopsychiatry, 66*(1), 17–31.

36. Kessler, R. C., et al. (1997). Lifetime co-occurrence of DSM-III-R alcohol abuse and dependence with other psychiatric disorders in the National Comorbidity Survey. *Arch Gen Psychiatry, 54*(4), 313–321.

37. Koob, G. F. (1996). Drug addiction: the yin and yang of hedonic homeostasis. *Neuron, 16*(5), 893–896.

38. Kreek, M. J., & Koob, G. F. (1998). Drug dependence: stress and dysregulation of brain reward pathways. *Drug Alcohol Dependence, 51*(1–2), 23–47.

39. Kreit, J. W. (2005). Antidepressant drug overdose. In M. P. Fink, et al. (Eds.), *Textbook of critical care medicine* (5th ed.). Philadelphia: Saunders.

40. Kron, F. W., Fetters, M. D., & Goldman, E. B. (2003). The challenging patient. *Clin Family Practice, 5*(4), 893–903.

41. Kruse, J. A. (2005). Ethanol, methanol, and ethylene glycol. In M. P. Fink, et al. (Eds.), *Textbook of critical care* (5th ed.). Philadelphia: Saunders.

42. Leevy, C. M., & Moroianu, S. A. (2005). Nutritional aspects of alcoholic liver disease. *Clin Liver Dis, 9*(1), 67–81.

43. Limper, A. H. (2004). Overview of pneumonia. In L. Goldman & D. Ausiello (Eds.), *Cecil textbook of medicine* (22nd ed.). Philadelphia: Saunders.

44. Mayo-Smith, M. F. (2003). Management of alcohol intoxication and withdrawal. In A. W. Graham, et al. (Eds.), *Principles of addiction medicine* (3rd ed.). Chevy Chase: Md: American Society of Addiction Medicine.

45. Mayo-Smith, M. F., et al. (2004). Management of alcohol withdrawal delirium. An evidence-based practice guideline. *Arch Intern Med, 164*(13), 1405–1412.

46. Mayo-Smith, M. F., et al. (1997). Pharmacologic management of alcohol withdrawal. *J Am Med Assoc, 278*(2), 144–151.

47. Mendes, L., & Loscalzo, J. (2001). Cardiomyopathy. In T. E. Andreoli, et al. (Eds.), *Cecil essentials of medicine* (5th ed.). Philadelphia: Saunders.

48. Miotto, K., et al. (2001). Gamma-hydroxybutyric acid: patterns of use, effects and withdrawal. *Am J Addiction, 10*(3), 232–241.

49. Mofenson, H. C., et al. (2005). Medical toxicology: ingestions, inhalations and Demerol and ocular absorptions. In R. E. Rakel & E. T. Bope (Eds.), *Conn's current therapy 2005* (57th ed.). Philadelphia: Saunders.

50. Mokhlesi, B., & Corbridge, T. C. (2003). Toxicology in the critically ill patient. *Clin Chest Med, 24*(4), 689–711.

51. Mokhlesi, B., et al. (2003). Adult toxicology in critical care part I: general approach to the intoxicated patient. *Chest, 123*(2), 577–592.

52. Mokhlesi, B., et al. (2003). Adult toxicology in critical care part II: specific poisonings. *Chest, 123*(2), 897–922.

53. Moore, R. D., et al. (1989). Prevalence, detection and treatment of alcoholism in hospitalized patients. *J Am Med Assoc, 261*(3), 403–407.

54. Moss, M., et al. (2003). Chronic alcohol abuse is associated with an increased incidence of acute respiratory distress syndrome and severity of multiple organ dysfunction in patients with septic shock. *Crit Care Med, 31*(3), 869–877.

55. Muskin, P. R., & Hasse, E. (2001). Personality disorders. In *Textbook of primary care medicine*. (3rd ed.). St. Louis: Mosby.

56. Myrick, H., et al. (2004). Diagnosis and treatment of co-occurring affective disorders and substance use disorders. *Psychiatr Clin North Am, 27*(4), 649–659.

57. Nestler, E. J. (2001). Molecular basis of long-term plasticity underlying addiction. *Natl Rev Neurosci, 2*(2), 119–128.

58. O'Connor, A. D., Rusyniak, D. E., & Bruno, A. (2005). Cerebrovascular and cardiovascular complications of alcohol and sympathomimetic drug abuse. *Med Clin North Am, 89*(6), 1343–1358.

59. O'Connor, P. G. (2004). Alcohol abuse and dependence. In L. Goldman & D. Ausiello (Eds.), *Cecil textbook of medicine* (22nd ed.). Philadelphia: Saunders.

60. O'Connor, P. G., Kosten, T. R., & Stine, S. M. (2003). Management of opioid intoxication and withdrawal. In A. W. Graham, et al. (Eds.), *Principles of addiction medicine* (3rd ed.). Chevy Chase, Md: American Society of Addiction Medicine.

61. Rao, R. B., & Hoffman, R. S. (2002). Substance abuse. In J. A. Marx, et al. (Eds.), *Rosen's emergency medicine: concepts and clinical practice* (5th ed.). St. Louis: Mosby.

62. Rayburn, W. F., & Bogenschutz, M. P. (2004). Pharmacotherapy for pregnant women with addictions. *Am J Obstet Gynecol, 191*(6), 1885–1897.

63. Regier, D. A., et al. (1990). Comorbidity of mental disorders with alcohol and other drug abuse: results from the Epidemiologic Catchment Area (ECA) study. *J Am Med Assoc, 264*(19), 2511–2518.

64. Reynolds, E. W., & Bada, H. S. (2003). Pharmacology of drugs of abuse. *Obstet Gynecol Clin, 30*(3), 501–522.

65. Rinder, H. M. (2001). Disorders of hemostasis: bleeding. In T. E. Andreoli, et al. (Eds.), *Cecil essentials of medicine* (5th ed.). Philadelphia: Saunders.

66. Rosenthal, R. A., & Kavic, S. M. (2004). Assessment and management of the geriatric patient. *Crit Care Med, 32*(4), s92–s105.

67. Samet, J. H. (2004). Drug abuse and dependence. In L. Goldman & D. Ausiello (Eds.), *Cecil textbook of medicine* (22nd ed.). Philadelphia: Saunders.

68. Satter, S. P., Petty, F., & Burke, W. J. (2003). Diagnosis and treatment of alcohol dependence in older alcoholics. *Clin Geriatr Med, 19*(4), 743–761.

69. Schoener, E. P., Hopper, J. A., & Pierre, J. D. (2002). Injection drug use in North America. *Infect Dis Clin North Am, 16*(3), 535–551.

70. Smith, J. W. (1995). Medical manifestation of alcoholism in the elderly. *Int J Addiction, 30*(13,14), 1749–1798.

71. Spickerman, F. (2004). The fine art of refusal. *Family Practice Management, 11*(2), 80.

72. Spies, C. D., et al. (2004). Altered cell-mediated immunity and increased postoperative infection rate in long-term alcoholic patients. *Anesthesiology, 100*(5), 1088–1100.

73. Stevenson, L. W. (2004). Diseases of the myocardium. In L. Goldman & D. Ausiello (Eds.), *Cecil textbook of medicine* (22nd ed.). Philadelphia: Saunders.

74. Stine, S. M., Greenwalk, M. K., & Kosten, T. R. (2003). Pharmacologic interventions for opioid addiction. In A. W. Graham, et al. (Eds.), *Principles of addiction medicine* (3rd ed.). Chevy Chase, Md: American Society of Addiction Medicine.

75. Stoelting, R. K. (1999a). Nonbarbiturate induction drugs. *Pharmacology and physiology in anesthetic practice* (3rd ed.). Philadelphia: Lippincott Williams & Wilkins.

76. Stoelting, R. K. (1999b). Drugs used for psychopharmacologic therapy. *Pharmacology and physiology in anesthetic practice* (3rd ed.). Philadelphia: Lippincott Williams & Wilkins.

77. Substance Abuse and Mental Health Services Administration. (2005). *Overview of findings from the 2004 National Survey on Drug Use and Health.* (Series H-27, DHHS Publication No. SMA 05–4061). Rockville, Md: Office of Applied Studies, NSDUH.

78. Swift, R. M. (2001). Drug abuse and dependence. In J. Noble, et al. (Eds.), *Textbook of primary care medicine.* St. Louis: Mosby.

79. Takeshita, J. (2004). Use of propofol for alcohol withdrawal delirium: a case report. *J Clin Psychiatry, 65*(1), 134–135.

80. Toombs, J. D., & Kral, L. A. (2005). Methadone treatment for pain states. *Am Family Physician, 71*(7), 1353–1358.

81. Vestal, R. E., et al. (1977). Aging and ethanol metabolism. *Clin Pharmacol Therapeutics, 21*(3), 343–354.

82. Wadland, W. C., & Ferenchick, G. S. (2004). Medical comorbidity in addictive disorders. *Psychiatr Clin North Am, 27*(4), 675–687.

83. Walsh, J. S. (2005). Personal conversations, Board Certified Addiction Medicine Physician Swedish Medical Center: Addiction Recovery Services, Seattle, Wash.

84. Walter, F. G., & Bilden, E. F. (2002). Antidepressants. In J. A. Marx, et al. (Eds.), *Rosen's emergency medicine: concepts and clinical practice* (5th ed.). St. Louis: Mosby.

85. Wakim-Fleming, J., & Mullen, K. D. (2005). Long-term management of alcoholic liver disease. *Clin Liver Disease, 9*(1), 135–149.

86. Ward, R. K. (2004). Assessment and management of personality disorders. *Am Family Physician, 70*(8), 1505–1512.

87. Watson, J. D., et al. (1993). Exertional heat stroke induced by amphetamine analogues. Does dantrolene have a place? *Anaesthesia, 48*(12), 1057–1060.

88. Weaver, M. F. (2005). Heroin and other opioids. *Up to Date.* Available at www.utdol.com.

89. Woodward, J. J. (2003). The pharmacology of alcohol. In A. W. Graham, et al. (Eds.), *Principles of addiction medicine* (3rd ed.). Chevy Chase, Md: American Society of Addiction Medicine.

90. Hopper, J. A., & Shafi, T. (2002). Management of the hospitalized injection drug user. *Infect Dis Clin North Am, 16*(3), 571–587.

CHAPTER 54

End-of-Life Care

Debra J. Lynn-McHale Wiegand and Laura D. Williams

"You matter to the last moment of your life, and we will do all we can not only to help you die peacefully, but to live until you die."

—Cicely Saunders

Death can and will come to each of us; for many it will happen in critical care. Critical care deaths represent the majority of hospital deaths, with more than half a million deaths each year.[8] The majority of patients who die in U.S. hospitals do so under circumstances in which decisions need to be made about how long to pursue life-extending treatments.[137] It is estimated that more than 90% of deaths in critical care are preceded by decisions to withhold or withdraw life-sustaining therapies (LSTs).[63,110]

Patients enter the acute care setting in physiologic crisis. Treatment is aggressive in an effort to be life-saving. Interventions are effective in stabilizing most critically ill or injured patients. However, it is estimated that as many as one in five patients dies in critical care.[8]

The last phase of life varies based on each person's illness trajectory and clinical course.[90,91] Patients may die quite unexpectedly after a sudden illness or injury or after a prolonged, progressive illness. Among those with forewarning of death, some may steadily and predictably decline, whereas others may have fairly long periods of chronic illness with episodes of acute crises, one of which may prove fatal, although an entirely different problem may intervene to cause death.[53] Palliative care is an important component of quality patient care and should be integrated along with LSTs throughout a person's illness (Figure 54-1). The goal of palliative care is to prevent and relieve suffering and support the best-possible quality of life for patients and their families, regardless of the stage of the disease or the need for other therapies.[102] Palliative care interventions are used to relieve pain, dyspnea, and restlessness, and facilitate the decision-making process while supporting patients and families. Palliative care expands traditional disease-model medical treatments and includes the goals of enhancing quality of life for patients and families, optimizing function, helping with decision making and providing opportunities for personal growth.[102] Box 54-1 contains strategies for incorporating palliative care into the care of critically ill patients.

PREDICTING DEATH IN CRITICAL CARE

At times it is clear to healthcare providers that patients will more than likely not survive their critical care stay. However, for many others, predicting who will live and who will die is often challenged by prognostic uncertainty. Over the past decade the development of clinical predictive models in critical care represents a significant advancement for clinicians, clinical investigators, critical care directors, and quality assurance managers. Complex models such as the Acute Physiology, Age, and Chronic Health Evaluation (APACHE II, III)[79,80]; Simplified Acute Physiology Score (SAPS) II[84]; and the Mortality Probability Model (MPM) II[85] produce probability estimates and allow adjustment to the severity of illness for a patient population. They have been developed and validated with large patient populations. The data and models must be valid and reliable for aggregated groups of patients to satisfy statistical and methodological requirements. However, they have not been validated for use in individual patient decision making. Each of these prognostic models has been used to compare observed outcomes to a case-mix-adjusted benchmark for hospital

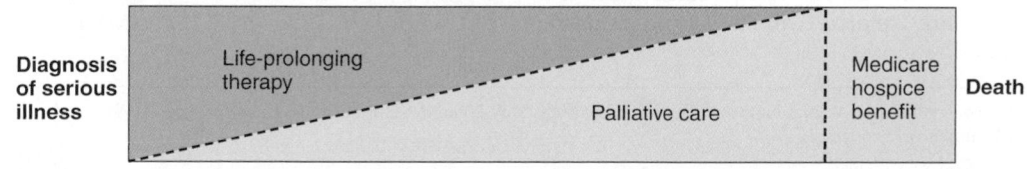

FIGURE 54-1 Palliative care integrated with life-sustaining therapy throughout a person's illness trajectory.

Box 54-1

Integration Strategies for Acute and Critical Care Settings Based on the National Consensus Guidelines for Quality Palliative Care's Clinical Practice Guidelines for Quality Palliative Care

DOMAIN 1: STRUCTURE AND PROCESSES OF CARE

- An interdisciplinary team, including the patient and family, develops an overall plan of care.
- The plan of care is based on the identified and expressed values, goals, and needs of the patient and family and is developed with professional guidance and support for decision making.
- Critical care providers know both the patient's and the family's understandings of the patient's condition and prognosis.
- Treatment decisions are based on goals of care, assessment of risk and benefit, best evidence, and patient and family preferences.
- Hospital-based policies, procedures, and guidelines are related to palliative care.
- Quality improvement programs evaluate the effectiveness of palliative care provided.
- Administration supports education and training regarding the integration of palliative care into critical care and is available to the interdisciplinary team.
- Relationships between palliative care and hospice services ensure continuity and the highest quality care across the illness trajectory.
- Resources are available to help the interdisciplinary team cope with the emotional impact of caring for dying patients and their families.

DOMAIN 2: PHYSICAL ASPECTS OF CARE

- The interdisciplinary team is knowledgeable and skilled at efficiently and effectively preventing and managing potentially distressing symptoms.
- Pain, dyspnea, anxiety, agitation, and other signs and symptoms of discomfort are quickly assessed and managed.

DOMAIN 3: PSYCHOLOGIC AND PSYCHIATRIC ASPECTS OF CARE

- Patients and families are assisted with psychologic and psychiatric issues.
- Grief and bereavement services are offered to patients and families.
- Family members at risk for complicated grief and bereavement are referred to expert psychiatric practitioners.

DOMAIN 4: SOCIAL ASPECTS OF CARE

- Family time together is encouraged.
- The healthcare team and the family meet regularly so that information can be shared, questions can be answered, and treatment goals can be discussed and reviewed.
- Discussions are focused on patient wishes and goals of care.
- Family meetings provide an opportunity to support the family and to facilitate the family decision-making process.

DOMAIN 5: SPIRITUAL, RELIGIOUS, AND EXISTENTIAL ASPECTS OF CARE

- The patient and family members' spiritual, religious, and existential concerns are assessed and addressed.
- Spiritual rituals are supported.
- Patients and families have access to pastoral care and to clergy of their own faith.

DOMAIN 6: CULTURAL ASPECTS OF CARE

- Patient and families members' cultural concerns are assessed and addressed.
- Interpreter services facilitate communication among the patient, family, and the interdisciplinary healthcare team.
- Patient and family rituals are supported.

DOMAIN 7: CARE OF THE IMMINENTLY DYING PATIENT

- Signs and symptoms of impending death are recognized and communicated to the patient and family.
- Care during the active dying phase focuses on promotion of comfort and support of the patient and family.
- Patients die in the setting of their choice.

DOMAIN 8: ETHICAL AND LEGAL ASPECTS OF CARE

- Adults with decision-making capacity direct their course of treatment.
- Children with decision-making capacity are given appropriate weight in decision making.
- If patients do not have decision-making capacity, previously expressed wishes, values, and preferences guide the decision-making process.
- Consultants such as specialists in ethical and legal issues are available to help as needed.

Modified from a poster presented at AACN's National Teaching Institute, May 2006, developed by P. Kalowes and D. Wiegand on behalf of AACN's Ethics Workgroup.

mortality, based on outcomes reflecting the efficacy of treatment.[152]

Studies using APACHE III, SAPS II, and MPM II within independent critical care databases have reported a predicted mortality significantly different from that observed.[57,152,153] Many explainable factors influence the accuracy of the predictions including that data collection must be accurate, reproducible, and interpretable. Nonetheless, exercise caution when using these data to enable appropriate and timely decisions to be made regarding the withdrawal or termination of treatments in critically ill patients.

Prediction models are inherently imperfect because they are in constant need of revision, thus APACHE version IV.[152] Older multivariable prediction models also are limited in that they are based on data obtained after admission to critical care. In addition, they do not provide information regarding the change in odds of dying after receiving critical care interventions; they are not deterministic.[8,9,17,79,92]

Another example of an earlier model used to demonstrate an inaccurate prediction of actual mortality risk was reported from the landmark Study to Understand Prognoses and Preferences for Outcomes and Risks of Treatments (SUPPORT) trial that examined patients' preferences for end-of-life care.[134] The SUPPORT model (modified from the APACHE II) showed the five study hospitals had the same adjusted mortality rates and the same associations of all predictive factors with mortality predictions. However, the SUPPORT model's performance with regard to finding a population that was likely to die within 6 months was inaccurate. For example, researchers found that within 1 week of a patient's death, it was predicted that the patient had a 50% chance of living 2 more months. Even on the day of death, it was estimated that patients had a 20% chance of living 2 more months. Although the SUPPORT model was a remarkably informative instrument, and probably useful in calibrating the effects of treatments or comparing the quality of life-sustaining care among hospitals or treatments, it is not a well-calibrated way to sort patients by their prognoses at 6 months because actual prognoses are quite uncertain for many terminal patients.[152]

Newer generation prognostic models, such as the APACHE IV[152] and an automated risk adjustment system recently developed for Veterans Affairs critical care units,[115] are more complex within precisely defined disease categories. The APACHE IV has excellent discrimination (aggregate predicted death and observed) compared with previous versions. Because of its accuracy for U.S. patients, APACHE IV can be used to benchmark critical care performance using aggregate standardized mortality ratios (SMRs) to assess quality of care and disease-specific SMRs to evaluate outcomes for patient subgroups.[152] In addition,

newer more accurate predictions may help patients and families make treatment decisions and bridge the abrupt transitions from life-prolonging care to palliative care. Although prognostic models have improved discrimination and individual accuracy, end-of-life decisions should not be based solely on predictive hospital survival, but should be made in the context of each patient's disease trajectory, quality of life, and treatment preferences.

END-OF-LIFE CONSIDERATIONS

Do Not Resuscitate Decisions

Do not resuscitate or allow natural death decisions are commonly made in critical care. Usually resuscitation decisions occur as a patient is nearing death and are made within the overall context of goals of care and treatment. Patients and their families need accurate information about the patient's medical condition, prognosis, and what resuscitation is, in order to make informed decisions. Ideally, resuscitation decisions in critical care are made after the patient, family, and health care team discuss the possible need for cardiopulmonary resuscitation (CPR) and the use of further aggressive life-sustaining interventions (i.e., advanced cardiac life support). Before discussing resuscitation with the patient and family, the healthcare team should consider the following questions:

- What is the likelihood of the need for resuscitation?
- What is the potential success of resuscitation?
- What are the patient and family members' understandings of resuscitation?
- What does or would the patient want?

Defining Life-Sustaining Therapy

LST has been defined as encompassing "all healthcare interventions that have the effect of increasing the life span of the patient."[112(p.3)] For example, LSTs may include mechanical ventilation, vasoactive agents, cardiac mechanical assist devices, renal replacement, nutrition, hydration, antibiotics, and blood replacement products. *Withholding LST* is defined as "the considered decision not to institute a medically appropriate and potentially beneficial therapy, with the understanding that the patient will probably die without the therapy in question."[109(p.1164)] *Withdrawal of LST* is defined as "the cessation and removal of an ongoing medical therapy with the explicit intent not to substitute an equivalent alternative treatment; it is fully anticipated that the patient will die following the change in therapy."[109(p.1164)] Technology should be used when necessary to accomplish the goals; its use should be minimized when the primary goal is achievement of a peaceful death.[113]

Defining Death

For decades the Harvard Criteria have been used to determine brain death.[10] These criteria include the following:

- Unreceptivity and unresponsiveness
- No spontaneous movement or spontaneous breathing
- No reflexes and the absence of elicitable reflexes
- As a confirmatory measure only, flat electroencephalograms (EEGs), taken twice within at least a 24-hour intervening period

Cardinal findings in brain death include coma or unresponsiveness, apnea, absence of cerebral motor responses to pain in all extremities, and absence of brain stem reflexes including pupillary signs, ocular movements, facial sensory and motor responses, and pharyngeal and tracheal reflexes.[129]

The President's Commission for the Study of Ethical Problems in Medicine and Biomedical and Behavioral Research served as a model for the adoption of the Uniform Determination of Death Act (UDDA).[11] According to the UDDA, "An individual who has sustained either irreversible cessation of circulatory and respiratory functions or irreversible cessation of all functions of the entire brain, including the brain stem, is dead." In addition to clinical findings, "a determination of brain death always requires a formal apnea test; depending on the mechanism of injury, the determination of brain death may also involve corroborative evidence, such as a cerebral perfusion study or an EEG."[109(p.957)] Patients' families should be aware that brain death testing is being performed and must be informed as soon as brain death is determined. They need to be told that brain death is death, with no chance of recovery. It is important to tell the family that patient movements may occur due to activation of spinal motor neurons.[64,117] The family should be given the opportunity to notify additional family members and to say final goodbyes before removal of all LSTs. The process is different from that of withdrawal of LST in that there is no withdrawal decision for the family to make.

Organ Donation

"Organ donation, with its ability to both improve the quality of life and potentially save lives, is a national healthcare priority."[41(p.81)] The organ donation process is initiated when death is imminent. Many patients and families receive tremendous comfort knowing that they can help others through organ donation. All hospitals who receive Medicare and Medicaid reimbursement are required to determine if the patient or family would be willing to donate tissues or organs.[52] Every death or imminent death in a U.S. hospital must be reported to an organ procurement organization (OPO) to meet the federal rules of the U.S. Department of Health and Human Services.[62] The OPO determines if the patient is an eligible donor as traditionally defined by meeting brain death criteria.

The OPO coordinator also assists with determining eligibility of a patient as a donor after cardiac death or as a non–heart beating organ donor. Donor criteria[95] for non–heart-beating organ donation include:

- A ventilator-dependent patient who has sustained a neurologic injury from which recovery is not possible, but who does not meet brain death criteria
- A severely ill patient receiving LST
- A patient who has had an unexpected cardiac arrest and from whom resuscitation has not been achieved

It is recommended that there be a decoupling process between discussions related to end-of-life decision making and organ donation. Thus organ donation discussions are separate from end-of-life discussions. Only the OPO coordinator or designated hospital requestor should approach the patient's family to discuss the possibility of organ donation. If the family decides to donate organs, the entire process is facilitated by the OPO coordinator working collaboratively with the critical care team.

ETHICAL PALLIATIVE AND END-OF-LIFE CARE

Creating an ethical environment is important in the provision of quality palliative and end-of-life care. Related ethical considerations in critical care include a patient's right to self-determination, family advocacy and decision making, utility or benefit versus burden of therapy, medical futility, withholding and withdrawing LST, use of neuromuscular blockade, and the principle of double effect related to analgesic administration.

A Patient's Right to Self-Determination

Autonomy is an essential principle in decisions related to palliative care and end-of-life care. Autonomy is defined as the individual determines his or her course of action in accordance with a plan chosen by himself or herself.[18] Respect for autonomy requires healthcare providers to obtain informed consent from patients before taking any action.[42] According to the

President's Commission for the Study of Ethical Problems in Medicine and Biomedical and Behavioral Research, the voluntary choice of a competent and informed patient should determine whether LST will be initiated, continued, or withdrawn, just as such choices provide the basis for other decisions about medical treatment.[112] Healthcare providers do not have the right to initiate and continue therapy that a patient does not desire.

Patients should be in control of all treatment decisions as long they have decision-making capacity. Sulmasy and colleagues[128] suggest that the following criteria should be used in determining decision-making capacity:

- The patient's judgment is intact.
- The patient can understand the nature of the procedure under consideration, its risks, benefits, and the consequences of deciding to accept or to forgo the procedure.
- The patient can communicate a decision.
- The patient can explain the reasons for a decision in a way that is consistent with his or her life history and previously held values.
- The patient's decision remains relatively stable over time.

During admission to critical care, important information needs to be ascertained to determine if patients have made their treatment preferences known such as through a written advance directive.[3] The Patient Self-Determination Act, part of the Omnibus Budget Reconciliation Act of 1990, was passed in an effort to encourage Americans to consider what they would and would not want toward life's end. It is estimated that only 15% to 25% of Americans have completed an advance directive.[21,60,73,99] The advance directive may be in the form of a living will or a durable power of attorney for healthcare. If the patient has an advance directive, a copy of the document should be obtained and placed in the patient's chart. Hospitals often have a system in place for the patient's advance directive to automatically be placed in the front of the patient's medical records. Computerized patient health information systems have facilitated the process to retrieve advance directive information.

The advance directive should be reviewed with the patient to see if the information is current and accurate. Patients with decision-making capacity have the right to change their minds and should be encouraged to communicate changes in treatment preferences.

Family Advocacy and Decision Making

Patients should be in control of all treatment decisions as long as they are able. Yet at the end of life, patients frequently no longer have that capacity

because of their illnesses, injuries, or treatments and a surrogate decision maker is needed. If the patient has a written advance directive, the individual identified who has durable power of attorney for healthcare (healthcare proxy) is the primary decision maker. All family members should be familiar with the designated healthcare proxy, and treatment decisions should be based on discussions the proxy had with the patient.

If the patient does not have a living will and has not identified a durable power of attorney for healthcare, the family is turned to for input regarding the patient's desired wishes. Even though a written advance directive may not have been executed, patients often have had discussions with family members about what they would or would not want, should their sense of well-being or personhood be affected. The family in essence then provides substituted judgment, in which a designee makes a decision based on what decision the patient would make. If the family does not know what decision the patient would make, the family provides a best interest decision, based on what they think the patient would want.

Families have found advance directives helpful when making decisions related to life-sustaining therapies.* Tilden and colleagues reported that written advance directives were most helpful to families making end-of-life decisions.[137]

Treatment discussions should always focus on what goals of care the patient would want. Conversations using words such as, "If your mother could talk to us, what would she tell us?" should be asked. It is of utmost importance that the surrogate or family speak from the patient's perspective, not from the perspective of the family members.

Benefit Versus Burden of Therapy

Historically, treatments were discussed as if they were ordinary or extraordinary. Both the President's Commission for the Study of Ethical Problems in Medicine and Biomedical and Behavioral Research[112] and the Guidelines on the Termination of Life-Sustaining Treatment and the Care of the Dying[131] recommended that all treatments—including nutrition, ventilation, dialysis, and others—should be determined based on the potential benefits versus burdens to the patient.

Determination of benefit versus burden is not a unilateral decision. It is essential that the patient (if able to participate in decision making), the surrogate or family, and the healthcare providers discuss the utility of treatment. Instrumental to these discussions are patient values, advance directives, and choices. Further, Sulmasy and colleagues distinguish between benefit and

---

*References 69, 96, 106, 130, 136, 137.

effectiveness of interventions. They state that effectiveness relates to the impact of the intervention on the biomedical good of the patient and is an objective determination made by the healthcare team, whereas benefit is much broader, encompassing any positive change in the patient condition (as the patient perceives it); it is a subjective determination.[128]

Medical Futility

Medical futility is a complex issue that often arises in critical care. Medical futility is defined as "any clinical circumstance in which physicians and their consultants, consistent with the available medical literature, conclude that further treatment [except comfort care] cannot, within a reasonable possibility, cure, ameliorate, improve or restore a quality of life that would be satisfactory to the patient."[66(p.26)] Another definition, suggested by Luce, is that treatment is considered futile when a patient cannot benefit from treatment, the patient's acute disorder is not reversible, it is projected that the patient will not survive the current hospitalization, or the quality of the patient's life following discharge will be poor.[94] Prendergast notes that there is no consensus definition of medical futility.[108]

Futility decisions come into play as goals of care increasingly become unachievable. As noted by Jecker, "Refraining from medically futile interventions is often the best way to care humanely for patients at the end of life."[72(p.287)] The realization of medical futility is usually a process that evolves over time. It is important that the family is involved in the process. The family should be informed as soon as the interdisciplinary team determines medical futility. On occasion, the family is not in agreement with the medical team's determination of futility and recommendations regarding patient care.[71] Futility guidelines may serve to help with these situations.[140] Guidelines include information related to the process for conflict resolution and may help all involved reach a compromise. Resources such as the palliative care team and the ethics committee may be helpful with these complex situations.

Withholding and Withdrawing Life-Sustaining Therapy

The President's Commission for the Study of Ethical Problems in Medicine and Biomedical and Behavioral Research provided essential direction for healthcare providers by stating that there is no moral difference between withholding and withdrawing LST.[112] Additional experts and professional associations, including the American Association of Critical-Care Nurses, American College of Physicians, American Thoracic Society, and the Society of Critical Care Medicine agree that there is no moral difference between withholding and withdrawing LST.[2,6,21,131,133]

The fundamental issue involved with both withholding and withdrawing is the efficacious use of the treatment and the patient's desire for the treatment. Each individual has the right to accept or refuse any treatment, including LST. There is no difference between deciding not to start a treatment or in deciding to stop a treatment. Consideration is given to the individual's desire for the treatment and the intended purpose of the treatment.

Time-limited interventions, especially in the face of uncertainty, can be trialed, in conjunction with palliative care interventions. Often a trial of treatment may be initiated for a patient with a plan for reevaluation and withdrawal of the treatment if it does not prove effective. From an ethical perspective, erring on the side of LST is a greater good than erring on the side of too little treatment or treatment that is withdrawn too quickly.[122] It is important to know that LSTs (e.g., intubation and ventilation) can be tried, but if they prove to be ineffective, they can be withdrawn. Thus if the appropriateness of LST is unclear, it should be initiated with the knowledge that if it proves to be futile, not beneficial, or disproportionately burdensome, it can later be stopped.[122]

Neuromuscular Blockade

Neuromuscular blockade should play no role in the care of patients for whom LST is withheld or withdrawn. Neuromuscular-blocking agents should be discontinued and time allowed for their clearance from the body before withholding or withdrawing therapy.

Healthcare providers have reported withdrawing LST from patients receiving paralytics.[48] "The use of paralytics in dying patients is disturbing because it is difficult, if not impossible, to adequately assess the comfort of patients who are paralyzed and because a paralyzed patient, unable to exert respiratory effort, cannot compensate for hypoxia resulting from either terminal weaning or extubation. Although appearing comfortable, the patient may experience respiratory distress or severe anxiety."[48(p.886)] The use of paralytics compromises the ability to monitor a patient for distress, eliminates opportunities for patient and family interaction, and guarantees patient death.[30]

The Principle of Double Effect

The principle of double effect "is invoked to justify claims that a single act having two foreseen effects, one good and one harmful [such as death], is not always morally prohibited if the harmful effect is not intended."[18(p.206)] The principle of double effect is an issue that may arise when providing care to dying patients. For example, pain medication is usually titrated to promote comfort. A secondary effect of the pain medication may be a decrease in blood pressure or respiratory rate. During end-of-life care, nurses and physicians administer pain medication to decrease discomfort; thus it is viewed as a beneficent act even though death may be hastened. This double effect is recognized as ethically justified by ethicists and professional standards of care.[4,131] The U.S. Supreme Court has also upheld the principle of double effect by supporting dying patients who obtain palliative care, where in some cases administration of analgesics may hasten death.[143]

PALLIATIVE SYMPTOM MANAGEMENT

Many seriously ill patients experience distressing symptoms. Family members from SUPPORT and the Hospitalized Elderly Longitudinal Project (HELP) studies reported that during the last 3 days of their lives, almost 40% of patients had severe pain, more than 50% of patients had severe dyspnea (excluding patients with colon cancer), and approximately 25% of patients had severe confusion.[93] In a study conducted by Tolle and colleagues, family members reported that 34% of dying patients were in moderate to severe pain during the last week of life.[139] More specific data from this study demonstrated that more hospitalized patients experienced moderate to severe pain during the final week of life (44%) as compared to individuals dying at home (34%) or dying in a nursing home (27%).[139] In a national study conducted by Puntillo and researchers, the majority of critical care nurses (78%) responded that in the unit where they worked, dying patients frequently (31%) or sometimes (47%) received inadequate pain medication.[114]

Symptom management is an essential aspect of all patient care. Managing symptoms is of primary importance in an effort to promote quality living to the very end and to promote peace and comfort during the dying process. Medications are administered and titrated to relieve symptoms. Anticipatory dosing is important. Anticipatory dosing refers to the initiation of medications in order to minimize symptoms that commonly occur at the end of life before the symptom is reported or displayed. If patients are already receiving continuous infusions of analgesics or sedatives (e.g., morphine, lorazepam [Ativan]), those medications are titrated to effect with consideration that patients may build up a tolerance, thus requiring high doses.

Pain

Pain is an unpleasant sensory and emotional experience associated with actual or potential tissue damage, or described in terms of such damage.[67] It is important to administer medications in anticipation of the possibility of pain and discomfort and titrate medications to effect. Pain can usually readily be assessed in an alert patient by using a numeric pain scale (0 to 10). Assessment of pain in the cognitively impaired or unconscious dying patient is more complex. Behavioral indicators such as agitation, restlessness, posturing, and facial expression as well as physiologic indicators including tachycardia, hypertension, tachypnea, diaphoresis, and mydriasis may indicate pain.[101] Instruments that include behavioral or physiologic indicators can be used to assess signs and symptoms of discomfort.[54]

Early, accurate detection of pain and quick management are essential.[44,45,100,148] A low-dose analgesic infusion can be administered to achieve patient comfort. Analgesic medications may include morphine, hydromorphone (Dilaudid), and fentanyl (Duragesic). Opiates are preferred based on potency, lack of a ceiling effect, and their concomitant mild sedative and anxiolytic properties.[101] Morphine is most commonly given intravenously as a continuous infusion. Morphine produces analgesia and often sedation; its half-life is 3 to 4 hours. Hydromorphone is a synthetic, highly soluble opioid; its half-life (2 to 3 hours) is a little shorter than that of morphine. Another synthetic opioid analgesic is fentanyl, a potent synthetic opiate with a short half-life of 1 to 2 hours.

The dose of the infusion can be increased based on signs and symptoms of pain. There are no maximum doses. At times two different medications may be needed to achieve patient comfort. Furthermore, there are a number of adjuvant analgesics that maximize patient comfort and distress, such as anticonvulsants, antidepressants, corticosteroids, local anesthetics and even baclofen (Lioresal), which helps relieve spasm-associated pain.[5] Clinical pharmacists, pain, and palliative care specialists are invaluable resources and can assist in managing pain.

Promoting comfort during the dying process is essential. It is important to ensure that the patient is in a comfortable position and is repositioned as needed to maintain comfort. Skin and mouth care, massage, hot and cold therapies including cool moist towels, fans, and warm compresses may promote comfort. Management of a fever with antipyretics also may be comforting.

The titration of analgesia for the cognitively impaired or unconscious dying patient is best guided by physiologic indicators and by careful observation for signs of distress.[101] According to Rubenfeld, "Unconscious patients, by definition, cannot perceive pain and therefore may not require sedation or analgesia."[118(p.448)] He also comments that "patients with diminished levels of consciousness also may not be able to manifest signs of discomfort."[118(p.448)] However, despite this uncertainty, it is ethical to err on the side of administering analgesia and sedation in an attempt to promote comfort rather than not treat patient distress.

Dyspnea

Dyspnea is a person's subjective awareness of altered or uncomfortable respiratory functioning.[25] Campbell describes respiratory distress as the physical or emotional suffering that results from the experience of dyspnea.[25] Alert patients should be asked to rate their perception of dyspnea, using a numeric scale (0 to 10) as a guide. Dyspnea in the cognitively impaired or unconscious patient can be assessed by observing the patient's respiratory rate, pattern, and use of accessory muscles, and by an auditory assessment of airway noises. Behavioral and physiologic indicators of respiratory distress may include tachycardia, tachypnea, use of accessory muscles, nasal flaring, paradoxical breathing pattern, fearful facial expression, grunting at end-expiration, and restlessness.[25] An instrument that includes behavioral or physiologic indicators can be used to assess signs and symptoms of dyspnea.[24]

Dyspnea may occur during the dying process, or during or after withdrawal of LST. Prevention and quick relief of dyspnea are essential. Breathing changes at the end of life may include an increase or decrease in respiratory rate, an increase in respiratory secretions, an increase in airway noises, and changes in breathing patterns. An increase in the respiratory rate may occur as the body attempts to meet oxygen demands. A decrease in respiratory rate may result from the dying process or as a secondary effect from medications. An increase in respiratory secretions may occur due to underlying pulmonary disease or may occur due to decreased contractility of the heart, resulting in a backup of fluid to the lungs. Airway noise may occur as muscles in the neck relax. Changes in a patient's breathing pattern may occur due to the dying process.

Preventing and managing dyspnea are important. Initiating an analgesic infusion (i.e., morphine) will physiologically promote pulmonary venodilation and may facilitate breathing at the end of life. Reducing intravenous fluids, administering diuretics, and administrating anticholinergic medications will decrease pulmonary secretions. Bronchodilators and benzodiazepines also may be effective in relieving dyspnea. Ensure that the patient is in a comfortable position, with the head of bed slightly elevated. Secretions may pool in the pharynx but can easily be suctioned to promote comfort. Oxygen use needs to be assessed on an individual basis.[19, 23]

Anxiety

Anxiety is a subjective feeling of apprehension, tension, insecurity, and uneasiness.[47] An alert patient should be asked to rate any anxiety as mild, moderate, or severe. Anxiety is difficult to assess in the cognitively impaired and may not be present in the unconscious patient. Signs and symptoms may include sweating, tachycardia, trembling, hyperventilation, restlessness, and agitation.[47]

Support should be provided to the greatest extent possible. Involvement of the family and other members of the healthcare team can provide additional patient support. Sedatives can be started and titrated as needed. Benzodiazepines (lorazepam, midazolam [Versed]) are commonly used to relieve anxiety. Tolerance can develop after several days; therefore, an increase in dosage may be needed to maintain symptom control.

Palliative sedation (also referred to as terminal or total sedation) is defined as sedating a patient to the point of unconsciousness and is used as a last resort to reduce suffering.[142] Palliative sedation is indicated when distressing symptoms (e.g., hallucinations, severe pain, etc.) cannot be managed with traditional pharmacologic agents. Continuous infusions of benzodiazepines are most commonly used for terminal sedation. Sometimes a barbiturate may be added if the patient continues to experience distressing symptoms despite the continuous infusion of a benzodiazepine. Patients may still be aware of their environment while receiving palliative sedation; therefore, communication with the patient and support are important. In addition, analgesic and sedative infusions for managing pain and anxiety are essential. Bispectral index (BIS) monitoring may be helpful in assessing sedation levels.

Delirium, Agitation, and Confusion

Dying patients may develop delirium, agitation, and confusion. Patients with delirium manifest a disturbance of consciousness characterized by an acute onset and fluctuating courses of impaired cognitive function so that their ability to receive, process, store, and recall information is impaired.[83] Patients with delirium may experience disorientation, distorted sensations, hallucinations, illusions, and delusions. The Confusion Assessment Method for the intensive care unit (CAM-ICU) can be used to assess delirium (see Chapter 9.)[46,83] Delirium may be accompanied by agitation and confusion.

Neuroleptic medications (i.e., haloperidol [Haldol]) have proven efficacy in the management of delirium.[142] Propofol (Diprivan) is a sedative and anesthetic medication that also can be considered. As mentioned, barbiturates can be administered if other medications are ineffective.

Patients at end of life experience a multiplicity of symptoms and syndromes, regardless of their underlying medical condition. Pain is the most obvious example, but others include dyspnea, anxiety, agitation, confusion, and delirium. Taken together, these and other symptoms add significantly to the suffering of patients and their families but can be treated or prevented if recognized early. Hence, it's important for critical care clinicians to assess and manage the symptoms that are known to occur in dying patients in order to facilitate a peaceful and good death for patients and families.

FAMILY CARE

Good communication is important between members of the interdisciplinary team and between the team and families. The President's Commission for the Study of Ethical Problems in Medicine and Biomedical and Behavioral Research identifies each patient's family as the best advocate for patients. Family members are directed to arrive at important patient decisions in collaboration with physicians and other healthcare professionals.[112]

Patients, Families, and the Healthcare Team

Patients and families need information and support as they travel the end-of-life course. A consistent member of the healthcare team should be identified and responsible for keeping the family informed.[105,151] Open communication is essential among the patient, family, and the interdisciplinary team.* As Levy notes, it is important that healthcare providers "communicate in an open, genuine manner about the truth of a patient's illness."[87(p.N57)] Box 54-2 contains suggestions related to delivering bad news.

Healthcare providers hold a key role in "planting seeds" by helping the patient and family understand the possibility that the patient might not survive.[104] Norton and Bowers also note the importance of the team presenting information together as a united group.[104] Family members need information that will help them to understand the patient's condition and prefer if healthcare providers are open, direct, honest, and realistic.[137] Treatment options should be discussed and the primary spokesperson for the interdisciplinary team should recommend a treatment option and explain the

rationale behind the option. When discussing treatment options, it is important to focus on goals of treatment. Avoid directly asking family members, "What do you want us to do?" Instead consider, "Based on Mr. Jones's condition, and what you have told me about your father, I think we should consider this. What do you think?" Once a decision has been made, ask, "Do you think this is what your father would want?"

It often takes time for the patient's surrogate or family members to understand the information provided. As discussions progress, continue to keep the conversations focused on what the patient would want. Together with the surrogate or family, determine a plan as well as a follow-up plan. If time permits (this depends on the severity of the patient's illness or injury) a gradual approach should be considered. This helps to avoid providing too much information or overwhelming the family.

Families "often struggle with concern that they are doing the right thing."[113(p.823)] Healthcare providers can help families through shared decision making.[16,144] Healthcare providers need to "use language that implies shared decision making [e.g., in our best clinical judgment, your loved one has essentially no chance to regain the quality of life you say he would want] in contrast to language that implies a completely neutral stance [e.g., it's up to you to decide]."[137(p.439)]

Tilden and researchers found that when decisions were made related to withdrawal of LST, family members tended to move through four phases that included recognition of futility, coming to terms, shouldering the surrogate role, and facing the question.[137] Family members usually came to terms when they realized that the ongoing medical treatments contributed to suffering.[137] McClement and Degner observe that nurses are extremely helpful in guiding patients and their family members to articulate their preferences for LST.[97]

Families have reported frustrations related to the inability to interact enough with their family member's physician.[1,105,138,151] The critical care nurse can help facilitate this process for the family.

Families need to be "aware of the possibility of death even as they are supported in their hope of recovery."[111(p.2735)] The healthcare team can help family members redirect their hope, moving from hoping for recovery to hoping for a comfortable death with as much dignity and meaning as possible.[40,104]

Healthcare Provider Conflict With Family Choices. Healthcare providers do not always agree with family choices. Abbott and colleagues reported that 46% of family members experienced conflict with healthcare providers.[1] The values of healthcare providers may conflict with the values of the surrogate decision maker or the family. Acknowledgment of the value differences and maintaining open dialog with the family are important.

---

*References 14, 39, 88, 89, 105, 106, 150, 151.

Box 54-2

Delivering Bad News

Giving bad news is never easy. Although we tend to think of delivering bad news in the context of end of life, in reality bad news is often delivered at various points over the illness continuum. The following steps may assist the healthcare provider as bad news is delivered.

1. Start off well.
   - Select a private location and a time that is good for the patient and family.
   - Ensure that key members of the interdisciplinary team are present (e.g., nurse, primary physician, palliative care specialist, etc.).
   - Before sitting down with the patient and family, determine the purpose of the discussion and identify who will facilitate the discussion.
2. Find out how much the patient and family know.

- Determine what the patient and family members' understandings are of the patient's condition.
- Clarify misconceptions.
3. Share the information.
   - Not too little, not too much
   - Be aware of language.
4. Respond to the patient and family.
   - What is said verbally
   - What is noticed nonverbally
5. Develop a plan.
   - Share possible options for "the next step."
   - Discuss pros and cons of the options.
   - With the patient and family, discuss a plan of care based on patient preferences.
6. Identify how the plan will be implemented.
7. Determine a time to talk again or a follow-up plan.

Modified from the work of Robert Buckman. Refer to Robert Buckman's textbook *How to Break Bad News: A Guide for Health Care Professionals* for further suggestions related to this difficult process.

Conflict can be constructive, uncovering differences in values and legitimate concerns that have been inadequately discussed.[146]

Disagreements may be effectively handled by negotiating with the family and the healthcare provider, agreeing to a time-limited trial of therapy.[108] Consistently keeping discussions focused on patient preferences for treatment may be helpful. Palliative care experts, pastoral care, or ethics consultations can be extremely helpful to families and staff during these difficult situations.

Family Conflict. Koch and colleagues found that when the patient and family disagreed on medical treatment goals it was helpful for the physician to discuss the issue with the patient in the presence of the family in an effort to resolve conflict.[81] The capable patient's opinion always takes precedence over the opinion of the family. Families or individual family members may not initially want to honor a patient's known wishes. Although they have the patient's best interest at heart, they may be influenced by their own need to prolong the patient's life.[70]

Families may be too distressed or embarrassed to discuss dissention and hostility that exists within their family unit.[138] Some family members may want treatments continued, whereas others may not. If often takes time for families to reach consensus. It is important to have frequent and open discussions with the family.

Family Meetings. Family meetings offer an opportunity for open dialog between the patient (if possible), the family, and the healthcare team. Family meetings should be set up in advance so that all key family members can be there. In addition, all key members of the interdisciplinary team should be present (primary nurse, physician, chaplain, social worker, member[s] of the palliative care team, etc.).[151]

It often is a good idea for the members of the interdisciplinary team to meet briefly before the family meeting. This permits time to discuss the purpose of the meeting, what will be discussed, who will facilitate the meeting, and share perspectives privately.

The critical care nurse usually works with the patient's family and physician to coordinate a date and time for the meeting. The critical care nurse usually determines a location close to the critical care unit, usually a private room, with enough chairs for everyone to sit.

It is important to make sure that everyone has their pagers and cell phones turned off. Healthcare providers (nurses, physicians, etc.) should prearrange for coverage by other members of the healthcare team so that the team's attention and time can focus on the meeting.

Usually the attending physician or intensivist facilitates the meeting. Although interns and residents may attend, they should not be responsible for facilitating.[87] Family meetings should start by asking everyone to introduce themselves. The facilitator should review the purpose of the gathering. The family is asked about its understanding of the family member's condition. This offers an opportunity for the healthcare team members to clarify any misconceptions.

It is important to clarify patient wishes or anticipated wishes. Questions can be asked about the patient's values and preferences for healthcare. The family can give a good sense of what the patient was like and what things he or she enjoyed doing, and has the best sense of what the patient would want done.

McDonagh and colleagues studied family meetings and found that physicians spoke 70% of the time and spent 30% of the time listening to families.[98] The researchers recommended giving families plenty of opportunity to talk during the meeting because the more time they had to speak, the more satisfied they were with the meeting.

At the end of the meeting, it is important to discuss what will likely happen next. The follow-up plan should include when the meeting facilitator or team will meet with the patient or family again and provide information as to how the patient or family can reach the facilitator if questions arise before the next meeting.[38]

Lilly found that early family meetings (held within 72 hours of patient admission to critical care) were effective in increasing family and healthcare provider consensus related to goals of patient care and early access to palliative care.[89] Early discussions of goals of care resulted in less CPR and decreased time from critical care admission to withdrawal of LST when death was determined to be inevitable.[59] Azoulay and Sprung recommended that "there should be a continuum of early information provision supplemented by intermittent family conferences when critical 'change in direction' decisions need to be made."[16(p.2324)]

WITHDRAWAL OF LIFE-SUSTAINING THERAPY

Withdrawal of Life-Sustaining Therapy—Is It an Option?

Variability exists related to willingness to forgo LST.[110] Physicians are not always willing to withdraw LST.[48,109] Faber-Langendoen found considerable variation in the willingness of physicians to withdraw ventilators from patients forgoing LST, with 15% of physicians almost never withdrawing ventilators from patients and 37% of physicians withdrawing ventilator therapy less than half the time.[48]

Using vignettes, Cook and colleagues found extreme variability in physician and nurse attitudes regarding withdrawal of LST.[37] In only 1 of 12 scenarios did more

than 50% of the healthcare providers make the same treatment choice. In 8 of 12 scenarios more than 10% of the respondents chose the opposite extreme. Thus the same patient may receive full aggressive intensive care from one healthcare provider and only comfort measures from another.

Christakis and Asch studied attributes of physicians associated with decisions to withdraw LST.[33] Internists were asked to respond to hypothetical vignettes, and again variability existed in the physician responses. All four vignettes described a critically ill and comatose patient for whom the decision to withdraw LST was in accord with the patient's previously stated goals and the family's current wishes, yet despite this almost half of the physicians (48%) were either neutral or unwilling to withdraw LST.

Thus differences in withdrawal of LST depend on the healthcare provider. Christakis and Asch found that physicians were more willing to withdraw LST if they were young, practiced in a tertiary care setting, and spent more time in clinical practice.[33] Physician specialty also may determine withdrawal of LST patterns, because internists and pediatricians in one study were more likely to withdraw ventilators than were anesthesiologists and surgeons.[48]

Healthcare providers have reported a reluctance to withdraw LST because of lack of comfort in acknowledging and implementing the decision, fear of litigation, fear of sanction by peer review boards, lack of training and experience, and lack of precision in patient prognostication.[81,82,126]

Withdrawal of Life-Sustaining Therapy—What Should Be Withdrawn?

Variability also exists in what type of LST is removed and how LST is removed. In a study conducted by Christakis and Asch, physicians reported that they preferred to withdraw therapy supporting organs that fail because of natural rather than iatrogenic causes, recently instituted rather than long-term treatment, therapy resulting in immediate rather than delayed death, and treatment resulting in delayed rather than immediate death when diagnostic uncertainty existed.[34]

Some physicians have reported that they prefer to withdraw all LSTs simultaneously.[124] Other physicians prefer to withdraw LST using a stepwise sequence, such as withdrawing vasopressor agents first, followed, if needed, by withdrawal of mechanical ventilation.[13,49,74,108,110]

Mechanical ventilation is probably the most difficult LST to withdraw as there is a direct link between removing the ventilator and the patient's death. Withdrawal of mechanical ventilation at the end of life is viewed as particularly problematic among physicians and nurses; many are reluctant to do it.[49,96] Decisions to withdraw mechanical ventilation tend to be late decisions, generally occurring only after other interventions are withdrawn.[29,49,74,110]

Withdrawal of Life-Sustaining Therapy—How Should It Be Withdrawn?

There is much variability in withdrawing mechanical ventilation. It can be withdrawn quickly or gradually, and the patient may or may not be extubated. In her survey of critical care physicians, Faber-Langendoen found that (33%) preferred terminal weaning, defined as a stepwise or gradual decreasing of ventilator support; extubation was the preferred method of withdrawal for 13% of the respondents, and the remainder (55%) of physicians used both methods, depending on clinical parameters and various other factors.[48] Wilson and colleagues reported that terminal weaning was common for the majority (83%) of patients.[149]

During terminal weaning, ventilatory assistance is withdrawn by changing the ventilatory mode and by decreasing the percentage of oxygen, the tidal volume, ventilatory rate, or the positive end-expiratory pressure; the process varies from provider to provider and may occur within minutes to hours or may extend to days.* It is unclear how decisions are made about ventilatory changes.[43] If terminal weaning is chosen, a limited time should be agreed on because terminal weaning that lasts for hours only prolongs the dying process and should be avoided.[51]

Another method of withdrawing mechanical ventilation is by discontinuing the ventilator and extubating the patient. Some healthcare providers routinely extubate patients during withdrawal of mechanical ventilation; others do not. Some have reported that they do not routinely remove the endotracheal tube during the process of withdrawing mechanical ventilation[27,29,56,119] because leaving the endotracheal tube in place prevents gasping and the risk of airway obstruction.[29,31,56]

Mayer and Kossoff reported that terminal extubation was performed in 43% (32 of 74) of patients for whom LST was being withdrawn.[96] Respiratory distress can be minimized and comfort promoted during and after extubation when adequate morphine is administered.[55,123] Gerber and Scott reported that signs of respiratory distress (e.g., stridor, obstruction) are transient and resolve quickly and spontaneously with simple maneuvers, such as repositioning or brief chin support in addition to morphine administration.[55] Rubenfeld and Crawford suggest that patients should be extubated on the rare occasion that they may be able to communicate with their family.[119]

Many healthcare providers believe that there is no single correct process for withdrawing mechanical ventilation that applies to all patients; each is unique to the patient.[108,120,121] Interestingly, the rationale that healthcare providers use for selecting terminal weaning or extubation as their preferred approach is similar and includes maximizing patient comfort and minimizing patient dyspnea. Although gradual and quick withdrawal of LST differs in directness and appearance, it is unclear whether one method should be recommended over another and, if so, on what basis.[48]

Preparing for Withdrawal of Life-Sustaining Therapy

Critical care nurses play a pivotal role during the withdrawal of LST that includes providing and reinforcing information about a patient's progress and prognosis to the patient's family; participating in the decision-making process regarding the discontinuation of LST; assessing and offering support to patients' families before, during, and after discontinuation of LST; preparing patients' families for discontinuation of LST; and managing or coordinating with physicians during discontinuation.[75] LST is withdrawn at a date and time determined by the patient or the patient's family. The critical care nurse should ask family members if they would like to be in the room when LSTs are discontinued or if they would like to come into the room immediately afterward. Family members may want to wait in the waiting room, a designated family room, or outside the patient's room. On occasion, family members want to be at the bedside; in this case, prepare them for what they might expect. Patients may gasp immediately after the endotracheal tube is removed. Assure the family that any signs of discomfort will be quickly treated. Families should be told that after mechanical ventilation is withdrawn, death is expected but not certain.[107,146]

During withdrawal of LST, critical care nurses administer and titrate analgesics, sedatives, and other medications to promote comfort. Daly and colleagues found that after withdrawal of mechanical ventilation, 64% of patients exhibited at least one sign of distress, with the two most common signs being labored breathing and upper airway noise or noisy respirations.[43] Mayer and Kossoff also found that after extubation, agonal or labored breathing was experienced by 59% of patients, and tachypnea occurred in 34% of patients.[96]

Truog and colleagues recommend anticipatory dosing before withdrawal of mechanical ventilation: "As a general rule, the doses of medication that the patient has been receiving hourly should be increased by two- or threefold and administered acutely before withdrawing mechanical ventilation."[142(p.2339)] Guidelines can be extremely helpful in guiding medication administration during the

---

*References 27, 29, 30, 31, 42, 51, 124, 149.

dying process.[22,26,147] The guidelines provide important information for bedside clinicians related to administration of morphine for pain and dyspnea; bronchodilators and diuretics for additional reduction of dyspnea; benzodiazepines to minimize anxiety, restlessness, agitation, or delirium; and anticholinergics to reduce the amount of pulmonary secretions.

If analgesics are not infusing and LST is being withdrawn, an infusion should be started. The Medication table below outlines initial infusion doses. In addition, a sedative is commonly initiated at the same time as the analgesic infusion. A sedative (i.e., midazolam) is titrated to comfort before withdrawing LST. Continuous infusions are recommended because they are easier to manage and have the advantage of maintaining a steady level of medication. Decisions should be made ahead of time regarding goals of interventions, what treatments will be removed, and how comfort and possibly distressing signs and symptoms will be prevented and managed.

Although analgesics and sedatives are administered before and after LST is withdrawn, the specific dose

MEDICATIONS USED TO TREAT PAIN AND ANXIETY IN END-OF-LIFE SITUATIONS

MEDICATION	ACTIONS	DOSAGE*	SPECIAL CONSIDERATIONS
Fentanyl (Sublimaze)	Increases pain threshold and alters pain reception by reducing sensory nerve stimuli through opiate receptor–site binding within the central nervous system	IV bolus: 50–100 mcg; Continuous infusion: 1–10 mcg/kg/hr	May cause bradycardia
Haloperidol (Haldol)	Produces a calming effect by blocking dopamine receptors and interrupting nerve impulse transmission.	IV bolus: 0.5–20 mg; Continuous infusion: 3–5 mg/hr	Causes dry mouth
Hydromorphone (Dilaudid)	Reduces pain stimuli from sensory nerve endings by binding opiate receptor sites in the CNS.	IV bolus: 0.3–1.5 mg; Continuous infusion: 0.2 mg/hr	Administer IV bolus slowly (over 2–5 minutes) to decrease risk of anaphylactoid reactions
Lorazepam (Ativan)	Induces anxiolytic and sedative effects by stimulating GABA receptors, which affects motor, sensory, cognitive, and memory functions.	IV bolus: 1–3 mg; Continuous infusion: 0.025–0.05 mg/kg/hr	May cause hypotension
Midazolam (Versed)	Induces anxiolytic and amnestic effects by binding to benzodiazepine receptors, thus increasing GABA effects.	IV bolus: 1 mg; Continuous infusion: 1–5 mg/hr	
Morphine	Decreases perception of pain and causes general CNS depression by binding opiate receptors in the CNS.	IV bolus: 2–10 mg; Continuous infusion: 0.05–0.1 mg/kg/hr	
Propofol (Diprivan)	Inhibits sympathetic nervous system activity: decreases vascular resistance	IV bolus: 1 mg/kg; Continuous infusion: 0.5–3 mg/kg/hr	Do nor leave hanging more than 6 hr
Pentobarbital		IV bolus: 150 mg; Continuous infusion: 3–5 mg/kg/hr	

Dosage data from reference 142.
CNS = Central nervous system, GABA = gamma-aminobutyric acid.
*These dosages are a reference point for starting the medication. All medications should be titrated for effectiveness in individual patients. There are no maximum doses in this patient population.

needed to relieve discomfort is unpredictable. Morphine has been administered in rates starting at 2 mg/hr, then titrated to comfort* and sedatives (diazepam, midazolam) have been administered in rates starting at 1 mg/hr, then titrated to comfort.† Studies have demonstrated that analgesics with or without sedatives are used in 65% to 86% of patients.[27,74,149] Those not receiving medications are usually deeply comatose.[149] Campbell and colleagues noted no difference in length of survival between patients receiving morphine and those who did not.[27]

PREPARING FOR THE END OF LIFE

Preparing for a patient's end of life is best done with great thoughtfulness. Particular attention should be given to the environment, the patient, and the patient's family. An important goal is to achieve the best possible death for the patient and the most compassionate care possible for the patient and family.[104,116]

Preparing the Environment

Patients should die in the same setting where care was provided. Families prefer consistency in healthcare providers during the dying process.[151] Preparing for family privacy is important. Priority should be given to full access for family members to be with the patient. Prepare the room so that there are plenty of chairs for family members. Try to create a peaceful environment.

Ideally patients should die in a location of their choice. Most patients die in critical care; however, on occasion, arrangements can be made for a patient to die at home with the support of hospice services. Every effort should be made to honor this if requested. The palliative care team or social worker can help with arranging patient transportation and coordinating care with the local hospice agency.

Preparing the Patient

Patients should be asked if they have any requests, which should be honored to the greatest extent possible. During the dying process comfort is the primary focus.

The patient's bed should be lowered and at a minimum the bottom side rails should be lowered. Nonessential monitors and equipment, unneeded catheters, and tubes should be removed from the room. All alarms should be shut off. Ensure that devices (i.e., automatic implantable cardioverter defibrillators) are inactivated.

Assist as needed to arrange for the hospital chaplain or the patient's clergy to have a final opportunity for a visit and prayers. Also ensure that cultural and religious end-of-life practices are honored.

Preparing the Family

Education and support should be provided that focuses on the goal of providing comfort and reducing suffering. Reinforce that the dying process is unpredictable and varies greatly. If families ask how long the dying process may take, explain that it varies and may take minutes to hours to days. If families do not want to be at the hospital during the dying process, set up a communication mechanism for keeping them informed. Families need to be prepared[78] for what will happen to the patient including changes in level of consciousness, breathing pattern, breathing sounds, coloration, changes in skin temperature, and possible reflexive movement of the patient's arms or legs.

The family may want to have children, extended family, and friends say final goodbyes. Prepare the children for what they will see. A pediatric clinical nurse specialist, palliative care specialist, or bereavement specialist may be a helpful resource in preparing children for visitation. Family members may even want the opportunity for visitation by a family pet. This process should be facilitated for the family if desired.

The family should be asked if they would like to participate in a final bath, massage, or rubbing lotion on the patient. They may want special music playing in the room. Families should have unrestricted presence at the bedside. Ensure that plenty of tissues are in the patient's room. If space is available, designate an area for families to go should they need a break or privacy.

Critical care nurses are well aware of the paramount role they hold in care of the dying: "We're with people in the most traumatic, beautiful, horrendous experiences in their lives but you can make a difference in someone's death."[7(p.61)] How a person dies has a lasting memory for family and friends. As a critical care nurse notes, "I know that's what they're going to remember. They're going to remember a lot about it for the rest of their lives and it's going to be really important."[7(p.61)]

CARE AT THE TIME OF DEATH

The patient and family may have preferences regarding which healthcare team members are present during the dying process. Nurses, physicians, clergy, and other members of the healthcare team should do their best to honor patient and family wishes. Family

---

*References 30, 32, 43, 50, 58, 74, 107, 108, 119.
†References 32, 50, 74, 107, 108, 127.

end-of-life cultural and spiritual preferences should be respected.

If possible, avoid transferring dying patients from critical care. Families have reported feeling abandoned when their dying family member was transferred.[151] Throughout the dying process the patient and family need to be assured that they will not be abandoned. The dying patient and the family need the utmost care and support throughout the process.

The critical care nurse plays an important role during active dying. The patient should be assessed frequently for signs or symptoms of pain, discomfort, or distressing symptoms. If symptoms develop, they should be treated quickly so that patient comfort is promoted. When this goal is achieved, further increases in sedation or analgesia are unnecessary and ethically problematic.[118]

Critical care nurses have reported that patients have a better quality of dying if they do not die alone.[15,65] Heyland and colleagues studied family members' satisfaction with care provided to dying patients in critical care.[63] Ninety one percent of family members reported that the patient was comfortable in the final hours of life. The majority of family members (88%) also felt supported by the healthcare team. Levy and researchers studied family members of patients who died in critical care and reported that pain was managed most or all of the time for 88% of patients, and 79% of patients died with dignity.[86]

BEREAVEMENT

Grief is a process that begins before the patient dies, continues after the loss, and is unpredictable. The combination of shock, grief, uncertainty, stress, and confusion may lead to varying emotional responses by family members.[76] How critical care nurses help families accept the death of a family member and deal with the initial stages of grief may influence their subsequent experience.[97] Critical care nurses should use available resources including pastoral care, palliative care, and bereavement specialists to help families.

Families should be sent home with information on how to access bereavement support services.[68] They also should be offered the opportunity to meet with a hospital physician, nurse, social worker, or clergy for a follow-up discussion.[35]

Consider sending condolence cards, conducting follow-up family telephone calls, and inviting family members to hospital memorial services. Family members have reported that it meant a lot to them to receive telephone calls and cards from hospital staff after the death of their loved one.[145] They also were helped by support they received from their pastor, family, and friends.[145]

END OF LIFE AND THE CRITICAL CARE NURSE

Providing quality palliative care and end-of-life care can be emotionally rewarding and draining. It is important that the interdisciplinary team support each other by acknowledging and supporting the care provided. Time off—even if it is just for a short break—is important after providing care to a dying patient and his or her family. Taking time with other colleagues to discuss the experience can be invaluable. Memorial services can help critical care nurses and other members of the interdisciplinary team find important closure in end-of-life care. Bereavement specialists can provide needed support to the critical care team.

Professional resources are available to assist critical care nurses in providing quality, ethical palliative care and end-of-life care (Box 54-3). These resources can be used to develop hospital-based palliative and end-of-life care guidelines. Treece and colleagues found that a standardized order form for withdrawal of LST was helpful for critical care nurses and physicians.[141] Protocols and guidelines can help guide palliative and end-of-life care.[28,36,61]

Palliative care specialists can also help to provide quality palliative and end-of-life care. In addition, ethics experts can assist with challenging end-of-life ethical dilemmas. Ethics committees can be consulted by the patient, family, or any member of the healthcare team if there are conflicts or dilemmas that need to be discussed.

CONCLUSIONS

A good or painless death has been a major human concern throughout history.[135] The availability of the critical care nurse "to assess symptoms, administer medications, and provide other forms of support and comfort may be the single most important component of effective palliative care for a critically ill patient."[103(p.N7)] Critical care nurses have described good end-of-life care as having the following characteristics[77]:

- Patient comfort and dignity are maintained
- Family members are involved
- Family members are given time to go through the grieving process
- Family is given opportunities for family rituals and goodbyes

"At one time, critical care and palliative care may have seemed to be inherently inconsistent. End-of-life care was simply a sequel to failed intensive care. This is no longer a workable paradigm. There is no reliable way to segregate patients who are dying from patients

---

Box 54-3

Palliative Care and End-of-Life Resources

AMERICAN ASSOCIATION OF CRITICAL-CARE NURSES

aacn.org

AACN Protocol for Practice: Palliative Care and End-of-Life Issues in Critical Care, 2006

Acute and Critical Care Choices Guide to Advance Directives, 2005

AMERICAN NURSES ASSOCIATION

ana.org

Position Statement: Nursing Care and Do-Not-Resuscitate (DNR) Decisions, 1992

Position Statement: Nursing and the Patient Self-Determination Act, 1991

Position Statement: Forgoing Nutrition and Hydration, 1992

Position Statement: Pain Management and Control of Distressing Symptoms in Dying Patients, 2003

HOSPICE AND PALLIATIVE NURSES ASSOCIATION

hpna.org

Position Statement: Providing Opioids at the End of Life, 2004

Position Statement: Value of Professional Nurse in End of Life Care, 2003

AMERICAN ASSOCIATION OF COLLEGES OF NURSING

aacn.nche.edu/elnec

End-of-Life Nursing Education Consortium (ELNEC) Project: Advancing End-of-Life Nursing Care

AMERICAN ACADEMY OF HOSPICE AND PALLIATIVE MEDICINE

aahpm.org

Position statement: Definition of Palliative Care, 2005

Position statement: Sedation at the end-of-life, 2002

Fast Facts

SOCIETY OF CRITICAL CARE MEDICINE

sccm.org

What are my choices regarding life support?

SCCM Statement on End-of-life Decisions

ROBERT WOOD JOHNSON FOUNDATION

promotingexcellence.org

Robert Wood Johnson Promoting Excellence at End-of-Life Program: Innovative Models and Approaches for Palliative Care: Promoting Excellence in Intensive Care and End-of Life Care, 2006

---

who will survive."[103(p.N7)] "Palliative care is not something that is offered because 'there is nothing we can do,'" it is an active, aggressive plan of care designed to alleviate patients' symptoms and meet the diverse needs of patients and patients' families."[132(p.34)]

REFERENCES

1. Abbott, K. H., et al. (2001). Families looking back: one year after discussion of withdrawal or withholding of life-sustaining support. *Crit Care Med, 29*(1), 197–201.
2. American Association of Critical-Care Nurses. (1990). *Position statement: withholding and/or withdrawing life-sustaining treatment.* Laguna Beach, Calif: The Association.
3. American Association of Critical-Care Nurses. (2005). *Acute and critical care choices: a guide to advance directives.* Aliso Viejo, Calif: The Association.
4. American Nurses Association. (2003). *Pain management and control of distressing symptoms in dying patients.* Washington, D.C.: The Author.
5. American Pain Society (APS). (2003). *Principles of analgesic use in the treatment of acute pain and cancer pain* (5th ed). Glenview, Ill: American Pain Society.
6. American Thoracic Society. (1991). Withholding and withdrawing life-sustaining therapy. *Ann Intern Med, 115,* 478–485.
7. Andrew, C. M. (1997). Optimizing the human experience: nursing the families of people who die in intensive care. *Intensive Crit Care Nurs, 3,* 59–65.
8. Angus, D. C., et al. (2004). Use of intensive care at the end of life in the United States: an epidemiologic study. *Crit Care Med, 32,* 638–643.
9. Angus, D. C., & Pinsky, M. R. (1997). Risk prediction: judging the judges. *Intensive Care Med, 23,* 363–365.
10. Anonymous. (1968). A definition of irreversible coma. Report of the ad hoc committee of the Harvard Medical School to examine the definition of brain death. *JAMA, 205,* 337–340.
11. Anonymous. (1981). Guidelines for the determination of death. Report of the medical consultants on the diagnosis of death to the President's Commission for the Study of Ethical Problems in Medicine and Biomedical and Behavioral Research. *JAMA, 246,* 2184–2186.
12. Anonymous. (1991). Withholding and withdrawing life-sustaining therapy. *Am Rev Respir Distress, 144,* 726–731.
13. Asch, D.A, et al. (1999). The sequence of withdrawing life-sustaining treatment from patients. *Am J Med, 107,* 153–156.
14. Azoulay, E., Pochard, F., & Kentish-Barnes, N. (2005). Risk of post-traumatic stress symptoms in family members of intensive care unit patients. *Am J Respir Crit Care Med, 171,* 987–994.
15. Azoulay, E. (2004). Nurse-assessed tool for evaluating death in the intensive care unit. *Crit Care Med, 32*(8), 1789–1791.
16. Azoulay, E., & Sprung, C. (2004). Family-physician interactions in the intensive care unit. *Crit Care Med, 232*(11), 2323–2328.
17. Barnato, A. E., & Angus, D. C. (2004). Value and role of intensive care unit outcome prediction models in end-of-life decision making. *Crit Care Clin, 20*(3), 345–362.
18. Beauchamp, T., & Childress, J. F. (2001). *Principles of biomedical ethics.* New York: Oxford University.
19. Booth, S., et al. (2004). Expert working group of the Scientific Committee of the Association of Palliative Medicine. The use

of oxygen in the palliation of breathlessness. A report of the Association of Palliative Medicine. *Respir Med*, 98(1), 66–77.

20. Braun, K. L., Onaka, A. T., & Horiuchi, B. Y. (2001). Advance directive completion rates and end-of-life preferences in Hawaii. *J Am Geriatr Soc*, 49(21), 1708–1713.

21. Brody, H. (1995). Withdrawing versus withholding therapy: still a pernicious distinction. *J Am Geriatr Soc*, 43, 716–717.

22. Brody, H., et al. (1997). Withdrawing intensive life-sustaining treatment: recommendations for compassionate clinical management. *N Engl J Med*, 336, 652–657.

23. Campbell, M.L (1998). *Forgoing life-sustaining therapy: how to care for the patient who is near death*. Aliso Viejo, Calif: American Association of Critical-Care Nurses.

24. Campbell, M. L. (2005). Psychometric testing of a respiratory distress observation scale (RDOS). *J Palliat Med*, 8(1), 201.

25. Campbell, M. L. (2004). Terminal dyspnea and respiratory distress. *Crit Care Clin*, 20(3), 403–417.

26. Campbell, M. L., Bizek, K. S., & Stewart, R. (1998). Integrating technology with compassionate care: withdrawal of ventilation in a conscious patient with apnea. *Am J Crit Care*, 7, 85–89.

27. Campbell, M., Bizek, K. S., & Thrill, M. (1999). Patient responses during rapid terminal weaning from mechanical ventilation: A prospective study. *Crit Care Med*, 27(1), 73–77.

28. Campbell, M., & Frank, R. R. (1997). Experience with an end-of-life practice at a university hospital. *Crit Care Med*, 25(1), 197–202.

29. Campbell, M. L., Hoyt, J. W., & Nelson, L. J. (1994). HealthCare ethics forum 94: perspectives on withholding and withdrawal of life-support. *AACN Clin Issues*, 5, 353–359.

30. Campbell, M., & Carlson, R. W. (1992). Terminal weaning from mechanical ventilation: ethical and practical considerations for patient management. *Am J Crit Care*, 1, 152–156.

31. Carlson, R. W., Campbell, M. L., & Frank, R. R. (1996). Life support: the debate continues. *Chest*, 109, 852–853. (letter to the editor).

32. Chan, J. D., et al. (2004). Narcotic and benzodiazepine use after withdrawal of life support: association with time to death? *Chest*, 12, 286–293.

33. Christakis, N. A., & Asch, D. (1995). Physician characteristics associated with decisions to withdraw life support. *Am J Public Health*, 85, 367–372.

34. Christakis, N. A., & Asch, D. A. (1993). Biases in how physicians choose to withdraw life support. *Lancet*, 342, 642–646.

35. Cist, A. F. M., et al. (2001). Practical guidelines on the withdrawal of life-sustaining therapies. *Int Anesthesiol Clin*, 39(3), 87–102.

36. Clark, E. B., et al. (2003). Quality indicators for end-of-life care in the intensive care unit. *Crit Care Med*, 31(9), 2255–2262.

37. Cook, D. J., et al. (1995). Determinants in Canadian health care workers of the decision to withdraw life support from the critically ill. *JAMA*, 273, 703–708.

38. Curtis, J. R. (2004). Communicating about end-of-life care with patients and families in the intensive care unit. *Crit Care Clin*, 20(3), 363–380.

39. Curtis, J. R., et al. (2003). Studying communication about end-of-life care during the ICU family conference: development of a framework. *J Crit Care*, 17, 147–160.

40. Curtis, J. R., et al. (2001). The family conference as a focus to improve communication about end-of-life care in the intensive care unit: opportunities for improvement. *Crit Care Med*, 29(2, suppl), N26–N33.

41. Daly, B. J. (2006). End-of-life decision making, organ donation, and critical care nurses. *Crit Care Nurse*, 26(2), 78–86.

42. Daly, B. J., et al. (1993). Withdrawal of mechanical ventilation: ethical principles and guidelines for terminal weaning. *Am J Crit Care*, 2, 217–223.

43. Daly, B. J., Thomas, D., & Dyer, M. A. (1996). Procedures used in withdrawal of mechanical ventilation. *Am J Crit Care*, 5, 331–338.

44. Desbiens, N. A., et al. (1996). Pain and satisfaction with pain control in seriously ill hospitalized adults: findings from the SUPPORT research investigations. *Crit Care Med*, 24(12), 1953–1961.

45. Desbiens, N., & Wu, A. W. (2000). Pain and suffering in seriously ill hospitalized patients. *J Am Geriatr Soc*, 48(5), S183–S186.

46. Ely, E. W., et al. (2001). Delirium in mechanically ventilated patients: validity and reliability of the confusion assessment method for the intensive care unit (CAM-ICU). *JAMA*, 286, 703–2710.

47. End of Life Nursing Education Curriculum (ELNEC). (2007). End of Life Nursing Education Consortium: Promoting Palliative Care in Critical Care Nursing: ELNEC-Critical Care Training Program. City of Hope and the American Association of Colleges of Nursing.

48. Faber-Langendoen, K. (1994). The clinical management of dying patients receiving mechanical ventilation: a survey of physician practice. *Chest*, 106, 880–888.

49. Faber-Langendoen, K. (1996). A multi-institutional study of care given to patients dying in hospitals: ethical and practice implications. *Arch Intern Med*, 156, 2130–2136.

50. Faber-Langendoen, K., & Bartels, D. (1992). Process of forgoing life-sustaining treatment in a university hospital: an empirical study. *Crit Care Med*, 20, 570–577.

51. Faber-Langendoen, K., & Lanken, P. N. (2000). Dying patients in the intensive care unit: forgoing treatment, maintaining care. *Ann Intern Med*, 133, 886–893.

52. Federal Register Final Rule: Conditions of participation for hospitals (42 CFR Part 482.45), (2000). Centers for Medicare & Medicaid Services, Department of Health and Human Services.

53. Field, M. J., & Cassel, C. K. (1997). *Approaching death, improving care at the end of life*. Washington, D.C.: National Academy Press.

54. Gelinas, D., et al. (2006). Validation of the critical-care pain observation tool in adult patients. *Am J Crit Care*, 15(4), 420–427.

55. Gerber, D. R., & Scott, W. E. (1996). Withdrawal of life support. *Crit Care Med*, 24, 1607–1608.

56. Gillagin, T., & Raffin, T. A. (1996). How to withdraw mechanical ventilation: more studies are needed. *Am J Crit Care*, 5, 323–325.

57. Glance, L. G., Osler, T. M., & Dick, A. W. (2002). Identifying quality outliers in a large, mutiple-institution datrabase by using customized versions of the Simmplified Acute Physiology Score II and the Mortality Probability Model II. *Crit Care Med*, 30, 1995–2002.

58. Hall, R. I., & Rocker, G. M. (2000). End-of-life care in the ICU: treatments provided when life support was or was not withdrawn. *Chest*, 118(5), 1424–1430.

59. Hall, R. I., Rocker, G. M., & Murray, D. (2004). Simple changes can improve conduct of end-of-life care in the intensive care unit. *Can J Anesth*, 51(6), 631–636.

60. Hanson, L. C., & Rodgman, E. (1996). The use of living wills at the end of life. A national study. *Arch Intern Med*, 156(9), 1018–1022.

61. Hawryluck, L. A., et al. (2002). Consensus guidelines on analgesia and sedation in dying intensive care unit patients. *BMC Med Ethics*, 3:3.

62. Health Care Financing Administration (1998). Medicare and Medicaid programs: hospital condition of participation; identification of potential organ, tissue and eye donors. Title 42, Vol 3. Washington, D.C.: Federal Register.

63. Heyland, D. K., et al. (2003). Dying in the ICU: perspective of family members. *Chest*, 124, 392–397.

64. Heytens, L., et al. (1989). Lazarus sign and extensor posturing in a brain-dead patient. Case report. *J Neurosurg*, 71, 449–451.

65. Hodde, N.M., et al. (2004). Factors associated with nurse assessment of the quality of dying and death in the intensive care unit. *Crit Care Med*, 32(8), 1648–1653.

66. Hudson, T. (1994). Are futile-care policies the answer? *HospHealth Netw, February 20*, 26–32.

67. International Association for the Study of Pain (IASP). International Association for the Study of Pain: definitions. www.iasp-pain.org.

68. Jackson, I. (1992). Bereavement follow-up service in intensive care. *Intensive Crit Care Nurs, 8*, 163–18.

69. Jacob, D. A. (1998). Family members' experiences with decision making for incompetent patients in the ICU: a qualitative study. *Am J Crit Care, 7*, 30–36.

70. Jacob, D. (1997). Family decision making for incompetent patients in the ICU. *Crit Care Nurs Clin North Am, 9*(1), 107–114.

71. Jacobs, B. B., & Taylor, C. (2005). Medical futility in the natural attitude. *Adv Nurs Sci, 28*(4), 288–305.

72. Jecker, N. S. (1995). Medical futility and care of dying patient. *West J Med, 163*, 287–291.

73. Jezewski, M. A., Meeker, M. A., & Schrader, M. (2003). Voices of oncology nurses: what is needed to assist patients with advance directives. *Cancer Nurs, 26*(2), 105–112.

74. Keenan, S. P., et al. (1997). A retrospective review of a large cohort of patients undergoing the process of withholding or withdrawal of life support. *Crit Care Med, 25*, 1324–1331.

75. Kirchhoff, K.T., et al. (2002). The vortex: families' experiences with death in the intensive care unit. *Am J Crit Care, 11*(3), 200–209.

76. Kirchhoff, K. T., Song, M., & Kehl, K. (2004). Caring for the family of the critically ill patient. *Crit Care Clin, 20*(3), 453–466.

77. Kirchhoff, K. T., et al. (2000). Intensive care nurses' experiences with end-of-life care. *Am J Crit Care, 9*, 36–42.

78. Kirchhoff, K. T., Conradt, K. L., & Anumandla, P. R. (2003). ICU nurses' preparation of families for death of patients following withdrawal of ventilator support. *Appl Nurs Res, 16*(2), 85–92.

79. Knaus, W., et al. (1991). The APACHE III prognostic system: risk prediction of hospital mortality for critically ill hospitalized adults. *Chest, 100*, 1619–1636.

80. Knaus, W., et al. (1985). APACHE II: a severity of disease classification system. *Crit Care Med, 13*, 818–829.

81. Koch, K. A., Rodeffer, H. D., & Wears, R. L. (1994). Changing patterns of terminal care management in an intensive care unit. *Crit Care Med, 22*, 233–243.

82. Kollef, M. H. (1996). Private attending physician status and the withdrawal of life-sustaining interventions in a medical intensive care unit population. *Crit Care Med, 24*, 968–975.

83. Kress, J. P., & Hall, J. B. (2004). Delirium and sedation. *Crit Care Clin, 20*(3), 419–433.

84. Le Gall, J. R., Lemeshow, S., & Saulnier, F. (1993). A new simplified acute physiology score (SAPS II) based on a European/North American Multicenter study. *JAMA, 270*, 2957–2963.

85. Lemeshow, S., et al. (1993). Mortality probability models (MPM II) based on an international cohort of intensive care unit patients. *JAMA, 270*, 2478–2486.

86. Levy, C.R., et al. (2005). Quality of dying and death in two medical ICUs: perceptions of family and clinicians. *Chest, 127*(5), 1775–1783.

87. Levy, M. M. (2001). End-of-life care in the intensive care unit: Can we do better? *Crit Care Med, 29*(2, suppl), N56–N61.

88. Lilly, C.M., et al. (2003). Intensive communication: four-year follow-up from a clinical practice study. *Crit Care Med, 31*(5, suppl), S394–S399.

89. Lilly, C.M., et al. (2000). An intensive communication intervention for the critically ill. *Am J Med, 109*, 469–475.

90. Lunney, J.R., et al. (2003). Patterns of functional decline at the end of life. *JAMA, 289*(18), 2387–2392.

91. Lunney, J. R., Lynn, J., & Hogan, C. (2002). Profiles of older Medicare decedents. *J Am Geriatr Soc, 50*, 1108–1112.

92. Lynn, J., et al. (1997a). Prognoses of seriously ill hospitalized patients on the days before death: implications for patient care and public policy. *New Horizons, 5*, 56–61.

93. Lynn, J., et al. (1997b). Perceptions by family members of the dying experience of older and seriously ill patients. *Ann Intern Med, 126*(2), 97–106.

94. Luce, J. M. (1997b). Withholding and withdrawal of life support from critically ill patients. *West J Med, 167*, 411–416.

95. Mahon, M. (2005). Non-heart-beating organ donation (donation after cardiac death). In Wiegand D., & Carlson, K. (Eds.), *AACN procedure manual for critical care*. Philadelphia: Saunders.

96. Mayer, S. A., & Kossoff, S. B. (1999). Withdrawal of life support in the neurological intensive care unit. *Neurology, 52*, 1602–1609.

97. McClement, S. E., & Degner, L. F. (1995). Expert nursing behaviors in care of the dying adult in the intensive care unit. *Heart Lung, 24*, 408–419.

98. McDonagh, J.R., et al. (2004). Family satisfaction with family conferences about end-of-life care in the intensive care unit: increased proportion of family speech is associated with increased satisfaction. *Crit Care Med, 32*(7), 1484–1488.

99. McKinley, E.D., et al. (1996). Differences in end-of-life decision making among back and white ambulatory cancer patients. *J Gen Intern Med, 11*, 651–656.

100. Medina, J., Puntillo, K. (Eds.). (2006). *AACN protocol for practice: palliative care and end-of-life care*. Boston: Jones and Bartlett.

101. Mularskski, R. A. (2004). Pain management in the intensive care unit. *Crit Care Clin, 20*(3), 381–401.

102. National Consensus Project for Palliative Care. (2004). *Clinical practice guidelines for quality palliative care*. Brooklyn, N.Y.: National Consensus Project for Quality Palliative Care.

103. Nelson, J. E., & Danis, M. (2001). End of life care in the intensive care unit: where are we now? *Crit Care Med, 29*(2), N2–N9.

104. Norton, S. A., & Bowers, B. J. (2001). Working toward consensus: providers' strategies to shift patients from curative to palliative treatment choices. *RINA, 24*, 258–269.

105. Norton, S.A., et al. (2003). Life support withdrawal: communication and conflict. *Am J Crit Care, 12*(6), 548–555.

106. O'Callahan, J. G., et al. (1995). Withholding and withdrawing of life support from patients with severe head injury. *Crit Care Med, 23*, 1567–1575.

107. O'Mahony, S., et al. (2003). Ventilator withdrawal: procedures and outcomes. Report of collaboration between a critical care division and a palliative care service. *J Pain Symptom Manage, 26*(4), 954–961.

108. Prendergast, T. J. (2000). Withholding or withdrawal of life-sustaining therapy. *Hosp Pract, 15*, 91–9295–102.

109. Prendergast, T. J., Claessens, M. T., & Luce, J. M. (1998). A national survey of end-of-life care for critically ill patients. *Am J Resp Crit Care Med, 158*, 1163–1167.

110. Prendergast, T. J., & Luce, J. M. (1997). Increasing incidence of withholding and withdrawal of life support from the critically ill. *Am J Respir Crit Care Med, 155*, 15–20.

111. Prendergast, T. J., & Puntillo, K. A. (2002). Withdrawal of life support: intensive caring at the end of life. *JAMA, 288*(21), 2732–2740.

112. President's Commission for the Study of Ethical Problems in Medicine and Biomedical and Behavioral Research. (1983). *Deciding to forgo life-sustaining treatment: a report on ethical, medical and legal issues in treatment decisions*. Washington, D.C: U.S. Government Printing Office.

113. Puntillo, K., & Stannard, D. (2006). The intensive care unit. In B. R. Ferrell & N. Coyle (Eds.), *Textbook of palliative nursing* (2nd ed., pp. 817–834). New York: Oxford University Press.

114. Puntillo, K.A., et al. (2001). End-of-life issues in intensive care units: a national survey of nurses' knowledge and beliefs. *Am J Crit Care, 10*(4), 216–229.

115. Render, M. L., et al. (2005). Variations in outcomes in Veterans Affairs ICUs with a computerized severity measure. *Crit Care Med, 33*, 930–939.

116. Rocker, G. M., & Curtis, J. R. (2003). Caring for the dying in the intensive care unit: in search of clarity. *JAMA, 290*(6), 820–822.

117. Rooper, A. H. (1984). Unusual spontaneous movements in brain-dead patients. *Neurology, 34,* 1089–1092.

118. Rubenfeld, G. D. (2004). Principles and practice of withdrawing life-sustaining treatments. *Crit Care Clin, 20*(3), 435–451.

119. Rubenfeld, G. D., & Crawford, S. W. (1995). Withdrawing life support: practice and principles. *Crit Care Alert, 2,* 89–96.

120. Salon, J. E. (1996a). Withdrawal of life support. *Crit Care Med, 24,* 1607.

121. Salon, J. E. (1996b). Life support: the debate continues. *Chest, 109,* 852. (letter to the editor.).

122. Schneiderman, L. J., & Spragg, R. G. (1988). Ethical decisions in discontinuing mechanical ventilation. *N Engl J Med, 318,* 984–988.

123. Siegel, M. D., & Ryder, A. (1996). Life support. The debate continues. *Chest, 109*(3), 852.

124. Smedira, N.G., et al. (1990). Withholding and withdrawal of life support from the critically ill. *N Engl J Med, 322,* 1891–1892.

125. Society of Critical Care Medicine (Task Force on Ethics). (1990). Consensus report on the ethics of forgoing life-sustaining treatments in the critically ill. *Crit Care Med, 18,* 1435–1439.

126. Solomon, M.Z, et al. (1993). Decisions near the end of life: professional views on life-sustaining treatments. *Am J Public Health, 83,* 14–23.

127. Sprung, C. L., et al. (2003). End-of-life practices in European intensive care units. The Ethicus Study. *JAMA, 290,* 790–797.

128. Sulmasy, D. P., FitzGerald, D., & Jaffin, J. H. (1993). Ethical considerations. *Crit Care Clin, 9,* 775–789.

129. Sullivan, J., & Severance-Lossin, L. (2005). Determination of death. In Wiegand, D., & Carlson, K. (Eds.), *AACN procedure manual for critical care*. Philadelphia: Saunders.

130. Swigart, V., et al. (1996). Letting go: family willingness to forgo life support. *Heart Lung, 25*(6), 483–494.

131. The Hastings Center. (1987). *Guidelines on the termination of life-sustaining treatment and the care of the dying*. Briarcliff Manor, NY: The Hastings Center.

132. Thelen, M. (2005). End-of-life decision making in intensive care. *Crit Care Nurse, 25*(6), 28–38.

133. The Society of Critical Care Medicine Ethics Committee. (1997). Consensus statement of the Society of Critical Care Medicine's Ethics Committee regarding futile and other possibly inadvisable treatments. *Crit Care Med, 25,* 887–891.

134. The SUPPORT Principal Investigators. (1995). A controlled trial to improve care for seriously ill hospitalized patients: The Study to Understand Prognoses and Preferences for Outcomes and Risks of Treatments (SUPPORT). *AMA, 274*(200), 1591–1597.

135. Thompson, J. E., & Thompson, H. O. (1985). *Bioethical decision making for nurses*. Norwalk, Conn: Appleton-Century-Crofts.

136. Tilden, V.P., et al. (2001). Family decision-making to withdraw life-sustaining treatments from hospitalized patients. *Nurs Res, 50*(2), 105–115.

137. Tilden, V.P., et al. (1999). Family decision making in forgoing life-extending treatments. *J Fam Nurs, 5*(4), 426–442.

138. Tilden, V.P., et al. (1995). Decisions about life sustaining treatment: impact of physicians' behavior on the family. *Arch Intern Med, 155,* 633–638.

139. Tolle, S. W., et al. (2000). Families reports of barriers to optimal care of the dying. *Nurs Res, 49*(6), 310–317.

140. Tomlinson, T., & Czlonka, D. (1995). Futility and hospital policy. *Hastings Center Rep, 25,* 28–35.

141. Treece, P.D., et al. (2004). Evaluation of a standardized order form for the withdrawal of life support in the intensive care unit. *Crit Care Med, 32,* 1141–1148.

142. Truog, R.D., et al. (2001). Recommendations for end-of-life care in the intensive care unit: the Ethics Committee of the Society of Critical Care Medicine. *Crit Care Med, 29*(12), 2332–2348.

143. *Vacco v. Quill*: Supreme Court, 1997.

144. Walter, S.D., et al. (1998). Confidence in life-support decisions in the intensive care unit: a survey of healthcare workers. *Crit Care Med, 26*(1), 44–49.

145. Warren, N. A. (2002). Critical care family members' satisfaction with bereavement experiences. *Crit Care Nurs Quart, 25*(2), 54–60.

146. Way, J., Back, A. L., & Curtis, J. R. (2002). Withdrawing life support and resolution of conflict with families. *BMJ, 325,* 1342–1345.

147. Weatherill, G. G. (1995). Pharmacologic symptom control during the withdrawal of life support: lessons in palliative care. *AACN Clin Issues, 6,* 344–351.

148. White, D. B., & Luce, J. M. (2004). Palliative care in the critical care unit: barriers, advances, and unmet needs. *Crit Care Clin, 20*(3), 329–343.

149. Wilson, W., et al. (1992). Ordering and administration of sedatives and analgesics during withholding and withdrawal of life support from critically ill patients. *JAMA, 267,* 949–953.

150. Wiegand, D. L. (2006a). Families and withdrawal of life-sustaining therapy. *J Fam Nurs, 12*(2), 165–184.

151. Wiegand, D. L. (2006b). Withdrawal of life-sustaining therapy after sudden, unexpected life-threatening illness or injury: interactions between patients' families, healthcare providers, and the healthcare system. *Am J Crit Care, 15,* 178–187.

152. Zimmerman, J.E., et al. (2006). Acute physiology and chronic health evaluation (APACHE) IV: hospital mortality assessment for today's critically ill patients. *Crit Care Med, 34*(5), 1297–1310.

153. Zimmerman, J. E., Draper, E. A., & Wagner, D. P. (2001). Comparing ICU populations: background and current methods. In W. J. Sibbald & J. F. Bion (Eds.), *Evaluating critical care*. New York: Springer Verlag.

Answers to Decision Point Questions

CHAPTER 4, PAIN AND SEDATION

Case Study 4-1, Part A: Acute Versus Chronic Pain

Decision point
What potential sources of *pain* can you anticipate during M.T.'s first 48 hours in the critical care unit?

Discussion. Potential sources of pain include tissue injury and trauma involving muscle-skeletal injuries, fractured ribs, lacerations and abrasions, pelvic stabilization, and head injury, as well as procedural pain related to airway manipulation, suctioning, and controlled ventilation.

Decision point
What potential sources of *discomfort* can you anticipate during M.T.'s first 48 hours in the critical care unit?

Discussion. Potential sources of discomfort can come from environmental factors (temperature, odors, sounds), emotional factors (fear, uncertainty, and anxiety), or physical factors (positioning, immobility, endotracheal tube and mechanical ventilation, orthopedic equipment, intravenous lines, indwelling catheter).

Case Study 4-1, Part B: Pharmacologic Interventions

Decision point
As M.T.'s nurse, what physiologic and emotional responses to pain and discomfort should you anticipate?

Discussion. Emotional responses include fear and anxiety that will affect the body's response to other stimuli, aggravating feelings of pain and discomfort. Physiologic responses are influenced by neuroendocrine and central nervous system activation. Patients may exhibit elevated blood pressure, tachycardia, and increased peripheral vascular resistance. This will place a burden on cardiovascular and respiratory systems, resulting in increased workload and a greater need for oxygen for tissues. It is important to remember that lack of physiologic response cannot be construed as absence from pain or discomfort. Lack of physiologic response may be related to comorbid or treatment factors associated with the patient's multiple injuries, equipment, and medications.

Decision point
To minimize physiologic and emotional consequences associated with pain and discomfort, what pain management interventions should you plan to initiate for M.T. and when should you start them?

Discussion. Interventions should begin with first contact. Minimize feelings of fear and anxiety by providing reassurance through your voice and through gentle touch. Manage the environment, minimizing noise and odors and offering music or guided imagery. Examine body alignment and turn or position frequently. Comfort and complementary therapies should be initiated early and continued throughout hospitalization. Concurrent with initiation of comfort measures and complementary therapies, the nurse should be administering medications for pain and sedation.

M.T. has demonstrated extreme inspiratory and expiratory chest movement, coughing, restlessness, and increased peak airway pressures. Patient-ventilator dyssynchrony and agitation are suspected. After ruling out other possible causes for M.T.'s symptoms, she is administered propofol.

Decision point
Identify potential side effects and methods to prevent or manage them.

Discussion. Side effects include sedation, confusion, respiratory depression, itching, nausea, constipation, or an ileus. All sedating agents, muscle relaxants, and opioid analgesic agents decrease gastric motility, predisposing M.T. to nausea, constipation, and possible ileus. M.T. is immobile, not taking food by mouth, and may be dehydrated, increasing her risk of side effect related complications. Altered level of consciousness, lethargy, sedation, and confusion are common side effects associated with many pain management medications. However, in M.T.'s case this risk is greater because of her head injury and rib fractures. Maximizing analgesia without increasing sedation is essential for this patient. The inclusion of basic comfort measures, complementary interventions, and analgesia will decrease M.T.'s risk of untoward events and complications related to her hospitalization and treatment regimen, while still providing optimal pain management.

Case Study 4-1, Part C: Co-Analgesics

Decision point
What method of assessing pain and sedation will be most appropriate for this patient?

Discussion. Self-report is the best method to assess pain and comfort. This patient probably cannot use a written scale; but may be able to respond to a verbal scale. The nurse can ask the patient to nod or blink when the nurse says the number that corresponds to her pain. If assessing pain using a number scale is beyond M.T.'s ability, you can ask if she is or is not in pain. If she cannot respond, behavioral and physiologic changes can be assessed. However, even though they may provide an indication of severe pain, they are not helpful in determining changes in pain or levels of comfort; and since behavioral and physiologic changes are affected by multiple factors such as fluid balance, body temperature, or current drug therapy, reliance on these variables to assess pain and discomfort is unreliable at best. When faced with a patient who is unable to communicate pain or discomfort, the nurse determines the need for pain relief interventions based upon knowledge of the probability that the patient is or is not in pain. In M.T.'s case, multiple extremity fractures will make any movement or positioning painful and fractured ribs will result in pain with each breath delivered by the ventilator.

Once M.T. has been medicated, it is also essential to monitor her sedation level. Sedation level is more reliable than respiratory rate and allows the nurse to detect potential problems early. When assessing sedation, it is best to use a standard sedation scale. Since M.T. is responsive and not receiving any neuromuscular blocking agents at this time, any of the sedation scales would be appropriate. However, if a neuromuscular blocking agent had been administered, we might want to add bispectral analysis to assess sedation levels. Bispectral analysis does not replace observational assessment by the nurse but is a useful adjunct.

CHAPTER 5, SYMPTOM MANAGEMENT

Case Study 5-1, Part A: Nausea, Vomiting and Diarrhea

Decision point
What risk factors does A.Z. have for experiencing nausea and vomiting?

Discussion. Crohn's disease can cause intestinal obstructions, which is most likely the cause of her nausea and vomiting. Her dehydration and fluid and electrolyte imbalances from diarrhea and vomiting are also perpetuating the symptoms. Lastly, she may have peritonitis related to Crohn's disease that would also trigger nausea and vomiting.

Decision point
What type of nausea and vomiting is most likely responsible for A.Z.'s symptoms?

Discussion. Several triggers may be stimulating her vomiting center. She most likely has an obstruction and possible fistula with inflammatory bowel disease such as Crohn's disease. Bowel obstruction activates serotonin and peripheral and vagus nerve response to the brain, activating the CTZ and VC. Inflammation is also present as evident by her febrile response. Histamine is released with an inflammatory response and triggers the CTZ, initiating a vomiting

response. Complications of her nausea and vomiting are severe dehydration and fluid and electrolyte imbalance, specifically hypochloremia, hyponatremia, and hypokalemia.

Case Study 5-1, Part B: Nausea, Vomiting, and Diarrhea

Decision point
What are the most likely risk factors for A.Z.'s persistent diarrhea?

Discussion. She most likely has an inflammatory bowel disorder that causes inflammation and malabsorption of nutrients. Diarrhea with hypermotility of the intestinal tract is associated with inflammatory bowel disease states. Complications associated with frequent diarrhea from Crohn's disease are electrolyte imbalances, dehydration, malnutrition, and fatigue. Depression and anxiety can also accompany the diarrhea symptoms because the frequency of stools may prevent the individual from leaving home, resulting in isolation (Economou, 2001).

Decision point
What are primary nursing concerns for A.Z. regarding her diarrhea and nutritional status?

Discussion. A.Z.'s inflammatory disease state is the most likely culprit of her diarrhea. Her 24-pound weight loss is most likely the result of inflammation within the lumen of her intestines inhibiting effective absorption of nutrients and water. Bacterial overgrowth and the presence of bile in the colon can occur with Crohn's disease and contribute to diarrhea. Protein loss in the diarrhea can create a state of hypoalbuminemia that will further exacerbate her diarrhea.

Case Study 5-1, Part C: Nausea, Vomiting, and Diarrhea

Decision point
Is A.Z. at risk of developing dyspnea as a symptom related to her acute admission?

Discussion. Absolutely. Any patient admitted acutely to the critical care unit is extremely stressed. Anxiety surrounding an unfamiliar environment can precipitate feelings of air hunger or dyspnea. In addition, A.Z. is very hypovolemic and tachypneic. Her oxygen requirements are increased because of her physiologic status that may cause her to begin to feel more short of breath. A.Z. may also have an infectious process developing in her abdomen—peritonitis—that may evolve into sepsis. She is at risk of developing acute respiratory distress syndrome (ARDS) that would also trigger dyspnea. Currently, her oxygen saturation is adequate on 4-L nasal cannula; however, dyspnea is a very subjective symptom; therefore ensuring emotional care along with support of A.Z.'s pulmonary system may prevent her from experiencing dyspnea.

Decision point
Is A.Z. at risk of developing delirium?

Discussion. Even though A.Z. is a young woman, she has several risk factors that place her at risk of developing delirium with her acute illness. She has an infection, metabolic and electrolyte imbalances from her diarrhea, nausea and vomiting, as well as possible hypoxemia. Efforts to correct her physiologic status will take time; however, asking her friend to sit closer to her and calm her through gentle conversation may be an effective intervention throughout A.Z.'s critical care stay.

CHAPTER 7, THERMOREGULATION

Case Study 7-1: Thermoregulation After Trauma

Decision point
What are the benefits of fever in R.A.?

Discussion. Fever has been associated with improved host defense in animal studies.[33] Interference in the ability to generate febrile response in animals has been associated with greater mortality. There are no randomized controlled trials in humans evaluating the effectiveness of fever as a host defense response.

Decision point
What are the consequences of fever?

Discussion. Fever is associated with increased metabolic demands that manifest as an increase in heart rate and oxygen consumption. Increased cardiopulmonary demands in patients with a history of cardiac and pulmonary disease may not be well tolerated. Although R.A. may tolerate the increased heart rate associated with fever, he may not be able to deliver enough oxygen to the tissues to meet the increased oxygen consumption associated with fever because of his pulmonary contusion.

Case Study 7-2: Malignant Hyperthermia

Decision point
What is the cause of Ms. P.P.'s MH?

Discussion. MH is associated with a genetic alteration in the ryanodine receptor and is inherited via autosomal dominant transmission. Triggers for MH include succinylcholine, anesthetic agents, and, in some cases, activities that increase core body temperature.

Decision point
What is the mechanism for the rise of Ms. P.P.'s core body temperature?

Discussion. Exposure to triggers leads to an increase in calcium released from the sarcoplasmic reticulum. The increased calcium causes the vigorous contraction of muscle, leading to increased heat production.

Decision point
What manifestations of malignant hyperthermia did Ms. P.P. display?

Discussion. Increased heart rate, elevated temperature, acidosis, muscle contraction, and increased carbon dioxide

production occur with MH. Manifestations do not always occur immediately with exposure to triggers; therefore patients that have received anesthesia may have manifestations that occur postoperatively.

CHAPTER 8, FAMILIES IN CRITICAL CARE

Case Study 8-1, Part A: Matching the Patient and Family's Needs

Decision point
How does theory help us explain what happened and how we could prevent such a situation?

Discussion. They are in crisis and trying to adapt to a level of functioning that will maintain their family system. Mrs. B. has a role in her family and is clearly struggling with the changes in that role. She feels threatened by the critical nature of her husband's illness. She has a need to feel accepted and safe in the critical care environment but her behavior alienates the staff. Understanding these changes and helping Mrs. B. aid her husband will assist both Mrs. B. and the staff to adapt to Mr. and Mrs. B.'s family crisis. In reflecting on Mrs. B.'s behavior, there is evidence that she has a need for honest information given in a timely manner. She appears to be seeking support from staff and has a need to be near her husband. Her behaviors only worsen when her presence at the bedside is limited by the staff. Mr. B. needs the support of his wife. However, he realizes that her behaviors are limiting his time with her.

Case Study 8-1, Part B: Matching the Patient and Family's Needs

Decision point
What evidence is available to formulate an effective plan of care to help this family?

Discussion. With her lack of understanding and her perceived limited information, Mrs. B. became very frustrated. A multidisciplinary conference, including Mrs. B., the physician, chaplain, social worker, nursing staff, and the clinical specialist, was held. The team developed a plan to provide information (i.e., daily at 1400, as needed based on Mr. B.'s condition, to include specific information about glucose and pain) and allow Mrs. B. to be with her husband at times that were best for her (a staff-wife contract was developed to address Mrs. B.'s need to be in husband's room outside of usual visiting hours). The hospital chaplain and social worker assisted her with other resources to help with some of her new responsibilities at home and to manage stress more appropriately. An experienced nurse served as a primary coordinator of care for this family. She monitored Mrs. B.'s response to the new interventions. The nurse acted as a liaison for staff on other shifts. Every day Mrs. B. was given a complete update by the nursing staff on Mr. B.'s condition that included a review of his glucose/insulin status and the effectiveness of the pain management plan.

Case Study 8-1, Part C: Matching the Patient and Family's Needs

Decision point

What outcomes might be expected as a result of this new plan of care?

Discussion. While this plan of care was not complicated, it was effective. Expected outcomes included assistance to help Mrs. B. gain insights into the overall plan of care, to reduce her anxiety, and to improve trust between this family and staff and, ultimately, a higher level of satisfaction with care.

CHAPTER 11, ACUTE CORONARY SYNDROMES

Case Study 11-1, Part A: Acute Coronary Syndrome

Decision point

What interventions should be instituted immediately?

Discussion. Cardiac monitoring along with pulse oximetry should be applied as intravenous access is obtained. A focused medical history, chest x-ray, and 12-lead ECG should be obtained. Oxygen by nasal cannula was applied since his SpO_2 was 90%. The ECG showed ST elevation (3 mm) in leads II, III, aV_F, I, and aV_L, indicating an acute inferolateral STEMI. The chest x-ray disclosed a normal-sized aorta, ruling out aortic dissection as a cause of the chest pain, and troponin and CK isoenzymes were sent to the lab for analysis. Heparin therapy was instituted, and clopidogrel (Plavix) was given; the institutional protocol directed the ED to initiate PCI process.

Decision point

Should fibrinolytic therapy also have been initiated to help improve Mr. C.'s outcome?

Discussion. Currently, PCI has been shown to be superior to fibrinolysis when considering outcomes of death, stroke, or reinfarction. The important variable is the amount of experience of the interventional cardiologist. The more experienced the provider, the better the patient outcomes.[4]

Case Study 11-1, Part B: Acute Coronary Syndrome

Decision point

Should Mr. C. have had a temporary pacemaker placed?

Discussion. His hemodynamic instability was corrected easily with volume resuscitation. If Mr. C. remained hypotensive and bradycardic, a pacemaker would have been indicated.

Case Study 11-1, Part C: Acute Coronary Syndrome

Decision point

How soon after initiation of atorvastatin therapy should Mr. C. have liver function tests performed?

Discussion. The usual time period is 3 months after initiation of therapy. The patient should be counseled about reporting muscle weakness or aching.

CHAPTER 12, HEART FAILURE

Case Study 12-1, Part A: Etiology of Heart Failure

Decision point

What signs and symptoms of heart failure was R.S. exhibiting?

Discussion. The signs and symptoms R.S. exhibited are difficulty breathing at rest, SO_2 of 82%, distended neck veins, S_3 gallop, 4+ pedal edema, rales, and pulmonary congestion on chest x-ray.

Decision point

What causes, risk factors, and lifestyle choices does R.S. have for heart failure?

Discussion. R.S. has a history of previous MI and poorly controlled hypertension. In addition, she has uncontrolled diabetes mellitus, is obese, and is African American. The lifestyle choices she has made that contribute to her decompensation are her nonadherence to prescribed medical therapy, including medications, and her continued consumption of a high-sodium, high-carbohydrate diet.

Case Study 12-1, Part B: Etiology of Heart Failure

Decision point

What pathophysiologic mechanism contributed to the left ventricular hypertrophy and left ventricular dysfunction?

Discussion. Ventricular remodeling was most likely triggered by the previous MI and then aggravated by neurohormone (norepinephrine, angiotensin II, and arginine vasopressin) release. Long-standing hypertension contributed to the increase in neurohormones, causing vasoconstriction and increased workload (and increased oxygen consumption) on the heart muscle.

Decision point

What pathophysiologic mechanism contributed to the fluid retention?

Discussion. Activation of the renin-angiotensin-aldosterone system causes release of aldosterone from the adrenal cortex. Aldosterone promotes sodium and water retention. In addition, arginine vasopressin (or antidiuretic hormone) promotes water retention.

Case Study 12-1, Part C: Etiology of Heart Failure

Decision point

What nonpharmacologic therapies are essential for R.S. after discharge?

Discussion. Self-care maintenance, including daily weight monitoring, following a low-sodium diet, daily physical activity, and taking her medications as prescribed, is essential to help her feel better and stay out of the hospital. In addition, self-care management activities, such as symptom recognition, must be taught and reinforced. Telephone follow-up by the critical care nurses will be instrumental to help her adjust to these lifestyle changes.

CHAPTER 14, CARDIAC SURGERY

Case Study 14-1, Part A: Coronary Artery Bypass Grafting

Decision point
What interventions should be implemented at this time?

Discussion. A warming blanket should be applied to increase J.P.'s temperature in an effort to promote hemostasis. Protamine 25-50 mg can be administered intravenously to reverse residual heparin effects from the operating room. A narcotic infusion could be used to treat potential pain, since propofol (Diprivan) does not have analgesic effects. A vasodilator (e.g., nicardipine [Cardene]) might also be initiated to decrease his MAP, thus reducing stress on cannulation sites and suture lines.

Case Study 14-1, Part B: Coronary Artery Bypass Grafting

Decision point
What interventions might be prudent at this point?

Discussion. A bolus of crystalloid (500-1000 ml) could be used to raise preload to improve his cardiac index, blood pressure, and SvO_2. If crystalloids are not successful in increasing filling pressures, albumin or hetastarch may also be used. A hematocrit would be helpful in determining if a blood transfusion is needed. If cardiac output remains low despite adequate preload, an inotrope (e.g., dobutamine or milrinone) may be used to stimulate increased contractility. Persistently low cardiac index or SvO_2, despite adequate volume resuscitation and moderate inotropic support, may necessitate IABP insertion.

Case Study 14-1, Part C: Coronary Artery Bypass Grafting

Decision point
What are important nursing interventions for J.P. after extubation?

Discussion. J.P. will need to have frequent evaluation of his pain, with administration of analgesics to facilitate increasing activity, such as getting up in a chair. He should be encouraged to use his incentive spirometer every 1 to 2 hours, and should be shown how to use a cough pillow for support of his sternal incision. As he begins oral intake with ice chips or clear liquids, he should be observed to assess for difficulty swallowing. His oxygen can be gradually weaned, while maintaining an SaO_2 greater than or equal to 92%. If he remains hemodynamically stable, his dobutamine drip can be weaned off.

J.P. remained stable overnight in critical care. His dobutamine was weaned off and his blood pressure and cardiac output remained adequate. He began oral pain medication (acetaminophen with oxycodone, 1 tablet every 4 hours PRN) and reported pain at a level of 2 out of 10 when he got out of bed to the chair. The next morning his pulmonary artery catheter, chest tubes, and Foley catheter were all discontinued and he was transferred to the telemetry unit.

CHAPTER 15, VALVULAR DISEASE AND SURGERY

Case Study 15-1, Part A: Acute Respiratory Distress and Pulmonary Edema

Decision point
When is the narrowed aortic valve considered to be critical?

Discussion. Critical aortic stenosis is defined as a peak systolic pressure gradient greater than 50 mm Hg or a valve area less than 0.8 cm^2, or less than one fourth of the normal aortic valve area (3.0 to 4.0 cm^2).

Decision point
What are key symptoms a patient with aortic stenosis should be taught to report to their healthcare provider?

Discussion. Key symptoms the patient should report are increased shortness of breath with exertion, angina, syncope, and signs of heart failure.

Decision point
How frequently should a patient with aortic stenosis be seen by their healthcare provider once the aortic valve orifice is 1.0 cm^2?

Discussion. Patients should be followed closely with echocardiograms at least yearly, and every 6 months if the aortic stenosis is severe.

Case Study 15-1, Part B: Acute Respiratory Distress and Pulmonary Edema

Decision point
Why would the pulmonary artery pressures be elevated in this patient?

Discussion. Pulmonary artery pressures would be elevated in this patient because of left ventricular hypertrophy and increased LVEDP needed to support the stroke volume.

Decision point
Is sinus tachycardia common following cardiac surgery? Why?

Discussion. Valvular heart disease is associated with atrial hypertrophy and the development of electrophysiologic changes in the area of the pulmonary veins in the left atrium contributing to atrial dysrhythmias. The postoperative incidence of atrial flutter and atrial fibrillation tends to be higher in these patients.

Case Study 15-1, Part C: Acute Respiratory Distress and Pulmonary Edema

Decision point
What discharge instructions should be provided for this patient?

Discussion. Discharge instructions should include similar information as other open heart surgery patients receive, as well as information on anticoagulation therapy and subacute bacterial endocarditis prophylaxis.

CHAPTER 16, VASCULAR EMERGENCIES

Case Study 16-1, Part A: Thoracic Aortic Dissection

Decision point
What interventions should be implemented at this time?

Discussion. R.B. was started on beta blockers to decrease blood pressure, HR, and the force of contraction, with the goal of preventing further extension of the aortic dissection. If beta-blocker therapy failed to achieve the target systolic blood pressure (i.e., 100-110 mm Hg), a vasodilator such as sodium nitroprusside (Nipride) or nicardipine (Cardene) may be needed. An arterial line was inserted to help guide therapy. Morphine sulfate was administered intermittently to help decrease the pain associated with the dissection. Frequent serial assessments were performed to evaluate for potential extension of the dissection. Since R.B. was exhibiting ischemic complications related to his Type B dissection, arrangements were made for a surgical consult as soon as possible.

Case Study 16-1, Part B: Thoracic Aortic Dissection

Decision point
What interventions should be performed at this time?

Discussion. R.B. received 1 unit of PRBCs for a hematocrit of 27%. His oxygen was increased to 4 L per nasal cannula, to achieve an SaO$_2$ of 97%. These actions ensured adequate oxygen was available for delivery to the tissues. The CSF drain was allowed to drain 20 ml of clear fluid, which reduced his CSF pressure to 8 mm Hg. He also received a bolus of 250 ml of albumin, which increased his MAP to 87 mm Hg. By increasing the incoming arterial pressure and decreasing the opposing pressure within the spinal column, perfusion to the spinal cord was enhanced. Following these interventions, R.B. was able to move both legs and reported no numbness in his lower extremities. His CSF drain was removed on postoperative day 3 and R.B. was transferred to the step-down unit.

CHAPTER 17, CARDIOMYOPATHY

Case Study 17-1, Part A: Etiology of Heart Failure

Decision point
Based on the above findings, what is the most likely etiology of D.P.'s heart failure?

Discussion. Based on D.P.'s medical history and clinical presentation, and using the WHO/ISFC classifications, the cause of HF could be dilated cardiomyopathy, hypertension, diabetes (metabolic cardiomyopathy), or a composite of multiple disease factors. By conventional practice, ischemic non–postmyocardial infarction cardiomyopathy must also be considered since HF could be the sequelae of loss of functioning myocytes, development of fibrosis, and subsequent left ventricular dysfunction and remodeling associated with hibernating myocardium from coronary artery disease.[39]

Case Study 17-1, Part B: Etiology of Heart Failure

Decision point
What diagnostic tests are key to determining etiology and developing an appropriate treatment plan?

Discussion. To determine if the etiology of D.P.'s HF is ischemic or nonischemic cardiomyopathy, differential testing is necessary. If the cardiomyopathy is determined to be ischemic in origin, testing for hibernating myocardium is necessary before a definitive treatment plan can be devised. Ultimately, in patients like D.P. who do not have a history of myocardial infarction to distinguish the two cardiomyopathies, SPECT might have value in determining perfusion defects, especially when the defects are large and severe; however, newer techniques (i.e., electron beam tomography, magnetic resonance imaging, and dobutamine stress tissue Doppler echocardiogram) might have improved sensitivity and specificity and better reproducibility.

Case Study 17-1, Part C: Etiology of Heart Failure

Decision point
Should the diffuse obstructive coronary artery disease found on coronary angiography be the primary focus of treatment to halt progression of D.P.'s cardiomyopathy?

Discussion. D.P.'s obesity, diabetes, and hypertension as well as the diffuse coronary artery disease are all important areas to address in the treatment plan. The coronary artery disease should be treated aggressively since it has been shown that coronary artery disease induced cardiomyopathy is improved with revascularization and medical management. Her hypertension and diabetes must also be controlled to diminish the effects on left ventricular remodeling and increased heart mass. And, regardless of the cause of the cardiomyopathy, evidence-based treatments for the management of heart failure should be instituted to halt the progression and decrease mortality (see Chapter 12, Heart Failure).

CHAPTER 18, HEART AND LUNG TRANSPLANTATION

Case Study 18-1, Part A: Post–Heart Transplant Care

Decision point
Is M.J. an appropriate heart transplant candidate?

Discussion. M.J.'s history includes the typical presentation for heart transplant evaluation—multiple CAD risk factors and progressive symptoms. Early optimal control of his DM and hypertension may have prevented or at least prolonged the period before onset of his CAD. Despite maximal medical therapy, however, his disease has progressed. He has recurrent angina and end-stage heart failure. His social history reveals that he has stopped smoking and is not abusing alcohol. He has adequate social support, but a family meeting would be important to evaluate his financial support (because he is on disability) and to determine if his wife's rheumatoid arthritis will significantly limit her ability to assist him in his posttransplant recovery period.

Case Study 18-1, Part B: Post–Heart Transplant Care

Decision point
What is your assessment of his overall status?

Discussion. M.J. is in fair condition despite relative bradycardia. His kidney function is probably a manifestation of relative ischemia intra- and postoperatively, plus exposure to cyclosporine.

Decision point
What interventions might be appropriate?

Discussion. Adding AV pacing to maintain a HR of 100 beats/min would probably help and would allow the epinephrine to be weaned off. Consideration of holding the cyclosporine for 1 day may also help the kidneys to recover. Elevated WBC count could be infection; however, he is afebrile. The leukocytosis could also be from the high-dose steroids. This parameter will need to be monitored and he should be examined for any sign of infection. M.J. also has hyperglycemia and should be treated with an insulin drip until this is well controlled. The hyperglycemia may be related to his preexisting DM, high-dose steroids, physiologic stress response, or an infection. Again, the search for possible infectious causes should proceed. M.J. can probably be weaned from mechanical ventilation and if possible extubated and placed on 40% oxygen via face mask.

CHAPTER 19, ACUTE RESPIRATORY FAILURE AND ACUTE LUNG INJURY

Case Study 19-1, Part A: Risk Factors for the Development of ALI/ARDS

Decision point
What risk factors does this patient have for development of ALI/ARDS?

Discussion. Traumatic chest injury, loss of consciousness with possibility of aspiration, multiple fractures (fat embolism), recent viral infection, middle lobe infiltrate, and smoking history.

Decision point
Are these risks a result of direct or indirect insults?

Discussion. The traumatic injury and fractures may be direct when there is contusion of the pleura or indirect when there

is a SIRS response. The viral infection may be direct when the viruses directly attack the pleura and indirect when the virus causes a SIRS response. All forms of pneumonia and smoking are direct results.

Decision point
What signs does the patient exhibit that show respiratory compromise?

Discussion. The patient exhibits decreased oxygen saturation, a chronic cough, increased sputum production, diminished respiratory excursion, tachypnea, elevated temperature, and tachycardia.

Case Study 19-1, Part B: Vital Signs

Decision point
What is the patient's *A-a* gradient, what is normal, and why is this important to know?

Discussion. The patient's *A-a* gradient is 156.18. His expected gradient is $[(35 + 10)/4] = 11.25$. The elevated *A-a* gradient indicates a lung etiology for the hypoxemia.

Decision point
What is the patient's P/F ratio, and does this patient have ALI or ARDS?

Discussion. The patient's Pa_{O_2}/Fi_{O_2} ratio is $58/0.36 = 161$, which is less than 200, so he has ARDS.

Decision point
What signs does the patient exhibit that show continued respiratory compromise?

Discussion. The patient is experiencing acute-onset, persistently decreased oxygen saturation with increasing Fi_{O_2} and bilateral lung infiltrates on CXR, indicative of edema.

Decision point
What changes should occur to the plan of care? What should the nurse monitor and report?

Discussion. The patient will need increased monitoring for respiratory failure, with transfer to a critical care unit. At this time, consider obtaining a pulmonary consultation. An assessment of nutritional status should occur. Nursing will need to provide assistance with activities of daily living, while monitoring for fatigue or respiratory failure. The nurse will be attentive to hydration needs and indicators of sepsis. The patient and family will need education on ARDS and the potential for intubation and mechanical ventilation.

Case Study 19-1, Part C: Additional Follow-up

Decision point
What is the P/F ratio for a patient who requires 1.0 Fi_{O_2} with a Pa_{O_2} of 72 mm Hg?

Discussion. $Pa_{O_2}/Fi_{O_2} = 72/1.0 = 72$.

Decision point
Based on the above P/F ratio, does the patient have ALI or ARDS?

Discussion. A P/F ratio less than 200 means that this patient is in ARDS.

Decision point

What are the recommendations for PEEP and plateau pressure limits according to the ARDSNet protocol for a patient on 0.7 FiO_2?

Discussion. The ARDSNet protocol recommends keeping PaO_2 between 55 and 80 mm Hg and end-inspiratory alveolar (plateau) pressure less than 30 cm H_2O and using a tidal volume of 6 ml/kg PBW, while manipulating PEEP and ventilator rate (maximum 35) to achieve arterial pH between 7.3 and 7.45. The ARDSNet table recommends PEEP of 10, 12, 14, or 20 mm Hg for a patient requiring 0.7 FiO_2, while measurement of the P_{flex} will determine a true PEEP need.

Decision point

What is the ARDSNet protocol recommended tidal volume for a patient with a predicted body weight of 80 kg?

Discussion. 80 kg $\times$ 6 ml/kg = maximum tidal volume of 480 ml.

CHAPTER 20, MECHANICAL VENTILATION AND WEANING

Case Study 20-1: PEEP

Decision point

What should be done to improve M.C.'s oxygenation status?

Discussion. The refractory hypoxemia and chest x-ray findings suggest acute respiratory distress syndrome (ARDS). The management of ARDS should focus on recruiting the lung with PEEP and preventing volutrauma. In M.C.'s case the PEEP level is too low and the tidal volume too high. The team recognizes this, and the V_t is decreased to 300 ml (i.e., 6 ml/kg lean body weight) and the PEEP is increased over the next hour to 15 cm H_2O. M.C. is also sedated with lorazepam intravenous boluses and fentanyl for analgesia, which helps her tolerate the ensuing anticipated hypercarbia. Her blood pressure is 110/60 mm Hg and heart rate 90 beats/min. Her next ABG result is as follows: pH=7.28, $PaCO_2$ = 67 mm Hg, and PaO_2 = 150 mm Hg.

Decision point

What should be done next?

Discussion. The hypercarbia is expected with these settings as a consequence of the reduced V_t. Oxygenation status is improved, suggesting lung recruitment. The next step is to decrease the FiO_2. The team's goal is to maintain an oxygen saturation of at least 90%. The PEEP level is maintained to ensure recruitment and prevent shear injury from repeated opening and closing of the lung during tidal breathing.

Case Study 20-2: Weaning

Decision point

How should these issues be addressed?

Discussion. Addressing the factors listed as impeding T.G.'s weaning progress will help ensure that T.G. is "ready" to

begin a weaning trial. The team decides to diurese T.G., infuse 1 unit of packed red cells, and provide a low-dose intermediate benzodiazepine for anxiolysis. Because the team believes the patient is fatigued, their goal is to decrease the patient's workload and provide respiratory muscle rest. T.G. is switched from the A/C mode to PSV at 17 cm H_2O. This level results in a V_t of approximately 400 ml and a respiratory rate of 18 breaths/min. Auto-PEEP resolves with the addition of albuterol nebulizer treatments and the change in ventilator settings. The team's plan is to provide "rest" for 12-24 hours and then reassess for resumption of weaning trials.

Decision point

Is she ready for extubation or is additional information needed?

Discussion. The team decides to extubate immediately because T.G. demonstrates no signs of wean trial intolerance (Box 20-9). The MICU protocol does not require obtaining an ABG before extubation. T.G. is extubated and placed on 2 L of O_2 per nasal cannula. Her oxygen saturation is 96%. 5 hours later she is transferred to the ward and is discharged on hospital day 9.

CHAPTER 21, THORACIC SURGERY

Case Study 21-1, Part A: Pulmonary Resection

Decision point

With a mass in the right apex of the lung, what additional signs and symptoms should be evaluated?

Discussion. Evaluation should also be made for any shoulder or back pain in this area along with an assessment of range of motion with the right arm. Depending upon the exact location via chest x-ray or computerized tomography, assess for pain in the area. If the mass has invaded through the visceral pleura and into the parietal pleura, the patient may describe chest wall pain or generalized pain/discomfort in this area.

Case Study 21-1, Part B: Pulmonary Resection

Decision point

What other disciplines should be involved in M.R.'s care? Provide your rationale.

Discussion. A nutritional consult would be appropriate since he has lost 20 pounds, has a body mass index of 20.9, has a history of alcohol intake, and will be scheduled for surgery. In addition, it would be helpful to have a pulmonary consult to optimize his pulmonary function before surgery, promote smoking cessation, and schedule him for "prehabilitation" with the pulmonary rehabilitation team.

Case Study 21-1, Part C: Pulmonary Resection

Decision point

Why would a temporary tracheostomy be placed in M.R.?

Discussion. A prophylactic tracheostomy will assist with secretion management and also assist in the weaning process from mechanical ventilation. Having a tracheostomy facilitates the team's ability to easily reestablish mechanical ventilation should he fail the initial weaning process (versus extubation and reintubation).

Decision point
What are the potential postoperative complications (pulmonary and nonpulmonary) M.R. may experience?

Discussion. M.R. is at high risk for pulmonary complications following surgery given his poor pulmonary function, smoking history, and the complexity of his surgical procedure.

Decision point
What issues may M.R. face in the immediate postoperative period?

Discussion. M.R. had an extrapleural completion pneumonectomy, which is a complex procedure. His fluid status will need to be closely monitored as will his oxygenation needs and secretion management (since he had difficulty in the first surgery). Also, since a redo-thoracotomy was performed and he had a rib removed with the first procedure, pain management will be critical. This will be especially important once he is extubated and beginning to ambulate and perform deep-breathing maneuvers.

Decision point
Given M.R.'s long and complicated hospitalizations, what issues may need to be addressed before discharge?

Discussion. M.R. continues to be debilitated at discharge. Potential services to be involved include pulmonary rehabilitation, physical therapy, and a nutritional consult. His oxygenation needs will need to be monitored upon discharge with hopes that he can become independent of supplemental oxygenation.

CHAPTER 22, HEAD INJURY AND DYSFUNCTION

Case Study 22-1, Part A: Head Injury and Dysfunction

Decision point
What is the patient's current GCS?

Discussion. GCS = 7.

Decision point
What caused the changes noted in M.P.'s pupils?

Discussion. The left pupil was larger than the right because of increased pressure on the left oculomotor nerve (cranial nerve III) caused by the SDH or SAH. Most likely it was caused by the SDH because after surgical evacuation of that hemorrhage, the pupils became equal in size. Sluggishness is also related to increased ICP; alleviation of the pressure caused by the SDH allowed the pupils to respond briskly.

Decision point
What clinical assessment criteria will the critical care nursing staff need to monitor on an ongoing basis?

Discussion. Vital signs; GCS and neuro assessments; signs of CSF leak, such as rhinorrhea; signs of seizure activity; pain and sedation control. ICP and CPP will also need to be monitored. Hypotension and hypoxia will require immediate intervention to avoid potentiating secondary brain injury.

Case Study 22-1, Part B: Head Injury and Dysfunction

Decision point
Why is it important that M.P. have only oral endotracheal and nasogastric tubes rather than nasal intubation?

Discussion. Patients with basilar skull fractures are at risk for tube insertion through the skull fracture into the brain parenchyma.

Decision point
What laboratory values are most important in M.P.'s care?

Discussion. ABGs, chemistry panel with particular attention to the serum sodium level, CBC, serum and urine osmolality, serum drug levels such as phenytoin and barbiturates. Serum lactate levels may be compared to jugular venous lactate levels; ongoing cerebral ischemia is present if the brain lactate level is higher than the serum lactate level.

Decision point
What interventions would be appropriately instituted for decreased $SjvO_2$ values?

Discussion. Appropriate interventions would include titration of FiO_2 to improve oxygenation, and evaluation for transfusion of PRBCs, fluids, and sedatives to increase cerebral oxygen delivery and decrease cerebral metabolic rate. Vasopressors may be indicated if the patient is hypotensive despite adequate fluid resuscitation.

Decision point
What additional interventions could be used to help control the patient's ICP?

Discussion. Nursing interventions include elevating the head of bed, ensuring that the head is aligned, and checking that the cervical collar is not too tight. Sedation before painful procedures such as suctioning might prevent ICP spikes. Limiting stimulating activities when the ICP waveform suggests poor compliance (P1 < P2) might also prevent dangerous spikes in ICP. A calm, quiet environment along with judicious use of analgesics and sedatives will prevent agitation and reaction to the environment, all of which exacerbate increased ICP. Medical interventions might include opening the ventriculostomy at all times to drain CSF and performing a hemi-craniectomy to allow room for the injured brain to swell without causing herniation.

Case Study 22-1, Part C: Head Injury and Dysfunction

Decision point
Why is it important to avoid hyperthermia in the care of M.P.?

Discussion. Hyperthermia is related to increased secondary brain injury and poor neurologic outcome in patients with TBI.

Decision point
What are the potential complications of barbiturate-induced coma?

Discussion. Decreased GI motility, decreased cough and gag reflexes, immunosuppression, myocardial depression, complications associated with immobility.

Decision point
What interventions should be in place to minimize long-term complications of TBI?

Discussion. The patient requires DVT prophylaxis; in the early postinjury phase sequential compression stockings are indicated. Later, when anticoagulation does not pose a risk for intracranial hemorrhage, low-molecular-weight heparin may be used. Frequent Doppler screenings for DVT should be ordered. Because of the increased caloric demands following TBI, the patient should receive enteral nutrition; ideally, jejunostomy feeding should be utilized to minimize risk of aspiration. Early and aggressive attempts to wean the patient from mechanical ventilation are important to minimize the risk of ventilator-associated pneumonia; extubation is indicated as soon as the patient is neurologically stable and able to protect the airway. Once the patient became alert, the lateral rotation bed was no longer appropriate. Changing the bed to one with a pressure-relieving mattress should be done to prevent development of decubitus ulcers. Physical therapy and occupational therapy should be involved early in the patient's care to assist with range-of-motion exercises and other activities to prevent joint contractures and muscle wasting.

CHAPTER 23, CEREBROVASCULAR DISORDERS

Case Study 23-1, Part A: Cerebrovascular Disorders

Decision point
What pathophysiology is associated with this stroke?

Discussion. Mrs. S.P. has had an aneurysmal SAH. The aneurysm has burst or leaked and blood has mixed with the CSF in the subarachnoid space. Her greatest risk during the first 24 hours is rebleeding, which could be fatal or cause loss of consciousness or major neurologic deficits. Her ventricles are most likely enlarged because the blood in the CSF has impaired the absorption of the CSF, resulting in hydrocephalus. In about 3 days, Mrs. S.P. will be at risk for vasospasm, which happens as a result of the blood surrounding the blood vessels, although the pathophysiology is not completely understood.

Decision point
What are the initial priorities for her care?

Discussion. The initial priorities for Mrs. S.P.'s care are ongoing assessment and management of oxygenation, neurologic status, intracranial dynamics, blood pressure, and pain. To minimize the risk of secondary injury, a nasal cannula is needed to increase the SaO_2 to 95% or better. Her drowsiness

may be related to hydrocephalus. A ventriculostomy may be needed to drain CSF and measure ICP. Initiation of nimodipine for the aneurysmal SAH plus a low-dose intravenous opioid for pain may decrease the blood pressure. However, if they are not effective, other anti-hypertensives may be needed. Dramatic increases or decreases in blood pressure are to be avoided. Mrs. S.P. needs minimal stimulation except for hourly assessments. She may also receive a loading dose of Dilantin as prophylaxis; however, the blood pressure must be monitored and the Dilantin given slowly to avoid hypotension. If Mrs. S.P. does not have a central venous catheter, fosphenytoin is preferable to phenytoin as it is less irritating to the tissues.

Case Study 23-1, Part B: Cerebrovascular Disorders

Decision point
What clinical signs and symptoms indicated the need for HHH therapy?

Discussion. Mrs. S.P. was in progressive vasospasm as evidenced by neurologic deterioration and increasing MCA mean flow velocities and MCA/ICA ratios on her daily TCD studies. While the nimodipine and HHH therapy may have initially stabilized her neurologically, the decreased level of consciousness, difficulty with numbers, right lower facial weakness, and dysarthria indicated deterioration. To decrease the risk of secondary injury and infarction related to vasospasm, she underwent angioplasty to restore blood flow to the area supplied by the constricted vessels.

Case Study 23-1, Part C: Cerebrovascular Disorders

Decision point
What signs and symptoms would indicate that Mrs. S.P. is not tolerating raising and clamping of the ventriculostomy?

Discussion. Signs and symptoms indicating that Mrs. S.P. is not tolerating raising and clamping of the ventriculostomy include increased ICP, decreased CPP, and a deterioration of the neurologic status, including but not limited to an increase in headache, a decrease in level of consciousness, decreased reactivity of the pupils to light, and impaired EOMs. Other signs would include leaking from the ventriculostomy site, enlarged ventricles on a non-contrast head CT, and improvement in neurologic status after lowering or opening of the ventriculostomy.

CHAPTER 24, SPINAL CORD INJURY

Case Study 24-1, Part A: Evidence-Based Management of a Patient With Traumatic Spinal Cord Injury

Decision point
What mechanisms of injury are likely to be associated with this injury?

Discussion. Since the moving vehicle broke the guardrail, repeatedly rolled down the hill, stopped abruptly, and ejected J.G., the mechanism of his injury is likely acceleration-deceleration. However, a number of other mechanisms are possible including hyperflexion, hyperextension, rotation, or axial loading. Based on J.G.'s clinical presentation, a hyperflexion injury may have fractured the vertebrae anteriorly, causing an anterior cord injury and disrupting posterior ligaments. Injury to the anterior cord results in damage to the corticospinal and spinothalamic tracts, the major voluntary movement and pain and temperature pathways. With ligamentous injury, the injury is unstable.

Decision point
What associated injuries are likely?

Discussion. With mechanisms of injury and traumatic SCI of this magnitude, a TBI is likely. J.G. remained conscious at the scene and during transport. Since he was found awake, talking, and confused following an acceleration-deceleration injury, he likely sustained a concussion. However, he needs to be closely monitored for deterioration in his level of consciousness that might occur with cerebral edema or hematoma formation. Other possible injures including facial and skull fractures, long bone fractures, and organ damage must be excluded.

Decision point
What are the initial priorities for his care?

Discussion. The initial priorities for J.G.'s care are oxygenation and circulation while maintaining immobilization of his spine. The bradycardia and hypotension with poikilothermia reflect neurogenic shock, which will require resuscitation with fluids, vasopressors, and gradual rewarming. Atropine may be needed as well. Failure to provide adequate oxygenation and perfusion or any movement of the spine may result in further neurologic deterioration.

Case Study 24-1, Part B: Evidence-Based Management of a Patient With Traumatic Spinal Cord Injury

Decision point
What are the priorities in caring for J.G. during his stay in critical care?

Discussion. The priorities of his care are as follows: (1) prevention of secondary neuronal injury; (2) stabilization of the spine; (3) weaning from mechanical ventilation; (4) minimizing the consequences of immobilization; and (5) initiating rehabilitation. Efforts toward prevention of secondary injury include completion of the methylprednisolone protocol; maintenance of the blood pressure within recommended parameters; adequate oxygenation; continued immobilization and stabilization with traction and then eventually surgical repair. Interventions to minimize the consequences of his immobility include a system-by-system approach to the sequelae of spinal cord injury. Aggressive pulmonary hygiene, nutrition, bowel and bladder management, gastrointestinal and thromboembolism prophylaxis, and an early rehabilitation approach, involving occupational and physical therapy, are imperative. Components of aggressive pulmonary hygiene include frequent repositioning, assisted (quad) coughing, mobilization, and adequate hydration. Interventions to assist J.G. and his family to cope with his deficits are also an integral part of his care and will help him achieve the best possible outcome.

A rotating bed or turning frame assists in decreasing skin breakdown until his spine is stabilized. However, skin must be assessed frequently, during repositioning, toileting, and hygiene measures. After spine stabilization and J.G. is no longer in traction, he must be turned every 2 hours at a minimum and his skin kept clean and dry. Assessment and protection of bony prominences, including the sacrum, ischial tuberosities, trochanters, heels, and elbows, are essential. Pressure from orthotic devices must be minimized and treated aggressively. Pressure-relieving mattresses may be beneficial as well but do not replace routine turning. While in a chair, a pressure-relieving seat cushion is mandatory and position changes, such as tilting back the wheelchair, must occur at least every 15 to 20 minutes. Meeting nutritional needs is mandatory.

Case Study 24-1, Part C: Evidence-Based Management of a Patient With Traumatic Spinal Cord Injury

Decision point
What is most likely occurring and what are the appropriate interventions?

Discussion. J.G. sustained his cervical spinal cord injury 1 month ago and he exhibits reflex activity, indicative of resolution of spinal shock. He is most likely experiencing AD, which places him at risk for myocardial infarction, stroke, or seizure. The nurse's first action is to raise the head of the bed and simultaneously assess for possible etiologies. Bladder or bowel overdistention is the most likely cause. If a protocol is in place or a house officer is available to initiate the order, the nurse may administer a short but rapid-acting anti-hypertensive such as orally chewed nifedipine (Procardia) or sublingual nitroglycerin while the stimulus for the AD is being determined. Catheterization yields 950 ml of cloudy, foul-smelling urine. Within 30 minutes of administering the anti-hypertensive and draining the bladder, the blood pressure returns to baseline and all symptoms resolve. A urinalysis and urine culture and sensitivity are sent to the lab for analysis and intermittent catheterizations are ordered every 6 hours until further notice.

CHAPTER 25, SPECIAL NEUROLOGIC PATIENT POPULATIONS

Case Study 25-1, Part A: Status Epilepticus

Decision point
Does the patient have any risk factors for developing SE?

Discussion. No specific risk factors for seizures, but lung cancer is one of the major forms of cancer that metastasize to the brain and S.B. does have past and current smoking history with chronic cough.

Decision point

Did the patient have any premorbid symptoms that might indicate neurologic pathology and a potential for seizure activity?

Discussion. The tingling on the right side of the face could be a related neurologic symptom.

Case Study 25-1, Part B: Status Epilepticus

Decision point

If you are concerned that S.B. is experiencing nonconvulsive SE, how would you determine if this is happening?

Discussion. Examine the patient closely for any types of motor activity that might indicate electrographic seizures, such as twitching of the face, hands, feet, ocular deviation, or nystagmus. As the propofol is weaned, the patient should gradually regain consciousness although considering the recent seizure activity, it may take several hours. Continuous EEG recording could diagnose ongoing seizure activity.

Case Study 25-1, Part C: Status Epilepticus

Decision point

What is happening to S.B.?

Discussion. S.B. is experiencing an acute neurologic deterioration. Because of the known left temporal lesion, a reasonable hypothesis would be that the patient has had a hemorrhagic event related to this site.

Decision point

What steps should the nurse take?

Discussion. After thoroughly examining the patient, the nurse should simultaneously call the physician and plan for a CT scan. ACLS protocols in critical care should be considered as the nurse keeps a close eye on the patient's hemodynamic status.

Decision point

What treatment plan for the next 24 hours might the nurse anticipate?

Discussion. If S.B. has had a hemorrhage, options include surgical evacuation or observation. The patient may need intracranial pressure monitoring with ventriculostomy, central line placement, and possibly an arterial line. The dilated pupil indicates that her left brain is under pressure and if the pressure is not alleviated, there is a potential for brain herniation and death by neurologic criteria. Her family will need considerable support during this crisis.

CHAPTER 27, LIVER DYSFUNCTION AND FAILURE

Case Study 27-1: Alcohol, Hepatitis, and the Liver

Decision point

What type of liver failure does the patient have?

Discussion. Given that the patient has a history of long-standing alcoholism and hepatitis C and ultrasound evidence of cirrhosis, he has acute on chronic liver failure, with decompensated cirrhosis.

Decision point

What other tests would be helpful in this case?

Discussion

1. Blood alcohol level and urine toxicology screen, to evaluate substance use/abuse.
2. Panculture of blood, urine, and ascitic fluid, as well as ascitic fluid total protein and glucose, to evaluate for infection.
3. Obtain urinalysis with urine electrolytes, total protein, and creatinine to evaluate underlying causes, besides hypovolemia, for the acute renal failure.

Case Study 27-2: A Diagnosis

Decision point

Based on the onset of symptoms and clinical data, what type of liver failure does the patient have?

Discussion. The patient has a rapid onset of jaundice, followed by mental alterations, and no prior history of liver disease, with severe hepatitis as evidenced by her elevated AST/ALT level. The patient has acute liver failure.

Decision point

What is your initial treatment plan for this patient?

Discussion

1. The patient is in stage 3 hepatic encephalopathy, with imminent danger of loss of airway protection and onset of coma. Consider sedation with propofol (Diprivan), and electively intubate/ventilate. Initiate cooling measures for induction of moderate hypothermia. Start lactulose administration.
2. Monitor and replace serum glucose and electrolytes.
3. Insert Foley catheter and monitor urine output and fluid status.
4. Monitor serum chemistry values with liver function tests, complete blood count, and coagulation values.
5. Consider radiographic tests: noncontrast CT of the head, ultrasound with Doppler evaluation of the abdomen to rule out alterations in hepatic or renal blood flow.
6. Contact and referral to a tertiary liver treatment/transplant center for emergency evaluation and management of liver dysfunction, and possible listing for liver transplantation.
7. Social work evaluation for evaluation and support of family members.

CHAPTER 28, PANCREATITIS

Case Study 28-1, Part A: Assessment and Management of Acute Pancreatitis

Decision point
What risk factors does J.D. have for the development of acute pancreatitis?

Discussion. Gallstone disease and the use of thiazide diuretics are his only known risk factors for the development of acute pancreatitis.

Decision point
What were the physical assessment findings with which J.D. presented to the emergency department? What is the rationale for the development of each?

Discussion. J.D. presented with abdominal pain, distention, nausea, and vomiting related to retroperitoneal inflammation and fluid sequestration. He had a fever and elevated WBC count related to inflammation/possible infection. His hypotension and tachycardia were related to retroperitoneal fluid losses. Possible pleural effusion and crackles to auscultation are related to fluid migration into the chest cavity. Tachypnea and decreased breath sounds may be related to hypoventilation with pain, guarding, and splinting with subdiaphragmatic fluid collection.

Case Study 28-1, Part B: Assessment and Management of Acute Pancreatitis

Decision point
What complications is J.D. likely experiencing?

Discussion. Hypovolemia with shock, respiratory insufficiency with hypoxemia, pancreatic necrosis, and possible renal dysfunction.

Decision point
What interventions are required for J.D.?

Discussion. Intubation with mechanical ventilation to achieve an improved level of oxygenation, volume resuscitation with normal saline or lactated Ringer's solution, insertion of a pulmonary artery catheter for further assessment and to guide volume resuscitation, monitor urine output and check serum creatinine level.

Case Study 28-1, Part C: Assessment and Management of Acute Pancreatitis

Decision point
What complications have now occurred in J.D.'s course?

Discussion. ARDS and infected pancreatic necrosis.

Decision point
What interventions do you anticipate for the problems previously identified for J.D.?

Discussion. For ARDS, ventilatory strategies need to be implemented to improve oxygenation but utilize lung protective strategies. Pancreatic necrosectomy with postoperative lavage and antibiotics are required to treat infected pancreatic necrosis.

Decision point
What is J.D.'s current complication and how should it be treated?

Discussion. Over the course of weeks he was identified as having multiple abscesses by CT scan. These were effectively percutaneously drained and he was treated with antibiotics. Because of severe ARDS, J.D. had difficulty being weaned from the ventilator and required a temporary tracheostomy. He slowly improved and was weaned, the tracheostomy was removed, and his infections resolved. He was discharged home after 5 months in the critical care and step-down unit.

CHAPTER 32, COMPLEX ACID-BASE DISORDERS AND ASSOCIATED ELECTROLYTE IMBALANCES

Case Study 32-1, Part A: Metabolic Acidosis

Decision point
Diagnose and determine the etiology of the acid-base disorder.

Discussion. This patient has a simple, compensated metabolic acidosis. The pH is low, the HCO_3^- is low, and the $Paco_2$ is low. There is appropriate compensation demonstrated by the fact that the measured $Paco_2$ of 16 mm Hg approximates the predicted $Paco_2$ calculated as follows (see Box 32-2, Step 2):

$$\text{Predicted Pao}_2 = (1.5 \times 6) + 8$$
$$= 9 + 8$$
$$= 17 \text{ mm Hg}$$

The *shortcut* can also be used to determine if this is a compensated metabolic acidosis. With full compensation, the $Paco_2$ approximates the last 2 digits of the pH. In this example, the $Paco_2$ of 16 approximates the last two digits of the pH 7.15.

Case Study 32-1, Part B: Metabolic Acidosis

Decision point
What are the manifestations of metabolic acidosis?

Discussion. Cardiovascular manifestations of metabolic acidosis in this case include hypotension attributable to arterial vasodilation and decreased responsiveness to endogenous catecholamines. Additionally, volume depletion from blood loss is also likely contributing to hypotension. The patient has altered mental status, which is a neurologic manifestation of metabolic acidosis. Respiratory manifestations include hyperventilation. The patient's respiratory rate was 34 breaths/min, which resulted in respiratory muscle fatigue requiring intubation and mechanical ventilation.

Decision point

What are the electrolyte imbalances associated with metabolic acidosis in this case?

Discussion. Hyperkalemia is the most concerning electrolyte imbalance in this case. The 12-lead ECG shows tall peaked T waves and prolongation of both the PR and QRS. This can be life threatening and requires immediate treatment before lethal ventricular dysrhythmias develop. Causes of hyperkalemia in this case include crush injury and muscle cell death with the release of intracellular potassium, acute renal failure, and metabolic acidosis. In metabolic acidosis hyperkalemia occurs as a result of transcellular K^+ and H^+ shifts (Figure 32-3). Hyperkalemia was treated with intravenous calcium, D_{50}, and sodium bicarbonate.

The calcium values are also impacted by the metabolic acidosis. The total calcium concentration is quite low, yet the ionized calcium concentration is normal. Remember, in metabolic acidosis ionized calcium levels increase because of changes in calcium-protein binding that result in a release of calcium from protein, thereby raising the ionized calcium level (Figure 32-4). When the pH is restored upward towards normal, the ionized calcium level will fall (pH and ionized calcium level are inversely related) and the patient could develop signs and symptoms of hypocalcemia.

Decision point

Was it appropriate to treat the metabolic acidosis with $NaHCO_3$?

Discussion. The patient had refractory hypotension despite volume replacement. In severe metabolic acidosis (arterial pH less than 7.20), hypotension secondary to arteriolar vasodilation and decreased cardiac contractility will occur. Increasing the pH with $NaHCO_3$ will likely improve hemodynamics transiently, but there is no evidence supporting improved survival when lactic acidosis is treated with bicarbonate therapy. However, this patient also needed the initial bolus of $NaHCO_3$ to treat symptomatic hyperkalemia (tall peaked T waves and widened QRS on the ECG). Dialysis was an appropriate treatment for metabolic acidosis in this patient with acute renal failure combined with lactic acidosis. Ongoing administration of sodium bicarbonate infusions would likely result in volume overload and pulmonary edema in this patient with acute renal failure.

Decision point

Was the bicarbonate drip preparation ordered correctly?

Discussion. No; the order stated to mix the bicarbonate drip as normal saline $1\,L + NaHCO_3$ 3 ampules and administer at 150 ml/hr. Administration of this drip would result in a hypertonic, hyperosmolar IVF, potentially causing acute hypernatremia and cerebral dysfunction. A better way to prepare the bicarbonate drip would be to mix D_5W $1\,L+3$ ampules $NaHCO_3$.

Decision point

Why did the patient have tetany?

Discussion. This is likely attributable to the sudden drop in the ionized calcium level after the administration of IV $NaHCO_3$ and a transient increase in the pH. Remember, pH and ionized calcium tend to be inversely related. By raising the pH, the ionized calcium level fell and the patient developed symptomatic hypocalcemia.

Case Study 32-2, Part A: Metabolic Alkalosis

Decision point

Interpret the blood gas and calculate the anion gap.

Discussion. P.G. exhibits metabolic alkalosis with compensation. The measured Pa_{CO_2} of 60 mm Hg approximates the predicted Pa_{CO_2}, calculated as follows (Box 32-2, Step 2):

$$\text{Predicted } PaCO_2 = 40 + 0.7(\text{Measurede } HCO_3^-$$
$$- \text{normal } HCO_3^-)$$
$$= 40 + 0.7(54 - 26)$$
$$= 40 + 0.7(28)$$
$$= 40 + 20$$
$$= 60 \text{ mm Hg}$$

The predicted Pa_{CO_2} matches the measured Pa_{CO_2}, confirming this is a simple metabolic alkalosis with compensation. The anion gap is calculated as follows:

$$Na^+ - (CI^- + HCO_3^-)$$
$$= 131 - (70 + 55)$$
$$= 131 - 125$$
$$= 6 \text{ mEq/L}$$

This normal anion gap of 6 mEq/L confirms that this is not a mixed acid-base imbalance.

Case Study 32-2, Part B: Metabolic Alkalosis

Decision point

What is the most likely etiology of the metabolic alkalosis?

Discussion. Metabolic alkalosis in this patient is due to protracted vomiting and the continued use of diuretics, despite volume depletion. There are two mechanisms of acid and chloride loss in this case study. There is loss of gastric hydrochloric acid from vomiting and loss of renal ammonium chloride caused by the diuretic. This is a chloride-responsive metabolic alkalosis.

Decision point

What are the manifestations of metabolic alkalosis in this case?

Discussion. Neuromuscular manifestations of metabolic alkalosis include numbness and tingling around her mouth and fingertips (paresthesias). This was due to a low ionized calcium level, which occurs with metabolic alkalosis. Remember, pH and ionized calcium level tend to be inversely related. This patient should be watched closely for seizures. Respiratory manifestations include a compensatory hypoventilation, resulting in an increased Pa_{CO_2} and a decreased Pa_{O_2}. This patient also developed electrocardiographic changes consistent with alkalemia—a prolonged QTc interval (>0.44 msec) on the 12-lead ECG that predisposes to the ventricular dysrhythmias (polymorphic ventricular tachycardia and ventricular fibrillation) that the patient developed.

Decision point
What are the electrolyte imbalances associated with metabolic alkalosis in this case?

Discussion. As typically occurs with metabolic alkalosis, there are numerous electrolyte imbalances in this case, including hypochloremia, hypokalemia, hypomagnesemia, hypophosphatemia, and a low ionized calcium level. These electrolyte deficits are, in part, caused by gastrointestinal and renal losses but are also due to transcellular electrolyte shifts.

Case Study 32-2, Part C: Metabolic Alkalosis

Decision point
How should the metabolic alkalosis and electrolyte imbalances be treated?

Discussion. The diuretic was stopped and the cause of vomiting (*E. coli* bacteremia and pyelonephritis) was treated to stop ongoing acid and volume losses. Replacement of volume deficits was accomplished with the administration of intravenous normal saline. Chloride deficits were replaced with chloride in the normal saline and in the potassium chloride the patient was given. It is critical to replace chloride in this patient to correct the metabolic alkalosis. In this volume- and chloride-depleted patient, the kidney will avidly reabsorb sodium in the form of sodium bicarbonate instead of sodium chloride. By replacing chloride, this allows the kidney to reabsorb sodium chloride and excrete the bicarbonate. The concurrent electrolyte imbalances (hypomagnesemia, hypokalemia, and hypophosphatemia) were also treated with aggressive intravenous and oral electrolyte replacement. Her ABG and electrolyte values were normalized within 48 hours after admission.

Case Study 32-3, Part A: Mixed Acid-Base Disorders

Decision point
Assess the acid-base status of this patient using the steps in Box 32-2.

Discussion
Step 1: Using the ABG, identify the most apparent disorder. The pH is normal but the Pa_{CO_2} is elevated. This signifies the presence of a mixed acid-base disorder. This is *not* compensation of a primary disorder. Remember, compensation does not return the pH to normal; therefore at least two acid-base disorders are present in this case. The elevated Pa_{CO_2} suggests a respiratory acidosis. This is consistent with the clinical presentation of this patient with shallow respirations.
Step 2: In the setting of a respiratory acidosis, the predicted HCO_3^- can be calculated to see if this is a compensated respiratory acidosis. In an acute respiratory acidosis, the HCO_3^- increases by 1 mEq for every 10 mm Hg increase in the Pa_{CO_2}. This patient's Pa_{CO_2} is 10 mm Hg above normal. If this was a

compensated respiratory acidosis, the HCO_3^- would be elevated, but it is within normal limits.
Step 3: Calculate the anion gap; $Na^+ - (Cl^- + CO_2)$. This patient's anion gap is calculated as follows: $131 - (70 + 28) = 33$ mEq/L. The high anion gap of 33 mEq/L confirms the presence of a metabolic acidosis.

This patient has a triple acid-base disorder: (1) respiratory acidosis caused by hypoventilation secondary to respiratory muscle fatigue (shallow respirations) because of hypokalemia and hypophosphatemia; (2) a high anion gap metabolic acidosis because of lactic acidosis from shock (BP 70/56 mm Hg) and volume depletion; (3) metabolic alkalosis secondary to hydrochloric acid loss from protracted vomiting. The patient's HCO_3^- level is normal in the setting of an elevated anion gap, which is the clue to the presence of a coexisting metabolic acidosis and metabolic alkalosis. Normally, when the anion gap is high, the HCO_3^- level is low (Figure 32-2). This is a chloride-responsive metabolic alkalosis; note the chloride concentration is only 70 mEq/L.

Decision point
What are the associated electrolyte imbalances and their cause?

Discussion. Hypochloremia, hypokalemia, and hypophosphatemia. These are due to protracted vomiting.

Decision point
How should the acid-base disorders be treated?

Discussion. The metabolic acidosis should be treated by improving tissue perfusion to reduce lactic acid production. In addition, an improvement in blood pressure will increase renal perfusion and enhance renal clearance of lactic acid; notice the BUN and creatinine levels are elevated. This patient needs intravenous fluids to restore intravascular volume, increase blood pressure, and improve tissue perfusion. If the patient is still hypotensive once the intravascular volume has been replaced, vasopressors can be administered.

The chloride-responsive metabolic alkalosis can be treated with volume replacement with normal saline, which will also replace chloride deficits. Additionally, hypochloremia can also be treated with KCl to replace both potassium and chloride. The vomiting, which is the primary cause of the metabolic alkalosis, must also be treated. This patient will require placement of a nasogastric tube to relieve gastric pressure as well as surgery to correct the small bowel obstruction.

The respiratory acidosis can be corrected by improving minute ventilation and administering O_2 for the accompanying hypoxemia. Because this patient will be undergoing surgery to correct the small bowel obstruction, she will require intubation and mechanical ventilation. Once on the ventilator, minute ventilation can be controlled by regulating the rate and tidal volume settings and improving ventilation to decrease the Pa_{CO_2}. In addition, the primary cause of the respiratory acidosis must be treated. The patient is hypoventilating because hypokalemia and hypophosphatemia cause respiratory muscle fatigue. The patient will require intravenous potassium and phosphate replacement. If not corrected, these electrolyte imbalances will make it very difficult to wean the patient from the ventilator postoperatively.

Case Study 32-3, Part B: Mixed Acid-Base Disorders

Decision point

Interpret the acid-base status after initial treatment.

Discussion. The pH is now low and the $Paco_2$ is higher than on admission, indicating a worsening respiratory acidosis. The bicarbonate level is normal and the anion gap is still elevated at 23 mEq/L. The patient still has a metabolic acidosis (high anion gap) and a metabolic alkalosis. However, the anion gap is decreasing: 33 mEq/L on admission and 23 mEq/L 3 hours after treatment. This confirms the metabolic acidosis is being corrected by volume replacement, resulting in improved tissue perfusion as evidenced by an increase in the blood pressure and falling BUN and creatinine levels.

The rise in $Paco_2$ from 49 to 69 mm Hg and the very low Pao_2 are consistent with acute respiratory failure. Immediate intubation and mechanical ventilation are required.

Case Study 32-3, Part C: Mixed Acid-Base Disorders

Decision point

Interpret the acid-base and electrolyte status of this patient before discharge.

Discussion. This patient now has a normal acid-base status. The pH is normal, the $Paco_2$ and the HCO_3^- are normal, and the anion gap is normal (12 mEq/L). The triple acid-base disorder the patient had on admission to the ED has been corrected. The electrolyte imbalances (hypokalemia, hypochloremia, and hypophosphatemia) have also been corrected. Additionally, the patient's renal function has normalized as evidenced by the BUN and creatinine values.

CHAPTER 33, ACUTE RENAL FAILURE

Case Study 33-1 Part A: Risk Factors for Developing Acute Renal Failure

Decision point

At this point, what are R.F.'s risk factors for developing ARF?

Discussion. His age, the physiologic stress of a prolonged period of hypotension, and a CT scan are all risk factors for the development of ARF. In addition, his surgery for repair of an abdominal aortic aneurysm (AAA) can be associated with serious blood loss. R.F.'s early vital signs showed hypovolemic shock, which can lead to ARF if not treated aggressively with fluids.

Decision point

What measure would you expect to carry out in the immediate postoperative period to help prevent ARF?

Discussion. Insertion of a central venous pressure (CVP) catheter, or preferably a pulmonary artery catheter (PAC), would allow the clinicians to measure R.F.'s volume status most accurately. His early vital signs, showing hypotension accompanied by obtundation, flat neck veins, and tachycardia,

provide a high index of suspicion for hypovolemia. The patient's AAA was successfully resected. Large volumes of fluid and many units of blood were given to try to compensate for the blood loss from the leaking aneurysm and the further blood loss experienced during the surgery. The priority in critical care during the recovery period would be to maintain or improve the patient's fluid status in order to preserve cardiac output and thus maintain adequate renal function. Having a CVP or PAC allows guidance of fluid replenishment by measuring filling pressures and, in the case of the PAC, the cardiac output, and helps minimize the risk of overloading the patient with fluid, leading to congestive heart failure or pulmonary edema.

Case Study 33-1, Part B: Determining Renal Status and Treatment Priorities

Decision point

What is the patient's current renal status, and what are your treatment priorities?

Discussion. The patient has prerenal failure. Because he has a PAC, focused efforts continue to replenish his volume should be continued. It is vital to establish fluid balance in order to supply adequate renal blood flow. He also has a base deficit as seen in his arterial blood gas results, which indicate that he is still low on fluid and becoming slightly acidotic. It is not appropriate to use diuretics at this time as fluid balance, or euvolemia, has not been attained.

Decision point

What are your treatment priorities?

Discussion. Prevention of contrast-induced renal damage is the highest priority especially given R.F.'s current renal status of intrarenal renal failure. In R.F.'s case, even nonionic contrast given without renal protection would almost ensure the complete loss of renal function. In addition to correct contrast selection of low molecular weight nonionic media by the radiologist, adequate hydration with iso-osmolar bicarbonate for at least 1 hour before the study is renal protective. In addition, free radical scavengers such as *N*-acetylcysteine might be considered among the most helpful of interventions to protect this patient's already compromised renal function. A solution containing iso-osmolar sodium bicarbonate added to the patient's hydration orders for at least 3 hours before contrast imaging might be considered. Alkalinizing the urine helps to minimize renal damage by inhibiting the formation of oxygen free radicals.

Case Study 33-1, Part C: Continuing Treatment Priorities

Decision point

What are your treatment priorities?

Discussion. Collaboration with the clinical nurse specialist or acute care nurse practitioner as well as the nephrology team can yield helpful problem solving for this patient requiring renal replacement therapy. First, the team must determine who can give informed consent for the insertion of the dialysis catheter. In this case the patient is unable to consent, a frequent dilemma in critical care. If the family of the patient is unavailable, the team social worker can be of enormous help in locating the family and in facilitating the communication of both the team's and the family's concerns to the others involved. Often the critical care nurse will need to be the coordinator of team members' activities, ensuring complete communication to all in difficult cases such as this.

Because his hemodynamics are unstable, R.F. is a better candidate for CRRT because it removes fluid slowly. At this point the patient would likely become a 2:1 assignment because of the increased complexity of his needs for renal replacement therapy. It would be a good idea to remove the Foley catheter to protect this compromised patient from urinary tract infection.

Decision point
What could you do to monitor the urine production without reinserting the Foley catheter since you want to minimize the patient's risk of infection after his renal insult?

Discussion. Realizing that his urine output may not stabilize for several days and the risk of UTI is great, you recommend either the patient void or the staff perform intermittent catheterization to drain the bladder, since the Foley catheter had been removed during his oliguric phase to prevent infection. It is still critically important to monitor urine production as the patient may go into the diuretic phase of recovery where he may lose as much as 3 L per day while the kidneys regain their concentrating function. This recovery may take weeks to months, so the patient will need to be educated about the need to stay well hydrated. While in the hospital, the need continues for strict measurement of I&O and daily weights because of the high likelihood of excess fluid loss during the diuretic phase of recovery from acute renal failure.

CHAPTER 34, GLYCEMIC CONTROL

Case Study 34-1, Part A: Abnormal Metabolism

Decision point
What risks for underlying diabetes did the patient exhibit?

Discussion. The patient's morbid obesity, ethnicity, weight distribution, history of hypertension, family history of CAD, and the fact that he is a smoker are risk factors for diabetes mellitus (DM).

Decision point
How quickly should the patient's glucose level be corrected and what are the risks associated with correcting the glucose level too quickly?

Discussion. The goal is to correct the glucose level by 50-70 mg/dl per hour. Correcting the glucose level too quickly can cause major fluid and electrolyte shifts, leading to potential cerebral edema.

Decision point
What additional challenges are present related to maintaining glycemic control?

Discussion. Multiple organ failures, including respiratory, cardiac, and renal failure. Potential infection as evidenced by the white blood cell count. No initiation of nutrition. Stress response of critical illness.

Case Study 34-1, Part B: Abnormal Metabolism

Decision point
What electrolyte shifts should you expect as the insulin infusion is initiated?

Discussion. Anticipate decreases in potassium, magnesium, and phosphorus levels. Electrolytes will need to be aggressively replaced to maintain levels within normal limits.

Decision point
Should the insulin infusion be transitioned to a subcutaneous regimen on initiation of enteral feedings?

Discussion. The tube feeding needs to reach goal infusion rate and insulin needs should be stable for at least 24 hours in order to accurately determine insulin requirements and initiate an appropriate subcutaneous regimen. In addition, patient tolerance and absorption of tube feedings should be stable before transition to subcutaneous insulin.

Case Study 34-1, Part C: Abnormal Metabolism

Decision point
Why is the insulin infusion continued another 2 hours after the initial dose of glargine?

Discussion. This allows the subcutaneous insulin to start absorption and create a steady state, before discontinuation of the infusion. Early discontinuation of the infusion would result in an elevated glucose level, making it more difficult to maintain adequate glycemic control.

Decision point
Identify interventions to avoid hypoglycemic episodes.

Discussion. Avoid bedtime insulin administration unless the bedtime glucose level is greater than 200 mg/dl. Ensure adequate and scheduled nutritional intake. Ensure enteral feedings and TPN are not discontinued or held without also discontinuing or decreasing the insulin infusion.

Decision point
Describe the educational requirements for L.W. as he prepares to be discharged home.

Discussion. L.W. will require the following areas of education: pathophysiology of DM and potential complications; how to determine insulin needs including basal/bolus management with CHO counting and correction management; self-administration of insulin; signs, symptoms, causes, and treatment of hyperglycemia and hypoglycemia; self-monitoring of blood glucose levels; medical nutrition for weight control; and awareness of DM as a chronic disease requiring coping and problem-solving skills.

CHAPTER 35, PITUITARY, THYROID, AND ADRENAL DISORDERS

Case Study 35-1: Diabetes Insipidus

Decision point

What are L.C.'s risk factor(s) for the development of DI?

Discussion. Depressed temporal skull fracture.

Decision point

Explain the results of the initial CBC, chemistries, and other tests.

Discussion. All test within normal limits except moderate amount of RBCs in urine (kidney injury).

Decision point

Explain the laboratory values 6 hours after admission to critical care.

Discussion

- Urinary output increased (no diuretics were given).
- Serum sodium level and osmolality elevated, specific gravity decreased reflect loss of free water.
- Hematocrit and hemoglobin levels decreased related to rehydration or possible retroperitoneal bleed.
- Lactate level increased with base deficit decreased, reflecting increased anaerobic metabolism.
- ABGs reflect metabolic acidosis with worsening oxygenation status.

Decision point

Explain the physician's orders.

Discussion. Aqueous vasopressin replacement was ordered to provide AVP loss related to hypothalamus-pituitary dysfunction. Fluid replacement with 0.45% normal saline allows for hypotonic rehydration since the serum sodium level is elevated.

Case Study 35-2: SIADH

Decision point

What other disease processes must be ruled out before SIADH can be confirmed?

Discussion. Adrenal insufficiency (primary or secondary), hypothyroidism, acute renal failure, and hyperglycemia, as all of these disease processes can lead to hyponatremia not related to SIADH.[26,64]

Decision point

What risk factors does R.D. have for the development of SIADH?

Discussion. R.D. recently stopped smoking and was prescribed a nicotine replacement patch. It has been documented that nicotine has been linked to the release of arginine vasopressin and the development of SIADH.[19] In addition, she was prescribed paroxetine for depression. Older patients started on selective serotonin reuptake inhibitors (SSRIs), such as paroxetine, have an increased possibility of the development of SIADH.[63]

Decision point

What additional information leads to the diagnosis of SIADH?

Discussion. The serum sodium level decreased from 129 to 112 mEq/L, the serum osmolality decreased from 282 to 258 mOsm/L, the urine sodium level is greater than the serum sodium level, the urine specific gravity 1.030, and the decreased urinary output is related to the action of AVP on the kidney tubules leading to reabsorption of water.

Decision point

Why is the sodium deficit calculated, and why is it important to replace sodium slowly?

Discussion. The sodium deficit should be calculated and then sodium should be replaced to increase levels no more than 1-2 mEq/L per hour over the first 2-4 hours, and then decreased to 0.5-1.0 mEq/L per hour as serum sodium concentration approaches 120 mEq/L.[64] The serum sodium level should not increase more than 12 mEq/day. If sodium is replaced too quickly, water will be pulled out of the brain, causing it to shrink quickly and possibly leading to osmotic demyelination syndrome, causing permanent paralysis (central pontine myelinosis).[64]

Decision point

Explain the rest of the physician's orders as they relate to the treatment of SIADH.

Discussion. Furosemide helps to increase urine output and blocks the action of ADH by limiting free water generation in the loop of Henle.[3,7,64] Demeclocycline, a tetracycline, is used to decrease the kidneys' response to ADH by impairing the generation and action of cyclic AMP.[3,64] Fluid restriction limits the amount of free water, and 3% NS is given to increase serum sodium level and prevent seizures.[3,7,64]

Case Study 35-3: Thyroid Storm

Decision point

What assessment parameters lead to a diagnosis of hyperthyroidism?

Discussion. Her chief complaints are diaphoresis, racing heart, nervousness, shortness of breath, fatigue, recent 20-pound weight loss, and a recent increase in pounding headaches. Tachycardia, hypertension, hyperthermia, and eventually pulseless ventricular tachycardia are all signs and symptoms of hyperthyroidism.[23,43,50]

Decision point

What risk factors does J.H. have that would predispose her to thyroid storm?

Discussion. She has possible undiagnosed hyperthyroidism. In addition, she has the following triggers that can lead to thyroid storm: hydrochlorothiazide, insulin, and a recent increase in aspirin intake.[23,50]

Decision point

Why did the physician order 40% face mask and TSH, T$_4$, and T$_3$?

Discussion. J.H. was placed on a 40% face mask because of the hypermetabolic state of thyroid storm, which increases oxygen demand as evidenced by her O_2 saturation of 88%.[23] Based on clinical presentation, the physician may suspect that J.H. has undiagnosed hyperthyroidism resulting in possible thyroid storm. Hormone levels (TSH, T_3, and T_4) will assist to diagnosis whether she has primary or secondary hyperthyroidism. However, diagnosis of hyperthyroidism is often based on clinical exam as thyroid hormone levels may take several hours to be completed.[50]

Decision point
Explain the laboratory values.

Discussion. Slight leukocytosis is common in thyroid storm or J.H. has an undiagnosed infection as she stated she had nausea and vomiting; elevated Ca^{++} levels are possibly a result of increased reabsorption of calcium from bone related to hyperthyroidism; elevated serum glucose levels are possibly a result of DKA or hyperthyroidism; elevated potassium levels and slightly decreased sodium levels possibly are a result of thyroid storm or developing DKA.

Decision point
Explain the physician's orders.

Discussion. PTU decreases TH synthesis and blocks peripheral conversion of T_4 to T_3. Propranolol (Inderal) is used to block the increased numbers of beta receptors and decrease adrenergic activity, which will decrease HR, palpitations, tremors, anxiety, and heat intolerance and can cause reduction in serum T_3 levels.[56] A beta blocker is considered the best treatment to alleviate the life-threatening complications of increased stimulation to beta and catecholamine receptors.[24,43] Dexamethasone is used to stabilize cell membranes and decrease peripheral conversion of T_4 to T_3.[23,24,44] These medications will be started before the results of the thyroid function tests are available as J.H.'s assessment verifies thyroid storm.

Decision point
Why did the physician use procainamide as the dysrhythmic agent for ventricular tachycardia instead of amiodarone?

Discussion. Procainamide is indicated for the treatment of recurrent ventricular tachycardia. In addition, amiodarone is not used in patients with diagnosed or suspected hyperthyroidism as it is an iodine-rich drug with a long half-life. Since the iodine would remain available for an extended time, it could lead to an increase in thyroid hormone production and worsening of thyroid storm.[37,41,53]

Decision point
Discuss how aspirin could have precipitated the thyroid storm.

Discussion. Salicylates enhance the conversion of T_4 to the physiologically active form of thyroid hormone, T_3. J.H. presented with tremors, increased heart rate, heat intolerance, shortness of breath, fatigue, and recent weight loss. In addition, she was taking a thiazide diuretic and insulin.

Case Study 35-4: Myxedema Coma

Decision point
What clinical symptoms would lead you to a diagnosis of myxedema coma?

Discussion. Decreased body temperature of 93° F, bradycardia, hypotension, nonpitting edema, large tongue, shallow respirations.

Decision point
Explain the physician's orders.

Discussion. ABGs are ordered to evaluate hypoxemia and hypercarbia, TSH and free T_4 to assess thyroid function, blood glucose to assess for hypoglycemia, cortisol level to assess adrenal function, electrolytes to assess sodium and potassium (hyponatremia and hyperkalemia), BUN and SCr to assess kidney function, urinalysis to determine possible infection before culture results, toxicology screen to rule out drug overdose as there is decreased metabolism of medications and question of suicide related to depression. Blood-urine-sputum cultures are drawn to rule out infection; levothyroxine IV should be given before TSH and free T_4 test as thyroid replacement is a life-saving priority.

Decision point
Explain why the physician ordered hydrocortisone, and why you would give it?

Discussion. The cortisol level of 10 mcg/dl falls within the normal range. Thyroid hormones are critical to metabolism, and the action of all other hormones is affected including cortisol.[14,34]

Decision point
Explain how the ventilator settings improved the ABGs.

Discussion. Tidal volume of 800 ml increases lung expansion, increasing surface area available for gas exchange. A rate of 20 will assist to blow off pCO_2 and correct the hypercapnia.

Decision point
Explain how the laboratory values verify the diagnosis of myxedema.

Discussion. The ABGs show that A.H. has hypercarbia and hypoxemia. Hypoglycemia, hyponatremia, and hyperkalemia all are common findings with myxedema. An increased TSH level with a decreased free T_4 level is a definitive diagnosis of myxedema. The TSH level of 39.9 microunits/L is approximately 10 times normal and the free T_4 level is almost negligible, which signals the inability of the thyroid gland to produce thyroid hormone. The BUN and serum creatinine levels are both elevated with a ratio of 25:1, which points to dehydration and possible renal insufficiency.

Decision point
What prompted the physician to order levofloxacin before culture results?

Discussion. A.H.'s urinalysis revealed concentrated, cloudy, foul-smelling urine with WBCs present, which is strongly suggestive of urinary tract infection. Also, serum WBCs are elevated to 18,000/mm^3. Infections in patients with myxedema coma can lead to further complications and should be treated promptly before culture results.

Case Study 35-5: Adrenal Insufficiency

Decision point
Discuss events of day 3 that place J.W. at risk for AI.

Discussion. J.W. has a temperature of 103° F and he returned to OR twice in 5 hours. J.W. experienced intermittent hypotension and hypoxia for several days.

Decision point
Discuss hemodynamic parameters as they relate to the diagnosis of AI.

Discussion. J.W. has the following readings: decreased CVP, decreased PCWP, decreased SVR, increased CO, continued hypotension despite fluids and vasopressors.[13,38,39,40,54] These readings are indicative of loss of the effects of cortisol (i.e., impaired pressor response to catecholamines resulting in hypotension). Glucocorticoids are needed for the cardiovascular system to respond to epinephrine, norepinephrine, and angiotension II.[39] On the other hand, these readings could also be attributed to the systemic inflammatory response syndrome (SIRS) or early sepsis response.

Decision point
Discuss ABGs and ventilator settings and what ventilator setting changes are needed.

Discussion. The ABGs reveal respiratory/metabolic acidosis; decreased Pa_{O_2} (71 mm Hg), decreased oxygen saturation (82%), and increased P_{CO_2} (50 mm Hg) are indicative of respiratory failure. In addition, it is possible that J.W. is developing acute respiratory distress syndrome. To increase oxygenation without increasing further damage to the alveolar membrane, lower tidal volumes to 4-6 ml/kg, increase FI_{O_2}, and allow for permissive hypercapnia.

Decision point
Discuss lab values as they pertain to AI.

Discussion. J.W. had increased potassium level (5.8 mEq/L) related to decreased ability to excrete potassium, decreased sodium level (129 mEq/L) related to inability to conserve sodium and inability to clear free water, and increased calcium level (12 mg/dl) related to the inability to form bone, allowing calcium to be reabsorbed into the bloodstream. He has decreased glucose concentration related to impaired gluconeogenesis.[38,52]

Decision point
Discuss the serum cortisol level.

Discussion. J.W. has experienced pain, fever, hypovolemia, hypotension, hypoxia, and tissue damage, all of which lead to a continuous release of corticotropin and glucocorticoid secretion with loss of diurnal variation.[39] Normal cortisol levels peak between 8:00 and 10:00 AM (5-23 mcg/dl) and are at their lowest around 4:00 to 6:00 PM. J.W.'s serum cortisol level at 6:00 to 10:00 PM (average 3-13 mcg/dl) was 22 mcg/dl. In multiple trauma patients, serum cortisol levels can be elevated greater than 30 mcg/dl for several days with a peak of 40-50 mcg/dl.[39]

Decision point
Discuss why the physician ordered a vasopressin drip.

Discussion. Vasopressin is an exogenous form of ADH. Catecholamine-resistant shock responds to this low-dose infusion that restores the physiologic concentration of vasopressin that may be depleted as a response to continuous stress.

Decision point
Why did the physician order dexamethasone before a corticotropin stimulation test?

Discussion. The physician suspects that AI is responsible for the vasopressor-resistant hypotension. Dexamethasone can be given before the corticotropin stimulation test as it will not interfere with the results of the corticotropin test.

Decision point
Explain how a corticotropin stimulation test is performed and why the test was ordered.

Discussion. This corticotropin test is performed by drawing a serum cortisol level. 250 mcg of synthetic corticotropin is administered IV. Serum cortisol levels are drawn at 30 and 60 minutes following the corticotropin administration. The corticotropin stimulation test is performed to determine if the HPA-adrenal axis is functioning. There should be a rise in the serum cortisol level following administration of exogenous ACTH. If no increase is noted, the diagnosis of primary adrenal insufficiency can be made, which reflects the inability of the adrenal gland to respond to ACTH.

Decision point
What would you expect the physician to order for the diagnosis of AI?

Discussion. The physician orders would include hydrocortisone 100 mg IV every 8 hours, which is considered to be a stress dose. Mineralocorticoids may need to be replaced in conjunction with hydrocortisone. Fludrocortisone can be given 0.1-0.2 mg every day. Aldosterone is secreted in response to renin-angiotension system stimulation as a result of hypotension. In primary AI, serum aldosterone levels may be decreased despite elevated renin levels.[5]

CHAPTER 36, BLOOD CONSERVATION AND BLOOD COMPONENT REPLACEMENT

Case Study 36-1, Part A: Blood Component Modification

Decision point
What blood components are indicated?

Discussion. Since D.A. was hypotensive, the massive transfusion protocol was initiated: 4 units of RBCs, 4 units of FFP, 1 pool of cryoprecipitate, and an apheresis platelet were rapidly transfused. The FFP and the RBCs were transfused through a blood warmer/rapid infuser and another EHP was drawn. She continued to experience coagulopathy after these additional blood components were transfused (INR 1.9, PT 19 seconds, hematocrit 27%, fibrinogen level

104 mg/dl, platelet count 92,000 cells/mm^3, hypotensive, and hypothermic at 35.2° C).

Decision point
Are there other therapies that should be considered at this time?

Discussion. It was decided to administer a dose of recombinant activated factor VIIa 4.8 mg IV to attempt to stop her bleeding and obtain hemostasis. Approximately 30 minutes later, her bleeding appeared to subside and her coagulation labs normalized. Her EHP following rFVIIa was as follows: INR 1.7, PT 18.2 seconds, hematocrit 29%, fibrinogen level 126 mg/dl, and platelet count 122,000 cells/mm^3.

D.A. continued to receive crystalloid boluses. A pulmonary artery catheter was placed to manage her fluid status (central venous pressure 18 mm Hg, pulmonary artery systolic pressure 42 mm Hg, pulmonary artery end-diastolic pressure 27 mm Hg, and pulmonary catheter wedge pressure 20 mm Hg).

Case Study 36-1, Part B: Blood Component Modification

Decision point
What are the complications of an incompatible blood transfusion?

Discussion. It is important to determine whether the patient received an incompatible blood component and to understand ABO/Rh compatibility, ensuring that the units transfused are compatible, if not identical, with the patient. Transfusion of ABO-incompatible blood may cause severe intravascular hemolysis as a result of an incompatible antigen on the transfused cells reacting with an antibody in the recipient's circulation. Severe hemolytic reactions may occur when as little as 10 ml of ABO-incompatible RBCs are transfused to a recipient.

Decision point
What is the nurse's role in assessing for an incompatible blood transfusion?

Discussion. Acute hemolytic transfusion reactions may be complicated to discern by symptoms alone. The nurse's primary role is to assess whether an incompatible blood transfusion occurred by determining whether a clerical error occurred at the time that the blood bank specimen was drawn or while identifying the patient at the time of transfusion.

Case Study 36-1, Part C: Blood Component Modification

Decision point
What laboratory studies should be obtained at this time?

Discussion. A transfusion reaction workup was performed at the blood bank with negative results. A direct antiglobulin test (DAT)/Coombs' test was also negative (Box 36-1). The testing pattern was not indicative of a warm-alloantibody or a drug-induced hemolytic anemia. Because of the absence of a previous transfusion history (other than transfusion on admit day 1) or a history of pregnancies, it was unlikely that an RBC alloantibody had formed.

Decision point
What investigations should be done to assist in determining the cause of her hemolysis?

Discussion. The outcome intervention would be to determine the cause of her hemolysis. Consider the following questions when trying to determine the cause for hemolysis:

- Are there mechanical reasons for the patient's hemolysis? For example, was a rapid infuser or a blood warmer used to administer the components? Was an incompatible IV fluid or medication administered with the components? Mechanical hemolysis can occur with transfusions when administered through a small needle or catheter, clogged IV line, or during rapid transfusion of blood components. Overheating, freezing, and transfusion of blood components with hypotonic (such as 5% dextrose in water) or hypertonic (e.g., 3% normal saline) solutions may cause hemolysis. Dextrose-containing solutions may cause clumping or hemolysis. Solutions containing calcium may cause clots to form. Mechanical hemolysis may be prevented if close attention is paid when handling and administering blood components. In this case, it was determined that all of the equipment used to transfuse the components was properly maintained and functioning appropriately. Medications were not administered through the same port or tubing as the components that were administered.

- Consider if the bacterium (*Clostridium perfringens*) causing the patient to be septic is responsible for her hemolysis. *Clostridium perfringens* infection is a rare cause of massive intravascular hemolysis considered early in treatment to prevent an otherwise rapidly lethal outcome. Bacterial infections can cause extrinsic nonimmune hemolytic anemia through several different mechanisms, such as damage from the release of bacterial products and infection. Examination of the peripheral blood smear may reveal a spherocytosis that develops within hours.[43] The diagnosis of clostridial sepsis should be entertained in patients who quickly become fatally ill with evidence of intravascular hemolysis.

CHAPTER 37, COAGULOPATHIES

Case Study 37-1, Part A: Coagulopathy Following Traumatic Injury

Decision point
What are the two major steps in hemostasis?

Discussion. The process of hemostasis has two major components: primary and secondary hemostasis. Primary hemostasis refers to the platelet response and formation of the platelet plug. Secondary hemostasis refers to the clotting cascade and formation of the fibrin clot.

Decision point
Where are most of the plasma coagulation factors produced?

Discussion. The liver produces the majority of clotting factors, including fibrinogen, prothrombin, and factors V, VII, IX, X, and XI.

Decision point

How is the hemostatic process activated in patients with trauma?

Discussion. Tissue trauma results in the release of tissue thromboplastin, which initiates the extrinsic pathway. The extrinsic pathway activates the intrinsic pathway and both work together to produce a clot.

Decision point

What ultimately happens to clots?

Discussion. During clot formation, the fibrinolytic system is activated to break down clots and reestablish blood flow through the affected vessels. This process occurs slowly so that vessel repair takes place before flow is established.

Case Study 37-1, Part B: Risk Factors for the Development of a Coagulopathy

Decision point

What were B.J.'s risk factors for the development of a coagulopathy such as DIC?

Discussion. B.J. suffered extensive trauma that results in the release of tissue factors and activation of the extrinsic pathway. In addition, he probably experienced hypothermia from exposure during the pre-hospital phase, during emergency care, and in the operating room. He received IV fluids and blood that may have been at room temperature or colder. He experienced hypovolemic shock and acidosis as a result of massive injury. He received multiple transfusions, but may be deficient in components.

Decision point

What nursing interventions can be used to minimize the risk of coagulopathy in the patient with extensive trauma?

Discussion. Steps can be taken to prevent hypothermia by minimizing exposure to the environment, warming IV fluids and blood, and warming the patient with blanket systems and other warming systems.

Decision point

What signs and symptoms did B.J. exhibit that were suggestive of coagulopathy?

Discussion. B.J. exhibited obvious oozing and bleeding from injury sites and signs of hypovolemic shock, including a labile blood pressure, tachycardia, poor peripheral perfusion, and low urine output.

Decision point

What laboratory values were indicative of DIC?

Discussion. In addition to clinical manifestations of bleeding, B.J. had multiple positive tests for DIC. The INR, aPTT, and thrombin time were elevated. Platelets and fibrinogen were depleted. Tests for fibrinolysis were positive.

Case Study 37-1, Part C: Treatment of the Coagulopathy

Decision point

What is considered to be the most important recommendation for the treatment of DIC?

Discussion. It is most important to treat the underlying disease process.

Decision point

What are the specific therapeutic effects of RBCs, FFP, and cryoprecipitate in the bleeding patient?

Discussion. Red cell mass provides hemoglobin and enhances oxygen-carrying capacity. FFP replaces fibrinogen and many other coagulation components to enhance blood clotting. Cryoprecipitate specifically provides fibrinogen and factor VIII. All provide needed volume in a hypovolemic patient.

Decision point

How is the effectiveness of blood and blood component therapy monitored?

Discussion. Serial assessments of key laboratory components such as hematocrit, aPTT, platelet count, and fibrinogen are used to guide therapy and assess effectiveness. These values are integrated with clinical manifestations of bleeding and overall patient assessment parameters.

Decision point

What physiologic processes make it possible to recover from DIC?

Discussion. Tissue fibrinolysis breaks down clots in the microcirculation, and leukocytes remove intravascular deposits, opening the vessels. The liver and bone marrow replace depleted clotting components.

CHAPTER 38, CARING FOR THE IMMUNOCOMPROMISED PATIENT

Case Study 38-1, Part A: Evidence-Based Management of the Immunocompromised Patient

Decision point

What does his admission lab work indicate?

Discussion. Clearly, S.E. is experiencing an infectious process, although the physical findings and diagnostic test results are not clearly definitive for a location or microbe. There is an acidosis, primarily of metabolic origin, but an intrapulmonary disorder is also present as indicated by a high normal carbon dioxide level when compensatory hyperventilation should be occurring.

Decision point

Given his symptoms, what diagnosis would be made?

Discussion. The presumed diagnosis of pneumonia is made.

Decision point
What are S.E.'s infection risks?

Discussion. S.E.'s infection risks are multifactorial, involving both intrinsic and therapy-related abnormalities of immune function. At the core of his current health problems is the underlying chronic illness of diabetes mellitus that impairs granulocyte function. The presence of malignancy is indicative of immunosurveillance failure. Normal immunosurveillance should detect cell mutations that are the precursors to malignant cell transformation. This impairment is at least partly related to the immunosuppressive medications used to prevent graft rejection after S.E.'s kidney transplant. These agents suppress the T-lymphocytic recognition and rejection of transplanted tissue, but may also impair recognition of malignant cells. Lymphoma is a recognized complication associated with immunosuppressive medications, and its involvement of the hematopoietic cells and lymph nodes indicates an even greater lymphocyte defect.[43]

Most chemotherapy agents destroy the rapidly dividing cells, which includes tumor cells as well as bone marrow, skin and mucous membranes. S.E.'s previous chemotherapy ending nine days ago caused predictable bone marrow suppression predisposing him to infection.[37] Chemotherapy-induced destruction of mucosal barriers has also resulted in oral mucositis. The open oral lesions may also contribute to a risk of infection for S.E., although his symptoms indicate that pneumonia is the predominant clinical problem. Most recently, S.E. received radiation therapy to the lung field, impairing normal alveolar macrophage function, and causing inflammation in the location of the tumor. Inflammation of the alveoli and bronchi can produce a chemical pneumonitis called "radiation pneumonitis," and also increase the risk for trapped secretions and development of infectious pneumonitis. The incidence of radiation pneumonitis peaks between three and six weeks after beginning therapy, matching the timing for S.E.'s symptoms.[10,23]

The most important risk factor influencing S.E.'s risk for infection is the granulocytic defects caused by his diabetes and chemotherapy. The severity of neutropenia and its timing are chemotherapeutic agent and dose specific.[37] S.E. received his last chemotherapy 9 days before admission and his particular treatment regimen produces moderate to severe neutropenia occurring between the seventh and fourteenth day after chemotherapy.[37] The exact date of onset for S.E.'s neutropenia is unclear since he presented with his white blood cell count already depressed; however, clinicians should be prepared to aggressively support S.E.'s infection while awaiting recovery of the white blood cell count, realizing that the current symptoms reflect a reversible critical illness that is related to a short-term immune deficit associated with therapy.[37] This patient presents with oral mucosal breakdown, also related to chemotherapy-induced mucosal injury. This complication tends to clinically follow the same timing as bone marrow suppression, but in addition to causing pain, it may be a source of systemic infection or cause significant inflammation that interferes with breathing.

The specific site of breath-sound and x-ray changes indicates predictable infection, given the existing tumor in the hilar lung region.

Case Study 38-1, Part B: Evidence-Based Management of the Immunocompromised Patient

Decision point
What interventions should be made at this time?

Discussion. Upon consultation with the oncology team, the critical care nurse can determine the probable time when the white blood cells should return, and develop an escalated respiratory assessment plan and monitoring of the white blood cell differential in anticipation of worsening respiratory symptoms.

Decision point
Provide an analysis of his neutropenia at this time.

Discussion. S.E. had a complete blood count with differential drawn in the emergency department, and the nurse examined the results upon arrival to critical care. The absolute neutrophil count is a reflection of the severity of granulocyte suppression and infection risk. S.E.'s total white blood cell count was 800 cells/mm^3. The differential reflected 40% neutrophils, 40% lymphocytes, and 20% monocytes. Absolute counts are calculated by the formula shown in Box 38-1 using S.E.'s counts.[7,37] This reflects a grade 3 neutropenia and, with the current evidence of infection, indicates the need for immediate hospitalization and emergent antimicrobial therapy. Other diagnostic tests indicative of immunocompromise may include immunoglobulin levels, complement protein levels, or tissue responses to intradermal antigens. Additional hematopoietic diagnostic tests to verify and stage S.E.'s malignancy or response to therapy may include bone marrow aspiration or biopsy, lymph node biopsy, or positron emission tomography (PET). Diagnostic tests, such as blood and excrement cultures, and computed tomography (CT) scans were performed to detect specific infections that were likely to cause S.E.'s clinical condition.[15]

Case Study 38-1, Part C: Evidence-Based Management of the Immunocompromised Patient

Decision point
What prophylactic steps would be taken to decrease S.E.'s risk for future infection?

Discussion. S.E. also has baseline health deviations of diabetes mellitus and kidney transplant, which have probably led to multiple previous episodes of infection. This patient may be colonized with abnormal or resistant microbes at the onset of his cancer therapy. Because of these high risks for preexisting infections and potential colonization, baseline polymicrobial cultures (bacteria, mycology, viral) of all body orifices and exudates would be beneficial.[15] The critical care nurse plays a crucial role in helping gather more knowledge about S.E.'s infection history, and current culture status. Nurses may be frequently required to culture orifices such as the throat, nose, or rectum. Since proper culturing technique is necessary to ensure optimal results, the critical care nurse should validate culture techniques, requirements for specialized medium, or special transport needed to enhance the accuracy of results.[27] For example, adequate blood volume for blood cultures (minimum of 3 ml) is essential for accurate culture results.[42] Infectious disease professionals also report that nasal washing is a more accurate technique than nasal swabs for diagnosis of respiratory syncytial virus (RSV) or influenza.[12] Patients who are already receiving antimicrobial therapy should have resin-bottle culture media used for anaerobic cultures so that the bloodstream antimicrobial agents do not interfere with culture results.[39] Some viral cultures must also be transported on ice. Antimicrobial therapy may include broader spectrum of coverage, or agents normally reserved for patients with polymicrobial infections with resistant organisms. This may include more liberal use of vancomycin, and medications less frequently given administered to other critically ill patients such as erythromycin, amphotericin, or ganciclovir. The experienced ICU nurse incorporates the special administration requirements for these less common antimicrobials in the plan of care.

S.E. presented on admission with mouth ulcerations most likely attributable to mucosal destruction from his recent chemotherapy treatment. Mucositis onsets between the fifth and fifteenth day after chemotherapy, and lasts about as long as the bone marrow suppression. If patients have preexisting periodontal disease, or oral hygiene is not performed conscientiously, the mouth can become a source of both systemic infection and pneumonia, especially if the patient is orally intubated.[13]

Decision point
Specifically, what interventions should be made to prevent oral infections?

Discussion. If possible, tooth brushing should be performed to reduce the incidence of periodontal infection.[31] Frequent oral rinsing with water, saline, or bicarbonate will also be effective at cleansing the mucosa.[13,31,40] Clinical evidence has shown that it is less important which solution is used for oral care than the frequency at which oral care is performed.[5] Research has also defined that colonization of the oral cavity contributes to the incidence of ventilator-associated pneumonia.[5,34] One study of oral care practices among critical care nurses showed great variability in the implementation of these evidence-based practices.[4] In one study of oral care practices in critical care, it was demonstrated that the nurse's knowledge of the importance of oral care in prevention of infection and improvement of patient outcomes was directly related to their prioritization of this practice.[16] The nurse can use this information to develop an oral assessment plan that allows for careful documentation of oral mucositis, and define an oral hygiene plan to prevent superinfection or ventilator-associated pneumonia with resistant organisms.

CHAPTER 39: BONE MARROW TRANSPLANTATION

Case Study 39-1, Part A: A Diagnosis of Acute Myelogenous Leukemia

Decision point
Why did the patient with AML have her stem cells collected for an autologous PBSC transplant?

Discussion. In this case, her cytogenetics showed moderate risk disease and an allogeneic stem cell transplant was the preferred therapy. Unfortunately, the patient's initial unrelated search failed to show any suitable donors. It was felt that finding a suitable transplant donor would be a difficult and lengthy procedure. Therefore autologous stem cells were collected in case a suitable donor could not be found. Although it is unusual to perform an autologous stem cell transplant on a patient with AML, it is done occasionally if the patient refuses an allogeneic transplant or a suitable donor cannot be found.

Decision point
Why were the parents or other family members not checked to see if they were a match before going to the unrelated donor?

Discussion. When searching for a related donor, only full siblings are tested to see if they are HLA compatible. Except in very rare circumstances, parents are not tested as they are usually haplo-matches or "half matched" because one half of the genetic material comes from one parent and the remaining half comes from the other. There are haplo-matched stem cell transplants, but few centers perform these difficult transplants.

Case Study 39-1, Part B: A Diagnosis of Acute Myelogenous Leukemia

Decision point
Why was vancomycin added before culture results were obtained?

Discussion. The patient had been neutropenic for several days. In addition, multiple barriers were breached attributable to her mucositis and her central line. Therefore the patient was at high risk to have a gram-positive infection. Coagulase-negative staph bacteremia is a common cause of neutropenic fevers in this patient population and tends to be sensitive only to vancomycin therapy.

Decision point
What other types of infections would the patient be at risk for acquiring?

Discussion. The patient is also at risk for fungal and viral infections. The patient is administered antiviral and antifungal prophylaxis by the transplant center protocols. If the fever had continued, the patient's antifungal therapy would have been adjusted. This patient had been receiving itraconazole solution, but was changed to Abelcet (liposomal amphotericin B solution) by the BMT center's protocol when she was unable to ingest oral medications. In addition, the antiviral agent (valacyclovir) was changed to IV formulation to ensure absorption. The patient was followed weekly for CMV reactivation by PCR and remained without detectable virus load.

Decision point

What special considerations related to her transplant need to be in place for this patient during critical care resuscitation?

Discussion. Most transplant patients have a central line placed before beginning their transplant regimen. However, if for some reason the patient is transferred to the critical care unit without one, a central venous catheter should be placed for safe administration of vasopressors and for monitoring central venous pressures. Not only would meticulous site preparation be necessary to prevent infection, but also the patient's platelets may need to be replaced with transfusion before insertion to avoid blood loss related to the procedure. Insertion of a Foley catheter to monitor urine output and adequacy of resuscitation also requires meticulous preparation before insertion and daily care to decrease the potential of infection. The patient's absolute neutrophil count (ANC) should be evaluated because placement in protective isolation may be necessary if the ANC levels are too low. Any healthcare team member or family member with a cold should not be allowed to care for the patient. Consistent oral care with normal saline rinses and aggressive pain management are essential for managing her mucositis. The patient should remain rousable and frequent neurologic assessment should occur every 4 hours because a change in level of consciousness could indicate an intracranial hemorrhage secondary to thrombocytopenia.

Case Study 39-1, Part C: A Diagnosis of Acute Myelogenous Leukemia

Decision point

Once she is stable following her critical care resuscitation, what care considerations related to her BMT need to be addressed?

Discussion. She needs to be showered or bathed daily to decrease the bacteria on the skin. Increased vigilance in skin care is imperative and notification to the BMT team of any new rashes is crucial. Close attention to immunosuppressive therapy is also critical. Blood levels of the P-glycoprotein inhibitor are measured twice weekly and doses are adjusted carefully to maintain a steady trough level. During the time the patient is unable to take oral medications, these medications are given IV to ensure absorption. aGVHD is variable in presentation and should be evaluated by both the BMT team and dermatology; daily assessments for new signs of multisystem aGVHD should be reported to the BMT team. The critical care nurses should remain in close contact with the BMT team to ensure the usual protocols are in place.

Decision point

Are patients ever admitted to the critical care unit for GVHD?

Discussion. Although these patients can be critically ill with aGVHD, they are usually managed on the BMT ward by specially trained nurses. Critical care unit admission may be necessary to manage severe systemic complications of aGVHD and infections that occur following the immunosuppressive therapy needed to control GVHD. The patient is at risk for fungal or viral pneumonias as well as the more common bacterial infections. A high level of suspicion for infection at early signs and symptoms is essential.

Decision point

How can the critical care nurse best support the patient and family during this unexpected complication?

Discussion. Since most patients and their families undergo BMT with high hopes of full recovery, any complication requiring critical care admission is emotionally stressful for all involved. Careful explanations about critical care routines and practices should occur so that the patient and family understand the plan of care and the critical care environment. Daily conversations with the intensivist to address goals for the day will keep them informed and able to influence decisions for care. Family members who provided care for the patient before transplant should be allowed to deliver care in the critical care unit as much as possible; this, too, allows them a sense of control during a very stressful time and keeps them close to their loved one. Advance directives should be explored early in the admission, and addressed frequently with the family should the patient continue to decompensate in such a way that a good outcome is unlikely.

CHAPTER 40, SHOCK AND END POINTS OF RESUSCITATION

Case Study 40-1, Part A: Resuscitating an Unstable Patient With Traumatic Injury

Decision point
What parameters indicated incomplete resuscitation?

Discussion. Initial review of the patient data indicates ongoing shock and the need for further resuscitation. This conclusion is based on the persistence of a metabolic acidosis (pH 7.20) with significant base deficit (BD) of −11 and elevated lactate concentration of 8 mg/dl. Despite the "normal" BP, tachycardia is persistent and systemic vascular resistance (SVR) is elevated, consistent with the compensatory mechanisms of hypovolemic shock. The presence of a mild hypothermia along with metabolic acidosis places this patient at further risk for coagulopathic bleeding. Tissue oxygenation may be further compromised because of impaired pulmonary gas exchange related to the presence of pulmonary contusion and rib fractures. This is evidenced by the significant shunt on ABG noted above. The PaO_2 is only 90 mm Hg on 100% FiO_2, resulting in a PaO_2/FiO_2 (P/F) ratio of 90.

Decision point
What types of fluids should have been used?

Discussion. Based on these findings, initial treatment strategies include the administration of 2 units of PRBCs and 4 units of FFP by fluid warmer to improve vascular volume and oxygenation as well as to correct coagulopathy. Calcium gluconate is given to treat hypocalcemia associated with transfusion of banked blood products that may worsen coagulopathy. Active and passive warming measures are initiated to correct hypothermia. Positive end-expiratory pressure (PEEP) is increased to 10 cm H_2O after volume resuscitation to recruit alveoli and improve oxygenation.

Decision point
What types of treatment might be expected in the immediate postoperative period?

Discussion. During this treatment and in the hours that follow, the multidisciplinary critical care team will continue to monitor the patient's response to therapy, using multiple endpoints of resuscitation to adjust treatment strategies. To do this effectively, the advanced practice nurse must have an understanding of shock, its treatment, and the endpoints of resuscitation that guide therapy.

Case Study 40-1, Part B: Treating Septic Shock

Decision point
What physiologic and global parameters suggest that this patient is in septic shock?

Discussion. In evaluating this patient, there are several physiologic and global parameters that indicate the presence of septic shock. The initial injuries, sustained shock, and resulting organ hypoperfusion place this patient at risk for infection. Most vulnerable are organs such as the intestine where intramucosal ischemia may result in translocation of intestinal bacteria to the circulatory system, triggering sepsis. In addition, the presence of an open abdomen and the invasive medical devices place the patient at risk for infection. Review of the patient data reveals fever, tachycardia, elevated CO/index, and low SVR. The ABG indicated persistent metabolic acidosis and oxygenation abnormalities as the Pao_2/Fio_2 ratio is 75. Worsening static lung compliance is also noted with bilateral infiltrates on CXR. Laboratory data show elevated glucose level, elevated prothrombin time, and elevated renal function parameters. Although a specific organism has not been localized, the patient exhibits evidence of systemic inflammatory response syndrome with failure of multiple organ systems. These systems include pulmonary, cardiovascular, hematologic, and renal.

Decision point
What are the priorities of care for this patient?

Discussion. Priorities of care for this patient are aimed at improving oxygenation of tissues compromised by hypoperfusion. Application of a lung-protective mode of ventilation may increase oxygenation through alveolar recruitment and reduction of pulmonary shunting while limiting the risks of alveolar shearing injury.[32] Preload indicators such as right ventricular end-diastolic volume index (RVEDVI), ejection fraction, and traditional indicators such as CVP and PACP indicate adequate preload at this time. However, this must be considered in light of how much resuscitation volume has already been received and the fact that septic patients require significant volume resuscitation because of fluid shifts from the intravascular space attributable to capillary leakage. The initiation of vasopressor and inotropic agents is required in this patient as efforts to improve perfusion through volume resuscitation alone were insufficient.[8,15,28]

Decision point
Which vasopressors are most appropriate for the patient in shock?

Discussion. The initiation of vasopressor and inotropic agents is indicated in patients refractory to fluid resuscitation. The ideal vasopressor agent for this patient is one that improves afterload through vasoconstriction as well as myocardial contractility. Norepinephrine is most likely to achieve these goals because of its combined alpha- and beta-sympathomimetic effects. Vasopressin may be considered as some data support the use of physiologic doses to replete endogenous vasopressin stores that are depleted in septic shock.[8,15,28] In the following sections of this chapter, the approach to resuscitation of the patient in shock will be discussed.

Case Study 40-1, Part C: Evaluating Organ-Specific Parameters

Decision point
Why are organ-specific parameters more informative than physiologic or global parameters?

Discussion. Global parameters tend to measure perfusion/oxygenation for the entire body; however, they are not sensitive to perfusion/oxygenation deficits of specific organ beds deprived of perfusion in shock. Organ-specific parameters (regional) are aimed at measuring restoration of perfusion to the end-organ (sublingual capnometry) or cell (tissue spectroscopy). Failure to fully resuscitate all organ systems may result in organ dysfunction and failure.

Decision point
What are three likely complications for someone who has been in uncompensated shock? What laboratory or clinical findings correlate with these complications?

Discussion. The persistence of uncompensated shock can result in complications from shock itself as well as from the therapeutic efforts to resuscitate the patient. In general, any patient is at risk for development of multiple organ system dysfunction and failure. In this patient there is risk for the development of intra-abdominal hypertension (IAH) related to intra-abdominal injury, reperfusion injury to the intestine, and intestinal swelling related to resuscitation fluid shifts.[71,81,121] The assessment findings for IAH are subtle and primarily involve elevation of intra-abdominal pressure (bladder pressure) above 12 mm Hg. If a gastric tonometer is present, reductions in intramucosal pH will be noted.[71] Changes in lung compliance, oxygenation, hemodynamics, and renal function will appear if IAH progresses to full-blown abdominal compartment syndrome (ACS). In addition to IAH, renal failure may result from hypoperfusion (prerenal) and resultant ATN. Indications of this condition include reduction in urine output and elevation of BUN and creatinine levels. Coagulopathy and bleeding may also occur. This is primarily associated with hypothermia, acidosis, and resuscitation with large quantities of crystalloid and banked blood products. Elevated PT and INR as well as bleeding from operative and injury sites indicate coagulopathy. While these complications may not always be avoided, they should be anticipated, so treatment may be instituted to limit the occurrence.

CHAPTER 41, OPTIMIZING HEMODYNAMICS: STRATEGIES FOR FLUID AND MEDICATION TITRATION IN SHOCK

Case Study 41-1, Part A: Causes of Hypertension

Decision point
To which parameter (HR, preload, afterload, or contractility) do you attribute J.Q.'s hypertension (158/86 mm Hg) on return from surgery?

Discussion. J.Q. is not extremely tachycardic so HR is probably not a primary factor. It is also doubtful that he has high preload after undergoing major surgery, and considering his cardiac history, elevated contractility is equally unlikely. Therefore the cause for his high BP is probably increased afterload. Vasoconstriction is common following cardiovascular surgery because of induced hypothermia to reduce oxygen demand, the absence of anti-hypertensive drug administration due to his NPO status for surgery, and catecholamine overdrive from the fight or flight state.

Decision point
What is your interpretation of each of these hemodynamic measures?

Discussion. Considering J.Q.'s age and health status, a CVP of 9 mm Hg while on mechanical ventilation is likely too low for him. A PAWP of 17 mm Hg, however, is probably acceptable, but may be reflecting ventricular ejection difficulties related to the high SVR more than an adequately filled vasculature. The CI is within normal limits.

Decision point
To what do you attribute J.Q.'s hypotensive state?

Discussion. The most likely reason for this change is warming (note the normalization of J.Q.'s temperature) and the reflexive fall in vascular tone. Without the high SVR, an occult hypovolemic state is uncovered, as seen by the drop in CVP and PAWP. Though both are within the "textbook normal" ranges, they are too low for a man of J.Q.'s age and cardiovascular status. (Note the low CI.) Hypovolemia is common following surgical procedures, especially those requiring aortic cross-clamping. This finding is secondary to fluid shifting and cardiopulmonary bypass related to hyperosmolar priming solutions that cause diuresis.

Case Study 41-1, Part B: The Etiology of the Hypotensive State

Decision point
From the above clinical profile, what do you interpret to be the etiology of this hypotensive state?

Discussion. From the elevated PAWP of 22 mm Hg (greater than 18 mm Hg), J.Q. is in cardiogenic shock. His CI of 1.8 L/min is critically low and he is maintaining his BP with a high SVR.

Decision point
What therapy is recommended at this time?

Discussion. Because of J.Q.'s postoperative status, an acute coronary intervention would be difficult at this time. There are several other options to consider, the most important of which is balancing oxygen supply and demand to reduce ischemia. J.Q.'s hemoglobin level should be evaluated and PRBCs infused if needed to reach a level of 12-14 g/dl. Ventilator adjustments should be considered to ensure an SaO$_2$ of greater than 90%. The restlessness he is experiencing should be managed with sedation and analgesic therapy to reduce oxygen consumption. His heart will need to have preload and afterload reduction to improve CI. Since his BP is low, it may be necessary to start an inotrope to support perfusion so that a vasodilator can be initiated. Note that J.Q.'s MAP is 75 mm Hg, so inotropes may not be required and should be avoided in light of the ventricular ectopy and MvO$_2$ increases they can induce. If used, a low dose should be started followed quickly by the vasodilator. Nitroglycerin would be a first choice because of J.Q.'s ischemia. Vasodilator therapy will reduce the PAWP, SVR, and MvO$_2$. It will also increase the CI. Once that occurs, inotropes should be weaned as soon as possible. Although IAB counterpulsation would be appropriate to achieve optimal hemodynamics if the above interventions are not successful, it would likely be considered too risky to insert because of J.Q.'s recent aortic surgery.

Case Study 41-1, Part C: Sources of Hypotension

Decision point
From this information, what is the source of J.Q.'s hypotension at this juncture?

Discussion. The lowered CVP and PAWP coupled with the abnormally low SVR (less than 900 dynes) indicate a distributive form of shock. Coupled with the elevated temperature, J.Q. is likely septic.

Decision point
What therapy is indicated to treat this form of shock?

Discussion. Early goal-directed therapy.

Decision point
What is your interpretation of these changes, and what interventions are appropriate?

Discussion. The ventilator requirements indicate refractory hypoxemia most likely a result of acute respiratory distress syndrome (ARDS). His faltering LOC and BP reflect ongoing SIRS and a need for vasopressive agents.

Decision point
What do these findings indicate?

Discussion. The ventilator requirements indicate refractory hypoxemia most likely due to the acute respiratory distress syndrome (ARDS). His faltering LOC and BP reflect ongoing SIRS and the need for vasopressive agents.

CHAPTER 42, TRAUMA

Case Study 42-1, Part A: Assessing the Patient's Trauma Circumstances

Decision point
What key pieces about this crash will assist the healthcare team in identifying injuries?

Discussion. This was a high-speed accident that occurred on a rural highway, implying that a lot of energy was transferred to her body during the crash. It was a rollover accident where the single occupant had used only a lap belt. Kinetic energy was concentrated around where the lap belt crossed her abdomen; acceleration-deceleration forces occurred when the vehicle rolled over, subjecting abdominal organs to repetitive shearing forces. This suggests that she may have significant abdominal injury. Although she states she did not lose consciousness, she was obtunded. This suggests that she may have hit her head or face on the steering wheel or windshield because her torso was not secured with a 3-point restraint. She did not require extrication, but because she was in a rural area there was a significant time delay before she was discovered and ultimately received care. Her hypotension was untreated for a prolonged time.

Decision point
What injuries are suspected in this patient?

Discussion. The circumstances of this high-speed MVC suggest that significant energy was absorbed by her abdomen and chest. Head and neck injuries are also likely because of the repetitive rollover and probability that her head hit the windshield. Her right tibia-fibula may have been fractured when the vehicle hit a tree and the floor of the jeep was forced up into her lower extremity.

Case Study 42-1, Part B: Determining Labs and Appropriate Diagnostic Tests

Decision point
What labs should be checked as part of the initial assessment in the emergency department?

Discussion. Hematocrit and hemoglobin, electrolytes, coagulation studies, liver enzymes, alcohol level, toxicology screen, pregnancy test, and blood gases.

Decision point
What is the most appropriate diagnostic test to assess for abdominal bleeding in this patient, and why?

Discussion. Either fast abdominal sonography for trauma (FAST) or diagnostic peritoneal lavage (DPL) is appropriate for this patient. Because she is hemodynamically unstable, it would be dangerous to take her to the CT scanner for a prolonged exam where she might be inaccessible to care. The FAST exam will show fluid collections in her pericardium, around her spleen and liver, and in her pelvis (probably blood). If the exam is initially negative, it should be repeated in 10–15 minutes to determine if slow bleeding has accumulated to the extent that it can be identified in the exam. The results of this test may be unreliable, however, as she is moderately obese. Consequently, a DPL might be done instead. This procedure is quickly performed after the patient's stomach and bladder have been decompressed. Not only does it identify if blood is present in the returned lavage fluid, but the presence of bacteria, food particles, bile, feces, and amylase would suggest that a hollow organ injury has occurred.

Decision point
What are the likely explanations for her hemodynamic profile in the critical care unit?

Discussion. The hemodynamic picture was confusing: while her filling pressures suggested hypovolemia, her SvO_2, DO_2I, VO_2I, and EDVI suggested that she had more than adequate volume to support excellent oxygen delivery. In fact, her consumption was low because her otherwise young and healthy heart and lungs and adequate hemoglobin were able to deliver more oxygen than her tissues required. The cause of these interesting hemodynamics was not sepsis, as would seem the most likely cause, but rather a lack of renal control of her blood pressure: because of her unusual bilateral renal injuries, she was lacking renin-angiotensin-aldosterone influences on her blood pressure. She was profoundly vasodilated, but had enough volume and a healthy heart to support adequate oxygen delivery to her tissues. The low SVR was disconcerting, however, as it provided no physiologic safety-net should she drop her blood pressure for any other reason. The surgeons ordered stress doses of IV hydrocortisone every 8 hours to simulate adrenal support, resulting in slight improvement of her SVR and blood pressure. (She required this support for several weeks before her adrenal function returned.)

Decision point
What are additional resuscitation and assessment priorities in the first hours following admission to critical care?

Discussion. Reversal of hypothermia is critical because lower body temperature increases hemoglobin's affinity for oxygen and contributes to coagulopathy. This is most efficiently done with warm blankets and IV fluids, convective warming blankets, and CAVR. The source of acidosis must also be addressed; in this case it is probably the need for continued resuscitation with fluids and pressors to ensure adequate perfusion of all organ beds. Evaluation of interventions can be done by frequently assessing ABDs, LA, or BD. Coagulation tests should be conducted as necessary until Hgb, platelets, PT, PTT, and fibrinogen are within normal levels. Ventilator inspiratory pressures, pulmonary compliance, ABGs, and repeat chest x-rays will determine if fluid overload or ARDS is present. Intra-abdominal pressure monitoring should be initiated to evaluate for ACS. The patient may develop early sepsis because of extensive contamination that occurred with her abdominal injuries. Close monitoring for persistent hypotension and elevation of WBC count would indicate that the patient is developing an infection. She will also require aggressive analgesia and sedation, with careful attention to their influence on her blood pressure.

Case Study 42-1, Part C: Follow-Up Care

Decision point
What is the most appropriate intervention for DVT prophylaxis in this patient?

Discussion. A sequential compression device on her uninjured leg is the safest choice since systemic anticoagulation was inappropriate because of bleeding risk. A temporary inferior vena cava filter might also be considered, but may be contraindicated because the patient had recurrent bouts of sepsis from multiple sources.

Decision point
Why was she losing weight despite tolerating her tube feedings well?

Discussion. Trauma patients are severely hypermetabolic for several weeks to months following significant injury, and they can quickly become catabolic as muscle stores are used to support energy demands. Because she is young with a high baseline resting energy expenditure, her metabolic needs are further increased. Recurrent bouts of serious infection placed further metabolic demands. Nutritionist consultation was essential to ensure that the appropriate enteral formula and supplementation were used to meet her needs. She was obese (admission weight was 201 pounds), but if not stopped, her weight loss could adversely affect her outcome.

Decision point
What signs and symptoms would the patient exhibit if she were experiencing PTSD?

Discussion. She would be anxious, fearful, and angry; she might have intense flashbacks of her crash. She might be withdrawn and unwilling to interact with family, friends, and caregivers. Physical symptoms might include shaking, headaches, and insomnia. Her family members might exhibit the same symptoms if they, too, were developing PTSD. Early assessment by social workers, chaplains, or psychiatrists should occur so that immediate interventions can be started, if needed.

CHAPTER 43, SYSTEMIC INFLAMMATORY RESPONSE SYNDROME AND MULTIPLE ORGAN DYSFUNCTION SYNDROME

Case Study 43-1, Part A: Evidence-Based Care of the MODS Patient

Decision point
Does L.M. show any signs of SIRS?

Discussion. The patient has four SIRS criteria: heart rate 104 beats/min, systolic blood pressure below 90 mm Hg, respiratory rate greater than 20 breaths/min, and a WBC greater than $12,000/mm^3$.

Decision point
What are appropriate interventions and further diagnostic tests for the patient at this time?

Discussion. The patient demonstrates uncompensated metabolic acidosis despite hyperventilation (pH 7.33 with HCO_3^- 14), suggesting hypoperfusion that requires fluid resuscitation. In addition to the maintenance IV infusion, one bolus of NS 500-1000 ml is indicated to see if this will improve the tachycardia and hypotension. The patient's PaO_2 is only 79 mm Hg on 3 L/min via cannula. It would be important to know his baseline PaO_2 to determine if this value represents his baseline. However, in the face of his metabolic acidosis and general distressed appearance, more oxygen is warranted. The dramatic change in his WBC count suggests a rapid consumption of mature WBCs, which is a particular concern in a patient with longstanding hepatic failure. Underlying infection should be suspected, and he requires pan cultures with initiation of broad-spectrum antibiotics after the cultures have been obtained. He should also be typed and crossed for possible blood transfusion since his admitting diagnosis is GI bleed and his platelet count has now dropped. Consideration should be given for placement of a Foley catheter and central venous catheter (CVC) to monitor fluid status. The CVC can also be used to track $ScvO_2$ as a resuscitation guide.

Decision point
What interventions should the critical care nurse anticipate in the event that the patient decompensates further?

Discussion. If oxygenation or his ability to protect his airway decompensates, the patient will require intubation and mechanical ventilation. Low tidal volume ventilation should be considered to minimize secondary pulmonary injury from barotraumas. If the patient remains hypotensive and the $ScvO_2$ remains below 70% despite fluid resuscitation, the patient will require additional fluids and the addition of vasopressors to keep his MAP higher than 65 mm Hg. Blood and blood component transfusions may be needed if he develops ongoing blood loss or coagulopathy. Continued monitoring of ABGs, lactic acid, Hgb, electrolytes, glucose, and coagulation factors will also be necessary.

Case Study 43-2, Part B: Evidence-Based Care of the MODS Patient

Decision point
How should his low $ScvO_2$ value be supported?

Discussion. Either dopamine or epinephrine can be added as a second vasopressor, but if these do not increase the patient's MAP, then dobutamine should be started for inotropic support of the cardiac output. His low Hct could also explain the low $ScvO_2$ value, and the patient should be transfused with PRBCs to improve oxygen-carrying capacity.

Because a Hct target of greater than 30 mg % has not been shown to improve outcome (and may, in fact, increase chances of pulmonary complications), the patient should be transfused to achieve an Hct between 25 and 30 mg %. Ventilator settings could also be adjusted, ensuring that settings that optimize Po_2 are achieved without compromising cardiac output. If the patient has significant secretions or atelectasis, a bronchoscopy may be needed to help clear his lungs and improve ventilation.

Decision point
What other interventions are needed to provide multisystem support of this critically ill patient with MODS?

Discussion. An insulin infusion should be started to maintain the patient's glucose levels between 100 and 120 mg/dl. A general surgery consult should be requested to rule out necrotizing fasciitis as a source of his overwhelming inflammatory response. A steroid infusion could be started as well. If monitoring of his urine output and chemistries suggests further progression toward acute renal failure, then CVVH could be initiated. DVT and stress ulcer prophylaxis should also be initiated per protocols. The patient could be considered for APC therapy; he meets criteria for more than one organ system failure, his platelets are greater than 30,000/mm^3, and he does not have a recent history of surgery or intracranial hemorrhage. Of concern, however, is the initial diagnosis of GI bleed and demonstration of ongoing blood loss as noted by his low Hct and, therefore, this agent is contraindicated

Case Study 43-1, Part C: Evidence-Based Care of the MODS Patient

Decision point
What additional interventions might be initiated to further support this patient?

Discussion. This patient developed a sudden tension pneumothorax, presumably from the high-pressure ventilation. Bilateral chest tubes should be placed for with immediate improvement. Ventilator pressures, Sao_2, $Scvo_2$, HR, and blood pressure should be constantly monitored. Dobutamine could be started to support cardiac contractility and vasopressin could be added for further blood pressure support. Additional PRBCs may also be given to support oxygen-carrying capacity if his Hct remains below 30 mg%. The patient's pain and sedation levels should be frequently addressed, and the infusions adjusted as necessary to provide maximum comfort and tolerance of mechanical ventilation. The unit's social worker and chaplain could be contacted to provide emotional support for the patient's family.

Decision point
Which organ systems became dysfunctional in this patient and what is his likely prognosis based on the number of dysfunctional organ systems?

Discussion. Two organ systems have failed, and three other systems are dysfunctional. The patient demonstrates dysfunction of his cardiovascular system (low blood pressure and poor $Scvo_2$ despite fluid resuscitation, multiple vasopressors,

and inotropic infusions) and his pulmonary system (refractory Pao_2 despite maximal ventilator settings). He appears to be developing early renal failure as noted by the poor urine output; measurements of BUN and Cr levels will help determine if his renal function continues to decline. He has metabolic failure as noted by the elevated serum lactate and glucose levels. His neurologic status is difficult to assess; however, a brief interruption of his sedative and analgesia infusion would allow for assessment of his level of consciousness. With two organ systems that are dysfunctional despite maximal support, his likely mortality is 54%; if the other three systems continue to worsen, his mortality will be 100%.

Final outcome: Because L.M.'s condition continued to decompensate, the patient was changed to Do Not Resuscitate (DNR) status following a conference with his wife and daughter. At 0115, they made the decision to withdraw support and he expired quickly thereafter at 0120. The final blood cultures confirmed *Vibrio vulnificus*.

CHAPTER 44, BURNS

Case Study 44-1, Part A: Assessing a Patient With a Thermal Flash Injury

Decision point
Given the extent of his burns, would it be appropriate to transfer him to a burn center?

Discussion. Yes. Physician-to-physician contact is made with the regional burn center and the accepting physician is determined. Nurse-to-nurse report is completed before transfer. Air transport is arranged, and T.W. is wrapped in clean, dry dressings. He is further insulated with wool blankets to maintain body temperature while in transit. A copy of all documentation, including the administration of tetanus prophylaxis, is sent with the patient. For airway protection and based on facial burns, the transport crew intubates the patient.

Case Study 44-1, Part B: Fluid Resuscitation, Wound Care, Pain Control, and Infection Prevention

Decision point
During the patient's fluid resuscitation, what parameters need to be monitored to determine adequacy of resuscitation?

Discussion. During the patient's fluid resuscitation, the following parameters need to be monitored: appropriate hypermetabolic response with a heart rate not to exceed 110–130 beats/min, maintenance of mentation unexplained by the infusion of analgesics or sedatives, and urinary output maintained within accepted parameters. Extremities must be routinely evaluated for diminution of pulses or onset of compartment syndrome.

Decision point
What burn wound and skin care interventions are indicated in the first 24 hours after injury?

Discussion. Detailed burn wound care is not necessary in the first 24 hours if the patient is to be transferred to a regional burn center or facility with definitive burn care; the patient should be covered with clean, dry sheets. In the absence of transfer, blisters >2 mm should be unroofed with manual debridement at a suitable time and covered with an appropriate antimicrobial solution such as Silvadene, Sulfamylon, Acticoat, or Silverlon. Protection from further tissue damage and skin breakdown starts immediately.

Decision point
What pulmonary complications is the patient most likely to experience in the first hours after injury? What are the signs and symptoms of these complications and how are the complications managed?

Discussion. If not already intubated, the patient needs to be observed routinely for potential development of airway obstruction; hoarseness, stridor, or changes in voice quality are primary indicators for developing airway difficulties. This can occur rapidly and with only subtle warning signs. Prophylactic intubation is the prudent choice whenever questioned.

Case Study 44-1, Part C: Wound Care and Pain Management After Grafting

Decision point
What are the signs and symptoms of graft failure?

Discussion. Grafts will be covered with dressing postoperatively. New-onset febrility should lead to the close observation of all burn wounds. An excised burn wound that is not pristine will increase the risk of colonization and graft loss. Non-adherent graft after wound dressings are taken off will appear dusky and needs to be removed, as it will not adhere after that time (typically at 7 days postoperative).

Decision point
What is the best way and when is the best time to initiate nutritional support for this patient?

Discussion. Nutritional support should be initiated at the earliest possible time in the hospital course, after giving priority to life-saving interventions and having developed the burn patient's resuscitation treatment plan. Resuscitation and nutritional support of nonsevere burns and those <20% TBSA may be first attempted orally. Severe burns, those >20% TBSA, and those failing to maintain requirements orally should receive nutritional support via small-bore feeding tube. Parenteral nutrition should be initiated only when refractory to all other treatment methods.

Decision point
How should this patient's ongoing pain be managed?

Discussion. In severe burns, pain will be continuous and basal rates of analgesia should be administered. This can be accomplished through continuous infusion of opiates supplemented with routine administration of methadone or other potentiators. Analgesics are administered intravenously because of the inconsistent absorption of the integument (intramuscular, subcutaneous, transdermal) or gut.

When able to tolerate enteral nutrition, oral (e.g., Percocet, Tylox) or sublingual (Actiq) analgesics can be administered with intravenous medications for acute pain. Proper analgesia before, during, and after potentially painful interventions will assist with compliance and the patient's ability to participate in care.

CHAPTER 45, MASS-CASUALTY COMPETENCIES

Case Study 45-1, Part A: The Mass-Casualty Incident

Decision point
In addition to the staff sent to help the critical care unit and ED, what are other sources of "reserve staff" that could help throughout the hospital as well as in the critical care area?

Discussion. Faced with the demands of a mass-casualty incident, critical care nurses and other hospital staff will be called upon to provide extraordinary service to their communities. Pressure and stress will be high. Casualties will be numerous and may include friends and neighbors. To help staff function at their highest potential, mass-casualty competencies should address the following: Preparedness will be enhanced by development of a critical care section concept of "reserve staff" identifying physicians, nurses, and other hospital workers who are (1) retired, (2) have changed careers to work outside of healthcare services, or (3) now work in areas other than direct patient care (e.g., risk management, utilization review). While developing the list of candidates for a unit-wide "reserve staff" will require limited resources, the reserve staff concept will only be viable if adequate funds are available to regularly train and update the reserves so that they can immediately step into roles in the hospital that allow regular hospital staff to focus on incident casualties.

Decision point
What other community resources can be used during an MCI?

Discussion. Mass-casualty preparedness can be greatly facilitated if hospitals work with community resources—school systems, churches, and employers—to include in their disaster plan prearranged supervision, shelter, and feeding for the families of those working in the hospital. These prearranged community support systems can be activated using public service announcements on radio and television stations. ICU managers should encourage each staff member to develop and maintain an effective coverage plan.

Decision point
What psychosocial stressors will be placed on the nurses who are working during this disaster?

Discussion. Facing long hours and the likelihood of limited communications, critical care nurses will not need the distraction of worrying and arranging for the needs of family members. In some communities, the network of an extended family or established group of friends provides "coverage" during an incident. In most communities, however, many staff members will not have any existing arrangements made to care for their families because of population immobility, or single-parent family status.

Those who have studied or experienced mass-casualty incidents have reported the enormous stress and pressure faced by healthcare workers. Effective response by these workers to the crisis requires that they have the necessary supportive services for themselves. These include access to vaccines, infection control advice, adequate rest and relief, and mental health counseling. In a sustained MCI, the inclusion of these resources in the disaster plan will assist staff in meeting the other demands that will be placed upon them.

Decision point
How might communications be supported, both to the general public and within the hospital?

Discussion. An MCI overloads the resources of the hospital(s), if not the whole community. Staff morale and effectiveness will be facilitated by developing clear information systems that use both telecommunications and a position-to-position cascade in the event that telecommunications are unavailable or overloaded. Such a cascade should be designated in terms of position, not person. The combination of hospital turnover, the multiple shifts of hospitals, and the reassignment of personnel during the incident have been found to undermine systems where the cascade specified names rather than positions.

Communications during an MCI are always complex and often intrusive. A unit communicator for external communications should be appointed in the MCI guidelines. Establishing a unit communicator who will provide necessary information to the hospital's main spokesperson may be helpful. In essence, this person will act as the information conduit for the unit. This will provide the other nurses freedom to provide necessary patient care and not be distracted by telephones ringing, family members calling, and news reporters seeking additional information.

Good internal communications are also essential. Hospitals and primary treatment areas such as a critical care unit need an ongoing, open channel of communication with emergency response teams who may have first awareness of the incident. Use of walkie-talkies may be helpful at times, but their use should be controlled as well. Concurrent transmission of multiple messages may create unintelligible cross-talk. Establishing a designated disaster channel for end users might prove to be useful.

As communications become more difficult, it may be necessary to establish dedicated "runners" who can serve as the crucial link between the critical care section and other parts of the hospital. Redundant backup capability must be built into the preparedness plan in case the usual means of communications are ineffective. The backup capability also requires regular testing.

The scale of the MCI will also create a demand for public information. In most cases, at least some of the information will not be readily available while the incident develops. We live in a mass media and multi-media culture. Every news and information source will seek access to the latest and most up-to-date information. Absent clear and credible information, speculation may reign and increase the stress and pressure of the incident, especially for those working in the critical care units. The appointment of a coordinator of media relations would relieve the staff so they are not distracted from their patient care priorities.

Finally, crowd control will be essential in a mass-casualty incident. There will be the sick and injured, relatives searching for each other, the "worried well," and the curious. To facilitate access to the hospital by nurses, physicians, and any "reserve staff" component, preparedness plans must include photo identification cards issued or authorized by the hospital. Before any incident, public safety officials must have information on the characteristics of authentic identification cards for each facility in the community. For "reserve staff" and predesignated volunteers, identification cards can be coded with number or letter systems so that public safety officials can readily identify those authorized to cross any crowd control perimeter.

Case Study 45-1, Part B: Triage and Patient Care Considerations

Decision point
What triage and patient care considerations should J.S. detail for her staff to help them prepare to receive multiple patients?

Discussion. Triage decisions affect the allocation of all available resources across the spectrum of care, from the scene to hospitals to alternate care sites. For example, emergency department access may be reserved for immediate-need patients; ambulatory patients may be diverted to alternate care sites (including nonmedical space, such as cafeterias within hospitals, or other nonmedical facilities) where "lower level" hospital ward care or quarantine can be provided.

- Only life-saving surgeries will be performed, and initial surgical care will aim to stabilize the patient. When more resources become available, additional surgery to fully treat injuries can occur.
- Intensive or critical care units may become surgical suites and regular medical care wards may become isolation or other specialized response units.
- Decontamination practices will change, so that only gross decontamination (e.g., removal of clothes) is performed.
- Needs of current patients, such as those recovering from surgery or in intensive care units, will become part of overall resource allocation.
- Elective procedures may have to be cancelled, and current inpatients may have to be discharged early or transferred to another setting. In addition, certain life-saving efforts may have to be discontinued.
- Usual scope of practice standards may not apply. Critical care nurses may have to function as physician extenders, and physicians may have to function outside their specialties. Credentialing of providers may be granted on an emergency or temporary basis. Baths, turning every 2 hours, line changes, and other critical care routines may need to be deferred until control is regained.
- Equipment and supplies will be rationed and used in ways consistent with achieving the ultimate goal of saving the

most lives (e.g., disposable supplies may be reused and rapid sterilization techniques may be necessary).

- There will be delays in hospital care because of backlogs of patients. Many disasters will cause a heavy demand and produce excessive waits for operating rooms, radiologic suites, and laboratory tests.
- Providers may need to make treatment decisions based on clinical judgment rather than diagnostic tests. For example, if laboratory resources for testing or radiology resources for x-rays are exhausted, treatment based on physical exam, history, and clinical judgment will occur.

Current documentation standards will be impossible to maintain. Providers may not have time to obtain informed consent or have access to the usual support systems to fully document the care provided, especially if the healthcare setting itself is damaged by the event. Computer charting and other electronic functions may be destroyed. Simple paper documentation of essential information will have to suffice. Triage efforts will need to focus on maximizing the number of lives saved. Instead of treating the sickest or the most injured first, triage focuses on identifying and reserving immediate treatment for individuals who have a critical need for treatment and are likely to survive. Resources are allocated to maximize the number of lives saved. Complicating conditions, such as underlying chronic disease, may have an impact on an individual's ability to survive. Critical care cannot be expended on the heroic efforts for patients with little chance of survival.

Case Study 45-1, Part C: Preparation for a Future Incident

Decision point
What suggestions might the staff nurses make to be better prepared for a future disaster of similar or larger magnitude?

Discussion. The unit might consider developing a specific disaster cart with basic survival supplies (such as batteries, water, flashlights) that could be immediately available should the need arise again. A place to stockpile critical burn care supplies would also be helpful. A one-page disaster charting document could be created to replace their current charting during such an event. Other suggestions might include the following:

- A supply of food and water for staff, patient, and families
- A staffing plan, should the crisis extend beyond a few hours
- Training of staff from nonacute care areas to support nursing staff (i.e., clinics)
- Clear communication of numbers of patients and estimated time of arrival to the unit
- A plan for quickly obtaining ventilators should additional equipment be required
- Triage arrangements with other hospitals that are quick to coordinate
- A plan for the hospital itself should it become unusable because of a disaster (fire, natural disaster, disease epidemic)

A review of ordering practices should be accomplished. The practice of ordering only the supplies needed for immediate use means that limited supplies will be depleted quickly. This situation will be compounded by same vendor/resource dependence. It will also be compounded by an event requiring large amounts of specialized supplies or care. Examples include mass-casualty events involving mostly children (substantial pediatric supplies needed) or demand for burn beds and related care.

Decision point
How might the special demands of an MCI change the way a hospital delivers patient care?

Discussion. Even if a hospital is among those still functioning, it may experience water, heating and cooling, and electricity shortages as well as communication problems.

- The provider-patient relationship may be interrupted.
- Providers may have service-specific assignments rather than patient group assignments (e.g., they would perform all intravenous infusions rather than provide all aspects of care for a group of patients).
- The hospital may need to exercise strict control of access to and from the hospital and diversion of ambulatory victims to alternative care sites.
- The emergency department should be protected to care for more critically injured victims (i.e., those who cannot walk to the hospital) who will arrive later.
- There may be a backlog in processing fatalities.
- Depending on the disaster, it may not be possible to accommodate cultural sensitivities and attitudes toward death. The hospital might start off receiving patients who are still alive, but expire shortly after. The number of fatalities may make it difficult to find and notify next of kin quickly. Transport to mortuary may be delayed and difficult. Standards for completeness and timeliness of death certificates may need to be lifted temporarily.

CHAPTER 46, CARING FOR THE PATIENT IN THE IMMEDIATE POSTOPERATIVE PERIOD

Case Study 46-1, Part A: Assessing Risk Factors of a Patient With Abdominal Aortic Aneurysm

Decision point
What are T.R.'s risk factors for his surgery and anesthesia?

Discussion. T.R.'s history is significant for cardiovascular disease (previous MI and stent placement), hypercholesterolemia, smoking, and diabetes. His history places him at high risk for the development of cardiovascular complications in the postoperative period. Additionally, he was treated with a beta blocker preoperatively (metoprolol), which further complicates his cardiovascular management. His alcohol use may have impaired his hepatic function. The surgical procedure is anticipated to exceed 3 hours, also increasing his risk for postoperative complications. His use of garlic supplements, if not stopped at least 2 weeks before surgery, may also increase his risk for bleeding and hypoglycemia.[30] His history of GERD and diabetes increases his risk of acid aspiration and potential pneumonia.

Case Study 46-1, Part B: Assessing and Managing a Postoperative Patient With Abdominal Aortic Aneurysm

Decision point
What is your interpretation of his postoperative status and what interventions are needed?

Discussion. While his PAP, PCWP, and CVP values are higher than normally observed, they are not uncommon given T.R.'s preoperative fluid resuscitation. Close monitoring is required because of his history of pulmonary and cardiac disease. It would be essential to correct his electrolyte disturbances to prevent any postoperative complications. He was given an insulin bolus of 2 units and regular insulin infusion initiated at 2 units per hour to maintain blood glucose level between 80 and 110 mg/dl. He begins shivering and comfort warming is initiated. His nausea is treated with dolasetron (Anzemet) 12.5 mg intravenously.

CHAPTER 47, CARING FOR THE CRITICALLY ILL PREGNANT PATIENT

Case Study 47-1, Part A: Stabilizing a Pregnant Patient With Premature Contractions

Decision point
What immediate interventions should be initiated?

Discussion. At this time, maternal bed rest in an optimal hemodynamic position should be anticipated to reduce maternal oxygen demands. Administration of supplemental oxygen is suggested. Blood pressure stabilization should be anticipated through use of vasodilator agents such as hydralazine (Apresoline), or with beta blockade through use of labetalol intravenously. Assessment and maintenance of maternal fluid status through intravenous fluid replacement should be anticipated. Maternal seizure prevention and maintenance should be anticipated with use of intravenous magnesium infusion to obtain a therapeutic serum magnesium level of 5-7 mg/dl.

Case Study 47-1, Part B: Monitoring, Assessing, and Managing a Compromised Pregnant Patient

Decision point
What physiologic and technical monitoring does the critical care nurse need to institute to monitor this pregnant patient and her fetus?

Discussion. Comprehensive maternal monitoring should be initiated, including temperature, heart rate, respiratory rate, blood pressure, and pulse oximetry. Ongoing maternal physical assessment to monitor overall physiologic status as well as assessment of contraction pattern is undertaken. Since contractions are occurring, continuous electronic fetal monitoring is undertaken to assess contraction pattern and fetal well-being.

Oxygen is provided at 15 L per face mask, and a radial arterial line and pulmonary artery catheter are placed. Hemodynamic data reveal cardiac output (CO) 4.0 L/min, pulmonary artery pressure (PAP) 48/30 mm Hg, pulmonary artery wedge pressure (PAWP) 28 mm Hg, systemic vascular resistance (SVR) 2860, and central venous pressure (CVP) 10 mm Hg. Arterial blood gas results include pH 7.34, $PaCO_2$ 25 mm Hg, PaO_2 70 mm Hg, bicarbonate 15 mEq/L, and SaO_2 92%.

Decision point
Which hemodynamic findings would suggest that this mother is compromised?

Discussion. Continued increases in maternal blood pressure and tachycardia outside of the expected range could herald hemodynamic compromise. Her CO is low while her PA and PACP are extremely elevated as is her SVR. CVP is normal. Her arterial blood gas demonstrates a metabolic acidosis. Presence of significant assessment findings such as continued headache, nausea, RUQ pain, decreased renal perfusion, and neurologic change could also indicate significant changes in maternal status.

Decision point
What interventions are needed to support her cardiovascular and pulmonary status?

Discussion. B.F. is electively intubated and provided with mechanical ventilation support on assist control, causing an increase in pulse oximetry to 98% and decrease in respiratory rate to 14 breaths/min. Diuresis is initiated with furosemide and aggressive blood pressure management continues with labetalol and very low dose nitroprusside.

Decision point
What findings would suggest that the fetus is compromised? What does the critical care nurse need to do to support the fetus and anticipate emergent delivery or C-section?

Discussion. Collaboration with obstetric colleagues is essential to determine changes in fetal tolerance of maternal status. Changes in fetal heart rate, variability, or pattern may herald the presence of fetal compromise. The critical care nurse should optimize maternal hemodynamic status and oxygenation in order to optimize uteroplacental perfusion. The obstetric and critical care nurses caring for the patient during this tenuous time must have excellent communication. Documentation must be comprehensive, timely, and cohesive. Nurses should ensure the presence of emergency supplies and equipment for both mother and fetus, as well as required equipment for emergent delivery.

Decision point
How should this pregnant patient's pain be managed in a way that is safe for the fetus?

Discussion. Pain should be assessed on a frequent and ongoing basis, using patient quotes and ratings of her comfort or discomfort. Nurses must work to establish a mutually acceptable pain management plan. Typically, management with incremental intravenous analgesics is undertaken. During labor or delivery, epidural analgesia may be employed. Regardless of the route of pain management, assessment of maternal and fetal impact is essential, and nurses should ensure the presence of reversal agents as well as emergency resuscitation equipment.

Case Study 47-1, Part C: Multidisciplinary Care After Emergency Cesarean Section

Decision point
What are three complications associated with pregnancy that the critical care nurse should anticipate? What are significant findings and interventions for each problem?

Discussion. Cardiopulmonary compromise. Significant findings include changes in maternal cardiac output, blood pressure, heart rate, peripheral perfusion, level of consciousness, pulse oximetry, and respiratory rate, effort, and effectiveness. Interventions include maternal positioning, fluid management, physiologic monitoring, pharmacologic support of cardiac output and blood pressure, oxygen administration, airway management and support, and prevention of aspiration, as well as mechanical support of ventilation if required.
　Fetal compromise. Significant findings include changes in fetal movement, activity, or heart rate baseline or patterns. Interventions include optimization of maternal cardiopulmonary status, analysis of fetal response to interventions, and preparations for emergent delivery if required.
　Venous thromboembolism. Significant assessment findings include changes in peripheral pulses, edema, capillary refill, color or temperature of extremity, presence of pain in extremities. Interventions include frequent position changes, leg and ankle exercises to reduce venous stasis, and administration of anticoagulation as ordered.

CHAPTER 49, CARING FOR THE CRITICALLY ILL ELDERLY PATIENT

Case Study 49-1, Part A: Evidence-Based Care of the Critically Ill Elderly Patient

Decision point
What are likely etiologies of R.S.'s initial episode of loss of consciousness?

Discussion. Postural hypotension, cardiac dysrhythmias, a transient ischemic attack, head injury secondary to a fall, medication complications, and hypovolemia caused by diarrhea.

Decision point
What impact will routine beta-blocker use have on R.S.'s physiologic response to his injury and hospitalization?

Discussion. Beta-blocking agents attenuate HR and other sympathetic responses to physiologic and psychologic stressors. Patients taking one of these drugs may be unable to mount an effective compensatory response despite the presence of hypotension or poor end-organ perfusion.

Decision point
What factors might be responsible for R.S.'s dwindling oxygen saturation?

Discussion. Aspiration, narcotic administration, supine positioning, fluid boluses.

Case Study 49-1, Part B: Evidence-Based Care of the Critically Ill Elderly Patient

Decision point
What musculoskeletal changes of aging predispose this patient to fractures?

Discussion. Aging is associated with osteoporosis, diminished muscular mass and strength, and drying of the joints. In addition, changes in gait, balance, and righting reflexes falls in the geriatric patient are a common event.

Decision point
What additional possible reason for R.S.'s hypotension, flushed skin, and altered level of consciousness is suggested by his cloudy, foul-smelling urine; flushed skin; and moderate temperature elevation?

Discussion. Urosepsis. Elderly patients have the highest incidence of sepsis of any age group. The respiratory and genitourinary tracts are the most common sources of infection.

Case Study 49-1, Part C: Evidence-Based Care of the Critically Ill Elderly Patient

Decision point
What are the probable effects of hypothermia on this patient?

Discussion. Added stress from shivering, slowed drug metabolism, poor circulation to already compromised skin, coagulopathies, delayed wound healing, immunosuppression, and increased cardiac and metabolic demands.

Decision point
What do you do in this situation?

Discussion. There is no simple answer to this question. Contacting the patient's primary physician can provide guidance. R.S. could have close relatives, such as a siblings or grandchildren, who are aware of his wishes. If time allows, a meeting of the ethics committee may shed light on additional options.

CHAPTER 50, CARING FOR THE CRITICALLY ILL PATIENT WITH A NEUROPSYCHIATRIC DISORDER

Case Study 50-1, Part A: Seeking the Cause of Abnormal Behavior

Decision point
Based on above information, what might account for J.C.'s restlessness and agitation?

Discussion. Her restlessness and agitation may be an adverse medication reaction; however, insufficient assessment data are available to arrive at this conclusion. Restlessness and agitation are nonspecific indicators. They are seen in severe anxiety, psychosis, mania, dementia, delirium, and some forms of depression.

Decision point
What additional assessment data do you need to plan J.C.'s care?

Discussion. Knowledge of J.C.'s medical history, recent medications, and social supports would be beneficial.

Decision point
What are J.C.'s most urgent nursing care needs?

Discussion. Safety and security top the list of most urgent needs. Try these simple nursing actions: Stop what you are doing. Quietly sit beside J.C.'s bed. Introduce yourself using a calm and reassuring voice. Patiently wait for J.C. to adjust to the novelty of your presence.

Case Study 50-1, Part B: A Review of Background Information and Medical Records

Decision point
What type of delirium is J.C. experiencing?

Discussion. She has symptoms of both hyperactive and hypoactive delirium, so her type is mixed delirium. A fluctuating level of consciousness is the feature of delirium that distinguishes it from dementia.

Decision point
What diagnoses does J.C. have that put her at risk for delirium?

Discussion. Multiple trauma, cognitive impairment, and hypertension put her at risk.

Decision point
What medications is J.C. taking that might predispose her to delirium?

Discussion. Nifedipine, furosemide, meperidine, and promethazine predispose J.C. to delirium. Dose adjustments are often necessary with older adults. For example, without a dose adjustment, promethazine can severely impair mentation in older adults, especially at night. To prevent nocturnal confusion, normal adult doses of promethazine (25 mg) should be halved (12.5 mg) for patients older than 75 years of age and quartered (6.25 mg) for patients over 90 years of age.[13]

Decision point
What are two major treatment goals for delirium?

Discussion. Treat the underlying cause and maintain patient safety.

Case Study 50-2: Drug Overdose

Decision point
What anticholinergic effects would you expect to see in K.E.?

Discussion. TCA toxicity causes altered mental status that can present as agitation, confusion, or lethargy. Other effects include dry mucous membranes, mydriasis, fever, and resting sinus tachycardia.

Decision point
What cardiac effects would you expect to see in K.E.?

Discussion. Early, transient hypertension occurs and should not be treated. It is followed by orthostasis and hypotension. In addition to sinus tachycardia, ECG changes include prolonged QRS complex, QT prolongation, and ventricular dysrhythmias. An ECG is considered the most important test to guide treatment.

Decision point
What central nervous system effects would you expect to see in K.E.?

Discussion. CNS excitation can produce symptoms that mimic acute anxiety, delusional psychosis, and mania. Hallucinations and paranoia may be present. Hyperreflexia, myoclonic twitches, and tremors can progress to seizure. Patients are comatose approximately 50% of the time. Depressed innervation to the gut yields decreased or absent bowel sounds. Similar to cocaine toxicity, extreme TCA overdose may result in respiratory depression requiring mechanical ventilation.

Decision point
What medications would you anticipate for TCA overdose?

Discussion. Sodium bicarbonate 1-2 mEq/kg to provide alkalization of the blood, which attenuates cardiotoxicity. Ventricular dysrhythmias refractory to sodium bicarbonate may be treated with lidocaine and/or magnesium sulfate. Class I-A, Class II, and Class III beta blockers are contraindicated. Direct alpha-agonists are used to treat persistent hypotension. Benzodiazepines are the drugs of choice for agitation, delirium, and seizures.

Decision point
What nursing interventions should you implement for K.E.?

Discussion. Suicide and seizure precautions should be started, and a quiet environment with minimal disruptions is critical. Monitoring of vital signs and cardiac rhythm is essential, and K.E. must be given opportunities to discuss his problems.

Decision point
What is K.E.'s prognosis?

Discussion. With prompt treatment, almost 100% of patients with TCA overdose survive.[38] Continued psychotherapy and treatment of underlying depression helps prevent recurrence.

CHAPTER 51, CARING FOR THE BARIATRIC PATIENT

Case Study 51-1, Part A: Defining Obesity

Decision point
What is J.W.'s BMI?

Discussion. 57.45 kg/m^2.

Decision point
Is J.W. considered extremely obese, super obese, or super-super obese?

Discussion. He is considered super obese because his BMI is greater than $50 \, kg/m^2$. If he were $<50 \, kg/m^2$ he would be considered extremely obese or morbidly obese, and if $>60 \, kg/m^2$ he would be considered super-super obese.

Decision point
Another way of defining obesity is by class of obesity. What class of obesity is J.W.?

Discussion. He is class III.

Decision point
What risk factors does J.W. have for the development of obesity?

Discussion. He had significant childhood obesity, as well as a family history of obesity and he is sedentary.

Case Study 51-1, Part B: Obesity-Related Traits and Complications

Decision point
What obesity-related complications does J.W. have?

Discussion
- Sleep apnea treated with nocturnal CPAP
- Hypercholesterolemia
- Hypertriglyceridemia
- Hypertension treated with beta blockers
- Degenerative joint disease in his feet and knees that requires use of a cane or walker for ambulation
- Significant back pain on standing or walking
- Chronic lower extremity edema with past episodes of cellulitis
- Gastroesophageal reflux disease with a small hiatal hernia
- Uncontrolled type 2 diabetes with a hemoglobin A_{1C} level of 8.2
- Left ventricular hypertrophy
- ''Fatty'' liver

Decision point
What common psychosocial obesity-related traits does he have?

Discussion. He is unmarried, lives alone, and did complete high school. He is unemployed as a result of his limited mobility. He does not date and has not had a significant relationship.

Decision point
What treatments has he tried to lose weight?

Discussion. The treatments he has tried include diet, exercise, and medical management with orlistat, all of which have failed.

Decision point
What criteria does J.W. meet for qualification for bariatric surgery?

Discussion
- His BMI is greater than $40 \, kg/m^2$.
- He has a significant number of obesity-related comorbidities.
- He is very motivated.

Case Study 51-1, Part C: Surgery and Its Complications

Decision point
What signs and symptoms of a leak did J.W. have?

Discussion. Anastomosis leaks are a complication of bariatric surgery. The clinical sepsis is evident. A persistent fever; increased white blood count; left shoulder, pelvic, or back pain; anxiety; restlessness; hiccups; unexplained tachycardia; and tachypnea are signs and symptoms. Other potential indicators of an anastomotic leak include bile drainage from the wound, unexplained oliguria, and a persistent tachycardia of 120 beats/min or greater for more than 4 hours.

Decision point
Why did he not complain of increasing abdominal pain?

Discussion. Abdominal pain is variable depending on the size of the patient, with some very large patients having little to no abdominal pain. In patients who do have pain, increasing pain can be an indicator.

Decision point
What other complications of surgery does this patient face postoperatively?

Discussion. Hypoventilation, pulmonary embolism, bleeding, sepsis, poor wound healing, wound infections, and renal failure.

Decision point
Given this patient's return to surgery, what special needs would he have had postoperatively?

Discussion. Anticipation of the course of events is critical and includes the following measures: accurate monitoring of his hemodynamic status, intake and output, and weight; immediate identification of a return of bile from his abdominal wound, indicating a possible continued leak; placing J.W. in or instituting rotational bed therapy to improve oxygenation; close monitoring of his blood glucose levels to lessen the development of further infection; monitoring his response to stress.

Decision point
What preventable complication did he develop?

Discussion. Skin care is critical in this patient. Use of dry washcloths in the folds of his skin and use of antifungal powder would have possibly prevented his skinfold secondary infections.

Decision point
What possible further complications might be anticipated related to his need for continued mechanical ventilation support?

Discussion. Given the risks associated in the obese for prolonged oxygen requirements and inability to wean coupled with his history of sleep apnea, there is the possibility of a tracheostomy requiring potentially longer tracheostomy tubes than standard. Furthermore, a change from propofol to lorazepam (Ativan) and the impact of both ultimately on his ability to wean should be considered. Also to be considered is his need for nutrition and accurate monitoring of his nutritional status.

CHAPTER 53, CHEMICAL DEPENDENCY

Case Study 53-1, Part A: Alcohol

Decision point
What predictors exist from admission about the possible severity of his withdrawal?

Discussion. The patient has repeated admissions for alcohol withdrawal in the past 2 years with known severe withdrawal events. He has been without alcohol for a given amount of time, possibly as long as 24 hours. He has previously experienced seizures and DTs with prior withdrawals. He drinks 18 to 20 beers and a fifth of vodka per day.

Decision point
Would you anticipate seizure activity with this withdrawal?

Discussion. You would anticipate it based on his history of prior seizures in withdrawal. He is also at risk for seizures because of his repeated withdrawal episodes in the past 2 years. In addition to benzodiazepines for withdrawal, anti-seizure medications should be instituted on admission.

Case Study 53-1, Part B: Alcohol

Decision point
From the information provided, you would estimate his CIWA score in the ED at what value?

Discussion
7 points for constant nausea, frequent dry heaves, and vomiting
7 point for drenching sweats
2 points for mild anxiety
7 points for tremor
23 points total

Decision point
At what level of CIWA points is it suggested that benzodiazepine therapy should begin?

Discussion. Most practitioners begin benzodiazepine therapy at a CIWA score of 8-10. Because this patient presents with a CIWA score of 23, he is classified as being in severe withdrawal on admission and will require a further determination of his CIWA score on admission to the medical-surgical floor to determine the effectiveness of the Ativan given in the ED.

On the nursing floor, a repeat CIWA reveals the following: vital signs are blood pressure 158/97 mm Hg; heart rate 128 beats/min; respiratory rate 24 breaths/min; oxygen saturation 96% on room air. He remains severely tremulous and continues to be diaphoretic. He remains nauseated but has stopped dry heaving. He denies visual or auditory disturbances though he reports having just talked with his brother at his bedside. When asked where his brother is, the patient states that he believes his brother is resting in the bed next to his. When asked where the bed is since the room is a single-patient room with one bed, he states he is not sure but he thinks that it is just outside the room in the hall. He has a slight tremor with his arms extended and states he is still feeling anxious as he believes he is in withdrawal and states he does not want to go through another bad withdrawal. He is oriented to person, time, and place. It has been an hour since his last dose of lorazepam.

Decision point
From the information provided, what would you estimate as his CIWA score?

Discussion
4 points for nausea
5 point for drenching sweats
2 points for mild anxiety
5 points for tremor
16 points total

Decision point
Does the CIWA score suggest that further benzodiazepine therapy should be administered?

Discussion. Though his score of 16 is less than in the ED he remains in moderate withdrawal. Since most benzodiazepine therapy is started at a CIWA score of 8-10, he remains in significant withdrawal and would warrant more lorazepam be administered.

Decision point
What would be the goal for this patient's therapy?

Discussion. The goal for this patient would be to have him medicated such that his withdrawal is maintained at a mild to minimal level without progression of his symptoms, indicating worsening of his withdrawal.

Decision point
What other therapies should be anticipated in this patient?

Discussion. The intravenous fluids should be continued for hydration. Since the patient is a great risk for seizure activity during this withdrawal, seizure prophylaxis would be indicated. Given his high alcohol intake, he should receive thiamine 100 mg IM on admission if it was not previously given in the ED. Therapy for his smoking should be considered. Independent nursing orders could include head of the bed elevated for aspiration prevention with monitoring of his vital signs and withdrawal symptoms after every medication administration as well as accurate intake and output measurements.

Case Study 53-1, Part C: Alcohol

Decision point
What is the basis for his somnolence after 24 hours?

Discussion. Because of his history of drinking, his age, and the need for increased doses benzodiazepines, it is likely he has more active drug than he is able to rapidly break down. This does not mean that he should stop receiving benzodiazepines because when he does wake up he will likely continue withdrawal, either from alcohol or from benzodiazepines, or both. Thus rather than stopping the drug altogether, he should receive very small amounts.

Decision point
Aspiration pneumonia places the patient at what additional risks?

Discussion. Given his history of alcoholism and tobacco use, he is at additional risk of a bacterial pneumonia and subsequent development of ARDS.

In critical care he is placed on a ventilator and given continuous sedation for prevention of planned extubation. His CIWA score drops to 2 and then 0 over the next 48 hours.

Decision point
What other potential complications could be anticipated?

Discussion. This patient is at risk of cardiac dysrhythmias, particularly atrial fibrillation and heart failure, because of his prolonged alcohol history. With his history of alcoholic pancreatitis, consideration should be given to evaluation of any abdominal tenderness found on assessment. He is also at risk of sepsis from his decreased ability to produce white blood cells. He is also at risk for gastrointestinal bleeding.

Case Study 53-2, Part A: Opiates

Decision point
What potential withdrawal states may impact his critical care stay?

Discussion. He is at risk of both alcohol withdrawal and opiate withdrawal, both of which will impact his critical care stay.

Decision point
Which withdrawal state can be fatal if untreated—alcohol or opiate?

Discussion. Alcohol can be fatal, even with treatment, if the patient goes into DTs. Opiate withdrawal, though excruciatingly painful and uncomfortable, will not place the patient at risk of death.

Decision point
What substances will not result in withdrawal states?

Discussion. Amphetamines and cocaine have no physiologic withdrawal but have a very high psychological withdrawal that will result in intense drug craving. In this case, his benzodiazepine use will not result in significant withdrawal given his use of Valium is reported to be intermittent and not regular. It would be highly critical to validate this use pattern as more regular use would result in withdrawal that will likely result in seizure activity. Also if benzodiazepines are used on a regular basis in the care of this patient, then over time he might be at risk of withdrawal.

Decision point
Would you anticipate seizure activity with this withdrawal?

Discussion. You would not anticipate it based on his history of alcohol use and no reported prior withdrawals. If it was discovered that his benzodiazepine use was more frequent than intermittent or his urine toxicology screen was positive for benzodiazepines, then there would be a definite seizure risk.

Decision point
What are the potential signs of alcohol withdrawal present on the initial assessment?

Discussion. Withdrawal symptoms could include nausea and dry heaves, profound diaphoresis, tremor with hands at rest, and elevated blood pressure and heart rate.

It is important to stress that this patient could also be experiencing these signs and symptoms from opiate withdrawal and from the pain and stress of the injuries sustained in the automobile accident. What is critical for the nurse to consider is whether these symptoms still remain or have worsened after other possible causes have been treated. Of significance is his BAL of 0.28 mg/dl, which, given his signs and symptoms, would lead you to consider his alcohol tolerance. In this patient, anticipating alcohol withdrawal is essential, and evaluating interventions and responses is pivotal in understanding the clinical picture.

Case Study 53-2, Part B: Opiates

Decision point
Is the label "drug seeker" appropriate?

Discussion. Because of his history of daily opiate use, he in fact may not be getting sufficient pain relief. Consideration could be given to administering more narcotic or adding adjunctive therapies such as NSAIDs to the treatment regimen. He would need to be evaluated for signs and symptoms of withdrawal, and his anxiety and nausea would need to be treated. It should be anticipated that this patient's perception and experience of pain will be more intense than that expected for a non-opiate user. He may sleep because of the benzodiazepines, and when they begin to dissipate, he in fact will be very uncomfortable.

Decision point
What nursing actions can be taken to help this patient?

Discussion. Reassurance that his pain will be treated is essential. He may sense or fear that he is not being treated fairly because of his drug use. He needs to know that the staff believe him and understand that he is experiencing real pain. This response may continue for a number of days into his admission. He also needs to know that his narcotics will be tapered off to prevent further withdrawal. Lastly, he needs a social worker or a drug and alcohol counselor to assist him in getting long-term treatment upon discharge from critical care.

Illustration Credits

CHAPTER 4

4-1, From Lewis SL, Heitkemper MM, Dirksen SR, et al: *Medical-Surgical Nursing: Assessment and Management of Clinical Problems,* ed 6, St Louis, 2007, Mosby.

CHAPTER 16

16-2, From Urden LD, Stacy KM, Lough ME: *Thelan's Critical Care Nursing,* ed 5, St Louis, 2006, Mosby.

CHAPTER 17

17-1, From Urden LD, Stacy KM, Lough ME: *Thelan's Critical Care Nursing,* ed 5, St Louis, 2006, Mosby.

CHAPTER 18

18-15, From Mora BN, Patterson GA: Lung preservation. In Baumgartner W, Reitz B, Kasper E, Theodore J (eds): *Heart and Lung Transplantation,* ed 2, Philadelphia, 2002, Elsevier.

CHAPTER 19

19-1, From McCance K, Huether S: *Pathophysiology,* ed 4, Philadelphia, 2003, Mosby; **19-4,** From Guyton A, Hall J: *Textbook of Medical Physiology,* ed 10, Philadelphia, 2002, Saunders.

CHAPTER 23

23-5, 23-10, 23-11, From Blumenfeld H: *Neuroanatomy through Clinical Cases.* Sunderland, Mass, 2002, Sinauer; **23-6, 23-14, 23-20, 23-21,** from Rengachary S, Ellenbogen, R: *Principles of Neurosurgery,* ed 2, Philadelphia, 2005, Mosby; **23-12, 23-16, 23-26,** From Layon A, Gabrielli A, Friedman W: *Textbook of Neurointensive Care,* Philadelphia, 2004, Saunders. **23-13, 23-27,** From Le Roux P, Winn HR, Newell D: *Management of Cerebral Aneurysms.* Philadelphia, 2004, Saunders; **23-17,** From Cho DY, Chen TC, Lee HC: Ultra-early decompressive craniectomy for malignant middle cerebral artery infarction. In *Surgical Neurology* 60:227–233, 2003; **23-22,** From Lewis SL, Heitkemper MM, Dirksen SR, et al: *Medical-Surgical Nursing: Assessment and Management of Clinical Problems,* ed 6, St Louis, 2007, Mosby; **23-28,** From Mohr J, Choi D, Grotta J, et al: *Stroke: Pathophysiology, Diagnosis, and Management,* ed 4, London, 2004, Churchill Livingstone.

CHAPTER 24

24-1, From Braddom R: *Physical Medicine and Rehabilitation,* ed 3, Philadelphia, 2007, Saunders; **24-13,** From Thibodeau GA, Swisher L: *Structure and Function of the Body,* ed 12, St Louis, 2003, Mosby; **24-14,** From Hall ED, Springer JE: Neuroprotection and acute spinal cord injury: A reappraisal. In *NeuroRX, The Journal of American Society for Experimental NeuroTherapeutics* 1(1):80–100, 2004; **24-15,** From AANN: *AANN Core Curriculum for Neuroscience Nursing,* ed 4, St Louis, 2004, Saunders; **24-16,** From Barker E: *Neuroscience Nursing: A Spectrum of Care,* ed 2, St Louis, 2002, Mosby; **24-18, 24-19,** From Wiegand DJLM, Carlson KK: *AACN Procedure Manual for Critical Care,* ed 5, St Louis, 2005, Saunders; **24-20,** Used by permission of Stryker, Kalamazoo, Mich; **24-22,** From Black JM, Hawks JH: *Medical-Surgical Nursing: Clinical Management for Positive Outcomes,* ed 7, St Louis, 2005, Saunders; **24-23,** From Lewis SL, Heitkemper MM, Dirksen SR, et al: *Medical-Surgical Nursing: Assessment and Management of Clinical Problems,* ed 6, St Louis, 2007, Mosby; **24-24, 24-28,** From Urden LD, Stacy KM, Lough ME: *Thelan's Critical Care Nursing,* ed 5, St Louis, 2006, Mosby; **24-26,** From Phipps W, Monahan F, Sands J, et al: *Medical-Surgical Nursing: Health and Illness Perspectives,* ed 7, St Louis, 2002, Mosby.

CHAPTER 25

25-1, 25-6, 25-11, Used with permission from Jenny Richardson, RN, MS; **25-5,** From Thibodeau GA, Patton KT: *Anatomy & Physiology,* ed 6, St Louis, 2008, Mosby; **25-7, 25-8, 25-15,** From Phipps W, Monahan F, Sands J, et al: *Medical-Surgical Nursing: Health and Illness Perspectives,* ed 7, St Louis, 2002, Mosby; **25-9,** From Black JM, Hawks JH: *Medical-Surgical Nursing: Clinical Management for Positive Outcomes,* 7th ed 7, St Louis, 2005, Saunders; **25-10,** Used with permission from the University of Chicago Press, Chicago; **25-12,** From www.dpd.cdc.gov/dpdx; **25-13,** From Garcia HH, Del Brutto OH: Imaging findings in neurocysticercosis. In *Acta Tropica* 87(1):73–75, 2003; **25-14,** From Phipps W, Monahan F, Sands J, et al: *Medical-Surgical Nursing: Health and Illness Perspectives,* ed 7, St Louis, 2002, Mosby.

CHAPTER 26

26-1, 26-2, From Phipps W, Monahan F, Sands J, et al: *Medical-Surgical Nursing: Health and Illness Perspectives,* ed 8, St Louis, 2007, Mosby.

CHAPTER 27

27-1, 27-2, From Thibodeau GA, Patton KT: *Anatomy & Physiology,* ed 6, St Louis, 2008, Mosby; **27-4,** From UCSD–The Liver Center/Center for Transplantation.

CHAPTER 28

28-1, From Thibodeau GA, Patton KT: *Anatomy & Physiology,* ed 6, St Louis, 2008, Mosby.

CHAPTER 35

35-1, Modified from and used by permission of Louis R. Stout; **35-2,** From Porterfield S: *Endocrine Physiology,* St Louis, 2001, Mosby.

CHAPTER 41

41-10, From Pinsky, M. R., & Vincent, J. L. (2005). Let us use the pulmonary artery catheter correctly and only when we need it. *Crit Care Med* 33(5), 1123-1124.

CHAPTER 43

43-2, From McCance K, Huether S: *Pathophysiology*, ed 5, Philadelphia, 2007, Mosby.

CHAPTER 44

All chapter photos by permission of Louis R. Stout except for **44-1,** From Jarvis C: *Physical Examination and Health Assessment*, ed 4, St Louis, 2004, Saunders.

CHAPTER 48

48-9, 48-10, 48-11, From Aehlert B: *Pediatric Advanced Life Support,* ed 2, St Louis, 2007, Elsevier/JEMS.

Index

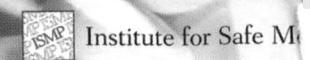

ISMP's List of *Error-Prone Abbreviations, Symbols*, and *Dose Designations*

The abbreviations, symbols, and dose designations found in this table have been reported to ISMP through the USP-ISMP Medication Error Reporting Program as being frequently misinterpreted and involved in harmful medication errors. They should NEVER be used when communicating medical information. This includes internal communications, telephone/verbal prescriptions, computer-generated labels, labels for drug storage bins, medication administration records, as well as pharmacy and prescriber computer order entry screens.

The Joint Commission on Accreditation of Healthcare Organizations (TJC) has established a National Patient Safety Goal that specifies that certain abbreviations must appear on an accredited organization's do-not-use list; we have highlighted these items with a double asterisk (**). However, we hope that you will consider others beyond the minimum TJC requirements. By using and promoting safe practices and by educating one another about hazards, we can better protect our patients.

Abbreviations	Intended Meaning	Misinterpretation	Correction
µg	Microgram	Mistaken as "mg"	Use "mcg"
AD, AS, AU	Right ear, left ear, each ear	Mistaken as OD, OS, OU (right eye, left eye, each eye)	Use "right ear," "left ear," or "each ear"
OD, OS, OU	Right eye, left eye, each eye	Mistaken as AD, AS, AU (right ear, left ear, each ear)	Use "right eye," "left eye," or "each eye"
BT	Bedtime	Mistaken as "BID" (twice daily)	Use "bedtime"
cc	Cubic centimeters	Mistaken as "u" (units)	Use "mL"
D/C	Discharge or discontinue	Premature discontinuation of medications if D/C (intended to mean "discharge") has been misinterpreted as "discontinued" when followed by a list of discharge medications	Use "discharge" and "discontinue"
IJ	Injection	Mistaken as "IV" or "intrajugular"	Use "injection"
IN	Intranasal	Mistaken as "IM" or "IV"	Use "intranasal" or "NAS"
HS	Half-strength	Mistaken as bedtime	Use "half-strength" or "bedtime"
hs	At bedtime, hours of sleep	Mistaken as half-strength	
IU**	International unit	Mistaken as IV (intravenous) or 10 (ten)	Use "units"
o.d. or OD	Once daily	Mistaken as "right eye" (OD-oculus dexter), leading to oral liquid medications administered in the eye	Use "daily"
OJ	Orange juice	Mistaken as OD or OS (right or left eye); drugs meant to be diluted in orange juice may be given in the eye	Use "orange juice"
Per os	By mouth, orally	The "os" can be mistaken as "left eye" (OS-oculus sinister)	Use "PO," "by mouth," or "orally"
q.d. or QD**	Every day	Mistaken as q.i.d., especially if the period after the "q" or the tail of the "q" is misunderstood as an "i"	Use "daily"
qhs	Nightly at bedtime	Mistaken as "qhr" or every hour	Use "nightly"
qn	Nightly or at bedtime	Mistaken as "qh" (every hour)	Use "nightly" or "at bedtime"
q.o.d. or QOD**	Every other day	Mistaken as "q.d." (daily) or "q.i.d. (four times daily) if the "o" is poorly written	Use "every other day"
q1d	Daily	Mistaken as q.i.d. (four times daily)	Use "daily"
q6PM, etc.	Every evening at 6 PM	Mistaken as every 6 hours	Use "6 PM nightly" or "6 PM daily"
SC, SQ, sub q	Subcutaneous	SC mistaken as SL (sublingual); SQ mistaken as "5 every;" the "q" in "sub q" has been mistaken as "every" (e.g., a heparin dose ordered "sub q 2 hours before surgery" misunderstood as every 2 hours before surgery)	Use "subcut" or "subcutaneously"
ss	Sliding scale (insulin) or ½ (apothecary)	Mistaken as "55"	Spell out "sliding scale;" use "one-half" or "½"
SSRI	Sliding scale regular insulin	Mistaken as selective-serotonin reuptake inhibitor	Spell out "sliding scale (insulin)"
SSI	Sliding scale insulin	Mistaken as Strong Solution of Iodine (Lugol's)	
i/d	One daily	Mistaken as "tid"	Use "1 daily"
TIW or tiw	3 times a week	Mistaken as "3 times a day" or "twice in a week"	Use "3 times weekly"
U or u**	Unit	Mistaken as the number 0 or 4, causing a 10-fold overdose or greater (e.g., 4U seen as "40" or 4u seen as "44"); mistaken as "cc" so dose given in volume instead of units (e.g., 4u seen as 4cc)	Use "unit"

Dose Designations and Other Information	Intended Meaning	Misinterpretation	Correction
Trailing zero after decimal point (e.g., 1.0 mg)**	1 mg	Mistaken as 10 mg if the decimal point is not seen	Do not use trailing zeros for doses expressed in whole numbers"
"Naked" decimal point (e.g., .5 mg)**	0.5 mg	Mistaken as 5 mg if the decimal point is not seen	Use zero before a decimal point when the dose is less than a whole unit

ISMP's List of *Error-Prone Abbreviations, Symbols,* and *Dose Designations*

The abbreviations, symbols, and dose designations found in this table have been reported to ISMP through the USP-ISMP Medication Error Reporting Program as being frequently misinterpreted and involved in harmful medication errors. They should NEVER be used when communicating medical information. This includes internal communications, telephone/verbal prescriptions, computer-generated labels, labels for drug storage bins, medication administration records, as well as pharmacy and prescriber computer order entry screens.

The Joint Commission on Accreditation of Healthcare Organizations (TJC) has established a National Patient Safety Goal that specifies that certain abbreviations must appear on an accredited organization's do-not-use list; we have highlighted these items with a double asterisk (**). However, we hope that you will consider others beyond the minimum TJC requirements. By using and promoting safe practices and by educating one another about hazards, we can better protect our patients.

Abbreviations	Intended Meaning	Misinterpretation	Correction
μg	Microgram	Mistaken as "mg"	Use "mcg"
AD, AS, AU	Right ear, left ear, each ear	Mistaken as OD, OS, OU (right eye, left eye, each eye)	Use "right ear," "left ear," or "each ear"
OD, OS, OU	Right eye, left eye, each eye	Mistaken as AD, AS, AU (right ear, left ear, each ear)	Use "right eye," "left eye," or "each eye"
BT	Bedtime	Mistaken as "BID" (twice daily)	Use "bedtime"
cc	Cubic centimeters	Mistaken as "u" (units)	Use "ml"
D/C	Discharge or discontinue	Premature discontinuation of medications if D/C (intended to mean "discharge") has been misinterpreted as "discontinued" when followed by a list of discharge medications	Use "discharge" and "discontinue"
IJ	Injection	Mistaken as "IV" or "intrajugular"	Use "injection"
IN	Intranasal	Mistaken as "IM" or "IV"	Use "intranasal" or "NAS"
HS	Half-strength	Mistaken as bedtime	Use "half-strength" or "bedtime"
hs	At bedtime, hours of sleep	Mistaken as half-strength	
IU**	International unit	Mistaken as IV (intravenous) or 10 (ten)	Use "units"
o.d. or OD	Once daily	Mistaken as "right eye" (OD-oculus dexter), leading to oral liquid medications administered in the eye	Use "daily"
OJ	Orange juice	Mistaken as OD or OS (right or left eye); drugs meant to be diluted in orange juice may be given in the eye	Use "orange juice"
Per os	By mouth, orally	The "os" can be mistaken as "left eye" (OS-oculus sinister)	Use "PO," "by mouth," or "orally"
q.d. or QD**	Every day	Mistaken as q.i.d., especially if the period after the "q" or the tail of the "q" is misunderstood as an "i"	Use "daily"
qhs	Nightly at bedtime	Mistaken as "qhr" or every hour	Use "nightly"
qn	Nightly or at bedtime	Mistaken as "qh" (every hour)	Use "nightly" or "at bedtime"
q.o.d. or QOD**	Every other day	Mistaken as "q.d." (daily) or "q.i.d. (four times daily) if the "o" is poorly written	Use "every other day"
q1d	Daily	Mistaken as q.i.d. (four times daily)	Use "daily"
q6PM, etc.	Every evening at 6 PM	Mistaken as every 6 hours	Use "6 PM nightly" or "6 PM daily"
SC, SQ, sub q	Subcutaneous	SC mistaken as SL (sublingual); SQ mistaken as "5 every;" the "q" in "sub q" has been mistaken as "every" (e.g., a heparin dose ordered "sub q 2 hours before surgery" misunderstood as every 2 hours before surgery)	Use "subcut" or "subcutaneously"
ss	Sliding scale (insulin) or ½ (apothecary)	Mistaken as "55"	Spell out "sliding scale;" use "one-half" or "½"
SSRI	Sliding scale regular insulin	Mistaken as selective-serotonin reuptake inhibitor	Spell out "sliding scale (insulin)"
SSI	Sliding scale insulin	Mistaken as Strong Solution of Iodine (Lugol's)	
i/d	One daily	Mistaken as "tid"	Use "1 daily"
TIW or tiw	3 times a week	Mistaken as "3 times a day" or "twice in a week"	Use "3 times weekly"
U or u**	Unit	Mistaken as the number 0 or 4, causing a 10-fold overdose or greater (e.g., 4U seen as "40" or 4u seen as "44"); mistaken as "cc" so dose given in volume instead of units (e.g., 4u seen as 4cc)	Use "unit"

Dose Designations and Other Information	Intended Meaning	Misinterpretation	Correction
Trailing zero after decimal point (e.g., 1.0 mg)**	1 mg	Mistaken as 10 mg if the decimal point is not seen	Do not use trailing zeros for doses expressed in whole numbers"
"Naked" decimal point (e.g., .5 mg)**	0.5 mg	Mistaken as 5 mg if the decimal point is not seen	Use zero before a decimal point when the dose is less than a whole unit